Rehabilitation
of the HAND
and UPPER
EXTREMITY

VOLUME 2

Rehabilitation *of the* HAND *and* UPPER EXTREMITY

SEVENTH EDITION

VOLUME 2

Terri M. Skirven, OTR/L, CHT
Director, Hand Rehabilitation Foundation; Director Emeritus, Hand Therapy, Philadelphia Hand to Shoulder Center, King of Prussia, PA

A. Lee Osterman, MD
Professor, Orthopaedic and Hand Surgery; Chairman, Division of Hand Surgery, Department of Orthopaedic Surgery, Thomas Jefferson University; President, The Philadelphia Hand to Shoulder Center, Philadelphia, PA

Jane M. Fedorczyk, PT, PhD, CHT
Director, Center for Hand and Upper Limb Health and Performance; Director, Advanced Practice Certificate in Hand and Upper Limb Rehabilitation; Clinical Professor, Department of Physical Therapy; Clinical Professor, Department of Occupational Therapy, Jefferson College of Rehabilitation Sciences, Jefferson (Thomas Jefferson University + Philadelphia University), Philadelphia, PA

Peter C. Amadio, MD
Lloyd A. and Barbara A. Amundson Professor of Orthopedic Surgery, Mayo Clinic, Rochester, MN

Sheri B. Feldscher, OTR/L, CHT
Director, Hand Therapy, Philadelphia Hand to Shoulder Center, Philadelphia, PA

Eon Kyu Shin, MD
Associate Professor, Department of Orthopaedic Surgery, Thomas Jefferson University Hospital, Philadelphia, PA

ELSEVIER

Elsevier
1600 John F. Kennedy Blvd.
Ste 1800
Philadelphia, PA 19103-2899

REHABILITATION OF THE HAND AND UPPER EXTREMITY,
SEVENTH EDITION

ISBN: 978-0-323-50913-8

Volume 1 ISBN: 978-0-323-76073-7
Volume 2 ISBN: 978-0-323-76074-4

Previous editions copyrighted 2011, 2002, 1995, 1990, 1984, 1978.

Library of Congress Control Number: 2019955465

Senior Content Strategist: Belinda Kuhn
Senior Content Development Specialist: Deidre Simpson
Publishing Services Manager: Catherine Jackson
Senior Project Manager: Daniel Fitzgerald
Designer: Maggie Reid

Printed in India

Last digit is the print number: 9 8 7 6 5 4 3

Working together
to grow libraries in
developing countries

www.elsevier.com • www.bookaid.org

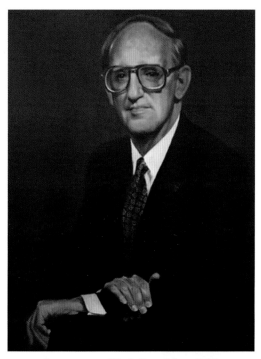

Lawrence H. Schneider, MD

MENTOR   TEACHER   COLLEAGUE   FRIEND

With affection and admiration, we proudly dedicate this seventh edition of *Rehabilitation of the Hand and Upper Extremity* to Lawrence H. Schneider, MD. His dedication to hand surgery is evident in his many accomplishments and awards. In contrast is his humility reflected in this quote from the article "The Remarkable Hand" in the Philadelphia Sunday Bulletin from 1976: "*I don't think my hands are any more important than anyone else's; actually, a laborer's hands are more important.*" Those of us who are fortunate to have worked with Dr. Schneider are well familiar with his sense of humor and practical nature. He along with colleagues James Hunter, MD, and Evelyn Mackin, PT, developed a unique model for the integrated management of hand and upper limb injured patients combining the specialties of hand surgery and hand therapy in a team-oriented approach at the Hand Rehabilitation Center, now the Philadelphia Hand to Shoulder Center. This philosophy of management has endured and been emulated and is clearly reflected in this seventh edition.

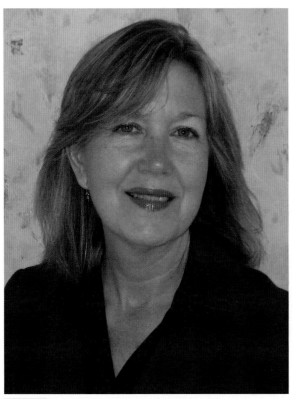

Terri M. Skirven, OTR/L, CHT
Editions 5, 6, 7

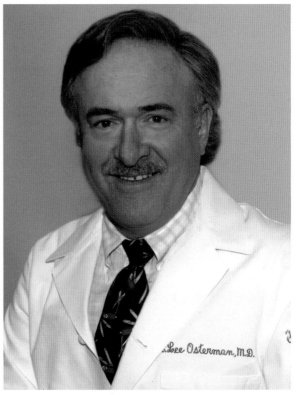

A. Lee Osterman, MD
Editions 5, 6, 7

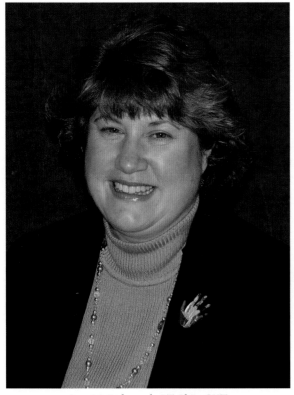

Jane M. Fedorczyk, PT, PhD, CHT
Editions 6, 7

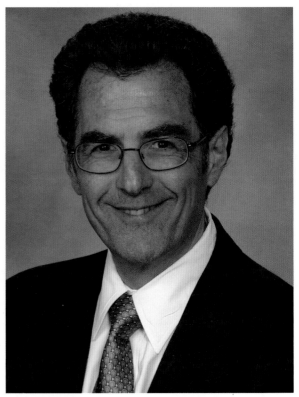

Peter C. Amadio, MD
Editions 6, 7

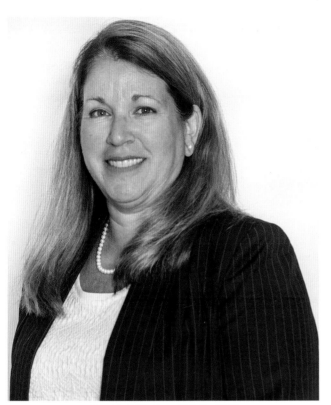

Sheri B. Feldscher, OTR/L, CHT
Edition 7

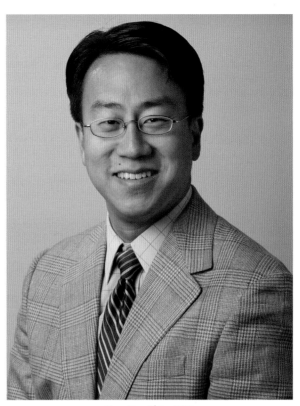

Eon Kyu Shin, MD
Edition 7

CONTRIBUTORS

The editors would like to acknowledge and offer grateful thanks for the input of all previous editions' contributors, without whom this new edition would not have been possible.

Joshua M. Abzug, MD
Associate Professor of Orthopaedics and Pediatrics, University of Maryland School of Medicine, Baltimore, Maryland

Daniel Acker, OTR, CHT
Clinical Coordinator, Occupational Therapy, Georgia Hand, Shoulder & Elbow, Atlanta, Georgia

Julie E. Adams, MD
Professor, Orthopedic Surgery, Mayo Clinic, Rochester, Minnesota; Professor, Orthopedic Surgery, Mayo Clinic Health System, Austin, Minnesota

Lori Algar, OTD, OTR/L, CHT
Doctor of Occupational Therapy, Hand Therapy Department, Orthopaedic Specialty Group, PC, Fairfield, Connecticut

Peter C. Amadio, MD
Lloyd A. and Barbara A. Amundson Professor of Orthopedic Surgery, Mayo Clinic, Rochester, Minnesota

Sarah Ashworth, OTR/L
Occupational Therapist, Rehabilitation Services, Shriners Hospital for Children, Philadelphia, Pennsylvania

Abdo Bachoura, MD
Hand Surgery Fellow, Philadelphia Hand to Shoulder Center, Philadelphia, Pennsylvania

Kathryn L. Baker, MS, OTR, CHT, USAF
Master of Science, Occupational Therapist, Certified Hand Therapist, United States Air Force, Colorado Springs, Colorado

Mary F. Barbe, PhD
Professor, Anatomy and Cell Biology, Temple University, Lewis Katz School of Medicine, Philadelphia, Pennsylvania

Nora Barrett, MS, OTR/L, CHT
Hand Therapist, Hand & Arm Therapy of Central Oregon, Bend, Oregon

Carrie Barron, MD
Director, Creativity for Resilience Program, Assistant Professor of Psychiatry, Dell Medical School—The University of Texas at Austin, Austin, Texas

Mark T. Bastan, PT, DPT, OCS, CMTPT, CSCS
Elite Physical Therapy, Providence, Rhode Island

Jeanine Beasley, EdD, OTRL, CHT, FAOTA
Professor, Occupational Therapy, Grand Valley State University, Grand Rapids, Michigan

Jeffrey A. Belair, MD
Assistant Professor, Radiology, Thomas Jefferson University, Philadelphia, Pennsylvania

Mark R. Belsky, MD, FAAOS
Clinical Professor of Orthopaedic Surgery, Tufts University School of Medicine, Medford, Massachusetts; Hand Surgeon, Newton-Wellesley Hospital; Former Chairman Orthopaedic Surgery, Newton-Wellesley Hospital, Newton, Massachusetts

Pedro K. Beredjiklian, MD
Professor of Orthopaedic Surgery, Sidney Kimmel Medical College at Thomas Jefferson University, Philadelphia, Pennsylvania

Sam J. Biafora, MD
Hand to Shoulder Associates, Arlington Heights, Illinois

Rebecca L. Birkenmeier, OTD, OTR/L
Assistant Professor of Occupational Therapy, College of Health Professions, Maryville University, St. Louis, Missouri

Anders Björkman, MD, PhD
Associate Professor, Department of Translational Medicine—Hand Surgery, Lund University, Malmö, Sweden

Susan Blackmore, MS, OTR/L, CHT, COMT-UL
National Director of Hand Therapy: Outpatient Division, Select Medical, King of Prussia, Pennsylvania

Michael J. Botte, MD
Co-Director, Hand and Microvascular Surgery Section, Division of Orthopaedic Surgery, Scripps Clinic; Orthopaedic Surgery Service, VA San Diego Healthcare System, La Jolla, California; Clinical Professor of Orthopaedic Surgery, Voluntary, Department of Orthopaedic Surgery, University of California, San Diego, School of Medicine, San Diego, California

David Bozentka, MD
Chief Hand Surgery, Orthopaedic Surgery, University of Pennsylvania Health System, Philadelphia, Pennsylvania

Anne M. Bryden, MA, OTR/L
Director of Clinical Trials and Research, Institute for Functional Restoration, Case Western Reserve University, Cleveland, Ohio

Matthew B. Burn, MD
Hand & Upper Limb Fellowship, Stanford University Medical Center, Redwood City, California

Katherine Butler, B Ap Sc (OT), AHT (BAHT), A Mus A (Flute)
Honorary Associate Professor, Department of Targeted Intervention University College London, London, Great Britain; Honorary Associate Professor, Faculty of Health, Education and Society, Plymouth University, Plymouth, Great Britain

Nancy N. Byl, PT, MPH, PhD, FAPTA
Professor and Chair Emeritus, Physical Therapy and Rehabilitation Science, University of California, San Francisco, San Francisco, California

Nancy M. Cannon, OTR, CHT
Occupational Therapist, Indiana Hand to Shoulder Center, Indianapolis, Indiana

Patti Carrillo, PT, DPT, FAAOMPT
Clinical Adjunct Professor, Doctor of Physical Therapy Program, University of Texas at El Paso, El Paso, Texas

Alexandria L. Case, BSE
Clinical Research Coordinator, Pediatrics and Orthopaedics, University of Maryland School of Medicine, Timonium, Maryland

Kevin Chan, MD, MSc, FRCSC
Clinical Assistant Professor, Orthopaedic Hand and Upper Extremity Surgery, Orthopedics Spectrum Health, Michigan State University College of Human Medicine, Grand Rapids, Michigan

Wayne W. Chan, MD, PhD
Assistant Professor, Department of
Orthopedics and Physical Rehabilitation,
University of Massachusetts Medical
School, Worcester, Massachusetts

Edward S. Chang, MD
Assistant Professor, Orthopedic Surgery,
Inova Health System, Fairfax, Virginia

James Chang, MD
Professor and Chief of Plastic Surgery,
Stanford University, Stanford, California

Ted Chapman, MS, OTR/L, CHT
Certified Hand Therapist, Occupational
Therapy, OhioHealth, Mansfield, Ohio

Adnan N. Cheema, MD
Resident Physician, Department of
Orthopaedic Surgery, University
of Pennsylvania, Philadelphia,
Pennsylvania

Neal C. Chen, MD
Interim Chief, Hand and Upper Extremity
Service, Orthopaedic Surgery,
Massachusetts General Hospital, Boston,
Massachusetts

Michael K. Cheng, PhD
Lecturer, Department of Psychiatry, University
of Toronto, Toronto, Ontario, Canada

Kevin C. Chung, MD, MS
Professor of Plastic Surgery and
Orthopaedic Surgery, Professor of
Plastic Surgery and Orthopaedic
Surgery, Chief of Hand Surgery,
Assistant Dean for Faculty Affairs,
Plastic Surgery, University of Michigan,
Ann Arbor, Michigan

Dan Conyers, CPO, FAAOP
National Clinical Director, Prosthetics,
Advanced Arm Dynamics, Beaverton,
Oregon

Shanna Corbin, MS, OTR/L, CHT
Occupational Therapist, Hand Therapy, The
Philadelphia Hand to Shoulder Center,
Philadelphia, Pennsylvania

Randall W. Culp, MD, FACS
Professor of Orthopaedic Surgery, Thomas
Jefferson University, Philadelphia,
Pennsylvania; Partner, Philadelphia
Hand to Shoulder Center, Wilkes Barre,
Pennsylvania

Farhad Darbandi, MD
Hand and Upper Extremity Surgery, The
CORE Institute, Phoenix, Arizona

Joseph M. Day, PT, PhD, OCS, CIMT
Assistant Professor, Physical Therapy,
University of Dayton, Dayton, Ohio

Lauren M. DeTullio, OTR/L, CHT
Assistant Director, Hand Therapy, The
Philadelphia Hand to Shoulder Center,
King of Prussia, Pennsylvania

**Rebecca Edgeworth Ditwiler, PT,
DPT, OCS**
Assistant Professor, School of Physical
Therapy and Rehabilitation Sciences,
University of South Florida Morsani
College of Medicine, Tampa, Florida

Carole Dodge, OTR/L, CHT
Supervisor/Clinical Specialist, Occupational
Therapy, Michigan Medicine, University
of Michigan, Ann Arbor, Michigan

Susan V. Duff, PT, OT/L, EdD, CHT
Certified Hand Therapist, Associate
Professor, Physical Therapy, Crean
College of Health & Behavioral Sciences,
Chapman University, Irvine, California

Brian Eckenrode, PT, DPT, OCS
Arcadia University, Glenside, Pennsylvania

Scott Edwards, MD
Hand and Upper Extremity Surgery, The
CORE Institute, Phoenix, Arizona

Bassem T. Elhassan, MD
Professor, Department of Orthopaedic
Surgery, Mayo Clinic, Rochester,
Minnesota

Melanie B. Elliott, PhD
Assistant Professor, Neurosurgery and
Neuroscience, Thomas Jefferson
University, Philadelphia, Pennsylvania

**Susan A. Emerson, MEd, OTR/L, CHT,
CEES**
Owner/Director, Rehab To Work Medical
Consultants, York, Maine

Mia Erickson, PT, EdD, CHT
Professor, Physical Therapy Department,
Midwestern University, Glendale, Arizona

Timothy Estilow, OTR/L
Clinical Specialist, Occupational Therapy
Department, The Children's Hospital
of Philadelphia, Philadelphia,
Pennsylvania

Roslyn B. Evans, OTR/L, CHT
Owner, Director, Indian River Hand and
Upper Extremity Rehabilitation, Vero
Beach, Florida

Frank Fedorczyk, PT, DPT, OCS
Salus Physical Therapy Tampa Bay, St.
Petersburg, Florida

Jane M. Fedorczyk, PT, PhD, CHT
Director, Center for Hand and Upper Limb
Health and Performance; Director,
Advanced Practice Certificate in Hand
and Upper Limb Rehabilitation; Clinical
Professor, Department of Physical
Therapy; Clinical Professor, Department
of Occupational Therapy, Jefferson
College of Rehabilitation Sciences,
Jefferson (Thomas Jefferson University +
Philadelphia University), Philadelphia,
Pennsylvania

**Lynne M. Feehan, BScPT, MSc(PT),
PhD, CHT**
Clinical Associate Professor, Department of
Physical Therapy, University of British
Columbia, Vancouver, British Columbia,
Canada

Sheri B. Feldscher, OTR/L, CHT
Director, Hand Therapy, Philadelphia
Hand to Shoulder Center, Philadelphia,
Pennsylvania

**Elaine Ewing Fess, OTD, MS, OTR,
FAOTA, CHT**
Adjunct Assistant Professor, School of Allied
Health and Rehabilitation, Indiana
University, Indianapolis, Indiana

**Denise Finch, OTD, OTR/L, CHT,
FAOTA**
Assistant Professor, Occupational Therapy,
MCPHS University, Manchester, New
Hampshire

**Annalisa Franzen, OTD,
OTR/L, CHT**
Hand Therapist, Philadelphia Hand
to Shoulder Center, Philadelphia,
Pennsylvania

**Kara Gaffney Gallagher,
MS, OTR/L**
Occupational Therapist, Hand Therapy,
King of Prussia Physical Therapy, King of
Prussia, Pennsylvania

Marc Garcia-Elias, MD, PhD
Consultant Hand Surgeon, Hand and Upper
Extremity Surgery, Institut-Kaplan,
Barcelona, Spain

Michael S. Gart, MD
Plastic & Reconstructive Surgery,
Hand & Upper Extremity Surgery,
OrthoCarolina Hand Center, Charlotte,
North Carolina

Michael P. Gaspar, MD, MBA
Associate Director of Research and Education, Philadelphia Hand to Shoulder Center, Surgeon-Scientist, Department of Orthopaedic Surgery, Thomas Jefferson University, Philadelphia, Pennsylvania

R. Glenn Gaston, MD
Hand Fellowship Director, OrthoCarolina, Charlotte, North Carolina

Bryce W. Gaunt, PT, SCS, CSCS
Director of Physical Therapy, Department of Physical Therapy, HPRC at St. Francis Rehabilitation Center, Columbus, Georgia

Michael J. Gerg, DOT, OTR/L, CHT, CEES, CWCE
Assistant Professor, Occupational Therapy Program, A. T. Still University, Arizona School of Health Sciences, Mesa, Arizona

Bryce T. Gillespie, MD
The Hand & Upper Extremity Center of Georgia, PC, The Shepherd Center, Atlanta, Georgia

Thomas J. Gillon, MD
Clinical Instructor, Orthopaedic Surgery, Thomas Jefferson University Hospitals, Sidney Kimmel Medical School, Philadelphia, Pennsylvania

Rachael Giordano, PT, DPT, OCS, CIDN
Elite Physical Therapy, Providence, Rhode Island

Sarah Glynn, PT, DPT, OCS
3 Dimensional Physical Therapy, Medford, New Jersey

Ronald Gonzalez, DO
Associate Professor, Hand and Upper Extremity Division, Department of Orthopaedics and Rehabilitation, University of Rochester Medical Center, Rochester, New York

Eduardo Gonzalez-Hernandez, MD
Private Practice, Miami, Florida

Joshua A. Gordon, MD
Hand and Upper Extremity Surgery, Hand and Microsurgery Medical Group, San Francisco, California

Michael B. Gottschalk, MD
Assistant Professor, Director of Clinical Research, Orthopedics, Emory University, Atlanta, Georgia

David J. Graham, MD, FRACS
Gold Coast University Hospital, Department of Orthopaedic Surgery, Southport, Queensland, Australia

Thomas J. Graham, MD
Director of Strategy & Innovation, Department of Orthopedic Surgery, NYU Langone Health, New York, New York

Elisabet Hagert, MD, PhD
Associate Professor, Department of Clinical Science and Education, Karolinska Institutet, Stockholm, Sweden

Douglas E. Haladay, PT, DPT, PHD
Associate Professor, School of Physical Therapy & Rehabilitation Sciences, University of South Florida, Tampa, Florida

M. Jake Hamer, MD
Co-Director, Hand and Microvascular Surgery Section, Division of Orthopaedic Surgery, Scripps Clinic, La Jolla, California

Douglas P. Hanel, MD
Professor of Orthopaedics and Sports Medicine, Department of Orthopedics and Sports Medicine, University of Washington Medical Center, Seattle, Washington

Susan D. Hannah, Med, BSc OT
Occupational Therapist, Altum Health, Surgical, Hand & Wrist Specialty Program, University Health Network; Lecturer, Occupational Therapy, University of Toronto, Toronto, Ontario, Canada

Dustin Hardwick, PT, DPT, PhD
Assistant Professor, School of Physical Therapy and Rehabilitation Sciences, University of South Florida Morsani College of Medicine, Tampa, Florida

Maureen Hardy, PT, MS, CHT
Hand Management Center, St. Dominic Hospital, Jackson, Mississippi

David C. Hay, MD
Kerlan-Jobe Orthopaedic Clinic, Cedars-Sinai Kerlan-Jobe Institute, Anaheim, California

Janet Holly, PT, MSc
Clinical Specialist in Pain Science, Senior Physiotherapist, The Ottawa Hospital Rehabilitation Centre; Clinician Investigator, Epidemiology, The Ottawa Hospital Research Institute, Ottawa, Ontario, Canada

Julianne Wright Howell, PT, MS, CHT
Self-Employed Hang/Upper Extremity Consultant, Saint Joseph, Michigan

Harry Hoyen, MD
Department of Orthopaedic Surgery, Cleveland MetroHealth Medical Center, Case Western Reserve University, Cleveland, Ohio

Larry Hurst, MD
Professor & Chairman, Orthopaedics, SUNY Stony Brook, Stony Brook, New York

Haroon Hussain, MD
Fellow, Hand Surgery, Philadelphia Hand to Shoulder Center, Philadelphia, Pennsylvania

David Hutchinson, PT, DSc
Director of Electrophysiologic Laboratory, Philadelphia Hand to Shoulder Centers, King of Prussia, Pennsylvania

Sidney M. Jacoby, MD
Professor of Orthopaedic Surgery, Department of Orthopaedic Surgery, Thomas Jefferson University Hospital, Philadelphia, Pennsylvania

Kathleen Kollitz Jegapragasan, MD
Department of Orthopedic Surgery, Mayo Clinic, Rochester, Minnesota

Christina Jerosch-Herold, MSc, PhD
Professor of Rehabilitation Research, School of Health Sciences, Faculty of Medicine and Health Sciences, University of East Anglia, Norwich, United Kingdom

Neil F. Jones, MD, FRCS
Distinguished Professor or Orthopedic Surgery, Distinguished Professor of Plastic and Reconstructive Surgery, University of California Los Angeles, Los Angeles, California

Sanjeev Kakar, MD, FAOA
Professor of Orthopaedic Surgery, Mayo Clinic, Rochester, Minnesota

Patrick M. Kane, MD
Director of Research, Philadelphia Hand to Shoulder Center; Assistant Professor, Department of Orthopaedic Surgery, Thomas Jefferson University, Philadelphia, Pennsylvania

Christos Karagiannopoulos, MPT, PhD, ATC, CHT
Assistant Professor, DeSales University, Doctor of Physical Therapy Program, Center Valley, Pennsylvania

Parivash Kashani, OTR/L
Hand Therapist, University of California Los Angeles Medical Center, Los Angeles, California

Vicki Kaskutas, OTD, MHS, OT/L
Associate Professor, Program in Occupational Therapy, Washington University School of Medicine, St. Louis, Missouri

Leonid I. Katolik, MD
Attending Surgeon, The Philadelphia Hand to Shoulder Center; Assistant Professor Orthopedic Surgery, Thomas Jefferson University School of Medicine, Philadelphia, Pennsylvania

Joseph R. Kearns, PT, DPT, OCS
Advanced Clinician II, Penn Therapy and Fitness, Good Shepherd Penn Partners, Philadelphia, Pennsylvania

Kenneth Kearns, MD
Attending Physician, Orthopaedic Surgery, Philadelphia Hand to Shoulder Center, Philadelphia, Pennsylvania

Michael W. Keith, MD
Professor of Orthopaedic Surgery, Biomedical Engineering and Physical Medicine and Rehabilitation, Case Western Reserve University; MetroHealth Medical Center, Cleveland VA Medical Center, Cleveland Functional Electrical Stimulation Center, Cleveland, Ohio

Martin J. Kelley, PT, DPT, OCS
Clinical Education Facilitator, Physical and Occupational Therapy, Good Shepherd Penn Partners, Philadelphia, Pennsylvania; Adjunct Assistant Professor, University of Pennsylvania Perelman School of Medicine, Department of Orthopaedics, Philadelphia, Pennsylvania

Jason S. Klein, MD
Orthopaedic Surgery, Shoulders and Elbow Surgery, W.B. Carrell Memorial Clinic, Dallas, Texas

L. Andrew Koman, MD
Professor and Chair, Department of Orthopaedic Surgery, Wake Forest School of Medicine, Winston-Salem, North Carolina

Scott H. Kozin, MD
Clinical Professor, Orthopaedic Surgery, Lewis Katz School of Medicine at Temple University; Clinical Professor, Orthopaedic Surgery, Sidney Kimmel Medical College at Thomas Jefferson University; Chief of Staff, Shriners Hospital for Children, Philadelphia, Pennsylvania

Jonathan Kretschmer, PT, DPT, MM
Physical Therapist, National Home Health Services, East Bay, Northern California; Founder and Owner, ptformusicians.com, San Leandro, California

Andrew F. Kuntz, MD
Assistant Professor, Orthopaedic Surgery, Perelman School of Medicine, University of Pennsylvania, Philadelphia, Pennsylvania

Donald Lalonde, HonsBSc, MSc, MD, FRCSC, DSc
Professor, Plastic Surgery, Dalhousie University, Saint John, Canada

Justine LaPierre, MS, OTR/L
Senior Occupational Therapist, Rehabilitation Department, Shriners Hospital for Children, Philadelphia, Pennsylvania

Paul C. Lastayo, PhD, PT, CHT
Professor, Physical Therapy & Athletic Training; Adjunct Professor, Health-Kinesiology-Recreation; Adjunct Professor, Orthopaedic Surgery, University of Utah, Salt Lake City, Utah

Marsha Lawrence, PT, DPT, CHT
University of Iowa Hospitals and Clinics, Rehabilitation Therapies, University of Iowa, Iowa City, Iowa

Matthew Lazinski, PT, DPT, OCS
Associate Professor, Physical Therapy and Rehabilitation Sciences, University of South Florida, Tampa, Florida

Melissa Lazinski, PT, DPT, DHSc, OCS
Associate Professor, Physical Therapy Department, Nova Southeastern University, Clearwater, Florida

Thanh Le, MD
Clinical Instructor, Department of Orthopaedic Surgery, Stony Brook Medicine, Stony Brook, New York

Marilyn P. Lee, MS, OTR/L, CHT, CLT
Hand-Upper Extremity and Lymphedema Specialist, Lahey Outpatient Center, Danvers, Massachusetts

Michael J. Lee, PT, DPT, CHT
Physical Therapist, Co-Owner - ProActive Physical Therapy, Tucson, Arizona

Steve K. Lee, MD
Associate Professor of Orthopaedic Surgery, Weill Cornell Medical College; Associate Attending Orthopaedic Surgeon, Hand & Upper Extremity Surgery, Hospital for Special Surgery, New York, New York

Brian G. Leggin, PT, DPT, OCS
Adjunct Assistant Professor, Department of Orthopedic Surgery, Perelman School of Medicine, University of Pennsylvania, Philadelphia, Pennsylvania

Matthew I. Leibman, MD, FAAOS
Director of Hand and Upper Extremity Sports Medicine, Newton-Wellesley Hospital, Newton, Massachusetts; Head Team Hand and Wrist Surgeon: Boston Red Sox, Boston Bruins, New England Patriots; Clinical Assistant Professor of Orthopaedic Surgery, Tufts University School of Medicine, Medford, Massachusetts

L. Scott Levin, MD, FACS
Paul B. Magnuson Professor of Bone and Joint Surgery; Chairman; Professor of Orthopaedic Surgery, Department of Orthopaedic Surgery; Professor of Surgery, Division of Plastic Surgery, Department of Surgery, University of Pennsylvania Health System, Philadelphia, Pennsylvania

Todd J. Levy, MS, OTR/L, CBIST
Clinical Specialist, Department of Occupational Therapy, Center for Rehabilitation, Children's Hospital of Philadelphia, Philadelphia, Pennsylvania

Zhongyu Li, MD, PhD
Professor, Department of Orthopaedic Surgery, Wake Forest School of Medicine, Winston-Salem, North Carolina

Bryan J. Loeffler, MD
Assistant Professor, Department of Orthopaedic Surgery, Atrium Health; Clinical Faculty, OrthoCarolina Hand & Upper Extremity Fellowship, OrthoCarolina, Charlotte, North Carolina

Andrew J. Lovy, MD
Assistant Professor, Department of Orthopaedic Surgery, Mount Sinai Hospital, New York, New York

John D. Lubahn, MD
Hand, Microsurgery and Reconstructive Orthopaedics, Erie, Pennsylvania

Ann M. Lucado, PT, PhD, CHT
Assistant Professor, Department of Physical Therapy, Mercer University, Atlanta, Georgia

Göran Lundborg, MD, PhD
Professor, Department of Translational Medicine—Hand Surgery, Lund University, Malmö, Sweden

Dianna Lunsford, OTD, MEd, OTRL, CHT
Associate Professor, Occupational Therapy, Gannon University, Ruskin, Florida

Cheryl Lutz, MS, OTR/L
Senior Occupational Therapist, Rehab Services, Shriners Hospitals for Children, Philadelphia, Pennsylvania

Joy C. MacDermid, BScPT, MSc, PhD
Professor, Physical Therapy, Western University; Co-Director Hand and Upper Limb Centre, Clinical Research Lab, St. Joseph's Health Centre, London, Ontario, Canada

Kyle MacGillis, MD
Clinical Instructor, Department of Orthopaedic Surgery, Stony Brook Medicine, Stony Brook, New York

Alexandra MacKenzie, OTR/L, CHT
Clinical Supervisor Hand Therapy, Hospital for Special Surgery, New York, New York

Norah Malkinski, OTR/L, CHT, CLT
Hand Therapist, Philadelphia Hand to Shoulder Center, Philadelphia, Pennsylvania

Kevin Malone, MD
Associate Professor, Case Western Reserve University School of Medicine, Chief of Hand and Upper Extremity Surgery, Department of Orthopaedic Surgery, University Hospitals Cleveland Medical Center, Cleveland, Ohio

Tambra Marik, OTD, OTR/L, CHT
Assistant Professor of Occupational Therapy, Medical University of South Carolina, Charleston, South Carolina

Elizabeth Anne McBride, MD
Orthopaedic Surgery Wake Forest School of Medicine, Winston-Salem, North Carolina

Philip McClure, PT, PhD, FAPTA
Professor and Chair, Physical Therapy, Arcadia University, Glenside, Pennsylvania

Claire McDaniel, MD
Resident Physician, Orthopaedic Surgery, John Hopkins University Hospital, Baltimore, Maryland

Corey Weston McGee, PhD, MS, OTR/L, CHT
Assistant Professor, Programs in Occupational Therapy and Rehabilitation Science, The University of Minnesota, Minneapolis, Minnesota

Pat McKee, MSc, OT(C)
Associate Professor Emeritus, Department of Occupational Science and Occupational Therapy, University of Toronto, Oakville, Ontario, Canada

Alison McKenzie, PT, MS, PhD
Professor, Physical Therapy, Chapman University Rinker Health Sciences Campus, Irvine, California

Kenneth R. Means, Jr., MD
Attending Physician, Curtis National Hand Center @ Medstar Union Memorial Hospital, Baltimore, Maryland

Shaun D. Mendenhall, MD
Assistant Professor of Surgery, Division of Plastic and Reconstructive Surgery, Department of Surgery, University of Utah School of Medicine, Salt Lake City, Utah

Wyndell H. Merritt, MD, FACS
Clinical Professor of Surgery, Division of Plastic & Reconstructive Surgery, Virginia Commonwealth University, Richmond, Virginia; Clinical Professor of Surgery, Department of Plastic & Maxillofacial Surgery, University of Virginia, Charlottesville, Virginia

R. Scott Meyer, MD
Chief, Orthopaedic Surgery, VA San Diego Healthcare System, La Jolla, California; Professor of Orthopaedic Surgery, Department of Orthopaedic Surgery, University of California, San Diego, School of Medicine, San Diego, California

Robyn Midgley, BSc(Hons) OT, AHT (BAHT), ECHT (EFSHT)
Hand Therapy Consulting, Private Practice, Johannesburg, Gauteng, South Africa

Nathan Miller, MD
Resident Physician, Division of Hand Surgery, Lehigh Valley Health Network, Allentown, Pennsylvania

Amy M. Moore, MD
Associate Professor of Surgery, Division of Plastic and Reconstructive Surgery, Washington University School of Medicine, St. Louis, Missouri

Steven L. Moran, MD
Professor of Plastic Surgery and Orthopedic Surgery, Mayo Clinic, Rochester, Minnesota; Staff Surgeon, Shriners' Hospital for Children, St. Paul, Minnesota

William B. Morrison, MD
Professor, Department of Radiology; Director, Division of Musculoskeletal and General Diagnostic Radiology, Thomas Jefferson University, Philadelphia, Pennsylvania

Surena Namdari, MD, MSc
Associate Professor of Orthopaedic Surgery, Sidney Kimmel Medical College, Thomas Jefferson University; Director of Shoulder and Elbow Research, Rothman Orthopaedic Institute, Philadelphia, Pennsylvania

Nancy Naughton, OTD, OTR/L, CHT
Doctor of Occupational Therapy, Certified Hand Therapist, Director of Occupational Therapy Hand Surgery Associates, Olyphant, Pennsylvania

Clayton Nelson, MD
Hand Fellow, Philadelphia Hand to Shoulder Center, Philadelphia, Pennsylvania

Jonathan Niszczak, MS, OTR/L, BT-C
Clinical Care Specialist, Bio Med Sciences Inc., Allentown, Pennsylvania; Occupational Therapist, Thomas Jefferson University Hospital Burn Center, Philadelphia, Pennsylvania

Christine B. Novak, PT, PhD
Associate Professor, Department of Surgery, University of Toronto, Toronto, Ontario, Canada

Kevin O'Malley, MD
Resident Physician, Orthopaedic Surgery, Georgetown University Hospital, Washington, DC

A. Lee Osterman, MD
Professor, Orthopaedic and Hand Surgery; Chairman, Division of Hand Surgery, Department of Orthopaedic Surgery, Thomas Jefferson University; President, The Philadelphia Hand to Shoulder Center, Philadelphia, Pennsylvania

Meredith Osterman, MD
Instructor of Orthopedics, Thomas Jefferson University, The Philadelphia Hand to Shoulder Center, Philadelphia, Pennsylvania

Lorenzo L. Pacelli, MD
Co-Director, Hand and Microvascular
Surgery Section, Division of Orthopaedic
Surgery, Scripps Clinic, La Jolla,
California

Tara L. Packham, OTReg.(Ont), PhD
Assistant Professor, School of Rehabilitation
Sciences, McMaster University, Hamilton,
Ontario, Canada

**Katherine R. Parrish, AGACNP, CNS,
CWS**
Burn Reconstructive Center, MedSTAR
Washington Hospital Center,
Washington, DC

Allan E. Peljovich, MD, MPH
The Hand & Upper Extremity Center of
Georgia, PC, The Shepherd Center,
Atlanta, Georgia

Karen M. Pettengill, MS, OTR/L, CHT
New England Hand Therapy Coordinator,
NovaCare Rehabilitation/Select Medical,
King of Prussia, Pennsylvania

Peter P. Pham, MD, MS
Resident, Department of Anesthesiology,
Emory University, Atlanta, Georgia

**Michael Piercey, PT, DPT, OCS, Cert.
MDT, CMPT, CSCS**
Lead Physical Therapist, Penn Therapy &
Fitness, Good Shepherd Penn Partners,
Philadelphia, Pennsylvania

Sarah N. Pierrie, MD
Clinical Faculty, Department of Orthopaedic
Surgery, San Antonio Military Medical
Center, JBSA-Ft Sam Houston, Texas

Katie Pisano, OTR/L, CHT
Certified Hand Therapist, Hand and Upper
Body Rehabilitation Center, Erie,
Pennsylvania

Benjamin F. Plucknette, DO, DPT
Philadelphia Hand to Shoulder Center,
Thomas Jefferson University Hospital,
Philadelphia, Pennsylvania

Marisa Pontillo, PT, PhD, DPT, SCS
Scientific Consultant, Department of
Orthopedic Surgery, Perelman School of
Medicine, University of Pennsylvania,
Philadelphia, Pennsylvania

Janet L. Poole, PhD, OTR/L, FAOTA
Professor and Director, Occupational
Therapy Graduate Program, University of
New Mexico, Albuquerque, New Mexico

**Ann Porretto-Loehrke, PT, DPT, CHT,
COMT, CMTPT**
Therapy Co-Manager, Therapy Department,
Hand to Shoulder Center of Wisconsin,
Appleton, Wisconsin

Hollie A. Power, MD
Clinical Lecturer, Division of Plastic Surgery,
Department of Surgery, University of
Alberta, Edmonton, Alberta, Canada

Eliza M. Prager, OTD, MSCI, OTR/L
Assistant Professor of Occupational Therapy,
College of Health Professions, Maryville
University, St. Louis, Missouri

Neal E. Pratt, PhD, PT
Emeritus Professor, Department of Physical
Therapy and Rehabilitation Sciences,
Drexel University, Philadelphia,
Pennsylvania

Matthew L. Ramsey, MD
Professor, Orthopaedic Surgery, Sidney
Kimmel College of Medicine at Thomas
Jefferson University, Philadelphia,
Pennsylvania

Christina M. Read, PT, DPT, CHT
Staff Hand Therapist/Fellowship
Director, Hand and Upper Extremity
Rehabilitation, University of Rochester,
Rochester, New York

Deborah K. Reich, PT, DPT, CHT
Hand Therapy, Philadelphia Hand
to Shoulder Center, Philadelphia,
Pennsylvania

Susanne Rein, MD, PhD, MBA
Department of Plastic and Hand Surgery,
Burn Unit, Hospital Sankt Georg, Leipzig,
Germany

Mark S. Rekant, MD
Associate Professor, Orthopaedic
Surgery, Thomas Jefferson University,
Philadelphia, Pennsylvania

David Ring, MD, PhD
Associate ean for Comprehensive Care,
Department of Surgery and Perioperative
Care, Dell Medical School—The University
of Texas at Austin, Austin, Texas

Annette Marie Rivard, PhD, OT(C)
University of Alberta, Edmonton, Alberta,
Canada

Marco Rizzo, MD
Professor of Orthopedic Surgery, Mayo
Clinic, Rochester, Minnesota

Birgitta Rosén, OT, PhD
Associate Professor, Department of
Translational Medicine—Hand Surgery,
Lund University, Malmö, Sweden

Phillip Ross, MD
Department of Orthopaedic & Sports
Medicine, University of Cincinnati,
Cincinnati, Ohio

David E. Ruchelsman, MD, FAAOS
Chief of Hand Surgery, Newton-Wellesley
Hospital; Director, Hand Surgery
Research & Education Foundation,
Newton, Massachusetts; Clinical
Associate Professor of Orthopaedic
Surgery, Tufts University School of
Medicine, Medford, Massachusetts

Casey Sabbag, MD
Orthopedic Surgery, Resident, Mayo Clinic,
Rochester, Minnesota

Chris Saporito, OTR/L, CHT
Certified Hand Therapist, Philadelphia
Hand to Shoulder Center, Philadelphia,
Pennsylvania

Rebecca J. Saunders, PT, CHT
Clinical Specialist, Research and Staff
Development; Curtis National Hand
Center, Hand Therapy Department @
Medstar Union Memorial Hospital,
Baltimore, Maryland

Luis R. Scheker, MD
Kleinert Institute for Hand and Microsurgery,
Associate Professor of Plastic and
Reconstructive Surgery, University of
Louisville, Louisville, Kentucky

**Karen S. Schultz, MS, OTR/L, CHT,
FAOTA**
Senior Consulting Therapist, N/A, Karen
Schultz Hand and Upper Limb Strategies;
President UE TECH Inc, Littleton,
Colorado

Jodi Seftchick, MOT, OTR/L, CHT
Senior Occupational Therapist, Centers for
Rehabilitation Services, University of
Pittsburgh Medical Center, Pittsburgh,
Pennsylvania

Michael Serghiou, OTR, MBA, BT-C
Clinical Care Specialist, Bio Med Sciences
Inc., Allentown, Pennsylvania

Gayle Severance, MS, OT/L, CHT
Hand Therapy Team Leader, Penn Therapy
and Fitness, Good Shepherd Penn
Partners, Philadelphia, Pennsylvania

Michael A. Shaffer, PT, ATC, OCS
Clinical Supervisor, Rehabilitation Therapies, University of Iowa Hospitals and Clinics, Iowa City, Iowa

Kshamata Shah, PT, PhD
Assistant Professor, Physical Therapy, Arcadia University, Glenside, Pennsylvania

Eon Kyu Shin, MD
Associate Professor, Department of Orthopaedic Surgery, Thomas Jefferson University Hospital, Philadelphia, Pennsylvania

Roger L. Simpson, MD, MBA, FACS
Director of the Burn Center, Division of Plastic Surgery, Nassau University Medical Center–Long Island Plastic Surgical Group, Garden City, New York

Catherine J. Sinnott, MD
Plastic Surgery Research Fellow, Plastic Surgery, Long Island Plastic Surgical Group, Garden City, New York

Bryan Sirmon, MD
Fellow, Hand Surgery, Philadelphia Hand to Shoulder Center, Philadelphia, Pennsylvania

Terri M. Skirven, OTR/L, CHT
Director, Hand Rehabilitation Foundation; Director Emeritus, Hand Therapy, Philadelphia Hand to Shoulder Center, King of Prussia, Pennsylvania

Beth Paterson Smith, PhD
Professor, Department of Orthopaedic Surgery, Wake Forest School of Medicine, Winston-Salem, North Carolina

Heather F. Smith, PhD
Director of Anatomical Laboratories, Department of Anatomy, Midwestern University, Glendale, Arizona; Visiting Scholar, School of Human Evolution and Social Change, Arizona State University, Tempe, Arizona

Thomas L. Smith, PhD
Professor Orthopaedic Surgery, Wake Forest School of Medicine, Winston-Salem, North Carolina

Elizabeth Soika, PT, DPT, CHT
Physical Therapist, Physical Therapy, Geary Rehabilitation and Fitness Center, Junction City, Kansas

Bryan Anthony Spinelli, PT, PhD
Assistant Professor, Thomas Jefferson University, Philadelphia, Pennsylvania

Angela Stagliano, PT, DPT, OCS, CSCS
Assistant Professor, School of Physical Therapy and Rehabilitation Sciences, University of South Florida Morsani College of Medicine, Tampa, Florida

Scott P. Steinmann, MD
Professor of Orthopedic Surgery, Mayo Clinic, Rochester and Austin, Minnesota

Susan Watkins Stralka, PT, DPT, MS
Consultant/Physical Therapist, Plymouth, Massachusetts

Adam B. Strohl, MD, FACS
Philadelphia Hand to Shoulder Center, Instructor, Orthopaedics; Instructor, Surgery–Plastic, Thomas Jefferson University Hospital, Philadelphia, Pennsylvania

Natania Streeter, OTR/L, CHT
Hand Therapy, Philadelphia Hand to Shoulder Center, Langhorne, Pennsylvania

Stephanie Sweet, MD
Clinical Assistant Professor, Orthopedic Surgery, Thomas Jefferson Hospital, Philadelphia, Pennsylvania

Jin Bo Tang, MD
Professor and Chair, Department of Hand Surgery, The Hand Surgery Research Center, Affiliated Hospital of Nantong University, Nantong, Jiangsu, China

John S. Taras, MD
University Orthopaedic Institute, Hahnemann University Hospital, Philadelphia, Pennsylvania

Kenneth A. Taylor, PT, DPT, OCS
Assistant Professor, Doctor of Physical Therapy Program, Gannon University, Ruskin, Florida

Raquel Cantero Tellez, PhD
Physiotherapy, Occupational Therapy, Tecan Hand Center, Rehabilitation, University of Málaga, Málaga, Spain

Michael A. Thompson, MD
Co-Director, Hand and Microvascular Surgery Section, Division of Orthopaedic Surgery, Scripps Clinic, La Jolla, California

Wendy Tomhave, OTR/L
Occupational Therapy/Clinical Research, Shriners' Hospital for Children, St. Paul, Minnesota

Rick Tosti, MD
Assistant Professor of Orthopaedic Surgery, Department of Orthopaedic Surgery, Thomas Jefferson University Hospital, Philadelphia, Pennsylvania

Kristin Valdes, OTD, OT, CHT
Associate Professor, Occupational Therapy, Gannon University, Ruskin, Florida

Joshua Vincent, PT, PhD
Adjunct Assistant Clinical Professor, School of Rehabilitation Sciences, McMaster University, Hamilton, Ontario, Canada; Clinical Expert, Workers Safety Insurance Board, Toronto, Ontario, Canada

Ana-Maria Vranceanu, PhD
Director, Integrated Brain Health Clinical and Research Program, Massachusetts General Hospital, Associate Professor of Psychiatry, Harvard Medical School, Boston, Massachusetts

Carol Waggy, PT, PhD, CHT
Assistant Professor, Human Performance-Physical Therapy, West Virginia University, Morgantown, West Virginia

Laura Walsh, MS, OTD, OT/L, CHT
Program Manager, Penn Therapy and Fitness, Good Shepherd Penn Partners, Philadelphia, Pennsylvania

Mark T. Walsh, PT, DPT, MS, CHT
Physical Therapist/Hand Therapist, NovaCare Rehabilitation, A Division of Select Medical, Somers Point, New Jersey

Lisa Smurr Walters, OTR, CHT
Advanced Arm Dynamics, Gulf Coast Center of Excellence, Houston, Texas

Dana Webb, PT, DPT, OCS, CSCS
Assistant Professor, School of Physical Therapy & Rehabilitation Sciences, University of South Florida, Tampa, Florida

Heather Weesner, OTR/L, CHT
Occupational Therapist, Certified Hand Therapist, Outpatient Orthopedic and Spinal Cord Injury University of Maryland Rehabilitation & Orthopaedic Institute, Baltimore, Maryland

Michael Weinik, DO, FAAPMR, FAOCPMR, FAANEM
Former Professor, Clinical Physical Medicine and Rehabilitation, Lewis Katz School of Medicine at Temple University, Philadelphia, Pennsylvania

Lawrence Weiss, MD
Chief, Division of Hand Surgery, Lehigh Valley Health Network, Allentown, Pennsylvania

Mary Whitten, MOT, OTR/L, CHT
Occupational Therapist, Physical Medicine and Rehabilitation, VA Connecticut Healthcare System, Newington, Connecticut

Gerald R. Williams, Jr., MD
John M. Fenlin, Jr., MD Professor of Shoulder and Elbow Surgery, Rothman Orthopaedic Institute; Professor of Orthopaedic Surgery, Sidney Kimmel Medical College at Thomas Jefferson University, Philadelphia, Pennsylvania

Matthew S. Wilson, MD
Clinical Instructor, Department of Orthopaedic Surgery, Thomas Jefferson University Hospital, Philadelphia, Pennsylvania

Brian R. Wolf, MD, MS
John and Kim Callaghan Chair in Sports Medicine, University of Iowa Hospitals and Clinics, Iowa City, Iowa

David M. Wolfe, OTR/L, CHT
Supervisor, Therapy Department, Philadelphia Hand to Shoulder Center, Philadelphia, Pennsylvania

Terri Wolfe, OTR/L, CHT
Director, Hand and Upper Body Rehabilitation Center, Erie, Pennsylvania

Kathleen E. Yancosek, OTR/L, CHT, PhD
Adjunct Faculty, Gannon University, Erie, Pennsylvania

Jeffrey Yao, MD
Associate Professor, Department of Orthopedic Surgery, Stanford University Medical Center, Redwood City, California

Imran Yousaf, MD
Clinical Researcher, Curtis National Hand Center, MedStar Union Memorial Hospital, Baltimore, Maryland

David S. Zelouf, MD
Assistant Professor, Department of Orthopaedic Surgery, Thomas Jefferson University Hospital; Attending Physician, Philadelphia Hand to Shoulder Center, Philadelphia, Pennsylvania

Miltiadis Zgonis, MD
Assistant Professor, Division of Sports Medicine, Department of Orthopedic Surgery, Perelman School of Medicine, University of Pennsylvania, Philadelphia, Pennsylvania

Dafang Zhang, MD
Attending Surgeon, Hand and Upper Extremity Service, Orthopaedic Surgery, Brigham and Women's Hospital, Boston, Massachusetts

FOREWORD

Forty-two years have passed since the publication of the first edition of *Rehabilitation of the Hand* edited by James Hunter, Lawrence Schneider, Evelyn Mackin, and Judith Bell. It is my privilege to write the Foreword for the seventh edition.

That volume, published in 1978, was based on the early meetings of our Symposium, "Surgery and Rehabilitation of the Hand." The Philadelphia Hand Center brought together surgeons and occupational and physical therapists involved in the care of patients with impairments of the upper extremity. Chaired by Hunter, Schneider, and Mackin, the meeting was eminently successful and has become an annual March event, now celebrating its 45th year in Philadelphia.

The idea of a close association between hand therapy and hand surgery as an ideal way to manage patient care for those with upper extremity impairments was recognized by Dr. Hunter early in his practice at Jefferson Medical College. He was further convinced as a civilian consultant in orthopedic surgery at Valley Forge U.S. Army Hospital from 1964 to 1971 and became a consistently strong and vocal advocate for hand therapy as a subspecialty for the occupational therapy and physical therapy community. This advocacy continued throughout his many years in practice. By 1967, with the addition of Evelyn Mackin PT, who worked closely with him in his practice, he was able to bring hand therapy directly to his own patients.

Evelyn Mackin proved to be an inspired choice as she was innovative and committed to bring the association of therapy and surgery to a successful collaboration. Mackin's enthusiasm and dedication inspired all who came into contact with her, and her remarkable achievements along with several colleagues led to the formation of the American Society of Hand Therapists (ASHT). Evelyn was an early President of that Society. She was a creator and the first editor of the *Journal of Hand Therapy*, a peer reviewed scientific journal.

While some textbooks on hand surgery were in print, there had been limited specific material for the therapist interested in hand care, making the first edition of *Rehabilitation of the Hand* a welcome addition to the literature.

Prior to my arrival in Philadelphia in 1969, I spent 2 years at the U.S. Army's Specialized Treatment Center for Orthopedic Surgery in Augusta, Georgia. That treatment center served as a hospital for Fort Gordon, an active Army training post, and had a large role as a center for soldiers injured in the Vietnam War. Evacuation channels were such that wounded military had immediate treatment in Vietnam and then were transferred to U.S. military hospitals. Wounded who required further care were then sent on to several hospitals at large military installations in the United States.

Those en route to our Center would reach us usually within 10 to 14 days of injury but with some arriving in as few as 72 hours. The 300 beds assigned to the Orthopedic Surgery Service afforded me an invaluable clinical experience.

In September of 1969, I arrived in Philadelphia to join Hunter and Mackin, and I found a thriving university-based practice with a recently established Hand Surgery Fellowship program. The Orthopedic Surgery service and the General Surgery service at Jefferson Hospital also provided junior residents with training.

Jim, Evelyn, and I, eager to establish a teaching program, put together a 2-day meeting that we called "Treatment of the Injured Hand." That meeting was held in a conference room at Jefferson Medical College in 1971. Surgeons and therapists were invited to participate in the program and blended well, suggesting to us that this could be a viable forum for future conferences.

Three years later we created a 3-day meeting on "Tendon Surgery in the Hand" with the sponsorship of the American Academy of Orthopedic Surgery, which led to the first "Surgery and Rehabilitation of the Hand Symposium" in 1976. That meeting preceded the first edition of *Rehabilitation of the Hand* 2 years later.

Subsequent editions benefitted from the contributions of Ann Callahan, MS, OTR/L, CHT, to the Editors list.

In the fifth edition Terri Skirven, OTR/L, CHT, and A. Lee Osterman, MD, assumed leadership of the Editorial Board.

For the sixth edition Skirven and Osterman added Jane Fedorczyk, PT, PhD, CHT, and Peter Amadio, MD, and for the current seventh edition (2021) they added editors Sheri Feldscher, OTR/L, CHT, and Eon Shin, MD.

The editors, in a massive effort, have put together a comprehensive two-volume text consisting of 125 chapters of up-to-date material. They have maintained the excellence established in past editions.

Under Terri Skirven's and Lee Osterman's guidance the March meeting has continued to draw a large number of therapists and surgeons. The meeting continues to evolve. Since 1999 a concurrent surgical symposium has been added. The meeting is held for therapists and surgeons in two concurrent venues. The teaching faculty continues to consist of world-renown specialists in upper extremity surgery and therapy.

On a personal note I would like to mention my gratitude to Andrew Cooney, CPA, who joined the group in 1986 and has been our Executive Director for 34 years.

Lawrence H. Schneider, MD

The first edition of *Rehabilitation of the Hand* was published in 1978, inspired at that time by the newly evolving practice of hand surgeons and hand therapists working together in the care of individuals with hand and upper limb injuries and conditions. The editors of this first edition—James Hunter, MD, Lawrence Schneider, MD, Evelyn Mackin, PT, and Judith Bell Krotoski, OTR, FAOTA, CHT—inspired generations of clinicians to emulate their partnership and achieve the standards of excellence exemplified in their text. This seventh edition is a testimony to the longevity and strength of professional interest and dedication inspired by these founding editors.

Underlying each successive edition of the text are the common threads of collaboration of surgeons and therapists and comprehensive management. As the knowledge base and clinical practice of hand surgery and therapy have expanded, so has the scope and size of the text, expanding from one volume to two and including not just the hand but the entire upper limb.

This seventh edition features a total of 125 chapters, 17 of which are new, with the returning chapters extensively re-organized and updated. We have invited many nationally and internationally known authorities to share their knowledge and expertise. Over 120 new authors have contributed to this edition with a blend of both expert clinicians and academic professionals including occupational therapists, physical therapists, certified hand therapists, nurse practitioners, orthopedic surgeons, plastic surgeons, physiatrists, psychiatrists, researchers and educators. As was the case for the sixth edition, emphasis is placed on evidence-based practice with each chapter supported with current references from peer-reviewed literature. The text is meant to be a comprehensive reference for practicing clinicians as well as students, residents, and fellows.

New chapters for this edition examine developing practice areas such as graded motor imagery, proprioception re-education, and platelet rich protein injections. Established practice areas are given a new look as in sensory relearning and the plastic brain. In fact, a recurrent theme in many chapters is the fact of cortical plasticity both in terms of the cortical changes that occur with injury and immobilization and in terms of prevention and re-education strategies in the rehabilitation of a variety of conditions.

Digital content is again included on the text companion website and updated with many useful surgery and therapy training videos, evaluation forms, patient education materials, and resources for clinicians and patients.

We have dedicated this seventh edition to Dr. Lawrence Schneider, a founding editor for the first edition of the text and for the second, third, and fifth editions. Dr. Schneider's practical nature and sense of humor are well known to those of us who are fortunate to have worked with him. Dr. Schneider along with colleagues James Hunter, MD, and Evelyn Mackin, PT, developed a unique model for the integrated management of hand and upper limb injured patients combining the specialties of hand surgery and hand therapy in a team-oriented approach at the Hand Rehabilitation Center, now the Philadelphia Hand to Shoulder Center. This philosophy of management has endured and been emulated and is clearly reflected in this seventh edition.

The publication of the seventh edition of *Rehabilitation of the Hand and Upper Extremity* is the result of the efforts of many individuals over more than 3 years and acknowledgements are due.

First and foremost, we thank the over 200 contributors, dedicated professionals all, who have shared their expertise and knowledge. We also wish to recognize and thank the many previous edition contributors whose work has been updated and expanded for this seventh edition. Our editors at Elsevier are most appreciated for their patience and persistence to see the text through to completion and publication. In particular, Dee Simpson, Senior Content Development Specialist, who managed the submission of manuscripts and the content editing process and deserves our thanks for what is a most difficult task considering the large pool of authors and number of chapters. Thanks to Project Managers Tara Delaney and Dan Fitzgerald, who kept the page proofing process on track; and Belinda Kuhn and Kristine Jones, Senior Content Strategists, who provided guidance along the way.

Thanks to Andrew Cooney, Executive Director of the Philadelphia Hand to Shoulder Center, who has provided support and encouragement during the work on the seventh edition as for prior editions.

Finally, we thank our family, friends, and colleagues for their support and patience over the more than 3 years it has taken to complete the text.

We are proud to present this seventh edition of *Rehabilitation of the Hand and Upper Extremity.*

Terri M. Skirven
A. Lee Osterman
Jane M. Fedorczyk
Peter C. Amadio
Sheri B. Feldscher
Eon Kyu Shin

CONTENTS

ONLINE SUPPLEMENTAL ELEMENTS

VIDEO CONTENTS

Frozen Shoulder: Surgery and Therapy

Michael Piercey, Martin J. Kelley, Andrew F. Kuntz

OUTLINE

CRITICAL POINTS

- Adhesive capsulitis may be classified based on the patient's irritability level (low, moderate, and high) to guide intervention decisions.
- Clinically, adhesive capsulitis can be divided into four stages, which may be complicated by extrinsic, intrinsic, or systemic causative factors.
- The hallmark of adhesive capsulitis on examination is a loss of passive range of motion in external rotation.
- An algorithmic approach offering conservative and surgical interventions can effectively address the adhesive capsulitis continuum as driven by the patient's response to treatment.

Adhesive capsulitis, also known as frozen shoulder, is poorly defined as a clinical condition with painful, restricted active and passive range of motion (ROM). Frozen shoulder syndrome was first described by Duplay[1] in 1872; however, it was not until 1934 in the classic article by Codman[2] that the term *frozen shoulder* was officially introduced into the orthopedic literature. In 1945, Neviaser[3] suggested that "the essential pathology is a thickening and contraction of the capsule which becomes adherent to the humeral head." With these findings, Neviaser[3] suggested that a more descriptive term based on the pathologic features be used, coining the term *adhesive capsulitis.*

Lundberg[4] further classified adhesive capsulitis into primary (idiopathic) and secondary adhesive capsulitis. Primary adhesive capsulitis is idiopathic, whereas secondary adhesive capsulitis can be attributed to a known intrinsic, extrinsic, or systemic cause.[4] More recently, Zuckerman and Rokito[5] proposed a classification schema defined by primary and secondary adhesive capsulitis (Fig. 70.1). Primary adhesive capsulitis and idiopathic adhesive capsulitis are considered identical and not associated with a systemic condition or history of injury.[5] Secondary adhesive capsulitis is that which is associated with a known cause. Three classes of secondary adhesive capsulitis exist: intrinsic, extrinsic, and systemic.[5] The intrinsic class includes rotator cuff pathology,

biceps pathology, glenohumeral arthritis, and acromioclavicular joint arthritis.[5] The extrinsic class includes proximal humerus fractures, cervical spine disease, myocardial infarction, stroke, and Parkinson's disease.[5] The systemic class includes hyperthyroidism, hypothyroidism, hypoadrenalism, and most notably, diabetes mellitus, which can also result in adhesive capsulitis.[5] Tertiary adhesive capsulitis can occur postoperatively or postfracture.[5]

Another proposed classification system is based on the patient's irritability level (low, moderate, and high) to guide intervention decisions.[6] (Table 70.1) Irritability reflects the tissue's ability to handle physical stress and is determined based on pain, ROM, and extent of disability.[6] Patients with low irritability have lower disability and less pain and have capsular end feels with little or no pain with over pressure; therefore, active and passive motion may be equal. These patients typically report stiffness, rather than pain, as a chief complaint. Patients with high irritability have significant pain, resulting in limited passive motion (caused by muscle guarding) and greater disability. These patients typically report pain rather than stiffness as a chief complaint. Although these criteria are not time based, most commonly, patients with early stage capsulitis have a high level of irritability, but patients in later stages have lower irritability.

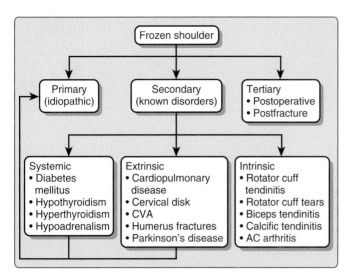

Fig 70.1 Proposed pathways for the development of adhesive capsulitis. *AC,* Acromioclavicular; *CVA,* cerebrovascular accident. (Copyright © 2007 by Lippincott Williams & Wilkins. Iannotti JP, Williams GR Jr, eds. *Disorders of the Shoulder: Diagnosis & Management.* 2nd ed. Philadelphia: Lippincott Williams & Wilkins; 2007.)

TABLE 70.1   Irritability Classification

	High Irritability	Moderate Irritability	Low Irritability
Pain level	High (>7/10)	Moderate (4–6/10)	Low (<3/10)
Night or resting pain	Consistent	Intermittent	None
Disability or outcome score (e.g., DASH, ASES, Penn Shoulder Score)	High disability	Moderate disability	Low disability
End-range pain	Pain before end ROM	Pain at end ROM	Min pain at end ROM with overpressure
ROM	AROM < PROM	AROM ~ PROM	AROM = PROM

AROM, Active range of motion; *ASES,* American Shoulder and Elbow Surgeons; *DASH,* Disability of the Arm Shoulder and Hand; *PROM,* passive range of motion; *ROM,* range of motion.

PATHOLOGY

The glenohumeral joint is an unconstrained joint with capsular surface area almost twice that of the humeral head. As such, a large capsular volume is necessary to allow the glenohumeral motion required during activities of daily living. At any one moment, only one fourth to one third of the humeral articular surface is in contact with the glenoid.[6] As a result, the shoulder relies heavily on soft structures for stabilization during ROM. Thus, contracture of any of the soft tissue stabilizers, be it the glenohumeral ligaments, the coracohumeral ligament, the shoulder capsule, or the rotator cuff musculature and tendons, can result in constriction of glenohumeral motion and the clinical picture of adhesive capsulitis.

Based on surgical dissections of patients with adhesive capsulitis, Neviaser[3] noted that the glenohumeral joint capsule was markedly thickened and adherent to the humeral head and associated with a paucity of synovial fluid within the glenohumeral joint. Histologic evaluation of the capsule demonstrates fibrotic changes with chronic inflammation as evidenced by perivascular infiltration with

TABLE 70.2   Stages and Physical Examination Findings in Adhesive Capsulitis

Stage	Physical Examination
1. Preadhesive	Near-normal ROM
	Pain at end points of motion
2. Freezing	Marked loss of motion
	Pain at end points of motion
3. Frozen	Marked loss of motion
	Less painful ROM
4. Thawing	Improved glenohumeral motion
	Painless ROM

ROM, range of motion.

mononuclear cells.[3] Neviaser's[3] early work also revealed decreased joint volume and obliteration of the axillary recess on shoulder arthrography in the setting of adhesive capsulitis.

More recently, arthroscopic evaluation of patients with primary adhesive capsulitis revealed a reduction in joint capacity with patchy synovitis, most consistently located in the rotator interval, but not the adhesions and axillary recess contractures that were present in the study by Neviaser.[7,8] Open exploration of patients with chronic adhesive capsulitis revealed thickening of the coracohumeral ligament and rotator interval tissue, with histologic analysis of resected capsular tissue demonstrating fibrosis and fibroid degeneration.[9] In another study, immunocytochemical analysis suggested active fibroblastic proliferation as the underlying pathologic process, mimicking the findings seen in Dupuytren's disease.[10] This was further supported by the presence of mRNA encoding for fibrogenic growth factors similar to those seen in Dupuytren's tissue.[11] Evaluation of the synovium has revealed marked increases in several cytokines, suggesting an upregulation of capsular fibroblasts, resulting in new collagen deposition.[12] In fact, a strong association between adhesive capsulitis and Dupuytren's disease has been suggested as patients with primary adhesive capsulitis have an eightfold increase in Dupuytren's disease compared with the general population.[13] Rodeo and associates[12] found a marked increase in several cytokines within the synovial tissue in patients with adhesive capsulitis, which suggests an upregulation of capsular fibroblasts and resultant new collagen production. Mast cells have also been found to be present in diseased tissue, and as regulators of fibroblast proliferation, these cells may also play an important role in the pathogenesis of adhesive capsulitis.[14]

Clinically, adhesive capsulitis can be divided into four stages[15] (Table 70.2). In stage 1, the preadhesive stage, patients present with painful active and passive range of motion (PROM) but without significantly decreased ROM. In this stage, symptoms typically have been present for less than 3 months, and pain is often described as achy at rest and sharp at end ROM, particularly at the end of external rotation with the arm at the patient's side.[16] Without significant loss of motion, patients are often misdiagnosed as having rotator cuff tendinitis and impingement. Arthroscopic examination during this early stage reveals a diffuse hypervascular synovitis, most commonly in the region of the rotator interval (Fig. 70.2). In stage 2, the "freezing" stage, patients present with a more profound loss of ROM secondary to capsular contracture and painful, proliferative synovitis. Even though this phase is represented by pain, examination under anesthesia reveals connective tissue changes resulting in loss of motion. Arthroscopic evaluation reveals a dense, tight capsule and hypertrophic synovium (Fig. 70.3). Stage 3 is the "frozen" phase when patients show a marked loss of ROM and increased joint stiffness but a decrease in pain. The decreased pain

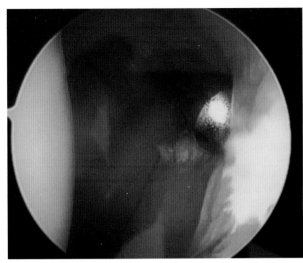

Fig 70.2 Synovitis within the rotator interval.

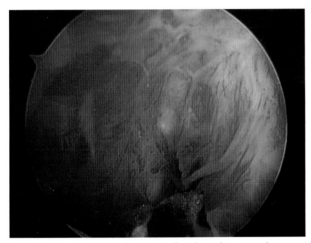

Fig 70.3 Proliferative synovitis extending into the posterior capsule, encompassing the entire glenohumeral joint.

experienced at this stage is caused by less synovitis and more mature adhesions. Patients in this stage have motion limited by established contracture as opposed to pain, with equal PROM on examination under anesthesia compared with when awake. Arthroscopic examination reveals a very thick, dense, low-volume capsule with limited synovitis. Stage 4, the "thawing" stage, is notable for the gradual resolution of symptoms with progressive improvements in ROM. There is also minimal pain during this final phase. Increased ROM is secondary to capsular remodeling and reestablishment of normal capsular volume.

Secondary adhesive capsulitis has many causative factors and can be generalized into three categories: extrinsic, intrinsic, and systemic. Specifically, patients with diabetes have been reported to have a fourfold increased risk of developing adhesive capsulitis.[17] It also appears that the duration of diabetes is an independent risk factor for the development of secondary adhesive capsulitis.[17,18] There has also been an association between the treatment of human immunodeficiency virus with antiretroviral therapies and the development of secondary adhesive capsulitis.[19,20] Patients with previous shoulder fracture or shoulder surgery and decreased glenohumeral joint ROM represent another spectrum of adhesive capsulitis. Although some patients have pure capsular stiffness from scarring or stiffening of the capsule, others have stiffness from joint incongruency, prominent hardware, malunion, or scarring between the deltoid and humerus.[21]

HISTORY AND PHYSICAL EXAMINATION

The diagnosis of primary adhesive capsulitis is a diagnosis of exclusion based on thorough history taking, physical examination, and appropriate imaging. A comprehensive history should include a patient-oriented shoulder outcome form, such as the constant score, the DASH (Disability of the Arm Shoulder and Hand), the SPADI (Shoulder Pain and Disability Index), the ASES (American Shoulder Pain and Disability Index), or the Penn Shoulder Score. A full upper quarter examination is performed to rule out cervical spine and neurologic issues. Three questions help to determine the current stage of the patient's adhesive capsulitis. First, "Can you sleep through the night?" The ability to sleep well indicates low irritability. Second, "Do you have more pain or stiffness?" Greater pain reflects active synovitis while stiffness indicates resolving synovitis and stage progression from stage 2 to 3. The third question, "Is it better or worse in the last 3 weeks?" can help determine if one is moving into or out of stage 2.

Pain is overwhelmingly the chief symptom on presentation. Motion loss may also be a symptom, but many times, even with profound stiffness, patients do not realize that they have lost motion. They simply believe that they cannot move the arm because it is painful. A history of trauma, both major and minor, can be an inciting factor; however, many patients do not recall any specific event. It is extremely common for patients to experience nighttime pain, pain when reaching behind the back, or pain when reaching away from the body. Scapular substitution frequently accompanies all active shoulder motion.[22,23] Passive motions are assessed supine to appreciate end-feel. Frequently, passive motions are very restricted because of pain at or before end range and muscle guarding can often be appreciated at end range. The clinician should be aware that muscle guarding can masquerade as a capsular end feel.[24] Acute left-sided shoulder pain may be a symptom originating from cardiac ischemia and should be considered during the evaluation.

Physical examination should include the cervical spine for referred pain secondary to radiculopathy or spondylosis, as well as other neurologic pathologies. After the cervical spine is cleared, the shoulder examination begins with inspection of the patient, both at rest and with motion. Atrophy, previous scars, and active motion can be observed for both shoulders to allow comparison of the involved side with the uninvolved side.

Glenohumeral motion is measured in planes of elevation, external rotation with the arm at the side, and internal rotation with the arm at the side, as a minimum. The hallmark of adhesive capsulitis on examination is a loss of PROM in external rotation, although active range of motion (AROM) and PROM will be lost in all planes, especially in stages 2 and 3. However, no matter what stage of the disease process the patient presents with, AROM equals PROM. Loss of motion of greater than 25% in at least two planes, a 50% loss of passive external rotation, or less than 30 degrees of external rotation is indicative of a patient with adhesive capsulitis.[10,22,23,25–33]

True evaluation of glenohumeral motion requires scapular stabilization to eliminate any compensatory scapulothoracic motion and thoracic extension. The tracking of the scapula during elevation can also be observed and compared with the uninvolved side because scapular substitution frequently may accompany active shoulder motion.[28,34] Passive motions should be assessed with the patient supine to appreciate the quality of the resistance to motion at the end of passive movement. Frequently, passive glenohumeral motions are restricted because of pain at or before end range. This can often be appreciated by muscle guarding. It is believed that muscle guarding can masquerade as a capsular end-feel.[24] Kelley and coworkers[24] examined six patients before manipulation both pre-and postanesthesia and revealed an increase in passive motion of 10 to 30 degrees during anesthetization in five of the six patients. A capsular end-feel was appreciated in all patients preanesthesia; however, this was a false interpretation. Partial improvement in motion related to diminished pain and muscle guarding has been reported after local or regional anesthetic.[35] The examination typically reveals significant global limitations of both active and passive elevation usually less than 120 degrees, but motion limitations are stage dependent.[3,10,25,35–37] The significant loss of passive external rotation with the arm at the side as well as loss of active and passive motion in other planes differentiates adhesive capsulitis from other pathologies. Although patients with rotator cuff tendinopathy may present with significantly restricted and painful active and passive motion, they rarely have significant restrictions of passive external rotation.[24]

Patients with adhesive capsulitis are considered to have normal strength and painless resisted motions; however, markedly reduced shoulder isometric maximal voluntary force has been reported in patients with adhesive capsulitis.[36–38] Objective shoulder strength measurements using a handheld dynamometer revealed significant weakness of the shoulder internal rotators[37,38] and elevators[36–38] in patients with adhesive capsulitis. Special tests such as impingement signs and Jobe's test are not helpful in differentiating adhesive capsulitis from rotator cuff tendinopathy because they require painful end-range positioning.[24]

Patients presenting in early stages of adhesive capsulitis have pain on palpation of the shoulder. ROM, particularly end ROM in external rotation, is painful secondary to the synovitis present within the rotator interval. The differentiating factor between stages 1 and 2 is that patients in stage 1 have nearly normal glenohumeral motion, whereas stage 2 patients show a loss of glenohumeral motion in multiple planes. Stage 3 patients have continued limitations in glenohumeral motion, but they report less pain than in earlier stages. Stage 4 patients will begin to gradually regain their shoulder function, with continued improvements in glenohumeral motion as the capsular contracture begins to resolve.

Differentiating early primary adhesive capsulitis from other pathologic conditions, such as rotator cuff pathology, can be quite difficult. However, the presence of signs of capsular irritation during the physical examination will help differentiate primary adhesive capsulitis from other possible underlying conditions.[16] Placing the arm at the patient's side and gently externally rotating the arm past the normal end point of motion will result in capsular stretching. In the presence of capsular pathology, the patient's pain will be reproduced but will not be present if rotator cuff pathology is the true pain generator. Another technique to distinguish between rotator cuff pathology and adhesive capsulitis is to perform a subacromial injection of local anesthetic. Injection of local anesthetic into the subacromial space should alleviate pain and improve motion if rotator cuff pathology is present but will have minimal effect to improve motion if caused by capsular contracture.

Postsurgical and posttraumatic stiffness can be complex to evaluate. Fractures of the proximal humerus, clavicle, or any of the other bony structures can lead to shoulder stiffness. Shoulder surgery of any type can also lead to shoulder stiffness. The cause of the stiffness may be from glenohumeral capsule contracture, scarring of the scapulohumeral interval, malunion, nonunion, avascular necrosis, prominent hardware, posttraumatic arthritis, infection, nerve palsy, or chronic dislocation. Although there is a wide range of potential underlying pathologies, evaluation should still begin with inspection and observation of ROM, both active and passive. Next, an assessment of rotator cuff strength and deltoid function is made. Then the quality of the glenohumeral motion is assessed to evaluate the presence or absence of crepitus during motion and whether the pain occurs throughout the ROM. The presence or absence of instability is also considered.

RADIOGRAPHIC STUDIES

Although plain radiographs are often included in the initial evaluation of a patient with shoulder pain, there are no radiographic findings diagnostic of adhesive capsulitis. Instead, the primary reason for obtaining plain radiographs for patients with idiopathic adhesive capsulitis is to rule out shoulder dislocation and to evaluate the glenohumeral joint space. Osteoarthritis of the glenohumeral joint can be quite painful and may limit glenohumeral ROM, thus making this the primary differential diagnosis when evaluating a patient with a stiff, painful shoulder. Plain radiographs will also allow evaluation for other secondary causes of adhesive capsulitis, such as fractures, calcifying tendinitis, and rotator cuff tear arthropathy.

Advanced imaging studies are not necessary to make the diagnosis of adhesive capsulitis. However, advanced imaging can aid in evaluating for secondary causes of adhesive capsulitis. In fact, Sher and colleagues[39] showed that performing magnetic resonance imaging (MRI) often results in a change in the primary diagnosis and the ultimate treatment plan. Most commonly, MRI allows for evaluation of soft tissue pathology, such as rotator cuff tears or biceps or labral pathology that serve as the underlying cause of pain and resultant decreased glenohumeral motion. The use of ultrasound is also becoming more common, even in the outpatient clinical setting. Ultrasonography has been proven effective in diagnosing adhesive capsulitis and allows for image-guided glenohumeral joint injection at the same time when clinically indicated.[40] Computed tomography (CT) typically is not obtained during the evaluation and treatment of adhesive capsulitis. However, CT may be of value in postsurgical and postfracture stiffness when a CT scan will allow for detailed evaluation of the glenohumeral joint and can also provide information regarding prominent hardware, bone loss, loose bodies within the joint, fracture malunion, and fracture nonunion.

TREATMENT

Multiple interventions have been studied, but definitive treatment remains unclear.[26,32,41–43] Unfortunately, comparison among studies is difficult because of varied inclusion criteria, differing protocols, and varied outcome assessment tools. One of the major difficulties in assessing efficacy is success criterion because the majority of patients with adhesive capsulitis significantly improve in approximately 1 year regardless of how they were treated. Successful treatment should not be defined by the return of "normal" motion but rather by significant symptom reduction, improved patient satisfaction, and improved functional ability. Therefore, the initial goal is pain reduction by influencing synovial tissue. Typically, as pain lessens, the patient moves well within the passive limits and "feels" greatly improved. The capsuloligamentous complex tissue length is restored and motion returns as dense fibrotic collagen remodeling occurs over time. Specific interventions and their evidence will be discussed and synthesized into a therapeutic intervention algorithm driven by the response to treatment. Within this algorithm, nonoperative measures are the first line of treatment for primary adhesive capsulitis. The goals of nonoperative management are twofold: pain relief and restoration and maintenance of glenohumeral motion. Adequate pain relief and physical therapy should be a part of all treatment regimens.

MODALITIES

Little data exist supporting the use of frequently used modalities such as heat, ice, ultrasound, or electric stimulation. Modalities may influence pain and muscle relaxation; therefore, they might enhance the effect of

TABLE 70.3 Treatment Strategies Based on Irritability Level

	High Irritability	Moderate Irritability	Low Irritability
Modalities	Heat, ice, electrical stimulation	Heat, ice, electrical stimulation	—
Activity modification	Yes	Yes	None
ROM and stretch	Short duration (1–5 sec) pain-free PROM → AAROM	Short-duration (5–15 sec) PROM → AAROM → AROM	End-range or overpressure, increase duration, cyclic loading
Manual techniques	Low-grade mobilization	Low- → high-grade mobilization	High grade mobilization, sustained hold
Strengthen	—	—	Low to high resistance through available ranges
Functional activities	—	Basic	High demand
Patient education	+	+	+
Other	Intraarticular corticosteroid injection	—	—

AAROM, Active assistive range of motion; *AROM,* active range of motion; *PROM,* passive range of motion; *ROM,* range of motion.

exercises and manual techniques. Hot packs can be applied before or during ROM exercises. Application of moist heat in conjunction with stretching has been shown to improve muscle extensibility.[44] This may occur by a reduction of muscle viscosity and neuromuscular-mediated relaxation.[31,45] Ice may be recommended for use upon completion of a prescribed exercise session to patients who experience undesired levels of soreness. Kurtaiş Gürsel and associates[46] demonstrated the lack of efficacy of ultrasound when compared with sham ultrasound in treating shoulder soft tissue disorders. Dogru and colleagues[47] studied the effects of therapeutic ultrasound as a treatment for adhesive capsulitis. Both groups received superficial heat and an exercise program. The treatment group received therapeutic ultrasound, whereas the control group received a sham ultrasound. After treatment, there was no difference when comparing the two groups in terms of ROM and patient satisfaction scales. Transcutaneous electrical nerve stimulation together with a prolonged low-load stretch resulted in less pain and improved motion in patients with adhesive capsulitis.[25] Cheing and coworkers[48] found that electroacupuncture or interferential stimulation in combination with stretching exercises were effective in treating patients with adhesive capsulitis compared with no treatment at all. Unfortunately, this study cannot rule out the exercise effect on improved outcomes. Recently, Jewell and associates[49] reported that ultrasound, massage, iontophoresis, and phonophoresis reduced the likelihood of favorable outcomes in the treatment of patients with adhesive capsulitis. Combining mobility and stretching exercises with modalities, such as short-wave diathermy, ultrasound, or electric stimulation, may help reduce pain and improve ROM.[24]

STRETCHING

Favorable outcomes have been reported in patients with adhesive capsulitis treated primarily with stretching exercises in therapy.[22,50,51] Stretching appears to influence pain and improve motion over time. Studies have shown that exercise results in improved ROM and outcomes; however, aggressive stretching may be counterproductive.[22,52] Griggs and associates[22] reported that 90% of patients classified as stage 2 idiopathic adhesive capsulitis demonstrated good outcomes when treated with supervised physical therapy and a home exercise program (HEP). Levine and coworkers[51] found that 89.5% of patients responded to nonoperative management when treated with a combination of physical therapy, nonsteroidal antiinflammatory drugs, and one or more corticosteroid injections. Diercks and Stevens[50] compared two groups of patients with adhesive capsulitis; one group was treated with "supervised neglect" and the other with "intensive physical therapy." Group 1 performed exercises not to exceed the pain threshold,

whereas group 2 performed active exercises up to and beyond the pain threshold, passive stretching, glenohumeral joint mobilization, and a HEP. Although both groups made significant improvement in pain and ROM (follow-up period, 24 months), 89% of the "supervised neglect" group achieved a constant score of greater than 80 compared to only 63% of the "intense physical therapy" group. An impressive finding among multiple studies is patient improvement and minimal or no difference in outcomes (at 3–6 months) in patients treated with a therapist directed HEP compared with other interventions.[27,32,53,54]

Applying the correct "dose" of stretching is important and based on the stage of adhesive capsulitis and the patient's irritability classification (Table 70.3). In patients with high irritability, low-intensity and short-duration ROM exercises are performed to simply alter the joint receptors input, reduce pain, decrease muscle guarding, and increase motion.[55] Regardless of how irritable a patient is, pain must be managed by an informed patient who is actively participating with therapy with exercise.[56] Three factors should be considered when calculating the "dose" or total amount of stress delivered to a tissue: intensity, frequency, and duration. The total end-range time[57,58] is the total amount of time the joint is held at or near end-range position. Total end-range time is calculated by multiplying the frequency and duration of the time spent at end-range daily and is a useful way of measuring the dose of tissue stress.[57,58] Intensity remains an important factor in tensile stress dose but is typically limited by pain. Traditional ROM exercises are considered lower forms of tensile stress, whereas the highest tensile stress doses are achieved by low-load prolonged stretching because total end-range time is maximized. Therefore, the goal with each patient is to determine the therapeutic level of tensile stress required based on his or her irritability level and response to treatment.

JOINT MOBILIZATION

Joint mobilization is a manual therapy technique to selectively influence the joint soft tissues depending on the technique or direction of translation. Classic theory describes the performance of low-grade mobilization (grades I and II) to influence pain. High-grade mobilization (grades III and IV) is performed to influence soft tissue length because the tissue is elongated. The capsuloligamentous complex should be viewed using the circle concept. The circle concept refers to all regions of the capsuloligamentous complex providing stability in all directions (e.g., anterior structures provide posterior stability and vice versa).[59] When this concept is applied to a shoulder with limited glenohumeral motion, improved extensibility of any portion of the capsuloligamentous complex results in improved motion in all planes. Johnson and coworkers[60] compared anterior with posterior glide mobilizations sustained for 1 minute at end range of abduction and external rotation in patients with adhesive capsulitis. They found greater improvement in external rotation motion in the group treated with posterior glides.

Several studies have examined the effect of joint mobilization in patients with adhesive capsulitis. Although there is evidence that it may be beneficial, there is little evidence to support that it is more efficacious than other forms of treatment.[27,28,60–62] Nicholson[61] found that patients treated with joint mobilization in addition to exercise did better than the group treated with just exercise when comparing abduction ROM; however, both groups significantly improved in ROM and pain reduction. Bulgen[63] found that patients significantly improved in ROM and pain reduction after 4 weeks of joint mobilization but not better than another group treated with corticosteroid injections. After 6 months, patients treated with joint mobilization did just as well as three other patients groups treated with corticosteroids, ice and proprioceptive neuromuscular facilitation, and HEP, respectively. One study treated one group with high-grade mobilizations and another with low-grade mobilizations without any other intervention for three sessions per week for 12 weeks. Outcome measures for both groups improved, and although the high-grade mobilization group did better, only few comparisons reached statistical significance, and the overall differences between the two interventions was minor.[28] This suggests that performing only low-grade mobilizations will bring about significant improvement in motion and function. This finding is surprising because low-grade mobilization is thought only to influence pain, not ROM; however, considering the pathology of adhesive capsulitis (synovitis), mobilization may influence the pain or mechanoreceptor, resulting in less pain, less muscle guarding, and improved ROM. Therefore, end-range can be achieved to ultimately assist with collagen remodeling.

Jewell and coworkers[49] performed a retrospective cohort study to determine if physical therapy interventions predicted meaningful short-term improvement in patients with adhesive capsulitis. They found bodily pain scores were more likely to improve in patients treated with joint mobilization. Clearly, some patients appear to react very favorably to joint mobilization demonstrated by their response to treatment. Further research is required to determine if certain patient characteristics respond to specific interventions such as joint mobilization.[24]

INTRAARTICULAR CORTICOSTEROID INJECTION

Corticosteroids can be administered by injection to dampen the inflammatory response in patients with adhesive capsulitis. There is substantial evidence to support that intraarticular corticosteroid injections provide significant improvement of symptoms in the first 4 to 6 weeks after injection.[26,32,41,42,54] Although no long-term differences can be attributed to corticosteroids, it is believed that the patient can be made more comfortable at rest and with functional movement while also potentially shortening the synovitis stage.

Steroids have long been used in the treatment of adhesive capsulitis secondary to their strong antiinflammatory and analgesic effects. Buchbinder and colleagues[64] showed that a short course of oral steroids resulted in improved pain scores, ROM, and overall shoulder function. A Cochrane Database review that analyzed the use of oral steroids for treatment of adhesive capsulitis showed "silver" level evidence that oral steroids provide significant short-term benefits in terms of pain relief and improved ROM; however, no evidence could be gathered to prove that this effect was maintained beyond 6 weeks.[64]

Many physicians favor the use of intraarticular steroid injections in an attempt to prevent the systemic side effects of oral steroid administration. A study comparing intraarticular corticosteroid injections alone with physical therapy alone showed that patients who received injections had better outcomes at 7 weeks but that there was no difference between the two groups at 26 and 52 weeks of follow-up.[42] Carette and colleagues[32] showed that the addition of intraarticular steroids to a physical therapy regimen resulted in statistically significant improvements in ROM and patient satisfaction outcome measures. A more recent study demonstrated short-term pain relief after corticosteroid injection for adhesive capsulitis; however, long-term pain relief was not found.[65] PROM improved in the short and long terms after injection.[65] Interestingly, another study found both short- and long-term benefits when the time to injection was shorter, suggesting early injection is more beneficial than delayed injection.[66] Finally, when it comes to low- versus high-dose intraarticular corticosteroid injection, Kim and colleagues[67] demonstrated equivalent pain relief with low-dose injection (20 mg of triamcinolone acetonide) compared with a higher (40 mg) dose.

Aside from corticosteroid injection, other medications and saline alone have been investigated in the treatment of adhesive capsulitis. Sodium hyaluronate has been shown to prevent peritendinous adhesions after flexor tendon injuries, which is thought to be secondary to its ability to minimize the inflammatory response.[68] However, Blaine and colleagues[69] studied the effects of intraarticular injections of hyaluronic acid compared with saline solution injections, and no statistically significant difference was found between the two groups when comparing ROM as an outcome measure. Capsular distention or brisement has also been used as a means to treat adhesive capsulitis. Corbeil and colleagues[70] performed a double-blinded, prospective study that looked at the effects of intraarticular corticosteroid injections with and without distention arthrography. Early pain relief was reported by 80% of the patients, but at 3-month follow-up, they did not find any improvements in ROM or pain relief in the capsular distention group. Likewise, Tveita and colleagues[71] found no benefit with the combination of intraarticular steroids and capsular distention compared with steroids alone six weeks after treatment. Conversely, Gam and colleagues[72] showed that patients who received intraarticular steroids and capsular distention had improved ROM compared with steroids alone. Vad and colleagues[73] prospectively evaluated the effects of capsular distention in patients who presented with stage 2 or 3 disease over a 2-year period. Patients who were in stage 2 showed statistically significant improvements in ROM, however those who presented in stage 3 failed to show any significant improvements.[73] This suggests that brisement may be more beneficial when reserved for patients presenting in the early stages of the disease process.[73] Watson and colleagues[74] showed that capsular distention may also have a role in treating patients with secondary adhesive capsulitis resulting from underlying rotator cuff pathology.

MANIPULATION UNDER ANESTHESIA

Manipulation under anesthesia is a commonly used treatment for patients with persistent adhesive capsulitis despite non-operative treatment. Placzek and colleagues[75] studied 31 patients who were treated with manipulation and followed them for 14 months. The patients showed a mean improvement in ROM of 84 degrees in abduction, 63 degrees in forward flexion, 58 degrees in external rotation, and 47 degrees in internal rotation. Patients also reported significantly improved pain scores, and there were no reported complications. Farrell and colleagues[76] looked at the long-term results of manipulation under anesthesia, with a mean follow-up period of 15 years. Patients had an average ROM improvement of 64 degrees in forward elevation and 44 degrees in external rotation. Of the 19 shoulders reviewed, 13 had no pain, and 3 had only slight pain. The benefits of manipulation under anesthesia are often seen relatively early, allowing for restoration of glenohumeral motion and improved functionality. In a 5-year follow-up study, Farrell and colleagues[76] showed that patients who benefited from manipulation obtained their 5-year follow-up ROM within the first 6 months after manipulation. Dodenhoff and colleagues[77] prospectively assessed the effects of manipulation under anesthesia on early recovery and return to activity. They found that patients had an increase of 60 degrees in abduction, 30 degrees in external rotation, and 40 degrees in internal rotation at 6 weeks of follow-up. In addition, patients had statistically significant improvements in their constant scores. Overall, 94% of the patients were satisfied with the procedure. However, Kivimäki and colleagues[53] performed a blinded, randomized trial with 1-year follow-up in which they compared manipulation under anesthesia with a HEP. They found that there was no statistical difference between the two groups, suggesting that patients who are properly instructed on how to perform a HEP will have a similar outcome as those treated with a formal manipulation. With regard to combining manipulation under anesthesia with intraarticular corticosteroid injection, Kivimäki and Pohjolainen[53] prospectively studied the effects of manipulation under anesthesia with and without intraarticular corticosteroid injection and found that there were no additional improvements in outcome measures with the addition of a corticosteroid injection. Finally, even though manipulation under anesthesia typically results in clinical improvement, a retrospective review of 730 patients (792 shoulders) who underwent manipulation over a 16-year period identified 141 shoulders (17.8%) that underwent revision manipulation because of persistent symptoms.[78] The authors found improved outcomes after repeat manipulation and suggested that repeat manipulation under anesthesia be considered in the setting of persistent symptoms despite an initial manipulation.

ARTHROSCOPIC SURGERY

Surgical treatment for adhesive capsulitis is typically reserved for patients with persistent symptoms for at least 6 months despite nonoperative management. Although manipulation under anesthesia has been shown to be effective in treating persistent adhesive capsulitis, the procedure does not allow for a controlled release of the pathologic tissue. Relative contraindications to manipulation include rotator cuff tear, chronic insulin-dependent diabetes, and osteopenia because of the fear of a humeral shaft fracture during the manipulation.[21] In these instances, arthroscopic surgery provides an excellent alternative that allows complete inspection of the glenohumeral joint and selective capsular release to address the true underlying capsular pathology. Warner and colleagues[79] showed that patients who were refractory to closed treatments and manipulation under anesthesia demonstrated statistically significant improvements in patient outcome scores and ROM after arthroscopic anterior capsular release. Ogilvie-Harris and Myerthall[80] performed an arthroscopic capsular release for diabetic patients with adhesive capsulitis and found statistically significant improvements in pain, external rotation and abduction ROM, and overall shoulder function. Ogilvie-Harris and colleagues[81] also compared manipulation under anesthesia with arthroscopic capsular release. Both groups showed similar improvements in ROM; however, the arthroscopic capsular release group had significantly better pain relief and restoration of shoulder function. Nicholson[82] prospectively studied the effects of arthroscopic release for adhesive capsulitis based on etiology. All groups showed significant improvements in ROM (forward elevation, external rotation, and internal rotation) and patient outcome scales, suggesting that the etiology does not have an effect on the outcome after arthroscopic capsular release. Berghs and colleagues[83] followed 25 patients after they underwent arthroscopic capsular release and found

significant improvements in ROM and patient outcome scales immediately after surgery. More important, these results were maintained at a mean of 14.8 months after surgery.[83] Ide and Takagi[84] confirmed that the improvements in motion and shoulder scoring systems that were seen in the first several months postoperatively were maintained at a mean of 7.5 years of follow-up. Holloway and colleagues[85] studied the effects of arthroscopic capsular release in idiopathic, postfracture, and refractory postoperative shoulder stiffness. All groups showed statistically significant improvements in patient outcome scores and ROM. However, the refractory postoperative stiffness group showed the least amount of improvement compared with the other groups.

PROPOSED INTERVENTION ALGORITHM

An algorithmic approach offering conservative and surgical interventions can effectively address the adhesive capsulitis continuum (Fig. 70.4). The patient is seen by the surgeon or physician and diagnosed with adhesive capsulitis or identified as having adhesive capsulitis by the therapist. The patient is given one of four treatment options based on the known pathology, evidence-based literature, and our experience. The patient is given the option to receive an intraarticular corticosteroid injection. Irrespective of this decision, all patients are referred to physical therapy for either a therapist-instructed HEP or to participate with supervised therapy. There is no clear evidence to predict which patients may need formal supervised therapy rather than simply a HEP. Therefore, we recommend this decision be made based on the physician and patient preference with input from the therapist after initial evaluation. Factors that may favor the recommendation of supervised therapy may include higher level of irritability, greater level of functional disability, multiple comorbid conditions, lower social support, lower educational level, or high patient fear and anxiety.

Regardless of which intervention is assigned, the patient is asked to return to the physician in 6 to 8 weeks to review the patient's progress. The algorithm is followed until the patient responds or is discharged. Gleyze and associates[86] suggest that patients participate with their individualized treatments for up to 3 months. Between 3 and 6 months, an intraarticular corticosteroid injection may be reconsidered in patients with limited progress.[86] If a patient does receive an intraarticular corticosteroid injection, usually only one or two are required to achieve the desired result.[79] A maximum of three intraarticular corticosteroid injections are considered for a single case of adhesive capsulitis.[79] Most patients respond positively to the interventions; however, some patients improve very slowly and continue to experience pain and functional deficits but are willing to continue with the HEP after the other conservative options are attempted. Approximately 7% to 10% of patients will fail to respond to conservative interventions and should consider a manipulation under anesthesia or arthroscopic capsular release.[22,87] This recommendation comes when the patient's symptoms and ROM are unresponsive to the various intervention options over a 6-month timeframe and quality of life continues to be compromised.[86] If the patient is unwilling to have a manipulation or surgery, she or he is discharged but encouraged to continue with a daily stretching program.

THERAPY INTERVENTION

When a patient is seen by a physical therapist a complete examination is performed. A key principle of this examination is to establish the patient's irritability level and determine an appropriate intervention strategy.[24] After a thorough evaluation, the therapist educates the patient about the pathology and the natural course of adhesive capsulitis while promoting a level of activity modification that encourages functional, pain-free ROM.[24] A physical therapist plays a crucial role

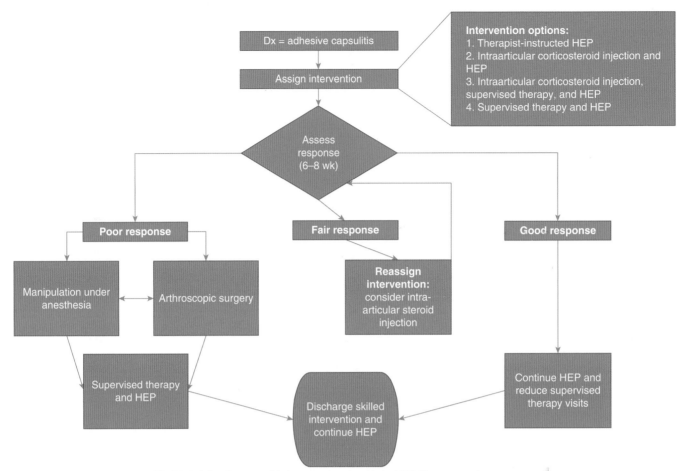

Fig 70.4 Adhesive capsulitis intervention algorithm. *HEP,* Home exercise program.

in educating the patient to ensure a proper understanding is achieved and to allay the fears of catastrophic illness while preparing the patient for an extended rehabilitation process.[88]

Gleyze and associates[88] suggest an intensive HEP with the supervision of a physical therapist to skillfully progress the program is most appropriate. All patients are instructed in a HEP based on their irritability level regardless if returning to participate with supervised therapy or completion of a HEP. For patients who are classified as having high or moderate irritability, the stretching time intervals are kept short (1–5 seconds). Although there is no evidence to support this recommendation, the patient is asked to perform each exercise at least 20 times per session, with three sessions per day. The fundamental exercises include pendulum exercise, passive supine forward elevation, passive external rotation with the arm in approximately 40 degrees in the plane of the scapula, active-assisted extension, active-assisted internal rotation, and active-assisted horizontal adduction (Fig. 70.5). These exercises primarily influence different regions of the synovial capsuloligamentous complex and have been used in supervised therapy and HEPs in patients with adhesive capsulitis.[22,32,52–54] Any exercise found to be too painful to perform should be held from the program and reintroduced as symptoms diminish. Patients with moderate irritability may be instructed to use an overhead pulley to improve elevation ROM. Patients classified with low irritability may also be instructed in the same exercises and overhead pulley; however, these patients will hold each stretch at their end-range for a longer duration (30 seconds). The overhead

pulley is performed with the elbow close to full extension and shoulder in forward flexion. This allows normal obligatory humeral internal rotation to occur. If the arm is raised with the elbow bent, the initial "forced" external rotation takes up all the capsuloligamentous complex slack, thereby limiting elevation (Fig. 70.6).

Patients who are prescribed to only perform a HEP are instructed to contact the physical therapist if pain increases or if the patient becomes uncertain of the proper exercise technique. Patients who demonstrate difficulty correctly performing the exercises independently are asked to return within 1 week to be sure they are doing them correctly.

If followed in supervised therapy, the patient is asked to perform the exercises for 1 week and then return for his or her next therapy appointment. The patient's response to the 1-week of HEP will assist in the determination of prognosis and appropriate treatment frequency. At the 1-week visit, the patient is asked to report any change in symptoms, with particular regard to night pain and ability to sleep. Before initiating the treatment, a reassessment of ROM is performed and compared with the initial examination. End-range "irritability" is determined with passive external rotation and elevation.

Treatment may begin with moist heat on the affected side with the patient supine and the arm placed in approximately 40 degrees of plane of the scapula abduction. After 5 minutes with heat, the patient begins to perform short-interval (5–15 second) intermittent passive external rotation stretching with the heat still applied for at least 20 repetitions (see Fig. 70.5C). After this exercise, passive external rotation motion is

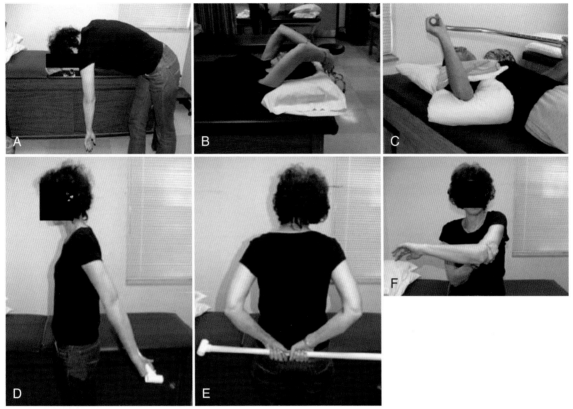

Fig 70.5 A, Pendulum. **B,** Passive supine forward elevation. **C,** Passive external rotation with the arm in approximately 40 degrees in the plane of the scapula. **D,** Active-assisted extension. **E,** Active-assisted internal rotation. **F,** Active-assisted horizontal adduction.

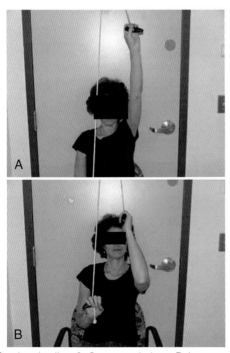

Fig 70.6 Overhead pulley. **A,** Correct technique. **B,** Incorrect technique.

reassessed. Patients often gain 10 to 15 degrees of motion, which suggests that muscle guarding and pain are the initial motion barriers. A patient with low irritability may find a minimal increase of motion (5 degrees), indicating the "fibroblastic wall" is the ROM barrier instead of pain. The patient performs passive supine elevation, undergoes joint mobilizations or gentle manual stretching, and then performs the remaining prescribed ROM exercises. Mobilizations are initially performed in the loose pack position anteriorly, inferiorly, and posteriorly. Traction and rotational oscillations are applied between translational glides to improve patient comfort and allow the stressed tissues an opportunity to recover.

Determining Treatment Frequency

Patients who are able to sleep through the night or have a significant overall reduction in irritability and decreased pain after the first week of the prescribed HEP have an excellent prognosis; it is recommended for these patients to be seen in therapy once a week or every other week. If minimal response is noted relative to pain and ROM after the 1-week period or if the patient presents to therapy with high or moderate irritability but is able to achieve a greater than 15 degrees gain in external rotation or elevation ROM during the treatment session, it is recommended for these patients to be seen in therapy twice a week. If the patient has increased irritability or further ROM loss, he or she may be referred back to the physician for a consideration of a glenohumeral intraarticular corticosteroid injection.

Treatment Progression

As pain and irritability improve, the grade of mobilization and intensity of stretching should increase. Mobilization positions are moved

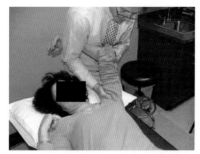

Fig 70.7 Inferior glenohumeral joint mobilization at end range.

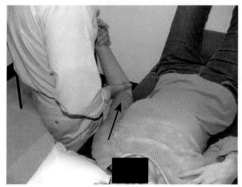

Fig 70.8 Inferior glenohumeral joint traction for rotator cuff interval contracture.

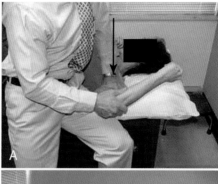

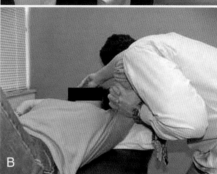

Fig 70.9 Glenohumeral joint mobilization for external rotation range of motion. **A,** Posterior glide. **B,** Anterior traction.

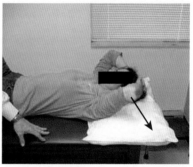

Fig 70.10 Quadrant stretch.

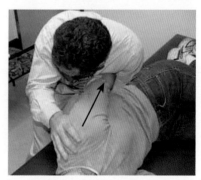

Fig 70.11 Inferior glenohumeral joint traction into extension and adduction.

from loose pack positions toward end range to further influence connective tissue length (Fig. 70.7). A hold–relax technique can be used near end range to maximize relaxation by reducing muscle guarding via antagonistic inhibition. Mobilization with movement is used to recruit agonist and inhibit antagonistic musculature. Specific mobilizations are performed to target the rotator cuff interval because contracture of this structure is often found with adhesive capsulitis (Fig. 70.8).[7,9,29,89] It is important to consider the rotator cuff interval because this structure limits external rotation and provides stability against inferior translation when the arm is adducted. External rotation motion can be improved with both anterior glides and posterior glides (Fig. 70.9).[60]

Patients are progressed to a quadrant stretch supine by placing their locked hands to the top of their head and allowing their elbows fall toward the surface (Fig. 70.10). This stretch is controlled by pectoral activity as the patient relaxes his or her shoulder while the arm moves into a slightly painful range. Patients are asked to bring their elbow forward after approximately 5 to 10 seconds and repeat 10 to 20 times. The intensity and duration of the stretching re based on irritability level, but painful aggressive stretching is avoided. The appropriateness of any stretch intensity is found when the pain of the stretch is eliminated upon leaving the end range. Patients with limited functional internal rotation are thought to have tightness of superior capsular structures in addition to posterior structures. Pouliart and coworkers[90] found a posterior superior ligamentous structure that limits internal rotation with the arm at the side; therefore, an inferior glide in adduction–extension and internal rotation can be performed to influence this structure (Fig. 70.11). To stretch the superior capsuloligamentous complex structures, the patient is placed sidelying with the involved hand on the hip and the elbow being gently pushed into adduction (Fig. 70.12). When irritability allows, the patient can be progressed to a sleeper stretch (Fig. 70.13). Caution must be taken to prevent an increase of irritability because these stretches may be very painful if an improper technique is used or if too aggressive.

At the end of each session, the therapist reassesses ROM with particular attention to external rotation and elevation. Before each subsequent session begins, ROM and end range reactivity should be assessed to note the sustainability of gains from the prior session. If the patient's symptoms worsen or remain highly irritable after the first four sessions, she or he is referred back to the physician for a glenohumeral intraarticular corticosteroid injection. After receiving a corticosteroid

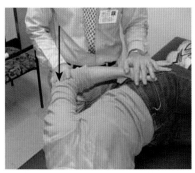

Fig 70.12 Superior capsuloligamentous complex adduction stretch.

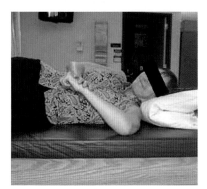

Fig 70.13 Sleeper stretch.

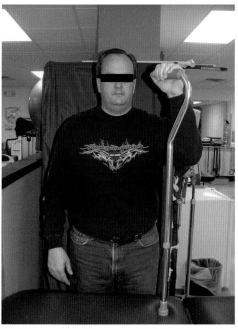

Fig 70.14 Low-load prolonged stretch into forward elevation.

injection, the patient is asked to perform only pendulum exercise several times a day to allow maximal medication effect without tissue provocation. After approximately 4 days, the patient may return to supervised physical therapy or the HEP (or both).

Constant reassessment of symptoms and modifying the "dosage" of tensile load is continued for 4 to 6 weeks. If the patient's symptoms continue to lessen, the concept of total end-range time is used so that low-load prolonged stretch is performed (Fig. 70.14). Cyclic loading exercises, such as tossing a weighted object into functional

internal rotation, can also be performed. As symptoms decrease, ROM improves, and the patient becomes more independent with the prescribed HEP and less reliant on therapist-introduced forces, and the duration between visits increases to one visit every 1 to 3 weeks. Discharge is considered when a patient demonstrates low irritability, minimal or no end-range pain, 10 degrees or less within session gains, and stagnant motion gain between visits. These criteria represent the presence of fibroblastic contracture, which will continue to improve and remodel with stretching home exercises. Some patients making slow progress may meet the discharge criteria but will be asked to return in 8 to 12 weeks for program progression.

SURGICAL INTERVENTION

Patients return to the referring physician every 6 to 8 weeks to monitor progress. As per the algorithm, if the symptoms are unresponsive to the various levels of treatment over time and quality of life is compromised, a manipulation or capsular release is offered. The vast majority of patients have improvement of shoulder pain and stiffness if given enough time. A small percentage continue to have dysfunction from loss of motion. Approximately 7% to 10% fail conservative treatment and require manipulation or capsular release.[22,87] If the patient is unwilling to have a manipulation or surgery, he or she is discharged but encouraged to continue with a daily stretching program.

For patients who have persistent loss of shoulder ROM but a decrease in joint irritation, an examination under anesthesia with manipulation and arthroscopic capsular release is performed. During the procedure, the patient's passive motion is recorded, and then the shoulder is gently manipulated. If full, symmetrical ROM is achieved, the procedure is completed. If any plane of motion continues to be restricted, arthroscopy of the patient's shoulder is performed. During arthroscopy, a circumferential capsulectomy and subacromial decompression are performed to achieve full passive motion (Fig. 70.15).

Patients begin therapy immediately after surgery, continued daily for at least the next 5 days. After a release, although decreasing inflammation is a priority, mobilization of the joint can be more aggressive than before surgery. Moreover, with the use of regional anesthesia and indwelling peripheral nerve catheters, patients are typically able to engage in physical therapy and home exercises with minimal discomfort or pain the first day after surgery. The final outcome after release is achieved at different times for different patients; however, significant gains in any persistent ROM restrictions are not typically noted beyond 6 months after surgery.

SUMMARY

Adhesive capsulitis is a commonly treated musculoskeletal problem, yet the etiology remains elusive. Patients present with a recognizable history, physical presentation, and natural course of recovery. Because multiple interventions have been investigated, we feel the adhesive capsulitis intervention algorithm (see Fig. 70.4) provides efficient options to maximize successful treatment. Corticosteroid intraarticular injections are favored in patients with high irritability or those who have not responded to supervised therapy or a HEP. Assessing the response to treatment determines the frequency of treatment and alternate interventions. The developed discharge criterion satisfies the short-term successes of significant pain relief, return of functional movement, and patient satisfaction. This is based on the belief that when pain in ameliorated, capsuloligamentous complex remodeling will occur over a prolonged period. Patients with recalcitrant adhesive capsulitis have the option of manipulation or capsular release (or both) in the unlikely event that conservative treatment is not successful.

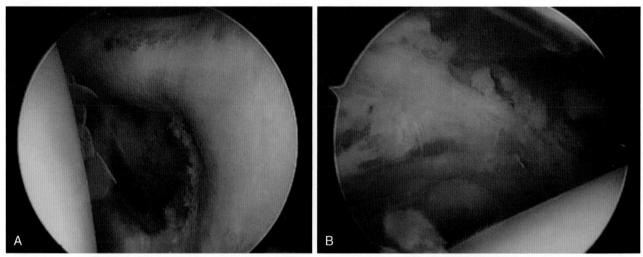

Fig 70.15 Arthroscopic photos of the glenohumeral joint following arthroscopic capsular release. **A,** Rotator interval release. Humeral head is to the *left,* and glenoid is to the *right.* Hyperemia is noted in the biceps tendon. **B,** Superior capsule release. Humeral head is at the *bottom right.* Mild hyperemia is noted in the superior labrum–biceps origin.

REFERENCES

1. Duplay S. De la péri-arthrite scapulo-humérale et des raideurs de l'épaule qui en sont la consequéce. *Arch Gen Méd.* 1872;(20):513–542.
2. Codman EA. *The Shoulder. Rupture of the Supraspinatus Tendon and Other Lesions in or About the Subacromial Bursa.* Boston: Private; 1934:216–224.
3. Neviaser JS. Arthrography of the shoulder joint: Study of the findings in adhesive capsulitis of the shoulder. study of the findings in adhesive capsulitis of the shoulder. *J Bone Joint Surg.* 1962;44-A:1321–1359.
4. Lundberg J. The frozen shoulder. Clinical and radiographical observations. the effect of manipulation under general anesthesia. Structure and glycosaminoglycan content of the joint capsule. Local bone metabolism. *Acta Orthop Scand.* 1969;(suppl 11959).
5. Zuckerman JD, Rokito A. Frozen shoulder: a consensus definition. *J Shoulder Elbow Surg.* 2011;20(2):322–325.
6. Cole BJ, Rios CG, Mazzocca AD, Warnerd JP. Anatomy, biomechanics, and pathophysiology of glenohumeral instability. In: Iannotti JPWG, ed. *Disorders of the Shoulder: Diagnosis and Management.* 2nd ed. Philadelphia: Lippincott Williams & Wilkins; 2007:281–312.
7. Wiley AM. Arthroscopic appearance of frozen shoulder. *Arthroscopy.* 1991;7(2):138–143.
8. Uitvlugt G, Detrisac DA, Johnson LL, Austin MD, Johnson C. Arthroscopic observations before and after manipulation of frozen shoulder. *Arthroscopy.* 1993;9(2):181–185.
9. Ozaki J, Nakagawa Y, Sakurai G, Tamai S. Recalcitrant chronic adhesive capsulitis of the shoulder. role of contracture of the coracohumeral ligament and rotator interval in pathogenesis and treatment. *J Bone Joint Surg.* 1989;71(10):1511–1515.
10. Bunker TD, Anthony PP. The pathology of frozen shoulder. A Dupuytren-like disease. *J Bone Joint Surg - British Volume.* 1995;77(5):677–683.
11. Bunker TD, Reilly J, Baird KS, Hamblen DL. Expression of growth factors, cytokines and matrix metalloproteinases in frozen shoulder. *J Bone Joint Surg - British Volume.* 2000;82(5):768–773.
12. Rodeo SA, Hannafin JA, Tom J, Warren RF, Wickiewicz TL. Immuno-localization of cytokines and their receptors in adhesive capsulitis of the shoulder. *J Orthopaedic Res.* 1997;15(3):427–436.
13. Smith SP, Devaraj VS, Bunker TD. The association between frozen shoulder and Dupuytren's disease. *J Shoulder Elbow Surg.* 2001;10(2):149–151.
14. Hand GCR, Athanasou NA, Matthews T, Carr AJ. The pathology of frozen shoulder. *J Shoulder Elbow Surg - British Volume.* 2007;89(7):928–932.
15. Hannafin JA, Chiaia TA. Adhesive capsulitis. A treatment approach. *Clin Orthop Relat Res.* 2000;(372):95–109.
16. Getz CL, Ramsey ML, Glaser DL, Williams GR. Adhesive capsulitis. In: Blaine TL,W, ed. *Shoulder Arthroscopy Monograph Series.* Rosemont, IL: American Academy of Orthopaedic Surgeons; 2006.
17. Thomas SJ, McDougall C, Brown IDM, et al. Prevalence of symptoms and signs of shoulder problems in people with diabetes mellitus. *J Shoulder Elbow Surg.* 2007;16(6):748–751.
18. Arkkila PE, Kantola IM, Viikari JS, Rnnemaa T. Shoulder capsulitis in type I and II diabetic patients: association with diabetic complications and related diseases. *Ann Rheum Dis.* 1996;55(12):907–914.
19. Grasland A, Ziza JM, Raguin G, Pouchot J, Vinceneux P. Adhesive capsulitis of shoulder and treatment with protease inhibitors in patients with human immunodeficiency virus infection: Report of 8 cases. *J Rheum.* 2000;27(11):2642–2646.
20. De Ponti A, Vigan MG, Taverna E, Sansone V. Adhesive capsulitis of the shoulder in human immunodeficiency virus-positive patients during highly active antiretroviral therapy. *J Shoulder Elbow surg.* 2006;15(2):188–190.
21. Romeo AA, Loutzenheiser T, Rhee YG, Sidles JA, Harryman DT, Matsen FA. The humeroscapular motion interface. *Clin Orthop Relat Res.* 1998;(350):120–127.
22. Griggs SM, Ahn A, Green A. Idiopathic adhesive capsulitis. A prospective functional outcome study of nonoperative treatment. *J Bone Joint Surg.* 2000;82-A(10):1398–1407.
23. Shaffer B, Tibone JE, Kerlan RK. Frozen shoulder. A long-term follow-up. *J bone Joint Surg.* 1992;74(5):738–746.
24. Kelley MJ, Shaffer MA, Kuhn JE, et al. Shoulder pain and mobility deficits: adhesive capsulitis. *J Orthop Sports Phys Ther.* 2013;43(5):1. https://doi.org/10.2519/jospt.2013.0302.
25. Rizk TE, Christopher RP, Pinals RS, Higgins AC, Frix R. Adhesive capsulitis (frozen shoulder): a new approach to its management. *Arch Phys Med Rehabil.* 1983;64(1):29–33.
26. Binder AI, Bulgen DY, Hazleman BL, Roberts S. Frozen shoulder: a long-term prospective study. *Ann Rheum Dis.* 1984;43(3):361–364.
27. Bulgen DY, Binder AI, Hazleman BL, Dutton J, Roberts S. Frozen shoulder: prospective clinical study with an evaluation of three treatment regimens. *Ann Rheum Dis.* 1984;43(3):353–360.
28. Vermeulen HM, Rozing PM, Obermann WR, le Cessie S, Vliet Vlieland T PM. Comparison of high-grade and low-grade mobilization techniques in the management of adhesive capsulitis of the shoulder: randomized controlled trial. *Physical therapy.* 2006;86(3):355–368.
29. Neer CS, Satterlee CC, Dalsey RM, Flatow EL. The anatomy and potential effects of contracture of the coracohumeral ligament. *Clin Orthop Relat Res.* 1992;280:182–185.

30. Reeves B. The natural history of the frozen shoulder syndrome. *Scand J Rheumatol.* 1975;4(4):193–196.

31. Wadsworth CT. Frozen shoulder. *Phys Ther.* 1986;66(12):1878–1883.

32. Carette S, Moffet H, Tardif J, et al. Intraarticular corticosteroids, supervised physiotherapy, or a combination of the two in the treatment of adhesive capsulitis of the shoulder: a placebo-controlled trial. *Arthritis Rheum.* 2003;48(3):829–838.

33. Kivimäki J, Pohjolainen T, Malmivaara A, et al. Manipulation under anesthesia with home exercises versus home exercises alone in the treatment of frozen shoulder: a randomized, controlled trial with 125 patients. *J Shoulder Elbow Surg.* 2007;16(6):722–726.

34. Rundquist PJ, Anderson DD, Guanche CA, Ludewig PM. Shoulder kinematics in subjects with frozen shoulder. *Arch Phys Med Rehabil.* 2003;84(10):1473–1479.

35. Quin CE. Frozen shoulder: evaluation of treatment with hydrocortisone injections and exercises. *Ann Phys Med.* 1965;8:5. PASSIM.

36. Sokk J, Gapeyeva H, Ereline J, Kolts I, Psuke M. Shoulder muscle strength and fatigability in patients with frozen shoulder syndrome: the effect of 4-week individualized rehabilitation. *Electroencephalogr Clin Neurophysiol.* 2007;47(4-5):205–213.

37. Leggin B, Kelley MJ, Pontillo M. *Impairments and Function in Patients with Frozen Shoulder Compared to Patients with Rotator Cuff Tendinopathy.* 2007.

38. Jrgel J, Rannama L, Gapeyeva H, Ereline J, Kolts I, Psuke M. Shoulder function in patients with frozen shoulder before and after 4-week rehabilitation. *Medicina.* 2005;41(1):30–38.

39. Sher JS, Iannotti JP, Williams GR, et al. The effect of shoulder magnetic resonance imaging on clinical decision making. *J Shoulder Elbow Surg.* 1998;7(3):205–209.

40. Tandon A, Dewan S, Bhatt S, Jain AK, Kumari R. Sonography in diagnosis of adhesive capsulitis of the shoulder: a case-control study. *J ultrasound.* 2017;20(3):227–236. https://doi.org/10.1007/s40477-017-0262-5.

41. Arslan S, Celiker R. Comparison of the efficacy of local corticosteroid injection and physical therapy for the treatment of adhesive capsulitis. *Rheumatol Int.* 2001;21(1):20–23.

42. van der Windt DA, Koes BW, Devill W, Boeke AJ, de Jong BA, Bouter LM. Effectiveness of corticosteroid injections versus physiotherapy for treatment of painful stiff shoulder in primary care: randomised trial. *BMJ.* 1998;317(7168):1292–1296.

43. Hazleman BL. The painful stiff shoulder. *Rheumatol Phys Med.* 1972;11(8):413–421.

44. Jrvinen TAH, Jrvinen TLN, Kriinen M, Kalimo H, Jrvinen M. Muscle injuries: biology and treatment. *Am J Sports Med.* 2005;33(5):745–764.

45. Safran MR, Garrett WE, Seaber AV, Glisson RR, Ribbeck BM. The role of warmup in muscular injury prevention. *Am J Sports Med.* 1998;16(2):123–129.

46. Kurtaiş Gürsel Y, Ulus Y, Bilgi A, Diner G, van der Heijden GJMG. Adding ultrasound in the management of soft tissue disorders of the shoulder: a randomized placebo-controlled trial. *Phys Ther.* 2004;84(4):336–343.

47. Dogru H, Basaran S, Sarpel T. Effectiveness of therapeutic ultrasound in adhesive capsulitis. *Joint, Bone, Spine.* 2008;75(4):445–450.

48. Cheing GLY, So EML, Chao CYL. Effectiveness of electroacupuncture and interferential electrotherapy in the management of frozen shoulder. *J Rehabil Med.* 2008;40(3):166–170. https://doi.org/10.2340/16501977-0142.

49. Jewell DV, Riddle DL, Thacker LR. Interventions associated with an increased or decreased likelihood of pain reduction and improved function in patients with adhesive capsulitis: a retrospective cohort study. *Phys Ther.* 2009;89(5):419–429. https://doi.org/10.2522/ptj.20080250.

50. Diercks RL, Stevens M. Gentle thawing of the frozen shoulder: a prospective study of supervised neglect versus intensive physical therapy in seventy-seven patients with frozen shoulder syndrome followed up for two years. *J Shoulder Elbow Surg.* 2004;13(5):499–502.

51. Levine WN, Kashyap CP, Bak SF, Ahmad CS, Blaine TA, Bigliani LU. Nonoperative management of idiopathic adhesive capsulitis. *J Shoulder Elbow Surg.* 16(5):569–573. https://doi.org/10.1016/j.jse.2006.12.007.

52. Diercks RL, Stevens M. Gentle thawing of the frozen shoulder: a prospective study of supervised neglect versus intensive physical therapy in seventy-seven patients with frozen shoulder syndrome followed up for two years. *J Shoulder Elbow Surg.* 2004;13(5):499–502.

53. Kivimäki J, Pohjolainen T. Manipulation under anesthesia for frozen shoulder with and without steroid injection. *Arch Phys Med Rehabil.* 2001;82(9):1188–1190.

54. Ryans I, Montgomery A, Galway R, Kernohan WG, McKane R. A randomized controlled trial of intra-articular triamcinolone and/or physiotherapy in shoulder capsulitis. *Rheumatology.* 2005;44(4):529–535.

55. Wyke B. The neurology of joints. *Ann R Coll Surg Engl.* 1967;41(1):25–50.

56. Gleyze P, Flurin P, Laprelle E, et al. Pain management in the rehabilitation of stiff shoulder: Prospective multicenter comparative study of 193 cases. *Orthop Traumatol Surg Res.* 2011;97(8):S203. https://doi.org/10.1016/j.otsr.2011.09.006.

57. McClure PW, Blackburn LG, Dusold C. The use of splints in the treatment of joint stiffness: biologic rationale and an algorithm for making clinical decisions. *Physical Ther.* 1994;74(12):1101–1107.

58. Flowers KR, LaStayo P. Effect of total end range time on improving passive range of motion. *J Hand Ther.* 2012;7(3):150–157.

59. Terry GC, Hammon D, France P, Norwood LA. The stabilizing function of passive shoulder restraints. *Am J Sports Med.* 19(1):26–34. https://doi.org/10.1177/036354659101900105.

60. Johnson AJ, Godges JJ, Zimmerman GJ, Ounanian LL. The effect of anterior versus posterior glide joint mobilization on external rotation range of motion in patients with shoulder adhesive capsulitis. *J Orthop Sports Phys Ther.* 2007;37(3):88–99.

61. Nicholson GG. The effects of passive joint mobilization on pain and hypomobility associated with adhesive capsulitis of the shoulder. *J Orthop Sports Phys Ther.* 1985;6(4):238–246.

62. Vermeulen HM, Obermann WR, Burger BJ, Kok GJ, Rozing PM, van Den Ende CH. End-range mobilization techniques in adhesive capsulitis of the shoulder joint: a multiple-subject case report. *Physical Ther.* 2000;80(12):1204–1213.

63. Bulgen DY, Binder A, Hazleman BL, Park JR. Immunological studies in frozen shoulder. *J Rheumatol.* 9(6):893–898.

64. Buchbinder R, Hoving JL, Green S, Hall S, Forbes A, Nash P. Short course prednisolone for adhesive capsulitis (frozen shoulder or stiff painful shoulder): a randomised, double blind, placebo controlled trial. *Ann Rheum Dis.* 2004;63(11):1460–1469.

65. Wang W, Shi M, Zhou C, et al. Effectiveness of corticosteroid injections in adhesive capsulitis of shoulder: a meta-analysis. *Medicine.* 2017;96(28):e7529. https://doi.org/10.1097/MD.0000000000007529.

66. Ahn JH, Lee D, Kang H, Lee MY, Kang DR, Yoon S. Early intra-articular corticosteroid injection improves pain and function in adhesive capsulitis of the shoulder: 1-year retrospective longitudinal study. *PM & R.* 2017. https://doi.org/10.1016/j.pmrj.2017.06.004.

67. Kim KH, Park JW, Kim SJ. High- vs low-dose corticosteroid injection in the treatment of adhesive capsulitis with severe pain: a randomized controlled double-blind study. *Pain Med.* 2017. https://doi.org/10.1093/pm/pnx227.

68. Liu Y, Skardal A, Shu XZ, Prestwich GD. Prevention of peritendinous adhesions using a hyaluronan-derived hydrogel film following partial-thickness flexor tendon injury. *J Orthop Res.* 2008;26(4):562–569.

69. Blaine T, Moskowitz R, Udell J, et al. Treatment of persistent shoulder pain with sodium hyaluronate: a randomized, controlled trial. A multicenter study. *J Bone Joint Surg.* 2008;90(5):970–979.

70. Corbeil V, Dussault RG, Leduc BE, Fleury J. Adhesive capsulitis of the shoulder: a comparative study of arthrography with intra-articular corticotherapy and with or without capsular distension. *Can Assoc Radiol J.* 1992;43(2):127–130.

71. Tveita EK, Tariq R, Sesseng S, et al. Hydrodilation, corticosteroids and adhesive capsulitis: a randomized controlled trial. *BMC Musculskeletal Dis.* 2008;(9):53.

72. Gam AN, Schydlowsky P, Rossel I, Remvig L, Jensen EM. Treatment of "frozen shoulder" with distension and glucocorticoid compared with glucocorticoid alone. A randomised controlled trial. *Scand J Rheumatol.* 1998;27(6):425–430.

73. Vad VB, Sakalkale D, Warren RF. The role of capsular distention in adhesive capsulitis. *Arch Phys Medicine Rehabil.* 2003;84(9):1290–1292.

74. Watson L, Bialocerkowski A, Dalziel R, Balster S, Burke F, Finch C. Hydrodilatation (distension arthrography): a long-term clinical outcome series. *Br J Sports Med.* 2007;41(3):167–173.

75. Placzek JD, Roubal PJ, Freeman DC, Kulig K, Nasser S, Pagett BT. Long-term effectiveness of translational manipulation for adhesive capsulitis. *Clin Orthop Relat Res.* 1998;(356):181–191.

76. Farrell CM, Sperling JW, Cofield RH. Manipulation for frozen shoulder: Long-term results. *J Shoulder Elbow Surg.* 2005;14(5):480–484.

77. Dodenhoff RM, Levy O, Wilson A, Copeland SA. Manipulation under anesthesia for primary frozen shoulder: effect on early recovery and return to activity. *J Shoulder Elbow Surg.* 2000;9(1):23–26.

78. Woods DA, Loganathan K. Recurrence of frozen shoulder after manipulation under anaesthetic (MUA): the results of repeating the MUA. *Bone Joint J.* 2017;99-B(6):812–817. https://doi.org/10.1302/0301-620X.99B6.BJJ-2016-1133.R1.

79. Warner JJ, Allen A, Marks PH, Wong P. Arthroscopic release for chronic, refractory adhesive capsulitis of the shoulder. *J Bone Joint Surg.* 1996;78(12):1808–1816.

80. Ogilvie-Harris D, Myerthall S. The diabetic frozen shoulder: arthroscopic release. *Arthroscopy.* 1997;13(1):1–8.

81. Ogilvie-Harris D, Biggs DJ, Fitsialos DP, MacKay M. The resistant frozen shoulder. manipulation versus arthroscopic release. *Clin Orthop Relat Res.* 1995;319:238–248.

82. Nicholson GP. Arthroscopic capsular release for stiff shoulders: effect of etiology on outcomes. *Arthroscopy.* 2003;19(1):40–49.

83. Berghs BM, Sole-Molins X, Bunker TD. Arthroscopic release of adhesive capsulitis. *J Bone Joint Surg.* 2004;13(2):180–185.

84. Ide J, Takagi K. Early and long-term results of arthroscopic treatment for shoulder stiffness. *J Bone Joint Surg.* 2004;13(2):174–179.

85. Holloway GB, Schenk T, Williams GR, Ramsey ML, Iannotti JP. Arthroscopic capsular release for the treatment of refractory postoperative or post-fracture shoulder stiffness. *J Bone Joint Surg.* 2001;83-A(11):1682–1687.

86. Gleyze P, Clavert P, Flurin P, et al. Management of the stiff shoulder. A prospective multicenter comparative study of the six main techniques in use: 235 cases. *Orthop Traumatol Surg Res.* 2011;97(8):S181. https://doi.org/10.1016/j.otsr.2011.09.004.

87. Murnaghan JP. Adhesive capsulitis of the shoulder: current concepts and treatment. *Orthopedics.* 1988;11(1):153–158.

88. Gleyze P, Georges T, Flurin P, et al. Comparison and critical evaluation of rehabilitation and home-based exercises for treating shoulder stiffness: Prospective, multicenter study with 148 cases. *Orthop Traumatol Surg Res.* 2011;97(8):S194. https://doi.org/10.1016/j.otsr.2011.09.005.

89. Omari A, Bunker TD. Open surgical release for frozen shoulder: surgical findings and results of the release. *J Bone Joint Surg.* 2001;10(4):353–357.

90. Pouliart N, Somers K, Eid S, Gagey O. Variations in the superior capsulo-ligamentous complex and description of a new ligament. *J Bone Joint Surg.* 2007;16(6):821–836.

Rehabilitation of Shoulder Instability

Michael A. Shaffer, Bryce W. Gaunt, Brian G. Leggin, Brian R. Wolf

OUTLINE

CRITICAL POINTS

- Shoulder instability constitutes a spectrum of disorders that includes laxity, subluxation, and dislocation.
- Immobilization has little effect on outcome after traumatic dislocation.
- The prognosis for nonoperative management of patients younger than 30 years of age after traumatic dislocation is poor.

- Rehabilitation is preferred over operative management in those with atraumatic instability.
- Controlling the rate at which range of motion is regained is important to adequately protect capsulolabral repairs of the shoulder from undue stress during the early and middle postoperative periods.

EPIDEMIOLOGY

Shoulder instability may affect 2% of the general population,[1] and shoulder dislocations account for 1% to 4% of annual emergency department (ED) visits.[2] These two statistics reveal the inherent instability of a joint with such a wide range of mobility requirements such as the human shoulder. At particular risk for instability events are young, active, male athletes or soldiers.[3–5] Male gender carries 1.64 to 2.64 times relative risk,[4,5] and in one series, male patients represented 71.8% of all patients presenting to an ED with a shoulder dislocation.[5] Patient age is also a significant predictive factor for shoulder instability with the highest incidence in the third decade of life. Nearly half of all dislocations occur in individuals between 15 and 29 years of age.[5] Some evidence suggests that it is the activities in which males participate that is the driving factor because the rate of shoulder instability is similar between genders if the same sports are evaluated.[6] Overall, dislocations among women become more numerous relative to their male counterparts with advancing age. Dislocations among older adults are often the result of falls at home, and relative to younger patients, carry increased risk for associated fracture, rotator cuff tear, and nerve injury.[7] Falling onto an outstretched hand or injuries sustained during sporting activities are the most common mechanisms of injury for young men.[5]

An anterior traumatic shoulder dislocation occurs when an external force exceeds the tensile strength of the anterior capsulolabral structures, typically with the shoulder in an abducted and externally rotated position.[8,9] Recurrent instability is a common complication after traumatic anterior shoulder dislocation, particularly among younger patients.[10] Two recent systematic reviews aggregated the rate of recurrence as 21%[3] or 39%, respectively, when analyzing all patients who had suffered an instability event. However, it may be more instructive to look at the recurrence rate among discrete subpopulations. Similar to the initial dislocation event, young active males carry a significantly higher rate of recurrent instability with an aggregated rate of 80% for patients in this demographic.[3] Not surprisingly, the rate of recurrence rises if structural damage extends beyond the anterior capsulolabral complex. Associated injuries such as bony injury to the humeral head[11] (Hill-Sachs lesions), acute or progressive loss of bone at the anteroinferior glenoid rim,[12,13] rotator cuff tears,[14] and the presence of axillary nerve injury[15] all have been associated with poorer outcomes or higher rate of recurrence.[13–15]

However, just as recurrence is partially driven by the extent of the injury, so too recurrent instability events produce progressive injury. Additional labral and ligamentous injury, bone loss, chondral defects, arthritic change, and pain all become more common with recurrent instability events.[16] The incidence of osteoarthritis in unstable shoulders may be as high as 55% with increasing prevalence for patients who were older at the time of their first dislocations, sustained their dislocations as the results of high-energy sports injury, or concomitantly sustained a glenoid defect.[17] However, arthropathy associated with instability might also be the result of operative stabilization procedures which either unintentionally or by design, limited external rotation (ER) range of motion (ROM).

ANATOMIC AND BIOMECHANICAL CONSIDERATIONS

Stability of the glenohumeral joint is maintained by a combination of static and dynamic restraints.[18] Static stabilizers include noncontractile structures such as the bony anatomy; capsulolabral and ligamentous complex; and negative intraarticular pressure, which produces a suction effect of the humeral head in the glenoid. Dynamic stabilization is the result of appropriately balanced contractions between a compressive force imparted by the rotator cuff muscles and long head of the biceps brachii against displacing forces produced by thoracohumeral muscles such as the deltoid and pectoralis major.[19] Periscapular muscles such as the trapezius, rhomboids, and serratus anterior are also crucial to allow the glenoid to serve as a base for the humeral head as the shoulder moves through an arc of motion. It is also important to remember that the scapula serves as the origin for the rotator cuff muscles, so any deviation of scapular position affects the length–tension properties of the rotator cuff muscles. Stability is ultimately provided through a well-coordinated balance between static structures and dynamic muscle activity.[19]

The rotator cuff provides stability of the glenohumeral through a combination of two mechanisms: concavity compression and counteracting the translational effects of the primary movers to essentially "steer" the humeral head on the glenoid.[20] In this way, the dynamic stabilizers of the shoulder joint create force couples. For example, coactivation of the subscapularis and infraspinatus provides an anteroposterior compressive force, pulling the humeral head into the glenoid. A coupling of forces also describes the relationship between the deltoid and the rotator cuff. Because of its origin and insertion, the deltoid produces a net superior translation of the humeral head. If activity of the deltoid is not balanced by the compressive effects of the rotator cuff, such as in the setting of a large rotator cuff tear, the resultant motion is superior humeral head translation and shoulder hiking rather than smooth, rotational elevation.[18] Finally, the balance between the serratus anterior and the trapezius illustrates another important force couple around the scapula important in shoulder instability. If an athlete with anterior shoulder instability cannot sufficiently retract his scapula, hyperabduction of the glenohumeral joint in the horizontal plane will result as the athlete tries to use his hand in the coronal plane. This would stress the anterior capsulolabral structures such as when trying to throw a baseball or make a tackle. The converse is true for patients with posterior instability who require serratus anterior function to sufficiently orient the glenoid to the sagittal plane to provide posterior support to the humeral head and avoid relative cross body adduction.

A review of the relative contributions and limitations of the static stabilizers provides an important base for understanding shoulder instability. Only 25% to 33% of the humeral head is in contact with the glenoid at any one time, lending to the common analogy of the golf ball (humeral head) sitting on a tee (glenoid). However, we shouldn't erroneously conclude that the articular surfaces have little bearing on shoulder stability, especially when one also considers the glenoid surface is, like the humeral head, convex in shape. In essence, it is the addition of the glenoid labrum that effectively makes the glenoid surface concave, deepening the socket by approximately 50% and increasing the contact area with the humeral head by 75%.[21] Further inspection of the joint surfaces reveals the humeral head and the glenoid are slightly retroverted toward each other, providing a small bony lip to prevent anterior instability. However, the degree of retroversion has important implications for posterior shoulder instability. Every degree past the normal 10 degrees of glenoid retroversion (relative to the plane of the

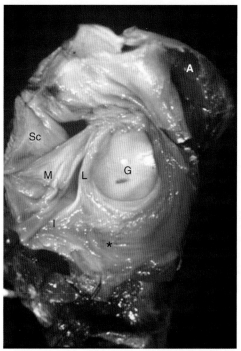

Fig. 71.1 Sagittal view of a cadaveric shoulder through the glenohumeral joint. The humerus has been removed to facilitate visualization of the ligaments. The main ligaments are located anteriorly. The labrum encircles the perimeter of the entire glenoid. *Asterisk* indicates the middle portion or pouch of the inferior glenohumeral ligament; *A,* Acromion; *G,* glenoid; *I,* anterior limb of the inferior glenohumeral ligament; *L,* labrum; *M,* middle glenohumeral ligament; *Sc,* subscapularis tendon.

scapula) leads to a 17% increase in the incidence of posterior instability.[22] Conversely, the incidence of anterior instability increases 20% for every additional 1 mm in coracohumeral distance.[23]

In addition to producing the concavity of the socket, the labrum is important as the attachment site through which the capsule attaches to the glenoid. The capsule of the glenohumeral joint contains thickened areas that form the glenohumeral ligaments (Fig. 71.1). These ligaments become taut at end ranges and thereby play an important role in stability of the shoulder at the extremes of the ROM positions where muscle forces decrease. The capsuloligamentous structures confer most of the stability of the shoulder at extreme ranges of motion. By contrast, the capsular structures are on slack in the midranges of motion, and dynamic stability provided by the shoulder musculature plays the more important role during typical daily activities In this way, the dynamic and static structures form a natural symbiosis to provide stability for normal daily activities that typically occur in midranges and athletic pursuits that often test the boundaries of shoulder stability.[18,19]

The main thickenings of the capsule are the glenohumeral ligaments (superior middle and inferior) and the coracohumeral ligament. These ligaments play distinctive roles for the control of anterior stability based on the position of the shoulder. The coracohumeral ligament and the superior glenohumeral ligament limit ER and inferior translation in adduction. The middle glenohumeral ligament limits ER and inferior translation in adduction and anterior translation in midabduction. The inferior glenohumeral ligament limits anterior, posterior, and inferior translation in abduction. The inferior glenohumeral ligament is designed with bands in the anterior and posterior aspects of the inferior aspect, with a patulous capsule in between that mimics a hammock.[24] Although it is simpler to think of each ligament restricting motion in a primary direction, the reality is that the posterior capsule also plays a role in controlling anterior displacement of the humeral head, a phenomenon frequently called the circle concept of shoulder stability.[25]

The key to a normal, stable articulation of the glenohumeral joint is to maintain the humeral head centered on the glenoid during motion. As will be explored in the next section, the difference between a "stable" shoulder and an "unstable" shoulder is not as obvious as it may seem.

Classification

One of the most important concepts to be understood for any joint is distinguishing between laxity and instability. The movements of any joint are constrained by the articulations of the bones and by the ligaments connecting them. The amount that two bones can slide or rotate upon each other depends on the relative position of the bones and the tension on the ligaments. This amount of movement is the laxity of the joint and is the amount of motion necessary for a joint's normal function. By contrast, instability is an abnormal, symptomatic translation of one joint surface relative to another. In the case of the shoulder, instability describes the humeral head translating excessively relative to the glenoid.

Disruption to either the static or dynamic glenohumeral restraints can manifest in a spectrum of clinical pathology ranging from subtle subluxation to shoulder dislocation. Classification of shoulder instability is important to tailor an individualized treatment programs for each patient. From a research standpoint, instability has been graded by the degree of separation of the joint surfaces, the angle of rotation of the joint, or strain or tension in joint structures.[8,9,24,26,27]

Becoming common among clinicians is a system based on four factors: the **f**requency of occurrences, the **e**tiology, the **d**irection of displacement, and the **s**everity of shoulder instability (FEDS).[28]

The frequency of instability events is an important component in establishing a rehabilitation plan. The most straightforward classification of frequency is simply acute or chronic. An *acute* episode of glenohumeral instability refers to the primary injury, whereas *chronic* instability usually refers to individuals who suffer recurrent episodes of instability.[29] Gaining a sense of the number of instability events and how atraumatic they are gives some indication about the severity of instability. For instance, learning a patient has had five recurrent instability events, and the most recent occurred while rolling over in her sleep communicates that this patient is quite unstable.

The cause of instability may be categorized as traumatic, atraumatic, microtraumatic, congenital, or neuromuscular.[29] Thomas and Matsen[30] originally introduced the acronyms TUBS and AMBRI to elucidate this concept. TUBS describes the patient with a **t**raumatic dislocation, **u**nidirectional, associated with a **B**ankart lesion, and typically requiring **s**urgery. A Bankart lesion refers to the detachment of the anterior–inferior capsulolabral complex from the glenoid rim. AMBRI describes a patient with **a**traumatic **m**ultidirectional instability (MDI) that is often **b**ilateral and typically responds well to **r**ehabilitation. If instability persists despite rehabilitation, then an **i**nferior capsular shift may be warranted. Although the TUBS and AMBRI mnemonics help simplify the injury pattern and the treatment, the binary choice of cause, either traumatic or atraumatic, may be overly simplistic and may not describe all variations of shoulder instability. The Stanmore classification system adds the possibility that shoulder instability may be caused by dyscoordinated muscle function even in a patient without any structural abnormality.[31]

The direction of instability refers to the displacement of the humeral head in relation to the glenoid and can be anterior, posterior, inferior, or even a combination of these.[29] Unidirectional instability occurs in only one of these directions. In a strict sense, the term MDI should be reserved to describe instability in at least two directions. But the most common, though likely incorrect, use of MDI is to describe a patient with shoulder pain and generalized ligamentous laxity without determining if the patient is truly unstable in two or more directions.[29] The distorted use of the term MDI and the use of a passive laxity assessment to diagnose a dynamic problem such as joint instability likely leads to an overestimation of the number of patients diagnosed with MDI.[32] By far, anterior instability is the most common direction, accounting for up to 98% of all patients with instability.[33,34] This is at least partially explained by the provocative position for anterior instability, a position where the arm is in a vulnerable position away from the body (abduction and ER), a position often encountered in sports (tackling an opponent, throwing an object), and a position where the demands of the sporting activity are quite high (high forces).

The severity of instability is relatively proportional to the level of injury to the capsulolabral structures. *Dislocation* is defined as complete separation of the articular surfaces leading to anatomical disruption and often requiring a reduction maneuver to restore joint alignment.[29] *Subluxation* is symptomatic instability without complete disruption of the articular surfaces. But in many cases, the instability is atraumatic in nature, and patients with subtle instability may complain of pain or a sense of looseness (or both). The prevailing theory of why these patients have pain is that the dynamic stabilizers are not able to completely offload lax static stabilizers that are innervated and relay pain when overly stressed or compressed.

TRAUMATIC INSTABILITY

Traumatic instability is usually the result of an uncontrolled high-velocity force applied at the end of the shoulder's ROM. The injurious force exceeds the tensile strength of the capsuloligamentous complex, resulting in a shoulder dislocation or subluxation. Between 85% and 95% of all traumatic shoulder dislocations occur in an anterior direction,[33,34] with injures nearly equally split between dominant (56%) and nondominant (44%) extremities.[34] During sports, 75% of anterior instability events occur when the shoulder is in the position of abduction and ER.[35] Other described mechanisms of injury include elevation with ER, direct blows, and falls on the outstretched arm.[36] For traumatic anterior shoulder instability, the most common anatomic injury is detachment of the anteroinferior portion of the labrum from the glenoid rim. This is the Bankart lesion and occurs from 78% to 100% of the time in series of traumatic anterior dislocations.[16,36,37] Bankart's lesion disrupts the concavity–compression effect during rotator cuff contraction and results in a 50% loss of the depth of the socket after detachment of the capsuloligamentous structures.[29] Although Dr. Bankart characterized the lesion bearing his name as the "essential lesion" leading to recurrent anterior instability, cadaver shoulders do not spontaneously dislocate after researchers produce a simulated Bankart lesion.[38,39] It is only when muscle forces, namely increased pectoralis major activity and decreased infraspinatus activity, are superimposed on the labral lesion that the humerus begins to translate anteriorly out of the socket.[40,41] Although the Bankart lesion is by far the most common injury, traumatic events can produce ruptures of the capsuloligamentous complex at other anatomic locations.[16] For instance, the humeral ligaments can avulse off the humerus (humeral avulsion of the glenohumeral ligaments [HAGL] lesion). There are also several variants of the Bankart lesion. For instance, the labrum, capsule, and anterior glenoid periosteum can avulse off the anterior aspect of the glenoid and heal or scar down significantly medial to the anatomic location. This is called an anterior labral periosteal sleeve avulsion (ALPSA) lesion. Another variant involves the labrum avulsing with an attached piece of the adjacent articular cartilage. This is a glenolabral articular disruption (GLAD) lesion. Because these injuries are uncommon compared with the usual Bankart lesion and because rehabilitation programs are fairly similar across the anterior stabilization procedures, we have chosen not to detail separate postoperative regimens for HAGL, ALSPA, and GLAD lesions later in this chapter.

Traumatic shoulder dislocations can also produce fractures of the humerus, glenoid, or both. The Hill-Sachs lesion is the most common fracture and defines impaction of the posterior aspect of the humeral head on the anterior glenoid.[42] There is not uniform agreement on how to measure Hill-Sachs lesions, but as the lesion gets larger, there is increased risk of this bony defect engaging the glenoid in abduction and ER (90/90 position), which can result in recurrent dislocation. In cases of engaging Hill-Sachs lesions, there are surgical procedures available to address the posterior humeral head, particularly in the setting of revision in which a previous soft tissue procedure failed to maintain shoulder stability. Surgical treatment of concerning Hill-Sachs lesions include tenodesis of the posterior rotator cuff into the humeral head defect (remplissage procedure), osteochondral grafting of the defect, or limited arthroplasty to this area.

Bony injuries to the anteroinferior glenoid are called bony Bankart lesions. The treatment for bony Bankart injuries most frequently involves primary repair of the bony fragment with the attached labrum. In cases of chronic or recurrent instability, the bony fragment off the glenoid can become fragmented, undergo attrition, or otherwise become smaller than the corresponding defect off the glenoid. Likewise, there can also be attritional loss of bone stock off the remaining intact glenoid with recurrent dislocations. In general, if the glenoid bone lesion encompasses 15% to 20% of the glenoid surface or when the bony Bankart fragment is deemed irreparable, stabilization surgery that addresses the bony deficiency (bone grafting, Latarjet or Bristow procedure) is the preferred method of treatment for these patients.[12,22] Underappreciated bone loss is one of the primary causes for failed stabilization surgery.[43–45]

Barring significant bony loss, the standard of care remains a trial of conservative management of the initial traumatic dislocation. Various nonoperative treatments, including shoulder immobilization, activity restriction, and exercise, have been advocated, but in general, the prognosis for young patients is considered to be poor with conservative management.[46] Surgical stabilization is becoming the treatment of choice in patients who are younger than 30 years of age and who are athletic.[47] Burkhead and Rockwood[33] conducted the seminal prospective study of 74 shoulders in 68 patients after traumatic dislocation. Patients performed a progressive strengthening exercise program emphasizing the rotator cuff, deltoid, and scapular stabilizers. Only 16% of the patients in this group had a good or excellent result.[33] The relative superiority of surgical stabilization as opposed to rehabilitation has stood the scrutiny of repeated analysis.[47,48] Prolonging the period of immobilization in internal rotation (IR) does not appreciably reduce the recurrence rate of subsequent instability after a traumatic dislocation. Hovelius and colleagues[49] reported the results of their landmark work, a prospective study of 255 patients (257 shoulders) with primary anterior shoulder dislocation who they have now followed out through 25 years. Patients in this cohort were randomized to either 4 weeks of strict immobilization or immobilization in a sling just until the patient felt comfortable. Regardless of the immobilization period, Hovelius and colleagues proved that recurrent instability is more common for younger patients with progressively less frequent recurrence with advancing patient age at the time of initial dislocation. At 25-year follow-up, regardless of immobilization, 38% of shoulders in patients who had been 12 to 25 years of age at the time of the original dislocation and 18% of patients who had been 26 to 40 years of age had undergone surgical stabilization. The authors concluded that patient age at

the time of initial dislocation was one of the most important factors in considering long-term prognosis after a traumatic anterior dislocation of the glenohumeral joint, surpassing gender or athletic participation in order of importance.[49]

Because of the relative ineffectiveness of immobilization of the shoulder in IR, other positions of immobilization after traumatic dislocation have been explored. Itoi and colleagues[50] demonstrated with magnetic resonance imaging (MRI) that Bankart's lesion is separated from the glenoid with the arm in IR but is approximated to the bone with the arm in 30 degrees of ER. An initial study revealed that patients were not comfortable with the arm in 30 degrees of ER. So the 3-week immobilization period was modified to a position of 10 degrees of ER for a clinical trial.[51] The ER group had a recurrence rate of 26%, whereas the recurrence rate for those immobilized in IR was 42%.[52] It is important to note that the average age of the patients in Itoi and associates' work was older than 30 years, so the results may not be generalizable to a younger athletic population. Patient age seems to be the most important variable when analyzing the relative success of immobilizing the shoulder in ER for 3 weeks after traumatic shoulder dislocation.[53] A study by Heidari and colleagues[54] that included patients up to 55 years of age (average age, 36 years) corroborated the results of Itoi and colleagues[52] and demonstrated a significant reduction of recurrent instability with ER immobilization. However, four other studies have failed to demonstrate any relative reduction of recurrent instability with ER immobilization when strictly analyzing patient populations younger than 30 years at the time of initial dislocation (average age, 25.2 years).[53,55–57] In addition, practically speaking, physicians shy away from ER immobilization because they are skeptical that patients will maintain an immobilization period of 3 weeks, particularly after the pain of the initial trauma has subsided. However, a recent meta-analysis did not find a significant difference in compliance with immobilization protocol between the ER and IR groups with average compliance of 71% of patients following the respective protocol.[58]

Of all studies examining nonoperative management of the primary, traumatic, anterior dislocator, Robinson and colleagues[59] have been the most explicit with regard to their physical therapy protocol. The rehabilitation program consisted of immobilization in a sling for 4 weeks. During this time, pendulum exercises and elbow ROM exercises were permitted three times daily. After sling removal at 4 weeks, patients were referred for a rehabilitation program consisting of active assisted shoulder ROM with limits of 90 degrees of elevation and 30 degrees of ER. After 6 weeks, patients were allowed unrestricted ROM except to continue to avoid terminal stretching. Isometric rotator cuff strengthening was performed at week 6, progressing to isotonic exercises at 12 weeks. Return to general fitness and noncontact sports was allowed at 12 weeks and return to competitive sports after 16 weeks. The authors of this chapter find Robinson and associates' protocol too conservative for practical use today, and although explicit about immobilization and exercises to restore ROM, we find the description of the strengthening exercises lacking. Therefore, from a historical perspective, the contribution of Robinson and associates is probably most important in terms of elucidating the natural time course of recurrent instability after traumatic dislocation. Of the original cohort of 252 patients (15–35 years of age), 150 (59.5%) patients had experienced a repeat dislocation or subluxation by the end of the 8-year study period. The mean time for the development of recurrent instability was 13.3 months. On survival analysis, recurrent instability had developed in 55.7% of the cohort by the end of 2 years, and 86.7% of all the patients with recurrence had their repeat instability event within a 2-year period.[59]

An athlete who sustains a dislocation during a competitive season poses a unique clinical dilemma.[42] Dickens and colleagues[60] prospectively studied 45 athletes from three different NCAA Division I

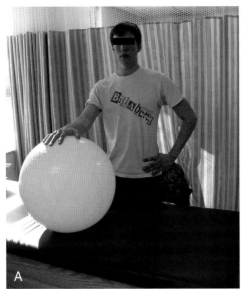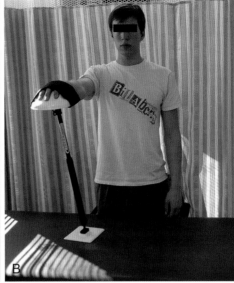

Fig. 71.2 Exercises using a large exercise ball (**A**) or an Upper Extremity Ranger (Rehab Innovations, Inc, Omaha, NE) after a period of immobilization after anterior shoulder dislocation (**B**).

institutions who sustained a traumatic dislocation playing a contact sport. Thirty-three (73%) of the athletes were able to return to sports within the same season with an average time loss of 5 days. Of athletes who returned to play, approximately two thirds (12 athletes, 64%) had, on average, 2.2 recurrent instability events that same season. Athletes who sustained a subluxation as their incident event were more than five times more likely to return to sport that season compared with athletes who had sustained a dislocation. Because the degree of anatomic disruption increases with the number of recurrences,[16] the athlete needs to be made fully aware of the risks before returning to play during the season in which he or she sustained an anterior dislocation.

Finally, clinicians must be aware that axillary nerve injury may result from traction of the humeral head resting on the axillary nerve after traumatic anterior inferior dislocation.[34] The reported incidence of axillary nerve injury after dislocation ranges from 5% to 54%, depending on the age of the patient studied and the extent of the diagnostic workup after dislocation. Neurologic complications after shoulder dislocation occur more frequently in patients 50 years of age and older and if the shoulder remains dislocated for longer than 12 hours. Patients with axillary nerve injury are rehabilitated in the same way as all patients after traumatic glenohumeral dislocation. In most cases, the injury is a neurapraxia, and deltoid function will gradually return over the course of 2 to 4 months.[14] The swallow tail sign, bilateral active shoulder extension, is a good clinical test to monitor recovery of axillary nerve function.

Authors' Preferred Rehabilitation after Traumatic Anterior Shoulder Dislocation–Subluxation

The authors strongly suggest that any significant shoulder subluxation or dislocation event be evaluated by a physician with radiography and other imaging as needed. An acute bony Bankart injury, in the authors' opinion, is best treated with early surgical management. Barring an obvious bony injury, nonoperative treatment begins with the shoulder immobilized in a standard sling for comfort and support after a traumatic anterior shoulder instability event. The duration of immobilization can be highly variable (2–21 days) depending on patient age, the degree of trauma necessary to displace the shoulder, and the number of preceding instability events. After immobilization, patients begin

active rehabilitation with exercises such as hand squeezes, elbow active ROM, and pendulum exercises. Some patients may experience apprehension, muscle guarding, or pain when initially performing pendulums. In these cases, it is prudent to support the arm while moving into forward elevation by performing closed-chain exercises such as dusting or a chair stretch (see Fig. 38.15). These exercises can be progressed to using a large exercise ball or an Upper Extremity Ranger (Rehab Innovations, Inc, Omaha, NE), which both require more control of the arm than a stable wall or chair (Fig. 71.2). when patients gain confidence with more passive movements, they may begin active assisted forward elevation with the opposite hand or exercise stick and ER with the arm supported in 45 degrees of abduction. Because ROM reliably returns, patients are cautioned to exercise only to tolerance and to not overstretch. When forward flexion has reached approximately 120 degrees, patients may begin posterior capsule stretching to help restore full elevation. Posterior shoulder stretches include extension, hand-behind-the-back IR, and cross-body adduction. Although isometric deltoid and rotator cuff contractions may have started previously, isotonic resistance in the form of elastic bands or dumbbells usually begins at this time. Resisted IR and ER with the arm adducted by the side are usually the first rotator cuff exercises (see Fig. 38.9). Rotator cuff strengthening will then be gradually progressed toward more functional positions such as internal and ER with the elbow supported and arm elevated away from the body (45–60 degrees) and then finally to approximately 90 degrees of elevation. Because abduction–ER is the most provocative position for patients with anterior instability, the progression for resisted elevation or elevated IR–ER usually begins in or anterior to the plane of the scapula and then progresses to the coronal plane. Because of the importance of retracting the scapula to orient the glenoid to the coronal plane and the necessity of a firm attachment site for the rotator cuff muscles, scapular strengthening exercises are also vital for the conservative management of anterior instability.[61] Scapular muscle retraining usually begins with scapular retraction at waist level with elastic resistance. Variations with the band fixed overhead (high rows) or near the floor (low rows) can be performed to recruit the other scapular retractors. Similar to rotator cuff strengthening, scapular retraction exercises against elastic resistance will eventually be progressed to positions with the arm elevated away from the side

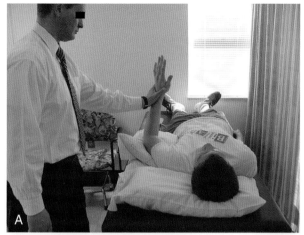

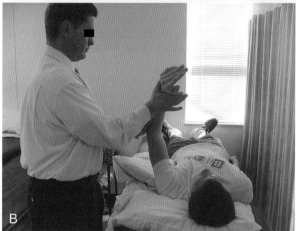

Fig. 71.3 Manual resistance used to promote co-contraction of the rotator cuff, deltoid, and scapular muscles. **A,** Manual resistance typically begins with the arm supported and performing alternating internal and external rotation. **B,** Progression is made to unsupported alternating abduction–external rotation and adduction–internal rotation.

such as horizontal abduction at 90 degrees of elevation (backhand). In the later stages of rehabilitation, prone scapular exercises (Hughston Clinic Exercises or The Letter Series) that have demonstrated a high level of electromyographic (EMG) activity can be used. Although these exercises elicit a high level of EMG activity, because the end position is often a combination of abduction and ER, they are also highly provocative for patients with anterior instability and should be added to the program with caution. Examples of exercises with high EMG activation but potentially provocative for patients with anterior instability include prone horizontal abduction with ER at 90 and 135 degrees, standing horizontal abduction with ER at 90 degrees of abduction with elastic resistance, and scaption with ER.[62]

Manual resistance is also very useful in this population to promote high levels of muscle activation within the ROM limits dictated by the therapist. All versions of proprioceptive neuromuscular facilitation such as rhythmic stabilization, alternating isometrics, and short-arc reversals can be used. Manual resistance typically begins with the arm supported and performing alternating IR and ER (Fig. 71.3A). Progression is made to unsupported alternating abduction–ER and adduction–IR (Fig. 71.3B).

To further enhance strength, dynamic control, proprioception, and endurance, the authors like to use the Bodyblade (Hymanson, Inc, Playa Del Ray, CA). With this fiberglass rod, patients maintain oscillations for various time intervals. The exercise progression begins

with the arm in nonprovocative positions at the side and working into more functional positions away from the body (Fig. 71.4). Controlling the oscillation of the blade requires co-contraction of the rotator cuff, deltoid, biceps, triceps, and scapular muscles. Buteau and colleagues[63] published a case report of a successful outcome using the Bodyblade in a patient after traumatic anterior shoulder dislocation.

Plyometric training using weighted balls can be used to enhance neuromuscular control, strength, and proprioception by reproducing the physiologic stretch-shortening cycle of muscle in multiple shoulder positions.[64] By catching and then throwing a weighted ball, the adductors and internal rotators are eccentrically loaded and elongated followed by the concentric shortening phase. Plyometric exercises create fast muscle contractions simulating athletic activity. For a patient undergoing rehabilitation after an anterior shoulder dislocation, we typically start with the arm in adduction and elbow bent to 90 degrees. The patient can simply toss the ball from one hand to the other. The exercise is progressed by gradually increasing shoulder ER and then by increasing the abduction angle, culminating in 90 degrees of abduction (Fig. 71.5). If an athlete is ever unable to tolerate the activity progression, he or she most likely will not be able to return to his or her sport without stabilization surgery. To return to sport, an athlete has to demonstrate full ROM, protective strength, and adequate neuromuscular control to engage in the necessary activities of his or her sport.

ATRAUMATIC INSTABILITY

The prevalence of atraumatic instability is unknown because the etiology is, by definition, void of a definite inciting event, and there is a broad spectrum of pathology ranging from mild pain with suspected micromotion to full dislocations when the patient actively moves her or his arm.[65] Patients with atraumatic instability have an enlarged joint capsule, the glenohumeral ligaments may be lax and thin, and the dynamic stabilizers (rotator cuff, deltoid, scapular muscles) may be weak or dyscoordinated.[66]

As mentioned previously, the terms *atraumatic instability* and *MDI* are often used interchangeably, meaning there is a wide variation in the definition of MDI in the literature.[32] Strictly speaking, the term *MDI* should be reserved for patients who have symptomatic instability in two or more directions.[32,67] In the clinical setting, the term *MDI* is most often used for patients who present with a positive sulcus sign indicating inferior laxity and some components of either anterior or posterior instability. This means the diagnosis of MDI is at least partially based on the examiner's ability to passively subluxate the shoulder even if the patient did not complain of symptomatic instability.[67,68]

Even more confusing than terminology or directions of instability, the central conundrum of atraumatic instability surrounds etiology.[67] There are three equally plausible yet not mutually exclusive causes of MDI. For instance, MDI may arise as the sequelae of a traumatic event.[68] Thus, one theory for the development of MDI is that of repetitive stress and progressive laxity in a previously injured shoulder. However, equally plausible is that the dynamic restraints are insufficient to counteract the stresses placed on the shoulder, resulting in injurious loads and gradually stretching out the passive restraints in a shoulder that had not previously suffered any isolated trauma. Indeed, patients with atraumatic shoulder instability have demonstrated deficits of joint position sense and decreases in other markers of proprioception compared with subjects without shoulder instability.[69] Finally, the authors of the Stanmore classification have postulated that dyscoordinated muscle firing may actually produce the destabilizing forces overloading the passive restraints.[31] Patients with MDI demonstrate differences in muscle firing patterns,[70] but it is unresolved if these abnormalities

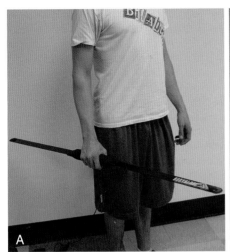
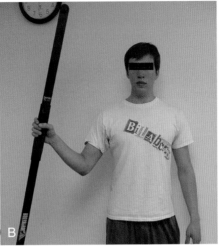
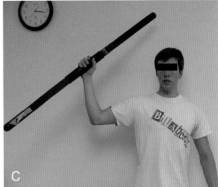

Fig. 71.4 The Bodyblade (Hymanson, Inc, Playa Del Ray, CA) is used to enhance strength, dynamic control, proprioception, and endurance. With this fiberglass rod, patients must sustain oscillations for various time intervals. The exercise can be performed with the arm in various positions starting in nonprovocative positions at the side (**A**) and working into more functional positions away from the body (**B** and **C**). Controlling the oscillation of the blade requires co-contraction of the rotator cuff, deltoid, biceps, triceps, and scapular muscles.

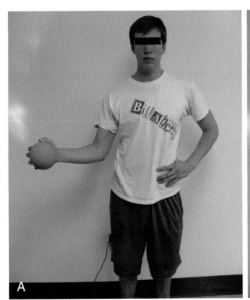
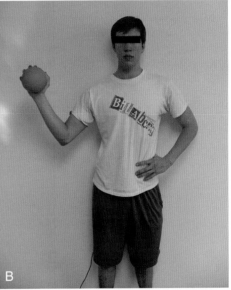

Fig. 71.5 Plyometric exercise creates a fast muscle contraction, simulating athletic activity. **A,** After anterior shoulder dislocation, exercises begin with the arm in adduction and elbow bent to 90 degrees. The patient can simply toss the ball from one hand to the other. **B,** The exercise is progressed by gradually increasing shoulder external rotation and then by increasing the abduction angle, culminating in 90 degrees of abduction.

are the underlying cause of the instability as the Stanmore classification suggests or if abnormal muscle firing results from being unable to completely constrain the center of humeral rotation on one part of the glenoid.[71] It is perhaps easier to think of any abnormality of muscle function as being an inability of the centering effect of the humeral head to balance the destabilizing effect of a contraction of a primary mover of the shoulder. But this line of thinking overlooks the very real possibility, particularly in patients with atraumatic instability, that their scapular position or periscapular muscle function is the underlying cause of their MDI.[72] Therefore, evaluation of scapular position and function is vital.[61,73] Another chapter of this text covers scapulothoracic evaluation and function in detail.

Although the vast majority of people with MDI seek medical attention because of involuntary subluxations and dislocations, a select group may have the ability to voluntarily subluxate their shoulders for secondary gain or psychiatric reasons.[65] EMG studies have identified several different abnormal firing patterns involving a combination of increased activation of the anterior deltoid and pectoralis major in conjunction with decreased activation of the posterior rotator cuff and serratus anterior.[74] Although individuals who voluntarily dislocate their shoulders are rare, understanding the muscle patterning involved may be helpful to understand instability that is out of the patient's control.

Some individuals who can voluntarily subluxate their shoulders are asymptomatic and do not require intervention. However, sorting the extent to which voluntarily subluxations contribute to a patient's reported symptoms is clinically difficult and time consuming for the medical team and is one of many reasons why a period of rehabilitation is preferable to rash surgical intervention.

The most commonly recommended treatment for atraumatic instability is nonoperative, with emphasis on rehabilitation of the dynamic stabilizers and activity modification.[33,65,75] Functional exercises that require coordination among multiple muscle groups have been recommended for retraining normal patterns of muscle activity in the patient with shoulder instability.[46] Occasionally, patients with atraumatic instability will come to the surgeon after MRI has already been performed. If the images demonstrate structural injury, then primary surgery is the preferred course. Otherwise, surgery in the form of an inferior capsular shift is reserved for patients in whom an extensive course of a well-designed rehabilitation program has failed and who continue to have shoulder symptoms.[33,65,76,77] In their seminal work on the topic, Burkhead and Rockwood[33] demonstrated that 80% of patients in a prospective series had good to excellent results with a strengthening exercise program emphasizing the rotator cuff, deltoid, and scapular stabilizers. Other authors have been less successful with nonoperative treatment for patients with atraumatic instability.[78,79] Misamore and associates[78] explicitly described an exercise program for MDI and prospectively followed patients for 7 to 10 years after enrollment. At the initial 2-year follow-up, 20 of 59 patients had already chosen surgical stabilization. In this series, most patients who reported success with the nonoperative program did so within 3 months. Patients were more likely to opt for surgery if their symptoms were more unilateral in nature, their instability affected their activities of daily living (ADLs), or they had more pronounced shoulder laxity. Of the 39 patients who did not have surgery, 19 still had pain or instability at 7- to 10-year follow-up. In their final tally, Misamore and associates[78] thought that only approximately one third of the 57 patients had a good or excellent result from nonsurgical intervention, well below the 80% success rate of Burkhead and Rockwood[33] despite a fairly similar exercise regimen and dosing (three times a day basis).

A recent systematic review of four clinical trials comparing exercise-based therapy with surgical stabilization has muddied the waters even further. The authors described all four trials as biased and of fairly low quality. In their opinion, stabilization surgery for patients with atraumatic shoulder instability was superior if impairment outcomes such as shoulder kinematic data and return to sport were evaluated. But a nonoperative exercise program was superior if one prioritized patient reported outcome measures such as the Constant score.[79]

Authors' Preferred Rehabilitation of Atraumatic Instability

The goal for exercise based rehabilitation of patients with atraumatic instability is to maximize the function of the dynamic stabilizers (i.e., rotator cuff, deltoid, scapular muscles) to allow functional movement patterns with the humeral head stabilized on the glenoid.

In extreme cases of instability, especially inferior subluxation, patients may be apprehensive about movement. In these cases, it is important to identify patterns of motion with which the patient feels stable to restore the patient's confidence in moving his or her arm. In a patient with inferior instability, ER in adduction will tighten the superior glenohumeral ligament complex and might allow the patient to begin raising his or her arm with increased confidence.[24] In addition, exercises which increase activation levels of the rotator cuff are emphasized. As an illustration of both principles, active elevation can be prescribed with the patient in the supine position (to minimize resistance), holding a towel in both hands with the forearms supinated and shoulders externally rotated (to pretension the superior capsule),

and asking the patient to pull the towel taught (activating the posterior rotator cuff). The resistance of gravity can be gradually added by increasing the angle of the table or adding pillows under the patient's head. The eventual goal is that the patient will be able to perform this activity in the upright position. The plane of elevation can be modified as appropriate for patients with more anterior instability (start with elevation closer to the sagittal plane) or more posterior instability type symptoms (start with elevation posterior to the plane of the scapula).

Similar to the rehabilitation program described for patients with traumatic instability, rotator cuff strengthening should begin in positions in which the shoulder is stable, usually beginning with the arm at the side and gradually working into more challenging positions of abduction and elevation. Resistance can be supplied by an elastic band and performed standing or with a dumbbell and performed in a sidelying position for internal and ER. When sufficient strength is achieved with the arm at the side, internal and external exercises are progressed away from the body into 45 degrees of elevation in the plane of the scapula with the arm supported on a table. A next step can be resisted elevation with the elbow bent to shorten the lever arm and moving through a limited arc of motion in the plane of elevation where the patient feels most stable (see Fig. 38.11). It is important not to neglect the scapular muscles and similar to the progression for patients with traumatic instability; we usually begin with scapular retraction exercises against elastic resistance at waist level and then progress to rows or horizontal abduction with the shoulder elevated to 90 degrees.

A theory of rehabilitation is to subject the shoulder to positions of instability during rehabilitation to elicit a reflexive muscular response which could be protective during unstable events.[20] Manual resistance is extremely effective in this patient population to help reestablish strength and proprioception. Rhythmic stabilization or manual perturbation training at a variety of glenohumeral angles, progressing from known to random patterns, from resistance applied proximal to distal to the glenohumeral joint, and from submaximal to maximal efforts, can be used to promote joint stability in functional positions.[65]

The Bodyblade (Hymanson, Inc, Playa Del Ray, CA) is a very useful tool for this patient population because the patient produces his or her own perturbations consistent with confidence and level of neuromuscular control. The rehabilitation clinician still controls the stresses placed on the shoulder based on the length of the blade, the positions of the shoulder, and the directions of perturbations that are prescribed. Individuals can gradually progress their challenges and move into sport-specific activities with the eventual goal of return to full participation when they have regained protective strength and the neuromuscular control necessary to keep the shoulder stable against the stresses imparted by their sport.

POSTERIOR INSTABILITY

Isolated posterior shoulder instability accounts for only 1% to 4% of all of shoulder dislocations.[80] In the acute setting, a posterior subluxation is usually the result of sports, electrocution, a seizure, or a fall on a forward flexed arm. Electrocution and seizures produce powerful contractions of the latissimus dorsi and teres major, producing a strong IR moment that displaces the humeral head posteriorly.[81] Among a young athletic population at the US Military Academy, male cadets were much more likely than female cadets to experience posterior instability with increased incidence when participating in wrestling and American football.[82] Increased glenoid retroversion beyond the normal 10-degree posterior angle of the glenoid has also been implicated as a risk factor.[22]

As in anterior dislocations, posterior dislocations may be associated with a posterior labral injury (reverse Bankart), capsuloligamentous tear, humeral head defect (reverse Hill-Sachs lesion), or posterior glenoid rim injury. Appropriate management is again determined after a careful assessment of the extent of the injury and the age and demands of the patient. In general, patients with posterior shoulder instability have a successful outcome with rehabilitation.[83] But a thorough nonoperative program must include eliminating uncontrolled seizures, restrained alcohol use to decrease the incidence of falls, and elimination of any voluntary subluxation. Patient compliance is necessary for a successful outcome, whether operative or nonoperative treatment is chosen. Substantial bony defects and recurrent instability despite appropriate rehabilitation are the strongest indications for surgical treatment. A posterior capsular shift is performed if capsular laxity is the only anatomic deficiency or posterior Bankart repair if the posterior labrum has been detached.[84]

SUPERIOR LABRUM ANTERIOR–POSTERIOR LESIONS

Andrews and colleagues[85] originally described detachment of the superior labrum in 73 young, throwing athletes with no history of a single episode of significant trauma. Snyder and colleagues[86] later attached the acronym SLAP (superior labrum anterior–posterior) to these findings, indicating an injury in the superior labrum and extending anterior to posterior. These authors reported on 140 injuries of the superior labrum, which represented 6% of shoulder procedures they performed over an 8-year period. In their series, the most common mechanism of injury (31%) was a fall or direct blow to the shoulder. The remainder arose from an episode of subluxation or dislocation (19%), pain when lifting a heavy object (16%), insidious onset of pain (14%), overhead racquet sports (6%), pain while throwing (6%), or no mechanism reported (8%).[87]

Repetitive overhead activity has also been hypothesized as a cause of SLAP lesions through two different potential mechanisms.[88] Andrews and colleagues[85] first theorized that SLAP lesions in overhead throwing athletes were the result of high eccentric activity of the biceps muscle, creating tension on the long head of the biceps tendon during arm deceleration in the follow-through phase of throwing. But then Burkhart and colleagues[89] hypothesized that a "peel-back" mechanism may actually be responsible for creating a SLAP lesion in overhead athletes. They believe that in a position of abduction and maximal ER, rotation of the shoulder causes a torsional force at the base of the biceps.[88] Illustrating the complexity of the mechanism of SLAP tears, the authors have demonstrated both increased tension and increased compression of the posterosuperior labrum with the shoulder in 90 degrees of abduction and full ER, a position that mimics the late cocking phase of overhead throwing.[88,90–92]

Superior labral anterior–posterior lesions have been classified into four distinct categories based on the labral injury and the stability of the labrum–biceps complex found at arthroscopy.[86] Subsequent authors added classification categories and specific subtypes.[93] Type I lesions denote fraying and degeneration of the superior labrum with a normal biceps tendon anchor. Type II lesions may have fraying of the superior labrum, but the hallmark is a pathologic detachment of the labrum and biceps anchor from the superior glenoid. In type III SLAP lesions, the superior labrum has a vertical tear analogous to a bucket-handle tear in the meniscus of the knee. The remaining rim of labral tissue is well anchored to the glenoid, and the biceps anchor is intact. A type IV pattern involves a vertical tear of the superior labrum extending into the biceps tendon. The torn biceps tendon tends to displace with the labral flap into the joint, whereas the biceps anchor itself remains firmly attached to the superior glenoid.[86] Last, a combination of two or more SLAP lesions may occur, with the most common presentation being types II and IV.[87]

Several special tests have been described to help determine the presence of labral pathology; however, no single test has demonstrated superior sensitivity or specificity to reliably determine the presence of a SLAP lesion. In addition, most studies evaluating the accuracy of special tests do not distinguish the type of SLAP lesion included. Keeping in mind that SLAP tears can be caused by several different mechanisms—eccentric loading of the biceps tendon, torsional stress of the biceps anchor via the peel-back mechanism, or compression of the posterosuperior labrum by the humeral head—it is unsurprising that a single special test would be unable to accurately detect all different varieties of SLAP tears. Furthermore, many patients with SLAP lesions present with concomitant pathology, making diagnosis difficult and complicating the ability of the medical time to create a hierarchy of the possible generators of a patient's pain. Because of the limitations of the physical examination, advanced diagnostic imaging plays an important role in the identification of SLAP tears, particularly for patients who are not progressing in rehabilitation. Magnetic resonance arthrography is currently the preferred imaging method to detect SLAP lesions.[94]

Patients with suspected SLAP lesions typically describe pain "deep inside" or "on the back" of their shoulder brought on by work or sport activity, reaching overhead, putting the shoulder in full abduction and ER (90/90, throwing position), or reaching up the back. Clinical presentation includes pain with overhead elevation, decreased IR or crossbody adduction ROM, decreased rotator cuff strength, and altered scapular mechanics.

Nonoperative management is generally preferred over surgery to address the loss of posterior shoulder flexibility, rotator cuff weakness, and scapular dyskinesis commonly associated with SLAP tears. Many patients respond positively to nonoperative management,[95] particularly those with lower demands, those older than 30 years of age, and those with type I lesions. The initial phase of nonoperative management consists of rest from the pain-producing activity, antiinflammatory medication, and stretching of the posterior capsule. These exercises include cross-body adduction and IR up the back with either the opposite hand or a towel. These stretches are generally very effective at improving posterior capsule flexibility.[96] Overhead athletes often require a more aggressive stretch, so the sleeper stretch is added (see Fig. 38.10).[97] This stretch can be performed in a sidelying or standing position with the involved arm against the floor or a wall.

When the pain begins to subside and patients demonstrate improvement of their posterior shoulder flexibility, we begin rotator cuff and scapular muscle strengthening as described earlier in this chapter. The same principle of starting with nonprovocative positions and working into more functional positions, such as a 90/90 throwing position, applies to the rehabilitation of patients with SLAP lesions. The exercise program for the overhead athlete needs to include trunk, core, and total arm strengthening exercises. We have found that most recreational athletes and patients who do not regularly perform heavy overhead lifting can return to their previous activities with rehabilitation. It is important that these patients are encouraged to continue their home programs and with the understanding that they may occasionally experience discomfort during or after stressful activities.

Unfortunately, the stresses of overhead throwing are such that many patients are not able to successfully return to throwing with rehabilitation alone.[98] However, the success rates of SLAP repair and return to throwing are only fair for position players (76%) and relatively poor (59%) for pitchers with progressively worse results as the competition level increases.[99] Major league athletes who are fortunate enough to return to activity end up pitching significantly fewer innings upon their return.[100] Poor outcomes have caused surgeons to consider augmenting or substituting SLAP repair by tenodesing the biceps tendon to the humeral head or shaft.[101] And yet the surgery with the best success for patient reported outcome measures without subsequently increasing the risk of postoperative stiffness is simple debridement of the SLAP tear.[102] The optimal management of SLAP tears, particularly in overhead athletes, remains an area of active debate among sports medicine professionals.

POSTOPERATIVE REHABILITATION OF CAPSULOLABRAL REPAIR OF THE SHOULDER

Optimal postoperative rehabilitation after capsulolabral repair of the shoulder requires the understanding and application of guiding rehabilitation principles while using guidelines that are specific to the surgical procedure performed and further individualized based on each patient's unique pathology, comorbidities, and specific functional demands.

GUIDING REHABILITATION PRINCIPLES

Successful rehabilitation after any orthopedic surgical procedure should depend on the appropriate application of stress to the repaired structures. Initially, reducing stress is required for healing followed by a progressive gradual increase in stress. However, as the rehabilitation proceeds, careful application of stress will promote healing but needs to be carefully controlled to protect the surgical repair. The American Society of Shoulder and Elbow Therapists (ASSET) has identified four principles of critical importance for the rehabilitation professional to understand to manipulate stress and facilitate healing in capsulolabral repairs of the shoulder and promote a safe return to function: (1) a basic understanding of the surgical procedure; (2) an understanding of the anatomic structures that must be protected, how they are stressed, and the rate at which they heal; (3) the identification and skilled application of the methods used during rehabilitation to manipulate stress to the surgical repair; and (4) identifying the appropriate length of immobilization and rate of return to full ROM.[103] These four principles form the foundation of the rationale for the specific rehabilitation guidelines, which are divided into three phases based on time since surgery (weeks 0–6, 6–12, and 12–24).

Guiding Principle 1: Understanding the Surgical Procedure

Because each surgical repair is unique, communication with the surgeon is important to become fully aware of the specifics of the surgical procedure and their impact on rehabilitation. Understanding the surgical procedure is important for the rehabilitation specialist because it provides knowledge about the extent of tissue damage and the method of surgical repair, both of which guide the speed and specific activities of rehabilitation.

Arthroscopic repairs for instability often are described as capsulolabral repairs (designating that both the capsule and labrum are repaired) or capsular plications (tensioning) either with or without a repair of the labrum. These general descriptions do not designate which part of the capsule or labrum was repaired (anterior, inferior, posterior, or a combination of these). Knowing which part of the capsule or labrum was repaired is vital because the repaired capsulolabral structures need protection from undue stress during rehabilitation and because the various parts of the capsulolabral complex are stressed by different planes of ROM. For example, a Bankart repair and anterior capsule plication would require extra protection during the restoration of ER ROM, whereas a posterior repair would require extra protection during IR and horizontal adduction. Detailed knowledge of the surgical procedure also allows the rehabilitation provider to gain knowledge of associated pathology such as bony lesions to the humerus or glenoid, rotator cuff tears, or SLAP lesions.

Arthroscopic anterior capsulolabral repair addresses anterior shoulder instability by repairing an unstable anteroinferior labrum,

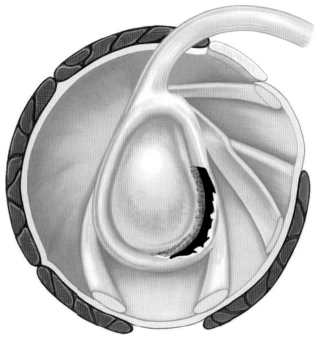

Fig. 71.6 A Bankart lesion. (From Gaunt B. arthroscopic capsular plication with or without Bankart repair. In: Gaunt B, McCluskey III G, eds. *A Systematic Approach to Shoulder Rehabilitation*. Columbus, GA: Human Performance and Rehabilitation Centers, Inc; 2012:290-321.)

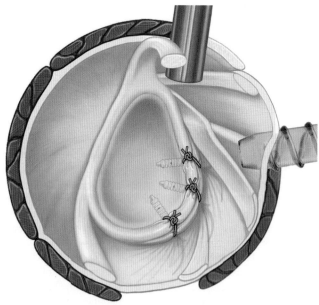

Fig. 71.7 A completed Bankart repair and capsular shift showing that the labrum has been stabilized and the capsule has been shifted 5 to 10 mm superiorly with each suture limb. (From Gaunt B. arthroscopic capsular plication with or without Bankart repair. In: Gaunt B, McCluskey III G, eds. *A Systematic Approach to Shoulder Rehabilitation*. Columbus, GA: Human Performance and Rehabilitation Centers, Inc; 2012:290-321.)

which is known as a Bankart lesion, back to the glenoid through the use of sutures or suture anchors (Fig. 71.6). In addition to a Bankart repair (Fig. 71.7), a capsular plication, which describes folding and suturing the capsule onto itself and/or stabilizing it to the labrum, is added as necessary to address permanent plastic deformation of the glenohumeral joint capsule that often accompanies recurrent anteroinferior dislocations. Similar procedures that restore normal tension to the capsule are performed in patients with inferior instability, posterior instability, and MDI.

Guiding Principle 2: Understanding the Structures That Require Protection During Rehabilitation, How They Are Stressed, and the Rate at Which They Heal

Arthroscopic capsulolabral repair involves a direct repair and retensioning of damaged capsular and possibly labral structures. The repaired tissues need protection from undue stress for an extended period of time to facilitate appropriate tissue healing.[104,105] It is well documented that specific portions of the capsule and labrum are selectively tensioned with specific glenohumeral motions.[24,26,27] A standard anterior capsulolabral repair, addressing laxity of the anteroinferior capsule, is most directly stressed by ER at all angles of abduction but particularly with the arm abducted to 90 degrees. If the repair is performed arthroscopically, the rotator cuff is not significantly disturbed and therefore does not need specific protection during rehabilitation. However, if an open procedure is performed in which the subscapularis is taken down, the suture line needs extensive protection from active IR and passive ER ROM during the first 6 postoperative weeks.

After the specifics of the capsulolabral repair are known, rehabilitation must only include activities that produce less stress to the healing tissues than the failure strength of the repair. The challenge for the rehabilitation professional is that the clinically detectable measures of tissue healing (e.g., pain, warmth, and swelling) are rather crude. To compound the situation, the stresses imparted by many rehabilitation activities remain unknown. An additional challenge is posed because patients generally return to demanding functional activities well before the repaired capsulolabral structures return to normal structural strength. Variations in the healing of the capsule, ligaments, and labrum as a result of factors such as health status, tissue quality, and extent of the injury must be carefully considered. Ligament healing times are often derived from animal research with few histologic studies in humans to guide progression of exercise after ligament injury. Ligament healing is thought to pass through the traditional phases of tissue recovery: inflammatory, proliferative, and remodeling and maturation phases.

We divided the rehabilitation process into three phases, each of a 6-week duration, because we believe that there are clinical milestones that occur at these times and our 6-week divisions partially reflect the three phases of tissue healing. Remodeling and final maturation of the tissue continues throughout the remainder of the formal rehabilitation process and may not be complete until 40 to 50 weeks after surgery. Understanding the effects age and comorbidities have possibly slowing the healing process is paramount for the proper application of these guidelines.

Guiding Principle 3: Identification and Skilled Application of Methods Used During Rehabilitation to Manipulate Stress to the Surgical Repair

Perhaps the single most important rehabilitation concept after arthroscopic anterior capsulolabral repair is that the healing capsulolabral structures must receive a gradual, measured, and therefore well-planned increase in stress. Each appropriate increase in stress is a stimulus for further proliferation and differentiation of fibroblasts. In a process analogous to Wolff's law of bone healing, the result is enhanced structural integrity of the capsulolabral complex as additional collagen fibers are laid down in response to controlled stresses. However, it is equally important to understand that if stress is applied inappropriately to the capsulolabral complex (during rehabilitation or ADLs), in terms of either magnitude or timing, the tissues are unable to adequately adapt,[106,107] resulting in damage to either the healing tissue or stabilizing material (sutures, anchors). During rehabilitation, three

mechanisms allow rehabilitation providers to manipulate stress to the surgical repair to positively affect patient outcome: (1) absolute ROM, (2) submaximal cyclic loading, and (3) dynamic stabilization.[103]

Initially, the structural integrity of the repair is based solely on the strength of the fixation method used during surgery. As time passes, the labrum begins to "heal" to the glenoid rim in the case of repair of Bankart's lesion, or plicated layers of the capsule begin to bind to one another in the case of a capsular plication. Excessive stretching must be avoided during ROM activities so as not to overload the structural integrity of these gradually healing tissues.[24,26,27] Additionally, much in the same way as micromotion may prevent bony union during fracture healing, submaximal cyclic loading[106,107] has the potential to disrupt the tenuous bond between soft tissue layers. Repeated submaximal stress of ligament plication in an animal model has been shown to negatively affect mechanical resistance properties, even as late as postoperative week 12.[106] Although it is unknown what effect the cyclic loading of rehabilitation interventions such as ROM and progressive functional activities have on the capsulolabral repairs, the rehabilitation provider should keep in mind that repeated submaximal tensioning of the repair during the remodeling phases of tissue healing may slowly stretch out the repair. Therefore, even though they are below the failure strength of the capsulolabral construct, repetitive submaximal stresses should be carefully controlled because they pose a potential threat to capsuloligamentous integrity. On the other hand, dynamic stabilization of a joint by the surrounding muscles provides protection of the surgical repair[8,9,41] by supporting the joint capsule, increasing joint compression forces,[41,108] and resisting joint displacement.[109] It is vital to understand that these three mechanisms (absolute ROM, submaximal cyclic loading, and dynamic stabilization) do not exist in isolation but are interrelated and are of paramount importance when selecting interventions for rehabilitation of the patient after capsulolabral repair.

Guiding Principle 4: Identifying the Appropriate Length of Immobilization and Rate of Return to Full Range of Motion

Strength of the arthroscopic anterior capsulolabral repair is tenuous through at least the first 12 postoperative weeks,[106] and more general reviews of ligamentous healing indicate that remodeling may continue through 40 to 50 weeks postoperatively. Therefore, controlling the rate at which ROM is regained is vitally important to adequately protect the surgical repair from undue stress during the early and middle postoperative period (~12 weeks). Gaining ROM too slowly may result in residual stiffness, whereas gaining ROM too quickly may result in recurrent laxity. Therefore, an initial period of controlled ROM is advised after arthroscopic anterior capsulolabral repair[103,110–112] to allow time for the surgically reattached labrum to bind to the glenoid and the plicated layers of capsule to heal to each other.

Strict immobilization (no glenohumeral ROM exercises and constant sling use) after arthroscopic stabilization of the shoulder began during the infancy of these procedures[113,114] when failure rates were high and surgical procedures were rapidly evolving. Current surgical methods use sutures and suture anchors to stabilize the labrum and retension the capsule.[43,110,115,116] Several studies demonstrated that using immediate staged ROM with contemporary surgical techniques yields a very low recurrence rate[110,116] and a quicker return to function compared with a 3-week period of immobilization.[110] Because of these studies, a range of 0 to 4 weeks of absolute immobilization is now commonly used after arthroscopic capsulolabral repair with sutures or suture anchors.[103,111,112]

Irrespective of immobilization period, the stability of the surgical repair is negatively affected by the patient regaining ROM too quickly any time during the first 2 to 3 months after surgery.[103,105,106]

TABLE 71.1	**Staged Range of Motion Goals for Arthroscopic Anterior Capsulolabral Repair**			
	PFE	**PER at 20 Degrees of Abduction**	**PER at 90 Degrees of Abduction**	**AFE**
POW 3	90 degrees	10–30 degrees	Contraindicated	NA
POW 6	135 degrees	35–50 degrees	45 degrees	115 degrees
POW 9	155 degrees	50–65 degrees	75 degrees	145 degrees
POW 12	WNL	WNL	WNL	WNL

AFE, Active forward elevation in the scapular plane; *NA,* not available; *PER,* passive external rotation; *PFE,* passive forward elevation in the scapular plane; *POW,* postoperative week; *WNL,* within normal limits.
Reprinted from Gaunt BW, Shaffer MA, Sauers EL, et al. The American Society of Shoulder and Elbow Therapists' Consensus Rehabilitation Guideline for Arthroscopic Anterior Capsulolabral Repair of the Shoulder. *J Orthop Sports Phys Ther.* 2010;40(3):155-168, with permission.

Controlling the speed of ROM gains is best accomplished through the use of staged ROM goals.[103,117] Staged ROM goals can be determined in at least two ways. The surgeon may have a preference based on factors such as the patient's specific injury, comorbidities, amount of natural laxity, surgical history, specific surgical technique (including type of fixation and arm position at the time of capsular plication), and his or her general philosophy. We offer a staged ROM table (Table 71.1)[103] as a general guideline for instances in which the surgeon provides no guidance. When using a ROM table, the goal is to have the patient comfortably obtain ROM to the specified angle. In some instances, little to no stretching is needed to achieve these staged ROM goals; in other instances, regular gentle stretching is required.

Although rehabilitation after all types of capsulolabral repair follows the same guiding rehabilitation principles, there are specific differences in the rehabilitation guidelines for procedures such as arthroscopic anterior capsulolabral repair, arthroscopic capsulolabral repair for MDI, arthroscopic posterior capsulolabral repair, SLAP repair, revision instability repair, open capsulolabral repair, and instability repair with bony augmentation caused by glenoid bone loss. In the remainder of this chapter, we will first detail rehabilitation guidelines for arthroscopic anterior capsulolabral repair. Using this guideline as a template, we will then briefly discuss alterations for use during rehabilitation after the aforementioned surgical procedures.

Guiding Principle 5: Understanding the Patient Variables That Affect Rehabilitation

Patient variables, such as age, activity level, hand dominance, generalized ligamentous laxity, personality type, and chronicity may play the largest role when it comes to setting up a postoperative rehabilitation plan for a patient with shoulder instability.

For example, because the recurrence rate is so much higher for younger patients, the rehabilitation progression, at least in theory, should progress more slowly. However, younger patients tend to be involved in competitive sports, which creates urgency for the rehabilitation program at certain times of the calendar year. By contrast, older patients usually do not have the approaching sports season to spur their rehabilitation and may need encouragement to overcome a learned fear of dislocating their shoulder and to move their shoulder to ensure they do not develop unintended postoperative stiffness.

The patient variables of hand dominance and activity level also intersect to significantly influence the postoperative rehabilitation. For instance, any loss of ER of the dominant shoulder in an abducted position negatively impacts the ability of the overhead athlete to return to his or her sport. Ensuring that the overhead athlete has enough ER ROM to return to his or her sport but not so much that he or she risks recurrence is a delicate balancing act for rehabilitation clinicians.

Finally, whether they occur together or in isolation, frequent preoperative instability events and excessive generalized ligamentous laxity necessitate a general slowing of the rehabilitation progression and greater caution as activities in more provocative positions are incorporated into the rehabilitation regimen.

SPECIFIC REHABILITATION GUIDELINE ARTHROSCOPIC ANTERIOR CAPSULOLABRAL REPAIR

The Appendix (online) contains The ASSET Consensus Rehabilitation Guideline for Arthroscopic Anterior Capsulolabral Repair.[103] ASSET's members are a multidisciplinary (physical therapy, occupational therapy, athletic training) group of rehabilitation professionals who practice in clinical, education, and research settings and specialize in shoulder and elbow rehabilitation. The best scientific evidence was used in the development of this guideline and general consensus among society members was used for instances in which the science was inconclusive or conflicting.

The guideline is divided into three phases based on general timeframes of capsulolabral healing. In addition, the Appendix lists specific criteria to achieve before progression to the next phase. Therefore, to progress from phase 1 to phase 2, both the timeframe and the progression milestones must be met. It is critical for the therapist to not only aim to meet these milestones but also to limit ROM within these timeframes to allow for optimal healing.

Successful rehabilitation after arthroscopic anterior capsulolabral repair includes no reports of pain nor recurrent instability, sufficient ROM to complete the desired task, and symmetrical strength and neuromuscular control of the rotator cuff and scapular musculature. Typically, we find that patients are able return to low-demand activities at postoperative months 2 to 4 and to very high-demand activities at 6 to 8 months.

These next few sections of the text will outline the modifications that we make from the ASSET Consensus Guideline for Arthroscopic Anterior Capsulolabral Repair (appendix) that we recommend for these specific conditions.

Posterior Capsulolabral Repair

Rehabilitation after repair for posterior instability uses the same guiding rehabilitation principles and the same methods to manipulate stress to the surgical repair as anterior capsulolabral repair. However, the part of the capsule that requires protection is obviously different; motions that are most stressful to the posterior repair are horizontal adduction, functional IR, and IR in both adduction and abduction.

Historically, a longer period of strict immobilization and a slower rehabilitation progression have been used for patients undergoing posterior instability repair compared with anterior repair. However, a recent prospective study of 200 contact and noncontact athletic shoulders undergoing arthroscopic posterior instability repair used early ROM and found 90% of patients were able to return to sport, including 64% returning to same level postoperatively with only 7% of patients demonstrating clinical symptoms of instability.[118] The timing of their rehabilitation regimen was not different from their anterior instability repair protocol, including controlled passive range of motion (PROM) within the first postoperative week, 4 to 6 weeks of sling use, light strengthening at 4 to 6 weeks, and return to sport approximately 6 months postoperatively. So it appears speed of rehabilitation for posterior stabilization is starting to mimic the speed of the more commonly performed anterior stabilization procedures with generally positive outcomes.

Although surgeon preference for immobilization varies more widely for posterior instability patients, most often patients are immobilized in a sling with or without an abduction pillow rather than a brace maintaining the shoulder in ER ("gunslinger" brace). Most of the sling immobilizer companies now offer immobilizers that hold the shoulder in neutral or slight ER to protect the posterior labrum and capsule during recovery. Regardless of the type of immobilization, it is important to educate the patient to avoid IR positions. During phase one, flexion ROM is restricted to less than 90 degrees to avoid load on the posterior capsule that occurs with overhead motions. Posterior capsule loading can be reduced during overhead elevation by using the plane of the scapula rather than sagittal plane elevation. IR ROM is limited for the first 4 to 6 weeks postoperatively. The degree of restriction varies by the surgeon and patient situation, but IR is typically limited to either 0 degrees or less than 30 degrees.

PROM and stretching may occasionally be needed during phase 2 rehabilitation to achieve full ROM. Compared with anterior stabilization procedures, only limited stretching is usually needed to achieve full ROM by postoperative week 12. More regular stretching can be used if a particular motion remains restricted. Discretion should be used when issuing direct posterior capsule stretches, such as cross-body adduction or the "sleeper" stretch, as part of a home program. The rehabilitation provider should prescribe posterior shoulder stretches when a moderate restriction of motion is present and should monitor progress closely to ensure ROM is not gained too quickly. Throwing athletes have more exacting demands, so normal flexibility must be restored, especially end-range IR and IR at 90 degrees of abduction.

Emphasis in phases 2 and 3 is on strengthening and neuromuscular control exercises. Early exercises are similar in patients with anterior and posterior stabilization because early exercises are performed in midrange angles in the plane of the scapula so as to avoid undue stress on either the anterior or posterior capsulolabral structures. Posterior repair necessitates avoiding load on the posterior capsule too soon or too quickly. For phase 2 to 3 exercises, this means delaying the initiation and speed of progression of closed-chain weight-bearing exercises. For example, exercises in the quadruped position are not begun until about 8 to 10 weeks after surgery, and then the amount of weight bearing with the arm in the forward flexed position should progress slowly. Closed-chain perturbation and unstable surface training are important progressions that require caution during this postoperative time period. When these activities are mastered, more unpredictable and faster loads can be introduced such as Plyoball chest passing and medicine ball drills progressing to activities such as controlled falling. The timeframes to complete functional progressions resulting in return activities that require large amounts of posteriorly directed force through the shoulder girdle, such as bench pressing, football, and wrestling, are highly variable depending on surgeon preference and patient situation but usually are not allowed before the 6th postoperative month.

Rehabilitation programs for patients whose posterior capsulolabral repair was performed via open incision are not significantly different from patients with arthroscopic repairs unless the infraspinatus is reflected during the repair. If the infraspinatus is surgically incised, no activation of the external rotators is allowed for the first 6 weeks postoperatively. Rehabilitation after open posterior stabilization is highly individualized and quite variable in the early postoperative period, so close communication among the surgeon, rehabilitation provider, and patient is vital.

Rehabilitation After Arthroscopic Repair for Multidirectional Instability

Rehabilitation after arthroscopic stabilization for MDI differs from anterior capsulolabral repair because MDI patients require retensioning of the posteroinferior capsule in addition to the anterior capsule. The typical patient who undergoes this procedure presents with general ligamentous laxity and the resultant decrease in proprioceptive abilities.[69] Because of the natural laxity in their connective tissues, MDI patients rarely have persistent ROM loss after surgery, and surgical repairs performed on MDI patients are thought to need more protection, especially during the early and middle postoperative periods. Therefore, patients with arthroscopic repair of MDI are often managed with a 2- to 4-week period of strict immobilization and then a slower ROM progression. Extra care should be taken to ensure that staged ROM goals are not exceeded and to recognize that MDI patients often reach their staged ROM goals with very minimal stretching. During all phases of rehabilitation, an extra emphasis should be placed on dynamic stability, neuromuscular control, and proprioception activities, ensuring that good control is mastered in nonprovocative positions before interventions are performed in positions that more directly stress the surgical repair. Neuromuscular control exercises can even begin during the later part of phase one rehabilitation with activities such as submaximal isometrics and rhythmic stabilization in a modified neutral position.

Rehabilitation After Superior Labrum Anterior–Posterior Repair

Postoperative rehabilitation after SLAP lesion debridement or repair is very similar to the rehabilitation after arthroscopic anterior capsulolabral repair. The primary difference is the need to minimize strain to the biceps anchor. Positions that create tension on the long head biceps origin should be avoided during the first 6 weeks after surgery, minimized for 10 to 12 weeks, and then advanced very slowly thereafter. These positions include shoulder extension, IR behind the back, and using the arm to carry or lift objects with the elbow extended. Additionally, it is vital that the repair must be protected from forces associated with the peel-back mechanism, of end-range ER with the arm in 90 degrees of abduction for 10 to 12 weeks after surgery, because of the large strain to the superior labrum in this position.[88,90-92] Biceps tenodesis or tenotomy is becoming a common treatment for patients with SLAP lesions in addition to or instead of SLAP repair. For patients with biceps tenodesis procedures, resisted elbow flexion or supination should be avoided for 6 weeks and deemphasized until 12 weeks postoperatively.

During phase 1 of rehabilitation, it is important to instruct patients in the precautions and rationale for the precautions listed earlier. The surgeon may request that ER ROM be limited to 45 degrees in patients who have evidence of a peel-back tear. Patients are expected to achieve full passive forward elevation approximately 6 weeks after surgery. Occasionally, light isometrics for the rotator cuff and deltoid are implemented at 3 to 4 weeks postoperatively.

During phase 2 of rehabilitation, which begins 6 weeks after surgery, rotator cuff, deltoid, and scapula strengthening exercises as described earlier in this chapter are initiated and become the primary focus of this stage of rehabilitation. It is important that strengthening, neuromuscular control, and proprioception exercises begin in non-provocative positions, emphasizing midranges and especially avoiding end-range ER. Emphasis is on strength development and smooth, controlled motions. PROM of the shoulder girdle should be carefully monitored at this time. Careful attention should be given to horizontal adduction and IR in abduction because flexibility of the posterior shoulder is so vitally important for the function of the shoulder, particularly for overhead athletes. These two motions are often restricted postoperatively, and it is important to remember that patients who sustain SLAP lesions often have preoperative tightness of the posterior shoulder. If cross-body adduction and IR ROM are limited, they should be gently stretched in a comfortable manner to restore normal motion. Finally, the target timeframe for full ER in abduction is 10 to 12 weeks after surgery so as to protect the repair from peel-back stresses earlier in the rehabilitation progression when the repair is still tenuous.

Phase 3 of rehabilitation, approximately 12 weeks after SLAP repair, is nearly identical to the phase 3 rehabilitation program for anterior capsulolabral repair. However, the final stage of rehabilitation for patients post SLAP repair is progressed more deliberately for overhead athletes. The rehabilitation clinician must ensure these athletes have the ability to control their shoulders during progressively higher loads at progressively higher speeds. Of particular importance is the ability to move from abduction with ER to IR with adduction because this is a common motion required for throwing sports, racquet sports, volleyball, and swimming. Return to competitive sports often takes 6 months or longer. Patients who must return to physically demanding work are gradually progressed to simulated work activities. Similar to overhead athletes, manual laborers must demonstrate the ability to control their shoulders during progressive challenges. Throughout rehabilitation, workers are educated on proper lifting mechanics, ergonomic modifications, and common sense use of their shoulder.

Open Capsulolabral Repair

Although the general principles and methods of repair are the same in both arthroscopic and open capsulolabral repair, it is important to understand the major differences between arthroscopic and open repair and the effect on rehabilitation. In general, patients undergoing arthroscopic repairs regain ROM more easily and with less risk of permanent ROM restriction than patients undergoing comparable open surgeries.[119] This is likely explained by the fact that open instability repair requires moderate to extensive tissue dissection of the subcutaneous and musculotendinous structures to gain access to the damaged capsulolabral structures, whereas arthroscopic repair minimizes tissue morbidity. Dissection through multiple tissue planes may lead to an increased likelihood of adhesions between adjacent tissue layers. Also, in open anterior and inferior capsulolabral repairs, exposure is achieved in part by either splitting the subscapularis in line with its fibers or completely detaching the subscapularis tendon, usually via a tenotomy just medial to its insertion to the lesser tuberosity. This tissue dissection affects rehabilitation in several ways. Most important, if the subscapularis is taken down or completely detached during the procedure, it presents another repaired structure and suture line that needs extensive protection from active IR and ER ROM during the first 6 postoperative weeks because subscapularis failure is a significant clinical problem, usually leading to complicated revision surgery. Although early passive ER with the arm in slight abduction is generally allowed, the surgeon will usually specify the limit of safe passive ER during phase 1 rehabilitation. The safe ROM is directly visualized at the time of open surgery and is typically the point at which the subscapularis suture line begins to receive

tension. If no limit is provided by the surgeon, 30 degrees of ER ROM is usually a safe range after open repair. If the subscapularis is split in line with its fibers, although ROM may be limited because of pain, no extra protection of the subscapularis is usually required, assuming adequate tissue quality.

Because of the tendency for long-term PROM limitations during rehabilitation of open capsulolabral repairs, early PROM is emphasized. Glenohumeral PROM is typically started within the first postoperative week and usually consists of both scapular plane elevation and passive ER. Although early PROM is emphasized, it *must* be done in a way that protects the healing anterior or inferior capsulolabral repair and subscapularis repair. Therefore, PROM should be performed regularly but not forcefully, and the same staged ROM goals used for arthroscopic anterior capsulolabral repair are used in this situation. More PROM is not necessarily better; ROM significantly greater than the staged goals is potentially detrimental to the surgical repair, and ROM significantly less than staged goals carries the risk of permanent ROM limitations. Phase 2 and 3 rehabilitation is virtually identical between open and arthroscopic capsulolabral repair except that passive ROM and flexibility interventions figure more prominently for patients with open repairs. If the subscapularis has been detached and repaired, then IR strengthening is not initiated until at least 6 weeks after surgery and then progressed very slowly thereafter.

Instability Repair with Bony Augmentation

Capsulolabral repair combined with bony augmentation of the glenoid caused by glenoid bone loss is becoming more common because of recognition of the relatively high risk for recurrent instability in patients with bone loss greater than 15% to 20% of the surface area of the glenoid.[12] Surgical procedures reconstitute the glenoid by transferring of part of the coracoid process with the conjoined tendon or a distal tibial allograft. Although the same general rehabilitation principles are used for rehabilitation of patients with bony procedures, the rehabilitation generally proceeds more slowly because these patients have usually sustained multiple dislocations and therefore have variable quality of the remaining soft tissues. In addition, the subscapularis often has to be addressed to allow direct visualization of the glenoid, and therefore postoperative subscapularis precautions are in effect. Clearly, rehabilitation must not disrupt the potential for bony healing. Load across the repair site must be limited because fibrous union or nonunion have been reported in 9.4% of patients in a systematic review of more than 1900 shoulders.[120] Because of the extensive and variable pathology that is often found in patients preoperatively, a wide range of postoperative outcomes is found in patients undergoing bony augmentation ranging from the ability to return to high-level activities to only being able to perform basic functional activities. Also, in coracoid transfer procedures, some loss of ER is expected, averaging 13 degrees in a large systematic review.[120] Therefore, regular communication needs to take place among the patient, surgeon, and rehabilitation professional so that all parties understand the restrictions, progression, and realistic outcome after surgery.

In patients who have good tissue quality and relatively few dislocations (<5), usually no change is needed from the standard rehabilitation guidelines for anterior capsulolabral repair other than a larger emphasis on achieving but not exceeding early ROM goals. For patients with fair to poor tissue quality or a high number of dislocations, the surgeon may choose to delay the start of glenohumeral PROM for several weeks and will often put strict ROM limits on elevation and ER. If the subscapularis is surgically detached to visualize the glenoid or if it is deficient and a pectoralis major tendon transfer is required, then extra protection is necessary as described in the section on rehabilitation after open capsulolabral repair.

Because of the loss of ER that is common after bony procedures, extra emphasis on PROM is needed; however, this must be performed in a *very gentle* manner to protect both the repaired capsulolabral structures and the bony transfer. We recommend frequent gentle stretching up to four to six times a day in this situation to improve ROM by repetition, *not* by stretching forcefully. The extra emphasis on stretching may need to continue for 3 to 4 months to maximize the patient's functional outcome. Rehabilitation activities in positions of abduction with ER as well as activities that result in large compressive loads through the glenoid, such as heavy weight training, should be performed only after close communication with the surgeon and only in select patient circumstances.

Revision Repair for Instability

Rehabilitation for patient after revision stabilization surgery should be highly individualized depending on a host of factors, such as the number of previous failed repairs, tissue quality, whether bone augmentation surgery was necessary, and other coexisting conditions such as generalized ligamentous laxity. In general, a slower rehabilitation program is warranted because, by definition, the patient has already failed previous surgery and at least one course of rehabilitation. The slower pace is meant to allow for more solid fixation to form between tissue layers during the early phase rehabilitation and for more complete restoration of strength and neuromuscular control during the latter phases. Appropriate modifications to the rehabilitation program might include one or more of the following: placing strict limits on the amount of PROM for ER or forward elevation during the first 6 to 12 weeks, delaying the initiation of ROM exercises up to 6 weeks, or delaying the start of strengthening until 3 to 4 months postoperatively.

Depending on the patient, return to advanced strengthening activities such as high-speed multiplanar exercises or return to sport activities that require end-range abduction with ER are delayed or might never be appropriate. Communication among the surgeon, patient, and rehabilitation clinician helps to determine appropriate restrictions and rehabilitation goals. The rehabilitation provider plays a vital role in repeated patient education throughout the rehabilitation process so that patients understand the importance of complying with this slower paced program.

SUMMARY

Shoulder instability is a common orthopedic disorder often requiring pre- or postoperative rehabilitation. For a joint with vast mobility requirements such as the human shoulder, the difference between normal laxity and instability is minimal. Pathologic shoulder instability can be classified by frequency, etiology, direction, and severity. Each component of this classification scheme provides its own clues as to the appropriate course of treatment and outcome. In general, the prognosis for nonoperative management of patients younger than 30 years of age who have sustained a traumatic dislocation is poor. In general, athletes are given "one chance to fail" with rehabilitation. If they have a repeat instability event, stabilization surgery, usually in the form of a Bankart repair, is performed and vastly reduces the likelihood of recurrent instability. By contrast, a long course of rehabilitation is generally preferred over operative management for patients who have developed atraumatic shoulder instability. More recent results have started to suggest that surgical stabilization, in the form of an inferior capsular plication, may also help to reduce the rate of recurrence for patients with atraumatic instability. Postoperative rehabilitation should be individualized based on patient factors such as the number of previous dislocations, associated pathology, type of stabilization procedure performed, and

patient goals and expectations. Controlling the rate at which ROM is regained is vitally important to adequately protect capsulolabral repairs of the shoulder from undue stress during the early and middle postoperative periods. Later stage rehabilitation should provide a gradual and measured return to the stresses the patient will encounter in ADLs, work, sport, and recreational activities. Successful rehabilitation for a patient with shoulder instability requires balancing the mobility necessary to achieve functional end-range positions against appropriate strategies of neuromuscular control, balancing the compressive effects of the rotator cuff against the displacing forces of the thoracohumeral muscles, and balancing the patient's ability to identify and avoid provocative positions while still possessing the confidence to perform all activities within his or her envelope of stability.

REFERENCES

1. Hovelius L. Incidence of shoulder dislocation in Sweden. *Clin Orthop Relat Res*. 1982;166:127–131. http://www.ncbi.nlm.nih.gov-/pubmed/7083659. Accessed December 10, 2017.
2. Mitchell C, Adebajo A, Hay E, Carr A. Shoulder pain: diagnosis and management in primary care. *BMJ*. 2005;331(7525):1124–1128. https://doi.org/10.1136/bmj.331.7525.1124.
3. Wasserstein DN, Sheth U, Colbenson K, et al. The true recurrence rate and factors predicting recurrent instability after nonsurgical management of traumatic primary anterior shoulder dislocation: a systematic review. *Arthrosc J Arthrosc Relat Surg*. 2016;32(12):2616–2625. https://doi.org/10.1016/j.arthro.2016.05.039.
4. Kardouni JR, Mckinnon CJ, Seitz AL. Incidence of Shoulder dislocations and the rate of recurrent instability in soldiers. *Med Sci Sport Exerc*. 2016;48(11):2150–2156. https://doi.org/10.1249/MSS.0000000000001011.
5. Zacchilli MA, Owens BD. Epidemiology of shoulder dislocations presenting to emergency departments in the United States. *J Bone Joint Surg Am*. 2010;92(3):542–549. https://doi.org/10.2106/JBJS.I.00450.
6. Peck KY, Johnston DA, Owens BD, Cameron KL. The Incidence of injury among male and female intercollegiate rugby players. *Sport Heal A Multidiscip Approach*. 2013;5(4):327–333. https://doi.org/10.1177/1941738113487165.
7. Paxton ES, Dodson CC, Lazarus MD. Shoulder instability in older patients. *Orthop Clin North Am*. 2014;45(3):377–385. https://doi.org/10.1016/j.ocl.2014.04.002.
8. Cain PR, Mutschler TA, Fu FH, Lee SK. Anterior stability of the glenohumeral joint. *Am J Sports Med*. 1987;15(2):144–148. https://doi.org/10.1177/036354658701500209.
9. Blasier RB, Guldberg RE, Rothman ED. Anterior shoulder stability: contributions of rotator cuff forces and the capsular ligaments in a cadaver model. *J Shoulder Elbow Surg*. 1992;1(3):140–150. https://doi.org/10.1016/1058-2746(92)90091-G.
10. Hovelius L, Rahme H. Primary anterior dislocation of the shoulder: long-term prognosis at the age of 40 years or younger. *Knee Surg Sport Traumatol Arthrosc*. 2016;24(2):330–342. https://doi.org/10.1007/s00167-015-3980-2.
11. Provencher MT, Frank RM, LeClere LE, et al. The Hill-Sachs Lesion: diagnosis, Classification, and Management. *J Am Acad Orthop Surg*. 2012;20(4):242–252. https://doi.org/10.5435/JAAOS-20-04-242.
12. Dickens JF, Owens BD, Cameron KL, et al. The Effect of subcritical bone loss and exposure on recurrent instability after arthroscopic Bankart repair in intercollegiate American football. *Am J Sports Med*. 2017;45(8):1769–1775. https://doi.org/10.1177/0363546517704184.
13. Shin SJ, Ko YW, Lee J. Intra-articular lesions and their relation to arthroscopic stabilization failure in young patients with first-time and recurrent shoulder dislocations. *J Shoulder Elbow Surg*. 2016;25(11):1756–1763. https://doi.org/10.1016/j.jse.2016.03.002.
14. Murthi AM, Ramirez MA. Shoulder dislocation in the older patient. *J Am Acad Orthop Surg*. 2012;20(10):615–622. https://doi.org/10.5435/JAAOS-20-10-615.

15. Robinson CM, Shur N, Sharpe T, Ray A, Murray IR. Injuries associated with traumatic anterior glenohumeral dislocations. *J Bone Joint Surg Am.* 2012;94(1):18–26. https://doi.org/10.2106/JBJS.J.01795.

16. Yiannakopoulos CK, Mataragas E, Antonogiannakis E. A Comparison of the spectrum of intra-articular lesions in acute and chronic anterior Shoulder instability. *Arthrosc J Arthrosc Relat Surg.* 2007;23(9):985–990. https://doi.org/10.1016/j.arthro.2007.05.009.

17. Hovelius L, Saeboe M. Neer Award 2008: arthropathy after primary anterior shoulder dislocation--223 shoulders prospectively followed up for twenty-five years. *J shoulder Elbow Surg.* 2009;18(3):339–347. https://doi.org/10.1016/j.jse.2008.11.004.

18. Abboud JA, Soslowsky LJ. Interplay of the static and dynamic restraints in glenohumeral instability. *Clin Orthop Relat Res.* 2002;400:48–57. http://www.ncbi.nlm.nih.gov/pubmed/12072745.

19. Matsen F a, Chebli C, Lippitt S, Collections S, Surgery J. *Principles for the Evaluation and Management of Shoulder Instability Selected The American Academy of Orthopaedic Surgeons*; 2007:647–659.

20. Day A, Taylor NF, Green RA. The stabilizing role of the rotator cuff at the shoulder - Responses to external perturbations. *Clin Biomech.* 2012;27(6):551–556. https://doi.org/10.1016/j.clinbiomech.2012.02.003.

21. Howell SM, Galinat BJ. The glenoid-labral socket. A constrained articular surface. *Clin Orthop Relat Res.* 1989;243:122–125. http://www.ncbi.nlm.nih.gov/pubmed/2721051.

22. Owens BD, Campbell SE, Cameron KL. Risk Factors for posterior shoulder instability in young athletes. *Am J Sports Med.* 2013;41(11):2645–2649. https://doi.org/10.1177/0363546513501508.

23. Owens BD, Campbell SE, Cameron KL. Risk Factors for anterior glenohumeral instability. *Am J Sports Med.* 2014;42(11):2591–2596. https://doi.org/10.1177/0363546514551149.

24. Turkel SJ, Panio MW, Marshall JL, Girgis FG. Stabilizing mechanisms preventing anterior dislocation of the glenohumeral joint. *J Bone Joint Surg Am.* 1981;63(8):1208–1217. http://www.ncbi.nlm.nih.gov/pubmed/7287791.

25. Flatow EL, Warner JI. Instability of the shoulder: complex problems and failed repairs: Part I. Relevant biomechanics, multidirectional instability, and severe glenoid loss. *Instr Course Lect.* 1998;47:97–112. http://www.ncbi.nlm.nih.gov/pubmed/9571407. Accessed November 16, 2017.

26. O'Connell PW, Nuber GW, Mileski RA, et al. The contribution of the glenohumeral ligaments to anterior stability of the shoulder joint. *Am J Sports Med.* 1990;18(6):579–584.

27. Terry GC, Hammon D, France P, et al. The stabilizing function of passive shoulder restraints. *Am J Sports Med.* 1991;19(1):26–34.

28. Kuhn JE. A new classification system for shoulder instability. *Br J Sports Med.* 2010;44(5):341–346. https://doi.org/10.1136/bjsm.2009.071183.

29. Cole BJWJ. *Anatomy, Biomechanics, and Pathophysiology of Glenohumeral Instability*; 1999.

30. Thomas SC, Matsen FA. An approach to the repair of avulsion of the glenohumeral ligaments in the management of traumatic anterior glenohumeral instability. *J Bone Joint Surg Am.* 1989;71(4):506–513. http://www.ncbi.nlm.nih.gov/pubmed/2703510. Accessed January 1, 2018.

31. Lewis A, Kitamura T, Bayley JIL. (ii) The classification of shoulder instability: new light through old windows! *Curr Orthop.* 2004;18(2):97–108. https://doi.org/10.1016/j.cuor.2004.04.002.

32. McFarland EG, Kim TK, Park H Bin, Neira C a, Gutierrez MI. The effect of variation in definition on the diagnosis of multidirectional instability of the shoulder. *J Bone Joint Surg Am.* 2003;85-A(11):2138–2144.

33. Burkhead WZ, Rockwood C a. Treatment of instability of the shoulder with an exercise program. *J Bone Joint Surg Am.* 1992;74(6):890–896.

34. Liu SH, Henry MH. Anterior shoulder instability. Current review. *Clin Orthop Relat Res.* 1996;323:327–337.

35. Baker 3rd CL, Uribe JW, Whitman C. Arthroscopic evaluation of acute initial anterior shoulder dislocations. *Am J Sports Med.* 1990;18:25–28.

36. Rowe CR. Acute and recurrent anterior dislocations of the shoulder. *Orthop Clin North Am.* 1980;11:253–270.

37. Taylor DC, Arciero RA, Taylor DC, Arciero RA. Pathologic changes associated with shoulder dislocations. Arthroscopic and physical examination findings in first-time, traumatic anterior dislocations. *Am J Sports Med.* 1997;25(3):306–311.

38. Speer KP, Deng X, Borrero S, Torzilli PA, Altchek DAWR. Biomechanical evaluation of a simulated Bankart lesion. *Surgery.* 1994;76(2):1819–1826.

39. Apreleva M, Hasselman CT, Debski RE, Fu FH, Woo SL, Warner JJ. A dynamic analysis of glenohumeral motion after simulated capsulolabral injury. A cadaver model. *J Bone Joint Surg Am.* 1998;80(4):474–480.

40. McMahon PJ, Lee TQ. Muscles may contribute to shoulder dislocation and stability. *Clin Orthop Relat Res.* 2002;(suppl 403):S18–S25. https://doi.org/10.1097/01.blo.0000031987.92980.86.

41. Labriola JE, Lee TQ, Debski RE, McMahon PJ. Stability and instability of the glenohumeral joint: the role of shoulder muscles. *J Shoulder Elbow Surg.* 2005;14(1 suppl):32–38. https://doi.org/10.1016/j.jse.2004.09.014.

42. Wang RY, Arciero RA, Mazzocca AD. The recognition and treatment of first-time shoulder dislocation in active individuals. *J Orthop Sport Phys Ther.* 2009;39(2):118–123.

43. Boileau P, Villalba M, Héry JY, Balg F, Ahrens P, Neyton L. Risk factors for recurrence of shoulder instability after arthroscopic Bankart repair. *J Bone Joint Surg.* 2006;88(8):1755–1763. https://doi.org/10.2106/JBJS.E.00817.

44. Balg F, Boileau P, Balg F, Boileau P. The instability severity index score. A simple pre-operative score to select patients for arthroscopic or open shoulder stabilisation. *J Bone Joint Surg - Br.* 2007;89(11):1470–1477.

45. Burkhart SS, Debeer JF, Tehrany AM, et al. Quantifying glenoid bone loss arthroscopically in shoulder instability. *Arthroscopy.* 2002;18(5):488–491.

46. Hayes K, Callanan M, Walton J, Paxinos A, Murrell G. Shoulder instability: management and rehabilitation. *J Orthop Sports Phys Ther.* 2002;32(10):497–509. https://doi.org/10.2519/jospt.2002.32.10.497.

47. Kirkley A, Werstine R, Ratjek A, Griffin S. Prospective randomized clinical trial comparing the effectiveness of immediate arthroscopic stabilization versus immobilization and rehabilitation in first traumatic anterior dislocations of the shoulder: long-term evaluation. *Arthroscopy.* 2005;21(1):55–63. https://doi.org/10.1016/j.arthro.2004.09.018.

48. Longo UG, van der Linde JA, Loppini M, Coco V, Poolman RW, Denaro V. Surgical versus nonoperative treatment in patients Up to 18 years old with traumatic shoulder instability: a systematic review and quantitative synthesis of the literature. *Arthrosc J Arthrosc Relat Surg.* 2016;32(5):1–9. https://doi.org/10.1016/j.arthro.2015.10.020.

49. Hovelius L, Olofsson A, Sandstrom B, et al. Nonoperative treatment of primary anterior shoulder dislocation in patients forty years of age and younger. a prospective twenty-five-year follow-up. *J Bone Joint Surg - Am.* 2008;90(5):945–952.

50. Itoi E, Sashi R, Minagawa H, Shimizu T, Wakabayashi I, Sato K. Position of immobilization after dislocation of the glenohumeral joint. A study with use of magnetic resonance imaging. *J Bone Joint Surg - Am.* 2001;83(5):661–667. http://www.ncbi.nlm.nih.gov/pubmed/11379734. Accessed January 21, 2018.

51. Itoi E, Hatakeyama Y, Kido T, et al. A new method of immobilization after traumatic anterior dislocation of the shoulder: a preliminary study. *J Shoulder Elbow Surg.* 2003;12:413–415.

52. Itoi E, Hatakeyama Y, Sato T, et al. Immobilization in external rotation after shoulder dislocation reduces the risk of recurrence. A randomized controlled trial. *J Bone Joint Surg.* 2007;89(10):2124. https://doi.org/10.2106/JBJS.F.00654.

53. Whelan DB, Litchfield R, Wambolt E, Dainty KN. Joint Orthopaedic Initiative for National Trials of The Shoulder (JOINTS). external rotation immobilization for primary shoulder dislocation: a randomized controlled trial. *Clin Orthop Relat Res.* 2014;472(8):2380–2386. https://doi.org/10.1007/s11999-013-3432-6.

54. Heidari K, Asadollahi S, Vafaee R, et al. Immobilization in external rotation combined with abduction reduces the risk of recurrence after primary anterior shoulder dislocation. *J Shoulder Elbow Surg.* 2014;23(6):759–766. https://doi.org/10.1016/j.jse.2014.01.018.

55. Finestone A, Milgrom C, Radeva-Petrova DR, et al. Bracing in external rotation for traumatic anterior dislocation of the shoulder. *J Bone Joint Surg Br.* 2009;91(7):918–921. https://doi.org/10.1302/0301-620X.91B7.22263.

56. Taşkoparan H, Kılınçoğlu V, Tunay S, Bilgiç S, Yurttaş Y, Kömürcü M. Immobilization of the shoulder in external rotation for prevention of recurrence in acute anterior dislocation. *Acta Orthop Traumatol Turc.* 2010;44(4):278–284. http://www.ncbi.nlm.nih.gov/pubmed/21252604. Accessed January 4, 2018.

57. Liavaag S, Brox JI, Pripp AH, Enger M, Soldal LA, Svenningsen S. Immobilization in external rotation after primary shoulder dislocation did not reduce the risk of recurrence. *J Bone Joint Surg Am Vol.* 2011;93(10):897–904. https://doi.org/10.2106/JBJS.J.00416.

58. Whelan DB, Kletke SN, Schemitsch G, Chahal J. Immobilization in external rotation versus internal rotation after primary anterior shoulder dislocation: a meta-analysis of randomized controlled trials. *Am J Sports Med.* 2016;44(2):521–532. https://doi.org/10.1177/0363546515585119.

59. Robinson CM, Howes J, Murdoch H, Will E, Graham C. Functional outcome and risk of recurrent instability after primary traumatic anterior shoulder dislocation in young patients. *J Bone Joint Surg Am.* 2006;88(11):2326–2336.

60. Dickens JF, Owens BD, Cameron KL, et al. Return to play and recurrent instability after in-season anterior shoulder instability: a prospective multicenter study. *Am J Sports Med.* 2014;42(12):2842–2850. https://doi.org/10.1177/0363546514553181.

61. Kibler W Ben, Sciascia A. The role of the scapula in preventing and treating shoulder instability. *Knee Surg Sport Traumatol Arthrosc.* 2016;24(2):390–397. https://doi.org/10.1007/s00167-015-3736-z.

62. Reinold MM, Escamilla RF, Wilk KE. Current concepts in the scientific and clinical rationale behind exercises for glenohumeral and scapulothoracic musculature. *J Orthop Sports Phys Ther.* 2009;39(2):105–117. https://doi.org/10.2519/jospt.2009.2835.

63. Buteau JL, Eriksrud O, Hasson SM, Buteau JL, Eriksrud O, Hasson SM. Rehabilitation of a glenohumeral instability utilizing the body blade. *Physiother Theory Pract.* 2007;23(6):333–349.

64. Swanik K, Lephart S, Swanik C, Stone D, Fu F. The effects of shoulder plyometric training on proprioception and selected muscle performance characteristics. *J Shoulder Elbow Surg.* 2002;11(6):579–586.

65. Guerrero P, Busconi B, Deangelis N, Powers G. Congenital instability of the shoulder joint: assessment and treatment options. *J Orthop Sports Phys Ther.* 2009;39(2):124–134. https://doi.org/10.2519/jospt.2009.2860.

66. Schenk TJ, Brems JJ. Multidirectional instability of the shoulder: pathophysiology, diagnosis, and management. *J Am Acad Orthop Surg.* 6(1):65–72. http://www.ncbi.nlm.nih.gov/pubmed/9692942. Accessed May 8, 2016.

67. Sher JS, Levy JC, Iannotti JP, Williams GR. Diagnosis of glenohumeral instability. In: 2nd ed. Iannotti JP, Williams GR, eds. *Disorders of the Shoulder: Diagnosis and Management.* vol. 1. Philadelphia: Lippincott Williams & Wilkins; 2007:339–367.

68. McFarland EG, Kim TK, Park H Bin, et al. The effect of variation in definition on the diagnosis of multidirectional instability of the shoulder. *J Bone Joint Surg Am.* 2003;85-A(11):2138–2144.

69. Edouard P, Gasq D, Calmels P, Degache F. Sensorimotor control deficiency in recurrent anterior shoulder instability assessed with a stabilometric force platform. *J Shoulder Elbow Surg.* 2014;23(3):355–360. https://doi.org/10.1016/j.jse.2013.06.005.

70. Kiss RM, Illyes A, Kiss J. Physiotherapy vs. capsular shift and physiotherapy in multidirectional shoulder joint instability. *J Electromyogr Kinesiol.* 2010;20(3):489–501. https://doi.org/10.1016/j.jelekin.2009.09.001.

71. LU Bigliani, Kelkar R, Flatow EL, Pollock RG, Mow VC. Glenohumeral stability. Biomechanical properties of passive and active stabilizers. *Clin Orthop Relat Res.* 1996;330:13–30. http://www.ncbi.nlm.nih.gov/pubmed/8804270.

72. Matias R, Pascoal AG. The unstable shoulder in arm elevation: a three-dimensional and electromyographic study in subjects with glenohumeral instability. *Clin Biomech.* 2006;21(suppl 1):52–58. https://doi.org/10.1016/j.clinbiomech.2005.09.014.

73. Watson L, Warby S, Balster S, Lenssen R, Pizzari T. The treatment of multidirectional instability of the shoulder with a rehabilitation programme: part 2. *Shoulder Elb.* 2017;9(1):46–53. https://doi.org/10.1177/1758573216652087.

74. Pande P, Hawkins R, Peat M, Pande P, Hawkins R, Peat M. Electromyography in voluntary posterior instability of the shoulder. *Am J Sports Med.* 1989;17(5):644–648.

75. Warby SA, Pizzari T, Ford JJ, Hahne AJ, Watson L. The effect of exercise-based management for multidirectional instability of the glenohumeral joint: a systematic review. *J Shoulder Elbow Surg.* 2014;23(1):128–142. https://doi.org/10.1016/j.jse.2013.08.006.

76. Neer CS, Foster CR. Inferior capsular shift for involuntary inferior and multidirectional instability of the shoulder. A preliminary report. *J Bone Joint Surg Am.* 1980;62(6):897–908. http://www.ncbi.nlm.nih.gov/pubmed/7430177.

77. Longo UG, Rizzello G, Loppini M, et al. Multidirectional instability of the shoulder: a systematic review. *Arthrosc J Arthrosc Relat Surg.* 2015;31(12):2431–2443. https://doi.org/10.1016/j.arthro.2015.06.006.

78. Misamore GW, Sallay PI, Didelot W. A longitudinal study of patients with multidirectional instability of the shoulder with seven- to ten-year follow-up. *J Shoulder Elbow Surg.* 2005;14(5):466–470. https://doi.org/10.1016/j.jse.2004.11.006.

79. Warby SA, Pizzari T, Ford JJ, Hahne AJ, Watson L. Exercise-based management versus surgery for multidirectional instability of the glenohumeral joint: a systematic review. *Br J Sports Med.* 2016;50(18):1115–1123. https://doi.org/10.1136/bjsports-2015-094970.

80. Perron AD, Jones RL. Posterior shoulder dislocation: avoiding a missed diagnosis. *Am J Emerg Med.* 2000;18(2):189–191. http://www.ncbi.nlm.nih.gov/pubmed/10750929.

81. Rouleau DM, Hebert-Davies J, Robinson CM. Acute traumatic posterior shoulder dislocation. *J Am Acad Orthop Surg.* 2014;22(3):145–152. https://doi.org/10.5435/JAAOS-22-03-145.

82. Lanzi JT, Chandler PJ, Cameron KL, Bader JM, Owens BD. Epidemiology of posterior glenohumeral instability in a young athletic population. *Am J Sports Med.* 2017;45(14):36354651772506. https://doi.org/10.1177/0363546517725067.

83. McIntyre K, Bélanger A, Dhir J, et al. Evidence-based conservative rehabilitation for posterior glenohumeral instability: a systematic review. *Phys Ther Sport.* 2016;22:94–100. https://doi.org/10.1016/j.ptsp.2016.06.002.

84. Bradley JP, Baker 3rd CL, Kline AJ, et al. Arthroscopic capsulolabral reconstruction for posterior instability of the shoulder: a prospective study of 100 shoulders. *Am J Sports Med.* 2006;34(7):1061–1071.

85. Andrews JR, Carson WG, McLeod WD. Glenoid labrum tears related to the long head of the biceps. *Am J Sports Med.* 1985;13:337–341.

86. Snyder SJ, Karzel RP, Del Pizzo W, Ferkel RD, Friedman MJ. SLAP lesions of the shoulder. *Arthroscopy.* 1990;6(4):274–279. http://www.ncbi.nlm.nih.gov/pubmed/2264894.

87. Snyder SJ, Banas MP, Karzel RP. An analysis of 140 injuries to the superior glenoid labrum. *J shoulder Elbow Surg.* 4(4):243–248. http://www.ncbi.nlm.nih.gov/pubmed/8542365. Accessed January 7, 2018.

88. Dodson CC, Altchek DA. SLAP lesions: an update on recognition and treatment. *J Orthop Sport Phys Ther.* 2009;39(2):71–80.

89. Burkhart SS, Morgan CD. The peel-back mechanism: its role in producing and extending posterior type II SLAP lesions and its effect on SLAP repair rehabilitation. *Arthroscopy.* 1998;14(6):637–640. https://doi.org/10.1016/S0749-8063(98)70065-9.

90. Pradhan RL, Itoi E, Hatakeyama Y, Urayama M, Sato K. Superior labral strain during the throwing motion: a cadaveric study. *Am J Sports Med.* 2001;29:488–492.

91. Jobe CM. Posterior superior glenoid impingement: expanded spectrum. *Arthroscopy.* 1995;11:530–536.

92. Walch G, Boileau P, Noel E, Donell T. Impingement of the deep surface of the infraspinatus tendon on the posterior glenoid rim. *J Shoulder Elbow Surg.* 1992;1:238–245.

93. Morgan CD, Burkhart SS, Palmeri M, et al. Type II SLAP lesions: three subtypes and their relationships to superior instability and rotator cuff tears. *Arthroscopy.* 1998;14(6):553–565.

94. Nam EK, Snyder SJ. The diagnosis and treatment of superior labrum, anterior and posterior (SLAP) lesions. *Am J Sports Med.* 2003;31(5):798–810. https://doi.org/10.1177/03635465030310052901.

95. Edwards SL, Lee JA, Bell J-E, et al. Nonoperative treatment of superior labrum anterior posterior tears improvements in pain, function, and Quality of Life. https://doi:10.1177/0363546510370937.

96. Balaicuis J, Heiland D, Broermsma ME, Thorndike C, Wood A, McClure PW. A randomized controlled comparison of stretching procedures for posterior shoulder tightness. *J Orthop Sport Phys Ther.* 2007;37:108–114.

97. Chepeha JC, Magee DJ, Bouliane M, Sheps D, Beaupre L. Effectiveness of a posterior shoulder stretching program on university-level overhead athletes: randomized controlled trial. *Clin J Sport Med.* 2017;0:1–7. https://doi.org/10.1097/JSM.0000000000000434.

98. Fedoriw WW, Ramkumar P, McCulloch PC, Lintner DM. Return to play after treatment of superior labral tears in professional baseball players. *Am J Sports Med.* 2014;42(5):1155–1160. https://doi.org/10.1177/0363546514528096.

99. Gilliam BD, Douglas L, Fleisig GS, et al. Return to play and outcomes in baseball players after superior labral anterior-posterior repairs. *Am J Sports Med.* 2018;46(1):109–115. https://doi.org/10.1177/0363546517728256.

100. Smith R, Lombardo DJ, Petersen-Fitts GR, et al. Return to play and prior performance in major league baseball pitchers after repair of superior labral anterior-posterior tears. *Orthop J Sport Med.* 2016;4(12):232596711667582. https://doi.org/10.1177/2325967116675822.

101. Chalmers PN, Monson B, Frank RM, et al. Combined SLAP repair and biceps tenodesis for superior labral anterior–posterior tears. *Knee Surg Sport Traumatol Arthrosc.* 2016;24(12):3870–3876. https://doi.org/10.1007/s00167-015-3774-6.

102. Schrøder CP, Skare Ø, Reikerås O, Mowinckel P, Brox JI. Sham surgery versus labral repair or biceps tenodesis for type II SLAP lesions of the shoulder: a three-armed randomised clinical trial. *Br J Sports Med.* 2017;51(24):1759–1766. https://doi.org/10.1136/bjsports-2016-097098.

103. Gaunt BW, Shaffer MA, Sauers EL, et al. The American Society of Shoulder and Elbow Therapists' consensus rehabilitation guideline for arthroscopic anterior capsulolabral repair of the shoulder. *J Orthop Sport Phys Ther.* 2010;40(3):155–168. https://doi.org/10.2519/jospt.2010.3186.

104. Nho SJ, Frank RM, Van Thiel GS, et al. A biomechanical analysis of shoulder stabilization. *Am J Sports Med.* 2010;38(7):1413–1419. https://doi.org/10.1177/0363546510363460.

105. McEleney ET, Donovan MJ, Shea KP, Nowak MD. Initial failure strength of open and arthroscopic Bankart repairs. *Arthroscopy.* 1995;11(4):426–431.

106. Hill AM, Jones IT, Hansen U, et al. Treatment of ligament laxity by electro thermal shrinkage or surgical application: a morphologic and mechanical comparison. *J Shoulder Elbow Surg.* 2007;16(1):95–100.

107. Wetzler MJ, Bartolozzi AR, Gillespie MJ, et al. Fatigue properties of suture anchors in anterior shoulder reconstructions: Mitek GII. *Arthroscopy.* 1996;12(6):687–693.

108. Karduna AR, Williams GR, Williams JL, Iannotti JP. Kinematics of the glenohumeral joint: influences of muscle forces, ligamentous restraints, and articular geometry. *J Orthop Res.* 1996;14:986–993.

109. Louie JK, Mote CD. Contribution of the musculature to rotatory laxity and torsional stiffness at the knee. *J Biomech.* 1987;20(3):281–300.

110. Kim SH, Ha KI, Cho YB, Ryu BD, Oh I. Arthroscopic anterior stabilization of the shoulder: two to six-year follow-up. *J Bone Joint Surg Am.* 2003;85-A(8):1511–1518. http://www.ncbi.nlm.nih.gov/pubmed/12925631.

111. Gibson J, Kerss J, Morgan C, Brownson P. Accelerated rehabilitation after arthroscopic Bankart repair in professional footballers. *Shoulder Elb.* 2016;8(4):279–286. https://doi.org/10.1177/1758573216647898.

112. Leggin BG, Sheridan S, Eckenrode BJ. Rehabilitation after surgical management of the thrower's shoulder. *Sports Med Arthrosc.* 2012;20(1):49–55. https://doi.org/10.1097/JSA.0b013e3182471f31.

113. Morgan CD, Bodenstab AB. Arthroscopic Bankart suture repair: technique and early results. *Arthroscopy.* 1987;3(2):111–122.

114. Johnson LL, Johnson LL. The shoulder joint. An arthroscopist's perspective of anatomy and pathology. *Clin Orthop Relat Res.* 1987;223:113–125.

115. Levine WN, Rieger K, McCluskey 3rd GM. Arthroscopic treatment of anterior shoulder instability. *Instr Course Lect.* 2005;54:87–96.

116. Bacilla P, Field LD, Savoie FH. Arthroscopic Bankart repair in a high demand patient population. *Arthroscopy.* 1997;13(1):51–60. http://www.ncbi.nlm.nih.gov/pubmed/9043604.

117. Phillips BJ, Gaunt BWKJ. What are the most important range of motion restrictions after shoulder surgery. In: Huxel Bliven K, ed. *Quick Questions in the Shoulder: Expert Advice in Sports Medicine.* Thorofare, NJ: SLACK, Inc.; 2015:147–152.

118. Bradley JP, McClincy MP, Arner JW, Tejwani SG. Arthroscopic capsulolabral reconstruction for posterior instability of the shoulder. *Am J Sports Med.* 2013;41(9):2005–2014. https://doi.org/10.1177/0363546513493599.

119. Hubbell JD, Ahmad S, Bezenoff LS, et al. Comparison of shoulder stabilization using arthroscopic transglenoid sutures versus open capsulolabral repairs: a 5-year minimum follow-up. *Am J Sports Med.* 2004;32(3):650–654.

120. Griesser MJ, Harris JD, McCoy BW, et al. Complications and re-operations after Bristow-Latarjet shoulder stabilization: a systematic review. *J Shoulder Elbow Surg.* 2013;22(2):286–292. https://doi.org/10.1016/j.jse.2012.09.009.

Examination and Management of Scapular Dysfunction

Philip McClure, Kshamata Shah

OUTLINE

CRITICAL POINTS

- Several tests have been developed to assess the function of the scapula and have been applied in multiple clinical studies. The measurement properties of some tests have been established, whereas others are still being investigated.
- The scapula should be assessed with most upper-quarter conditions, and the examination should include the scapula dyskinesis test, modified scapula assistance test, scapula reposition test, pectoralis minor length, thoracic kyphosis and flexibility, flexibility of the posterior capsule of the glenohumeral joint, and muscle performance testing for the primary scapular stabilizers: lower trapezius, middle trapezius, and serratus anterior.
- One key principle in designing a scapular exercise program is to match the difficulty of the exercise with the patient's level of motor control and strength. It is important to observe the patient posteriorly during exercise to ensure that he or she is able to maintain good scapular control.

EVALUATION AND MANAGEMENT OF SCAPULAR DYSFUNCTION

Scapular dysfunction is a common clinical problem, and proper scapular motion and stability is considered to be crucial to normal function of the shoulder. The scapula is required to serve as a stable base for glenohumeral function but is also required to move through a substantial arc of motion. This motion is required to maintain optimal muscle length-tension relationships and glenohumeral joint alignment and stability during elevation of the arm.

The goals of this chapter are to (1) describe normal and abnormal motion of the scapula, (2) discuss the relationship between scapular dyskinesis and shoulder pathology, (3) describe current examination techniques for identifying possible scapular pathology, and (4) describe intervention techniques for scapular pathology, including enhancing muscle performance, stretching, bracing, and taping.

Normal Scapular Motion

The basic anatomy of the shoulder girdle and the scapular muscles is covered in Chapter 4; therefore, this section focuses on describing scapular motion and the primary muscles and other factors controlling this motion. The terminology used to describe scapular motion is quite varied in the literature, and no definitive standard has emerged, but we have promoted using scapular and clavicular angles to accurately describe scapular orientation and position respectively. Three scapular rotations are typically used to describe scapular orientation,[1-3] and they are depicted Fig. 72.1A to C (upward and downward rotation, anterior and posterior tilting, and internal and external rotation).

Upward and downward rotation of the scapula occurs around an axis that is perpendicular to the plane of the scapula. Anterior and posterior tilting (sometimes called tipping[1]) occurs around an axis through the spine of the scapula. Posterior tilting involves the inferior angle of the scapula moving anteriorly and the superior border moving posteriorly. Internal and external rotation occurs around a vertically oriented axis, and external rotation involves the lateral border of the scapula moving away from the thorax. More precise biomechanical definitions of these axis systems are available in original sources.[3,4]

Scapular position on the thorax has been described in various ways using terms that correspond to superior–inferior or mediolateral translation of the scapula from its normal resting position between the second and seventh ribs. However, because the clavicle acts as a strut, the scapula remains at a fixed mediolateral position relative to the thorax (assuming an intact acromioclavicular [AC] joint and clavicle). Therefore, the rotational motion of the clavicle around the sternoclavicular joint into protraction–retraction and elevation–depression can be used to describe scapular position in two degrees of freedom.[5] The description of scapular position using these two clavicular angles can be likened to the identification of a point on the earth using two angles, longitude and latitude.[5] As shown in Fig. 72.1D and E, clavicular elevation and depression occur around an anterior–posterior axis through the sternoclavicular joint, and clavicular protraction and retraction occur around a vertical axis through the sternoclavicular joint. Therefore, the motions of "scapular elevation or depression" and "scapular protraction or retraction" really occur in conjunction with corresponding rotary motions at the sternoclavicular joint.

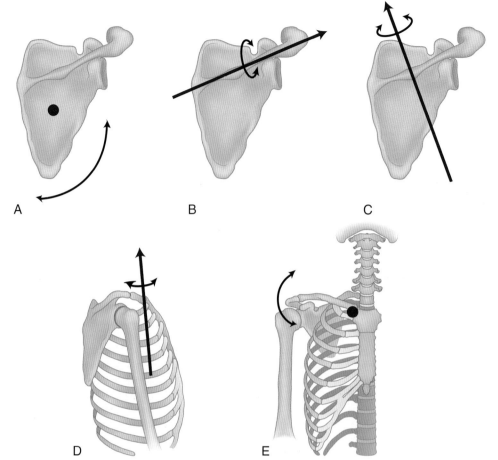

Fig. 72.1 Scapular and clavicular rotations used to describe motion. **A,** Scapular upward–downward rotation. **B,** Scapular anterior–posterior tilting. **C,** Scapular internal–external rotation. **D,** Clavicular protraction–retraction. **E,** Clavicular elevation–depression.

During elevation of the arm, there is a consistent pattern of scapular upward rotation, posterior tilting, and external rotation along with clavicular elevation and retraction. Fig. 72.2 shows the normal pattern for each of these motions in healthy participants derived using a sensor attached directly to the scapula via bone pins during arm raising and lowering in the scapular plane.[3] This figure shows each of the scapular and clavicular rotations separately with humerothoracic motion plotted along the *x*-axis.

As evidenced by Fig. 72.2A showing scapular upward rotation, in the early phase of elevation, there is a much greater contribution from the glenohumeral joint than the scapulothoracic joint to elevation. After 90 degrees of arm elevation, the contribution from the glenohumeral joint and the scapulothoracic joint become almost equal. While the scapula moves on the thorax, motion of the scapula is also intimately related to the motion at AC joint, which is the scapula moving relative to the clavicle. During arm elevation, the AC joint (scapula relative to clavicle) upward rotation contributes approximately 15 degrees of the total 50 degrees of motion of the scapula relative to the thorax.[6] Scapular upward rotation is controlled primarily by a force couple between the upper and lower trapezius and the serratus anterior.[7,8]

Posterior tilting (see Fig. 72.2B) and external rotation (see Fig. 72.2C) motions are nonlinear, with the majority of these motions not occurring until after 90 degrees of arm elevation. During arm elevation, posterior tilting motion of the scapula occurs almost exclusively at the AC joint, and less than 10 degrees of internal rotation at the AC joint occurs.[6]

A comprehensive review of the scapular muscle activity associated with posterior tilting and external rotation is beyond the scope of this chapter but is available.[9] The lower fibers of the serratus anterior and lower trapezius are positioned to produce posterior tilting, and the middle trapezius is positioned to produce external rotation. Weakness in these muscles after nerve injury has been clearly associated with scapular winging, which is attributable to excessive anterior tilting and scapular internal rotation.[10]

The clavicular retraction (see Fig. 72.2D) observed suggests the superior aspect of the scapula normally moves posteriorly during arm elevation while the scapula also moves superiorly as represented by clavicular elevation (see Fig. 72.2E). These motions are attributable to all parts of the trapezius muscle.[11]

ABNORMAL SCAPULAR MOTION (SCAPULAR DYSKINESIS)

A commonly observed abnormal pattern of scapular motion (scapular dyskinesis) is the premature or excessive scapular elevation that appears as *shrugging* (Fig. 72.3). This pattern has been associated with rotator cuff pain,[12] weakness,[13,14] and fatigue.[15] It has also been observed with loss of glenohumeral motion.[16,17] Therefore, excessive or early elevation of the scapula is a sign of scapular compensation for a weak rotator cuff or a stiff glenohumeral joint capsule (or both). This shrugging motion has been associated with increased upper trapezius activity.[18,19] Abnormal eccentric control of scapular rotation during

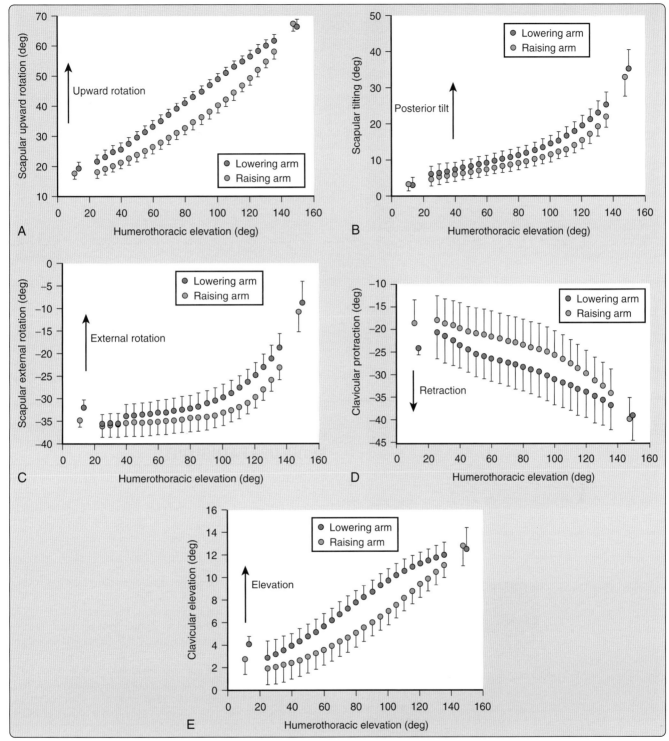

Fig. 72.2 Humerothoracic elevation (in degrees) during various scapular movements of arm elevation. **A,** Scapular upward rotation. **B,** Scapular posterior tilting. **C,** Scapular external rotation. **D,** Clavicle retraction. **E,** Clavicle elevation.

arm lowering may also occur. The normal pattern of scapular downward rotation during arm lowering is shown in Fig. 72.2B and can be seen to be quite linear, clinically this should appear as a smooth descent of the scapula during arm lowering. We have commonly observed poor eccentric control of this scapular downward rotation, which appears as a rapid "dumping" of the scapula instead of smooth downward rotation (Fig. 72.4). We are unaware of experimental documentation of this kinematic abnormality.

Another common form of scapular dyskinesis is *scapular winging* in which either the inferior angle or medial border of the scapula becomes more prominent. Inferior angle prominence or winging is associated with anterior tilting of the scapula, whereas medial border prominence is associated with excessive scapular internal rotation. We have documented these motion abnormalities in our lab on subjects with nerve injuries (Fig. 72.5) affecting the long thoracic nerve and serratus anterior muscle. Another source that may contribute to scapular winging is

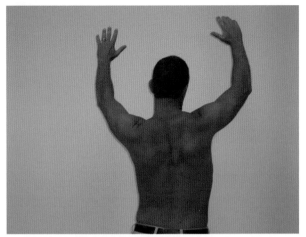

Fig. 72.3 Excessive scapular elevation "shrugging" associated with glenohumeral weakness or stiffness.

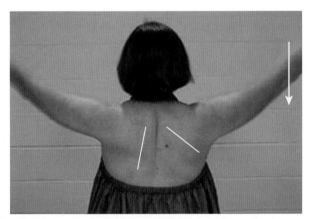

Fig. 72.4 Excessive and poor eccentric control of scapular downward rotation on the left side during arm lowering, known as "dumping."

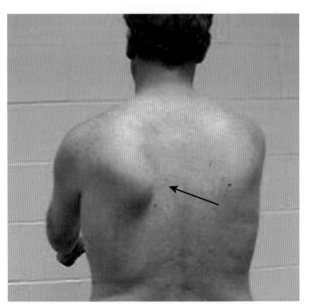

Fig. 72.5 Long thoracic nerve palsy and associated serratus anterior weakness producing scapular winging with anterior tilt and downward rotation on the left.

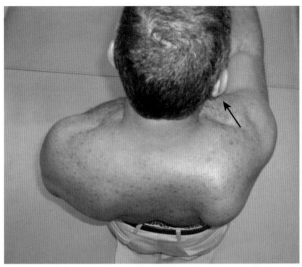

Fig. 72.6 Pectoralis minor tightness or overactivity producing anterior tilting of the scapula during arm elevation, which produces the appearance of winging.

the action of the pectoralis minor muscle. If this muscle is tight or overactive, it has the ability to tilt the scapula forward, producing winging of the inferior angle as well as scapular depression (Fig. 72.6). Borstad and Ludewig[20] have presented data suggesting that participants with tight pectoralis minor muscles demonstrate greater anterior tilting and scapular internal rotation.

IS SCAPULAR DYSKINESIS RELATED TO SHOULDER PATHOLOGY?

Recognition of the biomechanical role of the scapula in normal shoulder function has led to several clinical studies attempting to associate abnormal scapular motion, so-called "scapular dyskinesis," with shoulder pathology such as shoulder impingement[5,19,21–24] or instability.[25] These studies have included several methods of capturing scapular motion, including Moiré topography, electromechanical digitization, radiographic methods, magnetic resonance imaging (MRI), and electromagnetic tracking devices. Results of studies assessing three-dimensional scapular motion in those with pathology have been inconsistent. Participants with shoulder impingement have been found to demonstrate increased posterior tilting,[26,27] decreased posterior tilting,[19,24,21] decreased upward rotation,[19,21] increased upward rotation,[22,26] increased superior translation,[24,26] and increased internal rotation.[19,25] In addition to the variability of findings in these studies, the magnitude of differences between those with healthy shoulders and those with pathology is typically small, in the 3- to 5-degree range, and it is unclear whether these differences, although statistically significant, are really of clinical significance. Furthermore, studies that have examined shoulder kinematic changes after rehabilitation have not shown changes in scapular motion despite improvement of symptoms.[28–30]

The importance of the finding of scapular dyskinesis remains controversial and unclear. Conflicting evidence suggests that scapular dyskinesis could represent (1) normal variability in motion, (2) a mechanism initiating or perpetuating symptom, or (3) a potentially useful compensation. Several studies have suggested that the prevalence of scapular dyskinesis may be similar in those with and without shoulder symptoms suggesting normal variability in motion.[31,32] Other evidence has suggested that the presence of abnormal scapular motion may be associated with an increased risk of shoulder symptoms.[33,34]

Interestingly, two studies in overhead athletes have found a lower prevalence of shoulder symptoms in athletes with scapular dyskinesis, suggesting a possible protective effect.[32,35]

Therefore, despite some authors claiming a strong relationship between abnormal scapular motion and shoulder pathology,[36-38] the actual research evidence supporting this assertion is limited. Other clinical tests predicated on altering symptoms with manual scapula repositioning may hold promise in clarifying which patients truly have scapular dysfunction driving symptoms.[39-41]

Specific Nerve Injuries

The spinal accessory and long thoracic nerves are two nerves commonly injured that lead to scapular muscle dysfunction, primary winging and related shoulder disability. The spinal accessory nerve (cranial nerve XI) is derived from the ventral rami of C2, C3, and C4 and runs behind the sternocleidomastoid muscle and then more superficially over the levator scapula to innervate the trapezius muscle. Because of its relatively superficial course, it is more susceptible to injury. Spinal accessory nerve injury has been reported to occur after blunt trauma, traction, lymph node biopsy in the posterior cervical triangle, and radical neck dissection.[42] In the case of trapezius weakness, the shoulder appears depressed with the scapula translated laterally and the inferior angle rotated laterally, and winging is most apparent with frontal plane abduction to 90 degrees.[10]

The long thoracic nerve originates from the ventral rami of the C5, C6, and C7 cervical nerves. The nerve passes around the middle scalene muscle and then reaches the upper slip of the serratus anterior muscle and descends along its anterior surface. This nerve can be damaged from viral illness, repetitive trauma, stretching, or surgery. Long thoracic nerve injury produces weakness of the serratus anterior and results in primary winging most evident during sagittal plane elevation. The scapula is described as being superiorly elevated and medially translated, with the inferior pole medially rotated.

Friedenberg and associates[43] retrospectively reviewed 106 patients with either long thoracic or spinal accessory neuropathy with a mean follow-up period of 48 months. They found that with conservative care, 40 of 50 patients with long thoracic injury obtained a good outcome, whereas 37 of 56 patients with spinal accessory neuropathy obtained a good outcome. A traumatic injury mechanism was associated with a poorer outcome, but electrodiagnostic findings were generally not predictive of outcome.[43] With closed injuries, recovery is often spontaneous but may require up to 1 year. For patients in whom substantial weakness persists for longer than 6 months, surgical procedures may be warranted. Some authors have suggested that scapular winging is an important sign suggesting nerve injury and often misdiagnosed as other shoulder pathologies such as rotator cuff syndrome, glenohumeral instability, or AC joint dysfunction.[44] For more information on nerve injuries about the shoulder, see Chapters 50 and 51.

EXAMINATION

Evidence exists supporting the notion that altered scapular kinematics in a subset of persons may decrease the subacromial space and thereby may either contribute to subacromial impingement, or the altered kinematics may be a compensatory mechanism for the shoulder pathology.[19,45,46] In light of this, we need to be able to identify persons with scapular motion abnormalities. A scapular assessment measure should have clinical feasibility and acceptable reliability and validity and should assess dynamic, three-dimensional motion during concentric and eccentric loaded conditions, as would be present during athletics and occupational endeavors. Following is a description of existing clinical measures of scapular motion. Although we review the available

literature on several of the commonly used or cited scapula assessment measures, the end of this chapter contains a summary outline of assessment procedures used by these authors in the clinical setting.

Two-Dimensional Tests
Lateral Scapula Slide Test and Modifications of Linear Tests

Kibler[47,48] has described a measurement of scapular stability devised for use at static positions during arm elevation. The lateral scapular slide test involves taking a linear measure from the inferior angle of the scapula to the spinous process of the thoracic vertebrae and defines an "abnormality" threshold of 1.5 cm in side-to-side linear measurement difference in any of three test positions: with the arms resting at the sides, with the hands placed on the hips, and with the arms actively abducted to 90 degrees and internally rotated[48] (Fig. 72.e1). The reported reliability of this method was done on the actual linear measurements, not the difference in linear measures between sides at the different arm positions. Although Kibler cites a study reporting intertester reliability to be between 0.77 and 0.85, a replication of the original study found significant differences between the two testers on all Kibler measures.[49] Odom and associates[50] report interrater intraclass correlation coefficients ranging from 0.52 to 0.66 for the measurement of scapula side-to-side differences for participants with shoulder dysfunction and 0.75 to 0.80 for participants without shoulder impairment. The standard error of measurement (SEM) sometimes exceeded the mean value of the difference. Based on these results, the value of the difference in side-to-side scapular distance measurements with this technique was not found to be reliable in determining the presence and amount of scapular asymmetry. The researchers also stated that their reliability might be higher than that found by other researchers because all examiners received "considerable training" based on the knowledge of a person who studied with the test developer.

Other researchers have described modifications of the lateral scapular slide in the seated position,[51] using overhead upper extremity positions,[52] using string to measure linear distance, and calculating normalized scapular abduction (the linear distance from T3 to the inferior angle of the acromion divided by the scapular size).[53,54] The findings of these studies are inconsistent, but the use of a linear measure from the spinous process to a designated point on the scapula has inherent drawbacks irrespective of the reliability and validity issues. First, use of only linear horizontal or oblique measures along the thorax does not address displacement of the scapula's medial border or inferior angle away from the thoracic wall (winging). Additionally, in a study of 71 collegiate athletes who participated in one-arm-dominant sports, 52 of the 71 participants exhibited a difference of at least 1.5 cm on 1 or more of the three positions assessed for the lateral scapular slide test.[55] The calculated specificity of 26.8% in this study questions the usefulness of asymmetry as an indicator of pathology. In support of this finding, Nijs and coworkers[56] report no association between the results of the lateral scapular slide and measures of pain and disability in a group of 29 patients diagnosed with a shoulder disorder.

SICK Scapula Rating Scale

Based on the concept of the SICK scapula (scapular malposition, inferior medial border prominence, coracoid pain and malposition, and dyskinesis of scapular movement), linear measures of asymmetry have been described for use in throwers.[37] With the arms by the sides, three static measurements are taken: (1) inferior, which is the difference between the vertical height of the superomedial angle of the inferior scapula in centimeters and that of the contralateral scapula; (2) lateral displacement, which is the difference of the horizontal distance of superomedial scapular angle from midline between the inferior scapula and the contralateral scapula; and (3) abduction, which is the difference between scapulae in angular measure of the medial scapular border from a midsagittal plumbline using a goniometer. Based on these static measurements as well as subjective complaints and other clinical examination findings, a 20-point rating scale has been devised for use as a measure of severity of symptoms. The authors acknowledge, however, that superficial landmarks have less than optimal reliability but state that this scale is used as a qualitative measure of severity and progress assessment. A recent study performed on athletes performing repetitive overhead activities did support the assertion that static abnormalities with the arm at the side were associated with altered scapular kinematics found with dynamic movement, especially in the lower ranges of elevation.[39]

Visual Schemes

Although several authors[57,58] recommend assessing the scapula visually, and some even report statistics of abnormal scapula motion patterns,[59,60] they either do not provide operational definitions or fail to substantiate their assessment methods with reliability or validity studies. Bak and Faunl,[60] for example, observed scapulohumeral rhythm while standing behind competitive swimmers who were performing repeated abduction. They defined scapulothoracic instability as either scapular winging or asynchronous motion, but they offer no reliability of their assessment measures. In 2004, Bulut and colleagues[61] reported on the reliability of rating scapular position on 29 patients with shoulder pain. Two physical therapists rated scapula position as being either symmetrical or asymmetrical and described the scapula as normal, inferior angle winging, or medial border winging. Winging was operationally defined as being able to place the finger under respective location (inferior angle or medial border). Poor intertester reliability with κ coefficients ranging from −0.20 to 0.16 was reported for visual inspection of scapular position using this method and rating occurred only with static shoulder position with the arms by the side.

Classification System Developed by Kibler and Associates[40]

In contrast, rating during active arm elevation, operational definitions, and reliability measures are provided in a visual classification system reported by Kibler and associates,[40] who define scapular dyskinesis as "the observable alterations in the position of the scapula and the patterns of scapular motion in relation to the thoracic cage." They describe a system in which dyskinesis is categorized into three types: type I, inferior angle prominence; type II, medial border prominence; and type III, translation of the scapula superiorly with prominence of the superior medial border. These categories correspond to abnormalities occurring about the three scapular axes, respectively: transverse, vertical, and perpendicular to the scapular plane. A type IV category designates normal, symmetrical scapular motion. A reliability study was undertaken using this system[40] in which participants performed frontal and scapular plane elevation while being videotaped from behind. Tapes were subsequently reviewed and rated by two physicians and two physical therapists. κ coefficients were used to measure agreement. Interrater reliability was 0.42 between the physical therapists and 0.31 between the physicians. Intratester reliability was 0.5. Although these values are not high enough to support the use of their system as described, the authors suggest that with refinement, reliable visual analysis of scapular dysfunction may be possible.

Scapula Dyskinesis Test

We have developed a visually based test to identify abnormal motion called the scapular dyskinesis test (SDT) that has demonstrated validity[32] and has satisfactory reliability.[62] The SDT involves viewing the

---

BOX 72.1   Scapula Dyskinesis Test: Operational Definitions and Rating Scale

Definitions of Terms

Normal scapulohumeral rhythm: The scapula is stable with minimal motion during the initial 30 to 60 degrees of humerothoracic elevation; then it smoothly and continuously upwardly rotates during elevation and smoothly and continuously downwardly rotates during humeral lowering with no evidence of winging.

Scapular dyskinesis: either or both of the following motion abnormalities:

Dysrhythmia: Scapula Dyskinesis Test: Operational Definitions and Rating Scale demonstrates premature or excessive elevation or protraction, nonsmooth, or stuttering motion during arm elevation or lowering or rapid downward rotation during arm lowering.

Winging: There is posterior displacement of the medial border or the inferior angle of the scapula away from the posterior thorax.

Scapular Dyskinesis Rating Scale for Each Test Movement

N = *normal* motion: no evidence of abnormality

S = *subtle* abnormalities: mild pr questionable evidence of abnormality, not consistently present

O = *obvious* abnormalities: striking, clearly apparent abnormalities, evident on at least three of five trials (dysrhythmias or winging of 1 inch or greater displacement of the scapula from the thorax)

To determine the reliability of this system, 142 athletes competing in a collegiate sport that required repetitive overhead activity were recruited. This population was chosen because of the high incidence of shoulder pathology reported among athletes participating in sports requiring overhead arm use.[52-55]

---

exposed posterior thorax during elevation of the upper extremities in both the sagittal plane (flexion) and coronal plane (abduction) while grasping 3- to 5-lb dumbbells. Motion patterns are rated as having normal motion or as having "obvious" or "subtle" dyskinesis using the operational definitions in Box 72.1.

To determine the reliability of this system, 142 athletes competing in a collegiate sport that required repetitive overhead activity were recruited. This population was chosen because of the high incidence of shoulder pathology reported among athletes participating in sports requiring overhead arm use.[63-66] Each participant performed five repetitions of bilateral active weighted shoulder flexion and bilateral active weighted shoulder abduction (coronal plane) while they were videotaped from a posterior view. For participants weighing less than 150 lb, 3-lb weights were held. For those weighing 150 lb or more, 5-lb weights were held. The test movements were based on previous pilot studies by these researchers,[67] and Johnson[68] found that active movements with resistance resulted in abnormal scapular motion more often than static tests in participants with shoulder pathology.

All examiners underwent standardized training via a self-instructional PowerPoint presentation that included operational definitions, photographs, and embedded video examples. Six raters (three separate pairs consisting of two athletic trainers, two pairs of experienced physical therapists) independently viewed randomly selected videotaped athletes and rated their shoulders as having obvious dyskinesis, subtle dyskinesis, or normal motion (Fig. 72.7).

We found moderate interrater reliability (average $K_w = 0.54$ for video raters) in classifying scapular motion patterns as either normal or having subtle or obvious dyskinesis, which is a higher κ value than reported using the Kibler method.[40,69] Our system did not distinguish between subtypes of dyskinesis because we observed that the subtypes described in the Kibler method often occurred simultaneously. The SDT

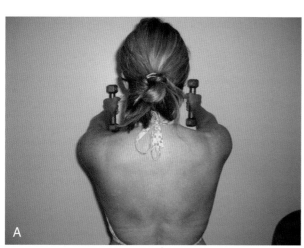 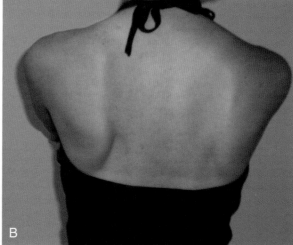

Fig. 72.7 Participant performing flexion with a 3-lb (1.4-kg) dumbbell. **A,** The scapular motion pattern was rated normal bilaterally. **B,** The scapular motion pattern was rated as having "obvious" dyskinesis on the left and "subtle" dyskinesis on the right.

also included loaded tasks, which can alter scapular kinematics.[19,70–72] There is also evidence that muscular fatigue, which may occur with repetition, directly affects scapulohumeral rhythm, and may result in compensatory increased rotation or destabilization of the scapula,[73] so we believe that repetitive motion is necessary for proper evaluation. More recent, comprehensive systematic reviews on the measurement properties of the SDT have demonstrated adequate reliability for the use of this test.[74,75]

To determine the validity of the SDT, athletes judged as having either "normal" motion or "obvious dyskinesis" underwent kinematic testing with an electromagnetic tracking system while performing weighted flexion and abduction, and the data from both groups were compared. Significant differences during arm elevation were found between the "normal" and "obvious dyskinesis" groups with the latter group demonstrating less scapular upward rotation less clavicular elevation and greater clavicular protraction. These alterations have previously been associated with subacromial impingement. The suprahumeral structures, namely the rotator cuff, subacromial bursa, and long head of the biceps, likely undergo greater compression with reduced upward rotation. Kamkar and colleagues[76] propose that upward rotation of scapula caused by serratus anterior activity is essential in preventing the humeral head from impinging on the acromion. The finding of less clavicular elevation in the dyskinesis group is consistent with the description of the SICK scapula syndrome in which the scapula appears clinically as a "dropped" or lower scapula on the involved side in symptomatic throwing athletes.[37] The scapulae in the dyskinesis group were more protracted than the normal group. Solem-Bertoft and associates[45] found a reduction in the opening width of the subacromial space with the scapula in a protracted position compared with a retracted position using MRI. Our finding of greater protraction in those with dyskinesis may be relevant to the compression of structures within the subacromial space. Furthermore, two recent studies found specific shoulder kinematic alterations such as decreased scapula external rotation and reduced posterior titling in patients with scapular dyskinesis as compared with those without dyskinesis.[77,78] They also report an increase in upper trapezius activity with arm elevation and lowering, suggesting a compensatory or causative mechanism to control the dyskinesis. The finding that shoulders visually judged as having dyskinesis have distinct alterations in three-dimensional scapular motion provides validity for the use of the SDT.

Under clinical conditions, use of the SDT is recommended using the test movements of repeated flexion and abduction, with the priority given to flexion if high irritability is encountered because this motion was more likely to evoke dyskinesis. To use this test, active elevation to at least 90 degrees is required. Although these authors found that weighted shoulder was more provocative than if done without weights, there are some instances when using weights is not feasible because of pain or significant weakness.

Symptom Alteration Tests

The aim of symptom alteration tests is to infer that scapular pathology exists if an improvement in symptoms is found when applying manual forces to the scapula during provocation testing. Three symptom alteration tests have been described. The Scapula Assistance Test was originally described by Kibler[48] as the application of a lateral and upward rotary force to the medial border of the scapula during arm elevation to determine if symptoms of impingement were reduced or abolished. By assisting upward rotation, this test was reported to facilitate the action of the scapular rotators, primarily the serratus anterior–lower trapezius force couple, to elevate the arm and simultaneously assess the effect on pain. No data were provided on this test; however, its concept provided the basis for further research regarding the potential identification of scapular pathology in those with shoulder pain.

Modified Scapula Assistance Test

Rabin and colleagues[41] have described the Modified Scapula Assistance Test in which posterior tilting was facilitated in addition to assisted upward rotation as described in the original Scapula Assistance Test. This modification was based on several studies that found reduced posterior tilting in those with symptoms of shoulder impingement.[19,23,46] The interrater reliability of the Modified Scapula Assistance Test was tested by two raters on 46 patients with shoulder pathology who were referred for physical therapy.[41] Patients were asked to rate their pain using a verbal numeric rating scale from 0 (no pain) to 10 (worst pain imaginable) to describe their symptoms during arm elevation in the scapular and sagittal planes. Arm elevation and rating were then repeated while the tester applied a posterior tilting force with one hand by pulling back on the superior aspect of the scapula and concurrently using the heel of the hand to apply a lateral and upward rotary force to the inferior angle. A 2-point decrease in pain was considered clinically

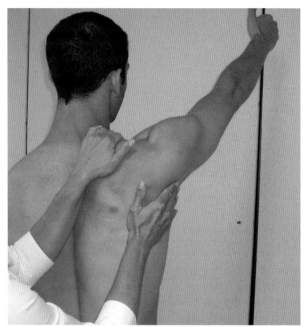

Fig. 72.8 Scapular assistance test. The clinician applies posterior tilting force through grasp on the superior border of scapula and applies upward rotation force through the inferior angle of the scapula as the participant elevates his arm.

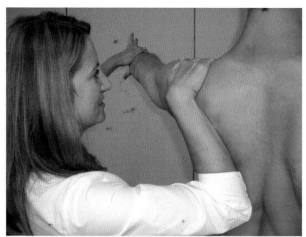

Fig. 72.9 Scapular reposition test. Clinician performing scapula reposition test by grasping the acromioclavicular joint superiorly and scapula posteriorly and then applying a posterior tilting and external rotation force to further approximate the scapula to the thorax. This is done during performance of the Jobe's "empty can" test, and diminished pain or a significant increase in strength is considered a positive test result.

significant.[79] κ values and percent agreement for elevation in the scapular plane and sagittal plane were 0.53 and 77% and 0.62 and 91%, respectively, indicating moderate reliability and thus making it acceptable for clinical use. These authors recommend performing the test using the patient's more painful arc of motion, either the scapular or sagittal plane (Fig. 72.8).

Scapula Retraction Test

The Scapula Retraction Test has been described as stabilization of the scapula in a retracted position on the thorax by manual application of force along the medial border of the scapula.[80] Kibler and colleagues[80] measured pain using a numeric rating scale and elevation strength using a handheld dynamometer during isometric shoulder elevation in the scapular plane with the scapula in its natural position and when manually retracted using the Scapula Reposition Test. This was performed in a group of 20 patients diagnosed with shoulder pathology and in 10 asymptomatic control participants. The researchers reported an increase in shoulder elevation strength using the Scapula Retraction Test position compared with testing with the scapula in its natural "rest" position in 100% of their patients. However, no warm-up trials were reported, and the natural position was always tested first, so strength gains may have been due to a practice or testing order effect instead of manual repositioning. In addition, this test was described using two examiners (one to apply the retraction and another to measure the strength using a dynamometer), which may be clinically impractical.[39]

Scapula Reposition Test

Smith and associates[81] have found decreased elevation strength with maximal scapular retraction, and these authors confirmed this finding during pilot testing. Therefore, we modified Kibler's test[80] by emphasizing posterior tilting and external rotation of the scapula but avoiding full retraction and named it the Scapula Reposition Test (SRT).[39]

The effect of the SRT on elevation strength and shoulder impingement was studied in 142 collegiate athletes who were engaged in sports requiring repetitive overhead movements.[39] As part of the examination, three tests for impingement (Neer,[82] Hawkins,[83] and Jobe[84]) were performed as originally described with the scapula in its natural resting posture. If the results of any of these tests were found to be positive for symptom provocation, the athlete was asked to rate his/her pain using a verbal numeric rating scale (VNRS) with 0 being no pain and 10 being the worst pain imaginable. Any pain provoking test was then repeated with the scapula manually repositioned using the SRT. The SRT was performed by grasping the scapula with the fingers contacting the AC joint anteriorly while remaining medial to the lateral acromial border. The palm and thenar eminence contact the spine of the scapula posteriorly with the forearm obliquely angled toward the inferior angle of the scapula for additional support on the medial border (Fig. 72.9) to encourage scapular posterior tilting and external rotation (inferior angle and medial border moved anteriorly toward the thorax) and approximate the scapula to a midposition on the thorax. As the SRT was applied, the impingement test(s) that originally provoked symptoms were repeated, and the athlete again rated his or her symptoms using the VNRS. Isometric elevation strength in the Jobe's test position (arm elevated to 90 degrees in the plane of the scapula and internally rotated by pointing the thumb down) was measured using a dynamometer (Microfet; Hoggan Industries, Draper, UT). Testing consisted of three repetitions of 5-second maximum isometric shoulder elevation contractions with the scapula in its natural position and with the scapula manually repositioned using the SRT.

Almost half of our athletes had a reduction in symptoms during impingement testing with scapular repositioning with a clinically significant strength in 26% of athletes with at least one positive shoulder impingement test result, which amounted to about 10% increase with the SRT. Strength gains may have been facilitated simply by providing a more stable proximal fixation for the muscles such as the deltoid and rotator cuff used to perform shoulder elevation[36] or may have been the result of an improved length–tension relationship of the rotator cuff or scapular musculature secondary to an altered scapular position. A finding of increased shoulder elevation strength with scapular repositioning may provide a clinical test to identify the subset of those with shoulder pathology that may benefit from interventions designed to improve scapular musculature function.

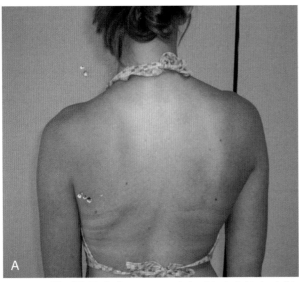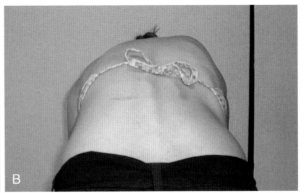

Fig. 72.10 A, Asymmetry of shoulder heights is visible with the patient in erect standing position. **B,** With flexion, a rib hump is present, confirming that the asymmetry is due to scoliosis rather than scapular pathology.

In the clinical setting, we recommend asking for a pain rating (0–10) during resisted shoulder elevation in the Jobe "empty can" position with the shoulder elevated to 90 degrees in the plane of the scapula and maximally internally rotated. Manual resistance may be applied directly or a handheld dynamometer can be used for more objective strength assessment. The Jobe test should then be repeated using the SRT. A finding of a 2-point decrease in pain rating or a significant increase in strength using the SRT denotes a positive test result and implies that suboptimal scapular orientation or position may be contributing to the patient's symptoms, which suggests the need for interventions addressing the scapula (discussed in the intervention section).

Muscle Performance

Muscle performance is evaluated using a make test and graded as normal, reduced, or markedly reduced compared with the uninvolved extremity[85] using the following operational definitions:

Normal (N): strong, with equal resistance applied as compared bilaterally

Reduced (R): mild to moderate deficit as compared bilaterally

Markedly reduced (MR): significant deficit as compared bilaterally (little to no resistance can be applied)

The muscles to be tested are the prime movers of the scapula, namely, the serratus anterior and the lower and middle trapezius. The testing positions have been described by Kendall and coworkers[86] and verified electromyographically as eliciting maximal muscle activity.[87,88]

Middle Trapezius

The patient is prone, and the shoulder is placed in a position of horizontal abduction and external rotation (thumb up) with scapula adducted towards midline. Pressure is applied against the forearm in a downward direction while the trunk is manually stabilized. Monitor the medial border of the scapula and grade on the ability to maintain scapular retraction (Fig. 72.e2).

Lower Trapezius

The patient is prone, and the arm is elevated overhead in line with the fibers of the lower trapezius with the scapula adducted. Downward resistance is applied proximal to the patient's wrist, and the medial border of the scapula is monitored. Strength is graded based on the ability to maintain scapular retraction (Fig. 72.e3).

Serratus Anterior

The patient is seated without back support, and the arm is flexed to 125 degrees in the sagittal plane. Resistance is applied proximal to the patient's wrist in the direction of extending the shoulder. Monitor the inferior angle of scapula and grade based on the ability of the serratus to hold upward rotation (Fig. 72.e4).

Posture

The relative height of the affected shoulder is observed from a posterior view. Although it has been stated that the dominant shoulder is often slightly lower than the nondominant shoulder,[86] a significant reduction in shoulder height, especially if seen in combination with winging of the scapula, may be indicative of the SICK scapula syndrome in which the scapula appears lower on the involved side.[37] Care should be taken to note if scoliosis is present, which may produce the appearance of a dropped shoulder that is unrelated to scapular pathology (Fig. 72.10). An "elevated scapula" has also been described as a type of impaired alignment in which the entire scapula and lateral portion of the clavicle are raised because of upper trapezius shortening.[89] Superior translation of the scapula during arm elevation (see Fig. 72.3) was shown to be present in a sample of persons who had recovered from unilateral shoulder pathology (adhesive capsulitis, frozen shoulder, impingement, rotator cuff tendonitis or tear), and this could be altered by tactile and verbal cuing, suggesting a motor control issue rather than reduced muscle length in this population.[16]

The patient should also be evaluated to determine if a forward head posture is present, as identified by the external auditory meatus being anterior to the lumbar spine. From the same sagittal view, shoulder protraction, defined as the acromion being anterior to the lumbar spine, should be noted (Fig. 72.11).[86] Kyphosis is observed for the upper, middle, and lower thoracic areas while viewing the patient from the side. The following segmental groups should be assessed: C7 through T2 (cervicothoracic junction), T3 through T5, and T6 through T10. Each segmental group should be rated as having either a normal kyphosis (no deviation), diminished kyphosis (a flattening of the normal convexity), or excessive kyphosis (an increase in the normal convexity) (Fig. 72.e5). A study of 80 participants found that those with increased kyphosis and rounded shoulders were more likely to have interscapular pain as were those with a forward head posture.[90] κ values measuring interrater reliability for shoulder and thoracic postural observation measures as described have been reported between 0.58 and 0.9.[91] In addition to spinal posture, intervertebral mobility of the cervical and thoracic spines should be assessed using spring testing (Fig. 72.e6), and spinal flexibility should be assessed.[91,92] McClure and colleagues[26] failed to find a difference in thoracic resting posture between those with and without shoulder impingement syndrome, but flexibility, not static posture may be a primary issue because mobility of the thoracic spine has been shown to vary significantly between those with healthy shoulders and those with shoulder pathology.[93]

Posterior Shoulder Tightness

Some authors have suggested that posterior shoulder tightness, reflected by limited glenohumeral internal rotation, is associated with scapular dysfunction.[37,94] Burkhart and associates[37] suggest that posterior capsular tightness may cause the scapula to rotate or

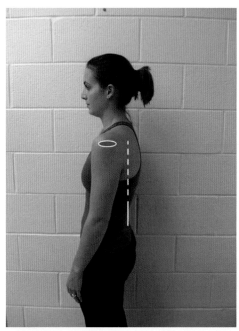

Fig. 72.11 Shoulder protraction is present, indicated by acromion location anterior to apex of lumbar spine.

protract excessively during follow-through of throwing or swinging, which involves a combination of adduction and internal rotation, and that scapular dyskinesis and tightness of the posterior capsule occur as part of a common syndrome in throwing athletes. They reported this finding in a group of symptomatic throwers, and it has been suggested that impingement of the posterior cuff may be exacerbated by scapular protraction. Borich and associates[94] studied participants involved in overhead sports with three-dimensional motion analysis and found that those with a glenohumeral internal rotation deficit had more anteriorly tilted scapulae during activities requiring arm elevation and internal rotation. Laudner and associates[26] studied 11 throwing athletes diagnosed with pathologic internal impingement and compared them with asymptomatic throwers. Somewhat in contrast, they found increased clavicular elevation and increased posterior tilting in symptomatic throwers. Thomas and coworkers[95] followed 36 high school female overhead athletes for a single competitive season and measured glenohumeral internal rotation and scapular upward rotation and scapula protraction. Overall, internal rotation decreased from pre- to postseason; however, the scapula upward rotation findings were inconclusive. Some athletes had an increase in upward rotation of the scapula, suggesting a protective mechanism, whereas some had a decrease in upward rotation, suggesting potentially detrimental effects. Therefore, there does appear to be a connection between posterior shoulder tightness (limited glenohumeral internal rotation) and scapular dyskinesis; however, the precise nature of the altered scapular motion is unclear.

Multiple measures of posterior shoulder tightness have been reported, including sidelying and seated horizontal adduction with the scapula blocked,[96,97] seated horizontal adduction,[98] supine internal rotation measured at 90 degrees of abduction,[99] and standing spinal level assessed with hand behind the back.[100,101] Only modest correlations between behind spinal level and internal rotation at 90 degrees of abduction were found ($r = 0.44$),[102] indicating that measurements taken in these varied positions likely assess the flexibility of different portions of the posterior shoulder. Using spinal level with the hand behind the back assesses the posterior–superior capsule, whereas internal rotation at 90 degrees assesses the posterior–inferior capsule.[103] Given this finding, we recommend that posterior shoulder tightness be assessed using both the standing spinal level and internal rotation at 90 degrees. When using the latter technique, it is critical to watch for the end of glenohumeral motion, which ends when the shoulder girdle lifts up, indicating compensatory scapulothoracic motion, which may mask a glenohumeral internal rotation deficit (Fig. 72.12).

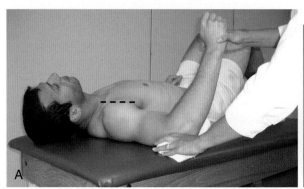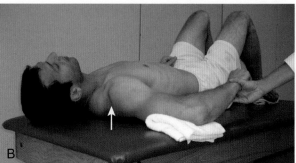

Fig. 72.12 Position for goniometric range of motion measurement of internal rotation as a measure of posterior capsule flexibility. **A,** End of glenohumeral internal rotation occurs when the shoulder begins to lift (beyond *dashed line*), signifying the end of glenohumeral motion. **B,** Incorrect positioning for goniometric internal rotation measurement allowing the scapula to lift from the plinth *(arrow)*.

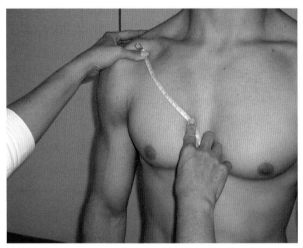

Fig. 72.13 Linear measure of pectoralis minor length using tape measure from the medial inferior angle of the coracoid process to the anterior inferior edge of rib 4 one finger-width lateral to the sternum.

Pectoralis Minor Tightness

It has been theorized that a forward shoulder posture, defined as a change in the resting position of the scapula in the sagittal or transverse plane, may over time lead to adaptive shortening of the pectoralis minor muscle by approximating its attachment sites on the coracoid process and ribs 3, 4, and 5.[86,104] Healthy participants with a relatively shorter pectoralis minor resting length demonstrated increased internal rotation of the scapula during arm raising and reduced posterior tilting at and above shoulder level than those with longer pectoralis minor lengths.[20] As previously discussed, these alterations in scapular kinematics have been found in persons with subacromial impingement and are thought to decrease subacromial space, resulting in increased compression on the rotator cuff and long head of the biceps tendons.[19,22,23] Recently, Borstad[104] has provided research supporting a relationship between resting normalized pectoralis minor length, thoracic kyphosis, and scapular internal rotation, finding that those with a relatively short pectoralis minor demonstrated increased scapular internal rotation. Because this research supports a relationship between pectoral length and scapular kinematics, measurement of pectoralis minor length is recommended. The problem one encounters, however, is that the simple traditional measure reported to represent pectoral muscle length using the distance from the posterolateral angle of the scapula to the table with the patient supine[105] have not been correlated with normalized pectoralis minor length and lacks diagnostic accuracy despite excellent reported intrarater reliability.[106] Taking a direct linear measure using either a measuring tape or Vernier caliper between the medial inferior angle of the coracoid process and anterior inferior edge of rib 4 one finger width lateral to the sternum was found to have acceptable intrarater reliability for clinical use. The Intrarater Correlation Coefficient (ICC) ranged from 0.82 to 0.87 in 26 adults without a history of shoulder pathology and was validated using comparison measures from an electromagnetic tracking device.[107] Borstad[107] describes palpation of these anatomic landmarks as follows: from the lateral concavity of the clavicle, palpate inferiorly in the deltopectoral groove for the medial inferior angle of the coracoid; then find the medial inferior aspect of rib 1 inferior to the sternoclavicular junction, and counting down to the anterior inferior edge of rib 4, one finger lateral to the sternum (Fig. 72.13). These authors have also used a PALM palpation meter to obtain the pectoralis minor length using the same landmarks because this device allows the clinician to circumvent other devices pressing into those with larger breast tissue. A pectoralis minor index (PMI) can then be calculated by dividing the pectoralis minor length in centimeters by the person's height in centimeters and multiplying by 100.[20] A PMI of less than 7.44 has been reported to indicate a relatively short pectoralis minor.[107]

Interestingly, some authors have suggested that surgical release of the pectoralis minor may be indicated in patients who fail to respond to a stretching program.[108,109]

Treatment

Because the etiology of scapular dysfunction appears to be multifactorial, the clinician should consider matching intervention strategies to the impairments identified during the examination process. A model based on matching treatment strategy to symptom irritability and identified impairments has been described and has demonstrated preliminary reliability and validity for classifying shoulder disorders.[110]

Muscle Strengthening

There is strong evidence that shoulder strengthening exercise is an effective treatment for several conditions, including shoulder impingement[111] and shoulder instability.[112] Most exercise programs for shoulder pathology should target both glenohumeral and scapulothoracic musculature, although the focus of this chapter is only scapular dysfunction.

One key principle in designing a scapular exercise program is to match the difficulty of the exercise with the patient's level of motor control and strength. Therefore, it is important to visually observe the patient from posterior during an exercise to make sure she or he is able to maintain good scapular control. This concept is particularly important in patients who may have well-developed glenohumeral muscles (e.g., the deltoid) but poor scapular control. These patients may be able to grossly accomplish the arm motion required in the exercise but be unable to adequately control the scapula. This situation would produce excessive stress on the glenohumeral tissues and even reinforce poor motor control patterns.[16] Another concept that often seems useful is to incorporate combined trunk and lower extremity movement to facilitate proper scapular motion. For example, hip and trunk extension can be combined to facilitate scapular retraction during arm extension or elevation.[36,113]

We present exercises as being early- (Fig. 72.e7), middle- (Fig. 72.e8), or late- (Fig. 72.e9) phase exercises. Exercises should be chosen and progressed based on the patient's ability to control the scapula as well as consideration of the healing phase of any injured or repaired tissue. Obviously, the simple variables to alter are the load and repetitions, but the speed and complexity of the motion should also be progressed. In general, early-phase exercises should keep the shoulder in a protected midrange or nonprovocative position, whereas late-phase exercises require end-range, more provocative positions.

Taping and Bracing

Although few studies have addressed the efficacy of shoulder taping, two case studies of patients with clinical symptoms of shoulder impingement have described the use of scapular repositioning as a diagnostic tool that reduced patients' symptoms.[114,115] Subsequent use of scapular taping was effective in symptom reduction and was used as part of a comprehensive intervention program. Additional studies have investigated the effect of shoulder taping in healthy participants,[116,117] professional musicians,[118] and persons with subacromial impingement.[117,119] Although taping did not produce significant electromyographic (EMG) changes in the scapular muscles of those with healthy shoulders,[120] it was successful in altering EMG activity of the scapular musculature in both symptomatic swimmers[119] and in professional violinists, half of whom were experiencing pain.[118] Taping has been effective in reducing thoracic kyphosis,[117,121] as well as increasing shoulder elevation and pain-free elevation range of motion (ROM) in the sagittal plane and in the plane of

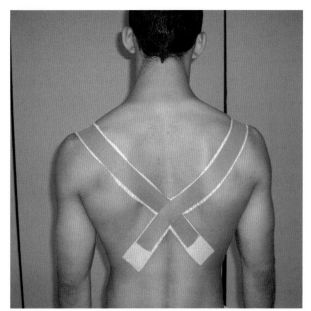

Fig. 72.14 Scapular taping with cover roll stretch applied beneath Leukotape (ERP Group, Laval, QC, Canada).

the scapula.[121] These findings are consistent with those of Kebaetse and coworkers,[122] who also reported increased shoulder elevation motion and a change in scapular position in the erect compared with slouched postures. Concomitant with enhanced ROM was increased elevation force at 90 degrees in the erect posture condition. This would logically lead one to believe that in symptomatic individuals with suboptimal scapulothoracic posture or motion, scapular taping may be an effective adjunct to enhance motor performance or reduce pain in a functional range of elevation. Taping has been described as "an adjunctive therapy to attempt to attain a more favorable scapular alignment and alleviate pain,"[115] and proposed mechanisms of action include improved scapular alignment, providing a low load-long duration stretch to tight structures about the shoulder, increased subacromial space, reduced tension in the subacromial tissues,[105] improved proprioception,[123] and improvement of joint positional faults.[124]

If either postural correction or the SRT reduces symptoms, scapular taping should be considered in the patient who has difficulty maintaining an optimal posture, requires a stretch to the anterior shoulder, or is unable to exercise without pain. The following procedure is a modification of the postural taping technique described by Greig and associates.[121] The modification allows additional approximation force over the inferior angle of the scapula to the thorax. Taping may be applied unilaterally or bilaterally, although these authors recommend bilateral taping to enhance thoracic spine extension (Fig. 72.14). Box 72.2 provides directions for the bilateral taping method.

The Spine and Scapula Stabilizing brace or S3 (Alignmed Inc., Santa Ana, CA) appears to work in a similar fashion as taping but should provide improved wearing tolerance over extended time periods because of the lack of adhesive contact with the skin (Fig. 72.15). Anecdotally, we have had favorable clinical experience using the S3 brace with patients, but further research should be done to determine widespread clinical efficacy.

Stretching

In patients with tight periscapular musculature or status post trauma or immobilization, limitations in scapulothoracic motion should be addressed using superior, inferior, medial, or lateral gliding or scapulothoracic distraction techniques (Fig. 72.16). Facilitatory techniques may be used in the early phase of rehabilitation programs in conjunction with scapular mobilization to promote isolated active scapular motion (see Fig. 72.37).

In addressing any loss of glenohumeral mobility in a patient with upper extremity symptoms, particular attention should be placed on tightness of the posterior shoulder musculature because this may affect scapular kinematics,[125,126] and adequate flexibility of the posterior capsule is recommended before the initiation of a shoulder strengthening program. Several methods of self-stretching have been described, including "cross-body stretch," in which the shoulder is elevated to approximately 90 degrees of flexion and pulled across the body into horizontal adduction with the opposite arm (Fig. 72.17)[127]; the "towel stretch," in which the glenohumeral joint is adducted, internally rotated, and extended while the hand now located behind the individual's back is pulled up by the opposite hand using a towel[29,128]; and a "sleeper stretch" that is accomplished by lying on the side to be stretched, elevating the humerus to 90 degrees on the support surface, and then passively internally rotating the shoulder with the opposite arm (Fig. 72.18).[37,128,129] A randomized study by McClure and colleagues[102] found that in healthy participants with limited internal rotation, the cross-body adduction method produced significant gains in internal rotation ROM after a 4-week intervention program of five 30-second stretches daily, whereas the "sleeper stretch" did not produce significant changes. For use in the clinic, manually assisted stretching techniques have been described in which the clinician manually stabilizes the scapula while the shoulder is passively adducted or internally rotated or performs posterior to anterior glides to stretch the posterior capsule (Fig. 72.19).[130] Postural exercises and mobilization techniques to facilitate cervical retraction and thoracic extension have also been described to improve shoulder elevation ROM[117] (Fig. 72.e10). Stretching of the pectoralis minor is also recommended to improve scapular kinematics during arm elevation, and Borstad and Ludwig[131] have used an electromagnetic motion tracking system and found that the unilateral corner stretch was most effective in elongating the pectoralis minor followed by a

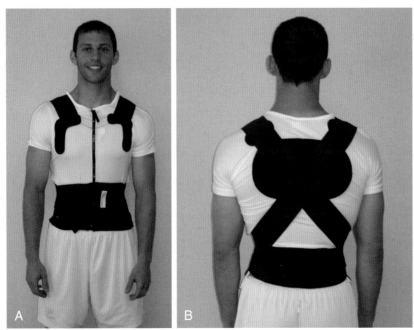

Fig. 72.15 The Spine and Scapula Stabilizing Brace (Alignmed, Inc.) incorporates a mesh fitted vest and adjustable Velcro straps (S3). **A,** Anterior view. **B,** Posterior view.

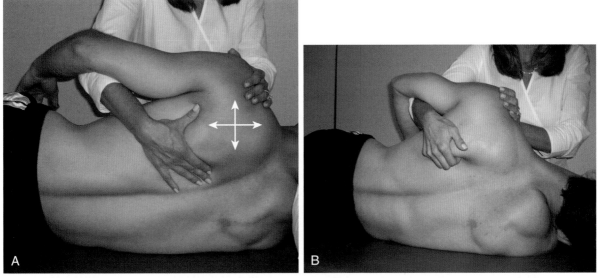

Fig. 72.16 Scapulothoracic mobilization. **A,** The *arrow* indicates that the scapula can be mobilized in superior, inferior, medial, and lateral directions. **B,** Scapulothoracic distraction.

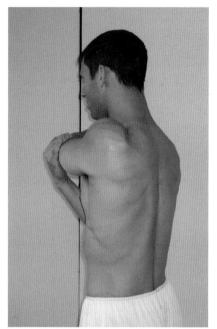

Fig. 72.17 Cross-body stretch.

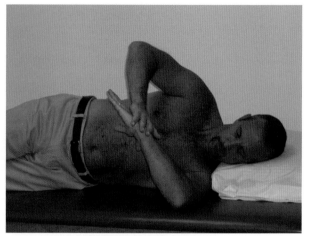

Fig. 72.18 Sleeper stretch.

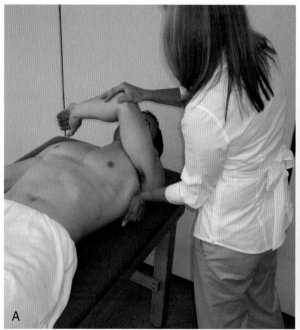

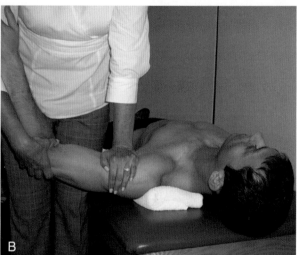

Fig. 72.19 A, Manual horizontal adduction stretch with scapula blocked. **B,** Anterior–posterior glide to stretch the posterior capsule of the glenohumeral joint.

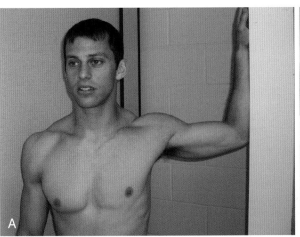 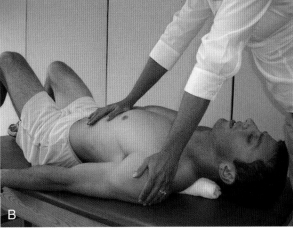

Fig. 72.20 A, Pectoralis minor corner stretch. **B,** Manual pectoralis minor stretch with the ribs stabilized and posteriorly directed pressure over the coracoid.

BOX 72.3 Recommended Guidelines for Examination and Management of Scapular Dysfunction

Examination

Visual Classification Using the Scapula Dyskinesis Test
- If the patient is able, active flexion with 3-lb (1.37-kg) dumbbells for persons weighing <150 lb (68 kg) or 5-lb (2.3-kg) dumbbells for persons weighing >150 lb
- If the patient is able, active abduction (coronal plane) with 3- or 5-lb dumbbells as above
- Rate as having
  - Normal motion
  - Subtle dyskinesis (inconsistent winging or dysrhythmia)
  - Obvious dyskinesis (obvious, consistent winging or dysrhythmia)

Symptom Alteration Tests
- Modified scapula assistance test
  - Perform active arm elevation (sagittal or scapular plane) with pain rating using a numeric rating scale (0–10).
  - Apply a posterior tilting force with one hand by pulling back on the superior aspect of the scapula and concurrently use the heel of the hand to apply an upward rotary force to the inferior angle. Reassess elevation range of motion and pain.
- Scapula reposition test
  - Perform Jobe's (empty can) test by isometrically resisting arm elevation in the scapular plane with the shoulder maximally internally rotated. Obtain pain rating using a numeric rating scale (0–10).
  - Lower the arm and then reposition the scapula using the scapula reposition test by grasping the scapula medial to the acromion with forearm, providing additional support obliquely over thorax to encourage posterior tilting and external rotation. Perform Jobe's test again to determine whether there is a decrease in pain or an increase in strength.

Muscle Performance
- Lower trapezius
- Middle trapezius
- Serratus anterior

Examination of Related Areas
- Pectoralis minor length
- Thoracic kyphosis or flexibility
- Posterior capsular flexibility of the glenohumeral joint

Treatment Principles

Muscle Strengthening
- Difficulty is matched to the patient's motor control and strength based on direct visualization of scapular control.
- Progress from protected midrange positions with arm supported or low resistance to end-range positions against gravity and resistance.
- Incorporate related areas such as hip and trunk during functional exercises.

Taping and Bracing
- Consider this alternative in patients whose symptoms are reduced with either postural correction or the scapula reposition test.

Stretching
- Pectoralis minor
- Posterior glenohumeral joint
- Posterior gliding, cross-body adduction, sleeper stretch, towel stretch
- Cervical retraction–upper thoracic extension program

---

manual stretch supine with a towel roll vertically placed over the thoracic spine (see Fig. 72.e10A). As a modification of the latter technique, these authors have additionally stabilized the lower ribs while applying downward pressure over the coracoid process (Fig. 72.20).

SUMMARY

Scapular dysfunction is a common clinical problem with many upper-quarter conditions, especially the shoulder. The scapula provides a stable base for glenohumeral function and upper extremity function. Therapists should examine for abnormalities in scapular motion and position to identify impairments in muscle performance and muscle length that create a suboptimal environment for scapular function. Examination tools have been developed to assist therapists with their assessment of the scapula. Additional research is needed to establish the clinical utility of these examination techniques, but current evidence suggests some useful therapeutic strategies to help resolve scapular dysfunction. Box 72.3, available on the companion website, provides a review of the clinical guidelines presented in this chapter.

REFERENCES

1. Ludewig PM, Cook TM, Nawoczenski DA. Three-Dimensional Scapular Orientation and Muscle Activity at Selected Positions of Humeral Elevation. *J Orthop Sports Phys Ther.* 1996;24(2):57–65.
2. Lukasiewicz AC, et al. Comparison of 3-dimensional scapular position and orientation between subjects with and without shoulder impingement. *J Orthop Sports Phys Ther.* 1999;29(10):574–583; discussion 584–586.
3. McClure PW, et al. Direct 3-dimensional measurement of scapular kinematics during dynamic movements in vivo. *J Shoulder Elbow Surg.* 2001;10(3):269–277.
4. Wu G, et al. ISB recommendation on definitions of joint coordinate systems of various joints for the reporting of human joint motion--Part II: shoulder, elbow, wrist and hand. *J Biomech.* 2005;38(5):981–992.
5. McClure PW, et al. Direct 3-dimensional measurement of scapular kinematics during dynamic movements in vivo. *J Shoulder Elbow Surg.* 2001;10(3):269–277.
6. Ludewig PM, et al. Motion of the shoulder complex during multiplanar humeral elevation. *J Bone Joint Surg Am.* 2009;91(2):378–389.
7. Bagg SD, Forrest WJ. Electromyographic study of the scapular rotators during arm abduction in the scapular plane. *Am J Phys Med Rehabil.* 1986;65(3):111–124.
8. Kronberg M, Nemeth G, Broström L-Å. Muscle Activity and Coordination in the Normal Shoulder. *Clin Orthop Relat Res.* 1990;257:76–85.
9. Phadke V, Camargo P, Ludewig P. Scapular and rotator cuff muscle activity during arm elevation: a review of normal function and alterations with shoulder impingement. *Rev Bras Fisioter.* 2009;13(1):1–9.
10. Kuhn JE, Plancher KD, Hawkins RJ. Scapular winging. *J Am Acad Orthop Surg.* 1995;3(6):319–325.
11. Johnson G, et al. Anatomy and actions of the trapezius muscle. *Clin Biomech.* 1994;9:44–50.
12. Scibek JS, et al. Shoulder kinematics in patients with full-thickness rotator cuff tears after a subacromial injection. *J Shoulder Elbow Surg.* 2008;17(1):172–181.
13. Paletta GA, et al. Shoulder Kinematics with Two-Plane X-Ray Evaluation in Patients with Anterior Instability or Rotator Cuff Tearing. *J Shoulder Elbow Surg.* 1997;6:516–527.
14. Yamaguchi K, et al. Glenohumeral motion in patients with rotator cuff tears: a comparison of asymptomatic and symptomatic shoulders. *J Shoulder Elbow Surg.* 2000;9(1):6–11.
15. Ebaugh DD, McClure PW, Karduna AR. Effects of shoulder muscle fatigue caused by repetitive overhead activities on scapulothoracic and glenohumeral kinematics. *J Electromyogr Kinesiol.* 2006;16(3):224–235.
16. Babyar SR. Excessive scapular motion in individuals recovering from painful and stiff shoulders: causes and treatment strategies. *Phys Ther.* 1996;76(3):226–238. discussion 239–247.
17. Jia X, et al. Clinical Evaluation of the Shoulder Shrug Sign. *Clin Orthop Relat Res.* 2008.
18. Kelly BT, et al. Differential patterns of muscle activation in patients with symptomatic and asymptomatic rotator cuff tears. *J Shoulder Elbow Surg.* 2005;14(2):165–171.
19. Ludewig PM, Cook TM. Alterations in shoulder kinematics and associated muscle activity in people with symptoms of shoulder impingement. *Phys Ther.* 2000;80(3):276–291.
20. Borstad JD, Ludewig PM. The effect of long versus short pectoralis minor resting length on scapular kinematics in healthy individuals. *J Orthop Sports Phys Ther.* 2005;35(4):227–238.
21. Endo K, et al. Radiographic assessment of scapular rotational tilt in chronic shoulder impingement syndrome. *J Orthop Sci.* 2001;6(1):3–10.
22. Graichen H, et al. Three-dimensional analysis of shoulder girdle and supraspinatus motion patterns in patients with impingement syndrome. *J Orthop Res.* 2001;19(6):1192–1198.
23. Hebert LJ, et al. Scapular behavior in shoulder impingement syndrome. *Arch Phys Med Rehabil.* 2002;83(1):60–69.
24. Lukasiewicz AC, et al. Comparison of 3-dimensional scapular position and orientation between subjects with and without shoulder impingement. *J Orthop Sports Phys Ther.* 1999;29(10):574–583; discussion 584–586.
25. Warner JJ, et al. Scapulothoracic motion in normal shoulders and shoulders with glenohumeral instability and impingement syndrome. A study using Moire topographic analysis. *Clin Orthop.* 1992;285:191–199.
26. McClure PW, Michener LA, Karduna AR. Shoulder function and 3-dimensional scapular kinematics in people with and without shoulder impingement syndrome. *Phys Ther.* 2006;86(8):1075–1090.
27. Laudner KG, et al. Scapular dysfunction in throwers with pathologic internal impingement. *J Orthop Sports Phys Ther.* 2006;36(7):485–494.
28. Camargo PR, et al. Effects of stretching and strengthening exercises, with and without manual therapy, on scapular kinematics, function, and pain in individuals with shoulder impingement: a randomized controlled trial. *J Orthop Sports Phys Ther.* 2015;45(12):984–997.
29. McClure PW, et al. Shoulder function and 3-dimensional kinematics in people with shoulder impingement syndrome before and after a 6-week exercise program. *Phys Ther.* 2004;84(9):832–848.
30. Turgut E, Duzgun I, Baltaci G. Effects of scapular stabilization exercise training on scapular kinematics, disability, and pain in subacromial impingement: a randomized controlled trial. *Arch Phys Med Rehabil.* 2017;98(10):1915–1923.e3.
31. Plummer HA, et al. Observational scapular dyskinesis: known-groups validity in patients with and without shoulder pain. *J Orthop Sports Phys Ther.* 2017;47(8):530–537.
32. Tate AR, et al. A clinical method for identifying scapular dyskinesis, part 2: validity. *J Athl Train.* 2009;44(2):65–173.
33. Hickey D, et al. Scapular dyskinesis increases the risk of future shoulder pain by 43% in asymptomatic athletes: a systematic review and meta-analysis. *Br J Sports Med.* 2018;52(2):102–110.
34. Clarsen B, et al. Reduced glenohumeral rotation, external rotation weakness and scapular dyskinesis are risk factors for shoulder injuries among elite male handball players: a prospective cohort study. *Br J Sports Med.* 2014;48(17):1327–1333.
35. Myers JB, Oyama S, Hibberd EE. Scapular dysfunction in high school baseball players sustaining throwing-related upper extremity injury: a prospective study. *J Shoulder Elbow Surg.* 2013;22(9):1154–1159.
36. Kibler WB, McMullen J. Scapular dyskinesis and its relation to shoulder pain. *J Am Acad Orthop Surg.* 2003;11(2):142–151.
37. Burkhart SS, Morgan CD, Kibler WB. The disabled throwing shoulder: spectrum of pathology Part III: the SICK scapula, scapular dyskinesis, the kinetic chain, and rehabilitation. *Arthroscopy.* 2003;19(6):641–661.
38. Burkhart SS, Morgan CD, Kibler WB. The disabled throwing shoulder: Spectrum of pathology part I: pathoanatomy and biomechanics. *Arthroscopy.* 2003;19(4):404–420.
39. Tate AR, et al. Effect of the Scapula Reposition Test on shoulder impingement symptoms and elevation strength in overhead athletes. *J Orthop Sports Phys Ther.* 2008;38(1):4–11.
40. Kibler WB, et al. Qualitative clinical evaluation of scapular dysfunction: a reliability study. *J Shoulder Elbow Surg.* 2002;11(6):550–556.
41. Rabin A, et al. The intertester reliability of the Scapular Assistance Test. *J Orthop Sports Phys Ther.* 2006;36(9):653–660.
42. Wright TA. Accessory spinal nerve injury. *Clin Orthop.* 1975;108:15–18.
43. Friedenberg SM, Zimprich T, Harper CM. The natural history of long thoracic and spinal accessory neuropathies. *Muscle Nerve.* 2002;25(4):535–539.
44. Srikumaran U, et al. Scapular Winging: a great masquerader of shoulder disorders: AAOS Exhibit Selection. *J Bone Joint Surg Am.* 2014;96(14):e122.
45. Solem-Bertoft E, Thuomas KA, Westerberg CE. The influence of scapular retraction and protraction on the width of the subacromial space. An MRI study. *Clin Orthop.* 1993;(296):99–103.
46. Graichen H, et al. Three-dimensional analysis of the width of the subacromial space in healthy subjects and patients with impingement syndrome. *AJR Am J Roentgenol.* 1999;172(4):1081–1086.
47. Kibler WB. Role of the scapula in the overhead throwing motion. *Contemp Orthop.* 1991;22:525–532.
48. Kibler WB. The role of the scapula in athletic shoulder function. *Am J Sports Med.* 1998;26(2):325–337.
49. Gibson MH, et al. A reliability study of measurement techniques to determine static scapular position. *J Orthop Sports Phys Ther.* 1995;21(2):100–106.

50. Odom CJ, et al. Measurement of scapular asymmetry and assessment of shoulder dysfunction using the Lateral Scapular Slide Test: a reliability and validity study. *Phys Ther.* 2001;81(2):799–809.

51. T'Jonck L, Lysens R, Grasse G. Measurements of scapular position and rotation: a reliability study. *Physiother Res Int.* 1996;1(3):148–158.

52. Davies GJ, Dickoff-Hoffman S. Neuromuscular testing and rehabilitation of the shoulder complex. *J Orthop Sports Phys Ther.* 1993;18(2):449–458.

53. DiVeta J, Walker ML, Skibinski B. Relationship between performance of selected scapular muscles and scapular abduction in standing subjects. *Phys Ther.* 1990;70(8):470–476. discussion 476–479.

54. Neiers L, Worrell TW. Assessment of Scapular Position. *J Sports Rehabil.* 1993;2:20–25.

55. Koslow PA, et al. Specificity of the lateral scapular slide test in asymptomatic competitive athletes. *J Orthop Sports Phys Ther.* 2003;33(6):331–336.

56. Nijs J, et al. Scapular positioning in patients with shoulder pain: a study examining the reliability and clinical importance of 3 clinical tests. *Arch Phys Med Rehabil.* 2005;86(7):1349–1355.

57. Paine RM, Voight M. The role of the scapula. *J Orthop Sports Phys Ther.* 1993;18(1):386–391.

58. Ellen MI, Gilhool JJ, Rogers DP. Scapular instability. The scapulothoracic joint. *Phys Med Rehabil Clin N Am.* 2000;11(4):755–770.

59. Rupp S, Berninger K, Hopf T. Shoulder problems in high level swimmers–impingement, anterior instability, muscular imbalance? *Int J Sports Med.* 1995;16(8):557–562.

60. Bak K, Faunl P. Clinical findings in competitive swimmers with shoulder pain. *Am J Sports Med.* 1997;25(2):254–260.

61. Bulut I, Fitzgerald GK, Irrgang JJ. Reliability of measuring shoulder range of motion, strength and scapular position. *J Orthop Sports Phys Ther.* 2004;34:A14.

62. McClure P, et al. A clinical method for identifying scapular dyskinesis, part 1: reliability. *J Athl Train.* 2009;44(2):160–164.

63. Lo YP, Hsu YC, Chan KM. Epidemiology of shoulder impingement in upper arm sports events. *Br J Sports Med.* 1990;24(3):173–177.

64. McMaster WC, Troup J. A survey of interfering shoulder pain in United States competitive swimmers. *Am J Sports Med.* 1993;21(1):67–70.

65. Soldatis JJ, Moseley JB, Etminan M. Shoulder symptoms in healthy athletes: a comparison of outcome scoring systems. *J Shoulder Elbow Surg.* 1997;6(3):265–271.

66. Wang HK, Cochrane T. A descriptive epidemiological study of shoulder injury in top level English male volleyball players. *Int J Sports Med.* 2001;22(2):159–163.

67. Tate A, McClure P, Neff N. Validity of a visual classification system for scapular motion. *J Orth Sport Phys Ther.* 2004;34:A42.

68. Johnson M. Development of a Model to Classify Scapular Motion: A Pilot Study. In: *Pennsylvania Physical Therapy Association: Annual Conference.* Pennsylvania: Seven Springs; 2001.

69. Landis JR, Koch GG. The measurement of observer agreement for categorical data. *Biometrics.* 1977;33(1):159–174.

70. McQuade KJ, Smidt GL. Dynamic scapulohumeral rhythm: the effects of external resistance during elevation of the arm in the scapular plane. *J Orthop Sports Phys Ther.* 1998;27(2):125–133.

71. Doody SG, Freedman L, Waterland JC. Shoulder Movements During Abduction in the Scapular Plane. *Arch Phys Med Rehabil.* 1970;51:595–604.

72. Warner JJP, et al. Scapulothoracic motion in normal shoulders and shoulders with glenohumeral instability and impingement syndrome. *Clin Orthop Relat Res.* 1992;285:191–199.

73. McQuade KJ, Dawson J, Smidt GL. Scapulothoracic muscle fatigue associated with alterations in scapulohumeral rhythm kinematics during maximum resistive shoulder elevation. *J Orthop Sports Phys Ther.* 1998;28(2):74–80.

74. Christiansen DH, et al. The scapular dyskinesis test: reliability, agreement, and predictive value in patients with subacromial impingement syndrome. *J Hand Ther.* 2017;30(2):208–213.

75. Lange T, et al. The reliability of physical examination tests for the clinical assessment of scapular dyskinesis in subjects with shoulder complaints: a systematic review. *Phys Ther Sport.* 2017;26:64–89.

76. Kamkar A, Irrgang JJ, Whitney SL. Nonoperative management of secondary shoulder impingement syndrome. *J Orthop Sports Phys Ther.* 1993;17(5):212–224.

77. Lopes AD, et al. Visual scapular dyskinesis: kinematics and muscle activity alterations in patients with subacromial impingement syndrome. *Arch Phys Med Rehabil.* 2015;96(2):298–306.

78. Huang TS, et al. Specific kinematics and associated muscle activation in individuals with scapular dyskinesis. *J Shoulder Elbow Surg.* 2015;24(8):1227–1234.

79. Farrar JT, et al. Clinical importance of changes in chronic pain intensity measured on an 11-point numerical pain rating scale. *Pain.* 2001;94(2):149–158.

80. Kibler WB, Sciascia A, Dome D. Evaluation of apparent and absolute supraspinatus strength in patients with shoulder injury using the scapular retraction test. *Am J Sports Med.* 2006;34(10):1643–1647.

81. Smith J, et al. Effect of scapular protraction and retraction on isometric shoulder elevation strength. *Arch Phys Med Rehabil.* 2002;83(3):367–370.

82. Neer CS, Welsh 2nd RP. The shoulder in sports. *Orthop Clin North Am.* 1977;8(3):583–591.

83. Hawkins RJ, Kennedy JC. Impingement syndrome in athletes. *Am J Sports Med.* 1980;8(3):151–158.

84. Jobe FW, Jobe CM. Painful athletic injuries of the shoulder. *Clin Orthop.* 1983;173:117–124.

85. Wainner RS, et al. Reliability and diagnostic accuracy of the clinical examination and patient self-report measures for cervical radiculopathy. *Spine.* 2003;28(1):52–62.

86. Kendall F, McCreary EK, Provance PG. *Muscles Testing and Function.* Baltimore: Williams and Wilkins; 1993.

87. Michener LA, et al. Scapular muscle tests in subjects with shoulder pain and functional loss: reliability and construct validity. *Phys Ther.* 2005;85(11):1128–1138.

88. Ekstrom RA, Donatelli RA, Soderberg GL. Surface electromyographic analysis of exercises for the trapezius and serratus anterior muscles. *J Orthop Sports Phys Ther.* 2003;33(5):247–258.

89. Sahrmann S. *Diagnosis and Treatment of Movement Impairment Syndromes.* St. Louis: Mosby; 2001.

90. Griegel-Morris P, et al. Incidence of common postural abnormalities in the cervical, shoulder, and thoracic regions and their association with pain in two age groups of healthy subjects. *Phys Ther.* 1992;72(6):425–431.

91. Cleland JA, et al. Interrater reliability of the history and physical examination in patients with mechanical neck pain. *Arch Phys Med Rehabil.* 2006;87(10):1388–1395.

92. Maitland GD. In: Maitland GD, et al., ed. *Maitland's Vertebral Manipulation.* 6th ed. Butterworth-Heinemann; 2001.

93. Meurer A, et al. [BWS-mobility in patients with an impingement syndrome compared to healthy subjects–an inclinometric study]. *Z Orthop Ihre Grenzgeb.* 2004;142(4):415–420.

94. Borich M, Bright JM, Lorello DJ, Cieminski CJ, Buisman T, Ludewigh PM. Scapular angular positioning at end range internal rotation in cases of glenohumeral internal rotation deficit. *J Orthop Sports Phys Ther.* 2006;36(12):926–934.

95. Thomas SJ, et al. Glenohumeral rotation and scapular position adaptations after a single high school female sports season. *J Athl Train.* 2009;44(3):230–237.

96. Tyler TF, Roy T, Nicholas SJ, Gleim GW. Reliability and validity of a new method of measuring posterior shoulder tightness. *J Orthop Sports Phys Ther.* 1999;29(5):262–269. discussion 270-4.

97. Myers JB, Oyama S, Wassinger CA, et al. Reliability, precision, accuracy, and validity of posterior shoulder tightness assessment in overhead athletes. *Am J Sports Med.* 2007;35(11):1922–1930.

98. Richards RR, An KN, Bigliani LU, et al. A standardized method for the assessment of shoulder function. *J Shoulder Elbow Surg.* 1994;3(6):347–352.

99. Awan R, Smith J, Boon AJ. Measuring shoulder internal rotation range of motion: a comparison of 3 techniques. *Arch Phys Med Rehabil.* 2002;83:1229–1234.

100. Mallon WJ, Herring CL, Sallay PI, et al. Use of vertebral levels to measure presumed internal rotation at the shoulder: a radiographic analysis. *J Shoulder Elbow Surg.* 1996;5:299–306.

101. Edwards TB, Bostick RD, Greene CC, et al. Interobserver and intraobserver reliability of the measurement of shoulder internal rotation by vertebra level. *J Shoulder Elbow Surg.* 2002;11:40–42.

102. McClure P, et al. A randomized controlled comparison of stretching procedures for posterior shoulder tightness. *J Orthop Sports Phys Ther.* 2007;37(3):108–114.

103. Gerber C, et al. Effect of selective capsulorrhaphy on the passive range of motion of the glenohumeral joint. *J Bone Joint Surg Am.* 2003;85-A(1):48–55.

104. Borstad JD. Resting position variables at the shoulder: evidence to support a posture-impairment association. *Phys Ther.* 2006;86(4):549–557.

105. Sahrmann S. *Diagnosis and Treatment of Movement Impairment Syndromes.* St. Louis: Mosby; 2002.

106. Lewis JS, Valentine RE. The pectoralis minor length test: a study of the intra-rater reliability and diagnostic accuracy in subjects with and without shoulder symptoms. *BMC Musculoskelet Disord.* 2007;8:64.

107. Borstad JD. Measurement of pectoralis minor muscle length: validation and clinical application. *J Orthop Sports Phys Ther.* 2008;38(4):169–174.

108. Hendrix ST, Hoyle M, Tokish JM. Arthroscopic pectoralis minor release. *Arthrosc Tech.* 2018;7(6):e589–e594.

109. Provencher MT, et al. Surgical release of the pectoralis minor tendon for scapular dyskinesia and shoulder pain. *Am J Sports Med.* 2017;45(1):173–178.

110. McClure PW, Michener LA. Staged approach for rehabilitation classification: shoulder disorders (STAR-Shoulder). *Phys Ther.* 2015;95(5):791–800.

111. Michener LA, Walsworth MK, Burnet EN. Effectiveness of rehabilitation for patients with subacromial impingement syndrome: a systematic review. *J Hand Ther.* 2004;17(2):152–164.

112. Burkhead WZ Jr, Rockwood CA Jr. Treatment of instability of the shoulder with an exercise program. *J Bone Joint Surg Am.* 1992;74(6):890–896.

113. Kibler WB, Press J, Sciascia A. The role of core stability in athletic function. *Sports Med.* 2006;36(3):189–198.

114. Schmitt L, Snyder-Mackler L. Role of scapular stabilizers in etiology and treatment of impingement syndrome. *J Orthop Sports Phys Ther.* 1999;29(1):31–38.

115. Host HH. Scapular taping in the treatment of anterior shoulder impingement. *Phys Ther.* 1995;75(9):803–812.

116. Cools AM, et al. Does taping influence electromyographic muscle activity in the scapular rotators in healthy shoulders? *Man Ther.* 2002;7(3):154–162.

117. Lewis JS, Wright C, Green A. Subacromial impingement syndrome: the effect of changing posture on shoulder range of movement. *J Orthop Sports Phys Ther.* 2005;35(2):72–87.

118. Ackermann B, Adams R, Marshall E. The effect of scapula taping on electromyographic activity and musical performance in professional violinists. *Aust J Physiother.* 2002;48(3):197–203.

119. Smith MJ, Sparkes V. The immediate effect of scapular taping on electromyographic activity of the scapular rotators in swimmers with subacromial impingement symptoms. In: *Physical Therapy in Sport International Conference: Enhancing Recovery and Performance in Sport.* Birmingham, UK; 2006.

120. Cools AM, et al. Scapular muscle recruitment patterns: trapezius muscle latency with and without impingement symptoms. *Am J Sports Med.* 2003;31(4):542–549.

121. Greig AM, et al. Postural taping decreases thoracic kyphosis but does not influence trunk muscle electromyographic activity or balance in women with osteoporosis. *Man Ther.* 2007.

122. Kebaetse M, McClure P, Pratt NA. Thoracic position effect on shoulder range of motion, strength, and three-dimensional scapular kinematics. *Arch Phys Med Rehabil.* 1999;80(8):945–950.

123. Robbins S, Waked E, Rappel R. Ankle taping improves proprioception before and after exercise in young men. *Br J Sports Med.* 1995;29(4):242–247.

124. Mulligan B. *Manual Therapy 'NAGS', 'SNAGS', 'MWMS' etc.* 5th ed. Wellington: Plane View Press; 1995.

125. Maitland GD. *Peripheral Manipulation.* 2nd ed. London: Butterworths; 1983.

126. Cook CE. *Orthopedic Manual Therapy.* Upper Saddle River, NJ: Pearson Education, Inc; 2007.

127. Bandy WD, Sanders B. *Therapeutic Exercise: Techniques for Intervention.* Baltimore: Lippincott Williams & Wilkins; 2001.

128. Weldon 3rd EJ, Richardson AB. Upper extremity overuse injuries in swimming. A discussion of swimmer's shoulder. *Clin Sports Med.* 2001;20(3):423–438.

129. Bach HG, Goldberg BA. Posterior capsular contracture of the shoulder. *J Am Acad Orthop Surg.* 2006;14(5):265–277.

130. Wilk KE, Meister K, Andrews JR. Current concepts in the rehabilitation of the overhead throwing athlete. *Am J Sports Med.* 2002;30(1):136–151.

131. Borstad JD, Ludewig PM. Comparison of three stretches for the pectoralis minor muscle. *J Shoulder Elbow Surg.* 2006;15(3):324–330.

Surgery Management of Complex Injuries of the Hand

Marco Rizzo, Casey Sabbag

CRITICAL POINTS

- Complex hand injuries can involve damage to skin, tendons, joints, bones, nerves, and blood vessels in varying degrees of severity.
- Advanced Trauma Life Support protocols should be prioritized on initial evaluation.
- Some of the most important aspects of management of complex injuries of the hand are prompt diagnosis, development of a treatment plan, and recognizing distracting or traumatic injuries to other body systems.
- A thorough history and physical examination may not always be possible because of other factors that impede communication (e.g., young children, altered mental status, intubated in field).
- Plain radiographs in two planes are an essential part of evaluation of complex hand injuries.
- Open fractures represent additional level of complexity to hand injuries.
- Patients with contaminated wounds require expedient delivery of intravenous antibiotics and thorough irrigation and debridement, preferably on an urgent basis.
- It is critical to maintain bone length and alignment.
- Perform multiple digit replantation using the structure-by-structure method.

- Identify all nerve, tendon, and or vascular injury before anesthesia induction if possible.
- Flexor tendon injuries can be repaired primarily or with use of graft techniques.
- Early active assisted range of motion is critical to prevent stiffness in patients with flexor tendon repairs.
- Stabilization of bony injuries can facilitate early active range of motion protocols in patients with complex hand injuries.
- When significant ischemia is present, it is urgent to prioritize restoration of blood supply.
- Tension free end-to-end repair of blood vessels is preferred.
- The goal of nerve repair is primary, end-to-end tension-free repair when possible. Vein autograft, allograft, and conduits are used when necessary.
- Many patients require soft tissue coverage if they have a large soft tissue defect, a wound with significant contamination requiring debridement, or risk of exposed hardware.
- Use delayed closure technique with wound vacuum-assisted closure when needed.
- Counsel patients on the importance of postoperative rehabilitation after a complex hand injury.

INTRODUCTION

Complex injuries to the hand are defined as injuries involving more than one group of tissues. The tissue systems involved may include bone, joints, tendon, ligament, vessel, nerve, and skin. A delicate balance of the anatomy and physiology exist within the hand. Complex hand trauma includes a wide spectrum of injury and can lead to significant morbidity and functional loss. Early diagnosis and thorough evaluation will help ensure prompt and optimal treatment.

The integrated system of tissue systems each serve a purpose in allowing the hand to be used. Bones provide structural support. Joints allow for motion of the hand and wrist, and the ligaments help maintain stability of the joints. Tendons arise from muscle bellies and insert into bone and facilitate motion of the bones and joints. Nerves supply signals to the complex coordination of intrinsic and extrinsic hand musculature and give sensory feedback. Skin provides an elastic protection of the deeper tissues from the outside world. The skin on the glabrous palmar surface is a specialized organ in itself with many special cell types, including Pacinian corpuscles for vibratory and pressure feedback. Blood vessels ensure the viability and nutritional status of these aforementioned structures.

Complex injuries to the hand can involve a multitude of mechanisms such as industrial accidents, high-pressure injections, high-energy trauma, burns, traumatic amputations, and crush injuries, just to name a few. The severity of trauma can often be obvious such as a complete or near-complete amputation. However, other injuries, such

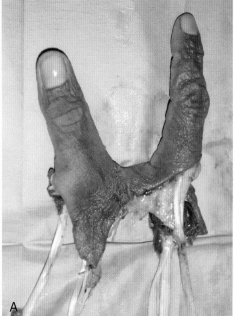
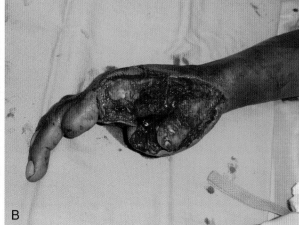

Fig. 73.1 A and **B,** A 54-year-old man who got his thumb and index finger caught in a conveyor. The zone of injury for this mechanism of injury is notoriously long, and attempted replantation was unsuccessful. He went on to have a groin flap for wound coverage.

as high-pressure grease-gun injections, can be deceptively benign at initial presentation. Multiple surgeries (both primarily and secondarily) are common, and therapy is a critical component in helping ensure optimal outcome. The timeline for recovery is likely prolonged. In addition, all stages of recovery are fraught with potential pitfalls. Because many of these injuries are contaminated and have skin loss, infection is a major concern. Stiffness, deformity, chronic pain, paresthesias, and functional loss can routinely result.[1]

Hand injuries are generally very common and represent nearly 30% of all traumas seen in emergency departments (EDs). Based on a classification system proposed by Campbell and Kay,[2] a recent study further examining the epidemiology of these injuries found that approximately 40% of hand trauma presenting to EDs are moderate to severe in nature.[3] Most injuries occurred in the domestic setting and affected young or middle-aged men. Trybus and coworkers[3] found that use of industrial machinery was associated with more severe injuries. In addition, the average total treatment time was nearly 3 months, and more than 60% of patients had some degree of permanent disability. This underscores the importance of a thorough evaluation, appropriate treatment, and team approach including the therapist, patient, and surgeon.

HISTORY AND PHYSICAL EXAMINATION

Combined hand injuries can be isolated to the affected extremity or may occur as part of multiple injuries. A systemic approach to evaluation of these patients will help ensure all components of the patient's trauma are diagnosed and avoid overlooking any aspects of the injury. In cases of high-energy accidents, the physician must be sure that there is no visceral or life-threatening head trauma. The patient's airway, breathing, and circulation need to be assessed and maintained. Profuse or uncontrolled bleeding from the extremity can be controlled in the acute setting by holding pressure on the wound or applying a tourniquet proximally.

Understanding the limits that come with patients who may be unresponsive, uncooperative, or sedated, a complete history and review of systems is essential in evaluating persons with extremity injuries. Hand dominance and employment of the patient should be included in the history. A good understanding of the patient's home life and age is also helpful

in deciding the best treatment. The mechanism of injury is important in predicting or raising suspicion of trauma to specific tissue groups.

An appreciation of patient comorbidities is helpful in predicting outcome and determining the best treatment options. These factors are important for preparing realistic treatment plans and avoiding medical and extremity related complications. For instance, persons with a significant cardiovascular history, pulmonary disease, or diabetes will inherit greater risk with longer anesthesia times. Success of microvascular reconstruction or replantation will be decreased in patients with peripheral vascular disease, diabetes, or inflammatory arthritis. Immune-suppressed patients often experience delayed healing and increased risk of infection.

The medication history of the patient can impact treatment. For instance, the use of anticoagulants can affect hemostasis. The social history also sheds important information regarding their other risk factors for failure of treatment and aid in decision making regarding treatment. Tobacco use is notoriously associated with diminished healing and failure of revascularization. Heavy use of alcohol or illicit drugs helps determine the risk for complications after treatment such as substance withdrawal that may occur during hospital admission or narcotic abuse or dependence that may occur as an outpatient. One of the major challenges of the health care provider team lies in understanding the commitment of the patient toward her or his recovery. More complex reconstructions often require closer follow-up periods and detailed rehabilitation to maximize their success. It is critical that the patient understand the importance of compliance and follow-up after the initial treatment. The optimal treatment for complex injuries may need to be catered to fit within these limitations.[4] With clear communication, the patient and health care provider can formulate the ideal initial treatment, establish follow-up care needs, and lay the groundwork for realistic outcome expectations.

The circumstances and details of the patient's injury can provide important information regarding complex hand injuries. For instance, the digit and the mechanism of traumatic amputation are important in predicting the success of reattachment. The rate of success of digit replantation is estimated to be 61%, and similarly, the rate of success of thumb replantation is 74%.[5] Avulsion injuries (Fig. 73.1) have a large zone of injury and are notoriously more difficult to reconstruct

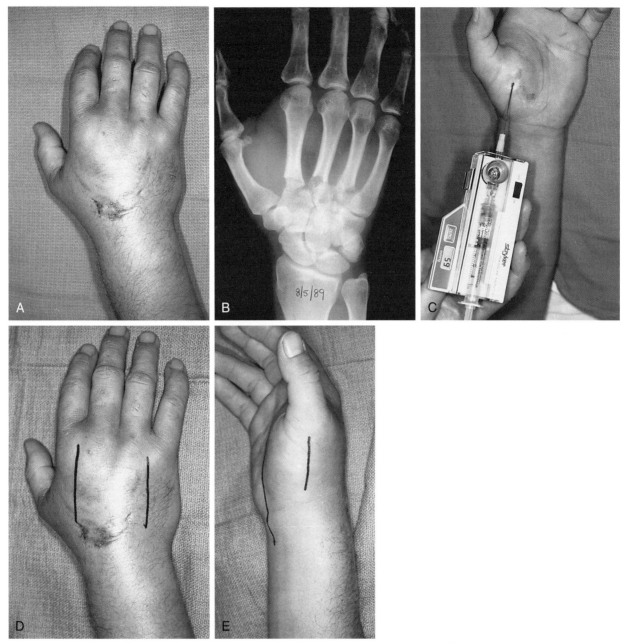

Fig. 73.2 A, Patient with a crush injury to the hand. **B,** Posteroanterior radiographs demonstrate fractures of the index, middle, and ring finger metacarpal bases. **C,** Compartment pressure measurements help to confirm clinical suspicion of compartment syndrome. **D** and **E,** Appropriate fasciotomy incisions are marked out.

compared with sharp amputations. Some injuries are more subtle. For instance, a crush injury may not show obvious deformity or skin defect but may lead to marked swelling and compartment syndrome (Fig. 73.2). High-pressure injections are also injuries that lead to significant morbidity and long-term functional loss.[6] Multiple surgeries are common, and the recovery is often prolonged. However, they often present as benign injuries with a small puncture wound, and their severity may be overlooked, which can compromise the overall outcome.

The timing, duration, and location of injury are essential. Contaminated wounds require urgent debridement to minimize the risk of infection. Some locations such as barnyards or other farm settings are notoriously dirty and require aggressive debridement. Contaminated wounds over 8 to 12 hours old may likely be left open and undergo serial debridement before contemplating formal closure to minimize

risk of infection. Definitive treatment of associated injures can be delayed until the wound is clean. Chemical injuries may occur in certain industrial settings, and it is important to understand special treatments. For instance, hydrofluoric acid contamination should be treated with copious irrigation followed by neutralization with calcium gluconate solution or infusion (or both). The duration of injury also carries special significance in limbs with compromised vascularity. Amputated fingers, hands, and arms require prompt treatment and revascularization. Although regionally and nationally dependent, digits are generally replanted in clean-cut amputations that involve the proximal digit, thumb amputations, multiple-digit amputations, and any digit amputation in a child.[7] Warm and cold ischemia times need to be considered. Traditional teaching suggests that these patients should be treated within 6 hours of injury. Finger replantations can usually be attempted within this time range. However, more proximal injuries

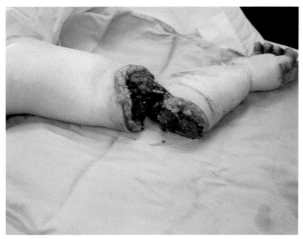

Fig. 73.3 A 4-year-old boy involved in a motor vehicle accident and near-complete amputation of the forearm. His warm ischemia time was approximately 8 hours. Despite successful reattachment, he went on to develop muscle necrosis and infection that necessitated amputation.

(e.g., forearm level) have a greater risk of failure because more muscle is at risk of developing ischemic damage (Fig. 73.3). The method of fixing multiple-digit amputation can be performed by either the structure-by-structure method (preferred) or the digit-by-digit method.[7]

Physical examination of patients with hand injuries should be performed in a systemic fashion to ensure that nothing be overlooked. However, the entire patient must also be assessed. Appropriate Advanced Trauma Life Support (ATLS) protocols should be used when applicable. A complete evaluation of the skin, bone, tendon, and nerves as well as perfusion of the extremity should be performed. The use of Doppler ultrasound is an important adjunct in determining vascular status of the hand at the level of the wrist and for each of the digital arteries. Some aspects of the physical examination may be limited by patient pain, unresponsiveness, or lack of cooperation. Additional injuries may be discovered when they are sedated or in the operating room. Although it does not preclude surgical intervention, in unconscious patients, complete exam information (e.g., a sensory examination) should be delayed until they are responsive and cooperative.

ANCILLARY STUDIES

Plain radiographs in at least two planes are an essential part of the evaluation of complex hand injuries. In addition to assessing the bones for fracture, these studies reveal the joint alignment and overall structural integrity of the extremity. Radiography may also demonstrate the presence of radiopaque foreign bodies or free air within the soft tissues. When clinically indicated, special views will help identify certain types of fractures. For instance, a radiograph of the wrist in an extended and ulnarly deviated position can help better show the scaphoid bone in the coronal plane. Oblique views can help show injuries of the metacarpal bones or carpal bones such as the hamate. Traction radiographs can also provide the surgeon with additional information regarding the fracture patterns.

Many complex injuries require immediate surgical attention for treatment of open or contaminated injuries. Time permitting, more specialized studies can be helpful in providing the caregiver with additional information. Computed tomography scans will show the bony anatomy in more detail and help confirm the presence of subtle fractures. Magnetic resonance imaging can help better evaluate the bone marrow, soft tissues, and presence of foreign material.

TREATMENT

Much of the decision regarding the course of treatment will be outlined by the surgeon and patient (when possible) in the preliminary evaluation. Before proceeding with treatment, it is important for the caregiver to educate and outline the plan. Factors such as the injury pattern, experience and expertise of the treating team, and patient's needs and preferences should contribute to formulation of the appropriate treatment plan.

Early treatment decisions of some of these injuries can help minimize the number of repeat surgeries and optimize the long-term outcome. For instance, the use of amputated or discarded parts for skin coverage or reconstruction of the bones, tendon, vasculature, or nerves of the hand can be helpful.[8,9] It is also important for the patient to have a realistic understanding of the details of rehabilitation and outcome. Although cosmetically pleasing, many digits after replantation may be stiff and painful and ultimately provide no functional improvement compared with an amputated digit.

The decision about definitive fixation, repair, or replantation may be delayed depending on the level and complexity of injury.[10] However, complex injuries often have associated wounds that require appropriate irrigation and debridement regardless of the timing of definitive fixation. This step is critical toward helping prevent infection and lay the foundation for good healing. Typically, the irrigation is performed with normal saline solution or sterile water. Although traditionally, there has been a tendency by many to use antibiotics in sterile saline solution, recent investigations have found no added benefit toward use of antibiotic saline solution for bacterial contamination. A detergent can be added in cases of chemical or industrial (e.g., grease, paint) infiltration. Aggressive sharp debridement of nonviable tissues is essential. Severely contaminated wounds often benefit from serial debridements. Obtaining cultures at the time of initial debridement helps identify infectious organisms and guides appropriate antibiotic treatment.

Musculoskeletal Injuries

Bones and joints make up the support structure for the hand and upper extremity. Fractures and dislocations can disrupt their function if they fail to heal or become malaligned. This can result in stiffness, pain, and diminished use of the hand. Fractures can have several characteristics. For instance, open fractures involve a violation in the skin, resulting in exposure of the bone. These fractures add a level of complexity to the patient's injury. They are associated with higher energy trauma and have a greater amount of soft tissue damage. As a result, there are increased incidences of infection, avascular necrosis, and diminished healing (Fig. 73.4). Intraarticular fractures extend into the joint and may result in joint incongruity and significant cartilage damage. These injuries carry a higher risk of developing joint stiffness, pain, and posttraumatic arthritis. Trauma involving disruption of the joints and ligaments can result in instability and incongruity. These injuries usually require ligamentous repair, reconstruction, or temporary pinning.[4,11]

The optimal treatment of complex fractures is based on multiple factors. Ultimately, surgical fixation is usually the best treatment for unstable fractures. Rehabilitation and early range of motion (ROM) will not likely be feasible until reconstruction of the skeleton is achieved. However, this must be balanced with the viability and cleanliness of the wound and soft tissue coverage. For instance, wounds with significant contamination and skin defects increase the risk to of exposed hardware to infection. Multiple surgical treatment options can be used, including plates and screws, Kirschner wires (K-wires), intramedullary pins, tension band wiring, and external fixation. Plates and screws tend to provide very rigid fixation and typically allow for early

ROM. However, use of this technique requires more extensive surgical dissection, which may result in devascularization, periosteal stripping, and slower wound healing. This may also increase the risk of infection. Alternatively, K-wires can be inserted percutaneously, obviating the need for extensive dissection. Unfortunately, the strength of fixation is typically less than that of open reduction and internal fixation. External fixation can be used either alone or in conjunction with pinning and enhance the rigidity of the construct (Fig. 73.5). External fixators will also allow access to the soft tissues while helping keep the bones aligned and maintain their length. External fixation may also be used as a temporary means of maintaining fracture reduction. For instance, if appropriate wound coverage and decontamination of the wound are achieved, more permanent or rigid hardware may then be used, thereby allowing early aggressive ROM. Unfortunately, K-wires and external fixation carry a higher risk of pin tract infection. Intramedullary fixation can be inserted with minimal soft tissue dissection and can also maintain bone length and alignment. However, intramedullary fixation has limited potential for rotational control. Studies evaluating outcomes of open fractures associated with complex injuries have shown that metacarpal injuries generally fared better than phalangeal fractures.[12] Fractures of the proximal phalanges or proximal interphalangeal joint with associated tendon injury carry a poor prognosis.

Maintaining bone length and alignment in the hand is extremely important. This allows for appropriate tension of the soft tissues. If the tendons require repair or reconstruction, this is best performed with the bone out to length. Although somewhat more forgiving, the same applies to the skin. Shortening is likely the result of either significant bone loss or comminution or angulation of the fracture. In the acute setting, a silicone or polymethyl methacrylate (PMMA) spacer can be used to maintain bone length while the soft tissue concerns and decontaminating the wound can be dealt with. Definitive fixation can later be performed using bone graft (Fig. 73.6).

The treatment of joint trauma can vary depending on the severity of the injury. A poorly healed, incongruent or arthritic joint will usually result in loss of motion and be a significant cause of pain and dysfunction. Whenever possible, repair or reconstruction is preferred. However, when not feasible, options include primary arthrodesis[13,14] (Fig. 73.7), implant arthroplasty,[13] and distraction arthroplasty (traction).[15,16] The ideal position of arthrodesis for a specific joint can vary depending on the joint, involved digit, and nature of the injury. Although exceptions apply, metacarpophalangeal joints typically are fused in slight flexion. Proximal interphalangeal joints are usually best positioned in a greater amount of flexion. Distal interphalangeal joints can be ideally fused between 0 and 15 degrees of flexion.

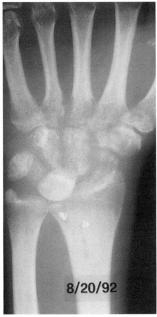

Fig. 73.4 A patient who developed carpal osteomyelitis and septic arthritis 6 weeks after open reduction for lunate dislocation. Follow-up anteroposterior radiograph demonstrated carpal osteopenia, erosions, and sclerotic appearance of lunate suggestive of osteonecrosis.

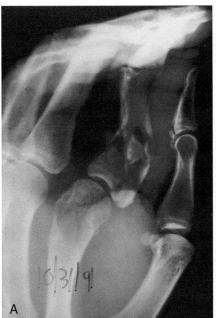
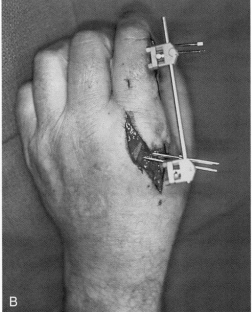

Fig. 73.5 A, A patient with an open comminuted fracture proximal phalanx index finger. **B,** He underwent application of external fixation from metacarpal to proximal phalanx. The fracture healed in satisfactory alignment; extensor tenolysis and dorsal proximal interphalangeal joint capsulotomy was required to restore range of motion.

Tendon Injuries

Tendons are commonly injured in complex hand injuries. Surgically, healing is facilitated by primary repair, reconstruction, or transfer. Reconstruction can be performed primarily using tendon grafts. Some investigators have advocated two-stage reconstruction in cases in which reconstruction was deemed necessary.[17,18] Tendon transfers with or without grafting can also be used in reconstructing severely injured tendons. Different zones of injury have been defined in both flexor and extensor tendon injuries. Each has prognostic implications. Generally speaking, tendon injuries in the fingers and hand carry a worse prognosis than those in the wrist and forearm. In particular, zone 2 flexor tendon lacerations are troublesome. Injuries within this zone can often involve both the flexor digitorum superficialis and profundus, and they occur within the tendon sheath, which can be constrictive to the repair. As a result, diminished excursion after repair is common. Repairs in this zone are also more prone to failure.

Much investigation has been done regarding tendon healing.[19-26] After repair, intrinsic and extrinsic mechanisms help assure healing. Intrinsic healing more likely occurs with early ROM. Thus, with controlled early motion, one can appreciate improved strength of repair and less scar tissue or adhesions. This underscores the importance (when possible) of bony stabilization and management of concomitant injuries so that early rehabilitation can be initiated. Whenever early motion cannot be initiated, the patient should be advised that a tenolysis will likely be necessary if stiffness results.

Many other factors play an important role in affecting tendon healing. Some are related to the surgical technique such as suture used for repair, strands across the repair, and tendon-to-tendon approximation. An additional factor is the integrity of the surrounding soft tissues.

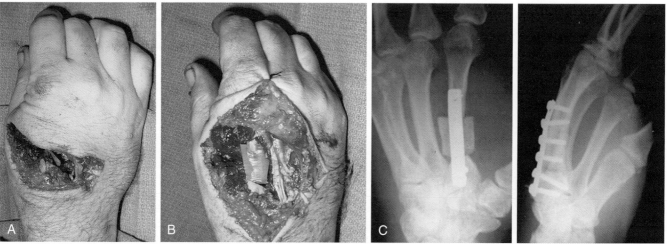

Fig. 73.6 Silicone spacer for metacarpal defect. **A,** Open fracture left index metacarpal with missing bone. **B,** Silicone spacer placed in metacarpal defect to maintain stability and metacarpal length. **C,** Four weeks later, the spacer was removed and replaced with a tricortical iliac crest graft and plate.

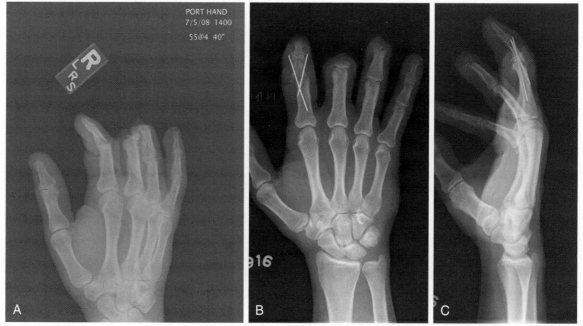

Fig. 73.7 **A,** A patient status after a saw injury with multiple injuries, including a proximal interphalangeal (PIP) joint obliteration and a near amputation of the index finger. Repair of the joint was not feasible. **B** and **C,** He underwent primary fusion of the PIP joint.

Tendons heal better and form fewer adhesions in a well-vascularized bed. On the flexor side of the hand, the integrity of the flexor tendon sheath and pulleys are important in optimizing hand function. In particular, the A2 and A4 pulleys should be preserved or reconstructed (Fig. 73.8) when treating a finger tendon injury.[17,27,28] Otherwise, the patient will likely experience bowstringing and limited motion.

Similar to many injuries in the hand, rehabilitation of these injuries is critical to ensuring optimal outcome. Several factors that affect the method and timing of therapy include the location of injury, method of repair or reconstruction, and associated injuries. Trauma that involves both the flexor and extensor tendons of the hand can be complicated by their differing rehabilitation protocols. More recently, early ROM exercises have been advocated to avoid tendon adhesions and have been proposed to contribute to earlier recovery of tensile strength and improved tendon nutrition.[29] These injuries are more likely to necessitate further surgery, such as tenolysis, after healing.

Vascular Injuries

Injuries to the blood vessels of the hand and upper extremity are common in complex hand trauma. The vessels are fairly close to the skin, especially in the digits, and are vulnerable to injury in complex trauma. The most commonly considered mechanism of injury to the arteries and veins is penetrating trauma. However, it is important to consider blunt trauma as a mechanism. Crush injuries can result in tears of the inner lining (intima) of the vessels, resulting in thrombosis (Fig. 73.9).

Physical examination of patients with vascular injury can vary from complete loss of perfusion to no perceptible deficit. A thorough understanding of the arterial anatomy will help the surgeon identify a lesion. At the level of the wrist, the radial and ulnar arteries provide the blood supply to the hand. They commonly communicate in the hand at the superficial and deep palmar arches. Thus, injury to one vessel may not show obvious diminished blood flow to the hand. Holding pressure and temporarily halting flow of the unaffected vessel can help discern injury of the other. In the digits, two neurovascular bundles, radial and ulnar, provide the innervation and perfusion. They lie superficial to and on either side of the flexor tendons. Thus, they are commonly injured when the tendon is lacerated. The dorsal aspects of the digits are rich in veins. Because of the collateral network and redundant blood supply, most isolated injuries to the hand are unlikely to cause limb-threatening ischemia. However, combined injuries are likely to injure more of the blood supply, risking the viability of the hand or fingers. In addition to obvious vessel disruption, increased sympathetic tone, certain patient medications, medical comorbidities, the patient's hemodynamic state, and social activities such as smoking contribute to the overall condition. When significant ischemia occurs, a special urgency is required to restore the blood supply to the affected area. Surgery to restore perfusion to the extremity is often detailed and requires significant anesthesia time. This should be weighed with the overall condition of the patient.

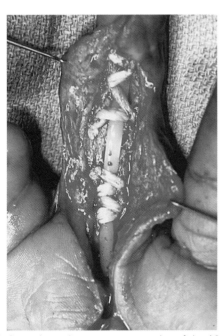

Fig. 73.8 Patient who underwent reconstruction of the A2 and A4 pulleys over a silicone rod. Ultimately, the patient underwent tendon grafting in a staged procedure.

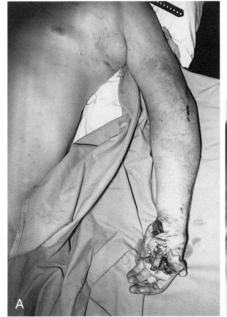
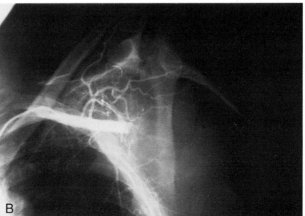

Fig. 73.9 A, A patient who sustained a roller crush injury to the hand. **B,** Arteriogram demonstrates occlusion of the axillary artery.

Although not always requiring revascularization, noncritical injuries may carry significant morbidity. The local tissues in these injuries are compromised, and infection and wound healing are concerns. In addition, nerve recovery may be diminished because of diminished local perfusion. Arteries that develop thrombosis (via blunt trauma or partial lacerations) carry of risk of future emboli. The surgeon should consider repair of noncritical blood supply in cases of associated nerve or significant soft tissue injury. Additional concerns regarding arterial injury include hematoma development, significant blood loss, and compartment syndrome.

On inspection, lacerations of arteries result in bright red, pulsatile bleeding. However, the clinical findings may be more subtle. The care provider should examine for a thrill, bruit, or expanding pulsatile hematoma. Ultrasound or arteriography can help better assess the integrity of the vasculature. A pulse oximeter, comparing with unaffected digits, can help raise suspicion of diminished perfusion. In addition, a relatively simple test is to pierce the pulp of the fingertip and assess the bleeding. Fingers with adequate perfusion will demonstrate bright red blood. In the finger, if there is disruption of the outgoing veins, arterial congestion may occur. Congested or inadequately perfused digits can demonstrate darker bluish appearance.

Indications for arterial repair are graded and must be weighed against the feasibility, patient comorbidities, and degree of ischemia. Critical and noncritical injuries with nerve or significant soft tissue injury that would benefit from improved perfusion should undergo arterial repair or reconstruction. Several principles of reperfusion need to be understood. Restoring bony stability and length is essential before arterial repair. When possible, shortening the bone will decrease the tension on the repair. Repair should be performed with microscopic instruments and under magnification. Damaged endothelium at the arterial ends must be trimmed away. Thrombus is excised, and the arterial ends are reapproximated. A tension-free repair will help ensure success of the anastomosis. An end-to-end repair is preferred. Reverse vein grafts from the forearm, leg, or wrist can be used in the presence of a gap. In the fingers, vein repairs are often necessary to ensure adequate outflow.

In cases of tissue necrosis, debridement is necessary. In the absence of infection, it is acceptable to allow the tissue to appropriately demarcate so that the level of debridement is appropriate. Resultant soft tissue defects can be treated with skin grafts or flaps.

Nerve Injuries

Nerve injuries are common in combined trauma. Similar to vessels, nerves can sustain trauma from laceration, crush, or avulsion mechanisms. Clinical manifestations of nerve injury include paresthesias, pain, and loss of motor function. Accurate early assessment of both motor and sensory function should be performed before administering anesthesia. This will establish a baseline examination. A proper neurologic examination requires that a patient be cooperative; in patients who are sedated or impaired, the physician may be unable to obtain a complete examination in the initial setting. Nerves that sustain blunt trauma may recover over time. This depends in part on the severity and duration of the compression as well as patient-related factors (e.g., patient age, comorbidities, tobacco use).

Nerves that are lacerated should undergo repair or reconstruction when feasible. This allows for proper nerve regeneration. It also helps prevent the formation of neuromas, which can often be painful. Repair can be done acutely or in delayed fashion. Repair within 5 to 7 days is considered delayed primary repair. Repair or reconstruction

of the nerve after 1 week is referred to as secondary repair.[30] Ideally, primary repair is preferred in the acute setting. However, if the zone of injury is somewhat difficult to determine at the time of initial surgery or if conditions are not favorable, delayed repair is the treatment of choice.

Primary repair is generally feasible in cases involving sharp, such as clean lacerations such from knives. The wound should be clean and free of contamination and, ideally, well vascularized. Similar to vessel repairs, bony stability is a prerequisite for nerve surgery. If secondary neurorrhaphy is required, tagging the nerve ends for later repair or reconstruction is helpful. Similarly, if the nerve is crushed or stretched (but in continuity), it should be marked for easier visualization at reoperation.[30,31] Neuromas within the nerve can form in these injuries, and they should be removed and trimmed to healthy nerve ends to facilitate repair or reconstruction. Nerve regeneration normally occurs at a rate of 1 mm per day, which translates to approximately 1 inch per month.

Nerve repair is best done under magnification with microscopy instruments. Epineural repair is the most commonly used method of coaptation. Similar to arterial and vein anastomoses, a tension-free repair is very important. Some degree of nerve mobilization is helpful in minimizing tension, but overmobilization has been shown to be detrimental to nerve healing.[32] Nerve grafting or use of nerve tubes (conduits) is indicated when a tension-free repair is not feasible.[31] Options for nerve grafts include the sural nerves and the medial and lateral antebrachial cutaneous nerves. Vein grafting and bioabsorbable nerve conduits have been shown to be effective in cases of small nerve gap.[33–36] In cases with large skin defects, nerve allograft or nerve branches within a pedicled or free flap used for skin coverage can be used as vascularized nerve grafts.[37]

Skin and Soft Tissue Defects

The skin is extremely important in protecting repairs of deeper structures from the outside environment and preventing infection. The integument is commonly injured in complex hand trauma. Severe skin injury or defect can result in deformity, contractures, and diminished sensation and circulation. Büchler[37a] described three zones of injury: (1) the obviously contaminated central zone with skin destruction; (2) an adjacent zone that is characterized by extensive devascularization of the skin and soft tissues; and (3) the peripheral zone, which is normal in appearance but can result in functional limitation.[38,39] Skin coverage can be performed immediately (or acute setting) or may be delayed.[39–41] Immediate coverage allows for earlier ROM and initiation of rehabilitation. Delayed coverage affords the opportunity to better clean out the wound and minimize colonization and subsequent infection. The use of wound vacuum-assisted closure (VAC) is helpful in minimizing edema and promoting wound bed granulation.[42] The suction of these devices stimulates angiogenesis into the wound and promotes healing. Options for definitive coverage include split- or full-thickness skin grafts (STSGs of FTSGs), local or rotational flaps, pedicled flaps, and free flaps. The use of bovine collagen matrixes has also been used to facilitate wound coverage.[43,44] The best option depends on multiple factors, including patient-related issues and anatomy, surgeon experience, and injury pattern. For example, the use of a pedicled reverse radial forearm flap would generally be contraindicated in a patient with an incomplete palmar arch. The reconstructive ladder provides guidelines for reconstruction of defects based on complexity (Box 73.1).

Skin grafts are the simplest method of wound coverage. They do require a well-vascularized bed to be inset into. Two main types exist: STSGs and FTSGs. STSGs are generally harvested with a dermatome and can cover large surface areas. They can be fenestrated to maximize their area of coverage. They do contract and can be associated with hyperpigmentation. Wound VACs or bolstering of the graft and immobilization are helpful in optimizing take of the graft in the immediate setting. FTSGs are more durable and less likely to contract. However, they carry a higher risk of failure. Factors that contribute to skin graft failure include hematoma formation, diminished blood supply to the wound, improper immobilization, infection, and gapping between the graft and the bed. Skin grafts are less favored for wounds with exposed nerves, arteries, or tendons.

As the complexity of the wound increases, flaps may be indicated. Examples include exposed bone or cartilage, tendon (without paratenon), hardware, nerves, and vessels. Local, regional, and distant flaps types are defined. In addition, the flaps may be pedicled (rotated on their blood supply) or free (transported with their blood supply for reattachment within area of the wound). In addition, flaps may be random (no named blood supply) or axial (with a named blood supply). Local random flaps have one side of the flap communicating with the wound are of limited usefulness in larger or complex defects. Examples include V-Y advancement flaps for finger defects.

Regional flaps are useful in covering larger wounds. They are used from the same extremity as the injury. Examples include the reverse radial forearm flap (Fig. 73.10), the first dorsal metacarpal flap, and the posterior interosseous flap. The first dorsal metacarpal flap can help cover dorsal wounds to the thumb and hand. The radial forearm flap can cover wounds of the dorsal and volar aspects of the hand, wrist, and forearm. Although the donor site can sometimes be closed primarily, an STSG is commonly needed to cover it. In addition, as previously mentioned, the flap requires sacrifice of the radial artery, and the patient should have collateral flow from the ulnar artery for this flap to be used.

The groin flap is an excellent example of a distant axial pedicled flap (Fig. 73.11). It is supplied by the superficial circumflex iliac artery and can be used to cover large defects.[45–48] It is fairly easy to raise and inset the flap, but care must be taken not to injure the lateral femoral cutaneous nerve that lies in the wound. Disadvantages include the patient is "attached" to the pedicle for 3 to 4 weeks, the flap is then partially or completely taken down, and rehabilitation is limited while the pedicle remains attached.

Free flaps are among the most versatile wound coverage options for surgeons. They can provide a large area of coverage and can fill deep defects, providing an aesthetically pleasing wound. They are performed in a single stage and thereby allow for early rehabilitation. The timing of free flaps has been classified as emergent (within the first 24 hours of injury) and early (within the first 72 hours after the injury). The necessity to perform free flaps on an emergent and early basis is indicated if there are bony injuries, exposed hardware, or exposed unrepaired tendons, nerves, or joints.[11] Examples include lateral arm (Fig. 73.12), latissimus, and gracilis flaps. The lateral arm flap has advantages in hand coverage because of its proximity, it also provides pliable skin coverage.[49] The gracilis flap can be harvested with its nervous attachment and undergo both vessel anastomosis and nerve repair at the insertion site to provide a functional muscle transfer.[21]

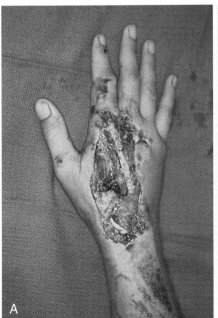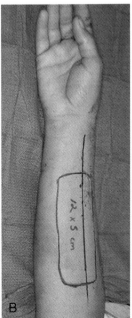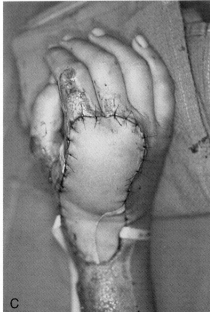

Fig. 73.10 Case example of a radial forearm flap. **A,** A patient sustained a wound with significant skin loss over the dorsal radial aspect of the hand. **B,** Landmarks for the flap harvest and dimensions are noted. **C,** The radial forearm flap is shown inset.

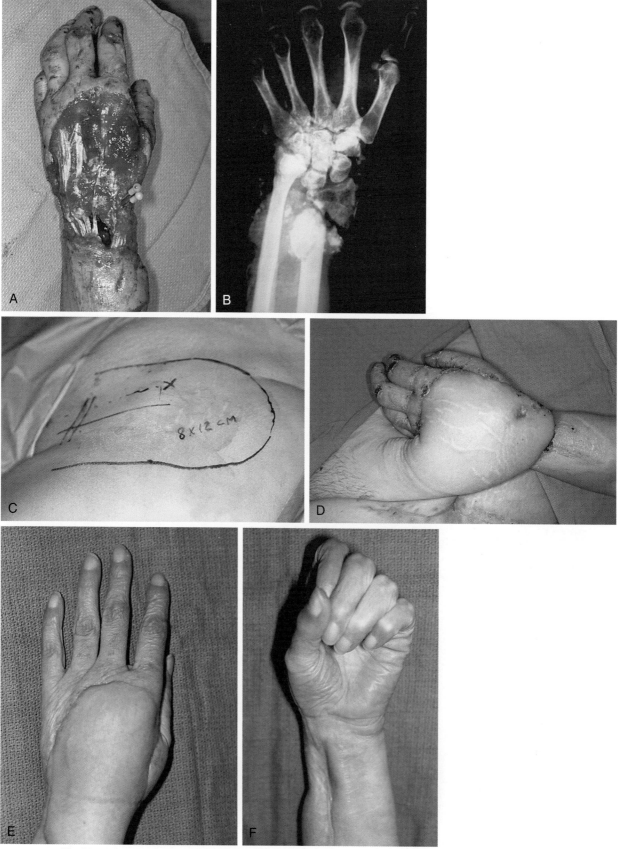

Fig. 73.11 A, A patient with a large dorsal defect over the hand with exposed tendons. **B,** Radiograph demonstrates highly comminuted distal radius fracture with significant bone loss. **C,** The flap is designed based on the superficial circumflex iliac artery. **D,** The flap is inset into the dorsum of the hand. **E,** The flap is shown after division. **F,** Finger range of motion after rehabilitation.

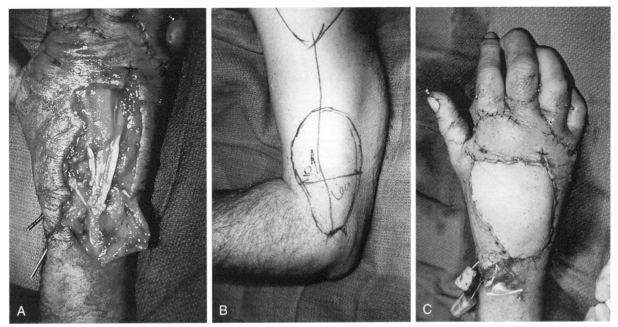

Fig. 73.12 A, A patient with a complex injury and significant skin defect. **B,** The design of the flap, which is anatomically based on the posterior radial collateral artery. **C,** The flap is inset over the dorsum of the hand after revascularization.

SUMMARY

Combined or complex injuries to the hand and upper extremity can be significant causes of long-term dysfunction and pain. Prompt diagnosis of all associated injuries and methodical treatment will help permit the earliest possible appropriate rehabilitation and allow for optimal outcomes.

REFERENCES

1. Abraham MK, Scott S. The emergent evaluation and treatment of hand and wrist injuries. *Emerg Med Clin North Am.* 2010;28(4):789–809. https://doi.org/10.1016/j.emc.2010.06.004.
2. Campbell DA, Kay SP. The hand injury severity scoring system. *J Hand Surg [Br].* 1996;21(3):295–298.
3. Trybus M, Lorkowski J, Brongel L, et al. Causes and consequences of hand injuries. *Am J Surg.* 2006;192(1):52–57.
4. McDonald 3rd AP, Lourie GM. Complex surgical conditions of the hand: avoiding the pitfalls. *Clin Orthop Relat Res.* 2005;(433): 65–71.
5. Hustedt JW, Bohl DD, Champagne L. The detrimental effect of decentralization in digital replantation in the United States: 15 years of evidence from the national inpatient sample. *J Hand Surg Am.* 2016;41(5):593–601. https://doi.org/10.1016/j.jhsa.2016.02.011.
6. Verhoeven N, Hierner R. High-pressure injection injury of the hand: an often underestimated trauma: case report with study of the literature. *Strategies Trauma Limb Reconstr.* 2008;3(1):27–33.
7. Tang JB, Wang ZT, Chen J, et al. A global view of digital replantation and revascularization. *Clin Plast Surg.* 2017;44(2):189–209. https://doi.org/10.1016/j.cps.2016.11.003.
8. Foo A, Sebastin SJ. Secondary interventions for mutilating hand injuries. *Hand Clin.* 2016;32(4):555–567. https://doi.org/10.1016/j.hcl.2016.07.006.
9. Neumeister MW, Brown RE. Mutilating hand injuries: principles and management. *Hand Clin.* 2003;19(1):1–15. v.
10. Tos P, Artiaco S, Titolo P, et al. Limits of reconstruction in mangled hands. *Chir Main.* 2010;29(4):280–282. https://doi.org/10.1016/j.main.2010.07.001.
11. Adani R, Tarallo L, Caccese AF, et al. Microsurgical soft tissue and bone transfers in complex hand trauma. *Clin Plast Surg.* 2014;41(3):361–383. https://doi.org/10.1016/j.cps.2014.03.002.
12. Hile D, Hile L. The emergent evaluation and treatment of hand injuries. *Emerg Med Clin North Am.* 2015;33(2):397–408. https://doi.org/10.1016/j.emc.2014.12.009.
13. Khouri JS, Bloom JM, Hammert WC. Current trends in the management of proximal interphalangeal joint injuries of the hand. *Plast Reconstr Surg.* 2013;132(5):1192–1204. https://doi.org/10.1097/PRS.0b013e3182a48d65.
14. Mangelson JJ, Stern P, Abzug JM, et al. Complications following dislocations of the proximal interphalangeal joint. *J Bone Joint Surg Am.* 2013;95(14):1326–1332.
15. Kapur B, Paniker J, Casaletto J. An alternative technique for external fixation of traumatic intra-articular fractures of proximal and middle phalanx. *Tech Hand Up Extrem Surg.* 2015;19(4):163–167. https://doi.org/10.1097/BTH.0000000000000102.
16. Nilsson JA, Rosberg HE. Treatment of proximal interphalangeal joint fractures by the pins and rubbers traction system: a follow-up. *J Plast Surg Hand Surg.* 2014;48(4):259–264. https://doi.org/10.3109/2000656X.2013.870909.
17. Samora JB, Klinefelter RD. Flexor tendon reconstruction. *J Am Acad Orthop Surg.* 2016;24(1):28–36. https://doi.org/10.5435/JAAOS-D-14-00195.
18. Sade I, Inanir M, Sen S, et al. Rehabilitation outcomes in patients with early and two-stage reconstruction of flexor tendon injuries. *J Phys Ther Sci.* 2016;28(8):2214–2219. https://doi.org/10.1589/jpts.28.2214.
19. Pauchard N, Pedeutour B, Dautel G. Graft reconstruction of flexor tendons. *Chir Main.* 2014;33(suppl):S58–S71. https://doi.org/10.1016/j.main.2014.05.007.
20. Asmus A, Kim S, Millrose M, et al. Rehabilitation after flexor tendon injuries of the hand. *Orthopade.* 2015;44(10):786–802. https://doi.org/10.1007/s00132-015-3160-6.
21. DeGeorge Jr BR, Becker HA, Faryna JH, et al. Outcomes of muscle brachialis transfer to restore finger flexion in brachial plexus palsy. *Plast Reconstr Surg.* 2017;140(2):307e–317e. https://doi.org/10.1097/PRS.0000000000003563.
22. Gulke J, Mentzel M, Krischak G, et al. Early functional passive mobilization of flexor tendon injuries of the hand (zone 2) : exercise with an exoskeleton compared to physical therapy. *Unfallchirurg.* 2017. https://doi.org/10.1007/s00113-017-0387-1.

23. Giesen T, Calcagni M, Elliot D. Primary flexor tendon repair with early active motion: experience in Europe. *Hand Clin.* 2017;33(3):465–472. https://doi.org/10.1016/j.hcl.2017.03.001.

24. Tang JB, Zhou X, Pan ZJ, et al. Strong digital flexor tendon repair, extension-flexion test, and early active flexion: experience in 300 tendons. *Hand Clin.* 2017;33(3):455–463. https://doi.org/10.1016/j.hcl.2017.04.012.

25. Frueh FS, Kunz VS, Gravestock IJ, et al. Primary flexor tendon repair in zones 1 and 2: early passive mobilization versus controlled active motion. *J Hand Surg Am.* 2014;39(7):1344–1350. https://doi.org/10.1016/j.jhsa.2014.03.025.

26. Puippe GD, Lindenblatt N, Gnannt R, et al. Prospective morphologic and dynamic assessment of deep flexor tendon healing in zone II by high-frequency ultrasound: preliminary experience. *AJR Am J Roentgenol.* 2011;197(6):W1110–W1117. https://doi.org/10.2214/AJR.11.6891.

27. Poggetti A, Novi M, Rosati M, et al. Treatment of flexor tendon reconstruction failures: multicentric experience with Brunelli active tendon implant. *Eur J Orthop Surg Traumatol.* 2017. https://doi.org/10.1007/s00590-017-2102-x.

28. Winspur I. The lost art of single-stage flexor tendon grafting. *J Hand Surg Eur Vol.* 2015;40(4):431. https://doi.org/10.1177/1753193415575985.

29. Dorf E, Blue C, Smith BP, et al. Therapy after injury to the hand. *J Am Acad Orthop Surg.* 2010;18(8):464–473.

30. Rasulic L. Current concept in adult peripheral nerve and brachial plexus surgery. *J Brachial Plex Peripher Nerve Inj.* 2017;12(1):e7–e14. https://doi.org/10.1055/s-0037-1606841.

31. Rbia N, Shin AY. The role of nerve graft substitutes in motor and mixed motor/sensory peripheral nerve injuries. *J Hand Surg Am.* 2017;42(5):367–377. https://doi.org/10.1016/j.jhsa.2017.02.017.

32. Means Jr KR, Rinker BD, Higgins JP, et al. A multicenter, prospective, randomized, pilot study of outcomes for digital nerve repair in the hand using hollow conduit compared with processed allograft nerve. *Hand (N Y).* 2016;11(2):144–151. https://doi.org/10.1177/1558944715627233.

33. Lee YH, Shieh SJ. Secondary nerve reconstruction using vein conduit grafts for neglected digital nerve injuries. *Microsurgery.* 2008.

34. Ahmad I, Akhtar MS. Use of vein conduit and isolated nerve graft in peripheral nerve repair: a comparative study. *Plast Surg Int.* 2014;2014:587968. https://doi.org/10.1155/2014/587968.

35. Kappos EA, Engels PE, Tremp M, et al. Peripheral nerve repair: multimodal comparison of the long-term regenerative potential of adipose tissue-derived cells in a biodegradable conduit. *Stem Cells Dev.* 2015;24(18):2127–2141. https://doi.org/10.1089/scd.2014.0424.

36. Agnew SP, Dumanian GA. Technical use of synthetic conduits for nerve repair. *J Hand Surg Am.* 2010;35(5):838–841. https://doi.org/10.1016/j.jhsa.2010.02.025.

37. Giusti G, Lee JY, Kremer T, et al. The influence of vascularization of transplanted processed allograft nerve on return of motor function in rats. *Microsurgery.* 2016;36(2):134–143. https://doi.org/10.1002/micr.22371.

37a. Büchler U. Hand surgery soft tissue defects. *Unfallchirug.* 1990;93(9):434.

38. Wharton R, Creasy H, Bain C, et al. Venous flaps for coverage of traumatic soft tissue defects of the hand: a systematic review. *J Hand Surg Eur.* 2017;42(8):817–822. https://doi.org/10.1177/1753193417712879.

39. Griffin M, Hindocha S, Malahias M, et al. Flap decisions and options in soft tissue coverage of the upper limb. *Open Orthop J.* 2014;8:409–414. https://doi.org/10.2174/1874325001408010409.

40. Mateev MA, Kuokkanen HO. Reconstruction of soft tissue defects in the extremities with a pedicled perforator flap: series of 25 patients. *J Plast Surg Hand Surg.* 2012;46(1):32–36. https://doi.org/10.3109/2000656X.2011.634562.

41. Ozbaydar M, Orman O, Ozel O, et al. Multiple extensor tendons reconstruction with hamstring tendon grafts and flap coverage for severe dorsal hand injuries. *Hand Surg Rehabil.* 2017;36(6):410–415. https://doi.org/10.1016/j.hansur.2017.07.004.

42. Moues CM, Heule F, Hovius SE. A review of topical negative pressure therapy in wound healing: sufficient evidence? *Am J Surg.* 2011;201(4):544–556. https://doi.org/10.1016/j.amjsurg.2010.04.029.

43. Carothers JT, Brigman BE, Lawson RD, et al. Stacking of a dermal regeneration template for reconstruction of a soft-tissue defect after tumor excision from the palm of the hand: a case report. *J Hand Surg [Am].* 2005;30(6):1322–1326.

44. Taras JS, Sapienza A, Roach JB, et al. Acellular dermal regeneration template for soft tissue reconstruction of the digits. *J Hand Surg Am.* 2010;35(3):415–421. https://doi.org/10.1016/j.jhsa.2009.12.008.

45. Scaglioni MF, Franchi A, Giovanoli P. Pedicled posteromedial thigh (pPMT) perforator flap and its application in loco-regional soft tissue reconstructions. *J Plast Reconstr Aesthet Surg.* 2017. https://doi.org/10.1016/j.bjps.2017.10.005.

46. Bajantri B, Latheef L, Sabapathy SR. Tips to orient pedicled groin flap for hand defects. *Tech Hand Up Extrem Surg.* 2013;17(2):68–71. https://doi.org/10.1097/BTH.0b013e31827ddf47.

47. Goertz O, Kapalschinski N, Daigeler A, et al. The effectiveness of pedicled groin flaps in the treatment of hand defects: results of 49 patients. *J Hand Surg Am.* 2012;37(10):2088–2094. https://doi.org/10.1016/j.jhsa.2012.07.014.

48. Al-Qattan MM, Al-Qattan AM. Defining the indications of pedicled groin and abdominal flaps in hand reconstruction in the current microsurgery era. *J Hand Surg Am.* 2016;41(9):917–927. https://doi.org/10.1016/j.jhsa.2016.06.006.

49. Ulusal BG, Lin YT, Ulusal AE, et al. Free lateral arm flap for 1-stage reconstruction of soft tissue and composite defects of the hand: a retrospective analysis of 118 cases. *Ann Plast Surg.* 2007;58(2):173–178. https://doi.org/10.1097/01.sap.0000232832.18894.2b.

Surgery Management for Replantation or Revascularization of the Hand

Neil F. Jones, David J. Graham, James Chang, Parivash Kashani

OUTLINE

CRITICAL POINTS

- Proper selection of candidates for replantation is very important. Although all attempts at reconstruction should be made, at times, the condition of the patient or the part may preclude successful replantation.
- Careful planning, meticulous operative technique, and intraoperative decision making are critical. One should adhere to the outlined sequence of steps for replantation.
- A well-vascularized replant with good soft tissue cover permits early range of motion to prevent tendon adhesions.

- Replantation in the upper extremity may be associated with a relatively high complication rate because of malunion or nonunion, joint stiffness, tendon adhesions, muscle contractures, poor sensory return, and cold intolerance.

Conclusion
- A replantation center provides comprehensive care for these complex injuries. Within the replantation center, close communication between the surgeon and hand therapist is essential.

Microsurgical techniques have made the salvage of devascularized digits, hands, and upper extremities possible. Trauma can result in either complete amputation or devascularization of parts. *Replantation* is the reattachment of a completely amputated part by restoration of arterial inflow and venous outflow, whereas *revascularization* is the restoration of arterial inflow, venous outflow, or both to an incompletely amputated part, no matter how small the point of attachment. This chapter focuses on the management of replantation; however, the principles presented also apply to revascularization.

The first successful replantation of an upper arm amputation was performed in 1962 by Malt and McKhann,[1] and the first successful replantation of an amputated thumb was performed in 1968 by Komatsu and Tamai.[2] Since then, replantation teams have been organized in major hospitals, and microsurgical techniques have become an integral part of the training of orthopedic and plastic hand surgeons.[3-5] The techniques of replantation in the upper extremity have been extrapolated to successful replantation of other parts of the body, including the lower limb,[6] the scalp,[7] the ear,[8] portions of the lip and nose, and the penis,[9] and have led directly to the evolution of elective microsurgical free tissue transfer.

Although success rates in microsurgery have risen, hand surgeons still need to critically evaluate the outcomes of replantation and revascularization. In some instances, a successful replantation or revascularization may lead to stiffness, insensibility, and pain, causing more dysfunction than immediate completion of the amputation. The purpose of this chapter is to outline principles in preoperative assessment and management, surgical technique, and postoperative therapy that will optimize overall hand function after traumatic amputation.

PREOPERATIVE ASSESSMENT AND MANAGEMENT

Transfer to a Replantation Service

Traumatic amputations and other severe hand injuries are best treated in a regional replantation center because of the availability of multiple hand microsurgeons and familiarity with preoperative, intraoperative, and postoperative protocols and clinical pathways. After the surgeon has decided, usually by telephone, that the patient and the amputated part are suitable for potential replantation, an established order of procedures is undertaken (Box 74.1). In many instances, it is difficult to assess the true severity of injury without direct examination. It is the policy of dedicated replantation centers to accept all possible candidates for evaluation of possible replantation.

The referring physician should ensure that hemorrhage from the amputation stump has been stopped by application of a pressure dressing and elevation. In cases of severe hemorrhage, fluid resuscitation is instituted. Tetanus prophylaxis is updated, and intravenous (IV) antibiotics are infused. The amputated part is then wrapped in sterile gauze moistened with saline solution, sealed in a plastic bag, and placed in a container of water and ice at a temperature of 4°C. The surgeon should also advise the referring physician as to the urgency of transfer of the patient and amputated part either by ambulance or, for major replantations, by helicopter. Radiographs of the part and the extremity are sent with the patient to save critical time in the receiving hospital.

Evaluation for Replantation Surgery

All transferred patients are received in the emergency department to be screened for other injuries. A rapid physical examination is performed to exclude any associated injuries. It is critical that life-threatening

---

BOX 74.1 Preoperative Checklist for Replantation

Telephone referral
Name, age, hand dominance, occupation
Mechanism of injury
Time of injury
Associated injuries
Medical history
Referring doctor and hospital
Coordinate transfer
    Via ambulance or helicopter
Instructions to transferring facility
    Ensure that patient is stable for transfer
    Apply pressure dressing to extremity
    Elevate extremity
    Update tetanus prophylaxis
    Administer cefazolin intravenously
    Wrap amputated part in wet sterile gauze; place in sealed plastic bag in container of ice and water
    Send radiographs with patient
Upon arrival in emergency department
    Review radiographs
    Type and screen
    Check complete blood count and pertinent laboratory test results
    Obtain operative consent for replantation and revascularization; completion amputation; transfusions; and possible vein, nerve, and skin grafts
In operating room
    General anesthesia or axillary block
    Warming blanket on operating table
    Aspirin suppository 325 mg per rectum
    Foley, intermittent pneumatic leg compression devices to prevent deep venous thrombosis
    Preparation of amputated part on back table: tagging of nerves, veins, and arteries

---

BOX 74.2 Amputations Suitable for Replantation

Thumb
Multiple digits
Transmetacarpal
Wrist
Forearm
Single digit in children

BOX 74.3 Absolute Contraindications to Replantation

Significant associated injuries
Multiple injuries within the amputated part
Systemic illness

BOX 74.4 Relative Contraindications to Replantation

Patient's age
Avulsion injuries
Prolonged warm ischemia time
Massive contamination
Psychological problems
Single-digit amputation in adults

---

concomitant injuries such as intracranial bleeding, cervical spine injury, and pneumothorax are ruled out. A member of the replantation team should obtain a careful history from the patient, including age, hand dominance, occupation, and preexisting systemic illness. Most important, a detailed description of the mechanism of injury usually allows the surgeon to determine whether the amputation was caused by a sharp transection or a crushing or avulsion mechanism. Radiographs of the amputated part and the proximal extremity should be obtained if they have not already been sent with the patient. It is important to exclude any associated fractures in the limb proximal to the level of amputation. Routine investigations include a chest radiograph, electrocardiogram, complete blood count, and electrolyte panel. Blood typing and cross-matching may be necessary for major limb replantations.

Replantation Decision Making
Indications

In general, any patient with a complete or partial amputation involving the upper extremity is a candidate for replantation or revascularization, but ideal candidates have sustained sharp, guillotine-type injuries of the thumb, multiple digits, hand, wrist, or forearm, and these wounds are only minimally contaminated (Box 74.2). However, the decision to proceed with replantation of an amputated part can be made only by an experienced microsurgeon or hand surgeon. Because the patient and family may expect a miraculous result, it is important that the physician referring such a patient to a replantation center explain that the

patient is being referred for evaluation by an experienced microsurgeon to determine whether replantation is possible rather than raising their hopes unrealistically. When faced with a difficult decision regarding replantation, the surgeon should consider whether the function of the hand can be improved by replantation compared with closing the amputation stump and fitting the patient with a prosthesis in the future. All patients undergoing possible replantation or revascularization must give consent for possible completion amputation.

Contraindications

Contraindications to replantation may be either *absolute* or *relative* (Boxes 74.3 and 74.4).

Absolute Contraindications

Significant associated injuries. Digital amputations are rarely associated with other major injuries, but major amputations of the arm are commonly associated with head, chest, and abdominal injuries. These may be life threatening and may preclude replantation of the upper extremity amputation.

Multiple injuries within the amputated part. Extensive damage along the digital arteries from a crush or avulsion mechanism may preclude replantation. If there is extensive crushing or degloving of the amputated part (Fig. 74.1) or if there are segmental amputations at multiple levels in the amputated extremity (Fig. 74.2), this will usually contraindicate replantation. Clinical inspection of the amputated part may be correlated with radiographs, which may reveal fractures at multiple levels.

Systemic illness. Finally, older adult patients with a history of a myocardial infarction, heart failure, chronic obstructive pulmonary disease, or poorly controlled insulin-dependent diabetes may not be candidates for prolonged surgery and anesthesia.

Relative Contraindications

Patient's age. Older adult patients may have significant systemic disease, but more important, the recovery of tendon and nerve function

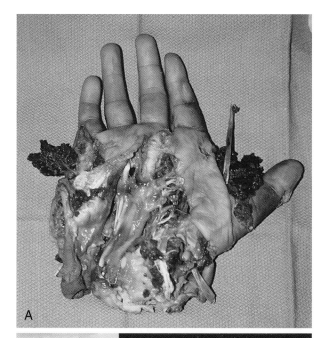

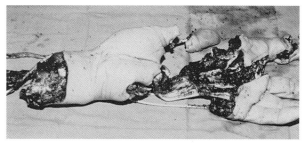

Fig. 74.2 A multiple-level injury is a contraindication to replantation.

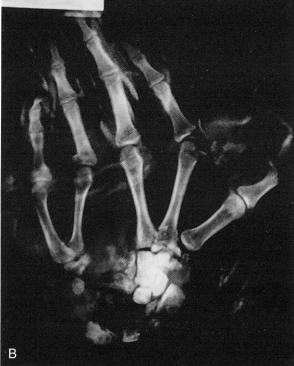

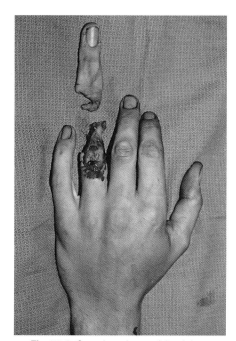

Fig. 74.3 Complete ring avulsion injury.

Fig. 74.1 A, This crush amputation of the hand is too extensively damaged to attempt replantation. **B,** Plain radiograph illustrates the extent of injury.

in the replanted digit is usually much poorer than in a younger patient; there is also the added risk of producing stiffness in the interphalangeal (IP) joints of adjacent uninjured fingers. Arteriosclerosis is relatively rare in the arteries of the upper extremity but can occasionally complicate the anastomoses of the radial and ulnar arteries during replantation at the wrist level in an elderly patient. Conversely, many older adult patients are quite active, and their hand function is critical to their activities of daily living (ADLs) and hobbies. The survival rate of replants in the older adult population is not dissimilar to that for adults.[10,11]

Replantation in young children may be more technically demanding because of the small caliber of the vessels and increased vasospasm,

but every effort should be made to replant a digit in a child because the digit will continue to grow. In addition, the results of the tendon and nerve repairs are much better than those in an adult.[12,13]

Avulsion injuries. With avulsion injuries, there is usually extensive damage to the digital arteries and digital nerves both proximal and distal to the level of amputation. Experimentally, injury to the digital artery has been shown to extend as far as 4 cm from the site of transection by electron microscopy compared with 0.8 cm under the operating microscope.[14] Avulsion amputations of the digits resulting from rodeo or water-skiing injuries are fairly obvious on clinical inspection, with long segments of the digital nerves or flexor and extensor tendons attached to the amputated digit. In contrast, the digital arteries are usually avulsed distally from within the digit, sometimes all the way to the trifurcation of the digital artery at the level of the distal interphalangeal (DIP) joint. Replantation will be successful only if a normal-appearing lumen of the distal digital artery can be found before the digital artery trifurcates and requires the use of interposition vein grafts or transposition of a neurovascular bundle from an adjacent digit.[15]

The most extreme example of an avulsion injury is the so-called ring avulsion injury. These injuries may range from circumferential lacerations at the level of the proximal phalanx with thrombosis or transection of the dorsal veins and both digital arteries to complete degloving of the soft tissue envelope of the digit or amputation of the digit through the DIP joint (Fig. 74.3). The simplest classification of ring avulsion injuries by Urbaniak and colleagues[16] consists of three categories (Box 74.5). This classification was subsequently expanded by Kay and colleagues[17] into four categories (Box 74.6).

BOX 74.5 Classification of Ring Avulsion Injuries by Urbaniak and colleagues[16]

Class I: adequate circulation
Class II: inadequate circulation
Class III: complete degloving or complete amputation

BOX 74.6 Classification of Ring Avulsion Injuries by Kay and colleagues[17]

Class I: circulation adequate with or without skeletal injury
Class IIa: arterial circulation inadequate; no skeletal injury
Class IIv: venous circulation inadequate; no skeletal injury
Class IIIa: arterial circulation inadequate with fracture or joint injury
Class IIIv: venous circulation inadequate with fracture or joint injury
Class IV: complete amputation

Arterial revascularization requiring interposition vein grafts usually is necessary for class IIa and IIIa injuries, whereas class IIv and IIIv injuries require venous anastomoses. Class IV complete degloving or complete amputations require a full replantation procedure. Approximately 75% of class II, III, and IV ring avulsion injuries can be successfully salvaged by revascularization or replantation.[16–18] A systematic review[19] of ring avulsion inquires has suggested that outcomes are superior for type I and II and that select type III injuries that can be treated with replantation. A type III injury has a tendency to produce a stiffer digit, with poorer two-point discrimination.

Prolonged warm ischemia time. Muscle is the one tissue most susceptible to ischemia and begins to undergo irreversible changes after 6 hours at room temperature. Because a proximal forearm or upper arm amputation contains significant muscle mass, it is vitally important that such amputations be cooled as quickly as possible and, if necessary, reperfused through arterial shunts to reduce the warm and cold ischemia times and allow successful replantation. Because the digits do not contain any muscle, they have a much longer ischemic tolerance. With multiple digital amputations, successful replantations after 33 hours of warm ischemia[20] and after 94 hours of cold ischemia[21] have been reported. A hand amputation was successfully replanted after 54 hours of cold ischemia.[22] Despite some authors reporting reasonable success rates for replantations with delayed presentations over 24 hours,[23] these represent extreme anecdotal cases, and every effort should be made to streamline transfer and preparation of patients.

Massive contamination. Radical surgical debridement precedes any major upper extremity replantation, but occasionally, massive contamination in farm injuries or by impregnation of all tissues by oil or grease in industrial injuries may prevent complete debridement and therefore preclude replantation because of the risk of infection and overwhelming sepsis.

Psychological problems. Self-inflicted amputations, usually of the hand or wrist, may precede a later successful suicide attempt. These patients definitely require an emergency psychiatric evaluation before any decision regarding replantation is made.[24]

Self-inflicted amputations may not be an absolute contraindication to replantation. Some reports of good early outcomes have been reported after such events.[25]

Single-digit amputations. Although a single-digit amputation should always be replanted in children, replantation of a single digit in an adult remains controversial.[26] Even though viability can be restored after amputation proximal to the proximal interphalangeal (PIP) joint, digital motion is compromised because of the adhesions associated with flexor tendon repairs in zone II, resulting in less than satisfactory flexion at the PIP and DIP joints. Replantation of an index finger amputation proximal to the PIP joint in an adult is almost universally unrewarding because the brain excludes the index finger and substitutes the middle finger for thumb–middle finger pinch. Similarly, replantation of a single middle finger, ring finger, or small finger may interfere with the motion of the other two fingers because of the common origin of the flexor digitorum profundus (FDP) tendons.[27] However, replantation of a single digit amputation through the middle phalanx distal to the insertion of the flexor digitorum sublimis (FDS) tendon[27,28] or through

the distal phalanx may provide excellent sensory return and full flexion at the PIP joint is maintained.[29,30]

A recent systematic review challenged the traditional view that distal digital replantation yields little functional gain, reporting a high success rate and good overall functional gains with distal replantation.[31]

SURGICAL TECHNIQUE

Preparation of the Amputated Part

If the surgeon decides that the patient and the amputated part fulfill the criteria for replantation, the amputated part and radiographs are taken to the operating room so that the amputated part can be prepared while the patient is still being made ready for anesthesia and surgery. The amputated part is cleaned with routine bactericidal solution and placed on a small operating table. If there is gross contamination, the part can be irrigated with sterile saline solution. All the structures in the amputated part are then identified and tagged, initially under loupe magnification and later under the operating microscope.

Skin Incisions

In an amputated digit, two midlateral incisions are made so that anterior and posterior skin flaps can be mobilized to provide access to the radial and ulnar neurovascular bundles.[16] For ring avulsion injuries, a single dorsal midline incision may sometimes be used. For arm and forearm amputations, the incisions are not placed directly overlying the nerves and arteries because it is likely that primary closure will not be possible, and it is better not to place skin grafts directly over the repaired arteries and nerves. Contused skin margins and any contaminated subcutaneous tissue are sharply debrided.

Debridement

In major forearm and upper arm amputations, it is difficult to determine how much of the muscle will eventually remain viable. Obviously contused, lacerated, or contaminated muscle must be sharply debrided. Carpal tunnel release and fasciotomies are usually required in upper arm and forearm amputations. These incisions are designed over the anterior and posterior forearm muscle compartments and over the second and fourth metacarpals to provide access to the intrinsic muscle compartments.

Tagging of the Neurovascular Structures

Under loupe magnification or the operating microscope, the two digital arteries and the radial and ulnar digital nerves are identified through the midlateral incisions and traced in a distal-to-proximal direction to identify the digital nerves and arteries at the level of the amputation. The two digital arteries and two digital nerves are identified with vascular clips to allow easier identification later in the procedure. We recommend tagging the nerve ends with medium-sized hemoclips and the arteries with small-sized hemoclips to differentiate these structures before coaptation or anastomosis. The digital nerves are cut 1 to 2 mm distal to the level of the amputation until a normal-appearing fascicular pattern is seen. Similarly, the digital arteries are cut with the microdissecting scissors and the vessel lumen dilated with a vessel dilator.

The dorsal skin flap is elevated distally in the plane between the subcutaneous tissues and the underlying extensor tendons to visualize the dorsal veins within the subcutaneous tissues. The dorsal skin is then elevated for 1 to 2 mm from the level of the amputation to identify two or three veins.

In upper arm and forearm amputations, the brachial, radial, and ulnar arteries, together with the median, ulnar, and radial nerves and several large subcutaneous veins, need to be similarly identified and tagged.

Preparation of Flexor and Extensor Tendons

The extensor tendon in the amputated digit does not usually retract and can be gently elevated from the underlying periosteum for a distance of 5 mm distal to the amputation. If the tendon end is ragged, it can be transected sharply with a scalpel. The FDP and FDS tendons may be apparent at the level of the amputation or may be found more distally in the digit, depending on the position of the hand at the time of amputation. The flexor tendon sheath will need to be incised to identify the two flexor tendons, but care should be taken to preserve at least 50% of the A2 and A4 pulleys to prevent postoperative bowstringing. The ends of the two flexor tendons should be cut sharply with a scalpel to debride any ragged or contaminated tissue. A core suture of 3-0 or 4-0 braided nylon may be placed into the FDP tendon before bony fixation of the amputated part because it may become more difficult to place this core suture later in the replantation sequence.

Bone Shortening and Fixation

Bone shortening is an integral component of replantation surgery in all upper extremity amputations because it potentially allows primary nerve repair and end-to-end vessel anastomoses. Depending on the level of amputation, the surgeon needs to decide whether bone shortening should be performed on the amputated part only, on the amputation stump only, or in both places. However, it is important to maintain the mobility of the metacarpophalangeal (MCP), PIP, and DIP joints and the insertion of the flexor and extensor tendons.

The periosteum on the amputated bone is elevated away from the bone end. A small hole is made in a piece of Esmarch's bandage or surgical glove, and the bone end is placed through this hole to protect the soft tissues during bony resection. The bone is then cut transversely using a power saw. In forearm amputations, the radius and ulna may need to be shortened 2.5 to 5 cm, and in upper arm amputations, the humerus may need to be shortened 4 to 8 cm to allow primary nerve and muscle repair.

Rigid internal fixation is the technique of choice in replantation surgery, primarily to allow early protected motion of the adjacent joints. Although Kirschner wire (K-wire) fixation is a rapid and simple technique, more rigid fixation will allow earlier and more aggressive postoperative therapy. For replantations through the phalanges, 90/90 intraosseous wiring[32] is used. In addition to 90/90 wire fixation (Fig. 74.4), longitudinal K-wires or plates can be used for transmetacarpal amputations. One should limit periosteal stripping in these cases, so wiring is usually preferred over plating. Rigid fixation of the radius and ulna requires 3.5-mm dynamic compression plates; 4.5-mm dynamic compression plates are necessary for rigid fixation of the humerus[33] (Fig. 74.5). These plates or intraosseous wires may be applied to the bone within the amputated part before fixation of the part to the amputation stump.

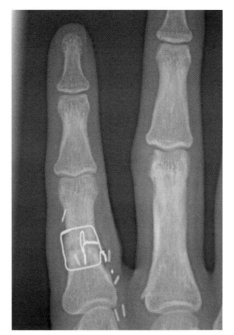

Fig. 74.4 Radiograph of 90/90 intraosseous wire fixation of the proximal phalanx in finger replantation.

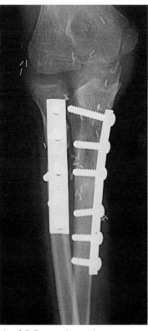

Fig. 74.5 Radiograph of 3.5-mm dynamic compression plate fixation of the radius and ulna in forearm replantation.

If the amputation passes through a joint, primary arthrodesis accomplishes both bony shortening and bony fixation. This is especially indicated in amputations of the thumb at the level of the MCP joint and amputations of the hand at the level of the radiocarpal joint. However, for amputations of the digit through the MCP joints, an alternative option is immediate placement of a silicone elastomer implant for arthroplasty to preserve motion at this joint.[34]

Hemostasis

Finally, hemostasis is achieved in the amputated part by bipolar coagulation because this is sometimes difficult to achieve after revascularization has been performed. Hemostasis is particularly important in transmetacarpal amputations, in which branches of the deep metacarpal arteries may bleed profusely, and in forearm amputations. The amputated part is now ready for replantation and is wrapped in gauze moistened with ice-cold saline solution until the patient is ready.

Preparation of the Amputation Stump

The patient is usually placed under general anesthesia. A urinary catheter must be inserted because of the length of the procedure. In addition, we routinely use stockings and intermittent compression devices on the legs to prevent deep venous thrombosis (DVT). The patient is covered with a heating blanket to maintain body temperature. A padded tourniquet is applied around the upper arm for preparation of the amputation stump for all amputations except those through the humerus itself. Debridement, identification, and tagging of all structures are performed exactly as described previously to prepare the amputated part. The flexor tendons may have retracted more proximally and, after retrieval, can be held out to a suitable length by transfixion with a 25-gauge needle. A similar core suture of 3-0 or 4-0 braided nylon can be placed in the proximal stump of the FDP tendon before replantation. After identification of the digital arteries, they can be mobilized more proximally into the palm. The ends of the digital arteries are then sharply cut with microdissecting scissors and the vessel lumen dilated with vessel dilators. The arteries are serially sectioned until a normal-appearing intima is seen under the operating microscope.

After debridement, identification, and tagging of all structures, the tourniquet is deflated to assess the force of arterial inflow. In transmetacarpal amputations, the ulnar artery may be released through Guyon's canal to expose the entire superficial palmar arch. Hemostasis is achieved in the proximal stump, especially in transmetacarpal amputations and in forearm and upper arm amputations.

Technique of Replantation

Although the following section describes the standard technique for replantation, revascularization procedures follow portions of this algorithm depending on the extent of injury. We advise using a sterile pen to compile a list of injured components. This provides a checklist for repair and, in multiple digit injuries, allows accurate recording of the injury and repair for decision making in postoperative therapy.

After the surgeon has established that there is good proximal arterial inflow and sufficient time (20 minutes) has elapsed since the previous tourniquet deflation, the tourniquet is reinflated to facilitate bony fixation and repair of the flexor and extensor tendons and digital nerves.

A definite sequence of repair during digital replantation has been advocated:

1. Bony fixation
2. Extensor tendon repair
3. Flexor tendon repairs
4. Nerve repairs
5. Arterial anastomoses
6. Venous anastomoses
7. Skin closure

However, the sequence of repair is now more related to the individual surgeon's preference.[35] It is logical to perform the bony fixation, flexor and extensor tendon repairs, and digital nerve repairs under the tourniquet and then complete the replantation with the digital artery anastomoses and dorsal vein anastomoses. Alternatively, the authors sometimes perform the venous anastomoses *before* releasing the tourniquet and performing the arterial anastomoses so that the venous anastomoses (extremely tedious) are done in a bloodless field. In cases of multiple digit amputations, the authors usually proceed with a structure-by-structure approach (fix all bones, then all tendons and so on) rather than a finger-by-finger approach.

Bone Fixation

The distal amputated part is aligned with the proximal stump, and rigid internal fixation is completed using compression plates for the humerus, radius, and ulna; longitudinal K-wires, 90/90 intraosseous wiring, or compression miniplates for the metacarpals; and 90/90 intraosseous wiring for the phalanges. Rigid fixation allows earlier postoperative therapy. Lee and associates[36] compared fixation methods for digital replantation. They concluded that there was no detriment to fixation with a single longitudinal K-wire, compared with dual wires, crossed wires, and intraosseous wiring. Newer fixation methods involving intramedullary headless compression screws have been advocated for metacarpal and proximal phalangeal fractures,[37] a concept that may prove of benefit in the setting of replantation and allow for earlier mobilization.[38]

Extensor Tendon Repair

The extensor tendon is then repaired using 4-0 nonabsorbable interrupted mattress or figure-of-8 sutures.

Flexor Tendon Repair

The hand is then turned over, and the volar periosteum is repaired with 5-0 absorbable sutures. Both FDP and FDS tendons are repaired if possible. The flat FDS tendon is repaired with interrupted mattress or modified Kessler sutures of 4-0 braided nylon. The two core sutures previously placed into the proximal and distal stumps of the FDP tendon are then tied, and the tendon repair is completed with a running circumferential suture using 6-0 monofilament suture. In both flexor tendons, a second horizontal mattress suture with 3-0 or 4-0 braided nylon is used to achieve a four-strand core repair that will allow early active motion.

Nerve Repair. The microscope is then brought into position, and the proximal and distal digital nerves are coapted by an epineurial repair using 9-0 or 10-0 nylon sutures. In more proximal amputations at the wrist, forearm, or upper arm level, a group fascicular repair of the median, ulnar, and radial nerves is performed, again using 9-0 nylon sutures. Obviously, the median, ulnar, and radial nerve repair should be performed without any tension at the site of repair, and this is usually possible because of the previous bony shortening.

Arterial Anastomoses

If the usual tourniquet time of 120 minutes has not been exceeded during bony fixation, extensor and flexor tendon repair, and the nerve repair, the venous anastomoses can be started under the tourniquet. Otherwise, the tourniquet is deflated, and the arterial and venous anastomoses are performed with the tourniquet down. If the digital arteries can be approximated under minimal tension using a double-approximator clamp, direct end-to-end anastomoses can be performed using interrupted 9-0 or 10-0 nylon sutures. If tension is excessive or if there is a definite segmental gap between the proximal and distal ends of the artery, interposition vein grafts will be necessary. In digital replantations, both digital arteries should be repaired, if possible, but most digits can be successfully replanted by anastomosis of only one digital artery. In the forearm, both the radial and ulnar arteries should be repaired.

Venous Anastomoses

Two or three dorsal veins in each digit are anastomosed end to end using standard microsurgical techniques, usually using 10-0 nylon sutures. If there is any tension whatsoever on the venous anastomoses when the proximal and distal stumps of the vein are introduced into the approximator clamp, interposition vein grafts should be considered. For transmetacarpal amputations and amputations at the level of

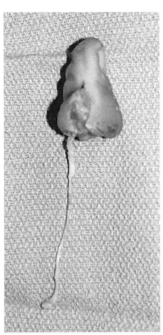

Fig. 74.6 Thumb replantation using interposition vein graft to distal ulnar digital artery.

the wrist, at least three or four dorsal veins should be anastomosed, approximately two veins for each artery.

Interposition Grafts. Interposition vein grafts may be required in three circumstances:

1. When bony shortening cannot be performed to preserve a functional joint.
2. In avulsion or crush injuries in which there is an extensive zone of injury along the artery.
3. In thumb amputations in which the ulnar digital artery is usually the dominant arterial blood supply to the thumb, it is necessary to hypersupinate the hand to perform an end-to-end anastomosis of the ulnar digital artery of the thumb. It is much easier to anastomose an interposition vein graft to the larger ulnar digital artery while the amputated thumb is on the back table (Fig. 74.6).

Vein grafts can be harvested from the volar aspect of the distal forearm for digital replantations or from the dorsum of the foot and lower leg for forearm vessels. Y-shaped vein grafts may be harvested to facilitate anastomosis of a single common digital artery to two digital arteries in adjacent digits.[39]

Many interposition vein grafts or arterial grafts can be anastomosed to the distal digital artery in the amputated part on a back table before bony fixation. Saha and associates[40] reported that there was no significant difference in the survival rates of dysvascular digits treated with a vein graft comparted with direct arterial repair and concluded that surgeons should have a low threshold to use vein grafts.

Reperfusion of the Amputated Part

After the arterial anastomoses or interposition vein grafts have been completed, the microsurgical clamps are released. All anastomoses are bathed with papaverine, and the extremity is irrigated with warm saline solution. Successful restoration of perfusion to the amputated digit or extremity is then assessed by return of turgor and color to the distal pulp and capillary refill in the distal phalanx. The patency of each arterial and venous anastomosis should then be tested using Acland's test,[41] stripping a segment of vessel with two-vessel dilators distal to the anastomosis, followed by release of the proximal vessel dilator.

Closure

When the surgeon is satisfied with perfusion of the extremity, the skin can be closed. Tight closure should be avoided because this will compress the venous outflow and lead to secondary venous thrombosis. Skin flaps can be transposed as Z-plasties, or small split-thickness skin grafts can be applied even directly over arterial or venous anastomoses or vein grafts. It is essential that dressings remain loose and are not applied circumferentially. Finally, the extremity is immobilized in a loose protective dorsal blocking plaster orthosis and is elevated.

Postoperative Care and Monitoring

After completion of the microsurgical anastomoses, a bolus of 40 mL of dextran 40 is given intravenously on release of the microsurgical clamps followed by a continuous infusion of dextran 40 at 25 mL/hr for 5 days (based on a 70-kg adult). Aspirin (81 mg) is given daily, and antibiotics are continued for several days at the discretion of the surgeon, depending on the degree of contamination. Heparin anticoagulation is not used in most replantations, except when there has been an extensive crushing injury or there have been prolonged difficulties restoring arterial inflow or venous outflow. The dose of continuous IV heparin is adjusted based on the activated partial thromboplastin time. However, heparin may cause hemorrhage within the replant itself,[42] producing edema and swelling, which may result in compression of the arterial or venous anastomoses and eventually secondary thrombosis. Furthermore, one must consider the systemic risks of anticoagulation for each patient individually. Buckley and Hammert[43] examined the evidence for anticoagulation after digital replantation and concluded that there is limited scientific evidence. However, they recommend using aspirin 325 mg/day for 5 days for standard replants and added subcutaneous low-molecular-weight heparin (LMWH) for DVT prophylaxis in immobile patients.

Levin and Cooper[44] remarked that "most surgeons agree that the most important factor in preventing arterial or venous thrombosis is excellent microsurgical technique, and although anticoagulants may be a useful adjunct, they can never substitute for a properly performed anastomosis." Efanov[45] reported that progressive tapering of IV heparin appeared to increase survival rates in finger replants, particularly for arterial insufficiency. Nikolis and associates[46] commented that in their initial series, the use of IV heparin was associated with a 3.59-fold increased risk of a complication and concluded that routine IV heparin is not warranted. A systematic review by Chen and associates[47] found no difference in replant success rates between LMWH and UFH, with a lower risk of bleeding and hypocoagulability after use of LMWH.

The patient should not be allowed to smoke because of the potentially detrimental effect of the vasoconstrictive mechanism of nicotine.[48] Experienced nursing staff should monitor the perfusion of the replant hourly for 72 hours by inspecting the color of the fingertip and the capillary refill. If the fingertip becomes pale with slow capillary refill, arterial thrombosis or vasospasm of the arterial inflow should be suspected. If the fingertip becomes swollen and blue with increased capillary return, this indicates venous congestion as a result of constrictive dressings or thrombosis of the venous anastomoses.

More objective techniques of postoperative monitoring of perfusion after replantation include temperature monitoring,[49] laser Doppler flowmetry,[50] transcutaneous Po_2[51] pulse oximetry,[52] and fluorescein injection. Differential temperature monitoring by comparison of the temperature of the replanted digit with an adjacent normal digit or the contralateral hand is one of the most common techniques. A temperature differential of 2°C or an absolute temperature of less than 30°C mandates immediate reexploration of the arterial and venous anastomoses.[49] A pediatric pulse oximeter probe loosely secured to the fingertip has proved to be the simplest technique for postoperative

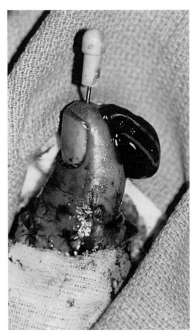

Fig. 74.7 Application of leeches for venous congestion.

monitoring and provides continuous oxygen saturation readings as well as the pulse rate within the digit.[52] Loss of the pulse indicates arterial occlusion, whereas a decrease in the oxygen saturation to less than 90% may indicate venous occlusion.

Reexploration of a Failing Replant

If clinical examination or a more objective monitoring technique suggests that perfusion of the replanted part is compromised, the surgeon should initially check that congealed blood within the dressings has not become constricting. All dressings should be removed, and if any sutures appear tight, these should be cut immediately. If color and capillary refill of the fingertip do not improve, the patient should be returned immediately to the operating room for reexploration of the arterial and venous anastomoses. If there is thrombosis or lack of flow, the anastomosis should be taken down and revised; however, this usually necessitates the use of an interposition vein graft. In cases of venous congestion in which no further venous anastomoses can be performed, the nail plate should be removed, the nail bed roughened, and heparin-soaked pledgets applied to promote venous bleeding.[53] Alternatively, serial application of leeches can occasionally salvage replants compromised by venous congestion (Fig. 74.7).[54] If leeches are used, it is imperative that third-generation cephalosporin antibiotics be administered as prophylaxis against *Aeromonas hydrophila* infection.

Replantation for Specific Levels of Amputation
Distal Phalanx

With sharp amputations through the distal phalanx, replantation may be a superior option to any other form of fingertip coverage. Although it can be technically demanding because of the small size of the distal digital arteries, it restores a virtually normal appearance to the finger or thumb, and the fingertip will regain very satisfactory sensation if the digital nerves can be approximated. A 0.028- or 0.035-inch K-wire is passed retrogradely through the distal fragment of the distal phalanx, and the amputated distal phalanx is partially sutured with one or two sutures along its palmar surface to temporarily stabilize the distal fragment. One digital artery and the two digital nerves are repaired under the operating microscope. The distal phalanx is then reduced, and the

K-wire is drilled antegradely to just beneath the articular surface of the distal phalanx or, if necessary, across the DIP joint into the middle phalanx.

Venous egress from the replanted distal phalanx may be a problem. Occasionally, after release of the tourniquet, a small dorsal vein can be identified just proximal to the nail fold, and a single venous anastomosis is performed. Alternative solutions to prevent venous congestion include removal of the nail plate and application of heparin-soaked pledgets, temporary application of leeches, or the creation of an arteriovenous anastomosis between the other distal digital artery and a proximal vein.[55] Finally, the dorsal skin and nail bed are loosely repaired.

Middle Phalanx

Good functional results can be achieved after replantation of digital amputations *distal* to the insertion of the FDS tendon on the middle phalanx. This is because PIP joint flexion is fully maintained, and the return of sensation is relatively good after repair of the digital nerves. The FDP tendon is repaired in a zone where it is the only tendon; thus, gliding is not restricted by scarring to the adjacent FDS tendon.

Proximal Phalanx

The results of replantation of amputations through the proximal phalanges are compromised by tendon adhesions in zone II. It is therefore essential to use the same meticulous technique to repair the FDP and FDS tendons in a replanted finger as in an isolated zone II flexor tendon repair. If K-wires are used in the bony fixation, they should not transfix the MCP or PIP joints so that early gentle passive range of motion (PROM) and active range of motion (AROM) exercises can be instituted.

If there is destruction of the articular cartilage at the PIP joint, arthrodesis of the PIP joint in a functional position is mandated. PIP joint arthrodesis can be accomplished by the same techniques of bony fixation used for replantation, preferably using 90/90 intraosseous wiring. The PIP joint of the index finger is usually arthrodesed in a position of 20 degrees of flexion, and the PIP joints of the middle, ring, and small fingers are positioned at angles of 30, 40, and 50 degrees, respectively.

In this region, the surgeon must consider the long postoperative rehabilitation and overall marginal functional outcome compared with completion amputation for each patient. PIP joint fusion commonly results in a stiff digit that may be bypassed in normal daily activities. If other fingers have associated injuries, including tendon lacerations, then single-digit amputations in this region should not be replanted to allow early rehabilitation of the remaining fingers (Fig. 74.8).

Multiple Digits

With multiple individual digital amputations, either through the proximal or middle phalanges, the surgeon can perform the replantation either in a digit-by-digit sequence or in a structure-by-structure sequence. In the first technique, all the structures in a single finger are repaired before proceeding to replant the subsequent digits. In the structure-by-structure technique, the same structure is repaired in all the replanted digits sequentially. For example, bony fixation of all the digits is performed followed by repair of all the flexor tendons and so on. Which technique is used depends on the surgeon's preference, but a structure-by-structure sequence may be faster and associated with a slightly improved survival rate.[56] If a structure-by-structure approach is selected, the digital arteries in each digit are repaired last so that repair of other structures is not obscured by bleeding.

Replantation should always be attempted when more than two digits have been amputated, even though the circumstances may be less

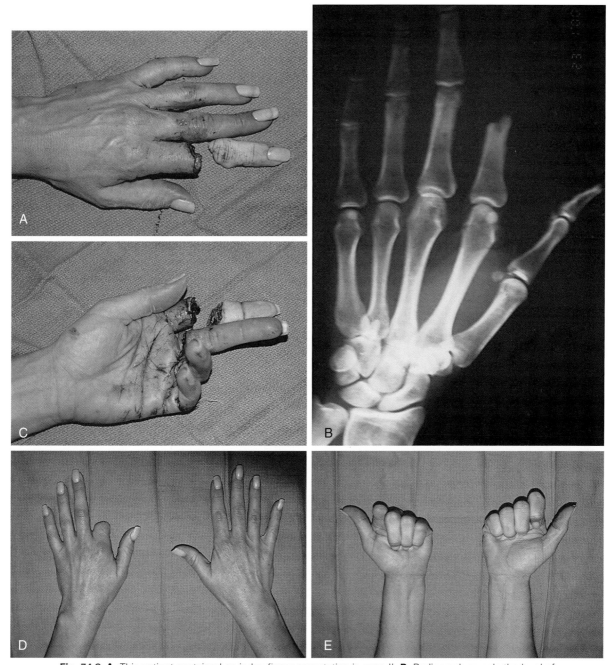

Fig. 74.8 A, This patient sustained an index finger amputation in zone II. **B,** Radiograph reveals the level of index finger amputation. **C,** Exploration of the middle finger revealed complete transection of the flexor digitorum profundus and flexor digitorum sublimis tendons in zone II. To allow optimal rehabilitation of the middle finger, the index finger was not replanted. **D,** Four months after left index finger completion amputation and left middle finger zone II flexor tendon repair (dorsal view). **E,** Four months after left index finger completion amputation and left middle finger zone II flexor tendon repair (volar view) showing excellent left middle finger range of motion.

than ideal. Such "salvage" replantations may involve substitution of an amputated digit to replace a more important digit that cannot be replanted. For example, if in a multiple-digit amputation, the thumb is so badly damaged that it cannot be replanted, one of the other digits can occasionally be replanted in the thumb position to provide a better functional reconstruction of the hand. Similarly, replacement of a longer amputated digit from the ulnar side of the hand may preserve more appropriate length of a digit on the more important radial side of the hand or may allow PIP joint motion to be maintained in the transposed

replanted digit.[57] Most important, vein grafts, nerve grafts, skin grafts, and even small free skin flaps or free joint transfers can be salvaged from a nonreplanted digit to reconstruct an adjacent digit.[58]

Thumb

Because the thumb contributes 40% to the overall function of the hand, all patients with thumb amputations should be considered candidates for replantation[59,60] (Fig. 74.9). Most thumb amputations occur at or distal to the MCP joint, and because the thumb is relatively unprotected

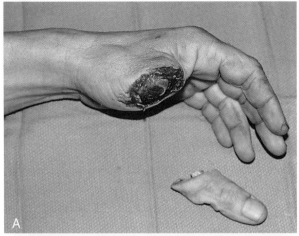

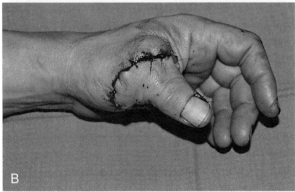

Fig. 74.9 A, Thumb amputation at the level of the metacarpophalangeal (MCP) joint. **B,** Immediate postoperative result of thumb replantation with MCP joint fusion.

by the other digits, avulsion amputations, such as in water-skiing or rodeo injuries, are relatively common.

Specific considerations for replantation of the thumb include the following:

1. Bony fixation of amputations through the MCP and IP joints
2. Use of interposition vein grafts to facilitate positioning of the thumb for completion of the arterial anastomosis
3. Use of immediate tendon transfers for avulsion injuries

If the thumb amputation involves disarticulation through the MCP or IP joint, bony shortening is performed on either side of the joint, and primary arthrodesis of the joint is performed using either crossed K-wires, tension-band wiring, or 90/90 intraosseous wiring in a position of function.

The ulnar digital artery of the thumb is usually the dominant arterial blood supply to the thumb, and it is usually much easier to anastomose an interposition vein graft end to end to the ulnar digital artery during preparation of the thumb on the back table. The vein graft can then be anastomosed to the radial artery on the dorsal aspect of the thumb–index finger webspace in a much more convenient position for completing the arterial anastomosis than having to hypersupinate the hand. If the radial digital artery to the thumb is of satisfactory caliber, this can also be repaired end to side to the same vein graft "upstream" to the anastomosis of the vein graft to the ulnar digital artery.

In avulsion injuries of the thumb, if the extensor pollicis longus and flexor pollicis longus tendons have been avulsed from their musculotendinous junction, immediate tendon transfers can be performed using the extensor indicis proprius to the extensor pollicis longus and the FDS from the ring finger to the flexor pollicis longus.

Transmetacarpal

Excellent functional results can be achieved after replantation of transmetacarpal amputations[61] (Fig. 74.10). Care must be taken during bony fixation to prevent malrotation of an individual digit because rotation at the metacarpal level translates into a greater functional deficit than a similar degree of malrotation further distally in the digit. Bony fixation can be achieved very simply by longitudinal K-wires in children or with rigid internal fixation with plates and screws in adults. At least 1 cm of bony shortening should be performed to prevent secondary intrinsic tightness in the fingers.

The carpal tunnel and Guyon's canal should be released prophylactically during the initial preparation of the amputation stump so that postoperative swelling does not result in compression of the median nerve or, more importantly, the ulnar artery. Finally, branches of the deep metacarpal arteries should be identified both in the distal amputated part and in the amputation stump, and these should be ligated to prevent postoperative hemorrhage and the development of hematoma after revascularization has been completed.

Wrist

Replantation at the transcarpal level is technically much easier than replantation of amputations across the palm or out in the digits because the radial and ulnar arteries and dorsal veins are much larger than the common digital and proper digital arteries and veins. Specific considerations for amputations at the level of the wrist include the technique of bony shortening, the need for fasciotomies of the intrinsic muscles, and whether primary nerve repair or delayed secondary nerve grafting is required.

There are three choices for bony shortening of amputations around the level of the wrist:

1. Partial or total carpectomy and primary arthrodesis of the wrist, which is especially indicated if the radiocarpal joint is destroyed or in a young working individual
2. Proximal row carpectomy if the distal articular surface of the radius is preserved
3. Shortening osteotomy of the radius and Darrach resection of the distal ulna if the level of amputation is just proximal to the distal articular surface of the radius

Depending on the time required to revascularize the hand and the degree of postoperative swelling, it is usually advisable to perform fasciotomies of the thenar, hypothenar, and interosseous muscle compartments of the hand.

Primary epineurial or group fascicular repair of the median, ulnar, and superficial radial nerves is optimal if bony shortening allows this option. Otherwise, the nerve ends should be tagged and group fascicular nerve grafting performed as a secondary procedure a few weeks later.

Forearm and Upper Arm[62,63]

More proximal amputations through the forearm and upper arm (Fig. 74.11) are rarely caused by a sharp, guillotine-type mechanism, and there is usually extensive damage to the adjacent muscles. Radical debridement of the muscles on the amputated part and on the stump is essential to prevent secondary infection and overwhelming sepsis. Debridement of forearm and elbow amputations should be performed under a sterile tourniquet, but a tourniquet cannot be used for amputations above the elbow. Fasciotomies of the anterior and posterior forearm compartments are an absolute necessity, and release of the transverse carpal ligament and fasciotomies of the intrinsic muscles in the hand may also be necessary if there is excessive swelling of the hand or if increased compartmental pressures are measured after reperfusion of the hand.

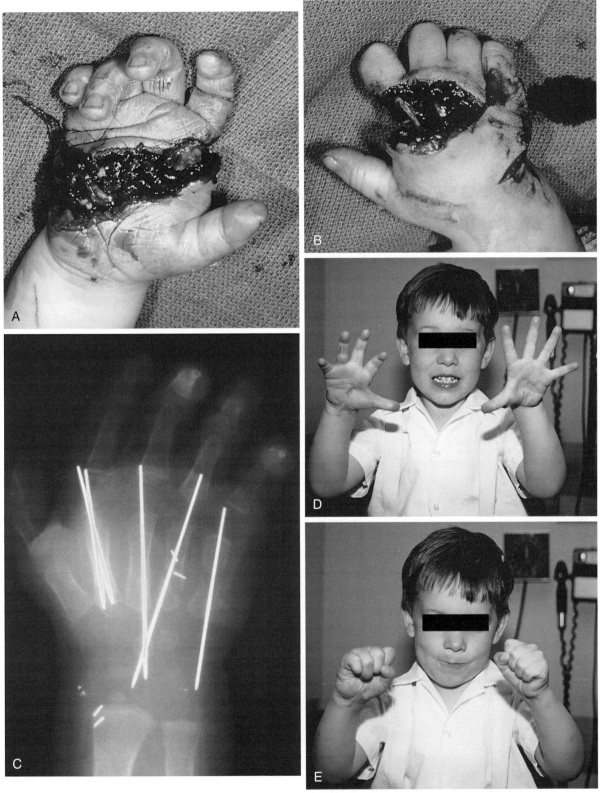

Fig. 74.10 A, Transmetacarpal near amputation with metacarpal fractures and devascularized fingers (volar view). **B,** Transmetacarpal near amputation with metacarpal fractures and devascularized fingers (dorsal view). **C,** Radiograph of longitudinal K-wire fixation of metacarpals. **D,** Postoperative view 2 years after revascularization. **E,** Postoperative view 2 years after revascularization showing full flexion.

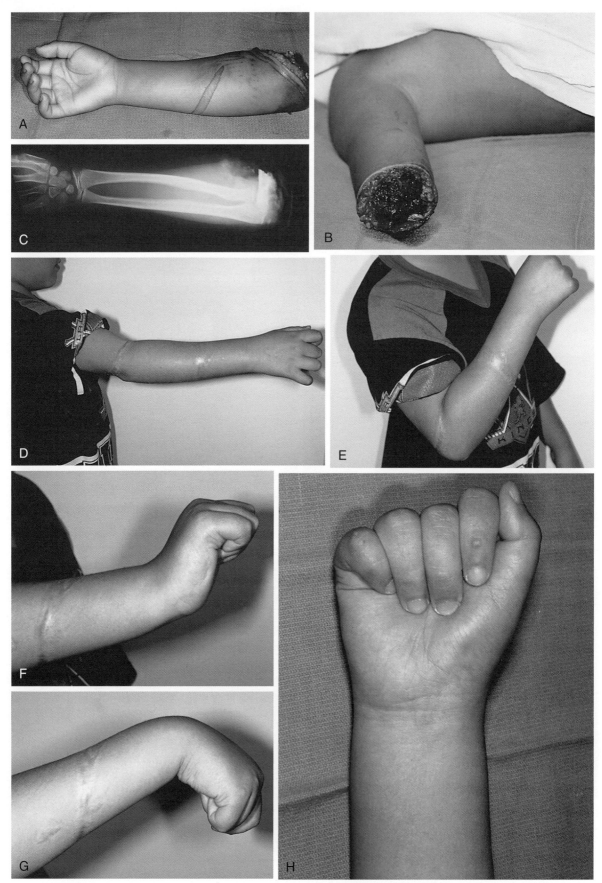

Fig. 74.11 A, This child sustained a sharp complete amputation of the right arm above the elbow. **B,** View of the proximal stump. **C,** Radiograph reveals the level of injury at the distal humerus. **D,** Postoperative result at 18 months showing excellent active elbow extension. **E,** Postoperative result at 18 months showing excellent active elbow flexion. **F,** Postoperative result at 18 months showing excellent active wrist extension. **G,** Postoperative result at 18 months showing excellent active wrist flexion. **H,** Postoperative result at 18 months showing excellent active finger flexion.

Arterial inflow must be reestablished as quickly as possible in amputations of the upper arm and forearm. If the ischemic time is relatively short, rigid bony fixation can be performed after radical debridement, followed immediately by arterial repair. The amount of bony shortening should be sufficient to allow primary repair of the median, ulnar, and radial nerves but may also facilitate skin closure over the vital structures. Rigid internal fixation is achieved with 4.5-mm dynamic compression plates for the humerus and 3.5-mm dynamic compression plates for the radius and ulna.

The arterial anastomosis is performed immediately after bony fixation, before the venous anastomoses are performed. After arterial inflow has been reestablished, the veins in the distal part are allowed to bleed to prevent this venous blood, which contains high concentrations of potassium and lactic acid, from reaching the systemic circulation and potentially triggering a cardiac arrest. Three to four venous anastomoses are then performed, but before release of the microsurgical clamps on the venous anastomoses, the patient is given IV sodium bicarbonate, again to neutralize the potential acidosis.

The flexor and extensor muscles or tendons are then repaired followed by epineurial or group fascicular repair of the median, ulnar, and radial nerves. If bony shortening was insufficient to allow primary nerve repair, the nerve ends should be tagged and sural nerve grafts performed as a secondary procedure.

The skin should be loosely approximated to cover the anastomoses and nerve repairs. If necessary, meshed split-thickness skin grafts can be harvested to provide complete coverage. Occasionally, an emergency free skin or muscle flap may be required to provide coverage of vital structures in amputations in which there has been extensive skin loss.

Unlike replantations in the hand, successful replantations through the forearm and upper arm may require a second-look operation 48 to 72 hours later to check for infection and to ensure that no further debridement of the wound is necessary. The best functional results are achieved with replantations through the distal forearm and wrist because the extrinsic flexor and extensor muscles remain innervated and satisfactory sensory return can be expected in young individuals.

Wide-Awake Replantation Surgery

Wide-awake surgery with local anesthetic, epinephrine, and no tourniquet has recently been popularized in hand surgery,[64] particularly for flexor tendon repair and tenolysis because direct dynamic assessment of tendon gliding can be performed intraoperatively. In the setting of an avascular digit, the use of epinephrine has historically been contraindicated. Wong and coworkers[65] have reported on five successful digital revascularizations and eight successful replantations using this technique. Four cases resulted in superficial necrosis, which healed by secondary intention.

POSTOPERATIVE THERAPY

Several principles apply to therapy after replantation and revascularization. First, these injuries occur suddenly, and the patient has no forewarning about the long-term consequences of the accident or the arduous task of rehabilitation that is ultimately required. The replantation team must anticipate the psychological needs of the patient. Second, each injury is unique; multiple structures in one digit may be involved, and the complexity of the injury and repair is multiplied if several digits are involved. Therefore, we have not found specific therapy protocols to be applicable. Instead, general guidelines can be established, but these need to be carefully individualized. It is critical that clear and continuous communication exist between the surgeon, the hand therapist, and the patient.

Postoperative rehabilitation for a patient with an amputation begins preoperatively with the decision to replant or revascularize. In certain situations, closure of the amputation with early hand therapy is a better alternative even though it may be technically possible to replant the digit.

During the operative procedure, postoperative therapy should be kept in mind as much as restoring blood flow. The most stable method of bone fixation is chosen to allow early motion protocols. As each tendon repair is performed, the surgeon should note the quality of the repair, the relationship of the repair site to pulleys, and the tension on the repair. PROM of the digit under direct visualization will provide the surgeon with valuable information about how aggressively to proceed with therapy. Tension on the nerve and vessel repairs should also be assessed. Finally, the quality of skin coverage (skin grafts, open wounds) will also influence the institution of postoperative therapy.

After the first week to 10 days, success of the replantation or revascularization is usually ensured, and attention can be directed toward regaining function. On the first postoperative visit (~7–10 days), the bulky dressing is removed, and the patient confronts the severity of the injury for the first time. It is vital to have the hand therapist present during this initial return visit. As the dressings are changed, the surgeon can discuss the injury and repair with both the patient and the therapist. Radiographs are reviewed, and the operative report is given to the therapist. Specific concerns, including arthrodeses, difficult tendon repairs, nerve repairs or vessel anastomoses under tension, and skin grafts are highlighted. An overall plan is developed with the hand therapist, and the patient participates in this process.

The rehabilitation strategies presented here are general guidelines. Each patient's treatment program is individualized based on numerous factors, including the following:

- Nature of the injury
- Fractures, type, and stability of skeletal fixation
- Joint mobility or arthrodesis
- Quality and tension of tendon repairs (flexors, extensors, or both)
- Quality and tension of nerve repairs
- Quality, tension, and location of arterial repairs
- Quality, tension, and location of vein repairs
- Skin: open wounds, skin grafts, and skin flaps

Treatment may also be altered based on the patient's general medical health, associated injuries, and the psychosocial status. Ugurlar and coworkers[66] found that patients who initiated rehabilitation quickly and participated well were able to overcome the depression experienced after amputation. They also reported better functional outcomes in patients who had a good compliance to therapy and performed their home exercises regularly and with appropriate frequency.

General Guidelines for Postoperative Therapy
Digital Replantation
Days 0 to 4

1. Elevate the hand on pillows above the level of the heart. Excessive elevation may decrease arterial flow and should be avoided.
2. Avoid exposure to cold. Keep the patient warm.
3. Instruct the patient on the risks of smoking.
4. A dorsal or volar protective orthosis should be fabricated if the postoperative dressing is changed.

Days 5 to 14. If a volar orthosis was originally fabricated, it should be replaced by a dorsal protective orthosis with the wrist in neutral position, MCP joints in 45 to 70 degrees of flexion, and the PIP and DIP joints in extension (Fig. 74.12). This position may not be attainable initially; therefore, the orthosis should be serially adjusted to obtain the optimal position.

Begin wound care when cleared by the surgeon. Surgeons usually prefer to perform the first dressing change. Dressings should be

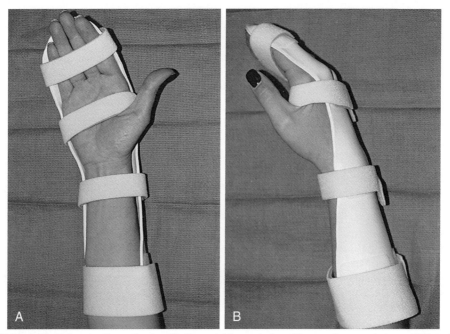

Fig. 74.12 A, Dorsal protective orthosis with the wrist in neutral position, metacarpophalangeal joints in 45 to 50 degrees of flexion, and proximal and distal interphalangeal joints in extension (volar view). **B,** Dorsal protective orthosis (dorsal view).

performed in a gentle and atraumatic manner to prevent vasospasm of the involved vessels. Dressing should be loose and nonadherent.

Begin early protective motion with passive wrist flexion to produce finger extension via the tenodesis effect and active wrist extension to produce finger flexion via the tenodesis effect. Perform AROM and PROM of all uninvolved fingers.

- Continue with wound care. Monitor for signs of infection.
- Continue with orthosis modification as needed.
- Upgrade home program as needed.

Days 14 to 21
1. Begin "place and hold" exercises (in intrinsic-plus and intrinsic-minus positions).
2. Continue with wound care.
3. Review and revise home program as needed.

Weeks 3 to 4
1. Continue with protected AROM and PROM exercises.
2. Begin scar massage if the wound has healed.
3. Begin light Coban wrap and retrograde massage only when cleared by the surgeon.

Weeks 4 to 5
1. Initiate composite finger flexion with the wrist in neutral position.
2. Initiate AROM and PROM exercises of the wrist beyond neutral position.
3. Continue with Coban wrap and retrograde massage.
4. May begin neuromuscular electrical stimulation (NMES) if cleared by the surgeon.

Weeks 5 to 6
1. Continue with scar management.
2. Begin composite wrist and finger flexion and extension exercises.
3. Begin gentle blocking exercises.
4. Begin differential tendon-gliding exercises.
5. Begin dynamic orthotic positioning of the fingers if indicated. Instruct the patient to check circulation with a dynamic orthosis and to increase wear time.
6. If flexor tightness is present, begin volar extension orthosis (Fig. 74.13) use at night.
7. Initiate light functional activities.

Weeks 6 to 12
1. Discontinue the protective orthosis at 6 weeks, except for protection when the patient is in public.
2. Continue light functional activities.
3. Progressively add light resistive exercises after 8 weeks.
4. Progress toward strengthening exercises.
5. Sensory evaluation can be performed at this time as a baseline to monitor nerve regeneration.

Weeks 12 and Later
1. Begin job simulation.
2. Continue with dynamic flexion and extension orthosis wear as needed to increase range of motion.
3. Sensory evaluation should continue every 5 to 6 weeks.

Thumb Replantation

Days 3 to 5
1. After the first postoperative dressing change, a dorsal protective thumb orthosis is fabricated with the wrist in neutral position (Fig. 74.14). The thumb should be positioned in abduction with no tension on replanted structures. If both flexor and extensors are involved, the flexor tendons should be favored over the extensor tendons. In other words, less tension should be placed on the flexor side because rupture of the flexor pollicis longus would require more extensive exploration and repair. Instruct the patient to elevate the hand.
2. Begin wound care.
3. Monitor the color and temperature of the replanted thumb.

Days 5 to 14
1. Begin gentle AROM and PROM of the wrist (gentle wrist flexion to about 10–15 degrees and extension to neutral position).
2. Begin PROM of the carpometacarpal (CMC) joint if repair sites are without tension.
3. Begin AROM of the CMC joint as the patient's tolerance improves with PROM exercises.
4. Begin passive MCP and IP flexion and active MCP and IP extension to the limit of the dorsal orthosis.

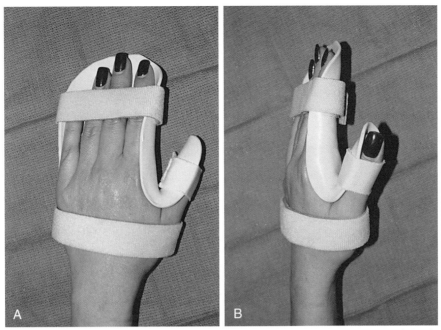

Fig. 74.13 A, Volar extension orthosis (dorsal view). **B,** Volar extension orthosis (lateral view).

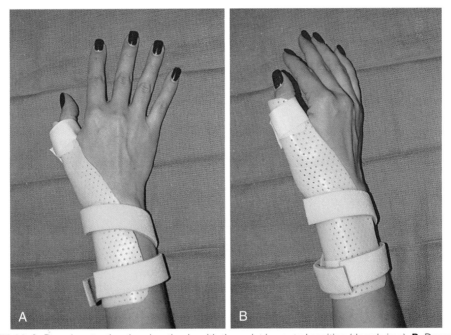

Fig. 74.14 A, Dorsal protective thumb orthosis with the wrist in neutral position (dorsal view). **B,** Dorsal protective thumb orthosis (lateral view).

Weeks 3 to 4
1. Begin active flexion of the MCP and IP joints and active extension to the limit of the orthosis.
2. After suture removal and if the wound has healed, begin scar massage.
3. Begin light Coban wrap and retrograde massage only when cleared by the surgeon.

Weeks 4 to 5
1. Initiate AROM and PROM of the wrist beyond neutral position.
2. Continue with Coban wrap.
3. Begin composite thumb motion at the CMC, MCP, and IP joints.

Weeks 5 to 6
1. Initiate NMES.
2. Begin gentle blocking exercises.
3. Begin light functional activities.
4. Discontinue the dorsal protective orthosis at 6 weeks except for protection when the patient is in public.

Weeks 6 to 12
1. Begin dynamic orthosis wear if there is any evidence of joint tightness.
2. Fabricate a first webspace orthosis if there is evidence of webspace tightness or incipient contracture.
3. Progressively add light resistive exercises after 8 weeks.
4. Continue with sensory reeducation and desensitization.

Weeks 12 and Later

1. Begin job simulation and return-to-work activities.
2. Continue with desensitization and sensory evaluation.

Hand Replantation

Days 2 to 7

1. Fabricate a dorsal protective orthosis with the wrist in neutral position, the MCP joints in 50 to 70 degrees of flexion, and the PIP and DIP joints in extension. Depending on the severity of the injury and the structures involved, the degree of MCP flexion may vary. For example, if the surgeon states that the nerve repairs and arterial anastomoses were under some tension, additional MCP flexion should be applied. Alternatively, if vein anastomoses or extensor tendon repairs were under tension, less MCP flexion should be applied. These considerations should be made on a case-by-case basis. Therefore, orthoses may require frequent adjustments to obtain the optimal position.
2. Begin passive finger flexion and extension to the limit of the orthosis.
3. Begin wound care.
4. Monitor the hand for any signs of infection or compromised circulation.

Days 7 to 14

1. Continue with early protective exercises.
2. Begin shoulder and elbow ROM exercises.
3. Instruct the patient on home exercises.

Weeks 3 to 4

1. Begin gentle retrograde massage of the digits.
2. Begin gentle tenodesis exercises if the wrist is not fused.
3. Begin intrinsic-plus and gentle intrinsic-minus exercises. Because of denervation of the intrinsics, the patient will not be able to actively assume the intrinsic-plus position.
4. Begin scar massage after sutures are removed.

Weeks 4 to 5

1. Continue with scar massage.
2. Begin gentle AROM exercises.

Weeks 6 to 8

1. Discontinue the dorsal protective orthosis at 6 weeks except for protection when the patient is in public.
2. Begin blocking exercises at the MCP and IP joints.
3. Begin NMES.
4. If there is evidence of flexor tendon tightness, fabricate a volar extension orthosis for use at night.
5. Continue with scar and edema management.

Weeks 8 and Later

1. Begin strengthening exercises.
2. Fabricate a dynamic orthosis if indicated.
3. Prevent intrinsic-minus contractures.
4. Begin sensory reeducation and evaluation.

Arm Replantation

Days 2 to 5

1. After the first postoperative dressing change, fabricate a dorsal elbow–wrist protective orthosis. The position of the orthosis depends on the injured structures involved, the severity and mechanism of the injury, and the surgery. Generally, the elbow is positioned in 70 degrees of flexion, the forearm in neutral pronation–supination, and the wrist in neutral to 25 degrees of extension. In the presence of median or ulnar nerve injury, the orthosis is extended distally to position the MCP joints in 50 to 70 degrees of flexion with the PIP and DIP joints in extension.

Weeks 1 to 2

1. If the vascular status is stable, begin PROM to the fingers, thumb, and wrist.
2. Instruct the patient to elevate the arm and to avoid dependent positions of the arm.
3. Begin wound care.

Weeks 2 to 3

1. Continue with edema management; may begin gentle Coban wrapping of the hand and the fingers if cleared by the surgeon.
2. Begin gentle AROM and PROM of the shoulder.

Weeks 3 to 4

1. Begin gentle PROM of the elbow and progress to gentle AROM.
2. Continue with antideformity static orthosis for the hand and wrist.
3. If evidence of loss of PROM of the fingers, begin dynamic orthosis wear.
4. Evaluate and train the patient for one-handed techniques to perform ADLs.
5. Because of the torque force on the forearm bones with supination and pronation, these movements need to be discussed with the surgeon.

Weeks 5 to 6

1. Continue with PROM, edema management, and ADLs.
2. Continue to monitor for contractures and deformities of the wrist and fingers.

Weeks 6 to 8

1. Discontinue the dorsal protective orthosis at 6 weeks except for protection when the patient is in public.
2. Continue with patient training for home ROM exercises and ADLs.
3. Initiate sensory evaluation and reeducation.

Weeks 8 and Later

1. Periodically reevaluate sensory function.
2. Begin NMES and biofeedback training if indicated.

Sturm and associates[67] reported on the rehabilitation of a hand replantation in a 55-year-old man. The authors commented that the Kleinert Institute Rehabilitation Treatment Guidelines alone often result in flexion contractures and reduced digit mobility. They advocated an early passive protocol, such as the Kleinert and modified Duran protocols, or active protocols for improved results. They also mentioned that having immediate access to a specialized replantation hospital, advances in modern technology and a clearer understanding of tissue healing in replantation likely contributed to their patients' positive outcome.

Complications

Replantation in the upper extremity may be associated with a relatively high complication rate because of the following:

Malunion and Nonunion

Whitney and colleagues[68] reported an overall 50% incidence of bony problems and a 16% rate of nonunion in digital replantations fixed with tetrahedral wiring or K-wires. However, this high complication rate may be reduced by better techniques of rigid internal fixation using 90/90 intraosseous wiring or miniplate fixation.

Joint Stiffness

Stiffness of the MCP, PIP, and DIP joints remains a problem because of edema and swelling in the replanted digit. The surgeon should avoid using longitudinal K-wires to transfix joints, and the hand therapist should begin gentle PROM exercises when the dressings are changed 5 to 7 days postoperatively. It is important to encourage AROM and PROM of the joints of adjacent noninjured digits; otherwise, these, too, can become stiff.

Tendon Adhesions

Replantations, especially at the level of the proximal phalanges and at the level of the wrist, are associated with restricted ROM because of adhesions around the flexor tendon repairs in zones II and IV. This problem can potentially be improved by meticulous repair of the flexor tendons and by early protected active flexion protocols for tendon rehabilitation. Secondary tenolyses or two-stage flexor tendon grafting may significantly increase the total AROM of a replanted digit.[69] Teoh[70] reported that improved functional outcomes in hand replantation correlate with reconstructive technique, appropriate debridement and shortening, stable bony fixation, strengthened tendon repair, quality nerve repair, extensive vascular anastomoses, complete skin coverage, and early intensive active rehabilitation.

Muscle Contractures

Intrinsic muscle contracture may develop after replantation proximal to the wrist. Ischemic contracture of either the forearm flexor or extensor muscles may compromise successful replantation at the forearm or elbow level. Intrinsic muscle contractures can be treated by release of a portion of the intrinsic tendon or by an intrinsic muscle slide. Loss of intrinsic muscle function can potentially be restored by conventional tendon transfers. Ischemic contractures of the forearm flexor or extensor muscles may be reconstructed by resection of the entire fibrotic muscle compartment and replacement with an innervated functioning free gracilis muscle transfer.

Sensory Return and Cold Intolerance

Sensory return[71] after upper extremity replantation depends on the level of amputation and whether bony shortening has allowed primary nerve repair. Replantation at the level of the middle phalanx is obviously associated with a better return of sensation than replantation at the level of the upper arm. Functional outcome, especially after major upper extremity amputations, depends on bony shortening to allow primary nerve repair and hopefully return of sensation in the hand and digits.[62,63] Wiberg and coworkers[72] showed a 30% loss of sensory fibres and a 60% loss of sympathetic nerve fibers after hand replantation based on skin biopsy. They also noted two-point discrimination was only present in patients younger than 40 years of age. Woo and associates[73] commented that a neuroma after digital replantation may best be treated by dorsal translocation of the nerve.

Alternatives to Replantation

The costs associated with replantation and often suboptimal results frequently leads to debate among hand surgeons as to the place of completion amputation and prosthetic fitting. Obviously, this varies greatly from a single-digit to a full-arm amputation. A systematic review of traumatic arm amputations[74] comparing replantation to amputation and prosthetic fitting concluded that replantation provides good function and higher satisfaction rates compared with a prosthesis regardless of the objective functional outcome. The authors commented that sensation and psychological well-being are the two major advantages over a prosthetic. These conclusions were supported by a large review in 2016.[75] Rider[76] compared the functional outcomes of replantation versus amputation for single fingertip amputations and reported better appearance, patient satisfaction, and functional outcomes in replantation but at a cost of longer hospitalization and out of work times. The study was performed in Japan, where aesthetics are particularly important.

CONCLUSION

Maximizing hand function after complete or incomplete amputation begins with the decision to replant or revascularize. Careful selection is based on predicted outcomes depending on the level of injury and the mechanism of injury. A replantation center provides comprehensive care for these complex injuries. Within the replantation center, close communication between the surgeon and hand therapist is essential.

REFERENCES

1. Malt RA, McKhann CF. Replantation of severed arms. *JAMA.* 1964;189:716.
2. Komatsu S, Tamai S. Successful replantation of a completely cut-off thumb. *Plast Reconstr Surg.* 1968;43:374.
3. Kleinert HE, Jablon M, Tsai T. An overview of replantation and results of 347 replants in 245 patients. *J Trauma.* 1980;20:390.
4. Tamai S. Twenty years' experience of limb replantation—review of 293 upper extremity replants. *J Hand Surg.* 1982;7:549.
5. Tark KC, Kim YW, Lee YH, Lew JD. Replantation and revascularization of hands: clinical analysis and functional results of 261 cases. *J Hand Surg.* 1989;14A:17–27.
6. Lesavoy MA. Successful replantation of lower leg and foot, with good sensibility and function. *Plast Reconstr Surg.* 1979;64:760.
7. Buncke HJ, Rose EH, Brownstein MJ, Chater NL. Successful replantation of two avulsed scalps by microvascular anastomoses. *Plast Reconstr Surg.* 1978;61:666–672.
8. Pennington DG, Pelly AD. Successful replantation of a completely avulsed ear by microvascular anastomosis. *Plast Reconstr Surg.* 1980;65:820.
9. Cohen BE, May Jr JW, Daly JS, Young HH. Successful clinical replantation of an amputated penis by microneurovascular repair. *Plast Reconstr Surg.* 1977;59:276–280.
10. Tatebe M, Erata S, Tanaka K, Kurahashi T, Takeda S, Hirata H. Survival rate of limb replantation in different age groups. *J Hand Microsurg.* 2017;9(2):92–94.
11. Cheng GL, Da-de P, Zhi-xian Y, et al. Digital replantation in children. *Ann Plast Surg.* 1985;15:325.
12. Daigle JP, Kleinert JM. Major limb replantation in children. *Microsurgery.* 1991;12:221.
13. Mitchell GM, Morrison WA, Papadopoulos A, O'Brien BM. A study of the extent and pathology of experimental avulsion injury in rabbit arteries and veins. *Br J Plast Surg.* 1985;38:278–287.
14. Alpert BS, Buncke HJ, Brownstein M. Replacement of damaged arteries and veins with vein grafts when replanting crushed, amputated fingers. *Plast Reconstr Surg.* 1978;61:17.
15. Pho R, Chacha P, Yeo K. Rerouting vessels and nerves from other digits in replanting an avulsed and degloved thumb. *Plast Reconstr Surg.* 1979;64:330.
16. Urbaniak JR, Evans JP, Bright DS. Microvascular management of ring avulsion injuries. *J Hand Surg.* 1981;6:25.
17. Kay S, Werntz J, Wolff TW. Ring avulsion injuries: classification and prognosis. *J Hand Surg.* 1989;14A:204.
18. Tsai TM, Manstein C, DuBou R, et al. Primary microsurgical repair of ring avulsion amputation injuries. *J Hand Surg.* 1984;9A:68–72.
19. Bamba R, Malhotra G, Bueno Jr RA, Thayer WP, Shack RB. Ring avulsion injuries: a systematic review. *Hand (N Y).* 2017.
20. Chiu HY, Chen MT. Revascularization of digits after thirty-three hours of warm ischemia time: a case report. *J Hand Surg.* 1984;9A:63.
21. Wei FC, Chang YL, Chen HC, Chuang CC. Three successful digital replantations in a patient after 84, 86 and 94 hours of cold ischemia time. *Plast Reconstr Surg.* 1988;82:346–350.
22. VanderWilde RS, Wood MB, Zeng-gui S. Hand replantation after 54 hours of cold ischemia: a case report. *J Hand Surg.* 1992;17A:217.
23. Lin CH, Avdyn N, Lin YT, Hsu CT, Lin CH, Yeh JT. Hand and finger replantation after prolonged ischaemia (more than 24 hours). *Ann Plast Surg.* 2010;64(3):286–290.
24. Stewart DE, Lowrey MR. Replantation surgery following self-inflicted amputations. *Can J Psychiatry.* 1980;25:143.
25. Davis SJ, Doyle MP. Major self mutilation leading to complete amputation of the hand during an acute psychotic episode. *CSS.* 2016;2(3):6–9.
26. Urbaniak JR. To replant or not to replant? That is not the question. *J Hand Surg.* 1983;8:507.

27. Urbaniak JR, Roth JH, Nunley JA, et al. The results of replantation after amputation of a single finger. *J Bone Joint Surg.* 1985;67A:611–619.

28. May JW, Toth BA, Gardner M. Digital replantation distal to the proximal interphalangeal joint. *J Hand Surg.* 1982;7:161.

29. Foucher G, Norris RW. Distal and very distal digital replantations. *Br J Plast Surg.* 1992;45:199.

30. Goldner RD, Stevanovic MV, Nunley JA, Urbaniak JR. Digital replantation at the level of the distal interphalangeal joint and the distal phalanx. *J Hand Surg.* 1989;14A:214–220.

31. Sebastin SJ, Chung KC. A systematic review of the outcomes of replantation of distal digital amputation. *Plast Reconstr Surg.* 2011;128(3):723–737.

32. Zimmerman NB, Weiland AJ. Ninety-ninety intraosseous wiring for internal fixation of the digital skeleton. *Orthopedics.* 1989;12:99.

33. Ikuta Y. Method of bone fixation in reattachment of amputions in the upper extremities. *Clin Orthop Relat Res.* 1978;133:169–178.

34. Wray RC, Young VL, Weeks PM. Flexible-implant arthroplasty and finger replantation. *Plast Reconstr Surg.* 1984;74:97.

35. Nissenbaum M. A surgical approach for replantation of complete digital amputations. *J Hand Surg.* 1980;65:58.

36. Lee SW, Lee DCL, Kim JS, Roh SY, Lee KJ. Analysis of bone fixation methods in digital replantation. *APS.* 2017;44(1):53–58.

37. Piñal F, Moraleda E, Rúas J, Guillermo H. Minimally invasive fixation of fractures of the phalanges and metacarpals with intramedullary cannulated headless compression screws. *J Hand Surg Am.* 2015;(40):692–700.

38. Peiji W, Qirong D, Jianzhong Q, Huayi W, Kailong Z, Nan Y. Intramedullary fixation in digital replantation using bioabsorbable poly-DL-lactic acid rods. *J Hand Surg Am.* 2012;37(12):2547–2552.

39. Jones NF, Jupiter JB. The use of Y-shaped interposition vein grafts in multiple digit replantations. *J Hand Surg.* 1985;10A:675.

40. Saha SS, Pandy A, Parwal C. Arterial segments as microvascular interposition grafts in venous anastomosis in digital replantations. *Indian J Plast Surg.* 2015;48(2):166–171.

41. Acland R. Signs of patency in small vessel anastomosis. *Surgery.* 1972;72:744.

42. Poole MD, Bowen JE. Two unusual bleedings during anticoagulation following digital replantation. *Br J Plast Surg.* 1977;30:267.

43. Buckley T, Hammert WC. Anticoagulation following digital replantation. *J Hand Surg Am.* 2011;36A:1374–1376.

44. Levin LS, Cooper EO. Clinical use of anticoagulants following replantation surgery. *J Hand Surg.* 2008;33A:1437–1439.

45. Efanov JI. Optimizing therapeutic anticoagulation for finger replantation: a retrospective analysis of outcomes. *J Hand Surg Am.* 2017;42(9):S43–S44.

46. Nikolis A, Tahiri Y, St-Supery V, et al. Intravenous heparin use in digital replantation and revascularization: the Quebec provincial replantation program experience. *Microsurgery.* 2011;31(6):421–427.

47. Chen YC, Chi CC, Chan FC, Wen YW. Low molecular weight heparin for prevention of microvascular occlusion in digital replantation. *Cochrane Database Syst Rev.* 2013;8(7).

48. Wilson GR, Jones BM. The damaging effect of smoking on digital revascularisation: two further case reports. *Br J Plast Surg.* 1984;37:613.

49. Stirrat C, Seaber AV, Urbaniak JR, Bright DS. Temperature monitoring in digital replantation. *J Hand Surg.* 1978;3:342–347.

50. Hovius SER, van Adrichem LN, Mulder HD, et al. Comparison of laser Doppler flowmetry and thermometry in the postoperative monitoring of replantations. *J Hand Surg.* 1995;20A:88–93.

51. Keller HP, Lanz U. Objective control of replanted fingers by transcutaneous partial O_2 (PO_2) measurement. *Microsurgery.* 1984;5:85.

52. Graham B, Paulus DA, Caffee HH. Pulse oximetry for vascular monitoring in upper extremity replantation surgery. *J Hand Surg.* 1986;11A:687.

53. Gordon L, Leitner DW, Buncke HJ, Alpert BS. Partial nail plate removal after digital replantation as an alternative method of venous drainage. *J Hand Surg.* 1985;10A:360–364.

54. Henderson HP, Matti B, Laing AG, et al. Avulsion of the scalp treated by microvascular repair: the use of leeches for post-operative decongestion. *Br J Plast Surg.* 1983;36:235–239.

55. Fukui A, Maeda M, Inada Y, et al. Arteriovenous shunt in digit replantation. *J Hand Surg.* 1990;15A:160–165.

56. Camacho FJ, Wood MB. Polydigit replantation. *Hand Clin.* 1992;8:3.

57. Chiu HY, Lu SY, Lin TW, Chen MT. Transposition digital replantation. *J Trauma.* 1985;25:440–443.

58. Alpert BS, Buncke HJ. Mutilating multidigital injuries: use of a free microvascular flap from a nonreplantable part. *J Hand Surg.* 1978;3:196.

59. Bieber EJ, Wood MB, Cooney WP, Amadio PC. Thumb avulsion: results of replantation/revascularization. *J Hand Surg.* 1987;12A:786–790.

60. Schlenker JD, Kleinert HE, Tsai T. Methods and results of replantation following traumatic amputation of the thumb in sixty-four patients. *J Hand Surg.* 1980;5:63.

61. Tonkin MA, Ames EL, Wolff TW, Larsen RD. Transmetacarpal amputations and replantation: the importance of the normal vascular anatomy. *J Hand Surg.* 1988;13B:204–209.

62. Russell RC, O'Brien BM, Morrison WA, et al. The late functional results of upper limb revascularization and replantation. *J Hand Surg.* 1984;9A:623–633.

63. Wood MB, Cooney WP. Above elbow limb replantation: functional results. *J Hand Surg.* 1986;11A:682.

64. Lalonde DH. Conceptual origins, current practice, and views of wide awake hand surgery. *J Hand Surg Eur Vol.* 2017;42(9):886–895.

65. Wong J, Lin CH, Chang NJ, Chen HC, Hsu CC. Digital revascularization and replantation using the wide-awake hand surgery technique. *J Hand Surg Eur Vol.* 2017;42(6):621–625.

66. Ugurlar M, Kabakas F, Purisa H, Sezer I, Celikdelen P, Ozcelik IB. Rehabilitation after successful finger replantation. *North Clin Istanbul.* 2016;3(1):22–26.

67. Sturm SM, Oxley SB, Van Zant S. Rehabilitation of a patient following hand replantation after near-complete distal forearm amputation. *J Hand Ther.* 2014;27:217–224.

68. Whitney TM, Lineaweaver WC, Buncke HJ, Nugent K. Clinical results of bony fixation methods in digital replantation. *J Hand Surg.* 1990;15A:328–334.

69. Jupiter JB, Pess GM, Bour CJ. Results of flexor tendon tenolysis after replantation in the hand. *J Hand Surg.* 1989;14A:35.

70. Teoh LC. Replantation Surgery – The reconstructive approach. *ANZ J Surg.* 2007;77(1):35.

71. Gelberman RH, Urbaniak JR, Bright DS, Levin LS. Digital sensibility following replantation. *J Hand Surg.* 1978;3:313–319.

72. Wiberg M, Hazari A, Ljunberg C, et al. Sensory recovery after hand reimplantation: a clinical, morphological, and neurophysiological study in humans. *Scand J Plast Reconstr Surg Hand Surg.* 2003;37(3):163–173.

73. Woo SH, Kim YW, Cheon HJ, et al. Management of complications relating to finger amputions and replantation. *Hand Clin.* 2015;31(2):319–338.

74. Otto IA, Kon M, Schuurman AH, Minnen P. Replantation versus prosthetic fitting in traumatic arm amputations: a systematic review. *PLoS One.* 2015;(9):10.

75. Pet MA, Morrision SD, Mack JS, et al. Comparison of patient-reported outcomes after traumatic upper extremity amputation: replantation versus prosthetic rehabilitation. *Injury.* 2016;47(12):L2783–L2788.

76. Rider D. A Retrospective study of functional outcomes after successful replantation versus amputation closure for single fingertip amputations. *J Hand Ther.* 2006;19(4):434–435.

75

Therapy Management of Complex Injuries of the Hand

Karen M. Pettengill

OUTLINE

CRITICAL POINTS

Skin and Superficial Soft Tissue

- What kind of closure or coverage has been used?
- How much protection does it need?
- Is healing expected to be by primary or secondary intention?
- What kind of dressing is appropriate?
- Are there signs of any complications in wound healing (e.g., infection, contamination)?
- Can problems be expected with wound contraction and secondary joint contracture or with adhesions?

Blood Vessels

- Which vessels were repaired?
- Does immobilization for other injuries adequately protect repaired blood vessels (2–4 weeks needed)?
- Is there a danger of arterial or venous insufficiency?

Nerves

- Which nerves were injured? Are there any nerve grafts?
- Were nerves repaired under tension?
- How much immobilization will be needed? (2–4 weeks of protection from excessive stress)?

Sensory Nerves

- Is there total loss of sensibility?
- What areas will need protection because of impaired sensibility?
- What will be the functional effects?
- Is there a need for desensitization or sensory reeducation?

Motor Nerves

- What muscle imbalance can be expected, and will orthotic repositioning be needed to improve function and prevent deformity?

Muscles and Tendons

- Which tendons were injured? What kind of repair was performed?
- Were both flexors and extensors injured? If so, how can each be protected and mobilized without endangering other injured structures?
- Is heavy scar formation expected (because of zone of injury, means of injury, or other factors)?

Bone and Articular Structures

- What structures were injured and need protection?
- What kind of fracture was sustained? How stable are the reduction and fixation? How will this affect the rate of healing, wound care, and mobilization programs?
- What is the optimum position of immobilization?

Inflammatory Phase

- Talk to the surgeon to find out what structures were injured and how they were repaired and what future surgical plans are.
- Teach the patient about injuries and provide help with set goals.
- Encourage uncomplicated wound healing.
- Protect all repaired structures. Mobilize *gently* if indicated.
- Control edema and pain.
- Prevent future problems: mobilize uninvolved joints.
- Address difficulties with activities of daily living (ADLs).
- Consider social services referrals.

Proliferative Phase

- Continue to do the following:
  - Communicate with the surgeon.
  - Educate the patient.
  - Manage wound, edema, and pain.
  - Mobilize uninvolved joints.
  - Address ADL difficulties.
  - Consider social services referrals.
  - Introduce scar massage and retrograde massage if not contraindicated.
  - Modify protection and mobilization as dictated by healing of involved structures. Identify potential joint contractures or other problems and modify splints and exercises as needed.
  - Introduce light activities.

Scar Maturation–Remodeling Phase

- Continue to do the following:
  - Communicate with the surgeon (focus on long-term goals and plans).
  - Educate the patient (focus on return to previous activities and work and on any future surgery).
  - Manage wound, scars, edema (more aggressively), and pain.
  - Mobilize uninvolved joints.
  - Address ADLs (address long-term needs).
  - Consider social services referrals.
- Modify orthosis and exercise programs as dictated by frequent evaluation.
- Progress to more demanding activities.
- Begin strengthening, dexterity, and endurance training.
- Begin job simulation and make specific plans for return to work.
- Begin sensory reeducation.

A complex injury encompasses multiple-system trauma: skeletal, neurovascular, and many soft tissue structures all may be involved. The injury may include amputation, crush, laceration, and avulsion in a single extremity and thus presents a difficult problem in management. Close cooperation among the patient, surgeon, and therapist is essential in this demanding course of treatment.

The goal of all hand rehabilitation is a hand that is functional and esthetically acceptable. All treatment efforts are in vain if, for any reason, the patient does not use his or her hand. From a psychological standpoint, the patient's difficulties with confronting the injury and reintegrating the hand into normal use must be recognized and addressed. From a physical standpoint, functional motion, strength, and sensibility to the hand must be restored. In both cases, the formation and remodeling of scar tissue must be controlled; uncontrolled scar can render a hand both unattractive and useless (Fig. e75.1).

Normal hand function requires strong tissue repairs with free gliding between neighboring structures. Scar tissue may adhere tissues to one another and prevent normal gliding; inadequate scar formation at the repair site will not withstand the demands of normal hand use. Therefore, management of a complex hand injury necessitates selective control of healing, ensuring stable, durable scar where strength is needed and long, mobile, elastic scar where motion between adjacent tissues is crucial.

The most difficult aspect of management in complex injuries is the coordination of treatment of the various systems and tissues injured. In addition to basic knowledge of hand anatomy, physiology, and kinesiology and a wide repertoire of therapeutic skills, the therapist must possess a thorough comprehension of the phases of normal and pathologic healing of each type of tissue injured and an understanding of the relationships between the various systems. When the complex injury is being treated, the key is careful examination of the individual systems and a treatment plan based on logical analysis of the problems identified.

Toward this end, this chapter first presents a review of wound healing and how healing can be influenced. The various tissues and special considerations for their treatment as dictated by anatomy, surgical-medical management, and mechanism of healing are then considered. This discussion is followed by a review of treatment modalities, giving more emphasis to techniques not covered in other chapters of this book. Guidelines for evaluation and treatment at each phase of healing are explored last.

WOUND HEALING

For full coverage of wound healing, readers are referred to Chapter 16, "Wound Classification and Management." The following description is very simplified and general.

All wounds, in any type of tissue, heal in a similar manner. The time frame given here applies to uncomplicated soft tissue healing. Times vary from one tissue to another and are never absolutely exact because healing is a continuum, and the phases overlap. In addition, complex injuries are characterized by untidy and extensive wounds, often contaminated or subject to other influences that considerably alter the timing of wound healing. The various tissues involved heal at different rates, which adds to the difficulty of evaluation and treatment planning.

The inflammatory phase of healing begins within hours of trauma and continues for at least 3 days, although it may persist for days or weeks, especially in complex injuries, and can be renewed in response to even a relatively minor trauma such as overuse of a newly healed structure. Hemostasis is established through initial vasoconstriction and coagulation, allowing formation of a fibrin clot that both limits loss of blood and provides a scaffold for further cell invasion. Local vasodilation permits the leakage of blood and plasma into the injured area, creating increased edema, heat, redness, and pain—the classic signs of inflammation. Inflammatory cells invade the wound. Macrophages remove bacteria and apoptotic cells from the area. Fibroblasts stimulate macrophage attraction.[1,2] Macrophages stimulate fibroblasts to begin epithelialization from the margins inward, usually completely covering small, clean wounds within 3 days. Early intercellular attachments are weak and easily disrupted.

The proliferative or fibroplasia phase begins at 3 to 4 days and lasts through 14 days. The wound matrix is formed through macrophage and fibroblast activity. Angiogenesis brings blood supply and nutrition to the area. Wound contraction is caused by fibroblast differentiation into myofibroblasts, which stimulate wound contraction.[1,2] Fibroblasts synthesize collagen at a rapid rate, but the tensile strength of the wound is still low, and excessive tension can rupture the fragile intercellular bonds.

The scar maturation and remodeling phase begins at day 8 and continues for at least 1 year, when the dynamic turnover of collagen provides for differentiation of scar to accommodate the tissue type and the stresses under which it is placed. Excessive mechanical loading early in this phase may prolong fibroblast synthesis of collagen, which could lead to hypertrophic scarring. Decreased mechanical loading slows collagen synthesis and stimulates apoptosis, thus controlling the rate of scar formation.[1,2] Mechanical loading can be exerted by excessive edema as well as compression or traction by external forces. Initially, all tissues involved in a wound develop a single, massive scar, with randomly oriented collagen fibers. In the remodeling phase, fibers reorient and scars assume some of the characteristics of the tissues being healed.

As noted earlier, controlled stress (compression or tension) and motion have been shown to influence collagen formation and organization, increasing strength of healing tissues and decreasing adherence between adjacent tissues.[3-10] However, it is not yet known how much stress is necessary and at exactly what time and manner it must be applied to any given type of scar tissue to produce a desired change. It is known that low levels of stress encourage cell migration and the orientation of new collagen fibers to allow tissue extensibility and gliding between adjacent tissues, whereas greater stress may cause tissue trauma or uncontrolled scar formation, leading to scar hypertrophy and adhesions. It also is known that in connective tissue, stress deprivation (such as occurs with immobilization after injury) predictably causes degenerative changes that lead to stiffness and deformity.[11-17]

During the inflammatory phase, efforts are directed toward controlling pain and edema and promoting uncomplicated wound healing. The patient is taught that orthoses, dressings, and gentle motion help prevent further damage by avoiding excessive physical stress to the injured tissues. Pain, exposure to cold, and even emotional stress all can impair oxygen perfusion of the wound microenvironment, thus lowering resistance to infection and slowing healing.[18] The resultant prolonged inflammatory response may lead to excessive fibrosis. During the proliferative and early remodeling phases, control of edema continues, and undue stress to the injured area is avoided. Depending on the nature of the injury and the tissues injured, some form of controlled stress may be started to further decrease edema and increase or maintain joint and soft tissue mobility. During the remodeling phase, the focus on mobility is increased gradually, and as healing allows, strengthening, dexterity training, and other intervention aimed toward return to former activity should begin.

Although the phases are described here in simple terms and as discrete entities, in reality, they overlap considerably[1,2,19] and involve simultaneous complex processes; treatment should always take this into account. For example, although as fibroplasia begins gentle controlled stress may be initiated, some inflammatory activity remains. Careful evaluation will reveal the signs of continued inflammation, and treatment is modified accordingly.

HEALING OF SPECIFIC TISSUES

Skin and Superficial Soft Tissue

Skin wounds heal relatively quickly, with a simple sutured wound tolerating mobilization within a few days. Sutures can be removed in 10 to 21 days, depending on the wound and the stresses to which it is subject. Grafts need more protection, the timing of which depends on the type of coverage. Areas left open and allowed to heal by secondary intention may take several weeks, depending on the size of the wound. See Chapter 16 and the references for further detail. Wound healing may be delayed by systemic disease such as diabetes[1,20,21] or hypothyroidism[1] or by other factors such as smoking,[22–24] age, tight bandages causing ischemia, excessive edema, or infection.[1]

Superficial scar management begins with early wound care, avoiding trauma that could prolong or exacerbate the inflammatory response and stimulate excessive scar formation. Treatment is aimed toward prevention of restrictive scar adhesions between superficial and deep soft tissues. If the skin is not allowed to glide normally over underlying tissues, motion may be severely limited. This is especially true of the dorsum of the hand, where the normal skin redundancy allows digit and wrist mobility.

Blood Vessels

Blood vessels require 1 to 2 weeks of protection. This generally is provided by the immobilization necessary for protection of other tissues. Bandages should be nonconstrictive. Close attention should be paid to signs of vascular insufficiency during this phase. Signs of arterial insufficiency include skin pallor, decreased temperature (measured with digit temperature probes or by touch), increased pain, sluggish capillary refill, and loss of pulse. Venous insufficiency is indicated by cyanosis and abnormally rapid capillary refill; with persistent venous insufficiency, temperature also may be reduced. Venous return can be assisted by elevation of the hand above heart level, which also assists lymphatic drainage and thus minimizes the compression placed on vessels by excessive edema. However, if arteries have been repaired, they should not be required to work too hard against gravity. If signs of arterial insufficiency are noted, elevation should be modified accordingly, as discussed subsequently in this chapter.

Nerves

Although healing at the site of nerve repair is similar to the healing of other tissues, the functional recovery of a repaired peripheral nerve involves the very different process of axonal regeneration, which is described in Chapter 40. Therefore, the suture site is protected according to the usual phases of soft tissue healing, but the return of sensory or motor function is expected to vary depending on the location of the injury.

The suture site of a completely transected and well-repaired nerve must be protected from excessive stress for 3 weeks. In general, orthoses should immobilize the joints distal and proximal to the repair without placing it under tension or direct compression or placing it at risk of adherence to adjacent tissues that will later restrict nerve gliding. An adherent nerve is subject to alternating compression and stretch, which may produce internal scar and impede transmission of nerve impulses. An example is the hyperflexed wrist after repair of median and ulnar nerves. The nerves may become adherent and compressed beneath the flexor retinaculum, and later attempts to regain wrist extension will subject the nerve to potentially harmful traction.

If the nerve is incompletely transected, is repaired under no tension, or is only contused, little or no immobilization may be needed. In fact, protected early mobilization of an intact but contused nerve may help restore gliding and prevent constriction and traction by scar adhesions. In the case of a digital nerve repaired along with flexor tendon repairs in zone II, early mobilization of the tendon will significantly improve the ultimate result, and clinically, this has not proven to compromise the sensory recovery. If the nerve was repaired under tension, limiting metacarpophalangeal (MCP) or proximal interphalangeal (PIP) joint extension may provide adequate protection while still allowing active or passive flexion. Bear in mind, however, that there is some early evidence in the literature[25] that early mobilization of repaired nerves may impair healing, so caution is necessary. Decisions to mobilize repaired nerves early should be made by therapist and surgeon together.

If a nerve was avulsed or a portion of the nerve was destroyed, leaving a gap, the nerve may be left unrepaired or may be grafted primarily or secondarily. In the first case, any insensate areas must be carefully protected. In the second case, the two suture sites must be protected appropriately.

After motor nerve injury, treatment considers the functional imbalance produced by loss of specific muscle function. Such imbalance can lead to development of secondary deformity during the lag time required for nerve regeneration. After sensory nerve injury, patients must be taught to protect insensate areas from injury.

In any nerve repair, exact end-to-end approximation of each severed axon is impossible to achieve, and a certain percentage of nerve function is therefore destined to be lost. Even if a nerve were perfectly repaired, with the two halves of each axon approximated precisely, axonal regeneration would take a long time (1–3 mm per day after a 3- to 4-week latent period[26]). Regeneration after crush injury is more rapid but may seem agonizingly slow to the patient. Sensory and motor function must be reevaluated frequently after peripheral nerve injury and the treatment plan adapted as needed. Because nerve regeneration is slow, this aspect of recovery can be neglected all too easily, to the great detriment of the patient.

After an amputation or other injury in which a nerve is transected and left unrepaired, neuroma formation is the inevitable result. Neuromas can be asymptomatic, but in many cases, they are quite painful. If not addressed promptly, a painful neuroma may become an enormous obstacle to functional recovery. Therefore, in the presence of unrepaired transected nerves, early prophylactic desensitization and protection of hypersensitive areas are advisable.

Muscles and Tendons

Detailed discussions of tendon healing and management are available elsewhere in this book and in the literature. The following is a simplified overview of tendon healing.

In the inflammatory phase, the repair site is weak, relying on the sutures to maintain continuity. In the proliferative phase, strength increases steadily as collagen is laid down. As noted previously, the quantity of collagen stabilizes by the end of fibroplasia. During the remodeling phase, destruction and replacement of collagen allows for stronger collagen cross-linking and differential reorientation of fibers. The parallel orientation of fibers within the tendon provides increased tensile strength, and the random orientation of peritendinous fibers allows tendon gliding.

The goal of tendon repair and rehabilitation is a strong repair that heals with a minimum of restrictive adhesion formation. As already noted, numerous studies[6,8,9,27] have demonstrated that the strength of the repair increases in response to controlled stress. For example, the strength of an immobilized tendon repair has been noted to decrease temporarily at 10 to 14 days,[28] but a tendon that is subject to some form of controlled mobilization develops an increased breaking strength while developing more pliable, gliding adhesions to the surrounding tissues.[6,8,27] Therefore, if an injured tendon is not mobilized until 2 weeks after repair to protect other healing structures, exercise should be very gentle because of the decreased strength of the juncture at this stage. If the tendon is first mobilized after 3 to 4 weeks, the repair will be somewhat stronger but still not as strong as in a tendon that was first mobilized within a day or two of repair.

In general, immobilized repaired tendons have sufficient strength to withstand gentle active motion at 3 to 4 weeks, and they can tolerate light resistance after another 2 to 3 weeks. Tendons that have been mobilized passively will be stronger when active motion is started at 3 weeks. However, these are general guidelines; the specifics of each case should be considered carefully in the timing of the progression of treatment. For example, repaired extensor tendons in zones I and II require 6 to 8 weeks of immobilization because of the unique anatomic features of that zone. Greater protection should be given if healing may be impaired by systemic conditions such as diabetes[20,21] or by habitual tobacco smoking,[22–24] or if flexor tendon vinculae have been damaged. If both flexor and extensor tendons are repaired, the program must be modified to prevent excessive stress to either tendon.

An injury to the richly vascularized muscle belly or musculotendinous junction heals more quickly and easily. Adhesions at this level can be strong but pose fewer problems than do tendon adhesions because in general, less gliding is demanded between muscle belly and surrounding tissues than between tendon and peritendinous tissues.

Bone and Articular Structures

As with other tissues, bone healing has three phases. During the inflammatory phase, a fracture hematoma forms and cellular debris is cleared away. The next phase can take considerably longer than the typical proliferative phase, depending on the location of the fracture. In this period, a soft tissue collar or *soft callus* develops and unites the fracture fragments, providing support for a fibrocartilaginous union. This callus, though joining fracture fragments, is not strong, forming what is known as a *clinical union*, not sufficiently solid to be visible on radiographs. Often, active and active-assisted motion of the joints adjacent to the healing bone is begun at this point because a clinically healed bone shows no motion at the site of fracture, and therefore controlled stress is safe. However, in many cases, radiographic healing must be seen to ensure stability in difficult fractures. Radiographic healing occurs during the remodeling phase when true cortical and cancellous bone is formed and gradually increases in strength in response to longitudinal and shearing stresses.

Remodeling may begin within a month and continue for several years. The healing rate of fractures varies widely depending on the bone and what part of the bone is affected. In the upper extremity, a fracture may be considered clinically healed at as early as 2 to 5 weeks or may require several months of immobilization. The type of fracture and fracture fixation naturally also affect the course of treatment. In fact, with open reduction and internal fixation using compression plates, primary bone healing can occur, in effect skipping the stage of callus formation. This may speed healing, and a sufficiently rigid fixation also will allow earlier motion of the involved bone.

Injured articular cartilage generally heals poorly, without regeneration of true hyaline cartilage. The result is an irregular joint surface, which opens up the possibility of posttraumatic arthritis. Because cartilage is avascular, nutrition is supplied entirely through diffusion and the contribution from the highly vascular perichondrium. In the absence of blood vessels in the cartilage itself, there can be no inflammatory response but instead a limited and unpredictable healing via chondrocyte activity. If the injury extends to the vascular subchondral bone, healing is aided by the inflammatory response of the injured bone and may actually improve the recovery of functional joint surfaces.

Ligaments present a different set of problems. In injured ligaments, scar tissue contraction can limit considerably the available motion of a joint. In addition, even if there is no direct ligament injury, inflammation of adjacent tissues can lead to fibrosis in an immobilized or edematous joint, thus diminishing ligamentous elasticity. Therefore, if joints must be immobilized, ligaments should be kept at the greatest length possible so that they do not shorten and produce joint contractures.

OVERVIEW OF TREATMENT TECHNIQUES

Patient Education

Many patients are overwhelmed by the gravity of a complex hand injury. Because the recovery of function depends on psychological and physical recuperation, patient education is crucial. From the first visit, patient education must be oriented toward both current status and future return to a normal way of life.

The complexity of the injury usually demands multifaceted and time-consuming therapy. The home program must be as clear and simple as possible so that the patient can and will follow through on his or her own. This means tailoring the program not only to the patient's physical needs but also to his or her psychosocial status. How extensive a program can the patient understand? How much time does the patient have during the day? What are the other demands on his or her time? Will the patient's health insurance cover everything desirable for therapy, or will limited coverage restrict the options open to him or her? The program is adapted as needed, beginning with a simple set of instructions. New elements are added as the patient becomes ready, and elements are deleted when no longer necessary. The home program strikes a balance between physical and psychosocial well-being; exercises must be performed often enough to meet physical needs but should not dominate the patient's life.

The home program is written out, demonstrated to the patient, and discussed thoroughly. The patient then reads the program and demonstrates to the therapist a full understanding of all instructions. This is repeated at each successive visit and with each addition or change to the program until the therapist is satisfied that the patient is following through well at home.

The patient may require therapy for months or years, with a series of surgical reconstructions and postoperative rehabilitation. Over time, some patients become dependent on hand therapy as a way of life. This dependence can be kept to a minimum or prevented altogether by careful patient education and early enlistment of family support. Referral to a psychologist or social worker also may be indicated. Such a referral can contribute immeasurably to the patient's successful recovery. Chapter 83 explores in greater depth the psychological effects of traumatic hand injuries.

Wound Care

Careful wound management can control scar formation and thus result in a more cosmetically acceptable hand with greater mobility and function. Detailed discussion of wound care can be found in Chapter 16. Only a few key points are included here.

Early wound care may include conservative debridement, removing only dead tissues that come away easily and avoiding trauma to the involved tissues. If a whirlpool is used for gentle debridement and cleansing, treatment time is short (from 5 to 20 minutes) to limit the time spent with the hand in a dependent position because this could increase edema. Careful thought is given to the water temperature, the level of agitation, and any additives to be used for their cleansing or antibacterial effects. Neither elevation nor active motion appears to affect postwhirlpool edema, but whirlpool temperatures have a significant effect.[29–31] A temperature of 32° to 35°C is recommended. Pulsed lavage is a modality that offers not only debridement but also facilitation of wound granulation.[1]

Whirlpools generally are contraindicated in the early care of grafts and flaps, when, in fact, it is often better to leave dressings undisturbed if possible to ensure that the graft or flap takes. When whirlpools are used, they should be of short duration (5 minutes), agitation should be kept low, and the water should not be too cold because this could produce vasoconstriction and ischemia.

Wounds with delayed healing may be treated with vacuum-assisted closure using VAC therapy (KCI, San Antonio, TX), also known as negative-pressure wound therapy or simply the wound VAC. This device, developed at Wake Forest University, applies negative pressure to the wound, draining excess fluids and exerting mechanical force on soft tissues. The mechanisms involved are not completely understood, but results have been good.[32]

Many more options for wound dressings are available now than in the past. Although a simple sutured wound is clean and often kept dry, many open wounds may be best treated with moist, occlusive dressings. The practice varies from center to center. It is best to follow the practice of the referring surgeon. See also Chapter 16.

Whether the wound is kept moist or dry, the goals are protection from undue stress and provision of the appropriate microenvironment for healing. Forceful removal of an adherent dressing can inflict trauma to the tissues and prolong the inflammatory response. This is especially important with grafts. Graft "take" involves the establishment of new vascular supply to the graft, and this tenuous developing circulation is easily disrupted. In addition, even after vascularity is established, the scar interface between graft and bed is weak in early stages. Therefore, shearing force and pressure must be avoided until at least 2 weeks after grafting. Several types of nonstick dressings on the market can prevent adherence to grafts or open areas and provide antibiotic protection as well (Fig. e75.2).

All gauze bandages should be nonconstrictive and wrapped in a figure-of-8 from distal to proximal to avoid creating a tourniquet with a circular wrap. Revascularizations, flaps awaiting division, free flaps and composite tissue transfers, and replanted parts present more difficult problems in dressing application, but in these cases, it is doubly important to avoid all constriction during the early stages when vascularity is being established. Skin color and temperature are monitored carefully for signs of ischemia or venous congestion after all microsurgical vascular procedures, and any problems are immediately reported to the attending surgeon.

Many patients with more simple wound care needs can perform dressing changes at home. External fixators are cleaned daily at the skin entrance sites by the patient using clean cotton swabs and hydrogen peroxide or a hydrogen peroxide solution. Some surgeons prefer to follow cleaning with application of antibiotic ointment, a light dressing, or both.

Patients should be instructed to monitor pin sites and all wounds for signs of infection: increased local redness or warmth, pain, or exudate. A fever also may be present. If the patient has any doubts, he or she should contact the therapist or doctor at once, and if the therapist identifies a possible infection, it should be reported immediately to the attending physician. A culture may be necessary to determine the appropriate antibiotic treatment.

Superficial Scar Management

Although the exact mechanism is still under investigation,[33] continuous pressure over a bulky superficial scar flattens it and may make it softer, more elastic, and more cosmetically acceptable to the patient.[34-41] In the hand, continuous pressure can be provided with elasticized gloves such as Jobst gloves (Jobst Co., Toledo, OH), with Coban elasticized paper bandage (3M Coban Self-Adherent Wraps; 3M Co., St. Paul,

MN), or for firmer and more localized pressure, with elastomer or gel sheets (mineral oil based or silicone gel).

There are two types of elastomer, both of which are applied quickly to allow time to set through a catalytic reaction. For the first type, the catalyst is added to a sticky liquid and thoroughly mixed before applying. For the second type, equal parts of two different putties are mixed in the therapist's hands. One of the two putties is the catalyst. As the elastomer sets, it forms an exact mold of the scar, and all the skin creases (Fig. e75.3). For the best results, the pad is worn constantly if possible and is held in place by a closely fitting orthosis or Coban wrapping. As the scar compresses over time, new molds must be made to accommodate changes.

A scar in a normally mobile area such as the palm or across the wrist is not a good candidate for elastomer unless the pressure is applied under an orthosis that holds the part immobile. When the wrist flexes and extends or when the hand is opened and closed, the scar moves and stretches, and the mold is no longer exact. In this case, gel sheets are preferable. Although these do not conform as exactly to the shape of the scar, they do provide very close pressure that is flexible and adapts to motion of the scar. Silicone gel sheets also serve to hydrate the scar.[33]

All of these materials or firm foam rubber also can be used to form a donut-shaped pad to protect a hypersensitive scar by transferring pressure to the surrounding area. In contrast, many patients find relief through the constant gentle pressure of a gel pad directly on the hypersensitive area.

Another method for prevention of hypertrophic scar is the constant application of paper tape during the first several weeks after surgery. The time and duration of application have not yet been defined, but several authors have recommended this treatment, which apparently reduces shearing forces that may contribute to hypertrophic scar formation.[33,42,43]

Some scars become badly adherent despite preventive efforts and thus limit motion by preventing gliding of the skin over deeper tissues. In these cases, deep transverse friction massage, crossing the grain of tightening connective tissue, will mobilize superficial scar by stretching its adhesions to underlying tissues. Heat applied before massage increases the extensibility of the tissues and thus increases the effectiveness of the massage. Bear in mind that vigorous massage too early in healing may cause hypertrophic scar formation and should therefore be avoided.

Keloid scars are often confused with hypertrophic scars but are in reality very different. Burd and Huang[44] summarized the differences as follows: hypertrophic scar is more common than keloid scar. It is not associated with race, whereas keloids are more common in those with darker pigmentation. Hypertrophic scars are always associated with trauma, but keloids can occur spontaneously. Keloids do not commonly cause skin or joint contracture, but hypertrophic scars do. Hypertrophic scars occur at the site of injury, but keloids may be more extensive. Hypertrophic scars usually resolve over time, and do not recur after surgery, but keloids do not resolve spontaneously and may recur after surgery. Hypertrophic scars occur at the site of injury regardless of anatomic location, but keloids are more common in certain anatomic regions. Finally, there are marked cellular differences between keloids and hypertrophic scars. This may explain why in clinical settings, pressure does not appear as effective in modifying keloid formation as it is in controlling hypertrophic scar.

In the case of amputations, residual digit care is an important part of scar management. The residual digit must be massaged frequently to soften scars and to prevent hypersensitivity caused by avoidance of contact (see subsequent section called Desensitization and Sensory Reeducation). "Dog ears" or corners must be softened and rounded

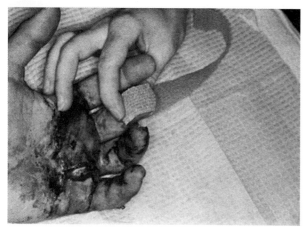

Fig. 75.1 Stump wrapping, step 1. A Coban 1-inch bandage is placed across the tip of the stump to apply conforming pressure.

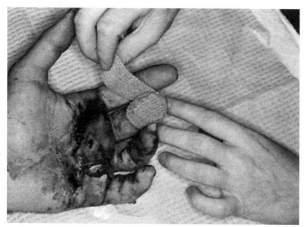

Fig. 75.2 Stump wrapping, step 2. After the tip is completely covered, the stump is wrapped from distal to proximal only as far as necessary to secure the wrapping.

because they may be either hypersensitive or bulky enough to impede sensibility. Pressure may be provided through Coban bandages with some form of pressure pad if necessary for unusually bulky or malformed residual digit. To wrap a residual digit, the therapist first wraps the Coban bandage across the tip, then back across to completely cover the tip, and finally in a figure-of-8 fashion, wrapped from distal to proximal only as far as necessary to anchor the wrapping (Figs. 75.1 and 75.2). Digit sleeves lined with a mineral oil–based gel are also commercially available, and they can be cut to fit an amputated finger.

In the case of all wrapping and pressure pads for scar control and protection, a balance must be struck between scar management and overprotection. The patient must grow accustomed to using an unprotected amputated digit, both to fully desensitize it and to use available sensibility. At some point, the constant pressure necessary for effective scar remodeling must be abandoned to allow greater function.

Desensitization and Sensory Reeducation

Although commonly viewed separately, desensitization and sensory reeducation programs often blend together in practice, and the two should be incorporated into the treatment of most patients with complex injuries (see Chapters 41 and 42). Neuromas and hypersensitive scars are a common outcome of complex soft tissue injuries. A prophylactic desensitization program may forestall severe hypersensitivity. It is easy to neglect sensory reeducation in a hand with

many other needs. Yet all efforts at gaining mobility will be wasted in a hand that is nonfunctional because of poor sensory return. Functional return depends on cortical "reprogramming," which can be enhanced through sensory reeducation.[26,45] There is some evidence of a correlation between cognitive capacity and functional return of sensibility.[46] Although some patients are innately very good at recovering function as sensibility returns, others require specific reeducation.

Edema Reduction Techniques

Edema control is crucial to controlling fibrosis and increasing mobility. The genesis and control of edema are covered in greater detail in Chapter 57; a simplified discussion follows here. The prolonged or renewed presence of inflammatory edema is a danger sign, in that inflammatory products stimulate fibrosis, which may ultimately limit mobility. If edema compromises vascularity, fibrosis also may result. In addition, excessive edema will limit mobility by its very bulk. When edema prevents full range of motion (ROM) for a long period, ligaments, skin, and other structures may shorten and thus permanently restrict mobility. During the normal inflammatory and proliferative phases, edema can be described as *pitting*. A fingertip pressed into the edematous area leaves a dent or pit that remains for at least several seconds. At this stage, edema is still relatively easy to mobilize. However, chronic inflammatory edema becomes "brawny" or fibrous and is difficult to mobilize.

In a traumatized hand, edema typically collects on the dorsum, where the skin is loose. Dorsal edema pulls the MCP joints into extension, which produces compensatory flexion at the interphalangeal (IP) joints and the wrist. Likewise, edema over the dorsum of the first webspace pulls the thumb into adduction. This is the classic wounded-hand position, which leads to severe joint contractures and functional limitations as fibrosis develops.

The most important means of edema control is early elevation of the hand above heart level, preferably with the whole extremity raised, with the hand above the elbow and the elbow above the heart. The patient should avoid using a sling because this rarely achieves acceptable elevation, and it positions the shoulder in adduction, internal rotation, and flexion and the elbow in flexion, putting the shoulder and elbow at unnecessary risk for stiffness and pain. Nighttime elevation must not be neglected; the patient should sleep with the hand supported on the chest or on pillows by the side, with the hand always above heart level.

Excessive elevation may be contraindicated in certain cases. After microsurgical procedures such as replantations, free flaps, or revascularizations, elevation above heart level may place too great a burden on the arterial anastomoses, resulting in ischemia. However, venous congestion may result from insufficient elevation. Therefore, the vascularity and the position of the extremity should be monitored carefully. Elevation also may be contraindicated in the presence of infection not yet controlled by antibiotics because elevation may aid proximal spread of the infection. When in doubt, the therapist always should consult the attending surgeon.

In the inflammatory phase, cold may be useful for reduction of edema, although this is more effective in combination with compression and elevation.

When healing structures develop sufficient strength, active and resistive exercise will aid in edema control. The intermittent compression produced by muscle contraction acts as a pump to assist the overburdened venous and lymphatic drainage systems. Elevation and active exercise can be combined in "pumping" exercises. Every waking hour, the patient may make 5 or 10 strong fists with his or her hand raised as high overhead as possible.

Prehension activities can be performed with the hand in elevation, and many patients find this a pleasant and motivating means of combining lightly resistive exercise with elevation. However, even lightly resistive tasks should be performed with caution because the patient may very easily overdo such activities in the early stages, provoking a renewed inflammatory reaction and thereby increasing, rather than decreasing, edema. If the patient reports that stiffness and edema seem to increase by bedtime, he or she may be overdoing some activity or exercise during the day.

External mechanical compression also aids edema reduction.[47-51] In the early inflammatory phase, when edema is acute and tissues are more reactive, the best treatment may be rest combined with compression. The entire hand can be wrapped snugly in bias-cut bandage over Dacron batting, supported with a plaster or plastic orthosis. Later, when inflammation has subsided, other methods are appropriate such as compressive wrapping or gloves, retrograde massage, or intermittent compression devices. To use an intermittent compression device, the patient inserts his or her hand and arm into a sleeve attached to a pneumatic pump, which alternately inflates and deflates the sleeve, applying intermittent pressure to the entire extremity to expel excess interstitial fluid. Caution should be exercised when these devices are being used because they have the potential for overstressing healing structures such as fractures. Infection and history of cardiac disease, high blood pressure, or kidney disease also may be contraindications. Pressure levels and inflation-to-deflation ratios should be monitored carefully and kept within the manufacturer's guidelines and the bounds of good clinical judgment. In general, 60 mm Hg is the pressure limit for the upper extremity, and the ratio of inflation to deflation time is 3:1.

For constant light compression, the hand can be gently wrapped in Coban elasticized paper tape to reduce edema. The 1-inch-wide bandage is wrapped from distal to proximal in a spiral manner, taking care not to stretch the tape but rather to lay it on. This avoids a tourniquet effect. Only a reliable patient should use compressive wrapping for edema control; he or she must check carefully for any signs of wrapping too tightly (e.g., cyanosis, cold or numb fingertips). Prefabricated finger sleeves are a convenient alternative.

Because it is difficult to wrap an entire hand with even pressure, sometimes gloves or an elasticized compression stockinette may be a better alternative. Several types of prefabricated gloves are available; if prefabricated gloves do not fit the patient because of edema or deformity, gloves can be custom made by one of several companies. All gloves should leave fingertips exposed to allow the patient to monitor fingertip color, sensibility, and temperature.

Ideally, gloves or compressive bandages should be worn continuously—day and night. They should be removed once a day for careful hygiene, and the patient should have spare gloves or bandages so they can be changed periodically. If gloves or bandages interfere with hand mobility, they should be removed for exercise or perhaps worn only at night.

As with all parts of the home program, the patient should demonstrate to the therapist that he or she understands precautions and can apply and remove gloves or dressings correctly. The patient should not wear compressive gloves or wrappings if he or she does not appear able to follow these instructions. Even with careful application by an experienced therapist, pressure gradation is affected by the amount of overlapping, the number of layers, and any joint motion that occurs while wearing pressure bandages.[52] Injudicious use may result in obstruction of capillary flow.

Retrograde massage may be performed several times a day for at least 5 minutes, preferably before exercises. It is more effective for mobile or pitting edema than for chronic, fibrous edema. Deep, firm, long strokes milk the excess interstitial fluid from distal to proximal.

An alternative means of edema control is manual edema mobilization, which is covered in Chapter 57. This approach is an adaptation of manual lymphatic drainage techniques. Edema may also be reduced by the use of electrical stimulation.

Active Range of Motion

Active exercise decreases overall stiffness and edema and preserves or increases gliding between tissue planes that otherwise would scar together. The patient should exercise not only the injured hand but also the entire upper extremity to prevent stiffness and weakness caused by disuse and protective positioning. Whole-body conditioning completes the program; after an injury that disrupts the normal pattern of life, the patient almost invariably becomes less active and less physically fit, with profound effects on his or her emotional outlook and health.

Exercises should be simple and comprehensive, moving all necessary structures. As much as possible, different motions should be combined into one exercise.

Blocking exercises involve stabilizing of the finger proximal to the joint being exercised, thus isolating motion to that joint. This promotes gliding of specific tendons and increases the ROM available at the isolated joint by exerting active force on tight soft tissue structures. For example, isolated distal interphalangeal (DIP) joint flexion requires differential gliding of the flexor digitorum profundus tendon while stretching tight oblique retinacular ligaments and the extensor mechanism.

Of all the digits, the thumb accounts for the greatest percentage of function in a normal hand. If the fingers are severely injured, the thumb carries a greater burden; thus, maximum thumb motion is critical. The functional value of the thumb results from its mobility in several planes; this mobility must be maintained or attained through exercises in all planes of motion.

Neuromuscular electrical stimulation may be used as an adjunct to active exercise. It can serve to reinforce a weak muscle contraction or provide a rhythm to exercise. Biofeedback also can aid in active and resistive exercise by encouraging a patient to use a stronger muscle contraction or to relax the antagonist muscles when co-contraction is a problem.

When initiating active motion, the healing of all affected tissues should be considered. That the tendon is ready for active motion does not mean the coexisting fracture is sufficiently stable; the therapist may want to encourage flexor tendon gliding but need to protect an extensor tendon repaired under tension.

Passive Range of Motion

Joints are passively ranged very gently at first, and later with greater firmness, to stimulate healing of joint structures and to stretch tightening soft tissues and thus increase available motion. Gentle traction should be applied to distract joint surfaces before moving the joint passively. This prevents compressive or shearing forces to the joint surfaces. Passive ROM should never be forceful or painful. More aggressive joint mobilization should not be performed without specific training in this skill.

The status of all healing tissues must be considered when performing passive range of motion (PROM); for example, passive finger flexion stretches the dorsal apparatus and joint structures, so extensor tendon healing must be sufficiently advanced to allow any such stretch. As a precautionary measure, adjacent joints can be held in protective positions during passive ranging (e.g., MCP and DIP joints maintained in extension during PIP flexion).

Continuous passive motion devices can be a valuable adjunct to therapy. Continuous passive motion devices assist in increasing and maintaining passive mobility, maintaining gliding between adjacent structures, stimulating nutrient diffusion to articular cartilage and tendons, and decreasing edema and pain.

During all exercise, but especially during PROM by the therapist, sharp or severe pain should be avoided. The patient should inform the therapist of any pain other than a stretching sensation or a mild ache or soreness; more severe pain indicates potential tissue damage.

Heat and Cold

Heat modalities can be effective adjuncts to passive and active ROM, either in combination with or preceding mobilization. Because of the relatively thin layers of insulating adipose tissue in the hand, superficial heat agents actually may increase temperatures of deeper structures, including joints, if applied at sufficiently high temperatures and for sufficiently long periods (≥20 minutes). Superficial heat agents include paraffin, heat packs, and fluidotherapy. Deeper heat is provided by ultrasound, which is discussed in Chapter 101. Cold can be provided through cold packs or ice. All heat and cold should be applied with caution in the hand with sensory or vascular compromise.

Local superficial heat application produces vasodilation and increased blood flow, which improve nutrition and may aid healing. Cold decreases muscle spasm and can reduce inflammatory edema if applied during early healing and for sufficient time. It can also control postexercise pain. Although the actual mechanism is not known, both heat and cold relieve pain, with some patients being more amenable to one than to the other. Therefore, it is often helpful to apply heat or cold before potentially painful treatments. Two caveats apply in the use of heat or cold to control pain during therapy. Cold may increase stiffness and therefore negate the benefits of pain relief, and either heat or cold may decrease a desirable pain response that would inform the therapist that the exercise is too vigorous.

In addition to decreasing pain associated with passive stretch, both heat and cold can increase extensibility of connective tissue, thus augmenting the effectiveness of stretch applied through orthotic positioning or exercise. The increased extensibility is temporary but allows the patient to safely and comfortably apply stretch, with an apparent cumulative effect over time. This phenomenon has been well demonstrated both clinically and through in vivo and in vitro study, but the exact mechanism is still open to question, as are the long-term results.[10]

The therapist must understand the cause of the underlying pain or stiffness and evaluate the patient's natural response to heat and cold in choosing the appropriate modality. Some patients find cold noxious and therefore prefer heat, but heat may increase inflammation. Hardy and Woodall[7] suggest the use of cold with compression to control pain and swelling or cold and stretch to control muscle soreness and spasm, as opposed to heat combined with low-load, long-duration stretch to address scar and myostatic contracture. Several authors[53–56] have provided excellent surveys of the current literature regarding the effects of heat and cold on pain, edema, and other responses to injury.

Orthotic Positioning

Static orthoses are used for rest and support, for protection, and to position for function and prevention of deformity. If possible, a resting orthosis in the early stages should position the wrist in 10 to 20 degrees of extension with 70 to 80 degrees of MCP flexion, 0 to 15 degrees of IP flexion, and thumb palmar abduction. This position counteracts the typical joint contractures of the injured hand, which produce a deformity of PIP joint flexion, MCP joint extension, thumb adduction, and wrist flexion. All injured structures must be taken into account and the orthosis design modified accordingly. For example, an extensor digitorum communis injury may demand greater extension of both wrist and MCP joints, but a coexisting MCP joint collateral ligament injury would need extra protection against lateral stress and carefully determined MCP joint flexion to prevent ligament healing in a shortened position.

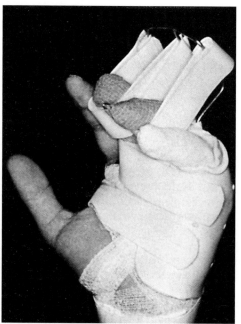

Fig. 75.3 This static progressive orthosis allows active motion of the fifth-digit interphalangeal joints while protecting a newly healed fifth-metacarpal head fracture by immobilizing the metacarpophalangeal joint. At the same time, serially adjusted, low-intensity static pull is exerted on the middle phalanges of the third and fourth digits to increase extension at the proximal interphalangeal joints. Note that a Kirschner wire immobilizes the fourth-digit distal interphalangeal (DIP) joint. The strap is therefore carefully positioned at the DIP joint level, rather than distal or proximal to the joint, to protect joint immobilization. The third digit is amputated at the DIP joint.

If edema is severe, postoperative orthoses are wrapped with Ace wrap or bias-cut bandage (3M Co., Minneapolis, MN), wrapped from distal to proximal in a figure-of-8 fashion to avoid the tourniquet effect of constrictive circular straps or bandages. Orthoses and straps also should be cut and modified to protect external hardware.

Passive stretch is most effective when applied with low intensity over a long period or at frequent intervals. Prolonged low-intensity stretch encourages increased length, not because the collagen fibers actually stretch but because as old fibers are degraded, the new fibers that replace them are laid down in response to the gentle tension. The new fibers are oriented in a manner that allows greater extensibility. Several authors[5,7,10,57] provide thorough reviews of the literature on connective tissue remodeling in response to stress.

Serial static, static progressive, and dynamic orthoses are the best means available for providing prolonged low-intensity stretch. Serial static orthoses are static orthoses that are periodically refabricated to accommodate for increases in available motion. Examples of these orthoses are periodically remade web stretchers and cylinder casts. Static progressive orthoses are adjusted by the patient as motion improves (e.g., serially adjusted flexion gloves). An orthosis that combines protective static orthotic positioning with static progressive orthotic positioning to increase joint motion is shown in Fig. 75.3. More information regarding orthoses designed to increase mobility can be found in Chapters 107 to 109.

No dynamic or serially adjusted orthosis should be used unless healing structures are clearly strong enough to withstand such stress, however gentle. Patients must understand precisely how to apply and remove orthoses, how long to wear them, and how to check for signs of incorrect fit or pressure problems. This is particularly important in an insensate hand.

When an orthosis is designed to increase motion, that motion should be measured at frequent intervals to determine the continuing utility of the orthosis. For example, when the PIP joint is being serially casted into extension, passive PIP extension is measured at each visit. In addition, if one of the goals of treatment is to maintain flexion through exercise between cast changes, active or passive flexion also should be measured. Thus evaluation ensures that casting continues only as long as it is effective and only if it does not compromise other desirable motion.

Prosthetics

Although it is beyond the scope of this chapter to discuss prosthetics, it should be noted that prosthetic planning and training begin very early. The residual limb or digit must be prepared and the appropriate prosthesis selected. Many types of prostheses are available, and the choice of prosthesis is crucial to the patient's functional and emotional recovery. See Chapters 77 and 78 for further discussion.

Muscle Strengthening

Effective strengthening exercise involves resistance that elicits the strongest muscle contraction that can safely be demanded. As strength increases over time, resistance likewise is increased as tolerated. Pain, edema, and strength must be monitored carefully to help determine the appropriate amount of resistance in a given session. If edema increased notably after exercise, for example, resistance would not be increased in the next session, and the exercise or activity could be modified to incorporate elevation. It is also possible that the patient performed too many repetitions while exercising independently, and he or she must be warned of the dangers of overworking the muscle.

Purposeful Activity

There is evidence in the literature supporting the concept that purposeful, goal-oriented activity elicits smoother, more efficient, and less effortful motion than do prescribed motions or exercises.[58-60] Many patients have great difficulty making a fist but when asked to transfer a handful of small objects from one container to another, they grasp firmly and with less difficulty or pain. In addition, activities performed in therapy or at home can be designed to incorporate functional motion of the entire body or upper quarter, thus promoting reintegration of the injured hand in daily activities.

With all activities, care must be taken to avoid overwork. Endurance should increase slowly to meet the demands of daily life.

Through job simulation, the patient can be observed performing work activities, and any necessary tool or task adaptations can be designed. The patient spends increasing amounts of time in therapy or in a home job-simulation program to improve endurance and to prepare for return to the rigors of a full workday.

Each patient has unique needs that must be carefully evaluated in planning return to work or avocational pursuits. The next section examines the evaluation and treatment of the special needs of injured workers.

REHABILITATION GUIDELINES FOR EACH PHASE OF HEALING

In the interests of simplicity, the following guidelines cover the three phases of wound healing as though all tissues in the hand were healing at the same rate. This is not the case in reality. Appropriate treatment depends on careful evaluation of the healing status of each individual tissue and the relationship between tissues.

Inflammatory Phase

The emphasis of treatment is on controlling edema and maintaining a healthy microenvironment for wound healing. At the same time, as much as possible, ROM is maintained.

In the first treatment session, the focus is on helping the patient understand the injury, making necessary orthoses, and introducing a simple home program. This session is usually tiring and confusing for the patient and thus should be kept short. If patients can be shown improvement in the first session (e.g., decreased discomfort, even a small increase in ROM), they may be more motivated in future therapy.

Before seeing the patient, the therapist should gather as much information as possible from the surgeon, including operative reports, precautions, and a look at the radiographs. Specific advice should be sought about unusual aspects such as special dressings or unfamiliar surgical procedures. The therapist should know exactly what structures should be immobilized or protected, in what positions, and the purpose of any orthoses or specific treatments requested by the surgeon.

Evaluation

In a complex injury, many tissues are involved, necessitating a comprehensive evaluation. A thorough medical, occupational, and psychosocial history is taken so that all factors can be considered in planning treatment. It may be helpful to take photographs or draw diagrams of the hand, including wounds, incisions, hardware, and amputations, as well as to indicate insensate areas or other special problems.

The wound is examined for width, length, depth, and characteristics such as granulation tissue, bleeding, contaminants, or exposed vital tissues. The therapist notes the presence of sutures or external fixators and signs of infection such as foul odor; thick exudate; or erythematous, warm skin surrounding the wound.

Edema is measured circumferentially rather than by volumeter because in the presence of open wounds, the hand should not be immersed in water except for any sterile whirlpools or soaks necessary for debridement. Edema should be monitored at the same point in each treatment session, preferably before treatment.

Range of motion is measured as allowed by applicable precautions or immobilization. Uninvolved joints should not be neglected, especially the shoulder and elbow if a sling has been worn.

Sensory status should be ascertained as far as possible. It is often better to delay a full objective sensory assessment until wound healing has progressed further and edema has subsided. Both pain and edema can interfere with examination, and a great change in sensory status is unlikely in the first week or so. Nonetheless, a good subjective screening is essential to alert the therapist to any insensate areas needing protection or any paresthesias or other signs of nerve compression. Such signs may indicate problems with bandaging, casting, or orthotic fabrication or may mean that a surgical decompression is needed. If the medical history does not explain the sensory findings and the therapist is unable to alleviate the symptoms by modifying the orthosis or dressing, the surgeon should be consulted immediately.

Pain should be assessed: is there constant pain, or pain only with motion? Is it sharp or dull? Is it relieved by elevation of the hand? An assessment of activities of daily living (ADLs) should begin in this stage, as the patient first encounters problems with using only one hand.

Treatment

Patient education is the most important element of early treatment. During the entire session, the therapist should explain and demonstrate, listen to the patient's questions and anxieties, and use every opportunity to set an example for home therapy. A referral to social services or communication with the family may be indicated at this time.

The patient must learn the difference between normal posttraumatic pain and discomfort and the sharp pain with motion that indicates excessive force. He or she must learn not to be afraid of dull pain and the feeling of mild stretch that accompanies early motion, but the patient must also realize that sharp or persistent pain is a danger sign.

Patients must be alert for the signs of fatigue and overwork and must also be aware that they cannot always rely on the body to tell them when they are overworking. Often, too many repetitions of an apparently innocuous and easy exercise produce great discomfort 1 or 2 days later. On the other hand, stiffness may be prolonged in a patient who skips exercise sessions, decreases repetitions because of normal postoperative pain or fatigue, or performs exercises with only half-hearted muscle contractions. If the patient learns at this stage to follow the home program exactly, without adding or subtracting, he or she will lay the foundation for a smooth recovery.

Because the patient has a lot of new information to absorb and is under the stress of pain and fatigue, the initial home program should be simple. A new element can be added to the program every session or so, giving the patient time to integrate each part in turn.

If the patient has a severe pain problem, the physician should be consulted to ascertain the cause of the pain and any possible intervention. Pain medication makes many patients drowsy and poses the risks of dependence and masking of pain, which is a useful danger sign. Electrical stimulation (either conventional transcutaneous nerve stimulation or interferential current) may be more helpful or appropriate than medication for some patients, especially those with chronic pain. Pain is always a difficult issue because a balance must be found between acceptable pain and pain that interferes with a patient's physical performance and emotional well-being.

If the hand is insensate, there may be no pain even with excessive pressure or motion. The patient can prevent inadvertent damage to the hand by avoiding overzealous pursuit of the home program.

Wound care includes whirlpools if necessary for debridement or cleansing of the wound, conservative manual debridement, and dressings, as well as pin care and monitoring of the wounds for signs of infection or unusual inflammatory response.

Edema control at this stage concentrates on elevation and active motion. If vessels were reconstructed, the referring surgeon should be consulted about limiting elevation to heart level to avoid overburdening fragile structures. Edema-reducing massage is restricted to areas where there are no open wounds and where massage will not disturb healing of adjacent tissues. Compressive wrapping may be contraindicated because of vascular compromise, grafts, flaps, or unusually unstable structures. In the presence of active infection, elevation above heart level, compressive wrapping, and massage all are contraindicated to avoid spreading the infection proximally.

One of the most challenging and therefore most exciting aspects of treatment planning is the choice of the structures to move actively or passively and those to protect and how to balance the needs of all the structures and tissues involved. This is where the therapist most surely demonstrates his or her skill at systematic and creative problem solving. Passive exercises generally should precede active exercises in each session so that weak or injured muscles are not working against excessive passive resistance from surrounding tissues. Likewise, edema-reduction techniques should be used as indicated to reduce the passive resistance of edematous tissues.

Exercises concentrate on preserving gliding of soft tissues and motion of all joints in which motion is not contraindicated, especially in areas where the nature of injury indicates there will be the greatest problems. This generally includes MCP joint flexion, PIP joint extension, wrist extension, and thumb palmar abduction, all of which are commonly limited after complex injuries with moderate to severe edema.

Uninvolved joints also should be moved through ROM to prevent problems secondary to disuse or protective positioning. This is the time to begin treatment to prevent shoulder and neck pain or stiffness. Exercise duration and frequency should be tailored to the tissue response noted in therapy. Some patients will fatigue easily and therefore need short, frequent exercise sessions, whereas others do better with less frequent, longer sessions to gain greater mobility.

Orthotic positioning will vary according to the individual injury but generally will be limited to static orthotic positioning to immobilize, rest, and support affected tissues. Dynamic orthotic positioning for protected early passive mobilization of tendons also may be indicated. If orthoses are fabricated during the patient's first visit, other treatment and evaluation should be kept to a minimum to keep the session short. ROM exercises may be performed before orthotic fabrication to decrease stiffness before applying the orthosis.

All patients benefit from discussion of problems they encounter in ADLs. Some will need adaptive equipment; others use adaptive techniques. The discussion itself is helpful because it focuses on the recovery of functional performance and reveals the patient's coping mechanisms.

Proliferative Phase

As the inflammatory response ends, treatment can be upgraded, focusing not only on continued wound care but also on managing scar and increasing motion. However, it must be remembered that the strength of healing wounds is still very low and that there is always the danger of provoking a renewed inflammatory response through excessive stress and resultant microscopic trauma.

Evaluation

Pain, wounds, and edema continue to be monitored, with changes in response to treatment particularly being noted. ROM is monitored with special attention to any developing joint contractures or restrictive adhesions.

A full sensory evaluation may be delayed until this period if indicated. Orthoses are checked closely for pressure problems and for changes in fit as edema decreases and dressings become less bulky. Each orthosis also should be reevaluated regularly to determine whether it still serves the patient well and whether the goals of the orthosis are still valid for the patient.

The therapist should frequently reassess the patient's comprehension and performance of the home program, any progress or problems with ADLs, and the adjustment to the stress of major trauma and its psychosocial consequences.

Treatment

Sutures are removed in this period, and as wounds heal, transverse friction massage is instituted for all scars, along with more extensive massage to decrease edema; for relaxation before or after exercise; for desensitization; and as a time for building patient–therapist rapport. A formal desensitization program also may begin.

If not contraindicated (e.g., in grafts, before 2 weeks), compression for edema may be initiated at this stage. Elastomer or other pressure pads should be fabricated as early as possible to influence collagen formation in its early stages.

If there are no contraindications and active motion is sufficient, the patient may begin light prehension tasks performed in elevation to control edema and begin functional hand use. Additional PROM exercises or orthoses may be needed because of developing joint contractures or adhesions that limit motion.

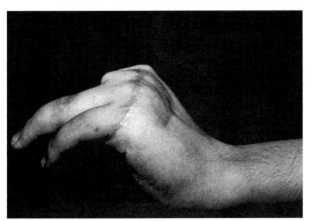

Fig. 75.4 In this child with revascularized ring and small fingers, active flexion could be limited by any of a number of factors. Joint stiffness or ankylosis and flexor or extensor tendon adhesions are the most likely causes.

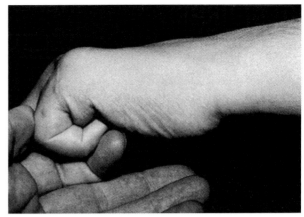

Fig. 75.5 Passive flexion of the small finger is complete, indicating that flexor tendon adhesions are the major culprit limiting active flexion of this finger.

While edema remains, the hand is still elevated when not active, but the need to elevate the hand or to wear orthoses or compressive wrappings should not interfere unduly with opportunities for active hand use. Problems will arise as the patient attempts to resume activities for the first time, and the therapist must address these problems promptly through adaptive techniques and equipment. Referrals to social services may assist the patient in psychosocial adjustment as the full effect of a severe injury becomes apparent.

Scar Maturation–Remodeling Phase

From this stage until discharge, therapy focuses on scar remodeling at all levels to strengthen repairs, to encourage gliding of soft tissues, and to improve function and cosmesis. For some patients, this may be an intermediate stage of preparation for further reconstructive surgery, but the ultimate goal is always the same: return to former vocational and avocational activities.

Evaluation

Until all wounds are healed in adjacent tissues still in earlier phases, the clinician must be alert to any signs of infection. Changes in edema in response to treatment should continue to be monitored.

Regular assessment of superficial scar and deep adhesions will reveal the relative success of scar management techniques and dictate changes in approach. With a complex injury, it is especially important to understand the etiology of any problems. For example, a deficit in digit extension could be a result of any of the following: adherence or shortening of long flexor tendons; secondary joint contractures; adherence, stretch, denervation, weakness, or rupture of long extensor tendons; denervation of the intrinsics; or pain. There also could be a combination of several problems. If the source of the limitation is not identified precisely, treatment cannot be effectively planned (Figs. 75.4 and 75.5).

Beginning approximately 6 to 8 weeks after a nerve repair, sensory examination may reveal regeneration. Monthly reexamination reveals not only regeneration but also the results of sensory reeducation. Progress of desensitization and sensory reeducation programs must be monitored closely because they require great dedication on the part of the patient.

As muscle strength, endurance, and dexterity begin to be addressed, periodic evaluation helps quantify progress and pinpoint problems. Toward the end of therapy, a functional capacity evaluation, possibly coupled with an onsite job assessment, helps determine the patient's readiness to return to work and dictates changes in discharge planning (see Chapters 119 and 120). The patient may have emotional and physical obstacles to overcome when returning to work; early identification may help with ultimate resolution of these difficulties.

Treatment

Management of cutaneous scar continues in this phase. Especially bulky or adherent scars should receive close attention; ultrasound may be initiated, and scar compression continues. As inflammatory edema subsides, heat modalities may be used safely as valuable adjuncts to exercise and soft tissue mobilization.

Active and passive ROM limitations become progressively harder to overcome in this phase. The rapidly remodeling scar tissue will become dense and restrictive if not subjected to stress of sufficient intensity, frequency, and duration. It is particularly important to identify problems through frequent evaluation and to adapt treatment accordingly. Some structures may have been immobilized before this phase; if motion is initiated now, the therapist can expect to encounter problems with adhesions and joint contractures secondary to immobilization.

Sensory reeducation begins and desensitization continues, facilitated also by functional activities. Muscle strengthening and endurance and dexterity training all start gradually, stepping up in intensity according to tissue healing and evaluation results (Figs. e75.4 and e75.5). In the later stages, job or activity simulation may begin. Training in ADLs focuses on specific problems as they emerge (Fig. 75.6).

A common problem is overwork, provoking an inflammatory response. Many patients, encouraged by their returning abilities, will overdo an apparently easy activity such as writing a letter; even 15 minutes of this light but repetitive prehension may not hurt today but could leave the hand edematous and sore tomorrow. This is especially true of resistive exercise; for example, patients must be warned not to use therapy putty or grip exercisers while watching television. The patient loses track of time and the number of repetitions. If, as in so many cases, there is no immediate pain or swelling, the patient does not even realize until the next day that he or she has overdone the exercise. One cannot emphasize too strongly to the patient that not only is this uncomfortable, but it also represents a step backward because the inflammatory response leads to further fibrosis. Cold, elevation, and a temporary decrease in exercise duration can alleviate the pain and edema, but prevention is infinitely preferable.

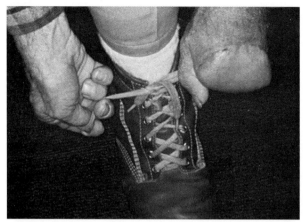

Fig. 75.6 In the absence of the second through fifth digits distal to the metacarpophalangeal joints, this patient regained functional prehension sufficient for independence in activities of daily living. His functional potential was particularly good because the injury was to his nondominant hand and spared the thumb.

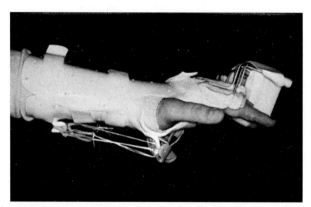

Fig. 75.7 A patient's hand shown after replant of long, ring, and small fingers followed by extensor and flexor tenolysis and metacarpophalangeal capsulotomies. Because the patient had complex orthotic positioning needs, one orthosis was designed to meet the two most pressing needs. A serial static extension to the proximal interphalangeal joints can be seen here, which exhibited a hard end feel.

Orthotic positioning in this phase focuses on increasing motion and function. Serial static, static progressive, and dynamic orthotic positioning provide prolonged low-intensity stretch, and dynamic orthoses assist weak motions while resisting antagonistic motions.

Because a hand with multiple injuries has such complex needs, it is all too easy to make orthoses of matching complexity. The patient is unlikely to wear large, complicated orthoses or follow confusing schedules involving many orthosis changes (Figs. 75.7 and 75.8). Higher priority needs should be addressed first and most aggressively, and the orthosis program should be changed as dictated by reevaluation.

During this stage, the patient may need to switch from traditional hands-on therapy to a work hardening or work conditioning program in preparation for return to work. Chapter 120 covers this important component of therapy.

SUMMARY

There are no easy formulas or protocols for rehabilitation after a complex injury. Each component of injury is assessed, and each intervention is designed both individually and in the context of the total picture. The psychosocial needs of the patient may be profound and

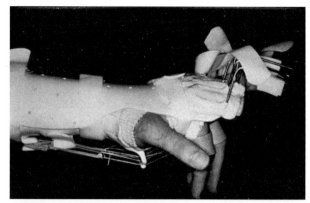

Fig. 75.8 This part of the orthosis (see Fig. 75.7) provided dynamic flexion to the metacarpophalangeal joints, which had a more elastic end feel.

must not be overshadowed by the physical injury. Key elements are the therapist's understanding of normal and pathologic healing of each injured tissue; logical and creative application of this knowledge to evaluation and treatment planning; and constant, close communication among patient, surgeon, and therapist. Although such cases may be daunting, it is the very challenge they present that makes them so rewarding when brought to a successful conclusion.

REFERENCES

1. Broughton 2nd G, Janis JE, Attinger CE. Wound healing: an overview. *Plast Reconstr Surg.* 2006;117:1e-S–32e-S.
2. Broughton 2nd G, Janis JE, Attinger CE. The basic science of wound healing. *Plast Reconstr Surg.* 2006;117:12S–34S.
3. Amadio P. Tendon and ligament. In: Cohen IK, Diegelmann RF, Lindblad WJ, eds. *Wound Healing: Biochemical and Clinical Aspects.* Philadelphia: W.B. Saunders Co; 1992:384–395.
4. Arem AJ, Madden JW. Effects of stress on healing wounds: I. Intermittent noncyclical tension. *J Surg Res.* 1976;20:93–102.
5. Cyr LM, Ross RG. How controlled stress affects healing tissues. *J Hand Ther.* 1998;11:125–130.
6. Gelberman RH, Woo SL, Lothringer K, et al. Effects of early intermittent passive mobilization on healing canine flexor tendons. *J Hand Surg [Am].* 1982;7:170–175.
7. Hardy M, Woodall W. Therapeutic effects of heat, cold, and stretch on connective tissue. *J Hand Ther.* 1998;11:148–156.
8. Hitchcock TF, Light TR, Bunch WH, et al. The effect of immediate constrained digital motion on the strength of flexor tendon repairs in chickens. *J Hand Surg [Am].* 1987;12:590–595.
9. Kubota H, Manske PR, Aoki M, et al. Effect of motion and tension on injured flexor tendons in chickens. *J Hand Surg [Am].* 1996;21:456–463.
10. Tillman LJ, Cummings GS. Biologic mechanisms of connective tissue mutability. In: Currier DP, Nelson RM, eds. *Dynamics of Human Biologic Tissues.* Philadelphia: F.A. Davis; 1992.
11. Akeson WH, Amiel D, Abel MF, et al. Effects of immobilization on joints. *Clin Orthop Relat Res.* 1987;219:28–37.
12. Cronan T. Effects of immobilization and mobilization on cartilaginous, bony, and soft-tissue structure: review of the literature. *J Burn Care Rehabil.* 1986;7:54–57.
13. Jozsa L, Thoring J, Jarvinen M, et al. Quantitative alterations in intramuscular connective tissue following immobilization: an experimental study in the rat calf muscles. *Exp Mol Pathol.* 1988;49:267–278.
14. Malaviya P, Butler DL, Boivin GP, et al. An in vivo model for load-modulated remodeling in the rabbit flexor tendon. *J Orthop Res.* 2000;18:116–125.
15. Shimizu T, Videman T, Shimazaki K, Mooney V. Experimental study on the repair of full thickness articular cartilage defects: effects of varying periods of continuous passive motion, cage activity, and immobilization. *J Orthop Res.* 1987;5:187–197.

16. Videman T. Connective tissue and immobilization. Key factors in musculoskeletal degeneration? *Clin Orthop Relat Res.* 1987;221:26–32.

17. Videman T, Eronen I, Candolin T. Effects of motion load changes on tendon tissues and articular cartilage. *Scand J Work Environ Health.* 1979;5:56.

18. Hunt TK, Hussain Z. Wound microenvironment. In: Cohen IK, Diegelmann RF, Lindblad WJ, eds. *Wound Healing: Biochemical and Clinical Aspects.* Philadelphia: W.B. Saunders Company; 1992:274–281.

19. Braakenburg A, Obdeijn MC, Feitz R, van Rooij IA, van Griethuysen AJ, Klinkenbijl JH. The clinical efficacy and cost effectiveness of the vacuum-assisted closure technique in the management of acute and chronic wounds: a randomized controlled trial. *Plast Reconstr Surg.* 2006;118:390–397: discussion 398-400.

20. Greenhalgh DG. Wound healing and diabetes mellitus. *Clin Plast Surg.* 2003;30:37–45.

21. Jazayeri L, Callaghan MJ, Grogan RH, et al. Diabetes increases p53-mediated apoptosis following ischemia. *Plast Reconstr Surg.* 2008;121:1135–1143.

22. Krueger JK, Rohrich RJ. Clearing the smoke: the scientific rationale for tobacco abstention with plastic surgery. *Plast Reconstr Surg.* 2001;108:1063–1073: discussion 1074-1067.

23. Manassa EH, Hertl CH, Olbrisch RR. Wound healing problems in smokers and nonsmokers after 132 abdominoplasties. *Plast Reconstr Surg.* 2003;111:2082–2087: discussion 2088-2089.

24. van Adrichem LN, Hovius SE, van Strik R, van der Meulen JC. The acute effect of cigarette smoking on the microcirculation of a replanted digit. *J Hand Surg [Am].* 1992;17:230–234.

25. Lee WP, Constantinescu MA, Butler PE. Effect of early mobilization on healing of nerve repair: histologic observations in a canine model. *Plast Reconstr Surg.* 1999;104:1718–1725.

26. Dagum AB. Peripheral nerve regeneration, repair, and grafting. *J Hand Ther.* 1998;11:111–117.

27. Aoki M, Kubota H, Pruitt DL, Manske PR. Biomechanical and histologic characteristics of canine flexor tendon repair using early postoperative mobilization. *J Hand Surg [Am].* 1997;22:107–114.

28. Mason J, Allen H. The rate of healing of tendons: an experimental study of tensile strength. *Ann Surg.* 1941;113:424.

29. Schultz K. The effect of active exercise on edema. *J Hand Surg.* American Volume. 1983;8:625.

30. Walsh M. Relationship of hand edema to upper extremity position and water temperature during whirlpool. *J Hand Surg.* American Volume. 1984;(9A):609.

31. Walsh M. Hydrotherapy: the use of water as a therapeutic agent. In: Michlovitz SL, ed. *Thermal Agents in Rehabilitation.* Philadelphia: F.A. Davis Company; 1986:119–139.

32. Argenta LC, Morykwas MJ, Marks MW, et al. Vacuum-assisted closure: state of clinic art. *Plast Reconstr Surg.* 2006;117:127S–142S.

33. Mustoe TA, Cooter RD, Gold MH, et al. International clinical recommendations on scar management. *Plast Reconstr Surg.* 2002;110:560–571.

34. Ahn ST, Monafo WW, Mustoe TA. Topical silicone gel for the prevention and treatment of hypertrophic scar. *Arch Surg.* 1991;126:499–504.

35. Baum TM, Busuito MJ. Use of a glycerin-based gel sheeting in scar management. *Adv Wound Care.* 1998;11:40–43.

36. Carr-Collins JA. Pressure techniques for the prevention of hypertrophic scar. *Clin Plast Surg.* 1992;19:733–743.

37. Costa AM, Peyrol S, Porto LC, et al. Mechanical forces induce scar remodeling. Study in non-pressure-treated versus pressure-treated hypertrophic scars. *Am J Pathol.* 1999;155:1671–1679.

38. Haq MA, Haq A. Pressure therapy in treatment of hypertrophic scar, burn contracture and keloid: the Kenyan experience. *East Afr Med J.* 1990;67:785–793.

39. Katz BE. Silicone gel sheeting in scar therapy. *Cutis.* 1995;56:65–67.

40. Rose MP, Deitch EA. The clinical use of a tubular compression bandage, Tubigrip, for burn- scar therapy: a critical analysis. *Burns Incl Therm Inj.* 1985;12:58–64.

41. Ward RS. Pressure therapy for the control of hypertrophic scar formation after burn injury. A history and review. *J Burn Care Rehabil.* 1991;12:257–262.

42. Atkinson JA, McKenna KT, Barnett AG, et al. A randomized, controlled trial to determine the efficacy of paper tape in preventing hypertrophic scar formation in surgical incisions that traverse Langer's skin tension lines. *Plast Reconstr Surg.* 2005;116:1648–1656: discussion 1657-1648.

43. Reiffel RS. Prevention of hypertrophic scars by long-term paper tape application. *Plast Reconstr Surg.* 1995;96:1715–1718.

44. Burd A, Huang L. Hypertrophic response and keloid diathesis: two very different forms of scar. *Plast Reconstr Surg.* 2005;116:150e–157e.

45. Lundborg G, Dahlin L, Danielsen N, Zhao Q. Trophism, tropism, and specificity in nerve regeneration. *J Reconstr Microsurg.* 1994;10:345–354.

46. Rosen B, Lundborg G, Dahlin LB, et al. Nerve repair: correlation of restitution of functional sensibility with specific cognitive capacities. *J Hand Surg [Br].* 1994;19:452–458.

47. Airaksinen O, Partanen K, Kolari PJ, Soimakallio S. Intermittent pneumatic compression therapy in posttraumatic lower limb edema: computed tomography and clinical measurements. *Arch Phys Med Rehabil.* 1991;72:667–670.

48. Ause-Ellias KL, Richard R, Miller SF, Finley Jr RK. The effect of mechanical compression on chronic hand edema after burn injury: a preliminary report. *J Burn Care Rehabil.* 1994;15:29–33.

49. Griffin JW, Newsome LS, Stralka SW, Wright PE. Reduction of chronic posttraumatic hand edema: a comparison of high voltage pulsed current, intermittent pneumatic compression, and placebo treatments. *Phys Ther.* 1990;70:279–286.

50. Van Geest AJ, Veraart JC, Nelemans P, Neumann HA. The effect of medical elastic compression stockings with different slope values on edema measurements underneath three different types of stockings. *Dermatol Surg.* 2000;26:244–247.

51. Veraart JC, Neumann HA. Effects of medical elastic compression stockings on interface pressure and edema prevention. *Dermatol Surg.* 1996;22:867–871.

52. Beach RB, Bell J. Ace, Coban and bias stockinette: pressures resulting from their use. *J Hand Surg.* 1983;8:627.

53. Michlovitz SL. Biophysical principles of heating and superficial heat agents. In: Michlovitz SL, ed. *Thermal Agents in Rehabilitation.* Philadelphia: F.A. Davis Company; 1986:99–118.

54. Michlovitz SL. Cryotherapy: the use of cold as a therapeutic agent. In: Michlovitz SL, ed. *Thermal Agents in Rehabilitation.* Philadelphia: F.A. Davis Company; 1986:73–98.

55. Newton RA. Contemporary views on pain and the role played by thermal agents in managing pain symptoms. In: Michlovitz SL, ed. *Thermal Agents in Rehabilitation.* Philadelphia: F.A. Davis Company; 1986:19–48.

56. Zarro VJ. Mechanisms of inflammation and repair. In: Michlovitz SL, ed. *Thermal Agents in Rehabilitation.* Philadelphia: F.A. Davis; 1986:3–118.

57. Cummings GS, Tillman LJ. Remodeling of dense connective tissue in normal adult tissues. In: Currier DP, Nelson RM, eds. *Dynamics of Human Biologic Tissues.* Philadelphia: F.A. Davis Company; 1992.

58. Lin KC, Wu CY, Trombly CA. Effects of task goal on movement kinematics and line bisection performance in adults without disabilities. *Am J Occup Ther.* 1998;52:179–187.

59. Ma HI, Trombly CA. The comparison of motor performance between part and whole tasks in elderly persons. *Am J Occup Ther.* 2001;55:62–67.

60. Trombly CA. Observations of improvement of reaching in five subjects with left hemiparesis. *J Neurol Neurosurg Psychiatry.* 1993;56:40–45.

76

Fingertip Injuries: Surgery and Therapy

Annalisa Franzen, Leonid I. Katolik

OUTLINE

CRITICAL POINTS

- Fingertip injuries are common and account for approximately 4% of all emergency department visits.
- Sequelae of fingertip injuries include scar contracture, cold intolerance, hypersensitivity, inadequate pulp volume, and stiffness in adjoining joints and adjacent digits with consequent long-term patient dissatisfaction or frank disability.

- Goals of management include preservation of functional length, durable coverage, preservation of useful sensibility, prevention of symptomatic neuromas, prevention of adjacent joint contractures, short morbidity, and early return to work or recreation.
- Most fingertip injuries require referral to a hand therapy unit for optimization of outcome and minimization of long-term sequelae.

Fingertip injuries are common and account for approximately 4% of all emergency department visits.[1,2] Significant costs are associated with treatment, lost work, and functional disability caused by these injuries. Furthermore, long-term sequelae of scar contracture, cold intolerance, inadequate pulp volume, and stiffness in adjoining joints and adjacent digits may lead to chronic patient dissatisfaction or frank disability.

Surgical options for the treatment of fingertip injuries span the spectrum from elegant simplicity to the absolute triumph of technology over reason.[3,4] Treatment decisions should ultimately be based on patient needs. These include preservation of functional length, durable coverage, preservation of useful sensibility, prevention of symptomatic neuromas, prevention of adjacent joint contractures, short morbidity, and early return to work or recreation.

Regardless of medical or surgical intervention, all fingertip injuries ultimately require referral to a hand therapy unit for optimization of outcome and minimization of long-term sequelae.

ANATOMY

For simplicity, we consider the fingertip as the digital unit distal to the insertion of the flexor digitorum profundus. It consists of the pulp, nail, and underlying phalanx.

The fingertip pulp is a closed space. Vertical fibrous septae anchor the pulp to the periosteum of the underlying phalanx. The pulp contains the distal arborization of cutaneous lymph vessels, as well as the terminal branches of the digital neurovascular system.

The nail unit provides support to the pulp during pincer grasp and tactile functions (Fig. 76.1). It consists of keratinized squamous cells produced by the germinal matrix at the base of the nail bed. The thin epithelium of the sterile matrix provides an adherent layer for firm nail attachment. It is in turn contiguous with the underlying periosteum of the distal phalanx. The eponychium forms the dorsal roof of the base of

the nail, and the paronychium is the lateral nail fold. The hyponychium is the junction of the nail bed and the fingertip skin distally.

SURGICAL CONSIDERATIONS

Fingertip injuries are typically caused by a crush or a crush–avulsion type of mechanism. They result in an injury spectrum consisting of

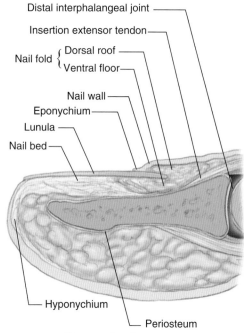

Fig. 76.1 The finger–nail unit.

disruption of the pulp, injury to the nail unit, and fracture of the underlying bone (Fig. 76.2).

Examination is best performed under loupe magnification, in a hemostatic field, and with the patient made comfortable. To this end, patients are offered a regional anesthetic. It is the authors' preference, for reasons of patient comfort, to administer wrist blockade rather than digital blockade. Multiplanar radiographs of the affected digit are then obtained. A finger cot tourniquet is applied. In the subacute setting, although the wound may initially be hemostatic, examination and debridement will shortly disrupt this. The wound is irrigated with sterile saline solution to clear blood and debris. Detailed and complete assessment is now possible. When the assessment is complete, the fingertip is dressed with nonadherent gauze, surgical sponges, and light

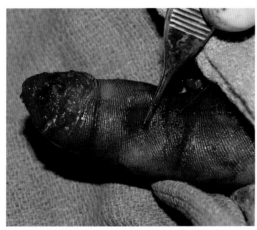

Fig. 76.2 Fingertip injury in 32-year-old truck driver with loss of pulp substance, open fracture through distal phalanx, avulsion of fingernail, and laceration of nail bed after a blunt injury.

compressive dressing. The bulky nature of this dressing generally provides adequate immobilization as well.

Fractures of the distal phalanx with fingertip injuries often involve significant comminution or bone loss. As such, operative intervention for the bony injuries alone is very uncommon.

Recall that the periosteum of the distal phalanx is contiguous with the sterile matrix, and disruption of the nail bed with tuft fractures is generally a certainty. If the overlying nail plate is not avulsed, surgical nail removal and repair of the nail bed is not performed. The overlying nail plate serves as an excellent occlusive dressing to allow for healing of the underlying matrix (Fig. 76.3). If the nail plate is disrupted or avulsed, it is removed, and meticulous nail bed repair is performed with fine absorbable (5-0 gut) sutures. The nail fold is then fixed using either the native nail plate or a contoured slip of sterile foil from the surgical wrapper (Fig. 76.4).

Linear skin lacerations may be easily repaired with fine absorbable suture. Stellate lacerations are loosely reapproximated. When the laceration involves the proximal or lateral nail folds, care must be taken to restore the anatomy without obliterating the underlying space.

The management of soft tissue loss of the fingertip with exposed bone has engendered tremendous controversy. The patient's work demands and the desire for restoration of appearance guide the choice of treatment. Microsurgical replantation, free tissue transfer, pedicled flap coverage, soft tissue advancement, cross-finger flap coverage, thenar flap coverage, and skin grafting have been described with varying degrees of success.[5-11] However, no single method is universally applicable. Indeed, no method guarantees prevention of the vexing sequelae of cold intolerance, tip sensitivity, or altered cosmesis.

Revision amputation is the most expeditious approach, but it involves shortening of the digit to the level of the head of the middle phalanx. While allowing for immediate soft tissue coverage, further shortening of an injured digit is not accepted by all patients (Fig. 76.5).

Simple shortening of exposed bone with a rongeur at the time of initial examination followed by dressing changes allowing for healing

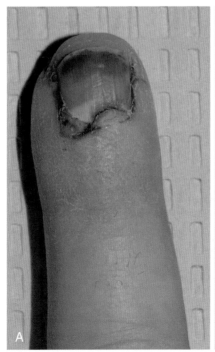
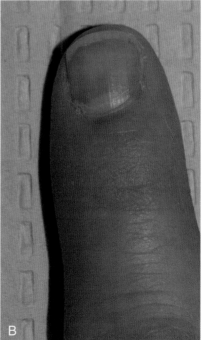

Fig. 76.3 Crush injury to the fingertip. **A,** Large subungual hematoma but without avulsion of nail from nail fold. This patient was treated with a tip protector orthosis for comfort, mobilization, and edema control. The injured nail fell off at 3 weeks, and at 9 months a new, normal-appearing nail was in its place (**B**).

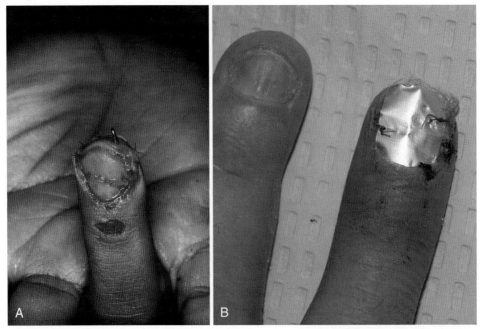

Fig. 76.4 A, linear laceration of the nail is approximated with fine gut sutures. **B,** It is commonly our practice to splint the nail folds and protect nail bed repairs with a "foil nail" made of sterile suture packaging. Note inset of the foil into the nail fold, secured proximally and distally with absorbable suture.

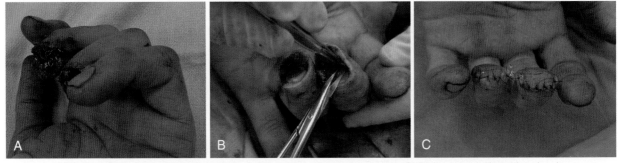

Fig. 76.5 Revision amputation. **A,** Patient with multiple digital amputations. **B,** Digits operatively explored and debrided, with neurectomies performed. **C,** Single-stage closure with local tissue.

by wound contraction and granulation allow restoration of satisfactory appearance and sensitivity. It avoids surgical intervention but generally entails a 3- to 4-week period in which meticulous wound care is required two to three times a day. Patients are instructed in dry dressing changes, secured with a lightly compressive wrap (Fig. 76.6). They may incorporate full use of the injured extremity into daily hand hygiene 3 days after the injury, including gentle cleansing of the amputated tip with a mild antibacterial soap.

More recently, the application of topical growth factors with dressing changes[12] has been shown to yield results superior to and less costly than surgical soft tissue reconstruction. It is unclear whether these offer any advantage to less technologically sophisticated wound care.

We have enjoyed great success with this method, but concerns over bone desiccation and osteomyelitis lead some to abandon this method except in the smallest of injuries.

Full-thickness skin grafting of pulp and tip defects enjoys limited benefit over simple healing by secondary intention. Although donor site morbidity is minimal, the fingers are immobilized for 7 to 10 days to allow for graft incorporation. A mature graft is relatively anesthetic, and graft contracture may lead to poor cosmesis.

Full-thickness pulp defects, with exposed bone or tendon, are typically not amenable to healing by secondary intention. These injuries have more recently been treated by us through a staged procedure involving the application of an acellular dermal matrix followed by full-thickness skin grafting at an interval of 3 weeks[13] (Fig. 76.7). This technique allows for preservation of length and contour but carries with it the costs of two procedures and a heavy expense for the acellular matrix template.

Homodigital flaps, such as the V-Y advancement flaps, have been in use for decades with little modification of the original technique described independently by Atasoy and Kutler[14,15] (Fig. 76.8). Tissue is advanced based on deep septal perforating vessels. There is no need for prolonged immobilization, and no donor site morbidity results. Clinically, however, the extent that tissue may be advanced distally is limited. Although advancement up to 10 mm is possible, considerable dissection is involved and possibly devitalization of septal perforators.[16]

The adipofascial "turnover" flap[17,18] is a reasonable option for coverage of large full-thickness defects to the dorsum of the fingers. This flap is based on constant dorsal cutaneous perforating vessels arising from the proper digital arteries at the level of the proximal interphalangeal

(PIP) joint. The flap may be extended to offer durable coverage to the entirety of the digit from the PIP joint to the fingertip dorsally. A full-thickness skin graft is applied over the flap while the donor site may be closed primarily (Fig. 76.9).

Heterodigital flaps such as thenar flaps and cross-finger flaps further expand the surgical armamentarium for fingertip reconstruction.[19,20] These are random flaps raised either at the base of the thumb or off the dorsal aspect of an adjoining digit. The injured digit is secured to this flap and sectioned 14 to 21 days later at a second surgery. The donor site is typically covered with a skin graft (Fig. 76.10). This iatrogenic syndactylization of two digits, often with the PIP joint in midflexion,

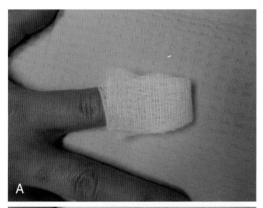

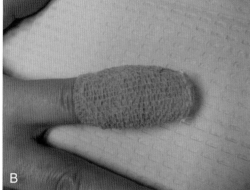

Fig. 76.6 A, A single, dry gauze is placed to cover the fingertip without excessive bulk. **B,** This is overwrapped with a light compressive dressing. This may easily be changed daily by the patient.

has an inherent propensity to lead to permanent flexion contracture. Although we have found these complications to be common, several authors assure us that this sequela is rare.[21]

Finger defect coverage using tissue perfused by the metacarpal artery system has become common in the past 2 decades. In 1990, Quaba and Davison[22] reported a series of finger defects that were covered by island skin flaps from the dorsal hand. These flaps were nourished by the palmar–dorsal vascular connection in the hand at the level of the metacarpophalangeal (MCP) joint just distal to the extensor tendon juncturae. Even in the extended fashion, however, these flaps generally reach only far enough to allow coverage of the nail bed.

Impressive advances in tip reconstruction have come from Asia, where an extreme primacy is placed on digital tip preservation. Lim and colleagues[9] described a spiral flap for digital tip defects. The flap is designed in a spiral shape and then extended to the fingertip in much the same way one would extend a spring with traction. The resultant proximal donor defect is covered with a skin graft. Amazingly, this group reports normal range of motion (ROM), normal sensation, and no cold intolerance. In an application of free tissue transfer expertise on an extremely small scale, Lee and coworkers[4] published an enormous series of fingertip defects that were reconstructed with pulp from the second toe. In addition to the microvascular anastomoses, these flaps are neurotized by digital nerve coaptation. Of the 854 flaps described, only three were outright failures, and there was a minimal revision rate. The authors report that static two-point discrimination averaged 8 mm. This two-point discrimination does not appear to be markedly better than that seen with healing by secondary intent. Operative time, cost, and the availability of an experienced microsurgical team preclude the recommendation of this option by us.

AUTHORS' RECOMMENDATIONS

We treat fingertip injuries with distal soft tissue loss by meticulous dressing changes to allow for wound contraction and healing by secondary intention. When bone is exposed, the treating physician must consider the importance of preserving functional length. Often the exposed bone may be rongeured to a level to allow for soft tissue closure.

For transverse amputations through the distal phalanx, homodigital advancement allows for restoration of contour and the

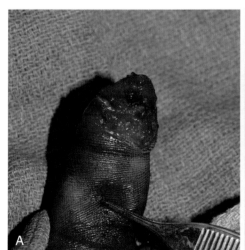
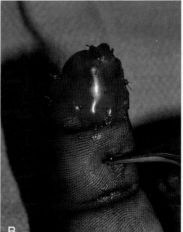
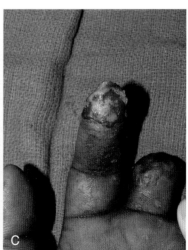

Fig. 76.7 Staged reconstruction of full-thickness pulp defect (**A**) with application of acellular dermal matrix (**B**). At 3 weeks, the matrix is ingrown and provides a suitable bed for skin grafting (**C**).

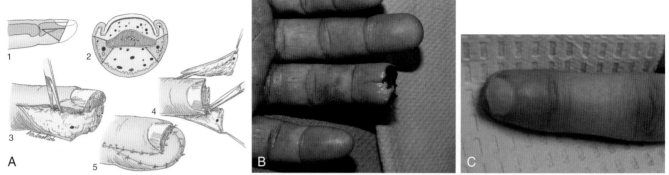

Fig. 76.8 A, Artist's rendering of V-Y advancement flap for fingertip coverage as described by Atasoy and Kutler. 1, Tip amputation injury. 2, Neurovascular bundles within the advancement flaps. 3, Flap mobilization through deep dissection. 4, Flap advancement. 5, Inset flaps at the fingertip with suture closure. **B,** Clinical case of 32-year-old patient with transverse amputation through distal phalanx. **C,** Four months after treatment with radial and ulnar V-Y advancement flap. (Reprinted with permission from Green D, Hotchkiss R, Pederson W, eds. *Green's Operative Hand Surgery*, 4th ed. Philadelphia: Churchill Livingstone; 1999, p. 1804.)

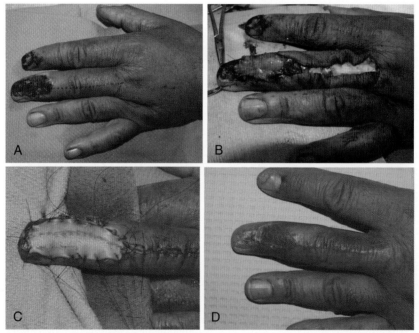

Fig. 76.9 Adipofascial turnover flap. **A,** Left hand of a 52-year-old craftsman after an auger injury. **B,** Adipofascial flap harvested from proximal finger and rotated distally based on perforating vessels at the level of the proximal interphalangeal joint. Coverage is obtained to the level of the fingertip. **C,** Full-thickness skin graft applied. **D,** Three months after surgery. The patient was self-employed and returned to work 10 days after surgery following removal of operative dressings. He continued with Coban wrap while at work.

provision of durable soft tissue coverage. Full-thickness soft tissue loss to the dorsum of the fingertip has been treated by us with dorsal metacarpal artery flaps. More recently, we have largely abandoned this technique in favor of the adipofascial turnover flap. Although we previously treated full-thickness injuries to the volar aspect of the fingertip with heterodigital flaps, we have now abandoned this technique in favor of staged reconstruction using acellular dermal matrix if pulp is avulsed to bone or with dressing changes, almost without regard for wound size. In our experience, defects greater than 1 cm^3 are still very easily and very satisfactorily treated in this fashion.

All injuries are followed weekly in the office for 3 weeks and then on a monthly basis for 3 months. Formal evaluation and treatment by a therapist is begun at the first visit.

THERAPIST'S MANAGEMENT

Evaluation

Evaluation of fingertip injuries should include a detailed history describing the method of injury and conservative or operative treatment. Access to radiographs and operative reports is helpful in guiding treatment of fractures and soft tissue injuries. The patient's health history is reviewed with particular attention to any factors that may interfere with healing, such as diabetes mellitus or smoking. Occupational and social history should be obtained to understand the patient's goals for return to work, recreation, and activities of daily living.

Acute fingertip injuries often present with a wound that may vary from a superficial laceration appropriate for simple wound care and dressing changes to an untidy wound requiring debridement, primary

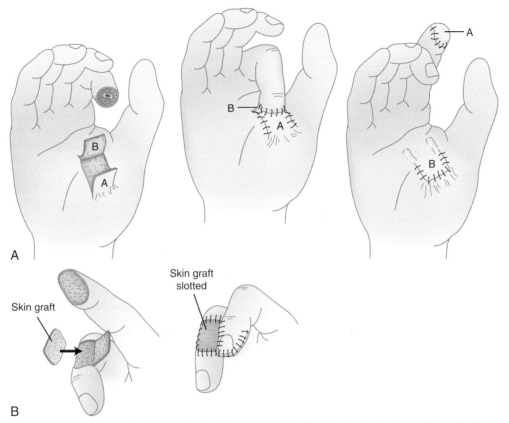

Fig. 76.10 A, Artist's sketch of thenar flap for tip reconstruction. **B,** Artist's sketch of cross-finger flap for tip reconstruction.

closure, or grafting. Documenting wound location, size, color, odor, and exudate at the time of initial evaluation and subsequent visits allows the therapist to monitor wound healing and adjust wound care accordingly. For injuries requiring pinning, pin sites and surrounding tissue are monitored for any signs of infection such as erythema or purulent drainage. Early recognition of these symptoms and communication with the referring physician allows for initiation of a suppressive antibiotic or pin removal if needed.

Many patients present with concomitant nail bed injuries. Nail growth is typically delayed for about 3 weeks after injury or repair.[23] Patients may present with a lump or thick nail ridge as the traumatized nail regrows after this initial latency period. This is caused by a sudden increase in growth over a period of about 50 days, which is often followed by a period of about 30 days of slowed growth before the nail grows at a normal rate.[23] The new nail typically grows at a rate of about 3 mm a month or 0.1 mm a day, given that no other factors delay healing.[24] For an intact but injured nail, the integrity of the nail bed should be noted. If the nail was injured or removed surgically, the surgeon may suture a small foil nail plate over the nail bed to protect the healing nail matrix (see Fig. 76.4). This should be protected until it falls off, usually within 2 to 3 weeks.

Edema is assessed to closed areas using circumferential measurements. Volumetric measurement may be useful to assess generalized edema if present in the hand, although cannot be used for injuries with open wounds or pins. For further information on assessment of edema, see Chapter 57.

Pain is often a primary complaint after these injuries because of the density of sensory endings along the distal phalanx. Patients also frequently present with *hypersensitivity* of the affected fingertip, a term that may be used to describe a variety of pain sensations resulting from normally non-noxious stimuli, including paresthesias, sensitivity to touch, and cold intolerance.[25] Pain can be rated using a numeric or visual analogue scale. Sensibility may be assessed using a two-point discriminator or Semmes-Weinstein monofilaments. For patients reporting cold intolerance, the Cold Intolerance Scale[26] may be useful to identify the types of activities causing intolerance and to rate the severity of symptoms.

Hyperesthesia, or increased sensitivity to touch, can be assessed by screening the patient's tolerance to moving light touch to closed areas. The Ten Test is a simple assessment that has been shown to be a valid and reliable method to accomplish this.[27] To perform this test with a fingertip injury, the examiner simultaneously strokes the affected finger and the equivalent area of the same finger on the unaffected hand. The patient compares sensation between hands by rating the stimulus from 1 to 10, a score of 1 indicating normal sensation and 10 indicating hyperesthesia. The same scale is then used to reevaluate changes in sensitivity over time.

Hypersensitivity may also be observed from general posturing of the hand. In some cases, patients may have developed a pattern of avoiding their affected digit. This may be assessed by observing patterns of functional use in the clinic or by asking them to perform grasp or pinch during the evaluation and documenting any tendency to divorce the finger from functional grasp and prehension.

Active range of motion (AROM) of the affected and unaffected adjacent joints should be assessed as permitted per the physician's prescription. Passive range of motion (PROM) may not be tolerated by the

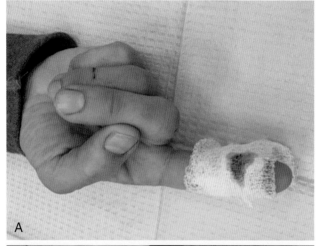

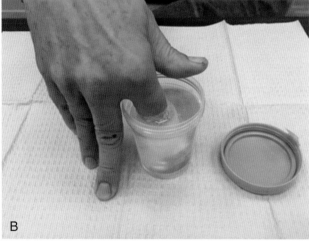

Fig. 76.11 A and **B,** An adherent dressing can be soaked in a sterile specimen container.

patient to the affected area initially. For patients requiring immobilization at the distal interphalangeal (DIP) joint, the PIP and MCP joints should be assessed for any restrictions in motion.

A patient-reported outcome measure should be selected that will capture functional limitations related to the patient's injury and demonstrate clinically meaningful changes in progress over time.[28] In addition to a standardized measure such as the Disabilities of the Arm, Shoulder and Hand (DASH),[29] a patient-specific measure, such as the Patient Specific Functional Scale (PSFS)[30] or Canadian Occupational Performance Measure (COPM),[31] may be useful for patients with fingertip injuries. The free response format of these measures allows the respondent to focus on a specific set of activity restrictions, such as difficulty with manipulation of small objects, managing fasteners, or typing, which may demonstrate more discreet changes in function related to a fingertip injury and can serve as a basis for comparison against other standardized measures.

Wound Care

Wounds and nail bed injuries with moderate exudate often present with adherent dressings that can be painful for the patient to remove. The dressing may be rinsed with saline or warm soapy water and removed by gently pulling the edges away from the wound. Wounds with significant adherence from dried drainage can be soaked in a sterile specimen container with saline and a disinfectant such as hydrogen peroxide or an iodine solution for 5 to 10 minutes to remove them more easily without

disturbing healing tissue (Fig. 76.11). This technique is not used for open draining wounds or with percutaneous pins to avoid contamination.

The nail bed or draining wound area is dressed with a sterile nonstick dressing, sterile gauze, and 1-inch Coban (3M Coban Self-Adherent Wraps, 3M Company, St. Paul, MN). Light dressings are used so as not to restrict motion. For fractures treated with pinning or with injuries to the terminal extensor tendon, a protective DIP extension orthosis may be needed (Fig. 76.12). A ⅛-inch thermoplastic material is preferable for these orthoses and can easily be remolded to accommodate changes in edema. If pins are present, the patient should be instructed in pin care. Preferences for pin care vary, and there is no consensus as to the best method[32]; however half-strength hydrogen peroxide has been shown to be effective[33] and is the authors' preference because full-strength hydrogen peroxide may dry pin sites excessively. Pin care is performed one or two times a day using a sterile cotton swab with a solution of 50% hydrogen peroxide and 50% saline to clean around the pin, with a separate swab to dry. Pins are padded with sterile gauze and gauze wrap (see Fig. 76.12). A tubular stockinette applied with a metal applicator may also be helpful to secure the dressing (see Fig. 76.12). Dressing changes several times daily may be required for wounds with moderate drainage, whereas dressing changes once daily may be sufficient for wounds with minimal drainage. Macerated wounds (Fig. 76.13) may require more frequent dressing changes and may need perforated orthosis material for sufficient aeration.

Scar Management and Stump Shaping

Scar management is initiated after wounds are healed. Patients are also instructed in stump shaping if bulging edges occur at the fingertip. A light figure-of-8 Coban wrap or digit compression sleeve may be used for shaping and can be worn during periods of rest or sleep so as not to interfere with hand use.[34] Gel-lined finger sleeves and elastic finger stalls are commercially available in various sizes and may be cut to the correct length for the affected finger (Fig. 76.14). These are issued with the instruction to avoid applying them too tightly and to monitor the finger for adequate circulation.

Desensitization

Hypersensitivity is a common result of a fingertip injury and should be addressed as soon as wounds have closed. The goal of *desensitization* is to decrease the painful response to touch at the fingertip and improve tolerance for functional use. The concept of desensitization is founded on Melzack and Wall's gate control theory of pain, which suggests that activation of large myelinated A fibers using touch and vibration can override signals from unmyelinated C fibers, which perceive pain.[35,36]

Lois Barber[37] developed a systematic approach to desensitization incorporating touch and vibration that has been used as the basis for several desensitization programs in the literature.[34,36] Barber's program, called the Downey Hand Center Sensitivity Test,[37,38] assesses tolerance for three sensory modalities: massaging various textures applied to dowels over the skin, immersing the hand into tubs of small particles, and applying vibration at various speeds using a handheld vibrator (Fig. 76.15). Patients rank 10 stimuli in each of these categories from most to least irritating, which is then used as the hierarchy for their individualized desensitization program. Patients begin desensitization with the stimuli that are slightly irritable but tolerable for them and progress in intensity with each modality as their tolerance improves, avoiding causing a painful response. The effect of the program is rated by the patient at regular intervals to track progress.

In Barber's program, dowel textures were applied at home for 10 minutes three or four times daily, and contact particles and vibration were used for 10 minutes each in the clinic. Patients progressed to

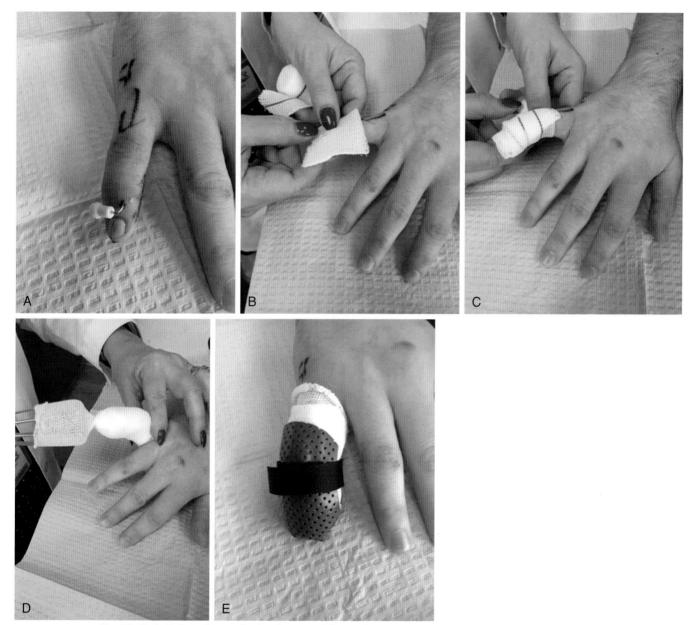

Fig. 76.12 A–E, Dressing application for a small finger distal interphalangeal joint fracture dislocation with pinning.

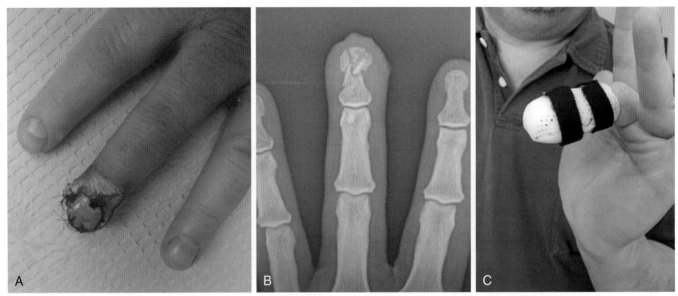

Fig. 76.13 A, Crush injury with a comminuted distal phalanx fracture and macerated wound. The wound is dressed with a nonstick sterile dressing, sterile gauze, and gauze wrap. **B,** A distal interphalangeal joint extension orthosis is fabricated with ⅛-inch perforated material to protect the distal phalanx. **C,** The patient performs active motion at his metacarpophalangeal and proximal interphalangeal joints to prevent stiffness.

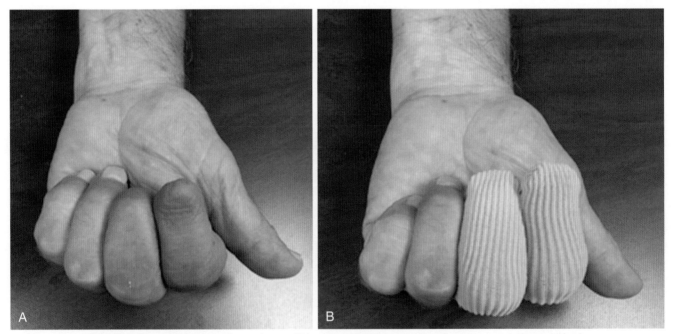

Fig. 76.14 A and B, Gel-lined finger sleeves. This patient with index and long fingertip amputations used gel-lined finger sleeves for shaping at night and for protection with certain work activities.

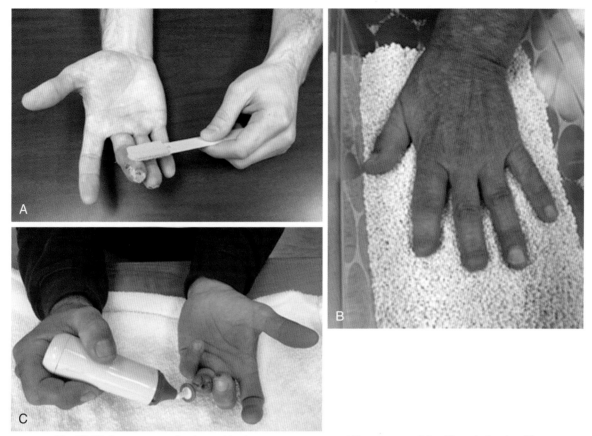

Fig. 76.15 Components of a desensitization program: textures (**A**), contact particles (**B**), and vibration (**C**).

the next texture after 2 to 3 weeks and received desensitization treatment for an average of 7 weeks.[37] Other studies have followed this model with favorable results for return of sensibility, grip strength, and return-to-work roles.[37] A cohort study using phase 1 of Barber's program proposed shorter duration of application of dowel textures (three times daily for 2–5 minutes or until the patient felt "numb" to the texture) and showed similar timeframes for progressing to the next texture (1–3 weeks) and a similar total time for treatment (6 weeks) with a significant effect on patients' reported pain and occupational performance.[36]

To encourage carryover of desensitization at home, patients can be provided with various textures applied to a tongue depressor (Fig. 76.15). These may be labeled in the order the patient should use them after establishing their personal hierarchy for desensitization. Patients may also select common household items to match the textures and contact particles demonstrated in the clinic. To apply vibration at home, patients can purchase a small handheld vibrator or use a vibrating tool such as an electric toothbrush to augment the in-clinic program, although these devices may not allow for adjustment of the cycles per second (cps) and therefore may not match the patient's specific level of need.

Fluidotherapy is a preparatory heat modality that may be particularly useful for desensitization once wounds are closed, as the digit is exposed to small particles and has the additional benefit of allowing motion to work on active tendon gliding. This modality cannot be used in the case of open wounds, pins, or a foil nail plate, and care should be taken to ensure temperatures are not too hot when applied to a fingertip with new skin or for patients with sensory deficits. Mirror box

therapy using visualization of the unaffected finger is also discussed as a desensitization strategy in the literature and may be a useful adjunct to the desensitization program.[39,40]

Desensitization is a gradual process that may take several weeks to months, and patients returning early to manual tasks may need protection for the hypersensitive fingertip until their tolerance improves. A gel-lined finger sleeve (see Fig. 76.14) is one method to protect the finger while allowing motion. The sleeve also provides light compression for edema control and softens scar. Patients should balance use of the sleeve with uncovered use of their fingertip and should be encouraged to wean off the sleeve as their tolerance for more resisted use improves. In some cases, patients may need a rigid orthosis for select work tasks if soft protection is not sufficient. Patients with cold intolerance may need gloves when working in cold environments or may need to insulate cold objects with rubber or other materials until the intolerance resolves.[41]

Mobilization and Strengthening

The DIP joint is less anatomically complex than other joints, and mobilization of fingertip injuries is often relatively simple. ROM can typically be initiated in the first week after injury or surgery. If the DIP joint is immobilized, patients are instructed in exercises to prevent stiffness in the adjacent joints, including isolated PIP–MCP motion and straight fisting. When ready to mobilize the DIP joint, patients perform active motion with tendon gliding and light grasp and prehension activities are incorporated into the therapy program to encourage normal patterns of use. Patients perform a home exercise program several times daily to maximize progress.

In some cases, patients will have developed a pattern of avoiding use of their affected digit and will need to "unlearn" this behavior. Buddy straps (Fig. 76.16) may be helpful to encourage normal functional use and may also be used to mobilize stiffness at the PIP joint. Patients avoiding use of their thumb can be instructed in bimanual pinch activities, such as folding a towel or picking up small objects, with the instruction to consciously incorporate the thumb tip into three-jaw pinch.

Therapy progresses with joint blocking exercises and PROM if limitations in motion persist. The DIP joint should be monitored for extensor lag and exercises should progress without causing or furthering a lag. In the case of ongoing tightness at the PIP or DIP, patients may benefit from use of elastic bands or a static progressive orthosis to provide a low-load stretch (Fig. 76.17). For principles of orthotic design for mobilization of joints, see Chapter 108.

Strengthening routines may be initiated with putty and functional grip and pinch exercises when appropriate. In addition to strengthening, the hand therapist assists patients with anticipated return to work by incorporating work simulation activities in the clinic. For example, patients who perform office work can trial their tolerance for typing with their affected finger using a keyboard in the clinic. Patients who perform manual labor may benefit from Baltimore Therapeutic Equipment simulated tool use to improve tolerance for various work tasks (Fig. 76.18). Simulating these tasks allow the therapist to problem solve with the patient to change the task or provide protection to the fingertip until tolerance improves.

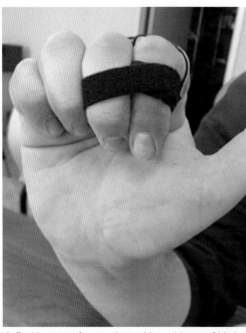

Fig. 76.16 Buddy straps for a patient with avoidance of his index finger following a crush injury and repair to the terminal extensor tendon.

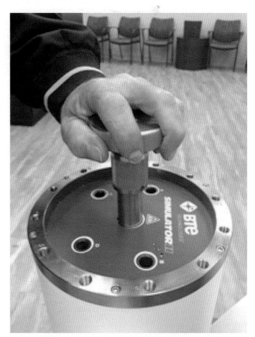

Fig. 76.18 Baltimore Therapeutic Equipment simulator to progress tolerance for tool use for a patient with an index fingertip injury returning to work in manual labor.

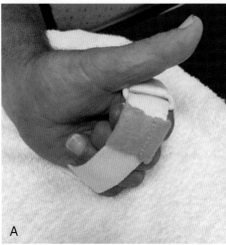 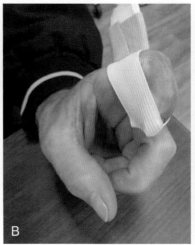 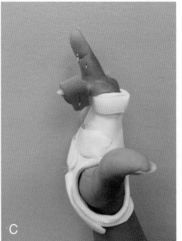

Fig. 76.17 A, Web strap for proximal interphalangeal (PIP) flexion. **B,** "PIP–DIP" strap for distal interphalangeal (DIP) flexion. **C,** Static progressive orthosis for DIP flexion.

SUMMARY

The fingertip makes up less than 0.25% of total body surface area. Injuries to this small unit, however, can be quite debilitating, affecting function of the adjacent digits and the entire hand. Surgical intervention seeks to restore a stable and durable soft tissue envelope. Issues such as stiffness and hypersensitivity are not predictably obviated with surgical intervention alone and can be addressed through early initiation of an effective therapy program.

REFERENCES

1. Bickel KD, Dosanjh A. Fingertip reconstruction. *J Hand Surg Am.* 2008;33(8):1417–1419.
2. Lemmon JA, Janis JE, Rohrich RJ. Soft-tissue injuries of the fingertip: methods of evaluation and treatment. An algorithmic approach. *Plast Reconstr Surg.* 2008;122(3):105e–117e.
3. Hirase Y, Kojima T, Matsui M. Aesthetic fingertip reconstruction with a free vascularized nail graft: a review of 60 flaps involving partial toe transfers. *Plast Reconstr Surg.* 1997;99(3):774–784.
4. Lee DC, Kim JS, Ki SH, et al. Partial second toe pulp free flap for fingertip reconstruction. *Plast Reconstr Surg.* 2008;121(3):899–907.
5. Alagoz MS, Uysal CA, Kerem M, Sensoz O. Reverse homodigital artery flap coverage for bone and nailbed grafts in fingertip amputations. *Ann Plast Surg.* 2006;56(3):279–283.
6. Han D, Hu HT, Jiang H. The subcutaneous pulp flap for fingertip defects. *J Hand Surg [Am].* 2008;33(2):254–256.
7. Hattori Y, Doi K, Sakamoto S, et al. Fingertip replantation. *J Hand Surg Am.* 2007;32(4):548–555.
8. Koshima I, Urushibara K, Fukuda N, et al. Digital artery perforator flaps for fingertip reconstructions. *Plast Reconstr Surg.* 2006;118(7):1579–1584.
9. Lim GJ, Yam AK, Lee JY, Lam-Chuan T. The spiral flap for fingertip resurfacing: short-term and long-term results. *J Hand Surg Am.* 2008;33(3):340–347.
10. Lin CH, Lin YT, Sassu P, Wei FC. Functional assessment of the reconstructed fingertips after free toe pulp transfer. *Plast Reconstr Surg.* 2007;120(5):1315–1321.
11. Ozyigit MT, Turkaslan T, Ozsoy Z. Dorsal V-Y advancement flap for amputations of the fingertips. *Scand J Plast Reconstr Surg Hand Surg.* 2007;1–5.
12. Freedman BM, Oplinger EH, Freedman IS. Topical becaplermin improves outcomes in work related fingertip injuries. *J Trauma.* 2005;59(4):965–968.
13. Katolik L, Roach J, Taras J. Use of Acellular Dermal Regeneration Template (ADRT) for soft-tissue reconstruction in hand injuries. *Combined Scientific Meeting of the American Society for Surgery of the Hand—British Society for Surgery of the Hand.* Westminster, UK: 2009.
14. Haddad Jr RJ. The Kutler repair of fingertip amputation. *South Med J.* 1968;61(12):1264–1267.
15. Shepard GH. The use of lateral V-Y advancement flaps for fingertip reconstruction. *J Hand Surg Am.* 1983;8(3):254–259.
16. Mehling I, Hessmann MH, Hofmann A, Rommens PM. V-Y flap for restoration of the fingertip. *Oper Orthop Traumatol.* 2008;20(2):103–110.
17. Braga-Silva J, Jaeger M. Repositioning and flap placement in fingertip injuries. *Ann Plast Surg.* 2001;47(1):60–63.
18. Laoulakos DH, Tsetsonis CH, Michail AA, et al. The dorsal reverse adipofascial flap for fingertip reconstruction. *Plast Reconstr Surg.* 2003;112(1):121–125; discussion, 126–128.
19. Lassner F, Becker M, Berger A, Pallua N. Sensory reconstruction of the fingertip using the bilaterally innervated sensory cross-finger flap. *Plast Reconstr Surg.* 2002;109(3):988–993.
20. Okazaki M, Hasegawa H, Kano M, Kurashina R. A different method of fingertip reconstruction with the thenar flap. *Plast Reconstr Surg.* 2005;115(3):885–888. discussion; 889–890.
21. Rinker B. Fingertip reconstruction with the laterally based thenar flap: indications and long-term functional results. *Hand (N Y).* 2006;1(1):2–8.
22. Quaba AA, Davison PM. The distally-based dorsal hand flap. *Br J Plast Surg.* 1990;43(1):28–39.
23. Zook EG. Understanding the perionychium. *J Hand Ther.* 2000;13:269–275.
24. Berker D, Baran R. Science of the nail apparatus. In: Baran R, De Berker, David AR, Holzberg M, Thomas L, eds. *Baran and Dawber's Diseases of the Nails and their Management.* 4th ed. Hoboken, NJ: John Wiley & Sons; 2012:15–57.
25. Packham T, Macdermid J, Michlovitz S, Cup E, Van de Ven-Stevens L. Cross cultural adaptation and refinement of an English version of a Dutch patient-reported questionnaire for hand sensitivity: the Radboud evaluation of sensitivity. *J Hand Ther.* 2017. https://doi.org/10.1016/j.jht.2017.03.003.
26. McCabe SJ, Mizgala C, Glickman L. The measurement of cold sensitivity of the hand. *J Hand Surg.* 1991;16:1037–1040.
27. Uddin Z, MacDermid J, Packham T. The ten test for sensation. *J Physiother.* 2013;59:132.
28. Valdes K, MacDermid J, Algar L, et al. Hand therapist use of patient report outcome (PRO) in practice: a survey study. *J Hand Ther.* 2014;27:299–308.
29. Hudak PL, Amadio PC, Bombardier C. The Upper Extremity Collaborative Group (UECG). Development of an upper extremity outcome measure: the DASH (disabilities of the arm, shoulder and hand). *Am J Ind Med.* 1996;29:602–608.
30. Stratford P, Gill C, Westaway M, Binkley J. Assessing disability and change on individual patients: a report of a patient-specific measure. *Physiother Can.* 1995;47:258–263.
31. Law M, Baptiste S, Carswell A, et al. *Canadian Occupational Performance Measure.* 5th ed. Ottawa: CAOT Publications ACE; 2014.
32. Lethaby A, Temple J, Santy-Tomlinson J. Pin site care for preventing infections associated with external bone fixators and pins. *Cochrane Database Syst Rev.* 2013:CD004551.
33. Patterson MM. Multicenter pin care study. *Orthopedic Nurs.* 2005;24:349–360.
34. Chu M, Chan R, Leung YC, et al. Desensitization of finger tip injury. *Tech Hand Up Extrem Surg.* 2001;5(1):63–70.
35. Melzack R, Wall P. Pain mechanisms: a new theory. *Science.* 1965;150:971–979.
36. Göransson I, Cederlund R. A study of the effect of desensitization on hyperaesthesia in the hand and upper extremity after injury or surgery. *Hand Ther.* 2011;16(1):12–18.
37. Barber L. Desensitization of the traumatized hand. In: Hunter J, Schneider LH, Mackin E, et al., eds. *Rehabilitation of the Hand and Upper Extremity.* 3rd ed. St Louis: Mosby; 1990:721–730.
38. Yerxa EJ, Barber LM, Diaz O, et al. Development of a hand sensitivity test for the hypersensitive hand. *Am J Occup Ther.* 1983;37:176–181.
39. Grünert-Plüss N, Hufschmid U, Santschi L, Grünert J. Mirror therapy in hand rehabilitation: a review of the literature, the St Gallen protocol for mirror therapy and evaluation of a case series of 52 patients. *Br J Hand Ther.* 2008;13(1):4–11.
40. Ramachandran V, Altschuler E. The use of visual feedback, in particular mirror visual feedback, in restoring brain function. *Brain.* 2009;132(7):1693–1710.
41. Carlsson IK, Edberg A, Wann-Hansson C, et al. Hand-injured patients' experiences of cold sensitivity and the consequences and adaptation for daily life: a qualitative study. *J Hand Ther.* 2010;23:53–62.

77

Acute Management of Upper Extremity Amputation

Michael S. Gart, Bryan J. Loeffler, R. Glenn Gaston

OUTLINE

CRITICAL POINTS

Principles of Targeted Muscle Reinnervation

- Multiple transfers of nonfunctional distal nerves to more proximal muscles to create "motor points" for amplification of distal nerve signals.
- Motor points allow for surface electromyographic recording of nerve signals and intuitive control of myoelectric prostheses.
- Additional motor points increase degrees of freedom in prosthetic control and enable simultaneous movements across multiple joints.
- Advanced pattern recognition algorithms can further increase the degrees of freedom available to the prosthetic user.
- Targeted muscle reinnervation has shown clinical promise in reducing or eliminating the formation of symptomatic neuroma.

Techniques for Targeted Muscle Reinnervation

- Targeted muscle reinnervation is indicated for patients with upper extremity amputations without more proximal nerve injury who seek either improvements in prosthetic control or treatment or prevention of symptomatic neuromas.
- It can be performed in the acute or delayed setting.
- Patterns of nerve transfers should be determined intraoperatively based on available donor nerves and recipient muscles.
- It is critically important to fully denervate the recipient muscle from its native innervation before reinnervating with a donor nerve in an end-to-end fashion.
- As with all nerve transfers, the donor nerve should be cut as distal as possible and the recipient nerve as close to the muscle as possible to allow tension-free coaptation, aggressive nerve trimming, and shorter time to reinnervation.
- Although end-neuroma resection is not essential, it is advisable when possible to remove any "mass effect" on the surrounding tissues.

Shoulder Disarticulation

- There is a high degree of impairment because of loss of shoulder, elbow, and wrist joints.
- Current prosthetics are difficult to manage and are highly nonintuitive.
- Nerve transfer patterns are highly variable because of the nature of these injuries and inconstant donor nerve and recipient muscle availability.

- The highest priority nerve function should be coapted to the clavicular head of the pectoralis muscle, when available.
- Elbow flexion should be prioritized first followed by a "hand close" signal.

Upper Arm Amputations

- Elbow disarticulation preserves the condyles, which allow for better prosthetic fitting and increased rotational stability; however, the residual limb is too long to accommodate an elbow joint prosthetic without significant limb-length discrepancy.
- Transhumeral amputation increases the length available for prosthetic elbow components but does not provide rotational stability and hinders prosthetic anchoring. In select patients, flexion osteotomy may be of benefit.
- When possible, humeral shortening osteotomy with preservation of the condyles may be a preferred alternative to maintain the benefits of both techniques.
- The distal median nerve is transferred to the short head of the biceps to generate a "hand close" signal.
- The distal radial nerve is transferred to the lateral head of the triceps to generate a "hand open" signal.
- The distal ulnar nerve is transferred to the brachialis to generate a fifth signal, which is often dedicated to wrist rotator control.

Forearm Level Amputations

- As with transhumeral amputations, the benefits of wrist disarticulation (improved prosthetic suspension and forearm rotation) and transradial amputation (increased length available for prosthetic wrist) must be considered.
- Patients with wrist disarticulation have lower rates of prosthetic usage than those with transradial amputations.
- The distal median nerve is transferred to the palmaris longus to generate a signal for thumb opposition.
- The distal ulnar nerve is transferred to the flexor carpi ulnaris to generate a pinch signal.
- The nerve to the supinator is transferred to the brachioradialis to "superficialize" and magnify the electromyographic signal for supination.
- Distal muscles with intact neurovascular pedicles can be transferred proximally as axial pattern flaps and used for additional motor points.

Transmetacarpal Amputations
- Current myoelectric prosthetics for the hand use nonintuitive muscle contraction patterns and can only generate "hand open" and "hand close" signals.

- The Starfish procedure transfers the interosseous muscles dorsally, bringing them closer to the skin for improved surface EMG detection.
- With this procedure, patients demonstrate the ability to control individual myoelectric fingers in a highly intuitive fashion.

INTRODUCTION

Major amputations of the upper extremity often result from traumatic injury when replantation is either not possible or not in the best interest of the patient because of extensive nerve or soft tissue damage, infection, vocational needs, or personal preference. In 2005, an estimated 1.6 million people in the Unites States were living with a major extremity amputation, a number projected to double by the year 2050.[1] Of these, more than half a million sustained an amputation of the upper extremity, with more than 40,000 limbs lost at or above the level of the hand.[1] Upper extremity amputation is most commonly the end result of high-energy trauma in the young, otherwise healthy patient population.[2–4] One population study demonstrated the incidence of upper extremity amputation at 1.9 per 100,000 person-years.[2] In contrast to the lower extremities, where a prosthesis functions as a load-bearing platform for ambulation, the dexterity, prehension, and degrees of freedom in the upper extremity are not as well replicated with existing prostheses.[4] One recent, large, multicenter study demonstrated a patient preference for replantation over revision amputation with prosthetic rehabilitation, a further testament to the limitations of current prosthetic technologies.[5] Innovations in surgical care and evolving technological advancements have great potential to make amputation and a prosthetic limb superior to limb replantation in some cases. Replantation and extremity salvage techniques are discussed in detail elsewhere in this text. Here, we discuss our approach to optimize function and minimize long term pain in patients who have sustained acute, nonsalvageable upper extremity amputations.

In general, the goals of amputation surgery should be to optimize residual limb length, prevent symptomatic neuroma formation, and provide stable soft tissue coverage to allow early prosthetic fitting, enabling return to work and daily activities. However, before performing definitive reconstructive surgery, the initial trauma of these devastating injuries requires acute management. These injuries can be not only limb sacrificing but often life threatening. At the time of initial management, meticulous irrigation and debridement with removal of all foreign material and devitalized muscle should be performed. A return to the operating room should be planned after the patient has been medically optimized for a definitive surgical procedure. The authors' philosophy when performing amputation surgery is to reconstruct the residual limb to facilitate prosthetic fit, minimize pain, and maximize prosthetic control. This represents a fundamental change from the approach of simply removing the damaged limb and then transferring care to a rehabilitation physician and prosthetist or orthotist. Over the past few years, the authors have applied techniques espoused by others and devised novel techniques to accomplish these goals while providing patients with an unparalleled ability to control increasingly advanced myoelectric prosthetic devices.

What follows is a discussion of preferred management strategies for upper extremity amputations by level, with an emphasis on nerve transfer techniques to provide patients with maximal prosthetic function while minimizing the formation of symptomatic neuromas. For the purposes of this chapter, we define acute management as occurring within 30 days of the initial injury, although the techniques discussed below can be performed at any time, even years after an amputation.

TARGETED MUSCLE REINNERVATION: BACKGROUND AND RATIONALE

Targeted muscle reinnervation (TMR) was developed by Dumanian and Kuiken in an effort to provide individuals with upper extremity amputations with improved control of a myoelectric prosthesis.[6–8] Initially developed for patients with shoulder disarticulation and transhumeral amputations,[6,8–11] the technique involves transfer of amputated nerve endings that formerly innervated distal upper limb muscles to proximal motor nerve branches that innervate muscles with redundant function. Conceptually, it can be thought of as switching the innervation of a residual proximal muscle to be under the control of one of the lost major nerves from the amputation. For example, in an above-elbow amputation, the two heads of the biceps are both present, and the median nerve function (grasp) has been lost. One can switch the innervation of one head of the biceps from the musculocutaneous nerve to the median nerve. This allows one head of the biceps to signal elbow flexion and the other to signal grasp in a highly intuitive manner. The newly reinnervated muscle is serving as a "biologic amplifier" to allow detection of a signal from previously lost nerves.

The end result is an amplification of motor signals from nerves that no longer serve a downstream function, enabling them to be detected by surface electrodes, which then control a myoelectric prosthesis. These additional motor signals are interpreted by the prosthesis at the skin level and converted into the corresponding motion(s). In the earlier example, when the patient attempts elbow flexion, one head of the biceps will contract, and when she or he thinks to close the amputated hand, the other head of the biceps will contract. This allows both functions to be independently detected and simultaneously performed by the prosthesis. The end result of TMR is a significant increase in the number of motor signals available for individuals with amputations, which in turn allows a greater amount of functional control of a myoelectric prosthesis at each amputation level.

Myoelectric Prosthetics

Prosthetic rehabilitation of individuals with upper extremity amputations is extensively covered in Chapter 78. In brief, current functional prosthetic devices (i.e., those not simply worn for aesthetic replacement of a missing limb) available to patients can be broadly characterized as body-powered or electric, although there are hybrid models available. Body-powered prosthetics use a system of cables and harnesses to convert movement at the shoulder into motion at the distal upper limb. Although these devices work well and are in wide use, they demand a certain level of physical strength from the patient and do not provide intuitive motion. Electric or "powered" devices use motors to generate movement and mostly consist of myoelectric prostheses. As described earlier, these devices use surface electromyographic (EMG) signals to control the distal limb (Fig. 77.1). There are, however, limitations to the capabilities of standard myoelectric prostheses, many of which have been addressed by advances in surgical technique and prosthetic technology.

Advantages of Targeted Muscle Reinnervation in Myoelectric Users

A conventional myoelectric prosthesis uses surface electrodes to detect EMG signals generated by muscle contractions in the residual limb and converts them to functional movements in the prosthesis. Conventional myoelectric prosthetics utilize a "direct control" algorithm, whereby independent muscle signals are paired 1:1 with a corresponding prosthetic motion. For example, a biceps muscle contraction in a patient with a transhumeral amputation would generate an EMG signal that causes flexion of the prosthetic elbow joint; similarly, a signal generated by triceps contraction will result in prosthetic elbow extension. If the patient then wants to open or close the hand, a "mode switch" function is required to

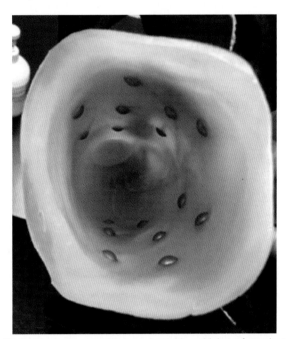

Fig. 77.1 Myoelectric prosthesis socket with multiple surface electrode array for electromyographic signal detection and pattern recognition.

convert the signals obtained from biceps and triceps contracture to close and open the hand, respectively. Simultaneous control of elbow and hand function is not possible. The primary limitation of direct control algorithms is readily apparent: the number of movements (i.e., degrees of freedom) in the prosthetic are limited by the number of distinct EMG signals that can be generated and independently detected. Mode switch requires a nonintuitive muscle contraction, manual switch, or other action that is cumbersome and delays performance of the desired action. Furthermore, conventional devices become less intuitive with more proximal amputation levels because proximal motor groups that control arm and forearm motion must now also control hand and wrist motion.

Targeted muscle reinnervation substantially increases the number of signals a patient can generate by transferring nonfunctional distal nerves into proximal motor branches, resulting in highly intuitive contraction of the recipient muscle by attempting to perform the function previously supplied by the donor nerve. In a patient with a transhumeral amputation, this expands the available motor signals from two (biceps and triceps) to four or five, depending on the level of amputation and number of available recipient muscles for the distal median, radial, and ulnar nerve remnants. Importantly, because two antagonistic signals are required for each degree of freedom (i.e., "flex and "extend" or "open" and "close"), the presence of four or more signals allows simultaneous control across multiple joints.[12]

Independent detection of these EMG signals is another limitation of conventional myoelectric devices. The ideal location for surface recording is directly over a superficial, independently controlled muscle, with limited "noise" from nearby, synergistic muscles, referred to as cross-talk.[13] Consider elbow flexion, a function mediated by multiple upper arm muscles. A conventional myoelectric device relies on EMG signal amplitude and is unable to discern a signal originating from the biceps or brachialis, which demonstrate significant cross-talk because of their proximity and synergistic function. As a result, only one pair of independent control sites is typically available in the residual limb (biceps–triceps or wrist flexors–extensors), which limits control of the prosthesis to one joint, or degree of freedom, at a time. Strategies to minimize cross-talk from nearby muscles can be employed such as adipofascial interposition flaps or allograft tissue interposition between muscles (Fig. 77.2). Separating muscles from one another using these

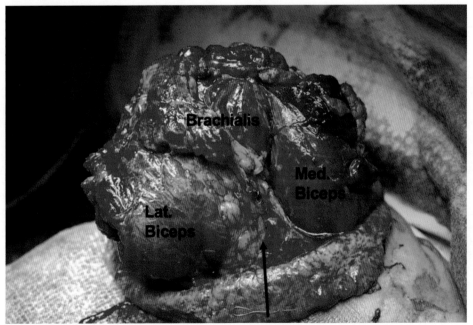

Fig. 77.2 Adipofascial interposition flap *(arrow)* for transhumeral amputation shown in the *inset* between the short (medial [Med.]) and long (lateral [Lat.]) heads of the biceps muscle.

techniques allows for cleaner signal detection by the prosthesis with less cross-talk.

Furthermore, as amputation levels move more proximal, conventional myoelectric control becomes less intuitive because of a lack of physiologically appropriate musculature.[13] Whereas a patient with a transradial amputation can control wrist and hand function using the wrist flexors and extensors, an individual with a transhumeral amputation must control the prosthetic hand with the biceps and triceps, an awkward and nonintuitive function. TMR makes prosthetic control more intuitive by providing signals for distal limb functions through nerves that previously controlled these functions in the native limb.

Although TMR addresses many of the limitations of conventional myoelectric prosthetics by increasing the number of available signals, reducing myoelectric cross-talk, and allowing intuitive control of prosthetic functions, the full functionality of the procedure is now being harnessed by advances in prosthetic control algorithms.

Advanced Pattern Recognition Algorithms

The distal nerves transferred in TMR surgery previously innervated several muscle groups acting across multiple joints. With surface electrodes relying on signal amplitude to dictate limb motion, the multiple functions of these nerves are grouped into a binary "on/off" signal that drives a single movement in the myoelectric limb. In the case of the median nerve, this grouping converts such diverse functions as thenar motor control, finger flexion, wrist flexion, and forearm pronation into one signal typically relegated to a "hand close" command. Conventional myoelectric "direct control" algorithms cannot take advantage of the rich neurologic information present at the TMR site.

High-density EMG recordings of multiple TMR sites have demonstrated the ability to discern intended movements through distinctive EMG pattern of signals despite a similar location and magnitude of EMG signal amplitude.[14] In a shoulder disarticulation patient after TMR, distinct patterns were identified for numerous wrist, hand, and finger motions and predicted intended motions with up to 8 degrees of freedom with an accuracy greater than 90%.[14] This served as the foundation for what is now commonly referred to as advanced pattern recognition (APR), or simply "pattern recognition." APR algorithms translate the aggregate signal from multiple surface EMG recordings into intended movements in the prosthetic limb. These algorithms use machine learning to align the patient's intended movements with patterns of EMG activity using a simple training exercise. In brief, the patient is asked by a computer program to attempt a series of movements, during which EMG signals are recorded from an array of surface electrodes. These patterns are then assigned to each movement, and when the same pattern is seen again, the prosthesis engages in the intended function. Pattern recognition algorithms allow patients to control elbow flexion–extension, wrist flexion–extension, wrist rotation, and multiple hand grasping patterns. This technology has exponentially increased the functionality of myoelectric prostheses by overcoming the "one muscle–one function" limitation of direct control algorithms and eliminating the confounding factor of EMG cross-talk by using a field of surface electrodes rather than discrete recording sites. In fact, cross-talk may even enhance the ability to identify discrete signals by its presence or absence across multiple recording sites.[15] TMR vastly improves the unique electrical pattern generated with an intended motion by harnessing the electrical signals of amputated nerves, which would otherwise be lost. Pattern recognition eliminates the need for a predictable pattern of nerve transfers because recordings are not based on known muscle topography. Pattern recognition can be used for any patient who has undergone TMR surgery, regardless of the strategy used for donor nerves and recipient muscles.

Targeted Muscle Reinnervation for Neuroma Control and Prevention

Approximately 25% of patients with upper extremity amputations will develop painful neuromas, which can be a source of significant discomfort even in the setting of a well-fitting prosthetic.[16–18] In the event of an amputation, the severed nerve ends are deprived of a scaffold along which to regenerate, culminating in a neuroma, the disorganized proliferation of axons and nerve connective tissue. In addition to improving prosthetic function for individuals with amputations, TMR has been demonstrated to reduce neuroma formation and reduce neuroma-related pain when performed as a primary or secondary intervention.[17,19] In theory, the coaptation of the distal nerve to a motor branch allows the regenerating axons to grow into the target muscle in an organized fashion, minimizing or eliminating neuroma formation. It is important to recognize that the recipient motor branch is transected (thus denervating the muscle) and then the donor nerve is coapted to it (thus reinnervating it) and that this is performed in an end-to-end fashion.

OPERATIVE TECHNIQUE FOR TARGETED MUSCLE REINNERVATION

Indications for Targeted Muscle Reinnervation

The ideal TMR patient is highly motivated and willing to comply with several months of therapy and prosthetic fitting postoperatively. Patients treated with TMR in the acute setting must be fitted with a body-powered or conventional myoelectric prosthesis while the nerve transfers mature and muscle reinnervation occur over several months. It is, however, worth emphasizing that whether or not a patient intends to use a myoelectric prosthesis, he or she may still benefit from TMR surgery by reducing or preventing the effects of neuroma pain. Neuroma pain can require chronic medication management and often precludes any prosthetic wear because of pain intolerance.

Targeted muscle reinnervation may be offered to any patient with any level of major upper extremity amputation who desires improved prosthetic control or as treatment or prevention of neuroma formation, provided the patient does not have a more proximal injury to the brachial plexus or spinal cord. Although it is widely accepted that outcomes of peripheral nerve surgery are improved in younger patients,[20] we have not found age to be a limiting factor in the success of TMR surgery. However, the correlation of age and TMR success is more difficult to study in this population given that the majority of patients with upper extremity amputations and patients who have undergone TMR are young people of working age, and older patients less commonly sustain these injuries.[1]

The importance of a good prosthetics team to the ultimate success of TMR cannot be overstated. Patients will work closely with their prosthetist and require several fittings and adjustments of their prosthetic during the postoperative period. Moreover, preoperative or even intraoperative consultation with the prosthetist can be very helpful in determining the appropriate length of residual limb or the need for angulation osteotomy to ensure a good prosthetic fit while maintaining adequate room for all of the necessary componentry.

Finally, the cost of a myoelectric prosthesis is significant and must be considered in the context of the patient's individual resources and insurance coverage. Many of the advances made in prosthetic technologies have been made possible with the help of robust government funding in light of recent military conflicts,[21] but the cost to an individual consumer can be very significant. Despite this, we believe in offering TMR as an option to patients regardless of their resources because the procedure appears to reduce or eliminate the formation of painful neuromas and keeps options open for patients in the future if myoelectric prosthetics become more affordable or routinely covered by insurance companies.

Technical Considerations for Targeted Muscle Reinnervation

When possible, patients should be examined preoperatively to determine the availability of viable proximal muscles that can be targeted as recipients for nerve transfer. In the delayed setting, the location of any Tinel's sign can be a clue to the location of the residual distal nerve stump and may indicate the length of donor nerve available for transfer. The ideal patient has a long residual limb, which will allow resection of any end neuroma and aggressive trimming of the traumatized nerve ends while still enabling tension-free coaptation.

In the setting of acute, traumatic amputation, preservation of limb length sufficient for prosthesis wear is critical. To preserve limb length in patients with proximal transradial or transhumeral amputations without sufficient soft tissue coverage, skin grafting, local flaps, or free tissue transfer should be used to maintain adequate bone length.[10,22] In addition to providing soft tissue coverage, free muscle or myocutaneous tissue transfer has also been described to import recipient muscle targets when native musculature is lacking.[23] When performed in a delayed fashion, a supple soft tissue bed will reduce the technical demands of a TMR procedure and facilitate prosthesis wear, but local or distant flaps can be used in combination.

It is critically important to fully denervate all recipient muscles from their native innervation before nerve transfer to dedicate each recipient muscle to the new, intended function. Reinnervation with a transferred nerve does not occur without denervation of the targeted muscle, which distinguishes TMR from simply burying a nerve ending into a muscle without denervating it. In addition, for segmentally innervated muscles, denervation of all branches to that muscle will allow for eventual generation of a pure signal from the donor nerve, thus reducing crosstalk. A nerve stimulator is used to confirm the identity of all motor branches before division and transfer (Video 77.1). Although we will outline the conventional pattern of nerve transfers by amputation level below, the pattern of nerve transfers used in each case should be determined by the availability of donor nerves and target muscles.[10] For example, a patient with a very proximal transradial amputation who has an intact elbow joint but lacks forearm musculature may require treatment with a "transhumeral" style of nerve transfers. Similarly, a patient with a very proximal transhumeral amputation may be treated with a "shoulder disarticulation" pattern of nerve transfers.

Intraoperatively, it is not critically important to excise the end neuroma if this would result in a significant amount of otherwise unnecessary dissection. In theory, after the proximal nerve input is removed, the neuroma should no longer function as a pain generator; however, neuromas are a well-described source of pain that can impair the ability to wear a prosthetic and may cause discomfort through a local "mass effect" on surrounding tissues (Fig. 77.3). An effort is made to resect the terminal neuromas unless the additional dissection necessary would pose unnecessary risk to the soft tissues or surrounding structures. Last, as with all nerve transfers, the time required for reinnervation should be minimized by following the principle of "donor distal, recipient proximal" and coapting the nerves as close as possible to the motor entry point on the recipient muscle.

MANAGEMENT OF UPPER EXTREMITY AMPUTATIONS BY LEVEL

Shoulder Disarticulation

Amputation through the level of the glenohumeral joint imparts significant disability to the patient and is fortunately a relatively uncommon event. Such a proximal amputation makes controlling a prosthesis extremely difficult and requires the user to lock one joint in a particular position before moving the other. This leads to unnatural

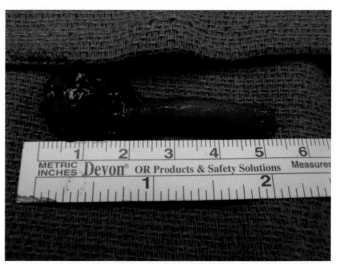

Fig. 77.3 Terminal neuroma after resection.

movements and a lack of coordination between the shoulder, elbow, and the hand–hook component. Current myoelectric devices for such proximal amputations rely on EMG signals generated by the pectoralis and latissimus muscles, limiting the device to two degrees of freedom at one time. To mode switch, patients must contract cervical muscles, making overall movement with a myoelectric prosthesis slow, cumbersome, and not intuitive. Not surprisingly, prosthetic rehabilitation of patients with shoulder disarticulation amputations is particularly challenging.

Targeted Muscle Reinnervation for Shoulder Disarticulation

Targeted muscle reinnervation in patients with shoulder disarticulations presents unique challenges because of the short length of available donor nerves, likelihood of distorted anatomy, and relative paucity of viable recipient muscle targets. The highly variable nature of this procedure is highlighted in a recent case series of 10 shoulder disarticulation TMR patients who underwent 7 different nerve transfer patterns compared with 16 consecutive transhumeral-level patients who all underwent identical procedures.[19]

The goals of the procedure are to generate four motor points to be used for elbow flexion–extension and hand open–close.[6,10,13] Although the precise pairing of nerves to muscles can vary from patient to patient, pattern recognition algorithms allow interpretation of any pattern of successful reinnervation. In other words, the exact nerve transfers performed are less important than how they are performed, and every effort should be made to produce a successful reinnervation. That said, there are some general guidelines we apply to these patients. Because elbow flexion is the highest priority function to regain in this patient population, we typically coapt the distal musculocutaneous nerve remnant to the clavicular head of the pectoralis major. The clavicular head is a reliable recipient muscle because of its distinct innervation and superficial location, facilitating surface electrode recording.[24] Our second priority is establishing a "hand close" signal through the remnant median nerve, which is coapted to the motor branch of the pectoralis major sternal head. An intraoperative assessment of the sternal head and its motor nerve branches can determine if this muscle can be split into two segments capable of independently accepting a nerve transfer. If there is a second discrete segment of the sternal head, the ulnar nerve is coapted here to provide a "hand open" signal (Video 77.2) Last, the radial nerve is preferentially transferred to the thoracodorsal nerve at its entry point into the latissimus dorsi to generate an elbow extension signal. If the sternal head of the pectoralis is not favorable for a dual nerve transfer or if the latissimus dorsi is injured, the serratus anterior or pectoralis minor can be used as alternative muscle targets.

Upper Arm Amputations

Amputations at or above the elbow joint present unique challenges to prosthetic rehabilitation in patients with the upper extremity amputations. Standard approaches to amputation at this level include elbow disarticulation and transhumeral amputation. Although elbow disarticulation preserves the humeral condyles, which aid in both suspension of a prosthetic and transmission of rotational forces to the forearm, there are drawbacks to this approach. Specifically, the additional length required for elbow componentry in the prosthesis results in a significant limb-length discrepancy, which is functionally limiting and aesthetically unacceptable. On the contrary, transhumeral amputation has the advantage of avoiding or minimizing limb-length discrepancies but with a less desirable limb–prosthesis interface. Prostheses for transhumeral amputation are fitted over the shoulder, restricting movement of the glenohumeral joint. The absence of condyles limits the ability to stabilize the prosthesis against humeral rotation.[25] In selected patients with longer residual limbs, humeral angulation osteotomy may address these limitations by improving rotational stability and obviating the need to include the shoulder joint in prosthetic fitting[25,26] (Fig. 77.4).

A third option, humeral shortening osteotomy, seeks to combine these advantages of elbow disarticulation and transhumeral amputation. Originally described in 2000, this technique uses a distal metaphyseal shortening osteotomy just proximal to the condyles, preserving them for prosthetic suspension and rotational stability while allowing additional length for a prosthetic elbow joint.[27] Patients with any level of bony amputation may benefit from TMR; however, preoperative consultation with the prosthetist should be considered because many patients would benefit from a revision amputation in conjunction with TMR.

Targeted Muscle Reinnervation for Transhumeral Amputation

The technique of TMR in patients with transhumeral amputations has evolved over time and is well-described in the literature.[9–11] The goals

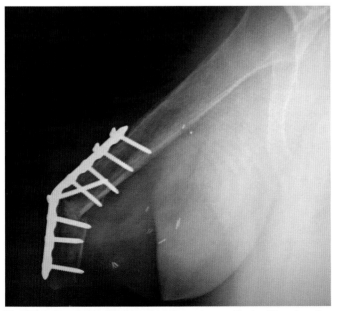

Fig. 77.4 Angulation (flexion) osteotomy in a patient with a transhumeral amputation, which assists with prosthetic load-bearing rotational stability.

of the procedure are to maintain the native innervation for elbow flexion and extension while providing additional, intuitive motor signals for downstream myoelectric prosthetic functions (Video 77.3). In its current form, TMR provides patients with transhumeral amputations with at least two additional motor signals, namely "hand open" and "hand close." With a third nerve transfer and pattern recognition technology, multiple additional functions can be generated, including forearm rotation, hand gestures, and the potential for wrist control.

Native elbow flexion and extension are maintained through the long head of the biceps brachii via the musculocutaneous nerve and two of the three heads of the triceps brachii via the radial nerve, respectively.[10] The signal for "hand open," a function typically carried out by radial nerve innervated muscles in the forearm, is generated by coapting the distal radial nerve to a motor branch to one of the three triceps heads. Classically, this coaptation is to the lateral head of the triceps, which is the most distally innervated of the three heads, but the choice of recipient is functionally irrelevant and should be selected for technical ease above all else.[10,11,28] Medial head of triceps reinnervation is less desirable because this muscle is deeper to the long and lateral heads of the triceps, and capturing a signal with a surface electrode is therefore more difficult.

The "hand close" signal, a function carried out in part by median nerve innervated muscles in the hand and forearm, is generated by coapting the distal median nerve to the short head of the biceps brachii muscle. Finally, patients with sufficient residual limb length are candidates for coaptation of the distal ulnar nerve to the brachialis muscle, creating a fifth signal.

In the original description of the procedure, adipofascial flaps were developed to be used as interposition material between the biceps and triceps heads to minimize cross-talk.[10,11] However, in light of advances in pattern recognition algorithms, this step may not be necessary in all cases.

Forearm-Level Amputations

Forearm-level amputations present both challenges and opportunities because they tend to sustain amputations as young, working age individuals. Although these patients are the most likely to have phantom limb pains and require neuropathic pain medications,[29] they are also the most likely of all patients with major upper extremity amputations to remain in the workforce[4,30] and use prostheses.[30]

There is no consensus about whether wrist disarticulation or transradial amputation provides better outcomes for patients who require removal of the hand. Similar to the earlier discussion of elbow disarticulation versus transhumeral amputation, there are advantages to—and proponents of—both techniques. Wrist disarticulation preserves the distal radioulnar joint and the distal forearm flare, improving forearm pronosupination and prosthetic device suspension. Moreover, the longer lever arm provides greater prosthetic control. However, the additional length required for wrist componentry in a prosthesis will result in a limb-length discrepancy, and the prominent radial and ulnar styloids can lead to pressure necrosis at the limb–prosthetic interface. Furthermore, patients with wrist disarticulations have been shown to have lower rates of prosthesis use than their transradial counterparts.[30]

A transradial amputation provides additional room for a prosthetic wrist component at the expense of reduced forearm pronosupination and shortened lever arm. Approximately 8 to 10 cm of ulnar resection seems to provide the most flexibility for prosthetic options, balancing forearm rotation and prosthetic control.[4] In general, the longer the residual limb, the greater amounts of forearm rotation are possible; however, at least 7 to 8 cm of distal radius should be resected to ensure adequate soft tissue coverage of the bone and room for prosthetic components.[31] For proximal forearm amputations, a minimum of 5 cm of residual ulna is required for adequate prosthesis fitting. Because of the significant functional differences presented by loss of the elbow joint, every effort should be undertaken to maintain length in proximal transradial amputation, including the use of local tissues and free flaps, when appropriate.

Targeted Muscle Reinnervation for Transradial Amputation

A technique for TMR to prevent or treat symptomatic neuromas in patients with transradial amputations has been described.[31] At our institution, we have developed a novel technique for transradial TMR to improve myoelectric prosthesis function in addition to neuroma control. Whereas traditional myoelectric techniques for patients with transradial amputations use the wrist flexors and extensors to drive distal prosthesis function, we applied the principles of TMR to incorporate thumb opposition, forearm pronosupination, and pinch. To generate a signal for thumb opposition, the distal median nerve is transferred to a superficial muscle belly in the residual forearm that is well-suited to surface EMG recording. The palmaris longus muscle meets these criteria and is our preferred target when available. The brachioradialis, flexor carpi radialis, flexor carpi ulnaris, and extensor carpi radialis longus are other potential targets because of their superficial locations and sites of motor branch innervation. Forearm rotation is increasingly limited as transradial amputation progresses more proximally. Therefore, to create an independent signal to control forearm rotation, the intact nerve branches to the supinator may be transferred to a more robust and superficially located muscle.

Although the supinator muscle and its innervation are typically intact with a transradial amputation, this muscle lies deep to the skin surface and is not readily detected by surface electrodes. To make this signal more superficial and robust for surface EMG detection, the nerve to supinator is transferred to the brachioradialis muscle. This allows for an additional signal to control a myoelectric wrist rotator (Video 77.4). Last, to obtain an independent signal for pinch function, the distal ulnar nerve remnant is transferred to the ulnar head of the flexor carpi ulnaris or other targeted muscle. In an attempt to limit cross-talk of multiple EMG signals in a small space, acellular dermal matrix products have been used as an interposition material to sequester muscles providing synergistic function (Fig. 77.5). A final postoperative photo demonstrating the location of surface EMG signals for each nerve transfer in a forearm TMR patient is demonstrated in Figure 77.6.

In addition, if muscles exist that maintain their neurovascular pedicle but their insertion or origin lies in the portion of the limb which is being amputated, these muscles may be preserved along with their neurovascular pedicle and transferred to the residual arm. Maintaining these muscles allows for additional intuitive signals to enhance prosthetic control and can also improve the residual soft tissue envelope. Pedicled muscle transfer in the amputation setting follows the principle of the senior author's "Starfish" procedure, which was originally described for use in partial hand amputation and is discussed later. An example of a "Starfish" procedure for the forearm is a distal forearm amputation performed with intact anterior interosseous artery and nerve to the pronator quadratus. The pronator quadratus is mobilized on the neurovascular pedicle to the residual forearm, where it can serve as an independent signal for forearm pronation as well as a soft tissue padding to cover the residual radius, ulna, or both.

Transmetacarpal Amputations

Currently available options for patients with partial hand amputations are limited. Although myoelectric prosthetics have the capacity for individual finger motion, surgical procedures described to date have yet to provide the requisite motor input to druive independent digital control. A typical myoelectric partial hand consists of two or three

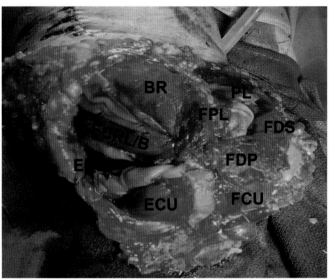

Fig. 77.5 Intraoperative view of completed transradial targeted muscle reinnervation procedure with acellular dermal matrix interposition grafts to isolate electrical signals and minimize electromyographic "crosstalk." *BR*, Brachioradialis; *Ecu*, extensor carpi ulnaris; *ECRB/L*, extensor carpi radialis brevis and longus; *EDC*, extensor digitorum communis, *FCU*, flexor carpi ulnaris; *FDP*, flexor digitorum profundus; *FDS*, flexor digitorum superficialis; *FPL*, flexor pollicis longus; *PL*, palmaris longus.

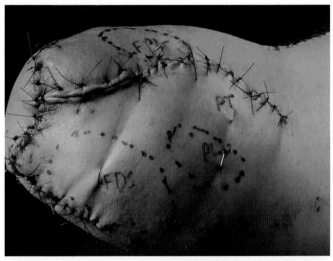

Fig. 77.6 Postoperative transradial targeted muscle reinnervation with signal fields for each underlying muscle marked at the skin surface can facilitate electrode placement for direct-control prosthetics. *FDS*, Flexor digitorum superficialis; *FPL*, flexor pollicis longus; *PL*, palmaris longus, *PT*, pronator teres.

surface electrodes that record signals from the intrinsic hand muscles or extrinsic forearm muscles (or both) to control hand open and close signals.[32] When the intrinsic muscles are used for surface recording, digital abduction triggers a "hand open" signal, and digital adduction triggers a "hand close" signal, neither of which is intuitive. Surface recording of the extrinsic muscles is not much better because wrist flexion produces a "hand close" signal and wrist extension triggers "hand open."[33]

"Starfish" Procedure for Transmetacarpal Amputations

To circumvent the limitations of myoelectric prosthetics for patients with partial hand amputations, the senior authors have developed the

"Starfish" procedure, which uses novel muscle transfers to enable intuitive control of independent digital function for patients with partial hand amputations.

In this procedure, the transmetacarpal amputation is performed 3 cm proximal to the native metacarpophalangeal (MCP) joint to optimize length of the myoelectric fingers and fit of the prosthesis. The volar and dorsal interosseous muscles are isolated on their neurovascular pedicles and transferred to the dorsal surface of the metacarpal bones, where they are sutured to periosteum to maintain their length and position (Fig. 77.7). The flexor tendon sheaths and volar plates are then interposed to minimize cross-talk between EMG signals.

Whereas preoperative surface EMG recordings could not detect adequate signals from individual interosseous muscle firing, patients are able to generate reliable, robust, individual signals for each digit after the procedure. Because the intrinsic muscles are natural flexors of the MCP joints, the signals generated intuitively control independent finger flexion. Remarkably, patients can demonstrate individual finger control with minimal or no prosthesis training because of the highly intuitive nature of these muscle transfers immediately after surgery (Video 77.5).

POSTOPERATIVE CARE AND CONSIDERATIONS

The residual limb is wrapped in a bulky, compressive dressing to minimize edema formation, and drains (if used) are pulled on the first postoperative day. Because the nerve transfers are performed to be tension free throughout a full range of motion, no immobilization of the residual limb is necessary. By convention, patients are typically admitted overnight for pain control or drain removal; however, in patients with adequate pain control and no drain in place, TMR can be performed in the outpatient setting.

After all incisions are fully healed and edema has resolved sufficiently, patients can resume wearing their original prostheses. Postoperative edema will typically allow for a proper fit of their original prostheses within 4 to 6 weeks of surgery.[34]

In our experience, symptoms of painful neuromas disappear or significantly reduce in the postoperative setting, but particularly in cases of delayed TMR, neuritic pain may temporarily increase in the early

postoperative period. Reinnervation of target muscles takes between 4 and 7 months on average to become clinically detectable,[35] but EMG signals with surface electrodes are often detectable by 6 weeks postoperatively if the transfers are performed at the level where the recipient nerve enters the muscle. In many patients, the earliest sign of reinnervation—before clinically detectable muscle contraction—is a feeling of generalized soreness in the target muscles and pain with palpation. This has been described in muscles undergoing reinnervation as the "tender muscle sign" and often precedes clinically detectable contractions.[36]

CONCLUSION

Ideal management of acute upper extremity amputations requires careful preoperative consideration to maximize the function of the residual limb. Limb length and residual soft tissue envelope are critical to the function of the limb and ability to fit a prosthetic. TMR surgery can be performed for patients with shoulder disarticulation down to amputations through the proximal hand, which allows for improved, intuitive control of a myoelectric prosthetic while minimizing the risk of painful neuroma formation. Following the principles of the "Starfish" procedure can allow for improved dexterity of prosthetic control as well as improved soft tissue envelope of the residual limb. Upper extremity amputation surgery should now be viewed as a reconstructive procedure rather than one of ablation.

REFERENCES

1. Ziegler-Graham K, et al. Estimating the prevalence of limb loss in the United States: 2005 to 2050. *Arch Phys Med Rehabil.* 2008;89(3):422–429.
2. Atroshi I, Rosberg HE. Epidemiology of amputations and severe injuries of the hand. *Hand Clin.* 2001;17(3):343–350 vii.
3. Freeland AE, Psonak R. Traumatic below-elbow amputations. *Orthopedics.* 2007;30(2):120–126.
4. Tintle SM, et al. Traumatic and trauma-related amputations: Part II: upper extremity and future directions. *J Bone Joint Surg Am.* 2010;92(18):2934–2945.
5. Pet MA, et al. Comparison of patient-reported outcomes after traumatic upper extremity amputation: replantation versus prosthetic rehabilitation. *Injury.* 2016;47(12):2783–2788.
6. Hijjawi JB, et al. Improved myoelectric prosthesis control accomplished using multiple nerve transfers. *Plast Reconstr Surg.* 2006;118(7):1573–1578.
7. Kuiken TA, et al. The use of targeted muscle reinnervation for improved myoelectric prosthesis control in a bilateral shoulder disarticulation amputee. *Prosthet Orthot Int.* 2004;28(3):245–253.
8. Kuiken TA, et al. Targeted reinnervation for enhanced prosthetic arm function in a woman with a proximal amputation: a case study. *Lancet.* 2007;369(9559):371–380.
9. Dumanian GA, et al. Targeted reinnervation for transhumeral amputees: current surgical technique and update on results. *Plast Reconstr Surg.* 2009;124(3):863–869.
10. Gart MS, Souza JM Dumanian GA. Targeted muscle reinnervation in the upper extremity amputee: a technical roadmap. *J Hand Surg Am.* 2015;40(9):1877–1888.
11. O'Shaughnessy KD, et al. Targeted reinnervation to improve prosthesis control in transhumeral amputees. A report of three cases. *J Bone Joint Surg Am.* 2008;90(2):393–400.
12. Kuiken TA, et al. Targeted muscle reinnervation for real-time myoelectric control of multifunction artificial arms. *Jama.* 2009;301(6):619–628.
13. Cheesborough JE, et al. Targeted muscle reinnervation and advanced prosthetic arms. *Semin Plast Surg.* 2015;29(1):62–72.
14. Zhou P, et al. Decoding a new neural machine interface for control of artificial limbs. *J Neurophysiol.* 2007;98(5):2974–2982.

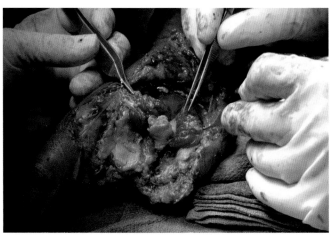

Fig. 77.7 Interosseous muscle *(color)* transposed to the dorsal surface of the metacarpal bones to improve surface electromyographic (EMG) detection. The flexor sheath and volar plate are sutured together and placed as an interposition graft to isolate the EMG signals from each muscle and minimize myoelectric cross-talk.

15. Scheme E, Englehart K. Electromyogram pattern recognition for control of powered upper-limb prostheses: state of the art and challenges for clinical use. *J Rehabil Res Dev*. 2011;48(6):643–659.

16. Geraghty TJ, Jones LE. Painful neuromata following upper limb amputation. *Prosthet Orthot Int*. 1996;20(3):176–181.

17. Pet MA, et al. Does targeted nerve implantation reduce neuroma pain in amputees? *Clin Orthop Relat Res*. 2014;472(10):2991–3001.

18. Soroush M, et al. Neuroma in bilateral upper limb amputation. *Orthopedics*. 2008;31(12).

19. Souza JM, et al. Targeted muscle reinnervation: a novel approach to postamputation neuroma pain. *Clin Orthop Relat Res*. 2014;472(10):2984–2990.

20. Verdu E, et al. Influence of aging on peripheral nerve function and regeneration. *J Peripher Nerv Syst*. 2000;5(4):191–208.

21. Zlotolow DA, Kozin SH. Advances in upper extremity prosthetics. *Hand Clin*. 2012;28(4):587–593.

22. Baccarani A, et al. Free vascularized tissue transfer to preserve upper extremity amputation levels. *Plast Reconstr Surg*. 2007;120(4):971–981.

23. Bueno Jr RA, et al. Targeted muscle reinnervation of a muscle-free flap for improved prosthetic control in a shoulder amputee: case report. *J Hand Surg Am*. 2011;36(5):890–893.

24. Lowery MM, et al. A multiple-layer finite-element model of the surface EMG signal. *IEEE Trans Biomed Eng*. 2002;49(5):446–454.

25. Neusel E, et al. Results of humeral stump angulation osteotomy. *Arch Orthop Trauma Surg*. 1997;116(5):263–265.

26. Marquardt E, Neff G. The angulation osteotomy of above-elbow stumps. *Clin Orthop Relat Res*. 1974;104:232–238.

27. de Luccia N, Marino HL. Fitting of electronic elbow on an elbow disarticulated patient by means of a new surgical technique. *Prosthet Orthot Int*. 2000;24(3):247–251.

28. Witoonchart K, et al. Nerve transfer to deltoid muscle using the nerve to the long head of the triceps part I: an anatomic feasibility study. *J Hand Surg Am*. 2003;28(4):628–632.

29. Tintle SM, et al. Reoperations following combat-related upper-extremity amputations. *J Bone Joint Surg Am*. 2012;94(16):e1191–1196.

30. Wright TW, Hagen AD, Wood MB. Prosthetic usage in major upper extremity amputations. *J Hand Surg Am*. 1995;20(4):619–622.

31. Morgan EN, et al. Targeted muscle reinnervation for transradial amputation: description of operative technique. *Tech Hand Up Extrem Surg*. 2016;20(4):166–171.

32. Tenore FV, et al. Decoding of individuated finger movements using surface electromyography. *IEEE Trans Biomed Eng*. 2009;56(5):1427–1434.

33. Atzori M, Muller H. Control capabilities of myoelectric robotic prostheses by hand amputees: a scientific research and market overview. *Front Syst Neurosci*. 2015;9:162.

34. Stubblefield KA, et al. Occupational therapy protocol for amputees with targeted muscle reinnervation. *J Rehabil Res Dev*. 2009;46(4):481–488.

35. Dumanian GA, Souza JM. Surgical techniques for targeted muscle reinnervation. Targeted muscle reinnervation: a neural interface for artificial limbs. In: Kuiken TA, Schultz Feuser AE, Barlow AK, eds. Boca Raton, FL: Taylor & Francis Group; 2014.

36. Lee EY, et al. The value of the tender muscle sign in detecting motor recovery after peripheral nerve reconstruction. *J Hand Surg Am*. 2015;40(3):433–437.

78

Rehabilitation of Upper Extremity Amputation and Prosthetic Training

Lisa Smurr Walters, Kathleen E. Yancosek, Daniel Acker, Dan Conyers

> *The world breaks everyone and afterward many are strong at the broken places.*
> Ernest Hemingway

OUTLINE

CRITICAL POINTS

- Amputation of an upper limb affects physical and psychological well-being and requires renegotiation of every aspect of daily life.
- An interdisciplinary team approach is essential to address the many needs of individuals with upper limb loss (ULL) or upper limb difference (ULD).
- Early initiation of rehabilitation creates an expectation of recovery and demonstrates the interdisciplinary team's commitment to facilitate the patient's return to independence.

- Education of the patient begins immediately and continues throughout the rehabilitation process.
- The therapist is instrumental in helping the patient develop a vision of independence that may include the integration of a prosthesis for a satisfying life after amputation.
- Connection to others with ULL or ULD is critical for acceptance and adjustment to limb loss.
- Early prosthetic fitting is associated with successful use of the prosthesis and a return to gainful employment.[1,2]

Working with individuals with upper limb loss (ULL) or upper limb difference (ULD) is rewarding and challenging. There are many facets of the rehabilitation process such as residual limb care, knowledge of mechanical operations of prosthetic equipment, behavioral health adjustments, phantom pain and sensations, adaptive equipment options, muscle retraining, and optimal use of a prosthesis for task accomplishments, as well as hand dominance transfer in the case of amputation of a dominant limb. This chapter provides guidelines to improve efficiency and uniformity in the delivery of rehabilitation services. Evaluation and rehabilitation differ among patients with major limb amputation (i.e., proximal to the wrist) and those with partial hand or partial finger amputations, and these differences are herein considered.

ETIOLOGY AND CLASSIFICATION OF UPPER LIMB AMPUTATIONS

Causes of amputation include vascular disease, trauma, and malignancy of bone and joint. Ninety percent of acquired upper limb amputation occurs from trauma involving machinery, explosives, projectiles, motor vehicle accidents, burns, electrical, and cold exposure injuries.[3–5] The majority of traumatic amputations occurs in young males, with one study[2] reporting a male-to-female ratio of 8:1; therefore, when appropriate, the pronoun "he" is used to refer to the singular tense of the individual with ULL or ULD.

The incidence of amputation in the United States is estimated at 185,000 per year.[6] The most recent prevalence data are derived from the National Health Interview Survey-Disability done in 1996, which did not separate upper from lower limb amputations. These data reported 1.2 to 1.9 million people in the United States living with an amputation.[7] Multistate probabilistic models estimated prevalence of amputation in the United States to be upward of 3 million people by 2050.[8]

INTERDISCIPLINARY TEAM APPROACH

Amputation of an upper limb affects physical and psychological well-being and requires renegotiation of virtually every aspect of daily life. Surgeons are responsible for initial management of the patient with ULL; however, a physiatrist leads the care for rehabilitation and guidance through prosthetic selection, as well as long term management. Addressing the many needs involved is best accomplished through an interdisciplinary care team approach.[9–11] A physiatrist familiar with specialized knowledge in upper limb amputations is at the helm of this team with the patient at the center. Team members include family members or caregiver, surgeon(s), case manager, occupational or physical therapist, behavioral health provider, prosthetist, and peer mentor or peer visitor.[11] Some centers and facilities hold amputation clinics to promote an interdisciplinary team approach to care; however, if this format is not available, it becomes critical (at a bare minimum) to develop open lines of communication among the physician, patient, therapist, and prosthetist.[12]

Patients with major limb amputation are evaluated by each discipline of the interdisciplinary team. Results of these evaluations are shared with other team members to determine an interdisciplinary rehabilitation plan designed to meet the patient's functional goals.[11] At the point in the process when prosthetic recommendations and treatments are being formed and executed, the prosthetist, therapist, and patient form the nucleus of the team. The patient drives the process with his goals and functional needs, whereas the prosthetist and therapist develop treatment plans to foster timely progress. Patients may disclose issues regarding pain, range of motion (ROM) limitation, psychological struggles, sleep challenges, family dynamics, or work and social integration concerns. As relevant to the patient's care, these issues should be shared with all interdisciplinary team members.

PATIENT EVALUATION

The initial encounter includes a thorough interview, formal physical evaluation, and patient education. The mechanism of injury is noted as well as any comorbidities that occurred at the time of amputation, such as multiple amputations, bone injuries, soft tissue injuries or deficits, nerve damage or injury, loss of consciousness or diagnosed brain injury, burns, visual deficits, vestibular injuries, or hearing loss. Comorbidities are common in patients who have sustained amputations by trauma.[13]

The initial interview includes a discussion of the patient's desired functional goals; vocational responsibilities; avocational interests; cultural factors; level of family or caregiver support; spiritual support; roles and responsibilities at home, work, and in the community; accessibility to resources and services; and financial limitations or constraints. Additionally, a learning assessment is administered to evaluate language barriers, educational level, and the patient's preferred learning style.[11] The presence of residual limb pain, phantom limb pain, and phantom limb sensation is assessed. Pain level is documented with note made of the type, duration, location, and intensity. The patient's familiarity with other persons living with amputation is determined, providing insight as to the patient's exposure to and level of understanding of others with ULL or ULD.

The current level of functioning in activities of daily living (ADLs) is evaluated, and an assessment of cognitive status is administered because it influences recommendations regarding prosthetic prescription. Advanced prosthetic designs require a higher cognitive aptitude to operate.[14]

Measurements are taken of residual limb length, shape, distal soft tissue integrity, presence of edema, areas of sensitivity or potential neuromas or heterotrophic ossification about the residuum that may impact wear of prosthesis or use of the residual limb in ADLs; open or healing wounds (if present), characteristics of other scars; upper trunk and neck mobility; ROM of remaining joints; sensation; and proximal residual limb muscle strength as well as muscle strength in the nonaffected, intact limb, if appropriate. In the case of a traumatic amputation, the surgical report is reviewed to determine what surgical

treatments were performed to address bony structures, cut ends of bones, nerve tissue management, and muscle treatments by myodesis or myoplasty. Strength, dexterity, sensation, and ROM are evaluated as well as the presence of overuse symptoms in the contralateral upper limb. It is common for individuals who have lived with ULL or ULD to experience overuse symptoms in the contralateral limb as a result of excessive reliance or from the use of poor body mechanics to complete necessary functional tasks.[11]

EDUCATION AND RESOURCES

Education begins early and continues throughout the course of rehabilitation. The patient and family should be given information on the program, expected outcomes, realistic goals, pain management, residual limb and postoperative wound healing management, options regarding upper limb prostheses, review of expected training timelines, available community and nonprofit resources to assist as the patient integrates back into the community, and caution regarding the risk of overuse injury in the contralateral limb. Expectations, goals, progression toward discharge from care, and the importance of compliance and motivation in promoting optimal outcomes are all discussed.[15] A vision of independence is developed that may or may not include the integration of a prosthesis for a satisfying life after amputation. An attitude of optimism and encouragement is critical because this initial meeting is often overwhelming to the patient and family members. The Amputee Coalition has resources for individuals with ULD or ULL and their family members and also has a written publication, *InMotion*, which is very helpful to individuals learning to cope with ULL or ULD. Last, the patient and family are advised of the importance of self-advocacy, which is often necessary to obtain insurance authorization for a prosthesis.

Behavioral Health Implications

A patient experiences a variety of emotions, such as helplessness, hopelessness, anger, social isolation, and fear of the future.[12] Patients vary in response based on emotional resources and coping abilities.[16] Family and friends alleviate some aspects of stress by their support.[17] If amputation was caused by trauma, additional concern is warranted, and these patients may require further evaluation by a psychiatrist for posttraumatic stress conditions.[18]

Individuals with upper limb amputation were more likely than the general population to screen positive for depressive symptoms and posttraumatic stress disorder (PTSD).[19–21] Walsh and coworkers[22] published results of a study of 263 consented prospective patients with upper limb amputation who completed a customized wellness inventory. The Walsh study also suggested that pain affects PTSD and depressive symptoms because it impacts positive emotions and postinjury activity. The majority of these participants had partial hand amputation. Unpublished results from this same study identified that there were no significant differences between emotional reaction scores for individuals with above-elbow and below-elbow amputations.[23] A 2010 study found individuals from both Vietnam and Operation Enduring Freedom and/or Operation Iraqi Freedom with unilateral ULL reported lower levels of adjustment to life with a prosthesis.[21] Furthermore, individuals with partial hand amputation were even more likely to screen positive for these psychological changes. Elliott and coworkers[24] found that individuals who are less resilient tend to engage in avoidant coping behavior, which is prospectively predictive of higher PTSD and depression.

Results of survey research[25] performed with 44 patients with amputations (10 upper limb) to determine factors influencing coping with life using a prosthesis revealed that the coping strategy and level of adjustment varied with age and mechanism and site of amputation.

Other studies have contradictory findings.[26,27] Van Dorsten[18] proposes a three-stage adjustment process of survival, recovery, and reintegration. He suggests that this process coincides with rehabilitation stages of preprosthetic, prosthetic, and vocational rehabilitation phases.

The many hours that patient and therapist spend together create a strong therapeutic bond, which is instrumental in the adjustment to amputation. The following are suggested actions to incorporate into rehabilitation programs:

- Provide adaptive equipment and training in adaptive strategies to expedite a return to independence.
- Encourage establishment of habits, patterns, and routines to facilitate a sense of control and influence over situations.
- Discuss body image issues as they relate to physical ability; listen empathetically and give positive feedback.
- Engineer success at each rehabilitation session to bolster self-confidence.
- Reinforce identity through occupation-based therapy activities to offset the (temporary or permanent) loss of familiar life roles.
- Introduce the patient to others with similar levels of ULL or ULD (peer visitation).
- Monitor changes in pain intensity and provide education regarding the relationship between pain and mood.[26]

PEER SUPPORT AND PEER MENTOR

Individuals with ULL commonly feel fearful when anticipating a lack of acceptance by friends or family, a loss of function, and an alteration in body image. Involvement of a carefully selected and appropriate peer visitor who can demonstrate healthy adaptation to ULL is helpful. Meeting someone with a like-level amputation provides an opportunity for the individual who recently experienced limb loss to talk about personal issues and to begin to learn new ways to solve common challenges in everyday life from someone who is similar to them physically. Additionally, peer support programs are often helpful to provide a sense of hope in recovery and to demonstrate the potential to return to normalcy in life. The Amputee Coalition (AC) website has resources to request a peer visitor and to find peer support programs in the individuals' local area. A powerful resource is a peer-visitor (certified through the AC) who serves as a role model of someone living and dealing with amputation (Box 78.1).

PAIN MANAGEMENT

Pain adversely affects quality of life. The cause of pain after upper limb amputation is likely multifactorial and is best managed through a multidisciplinary approach. Residual limb pain, phantom limb pain, and phantom limb sensation are three separate conditions that may be experienced individually or all together. The care team must teach the patient to distinguish between each. Residual limb pain is felt as pain in the remaining limb and is expected. It is experienced by 60% of individuals with amputation.[26] When recalcitrant, the most common cause is a painful neuroma.[28] Phantom limb pain is perceived pain in the portion of the limb that is no longer present. Phantom limb pain is described as "stabbing" (24.3%) or "pins and needles" (20.5%).[29] This type of pain is experienced in more than 40% of patients 1 year after amputation and is more challenging to treat because the cause is not clearly understood. Central nervous system processing and peripheral nerve mediation are suspected to play a role in phantom limb pain.[11]

Phantom limb sensation is a perceived nonpainful sensation in the amputated limb. Phantom limb sensation may be described as proprioception of the missing limb, temperature variations, itching, pressure, and tingling.[28] The cause of phantom sensation, like phantom limb pain, is not clearly understood and is often perceived long term after amputation.[30] Fear and anxiety in response to sensations in a limb that

---

BOX 78.1 Recommended Resources for Therapists and Patients

Patient and Therapist Resources
- Adaptive Sports Foundation: https://www.adaptivesportsfoundation.org
- Amputee Coalition: https://www.amputee-coalition.org
- Arm Dynamics: https://www.armdynamics.com
- Challenged Athletes Foundation: https://www.challengedathletes.org
- Disabled American Veterans: https://www.dav.org
- International Society for Prosthetics and Orthotics: https://www.ispoint.org
- Handwriting for Heroes from Loving Healing Press: https://www.lh-press.com
- *One-Handed in a Two-Handed World* (book) by Tommye K. Mayer
- Limbless Association: http://www.limbless-association.org
- Limbs for Life Foundation: http://limbsforlife.org
- O&P Amputee Info and Resources: http://www.oandp.com/resources/patientinfo
- The O&P Edge: https://opedge.com

Manufacturer and Vendor Resources
- Coapt, LLC: https://www.coaptengineering.com: manufacturer of pattern recognition, an advanced prosthetic technology
- College Park: https://www.college-park.com: manufacturer of prosthetic components
- Infinite Biomedical Technologies: https://www.i-biomed.com: manufacturer of pattern recognition, an advanced prosthetic technology, and other prosthetic componentry
- Hosmer-Dorrance: https://www.hosmer.com: manufacturer of prosthetic and orthotic components
- Liberating Technologies, Inc: https://www.liberatingtech.com: supplier of upper limb prosthetic components to include the Boston Digital elbow and M-Fingers
- Motion Control: http://www.utaharm.com: manufacturer and supplier of mostly upper limb externally powered components to include the Utah Arm, Electric Terminal Device, ETD2, and TASKA terminal devices
- Naked Prosthetics: https://www.npdevices.com: manufacturer and vendor of body-powered prostheses for partial finger or partial thumb amputations
- Otto Bock North America: https://www.ottobockus.com: manufacturer and vendor of vast prosthetic and orthotic components for lower and upper extremity amputations to include the DynamicArm and Bebionic terminal device
- Point Designs: https://www.pointdesignsllc.com: manufacturer of heavy duty passive digits for individuals with partial hand or partial finger amputations
- Texas Assistive Devices (TAD): http://www.n-abler.org: manufacturer of upper limb prosthetic components for individuals with hand dysfunction and amputation
- Therapeutic Recreation Systems Inc: https://www.trsprosthetics.com: manufacturer of body-powered and activity-specific components
- Touch Bionics by össur: http://touchbionics.com: vendor of externally powered prosthetic hands and digits as well as passive functional prosthesis
- ToughWare Prosthetics: https://www.toughwareprx.com: engineering and design company focused on inexpensive but rugged body-powered prosthetic componentry

---

is no longer there may cause misinterpretation of phantom limb sensation *as* pain. Informing patients that phantom limb sensations are normal helps to alleviate anxiety.

Musculoskeletal pain may occur in areas other than the residual limb such as the neck, shoulders, back, or contralateral limb. This type of pain may be related to overuse issues or associated with prosthetic use and is aggravated by abnormal biomechanical stresses to joints and muscles as well as advancing age.

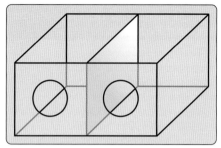

Fig. 78.1 Ramachandran mirror box used for managing phantom limb pain.

A prophylactic approach to manage pain before rehabilitation is recommended, and nonpharmacologic approaches should be included as an adjunct for a multimodal approach to managing the complex pain syndromes associated with ULL.[11] Nonpharmacologic modalities include transcutaneous electrical nerve stimulation, scar mobilization, relaxation, biofeedback, graded motor imagery, desensitization, and socket modification if the patient has a prosthesis that is determined to be a pain source.[10,11]

Use of a Ramachandran mirror apparatus (mirror box) has been shown to lessen the magnitude of phantom limb pain.[31,32] Finn and associates[33] reported that mirror therapy reduced the severity and duration of daily episodes of phantom limb pain in a randomized control trial with unilateral, upper limb male amputees. Mirror therapy should occur in a quiet, nondistracting environment. It is performed with a commercial mirror box (available through NOI Group, http://www.noigroup.com/en), a custom mirror box (Fig. 78.1), or a portable 24- × 30-inch mirror. The mirror or mirror box is positioned at midline, facing toward the patient's contralateral, intact limb. The residual limb is positioned behind the mirror so that view of it is obstructed. The patient is instructed to look into the mirror and watch the reflection of the intact limb, which now visually appears to be the missing limb. This illusionary image of the amputated limb provides feedback to the brain, closing the "broken" sensorimotor circuit of the hand to the brain. The patient spends 15 minutes per session making limb motions in front of the mirror while watching the reflection of movements produced by the intact limb. To avoid triggering a pain memory, patients are instructed to avoid movement in positions that cause pain. A patient who reports feeling his phantom limb in a cramped and awkward position of discomfort is encouraged to mimic the motions to relieve the perceived cramp with his sound hand and arm or to reverse the contorted posture.

CARING FOR THE RESIDUAL LIMB

After the postoperative dressing is removed, the residual limb is wrapped with an elastic wrap in a figure-of-8 formation. The wrap is removed and reapplied every 3 hours. More compression is applied distally and less proximally to promote a tapered shape of the residuum needed for prosthetic fitting.

The patient progresses from an elastic wrap to an elastic stockinette. The stockinette is sewn closed in the middle and applied in a double-layer fashion. Alternatively, the stockinette can be applied halfway, twisted at the bottom, and doubled back over the limb. When the residual limb is well healed (sutures removed with definitive wound closure), the patient may progress to a silicone gel–lined shrinker. Edema levels fluctuate over the course of recovery as the limb matures to final resting volume. Advise the patient to keep a compressive garment on the limb at all times, other than for cleaning, wound debridement, or

preprosthetic training (i.e., 23 hours/day, 7 days a week for approximately 1 year postamputation).

Although immediate postoperative fittings of an initial prosthetic device are performed in some settings, it is difficult to navigate the funding labyrinth that may exist to make use of this resource in an effective way. When circumstances are ideal for an immediate postoperative prosthetic procedure, care should be taken to choose prosthetic designs that limit pressures on the sutures, which may be caused by the movements and forces required to operate a cable-driven or body-powered prosthesis.

Caring for the residual limb includes desensitization. A fully desensitized limb is necessary to tolerate routine wear and effective use of a prosthesis. Desensitization is not considered a system of "toughening up" the residual limb for this erroneously implies aggressive exposure to materials and media. Desensitization incorporates textures, contact particles, and vibration.[34] Desensitization begins with gentle limb massage, light rubbing, percussion, and tapping the limb for 10-minute sessions twice daily. The desensitization program is advanced by exposure of the residual limb to the following materials: cotton, silk, burlap, polyester, nylon, and Velcro. Materials of graded textures can be attached to dowels to aid in application. Particle immersion involves the patient placing the limb into a container of various media such as cotton balls; uncooked pinto beans, rice, and macaroni; and small and large pebbles. During immersion activities, patients benefit from gentle weight bearing onto the limb. Eventually, patients tolerate vibration to the limb.

Range of Motion, Strengthening, and Body Conditioning

Patients with amputations at or above the transhumeral level benefit from scapular, shoulder, and chest motions to create excursion necessary to position and operate the prosthesis. All motions are included in a ROM program. After suture removal, begin training musculature in preparation for prosthetic use.

Conditioning the entire upper body aids in tolerance of the weight and stress of using a prosthesis and prepares the patient to use the remaining limb in daily activities. Scapular stabilization exercises and proximal residual limb muscle strengthening are critical regardless of the level of amputation. Some creativity is required to identify strategies to affix resistance bands to a patient's residual limb. Use of wrist cuffs with D-rings such as MediCordz Wrist wrap (NZ Manufacturing, Tallmadge, OH) or TheraBand CLX Consecutive Loops (TheraBand, Akron, OH) are useful for strengthening a patient's residuum. Strengthening begins with isometric exercises and progresses to kinetic and then to plyometric exercises as appropriate. Resistance and repetitions are adjusted based on the patient's overall fitness level and baseline strength. If a patient and the rehabilitation team have determined it most appropriate to start with a myoelectric prosthesis, muscles of the residuum must possess strength and endurance for efficient operation. This is done through use of an electromyographic (EMG) biofeedback system, such as the Otto Bock (Austin, TX) "MyoBoy" or the Motion Control (Salt Lake City, UT) "Myo-lab."

A training program targeted at core strengthening, balance, flexibility for the entire body, and cardiovascular endurance is important. If a patient has bilateral upper limb absence, the patient will use the body and lower limb in unique ways to make up for the loss of upper limbs, so a flexibility and strengthening program for the lower extremities is designed to facilitate task accomplishment.[35] Core stabilization exercises are also necessary to promote distal mobility, improve balance, and protect the low back particularly when using a prosthesis. Yoga is an effective low-impact form of exercise to improve posture, balance, and strength. A general cardiovascular program should be introduced after the patient is medically cleared and pain is well controlled. Operation of a prosthesis requires increased energy demands and patient weight management is critical for consistent device fit and function.

Exercises such as walking, recumbent cycling, elliptical, jogging, rowing, and swimming are all possible but may require some activity modifications.

PROSTHETICS

To mitigate common, unrealistic expectations of the capabilities of a prosthesis, the team must manage the expectations of the patient as early as possible when discussing prosthetic options.[36] A prosthesis is considered a tool and cannot replace the multitude of movements, functions, and capabilities of the human hand. A prosthesis can be used to complete certain activities and can be removed as desired. Valuable benefits associated with prosthetic use are (1) protection of a painful or sensitive residual limb, (2) limb protection from repetitive stress injuries,[37] and (3) reduction in phantom limb pain.[38]

Ideally, the patient is fit with a prosthesis as soon as the residual limb is healed and tissues can tolerate mechanical stress; however, this "ideal" is often not feasible because of current health care authorization and funding practices, which may delay prosthetic fitting.[39] Early fitting is associated with successful prosthesis use and a return to gainful employment.[2,40,41] The desired end state of both prosthetic and rehabilitative care is to return the individual to the most reasonable level of self-sufficiency.

There are up to six different prosthetic options for ULL and ULD. The types of prosthetic options include (1) no prosthesis, (2) passive prosthesis, (3) body-powered prosthesis, (4) externally controlled prosthesis, (5) hybrid prosthesis, and (6) activity-specific prosthesis. It is crucial for a patient to meet with a skilled upper limb prosthetist to discuss his options based on the level of amputation. This helps him make an informed decision on the best type of device to start with, if any device at all. Therapists with experience in prosthetics can help with this education process as can experienced prosthesis users acting as peer support to the patient. One significant factor in upper extremity device abandonment is the patient's lack of participation choosing which device he would like to use.[42]

No Prosthesis

Current commercially available prostheses are not capable of restoring sensation; however, there is a great deal of research and development directed at this aspect of prosthetics. Use of no prosthesis is an acceptable option because the native sensation in the residual limb is not covered or masked by a prosthetic device. The challenges of not wearing a prosthesis include limited grasping ability, particularly for bimanual tasks, and an increased reliance on an intact limb, if one is present, which increases the risk of overuse injury.

Passive Prosthesis

This option may generally be chosen for cosmetic purposes, although some function is possible to assist in low-demand bimanual tasks; fewer involved components make it potentially lightweight.[43] High-definition solutions are created to mimic the patients anthropomorphic form and color and can be so detailed that prosthetic representations of hair, skin markings, and nails appear natural. Aesthetic solutions are typically made from silicone materials and are customized to match the patient. Low-definition solutions can also be custom made from silicone but with less attention to the exact duplication of appearance of the patient's contralateral side (or carefully selected model for bilateral involvement). These solutions are typically used as an alternative to a high-definition solution, when the patient's activities or environment may put a high-definition solution at risk for damage. Additionally,

there are low-definition solutions that are made of other materials, such as PVC (rubber, vinyl, plastic), that can be incorporated into the passive prosthetic solution.

For treatment of partial hand amputation, this solution assists the patient to develop an awareness of what functions may be absent or compromised by the missing parts of the hand. Many patients adopt this solution as a way to mitigate social awkwardness but rely on other solutions for tasks that demand dexterity or active grasp.

Positionable joints for hand, wrist, elbow, and shoulder joint movements are manufactured by a number of companies in the prosthetics industry. Some of these joints can be covered with the types of "passive" solutions discussed earlier to create a passive prosthesis that can be positioned to a variety of angles, postures, or stances to effect passive "grip" or stabilization of objects.

For partial hand amputations, these solutions include a variety of approaches to creating joint movements and stability to achieve a functional position that is stable enough to rely on for certain tasks. Friction, locking, ratcheting, and linked joints are all available to align onto a socket that is fitted comfortably and securely to the patient's remaining hand anatomy.

Body-Powered Prosthesis

This option is activated by upper limb and upper body movements that transmit force through a cable system which in turn effects movement in prosthetic components such as the shoulder, elbow, wrist, and terminal device (TD).

For the partial hand level, this body movement can be a prosthetic linkage between remnant movements of a finger segment, as well as potential wrist movements, that will influence movements of the prosthetic components. These solutions are often difficult to maintain an anthropomorphically correct size because only a few of the options currently available can be customized to the patient's own measurements.

Externally Powered Prosthesis

The most common form of an externally powered prosthesis is "myoelectric," which merely describes one of several control input options for the rehabilitation team to consider. In the myoelectric control input system, electromuscular activity is detected (and amplified) by surface electrodes within the socket, called myosites. Other externally powered control schemes include control input using force-sensing resistors, linear potentiometers, linear transducers, inertial motion units, and pull and push switches, as well as servo- and switch-operated control inputs.[44]

These systems rely on a battery configuration to power the motors in each joint that is powered. Modern externally powered systems also rely on a processor and software to interpret the control input signals that the patient directs to the components.[45] These signals and control schemes can be electronically monitored and adjusted by trained members of the rehabilitation team. In some instances, adjustments or control strategies and grip patterns can also be managed through software by the patient. More systems are gravitating toward "app" control platforms that the user can manage on a smart phone.

For partial hand solutions of this type, the most common design includes motorized digits that are controlled through a processor and powered by a battery. Control inputs vary depending on the goals of appearance, space considerations within or on the prosthesis, the patient's native electromyography signal strength, and his ability to separate muscle signals for discreet control of digits moving in two directions.

Hybrid Prosthesis

The hybrid prosthesis is a unique option that combines elements from different types of devices, typically composed of a mix of body-powered and externally powered components. Generally, the prosthetic elbow is body powered (manual lock or passive friction), and the wrist, hand, or hook TD is electrically powered.[46] Systems in which the elbow is externally powered, and the wrist or TD is body powered do exist, but these are designed with respect to other criteria that may present with the patient's goals, physicality, and environment.

The hybrid system for amputations at and proximal to the elbow offers the potential of weight and cost savings if the patient is able to initiate body-powered control over at least one of the prosthetic components. Although there can be numerous reasons to select a hybrid prosthesis, the hybrid may be a solution for a patient who only has enough strength and ROM to initiate excursion of a harness and cable control input that is sufficient to operate one prosthetic function but not a second or third function.

Activity-Specific Prosthesis

This prosthetic option engages the creativity of the patient and rehabilitation team. The simplest way to represent this option is to suggest that it fills in the gaps for activities or tasks that any of the other prosthetic options cannot fill. The activity specific prosthesis is customized to address both vocational and avocational tasks. Many manufacturers create TDs and attachments that offer recreational and work-specific tools that can be incorporated into an existing prosthesis or combined into a unique stand-alone prosthesis to address factors related to a specific activity. When a ready-made solution does not exist, the creativity of the team in producing custom solutions is critical.

Factors Influencing Prosthesis Selection

Ideally, the therapist, patient, and prosthetist work together to select the best choice of prosthesis.[9] The following factors are considered in the decision: comorbidities (impaired cognitive abilities, multiple-limb amputations, orthopedic injuries), motivation to learn and use a prosthesis, preferences for cosmesis and function (two common goals that are often at odds with each other when it comes to the prosthesis),[39] residual limb attributes (length, ROM, skin integrity, strength), hand dominance, life roles (work, home, community, leisure), and financial resources related to covering inherent costs.[44] The general consensus among individuals with amputations and professionals involved in prosthetic rehabilitation is that the order of importance of the features of a prosthesis are comfort, function, and cosmesis[46,47]; however, each patient's unique preferences and priorities must be considered. A prosthesis that meets the majority of the patient's needs and goals is an ideal starting place for a prosthetic prescription. Additionally, one prosthesis may not meet all the needs that a patient has; therefore, a secondary prosthesis may be warranted to meet new goals and pursuits after mastery and use of the first device have been demonstrated.[14] Over the course of rehabilitation, patients begin to pursue recreational and avocational goals, and the team then explores if additional adaptations or prosthetic solutions are indicated.

Historically, it was common clinical practice to start with a body-powered prosthesis instead of myoelectric; this has evolved into standard of care for many facilities and has been adopted by insurance authorization entities, yet this may not be appropriate.[39] Rather, a comprehensive interdisciplinary team approach should be taken to understand a patient's desired goals and the environment where he spends most of his time to determine which is the most appropriate initial device.

Because of the added weight of the necessary prosthetic componentry, the challenge of achieving optimal fitting and function increases progressively with higher amputation levels. This may lead to a decreased likelihood of the patient choosing to wear a prosthetic

solution.[48] To help with adjusting to the wear and operation of a prosthesis, an initial "test socket" or "check socket" is created before fabrication of the final model. The prosthetic componentry is connected to the test socket to create a preparatory prosthesis to permit early prosthetic training.

As the patient's strength and skill improve, the prosthetist adjusts the control options and input characteristics of the prosthesis regardless of which prosthetic option is being fit. It is especially important for the prosthetist and therapist to work closely together when an externally powered prosthesis is selected because of the ongoing adjustments to fit, function, electronic control inputs, and microprocessor changes that are crucial to result in a well-functioning prosthesis. The therapist must have a comprehensive understanding of the chosen prosthesis to adequately train the patient in prosthetic use and to work with the prosthetist to choose the ideal input and control schemes.[49] The therapist is also helpful in identifying socket or prosthesis design issues, alignment, and control challenges that decrease patient function during prosthesis use.

Prosthetic Components

Depending on the level of amputation and type of prosthetic solution chosen, a prosthesis may have the following components: socket, frame, TD, wrist unit, forearm section, elbow unit, humeral section, shoulder unit, harness, and suspension elements.

Socket

The socket is the portion of the prosthesis that intimately encases the residual limb or intimately contours to the chest and back in patients with interscapulothoracic or glenohumeral disarticulation limb absences. Generally, sockets are made of thermoplastic polymers and are constructed according to characteristics of the residuum (length, girth, scar tissue, shape) and the patient's intended future use. Silicone is becoming a more common socket material and can be useful in addressing scar tissue or sensitive skin that remains on the residuum. Prosthetists consider socket design factors based on the goal of creating the prosthesis to withstand rotary and axial forces. Sockets are designed to distribute force over a large enough area to improve comfort and not impede proximal joint motion. Sockets can be suspended through a combination of harnessing systems, suction or vacuum systems, or anatomic contouring. It is also possible to create a shuttle–lock interface using a silicone or gel sleeve that rolls onto the residuum and then anchors to the distal area of the socket. Socket comfort and stability are directly related to long-term wear and use of a prosthesis and is therefore critical in constructing an acceptable and functional prosthesis. A well-executed socket becomes the foundation of a properly designed and fitted prosthesis.[50]

Frame

The purpose of a frame is to provide rigidity to the socket in key areas where the inner socket should not have flexibility, to protect the internal components of a device, and to connect all of the components to the socket in a way that preserves the alignment of the parts relative to the patient. Depending on the level of amputation and the type of prosthetic solution, a frame may or may not be required. Some levels of partial finger, hand, and transradial amputations may not require a frame and may suspend directly off of the residuum through suction.

Terminal Devices

The TD is the distal-end component that essentially replaces the amputated or missing hand. Available options depend on the chosen power source and control inputs. Two primary options are hooks and hands, both of which provide fixed prehension. A split-hook TD provides

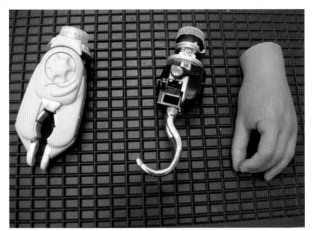

Fig. 78.2 Electric terminal device options: Greifer (Otto Bock Austin, TX) *(left)*, electric terminal device (Motion Control, Salt Lake City, UT) *(middle)*, and hand with a silicone sleeve covering *(right)*.

precise grasping; allows relatively good visibility of objects during grasp; and is potentially lightweight, reliable, and affordable. An externally powered hook can generate significant grip forces, and an externally powered hand TD can be cosmetically appealing and can offer a pinch force that is usually stronger than that of the voluntary opening split-hook TD.

A body-powered prosthesis with a split-hook TD can be designed to voluntarily open or close. The voluntary open option is more common. The patient places tension through a harness on to a cable system by motions such as scapular protraction, shoulder forward flexion, and elbow extension, which open the TD. The amount of pinch force between the hook tines comes from rubber bands or springs. A voluntary closing system is the reverse of the voluntary open. The hook remains open at rest secondary to spring tension and closes when body movements create tension that is placed on the cable. This requires constant tension on the cable to sustain the grasp of an object between the split-hook TD, or the patient may choose to use a lock for situations when the TD needs to maintain grasp tension over time, for example, when carrying objects.[51]

A body-powered prosthesis can have a mechanical hand as a TD. Adjustable springs, rather than rubber bands, create grasping force. The hand TD on a body-powered prosthesis typically has less pinch strength than a body-powered hook and requires substantial effort to open.

An electrically powered prosthesis can also accommodate a hook or hand TD (Fig. 78.2). It is highly recommended that a patient be fit with both a hook and hand TD to provide more functional capabilities and guarantee that the patient will not lose function should a TD need to be sent in for repair. Many patients have a variety of TDs and select the most appropriate one for each task or activity. Terminal devices are not typically prescribed for partial hand amputation.

Shoulder, Elbow, and Wrist Units

The shoulder, elbow, and wrist joints may be controlled through harness and cable activation, passive friction, external power and can use mechanical, electro-mechanical, or active locking mechanisms. The mechanically locking elbow unit is the most common. In this configuration, the patient uses shoulder extension, abduction, and slight depression to activate the lock in one of many preset positions. Shoulder units can also be configured to operate with passive friction or active locking. The shoulder is generally prepositioned in preparation for a task, and then the patient continues to operate the elbow and TD

in sequence. Some configurations allow for simultaneous control of elbow and TD (or wrist), and these systems can create a more fluid natural appearance when operated by a skilled, well-trained patient.

The wrist unit serves as a critical interface with the TD and allows rotation, which substitutes for movements of supination and pronation. Some wrist configurations may provide wrist flexion–extension or ulnar deviation–radial deviation, depending on the device. Wrist rotation allows the patient to orient and preposition the TD and improve access to different planes and positions, leading to a more natural accomplishment of tasks. Various wrist units provide a quick disconnect option to allow changing to different TDs. When a wrist unit is controlled passively, through a constant friction or locking design, the patient either uses the contralateral limb or a fixed object to apply pressure to manually rotate the TD. It is important to watch for and correct proximal compensatory movements that the patient may use to substitute for forearm rotation.

Harnessing Systems

A harnessing system connects the prosthesis to the body and "harnesses" body movements to operate prosthetic components through tension on the prosthetic cabling. Harnesses are configured in numerous ways based on amputation level and characteristics of the residual limb. Popular harness formations are figure-of-9, figure-of-8, and chest-strap designs. Harness systems for patients with amputation at the transhumeral level may fit tighter than systems for transradial amputation levels; this may be necessary to capture more excursion (total of 4.5 inches of cable travel).[48] Prosthetists use rings and straps to configure a harness that creates suspension and captures excursion from the body to transfer to the cabling system. The harnessing provides some semblance of proprioceptive feedback when there is adequate resistance felt through the system.[50] It is important to be familiar with the harnessing system to appropriately train the patient in donning and doffing procedures.

Options Based on Level of Amputation
Wrist Disarticulation Limb Absence

Prosthetic solutions for wrist disarticulation come from all six prosthetic options covered earlier in this chapter. Low-profile prosthetic componentry is necessary to provide a functional TD while at the same time not creating a limb-length discrepancy with the intact limb. If an externally powered prosthesis is chosen, an electric wrist rotation unit is not an option because of the space needed to place it. Several manufacturers offer an electric hand that is configured to a shorter architecture to eliminate length asymmetry. If the wrist styloids remain anatomically adequate for suspension, a self-suspending socket design should be considered to permit maximum forearm rotation regardless of the prosthetic type that is chosen.

Transradial Limb Absence

A patient with transradial amputation can be fit with any of the six prosthetic options. Initial prosthetic solutions typically start with either a body-powered or an externally powered prosthesis. The optimal residual limb length is 10 cm proximal to the ulnar styloid.[11,52] The residual limb is encased in a socket that is connected via a harness (for body powered) or self-suspending (for myoelectric or body powered). The Transradial Anatomically Contoured (TRAC) Interface is a type of self-suspension socket that combines design principles from two previous traditional sockets known as the Muenster socket and the Northwestern University Supracondylar Suspension Technique. The TRAC interface contours intimately to the residuum and generally allows greater elbow ROM than other self-suspending socket techniques.[53]

Elbow Disarticulation Limb Absence

The elbow disarticulation prosthetic solution can also come from any of the six options. The challenge of fitting this level is to work toward a prosthesis that is constructed to match the length of the sound side. This is typically done by either lowering the elbow joint center and shortening the prosthetic forearm or by using elbow hinges that are configured external to the anatomical elbow joint, called "externally locking hinges."[52] A harness and cable system is typically necessary for elbow control, but TD operation can come from the other options available. Suspension is commonly achieved with a self-suspending design with the socket suspending over the remaining humeral epicondyles.

Transhumeral Limb Absence

Transhumeral prosthetic solution can come from any of the six options. A patient with a transhumeral limb absence may choose to wear a harness system regardless of the primary power source and control input of the prosthesis to increase stability and comfort while using the prosthesis. The trim line of the socket may be cut out below the acromion if the residual limb is long enough. The optimal residual limb length is 14 cm proximal to the olecranon.[52]

Four common prosthetic elbow components are prescribed: (1) DynamicArm (Otto Bock, Austin, TX), (2) UtahArm3 (Motion Control, Salt Lake City, UT), (3) Boston Digital Arm System (Liberating Technologies, Inc, Holliston, MA), and (4) Espire Elbow (College Park, Warren, MI). These externally powered prosthetic solutions offer on-board microprocessors, may allow simultaneous operation of components via many control options, and facilitate more natural upper limb movements. Hybrid options are also available. The preference of one system over the other is generally not predetermined. When prescribing a system, upper limb prosthetists consider associated details that will best meet the patient's rehabilitation goals. It is important to know the details of each of these prosthetic systems. Each company provides valuable information online (see Box 78.1).

Glenohumeral Disarticulation

All six prosthetic options are considered for the glenohumeral limb absence. Creative prosthetic designs are needed at this amputation level to facilitate motion because little scapular abduction can be achieved. Socket designs for this level include the "Micro-Frame," "Sauter," "X-frame," and others. A chin-activated control (body powered or externally powered) can be mounted and used to control several elements of a prosthetic solution as well as several control input options. At this level, the complexity of properly considering body-powered, externally powered, and hybrid solutions is critical to match the anatomy, goals, and tolerances of the patient to the prosthetic solution. Upper limb prosthetic specialists are best suited to address these complex systems. Researchers continue to explore the treatment of patients with targeted muscle reinnervation (TMR) in persons with transhumeral and higher level amputations.[54,55] Results presented of six participants (three with glenohumeral disarticulation and three with transhumeral level amputations) showed improved functional use of a prosthesis after undergoing TMR.

Interscapulothoracic Limb Absence

All six prosthetic options are carefully considered for the interscapulothoracic limb absence by the skilled upper limb prosthetist. Because of the substantial weight of the prosthetic componentry of a body-powered or externally powered prosthesis and the difficulty in donning and operating the prosthesis, which requires multiple steps to control shoulder, elbow, wrist, and hand (as well as heat build-up during wear time), some patients choose "no prosthesis" or a "passive" prosthesis.[48,53] The MicroFrame interface is a popular design engineered to address socket comfort and stability to counter those common resistances to prosthetic use.[52]

PARTIAL FINGER AND PARTIAL HAND CONSIDERATIONS

There are additional considerations when treating patients with a partial hand amputation (amputation distal to the wrist), which constitute approximately 91% of all upper limb amputations.[4]

Partial Hand and Partial Finger Absence

Partial hand prosthetic solutions can be expected to come from all six prosthetic options. Although "no prosthesis" was possibly the most common treatment for millennia, passive solutions became more popular as companies specializing in anaplastology began to offer solutions. Today, body-powered, externally powered, hybrid, and activity-specific solutions are becoming more readily available as more manufacturers enter this market space. The challenge with partial hand prosthetic solutions, such as partial finger prosthetics, is the constraint of creating anthropomorphically appropriate prosthetic component sizes for such a small anatomical structure. As these solutions develop, the manufacturers are putting increasing focus on making small parts that are also robust enough to carry and hold objects of significant weight. One such manufacturer, Point Designs LLC (Louisville, CO), has developed a full finger prosthesis that has a load rating of 100 pounds and is appropriate for individuals with amputations through the metacarpophalangeal (MCP) joint (see Box 78.1). For limb absences that are quite proximal in the hand structure, there is even a transcarpal externally powered solution.

Depending on the level of partial finger amputation, prosthetic solutions range from passive to body powered. High- and low-definition prosthetic restorations are common solutions based on the inherent challenges of fitting small anatomical structures. One manufacturer, Naked Prosthetics (Olympia, WA) creates an innovative solution that captures remnant movements in the remaining structures of the absent finger to create linked movements in the prosthetic portions of the digit (see Box 78.1). At this time, no externally powered solutions exist for true partial finger absences. One could argue that a "hybrid" solution can be created by combining some elements of the passive and body-powered solutions. Activity-specific prostheses are a common request when patients present with dexterous needs for specific tasks that require creative solutions.

A "PROSTHOSIS" AS A TEMPORARY PROSTHESIS

A "prosthosis" (a prosthesis and orthosis) can be designed and fabricated out of a low temperature thermoplastic. A "prosthosis" can provide the patient with an opportunity to experience what a passive prosthesis may be able to restore (Fig. 78.3). A temporary prosthosis has value because it immediately compensates for a loss by restoring length to the limb to allow two or three points of contact on an object or restores a webspace to allow certain functional grasps. It also provides for a trial of various joint angles and finger lengths to evaluate the right balance to restore function. This prototypical prosthosis is then used by the patient daily for functional tasks, such as writing (Fig. 78.4) or handling money (Fig. 78.5). If the prosthosis concept is helpful, this information can be shared with the prosthetist for future considerations in prosthetic design. Success with a prosthosis may facilitate patient participation in the choice of his device and provides the team with objective information to justify reimbursement for a more durable, permanent version of a device to be fabricated by the prosthetist.

Other authors have reported using simple passive rigid orthoses, fabricated from plastic or silicone to restore function by restoring length to a finger as well.[56–59] To restore thumb function, Dewey and associates[60] published a single case study of a partial thumb amputation after a hand burn and described success with provision of a thermoplastic opposition post. Specific fabrication instructions are described in this article.

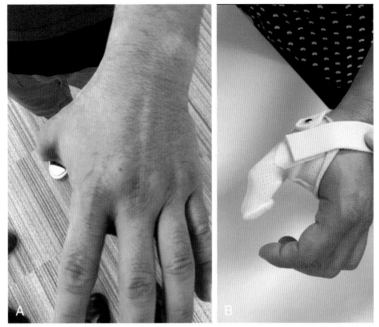

Fig. 78.3 A, Patient with partial thumb amputation. **B,** Thumb prosthosis designed to restore webspace and tip and tripod pinch. (Courtesy of Daniel Acker, OTR, CHT.)

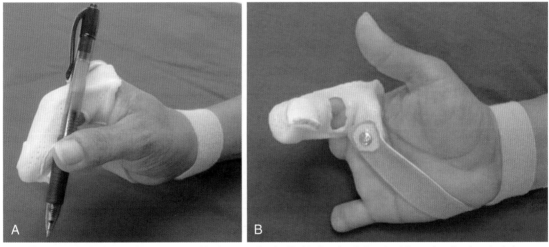

Fig. 78.4 A, Patient holding a pen with the prosthosis. **B,** Notice the "piggyback" on the distal end of the prosthetic finger. This allows for a third point of contact to control the pen more effectively. (Courtesy of Daniel Acker, OTR, CHT.)

To fabricate the prosthosis, the preferred thermoplastic material is ³⁄₃₂ -inch perforated Orfit Classic (Orfit Industries, Antwerp, Belgium). The therapist uses her or his own finger, termed the mock finger, to simulate and determine the optimal length of the prosthosis and appropriate joint angles that need to be restored on the patient's residual digit or hand. A strip of Orfit (Orfit Industries America, Jericho, NY), as wide as the mock finger and twice as long, is applied and wrapped length wise, parallel to the long finger bones, around the mock finger in a volar to dorsal approach (Fig. 78.6). The plastic is formed to the mock finger, pinching the excess material on the sides, thus welding the seams together (Fig. 78.7A). The remaining excess is cut off (Fig. 78.7B). The mock finger is positioned at exactly the joint angles determined initially (Fig. 78.8). The thermoplastic mold is removed from the mock finger. The prosthosis can either be mounted on a hand orthosis formed on the patient or suspended on the remaining digit of

the patient using tape or straps (Fig. 78.9). The finger pad of the prosthosis can be heated and flattened slightly and then scuffed with a file to produce a more uniform, tackier surface to hold onto objects.

ESSENTIAL FUNCTIONS OF THE HAND AFTER PARTIAL HAND AMPUTATION

Each patient retains a certain measure of hand function. And although there is no single standardized test that comprehensively measures all of the many hand functions (described below), the clinician should observe the patient's ability to perform activities with the residual, partial hand. Suggested tasks to observe include: squeezing a dynamometer, wet sponge, washcloth, or full size paper towel (power); grasp, pick up, and release a standing can from a tabletop (cylindrical); grasp, lift, and release a bucket handle (hook); grasp and release a baseball or

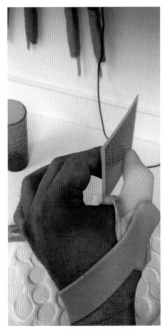

Fig. 78.5 Patient using a prosthosis for tip pinch such as handling cards, bills, or paper. (Courtesy of Daniel Acker, OTR, CHT.)

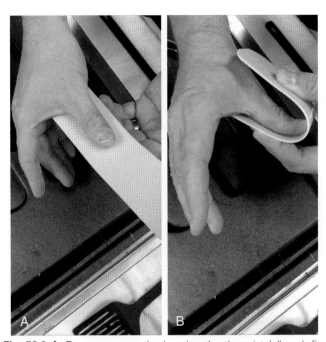

Fig. 78.6 A, To create a prosthosis using the therapists' "mock finger," use a thin thermoplastic material to mold a strip around a similar thumb size and desired position of another person. **B,** Make sure to leave ample material at the proximal end for stability. (Courtesy of Daniel Acker, OTR, CHT.)

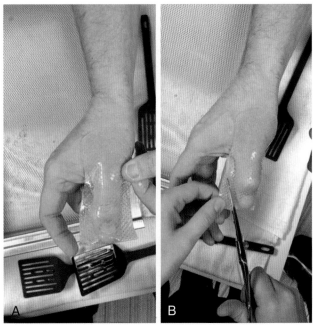

Fig. 78.7 A, Mold the thermoplastic material around the "mock finger" by pinching the material closed to form a very tight contour around the entire finger. **B,** While the material is still warm, cut the edges off down to the seam to re-create a thermoplastic finger. (Courtesy of Daniel Acker, OTR, CHT.)

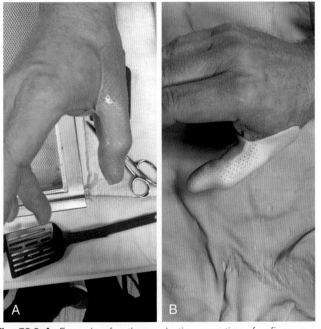

Fig. 78.8 A, Example of a thermoplastic re-creation of a finger on a sound hand with the missing joint(s) positioned at the predetermined joint angles. **B,** This thermoplastic device can be transferred to the hand of an individual with partial thumb loss. (Courtesy of Daniel Acker, OTR, CHT.)

softball (spherical); grasp a screwdriver and turn a screw (lateral grip); grasp the spine of a 1-inch book and pick the book up perpendicular to the tabletop (lumbrical function); grasp, pick up, manipulate, and release a coin (tip pinch, tripod pinch, shift, translate, rotate); and grasp and insert a key into a door lock (key pinch).

Tubiana and associates[61] define "prehension" as "all of the functions that are put into play when an object is grasped by the hands; intent, permanent sensory control, and a mechanism of grip." Additionally, Exner[62] identifies patterns of object manipulation separate from grasp, called "in-hand manipulation." After the hand grasps or pinches an object such as a tool, it then often needs to manipulate and reposition the object within the hand for further use.

There are essentially nine grasp and pinch prehension patterns and three in-hand manipulation functions identified, which the human hand performs during common ADLs.[62-67] These 12 prehension and manipulation functions are described as follows.

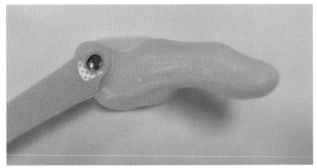

Fig. 78.9 Anchor strapping to prosthosis near the base of the carpometacarpal and guide strap anterior to posterior around the wrist to the dorsal aspect of the prosthosis. (Courtesy of Daniel Acker, OTR, CHT.)

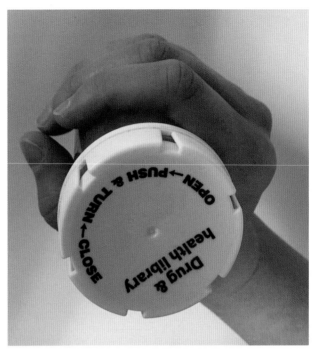

Fig. 78.11 Cylindrical grasp. (Courtesy of Daniel Acker, OTR, CHT.)

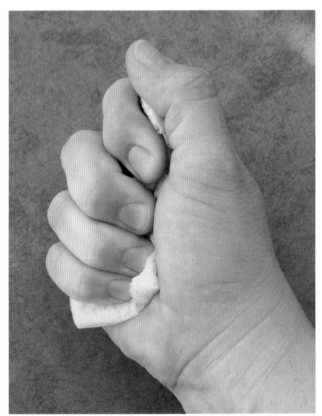

Fig. 78.10 Power grasp. (Photo courtesy of Lisa Smurr Walters, OTR, CHT.)

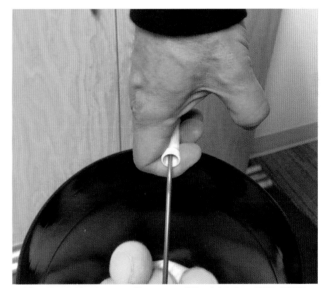

Fig. 78.12 Hook grasp. (Courtesy of Daniel Acker, OTR, CHT.)

Grasps

1. *Power*: The ability of the index, long, ring, and small fingers to compress an object against an opposed thumb and palm (Fig. 78.10).
2. *Cylindrical*: The palm contacts the object with the thumb in direct opposition and abduction as if holding a glass. This grip involves a combination of extrinsic flexor activity, lumbricals, and palmar interossei to help the fingers contour around a cylinder shape (Fig. 78.11).
3. *Hook*: The interphalangeal joints of the index, long, ring, and small fingers are flexed with the MCP joints extended. The extrinsic flexor tendons are most active in this grip, usually around an object with a small diameter such as a handle (Fig. 78.12).
4. *Spherical*: The index, long, and ring fingers are abducted, and the thumb is opposed and abducted to contour around an object with a round shape. This grasp involves a combination of extrinsic flexors and intrinsic muscle control so that the fingers can contour to the object. The dorsal interossei need to be active along with the extrinsic flexors, which is not a common action (Fig. 78.13).
5. *Lateral, directional, or power precision*: The object is stabilized by power of the long, ring, and small extrinsic flexors. The index finger and abducted thumb control and rotate the object with tip pinch (Fig. 78.14).[68]
6. *Lumbrical*: The intrinsic muscles of the index, long, ring, and small fingers are most active in this grip, flexing the MCP joints to contact the object at the distal ends of the fingers and thumb. The palm is not involved. This grip is used when the fingers need to hold onto a larger, flat object (Fig. 78.15).

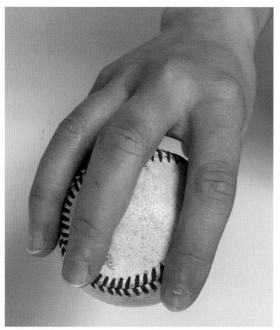

Fig. 78.13 Spherical grasp. (Courtesy of Daniel Acker, OTR, CHT.)

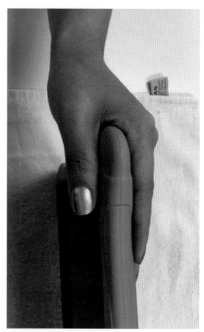

Fig. 78.15 Lumbrical grasp. (Courtesy of Daniel Acker, OTR, CHT.)

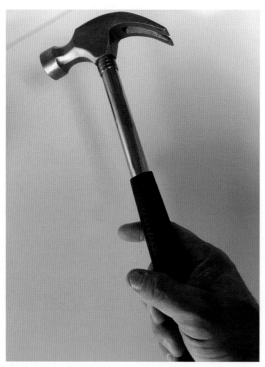

Fig. 78.14 Lateral, directional, or power-precision grip. (Courtesy of Daniel Acker, OTR, CHT.)

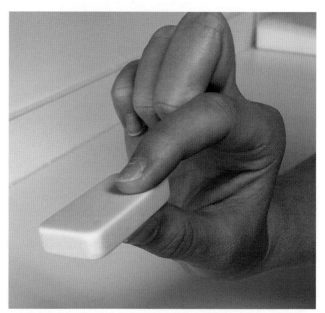

Fig. 78.16 Tip pinch. (Courtesy of Daniel Acker, OTR, CHT.)

Pinches

1. *Tip:* The thumb and one other fingertip contact the object. Usually this is used to pinch or hold a very small object and typically between the fingers of the radial hand (Fig. 78.16).
2. *Tripod:* The thumb and two other fingertips contact the object usually used to create a larger surface area and provide three points of pressure to manipulate the object if needed (Fig. 78.17).
3. *Key or lateral:* The hand is closed in a fist to provide a more stable mass to pinch against. The thumb contacts the proximal–lateral part of one or more of the fingers. The object is pinched between the thumb and the index finger. This pinch is for power, such as turning a key in a lock (Fig. 78.18).

In-Hand Manipulation

1. *Translation:* The object is actively moved within the hand, from the palm to the tips of the fingers and vice versa.
2. *Rotation:* The object is actively rotated in any direction, being repositioned by the fingertips.
3. *Shift:* The object is actively moved from the ulnar side of the hand to the radial side of the hand and vice versa.

The Functional Dexterity Text requires patients to manipulate 16 wooden pegs using tripod pinch and rotation of the pegs on a square board.[69] Inter- and intrarrater reliability and construct validity are established and confirmed by other authors.[70]

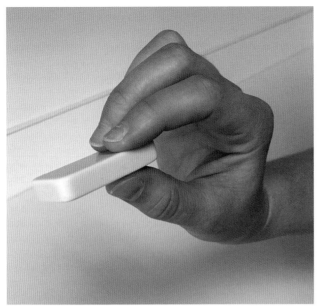

Fig. 78.17 Tripod pinch. (Courtesy of Daniel Acker, OTR, CHT.)

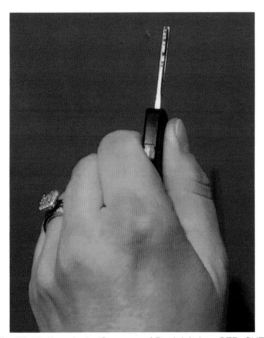

Fig. 78.18 Key pinch. (Courtesy of Daniel Acker, OTR, CHT.)

AMPUTATION CONSIDERATIONS EXPLORED BY DIGIT LEVEL

The radial side of the hand contributes to 60% of the overall grip strength, whereas the ulnar side of the hand produces 40%.[71] Each digit works in concert with the others to produce movement synergies, or predictable patterns of motions and postures needed for prehension[72]; however, each finger also has a unique skill it contributes to hand function.[68]

Ray Resection

The ray resection, pioneered by Bunnell in the 1920s, is a surgical approach involving partial or complete removal of a ray to restore hand function and improve aesthetics, particularly in individuals with a

short amputation of the proximal phalanx. In 2015, Blazar and Garon[73] reported improved patient satisfaction after single-ray resection with a reduction of grip and pinch strength of 15% to 30%.

Proximal Phalanx Amputations

Amputation at the proximal phalanx level can be very challenging to securely suspend a prosthesis depending on the length of the remaining residual digit(s). Pillet and associates[74] recommend a length of 1.5 cm, measured from the MCP crease, for adequate fixation of a passive prosthesis on the residual finger; otherwise, suspension will involve use of glove with adjacent fingers and the palm included. If at least ½ inch of the proximal phalanx remains and the patient regains at least 45 degrees flexion and 10 degrees of extension at the MCP joint, the patient may be a candidate for MCP body-powered prosthesis (Naked Prosthetics). If the amputation occurs near the base of the proximal phalanx, the ability of the remaining segment to participate in meaningful grasp and hold is minimal, and the resulting gap (particularly when the long or ring finger is involved) often allows small objects to fall out of the palm.[75]

Distal Phalanx Amputations

The distal phalanx provides normal finger length and pulp to pulp pinch, so loss at this level may be functional and aesthetic. Depending on the type of device, restoration of length can assist the patient to operate a computer keyboard, play an instrument or sport, or possibly restore tip pinch. Passive, or silicone, prostheses may not restore the same mechanical stability of the natural fingertip. Pillet and associates[74] recommend the fabrication and application of a small dorsal thermoplastic orthosis to be worn over the prosthesis to improve mechanical strength and stability. Take caution when fabricating an orthosis over a passive silicone prosthesis. Application of a barrier, such as a latex glove with an external thin layer coating of petroleum jelly or lotion, should be applied over the prosthesis to prevent adherence of low temperature thermoplastic directly to the prosthesis material.

Thumb Amputations

The American Medical Association considers the thumb to generate 40% of the hand's overall function. The thumb is unique because the carpometacarpal (CMC) joint of the thumb is much more mobile than the CMC joint of the small finger. It can adduct and oppose the remaining fingers so that it is parallel to the plane of the metacarpals. This movement positions the thumb to assist with tip and tripod pinches and creates a webspace, increasing the hand's power grasp and aperture width to hold a cylinder.[76]

The thumb is essential for power, cylindrical, spherical, directional, and lumbrical grips as well as tip, tripod, and key pinches. Decreased thumb length lessens opposition proportionally and reduces the necessary counterpressure needed to maintain grip on objects held with the thumb in opposition.[74] Amputation of the thumb at the distal phalanx results in decreased opposition to all the fingers and decreased ability to hold objects that the fingers cannot encircle.[74] Amputation of the thumb proximal to the MCP joint reduces thumb length beyond being able to assist with pinches and significantly decreases the webspace.[77] A prosthetic thumb, or a temporary post (prosthosis), is used to restore opposition of the thumb to the remaining fingers; this enables the application of pressure to an object being manipulated and may be created with enough length and contour to produce a webspace for holding a cylinder. Clinically, it can be a challenge to suspend and secure the prosthosis in place without hindering CMC joint ROM.[57]

Index Finger Amputations

The index finger is functionally important because it easily pinches against an opposed thumb in the sagittal plane, has a very mobile tip for repositioning objects because of intrinsic muscles that can abduct and adduct to meet the thumb,[78] and produces as much as 25% of the hand's available grip strength.[71,79]

Loss of significant length to the index finger impairs tripod pinch because of the inability to match fingertips with the adjacent long finger as two parts of the tripod pinch. Loss of the entire index finger ray does not impair the ability for the hand to produce a webspace but does affect handling of an object because of a lack of a full distal transverse arch. Lack of a full, stable distal transverse arch can affect the ability of the arm to forcefully pronate.[80] Additionally, with most of the index finger amputated, directional grip is affected because the index finger is no longer rotating the handle of the tool as the long, ring, and small fingers grasp with power. Therefore, loss of the index finger affects grip strength and directional grip handling as well as forcing the hand to shift its tripod functions past the center axis of the hand to the long finger ray.[81] Index finger amputation combined with any loss of the long finger is considered the most impairing partial hand injury possible.[78]

Long or Middle Finger Amputations

The long finger is the center axis of the hand[82] and produces the most power of any other finger (35% of grip strength).[71,79] Partial or total loss of a middle phalanx interferes with lateral or key pinch[74] and tripod pinch if the radial side of the hand is involved. Multiple digit amputations at the level of the middle phalanx of rays 2 to 5 impair all grasp patterns. A passive, body-powered, or activity-specific device may restore length and protect painful residual digits; thus, the patient regains the ability to use the intact thumb to oppose against prosthetic fingers to hold objects. Restoration of grip strength with a prosthesis will vary based on the type of device selected and the residual digit length. Current commercially available partial finger devices cannot restore normal grip, but passive prostheses generally restore the ability to hold light objects.[74]

Because of poor results, it is not current surgical practice to replant a long finger at the level of the proximal phalanx.[83] If the long finger is amputated at the middle phalanx, strength is lost in key pinch.[74] Amputation at this level also results in a void in the center of the finger span and impairs tripod pinch because the tip of the index finger no longer matches up to the tip of the long finger. Small objects easily fall out of the hand. In the absence of the tip of the long finger, it becomes more difficult to hold an object with tripod pinch because the index finger must be repositioned toward the center of the hand, and the ring finger must also adduct to the center of the hand. Tripod pinch can be achieved in this fashion, but it is not as effective and requires labored intrinsic muscle function. Clinically, with loss of a portion of the long finger, efforts should be made to fill the void in between the ring and index fingers and to consider a prosthesis that extends the long finger to return a form of radial hand structure. This can restore some contribution to tripod pinch with the index finger.

Ring Finger Amputations

The ring finger contributes 25% to 26% of the hand's grip strength.[71,79] With both palmar and dorsal interossei intrinsic muscles, the ring finger can both abduct and adduct. However, it does not cross the center, or third ray of the hand, during adduction, so its contribution to tripod pinch after long finger amputation requires the thumb to flex across the palm to meet the ring finger. The ring finger is arguably the least valuable finger functionally in the hand.[68] It appears to be at its best when working in concert with the small finger, as in lumbrical grasp.[68]

Amputation of the ring finger at the level of the middle phalanx allows the long finger to ulnarly deviate over time, causing reduced stability during key pinch.[74] If the radial hand is still intact after loss of most or all of the ring finger, functional retraining may not be as extensive.

Small Finger Amputations

The small finger has matching hypothenar muscles to the thumb, although the CMC joint of the small finger is not as mobile as the thumb. The primary function of the small finger is its ability to abduct away from the hand, creating span within the fingers, which creates stability when weight bearing through an open palm.[68] The small finger CMC joint can flex up to 25 degrees and adduct the metacarpal, allowing it to contour objects during grip to stabilize an object.[68] Adduction and opposition of the fifth metacarpal also aids in cupping ability during grip. Additionally, the small finger produces up to 15% of the grip power in a normal hand.[71,79] In an uninjured hand, pinch and in-hand manipulation are performed primarily by the three radial fingers, so loss of the small finger does not typically impair small object prehension.[68]

Loss of most of the small finger causes a small decrease in grip strength and possibly loss of stability in weight bearing. Loss of the entire small ray can significantly affect stability during weight bearing through the hand as well as when handling a cylinder-shaped object. In the case of small finger amputation at any level, the patient will still exhibit most of the grasps and pinches and will still be proficient with in-hand manipulation of an object, so functional retraining may be minimal.

RESIDUAL LIMB MANAGEMENT AFTER PARTIAL HAND AMPUTATION

When working with individuals with partial finger or partial hand amputation, the information on residual limb management previously presented applies. For partial finger amputation, it is recommended that elastic compression wrap be applied in a figure of eight pattern over the residual finger with slightly more pressure distally and at the corners of the residual finger to prevent the development of "dog ears." Patients may progress to use of digi-caps (Silipos Holding LLC, Niagara Falls, NY) as appropriate to stabilize residual limb volume and protect sensitive residual fingers. Edema management can be particularly challenging because of often unique residual limb shapes. Custom compression gloves such as Jobst (BSN Medical, Charlotte, NC) may help stabilize limb volume. Patients should follow the same wearing schedule as previously recommended.

RANGE OF MOTION AND STRENGTHENING CONSIDERATIONS

As with major upper limb amputation management, restoring ROM to proximal joints and the surrounding digits of the residual fingers or hand is critical for function. Stretching should focus on composite extrinsic tightness and intrinsic tightness. With the presence of generalized edema and limited hand motion after a traumatic amputation of a complete or partial finger(s) or partial hand amputation, the remaining interosseous muscles are prone to adaptive shortening compared with the lumbrical muscles in the intact, contralateral hand.[84] Additionally, there have been multiple studies related to chronic pain that demonstrate changes in the motor representation of the brain as a result of decreased or limited joint motion. Motor areas that are used enlarge, whereas those that go unused lose cortical representation.

Patients with partial finger or partial hand amputations may develop compensatory motor patterns in the residual hand akin to a fear avoidance behavior, in which the patient may describe fear of using the residual hand or fingers. These fears may be related to pain as a result of hypersensitivity, development of a neuroma, or a pain memory. In such situations, it is prudent for the team to identify the underlying cause and provide appropriate and swift intervention such as desensitization and buddy taping the residual finger to an uninjured finger to encourage use.

To strengthen the intrinsic muscles, residual digit abduction and adduction exercises should be included with the goal of increasing ROM in either direction of motion that demonstrates a deficit. Isolated isometric strengthening of the residual intrinsic hand musculature, functional intrinsic strengthening (Box 78.2), as well as proximal muscle strengthening as described previously in the chapter are included. Goals for hand strengthening should consider digit deficit in relation to the contribution each digit has on overall hand grip strength.

RETRAINING PREHENSION IN THE PARTIAL HAND AMPUTEE

During the initial evaluation, it is beneficial to test the patient's dexterity, particularly if the dominant hand is involved, to establish a realistic rehabilitation goal to improve nondominant hand dexterity. If the radial portion of the patient's hand is intact and sensate to some degree, it is appropriate to administer the Box and Blocks Test to determine gross manual dexterity as well as the 9-Hole Peg Test to determine fine manual dexterity. There are no published norms for the use of either of these tests in the partial hand amputation population; however, when assessing and monitoring improvement in nondominant hand dexterity, these tests can be useful. Testing results of the affected hand help to show improvement in dexterity, which may indicate decreased pain or sensitivity in the residual hand or change in patient confidence with use of the residual hand anatomy.

It is important for the patient to retrain as much hand function as possible, regardless of the prosthetic device decision. Retraining should occur when the patient has enough sensate and moveable remaining hand to perform some or all of the 12 essential functions previously discussed as appropriate to perform ADLs. If the remaining hand has enough function from the radial three fingers to form a radial hand (thumb, index finger, long finger), then quite a few of the 12 functions can be retrained.

Retraining In-Hand Manipulation
Translation
The patient places a tennis ball in the palm and then moves it to the tips of the thumb and two other remaining fingers in a tripod posture. The patient holds the hand up vertically from the table to avoid compensating by rolling the ball to the fingertips to finish. As proficiency with a tennis ball improves, a golf ball and then a quarter can be used. Another useful exercise is to have the patient hold three or more small objects in the hand such as a coin, a key, or a poker chip and call out an object, requiring the patient to translate that object past the others and place it on the table while still maintaining grip of the remaining objects. As the patient becomes more proficient with these objects, all coins can be used because translating a coin from other coins in one's palm is a common daily task for anyone who must handle money.

Rotation
The same objects that retrain translation can be used for retraining rotation. Initially, the patient starts with a tennis ball with five numbers written on it. The patient is to hold the tennis ball using a tripod pinch pattern and rotates the ball, trying to find each of the five numbers one at a time. As the patient becomes more proficient, he should repeat this with a golf ball and then a dice.

Hand Dominance Transfer
More than half of all unilateral upper limb amputations affect the dominant side.[15] These patients automatically begin hand dominance transfer to complete necessary ADLs. Current prostheses lack the sophistication to enable proficiency in fine-motor tasks and in-hand manipulation; therefore, the intact limb is often used for tasks such as buttoning, writing, applying make-up, shaving, brushing teeth, and manipulating small objects such as coins. Therefore, it is imperative that the patient begin a fine-motor training program to enhance dexterity and coordination and improve functional task proficiency in ADLs with the nondominant hand. Additionally, it is the experience of the authors that patients will find tasks more manageable if they are encouraged to learn to use the nondominant hand as the primary mover instead of the amputated dominant hand. For example, when holding a hammer and nail, the patient will most likely experience more success using the nondominant hand to hold the hammer and using the residual fingers or a prosthesis, with a hook type TD, to hold a nail and drive it through a board or wall. The sound limb provides natural force regulation and strength to swing the hammer and the hook or residual fingers are beneficial to stabilize the nail when initially hammering. Initially, use of the nondominant hand may be described as "awkward" by the patient; therefore, task repetition is essential to create new motor pathways in the brain.

Handwriting is a specialized and highly integrated fine-motor coordination activity that must be trained via directed penmanship exercises.[13,51] Adequate time is given to facilitate proficiency in handwriting, which restores a sense of dignity when a patient can independently fill out forms and sign his own name again (Fig. 78.19). A 6-week handwriting training manual was developed for use with military patients with ULL and is available through Loving Healing Press (Ann Arbor, MI). An experiment in which 21 nonimpaired participants repeated a handwriting task every day for 4 weeks using their

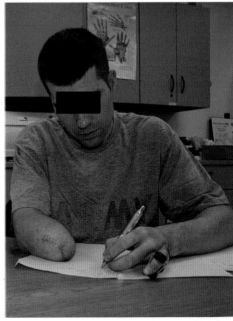

Fig. 78.19 Change of hand-dominance activity for handwriting task.

BOX 78.2 Activities to Strengthen the Intrinsic Muscles of the Hand

- Roll small putty balls with thumb and fingers
- Wrap rubber bands around Jenga pieces to build different shapes
- String beads
- Place rubber band around all digits and stack and unstack cups into pyramids
- Stamp putting
- Squeeze water out of plastic bottles
- Squeeze spray bottles
- Cut resistive materials with scissors
- Play tug-of-war

BOX 78.3 Recommended Adaptive Equipment Considerations[a]

- Nonslip grip materials such as Dycem (Dycem, Ltd, Warwick, RI)
- Electric toothbrush or Water Pik
- One-handed ("tuning fork") dental flosser
- Electric razor
- Modified long-handled sponges, wash mitts, wall mounted hands-free back scrubbers, or long shower loofah sponge
- One-handed nail clippers and nail brushes with suction cups for mounting
- Zipper pulls or key rings for zipper pulls
- Button hook
- Elastic shoe laces or LockLaces (Positive Distributions LLC, Durham, NC)
- Universal or quadriplegic cuffs
- Rocker Knife, such as Maddox Verti-Grip Rocker Knife (The Wright Stuff, Crystal Springs, MS)
- Knork (Knork, Newton, KS), which is a combination utensil of a fork and knife
- One-handed cutting board
- Multipurpose or electric jar, bottle and can openers
- Electric hands-free can opener
- Foam tubing to build up handles, utensils, and writing instruments
- Sling backpack
- Spring action scissors, such as Fiskars Softouch spring action scissors (Fiskars Brand, Inc, Middleton, WI)
- Voice recognition software or Livescribe (Livescribe, Inc, Oakland, CA) pen
- Voice Activated Bluetooth headset
- Toileting aids such as bidets
- Items can be mounted to stable surfaces to provide ease of accomplishing tasks
- Toothbrushes and eating utensils can be mounted on a thigh cuff

[a]This list is not exhaustive.

nondominant hand demonstrated that all adult participants ages 20 to 56 years gained proficiency in handwriting using their nondominant hand with no decrement because of increasing age.[85]

Functioning without a Prosthesis: Adaptive Equipment and Activity Modifications

It is important for individuals with ULL or ULD to be able to perform meaningful ADLs and instrumental activities of daily living (IADLs) with maximum independence with or without the use of a prosthesis. Time and attention should be spent to train the patient how to perform basic self-care ADLs with their residual limbs, when possible. Any deficits in the areas of personal hygiene, dressing and eating should be initially addressed if deficits were noted at the initial evaluation. Restoring a sense of independence in these areas provides the patient immediate success, aids in self-image, and fosters a sense of control.

Completion of an adaptive equipment evaluation is warranted within the first few visits for most patients with ULL or ULD. Adaptive equipment is also beneficial to reduce awkward body mechanics and use of compensatory patterns with either the intact or involved limb(s), which is important from a long-term health perspective because individuals with ULL or ULD are at a higher risk of developing overuse type injuries as a result of limb loss.[86]

The patient is educated and trained in the use of adaptive equipment, activity modification, work simplification, and energy conservation as appropriate to facilitate optimal performance. Analysis and recommendations are based on changes to the person, task, or environment. Even a successful prosthetic user does not always wear his prosthesis and therefore needs to be trained in one-handed living techniques. A list of the recommended items, considerations, and resources is offered in Box 78.3.

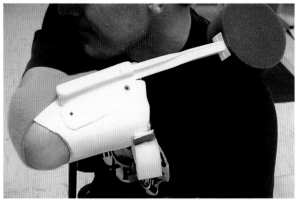

Fig. 78.20 Modification of a long-handled sponge for use in personal hygiene.

Eating

A sense of well-being is related to being able to feed oneself. To cut food, a variety of one-handed cutting devices are available (see Box 78.3). To open containers, the patient can be shown how to use his teeth. Dycem placemats (Performance Health, Bolingbrook, IL) can be placed under plates and bowls to keep them from moving around on the table or tray surface. Using a straw for drinking is helpful so the intact limb is free to maintain grasp of an eating utensil. The patient can use the residual limb as an assist; for example, a patient may steady a beverage bottle in the antecubital fossa or axilla on the amputated side while using the intact hand to open the bottle top.

Personal Hygiene

Patients should be encouraged to bathe or shower as soon as they are medically cleared to do so. A shower bag can be used to cover the residual limb and protect postoperative surgical dressings, if necessary. Patients are taught to set up all products before starting their hygiene routine. Patients with amputations at and above the transhumeral level are advised to use a shower seat and grab bars because balance reactions may be compromised and create a risk of falling. Female patients are instructed to sit down while shaving their legs to avoid falling. To avoid awkward posturing of the wrist and elbow when shaving axillary hair of the intact limb, female patients with glenohumeral disarticulations are advised to have laser hair removal. Soap and shampoo bottles that operate with a pump rather than a flip top or screw cap are recommended because they are easier to manage with one hand. To reach hard-to-reach areas such as the back or intact limb, a wall-mounted back scrubber, long loofah back strap, or a modified long-handled sponge (Fig. 78.20) should be considered.

Dressing

Patients are advised that loose-fitting athletic clothes and nonslip sandals or slipper shoes are most efficient at the onset after injury. One-handed management of buttons, snaps, zippers, and shoe tying is taught and can be practiced with dressing boards, loose clothes over own clothes, and then personal clothing. Button hooks, modified shoelaces, and Sock-Aid devices are used as necessary. Male patients may practice how to tie a dress tie with a prosthesis, or it may be appropriate to consider clip-on ties or zipper ties that close with a hidden zipper. Female patients should practice donning and doffing bra and hosiery; use of sports bras, magnetic bra clips, or the Buckingham Bra Angel (Performance Health, Warrenville, IL) can be useful. Adaptive clothing lines are also commercially available, although options are somewhat limited because most are in manufacturing infancy.

TABLE 78.1	Recommended Muscle Sites for Operating Dual Site Externally Powered Prosthesis	
Amputation Level	**Muscle**	**Component Control Output**
Interscapulothoracic	Clavicular or sternal pectoralis	Elbow flexion or Forearm pronation or TD close
	Trapezius, infraspinatus, rhomboid, or latissimus dorsi	Elbow extension or Forearm supination or TD open
Glenohumeral disarticulation	Clavicular or sternal pectoralis	Elbow flexion or Forearm pronation or TD close
	Infraspinatus or teres minor	Elbow extension or Forearm supination or TD open
Transhumeral	Biceps or coracobrachialis	Elbow flexion or Forearm pronation or TD close
	Triceps	Elbow extension or Forearm supination or TD open
Midlength or short transradial	Forearm flexors	Forearm pronation or TD close
	Forearm extensors	Forearm supination or TD open
Long transradial or wrist disarticulation	Forearm flexors	TD close
	Forearm extensors	TD open

TD, Terminal device

Preparing for Myoelectric Control

If the patient and rehabilitation team have determined that an externally powered myoelectric prosthesis is the most appropriate device, myosite strengthening begins to prepare the patient for control of the device. If the prosthetist has already identified the patient's myosites, the therapist should be knowledgeable of the location of the sites. If the prosthetist has not identified the site, the operative report should be reviewed to learn how the surgeon stabilized muscles over the distal bone. Two procedures are done: myoplasty involves muscle-to-muscle closure, and myodesis involves the attachment of muscle to periosteum or bone, which is the preferred surgical procedure for patients at all levels of amputation.[52] The process of operating the prosthesis is explained (i.e., how firing muscles separately is necessary to control distinct motions of the prosthesis). In a traditional myoelectric prosthesis, two antagonistic muscles are identified that are capable of producing distinguishable contractions using a biofeedback machine, such as MyoLabII (Motion Control, Salt Lake City, UT) or Myoboy (Otto Bock, Austin, TX) to read surface EMG output. The sites on the muscle that produce a strong signal are marked using an indelible pen (Table 78.1) and biofeedback equipment is used to train the identified myosite to produce separate and strong signals with minimal patient exertion.

Prosthetic Training

Upon receiving the prosthesis, the patient receives training regarding care, operation, and use. This education may be done by the prosthetist at the time of prosthetic delivery, and it is immensely helpful for the therapist to attend this session so that reinforcement of education is consistent. This process varies in length and scope depending on amputation level and type of prosthesis prescribed.

Donning and Doffing Prosthesis and Wear Schedule

The patient is taught how to independently put on and remove the prosthesis. Failure to master this first step can lead to rejection of the prosthesis. The higher the level of amputation, the more instruction and assistance are needed. Body image issues must be respected by providing a private area where the patient may remove upper body clothing to don the prosthesis, as needed. A thin cotton shirt may be worn underneath the harnessing system to prevent skin chafing, irritation, and perspiration caused by harnessing components.[87]

There are different methods to don a prosthesis, which the prosthetist typically covers with the patient at the time of device delivery. Some patients push into a prosthesis using a wet fit (use of specific lubricant) or dry fit (may include use of socks or talcum powder); others pull into a prosthesis using a special pull sleeve made of a low-friction material that covers the residuum as it is placed into the socket. When inside the socket, the pull sock is drawn out through a hole by way of an attached lanyard. This action pulls the residual limb snugly into the socket to ensure optimal skin-to-electrode contact. Limited anatomic suspension at the transhumeral amputation level necessitates the addition of an air-release valve to create a vacuum seal.

Before taking the prosthesis home, the patient must be educated in a device wear schedule. A recommended wear schedule is 30-minute sessions three times per day with advancement each day by 30 minutes.[88] A patient with limited sensation or extensive scarring of the residuum follows a modified schedule with 20-minute increments and advances through the schedule at half the suggested rate. The patient is instructed to remove his prosthesis; examine his residuum for redness, irritation, blistering, and maceration; and clean the residuum with antibacterial soap. The patient should discontinue wear and contact the prosthetist if redness persists 20 minutes after removal of the prosthesis.

TABLE 78.2	Suggested Activities for Instrumental Activities of Daily Living Prosthetic Training			
Yard Work	**Home Maintenance**	**Shopping**	**Meal Preparation**	**Child and Pet Care**
Use tools such as a shovel, wheelbarrow, hedge clipper, or rake.	Use tools such as a vacuum, step stool, broom, or laundry basket.	Use items such as a shopping basket, cart, wallet, or purse.	Use tools such as a spatula, cutting knife, pots and pans, can opener, or electric mixer.	Use items such as a leash, brush, bowls, diaper, stroller, or bottle.
Rake leaves.	Repair pipes of "leaky" sink.	Shop for groceries or clothes.	Cut food items to make a salad.	Hold a child or pet.
Shovel snow.	Replace a light bulb.	Manage bagged items.	Mix pancake batter and flip pancakes on hot griddle.	Feed a child or pet.
Plant flowers or seeds in a garden.	Change bed sheets.	Manage items and money exchange at a self-checkout counter.	Wash, dry, and put away dishes.	Take a pet or child for a walk.
Trim bushes or shrubbery and discard lawn waste.	Iron and hang dress clothes.	Carry food tray at a multirestaurant food court.	Mix cupcake batter, place paper liners in a baking tin, and pour batter.	Bathe, dry, and groom a child or pet.

Gross Motor Movements

Addressing gross motor movements before beginning controls training helps to foster adjustment to the initial shock of the weight and stress associated with prosthetic wear. Static and dynamic postures are practiced in front of a mirror, and body awareness principles are reinforced so patients know how to correct awkward postures and body asymmetry.[13,51] Patients repeat proximal upper body movements to get comfortable with their changed body dynamics.

With amputations above the wrist, wearing the prosthesis will have an effect on the patient's gait.[89] The patient with a transradial amputation likely postures in stiff elbow flexion and pronated forearm and avoids normal arm swing. The patient with transhumeral or higher amputation likely elevates the shoulder and laterally flexes the trunk to compensate for imbalance caused by missing limb weight. The therapist should incorporate gait analysis and correct awkward postures and asymmetry as part of the therapy program. If the patient consents, it is also helpful to record the patient during training, review the video with the patient, and provide the patient with feedback on awkward postures and body asymmetries.

Controls Training

Controls training involves teaching the patient basic device operation and control in different planes. Training progresses in the following ways: standing to sitting, from the prosthetic side of the body to midline and then across the body, and from table-top height to overhead and floor levels. Regardless of the device type, all patients must master basic control operations of the device. During this phase of training, tasks are simple and repetitive, although variety is possible by using objects of different sizes, shapes, densities, and weights. Because tactile sensation cannot be reproduced through current commercially available prosthetic technology, patients must rely on vision to know where the device is in relation to the environment or an object. Two main themes of controls training are joint positioning and force regulation.

Joint positioning involves instructing the patient how to position joint components in different planes of space for function and how to preposition joints to optimize body mechanics during task performance. If the device is designed with locking joint components (i.e., shoulder, elbow, wrist, or digit joints), patients are taught how to unlock and lock each joint component as appropriate.

Force regulation involves training the patient how to regulate residual limb movements to adjust to the size and shape of objects during grasp, particularly when using an externally powered prosthesis. The goal is for the patient to learn the degree of muscle contraction needed to operate the TD or powered fingers for grasp of small or large, soft or hard, light or heavy objects for task performance. This skill allows the patient to regulate a contraction to slightly open a TD or powered fingers to grasp a pencil or open widely to grasp a soda can. To regulate grasp pressure, objects of various densities can be used such as marshmallows, dry cereals, hard candies, potato chips, wooden blocks, and cotton balls. This training develops control of TD pressure.

A variety of activities can be used to build skill with the use of the prostheses. These activities can be modified to be more challenging by working at different heights and across the body or by introducing a speed or repetition challenge. Examples of activities include stacking blocks on a flat surface, picking up pencils from a table and placing them in a cup, moving marshmallows and potato chips from one bowl to another, picking up cones from the floor and placing them on a table, and pouring water from one cup to another or into ice cube trays.

Functional Use with a Prosthesis

When the patient demonstrates basic control mastery of his prosthesis, the focus of training shifts to learning to use the prosthesis as an assistive tool during functional activities. The goal is to teach the patient how to safely integrate the prosthesis during bimanual task performance as well as maximize independence in functional tasks. Training begins with performance of basic ADLs, such as dressing, eating, and progresses to performance of IADLs such as shopping, home maintenance, and child and pet care with the use of the prosthesis (Table 78.2).

Functional training should be guided by the patient's desired goals with the prosthesis. Examples of treatment activities include brushing teeth, managing buttons and zippers on clothing particularly as it relates to toileting, cutting food with knife and fork, light meal preparation tasks, washing dishes, removing and replacing trash bags from trash cans, sweeping or mopping a floor, carrying bags, wrapping a package, diapering a baby, making a bed, and placing groceries in cupboards. When the patient performs these tasks, the prosthesis is used as an assisting limb.[90] For example, in the task of teeth brushing, the prosthesis is used for holding the toothbrush while the sound limb squeezes the toothpaste onto the brush. Each task is analyzed, and the prosthesis is incorporated as appropriate. There are useful ADL checklists available to evaluate a patient at this phase of rehabilitation.[90] The patient's ability to move in a smooth, coordinated way while accomplishing an ADL is evaluated.

Throughout ADL and IADL task performance, the patient is provided verbal, visual, or tactile cues and feedback regarding body mechanics and body postures during task performance. The therapist must communicate regularly to the prosthetist any emerging difficulties with the fit and function of the prosthesis. Adjustments may be needed by the prosthetist to modify the device to optimize function.

To achieve the goal of full integration of a prosthesis into the patient's movement repertoire, the training process is thought of as "rehabituation." The focus is on developing new motor patterns that eventually become habits. Motor learning principles are commonly used in rehabilitation. Motor learning requires neuroplasticity at the central and peripheral levels of the nervous system. Treatment interventions are organized according to three phases: (1) skill acquisition, (2) skill retention, and (3) skill transfer. During skill acquisition, verbal and hands-on feedback are given to foster correct movement patterns. During skill retention training, the focus is placed on repetitive practice of movements and attention to the quality of performance. During the skill transfer stage, only perfect movement patterns are accepted until they are automatic. The advanced training phase of rehabilitation is used to broaden the application of rehearsed movements.[91]

Advanced Training

The following factors indicate that a patient is ready to progress to advanced prosthetic training: (1) mastery of all basic prosthetic operations has been achieved, (2) the prosthesis can be comfortably worn for 6 or more hours, (3) the residuum can withstand additional stressors placed by heavier functional tasks, and (4) motivation to use the prosthesis for advanced skill acquisition is evident.

Advanced rehabilitation is aimed at facilitating efficient and well-defined movements with consistent and correct control. At this stage in recovery, both the challenge and the reward of independence are elevated. The following are five distinctions of this training stage[51]:

1. *Individualized:* The patient's unique interests, abilities, and goals are incorporated.
2. *Includes tool use:* Tools and appropriate TDs necessary to interface with tools such as carpentry tools, kitchen cooking utensils, musical instruments, and yard and garden tools are introduced.
3. *Inherent complexity.* Training tasks are engineered to be multistep, complex, and challenging. Often this distinction is best made by working outside the confines of the therapy clinic.
4. *Prosthesis preference:* If the patient receives more than one prosthesis, this stage of rehabilitation allows for patient selection of his preferred prosthesis.
5. *Tangible product or defined outcome:* A therapeutic goal is established that results in completion of a project, so the patient has a tangible (take-home) product. Alternatively, the goal may be a defined outcome such as a changed tire or repaired sink.

Return to Driving, Work, and Leisure Pursuits

During this advanced phase of rehabilitation, return to work and leisure goals are pursued. If independence in driving is a goal, available options are discussed. The Association for Drivers Rehabilitation Specialists[92] recommends automatic transmission, modification to gear shifts and secondary controls (turn signals, lights, windshield wipers), reduced-effort steering, and possibly steering-assist devices. Patients are advised to check with the Department of Motor Vehicles in their state for information about reporting amputation and vehicle modifications.

Early after amputation, a patient contemplates his ability to return to work and hobbies. Although discussions on these topics occur early in recovery as part of the prosthetic prescription process, it is appropriate to actively pursue these goals during this final phase of rehabilitation. If a patient is returning to his previous occupation, the therapist can accompany him to his work environment for a job-site analysis; if

this is not feasible, work tasks are simulated during the therapy session. A patient may use the life-altering experience of amputation to make a vocational change. A decision to switch jobs often demands additional schooling or training.[10] Consultation with a vocational rehabilitation specialist may be warranted, and in cases in which the patient has been injured on the job, vocational rehabilitation services may be available through the state. Referral to such services should occur once the patient has maximized rehabilitation with a primary prosthesis. In cases in which the patient and team have determined that the patient is not a candidate for a prosthesis or that no prosthesis is the best option, the patient may be referred to vocational rehabilitation services. Because a patient's livelihood equates with financial security, anxiety often pervades vocational decisions. It is important to encourage him to remain goal-directed and focused while emphasizing that no decision ever has to be final. This lightens emotional tension surrounding his choices, gives him permission to change his mind, and confirms willingness to redirect therapy goals if necessary.

BILATERAL UPPER LIMB ABSENCE REHABILITATION

Patients who sustain bilateral limb loss require more intensive rehabilitation, but rehabilitation principles and phases of rehabilitation remain the same as with unilateral amputation. The U.S. Department of Veterans Affairs and US Department of Defense developed a comprehensive clinical practice guideline on the management of patients with upper limb amputation that includes strategies to rehabilitate individuals with bilateral ULL.[11]

Rehabilitation requires creative strategies, exploration of environmental modifications, and a thorough assessment of adaptive equipment options to regain or maximize independence in ADLs and IADLs. Patients commonly attempt manual tasks using the feet or mouth because sensation is often still intact. A training program to develop foot manipulation skills can be integrated into therapy. The patient begins using the feet to work resistive exercises putty between the toes, placing pegs into a peg board with the feet or toes, and then on to manipulating household objects with feet. The patient can work in front of a mirror to facilitate visualization of motions until proprioception and sensory feedback increase. Patients are trained how to use waterless sanitizer liquid from a pump bottle to clean their feet and maintain a healthful living environment.

Patients are encouraged to trial prostheses to enhance function. Most individuals with bilateral ULL or ULD wear at least one prosthesis, typically on the shorter limb. The best device option is determined by the treatment team and is based on the patient's goals. The majority of prosthetists, therapists, researchers, physicians, and engineers who work with individuals with ULL or ULD agree that function is the most important factor for successful prosthetic use.[47] Previously described prosthetic training methods are modified as needed to meet the unique needs of patients with bilateral upper limb amputations. The patient is advised that (1) his loss of surface body area increases body temperature, (2) the experience of overheating and sweating more intensely is normal, and (3) his body will adjust over time. Increased perspiration also impacts device wear and tolerance. Over-the-counter and prescription antiperspirants are available such as Certain Dri (Clarion Brands, LLC, Trevose, PA) and Drysol (Seaford Pharmaceuticals, Inc, Mississauga, Ontario, Canada), respectively, to address hyperhidrosis.

It is important to pay attention to family dynamics that may reinforce dependency. Family members must be educated that the goal of rehabilitation is a return to independence. They will need guidance regarding the part that they play in supporting the goal of independence.

TABLE 78.3	**Prevention and Management Strategies for Common Limb Complications**	
Complication	**Prevention**	**Management**
Poor wound healing	Educate and encourage proper nutrition, sleep hygiene, general cardiovascular activity; discourage tobacco use	Slow down timeline of rehabilitation to accommodate healing rate
Wound infection	Provide proper wound care, clean and dry dressings; educate patient on sterile and clean procedures; teach patient to be watchful for signs of infection	Provide encouragement to complete course of antibiotic therapy, watch carefully for future recurrence, engage in gentle exercises that do not stress residual limb
Inadequate soft tissue coverage	Unable to prevent this condition	Educate patient to check limb regularly for sores, adjust wear schedule, encourage myoelectric prosthesis
Redundant soft tissue coverage	Unable to prevent this complication	Wrap limb at all times to avoid "dog-ear" appearance, teach patient to check for invagination and to clean distal limb to prevent infection, keep muscles of residual limb toned by isometric exercises
Hypersensitivity	Engage in desensitization program; limit scar adherence at distal limb–suture line; keep tissues pliable	Motivate patient to engage in regular desensitization or TENS; rule out painful neuroma and refer to physician if suspected
Tissue contracture	Provide regular ROM to upper extremity joints; keep scar tissue pliable and nonadherent through massage and silicone scar conformers	Wear an orthosis; apply modalities, massage, progressive stretch-hold exercises
Heterotopic ossification	Avoid excessive weight bearing and weight lifting in early postoperative care	Check limb regularly, keep surgeon and physiatrist aware of progression of clinical manifestations, alert prosthetist to consider socket modification, modify wear schedule, educate patient about the condition

ROM, Range of motion; *TENS,* transcutaneous electrical nerve stimulation.

Clothing Modifications

Depending on the level of amputation and if multiple limbs are involved, clothing modifications may be beneficial to return to independence with dressing. Purchasing clothing one size larger is also helpful to maximize independence in dressing. Buttons on dress shirts or pants can be modified to close with Velcro while still preserving the buttoned appearance. Stiff loops can be sewn into the side panels of undergarments, sock, pants, or shorts so the patient can use the residual limb(s) to pull items up during dressing or toileting. Long sleeves can be inverted to hang on the inside of the clothing and tucked into pants if desired. Suit or jacket sleeves can be folded over and tacked to the upper sleeve, or some tailors can design a means to temporarily fold jacket sleeves so that the patient can still wear the jacket normally with a prosthesis. It is helpful to work with the prosthetist to come up with a clothing modification pattern on a single piece of clothing that works for the patient and provide the patient with the pattern so he can work with a local tailor to make necessary clothing modifications and alterations.

Environmental Modifications and Adaptive Equipment

Setting up the environment is critical. Environmental control units for electric household operations such as light switches, garage doors, and the television are very helpful. Other recommended accommodations include robotic vacuum cleaners, touch-pad switches, motion-sensor lighting, and doorknob extenders to create lever door handles.[51]

POTENTIAL COMPLICATIONS

The pace of rehabilitation is influenced by the patient's overall medical condition and management. Generally, rehabilitation involves a balance between moving quickly to capture the patients' motivation and moving slowly to accommodate the delicate tissue response to injury and amputation, taking care to avoid potential complications. Complications can delay, interrupt, or extend rehabilitation. Common limb complications include poor wound healing, wound dehiscence secondary to infection, inadequate or excessive soft tissue coverage, hypersensitivity, painful neuroma, hypertrophic scar formation, skin and soft tissue contracture, and heterotopic ossification.[87] The risk of delayed healing and complications is increased if the patient has cardiac disease, diabetes, and malignancy.[12] Smoking also increases the risk of wound infection after amputation.[93]

It is important that the interdisciplinary team takes action at the first sign of complications. Patient education regarding risk factors and prevention is essential (Table 78.3). With this information, the patient can adjust his lifestyle and be an active participant in his recovery.

CONCLUSION

Rehabilitation after ULL is a challenging process marked by successive accomplishments of milestones; the journey requires an interdisciplinary approach. The therapist plays a unique and critical role on the treatment team. It is the therapist who is responsible for the patient's return to independence and participation in the roles and responsibilities in his family, workplace, and social networks. The therapist must be fully knowledgeable and current regarding preprosthetic and prosthetic training and technology. Successful integration of the prosthesis in the patient's performance of daily activities hinges on the skill of the therapist in providing training that is individualized, motivating, and meaningful to the patient. Patients who receive training are more skillful and efficient in prosthetic use than those who are untrained.[94] Rehabilitation, early prosthetic fitting, and counseling are correlated with optimal benefits to the patient.[95] Reward and encouragement of the patient at each milestone serve as motivation to proceed.

REFERENCES

1. Kejilaa GH. Consumer concerns and the functional value of prostheses to upper limb amputees. *Prosthet Orthot Int.* 1993;17:157–163.
2. Gaine W, Bransby-Zachary M. Upper limb traumatic amputees, review of prosthetic use. J Hand Surg Br. 22B:73–76.
3. Lamb D, Law H. Upper-limb deficiencies in children. In: *Prosthetic, Orthotic, and Surgical Management*. Little Brown and Co.
4. Dillingham T, Pezzin L. Limb amputation and limb deficiency: epidemiology and recent trends in the United States. *South Med J.* 95:875–883.
5. Astroshi I, Rosburg H. Epidemiology of amputations and severe injuries of the hand. *Hand Clin.* 2001;17:343–350.
6. Owings M, Kozak L. Ambulatory and inpatient procedures in the United States, 1996. *Vital Health Stat.* 1998;13(139):1–119.
7. Hubbard S. Upper limb and prosthetics epidemiology, evidence, and outcomes. In: *Textbook of Military Medicine, Care of the Combat Amputee.* Bordon Institute, Office of the Surgeon General, Department of the Army; 2010.
8. Ziegler-Graham K, MacKenzie, EJ, Ephraim PL. Estimating the prevalence of limb loss in the United States: 2005 to 2050. *Arch Phys Med Rehabil.* 89:422–429.
9. Esquinazi A. Amputation rehabilitation and prosthetic restoration: from surgery to community reintegration. *Disability Rehabil.* 2004;26:831–836.
10. Davidson J, Jones L, Cornet J, Cittarelli T. Management of the multiple limb amputee. *Disability Rehabil.* 2002;24:688–699.
11. VA/DoD clinical practice guideline for the management of upper extremity rehabilitation.
12. May B. Amputation. In: O'Sullivan S, Schmitz T, eds. *Physical Rehabilitation.* F.A. Davis Company; 2007.
13. Smurr L, Yancosek K, Ganz O. Managing the upper extremity amputee: a protocol for success. *J Hand Ther.* 2008;21:160–176.
14. Resnik L, Acluche F, Lieberman-Klinger S, Borgia M. Does the DEKA Arm substitute for or supplement conventional prostheses. *Prosthet Orthot Int.* 2017.
15. Edelstein J. Upper limb amputations. In: May B, ed. *Amputations and Prosthetics. A Case Study Approach.* F.A. Davis Company; 2002:236–254.
16. Hannah S. Psychosocial issues after a traumatic hand injury: facilitating adjustment. *Int J Rehabil Resour.* 2011;24:95–103.
17. Ligthelm E, Wright S. Lived experience of persons with an amputation of the upper limb. *Int J Orthop Trauma Nurs.* 2014;18:99–106, V.
18. Van Dorsten B. Integrating psychological and medical care: practice recommendations for amputation. In: Meier R, Atkins D, eds. *Functional Restoration of Adults and Children with Upper Extremity Amputation.* Demos Med Pub; 2004:73–88.
19. Desmond DM. Coping, affective distress, and psychosocial adjustment among people with traumatic upper limb amputations. *J Psychosom Res.* 2007;62:15–21.
20. Darnall BD, et al. Depressive symptoms and mental health service utilization among persons with limb loss: results of a national survey. *Arch Phys Med Rehabil.* 2005;86:650–658.
21. Reiber GE, et al. Service members and veterans with major traumatic limb loss from Vietnam war and OIF/OEF conflicts: survey methods, participants, and summary findings. *J Rehabil Res Dev.* 2010;47:275.
22. Walsh MV, et al. Resilience, pain interference, and upper limb loss: testing the mediating effects of positive emotion and activity restriction on distress. *Arch Phys Med Rehabil.* 2016;97:781–787.
23. Kearns N, Jackson W, Elliott T, Ryan T, Armstrong, T. Differences in level of upper limb loss on functional impairment, psychological well-being, and substance use: a brief report. *Rehabil Psychol.* 63(1):141.
24. Elliott T, Hsiao Y, Kimbrel N. Resilience, traumatic brain injury, depression, and posttraumatic stress among Iraq/Afghanistan war veterans. *Rehabil Psychol.* 2015;60:263–276.
25. Gallagher P, Maclachlan M. Psychological adjustment and coping in adults with prosthetic limbs. *Behav Med.* 1999;25:117–127.
26. Pucher I, Kickinger W, Frischenschlanger O. Coping with amputation and phantom limb pain. *J Psychosom Res.* 1999;46:379–383.
27. Frank R, Kashani J, Kashani S. Psychological response to amputation as a function of age and time since amputation. *J Psychiatry Br.* 1984;144:493–497.
28. Kobiela Ketz A. Pain management in the traumatic amputee. *Crit Care Nur Clin N Am.* 2008;20:51–57.
29. Wartan S, Hamann W, Wedley J, McColl I. Phantom pain and sensation among British veteran amputees. *Br J Anaesth.* 78:100–108.
30. Flor H, Nikolajsen L, Staehelin Jansen T. Phantom-limb pain: a case of maladaptive CNS plasticity? *Neuroscience.* 2006;7:873–879.
31. Ramachandran V, Hirstein W. The perception of phantom limbs: the D.O. Hebb Lecture. *Brain.* 1998;121:1603–1630.
32. Chan B, et al. Mirror therapy for phantom limb pain. *N Engl J Med.* 2007:2206–2207.
33. Finn SB, et al. A randomized, controlled trial of mirror therapy for upper extremity phantom limb pain in male amputees. *Front Neurol.* 2017;8:267.
34. Chu M, Chan R, Leung Y, Fung Y. Desensitization of finger tip injury. *Tech Hand Up Extr Surg.* 2001;5:63–70.
35. Garza P. Case Report: Occupational therapy with a traumatic bilateral shoulder disarticulation amputee. *Am J Occup Ther.* 1986;40:194–198.
36. Melton DH. Physiatrist perspective on upper-limb prosthetic options: using practice guidelines to promote patient education in the selection and the prescription process. *JPO J Prosthet Orthot.* 2017;29:40–44.
37. Burger H, Vidmar G. A survey of overuse problems in patients with acquired or congenital upper limb deficiency. *Prosthet Orthot Int.* 2016;40:497–502.
38. Jones L, Davidson J. Save that arm: a study of problems in the remaining arm of unilateral upper limb amputees. *Prosthet Orthot Int.* 1998;22:216–223.
39. Melton D. Physiatrist perspective on upper-limb prosthetic options: using practice guidelines to promote patient education in the selection and prescription process. *JPO J Prosthet Orthot.* 2017;29.
40. Postema SG, et al. Upper limb absence: predictors of work participation and work productivity. 97:892–899.
41. Kejilaa G. Consumer concerns and the functional value of prostheses to upper limb amputees. *Prosthet Orthot Int.* 1993:157–163.
42. Biddiss E, Chau T. Upper limb prosthetics: critical factors in device abandonment. *Am J Phys Med Rehabil.* 2007;86:977–987.
43. Fraser C, Fraser CM. An evaluation of the use made of cosmetic and functional prostheses by unilateral upper limb amputees. *Prosthet Orthot Int.* 1998;22:216–223.
44. Miguelez J. Critical factors in electrically powered upper-extremity prosthetics. *J Prosthet Orthot.* 2002;14:36–38.
45. Geethanjali P. Myoelectric control of prosthetic hands: state-of-the-art review. *Med Devices Auckl.* 2016;9:247–255.
46. Meier III R, Esquenazi A. Prosthetic prescription. In: Meier R, ed. *Functional Restoration of Adults and Children with Upper Extremity Amputation.* Demos Med Pub; 2004:159–164.
47. Schultz A, Baade S, Kuiken T. Expert opinions on success factors for upper-limb prostheses. *J Rehabil Res Devel.* 2007;44:483–490.
48. Stark G, LeBlanc M. Overview of body-powered upper extremity prostheses. In: Meier R, Atkins D, eds. *Functional Restoration of Adults and Children with Upper Extremity Amputation.* Demos Med Pub; 2004:175–186.
49. Lake C, Miguelez J. Comparative analysis of microprocessors in upper limb prosthetics. *J Prosthet Orthot.* 2003;15:58–65.
50. Michael J. Externally powered prostheses for the adult transradial and wrist disarticulation amputee. I. In: Meier R, Atkins D, eds. *Functional Restoration of Adults and Children with Upper Extremity Amputation.* Demos Med Pub; 2004:187–197.
51. Smurr L, et al. Occupational therapy for polytrauma casualty with limb loss. In: *Textbook of Military Medicine, Care of the Combat Amputee.* Bordon Institute, Office of the Surgeon General, Department of the Army; 2010.
52. Lake C, Dodson R. Progressive upper limb prosthetics. *Phys Med Rehabil Clin N Am.* 2006;12:49–72.
53. Miguelez J, Lake C, Conyers D, Zenie J. The Transradial Anatomically Contoured (TRAC) Interface: design principles and methodology. *J Prosthet. Orthot.* 2003;15:148–157.
54. Kuiken T. Targeted reinnervation for improved prosthetic function. *Phys Med Rehabil Clin N Am.* 2006;17:1–13.

55. Miller L, Stubblefield K, Lipschultz R, Lock B, Kuiken T. Improved myoelectric prosthesis control using targeted reinnervation surgery: a case series. *IEEE Trans. Neural Syst. Rehabil Eng.* 2008;16:46–50.

56. Kuret Z, Burger H, Vidmar G, Maver T. Impact of silicone prosthesis on hand function, grip power and grip force tracking ability after finger amputation. *Prosthet Orthot Int.* 2016;40:744–750.

57. Jain A, Walker F, Makkad S, Ugrappa V. Three-part mold technique for fabrication of hollow thumb prosthesis: a case report. *Prosthet Orthot Int.* 2016;40:756–762.

58. Goyal A, Goel H. Prosthetic rehabilitation of a patient with finger amputation using silicone. *Prosthet Orthot Int.* 2015;39:333–337.

59. Jacob P, Shetty K, Garg A, Pal B. Silicone finger prosthesis: a clinical report. *J Prosthodont.* 2012;21:631–633.

60. Dewey WS, et al. Opposition splint for partial thumb amputation: a case study measuring disability before and after splint use. *J Hand Ther.* 2009;22:79–87.

61. Tubiana R, Thomine J, Mackin E. Movements of the hand and wrist. In: *Examination of the Hand and Wrist.* Mosby; 1996:40–125.

62. Exner C. Development of hand functions. In: Pratt Allen, ed. *Occupational Therapy for Children.* Mosby; 1989:33–45.

63. Napier J. The prehensile movements of the human hand. *J Bone Jt Surg.* 1956;38(B):902–913.

64. Landsmeer J. Power grip and precision handling. *Ann Rheum Dis.* 1962;21:164–170.

65. Pont K, Wallen M, Bundy A. Conceptualizing a modified system of classification of in-hand manipulation. *Aust Occup Ther J.* 2009;56:2–25.

66. Elliot J, Connolly K. A classification of manipulative hand movements. *Dev Med Child Neurol.* 1984;26:283–296.

67. Vergara M, Sancho-Bru J, Gracia-Ibanez V, Perez-Gonsalez A. An introductory study of common grasps used by adults during performance of activities of daily living. *J Hand Ther.* 2014;27:225–234.

68. Moran S, Berger R. Biomechanics and hand trauma: what you need. *Hand Clin.* 2003;19:17–31.

69. Aaron D, Stegink-Jensen C. Development of the Functional Dexterity Test (FDT): construction, validity, reliability, and normative data. *J Hand Ther.* 2003;16:12–21.

70. Sahin F, Atalay N, Akkaya N, Aksoy S. Factors affecting the results of the functional dexterity test. *J Hand Ther.* 2017;30:74–79.

71. MacDermid J, Lee A, Richards R, Roth J. Individual finger strength: are the ulnar digits powerful? *J Hand Ther.* 2004;17:364–367.

72. Thakur P, Bastian A, Hsiao S. Multidigit movement synergies of the human hand in an unconstrained haptic exploration task. *J Neurosci.* 2008;28:1271–1281.

73. Blazar PE, Garon MT. Ray resections of the fingers: indications, techniques, and outcomes. *J Am Acad Orthop Surg.* 2015;23:476–484.

74. Pillet J, Didierjean-Pillet A, Holcombe LK. Aesthetic hand prosthesis: its psychological and functional potential. In: Skirven T, Osterman L, Fedorczyk J, Amadio P. eds. *Rehabilitation of the Hand and Upper Extremity 1282–1292 (Elsevier).*

75. Care of the Combat Amputee. In: Lenhart MK, ed. *Textbooks of Military Medicine.* Bordon Institute, Office of the Surgeon General, Department of the Army; 2009.

76. Imbinto I, et al. Treatment of the partial hand amputation: an engineering perspective. *IEEE Rev. Biomed. Eng.* 2016;9:32–48.

77. Shin A, Bishop A, Berger R. Microvascular reconstruction of the traumatized thumb. *Hand Clin.* 1999;15:347–371.

78. Kuret Z, Burger H, Vidmar G. Influence of finger amputation on grip strength and objectively measured hand function: a descriptive cross-sectional study. *Int J Rehabil Res.* 2015;38:181–188.

79. Talsania JS, Kozin SH. Normal digital contribution to grip strength assessed by a computerized digital dynamometer. *J Hand Surg Br Eur.* 1998;23:162–166.

80. Murray J, Carman W, MacKenzie J. Transmetacarpal amputation of the index finger: actual assessment of hand strength and complications. *J Hand Surg.* 1977;2:471–481.

81. Bhat A, Narayanakurup JK, Kumar B, Nagpal PS, Kamath A. Functional and cosmetic outcome of single-digit ray amputation in hand. *Musculoskelet Surg.* 2017;101:275–281.

82. Biggs J, Horch K. A three-dimensional kinematic model of the human long finger and the muscles that actuate it. *Med Eng Phys.* 1999:625–639.

83. Soucacos P, et al. Current indications for single digit replantation. *Acta Orthop Scand Suppl.* 1995;264:12–15.

84. Colditz JC. Clinical pearl. *Interosseous Muscle Tightness Testing.* 2012;19.

85. Walker L, Henneberg M. Writing with the non-dominant hand: cross-handedness trainability in adult individuals. *Laterality.* 12:121–130.

86. Burger H, Gaj V. A survey of overuse problems in patients with acquired or congenital upper limb deficiency. *Prosthet Orthot Int.* 2016;40:497–502.

87. Levy C, Bryant P, Spires M, Duffy D. Acquired limb deficiencies. *Troubleshooting Arch Phys Med Rehabil.* 2001;82:S25–S30.

88. Atkins D, Edelstein J. Training patients with upper-limb amputations. In: Carroll K. Edelstein JE, eds. In Prosthetics and Patient Management, A Comprehensive Clinical Approach Slack, Inc; 2006:167–177.

89. Yancosek K., Schnall B, Baum B. Impact of upper limb prosthesis on gait: a case study. *J Prosthet Orthot.* 20:163–166.

90. Atkins D. Functional skills training with body-powered and externally powered prostheses. In: Meier R, Atkins D, eds. *Functional Restoration of Adults and Children with Upper Extremity Amputation.* Demos Med Pub; 2004:139–157.

91. Fitt P, Posner M. *Human Performance.* Brookes/Cole Publishing; 1967.

92. Association for Driver Rehabilitation Specialist.

93. Sorensen L. Wound healing and infection in surgery: the pathophysiological impact of smoking, smoking cessation, and nicotine replacement therapy: a systematic review. *Ann Surg.* 2012;255:1069–1079.

94. Lake C. Effects of prosthetic training on upper-extremity prosthesis use. *J Prosthet Orthot.* 9:3–9.

95. Gaine WJ, Smart C, Bransby-Zachary M. Upper limb traumatic amputees, review of prosthetic use. *J Hand Surg Br Eur.* 1997;22B:73–76.

79

Hand and Upper Extremity Transplantation: Surgical and Therapy Management

L. Scott Levin, Gayle Severance, Todd J. Levy, Shaun D. Mendenhall, Laura Walsh

OUTLINE

CRITICAL POINTS

- Hand transplantation requires an interdisciplinary team centered on the patient and caregiver(s). Psychosocial factors, physical factors, and the goals and expectations of the patient must be carefully considered from patient selection through rehabilitation.
- Working with a hand transplant patient is both fulfilling and challenging. Hand therapy program development, team collaboration, assessment, intervention, patient education, and orthosis fabrication is both time intensive and labor intensive. It requires study, creativity, and patience.

- Functional outcome is largely based on level of transplant, the rate and level of sensorimotor recovery, and patient compliance. Distal transplants demonstrate faster and more complete recovery of strength and sensation than midforearm and proximal transplants.
- Monitoring for rejection and ensuring safety are paramount. Frequent limb inspection is necessary. Early on, patients and caregivers must learn how to inspect the new limbs for signs of rejection and to protect insensate and sensory diminished skin from injury. Children are especially vulnerable to injury.

MEDICAL-SURGICAL

Introduction

Vascularized composite allotransplantation (VCA) refers to the transplantation of multiple tissue types together as a single functional unit such as a hand or face, which contains bone, muscle, fat, vessels, nerves, and skin.[1] VCA performed to date includes the hand, arm, thumb, face, abdominal wall, scalp and calvarium, knee joint, anterior neck, larynx, penis, and uterus. Beginning in 1998 with the first successful hand transplant,[2] the modern era of VCA has been a worldwide effort with transplants and research taking place on nearly every continent of the world.[3] Since then, many major milestones have been reached in this growing field, including the world's first bilateral hand transplantation in a child performed by our team at the Children's Hospital of Philadelphia in 2015.[4–8] This chapter reviews the key historical, surgical, and rehabilitation considerations of hand and upper extremity VCA.

Hand and Upper Extremity Transplantation

With approximately 150 transplants in more than 100 patients worldwide, transplantation of the hand and upper extremity has become by far the most widely performed VCA to date.[3] The first modern-era hand transplant occurred in Lyon, France, when Jean-Michel Dubernard led a team of international surgeons in a unilateral dominant hand transplant in 1998.[2] Patient noncompliance with immunosuppression led to rejection of this allograft and the subsequent need for transplant removal, but long-term success was found in the second modern-era

hand transplant 4 months after the first.[9] Dr. Warren Breidenbach and his team led this transplant in Louisville, which would become the longest VCA in the world currently at nearly 18 years posttransplant. Since then, many bilateral transplants and even above-elbow transplants have been performed worldwide, which have demonstrated technical success and excellent functional outcomes in select patients. Patient survival has been good with only one patient death from isolated upper extremity transplantation in the worldwide experience.[10] The 5-year allograft survival rate for upper extremity transplants approaches 90%,[3,11] which is better than that of other deceased donor solid organ transplant (SOT), with the best outcomes reported for heart transplants at a 75% 5-year survival rate.[12,13]

Functional outcomes of hand transplantation have been promising. Nearly all hand transplant patients recover protective sensation of the hand and 84% recover discriminative touch.[14] Motor function is more dependent on the level of the transplant with wrist-level transplants generally obtaining the best functional outcomes. Nevertheless, even above-elbow transplants can regain meaningful function.[15] Outcomes data from the International Registry on Hand and Composite Tissue Allotransplantation (IRHCTT)[16] and others demonstrate an overall trend toward continued functional improvement over the life of the allograft.[14,17] Of note, starting just 1 year after transplant, the Disability of the Arm, Shoulder and Hand (DASH) scores are on average better for transplants than for prosthetic users.[14,17,18]

As with SOT, VCA outcomes have been tempered by the sequelae of lifelong immunosuppression, including opportunistic bacterial, fungal, and viral infections; metabolic complications; and malignancies.[19,20] Because these transplants are not lifesaving but quality of life enhancing, the benefits of improved function and appearance must be carefully weighed with the complications of immunosuppression.

Ethical Considerations

Vascularized composite allotransplantation has had significant ethical implications since its inception.[21–23] Traditionally, VCAs have been considered non-lifesaving but quality of life–enhancing procedures. Therefore, one of the biggest ethical dilemmas for VCA is weighing the risks of lifelong immunosuppression with the benefits of improved function, appearance, and independence that transplantation offers. With children, this is obviously a bigger dilemma because with longer exposure to immunosuppression, the risks of untoward side effects are greater.

Some authors have recently argued that VCA are actually lifesaving, thus tipping the risk-to-benefit ratio.[24] In this view, the concept of "social death" is introduced, which includes ostracism, social isolation and loneliness, and loss of personhood and a worthwhile life.[24] People with social death have higher mortality rates, suicidal ideation, and attempts. Those with severe disfigurement, including amputations (especially quadrimembral amputations and facial disfigurement), are at high risk for social death and therefore can have a lifesaving benefit from VCA. The concept of social death should be considered with screening children for hand transplantation and other VCAs.

Psychosocial Considerations

Psychosocial considerations are extremely important for successful VCA in adults and children. The worldwide experience in adult hand transplantation has demonstrated that one of the biggest risk factors for allograft failure is patient noncompliance with medication and therapy.[3,25,26] A psychosocial subcommittee including social workers, psychologists, and psychiatrists should be involved in the screening process to help determine if a candidate has the psychological stability and resilience needed to cope with the vigorous demands of postoperative therapy, medical treatment, and close follow-up. Strong family and social support are paramount for obtaining a successful outcome in upper extremity VCA.

SURGICAL CONSIDERATIONS

Surgical Team

There are a number of important surgical considerations in hand transplantation. It is important to develop a surgical team familiar with upper extremity surgery and microsurgery. The team must dedicate themselves to the significant time commitment required for preoperative planning, surgical rehearsals, the lengthy transplant operations, and the potential for vascular compromise and urgent reexploration in the operating room (OR). The team must be willing to be available at all times and to expeditiously return home if travelling as soon as an appropriate donor is found.

Procedure

Donor Operation

After a donor is found and the decision is made to proceed with transplant, the donor procurement team consisting of two hand transplant surgeons and a SOT surgeon usually travel by air to the donor hospital. The team meets with other transplant surgeons who will be procuring solid organs and devises a plan as to the order of procurement. Ideally, the hand team goes first and under tourniquet control quickly identifies the brachial artery and major nerves and then performs a guillotine

amputation either through the elbow if the transplant will be distal or transhumeral if the transplant will be more proximal. The limbs are flushed with UW cold storage solution and packaged, and the team travels back to the recipient location. The donor limbs are then dissected on the back table of the recipient OR, tagging all key structures for transplant.

Recipient Operation

After communication is received from the donor team that the limbs are suitable for transplant, the recipient patient is taken to the OR and prepared for transplant by placement of appropriate central venous lines and indwelling nerve block catheters. Dissection of the residual limbs is then performed by identifying all key vessels, nerves, tendons, muscles, and bones for transplant. The bones are then prepared for osteosynthesis. Our team uses custom three-dimensional printed osteotomy cut guides from Materialise (Leuven, Belgium) that attach to the recipient and donor that enable precise and time-efficient osteotomies and plating of the donor and recipient bones together.[6]

Transplant Operation

After preparation of the recipient and donor limbs, the hand allografts are brought to the recipient limbs and the transplant proceeds. Osteosynthesis is performed with plates and screws. If the ischemia time is low up until this point, the extensor tendons and deep flexors can be repaired followed by arterial anastomoses and revascularization. If the ischemia time is not favorable, revascularization can take place immediately after bony fixation. Tenorrhaphy of the flexor and extensor tendons of the wrist, thumb, and digits is then performed while keeping the wrist in 30 degrees of extension and hand in a fist to ensure appropriate tension of the tendons. This is followed by repair of the nerves. Interdigitating skin flaps are closed with excess donor skin included for accommodation of swelling and subsequent biopsies.

Level-Specific Details

Upper extremity transplants have taken place from the shoulder joint down, with the most predictable results being those performed below the elbow. In our experience with three bilateral transplants, we have performed four at the proximal forearm level and two at the distal forearm–wrist level.[5,27,28] For the proximal forearm–level transplants, we prefer to excise the proximal muscle stumps of the common flexor and extensor origins and to transplant the entire donor flexor and extensor origins onto the recipient's epicondyles. This essentially becomes a functional muscle transfer because the muscles are reinnervated with time. This technique avoids coapting muscles at the belly level with the associated scarring and poor excursion. With this technique, it usually takes 3 or more months before any active movement of the wrist or fingers return because this requires reinnervation. At the distal forearm–wrist level, active wrist and finger movements are possible right away. With above-elbow transplants, similar to proximal forearm transplants, focus should be on protecting the joints from contractures and stiffness while reinnervation takes place.

EARLY POSTOPERATIVE MONITORING

Posttransplantation surveillance includes daily physical examination of the limbs as well as continuous pulse oximetry to monitor tissue perfusion. Weekly skin biopsies are performed and graded by the 2008 Banff criteria.[29] The patients receive standard transplant antimicrobial prophylaxis with valganciclovir and trimethoprim–sulfamethoxazole. The patients are required to be on lifelong immunosuppression regimen, but research is ongoing to minimize the dependency.

ADULT REHABILITATION PROGRAM

Introduction

Hands represent a fundamental part of human identity, the body's tools for work, leisure, self-care, social interactions, and communication.[30] For people with upper extremity limb loss, recent advances in science, medicine, and rehabilitation offer new opportunities, including prosthetics, targeted muscle reinnervation, and hand transplantation. Individuals with limb loss pursue VCA as a way to recover their sense of wholeness and restoration of body integrity. There is a desire to improve functionality and strength, enjoy the skill and intimacy provided by the sense of touch, and even the power to improve their lives and add closure to the event that caused them to lose their limb(s)[25,26,31] (see Chapter 83, "Psychological Issues After Hand Trauma"). Therapists working in VCA work closely with patients and the medical -surgical team to help bring these goals to fruition.

Hand Transplant Team

Vascularized composite allotransplantation brings together an interdisciplinary team to manage the medical, psychological, and functional components of a procedure aimed to improve the quality of life for a person with upper extremity limb loss.[32] This team is composed of specialists in surgery, medicine, nursing, pharmacy, social work, psychology or psychiatry, nutrition, organ donation organizations, administration and financial planning, occupational therapy, physical therapy, and more.[28,33,34] The hand therapist aids the team in the selection of the VCA candidate through patient education and skilled therapeutic assessment and then guides the patient through her or his posttransplant rehabilitation. The role of the hand therapist is distinct because of the extensive amount of time spent with the patient and the intimate nature of the therapeutic relationship. Navigating this therapeutic relationship takes extensive planning, frequent adjustments, and a great deal of patience and understanding.[28]

Therapy Program Planning

In developing a VCA program, therapists should familiarize themselves with the unique aspects of this patient population by reviewing the literature, practice specialized orthosis fabrication, and inventory necessary intervention and assessment tools (Fig. 79.1). Therapists should connect with other hand transplant centers, the American Society for Reconstructive Transplantation, and the IRHCTT for guidance and collaboration.

The IRHCTT is the largest database and research initiative for the collection of information on composite tissue allotransplant and provides a comprehensive overview about what is happening in this field of transplantation medicine. This group developed the Hand Transplant Score System (HTSS),[35] a multidisciplinary tool that collects data in six areas: appearance, sensation, movement, psychological and social acceptance, daily activities, and patient satisfaction and general well-being (Fig. E79.1).[16] The patient's score is reported annually, and the hand therapist may assist in gathering data. The HTSS provides useful information on postoperative outcomes. However, the data are hampered by inconsistent benchmarks. Participation is voluntary so representation is incomplete, and patients are not matched in length of time since transplantation and transplant level.[11]

Candidate Therapy Evaluation

Potential candidates and family or caregivers present to the transplant medical center for a multidisciplinary team evaluation. This is regarded as one of the most important components of the transplant program. The therapy section of the candidate intake process includes three parts: candidate interview, a physical and functional evaluation, and therapy program education.

Candidate Interview.

The interview addresses the candidate's health literacy regarding transplant.[36] The conversation includes the patient's motivation and goals for transplant surgery and his or her expectations for recovery, with respect to both the timeline and the level of function. It is important to review the patient's perceived functional level both pre- and postamputation, previous experience and compliance with therapy, history of pain and management strategies, and family and social support.[3,33] Experience with prosthetics is required, and programs must examine the candidates' habits and functional successes or failures with these devices. Quality of life outcome measures may be used to facilitate the candidate interview. The DASH[37] and Short Form 36[38] are two outcome measures commonly reported in hand transplant,[28,32,34,39] as well as the HTSS daily activity section.[28] (See Chapter 14.)

Physical and Functional Evaluation

Physical and Functional Evaluation Instruments for evaluation of upper extremity function pre- and posttransplant should be comprehensive; should be reliable for comparison between transplant centers and for longitudinal comparison for the same patient; and should consider impairment, activities, and participation.[40] However, there are no universally accepted evaluation process, no condition-specific validated tool, and no uniform guidelines for hand transplantation or amputation.[11,40,47] No instrument exists to measure the full measure of the impact of hand loss.[25] Rather, a battery of established, general assessments and standardized tools have been used by the various transplant centers with some uniformity both pre- and posttransplant. (For information on sensibility and dexterity tests, refer to Chapters 10 and 11.) However, there is growing attention and collaboration in the VCA community to address this issue. During the candidate assessment, a baseline physical assessment records range of motion (ROM), strength, sensation of residual limbs, limb size and edema, and notations about skin and scar. The candidate's history of pain, including any experience with PLP, should be discussed as well as the patient's coping strategies. Previously mentioned quality of life outcome measures and the Carroll Upper Extremity Function Test,[48] the Sollerman Hand Function Test,[49] and the Action Reach Arm Test[50] are the most common tools used by transplant centers to measure function. We prefer the Sollerman test and have patients perform it with prosthetics or with their residual limb based on their normal daily routines (Fig. E79.5). Patients with lower extremity amputations should have a physical therapy assessment for gait, balance, core strength, and endurance.

Therapy Program Education

Program education covers the physical and psychosocial factors related to the rehabilitation process. The candidate and family or caregiver need to be fully aware of the extensive time requirements for therapy, the day-to-day expectations and responsibilities, and the known functional outcomes in hand transplant. The following information serves as a reference for the therapist in their process to educate individuals considering VCA as an option for functional recovery after limb amputation.

Therapy Treatment Time. Adult patients are required to stay local to the transplant medical center for up to 3 months after surgery to establish medical and pharmacologic stability and initiate specialized therapy programs.[28,40,41] Initially, the patient spends 1 to 3 weeks in the acute care hospital. Therapy begins within the first postoperative week and is dependent on the level of transplant. In the acute care setting, the patient is seen 5 to 7 days a week from 2 to 8 hours a day.[14,28,39,40,42] This encompasses hand therapy and inpatient occupational therapy

Range of motion	Edema
• Goniometry • Kapandji scale	• Volumetry • Circumferential and figure-of-8 method

Strength	Pain
• Dynamometry • Pinch meter dynamometry • Manual muscle testing • Physical therapy assessments for gait, balance, strength, and posture	• Numeric Rating Scale (NRS) • Visual Analog Scale (VAS)

Sensibility	Dexterity and coordination
• Semmes-Weinstein Monofilament Test • WEST (Weinstein Enhanced Sensory Test) • Hot–cold discrimination • Shape Texture Identification Test (STI) • Two-point Discrimination Test • Modified Moberg Test • Vibration (256 Hz)	• 9-Hole Peg Test • Box and Blocks • Purdue Peg Board • Minnesota Rate of Manipulation

Nerve regeneration	Activities of daily living
• Tinel's sign	• Observation

Function	Quality of life and participation
• Carroll UE Function Test • Sollerman Hand Function Test • Action Reach Arm Test • Jebsen Hand Function Test	• Hand Transplant Score System • Disability of Shoulder, Arm and Hand • Short Form 36 Health Survey • EQ-5D • Patient Satisfaction Function Scale • Michigan Hand Questionnaire • Patient Reported Outcome Measurement System (PROMIS) • Lawton ADL/IADL Questionnaire • Brief Symptom Inventory

Fig. 79.1 Assessment tools used in adult hand and upper extremity vascularized composite allotransplantation. *ADL,* Activity of daily living; *IADL,* instrumental activity of daily living; *UE,* upper extremity. (Data from references[28,34,35,39,40].)

and physical therapy, particularly if the patient has lower extremity amputations. Time accounts for direct intervention, fabricating orthoses and adaptive tools, activity of daily living (ADL) and transfer training, working with the team, and instructing caregivers. There is a high level of physical and emotional fatigue for the patient. Frequent breaks are necessary for the patient's comfort and other needs, including personal care, toileting, meals, and nursing and medical priorities. After the patient is discharged from the hospital, she or he continues with daily outpatient hand therapy. For patients with comorbid lower extremity amputations, a brief inpatient rehabilitation stay may be necessary to improve safety with gait and transfers.

After the patient returns to his or her hometown, he or she continues with outpatient hand therapy. Frequency of visits may be reduced depending on the level of transplant, nerve regeneration, and the patient's functional level. During the first postoperative year, patients are required to return to the transplant medical center every few months to assess their health and functional recovery. This decreases to annual visits thereafter.[28,41]

Caregivers. A consistent and reliable caregiver should be identified as a part of the candidate selection process. The caregiver is the single most important person for the patient in the weeks and months after surgery. Patients, particularly those receiving bilateral or proximal transplants, are unable to use their new limbs for weeks to months after surgery. Comorbid lower extremity amputations further limit independent function. Caregivers perform intimate tasks such as bathing and personal hygiene. They assist with feeding, medications, and managing orthoses and prosthetics. Most important, the caregiver is a vital emotional support system (Fig. E79.2). Initially, these are important and possibly difficult facts for the patient and caregiver to learn and accept but are also critical for postoperative success.

Outcomes. Outcome is largely based on the level of transplant and the rate of nerve regeneration and sensorimotor recovery. Transplant levels are frequently referred to as distal and proximal. Distal transplants refer to transplantation at the distal forearm or wrist–hand level, and the patient maintains her or his native forearm musculature.[43] By maintaining the native forearm extrinsic muscles, motor recovery may occur in days to weeks. Neural regeneration has a short distance to travel, leading to a higher likelihood to recover some intrinsic motor function and two-point discrimination.[11] Proximal level transplants occur at the proximal third of the forearm or above and are reliant on reinnervation of donor extrinsic muscles,[43] delaying sensorimotor recovery for several weeks to months. The greater distance needed for nerve reinnervation affects the quality of this recovery.[44] Sensation and muscle strength may be weaker, and the distant intrinsics are less likely to recover.[11] In a 2016 report, the IRHCTT collected data from 56 patients (25 unilateral and 31 bilateral) with a majority of cases being considered as distal. Patient survival in hand transplant is 96%, and graft survival is 82%. A total of 74% experienced at least one rejection episode in the first year. All patients recover protective sensation, 90% tactile sensibility, and 82% partial discrimination. Functional recovery is optimistic and summarized as VCA patients regaining independence in most ADLs.[45] A 2010 IRHCTT report noted intrinsic function return in 57% of the patients ranging from 9 to 15 months posttransplant and 75% reported improved quality of life compared with pretransplant function, including a level of independence enabling independent living and some returning to full time occupation[14] (Fig. E79.3). Nevertheless, Kumnig and associates[26] note that some patients commented on feeling less function than hoped for, frustration over the length of rehabilitation and recovery, and side effects of medications, and some have episodes of anxiety and depression, further validating the need for careful candidate screening and communication. Kumnig and associates[26] describe pain as one of the most acutely stressful aspects of traumatic injury. Phantom limb pain (PLP) occurs in more than 60% of amputations, negatively impacting postamputation adaptation, and transplant candidates with PLP are at higher risk of PLP persisting after hand transplant. Transient pain related to nerve regeneration is possible in hand transplantation.

Graft Appearance and Acceptance. The medical team reviews the matching protocol with the patient, but the hand therapist should be ready to address concerns about postsurgical cosmesis to help the patient accept the new limbs as his or her own. The grafted limb is visible to the patient and others. An inability to accept the new limb may complicate the psychological integration of the new body part and raise the risk of noncompliance, which can result in impaired function, rejection episodes, and even graft loss.[26,46] Aesthetic considerations to match the donor and recipient include gender, height, weight, race, and skin tone and avoidance of identifying markers such as tattoos. After transplant, the suture line clearly delineates the graft from the native limb. Postoperative sutures, edema, trophic changes, and some variability between the donor and recipient should be expected. Over time the graft may modify closer to the patient's native appearance (Fig. E79.4). Some skeletal deformities related to uneven motor recovery may develop. Therapy intervention, orthoses, and the patient's compliance with rehabilitation help to minimize deformities and improve function. Surgeons may perform revision procedures for cosmesis to address motor deficits and imbalances and tendon adhesions.[11]

Therapist's Assessment and Recommendation

The candidate assessment process helps the therapy team make its recommendation to the transplant team by helping to answer the essential question: is this person a good rehabilitation candidate? This question requires consideration of several factors. Is the patient physically ready for the rigorous postoperative rehabilitation, and if not, what is recommended to address the physical limitations? For instance, a patient with lower extremity amputations may still be using his or her residual upper extremity for balance on stairs and transfers, and a referral

to physical therapy may be beneficial. Psychological factors may be revealed during the therapy interview. Was the candidate compliant with therapy in the past, and is she or he motivated for a long-term commitment to rehabilitation? Has the patient used strategies for acceptance, flexibility, and problem solving after amputations that will again be necessary after transplant surgery? Are the patient's expectations for functional recovery realistic and achievable given what is known about transplant outcomes, and does the patient acknowledge the initial postsurgical functional regression, protracted recovery, and potential limitations in his or her expectations? What are the status and ability level of the caregiver? Does the patient have strong family or social support?[26,32] It is desirable for the patient to be at least 1 year out from amputation so she or he has had time to participate in rehabilitation to recover from the initial trauma or illness, practice with prosthetics, manage pain issues, and address the psychological trauma from losing a limb. These matters influence the patient's participation and success in the transplant rehabilitation and should be considered in the pretransplant evaluation.

ADULT POSTTRANSPLANT THERAPY

Therapy after adult transplantation begins as early as day 1 after surgery up to day 6.[28,39,40,51–55] The specific timing is determined by the hand surgeons and hand therapists. Reported timelines vary regarding progression. Some are described in days, weeks, or months,[39,53–55] whereas others refer to periods of time[40] or phases of progression[28,39] or do not outline therapy progression and advancement at all. The stages of biological healing are fairly universal, but given the variability in the number of limbs, level of transplant, and surgical and medical considerations, looking at intervention in a timeline of weeks can be arbitrary and misleading.[28] The authors of this chapter suggest treatment progression for the hand transplant patient in phases and discuss the different interventions for proximal versus distal level transplants. Yet regardless of the phase or level, it is important to understand that all transplants are susceptible to rejection at any time, and the hand transplant patient and all team members, including the hand therapist, must be able to recognize the signs of rejection.

Monitoring for Rejection

Similar to those undergoing SOT, hand transplant patients are on a combination of immunosuppression medications. However, Schneeberger and associates[56] explain that unlike SOT, hand transplant is composed of heterogeneous tissue, including skin, bone, muscle, cartilage, tendon, nerve, vessels, and subcutaneous tissue. The skin is highly immunogenic and is therefore the main target of the body's autoimmune response. For this reason, the skin on the new transplanted limbs should be closely monitored for graft rejection. This can be done by visual inspection and directed skin punch biopsy.[56] This allows for earlier detection and successful treatment with oral or intravenous steroids and topical or oral tacrolimus.[47,56] It should be noted that reported acute rejection (AR) occurs in 85% of hand transplant recipients in the first year, and a majority have occurred when a patient was noncompliant or the intensity of immunosuppression was decreased because of side effects or other reasons.[14]

The hand therapist has frequent opportunities for visual and physical inspection of the grafts, so it is important to recognize the signs of AR and work with the patient and caregiver to perform frequent skin checks. Early clinical manifestations of AR may be a diffuse or focal pattern of erythematous maculopapular lesion or rash. Typical patterns will present over the dorsal aspects of the forearm and hands[56–58] (Fig. 79.2). Careful inspection is needed to detect subtle presentations and on skin that is of darker tone. Palmar presentations have been

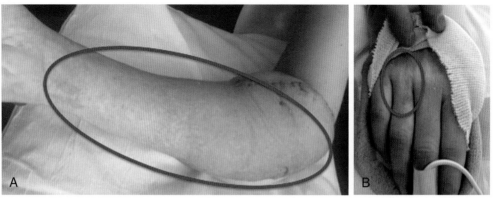

Fig. 79.2 Early clinical manifestations of acute rejection on the forearm (A) and on the hand (B). Diffuse and focal pattern of erythematous maculopapular lesion.

associated with mechanical stress.[59] Atypical presentation involves the development of papular rash, scaling and the development of hard, leathery skin. There may be nail dystrophy or nail loss.[56,57] Not all skin changes indicate rejection. Infectious or allergic inflammatory skin diseases are common in immunosuppressed patients and can mimic AR both clinically and histologically.[58] Regardless, any abnormalities should be immediately reported to the medical team. Therapy may proceed during treatment for rejection unless otherwise advised by the medical-surgical team.

Initial Phase

The initial phase of hand therapy begins during the first postoperative week in the hospital setting and may last up to 4 weeks.[28,39] As previously stated, the patient is seen 5 to 7 days a week from 2 to 8 hours a day.[28,39,40,42,60] The amount of treatment time is established by each individual program based on bilateral versus unilateral transplant, level of transplant, and the patient's overall therapy. The primary goals at this time are protection; proper positioning; safe ROM of the transplanted upper extremity(s); wound and skin inspection; edema control; pain management; and education of the patient, caregiver, and nursing personnel.[28,39,40,61] Bony fixation, musculotendon balance, and soft tissue and vascular integrity must be considered. The main focuses of therapy during this phase are orthosis fabrication and adjustments and ROM. The balance for graft protection and safe ROM is determined with consultation among the hand therapists and the hand surgeons. Additional collaboration among the hand surgeons, nursing staff, and the hand therapist along with the entire team is vital to an optimal outcome throughout the rehabilitation process.[28,39] In particular, nursing personnel provide 24-hour care and are essential to helping with ROM, positioning, and orthotic intervention. Nursing, patient, and patient caregiver education regarding orthosis donning and doffing and ROM exercises are necessary during this phase.

Orthotic Intervention

Particularly in the early phases, orthotic fabrication is labor intensive and time consuming, often requiring frequent alterations because of bandages, fluctuations in edema, skin and tissue integrity, patient comfort, and functional adaptations. Over time, additional orthoses for function and positioning may be required depending on the quality of motor return, especially in a proximal-level transplant. Wearing orthoses can be frustrating for patients, but compliance is essential to protect the new limbs through the acute healing and neuroregeneration phases. O'Brien[62] advises therapists to consider the long duration for which patients must wear some form of orthosis. It is important to

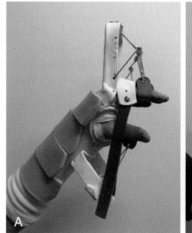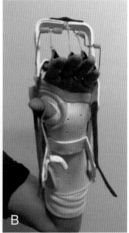

Fig. 79.3 (A) Lateral view and (B) volar view of the "Crane Outrigger" orthosis used for distal hand transplants.

consider not only the protective nature but also the comfort and aesthetics to enhance compliance. Additionally, therapy sessions should offer examples and practice in adapted activities that do not compromise the orthotic regimen. The hand therapist must train the patient, caregivers, and nursing on how to don and doff the orthosis and the wearing schedule, and team members should support the therapy plan for orthotic intervention.

Distal Transplants. The Crane Outrigger orthosis was first described by Chesher and coworkers[63] for use in proximal interphalangeal (IP) joint replacements and later used for hand replants[64,65] (Fig. 79.3). This custom orthosis was adopted for use in distal hand transplants when the patients maintain their own extrinsic forearm musculature for early active motion. The unique design permits safe early tendon gliding with an outrigger system that provides passive IP extension and allows active digital flexion, with minimal and near consistent tension throughout the arc of motion. Early on, the patient or therapist may reduce some of the tension to flexion by manually assisting the outrigger system through the arc of motion. The presence of a lumbrical blocking bar prevents claw deformity.[64,65] We suggest a slight adjustment of the arc of the lumbrical blocking bar to meet the height difference of each digit so as to avoid undue stress on the muscle–tendon length of the long finger in relationship to the small finger. During downtime and sleep, a static forearm-based orthosis should be used. This static orthosis positions the wrist at 20 degrees of extension and the hand in an intrinsic-plus position with the metacarpophalangeal (MCP) joints in 50 degrees of flexion, the IP joints in extension, and the thumb in palmar abduction.

Proximal Transplants. The Crane Outrigger orthosis is not used in the proximal-level transplant because initially, there is no active motor to the fingers, and by the time neuromotor regeneration occurs for proximal transplants, protecting the tendon anastomosis is no longer necessary. Therefore, full arm static protection is required for the proximal level transplants (Fig. E79.6). When the transplant is close to the elbow joint, it is important to prevent tension or compression of vascular structures, especially in the presence of postoperative edema. Generally, the elbow is positioned at 30 degrees flexion, the forearm in neutral (if possible), the wrist at 20 degrees of extension, the MCP joints in 50 degrees of flexion, the IP joints in extension, and the thumb in palmar abduction. For ease of fabrication and donning and doffing, the orthosis can be fabricated in two sections, a proximal and distal section. The proximal section begins at the upper arm and ends distally at wrist, whereas the distal section begins at the forearm and includes the wrist and hand. The distal section is fabricated to fit over the proximal section. The sections overlap at the forearm level.[28] Padding and soft straps are recommended to eliminate pressure.

Edema Management

Edema may be monitored and measured via circumferential measurements. An OR marker may be used on the skin to identify consistent measurement points. It is advisable to avoid mechanical stress to the delicate skin, prevent unsafe accessory motions, and maintain easy access to the grafted limb for skin inspection. Therefore, it is our opinion that during this early phase, edema garments such as compression sleeves and gloves should be limited or not used at all. Kinesio taping and manual lymphatic drainage massage over the new grafted limb is not recommended. Instead, the limb should be positioned in comfortable elevation to promote lymphatic flow and edema control.

Range of Motion and Exercise

In discussing exercises after nerve transfers, Kahn and Moore[66] suggest, based on their research, that physical activity encourages functional motor and sensory recovery, and maintaining muscle activity with active and passive exercise may increase trophic factors to be released on regenerating motor neurons. They report that low-intensity exercise has been found to increase the length of regenerating axons after peripheral nerve repair but caution that intense training may have negative effects and care should be taken not to overwhelm a recovering muscle.[66]

Distal Transplants. Transplant at the distal level is treated much like a replantation[54,61] in which active protective ROM may be initiated immediately.[39,40] Early ROM is started as soon as the recipient's native extrinsic flexors and extensors are working while in the crane orthosis.[39,40] It has been determined that active tension on the tendon repair is important to allow proximal movement that may not happen with passive movement alone.[67] In addition to ROM of the fingers with the Crane Outrigger orthosis, active assisted range of motion (AAROM) of the shoulder and elbow in all planes and passive range of motion (PROM) of wrist in a tenodesis pattern is initiated in the first postoperative week as cleared by the surgeons.

Proximal Transplants. Clearance for ROM is based on the transplant level; the strength of the bony fixation; and musculotendinous, soft tissue, and vascular integrity. For instance, when connection is close to the elbow, the surgical team initially may impose ROM limits at the

elbow to avoid compression or stretch of vascular structures. In the case of a midhumeral transplant, shoulder passive/active assisted/active range of motion (P/AA/AROM) may not be safe initially, whereas with a midforearm transplant, shoulder ROM is typically safe. Regardless of the level, after clearance is given to move and use the shoulder, the patient will require assistance with motion because of the weight of the new arm(s) and orthoses and to limit stress on the attached structures. Initially, in cases in which the connection is close to the elbow, the orthosis is removed for PROM of the elbow, forearm, wrist, and digits. Wrist and digit PROM is performed in a tenodesis pattern.

TRANSFERS AND AMBULATION

In the acute care setting, physical therapy and occupational therapy play a vital role in functional mobility training.[28,39] The patient must be able to safely transfer either independently or with the help of a caregiver to a wheelchair, toilet, and car before discharge from the hospital to attend outpatient therapy. In addition to transfers, ambulation training is needed because the weight of the new arm(s) may throw off balance more than anticipated, particularly if the transplant is bilateral or when lower extremity prosthetics are used for ambulation.[28] Until the patient is cleared by the surgeon to ambulate without protection, orthoses, platform walkers, or adapted slings are used for protecting the upper extremity and for safe mobility, and this is most important for proximal-level transplants[28] (Fig. E79.7).

Cortical Retraining, Sensory Retraining, and Functional Use

Cortical reorganization, after longstanding deafferentation and deefferentation, is partially reversible. In the case of a hand transplantation patient, this continues for at least 2 years.[68] This is discussed in more detail later in this chapter. Encouraging the patient to accept the new hand(s) as her or his own, particularly during therapy sessions and ROM exercises, is key to successful acceptance and cortical reorganization. Guiding the patient to touch the new hand(s) to her or his sensate skin may help initiate the patient's acceptance of the new hands as her or his own.[28] Sensory retraining strategies should be used to aid in cortical retraining and functional hand use. (See Chapter 42, "Sensory Relearning and Brain Plasticity.") Viewing the hand improves tactile discrimination and facilitates perception, which seems to modulate somatosensory cortical processing. Associations between visual and tactile stimuli from the external environment are foundational to behavior.[69] Additionally, stimulating the nerve endings with various textures is important to help relearn tactile sensation.[61]

A universal cuff or modifications to the orthoses will allow for practice of light functional use of the arms such as feeding, using the call bell, and phone and computer use (Fig. E79.8). This is the patient's first sense of independence since the transplantation procedure[28] and aids in position sense and cortical integration. In the case of a proximal-level transplant, the patient must first be cleared for AROM to the elbow.

Electrical Stimulation

Electrical stimulation has been described for use with hand and upper extremity transplant patients to facilitate muscle activity. Caution must be observed given that without recovery of skin sensation and muscle innervation, skin integrity might be compromised. Electric stimulation can only produce contractions of denervated muscles when a direct current (DC) is used. A denervated muscle will not contract with electric stimulation such as used for neuromuscular electrical stimulation (NMES). DC current is direct and much stronger than NMES.[70]

Cameron[70] recommends that electrical stimulation may be initiated after the patient regains protective sensation to the skin where the electrodes would be placed and when there is a trace of muscle action. NMES of the proximal nerve branches on the native skin above the anastomosis may be considered.[61] In addition to NMES, transcutaneous electrical nerve stimulation (TENS) can be used for pain management, but the TENS pads should not be placed on denervated skin.

Intermediate Phase

This phase begins when the patient is discharged from inpatient hospitalization to a transitional outpatient living facility. The patient is scheduled for outpatient hand therapy for 2 to 6 hours, Monday through Friday depending on the program. During this phase, PROM is continued, and active assisted (A/A) and AROM are based on the biological healing, neuromotor recovery, and the surgeon's clearance for activity. In addition to outpatient therapy, unilateral hand transplant patients should be educated on a home exercise program (HEP) using the noninvolved hand to perform ROM on the involved hand. With bilateral hand transplant patients, the caregiver is instructed in the HEP and assists the patient. Upper extremity proximal and core strengthening are needed to support the weight of the new limb(s). Orthosis adjustments continue, and ADL training is ongoing (see Fig. E79.8). The hand therapist continues to monitor motor regeneration, adapting exercises to facilitate muscle activation being mindful to prevent strain, fatigue, and maladaptive movement patterns. It is about this time that patients may start to show impatience with the slow process of neuromotor regeneration. Emotional support and careful selection of successful and meaningful activities are important to keep the patient motivated and engaged. The patient might also need outpatient physical therapy for continued refinement with gait, balance, and transfers.

When there is sufficient motor recovery with active wrist control, the patient is transitioned to a hand-based lumbrical blocking orthosis (anticlaw or helmet orthosis) after a 2 out of 5 motor strength is appreciated.[28] This dorsal-based orthosis blocks digit 2 to 5 MCP joints at approximately 45 degrees of flexion, with the IP joints and wrist free, and holds the thumb in functional abduction[64,65] (Fig. E79.9). This low-profile orthosis promotes active wrist extension and flexion for normal grasping and tenodesis function.[64] For patients with a distal amputation and transplantation, this dorsal anticlaw orthosis may be started as early as 3 to 4 weeks after surgery. Patients are encouraged to wear this orthosis up to 1 year until intrinsic function returns or there is an adequate muscle balance or inherent stiffness to prevent a claw deformity.

Late Phase

This phase begins when the patient is medically stable to return home. The hometown therapist must be carefully selected by both the initial treating therapist and the surgeon's network. When possible, the hometown therapist should be invited to visit and observe therapy while the patient is at the transplant site and develop a plan for exchanging information and progress reports. Video conferencing is a useful way for the patient and therapy teams to collaborate. To ensure consistency of care, the hand therapy team at the transplant location needs to provide support and education to the hometown therapist, and communication between the groups is vital for the patient's success.

Over the coming weeks and months, motor and sensory training should continue based on neuroregeneration. Recovery to the extensors and flexors of the newly grafted limb will be unbalanced, and the extrinsic muscles will overpower the smaller, more distal intrinsics. Interventions should include motor control strategies such as biofeedback, coactivation, and isometric exercises and should be integrated into meaningful tasks. Engaging the patient in sensory retraining

further enhances motor control and functional use of the new limb(s). In some cases, sensory recovery can be painful for some transplant patients, and pain management techniques such as graded motor imagery may be useful (see Chapters 96 and 100).

It is important that the patient resumes her or his previous community, avocational, and vocational roles as soon as possible. The emphasis of therapy at this stage is on achieving independence with ADLs, functional training, home and workplace adaptations, community mobility or driving, and social and leisure pursuits.

Reassessment

During the first postoperative year, the patient may return every few weeks or months as determined by the medical team. The therapist meets with the patient to assess progress. But it is at the annual visit that a full formal assessment should be performed using the battery of tests previously discussed, and the HTSS score should be reported to the IRHCTT. For the patient, reassessment can be a stressful experience. Patients want to know how they are doing compared with other transplant patients, and they may find the assessment's standardized activities challenging and a poor representation of their progress and skills. This further validates the argument for developing a better battery of assessment tools for this population. In addition to standardized assessments, time should be allocated to allow patients to demonstrate their self-identified accomplishments and consult with the therapy team on future strategies that aid in their recovery and keep them motivated, engaged, and compliant with therapy (see Chapter 105).

SPECIAL CONSIDERATIONS FOR PEDIATRIC TRANSPLANT PATIENTS

Hand and upper extremity VCA can provide children a unique opportunity to enrich their developmental experiences and develop a more fully integrated body schema. The decision for transplantation requires an interdisciplinary team centered not only on the child but also his or her family. Many children enjoy excellent quality of life with or without upper extremity prosthetics or allografts. This section presents unique selection and therapeutic considerations for children based on insights gained from the first successful pediatric bilateral hand transplantation and extrapolation from adult cases and other pediatric reconstructive procedures. Z.H. is a 10-year-old boy who underwent quadrimembral amputation at the age of 2 years related to sepsis. His right upper limb was amputated at the radiocarpal joint and the left upper limb at the distal radius, preserving some movement at the wrist. He abandoned upper extremity prosthetics and had been taking immunosuppression agents for a kidney allograft, mitigating some of the risk of hand transplantation. He received hand allografts at 8 years of age.[5]

Development and Neuroplasticity

The experience-dependent nature of brain development[71–73] suggests some potential unique benefits when surgical and rehabilitative restoration of hands occurs during childhood. Transplantation during childhood might afford enriched physical and social experiences during possible "critical" or "sensitive"[73] periods of development and a longer period of time to benefit from the allografts. Sensate hands play a role in precision movements and daily activities[74–77] and social integration.[78,79] Generally, functional outcomes of nerve repair are better in children[79–81] and are associated with less maladaptive neuroplasticity in the form of neuropathic pain.[80,82] Replantation has been successful in children,[81–83] although there are higher success rates reported in adult replantation possibly related to injury mechanism, technical demand,[84] or a greater incidence of performing the procedure.

Before Z.H.'s case, evidence of cortical reorganization in children after reconstructive surgeries was indirect. Previously, cortical reorganization was observed with sensorimotor recovery after toe-to-thumb transfer in young adults,[85] and functional outcomes of childhood digital transposition[86,87] suggested neuroplasticity. Free-gracilis grafts to the masseteric nerve plus motor therapy restored smiles for children with facial nerve palsy. Their ability to smile without biting likely occurred through brain plasticity.[88–90] Neuroimaging studies have demonstrated cortical plasticity after facial reanimation surgery in subjects ranging in age from 9 to 85 years.[91,92] Changes in Z.H.'s somatotopic map after amputation reversed after sensory input from transplantation.[93] This massive cortical reorganization was associated with therapy aimed at shifting pretransplantation movement patterns to active hand movements.

Pediatric Patient Selection and the Pretransplantation Process

The interdisciplinary team must be prepared for many pediatric-specific challenges. The child and family are committing to a lifetime of frequent medical visits, bloodwork, skin biopsies, and daily medications as well as demanding therapy. The process will result in missing some school and social experiences. Social workers and pediatric psychologists play a critical role. Although transplantation during childhood presents unique opportunities for functional and social gain, it also introduces a longer period of risks associated with lifetime immunosuppression, as well as chronic rejection and unknown allograft lifespan.[5] Research on SOT suggests that nonadherence to immunosuppression regimens is particularly high in adolescents,[94,95] and increased support is needed when pediatric hand recipients transition from being completely dependent on caregivers to increasing their health care and self-management.

Patients interested in transplantation should first thoroughly explore prosthetics with a prosthetist and a pediatric therapist. Although many options are available to suit the specific needs and preferences of children, patients wear prosthetics part time, and artificial sensibility is not commercially available at the time of this publication. Prosthetic use is selective and variable during childhood. Egermann and associates[97] found preferential use of prosthetics for indoor play and cycling. Myoelectric prosthetics lack the durability required by many children for outdoor play, rough-and-tumble play, and weight bearing tasks. Adolescents may prefer to use prosthetics for eating in public, socializing, and light house work and often choose not to wear body-powered hooks suited for heavy work and play.

General prosthetic abandonment rates are as high as 45% and are reported to be higher in children than adults, especially when initially fitted after 2 years of age.[98–100] Although myoelectric prosthetics appeal to children,[101] they do not clearly increase acceptance.[100,101] Sjöberg and coworkers[102] reported myoelectric prosthetic abandonment as low as 19% over a 17-year follow-up period for children first fitted with passive prosthetics in infancy. However, many became "part-time," "sporadic," or "occasional" users. Many children with unilateral upper extremity loss abandon prosthetics in favor of using their sensate residual limb.[103] Bilateral amputation and level of amputation introduce other complex variables.

After transplantation, Z.H. incorporated his hands into a variety of activities throughout the day, including dressing, writing, playing baseball, and toileting, thus demonstrating transplantation as a unique alternative. His progress has demonstrated the feasibility and potential for VCA in children. Thus, if prosthetics do not satisfy the family or child, an interdisciplinary pediatric team can help them consider transplantation. Ethicists must be involved in the risk-to-benefit analysis. All candidates should undergo psychological and psychiatric screenings and assessment of family support.[104] The hand therapist should discuss behavioral observations and the demands of the individualized

rehabilitation plan with the team. For example, considering the challenge of engaging children with hemiparesis in therapy and their relative independence, the benefits of transplantation for a child with unilateral amputation might not outweigh the risks. Children are particularly vulnerable to exploitation. The potential for public and media interest in hand transplantation must be discussed with the child and family. A psychologist should be involved in the process to obtain the child's assent and caregiver consent. The team should consider the goals, expectations, and quality of life of the child and caregivers.

Careful patient selection is imperative to ensure functional outcomes and to mitigate risks of injury. Risk of injury is particularly high when there is a mismatch between developmental skills and task demands.[105] The demands of transplantation rehabilitation are high. The child is required to sit still for hours at a time during orthotic fabrication and assessment tests. Biofeedback and functional training exercises require a high degree of attention and patience. The child is particularly susceptible to injury while allografts are insensate and while adjusting to the weight of the allografts. Studies suggest that high emotional reactivity, inattention, and hyperactivity may also increase risk of injury in children.[105–107] The team should consider each candidate's ability to meet the demands of rehabilitation.

Candidate's Therapy Evaluation

A pretransplantation therapy evaluation can determine baseline abilities and the potential benefit of allografts. The therapist should note the child's demeanor and ability to follow directions. Patient- and caregiver-reported outcome measures (PROs) are important to elucidate potential gains.[104] The Pediatric Evaluation of Disability Inventory computerized adapted test (PEDI-CAT) assesses a variety of life skills from the caregiver's perspective. The Canadian Occupational Performance Measure[108] can ascertain the family's goals. The PROMIS (Patient-Reported Outcomes Measurement Information System)[109] and The Pediatric Outcomes Data Collection Instrument (PODCI)[110] assess relevant domains of function and quality life. Lerman and associates[111] found the PODCI's functional scales insensitive to prosthetics for children with unilateral upper extremity deficiencies, presenting a unique opportunity to study the impact of transplantation. The PODCI also assesses the family's expectations and how they feel about the child's current physical condition; these are important aspects of the risk-to-benefit analysis.

The Box and Block test is a brief test of gross motor dexterity with pediatric normative data.[112] The child can use his or her residual limbs bilaterally to complete the test before transplantation. After surgery, the test can be quickly administered using standardized procedures to track progress of each hand. Functional tests such as the Sollerman Hand Function Test[49] and the Carroll Quantitative Test of Upper Extremity Function[48] are less appropriate for children. The authors use the GOAL (Goal-Oriented Assessment of Life Skills)[113] and a modified version of the Jebsen-Taylor Hand Function Test[114]; however, the utility of these tests for pediatric hand transplantation remains unclear. New functional tests might be required as this field develops and expands. Occupational or activity profiles might help anticipate motivating interventions and track progress.

Rehabilitation

When restoration of motor control is the goal, as opposed to reducing disability by compensation, therapy should be strategic, intense, and aimed at neuromotor control. Cortical plasticity after reconstructive surgery is responsive to experience,[90,115–117] and practicing specific movements changes the brain specifically.[118–121] Gaser and associates[122] showed grey matter volume changes in the primary motor cortex representing the hand commensurate with intensity of piano playing. Although motor training changes cortical networks rapidly,[118] skill retention and associated plasticity require long-term training in adults.[119,123] In monkeys, motor training over years leads to greater skill and corresponding changes in the motor cortex.[120,123] Z.H. developed compensatory motor strategies between the age of 2 and 8 years and could have had no memory of having hands. With intense therapy, he transitioned from using the allografts passively (e.g., pressing them together against objects for carrying, using proximal movements to push and pull objects) to using active prehensile patterns.

Z.H.'s initial therapy schedule was arduous and tailored to the attention span, occupations, and emotions of a child. Therapy was initiated 6 days after surgery and provided daily for 5 weeks in acute care and then 2 weeks in inpatient rehabilitation.[5] The quality of therapy closely resembled outpatient hand therapy. The team must secure appropriate resources before transplantation. Four occupational therapists worked with Z.H., often in teams, and were on call at all times. He spent most of each day in therapy with time allotted for naps, patient–caregiver bonding, and Child Life activities. Pediatric therapists used play and peer interactions to improve fine-motor skills[124] and addressed balance and mobility. A daily therapy progress report was provided to the surgical team with pictures and videos, and the therapist attended morning rounds to collaborate and ensure that the dressings accommodated his orthoses and functional rehabilitation.

Z.H. transitioned to a day hospital program in his community, where he received therapy and schooling 5 days per week and then outpatient occupational therapy. Therapy is ongoing at 2 years after surgery. Therapists from the transplantation center continue to follow Z.H. and collaborate with the medical team to target therapies. The authors suggest continuing therapy and minimizing compensatory motor strategies for 2 years after plateau of sensorimotor function and cortical plasticity. Collaboration between transplant center therapists and local therapists is especially important given the pediatric subspecialty care required.

The rehabilitation program should use neurorehabilitation, biomechanical, and occupational frames of references. Safety is paramount because children are likely to overestimate their readiness to walk, run, play, or cook. Goals must include balance and regard for obstacles and heat sources. Orthoses can prevent clawing and protect against falls and compromising positions while sleeping. Early therapy includes edema and wound care. Many children mouth their hands. When Z.H. bit a nail off his insensate hand shortly after surgery, Chewy Tubes were fixed to an orthosis (Fig. 79.4) to provide a safe outlet for this behavior.

Therapy for Z.H. focused on integrating his hands into his body schema and transitioning from adaptive bilateral residual limb patterns to using hand movements for daily activities.[5] The use of age-appropriate, child-centered occupations is important to fully engage the child in therapy. Purposeful, goal-directed activities improve motor performance in adults and children.[125,126] The therapist can identify meaningful activities and use Takata's developmental hierarchy of play to facilitate skilled therapy[127] as well as bedside and home programs. Occupational therapists occasionally facilitated compensatory movements to ensure successful participation in meaningful activities.[5]

Neurorehabilitation for Z.H. involved biofeedback, lateralization training, motor imagery, repetitive movement, and electrical stimulation. His mother helped him engage in therapy and connect with his hands. For months, only native extrinsic muscle spindles provide proprioceptive feedback from hand movements. Biofeedback is used to substitute visual and auditory feedback for somatosensory information. Sensory substitution can enhance recovery from nerve injury (Lundbord) and hand transplantation in adults.[117] The handheld Saebo MyoTrac Infinity unit provided visual and audio feedback from forearm myoelectric activity at the bedside. Z.H. watched and listened as

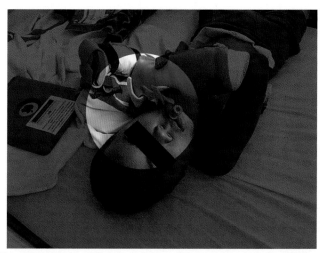

Fig. 79.4 Z.H. is pictured accessing Chewy Tubes to safety redirect mouthing behaviors from his insensate hands. The T-shaped oral Chewy Tubes were attached to his dorsal forearm-based intrinsic-plus protection orthosis using ribbon-shaped strips of Aquaplast orthosis material.

he moved his digits. Finger flashlights and puppets enhanced visual feedback (Video 79.1). Z.H. used the Biometrics E-LINK system for immediate biofeedback using computer games with joint movement sensors. In the absence of somatosensation, the therapist must help the child view his or her hand and computer screen simultaneously (Video 79.2). The team must consider topical immunosuppression drugs and fragile skin before applying adhesives or electrical stimulation.

The biomechanical approach includes protective and functional orthoses similar to those used for adult transplantations. Early dynamic mobilization is unlikely to suit pediatric transplantation patients. For example, the weight and resistance of a crane orthosis could have hindered Z.H. in the months after transplantation. Considering the relative capacity of a child to participate in therapy, the therapist must cautiously consider each orthosis. Z.H. wore intrinsic plus orthoses to facilitate movement and prevent clawing before reinnervation of intrinsic muscles. Inconsistent with principles of tenodesis, IP joint flexion improved while MCP joints were blocked in flexion. This might have been the result of muscle length–tension curves affected by the surgery. Therapists should experiment to determine functional positions. The hand-based helmet anticlawing orthosis slipped and the figure-of-8 orthosis did not accommodate edematous changes. A hand-based dorsal–volar intrinsic-plus orthosis was designed to improve fit and maximize Z.H.'s view of his hands for biofeedback (Fig. 79.5). About 4 months posttransplantation, Z.H. used dynamic MCP orthoses to assist index and middle finger flexion for radial digital grasp.

Ongoing Assessment of Progress and Plan

Sensorimotor assessment should be continuous and flexible. At first, goniometry was not practical to capture Z.H's small, unsustainable movements. A portable kinematic measurement system might reveal early progress. Results of PROs should be interpreted together with observation-based measures, with attention to discrepancies. The intensity of transplantation can introduce bias to clinicians, patients, and caregivers because all are heavily invested in the outcome. The Box and Block test was useful to understand Z.H.'s progress. By 12-months posttransplantation, his score using each hand was better compared with his pretransplantation bilateral strategy, demonstrating improved gross motor dexterity and new prehensile skills. The 9-Hole Peg Test also showed progress over time. Adult somatosensory measures can

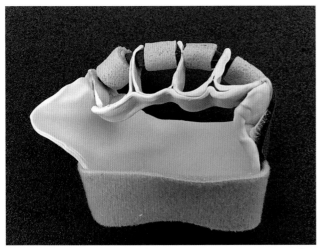

Fig. 79.5 Hand-based dorsal–volar intrinsic-plus orthosis. TailorSplint (⅛-inch thick) material was used to fabricate a dorsal metacarpal shell with volar proximal phalangeal bar. Orthosis material was pulled through the digit webspaces in a volar direction. The material was flattened with jeweler's pliers and then hole punched to create a scaffold for loop strap.

be used, but children are likely to require more breaks because of the sustained attention required of these tedious tests.

At 2 years posttransplantation, Z.H. continues to make progress with therapy. Measures of dexterity, sensation, ADL function, and caregiver reported outcomes remain favorable and correspond to changes in the brain. Long flexor pull-through and intrinsic muscle strength have improved. (See Video 79.3 for examples of function from 11 to 25 months posttransplantation.) Other details of 18-month outcomes were previously published.[5] Given hand transplantation is a new option for children, the therapist should be prepared for unexpected challenges and work collaboratively with other team members both within and between centers to develop innovative approaches to enhance therapeutic success. Further data from future pediatric cases are needed to inform progress in assessments and interventions to optimize patient selection and functional outcomes in pediatric hand transplantation.

SUMMARY

Working with hand and upper extremity VCA is a unique opportunity that takes a multidisciplinary team approach tapping into medical, surgical, psychological, and rehabilitation foundations. For hand therapists, it requires a broad knowledge base and wide skill set from creative orthosis design, proficiency in therapy assessments, purposeful intervention, and insightful psychosocial support. The interdisciplinary team must place the patient and family and caregivers at the center during careful consideration of patient selection as well planning the surgical and rehabilitative approach. The hand therapist should participate in the worldwide VCA community to help develop outcomes assessments and treatments.

REFERENCES

1. Tintle SM, Potter BK, Elliott RM, Levin LS. Hand transplantation. *JBJS*. 2014;2.
2. Dubernard JM, Owen E, Herzberg G, et al. Human hand allograft: report on first 6 months. *Lancet*. 1999;353:1315–1320.
3. Shores JT, Brandacher G, Lee WPA. Hand and upper extremity transplantation: an update of outcomes in the worldwide experience. *Plast Reconstr Surg*. 2014;135. 351e–60e.
4. Amaral S, Levin LS. Pediatric and congenital hand transplantation. *Curr Opin Organ Transplant*. 2017;22:477–483.
5. Amaral S, Kessler SK, Levy JT, et al. 18-month outcomes of heterologous bilateral hand transplantation in a child: a case report. *Lancet Child Adolesc Health*. 2017;1:35–44.
6. Galvez JA, Gralewski K, McAndrew C, Rehman MA, Chang B, Levin LS. Assessment and planning for a pediatric bilateral hand transplant using 3-dimensional modeling: case report. *J Hand Surg Am*. 2016;41:341–343.
7. Gurnaney HG, Fiadjoe JE, Levin LS, et al. Anesthetic management of the first pediatric bilateral hand transplant. *Can J Anaesth*. 2016;63:731–736.
8. Momeni A, Chang B, Levin LS. Technology and vascularized composite allotransplantation (VCA): lessons learned from the first bilateral pediatric hand transplant. *J Mater Sci Mater Med*. 2016;27:161.
9. Jones JW, Gruber SA, Barker JH, Breidenbach WC. Successful hand transplantation. One-year follow-up. Louisville Hand Transplant Team. *N Engl J Med*. 2000;343:468–473.
10. Iglesias M, Leal P, Butron P, et al. Severe complications after bilateral upper extremity transplantation: a case report. *Transplantation*. 2014;98:e16–e17.
11. Shore JT, Malek V, Lee WPA, Brandacher G. Outcomes after hand and upper extremity transplantation. *J Mater Sci Mater Med*. 2017;28:72.
12. Scientific Registry of Transplant Recipients (SRTR) 2012 Annual Data Report; 2012. https://srtr.transplant.hrsa.gov/annual_reports/2012/Default.aspx. Accessed January 1, 2018.
13. Mendenhall SD, Schmucker RW, De la Garza M, Lutfy J, Levin LS, Neumeister M. Osteosynthesis in forearm transplantation using a novel ulnar-shortening osteotomy system for simultaneous both bone fixation. *Vascularized Composite Allotransplantation*. 2015;2:53–59.
14. Petruzzo PM, Lanzetta J, Dubernard M, et al. The international registry on hand and composite tissue transplantation. *Transplantation*. 2010;90:1590–1594.
15. Cavadas PC, Ibanez J, Thione A, Alfaro L. Bilateral trans-humeral arm transplantation: result at 2 years. *Am J Transplant*. 2011;11:1085–1090.
16. International Registry for Hand and Composite Tissue Transplantation. https://www.handregistry.com. Accessed October 1, 2017.
17. Landin L, Bonastre J, Casado-Sanchez C, et al. Outcomes with respect to disabilities of the upper limb after hand allograft transplantation: a systematic review. *Transpl Int*. 2012;25:424–432.
18. General, Department of Veterans Affairs Office of Inspector. Healthcare Inspection Prosthetic Limb Care in VA Facilities; 2012. http://www.va.gov/oig/pubs/VAOIG-11-02138-116.pdf. Accessed Dec 16, 2017 .
19. Pomahac B, Gobble RM, Schneeberger S. Facial and hand allotransplantation. *Cold Spring Harb Perspect Med*. 2014;4.
20. Khalifian S, Brazio PS, Mohan R, et al. Facial transplantation: the first 9 years. *Lancet*. 2014;384:2153–2163.
21. Simmons PD. Ethical considerations in composite tissue allotransplantation. *Microsurgery*. 2000;20:458–465.
22. Rohrich RJ, Longaker MT, Cunningham B. On the ethics of composite tissue allotransplantation (facial transplantation). *Plast Reconstr Surg*. 2006;117:2071–2073.
23. Barker JH, Brown CS, Cunningham M, Wiggins O, Furr A, Maldonado C, Banis JC. Ethical considerations in human facial tissue allotransplantation. *Ann Plast Surg*. 2008;60:103–109.
24. Bramstedt KA. A lifesaving view of vascularized composite allotransplantation: patient experience of social death before and after face, hand, and larynx transplant. *J Patient Exp*. 2017: 2374373517730556.
25. Kumnig M, Jowsey SG, DiMartini AF. Psychological aspects of hand transplantation. *Curr Opin Organ Transplant*. 2014;19:188–195.
26. Kumnig M, Jowsey SG, Moreno E, Brandacher G, Azari K, Rumpold G. An overview of psychosocial assessment procedures in reconstructive hand transplantation. *Transpl Int*. 2014;27:417–427.
27. Foroohar A, Elliott RM, Fei DR, et al. Quadrimembral amputation: indications and contraindications for vascularized composite allotransplantation. *Transplant Proc*. 2011;43(9). 5521–3528.
28. Severance G, Walsh L. Rehabilitation after bilateral hand transplantation in the quadrimembral patient: review and recommendations. *Tech Hand Up Extrem Surg*. 2013;17:215–220.

29. Schneider M, Cardones AR, Selim MA, Cendales LC. Vascularized composite allotransplantation: a closer look at the Banff working classification. *Transpl Int.* 2016;29:663–671.

30. Ladds E, Radgrave N, Hotton M, Lamyman M. Systematic review: Predicting adverse psychological outcomes after hand trauma. *J Hand Ther.* 2017;30(4):407–419.

31. Durmont M, Sann L, Gazarian A. Bilateral hand transplantation: supporting the patient's choice. *J Plast Reconstr Aesthet Surg.* 2017;70:147–151.

32. Jowsey-Gregoire SG, Kumnig M, Morelon E, et al. The Chauvet 2014 meeting report: psychiatric and psychological evaluation and outcomes of upper extremity grafted patients. *Transplantation.* 2016;100:1453–1459.

33. Amirlak B, Gonzales R, Gorantla V, et al. Creating a hand transplant program. *Clin Plastic Surg.* 2007;34:279–289.

34. Gordon CR, Siemionow M. Requirements for development of hand transplantation program. *Ann Plast Surg.* 2009;63:262–273.

35. Lanzetta M, Petruzzo P. A comprehensive functional score system in hand transplantation. In: Lanzetta M, Dubernard JM, eds. *Hand Transplantation.* Milan: Springer-Verlag; 2007:355–362.

36. Kumnig M, Jowsey-Gregoire SG. Key psychological challenges in vascularized composite tissue allotransplantation. *World J Transplant.* 2016;6(1):91–102.

37. Hudak Pl, Amadio PC, Bombardier C. The Upper Extremity Collaborative Group (UECG). Development of an upper extremity outcome measure: the DASH (disability of the arm shoulder and hand). *Am J Ind Med.* 1996;29(6):602–608.

38. Ware JE, Kosinski M, Keller SD. *SF-36 Physical and Mental Health Summary Scales: A User's Manual.* New England Medical Center Boston: The Health Institute; 1994.

39. Bueno E, Benjamin MJ, Sisk G, et al. Rehabilitation following hand transplantation. *Hand.* 2014;9:9–15.

40. Bernardon L, Gazarian A, Petruzzo P, et al. Bilateral hand transplantation: functional benefits assessment in five patients with a mean follow-up of 7.6 years. *J Plast Reconstr Aesthet Surg.* 2015;68:1171–1183.

41. Kaufman CL, Ouseph R, Marvin MR, et al. Monitoring and long-term outcomes in vascularized composite tissue allotransplantation. *Curr Opin Organ Transplant.* 2013;18:652–658.

42. Ninkovic M, Weissenbacher A, Gabl M, et al. Functional outcome after hand and forearm transplantation: what can be achieved? *Hand Clin.* 2001;27:455–465.

43. Haddock NT, Chang B, Bozentka DJ, Steinberg DR, Levin SL. Technical implications in proximal forearm transplantation. *Tech in hand and upper extrem surg.* 2013;17:228–231.

44. McClelland B, McCabe S, et al. Proximal forearm transplantation for below elbow amputations: rational and surgical technique. *VCA.* 2015;2(1):26–28.

45. Petruzzo P, Dubernard JM, Lanzetta M. International registry on hand and composite tissue transplantation. *VCA.* 2016;3:7.

46. Petruzzo P, Lanzetta M, Dubernard JM, et al. The International Registry on Hand and Composite Tissue Transplantation. *Transplantation.* 2008;86:487.

47. Murphy BD, Zuker RM, Borschel GH. Vascularized composite allotransplantation: an updated on medical and surgical progress and remaining challenges. *J Plast Reconstr Aesthet Surg.* 2013;66:1449–1455.

48. Carroll D. A quantitative test of upper extremity function. *J chronic dis.* 1965;18(5):479–491.

49. Sollerman C, Ejeskär A. Sollerman hand function test: a standardised method and its use in tetraplegic patients. *Scand J Plast Reconstr Surg Hand Surg.* 1995;29(2):167–176.

50. Lyle RC A performance test for assessment of upper limb function in physical rehabilitation treatment and research. *Int J Rehabil Res.* 1981;4:483–492.

51. Schuind F, Abramowicz D, Schneeberger S. Hand transplantation: the state-of-the-art. *J Hand Surg. European Volume.* 2007;32E(1):2–17.

52. Ravindra K, Buell J, Daufman C, et al. Hand transplantation in the United States: Experience with 3 patients. *Surgery.* 2008;144:138–144.

53. Piza-Katzer H, Ninkovic M, Gabl P, Ninkovic M, Hussi H. Double hand transplantation: functional outcome after 18 months. *J Hand Surg.* 2002;27B(4):385–390.

54. Jones J, Gruber S, Barker J, Breidebach W. Successful hand transplantation. *N Engl J Med.* 2000;343:468–472.

55. Dubernard J, Petruzzo P, Lanzetta M, et al. Functional results of the first human double-hand transplantation. *Ann Surgery.* 238: 128–136.

56. Schneeberger S, Khalifian S, Brandacher G. Immunosuppression and monitoring of rejection in hand transplantation. *Tech Hand UE Surg.* 2013;17:208–214.

57. Sarhane KA, Tuffaha SH, Broyles JM, et al. A critical analysis of rejection in vascularized composite allotransplantation: clinical, cellular, and molecular aspects, current challenges and novel concepts. *Front Immunol.* 2013;4:406.

58. Fisher S, Lian CG, Kueckelhaus M. Acute rejection in vascularized composite allotransplantation. *Curr Opin Organ Transplant.* 2014;9:531–544.

59. Wessenbacher A, et al. Hand transplant in its fourteenth year: the Innsbruck experience. *VCA.* 2014;1:11–21.

60. Petruzzo P, Dubenard JM. The international registry on hand and composite tissue allotransplantation. *Clin Transpl.* 2011:247–253.

61. Jablecki J, Syrko M, Arendarska-Maj A. Patient rehabilitation following hand transplantation at forearm distal third level. *Orthop Traumatol Rehabil.* 2010;6(12):570–580.

62. O'Brien L. The evidence on ways to improve patient's adherence in hand therapy. *J Hand Ther.* 2012;25(3):247–250.

63. Chesher SP, Schwartz KS, Kleinert HE. A new early mobilization splint for proximal interphalangeal joint replacements. *J Hand Ther.* 1988;1:200–203.

64. Scheker L, Chesher S, Netscher D, Julliard K, O'Neill L. Functional results of dynamic splinting after transmetacarpal, wrist, and distal forearm replantation. *J Hand Ther (British and European).* 1995;20B:584–590.

65. Scheker LR, Hodges A. Brace and rehabilitation after replant and revascularization. *Hand Clin.* 2001;17:473–480.

66. Kahn LC, Moore AM. Donor activation focused rehabilitation approach: maximizing outcomes after nerve transfers. *Hand Clin.* 2016;32:263–277.

67. Evans R, Thomson DE. The application of force to the healing tendon. *J Hand Ther.* 1993:6266–6284.

68. Brenneis C, Loscher N, Egger T, et al. Cortical motor activation patterns following hand transplantation and replantation. *J Hand Surg* (British and Europe). 2005;30(5):530–533.

69. Hansson T, Nyman T, Bjorkman A, et al. Sights of touching activates the somatosensory cortex in humans. *Scan J Plast Reconstr Surg Hand Surg.* 2009;43:267–269.

70. Cameron M. Introduction to electrotherapy. In: Cameron M, ed. *Physical Agents in Rehabilitation, an Evidence-Based Approach to Practice.* 5th ed. St. Louis: Elsevier; 2018:219–236.

71. Greenough WT, Black JE, Wallace CS. Experience and brain development. *Child Develop.* 1987:539–559.

72. Hubel DH, Wiesel TN. The period of susceptibility to the physiological effects of unilateral eye closure in kittens. *J Physiol.* 1970;206(2):419–436.

73. Knudsen EI. Sensitive periods in the development of the brain and behavior. *J Cogn Neurosci.* 2004;16(8):1412–1425.

74. Cooper J, Majnemer A, Rosenblatt B, Birnbaum R. The determination of sensory deficits in children with hemiplegic cerebral palsy. *J Child Neurol.* 1995;10(4):300–309.

75. Duff SV. Impact of peripheral nerve injury on sensorimotor control. *J Hand Ther.* 2005;18(2):277–291.

76. Augurelle AS, Smith AM, Lejeune T, Thonnard JL. Importance of cutaneous feedback in maintaining a secure grip during manipulation of hand-held objects. *J Neurophysiol.* 2003;89(2):665–671.

77. Ebied AM, Kemp GJ, Frostick SP. The role of cutaneous sensation in the motor function of the hand. *J Orthop Res.* 2004;22(4):862–866.

78. Ackerman JM, Nocera CC, Bargh JA. Incidental haptic sensations influence social judgments and decisions. *Science.* 2010;328(5986):1712–1715.

79. Lundborg G. Nerve injury and repair–a challenge to the plastic brain. *J Peripher Nerv Syst.* 2003;8(4):209–226.

80. Atherton DD, Taherzadeh O, Elliot D, Anand P. Age-dependent development of chronic neuropathic pain, allodynia and sensory recovery after upper limb nerve injury in children. *J Hand Surg (European Volume).* 2008;33(2):186–191.

81. Saies AD, Urbaniak JR, Nunley JA, Taras JS, Goldner RD, Fitch RD. Results after replantation and revascularization in the upper extremity in children. *JBJS.* 1994;76(12):1766–1776.

82. Taras JS, Nunley JA, Urbaniak JR, Goldner RD, Fitch RD. Replantation in children. *Microsurgery.* 1991;12(3):216–220.

83. Mohan R, Panthaki Z, Armstrong MB. Replantation in the pediatric hand. *J Craniofac Surg.* 2009;20(4):996–998.

84. Kim JY, Brown RJ, Jones NF. Pediatric upper extremity replantation. *Clin Plast Surg.* 2005;32(1):1–0.

85. Ni Z, Anastakis DJ, Gunraj C, Chen R. Reversal of cortical reorganization in human primary motor cortex following thumb reconstruction. *J Neurophysiol.* 2010;103(1):65–73.

86. Kozin SH. Pollicization: the concept, technical details, and outcome. *Clin Orthop Surg.* 2012;4(1):18–35.

87. Lightdale-Miric N, Mueske NM, Lawrence EL, et al. Long term functional outcomes after early childhood pollicization. *J Hand Ther.* 2015;28(2):158–166.

88. Marre D, Hontanilla B. Brain plasticity in Möbius syndrome after unilateral muscle transfer: case report and review of the literature. *Ann Plast Surg.* 2012;68(1):97–100.

89. Lifchez SD, Matloub HS, Gosain AK. Cortical adaptation to restoration of smiling after free muscle transfer innervated by the nerve to the masseter. *Plast Reconstr Surg.* 2005;115(6):1472–1479.

90. Manktelow RT, Tomat LR, Zuker RM, Chang M. Smile reconstruction in adults with free muscle transfer innervated by the masseter motor nerve: effectiveness and cerebral adaptation. *Plast Reconstr Surg.* 2006;118(4):885–899.

91. Buendia J, Loayza FR, Luis EO, Celorrio M, Pastor MA, Hontanilla B. Functional and anatomical basis for brain plasticity in facial palsy rehabilitation using the masseteric nerve. *J Plast Reconstr Aesthet Surg.* 2016;69(3):417–426.

92. Garmi R, Labbé D, Coskun O, Compère JF, Bénateau H. Lengthening temporalis myoplasty and brain plasticity: a functional magnetic resonance imaging study. *InAnnales de Chirurgie Plastique Esthétique.* 2013;58(4):271–276. Elsevier Masson.

93. Gaetz W, Kessler SK, Roberts TPL, et al. Massive cortical reorganization is reversible following bilateral transplants of the hands: evidence from the first successful bilateral pediatric hand transplant patient. *Ann Clin Transl Neurol.* Manuscript accepted 2017

94. Dobbels F, Ruppar T, De Geest S, Decorte A, Damme-Lombaerts V, Fine RN. Adherence to the immunosuppressive regimen in pediatric kidney transplant recipients: a systematic review. *Pediatr Transplant.* 2010;14(5):603–613.

95. Fine RN, Becker Y, De Geest S, et al. Nonadherence consensus conference summary report. *Am J Transplant.* 2009;9(1):35–41.

96. Deleted in review.

97. Egermann M, Kasten P, Thomsen M. Myoelectric hand prostheses in very young children. *Int Orthop.* 2009;33(4):1101–1105.

98. Biddiss EA, Chau TT. Upper limb prosthesis use and abandonment: a survey of the last 25 years. *Prosthet Orthot Int.* 2007;31(3):236–257.

99. Scotland TR, Galway HR. A long-term review of children with congenital and acquired upper limb deficiency. *Bone Joint J.* 1983;65(3):346–349.

100. Toda M, Chin T, Shibata Y, Mizobe F. Use of powered prosthesis for children with upper limb deficiency at Hyogo Rehabilitation Center. *PloS One.* 2015;10(6). e0131746.

101. Kruger LM, Fishman S. Myoelectric and body-powered prostheses. *J Pediatr Orthop.* 1993;13(1):68–75.

102. Sjöberg L, Lindner H, Hermansson L. Long-term results of early myoelectric prosthesis fittings: A prospective case-control study. *Prosthet Orthot Int.* 2017: 0309364617729922 (Epub ahead of print).

103. Zlotolow DA, Kozin SH. Advances in upper extremity prosthetics. *Hand Clinics.* 2012;28(4):587–593.

104. Tintle SM, Potter BK, Elliott RM, Levin LS. Hand transplantation. *JBJS Reviews.* 2014;2(1).

105. Rivara FP. Developmental and behavioral issues in childhood injury prevention. *J Dev Behav Pediatr.* 1995;16(5):362–370.

106. Hoarea P, Beattieb T. Children with attention deficit hyperactivity disorder and attendance at hospital. *Eur J Emerg Med.* 2003;10(2):98–100.

107. DiScala C, Lescohier I, Barthel M, Li G. Injuries to children with attention deficit hyperactivity disorder. *Pediatrics.* 1998;102(6):1415–1421.

108. Law M, Baptiste S, McColl M, Opzoomer A, Polatajko H, Pollock N. The Canadian Occupational Performance Measure: an outcome measure for occupational therapy. *Can J Occup Ther.* 1990;57(2):82–87.

109. Cella D, Yount S, Rothrock N, et al. The Patient-Reported Outcomes Measurement Information System (PROMIS): progress of an NIH Roadmap cooperative group during its first two years. *Medical care.* 2007;45(5 suppl 1):S3.

110. Daltroy LH, Liang MH, Fossel AH, Goldberg MJ. The POSNA pediatric musculoskeletal functional health questionnaire: report on reliability, validity, and sensitivity to change. *J Pediatr Orthop.* 1998;18(5):561–571.

111. Lerman JA, Sullivan E, Barnes DA, Haynes RJ. The Pediatric Outcomes Data Collection Instrument (PODCI) and functional assessment of patients with unilateral upper extremity deficiencies. *J Pediatr Orthop.* 2005;25(3):405–407.

112. Jongbloed-Pereboom M, Nijhuis-van der Sanden MW, Steenbergen B. Norm scores of the box and block test for children ages 3–10 years. *Am J Occup Ther.* 2013;67(3):312–318.

113. Miller LJ, Oakland T, Herzberg DS. *Goal-Oriented Assessment of Lifeskills*; 2015.

114. Taylor NE, Sand PL, Jebsen RH. Evaluation of hand function in children. *Arch Phys Med Rehabil.* 1973;54(3):129.

115. Anastakis DJ, Chen R, Davis KD, Mikulis D. Cortical plasticity following upper extremity injury and reconstruction. *Clin Plast Surg.* 2005;32(4):617–634.

116. Giraux P, Sirigu A, Schneider F, Dubernard JM. Cortical reorganization in motor cortex after graft of both hands. *Nat Neurosci.* 2001;4(7):691–692.

117. Lanzetta M, Perani D, Anchisi D, et al. Early use of artificial sensibility in hand transplantation. *Scand J Plast Reconstr Surg Hand Surg.* 2004;38(2):106–111.

118. Classen J, Liepert J, Wise SP, Hallett M, Cohen LG. Rapid plasticity of human cortical movement representation induced by practice. *J Neurophysiol.* 1998;79(2):1117–1123.

119. Karni A, Meyer G, Jezzard P, Adams MM, Turner R, Ungerleider LG. Functional MRI evidence for adult motor cortex plasticity during motor skill learning. *Nature.* 1995;377(6545):155–158.

120. Picard N, Matsuzaka Y, Strick PL. Extended practice of a motor skill is associated with reduced metabolic activity in M1. *Nat Neurosci.* 2013;16(9):1340–1347.

121. Nudo RJ, Wise BM, SiFuentes F, Milliken GW. Neural substrates for the effects of rehabilitative training on motor recovery after ischemic infarct. *Science.* 1996;272(5269):1791.

122. Gaser C, Schlaug G. Brain structures differ between musicians and non-musicians. *J Neurosci.* 2003;23(27):9240–9245.

123. Matsuzaka Y, Picard N, Strick PL. Skill representation in the primary motor cortex after long-term practice. *J Neurophysiol.* 2007;97(2):1819–1832.

124. Case-Smith J. Effects of occupational therapy services on fine motor and functional performance in preschool children. *Am J Occup Ther.* 2000;54(4):372–380.

125. Hétu S, Mercier C. Using purposeful tasks to improve motor performance: does object affordance matter? *Br J Occup Ther.* 2012;75(8):367–376.

126. Sakzewski L, Gordon A, Eliasson AC. The state of the evidence for intensive upper limb therapy approaches for children with unilateral cerebral palsy. *J. Child Neurol.* 2014;29(8):1077–1090.

127. Peck–Murray JA. Utilizing everyday items in play to facilitate hand therapy for pediatric patients. *J Hand Ther.* 2015;28(2):228–232.

80

Management of Skin Grafts and Flaps: The Surgeon's Perspective

Adam B. Strohl, L. Scott Levin

OUTLINE

CRITICAL POINTS

- Advances in wound care, flap design, and microsurgical techniques that include an ever expanding armamentarium of free tissue transfer, postoperative management, and rehabilitation protocols have allowed for the continued improvement in reconstructive surgery of the upper limb.
- Soft tissue reconstruction options include primary closure, delayed primary closure, healing by secondary intention, skin grafting, local tissue transfer, free tissue transfer, and any combination

of these techniques. Free tissue transfer, by definition, includes vascularized tissue such as skin, muscle, bone, fascia, or a combination of thereof that is dependent on a vascular pedicle for survival after transfer.
- An algorithmic approach to reconstruction of the upper extremity treatment of upper is based on the extent and severity of the bone and soft tissue injury or defect, the functional needs of the patient, medical comorbidities, and the availability of required tissues.

INTRODUCTION

Reconstructive surgery of the upper extremity has developed significantly over the past 6 decades after introduction of the operating microscope by Jacobsen in 1960. Microsurgical techniques as well as the continuous development of new tissue transfers have greatly enhanced the armamentarium of reconstructive surgeons.[1] The continuing evolution of wound management has facilitated a more optimal environment that promotes wound healing, rehabilitation, and recovery. Reconstructive surgery has evolved from the practice of simply providing soft tissue coverage for traumatic defects to a complex algorithmic process of wound management and optimization of function. This pathway involves thorough clinical assessment, evaluation of individual functional and social needs of the patient, creation and implementation of a surgical plan, and structured postoperative management using appropriate rehabilitation protocols. The algorithmic approach offers a reconstructive ladder for the evaluation and treatment of wounds, ranging from acute traumatic injuries to various chronic conditions, including osteomyelitis, nonhealing wounds, and defects resulting from tumor resection.[2,3] This reconstructive ladder directs the surgeon to the indicated reconstructive surgical approach based on the extent and severity of the wound, the functional needs of the patient, and the availability of required tissue elements. The initial goal of the reconstructive surgeon is the reconstitution of the soft tissue envelope, providing a well-vascularized, healthy environment to facilitate localized healing.[3] After this has been achieved, therapists can maximize outcomes, prevent secondary complications, and restore the patient's function. With successful recovery and healing, the reconstructive surgeon can attain the ultimate goal of optimizing rehabilitation based on individual needs, thus maximizing functional restoration and providing patients with the opportunity for

rapid social reintegration and the overall improvement of their quality of life. This chapter discusses an algorithmic approach to reconstruction of the hand and upper extremity, providing examples of reconstructive options for surgical problems, ranging from skin grafts, to local tissue flaps, to advanced free tissue transfer.

PATIENT ASSESSMENT

The first step in developing a reconstructive strategy is the assessment of the patient. The surgeon must recognize the clinical reconstructive needs of the patient based on the severity of a traumatic injury, the extent and complexity of a chronic wound, or a malignant tumor requiring resection. Important considerations include age, significant medical morbidities, pre-injury functional status, occupation, dominance of the extremity involved, psychosocial considerations, and individual patient motivation and compliance. In patients with acute traumatic injuries of the upper extremity, a thorough clinical evaluation is necessary to first rule out the presence of other significant life-threatening conditions or injuries that will alter rehabilitation capacity.[4] For chronic wounds, it is essential to identify and address causative factors such as malnutrition and vascular insufficiency. With wounds secondary to malignancy, the determination must be made whether additional resections will be needed as well as the need for chemotherapy or radiation therapy, which have deleterious effects on wound healing. In the cases of traumatic injury when a patient is hemodynamically stable, an assessment of the extremities can occur. Evaluation of the hand and upper extremity involves a systematic approach to the extremity as a functional organ.[1,4] Complete examination includes gross visual inspection, evaluation of limb perfusion, assessment of passive and active motion, and a review of neurologic function. Imaging studies, such as radiography, ultrasonography, computed tomography, magnetic resonance imaging, or angiography, are incorporated as indicated to further establish the extent of soft tissue, bone, and vascular involvement. After the clinical needs of the patient and deficits from the wound have been clearly established, a surgical management strategy can be created to optimize the reconstruction, postoperative management, and the functional rehabilitative goals of the patient.

MANAGEMENT STRATEGY

The first step in surgical wound management is exploration, irrigation, and meticulous debridement.[4] Adequate debridement of all nonviable tissues is required to establish a healthy environment for healing and to decrease the risk of potential infection. In severe injuries, it can help to determine whether or not a limb should be savaged or amputated. Underlying injuries to vital structures must be identified and repaired. Neurovascular injuries need to be repaired either primarily or with the use of shunts in cases of vascular injury and prolonged ischemia. Fractures must be identified, irrigated, debrided, and then stabilized with internal or external fixation. Tendon injuries should be repaired primarily, if possible, or prepared for more extensive future reconstruction as a staged procedure. All of these interventions will likely have bearing on postoperative rehabilitation and associated restrictions that therapists will need to be informed of to optimize outcomes. After repair of these underlying vital structures, soft tissue coverage becomes the next consideration. Soft tissue reconstruction options include primary closure, delayed primary closure, healing by secondary intention, skin grafting, local tissue transfer, free tissue transfer, or any combination of these techniques. The "reconstructive ladder" is a simple, metaphorical concept of these increasing levels of complexity and required skill that helps facilitate reconstructive options[2] (Fig. 80.1). By no means, though, is the reconstructive surgeon restricted to attempting the lower rungs of the ladder before using more advanced techniques of the higher rungs. This concept has been alternatively suggested as the "reconstructive elevator" with decision making being based on surgeon's experience and specifics of the wound.

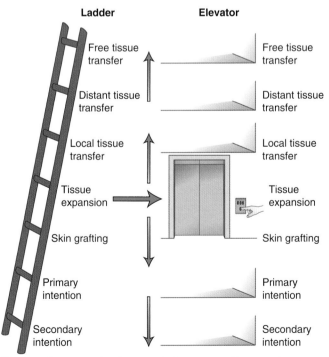

Fig. 80.1 Reconstructive ladder and elevator to guide wound coverage management.

Primary Wound Closure

Primary wound closure simply involves approximating the wound edges. This is accomplished with the use of sutures, staples, tapes, or skin glue, as a single or multilayered repair. *Delayed* primary closure suggests a delay in the repair, such as waiting for associated edema to resolve sufficiently to allow for direct skin closure or to reassess soft tissue viability before closure. Delayed primary closure can be a useful technique for fasciotomy wounds after decompression of a muscle compartment. If motion at the joints adjacent to the wound might place tension forces on the incision or underlying musculoskeletal injury indicates, a custom fabricated orthosis may be considered. It is always important that such orthoses and dressings in general do not place excessive external compression on the incision or skin flaps.

Healing by Secondary Intention

Healing by secondary intention refers to leaving a wound open and allowing it to heal spontaneously through contraction and reepithelialization. Use of the method is based on wound size and whether or not there are exposed structures or hardware. In the hand and upper extremity, healing by secondary intention can be successfully applied to small wounds (with acceptable results) such as fingertip injuries involving less than a 1.5-cm defect, without exposed underlying bone. Healing of larger hand and upper extremity wounds by secondary intention, however, can result in significant scar formation and contracture, with subsequent limitations in range of motion (ROM) and function. Proper wound care should involve regular cleansing to prevent infection and to dislodge superficial debris along with the application of topical emollient to prevent wound desiccation.

Negative-pressure wound therapy (NPWT) uses a vacuum dressing changed in cyclical fashion to facilitate wound closure by removing blood and serous fluid, decreasing bacterial burden, and increasing microperfusion at the wound bed.[5] The porous "sponge" dressing achieves this while deforming the wound into a smaller shape. Some wounds treated in this manner can eventually reepithelialize completely when small enough or can be closed later with another method of reconstruction.

Skin Grafts

A skin graft is a harvested segment of epidermis and dermis that has been elevated and separated completely from its blood supply. The first reported transfer of skin was credited to Reverdin in 1870,[6] but skin grafting did not become common until the invention of the dermatome by Padget[7] during World War II. The dermatome simplified the method of elevating a skin graft, providing a reliable instrument for consistently harvesting a graft of a desired size and depth. The dermatome remains the primary tool used today for harvesting skin grafts. With the increased use of skin grafts, it was recognized that their early use for wound coverage could retard the extent of wound contracture, thus limiting deformity and functional disability.[8]

Skin grafts can either be full thickness or split thickness. All skin grafts heal by a well-studied progression of vascular perfusion whereby nourishing blood vessels will grow from the wound bed through the dermis of the graft. These phases are referred to as plasmatic imbibition, inosculation, and neovascularization.[8]

A full-thickness skin graft (FTSG) is a segment that includes the epidermis and entire dermis. An FTSG resembles normal skin more closely, including texture, color, and potential for hair growth. Am FTSG demonstrates the greatest amount of primary contracture but the least amount of secondary wound contracture. That is, after the harvest of an FTSG, it quickly contracts and appears much smaller because of the abundance of elastin fibers in the dermis. However, when the full-thickness graft is applied to a wound defect early, it maintains its size and can significantly limit contracture of the wound.

Full-thickness skin grafting do have limitations though. Given its thickness that blood vessels must traverse to support its "take," there is a slightly greater risk of nonadherence of the graft. Additionally, donor site availability must be considered before full-thickness skin harvest. The donor site of an FTSG must be amenable to primary closure, or the created donor defect may require an additional skin grafting, local flap, or other means of coverage.

A split-thickness skin graft (STSG) consists of the entire epidermis and a variable portion of the dermis, most often harvested currently with a mechanical dermatome. An STSG has less primary contraction at harvest but is susceptible to more secondary contraction as the wound matures with healing. Increasing the thickness of the dermal component impedes secondary contraction but also increases risks of nonadherence as previously explained. STSGs typically do not contain sweat glands, sebaceous glands, and hair follicles in their thin dermis. As a result, the healed graft will be often dry, brittle, and hairless as opposed to FTSGs, which contain these structures.

An STSG can be either meshed or unmeshed. STSGs are typically meshed at ratios ranging from 1:1 to 3:1, with the ratio selected depending on the size of the defect needed to be grafted and the skin available for grafting. Meshing of the harvested skin graft facilitates expansion of the graft for coverage of more extensive wound defects. An STSG also may be left unmeshed and used to cover a wound as a sheet graft. A sheet graft avoids the meshed-pattern scarring associated with meshed skin grafts, thus resulting in a better aesthetic appearance.

Skin grafts may be secured to the margins of the wound with sutures, staples, tape, or skin glue. After the graft has been secured, the wound dressing and the postoperative management take precedence for the survival of the transferred skin graft. Various potential postoperative complications can lead to the demise of a skin graft. The best method for avoiding graft failure is prevention through meticulous postoperative management. The number one reason for failure of a skin graft is hematoma or seroma beneath the graft, thereby interfering with the delicate stages of skin graft healing and leading to loss of graft. Shearing of the skin graft can disrupt the fragile, early vessels supporting the graft. Prevention includes assuring hemostasis and application of well-placed postoperative dressings. Dressings over a skin graft must provide lubrication to prevent desiccation, appropriate compression to eliminate the potential space between the skin graft and the wound bed, and local immobilization to prevent shearing of the graft. This is best achieved by placing a lubricating (petrolatum) gauze such as Adaptic or Xeroform directly over the skin graft followed by cottonoid layering saturated in mineral oil. Securing these layers is essential to prevent shear and can be achieved by multiple means such as staples, circumferential dressing, tie-over bolster, or NPWT via vacuum-assisted dressing. Concave wounds often require a tie-over bolster to compress the graft evenly into the wound bed. Postoperative immobilization of nearby joints might be necessary to enhance skin graft adherence by preventing shear.

Postoperative Follow-up and Management

The dressing over an upper extremity skin graft typically is removed in 4 to 7 days, and the wound is reevaluated. By this time, the skin graft should be adherent to the wound bed, but continued wound care is still required to protect the reconstruction. It remains important to maintain a moist and lubricated environment to prevent the persistent risk of desiccation of the skin graft and to facilitate complete healing. This is accomplished with either continued wet-to-wet dressing changes or the application of a lubricating agent such as an antibacterial ointment (e.g., bacitracin) or other petroleum-based emollient. Typically, normal hygiene practices can resume with caution against scrubbing of the graft. After epithelialization of the skin graft is recognized, serial

application of a moisturizing cream, such as Eucerin or the equivalent, in combination with gentle massage, can be initiated to facilitate progressive contoured scar maturation with flattening of the grafted surface and improve the overall cosmetic results. Rehabilitation of the upper extremity can then often be and advanced depending on the associated neurovascular, tendon, and bone injuries.

Management of the Skin Graft Donor Site

There are various methods for skin graft donor site management. Donor sites from FTSGs are treated as any other primarily closed incision. The donor site of an STSG has exposed dermis with sensitive nerve endings and is moist in the early period. Occlusive dressings such as OpSite (Smith and Nephew) or Tegaderm (3M Medical) can be applied at time of harvest to contain fluid production. Nonocclusive options include application of petroleum-impregnated dressing, such as Xeroform, at time of harvest and allowing it to desiccate as a "pseudo-eschar" until reepithelialization occurs. Reepithelialization of the graft donor site typically occurs in approximately 1 to 2 weeks. If fluid collects beneath the dressing, it is simply drained with a needle and the dressing patched with an additional OpSite, or the entire dressing is changed. After complete reepithelialization of the donor site, dressings are discontinued, and the healing bed can be treated for dryness as needed, using a moisturizing lotion such as Eucerin or an equivalent. Discoloration of the STSG donor site is common and should be protected with sunscreen. An STSG donor site can be reharvested in the future after epithelization has occurred, typically if all other donor sites are harvested or unavailable.

Skin Substitutes

Multiple dermal skin substitute products are commercially available to assist in wound coverage.[9] Acellular dermal matrices are available as allograft from human cadavers (i.e., Alloderm; BioHorizons, Birmingham, AL) or xenograft from other species such as porcine (i.e., Strattice; Allergan, Madison, NJ). Bioengineered wound technologies are available as well that can assist in covering exposed bone, tendon, and neurovascular structures. The most commonly used synthetic skin substitute is Integra Dermal Regeneration Template (Integra LifeSciences, Plainsboro, NJ), which is a bilayer composed of a protective, removable silicone layer and a scaffold layer of bovine collagen and chondroitin sulfate. All of these products allow for neovascularization and ultimately incorporation into the recipient wound bed.[9] Secondary skin grafting may be necessary after a mature, vascularized wound bed is achieved with coverage of underlying structures.

Postoperative management of skin substitutes is similar to that of skin grafts. Dressings are used to prevent shear and disturbance of early angiogenesis. Orthoses may be used to help stabilize and minimize disruption of the wound. Topical ointments or moist gauze is often used to prevent desiccation of these products along with surveillance for infection.

Local Tissue Transfer

Skin grafts are not appropriate for all wounds. When traumatic defects of the upper extremity involve significant soft tissue loss, a more complex reconstructive approach is required. These wounds typically involve exposure of underlying vital structures such as blood vessels, nerves, tendons devoid of paratenon, bones stripped of periosteum, or wounds with insufficient vascularity to support a skin graft. The next step in the algorithmic approach to reconstruction of the upper extremity, is of local, vascularized tissue.. Local tissue transfer refers to the dissection, elevation, and transfer of skin, combined with a varied amount of underlying tissue, potentially including subcutaneous tissue, fascia, muscle, nerve, tendon, and occasionally bone. During the elevation of a local tissue flap, the local blood supply supporting the flap is preserved. This undivided portion of the flap containing the vascularity required for flap survival is labeled the pedicle. The pedicle contains an artery and its respective venae comitantes. A local flap can close a local tissue defect, establishing a well-vascularized, healthy environment to potentiate healing of the associated underlying injuries. Local tissue flaps are labeled according to the layers of tissue used, the pattern of the blood supply, and the type of mobilization required.

Skin Flaps

Using a local skin flap for reconstruction of an upper extremity defect refers to transferring adjacent skin and subcutaneous tissue into a wound to supply coverage and closure. A skin flap design is based on the local vascular anatomy of the skin and its type of movement. An axial pattern flap is a single-pedicle skin flap with an anatomically established arteriovenous system along its longitudinal axis.[10] An island flap is an axial pattern flap in which the skin bridge has been separated, leaving only the vascular pedicle intact at the base much like a balloon on its string.[10,11]

For historical relevance, a random pattern flap referred to local skin flap without a specifically named arteriovenous system. This term is now archaic because we now know that all viable flaps require some sort of vascular anatomy. Perfusion of specific tissue territories by axial vessels throughout the body have been identified and labeled as angiosomes.[12] On an even smaller scale, individual perforating vessels from these larger vessels supply a finite tissue territory now known as perforasomes.[13]

Skin flaps are also classified by mobilization techniques: rotation, advancement, and transposition. Rotation flaps pivot around a fixed point in a planned arc to reach a wound defect (Fig. 80.2). An advancement flap advances from the donor site to the recipient wound bed in a unidirectional vector without any rotation (Fig. 80.3). Transposition flaps move laterally and sometimes over an intervening peninsula of

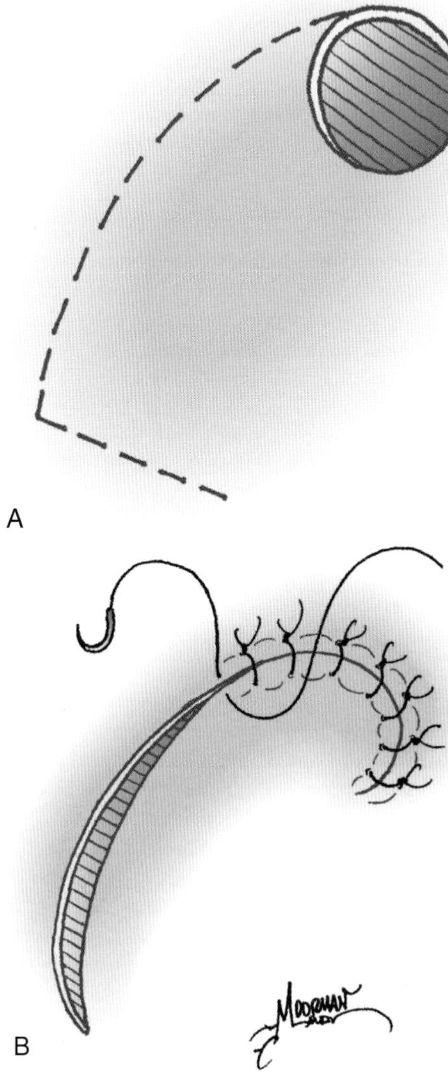

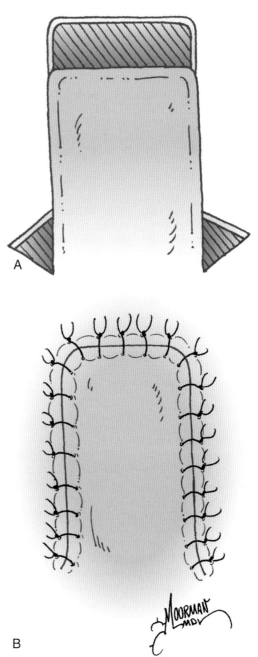

Fig. 80.2 A and **B,** Rotation flap. **A,** The flap is designed to arc away from the defect and thereby recruit the tissue flap in a subcutaneous or subfascial plane. **B,** The flap is rotated along the arc to fill the original defect and secured into position with sutures.

Fig. 80.3 A and **B,** Advancement flap. **A,** A long rectangular flap is designed to match the width of the original defect (top of figure) and "Burow's triangles" are excised along its base to allow for easier advancement. **B,** The flap is advanced in a subcutaneous or subfascial plane to fill the defect and secured into place with sutures.

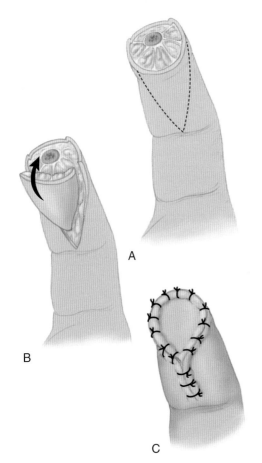

Fig. 80.4 V-Y advancement flap. **A,** Fingertip injury with planned V-shaped volar incision. **B,** Elevation of volar flap. **C,** Distal advancement of volar flap and closure in a Y pattern.

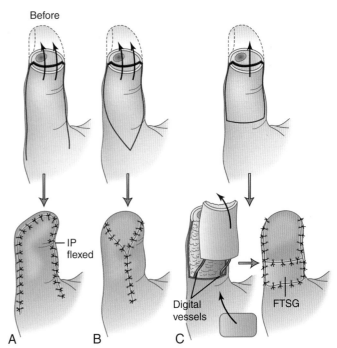

Fig. 80.5 Volar advancement Moberg flap for thumb tip reconstruction. **A,** Original description based on both radial and ulnar digital neurovascular bundles, allowing distal advancement. **B,** Modification with proximal extension and V-to-Y closure. **C,** Islandized flap based on radial and ulnar digital neurovascular bundles, known as O'Brien modification. Secondary proximal defect covered with full-thickness skin.

intact skin. Numerous accounts of local flaps are well described in the literature; local flaps are traditionally valuable and versatile options in the reconstruction of many upper extremity defects at all levels: the fingers, hands, forearm, and upper arm.

Digital Reconstruction

Fingertip injuries involving a surface area of less than 1.5 cm, without exposure of bone or vital structures, can be allowed to heal by secondary intention with proper wound care. Moist dressings should be applied until the wound has reepithelialized. In fingertip injuries involving a surface area defect greater than 1.5 cm or digital defects with exposed underlying vital structures, a soft tissue reconstruction is often needed. The reconstructive goal is to achieve wound closure and restore digital sensibility. The selection of a particular surgical procedure is individualized to the patient based primarily on the wound size, location of the wound defect, adjacent tissue injury, and specific digit.

V-Y Advancement Flap. The volar V-Y[14–16] or lateral V-Y[17] advancement flaps are skin flaps indicated for small fingertip injuries. These flaps offer a reconstructive dimension of 1 to 1.5 cm. After appropriate debridement of the injured tissues, the volar V-Y flap is created by making an apex-proximal triangular skin incision(s) just below the defect. The subcutaneous tissue is preserved, and the fibrous septae from the pulp to the periosteum are released. The dissected V-shaped flap is then advanced distally to cover the defect and subsequently closed in a Y-pattern with sutures (Fig. 80.4).

Volar Advancement Moberg Flap. Defects of the pulp of the thumb too large for coverage with a V-Y advancement flap may be

closed using a Moberg flap. Moberg's volar advancement flap may be advanced a distance of 1.5 to 2.0 cm and used to cover a traumatic defect involving the entire volar surface of the thumb.[18] This flap is based on both radial and ulnar neurovascular bundles that are unique to the thumb, which has additional dorsal blood supply. The Moberg flap is created by making midlateral incisions below the fingertip defect. The neurovascular bundles are preserved within the flap design, and the volar flap is then mobilized and advanced distally to cover the defect (Fig. 80.5). This is a reliable, sensate flap that restores sensibility to the pulp. Multiple modifications have been described to aid in mobility, including adding a proximal back cut and even creating an island flap known as O'Brien modification.

Cross-Finger Flaps. A cross-finger flap relies on tissue being transferred from an adjacent digit. The process of inosculation allows growth of new blood vessels from wound bed into the transferred flap. A conventional cross-finger flap uses an elevated skin flap from the dorsal aspect of one finger to cover an open volar or tip wound with exposed tendon or bone of an adjacent finger.[19] The donor site is then covered with a skin graft (Fig. 80.6). A reverse cross-finger flap requires dissecting an additional adipofascial flap beneath the full-thickness skin flap. The adipofascial flap is used to cover a dorsal wound defect of an adjacent finger.[20] The full-thickness skin flap is then reinset over the donor defect and a skin graft is placed over the transferred adipofascial flap on the dorsal surface of the reconstructed digit. Each of these flaps can cover a digital defect up to 2 cm. Additional soft tissue injury to adjacent digits may preclude the use of a cross-finger flap.

Postoperative care for the skin graft is based on principles previously described in this chapter. Caution is emphasized to the patient while the two digits are "attached" by the skin flap, often protected by bulky dressing or an orthosis. After a period of 2 to 3 weeks after the first stage, the flap is then divided at its base of the donor digit and inset

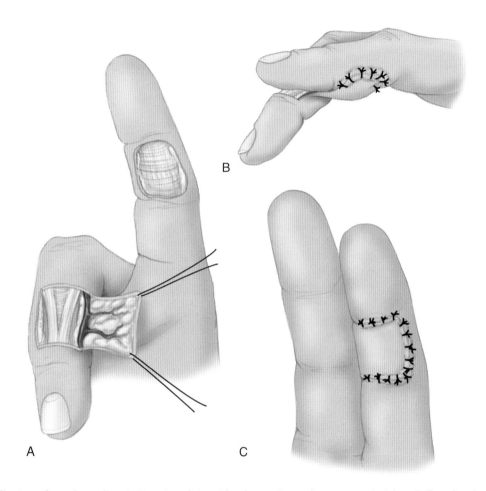

Fig. 80.6 Cross-finger flap. **A,** Elevation of dorsal flap from adjacent finger to match defect. **B,** Transfer of the flap to the defect. **C,** Suture closure of the flap. The donor site is covered with a skin graft.

in to the reconstructed digit. Hand therapy is initiated early to maintain optimal ROM and function.

Digital Island Flaps. Digital island flaps are excellent reconstructive tools for covering either distal or proximal digital defects up to 2.5 cm, overlying exposed joints or tendons (Fig. 80.7). A skin flap is created in a pattern indicated by the local defect and then harvested based on the proper digital artery and vein.[21] The associated proper digital nerve can be included to add sensibility to the reconstructed flap or preserved in its natural anatomic state. These flaps can be based on anterograde blood flow of the digital artery or even retrograde flow from the other digital artery of the digit crossing bridging vessels, known as a reverse digital island flap. Homodigital island flaps are based on the donor site from the same digit, whereas heterodigital island flaps are transferred from an adjacent digit. The flap is secured in to place, and the donor site is usually reconstructed with a small FTSG.

Postoperative Management of Local Tissue Flaps for Digital Reconstruction

For these various flaps used to reconstruct digits, the wounds are covered with a nonconstricting, nonadherent dressing and often further protected with an overlying orthosis, such as cap splint. These flaps are monitored for viability, swelling, and venous congestion. After 2 weeks, sutures are usually removed, and motion can be initiated depending on associated bone or tendon repairs. After the wound has achieved stable healing, additional modalities for edema control and desensitization may be added to the therapy regimen.

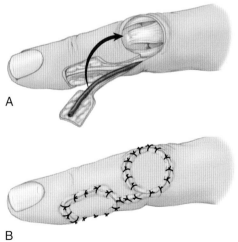

Fig. 80.7 Digital island flap. **A,** Dissection and elevation of skin flap based on the proper digital artery and vein, designed to cover the illustrated defect over the dorsal surface of the proximal interphalangeal joint. **B,** Rotation of the island flap to cover the defect and closure of the donor site with a skin graft.

Muscle, Musculocutaneous, and Fasciocutaneous Flaps

Muscle, musculocutaneous, and fasciocutaneous flaps are more complex reconstructive procedures used for full-thickness wound defects of the upper extremity. If vital structures, such as tendons, blood vessels, nerves, and bone, are exposed, these injuries require vascularized soft tissue coverage to optimize healing. Additionally, hardware for fracture fixation or joint implants is susceptible to bacterial biofilms and must be protected with vascularized soft tissue.

These flaps can be designed with variable layers of tissues dictated by the wound defect and reconstructive needs. Size limitations of particular flaps can preclude their use for certain defects. For wounds that have partial areas without exposed structures, flap reconstruction can be combined with other techniques previously described such as skin grafts. Muscle, musculocutaneous, and fasciocutaneous flaps, either harvested and used as local flaps or as free tissue transfers, can provide sufficient healthy tissue bulk to cover and fill large wound defects. These soft tissue flaps are based on reliable vascular anatomy and are versatile tissue transfers.[20] Muscles transferred with their motor innervation can even be used for reanimation of function. The upper extremity offers several excellent choices for local tissue transfers.

Postoperative Management of Local Tissue Flaps

At the time of the operation, the local tissue flap is protected with a sterile dressing and a supportive orthosis at the appropriate joint level. A "window" is often cut out of the dressing over the created flap to allow direct visualization of the reconstruction in the immediate postoperative period. This allows for clinical observation of the tissue vascularity, which is monitored by color, skin turgor, and capillary refill. Pallor or delayed capillary refill may represent lack of arterial blood flow within the flap, whereas darkened discoloration or brisk capillary refill suggests venous congestion. Each of these clinical findings suggests potential flap failure and the need for surgical reexploration and revision. Postoperatively, the reconstructed upper extremity is elevated on a couple of pillows or a prefabricated foam wedge commercially designed for limb elevation. Elevation is of utmost importance to prevent upper extremity swelling, which increases pressure on compressible veins, thereby decreasing venous outflow and leading to congestion. The tissue pressure seen as venous congestion can overwhelm arterial inflow and microvascular perfusion, leading to thrombosis or cell death. Upon discharge home, elevation is continued, and orthoses are left intact to maintain support and protection, facilitating complete healing of the reconstruction.

Indwelling drains are used to eliminate fluid, which can add pressure on the flap and incisions. The patient or a home health care agency can monitor operative drains at home, where output is measured and recorded over 24-hour periods. The drains are removed at clinic follow-up when the reported output falls below a minimum volume determined by the surgeon over a 24-hour period. Sutures or staples are removed at approximately 2 weeks postoperatively, and an early rehabilitation protocol is instituted to facilitate functional restoration. The intensity and timing of the postoperative rehabilitation therapy depend on the extent and specific nature of the structural injuries.

During the first few weeks of recovery, new blood vessels are growing from the underlying wound bed into the flap. Eventually, the perfusion of the flap is not solely provided by the vascular pedicle that allowed its initial transfer. Such flaps can often be reliably reelevated for debulking or secondary stages of reconstruction within a few months. Cognizance of the pedicle remains important tand avoidance of its division is desirable when possible.

Free Tissue Transfer

Reconstruction of an upper extremity wound defect using a local regional tissue flap is not always feasible. Local tissue transfer may be limited because of the wound location, defect size, or regional donor site deficiencies. A vascular pedicle may not be long enough to reach a particular defect, or the defect may be too large to cover completely with local tissue. In these instances, the reconstructive surgeon looks to the highest rung of the reconstructive ladder, free tissue transfer.

Autologous free tissue transfer or *free flap* refers to the transplant of tissue from one location of the body to another. This is achieved by using an operating microscope and techniques of microsurgery to perform small-vessel anastomoses between the pedicle of the transferred free tissue flap and the prepared local recipient vessels near the defect site.

Microsurgery for extremity reconstruction began almost 6 decades ago with the introduction of the operating microscope for anastomoses of blood vessels, described by Jacobson.[22] The operating microscope was first used to repair injured digital arteries, which began the age of digital replantation in the 1960s.[23,24] In the 1970s, the use of the microscope was expanded to microsurgical composite free tissue transplantation.[25] Composite free tissue transplantation is the harvesting and transfer of a composite (or collection) of tissues, including muscle, fascia, skin and subcutaneous tissue, nerve, tendon, bone, or any combination of these. The vascular inflow and outflow of the harvested free tissue flap is preserved for anastomosis with the local blood supply. Efforts of the modern microsurgeon have expanded from just providing soft tissue bulk for coverage of a wound defect to the ultimate reconstructive goal of full functional restoration.[26]

Free tissue transfer continues to play an increasingly vital role in the reconstruction of upper extremity complex wounds. Free tissue flaps, dissected as muscle, musculocutaneous, or fasciocutaneous flaps, can be harvested out of the zone of injury and transferred to a distant extensive wound, providing healthy tissue for coverage and optimizing the healing potential. Free tissue transplantation offers many advantages, primarily including early mobilization and rehabilitation. Free flaps also offer the possibility of using composite free tissue transplantation, as a single-stage procedure, even in the emergency setting.[27]

Free muscle flaps can provide potential restoration of specific upper extremity motor function and sensibility.[34] For example, after Volkmann's contracture of the forearm, flexion of the fingers is lost because of the ischemic injury associated with this local traumatic event. In this instance, a free functional muscle such as gracilis muscle may be harvested with its motor nerve and transferred as an innervated free muscle flap to restore finger flexion. Similarly, an innervated latissimus dorsi free muscle flap may be used to restore elbow flexion in individuals lacking elbow function secondary to traumatic injury or congenital anomaly. A cutaneous sensory nerve also may be preserved with a harvested free fasciocutaneous flap and used to create a neurosensory flap, potentially restoring sensibility to a particular area. Free tissue reconstruction also allows for transfer of whole or partial toes to the hand for restoration of functional grasp and pinch.

Numerous excellent free flaps are available for reconstruction of upper extremity wound defects, each indicated by the size and deficiencies of the particular wound. Several muscle, musculocutaneous, and fasciocutaneous flaps can be used for either local tissue transfer or as free flaps for upper extremity reconstruction, including the radial forearm flap, lateral arm flap, parascapular and scapular flaps, and the latissimus dorsi flap.

Postoperative Management of Free Flaps

After free tissue transfer, the free flap is protected with sterile dressings and a supportive orthosis with care to prevent any pressure on the vascular pedicle and anastomoses. A window in the dressing is created over the reconstruction to allow for meticulous postoperative clinical observation. Physical examination includes flap color, skin turgor, capillary refill, and surface Doppler signals for arterial and venous flow. Additional technologies are available for flap monitoring. Commercially available implantable Doppler devices are placed on the vascular pedicle and allow for instantaneous audible assessment of flow through the vessels. Another device monitors continuous skin oxygenation through a skin surface probe on the flap island and allows for trending data and abrupt disruptions in perfusion. Loss of the signal suggests vascular compromise and impending failure of the free flap unless addressed expeditiously in the operating room. Thrombosis of either venous or arterial anastomoses that is recognized early can undergo emergent thrombectomy and revision of anastomosis with potential salvage of the free flap. The most reliable method of accurate free flap monitoring remains clinical observation and physical assessment.

Donor sites are often closed primarily but occasionally require skin grafting or adjacent tissue transfer. Additionally, harvest of bone, such as fibula or medial femoral condyle, may require assistive devices for walking, gait training, or orthoses in the short term. Depending on the underlying injuries to vital structures, such as tendons or bone, early rehabilitation, including occupational therapy and social reintegration, can now be initiated. Neovascularization occurs as well in the weeks after free flap reconstruction and allows for reliable re-elevation for additional reconstructive procedures or further contouring of the flap at a later stage.

Common Flaps for Reconstruction of the Upper Extremity

Radial Forearm Flap. The radial forearm flap is a fasciocutaneous flap harvested from the volar forearm based on the radial artery and concomitant veins[28] (Fig. 80.8). This flap offers the reconstructive surgeon an excellent option for coverage of defects requiring thin, pliable tissue. The radial forearm flap can be raised on its pedicle and rotated locally. When based on antegrade flow, it can be rotated to cover forearm or elbow defects. When based on retrograde flow, the reverse radial forearm can cover hand and wrist wounds. Additionally, this flap can be harvested as a free flap or combined with the palmaris longus tendon or part of the brachialis tendon for associated tendon reconstruction, a portion of the radius for bony reconstruction,[29] or the lateral antebrachial cutaneous nerve to establish an innervated sensate flap. A variation of this flap harvest is the use of the antebrachial fascia only to provide a gliding surface or closure of a wound. The disadvantages of this procedure are the sacrifice of a major forearm artery, and the unsightly donor harvest site, which often requires a skin graft for coverage for sizeable skin paddles. An Allen's test should be performed before the procedure and temporary occlusion of the radial artery should be performed intraoperatively before division of the artery using a microvascular occluding clamp to ensure adequate hand perfusion from the ulnar artery.

Posterior Interosseous Flap. The posterior interosseous flap is a fasciocutaneous flap that can be used as a reverse pedicled local tissue transfer based on the posterior interosseous artery, which is located between the extensor carpi ulnaris and extensor digiti minimi. It can be used to cover distal defects of the wrist, dorsal hand, and first webspace. A reconstructive dimension of 8 × 15 cm may be elevated and rotated, but any skin island greater than 4 cm wide requires a skin graft for closure of the donor site. This flap is dissected and harvested

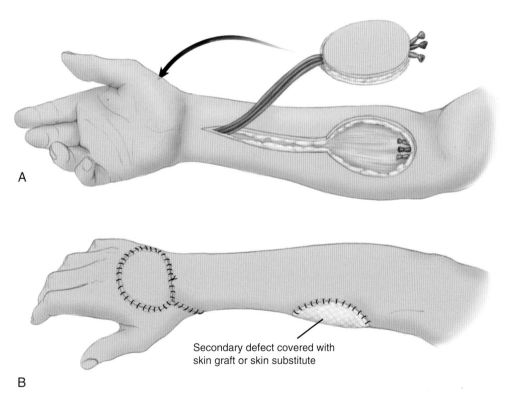

A

B

Secondary defect covered with skin graft or skin substitute

Fig. 80.8 Radial forearm flap. **A,** Elevation of the fasciocutaneous flap based on the radial artery and veins, designed to cover a wound defect on the dorsum of the hand. **B,** Rotation of the flap distally and suture closure. Coverage of the donor site with a skin graft.

from the proximal dorsal forearm, rotated distally, and secured into the defect. Preservation of major arteries to the hand is a significant advantage of this flap. A disadvantage of this flap is hair growth on the skin island, which may be problematic for palmar reconstruction. One must be cognizant of the location of the posterior interosseous nerve and be careful to avoid injury to this nerve.

Lateral Arm Flap. The lateral arm flap is an excellent flap for reconstruction of upper extremity soft tissue defects. This flap can be used as a local pedicled flap or free flap based on antegrade flow through the posterior radial collateral artery. Retrograde flow through interosseous recurrent artery at the distal humerus allows for rotation of a reverse lateral arm flap to cover elbow and proximal forearm wounds. The lateral arm flap can be harvested as an innervated cutaneous flap with a reconstructive dimension of up to 15 × 18 cm. It may be harvested as an osteocutaneous flap using a portion of the lateral column of the humerus and may include a fasciocutaneous forearm extension for additional surface area or a tendon strip from the triceps, depending on the individual needs for reconstruction.[30] As a free flap, the lateral arm flap may be further used for coverage of defects involving the dorsum of the hand or the first webspace after contracture release.

Groin Flap. The groin flap is an axial pattern flap that provides a reliable surgical option for reconstruction of distal upper extremity injuries. This flap is most often elevated as a pedicle flap based on the

superficial circumflex iliac artery and concomitant veins and then used to cover either hand or forearm defect[31] (Fig. 80.9). The donor defect may close primarily, or it may require a skin graft for coverage depending on the size. The arm is brought in proximity to the groin to allow for inset of the flap into the defect. After the flap is secured to the defect, the upper extremity must be immobilized to eliminate tension on the vascular pedicle. Immobilization of the flap may be achieved with circumferential dressings, tape, or supportive orthoses and carefully maintained as an outpatient.

The patient then returns in approximately 3 weeks for surgical division of the vascular pedicle at the torso and final contouring and insetting of the flap. Before division of the flap, gentle ROM of the uninvolved digits should be performed. Shoulder and elbow stiffness can be seen as a result of this flap and associated immobilization but often responds to therapy after division of the flap from the groin.

This flap can also be harvested as a free flap based on the superficial circumflex iliac perforator, known as an SCIP flap, and offers another choice of thin, pliable fasciocutaneous reconstruction.

Parascapular and Scapular Flaps. The parascapular and scapular flaps are cutaneous flaps based on a branch of the circumflex scapular artery of the posterior shoulder[32] (Fig. 80.10). Each of these flaps has a reconstructive dimension of about 10 × 25 cm. A parascapular or scapular flap can be rotated locally and used as a pedicled flap for coverage of shoulder or proximal, posterior arm defects. This flap can be harvested and transplanted as free flap for coverage of both forearm and dorsal hand defects.[33] Parascapular and scapular flaps also provide the reconstructive surgeon the opportunity to incorporate additional fascial extensions to provide gliding surfaces for associated tendon repairs, if necessary, or include a portion of scapular bone for reconstruction of segmental forearm defects.

Latissimus Dorsi Flap. The latissimus dorsi flap is an excellent reconstruction option for the coverage of large surface area defects. This flap may be harvested as a muscle only or musculocutaneous flap and used as a pedicled tissue transfer to cover significantly large local defects of the shoulder and upper arm or as a free flap to cover extensive distal upper extremity wounds. The latissimus dorsi flap is harvested based on the thoracodorsal artery and concomitant vein[34] and contoured to fit the defect (Fig. 80.11). The thoracodorsal nerve can be harvested as well for functional animation of this muscle after transfer, both pedicled for elbow flexion or coapted to a donor motor nerve elsewhere. This flap has a very large surface area of up to

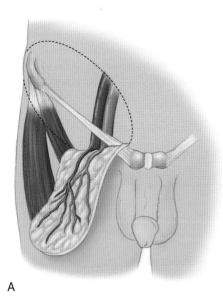

A

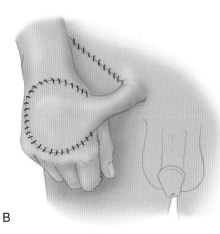

B

Fig. 80.9 Groin flap. **A,** Elevation of the groin flap. **B,** Contouring the flap as a tube for coverage of a complex degloving hand injury.

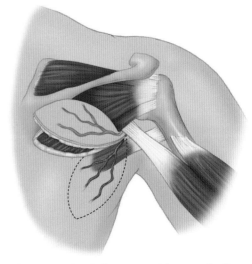

Fig. 80.10 Surgical anatomy of the scapular flap.

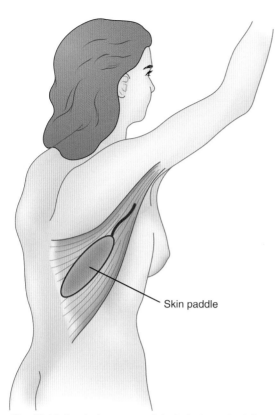

Fig. 80.11 Surgical anatomy of the latissimus dorsi flap.

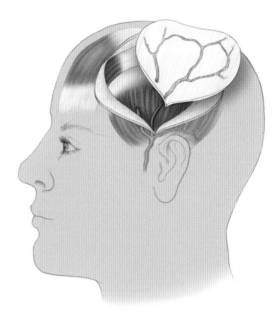

Fig. 80.12 Surgical anatomy of the temporoparietal fascial flap.

20 × 35 cm, depending on the size of the individual and amenable to immediate skin grafting at the reconstruction site. Fluid accumulation or seroma at the donor site can be seen, and therefore drains are often used until well healed. Functional deficits after latissimus dorsi harvest are minimal for most patients except potentially for those in overhead athletics or with bilateral harvest of muscles.

Serratus Muscle and Fascial Flap

The serratus flap is harvested as a muscular or fascial flap with or without a skin island based on the serratus vascular arcade originating from the subscapular artery. This flap has a reconstructive dimension of about 10 × 18 cm and provides the reconstructive surgeon with another versatile option for repairing upper extremity defects requiring thin pliable tissue or gliding tissues for associated tendon reconstructions. Vascularized ribs may be harvested with this flap for additional bony reconstruction. Multiple slips of muscle can be neurotized by the long thoracic nerve for functional animation as well.[35]

Temporoparietal Fascial (TPF) Flap

The temporoparietal fascial flap (TPF) consists of thin, supple fascia, harvested as a free flap, based on the superficial temporal artery and vein for the scalp[36,37] (Fig. 80.12). This flap has a reconstructive dimension of 8 × 15 cm and is often used for defects of the dorsal hand, palm, and digits. The TPF flap conforms nicely to the contour of a wound surface but requires the addition of a skin graft for completion of the surface coverage. Appropriate dressings are required for maintenance of a moist environment to facilitate skin graft survival and healing.

Gracilis Flap

The gracilis flap can be harvested as a muscle or musculocutaneous flap and transplanted to the upper extremity as a free tissue transfer. This flap is based on the terminal branch of the medial femoral circumflex artery and concomitant veins[38,39] and can be used to cover

defects up to 6 × 25 cm. The gracilis muscle also can be harvested with a motor branch of the obturator nerve and used as an innervated free muscle flap to restore flexor function to the upper extremity[38] (Fig. 80.13). Common functional uses of the gracilis are reconstruction for Volkmann's contracture to restore digit flexion and for brachial plexus injury to restore flexion or extension of the elbow or digits.

Fibula Flap

The fibula flap involves the harvest of bone, with or without a skin paddle or muscle, for reconstruction of segmental defects of the shoulder, humerus, radius, ulna, wrist, and metacarpal associated with soft tissue loss. Choice of stabilization is critical to assure reconstructive success. This flap is based on the peroneal artery and veins and can include a segment of fibula up to 26 cm.[40] The proximal and distal 6 cm of the fibula are preserved to maintain stability of knee and ankle. A skin island with a reconstructive dimension of 8 × 15 cm may be included based on septal perforators from the peroneal vascular pedicle (Fig. 80.14). The donor site may or may not require a skin graft for closure, depending on the size of the skin paddle harvested. Periosteum-preserving osteotomies can be made in the harvest bone to allow for multiple configurations of bony reconstruction.

Anterolateral Thigh Flap

The anterolateral thigh (ALT) flap allows for a large fasciocutaneous skin island based on the descending branch of lateral femoral circumflex artery.[41,42] Islands can be as large as 25 cm wide but would require skin grafting for closure of the donor site. For upper extremity reconstruction, the ALT flap is harvest as a free flap (Fig. 80.15). Vastus lateralis muscle may be included with the design of the flap to obliterate dead space. Additionally, local vascular anatomy of the donor site allows for potential inclusion of tensor fascia lata muscle, which can be useful for tendon reconstruction. Multiple perforator anatomy permits multiple separate skin islands as well for complex reconstruction involving more than one defect nearby.

Medial Femoral Condyle Flap

The medial femoral condyle flap provides a segment of corticocancellous from the medial leg based on the descending genicular artery.[42] A small skin island for coverage or more often monitoring purposes

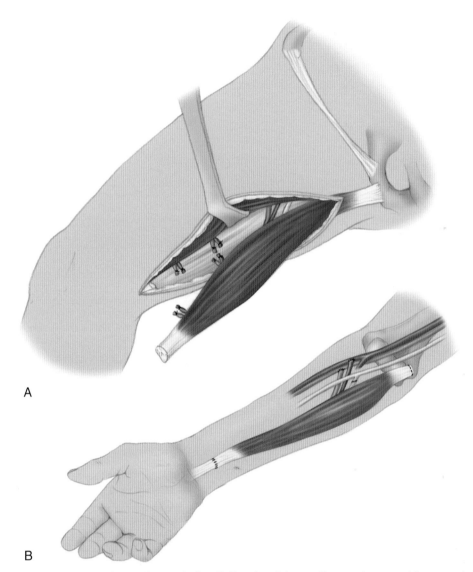

Fig. 80.13 A, Elevation of a gracilis muscle flap. **B,** Transfer of the gracilis as an innervated free muscle flap to restore flexor function to the upper extremity.

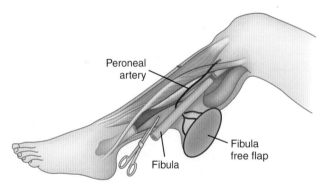

Fig. 80.14 Surgical anatomy of fibular flap with skin island.

can be included with the flap. This flap has been used most commonly for scaphoid nonunion reconstruction as well as long bone nonunion including the clavicle and humerus and forearm. A variation of the flap allows for harvest of cartilage-bearing trochlea from the knee as well, known as the medial femoral trochlea flap. This flap requires free tissue transfer to the defect.

SUMMARY

Advances in applied anatomy and therapy have expanded choices for reconstruction of the upper extremity. These advances have been facilitated by the addition of new flaps and the increasing use of functional free tissue transfer. Surgeons should use the reconstructive ladder or elevator

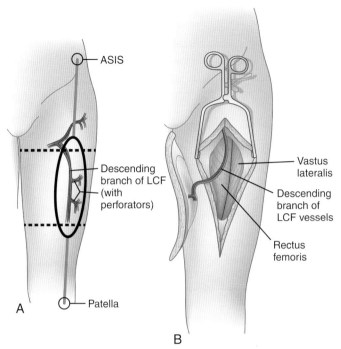

Fig. 80.15 Anterolateral thigh flap anatomy. **A,** Flap design. **B,** Flap elevation. The *black dotted lines* depict the central third of the thigh pertaining to highest density of perforating vessels to skin. *LCF,* Lateral circumflex femoral vessels.

for the treatment of upper extremity wounds. The extent and severity of the wounds coupled with the functional needs of the patient and availability of required tissues elements directs the reconstructive surgeon to the most appropriate option(s). The reconstructive options, surgical techniques, and postoperative pearls described in this chapter are used daily in practice. They offer excellent reconstructive management strategies for facilitating healing and optimizing functional rehabilitation.

REFERENCES

1. Germann G, Sherman R, Levin LS. *Decision-Making in Reconstructive Surgery: Upper Extremity.* New York: Springer; 2000.
2. Levin LS. The reconstructive ladder: an orthoplastic approach. *Orthop Clin North Am.* 1993;24:393–409.
3. Chim H, Ng ZY, Carlsen BT, Mohan AT, Saint-Cyr M. Soft tissue coverage of the upper extremity. *Hand Clin.* 2014;30:459–473.
4. Panatton JB, Ahmed MM, Busel GB. An ABC technical algorithm to treat the mangled upper extremity: systematic surgical approach. *J Hand Surg Am.* 2017;42: 934e1–e10.
5. Nie B, Yue B. Biological effects and clinical application of negative pressure wound therapy: a review. *J Wound Care.* 2016;25(11):617–626.
6. Klasen HJ. *History of Free Skin Grafting.* Heidelberg: Springer-Verlag; 1981.
7. Padget EC. Skin grafting in severe burns. *Am J Surg.* 1939;43:626–631.
8. Fisher JC. Skin grafting. In: Georgiade GS, Reifkohl R, Levin LS, eds. *Plastic Maxillofacial and Reconstructive Surgery.* 3rd ed. Baltimore: Williams & Wilkins; 1997.
9. Haddad AG, Giatsidis G, Orgill DP, Halvorson EG. Skin substitutes and bioscaffolds: temporary and permanent coverage. *Clin Plast Surg.* 2017;44(3):627–634.
10. Fisher J, Gingrass MK. Basic principles of skin flaps. In: Georgiade GS, Reifkohl R, Levin LS, eds. *Plastic Maxillofacial and Reconstructive Surgery.* 3rd ed. Baltimore: Williams & Wilkins; 1997.
11. Bashir MM, Sohail M, Shami HB. Traumatic wounds of the upper extremity: coverage strategies. *Hand Clin.* 2018;34:61–74.
12. Taylor GI, Palmer JH. The vascular territories (angiosomes) of the body: experimental study and clinical applications. *Br J Plast Surg.* 1987;40:113–141.
13. Saint Cyr M, Wong C, Schaverien M, Mojallal A, Rohrich RJ. The perforasome theory: vascular anatomy and clinical implications. *Plast Reconstr Surg.* 2009;124(5):1529–1544.
14. Atasoy E, Iokimidis E, Kasdan L, Kelinert HE. Reconstruction of the amputated finger tip with a triangular volar flap: a new surgical procedure. *J Bone Joint Surg Am.* 1970;52:921–926.
15. Tranquilli-Leali LE. Ricostruzione dellapice delle falangi ungeali mediante autoplastica volare peduncolata per scorrimento (Reconstruction of the fingertip by a medial volar flap). *Infort Traum Lavoro.* 1935;1:186–193.
16. Geissendorffer H. Beitrag zur Fingerkuppenplastik (Thoughts on fingertip plasty—first description of a lateral V-Y flap). *Zbl Chir.* 1943;70:1107–1108.
17. Kutler W. A new method for fingertip amputation. *JAMA.* 1947;133:29–30.
18. Moberg E. Aspects of sensation in reconstruction of the upper limb. *J Bone Joint Surg Am.* 1964;46:817–825.
19. Cronin TD. The cross-finger flap: a new method of repair. *Am Surg.* 1951;17:419–425.
20. Atasoy E. Reversed cross-finger subcutaneous flap. *J Hand Surg.* 1982;7:481–483.
21. Kojima T, Tsuchida Y, Hirasé Y, Endo T. Reverse vascular pedicle digital island flap. *Br J Plast Surg.* 1990;43:290–295.
22. Jacobson JH. Microsurgery and anastomosis of small vessels. *Surg Forum.* 1960:243–245.
23. Buncke CM, Schultz WB. Experimental digital amputation and replantation. *Plast Reconstr Surg.* 1965;36:62–70.
24. Kleinert HE, Kasden M, Romero JL. Small blood vessel anastomosis for salvage of severely injured upper extremity. *J Bone Joint Surg Am.* 1963;45A:788–796.
25. Serafin D, Buncke HJ. *Microvascular Composite Tissue Transplantation.* St Louis: Mosby; 1979.
26. Godina M. Early microsurgical reconstruction of complex trauma of the extremities. *Plast Reconstr Surg.* 1986;78:285–292.
27. Lister G, Shecker L. Emergency free flaps to the upper extremities. *J Hand Surg.* 1988;13A:22–28.
28. Soutar D, Tanner NS. The radial forearm flap in the management of soft tissue injuries of the hand. *Br J Plast Surg.* 1984;37:18–26.
29. Cormack GC, Duncan MJ, Lamberty BG. The blood supply of the bone component of the compound osteo-cutaneous radial artery forearm flap: an anatomical study. *Br J Plast Surg.* 1986;39:173–175.
30. Katsaros JM, Schusterman M, Beppu M, et al. The lateral upper arm flap: anatomy and clinical applications. *Ann Plast Surg.* 1984;12:489–500.
31. McGregor IA, Jackson IT. The groin flap. *Br J Plast Surg.* 1972;25:3–16.
32. Urbaniak JR, Koman LA, Goldner RD, et al. The vascularized cutaneous scapular flap. *Plast Reconstr Surg.* 1982;69:772–778.
33. Barwick WJ, Goodkind DJ, Serafin D. The free scapular flap. *Plast Reconstr Surg.* 1982;69:779–787.
34. Bartlett SP, May Jr JW, Yaremchuk MJ. The latissimus dorsi muscle: a fresh cadaver study of the primary neurovascular pedicle. *Plast Reconstr Surg.* 1981;67:631–636.
35. Manktelow RT, McKee NH. Free muscle transplantation to provide active finger motion. *J Hand Surg.* 1978;3:416–426.
36. Brent B, Upton J, Acland RD, et al. Experiences with the temporoparietal fascial free flap. *Plast Reconstr Surg.* 1985;76:177–188.
37. Chowdary RP, Chernofsky MA, Okunski WJ. Free temporoparietal flap in burn reconstruction. *Ann Plast Surg.* 1990;25:169–173.
38. Giordano PA, Abbes M, Pequignot JP. Gracilis blood supply: anatomical and clinical re-evaluation. *Br J Plast Surg.* 1990;43:266–272.
39. Harii K. Microvascular free flaps for skin coverage: indications and selection of donor sites. *Clin Plast Surg.* 1983;10:37–54.
40. Wei FC, Chen HC, Chuang CC, Noordhoff MS. Fibular osteoseptocutaneous flap: anatomical study and clinical applications. *Plast Reconstr Surg.* 1986;78:191–200.
41. Wei FC, Jain V, Celik N, Chen HC, Chuang DC, Lin CH. Have we found an ideal soft-tissue flap? *Plast Reconstr Surg.* 2002;109(7):2219–2226.
42. Friedrich JB, Pederson WC, Bishop AT, Galaviz P, Chang J. New workshorse flaps in hand surgery. *Hand.* 2012;7(1):45–54.

81

Medical and Surgical Management of Burns of the Upper Extremity

Roger L. Simpson, Catherine J. Sinnott

CRITICAL POINTS

- Thermal burns to the upper extremity constitute a major injury and source of disability despite the disproportionately small body surface area involved.
- The depth of burn injury predicts the course of treatment and the degree of functional recovery. Correct assessment is essential.
- Early excision and grafting of deep burns is preferred.
- Burn contraction and surface contour determine therapy planning and plateaus.
- The quality of the burn scar, its response to therapy, and the expected functional outcome suggest the timing and extent of the burn scar reconstruction.

In the United States in 2015, approximately 486,000 people received treatment for a burn injury, of whom 40,000 required hospitalization.[1,2] Of burned patients admitted to the hospital, it is reported that between 54% and 80% have a burn injury involving the upper extremity.[3–5] Flame burns are the predominant cause of burn injury in adults admitted to hospitals. Scald burns from hot liquids are the most common cause of burn injury in children; 45% of children sustaining burns are younger than 5 years of age. Work-related burn injuries account for almost one third of burn-related hospital admissions.[4]

Burns of the hand and upper extremity result in permanent functional and aesthetic deformities. The extent of the deformity is directly related to the severity of the initial injury.[6] Thermal burns to the hand constitute a major injury despite the disproportionately small body surface area involved. Proper evaluation, assessment of burn depth, and coordinated management of the burned upper extremity can improve the level of functional return and shorten the period before a return to productivity and work.[7,8]

ACUTE PERIOD

Understanding the cause of the burn as well as the length of contact time plays a significant role in assessing the depth of the injury, the recovery time, the plan for treatment, and the anticipated level of functional recovery. A burn wound heals by reepithelialization if the depth of injury is confined to the dermis or epidermis. The concentration of uninjured hair follicles, neural elements, and sweat glands within the unburned dermis determines the speed of reepithelialization. The greater the remaining concentration of these uninjured adnexal elements in the dermis, the faster the burn wound will heal and the better the quality of the resultant burn scar. Complete loss of the dermis in full-thickness burns requires skin resurfacing if the surface area is large enough. The quality of a healed burn scar will influence the degree of

functional return. Correct assessment of the depth of injury is the first step in managing the upper extremity burn.

Burn care involves a team management approach. A total patient care plan must be established within the first 24 hours. The physicians are responsible for resuscitation and the management plan. The nursing staff coordinates and implements dressing change protocols and family interaction. Their constant patient contact allows the nurses to provide physicians with the information necessary to make appropriate decisions regarding pain management, times of dressing change, therapy, and periods of needed rest. Occupational and physical therapists coordinate a plan for orthosis design and use and exercise. Close interaction with the staff is a part of the daily plan. Nutritionists plan the appropriate calorie and protein content and coordinate with nurses and physicians regarding ongoing procedures. The social service professional plays a significant role in establishing benefits for the patient and answering insurance coverage and job-related questions. Many others play a role in the medical and surgical care of the patient. Management strategies are formulated in twice-weekly multidisciplinary conferences. The patient and family are immediately aware of the treatment plan as well as the changing goals for optimum functional improvement. Strict attention to upper extremity function during total patient care is a responsibility of all involved in the treatment of the burn patient.

Assessment

The initial extent of the total burn injury is assessed using the "rule of nines."[9,10] The total body surface area (TBSA) burned is estimated using this easily reproducible protocol. This information predicts the overall severity of the burn injury and estimates early patient fluid resuscitation. The upper extremity constitutes 9% of the TBSA; the hand itself represents 3%.[3,11] The depth of burn injury and the total surface area and location involved predict the course of treatment and

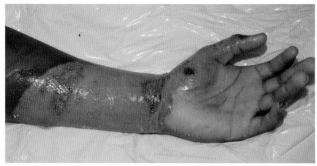

Fig. 81.1 Superficial second-degree burn depth that is expected to heal within 10 days with minimal long-term scarring.

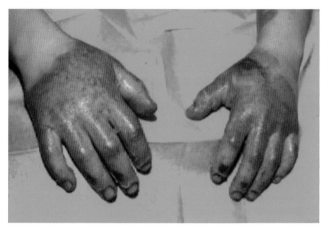

Fig. 81.2 Deep second-degree burn of both hands with moderate-thickness eschar.

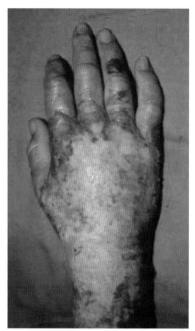

Fig. 81.3 Third-degree burn with eschar and full-thickness loss of tissue.

the functional recovery. This assessment also conveys early valuable information to the patient and family concerning time of recovery.

A first-degree burn is confined to the epithelial layer of skin, producing erythema and mild discomfort. The injured area is red, and blisters are usually not present on examination. Full function remains, reduced, however, by the acute pain. Symptoms of pain and swelling are of short duration. Topical application of a soothing moisturizer to the exposed surface of the burned area reduces the pain. Reepithelialization begins within 48 hours. No visible or restrictive scar results.

By definition, second-degree burn injury penetrates the dermis (Fig. 81.1). These levels of injury are classified into superficial second-degree and deep second-degree burn. The superficial second-degree injury involves the upper level of the dermis and is expected to reepithelialize within 10 to 14 days with topical wound care.[12] The appearance of the burn is characterized by blisters, intact or ruptured, a thin eschar, and severe pain. The periphery shows an erythema as the level of burn injury becomes progressively more superficial at a distance from the point of contact.

The deep second-degree injury extends to the depth of the dermis, injuring a progressively greater concentration of the adnexal hair follicles and sweat glands. This reduces the ability for reepithelialization and results in delayed healing—taking between 14 and 21 days to completely resurface the burn. The appearance of this injury, in contrast to the superficial second-degree burn, shows the absence of blisters and sometimes a moderate-thickness eschar (Fig. 81.2). Immediate pain is less intense because the superficial nerve endings are injured by the burn at this depth. The quality of the resultant burn scar after this depth of injury can be poor, increasing the risk of later hypertrophy and secondary scar contracture.

The specific location of injury also helps guide the management plan. Areas of thin skin, flexion and extension creases, and fine joints of the fingers are severely affected by the persistent inflammation of slowly healing wounds and the resultant restricting scars. When poor-quality healing or hypertrophic scarring is anticipated, early resurfacing with better quality skin must be considered.

Full-thickness, or third-degree, burn injury destroys the entire depth of dermis and with it the potential for reepithelialization and wound healing. The presence of a thick inelastic eschar clinically defines the depth of injury (Fig. 81.3). Initially, the burn surface is not painful. Skin graft resurfacing is indicated because no spontaneous epithelialization is possible. Early grafting reduces the morbidity of anticipated contracture and subsequent reduction of function. The small joints of the hand are extremely sensitive to any degree of skin or scar restriction.

A fourth-degree burn results from prolonged thermal contact and involves the soft tissue and underlying tendon, muscle, joint, and bone.[4] The injured tissue at this depth is charred. Prolonged hot liquid immersion, extended flame contact, and electrical burn injury may show this depth of tissue destruction. Extensive reconstructive procedures and, more often, amputation may be required.

Hand burns are often of mixed depth (Fig. 81.4). Superficial areas of injury will heal spontaneously by epithelialization, whereas deeper areas require resurfacing to prevent functional loss. The treatment plan must be individualized after careful burn assessment. The management goal is to resurface all burns that are not expected to reepithelialize within 14 to 21 days with suitable quality skin grafts.[13] Burns that will reepithelialize sooner are carefully assessed for improvement daily.

Although the depth of burn is important, additional information concerning the injury permits the treatment team to plan more precisely. The source of the thermal injury is extremely important. A scald injury traditionally produces a burn more homogeneous in depth and appearance. Knowledge of the temperature of the scalding liquid and the length of the contact time helps to better define the depth of injury. Water at 158°F causes full-thickness injury to a child's skin within 1 second.[9] Lower temperatures also produce equal-depth burn if the

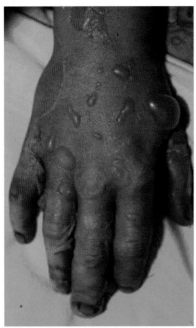

Fig. 81.4 Mixed deep and superficial second-degree burns. The burn injury is deeper where the skin of the hand has a thinner dermis.

TABLE 81.1	Time Needed for Hot Water Immersion to Produce Third-Degree Burns[9]	
Temperature (°F)	**Time**
158	1 sec
150	2 sec
140	10 sec
130	30 sec
127	1 min
120	10 min

contact time is prolonged. Liquid with fat or grease added retains greater heat, producing a deeper burn in less time (Table 81.1). The flame from a house fire will generate temperatures of 1100° to 1500°F. Contact with burning substances or ignition of clothing often produces a full-thickness burn injury immediately on contact.

The thickness of the skin in the involved area of burn also plays a very significant role. The thickness of the dermis in the injured area determines the speed with which the skin can reepithelialize. The depth of injury relative to the skin thickness also predicts the quality of the healing process. The skin of the dorsum of the finger, the dorsum of the hand, the volar wrist, and the inner arm represents relatively thin dermal thicknesses. A deep second-degree burn at any of these levels is associated with delayed epithelialization and a poor-quality restricting burn scar. Scar breakdown, fibrosis, and injury in proximity to joints compromises function because of associated joint contracture and restricted motion. The same source and contact time of the burn injury applied to the palm, however, may be associated with a more rapid epithelialization with no functional long-term restriction owing to the rich concentration of adnexal elements in the dermis of palmar skin. The quality of the skin at the level of injury is another major factor in determining the outcome.

The severity of the burn is determined by the combination of the temperature of the source, time of contact, thickness of the skin, and area of the burn injury. This information and the early appearance on examination permit decision making for either continuation of conservative management or an early plan for excision and grafting of the wound. The goal of burn management is maximum restoration of function with stable soft tissue coverage in the earliest possible time.[14,15]

The management of each burn injury must be individualized. Patient compliance, understanding the type of work the patient performs, and overall burn size are key factors in the management plan. The experience of the surgeon and therapist in evaluating the progressing clinical picture and the expected outcome are extremely important parts of the initial treatment protocol.

Acute Management

Admission to a burn treatment facility is indicated for second-degree burns more than 10% to 15% of TBSA and for third-degree injuries as small as 3% TBSA. Patients requiring resuscitation or those having smaller areas of burn requiring specialized care meet the criteria for hospital admission as well.[2] A large number of minor burn injuries are also treated on an outpatient basis in major centers or physicians' offices. Initial management involves evaluation of the burn wound severity and the selection of a treatment plan. The burn surface is cleaned, and all foreign debris is removed. Broken blister epithelium is debrided. When blisters are intact, the treating physician is faced with a decision to either debride the blisters or leave them intact until the next dressing change.[16,17] As a matter of protocol, when the blisters are covered by thin epithelium, they are debrided along with the exudate. Blisters in the palm are usually covered by a thicker epithelium. These blisters are incised, the viscous fluid is removed, and the epithelium is used for resurfacing the wound as a biological dressing. This provides effective wound coverage, diminishes pain, and creates an ideal environment for epithelialization below. For wounds without epithelial coverage, an impregnated gauze dressing or temporary skin substitute may be used as temporary coverage with dressing changes at 24 to 48 hours.

A more extensive burn injury requiring fluid resuscitation produces local and often generalized edema.[18] An orthosis should be applied immediately to maintain joint position of the wrist in extension at 30 degrees and the metacarpophalangeal (MCP) joint at 90 degrees of flexion to protect ligament tension. The interphalangeal (IP) joints are positioned in full extension (Fig. 81.5).[14,15] This extended position decreases tension on IP joint capsules, ligaments, and the overlying burned skin. The extended position also reduces the risk of exposure of the extensor tendon through the severely injured thin skin covering the proximal interphalangeal (PIP) or the distal interphalangeal (DIP) joint.

Fibrosis and persistent small-joint inflammation are a cause of postburn stiffness and joint contracture. The longer the burn wound remains unhealed, the longer inflammation around the small joints of the hand continues. Inflammation is the source of progressive scar formation and restriction of motion.[19] Intensive hand therapy during the acute period is scheduled at least twice daily, with the nursing staff continuing exercises intermittently between dressing changes. Pain, high levels of sedation, and significant swelling may preclude full active or passive joint motion. Continuous passive motion devices can be used in an attempt to maintain overall range until the patient can participate in active exercises.[7] Compliance, however, is often altered by pain, dressings, and stiffness, and goals are all too often incompletely met during the acute period.

Most patients with burns of the upper extremity have additional areas of burn injury. More than 50% of nonfatal burns involve the upper extremity.[4] The burn patient is assessed for the extent of the total burn injury. Airway patency and fluid resuscitation are first ensured. When the patient's emergent condition is stabilized, management of the upper extremity becomes an active part of the overall burn care. Evaluation

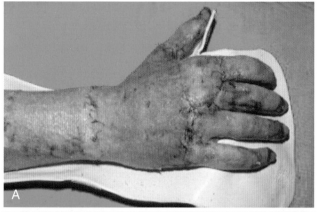

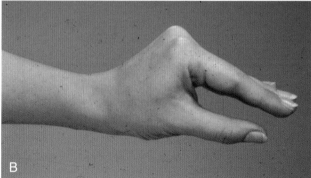

Fig. 81.5 **A,** Universal orthosis used to protect ligaments and fine joint capsules. **B,** Metacarpophalangeal joints at 90 degrees and interphalangeal joints in full extension.

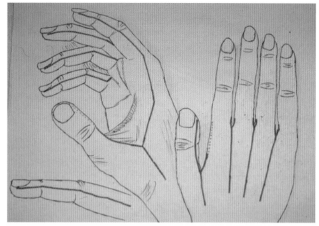

Fig. 81.6 Diagram of escharotomy procedures for immediate decompression of swelling of the hand from deep or circumferential burn injury.

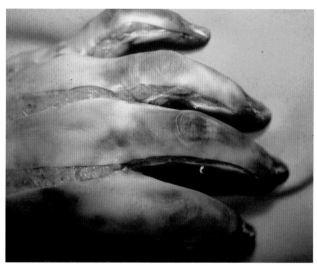

Fig. 81.7 Escharotomy was performed in a timely manner, but severe tissue injury resulted in necrosis of the fine soft tissue distally.

of the hand and upper extremity begins with an appreciation for the presence of constricting or compartment swelling. Observation of the extremity with dressings removed is essential. Circumferential burns of the hand, fingers, and extremity will increase venous pressure and begin acting as a tourniquet. Combined with an increase in soft tissue swelling, compartment pressure may progressively increase above 30 mm Hg, causing compartment syndrome and tissue necrosis. An initial clinical diagnosis may be sufficient when the pattern of burn involvement is extensive and deep.[20] Burn injury, however, may show progressive swelling with slowly increasing pressure and less acute signs of compartment syndrome. Clinical signs of severe distal swelling despite elevation, progressive loss of sensibility, intrinsic negative posturing of the hand, and constant unrelenting pain suggest increased compartment pressures.

Increased pressure from the circumferential burn or the expectation of an impending compartment syndrome as edema increases indicates the need for an emergency escharotomy (Fig. 81.6).[20,21] The axial escharotomy incisions of the fingers and the upper extremity result in immediate reduction of pressure.[22] Individualized compartment releases in the hand by fasciotomy, including the intrinsic muscles, may also be necessary to achieve pressure reduction.[23] Escharotomy is, however, not a guarantee of tissue survival. The origin of the burn and length of exposure may be too extensive for soft tissue survival of the distal digits (Fig. 81.7). Clinical observation of progressive distal swelling, intracompartment measurements, and pulse oximetry have been used to evaluate these conditions.[24] The application of an enzymatic preparation capable of lysing the burn eschar within hours, obviating the need for surgical debridement is a promising alternative to early escharotomy.[25] The enzyme has an affinity for burned necrotic tissue and does not damage healthy skin. The circumferential pressure can be relieved; however, close observation during the hours of application is critical.

The thin dorsal skin of the hand and fingers is often involved in deep burns of the extremities based on initial protective motions such as firm fist making or covering the face from the heat source. Immediate management of all burns includes surface lavage of all debris and debridement of loose nonviable epithelium and blisters. Topical silver sulfadiazine antibacterial cream is applied with soft bulky nonconstricting gauze dressings, contoured to the burned areas of the extremity. Custom-fitted orthoses are fabricated at the bedside to maintain individual functional positions and to protect the small joints.

Management of second-degree burns of the extremity is guided by burn depth and area of involvement. Conservative management with dressing changes, whirlpool, and active and passive range of motion (PROM) exercises provided by a therapist is appropriate for burns that are expected to heal satisfactorily in a defined period of time. Early excision and grafting are advocated for those injuries for which no healing, or poor-quality healing is anticipated.

Several authors have advocated delayed excision of deep second-degree and even limited third-degree burns of the hand, allowing additional time for epithelialization to occur.[26] In a selected group of patients with deep second-degree burns, Salisbury and Wright[13] showed that intensive hand therapy produced functional results similar to those achieved in hands in which the burns were excised and grafted

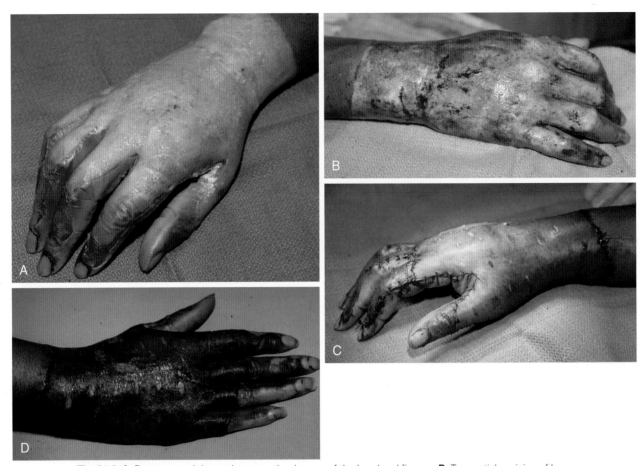

Fig. 81.8 A, Deep second-degree burns on the dorsum of the hand and fingers. **B,** Tangential excision of burn eschar to punctate bleeding in the dermis. **C,** Designed application of a split-thickness skin graft. **D,** Supple graft at 3 months with expected hyperpigmentation.

early in their course. Patient compliance is essential in these circumstances. Third- and second-degree burns of the hand and fingers that are not expected to epithelialize within 14 days are excised early and immediately skin grafted. This has resulted in a predictable return to function and decreased long-term stiffness. Reports of continued conservative dressing management of selected deep second-degree burns of the hand in the compliant patient also show epithelialization occurring with resultant good motion, decreased pain during management, and no reports of hypertrophic scarring. One such treatment uses an occlusive dressing consisting of Silvadene applied to the burn and the hand placed into a large glove. The moist environment decreases the pain and allows the patient to continually put the hand and fingers through a full range of motion (ROM).[27]

Direct tangential excision or full-thickness excision is indicated for burns that cannot heal by reepithelialization.[28,29] Early excision is preferred as soon as possible after the decision to excise is reached and the patient is stable for anesthesia.[30] Tangential excision under tourniquet control removes all injured tissue, leaving only viable dermis or a well-vascularized bed for a skin graft (Fig. 81.8). If the burn injury involves the entire dermis and has produced thrombosis of the subdermal vessels, the plane of excision must be deeper. In the hand, all attempts are made to excise above the venous–cutaneous nerve plane of the dorsum if possible. Excision involves surgical judgment to ensure complete resection of nonviable burn tissue. This plane is characterized by white, areolar, soft, pliable tissue. When complete excision is achieved, the tourniquet is deflated, rand the wound is observed for the quality and quantity of the dermal or subcutaneous bleeding.

Questionable areas are reexcised until all nonviable tissue is removed. Hemostasis is obtained, temporary pressure dressings are applied, and the hand and extremity are elevated as preparations are made for skin graft harvest.

When hemostasis is complete, the skin graft is applied to the bed. Sheet grafts, pie crusted for drainage and contour, generally measuring approximately 0.012 inches in thickness for the average adult, are preferred for the hand and fingers. Resurfacing a child's hand requires thinner grafts. Meshed grafts in ratios of 1:1.5, 1:2, or 1:3 may be used to minimize harvest from the available remaining noninjured skin. Conservation of donor skin is critical when the patient has sustained injuries over more than 50% of the body's surface. The interstices of these meshed grafts heal by epithelialization over excised burn scar and are subject to somewhat greater contraction than the sheet graft. If the wound is initially thought unsuitable for graft coverage, application of a topical skin substitute or allograft cadaver skin or frequent dressing changes are preferable to immediate grafting. Delayed secondary grafting if indicated will reduce the risk of graft loss on a less than optimal recipient bed.

The skin graft is applied to the bed with the hand in the functional position of gentle flexion of the fingers and wrist extension.[31] The graft is secured with sutures, staples, or fibrin glue (or a combination).[32–34] An interface dressing is used followed by a bulky soft dressing and an immobilizing orthosis. Vacuum-assisted closure (VAC) is a technique of wound management, used by some, that seals the wound with a foam dressing and applies negative pressure to the wound. The vacuum pressure can be applied continuously to the skin-grafted site. Use of the

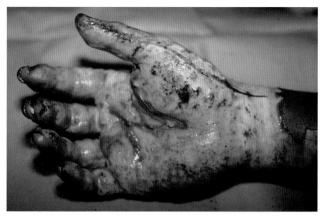

Fig. 81.9 Palmar burns are managed conservatively until the depth of injury is fully demarcated.

VAC dressing supports the graft, prevents shear forces, and is reported to be associated with a lower need for secondary grafting.[35–37]

Initially, skin graft observation and assessment are performed at 48 to 72 hours after the acute excision and grafting, depending on the confidence in the hemostasis obtained. If no fluid collections are noted, the next dressing change can be at postoperative day 3 to 5. Hand therapy begins at 4 to 5 days after grafting, when graft adherence is secure.[38] Exercises consist of active and gentle PROM. Orthoses are designed with an emphasis on wrist extension and MCP joint flexion. Dynamic orthoses may be used when the graft is stable and active range of motion (AROM) is slow to return because of stiffness or lack of compliance. Pain management is an essential part of the therapy plan. (See Chapter 82 for an in-depth discussion of therapy for burned hands.)

Burns of the palm often require a more conservative management plan (Fig. 81.9). The specialized skin of the palm and volar aspect of the fingers has a thick epidermis and a dermis rich in adnexal elements. Burn depth is based on palmar skin thickness and contact time. A protective clenched fist flexion response to injury may permit high-quality reepithelialization in a shorter than expected time. More conservative treatment is suggested until the depth of the palmar burn is fully defined. When the palmar burn is full thickness, resurfacing is indicated to prevent the functional loss brought about by late palmar and digital joint contracture.

Advocates for resurfacing of the palm with either full-thickness or split-thickness skin have based their decisions on long-term wound hypertrophy, recurrence of contractures, and development of burn syndactyly.[39–42] A split-thickness graft offers the best alternative in the acute burn wound. This thinner graft take is often better because of the shorter time to revascularization and the ability to resurface larger areas. No appreciable difference was seen in long-term contracture results in deep palmar burns.[43] Full-thickness grafting can be reserved for later reconstructive procedures when there is less of a risk of graft loss.[40]

RECONSTRUCTIVE PERIOD

The quality of the burn scar influences the ease of return of hand and extremity motion. A poor-quality thick scar is associated with stiffness that is more pronounced after sleep or inactivity. Improvement in scar quality as softening occurs over the first 6 to 12 months updates the prognosis for improved or full-joint function. Strict attention to anticipated time of healing of the initial burn wound, scar fibrosis and thickening, proximity of the injury to fine joints, age, and occupation help predict return to function. Early resurfacing of a deep burn injury with a better quality skin produces a better long-term result.[30,44–46]

The following case study outcome defines the practical meaning of quality results in burns of the hand.

A 19-year-old man was admitted to the burn center when he sustained burns to the dorsal aspect of both hands and fingers while working on a car engine. The entire dorsal aspect of both hands and fingers were noted to have deep second-degree burns with extension onto the thenar eminence and distal wrist. Left and right hands were similar in involvement. The palmar surfaces were not burned. There was no suggestion of compartment syndrome or increased pressure. A decision was made to excise the deep burns early with immediate skin graft resurfacing, beginning with the right hand and 48 hours later with the left.

All fingers and the dorsum of the right hand and wrist underwent an uncomplicated excision and graft procedure. Graft take was complete. Just before scheduling the left hand for a similar procedure, the treating physician decided to allow more time for reepithelialization rather than grafting the left hand. The management plan was changed. The left hand had completely epithelialized by the 20th postburn day. The patient showed excellent compliance in therapy and achieved full flexion of all digits of both hands. He returned to his work as an auto mechanic approximately 4 months after his injury.

At 6 months postdischarge, during routine follow-up examination, this patient provided a serious insight into the quality of burn healing (Fig. 81.10). He noted that the right hand showed no stiffness on awakening, and he had a full ROM of all digits. He was comfortable and had no pain in making a fist. The stability of the right-hand grafts was excellent, and he described no wound breakdown since the graft had been applied. He had no trouble going about his work, even sustaining frequent superficial injuries against the engine block. The left hand, however, was extremely stiff in the morning, taking up to 20 minutes for him to overcome the stiffness in the small joints and obtain full flexion. The left hand had a constant general aching, and wound breakdown in response to minor trauma was frequent. The appearance of the left hand showed parchment-like burn scar and contracted web syndactyly as opposed to the smooth, well-pigmented graft on the right hand.

The patient did not want to undergo a secondary procedure unless necessary for unstable scarring or web restriction. The patient achieved full coverage of the burn wound of both hands and, with therapy, achieved full AROM and PROM. The difference in quality of the function of the healed burn wounds is clearly appreciated in this patient interview. Appreciation of expected wound quality is an important part of decision making during the acute period.[47] The notion that if the wound becomes hypertrophic or unstable, then one can always return for resurfacing is not valid. The fibrosis, soft tissue shortening, and tendon imbalance that occur cannot be improved satisfactorily after long-standing stiffness and decreased motion (Fig. 81.11). Early aggressive wound management based on a thorough knowledge of wound healing decreases many of the problems seen in the reconstructive period.

Basic principles in planning burn scar reconstruction involve a serious appreciation of forces of contraction.[48–51] Understanding how the contracture developed increases the possibility that a reconstructive procedure will be successful, avoiding an early recurrence and its associated functional restriction. These principles assume that the burn scar is well healed and fully mature and that all therapy has reached the maximum level of improvement.

Montandon and colleagues[52] write that a scar or skin graft continues to contract until it meets an opposite and opposing force.[53,54] This is an essential principle in appreciating postburn hand and extremity reconstruction. Scar and graft contraction progresses over the first 3 months of maturation. The surface over which a contracting burn scar lies also influences the contraction process. Scar over concave surfaces meets less resistance than that over convex surfaces, allowing greater

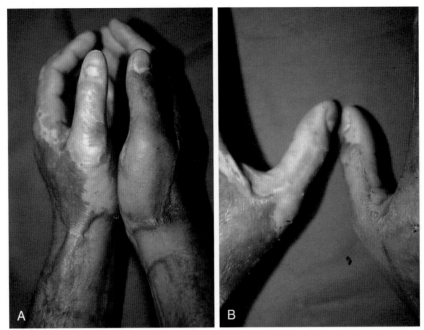

Fig. 81.10 A, Significant functional difference between the grafted right hand and the epithelialized left hand after a deep second-degree burn. Note the parchmentlike epithelium, the hypertrophic scarring, and the loss of pigmentation on the left. **B,** Note the poor-quality scar and the contracting webspace associated with secondary healing on the left compared with skin graft resurfacing on the right.

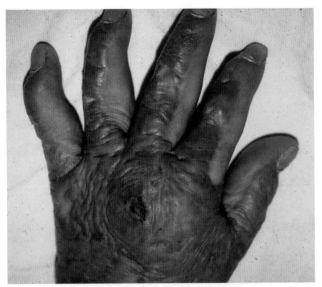

Fig. 81.11 Extensive fibrosis and hypertrophic scarring has resulted from delayed healing of this deep second-degree burn. The resultant stiffness will be permanent.

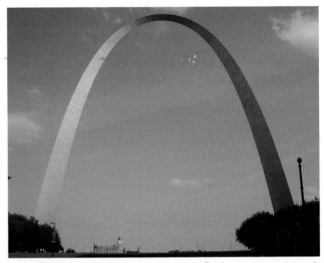

Fig. 81.12 Surface contour is essential. Resistance to contraction is diminished along a concave surface; resistance to contraction is increased on convex surfaces.

migration of the scar and webbing (Fig. 81.12). Examples include axillary contractures, distal migration of the dorsal finger webs, and flexion contractures on the volar wrist and antecubital surface of the elbow (Fig. 81.13). The quality of the scar, its response to therapy, and the expected functional result based on the contour of the area in question help determine the timing, planning, and extent of the burn scar reconstruction.[55]

A burn scar is always synonymous with a skin deficit. In planning a reconstructive procedure, the deficit of soft tissue after scar release is always larger than expected. A diagram of the original burn injury surface helps to anticipate the reconstruction defect. A generous overcorrection with skin graft alone does not ensure a successful reconstruction because the forces of contraction are governed by the surface characteristics of the area. Adding more skin grafts to the release of a severe axillary contracture does not guarantee that restriction of the arm abduction will not recur. External orthosis application and the early return of abduction and extension motion adds resistance to the contractile forces. The graft will simply continue to contract until it meets the precise opposing force, also determined by surface characteristics and the resistance applied by motion.

Palmar Contractures

The resting posture of the hand normally maintains the fingers and wrist in slight flexion. Moderate to deep burn injury across the volar

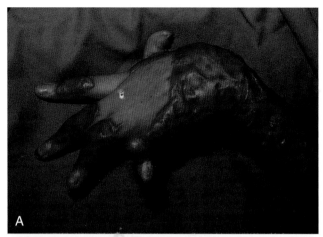

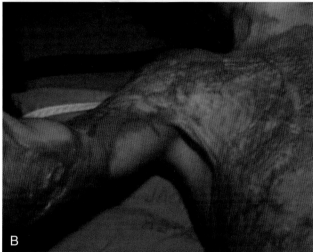

Fig. 81.13 A, Burn scar on concave flexor surfaces of the digits and the wrist result in increased forces of contraction. **B,** The anterior axillary fold contracts easily on its concave surface caused by decreased resistance.

wrist, the palm, and the palmar surface of the digits can easily produce a flexion contracture if the details of proper treatment are neglected (Fig. 81.14). Palmar burns that heal by epithelialization or even those that require skin graft coverage have a common tendency to contract, producing flexion deformities. ROM and stretch exercises as well as the use of sequential orthoses or dynamic orthoses during the period of scar maturation can counter the forces of contraction and result in well-balanced motion. Failure to satisfactorily improve this flexion deformity as the burn scar matures prompts consideration for early scar contracture release, resurfacing the deficit, and renewed hand therapy to restore ROM.

Flexion contraction that progresses despite the use of extension orthoses results in secondary joint contractures as the burn scar matures and contracts. Pain with orthosis use and the inability to obtain full extension of the digits progressively reduce the amount of passive stretch that can be tolerated. The contraction becomes permanent and reduces motion and function. Surgical reconstruction is indicated before further joint contraction is appreciated. Radiographic examination is obtained before reconstruction to verify the alignment of the joint surfaces. Kurtzman and coworkers[56,57] classified PIP joint contractures based on their degree of skin deficit and joint narrowing. More severe and longstanding flexion contractures may require joint release in addition to resurfacing of the volar skin deficit. Arthrodesis must be considered in those fingers in which secondary joint destruction precludes full extension despite adequate soft tissue release.

Complete soft tissue release perpendicular to the direction of maximum contracture is indicated. A transverse incision in the finger from midaxial to midaxial point is often necessary to release all tissue tension.[58] Passive stretch of the contracted joint after soft tissue release defines existing tension. Complete excision of contracted scar is usually not indicated because residual hypertrophic burn scar will mature and soften when the tension forces are released.[59] Resurfacing of the deficit is often achieved using full-thickness skin graft.[60] When contracture release involves exposure of tendon, a local flap, if available, is the procedure of choice.[49,61–64] Soft bulky dressings and extension positioning continue during the postgrafting period. After adequate release

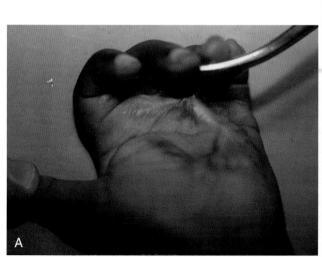

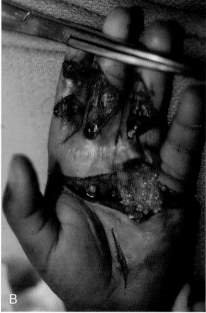

Fig. 81.14 A, Palmar contractures result in significant soft tissue deficit. Burn contractures in the palm necessitate the addition of skin. **B,** Note the very significant tissue deficit resulting from complete release of burn scar contractures.

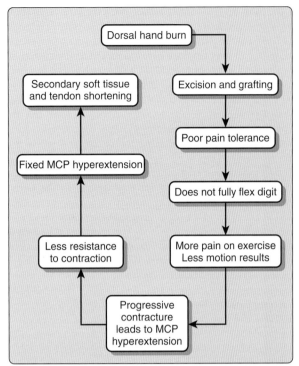

Fig. 81.15 Metacarpophalangeal (MCP) hyperextension deformities may be prevented by early initiation of hand therapy. Range of motion and passive stretch flexion exercises diminish contraction before secondary soft tissue shortening.

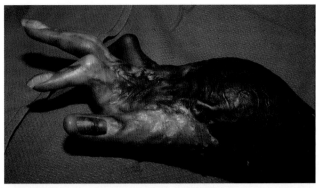

Fig. 81.16 Intractable hyperextension deformities at the metacarpophalangeal joints with secondary proximal interphalangeal flexion deformities.

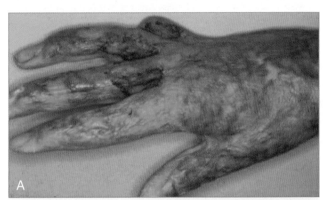

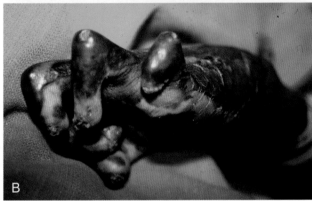

Fig. 81.17 A, Pseudoboutonnière deformities of the ring and small fingers after burn injury result from secondary proximal interphalangeal (PIP) after following fixed metacarpophalangeal hyperextension. B, True boutonnière deformities are caused by exposure or attenuation of the central slip and capsule over the PIP joint.

of a contracture in children was established, longitudinal growth did not necessarily produce a recurrence of the contracture. Active extension exercises increase the resistive forces against the graft contraction, diminishing the rate of recurrence.

Dorsal Hand Burns

Maturing dorsal hand burns are characterized by restricted flexion and pain. Rehabilitation begins in the acute period with early motion and excision of the burn for deep second-degree or full-thickness injury. The relatively thin dorsal skin of the hand and digits contracts when thermally injured, making digital flexion difficult and producing extension deformities. Achieving maximum flexion at the MCP joints increases resistive force over the dorsum of the hand and is the best prevention against extension contractures. AROM, passive stretch into flexion, and dynamic flexion orthotic positioning are used to increase flexion of the fingers during wound healing and maturation.[7] This progressive flexion increases the force over the dorsum of the hand and is strong enough to prevent extension contractures. Failure to achieve progressive improvements in flexion results in hyperextension deformities of the MCP joints and secondary flexion deformities at the PIP joints (Fig. 81.15). This deformity occurs more easily in the ring and small fingers because of the greater degree of their metacarpal flexion into the palm at the metacarpal–hamate articulation.[65,66]

The ability to overcome hyperextension stiffness across the dorsum of the hand and fingers demands persistence, compliance with therapy, and tolerance of pain. Some patients, despite analgesia and encouragement, cannot or will not achieve sufficiently improved digital flexion at the MCP level necessary to overcome the increasing forces of contraction. As the dorsal graft or reepithelializing burn scar continues to contract until it meets an equal and opposing resistive force, the MCP joint extension contraction steadily increases toward a fixed contracture deformity (Fig. 81.16). The fourth and fifth metacarpals descend

progressively into palmar flexion, creating a more concave dorsal surface at the MCP joint level. This pattern of ring and small metacarpal descent differs from the stable nonflexing index and long carpal metacarpal carpal (CMC) joints—the fixed unit of the hand. This accentuated hyperextension is more prominent on the ring and small fingers. Resistance to graft contraction is therefore further reduced. If this cycle is not broken, fixed MCP joint hyperextension results followed by secondary flexion deformities at the PIP joints. The PIP joint deformity in these cases originates from MCP joint hyperextension and not from direct injury to the central slip over the PIP joint. Because these PIP joint flexion changes are secondary, this deformity is termed *pseudo*boutonnière deformity, as opposed to a true boutonnière deformity resulting from primary deep tendon injury at the PIP joint level[65] (Fig. 81.17).

Reconstruction of MCP joint extension contractures begins as hand therapy reaches a plateau. The dorsal soft tissue contracture is released transversely, including the MCP joint capsules when indicated, and the deficit is covered with a split-thickness skin graft.[67] Postoperative orthosis application following the graft application and the use of dynamic flexion orthoses after the graft has securely taken (5–7 days) will maximize improvement of the extension deformity. However, these results depend on the overall suppleness of the released MCP joint and the continued ability to overcome capsular and soft tissue contraction.

Longstanding extension contractures over the dorsum of the hand, if unresolved, produce fixed hyperextension MCP joint deformities. Simple release of the overlying contracted skin may not reduce the entire soft tissue tension present at the capsule level and along the longitudinal extensor tendons. Forced passive stretch of the MCP joint may achieve the desired degree of flexion. Kirschner wire pin fixation can hold the MCP joint near 90 degrees if the surgeon anticipates significant residual tension in the longitudinal contraction of the extensor tendons over the dorsum. This unresolved extrinsic extensor tightness favors recurrence of the hyperextension deformity, frequently within weeks of the contracture release. In this instance, a relative discrepancy persists between skeletal length and available soft tissue. This balance must be restored for maximum motion improvement.

Fixed MCP joint extension contractures caused by soft tissue shortening after burn injury can only be resolved by lengthening the foreshortened composite soft tissue or shortening the skeleton length, returning this soft tissue to skeletal ratio to 1:1. Available techniques for these intractable deforming contractures include metacarpal shortening, MCP joint replacement, arthrodesis (skeletal length shortening), and extensor tendon lengthening with dorsal flap reconstruction (composite soft tissue elongation). An advanced technique using a tissue expander placed *below* the extensor tendons stretches these tendons as well as the overlying soft tissue and skin graft, creating a composite soft tissue expansion and returning the skeletal–soft tissue length ratio to normal. Slow, progressive inflation of the expander reduces the risk of expander extrusion and complication even in burn-scarred soft tissue. On removal of the expander, release of the dorsal MCP joint capsule beneath the flap permits passive flexion to 90 degrees with no restriction from the now longitudinally elongated extensor tendon. A dynamic orthosis protocol permits the extensor tendon to rebalance itself against normal MCP joint flexion exerted by the patient. The strength of this unrestricted digital flexion is now sufficient to bring about a lasting resolution to the extension contracture. The overlying skin and soft tissue remain stable and significantly less contracted when the force of flexion is unrestricted.[68]

Deep burns occurring over the PIP joints may produce secondary extension contractures or may result in true boutonnière deformities, depending on the depth of involvement. The dorsal skin is extremely thin, and exposure or injury to the underlying extensor tendon is common in patients sustaining deep flame burn injuries. A full extension orthosis of the IP joints protects the tendon from exposure in the acute period depending on the original depth of injury. Early graft resurfacing provides quality tissue if the underlying tendon was not injured.

Injury or exposure of the central slip of the extensor tendon overlying the PIP joint progressively results in a true boutonnière deformity. If the quality of the overlying skin remains poor, arthrodesis of the PIP joint into an optimum position of function shortens the skeleton length relative to the available, often unstable, soft tissue. Multiple procedures for soft tissue reconstruction of a postburn boutonnière deformity have been described.[49,69–71] When the overlying skin quality is good, results of tendon reconstruction are fair at best. Stiffness and tendon imbalance persist. Late complications are related to overlying poor-quality skin breakdown and unresolved joint

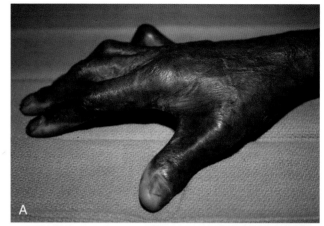

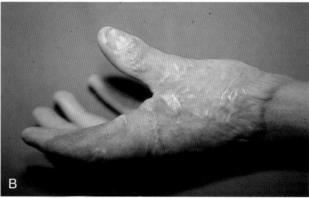

Fig. 81.18 A, Mild postburn contracture of the first dorsal thumb index webspace. **B,** Progressive loss of thumb abduction with more severe web contracture.

stiffness. Arthrodesis of the PIP joint is a reproducible procedure that improves function of the hand and, by shortening, decreases soft tissue tension and stable wound coverage.

Thumb Index Web Contractures

Contracture of the first webspace of the hand results in reduction of thumb abduction and opposition (Fig. 81.18).[72] When contraction progresses, static and dynamic orthoses become less effective in preventing further deformity because the force of positioning the thumb metacarpal is dissipated by the secondary radial deviation of the MCP joint of the thumb. Secondary contracture and stiffness of the first dorsal interosseous muscle, fascia, and the metacarpal trapezial joint can result in a more severe restriction of function.[73,74]

The classification of the thumb index web contracture can be based on the severity of injury.[75,76] A simple web-band contracture, often resulting from a palmar burn, restricts only abduction. With minimal or no burn on the dorsal skin, a simple lengthening Z-plasty is usually sufficient to cover the deficiency. When dorsal *and* palmar surfaces show burn scarring, the anticipated deficit often exceeds the soft tissue gain provided by a Z-plasty local flap. A three-dimensional reconstruction may be indicated to lengthen the scar and regain depth of the web (Fig. 81.19) A double Z–V–Y advancement is suitable coverage for the moderate contracture deficit. A tighter web contracture is characterized by a greater skin deficit, exceeding the lengthening possibility with local flap tissue alone. Release of the contracture and resurfacing with full- or split-thickness skin grafts permits maximum functional return in these cases.[74,77–83]

Very severe burns of the first webspace can involve contraction of the first dorsal interosseous muscle, fascia, and even the joint capsule

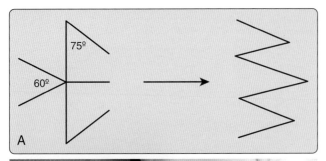

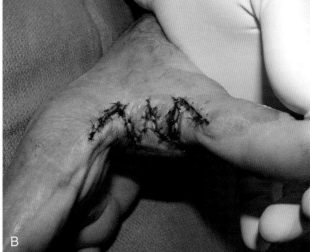

Fig. 81.19 A, Design of interdigitating flaps to lengthen the scar contracture and deepen the webspace. These flaps are most successful in contractures showing little skin deficit. **B,** Restoration of web contour and depth with tissue rearrangement.

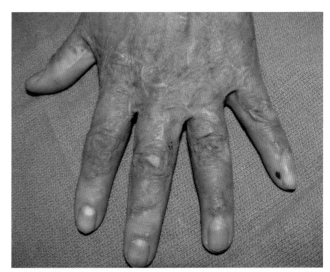

Fig. 81.20 Burn scar syndactyly showing distal migration of the dorsal burn scar, distorting the webspaces.

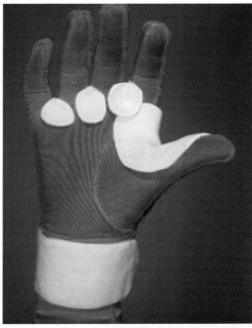

Fig. 81.21 Compression gloves or gauntlets provide pressure on the dorsal hand burns. Webspace conformers (placed beneath the glove) also play a role in softening contracting and hypertrophic scars.

of the metacarpal trapezial joint. The thumb is slowly pulled into the plane of the palm with severe restriction in all directions of motion. The release of the skin deficit contractures; muscle fascia; and, if needed, the CMC joint capsule, permits the return of the thumb to a functional position. Flap coverage is then necessary (radial forearm, free flap, groin, random) to reliably resurface the large defect and possible basal joint exposure.[84,85]

A basal joint arthroplasty with resection of the trapezium and creation of metacarpal support can increase the ROM in the severely contracted metacarpal. The skeletal length of the thumb ray is thereby shortened, restoring the soft tissue to skeletal ratio and allowing greater motion within the contracted soft tissue envelope.

Maintenance of joint position after contracture releases ensures good graft or flap contact to the underlying bed. The immobilization of the area is maintained for 5 to 10 days until complete graft take or flap stability permits motion without risk of shear. Positioning of the thumb index webspace has been described using pin fixation or an external fixator in the more severe cases.

Burn Syndactyly

Burn syndactyly is anticipated on any concave web surface where scar or graft has been pulled distally by contraction forces (Fig. 81.20). This distal migration continues until the scar has reached its maximum tension against resistance. Acute burn injuries of the dorsal hand and fingers often produce burn syndactyly in the webspaces as scar contraction matures. In deep dermal burns that are allowed to reepithelialize over time, burn syndactyly reconstruction is part of the future reconstructive plan. In deep hand burns that are excised and grafted, injury extending into the web and dorsally onto the digits ensures web

syndactyly deformity during the healing and maturing period. The details of early skin grafting should include the application of deep darts from the dorsal to volar aspect of the web in an attempt to break the anticipated straight-line contraction of the graft interface with healthy soft tissue. Application of a dart elongates the graft surface. This technique may not be sufficient to counterbalance the distal pull of the contracting graft that advances the soft dorsal skin distally toward the digit, creating a prominent dorsal hood.

Pressure garments with conformers inserted into the web exert extrinsic pressure in an attempt to restrict the distally migrating contraction (Fig. 81.21). This pressure is maintained until the wound is mature. Any residual burn syndactyly can be reconstructed at that time.[86] A neglected burn, allowed to heal mostly by secondary intention, may produce a tight web between digits with severe functional motion restriction.

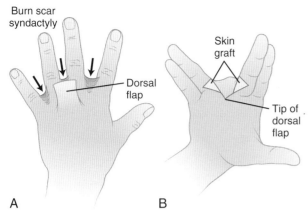

Fig. 81.22 **A,** Burn scar syndactyly reconstruction using reliable dorsal flaps. **B,** Lateral-based skin deficits require full-thickness skin grafts.

Many techniques of reconstruction have been described, varying according to the location and extent of the skin deficit. A simple midline split with placement of the skin graft simply recreates the original contraction pattern; recurrences are therefore common. Local flap rotations may be sufficient for the minimal syndactyly web. The basic principle of skin deficit must not be underestimated. The use of a dorsal flap physically separating portions of the skin graft usually re-creates the dorsal web slope and offers significant protection against recurrence (Fig. 81.22). The composite tissues in the dorsal flap show less contraction than skin grafts. Placing the skin graft against the lateral and medial aspect of the digits, separated by the dorsal flap, will partially protect the web from future distal scar migration and recurrent contraction (Fig. 81.23). Pressure garments and conformers are continued until scar maturation is complete (~12 months).

Distal Finger Burn Contractures

Burn scar contracture over the middle and distal phalanges often results in extension contractures of the DIP joint and deformities about the nail and eponychial area.[87] When the contracture is present, active exercise and passive stretch are not completely successful in restoring full flexion. Pain is often a symptom of the sensitive DIP joint being pulled into hyperextension. Release of the contracture centered over the DIP area is preferred with either graft or flap coverage.[88,89] The deformity of the eponychial fold from longitudinal contraction causes proximal migration of the nail fold (Fig. 81.24). Restoring the curvature of the nail cuticle from extrinsic contracture requires release across the DIP area, perpendicular to the line of contraction. Improvement of motion and a restored nail fold often result.[90] Direct burn injury may, however, result in destruction of the nail matrix, which cannot be restored by simple resolution of the contracture. Techniques at postburn reconstruction of the entire nail and nail matrix have produced only fair results.[91,92]

Elbow and Axillary Contractures

Kurtzman and Stern[56] classified elbow flexion contractures into extra- and intraarticular contractures. The extraarticular contractures may involve the skin, possibly tendon structures, and the underlying joint capsule (Fig. 81.25). Scar contraction at the level of the capsule is not fully appreciated until all the overlying structures are first released. The complete antecubital release is approached by a horizontal midaxial-to-midaxial incision.[93] With maximum elbow extension achieved

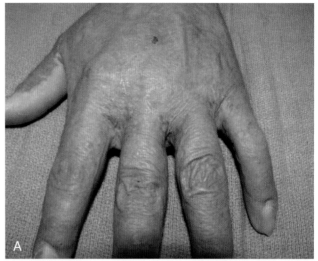

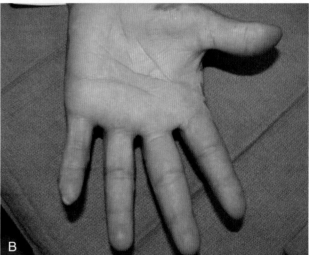

Fig. 81.23 **A,** Syndactyly reconstruction with flaps and grafts showing restoration of web position and slope. **B,** Proper creation of web depth shows accurate contour on the palmar surface.

and a stable soft tissue base present, a split-thickness skin graft can be applied. Extension positioning is maintained with an orthosis until full graft take is appreciated. Passive stretch and use of a dynamic orthosis can apply even greater force to improve extension after the graft is stable.[94] If the elbow joint is exposed during deep multilevel contracture release, local or regional composite flap reconstruction is required.[95] Release to within 30 degrees of full extension permits most activities of daily living.[56]

Heterotopic ossification occurs in about 3.5% of all burns of the upper extremity.[56,96,97] X-ray examination before contracture release will document the presence of heterotopic ossification. Resection after maturation of the bone formation is possible with difficulty. Indications for surgery include failure of improvement of elbow motion, inability to reach the mouth or perineum, and a total ROM of less than 50 degrees. Injury to articular cartilage and nerve compression about the elbow is common. Surgical correction usually at about 18 months postinjury has resulted in an improved ROM and absence of recurrence.[98]

Contractures of the anterior axillary or posterior axillary fold result in restricted abduction, flexion, and extension of the shoulder. Restriction and progressive loss of motion, refractory to therapy,

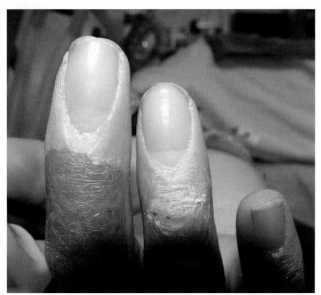

Fig. 81.24 Proximal nail fold contracture at the distal interphalangeal joint. Addition of full-thickness skin graft will decrease tension and restore paronychial contour.

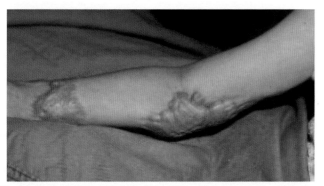

Fig. 81.25 Extraarticular contracture of the elbow precluding full extension. Fibrosis of the surrounding soft tissue is appreciated.

indicate the need for early scar release.[99,100] In some cases, the central portion of the axilla is spared from burn injury and contraction. The concave surfaces of the anterior and posterior folds allow progressive contraction because full abduction is often limited by pain. (Fig. 81.26).[101] Release of the contracted axillary fold perpendicular to its axis and use of split-thickness skin grafting extending into the axilla and beyond the folds allow for early active abduction and stretch when the graft is secure. Release often must be carried on to the lateral chest wall to include the pectoralis fascia if that portion participates in the contracture.

When the soft tissue of the axilla is also contracted, successful long-term release is difficult. Resurfacing the axilla after complete release requires an abduction orthosis until active stretch is possible. The large surface area of graft in this case is associated with recurring contracture on both the anterior and posterior surfaces. Secondary release once the skin graft is mature and abduction has been maximized is common. Lateral chest wall flaps, fasciocutaneous flaps, or distant muscle flaps will reduce the rate of recurrent contracture significantly in the more severe cases.[102–104]

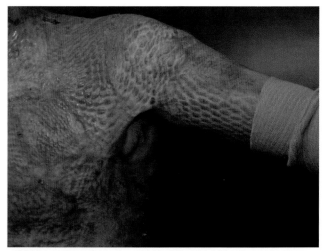

Fig. 81.26 Axillary burn scar will contract along the concave surface, resulting in functional restriction to abduction.

Tissue Expansion

The use of tissue expansion in burn reconstruction can replace deficient soft tissue with donor skin and subcutaneous tissue of similar color, thickness, and texture.[68,105] Resection of unstable or unsightly scars is possible by advancement of the expanded, better quality, sensate skin. An attempt is always made to hide the resultant scars in concealed sites when possible. Longitudinal defects lend themselves better to expansion reconstruction than do wide horizontally oriented burn scars on the upper extremity. The broad lateral-based flaps have a more reliable base circulation. Excessive tension in the expanded flap after advancement necessitates a staged reconstruction of the burn scar. It is prudent to not resect the entire scar until the expanded flap is completely advanced and its tension assessed.[106]

Composite tissue expansion can address deficiencies of the burn scarred hand as well as secondary foreshortening of the underlying tendons. This is often seen when longstanding hyperextension deformities of the MCP joints are present after dorsal burn contraction. An expander placed below the extensor tendons will stretch both the tendons and the overlying burned skin, allowing for a second-stage release of the MCP joint capsules, bringing the digits into flexion (Fig. 81.27). Fabrication of a dynamic orthosis will maintain the correct finger position as the extensor tendons rebalance.[66]

SUMMARY

Management of burned upper extremities begins with attention to detail during the acute injury phase. Appreciation of burn depth, potential for contraction, and loss of function indicate an aggressive approach of burn excision and resurfacing. Therapy plays a significant role in preventing early burn deformity and in maximizing functional return after closure and resurfacing of the burn wound.[107] When this management has reached maximum improvement, a decision concerning the need for reconstructive procedures must be weighed against the benefit of functional gain. Burn scar is synonymous with *skin deficit,* and the concave and convex surface contours play a significant role in planning the successful reconstructive procedure. Attention to these details prevents secondary contracture where possible. Maximum functional return of the upper extremity with quality skin coverage is the goal for each thermally injured patient.

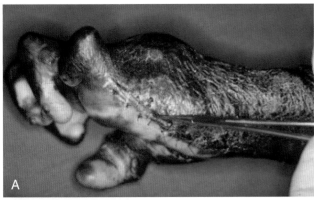

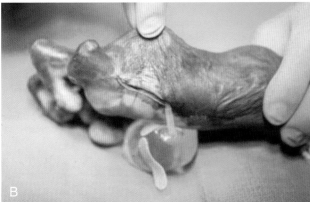

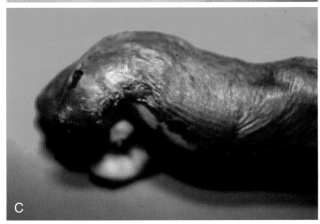

Fig. 81.27 A, Intractable fixed metacarpophalangeal(MCP) hyperextension produced by a contracted burn scar and secondary shortening of the extensor tendons. Tissue expansion will stretch the dorsal burn scar and lengthen the extensor tendons. **B,** Completion of expansion with ample dorsal skin and lengthened tendons permitting MCP joint flexion. **C,** Release of all layers of contraction permits active flexion at the MCP joints.

REFERENCES

1. American Burn Association. *Burn Incidence Fact Sheet*; 2017. Available from: http://ameriburn.org/who-we-are/media/burn-incidence-fact-sheet/.
2. Hartford CKG. Care of outpatient burns. In: DN H, ed. *Total Burn Care*. 3rd ed. Philadelphia: Saunders; 2007:67.
3. Pruitt BWS, Mason AD. Epidemiological, demographia, and outcome characteristics of burn injury. In: DN H, ed. *Total Burn Care*. 3rd ed. Philadelphia: Saunders; 2007.
4. Tredget EE. Management of the acutely burned upper extremity. *Hand Clin*. 2000;16(2):187–203.
5. Kamolz LP, Kitzinger HB, Karle B, Frey M. The treatment of hand burns. *Burns*. 2009;35(3):327–337.
6. Kowalske K. Outcome assessment after hand burns. *Hand Clin*. 2009;25(4):557–561.
7. Barillo DJ, Harvey KD, Hobbs CL, Mozingo DW, Cioffi WG, Pruitt Jr BA. Prospective outcome analysis of a protocol for the surgical and rehabilitative management of burns to the hands. *Plast Reconstr Surg*. 1997;100(6):1442–1451.
8. Sheridan RL, Hurley J, Smith MA, Ryan CM, Bondoc CC, Quinby Jr WC, et al. The acutely burned hand: management and outcome based on a ten-year experience with 1047 acute hand burns. *J Trauma*. 1995;38(3): 406–411.
9. Boswick JJ. *The Art and Science of Burn Care*. Rockville, MD: Aspen; 1987.
10. Lee J, Herndon DN. The pediatric burned patient. In: Herndon D, ed. *Total Burn Care*. 3rd ed. Philadelphia: Saunders; 2007.
11. Rossiter ND, Chapman P, Haywood IA. How big is a hand? *Burns*. 1996;22(3):230–231.
12. Zawacki BE. The natural history of reversible burn injury. *Surg Gynecol Obstet*. 1974;139(6):867–872.
13. Salisbury RE, Wright P. Evaluation of early excision of dorsal burns of the hand. *Plast Reconstr Surg*. 1982;69(4):670–675.
14. Boswick Jr JA. Management of the burned hand. *Orthop Clin North Am*. 1970;1(2):311–319.
15. Boswick Jr JA. Rehabilitation after burn injury. *Ann Acad Med Singapore*. 1983;12(3):443–448.
16. Heggers JP, Ko F, Robson MC, Heggers R, Craft KE. Evaluation of burn blister fluid. *Plast Reconstr Surg*. 1980;65(6):798–804.
17. Robson MC, Heggers JP. Evaluation of hand frostbite blister fluid as a clue to pathogenesis. *J Hand Surg Am*. 1981;6(1):43–47.
18. Edgar DW, Fish JS, Gomez M, Wood FM. Local and systemic treatments for acute edema after burn injury: a systematic review of the literature. *J Burn Care Res*. 2011;32(2):334–347.
19. Ogawa R. Keloid and hypertrophic scars are the result of chronic inflammation in the reticular dermis. *Int J Mol Sci*. 2017;18(3).
20. Wong L, Spence RJ. Escharotomy and fasciotomy of the burned upper extremity. *Hand Clin*. 2000;16(2):165–174, vii.
21. Salisbury RE, Taylor JW, Levine NS. Evaluation of digital escharotomy in burned hands. *Plast Reconstr Surg*. 1976;58(4):440–443.
22. de Barros MEPM, Coltro PS, Hetem CMC, Vilalva KH, Farina JAJ. Revisiting escharotomy in patients with burns in extremities. *J Burn Care Res*. 2017;38(4): e691–e8.
23. Salisbury RE, McKeel DW, Mason Jr AD. Ischemic necrosis of the intrinsic muscles of the hand after thermal injuries. *J Bone Joint Surg Am*. 1974;56(8):1701–1707.
24. Bardakjian VB, Kenney JG, Edgerton MT, Morgan RF. Pulse oximetry for vascular monitoring in burned upper extremities. *J Burn Care Rehabil*. 1988;9(1):63–65.
25. Krieger Y, Rosenberg L, Lapid O, Glesinger R, Bogdanov-Berezovsky A, Silberstein E, et al. Escharotomy using an enzymatic debridement agent for treating experimental burn-induced compartment syndrome in an animal model. *J Trauma*. 2005;58(6):1259–1264.
26. Krizek TJ, Flagg SV, Wolfort FG, Jabaley ME. Delayed primary excision and skin grafting of the burned hand. *Plast Reconstr Surg*. 1973;51(5):524–529.
27. Coffey MJ, Thirkannad SM. Glove-gauze regimen for the management of hand burns. *Tech Hand Up Extrem Surg*. 2009;13(1):4–6.
28. Beasley RW. Principles and techniques of resurfacing operations for hand surgery. *Surg Clin North Am*. 1967;47(2):389–413.
29. Janzekovic Z. A new concept in the early excision and immediate grafting of burns. *J Trauma*. 1970;10(12):1103–1108.
30. Omar MT, Hassan AA. Evaluation of hand function after early excision and skin grafting of burns versus delayed skin grafting: a randomized clinical trial. *Burns*. 2011;37(4):707–713.
31. Burm JS, Chung CH, Oh SJ. Fist position for skin grafting on the dorsal hand: I. analysis of length of the dorsal hand surgery in hand positions. *Plast Reconstr Surg*. 1999;104(5):1350–1355.

32. Buckley RC, Breazeale EE, Edmond JA, Brzezienski MA. A simple preparation of autologous fibrin glue for skin-graft fixation. *Plast Reconstr Surg.* 1999;103(1):202–206.

33. Kubo T, Hosokawa K, Haramoto U, Takagi S, Nakai K. A simple technique for fibrin glue application in skin grafting. *Plast Reconstr Surg.* 2000;105(5):1906–1907.

34. McGill V, Kowal-Vern A, Lee M, Greenhalgh D, Gomperts E, Bray G, et al. Use of fibrin sealant in thermal injury. *J Burn Care Rehabil.* 1997;18(5):429–434.

35. Adamkova M, Tymonova J, Zamecnikova I, Kadlcik M, Klosova H. First experience with the use of vacuum assisted closure in the treatment of skin defects at the burn center. *Acta Chir Plast.* 2005;47(1):24–27.

36. Scherer LA, Shiver S, Chang M, Meredith JW, Owings JT. The vacuum assisted closure device: a method of securing skin grafts and improving graft survival. *Arch Surg.* 2002;137(8):930–933; discussion 3–4.

37. Webster J, Scuffham P, Stankiewicz M, Chaboyer WP. Negative pressure wound therapy for skin grafts and surgical wounds healing by primary intention. *Cochrane Database Syst Rev.* 2014;(10):CD009261.

38. Richard RL, Miller SF, Finley Jr RK, Jones LM. Comparison of the effect of passive exercise v static wrapping on finger range of motion in the burned hand. *J Burn Care Rehabil.* 1987;8(6):576–578.

39. Pensler JM, Steward R, Lewis SR, Herndon DN. Reconstruction of the burned palm: full-thickness versus split-thickness skin grafts--long-term follow-up. *Plast Reconstr Surg.* 1988;81(1):46–49.

40. Simpson RL. Skin grafts for the burned palm in children. *Plast Reconstr Surg.* 1988;82(4):728.

41. Chandrasegaram MD, Harvey J. Full-thickness vs split-skin grafting in pediatric hand burns--a 10-year review of 174 cases. *J Burn Care Res.* 2009;30(5):867–871.

42. Engelhardt TO, Djedovic G, Pierer G, Rieger UM. The art of skin graft inset in the treatment of full-thickness burns and postburn contractures in the pediatric palm. *J Burn Care Res.* 2012;33(4):e222–e224.

43. Prasetyono TO, Sadikin PM, Saputra DK. The use of split-thickness versus full-thickness skin graft to resurface volar aspect of pediatric burned hands: a systematic review. *Burns.* 2015;41(5):890–906.

44. van Zuijlen PP, Breederveld RS, Tempelman FR, Vloemans JF. The treatment of hand burns: timing of debridement and grafting. *Burns.* 2010;36(3):438; author reply 40.

45. Williams N, Stiller K, Greenwood J, Calvert P, Masters M, Kavanagh S. Physical and quality of life outcomes of patients with isolated hand burns--a prospective audit. *J Burn Care Res.* 2012;33(2):188–198.

46. Tredget EE, Shupp JW, Schneider JC. Scar management following burn injury. *J Burn Care Res.* 2017;38(3):146–147.

47. Schneider JC, Holavanahalli R, Helm P, O'Neil C, Goldstein R, Kowalske K. Contractures in burn injury part II: investigating joints of the hand. *J Burn Care Res.* 2008;29(4):606–613.

48. Parks DH, Evans EB, Larson DL. Prevention and correction of deformity after severe burns. *Surg Clin North Am.* 1978;58(6):1279–1289.

49. Brown M, Chung KC. Postburn contractures of the hand. *Hand Clin.* 2017;33(2):317–331.

50. Goverman J, Mathews K, Goldstein R, Holavanahalli R, Kowalske K, Esselman P, et al. Adult contractures in burn injury: a burn model system National Database Study. *J Burn Care Res.* 2017;38(1):e328–e336.

51. Goverman J, Mathews K, Goldstein R, Holavanahalli R, Kowalske K, Esselman P, et al. Pediatric contractures in burn injury: a burn model system National Database Study. *J Burn Care Res.* 2017;38(1): e192–e199.

52. Montandon D, D'Andiran G, Gabbiani G. The mechanism of wound contraction and epithelialization: clinical and experimental studies. *Clin Plast Surg.* 1977;4(3):325–346.

53. Peacock E, Van Winkle W. *Surgery and Biology of Wound Repair.* Philadelphia: WB Saunders; 1970.

54. Peacock Jr EE, Madden JW, Trier WC. Some studies on the treatment of burned hands. *Ann Surg.* 1970;171(6):903–914.

55. Sorkin M, Cholok D, Levi B. Scar management of the burned hand. *Hand Clin.* 2017;33(2):305–315.

56. Kurtzman LC, Stern PJ. Upper extremity burn contractures. *Hand Clin.* 1990;6(2):261–279.

57. Kurtzman LC, Stern PJ, Yakuboff KP. Reconstruction of the burned thumb. *Hand Clin.* 1992;8(1):107–119.

58. Salisbury REP,BA. *Burns of the Upper Extremity.* Philadelphia: WB Saunders; 1976.

59. Parrett BM, Donelan MB. Pulsed dye laser in burn scars: current concepts and future directions. *Burns.* 2010;36(4):443–449.

60. Park S, Hata Y, Ito O, Tokioka K, Kagawa K. Full-thickness skin graft from the ulnar aspect of the wrist to cover defects on the hand and digits. *Ann Plast Surg.* 1999;42(2):129–131.

61. Groenevelt F, Schoorl R. Cross-finger flaps from scarred skin in burned hands. *Br J Plast Surg.* 1985;38(2):187–189.

62. McLean NR, Clarke JA. Resurfacing of the severely burned hand with a radial forearm flap. *Burns Incl Therm Inj.* 1985;11(5):371–373.

63. Pribaz JJ, Pelham FR. Use of previously burned skin in local fasciocutaneous flaps for upper extremity reconstruction. *Ann Plast Surg.* 1994;33(3):272–280.

64. Schoofs M, Bienfait B, Calteux N, Dachy C, Vandermaeren C, De Coninck A. The forearm fascia flap. *Ann Chir Main.* 1983;2(3):197–201.

65. Simpson RL. Post burn boutonniere deformity. In: Kasden MAP, Bowers WH, eds. *Technical Tips for Hand Surgery.* St. Louis: Mosby; 1994.

66. Simpson RL, Flaherty ME. The burned small finger. *Clin Plast Surg.* 1992;19(3):673–682.

67. Graham TJ, Stern PJ, True MS. Classification and treatment of postburn metacarpophalangeal joint extension contractures in children. *J Hand Surg Am.* 1990;15(3):450–456.

68. Simpson R. The use of tissue expansion in reconstructive upper extremity surgery. In: Tubiana R, ed. *The Hand. 5.* Philadelphia: WB Saunders; 1999.

69. Grishkevich VM. Surgical treatment of postburn boutonniere deformity. *Plast Reconstr Surg.* 1996;97(1):126–132.

70. Groenevelt F, Schoorl R. Reconstructive surgery of the post-burn boutonniere deformity. *J Hand Surg Br.* 1986;11(1):23–30.

71. Larson DL, Wofford BH, Evans EB, Lewis SR. Repair of the boutonniere deformity of the burned hand. *J Trauma.* 1970;10(6):481–487.

72. Kessler I. Etiology and management of adduction contracture of the thumb. *Bull Hosp Jt Dis Orthop Inst.* 1984;44(2):260–275.

73. Mehrotra ON. Restoration of grasp and pinch in a burnt hand by pollicization of an island flap taken from the same finger. *Aust N Z J Surg.* 1977;47(6):806–810.

74. Meyer RD, Gould JS, Nicholson B. Revision of the first web space: technics and results. *South Med J.* 1981;74(10):1204–1208.

75. Stern PJ, Neale HW, Carter W, MacMillan BG. Classification and management of burned thumb contractures in children. *Burns Incl Therm Inj.* 1985;11(3):168–174.

76. Yuste V, Delgado J, Agullo A, Sampietro JM. Development of an integrative algorithm for the treatment of various stages of full-thickness burns of the first commissure of the hand. *Burns.* 2017;43(4):812–818.

77. Bhattacharya S, Bhatnagar SK, Pandey SD, Chandra R. Management of burn contractures of the first web space of the hand. *Burns.* 1992;18(1):54–57.

78. Dmitriyev GI, Petrov SV. Surgery for adduction contracture of the thumb after burn. *Acta Chir Plast.* 1989;31(4):236–242.

79. Hallock GG. The radial forearm flap in burn reconstruction. *J Burn Care Rehabil.* 1986;7(4):318–322.

80. Housinger TA, Ivers B, Warden GD. Release of the first web space with the "goalpost" procedure in pediatric burns. *J Burn Care Rehabil.* 1993;14(3):353–355.

81. Jin YT, Guan WX, Shi TM, Quian YL, Xu LG, Chang TS. Reversed island forearm fascial flap in hand surgery. *Ann Plast Surg.* 1985;15(4):340–347.

82. Scheker LR, Lister GD, Wolff TW. The lateral arm free flap in releasing severe contracture of the first web space. *J Hand Surg Br.* 1988;13(2):146–150.

83. Sharpe C. Tissue cover for the thumb web. A review. *Arch Surg.* 1972;104(1):21–25.

84. Araico J, Valdes JL, Ortiz JM. An internal wire splint for adduction contracture of the thumb. *Plast Reconstr Surg.* 1971;48(4):339–342.

85. Harnar T, Engrav L, Heimbach D, Marvin JA. Experience with skeletal immobilization after excision and grafting of severely burned hands. *J Trauma.* 1985;25(4):299–302.

86. Gorham K, Hammond J. An improved web-space pressure technique to prevent burn syndactyly. *J Burn Care Rehabil.* 1991;12(2):157–159.

87. Alsbjorn BF, Basse P. Surgical relocation of retracted eponychion. *Acta Chir Plast.* 1991;33(2):110–113.

88. Achauer BM, Welk RA. One-stage reconstruction of the postburn nail-fold contracture. *Plast Reconstr Surg.* 1990;85(6):937–940; discussion 41.

89. Hayes CW. One-stage nail fold reconstruction. *Hand.* 1974;6(1):74–75.

90. Donelan MB, Garcia JA. Nailfold reconstruction for correction of burn fingernail deformity. *Plast Reconstr Surg.* 2006;117(7):2303–2308; discussion 9.

91. Ngim RC, Soin K. Postburn nailfold retraction: a reconstructive technique. *J Hand Surg Br.* 1986;11(3):385–387.

92. Spauwen PH, Brown IF, Sauer EW, Klasen HJ. Management of fingernail deformities after thermal injury. *Scand J Plast Reconstr Surg Hand Surg.* 1987;21(3):253–255.

93. Breen TF, Gelberman RH, Ackerman GN. Elbow flexion contractures: treatment by anterior release and continuous passive motion. *J Hand Surg Br.* 1988;13(3):286–287.

94. Weiss AP, Sachar K. Soft tissue contractures about the elbow. *Hand Clin.* 1994;10(3):439–451.

95. Salinas Velasco VM, Garcia-Morato V, Fregenal Garcia FJ. Burn of the elbow: the role of the radial forearm island flap. *Burns.* 1992;18(1):71–73.

96. Elledge ES, Smith AA, McManus WF, Pruitt Jr BA. Heterotopic bone formation in burned patients. *J Trauma.* 1988;28(5):684–687.

97. Agarwal S, Loder S, Levi B. Heterotopic ossification following upper extremity injury. *Hand Clin.* 2017;33(2):363–373.

98. Gaur A, Sinclair M, Caruso E, Peretti G, Zaleske D. Heterotopic ossification around the elbow following burns in children: results after excision. *J Bone Joint Surg Am.* 2003;85-A(8):1538–1543.

99. Greenhalgh DG, Gaboury T, Warden GD. The early release of axillary contractures in pediatric patients with burns. *J Burn Care Rehabil.* 1993;14(1):39–42.

100. Sison-Williamson M, Bagley A, Petuskey K, Takashiba S, Palmieri T. Analysis of upper extremity motion in children after axillary burn scar contracture release. *J Burn Care Res.* 2009;30(6):1002–1006.

101. Lester ME, Hazelton J, Dewey WS, Casey JC, Richard R. Influence of upper extremity positioning on pain, paresthesia, and tolerance: advancing current practice. *J Burn Care Res.* 2013;34(6):e342–e350.

102. Achauer BM, Spenler CW, Gold ME. Reconstruction of axillary burn contractures with the latissimus dorsi fasciocutaneous flap. *J Trauma.* 1988;28(2):211–213.

103. Hallock GG. Regional fasciocutaneous flaps for the burned axilla. *J Burn Care Rehabil.* 1991;12(3):237–242.

104. Hallock GG. A systematic approach to flap selection for the axillary burn contracture. *J Burn Care Rehabil.* 1993;14(3):343–347.

105. Wagh MS, Dixit V. Tissue expansion: concepts, techniques and unfavourable results. *Indian J Plast Surg.* 2013;46(2):333–348.

106. Borenstein A, Yaffe B, Seidman DS, Engel J. Tissue expansion in reconstruction of postburn contracture of the first web space of the hand. *Ann Plast Surg.* 1991;26(5):463–465.

107. Hwang YF, Chen-Sea MJ, Chen CL. Factors related to return to work and job modification after a hand burn. *J Burn Care Res.* 2009;30(4):661–667.

82

Therapy Management of the Burned Hand and Upper Extremity

Ted Chapman, Michael Serghiou, Jonathan Niszczak

OUTLINE

CRITICAL POINTS

Skin and Scar Tissue
- Basal cells line the epidermal appendages, allowing for re-epithelialization of superficial burn wounds.
- Therapy management of a burned hand and upper extremity is a "scar tissue issue" with an overarching goal to prevent and correct burn scar contracture and deformity.
- With ill-managed burn scar contracture, the "position of comfort" will become the "position of contracture" (see Fig. 82.3).

Evaluation and Treatment
- Pain is often a major obstacle in preventing and correcting burn scar contractures; although pain is relevant to treatment, therapy cannot be withheld.
- Constant attention is required to maintain accurate evaluation and assessment of the burn injury because the wound (and later scar) will change significantly during the maturation process.

- A through and comprehensive evaluation is required; special attention must be paid to the entire skin healing process as required for functional mobility and joint integrity.

Scar Management
- Compression garments are required for skin-grafted areas and burn wounds taking more than 21 days to heal and recommended when healing takes more than 14 days to heal.
- Full-thickness burn injury involving the radial or ulnar aspect of the hand requires close monitoring of range of motion and treatment to minimize burn scar contracture of small finger metacarpophalangeal and interphalangeal joints and the thumb first dorsal webspace.
- Effective scar management should limit hypertrophic scar contracture and should allow for optimal functional recovery.

SKIN ANATOMY AND FUNCTION

Burn injury primarily involves damage to the skin and disruption of its physiologic function. An understanding of the normal anatomy and function of the skin is basic to the understanding of burn management.

The human integumentary system is the largest of the body's 11 organ systems, making up approximately 15% of the total body weight and covering 100% of total body surface area (TBSA).[4] The integument is unique in being one piece of tissue that encapsulates and protects all the other organs of the body while resisting mechanical shear forces and allowing for unrestricted flexibility throughout the body.[4,5] The integument can be characterized as a viscoelastic, nonlinear, anisotropic (directional orientated) tissue with an ability to preserve homeostatic control and the future capability to restore homeostatic control.[5,6] The integumentary system communicates and works interdependently with the other 10 organ systems to regulate and control the body by maintaining and regaining homeostasis to stabilize health and function. The skin is considered a mirror of general health because upon the body's losing the skin's protection and homeostatic control, there are often accompanying multiorgan system complications or failures throughout the body.[5,7,8]

Anatomically, the integument is a complex organ system consisting of the skin and its embedded accessory appendages (Fig. 82.1). The skin is formed by two distinct layers. The thin external covering is the epidermis, and the deeper layer of the skin is the dermis. The hypodermis, also known as the subdermal layer, is not technically part of the skin and is primarily composed of adipose tissue.[4,5,7]

Epidermis

The epidermis is a paper-thin covering of the skin varying in thickness from approximately 0.07 on the eyelids to 0.12 mm on the forearm and 1.6 mm on the palms of the hands.[4] The epidermal layer is avascular and receives its support and nourishment through diffusion from the underlying papillary dermis. This thin external layer consists of tightly packed stratified squamous cells that progressively migrate to the surface of

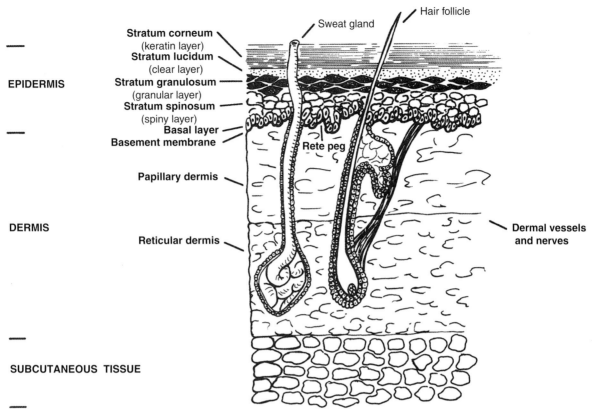

EPIDERMIS
- Stratum corneum (keratin layer)
- Stratum lucidum (clear layer)
- Stratum granulosum (granular layer)
- Stratum spinosum (spiny layer)
- Basal layer
- Basement membrane

DERMIS
- Papillary dermis
- Reticular dermis

SUBCUTANEOUS TISSUE

Sweat gland
Hair follicle
Rete peg
Dermal vessels and nerves

Fig. 82.1 Anatomy of the skin. Normal skin has an epidermis that is composed of five layers. The basement membrane separates the dermis from the epidermis. The cells of the epidermal basal layer continue into the dermis as they line the hair follicles and other skin appendages. (From Greenhalgh DG, Staley MJ. Burn wound healing. In: Richard RL, Staley MJ, eds. *Burn Care and Rehabilitation Principles and Practice.* Philadelphia: FA Davis; 1994:81; with permission.)

the skin while differentiating from living basal cells to flattened dead keratinized cells that are continually shed. The primary purposes of the epidermis include protection, water proofing, and regeneration. Most of the cells of the epidermis consist of dead, fully keratinized skin cells and deep living basal cells. The other remaining cells of the epidermis include melanocytes that produce pigment, immune-competent Langerhans cells, and Merkel tactile touch receptors. These specialized cells and epidermal appendages help protect the body from harm.[4,5,7]

The thin epidermis is composed of five cellular layers, or stratums, and is illustrated in Figure 82.1: corneum, lucidum, granulosum, spinosum, and germinativum or basal layer. The most superficial layer is the stratum corneum. The skin cells in this layer lack a nucleus because the cytoplasm is replaced by keratin. Therefore, this layer consists of several layers of flattened, dead, dry, flaky cells of keratin that protect and waterproof the skin. Fingernails are keratinized epidermal cells and provide durable dorsal protection of the fingertips.

The second layer of the epidermis is the stratum lucidum. This clear layer got its name from its translucent appearance under the microscope. This layer is primarily found on the palms of the hands and the soles of the feet, providing skin thickness and reducing friction and shear forces between the stratum corneum and stratum granulosum.

The third layer is called the stratum granulosum, which consists of one to three layers of cells in transition from being alive to becoming dead. While the superficial layer of cells is dying, the deeper layer of cells is alive. When fibrous protein granules, called keratin, begin to appear within the basal cells, the layer becomes known as the stratum granulosum. The stratum granulosum helps with water retention to prevent dehydration.

The fourth layer is called the stratum spinosum and is the thickest layer of the epidermis. This layer is often referred to as the "spinous" layer where keratinization begins within the basal cells, as they form into keratinocytes from the inside out. This layer contains several layers of polyhedral-shaped cells that flatten as they get closer to the stratum granulosum. The spinous layer protects the basal layer and contains free nerve endings for sensing pain and temperature.

The fifth and deepest layer of the epidermis is the stratum germinativum or basal layer. This single layer of basal cells rests on the basement membrane and gives rise to all the cells of the epidermis. Together, the basal and spinous layers are mitotically active, enabling the epidermis to keep pace with the continuous loss of surface layer cells as well as providing it with regenerative properties when injured. Throughout the basal layer, the cells divide to form new basal cells, which undergo keratinization while migrating to the surface of the skin. Depending on the thickness of the skin, this migration process from the basal layer to the base of the stratum corneum takes about 2 weeks. It takes another 2 weeks for the cells to reach the surface where the fully keratinized cells are continually shed. The cells of the basal layer project deep into the dermis and they line the hair follicles and other skin appendages.[4,5,9]

Epidermal Appendages

Epidermal appendages are derived from epidermal tissue, and no new appendages are formed after birth. Appendages of the skin significantly affect the function and physiology of the integumentary system and are a deep source of epidermal cells, often projecting deep into the underlying dermis of the skin. Epidermal appendages include hair follicles, fingernails, sebaceous glands, and apocrine and eccrine sweat glands, which allow the skin to function well with regards to touch, temperature, sensation, excretion, perspiration, and thermoregulation.[4,5,7] The basement membrane of the appendages is lined with mitotically active basal cells that allow for rapid re-epithelialization of superficial wounds.[5,7,9] Figure 82.1 presents a diagram showing the basal layer as the primary layer of cells responsible for the re-epithelialization phase of wound healing. It should be noted that epidermal regeneration can occur in injuries to the skin where the epidermis and areas of the dermis have been destroyed, as long as sufficient amounts of epidermal appendages remain viably intact. Responsively, the basal cells that line the appendages proliferate and re-create the different cellular layers of the epidermis.[10]

Basement Membrane

The basement membrane, or rete pegs region, is the interface between the epidermis and dermis and consists of epidermal ridges that fit intimately with dermal papillae, which are projections from the subjacent papillary dermis. This rete pegs region identified in Figure 82.1 is where the epidermal ridges and dermal papillae merge to form a series of hills and valleys, which serve as a reservoir of skin and help resist mechanical shear forces between the epidermis and dermis. Upon sustaining injury to this area or below, it is common to see minimal epidermal regeneration. After a burn injury, newly skin grafted areas along with recently regenerated epidermis often lack these rete pegs interconnections for an extended period of time, making these newly healed areas prone to abrasion and lesions with only minor shear forces.[4,10,11]

Dermis

Beneath the epidermis is the deeper layer of the skin called the dermis. The average thickness of the dermis is 1 to 2 mm, and depending on its location, it can be 15 to 40 times thicker than that of the epidermis.[4] The dermis is a multicomponent structure composed of intertwined networks of small blood vessels and lymphatics; elastin, nerve, and collagen fibers, and it encloses the hair shafts and ducts of sweat and sebaceous glands (see Fig. 82.1).

The two layers of the dermis provide nutrition to the epidermis and tensile strength for the skin. The papillary dermis is the thinner and more superficial layer, and the reticular dermis is the thicker layer that merges with the subcutaneous connective tissue. The papillary layer consists of loosely organized bundles of collagen and elastic fibers with vascular eminences or dermal papillae that rise up into the epidermis. The reticular layer is the deeper layer of the dermis and consists of densely packed collagen bundles. The collagen and elastin fibers in both layers are organized in a reticular basket weave pattern. The subcutaneous tissue is primarily composed of adipose tissue, or subcutaneous fat, and although it is deep to the skin, it is not actually part of the skin. This adipose layer provides protective cushioning to underlying tissue structures.[4,5,7]

Sensory Receptors

Somatosensory nerve receptors of the skin are located in the epidermis and the dermis with the majority of the receptors located in the dermis. Figure 82.2 presents a diagram of various nerve endings in the skin of the fingertip. These somatosensory receptors provide immediate pain, itch, touch, hot, cold, pressure, and vibration sensations to the body. The free nerve endings are found in the epidermis and dermis and function as pain and itch receptors. Merkel's disk receptors are touch receptors and are located in the stratum spinosum and basal layers of the epidermis. Meissner's corpuscles are also touch receptors and are situated just below the epidermis in the papillary dermis. Ruffini's corpuscles detect stretching and tension and are warm receptors and Krause's end bulbs are cold receptors, both found in the papillary

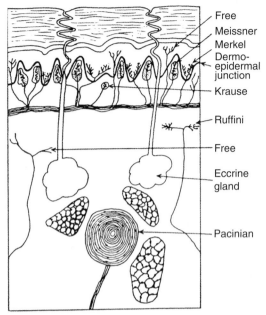

Fig. 82.2 Diagram showing various nerve endings in the skin of the fingertip. (From Eady RAJ, Leigh IM, and Pope FM: Anatomy and organization of human skin. In Rook A, Wilkinson DS, and Ebling FJG [ed]: *Textbook of Dermatology*, Volume 1, 6th edition, Oxford, John Wiley and Sons Inc, 1998, pp 37-111; with permission.)

dermis. Finally, the pacinian corpuscles are pressure and vibration receptors and are detected in the reticular dermis.[4]

Functions of the Skin

The principal purpose of the integumentary system is to protect all of the other organ systems of the body and maintain homeostasis. The outer epidermal covering serves as the first line of defense in protecting the body from harm by functioning primarily as a physical barrier between the external environment and the internal structures of the body. The thin exterior epidermal layer of keratinocytes protects against infection. When the epidermis is injured, it re-epithelializes quickly to prevent invasion of outside agents. This rapid healing process prevents excessive fluid loss. As a semi-impermeable barrier to fluid loss, the skin controls evaporation and conserves bodily fluids to support homeostasis and maintains essential nutrients within the skin and body. To maintain this function, the sebaceous glands secrete an oily waxy substance called sebum, which waterproofs and lubricates the hair and skin surface, keeping it soft and pliable.[4,5,7]

The epidermal layer also functions as the primary source of vitamin D production and metabolism for the body. With short-term exposure to sunlight, somatosensory light receptors in the skin promote metabolic synthesis of vitamin D. Concurrently, these receptors encourage melanocytes in the basal layer to produce pigmentation called melanin to protect the body from ultraviolet rays.[4,5,7]

The dermal layer functions as a blood reservoir that enables the skin to regulate body temperature. Blood flow to and from the skin (perfusion and constriction) is controlled via the nervous system. Blood vessels in the skin can hold and release heat to maintain a constant body temperature. Body temperature regulation occurs via the nervous system controlling dermal blood flow to and from the skin along with excretions by sweat glands to keep the body cool when it is warm. Secretions from sweat glands also control skin pH to prevent dermal infections, whereas Langerhans cells make up a portion of immunologic function. The collagen within the dermis gives the skin its durability and tensile strength. The deeper subdermal layer encompasses adipose tissue, providing insulation and protective cushioning against trauma to underlying structures of the body. The skin of the upper extremity and hand is anisotropic with directional strength and extensibility, allowing the body fluid movement and function by way of motor, process and social interaction skills, physical appearance, and personal identity through interaction in time and the contextual environment.[4–7]

BIOMECHANICS AND BIORHEOLOGY OF SKIN AND SCAR

Severe burn injury is physical trauma to the integumentary system and physiological insult to multiple organ systems because the skin's protective and homeostatic properties are compromised, especially when the extent of burn injury involves 20% or more of the person's TBSA.[12] After a severe burn injury, wound contracture is a normal part of healing as the elastic physical behavior of pliable skin is replaced by skin grafts and inelastic scar tissue, which can lead to the development of debilitating contractures and hypertrophic scar.[13,14] Throughout the course of acute, intermediate, and long-term rehabilitation, the primary responsibilities of the therapist are to prevent and correct burn scar contracture (BSC) and deformity and to minimize hypertrophic scarring.

The skin forms the external protective covering of the body, and its pliability and flexibility allow for unrestricted movement of the hands and upper extremity. The skin is often described as having regenerative, viscoelastic, and tensile strength properties.[14] Although the epidermis and its accompanying appendages provide the regenerative properties in superficial wounds via re-epithelialization, the role of the epidermis is less significant as it relates to the biophysical behavior of the skin. Thus, the primary biophysical behavior of the skin occurs in the dermis, particularly the deeper reticular layer, among the collagen and elastic fibers and the lubricative amorphous ground substance.

Weber and Davis[15] state: "Hand therapy is behavioral modification of the fibroblast during the healing response." Therefore, to respond effectively and efficiently in managing the biological formation of scar tissue, the therapist must understand the biomechanical and biorheological principles underlying skin and scar. Burn scar begins to form early in the proliferative stage of wound healing, which begins approximately 5 to 7 days after injury.[13,14] During this stage, the extensibility of burn scar must be managed determinedly while it is being produced and throughout the remodeling phase. Early therapy intervention is imperative and should be based on the principles discussed in this section. From this foundational perspective, the tissue of the skin is characterized as a composition of three viscoelastic components of collagen, elastin, and ground substance.

Collagen fibrils are long, individual (nonbranched), and coiled at rest in an omnidirectional orientation and are resistant to stretch, which makes them responsible for the tensile strength of skin and scar.[14] Normal skin is maintained in a state of constant tension via elastic fibers in accordance with Langer's lines of the body, which represent lines of maximal tension. The elastic fibers in normal skin are partly responsible for the bundling of collagen, but because very little elastin is redeveloped in scars, it is unclear as to what causes the whorl-like configuration of burn scar collagen. In a relaxed state, collagen appears relaxed, loose, and convoluted. In the normal dermis, the collagen fibers rest in bundles, but in pathologic burn scar, the collagen fibers form in a random oriented whirl or coiled state.[14] In response to the scar tissue's disoriented, coiled, shortened state, the primary patient intervention is "stretching" the burn scar to regain tissue length to improve range of motion (ROM) and function.

According to Brand, the human body responds to internal and external stretching forces in one of three ways: (1) the force is suboptimal, and the tissues atrophy or contract and shorten, such as constant relaxation without tension; (2) the force is excessive, and the tissue breaks and ruptures, or micro-tears occur, such as the constant cyclical tension of creep; and (3) the optimal force is adequately applied and held for a prolonged period of time (stress–relaxation), resulting in tissue hypertrophy, lengthening by growth to a new satisfying resting length with new homeostatic control over movement of the area. As the skin and scar mature at this new length, the tissue becomes able to tolerate additional internal stress–strain forces.[16–18] To understand these principles and properties of skin and scar, Table 82.1 provides a glossary of definitions and terminology regarding the concepts of biomechanical creep and biorheological growth.

Relaxation: Position of Comfort => Position of Contracture

The biophysical properties of the healing wound and subsequent maturing scar are an important determinant of hand function after burn injury. A relaxing response to contracting scar tissue throughout the course of recovery, without the application of an opposing force, can lead to atrophy, contracture, and deformity. Brand[17] states that when "a range of motion is not used regularly, it is gradually lost." The process of allowing the severely burned hand and upper extremity to be comfortably positioned while being subject to the contractile forces of wound closure results in continual contraction in a shortened direction, especially when there is protracted wound healing greater than 21 days. Scar is new connective tissue that is structurally and biomechanically isotropic, meaning that at all time points of healing, collagen fibers have no orientation and no functional direction.[6] Thus, there is a lack of orientation and direction of new scar caused by less than optimal opposing tension, and there is no internal resistive stress. Subsequently, an unopposed position of comfort without tension leads to progressive BSC throughout recovery.

Thus, impeding BSCs are partly caused by the tissue losing its directional functional strength, which results in a loss of ROM and function of the hand and upper extremity, which can lead to severe contractures and disability. Allowing a burn survivor to respond to an ensuing BSC with a comfortable relaxed posture throughout normal wound contraction, scar formation, and remodeling will result in contractile forces that reduce tissue extensibility. As a result, minimal to no orientation of collagen fibers or lengthening occurs throughout the remodeling phase as BSCs form (Fig. 82.3).

Creep: Biomechanical Force

Biomechanical creep is the application of cyclical tension to an area of tissue causing a change in the position of the tissue. This change in position of the tissue can result in a temporary stretch, deformed lengthening, or terminal extensibility. The application of tension to lengthen tissue is often illustrated using a stress–strain or length–tension curve (Fig. 82.4).[17] Whereas tension is a biomechanical action to lengthen the tissue, stress and strain are reactions to the force being applied to lengthen the tissue. Stress is the internal resistive force to the applied tension, and strain involves resistive shear forces as slippage of short fibers slide on each other as they unfold, align, and elongate in response to the applied force.[19]

Tissue creep applies cyclical force to the tissue, resulting in temporary elastic physiological lengthening, permanent lengthening by nonphysiological plastic change from slippage of bonds between collagen fibers, or terminal relief of cyclical tension by the fibers rupturing.[19] With reference to the length–tension curve in Figure 82.4, temporary lengthening is represented by the *a, b,* and *c* regions of the curve, and

TABLE 82.1	Definitions of Biomechanical and Biorheological Terminology
Term	**Definition**
Burn scar contracture	Replacement of skin with pathologic neoconnective tissue that begins to shorten within 5–7 days postinjury, causing insufficient extensibility and length of scar tissue, resulting in loss of movement or tissue alignment of an associated joint or anatomic structure
Biorheology	Study of deformation or flow of living tissue that exhibits a time-dependent response to force
Rheo	The science of flow, which does not emphasize deformation
Load	Force
Tension	Directed force pulling on an area of tissue to elongate its length
Stress	Force per unit area or stress per area
Strain	Change in length of tissue, or elongation
Strain rate	Change in strain over time
Extensibility	The ability to be extended or lengthened; strain or length at failure
Stiffness	Change in stress or change in strain
Displacement	Change in position associated with movement
Creep	Cyclical tension for acute time, leading to displacement
Stress–relaxation	Cyclical tension induced displacement held in place by noncyclical tension for prolonged time, leading to a decrease in tension
Compression	Directed force compressing an area of tissue to condense its size

Adapted from Richard et al,[1] Brody,[6] Richard and Staley,[14] Dunn et al,[20] Jacobs,[25] and Copley.[23]

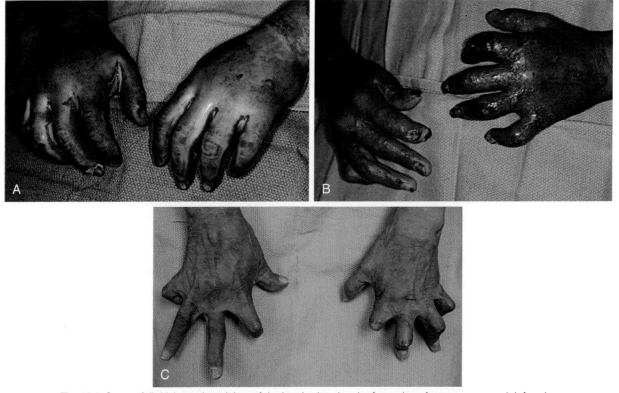

Fig. 82.3 Severe full-thickness burn injury of the hands showing the formation of contractures and deformity via relaxation without optimal stress throughout the acute (**A**), intermediate (**B**), and long-term (**C**) phases of recovery. Notice how the position of "comfort–relaxation" becomes the position of contracture.

plastic change and terminal relief are depicted from the yield point at the peak of the curve through the *d* region until rupture occurs. The cyclically applied tension induces an internal resistive stress response within the tissue causing a change in the position of the collagen fibers as they align, elongate, and begin to strain. Through this straining process, the collagen fibers accumulate and draw tight and taut in response to the direction of the applied tension.[6,14,16,17,20] Throughout the phases of the length–tension curve depicted in Figure 82.4, greater and greater amounts of cyclical tension are applied to the skin and scar, which yields less and less tissue length. As the tension increases,

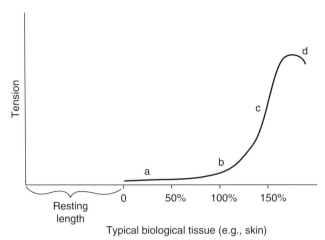

Fig. 82.4 Length–tension curve for skin. (From Brand PW, Hollister AM, Thompson DE. Mechanical resistance. In: Brand PW, Hollister AM, eds. *Clinical Mechanics of the Hand.* 3rd ed. St. Louis: Mosby; 1999:234; with permission.)

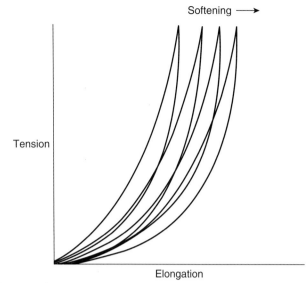

Fig. 82.5 Successive length induction of skin and scar tissue with the ability to rapidly restore homeostatic control of its resting length. (From Brody G. The biomechanical properties of tissue. In: Rudolph R, ed. *Problems in Aesthetic Surgery: Biological Causes and Clinical Solutions.* St. Louis: CV Mosby; 1986:54; with permission.)

collagen fibers respond by accumulating and aligning together in the direction of the applied force, creating internal resistive stress and tensile strength.[13,14,16,17,20] The tensile strength and internal resistive stress response of the tissue resist being pulled apart.

With creep, the applied cyclical tension continues over time until shorter collagen fibers gradually slip and slide on each other, which is followed by microtearing; if not completely ruptured, the tissue becomes stretched and deformed in a permanent way, known as a non-physiological plastic change.[14] When the breaking point of the tissue is reached, the tissue is said to have reached terminal extensibility.[19,20] Within the principle of creep, if the cyclical tension is not halted, then the biological tissue has a definite limit in its ability to resist being pulled apart, which begins to occur at the tissue's yield point.

As cyclical tension persists, some of the taut and tight fibers can rupture and breakdown, causing a permanent plastic change.[14,16,17,19] The threshold of the tissue is exceeded when its internal resistive stress limit is surpassed and the tissue continues to yield length until it finally reaches its terminal breaking point.[6,14,16,17,20] The tissue tears apart because it simply lacks any additional ability to extend or lengthen, and if the force is too great, then there is not enough response time for tissue to grow. Therefore, in and of itself, biomechanical creep leads to a progressive change in displacement, resulting in biomechanical elongation with a definite terminal limit at which tissue tearing, rupture, and failure occur.[6,16,17] Of note, "aggressive ROM," traction devices, and dynamic hinge orthoses can potentially lead to microtearing of tissue and ensuing inflammation and proliferation of fibroblasts and further thickened short scarring.[13,16,17,19,21,22]

Successive Length Induction

Repeated exercise, such as the use of reciprocal pulleys, harness the principle of successive length induction. This biomechanical lengthening process is also called preconditioning and in engineering terms, load cycling. With this biophysical lengthening principle, for each repetition that the body segment is moved, the skin and scar tissue elongate more and more as the tension lessens and internal resistive stress diminishes (Fig. 82.5). Only after repeated cycling (reportedly 6–10) does the tissue reach a steady state at which no further elongation will occur unless the cycling routine is changed.[14] A frequent saying in burn rehabilitation is, "If it's white, then it's tight," meaning that when the skin is gently and repeatedly stretched to the point of early blanching, it is stimulated to lengthen.[16]

The principle of successive length induction illustrated in Figure 82.5 is an important concept for management of burned hands and upper extremities. Before any application of prolonged positioning to oppose contracting scar tissue, the optimal tissue length should be gained through repeated cycles of tissue elongation. With successive length induction, directional tension is applied to the tissue, and collagen fibers accumulate and align parallel to one another in the direction of the applied force.[14,16,17]

Internal and external loading can be used to provide cyclical or noncyclical tension to tissue. For example, internally, muscle contraction can be used to load the tissue during activities of daily living (ADLs), instrumental activities of daily living (IADLs), active range of motion (AROM), or active assisted range of motion (AAROM) exercises that provide directed force or tension to the tissue. However, the application of AAROM, passive range of motion (PROM), positioning, and orthoses are often superior to muscles that soon fatigue, and clients often consciously or unconsciously seek the position of comfort and forget to contract the muscle.[17] With the use of positioning devices and orthoses, Brand[17] states that it is "not so much to pull harder than the muscles but to maintain the tension longer." Both internal and external forces are load-inducing forces that provide tension to the tissue that elicits an internal resistive stress response that the client can typically feel within the tissue.[17] Externally loading the tissue with positioning, orthoses, or casting can provide prolonged noncyclical tension for the tissue.

Strain Rate

Another important principle to consider when applying treatment interventions is strain rate. Strain rate is the amount of tissue elongated per unit time. Strain rate is how fast or slow the tension is applied to elongate the tissue (Fig. 82.6). Basically, the more quickly the force is applied to strain the tissue to gain length, then the greater the force required and the greater the internal resistive stress. Brand[17] states that the application of tension too rapidly can cause micro-tearing and tissue rupture. However, if the same directed force is applied slowly, tissue injury can be avoided. Therapeutically, the therapist can better form trust and compliance with the burn patient if an adequate amount of

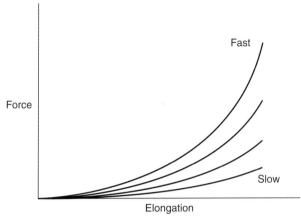

Fig. 82.6 Reaction of tissue at different strain rates. Notice the same endpoint of tissue elongation for fast or slowly applied force, but there is a greater amount of force required when a faster rate of force is applied. (From Richard RL, Staley MJ. Biophysical aspects of normal skin and burn scar. In: Richard RL, Staley MJ, eds. *Burn Care and Rehabilitation Principles and Practice.* Philadelphia: FA Davis; 1994:66; with permission.)

time is used to attain the desired amount of tissue length using less force, a reduced strain rate, and less pain.[14,17]

Stress–Relaxation: Biomechanical Tension-Biorheological Flow and Growth

The literal meaning of the term *biorheology* from the Greek root *rheo* is the science of flow, which does not emphasize the deformation caused by applied tension.[23,24] Within the *Quick Reference Dictionary for Occupational Therapy* (2nd edition), Jacobs[25] defines flow as "optimal experience," also without emphasizing deformation. Likewise, the concept of stress–relaxation emphasizes the optimal behavior of tissue flow and growth that occurs over time while deemphasizing the initial stress required to produce the deformed state needed for growth to occur. Because skin and scar and all viscoelastic tissues of the body exhibit a time-dependent response to stress,[6,14] there are significant differences between the shortening that occurs with ongoing contraction of unopposed burn scar, the acute episode of biomechanical creep, and the optimal behavior of biorheological growth that occurs with stress–relaxation over a prolonged period of time.

The prevention and correction of BSC uses the principle of stress–relaxation to oppose contracting scar and encourage tissue growth. Burn scar tissue that appears taut and under tension when positioned at end range or when an orthosis is first applied gradually becomes relaxed at follow-up a few hours or days later. This is an example of stress–relaxation. This principle of stress–relaxation has three consecutive stages: (1) acute application of cyclical tension until optimal tissue length is obtained, (2) fixed displacement and positioning of the lengthened tissue with noncyclical tension, (3) diminishing tension and tissue relaxation, and (4) growth over time.

Within the concept of stress–relaxation, there is an acute change in the direction, displacement, and placing and holding of the tissue in a lengthened position followed by a prolonged period of time. The outcome of uniting optimal "acute stress" with "chronic relaxation" is biosynthesis of fibrillar collagen or tissue growth. Therefore, stress–relaxation is a corollary and physiological consequence of the early physiological phase of creep.[24] United together, the physiological or elastic phase of creep is used to create the initial "stress" required within the concept of "stress–relaxation." This union between acute and chronic time is used to change the directional forces of the tissue.

Brand[17] states that the optimal tension occurs about midway into the elastic or physiologic portion of creep in the upper *b* and lower to mid *c* areas of the curve in Figure 82.4, making creep a required forerunner for biological growth. Cyclical tension is often applied using the preconditioning principle of successive length induction until "optimal tension–length" is obtained (see Fig. 82.5). The scar tissue begins to form in a different direction, thus becoming more anisotropic (oriented) and less isotropic (disoriented).

Wound contraction is a normal part of wound healing. Upon wound closure, a newly healed area at risk for BSC continues to shorten and assumes a comfortable homeostatic resting length. Often, early BSC can be measured as a 5- to 10-degree loss in ROM that can quickly worsen if not managed well. A new and more functional resting length for the contracted tissue can be obtained by using stress–relaxation to change the direction of the forces that shape the scar tissue. Initially applying tension (directed force) will oppose the contracture. This tension, if optimal, is the opposing-force needed to change the direction of the forces influencing tissue formation from a shortening direction to a lengthening direction. The scar tissue begins to form in a different direction, thus becoming more anisotropic (oriented) and less isotropic (disoriented).

As the tension is applied, the tissue begins to deform from its current resting length. This deformation is when the collagen unfolds, orients, aligns, and straightens in the direction of the applied tension along with slipping and shearing between fibers as they become taut and under tension. To prevent excessive microtearing, the applied tension needs to be optimal. Although this "deformation" phase is not typically emphasized in "stress–relaxation," it is critically needed because it serves as the precursor for tissue growth and extensibility.[6,16,17,19]

The acutely applied cyclical tension becomes noncyclical by positioning the tissue in an elongated state. This changed position is then held in place by noncyclical tension for a prolonged period of time. Here, the key to success is directed force under control, not force out of control. Biorheological flow is when noncyclical tension diminishes over time. This relieving flow of tension is the "relaxation" portion of the concept of stress–relaxation. Of note, when the elongated tissue length is gently positioned for a prolonged period of time, relief of internal resistive stress occurs by the externally applied tension being diverted, dissipated, and distributed throughout the length and area of the positioning device, orthosis, or cast.[16,17,22] The car jack depicted in Figure 82.7 illustrates how the tissue is halted by an equally opposed external force. Subsequently, this optimal noncyclical tension is positioned for a prolonged period of time.[6,16,17,24] In response, "stress" departs the tissue as the tissue enters into "relaxation" for an extended period of time, creating the potential for tissue accommodation and biological growth.[6,16,17] Thus, the tissue finds relief by leaving the initially applied cyclical tension in the past along with its accompanying internal resistive stress.[6] The clocks in Figure 82.7B represent a prolonged period of time, and the *green undulating curvature line* denotes future flow in the form of tissue growth after a prolonged period of time.[6] Brand[6,19] states that there is no easy way to measure tissue growth, and theoretically, repeated episodes of stress–relaxation can occur indefinitely.

The tissue goes beyond unfolding, aligning, and straightening and unassumingly submits to prolonged positioning by growing into a new resting length position via biosynthesis of fibrillar collagens. In response, stress–relaxation transforms the tissue through biorheological flow, and after an extended time, the experience of growth is seen clinically. This new length is needed for the tissue to maintain homeostatic control over the new resting length of the tissue.

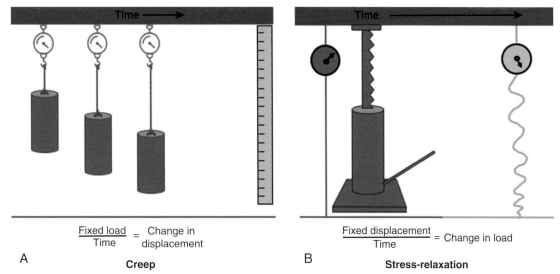

$$\frac{\text{Fixed load}}{\text{Time}} = \frac{\text{Change in}}{\text{displacement}}$$

A   **Creep**

$$\frac{\text{Fixed displacement}}{\text{Time}} = \text{Change in load}$$

B   **Stress-relaxation**

Fig. 82.7 Pictorial representation of creep (**A**) and stress–relaxation (**B**). Colors indicate changes over time with *blue* indicating the past, *green* indicating the future, and *red* indicating the present. **A,** Within the creep perspective, *blue* represents the constant application of tension over time as the past cyclical tension remains continually present within the tissue over acute time, and the *green* measuring stick connotes a definite terminal limit since the breaking point of tissue can be measured. **B,** From the perspective of stress–relaxation, the acutely applied tension immediately becomes noncyclical, and this past tension rapidly dissipates over prolonged time. *Green* shows the capability for tissue extensibility via biorheological flow and growth. (Modified from Brody G. The biomechanical properties of tissue. In: Rudolph R, ed. *Problems in Aesthetic Surgery: Biological Causes and Clinical Solutions.* St. Louis: CV Mosby; 1986:51; with permission.)

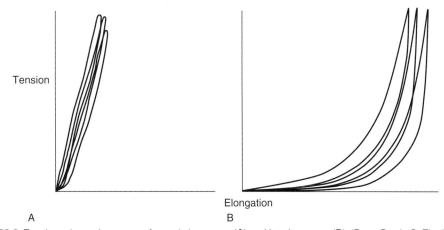

Fig. 82.8 Tension–elongation curves for early burn scar (**A**) and late burn scar (**B**). (From Brody G. The biomechanical properties of tissue. In: Rudolph R, ed. *Problems in Aesthetic Surgery: Biological Causes and Clinical Solutions.* St. Louis: CV Mosby; 1986:55; with permission.)

Dunn and colleagues[20] studied scar tissue with regards to "stiffness" and "extensibility" and explained that early burn scar and late burn scar are equally stiff with differing extensibility. When scar tissue is managed well throughout long-term rehabilitation, late burn scar will have more length and extensibility than early burn scar. The late burn scar does not demonstrate less stiffness.[20] Both early and late burn scar tissues are equally stiff at their final lengths with both early and late burn scar stress–strain slopes similar and curves becoming vertically parallel as they approach comparable yield points (Fig. 82.8). After a chronic period of 1 year, the burn scar tissue exhibits improved extensibility, not improved stiffness. Whereas the early burn scar was inextensible, the late burn scar is more extensible.[6,20]

EVALUATION AND TREATMENT

Burn Wound Severity: Extent, Location, and Depth
Burn Extent

The physician determines the severity of a burn injury by estimating the extent, location, and depth of the burn injury. In determining the size of the burn injury, the majority of physicians use the Lund and Browder chart to estimate percent TBSA burn.[13] The chart is used to assign and record the location and depth of the burn injury among 10 body surface area regions. The location and depth of the burn wounds are recorded on the Lund and Browder body diagram chart by shading in partial-thickness loss (PTL) and full-thickness loss (FTL) areas. The PTL and FTL percentages are summed to provide the extent of the

TABLE 82.2   Burn Wound Terminology and Classification

Depth of Burn	Depths of Tissue Involved	Appearance	Pain	Edema, Healing, and Scarring
Epidermal (first degree)	Involves epidermis with an irritated papillary dermis	Erythematous, pink, or red, or deeply tanned; dry; no blisters	Delayed pain; tender	Minimal to no edema, spontaneous healing via re-epithelialization, no scarring
Superficial partial thickness (superficial second degree)	Involves both the epidermis and extends into papillary dermis	Bright pink or red, mottled red; moist surface, weeping or glistening, intact blisters; erythematous and blanching with brisk capillary refill	Painful; sensitive to light touch, exposure to air currents, and changes in temperature	Moderate edema, spontaneous healing via re-epithelialization, minimal to no scarring (discoloration)
Deep partial thickness (deep second degree)	Involves the epidermis and papillary dermis and extends into the reticular dermis	Mixed red, wet surface, waxy white or cream colored beneath broken blisters, blanching with slow capillary refill	Sensitive to pressure; insensitive to light touch or soft pin prick	Marked edema, heals slowly (takes >3 weeks to heal), risk for excessive scarring
Full thickness (third degree)	Involves death of the entire depth of the skin, both the epidermis and the dermis	White (ischemic), charred, tan, yellowish-brown, reddish-brown; hemoglobin fixation; thrombosed vessels; dry, parchment-like, leathery, rigid; no blanching	Anesthetic; insensate	Marked edema with depressed area; must heal from the wound margins or by skin grafting or scarring
Subdermal (fourth degree)	Necrosis of skin and involves deep tissue below the level of the dermis such as nerve, muscle, tendon, or bone	Charred area; subcutaneous tissue evident	Anesthetic; insensate	Soft tissue defect with edema in surrounding area; risk for muscle, tendon, or bone necrosis and neurologic involvement; scarring

Adapted from Hedman et al,[13] Germann et al,[8] Lewis et al,[27] and Johnson.[28]

burn injury by percent TBSA. For instance, a 33% TBSA flame burn with 13% FTL to bilateral upper extremities and hands and 20% PTL to the face and anterior trunk. With burn severity involving greater than 20% TBSA, the physician uses the TBSA percentage to calculate lifesaving resuscitation needs.[12,13] After fluid resuscitation, and within approximately 36 to 72 hours postburn, the extent and location of burn injury remains relatively unchanged; however, the depth of burn injury is more precisely determined as edema begins to subside and the classification of burn wounds become more clearly demarcated. It should be noted that in accordance with the Lund and Browder chart, the right and left upper extremities account for 20% of the TBSA, with each arm equating to 4%, each forearm 3%, and each hand 3%.[13]

Burn Location

The location of burn injury is an important component in determining burn severity. The Lund and Browder visual representation can be further appreciated by segmenting the 10 general body regions into 33 segmented body surface areas which yields 16 anterior segments and 17 posterior segments. Together, the right and left upper extremities make up 12 of the 33 body segments. Along with the initial focus on burn extent, resuscitation, monitoring end-organ perfusion, and edema management procedures, the therapist uses the completed Lund and Browder chart to begin assessing burn location sites to determine skin recruitment areas or cutaneous functional units (CFUs) at risk for scar contracture and deformity. During the initial evaluation of the burned hand and upper extremity, the location and depth of burn injury assists the therapist in determining therapy time and resource allocation. Even though burn injury to the hands represents a small extent of TBSA, it is considered a major burn by the American Burn Association (ABA) because of the significant impact hands have on functional and aesthetic outcome.[26]

Burn Depth

Historically, burns have been classified into degree categories (i.e., first, second, third, and fourth). More recently, however, burns have been classified

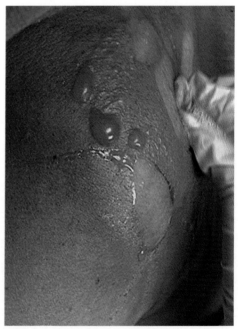

Fig. 82.9 Superficial partial-thickness burn with intact blisters.

by depth in relation to the tissues involved. Table 82.2 describes the classification of burn injury by depth in relation to the tissues involved: epidermal, superficial partial thickness, deep partial thickness, full thickness, and subdermal.[8,13,27,28] For example, a sunburn is a standard epidermal burn that irritates the papillary dermis with delayed pain and typically heals in 3 to 6 days with no scarring and contracture.[29] Superficial partial-thickness burns are deeper than a sunburn extending through the epidermis into the papillary dermis (Fig. 82.9). They are painful and best treated with daily dressing changes, and if further trauma and infection are avoided, the wound will heal spontaneously by re-epithelialization (Fig. 82.10).

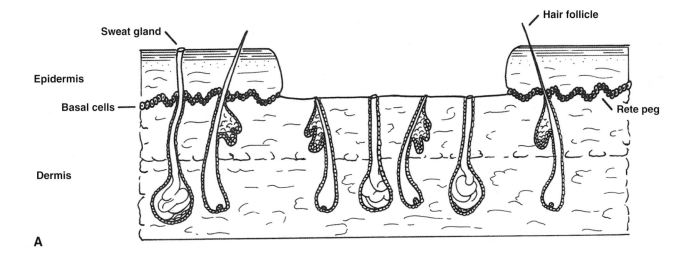

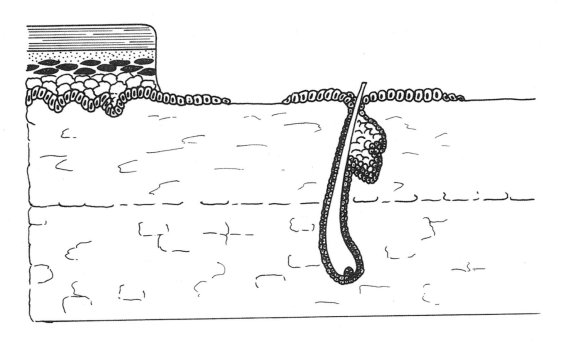

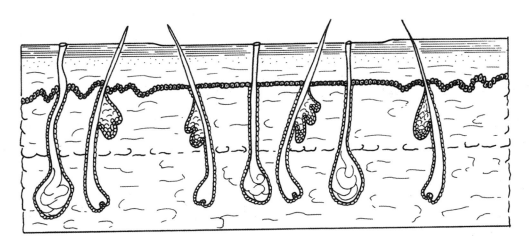

Fig. 82.10 A, After a partial-thickness injury, some of the dermis and its skin appendages remain intact and viable. **B,** The basal cells adjacent to the wound and in lining the appendages lose cell–cell contact inhibition and migrate across the viable wound surface. Migrating cells are replaced by proliferating basal cells at the wound edge and in the appendages. **C,** After migrating epidermal cells meet, cell–cell contact inhibition stops migration. Basal cells differentiate to re-create the different layers of the epidermis. The healed skin blisters easily because the rete pegs region does not redevelop for several months. (From Greenhalgh DG, Staley MJ. Burn wound healing. In: Richard RL, Staley MJ, eds. *Burn Care and Rehabilitation Principles and Practice*. Philadelphia: FA Davis; 1994:84; with permission.)

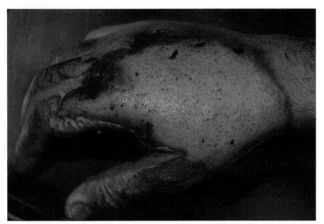

Fig. 82.11 Deep partial-thickness burn of the dorsal right hand.

A superficial partial-thickness burn can heal with minor color and texture changes but does not develop scarring.[30] In contrast, a deep partial-thickness injury results in loss of the epidermis and papillary dermis and extends into the reticular dermis (Fig. 82.11). This depth of burn is insensitive to light touch but sensitive to pressure, requires increased time to heal, and can create severe hypertrophic scarring.[13,31] Deep partial-thickness burn is best treated with early excision and grafting.[32] Figure 82.12 illustrates how the healing of skin grafts can be divided over three timed phases.

A full-thickness burn involves death of both the epidermis and dermis and is insensate[13] (Figs. 82.13 and 82.14). A full-thickness burn must heal from the wound margin and if larger than 3 cm in diameter is best treated with early excision and grafting to prevent significant scarring.[13,32] Subdermal burns involve tissue below the level of the dermis such as muscle, nerve, tendon, or bone and should be treated promptly by debriding devitalized tissues, ensuring exposed bone and tendons are covered by soft tissue and skin grafting to prevent significant scarring[13,32] (Fig. 82.15). Subdermal burns often require more extensive soft tissue coverage, such as full-thickness skin graft, rotational, cross-finger, or free flap, to provide protective covering of underlying exposed structures.

Burn injury to the hand occurs in more than 80% of all severe burns, and the upper extremity is involved in 89% of burns, making it the most common anatomically burned area of the body.[8] Therefore, knowledge of location and the character of the skin at the site of injury is imperative in determining the depth of the injury. For example, the palmar skin, with its thick epidermal layers, can endure greater thermal energy than the dorsal skin. However, in the presence of a deep palmar burn, very severe scarring and contracture typically ensue, and this should be considered in the design of orthotic and casting interventions (Fig. 82.16). Whether dorsal or palmar, small burns of the hand can result in severe impairment and functional limitations.[8]

Dorsal hand burns are predominantly involved in flame and flash flame explosive injuries, and deep burn injuries to the palm occur more frequently with war explosions, chemical exposure, friction burns, or high-voltage injuries.[8] Before surgical excision of full-thickness eschar to the dorsal skin of the hand, if tendon involvement is suspected, precautions should be taken as if tendon involvement were definitive.[8,13] The dorsal skin of the hand is thin and extensible with a fairly thin subdermal layer of fatty tissue with the most crucial areas over the proximal interphalangeal (PIP) and metacarpophalangeal (MCP) joints.[8] These characteristics allow for maximal tendon excursion and joint mobility but provide minimal protection. As seen in Figure 82.3B, the

skin over the PIP joint is especially thin, making it one of the most common sites for tendon exposure.[8,13,33] Rupture of the central slip with PIP joint exposure is one of the most common complications after deep dorsal hand burns. Hunt and Sato[34] found that damage to the extensor tissue over the PIP joint resulted in the worst functional outcomes. The paratenon brings blood supply and permits movement, but exposed tendons can dry and desiccate very quickly, so if suspected or confirmed, care must be taken to protect the integrity of the tendon.[8,33] Tendon exposure, or failure of skin graft adherence over these areas, typically leads to exposure of the joint with high risk for rupture of the central slip with PIP joint exposure, which leads to infection, cartilage erosion, and joint deformity, as shown in Figure 82.3.[8,13] Until durable tissue coverage is achieved, the tendon must be prevented from drying out by maintaining a moist environment with antibiotic ointments and petroleum-based gauze.[13]

Clinical Relevance

The severity of burn injury acutely impacts survival and surgical considerations. In addition, the extent, location, and depth of burn injury largely influence rehabilitation functional and aesthetic outcomes.[35] The biological formation of BSC, hypertrophic scarring, and overall long-term functioning are directly attributable to how the therapist is able to help the individual respond to and manage his or her severely burned hand and upper extremity.[13]

In the management of the burned hand and upper extremity, the therapist is chiefly responsible for promoting wound healing, protecting healing wounds, and preventing and correcting BSC, deformity, and hypertrophic scarring.[13] Throughout the course of recovery, the therapist remains directly involved in the care of the burned individual from the acute open wound phase through the intermediate wound healing and early scar remodeling phase and far into the long-term scar remodeling and maturation phase. The length of time in which the therapist will follow the burned individual depends on the severity of the burn wounds, contractures, and hypertrophic scarring.[36] In general, most of a therapist's time and resources are spent on burned survivors who heal by skin graft and scar.

During the acute phase, the therapist typically uses the following methods to evaluate the burn wounds over time: Lund and Browder to assess burn wound severity, along with the number of days since burn injury or postburn day, number of days since surgical excision and grafting or postoperative day, and hand edema measurements using either figure-of-8 method or volumetric measurements (see Chapter 57). During the acute phase, the therapist's focus is on edema management and wound protection along with remaining acutely aware of the number of days required to achieve wound closure. Also, during the acute phase, ROM is typically within normal limits unless there is a preburn physical limitation in movement, which the therapist should document in the patient's chart.

The therapist must track and record the number of days for wounds to heal, especially areas at risk for BSC and limitations in ROM. Deitch and associates[31] indicate that the length of time to accomplish wound closure was the single most important factor in predicting the formation of hypertrophic scar. The results of their study indicated that 78% of the burn injuries requiring greater than 21 days to heal developed hypertrophic scar. Because of this risk for scarring, skin grafting is advised for the burned individual whose wounds will not heal within 3 weeks of injury.[37] Furthermore, Deitch and associates[31] recommend that the application of force such as compression be mandatory for burn wounds that require more than 21 days to heal or skin grafting.[31,37] Deitch and associates[31] further recommend the application of force to be used in burn wounds that take between 14 and 21 days to heal.

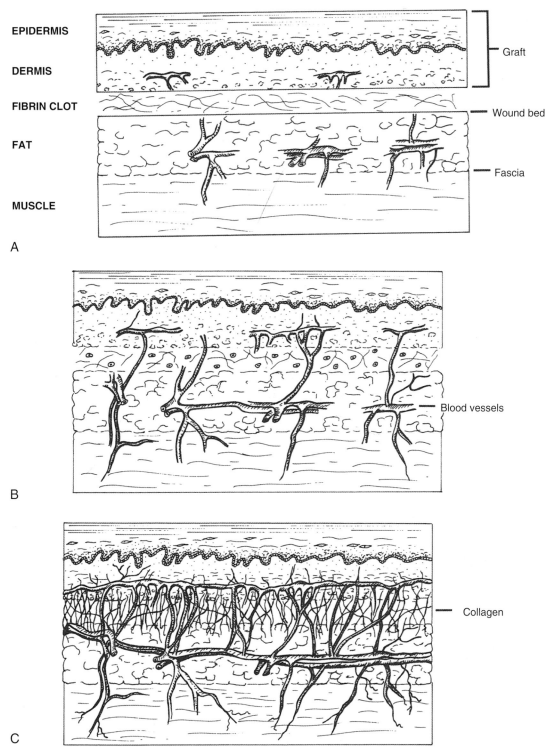

EPIDERMIS

DERMIS

— Graft

FIBRIN CLOT

— Wound bed

FAT

— Fascia

MUSCLE

A

— Blood vessels

B

— Collagen

C

Fig. 82.12 The healing of skin grafts involves three phases. **A,** During the initial phase of serum imbibition, the graft is whitish-pink and held on the wound bed with staples or sutures and weak fibrin bonds. The cells survive by diffusion of nutrients from the wound bed serum fluid. **B,** At 24 to 48 hours, new capillaries invade the skin graft as anastomosis occurs; the graft becomes pink, marking the phase of revascularization. **C,** The graft becomes pinkish-red during days 4 and 5 when organization starts, and collagen linkages are made between the wound bed and the graft to create firm adherence. (From Greenhalgh DG, Staley MJ. Burn wound healing. In: Richard RL, Staley MJ, eds. *Burn Care and Rehabilitation Principles and Practice*. Philadelphia: FA Davis; 1994:88; with permission.)

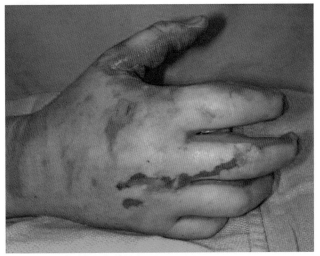

Fig. 82.13 Full-thickness burn of the hand.

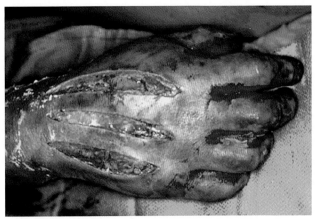

Fig. 82.14 Full-thickness burn with dorsal hand escharotomies.

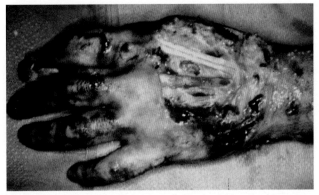

Fig. 82.15 Subdermal burn trauma of the dorsal hand with exposed extensor tendons.

Throughout the late acute and early intermediate phase, the focus remains on promoting and supporting wound healing. The therapist assists with wound care of the hand and upper extremity while protecting wounds and skin grafts to promote graft adherence and minimize risk for graft loss caused by mechanical shear forces. As the proliferative repair stage of wound healing subsides, the skin and scar tissue remodeling phase commences. In this stage, tissue remodeling, realignment, and elongation are encouraged by applying

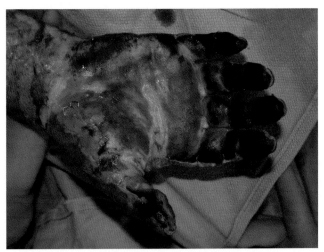

Fig. 82.16 Deep palmar burn.

tolerable gentle tension to contracting collagen fiber scars and gentle compression to areas at risk for hypertrophic scarring. Throughout the intermediate phase, ROM is closely monitored while using contracture management techniques such as encouraging ADL performance, exercise, positioning, and orthotic use.[13] Additionally, upon wound closure, the therapist begins describing the appearance of the healed wounds using a scar assessment tool such as the Vancouver Scar Scale. Scar and contracture management will continue throughout long-term rehabilitation.[38]

Edema: Postburn Assessment and Treatment

Extensive tissue edema develops after severe thermal injury.[12,39] The acute postburn swelling pattern involves marked bloating of the skin on the dorsal surface of the hand (see Fig. 82.3A). This marked edema results in flattening of the hand and loss of the longitudinal and transverse arches.[11,13,40,41] Postburn hand edema is caused by an increase in vascular permeability combined with a shift of fluids to the extravascular space. Edema is minor and transitory in superficial partial-thickness hand and upper extremity burns in which there is less than 20% TBSA involvement and minimal fluid is leaked into the extravascular space. However, in deep partial-thickness and full-thickness hand and upper extremity burns, in which there is involvement of greater than 20% TBSA, marked edema formation is more severe and lingering because of both increased capillary permeability and the massive fluid loads often required to maintain intravascular volume.[11,42]

The assessment and treatment of edema differs throughout each of the three stages of wound healing. The stages consist of the inflammatory phase, which begins at injury and lasts 3 to 5 days; the proliferative or fibroplastic phase, which can last 2 to 6 weeks depending on the depth of injury and wound closure method; and the maturation or remodeling phase, which begins upon wound closure and can last from 6 months to 2 years.[43] Edema management should remain a priority throughout the inflammatory, proliferative, and maturation stages of recovery to maintain tissue perfusion, prevent wound conversion, minimize residual stiffening of the soft tissue, and minimize loss of tendon glide and joint mobility. Depending on the location and depth of the burn injury, techniques for reducing edema differ for each of the three stages of wound healing. Therefore, it is essential to monitor the severity and progress of hand or upper extremity edema throughout recovery to prevent stagnation of protein rich fluid in the interstitium, which in turn can form into a fibrotic tissue state with subsequent stiffness.[42,43]

Assessment

Measuring hand edema throughout the stages of healing and recovery is an important aspect of the therapist's evaluation. Postburn edema affects all areas of the body and is particularly troublesome in the hands. Upon initial inpatient evaluation, the therapist will typically assess hand and upper extremity edema using the figure-of-8 method for the hand and the upper extremity on a subjective scale as minimal, moderate, or severe. Treatment consists of elevation and ROM exercises. Edema in the inflammatory phase of wound healing is mainly water and electrolytes—soft, and easy to mobilize as the wound prepares for healing.[43] With that, edema usually dissipates at the end of the inflammatory phase and with wound closure during the proliferative phase of healing.[42] However, if the edema persists or worsens beyond 7 to 10 days, the therapist should obtain baseline edema measurements to monitor the effects of treatment over time.[44]

To objectively assess the size of the hand and wrist a valid, reliable, timely, and clinically practical technique is necessary to monitor severity and progress over time.[45] There are several standardized clinical assessment methods used to accurately assess the increased size of hand or digit. Currently, the most commonly used methods to objectively assess postburn hand edema include volumetry, circumferential, and figure-of-8 measurement (see Chapter 57). Volumetry is a reliable and valid measurement technique and can be efficacious in an outpatient clinic; however, it is time consuming and clinically impractical to administer in an inpatient or intensive care unit setting.[41,45] The circumferential method uses a flexible tape measure or circumferential finger gauge and is more time efficient but lacks intra- and interrater reliability because of variations in reference landmarks among therapists as hand edema changes over time. Moreover, the circumferential method is a single-plane measurement that does not adequately reflect the volume and size of the hand and wrist.[45] The figure-of-8 tape measure method requires minimal equipment; is simple to perform; and is time efficient, low cost, and effective in demonstrating reliability and validity.[41,45]

Treatment

The most important principle in the acute management of a burned hand and upper extremity is maintenance of tissue perfusion, which is assured by adequate fluid resuscitation and removal of any mechanical obstruction of arterial and venous flow to the extremity and hand.[42] Acutely, if the hand is placed in a dependent position, then the presence of lingering hand edema can limit end organ perfusion to the skin causing partial-thickness loss to convert to a full-thickness loss.

Edema progressively increases during the first 48 hours postburn, and so can the pressure within the compartments of the arm, forearm, and hand.[42,46] Therapists involved in the treatment of these hands must be aware of the early signs of vascular insufficiency because edema can be compounded by the tourniquet effect of an underlying circumferential burn eschar, and the potential for vascular insufficiency resulting in tissue ischemia is great.[11,42] Consequently, excessive intracompartmental hand and forearm pressures can impair arteriovenous function.

Edema must be monitored carefully during the first 48 hours postburn to ensure that the hand is adequately perfused. Palpable radial and ulnar pulses should be monitored to ensure forearm and hand perfusion, but their presence does not always guarantee adequate flow into the hand. If a Doppler ultrasound flow meter is available, then examination should be done to determine flow in the palmar arch. If vascular insufficiency is suspected, the patient's physician should be notified immediately, all dressings should be removed, and the upper extremity should be elevated. Escharotomies are performed immediately if vascular insufficiency is confirmed.[11,42]

If palpable radial and ulnar pulsations cease or if the flow in the palmar arch is lost on ultrasonic examination, then decompression is performed. If warranted and escharotomies of the hand are not performed, then intrinsic muscle ischemia can occur with a resultant intrinsic-minus deformity. In cases of electrical injuries, fasciotomies are often mandatory because the primary injury is usually in the muscle, and sensory deficit in the distribution of the median or ulnar nerve is an indication for decompression of the involved nerve.[42] If a pulse is present, then adequate vascular sufficiency exists, and the limb should be elevated, exercised, and checked hourly for continued evidence of perfusion.[41,42]

The treatment of hand burn edema is of paramount importance throughout each phase of recovery especially if it persists beyond the inflammatory phase of recovery.[40,42] The majority of edema resolves during the acute inflammatory phase as the initial physiological response to burn injury and fluid resuscitation ends.[13] During the proliferative phase of wound healing, repair of the injured tissue is initiated and completed primarily through epidermal, dermal, and skin graft healing.

Edema that progresses into the fibroplasia phase is of particular concern to the therapist.[43] Prolonged postburn edema of the hand and forearm can result in devastating physiological changes that can lead to decreased joint motion and limit the overall function and dexterity of the hand.[45,46] Early intervention is applied to prevent this edema from becoming an ongoing problem. The edema fluid will begin to become more viscous and referred to as exudate because of an increase in protein-rich content. This can lead to dense fibrosis and thickening of the tissues, leading to underlying adhesions of tendon and sheaths, joint capsules, synovial membranes, and fascial layers.[43] The consequences of prolonged hand edema can result in chronic pain and the formation of extensive scarring leading to adhesions, disfigurement, and debilitating contractures.

During the fibroplastic or repair stage of healing, burn wounds heal or become nearly healed. It is typically during this proliferative phase of healing that clients begin to become more responsive and oriented to person, place, time, and situation. The client's improved responsiveness allows her or him to participate in the process of actively mobilizing edema with AROM exercises, ADL performance, continuous elevation, and compressive wraps. The therapist should practice caution when using self-adherent elastic compression wraps such as Coban Ace wraps to the hands and forearms. If compression is applied too early or incorrectly, elastic wraps can contribute to vascular compromise or skin graft loss caused by mechanical shearing. The wrap should be applied uniformly and must not have greater compression proximally than distally.[13] Therapists should frequently monitor vascularity for areas receiving compressive wrap treatment. While performing ambulatory activity as an inpatient, dependent positioning of the hands and upper extremity can be avoided by applying a cross-tube of PVC pipe or bar to an intravenous (IV) pole for the client to grasp on to with his or her hands or rest his or her hands on during ambulation.

During the transition from the intermediate to the early phase of long-term rehabilitation, longstanding edema can become chronic, resulting in the need for extended use of compression wraps or edema gloves to manage gains made in edema reduction (Fig. 82.17). Continual use of Tubigrip, self-adherent wrap, and edema gloves are typically used to keep edema from progressing throughout the maturation stage of healing and long-term rehabilitation. If edema persists through this stage, it will often become hard, thick, and brawny. Readers are referred to Chapter 57 for further edema management techniques that will effectively mobilize chronic edema.

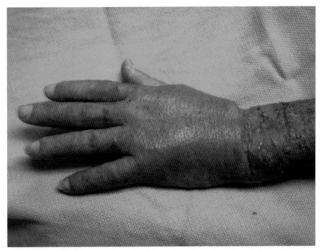

Fig. 82.17 Chronic hand edema primarily caused by circumferential fascial excision proximal to the hand resulting in compromised venous flow.

Positioning the Hand and Upper Extremity

Effective positioning of the severely burned hand and upper extremity is essential in achieving three of the main rehabilitation goals: decreasing edema, protecting healing wounds, and preventing and correcting BSC and deformity. Although each of these aims is often treated simultaneously, one is usually of primary concern during each phase of rehabilitation. Therefore, the primary, secondary, and tertiary purposes of positioning change as the patient progresses from the acute, intermediate, and long-term phases of rehabilitation.

Acute Phase

Acutely, optimal positioning of the hand and upper extremity is important for managing edema. In cases of severe thermal injury, during the initial 36 hours, it is important to monitor for signs and symptoms of vascular insufficiency or compartment syndrome.

Throughout the first 3 days after burn injury, the primary purpose of positioning is to reduce edema throughout the upper extremity to improve survivability of the burn wound zone of stasis until the patient is stabilized and edema subsides to a manageable level. The optimal position to manage edema of the upper extremity is placing the hand slightly higher than the elbow and the elbow slightly higher than the shoulder.[13,43] Elevation is especially helpful when initiated immediately postburn or upon admission to the hospital. Elevation uses gravity to facilitate venous and lymphatic flow out of the burned hand, helping to decrease the hydrostatic pressure in the blood vessels, which in turn decreases the capillary filtration pressure at the arterial end.[43] Positioning of the hand and upper extremity in a dependent position at night must be avoided. Elevation at night will assist with sustaining the edema-reducing benefits of activity performed throughout the day.[13]

Intermediate Phase

The primary purpose of positioning during the intermediate phase is to help protect healing wounds, skin grafts and exposed tendon, joints, and bone, if any.[13] Replacing lost dermal elements with excision and grafting followed by healing within 21 days postgrafting to include the edges of the grafts can greatly assist with preventing BSC and deformity.[47,48] The secondary and tertiary reasons for positioning during the intermediate phase are preventing peripheral neuropathies, providing anticontracture alignment of joints and joint structures, preventing and correcting BSCs by aligning and shaping reparative scar formation, and reducing edema.

Long-Term Phase

At the later stages of the intermediate phase and throughout the long-term phase of rehabilitation, the primary purpose of positioning is the prevention and correction of BSC and deformity. Positioning is used to prevent BSC by inducing optimal opposing tension against the forces of scar contraction during scar formation and remodeling.[47] Positioning for elongation requires maintaining tissue at an optimal length short of its breaking point, and over time, stress becomes relaxation with added tissue extensibility (see Fig. 82.7B).

Positioning the hand and upper extremity, with or without orthoses, is not a complicated concept to learn and understand; however, it can be terribly difficult to implement in practice. This difficulty is evident in that mortality rates are low, but morbidity rates remain high. Currently, 96.7% of burn patients survive and transition through the acute and intermediate phases of recovery and into long-term rehabilitation with many survivors sustaining serious scarring and lifelong physical impairment and disabilities.[49] A commitment to effective positioning throughout all phases of rehabilitation can minimize physical impairment but can be very challenging to implement and maintain and could be a reason morbidity rates remain high. With clear hindsight, therapists ultimately know that "the position of comfort will become the position of contracture." Therefore, in knowing this truism, therapists should be encouraged to sustain forethought and commitment to the dictum that "the position of optimal discomfort is the genesis toward preventing and correcting contracture and deformity."[2] In knowing the advantages of gentle prolonged tension with positioning, the therapist should encourage his or her patient to endure the short-term discomfort needed to achieve a new long-term comfortable resting length of skin and scar tissue that is more extensible and functional. Thus, avoiding the need for surgical releases and reconstruction.

Whether the patient is in a bed or chair or ambulating, the therapist will need to implement creative and diverse orthotic and nonorthotic techniques to optimally position the hand and upper extremity. Some of the nonorthotic ways include foam wedges; pillows; silicone-filled pillows; bedside tables; metal troughs attached to the bed or chair; and metal, plastic, or thermoplastic arm troughs suspended from a trapeze mechanism or an IV pole[50-53] (Fig. 82.18). Some of the common ways to position the hand and upper extremity using orthoses are discussed in the orthotic intervention section of this text.

Positioning the upper extremity can be restrictive or unrestrictive. With good education and clear instruction, an adult patient without learning difficulties can understand the purpose of positioning and orthotic use to manage scar contracture and is usually cooperative in following a positioning plan.[54] However, when the burn patient is a child or the patient has learning difficulties, she or he typically does not have the ability to comprehend the purpose of positioning and orthotics. Therefore, the staff, parents, or caregivers often create diverse methods to assist the child with tolerating and enduring the discomfort of positioning, orthoses, and exercise such as distraction, play, and other creative treatment techniques.

Shoulder and Axilla

At the expense of stability, the shoulder complex allows the upper extremity a wide range of mobility. Its articulations are loose; therefore, consistent positioning of the upper extremity throughout recovery from severe burn injury is important for maintaining and regaining mobility. For severe burn injury to the anteroposterior lateral trunk, axilla, and medial upper extremity, the recommended position for

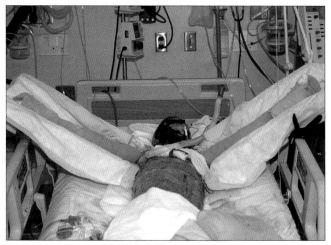

Fig. 82.18 Shoulder positioning. (From Serghiou MA, Ott S, C, Cowan A, et al. Burn rehabilitation along the continuum of care. In: Herndon DN, ed. *Total Burn Care*. 5th ed. Philadelphia: Elsevier; 2018:476–508; with permission.)

the shoulder axilla complex is 90 to 110 degrees of abduction with 15 to 20 degrees of horizontal adduction, forward flexion, and maximal external rotation.[13,51] This crucifix position with some shoulder flexion unfolds the inferior capsular ligament between the necks of the scapula and humerus, preventing tightness of deep tissues of the shoulder joint capsule. External rotation of the humerus with shoulder abduction is important because shoulder abduction alone can cause impingement of the rotator cuff musculature between the acromion of the scapula and greater tubercle of the humerus. Externally rotating the glenohumeral joint allows the greater tubercle to clear the acromion and helps to counteract anticipated deformities of internal rotation and adduction to maintain elongation of soft tissues of the shoulder complex. Placement in horizontal adduction anatomically reduces the potential for traction on the brachial plexus.[13,50–53] Lester and coworkers[51] demonstrated that shoulder positioning of 150 degrees for 2-hour increments is safe and well tolerated. Therefore, to maintain and regain the movements of the shoulder complex, skin and scar recruitment lengthening exercises followed by periodic shoulder positioning at 150 degrees throughout the day are encouraged. Shoulder positioning alternates between the crucifix pose (90–110 degrees), which maintains functional length of deep tissues, and the victory pose (~150 degrees), which opposes contracting burn scar by lengthening the more superficial skin and scar tissue areas that allow for optimal functional extensibility.

Elbow and Forearm

Acutely, the basic position of the elbow is extension with the elbow slightly elevated above the shoulder and heart. Severe burn injury involving the anterior arm and forearm often leads to limited skin recruitment required for elbow extension, resulting in a flexion contracture. Severe burn to the loose skin on the posterior aspect of the elbow can lead to joint exposure. Therefore, full elbow extension, short of terminal extension, is the protective position for the elbow. If the elbow joint is exposed posteriorly, extension is often maintained with an orthosis for several weeks until durable tissue coverage is achieved. If the joint is not exposed and not suspected of becoming exposed, then mobilization with progressively increasing elbow ROM can begin very soon after the burn injury. As with the shoulder, the elbow is integral to positioning of the hand for function, and elbow movement to full or near-full flexion with 100° arc of motion is more important for overall function than range to full or near-full extension.[50–53]

Forearm rotation is essential for accurate hand placement and function and is usually maintained postburn injury because minimal skin recruitment is needed for pronation and supination. However, pronator and supinator musculature is often injured in severe electrical burns to the upper extremity. Depending on the location and severity of the injury, the forearm can be positioned in neutral or in slight supination using orthoses or other devices designed by the therapist.[52–53]

Wrist and Hand

Managing the severely burned hand requires a thorough understanding of the effects of burn injury to the dorsal and palmar surfaces of the wrist, hand, and underlying structures. Superficial hand burns result in minor, transient edema and should be positioned to reduce edema but typically do not require orthoses. Because superficial partial thickness wounds heal by re-epithelialization, there is minimal to no risk for BSC.[50] In the presence of partial thickness burn injury, it is important to allow frequent skin mobility and joint movement, as seen in the performance of functional activity, in order to prevent joint stiffness and the potential for skin contracture development.

Deep partial-thickness and full-thickness injuries exhibit more severe and prolonged postburn edema. The overall appearance of a severely burned edematous hand is an intrinsic-minus posture (see Fig. 82.3A). A more specific description of this deformed posture is marked dorsal hand edema that has recruited all available extensible skin complicated by tight restrictive eschar causing the hand to assume an antifunctional position with wrist flexion, MCP joint hyperextension, interphalangeal (IP) joint flexion, thumb radial adduction, and thumb IP joint flexion. Acutely, during lifesaving fluid resuscitation, the intrinsic-minus posture of the hand is primarily caused by edema. However, during the late intermediate and long-term phases of rehabilitation, the cause of the intrinsic-minus deformity is no longer edema but the loss of extensible tissue caused by pliable dorsal hand skin being replaced by burn scar tissue throughout the dorsum of the hand. The unopposed force of scar contracture is usually the cause of long-term burn scar intrinsic minus deformity.

Acute positioning of the hand after deep partial-thickness and full-thickness burn injury is for edema control. Typically, within 36 to 72 hours hand edema subsides to a manageable level. Other than the initial 5 to 7 days postoperative excision and grafting or exposed deep structures, it is recommended that the wrist and hand be exercised routinely and self-care functional activity be encouraged as tolerated. The wrist and hand with deep partial-thickness and full-thickness injury should be maintained in a position that opposes impending scar contracture when not performing activity and exercises.

The recommended functional position of the wrist is extension. Wrist extension is essential to control the position of the fingers to prevent intrinsic-minus posturing. With or without a wrist orthosis, the wrist is maintained in an extended position, which allows the MCP joints to fall into flexion because of the normal tenodesis action of the hand and fingers. At night, the severely burned hand is typically placed in a volar forearm-based orthosis resembling an intrinsic-plus position with the wrist between 0 and 30 degrees of extension, 70 and 80 degrees of MCP flexion, and the IP joints in full extension.

ORTHOTIC INTERVENTION

Orthotic intervention is integral in protecting healing wounds and grafts, directing forces, and aligning collagen throughout the management of burn injury to the hand and upper extremity.[55] Orthoses are primarily used to protect healing wounds and grafts and to prevent and correct BSC and deformity to achieve optimal functional outcomes at the conclusion of rehabilitation. In addition to the destruction of the skin, severe burns to the hand and upper extremity can affect deep

BOX 82.1 Purposes of UE Orthoses

Hand and upper extremity orthoses are often used to:
- Reduce edema during the acute emergent phase (0–72 hours postinjury)
- Protect healing skin grafts or flaps
- Protect exposed tendons or joints
- Prevent and correct contractures
- Remodel and shape the formation of scar tissue
- Correct joint alignment
- Improve or maintain ROM
- Provide resistive strengthening of weak muscles
- Assist weak or partially innervated muscles to facilitate function
- Provide functional positioning to allow for movement and ADL performance

ADL, Activity of daily living; *ROM,* range of motion.
Adapted from Daugherty MB, Carr-Collins JA. Splinting techniques for the burn patient. In: Richard RL, Staley MJ, eds. *Burn Care and Rehabilitation: Principles and Practice.* Philadelphia, FA Davis;1994:242-323.

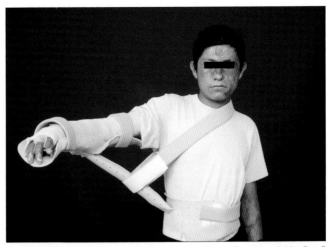

Fig. 82.19 The "airplane splint" orthosis. (From Serghiou MA, Ott S, C, Cowan A, et al. Burn rehabilitation along the continuum of care. In: Herndon DN, ed. *Total Burn Care.* 5th ed. Philadelphia: Elsevier; 2018:476–508; with permission.)

structures such as tendons, muscles, joints, nerves, and vessels. Therefore, the therapist must know the anatomy and kinesiology of the entire upper extremity as well as the basic principles of orthotic fabrication (see Chapters 106 to 109).

Box 82.1 lists a variety of purposes for which upper extremity orthoses might be fabricated.[56] The therapist should have a good understanding of mechanical force systems, the importance of distributing pressure across larger surface areas, increasing mechanical advantage, strap placement, rotational and translational forces, reciprocal parallel forces or three-point fixation, and torque effect. Each of these factors can assist greatly in preventing and correcting BSCs while preventing pressure areas, mechanical shear forces, subluxation, dislocation, and other injuries to the joints and skin and scar areas being treated. After they have been designed, fabricated, fitted and tested, orthoses should:
- Not migrate or shift causing kinetic friction and shearing
- Not cause pain
- Not occlude wound drainage
- Be purposeful
- Be cosmetically appealing
- Be easily applied and removed
- Be light weight and low profile

Keeping all of these principles in mind during the construction and management of orthoses can help improve the patient's satisfaction, adherence, and compliance with orthotic wear schedules. Careful attention to the patient's complaints about an orthosis can provide very useful clues as to ways to improve fit and wear tolerance.[18]

As a guiding resource for using custom fabricated orthoses in managing burn patients, Richard and coworkers[57] published an *Atlas and Compendium of Burn Splints* organized from head to toe describing more than 90 orthoses used to protect healing wounds, prevent and correct BSC, and minimize hypertrophic scarring throughout the acute, intermediate, and long-term phases of burn rehabilitation. The *Atlas and Compendium* describes the orthoses and the materials used in the fabrication along with instructions, advantages, disadvantages, indications, precautions, contraindications, and references. This comprehensive guidebook of orthoses includes all known upper extremity orthoses used to manage burn patients and can be used to generate new ideas and improved methods.[57]

Generally, edema peaks within 36 to 48 hours postburn.[46] When applying orthoses during these initial 48 hours, caution should be taken to avoid further compromising the vascularity of the injured hand. Orthosis straps can have a tourniquet effect and increase interstitial pressures within the anatomic compartments.[11,42] In cases of persistent edema, the hand can be elevated and positioned in the intrinsic-plus position within a burn hand orthosis to aid in preventing deformity and reducing edema.

Immediately after grafting, the upper extremity often requires an orthosis and appropriate positioning to protect the grafted sites and prevent the development of contractures.[52,53] Full-thickness burns that result in tendon or joint exposure require immediate and constant immobilization with an orthosis Kirschner wire fixation by the physician until durable tissue coverage is achieved. In the case of an electrical burn to the upper extremity in which peripheral nerve damage is affecting hand function, the therapist should position and protect the involved joints to prevent anticipated muscle–tendon tightness, joint stiffness, and deformities.[11,50,56,58]

Shoulder and Axilla Orthoses

Acutely, the upper extremity positioning program focuses on reducing edema through elevation. Failure to reduce edema in the first 48 to 72 hours can contribute to the development of a fixed deformity, resembling an intrinsic-minus hand. Additionally, improper elevation techniques of the upper extremity can lead to soft tissue calcification, increased bone density, and compressive neuropathies. Positioning of the shoulder can be achieved with custom orthoses, prefabricated abduction pillows, silicone-filled pillows, bedside tables, foam arm troughs, metal abduction troughs, and thermoplastic slings suspended from a trapeze mechanism. The use of orthoses to position the shoulder and axilla becomes more intensive as scar contractures develop along with increased risk for loss of functional motion. Airplane orthoses are used to prevent and correct axillary contractures, and postoperatively they are used to protect grafts and reconstructive procedures (Fig. 82.19). To accommodate wound dressings and promote healing, a three-piece airplane orthosis can be fabricated. Additional modifications are often required if the patient has a residual limb from amputation. Prefabricated airplane orthoses come equipped with mechanisms that allow for adjustments depending on available shoulder ROM. A figure-of-8 axillary wrap can be used in conjunction with an airplane orthosis to provide compression for axillary contour and elongation of skin surfaces (Fig. 82.20). For contracture management of the shoulder to be successful, the positioning program must be supplemented by ROM and strengthening exercises.[50,53,56,58–60]

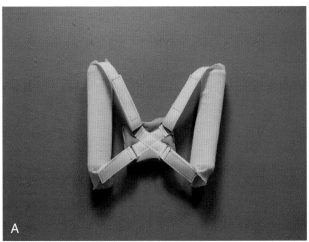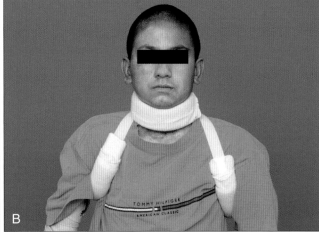

Fig. 82.20 A and **B,** The "figure-of-8" axillary wrap. (From Serghiou MA, Ott S, C, Cowan A, et al. Burn rehabilitation along the continuum of care. In: Herndon DN, ed. *Total Burn Care.* 5th ed. Philadelphia: Elsevier; 2018:476–508; with permission.)

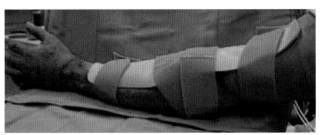

Fig. 82.21 Elbow extension orthosis.

Elbow Orthoses

Acutely, to manage upper extremity edema, elevation slightly above the shoulder and elbow extension is the desired position. Severe burn injury involving the elbow can result in flexion contracture and threaten posterior exposure of the joint. Therefore, full extension is the protective position for the elbow. If the posterior elbow joint is exposed, then extension needs to be rigidly maintained with an elbow extension orthosis for several weeks until durable tissue coverage is achieved. If the joint is not exposed, mobilizing the elbow is encouraged to maintain or improve elbow flexion and is begun within 48 hours after burn injury.

Depending on the location and severity of the injury, the forearm can be positioned in neutral or slight supination. Static elbow orthoses can be custom fabricated by the therapist using thermoplastic or other materials (Fig. 82.21). They may be fabricated as indicated over dressings and used immediately after surgery to protect healing grafts of the arm. Static progressive and dynamic elbow extension or flexion orthoses can be used to provide prolonged gentle sustained stretch and assist in the correction of contractures.[53,56,58,61]

Wrist Orthoses

Throughout recovery, while exercise and ADL performance are encouraged, the therapist should consider fabricating a wrist orthosis to provide stability and allow for improved function with grasp and pinch activities. Wrist orthoses may be custom fabricated by the therapist in cases of contractures, neurologic impairment, and weakness.[18,56,58] The design of the wrist orthosis often varies depending on the presence and location of wound and scar and pain or hypersensitivity and can be either dorsal or volar based. As wounds continue to heal and scar becomes shortened, taut, and hypertrophic, the therapist should assess the need for specialized orthoses to counteract the contractile forces limiting tissue extensibility. Contracting scar, if not attended to with an opposing force, can lead to the development of hand and wrist deformities with functional deficits.

Burn Hand Orthoses: Antideformity Position

Optimal positioning for a severely burned hand 72 hours postburn injury is the intrinsic-plus position with the wrist in 0 to 30 degrees of extension, 70 to 80 degrees of MCP joint flexion, and the IP joints in full extension with the thumb in a combination of carpometacarpal (CMC) joint palmar–radial abduction.[53,58] Hands having tendon or joint exposure should always be immobilized to prevent desiccation and tendon rupture until durable tissue coverage is achieved. Wounds with exposed tendon or bone should be assessed daily, and exercise should be performed as directed by the referring physician under the direct supervision of the therapist.[62] Alternately, if tendon and joint exposure is not suspected over the dorsum of the hand and fingers, some therapists advocate for the position of wrist 0 degrees, MCP joints at 80 degrees, and IP joints in slight flexion (~30 degrees), deeming the position to be "safe" and suggesting that this position helps to regain extensibility of skin and scar folds covering the dorsal IP joints, allowing for composite finger flexion. If the volar thumb web space sustained no burn injury or superficial partial-thickness injury, then the thumb should be positioned in palmar abduction with the finger MCP joints flexed and IP joints extended. If the dorsal and volar aspects of the thumb webspace have deep partial-thickness or full-thickness wounds, then the thumb should be positioned halfway between radial and palmar abduction with the finger MCP joints flexed and IP joints extended.

The antideformity intrinsic-plus position is often achieved by fabricating a custom hand burn orthosis (Fig. 82.22) or applying a prefabricated hand burn orthosis and securely fitting it with straps or gauze wrap. This orthosis opposes the intrinsic-minus posture of the wrist and hand to minimize the risk for BSC and joint contracture by preserving and regaining the tissue extensibility needed for functional movement.[50–53] However, this position is not sustained if the strapping or gauze wrap is applied incorrectly because this orthosis has a tendency to slip distally as the hand slides proximally reassuming the deformed position, especially the small finger.[56,57] Therefore, the placement and maintenance of the hand in an antideformity intrinsic-plus position for a prolonged period of time requires a well-fitting orthosis with the strapping being critical

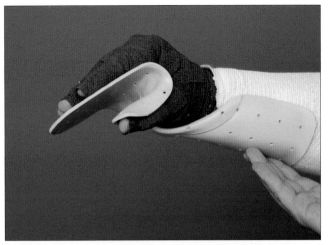

Fig. 82.22 Burn hand orthosis. (From Serghiou MA, Ott S, C, Cowan A, et al. Burn rehabilitation along the continuum of care. In: Herndon DN, ed. *Total Burn Care.* 5th ed. Philadelphia: Elsevier; 2018:476–508; with permission.)

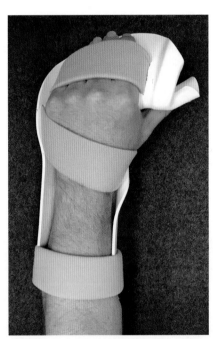

Fig. 82.23 Burn hand orthosis with diagonal dorsal hand strapping to prevent hand from slipping and sliding out of the intrinsic-plus position.

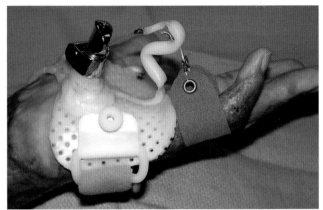

Fig. 82.24 Cobra design static progressive small finger metacarpophalangeal joint flexion orthosis.

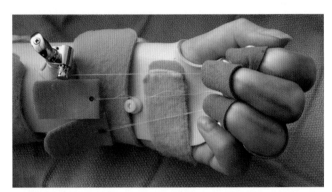

Fig. 82.25 Static progressive composite finger flexion orthosis. Note the blanching tightness of the dorsal scar to help restore dorsal interphalangeal skin and scar fold extensibility.

for optimal fit[18] (Fig. 82.23). At least three dorsal-based straps should be used to secure the hand within the orthosis. The proximal forearm strap secures the distal forearm within the trough of the orthosis. The middle strap is the key to preventing the orthosis from slipping distally and the hand from sliding proximally; it should be snugly fit and well conformed to the wide surface area along the first metacarpal before running diagonally from the dorsoradial aspect of the hand to the distal ulnar aspect of the hand. It is very important to note that the strap must conform fully with the first metacarpal area and does not bridge over the radial aspect of the hand. Often the strap has to be threaded through a slot in the orthosis for it to conform properly. When the middle strap is secure, the distal strap is conformed to the dorsal fingers just distal to the MCP joints to maintain MCP and IP joint position. This technique helps prevent small finger MCP joint hyperextension and IP joint flexion, or the "ulnar claw deformity." This impending dorsal ulnar hand scarring often requires treatment with a static progressive orthosis to correct the BSC (Fig. 82.24).

If the dorsal hand skin and scar contracture remains fixed at a shortened length and is not improving as expected, then a static progressive composite flexion orthosis can be fabricated to correct scar length and prevent subsequent underlying ligamentous contractures of the MCP and IP joints[18,57] (Fig. 82.25). The wear schedule will vary as indicated from full-time use to full-time use with removal for exercise and ADL performance to nighttime only use.

Dorsal Metacarpophalangeal Joint Hyperextension Block Orthosis

Severe burn injuries to the dorsum of the hand can cause "palmar planus," also referred to as flat palmar arch deformity. As scar causes the hand to contract dorsally, the arches of the palm flatten, making it difficult to flex the MCP joints for grasping.[62] Flattening of the palmar arches often occurs with an intrinsic-minus hand contracture in which the skin and scar on the dorsum of the hand become tight and lose extensibility; consequently, the MCP joints hyperextend, and the IP joints assume a flexed position.[11] A dorsal MCP joint block orthosis can be fabricated with the MCP joints positioned in flexion and serially adjusted to further improve MCP joint flexion. The purpose of this orthosis is to place the hand in a more functional position for grasping.

First Web C-Bar Orthosis

To prevent a first webspace contracture, a C-bar orthosis should be fabricated to maintain the first web opening and functionally position the thumb CMC joint for the performance of opposition and grasp. The orthosis can be serially adjusted to increase the first webspace.[56–58]

Carpometacarpal Antideformity Orthosis

Subluxation of the thumb CMC joint can occur in cases of deep palmar or dorsal burn injuries when thick immature scar contracts and pulls the thenar and hypothenar eminence toward the center of the palm leading to a cupping deformity. A hand-based CMC antideformity orthosis or a first and fifth palmar contracture orthosis can be fabricated to stabilize the joint in a functional position and allow the thumb to correctly oppose during functional activities.[57,63]

Metacarpophalangeal and Interphalangeal Joint Flexion Orthosis

Contracting scars on the dorsal surface of the hand can affect hand function and lead to joint tightness and hyperextension deformities. When tightness of the joints and the dorsal skin is detected, the therapist can fabricate a dynamic flexion orthosis for the MCP joints[64] or a composite dynamic MCP–IP joint flexion orthosis.[57] Elastic band traction, monofilament line, and finger slings are attached to a volar forearm-based wrist orthosis to improve MCP joint flexion. PIP joint flexion can be included as well by attaching a hook to the fingernails. To produce PIP joint flexion, a pulley can be created by attaching a D-ring to the distal aspect of the orthosis. Monofilament is attached to the fingernail hook, threaded through the D-ring and attached proximally with elastic bands. Another D-ring, acting as a tunnel for the monofilament lines to go through, can be attached on the volar wrist orthosis over the proximal palmar crease surface to promote full distal interphalangeal (DIP) joint flexion.[65] Because of the volar placed traction, dynamic flexion orthoses prevent functional hand use. Dynamic flexion orthoses are used intermittently throughout the day and are removed for exercise and ADL performance. Frequent adjustments of the orthosis are required to maintain a 90-degree angle of pull.[18] This angle is important to prevent inappropriate translational, rotational, and shear forces that can result in joint compression, distraction, shearing, and pressure sores caused by uneven distribution of forces through the finger slings.[18] Traction provided by the elastic bands should be between 100 and 300 g and can be measured with a spring tension scale. Skin and scar areas should be assessed often to ensure that the orthosis is not causing blistering because of mechanical shear forces. (For more information, see Chapter 108.)

Metacarpophalangeal and Interphalangeal Extension Orthosis

Scar contracture on the volar surface of the hand and fingers can lead to flexion contractures of the MCP and IP joints. To prevent these disabling contractures, a dorsal forearm-based dynamic extension orthosis can be fabricated. A similar orthosis is fabricated when the burn injury is complicated by accompanying radial nerve injury.[65] The dynamic MCP joint extension orthosis involves the fabrication of a dorsal wrist orthosis extending just distal to the metacarpal heads. A digital extension outrigger and a thumb MCP joint extension outrigger are attached to the dorsal orthosis; the dynamic traction is provided through finger slings on the proximal phalanges of all digits. The slings are connected to monofilament line and rubber bands, which in turn connect to a D-ring on the forearm surface of the orthosis. If the volar scar contractures involves the IP joints, then the dorsal orthosis is constructed to extend over the dorsum of the proximal phalanx, ending just distal to the head of each proximal phalanx.[66] The dynamic extension orthosis allows for the functional use of the hand during ADL performance.

Devastating burn injuries to the upper extremity can require many different orthoses in the rehabilitation process. Circumferential injuries to the hand often require both flexion and extension orthoses which, in some cases, can become a burden for the patient to carry around.

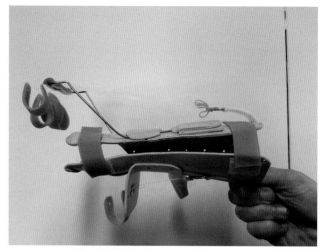

Fig. 82.26 The "super splint" orthosis.

A diverse multipurpose orthosis such as the "super splint" includes a forearm-based ulnar or radial gutter–type orthosis that can accommodate outriggers for both flexion and extension along with a thumb outrigger, thus eliminating the need for multiple dynamic orthoses to treat the injured hand[67] (Fig. 82.26).

Finger Gutter or Trough Orthoses

Fingers can sustain very severe injuries that require special attention and custom orthoses. Scar contractures on the dorsal or volar surface of the digits can be addressed with custom-made or prefabricated spring-loaded IP joint orthoses. The dynamic tension provided by the spring mechanism must be carefully monitored by the therapist and adjusted as needed to prevent excessive damaging and painful forces exerted on the digits.[16–18]

A finger gutter, also referred to as a canoe or trough orthosis, can be fabricated to immobilize the affected IP joints in extension to prevent deformity or protect an exposed tendon of the dorsum of the fingers. This orthoses is essential when tendon, bone, or joint exposure is present or suspected as a result of a deep burn to the dorsal fingers and is used until durable soft tissue coverage is achieved.[57,62] It can also be fabricated and serially adjusted to correct a PIP or DIP joint contracture, using a dorsal, volar, radial, or ulnar design. Finger gutters can be applied before and in conjunction with forearm-based orthoses.[62] A three-point extension orthosis or serial cast can also be fabricated to serially correct PIP joint flexion contractures.[68] A dorsal finger gutter or figure-of-8 orthosis is helpful for PIP joint hyperextension deformity.[11]

Severe dorsal hand burns can cause damage to the extensor tendon mechanism and central slip at the level of the PIP joint. The resulting boutonnière deformity presents as flexion of the PIP joint and hyperextension at the DIP joint.[62] A finger gutter orthosis used at the first sign of tightness can help prevent these contractures. Orthoses should be worn continuously and removed only in the presence of a therapist for supervised exercise. If the central slip is ruptured, then complete immobilization of the PIP joint is required. Complete immobilization of the PIP joint during the wound healing phase can lead to the production of a strong scar, creating a pseudo tendon that can support the PIP joint in extension.

Proximal Interphalangeal Joint Hyperextension Block Orthosis ("Figure-of-8")

Immature contractile scar anterior to the flexion axis of the PIP joint can create an imbalance of forces within the digit's intrinsic and

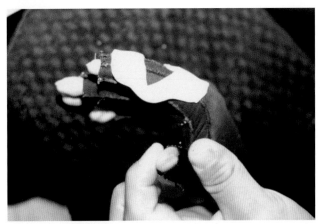

Fig. 82.27 Proximal interphalangeal hyperextension block "figure-of-8" orthosis.

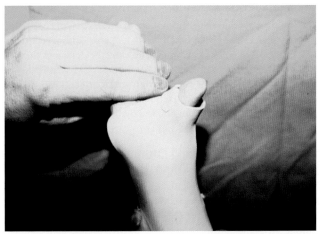

Fig. 82.28 Thumb spica anticupping orthosis.

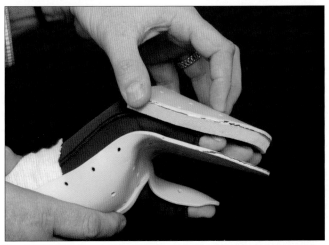

Fig. 82.29 The "sandwich splint" orthosis; the fingers are in flexion. (From Serghiou MA, Ott S, C, Cowan A, et al. Burn rehabilitation along the continuum of care. In: Herndon DN, ed. *Total Burn Care*. 5th ed. Philadelphia: Elsevier; 2018:476–508; with permission.)

extrinsic musculature that results in a swan-neck deformity. This deformity presents as hyperextension of the PIP joint and flexion of the DIP joint. A "figure-of-8" orthosis or prefabricated Murphy Ring Splint (North Coast Medical) can be used to correct mild contractures[11] (Fig. 82.27). Serial casting can be used for severe contractures before the use of such an orthosis. These orthoses block PIP joint hyperextension and allow for PIP joint flexion during ADL performance. They are worn until healing of the involved structures occurs and contractile scars have matured.

Mallet Finger Deformity Orthosis

Injury to the extensor tendon over the DIP joint can lead to the development of a mallet deformity characterized by a loss of DIP joint extension with a posture of flexion at the DIP joint.[11] If tendon exposure or rupture occurs, the DIP joint is completely immobilized for up to 6 to 8 weeks in a DIP joint extension orthosis.[69]

Thumb Spica Anticupping Orthosis

Cupping of the palm can occur in cases in which the hand has sustained a deep partial-thickness or full-thickness palmar burn that takes longer than 3 weeks to heal. Palmar scar bands pull the thenar and hypothenar eminences on the volar surface of the hand toward each other, creating a "cupping effect" in the hand. The thumb can begin to hyperextend at the MCP joint, which can lead to further injury such as joint subluxation or, in severe cases, dislocation.[62] A forearm or hand-based thumb spica anticupping orthosis can be designed to stretch the palm (reverse the "cupping effect") and position the thumb appropriately for function[57] (Fig. 82.28). Silicone or elastomer inserts are often applied underneath the orthosis to help soften the scar causing the palm deformity. The orthosis is serially adjusted until correction is achieved.

"Sandwich" or Bivalved Orthosis

When the hand is positioned in the antideformity orthosis, the IP joints should be positioned in neutral (0 degrees). In cases in which compliance is difficult (i.e., pediatrics), the IP joints can assume a flexed position, which in turn can lead to pressure points on the fingertips or flexion contractures of the IP joints. A "sandwich" or bivalved orthosis can be fabricated to prevent this problem. This orthosis consists of a volar antideformity burn orthosis and a dorsal thermoplastic shell, padded with foam and placed over the dorsum of digits 2 to 5 extending from the proximal phalanges (clearing the MCP joints) to the fingertips of digits 2 to 5 (Fig. 82.29). In cases in which orthosis migration is an issue, the dorsal component of the orthosis can extend to the forearm.[56,57,70] The dorsal component must be padded to prevent pressure points on the dorsum of the fingers. Another way to create the "sandwich" effect and maintain the fingers in extension is to simply use dorsal and volar hand-based foam shells and an elastic wrap to include all digits, excluding the thumb.[70]

Palmar Extension Orthosis

Severe circumferential burn injuries to the hand mandate the fabrication of an orthosis that positions the hand in extension. The resting pan extension orthosis (Fig. 82.30) provides wrist extension, thumb radial–palmar extension, and MCP and IP joint extension.[13,57–58] All digits are positioned in abduction within the orthosis to prevent syndactyly of the finger webspaces. The range of extension provided should be enough to cause blanching of the skin. This orthosis assists in prevention of palmar contractures and syndactyly of all webspaces and maintains the excursion of the extrinsic flexor musculature. This orthosis should be alternately worn with the antideformity burn hand orthosis at set intervals throughout the day and night to manage the contractures and maintain the excursion of both the agonist and antagonist musculature. A dorsal resting pan extension orthosis can be designed to position the hand as described previously and avoid contact with the painful and sensitive volar hand surface.[56]

Another orthosis used to prevent flexion contractures of the wrist, palm, fingers, and thumb webspace is the slot-through orthosis with a

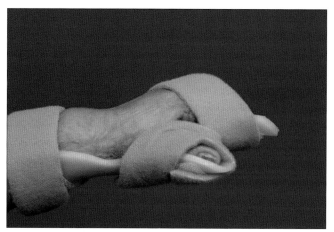

Fig. 82.30 Resting pan extension orthosis. (From Serghiou MA, Ott S, C, Cowan A, et al. Burn rehabilitation along the continuum of care. In: Herndon DN, ed. *Total Burn Care*. 5th ed. Philadelphia: Elsevier; 2018:476–508; with permission.)

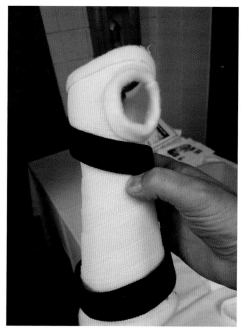

Fig. 82.32 Wrist extension fiberglass cast.

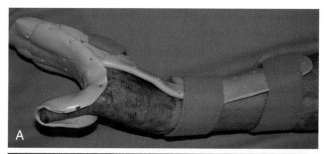

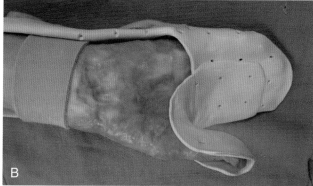

Fig. 82.31 Slot-through orthosis with a C-bar attached. **A,** Radial view **B,** Volar view.

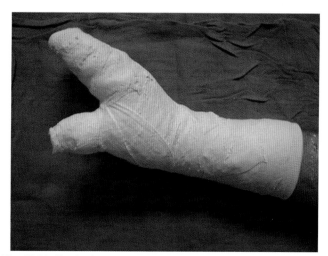

Fig. 82.33 Hand extension serial casting for severe palmar contracture.

C-bar attached (Fig. 82.31). This slot-through orthosis positions and maintains scar on the palmar surface of the hand at an optimal length for a prolonged period of time to manage contractures of the palm.[13,57]

SERIAL CASTING

Serial casts provide end-range positioning for long-duration to contracted scar tissue. Brand developed the concept when treating patients with leprosy who had long-standing contractures of the ankle, feet, and hands. Brand's method uses plaster of paris total contact casts to produce tissue realignment and "growth."[16,17,19,71] He states that cast application without padding prevents cast migration by providing a more formed fit, therefore reducing the occurrence of pressure sores and blisters caused by localized compression or shear forces. Along with Brand, Bell-Krotoski[22] has presented her clinical experience using serial plaster casting for tissue remodeling and correction of contractures to

include improving ROM of the PIP joint. Bennett and coworkers[72] have described ROM increases in several joints with serial casting.

This technique has been adopted in burn rehabilitation with both plaster of paris or fiberglass cast tape used (Fig. 82.32). Plaster of paris is a quick-setting gypsum plaster that is often preferred because of its conformity, but fiberglass cast material is preferred because it can be less bulky, lighter, and more durable. Casting is especially useful for patients who are unable to comply with removable thermoplastic orthoses. Moreover, plaster and fiberglass cast tape are less expensive and more accessible than thermoplastic material in many parts of the world. Recently, Deltacast Polyester conformable Cast Tape has become available and shows great potential in children with burns. This material is flexible and can be univalved to be used as a total contact orthosis. All types of casts can be outfitted with traction components to provide static progressive or dynamic tension.

In treating severe BSC of the hand, serial casts are often applied to manage dorsal based BSC when passive MCP flexion is less than 30 to 45 degrees and applied to palmar BSC when passive MCP extension is less than −40 degrees (Fig. 82.33). Upon initial application, the cast should be changed the next day to assess the patient's skin and scar areas. If there are no skin and scar complications noted during inspection, then a new cast is reapplied and changed every 2 to 7 days. Skin and scar areas with loss of protective sensation can be serial casted; however, the therapist must have expertise in the application and wear of the cast. When considering application of a cast, one must carefully assess the skin. The presence of small- and medium-sized wounds is not a barrier to serial casting. However, the wound should be clean, free of infection, and dressed appropriately beneath the cast. For patients with wounds, the casts are changed more frequently (every 1–2 days). Before applying the cast, wounds are often dressed using antibiotic ointments and minimal gauze. Compression garments, whether custom or prefabricated, should not be worn beneath the casts because the seams can cause pressure sores to newly healed fragile skin and scar, and the garment can be damaged during cast removal. ROM should be assessed before the application of any cast and after removal to determine the effectiveness of casting treatment.[73,74]

RANGE OF MOTION

Postburn edema, pain, and open wounds can significantly impair the patient's ability to functionally move her or his hand and upper extremity. Before initiating a mobilization plan to prevent and correct scar limiting ROM deficits, baseline goniometric measurements are recorded and used to track both losses and gains in ROM over time. Based on location and depth of burn injury, an extensive goniometric evaluation of AROM, PROM, and total active motion (TAM) should be conducted using standardized methodology to record measurements to communicate findings and changes for the therapist, patient, and burn team clinicians to ensure optimal outcomes.[75]

Therapists should avoid using the term "within functional limits" when collecting measurements of the hand and upper extremity because functional ROM of one joint can be enough to perform a certain task but it can be insufficient to perform other tasks when all planes of motion are taken into consideration. Furthermore, for a burned area of the upper extremity that is at risk for BSC, it is important to record even minimal losses in ROM.

It has been determined that assessing joint ROM with a goniometer or hand movement with linear or scale measurements can provide accurate, objective measures in the burn population.[76,77] Evaluation of PROM is completed in a protective manner when the integrity of the soft tissue structures is compromised. TAM, as per the American Society for Surgery of the Hand, has been found to be useful in evaluating burned hand function; it allows more effective communication between the hand therapist and hand surgeon about the true length and extensibility of the scar across multiple joints and provides an accurate perspective on the cumulative functional motion of the burned hand.[78,79] If the patient's medical status allows, immediate mobilization of the hand and upper extremity is recommended to prevent functional movement limitations later in recovery. The therapist should design an exercise program that focuses on purposeful and meaningful use of the hand and upper extremity. Patients are encouraged to actively learn and participate in the management of their scar and ADLs.

Exercise in the rhythm of music has shown to significantly improve both active and passive ROM in young children with severe burns.[80] In this study, young children were given a variety of musical instruments with play activities. The children mimicked the movements of enjoyable music while the therapist encouraged them to perform hand and upper extremity movements.

During the acute phase of rehabilitation, gentle AROM and tendon gliding exercises create a muscle-pumping action that is effective in reducing edema and in addition will help to minimize adhesion formation. Additionally, active exercises of at least 25 repetitions every waking hour of the shoulder, elbow, wrist, and hand will allow for more efficient drainage of distal edema and prevent stagnation of proximal tissue fluids that can result from disuse.[43]

After an excision and grafting procedure, it is necessary to immobilize the hand and upper extremity for a period of time; typically this is 5 to 7 days but varies depending on the location of the grafting procedure and the type of graft used. Earlier excision and autografting of the hand have been shown to accelerate recovery time, improve functional outcomes, and shorten the rehabilitative process.[81]

Functional use of the hand should be encouraged throughout the intermediate and long-term phases of rehabilitation. The exercise program should be carefully monitored to ensure that exercises are performed correctly. During exercise performance, the therapist should observe for blanching of the scar to ensure that the tissue is being exercised at its longest length. Upon seeing a blanching white appearance of the scar, the patient should be encouraged to perform and maintain the movement within his or her tolerance. A good motto is "When it's white, it's tight" (see Figs. 82.25 and 82.31B). Forceful and "aggressive" PROM exercises can lead to traumatic inflammation, which increases the density of the contracture and must be avoided. Aggressive PROM is not necessary and often leads to excessive pain and noncompliance with the exercise program.[17,62] The therapist should interpret a physician order for "aggressive ROM" as meaning "prolonged gentle stretching and lengthening." For circumferential full-thickness burned fingers, unrestricted exercise of the PIP and DIP joints is not permitted because of the risk of ischemic necrosis and disruption of the central slip of the extensor mechanism.

When managing contractures, the therapist should remain focused on the application of gentle low-load, long-duration stress. In general, managing a patient at risk for BSC of the hand and upper extremity involves a daily routine of frequent exercise, ADL performance, and prolonged positioning of scar tissue at its optimal length throughout the day. Gains made in ROM and tissue extensibility must be maintained throughout the night with optimal orthotic positioning until patient goals are met.

STRENGTH, CONDITIONING, AND ACTIVITIES OF DAILY LIVING TRAINING

Management of the burned hand requires a comprehensive approach. Recent data have demonstrated that resistive exercise training performed on children and adolescents with severe burns with a TBSA of 49% (≥15%) can achieve similar strength capacity as their unburned matched counterparts at 6 months postinjury.[82] Resistive exercises and activities that challenge hand and finger dexterity should be increased in pace with the patient's tolerance.

Cronan and colleagues[83] reported that because muscle tissue is one of the most mutable tissues in the body, a burn injury can affect the musculoskeletal system as well as the skin. In a study of burn patients returning to work, Cronan and colleagues[83] demonstrated that patients given isokinetic exercise in addition to isometric and isotonic exercise were found to produce a better test outcome than those receiving isometric and isotonic exercise training only. Cronan and colleagues[83] stated that therapy must involve training of both slow-twitch and fast-twitch fibers. They explained that fatigue results from improper training of slow-twitch fibers and that joint pain after increased activity or the inability to perform certain workloads for extended periods can be caused by improper training of fast-twitch fibers. Training involved the use of isokinetic exercise equipment. Cronan and colleagues[83] stated that light submaximal contraction selectively recruits slow-twitch fibers, moderate submaximal contraction adds fast-twitch fibers, and maximal contraction leads to an "all-or-none" recruitment of both fiber types.

Critically important for therapists working with burn patients is the impact of the injury to the entire body and unaffected extremity. Therefore, the unburned hand should be included in the therapy program. In a study of hand function after major burns, Covey and colleagues[84] found that the unburned hand can show impairments in strength, TAM, and coordination at the time of hospital discharge. Within 3 months after discharge, all study participants had normal TAM, and most had achieved normal grip strength and coordination; however, some required as long as 12 months after discharge to regain normal strength and coordination.

In addition to weakness that can occur as the result of any hospitalization, many metabolic disorders, including altered protein kinetics with muscle weakness, result from burn injury. The hypermetabolic state of burns promotes excessive caloric demands and alters the aerobic and muscle-building capacity of the body. Investigators compared muscle dysfunction in burn-injured rats in the absence of apparent immobilization with muscle dysfunction after immobilization alone.[85] Their findings suggest that muscle dysfunction after immobilization alone occurs primarily as the result of loss of muscle mass, whereas muscle dysfunction after burn injury on days 1 to 7 is a result of a decline in specific tension and at day 14 is the result of a decline in specific tension and muscle mass. Research on rats with 40% TBSA scald burns showed that although the muscles directly beneath the burned skin were not damaged by the burn, they demonstrated dramatic apoptotic (cell death initiated by the cell itself) changes.[86] Apoptosis was also confirmed at muscle sites distant from the injury. These changes peaked at postburn days 3 and 7, indicating to the investigators the need for early and continuous intervention. Hand burn injuries predominantly impact ADLs and can impact the burn survivors' ability to fully recover from their injury. Therapeutic interventions should be focused on restoration of full function, and adaptive devices should only be provided as a temporary intervention; the focus of treatment must always be on the restoration of full AROM and strength in all capacities.

PAIN MANAGEMENT

Burn pain is characterized as one of the most complex processes impacting the skin. The instant pain that follows a burn injury is caused by stimulation of skin nociceptors that respond to heat (thermoreceptors), mechanical distortion (mechanoreceptors), and a cascade of chemical stimuli that can be both exogenous and endogenous. Nerve endings that are destroyed will not transmit pain, yet those that remain undamaged and exposed will generate pain throughout the course of rehabilitation. This pain further promotes both a primary (nociceptor) and a secondary (peripheral) hyperalgesia response that can impact all phases of pain, including procedural pain, resting pain, and breakthrough pain. The experience of pain has been found to be a mediating risk factor for posttraumatic stress disorder (PTSD) in both pediatric and adult burn patients.[87]

The use of opioids and other pain medications will not cause dependence if adequately administered and tapered when pain levels decrease. Pain and depression seem to be linked in such a way that they can cause each other. Also, acute pain at the time of discharge seems to produce long-term suicidal ideation, in which there is a reciprocal relationship between pain and depression or anxiety, and after discharge, many burn survivors have significant sleep problems that can be secondary to PTSD symptoms, depression, itch, or pain.[88] Sleep can also affect burn pain level because patients with more disturbed sleep tend to require more analgesics; it should be noted that the pain

level experienced during the day might not predict a night of disturbed sleep. However, the inability of the individual to manage both the pain of daily therapy and loss of sleep will often require a comprehensive pharmacological approach.

Burn patients are often attempting to overcome their fear of pain, disfigurement, and loss of function. The therapist should attempt to captivate and motivate burn patients by consistently providing them with ongoing education and setting goals to pursue rather than creating more fear. As a change agent, the therapist has the capability to provide patients with hope by gently helping them place fears under control.

SENSATION

After a significant burn injury, it is common to observe loss of specialized skin functions or peripheral nerve functions, which subsequently impact sensation. It has been documented that perhaps the best predictor of cutaneous sensory loss is the depth of the burn injury. Additionally, Ward and Tuckett[89] reported that patients who underwent grafting demonstrated impaired or absent responses to sharp–dull, hot–cold, and light touch stimuli over the grafted sites. Therapists should anticipate some level of short- or long-term impaired sensation when treating hand burns. Ward and Tuckett[89] tested the recovery of sensation after third-degree hand burns and found that participants rarely achieved perfect discrimination, and, in some cases, protective sensation was absent. Holavanahalli and coworkers[90] studied patients who survived major burn injuries and reported that problems with hot–cold temperature and sensory loss can persist decades after the injury. Today, as people survive large burn injuries, it is very important that they seek treatment for their sensory sequelae long after the completion of rehabilitation. Electrical injuries to the upper extremity are often the most devastating in terms of reduced sensation to the hand. In many cases after such injuries, patients are unable to perceive cutaneous touch or pressure in the hand, particularly in the median nerve distribution.[91] Acutely, a formal evaluation of sensation is not possible because of the presence of wounds. As the patient progresses in recovery and wounds close, a thorough sensory evaluation can and should be performed.[90] Standardized measures should be used to assess and reassess cutaneous sensation to track the patient's sensory recovery. Wound depth, history of skin grafting, the stage of scar maturation, and scar hypertrophy should be considered during the sensory evaluation.[89] The primary and protective sensations of touch, temperature, and pain should be tested first. Testing the primary sensations requires light touch testing, temperature recognition, and sharp–dull testing methods. If the primary sensations are found lacking, then discriminatory testing is not indicated. Screening of the discriminative sensations can be achieved using monofilament testing and static two-point discrimination. One objective way to measure cutaneous sensibility is through threshold testing using monofilaments.[92] Two-point discrimination testing assesses the patient's functional hand sensibility as it relates to the ability to perform fine tasks. Functional tests, such as the Dellon modification of the Moberg pickup test, which assesses for stereognosis or object recognition, can be used during sensibility testing. It is vital to use sensory reeducation and desensitization interventions in therapy as indicated to help the patient reach maximum potential sensory recovery.[93]

SCAR MANAGEMENT

Scar Assessment

Currently, research is focusing on the development of a comprehensive objective measure to assess burn scars; however, a single tool that objectively measures the volume, pliability, and color of the scar has

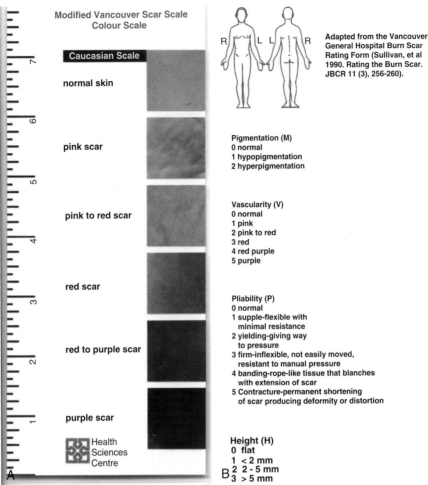

Fig. 82.34 An example of the Modified Vancouver Scar Scale, which is used to assess hypertrophic burn scars. **A**, Front. **B**, Back.

yet to be developed.[94,95] The Vancouver Burn Scar Assessment is a subjective tool that rates the burn scar in terms of its pigmentation, vascularity, pliability, and height and is currently the most widely used tool to rate burn scar (Fig. 82.34). More recently, several new scales have been developed to increase the reliability of subjective assessment and provide construct validity including the Modified Vancouver Scar Scale (MVSS), Patient and Observer Scar Assessment Scale (POSAS), Burn Specific Health Scale (BSHS), and Matching Assessment of Photographs and Scars (MAPS).[95–97] Even though a comprehensive objective measure for rating burn scars remains elusive, a variety of individual objective tools are currently available. Scar thickness and height can be measured through the use of noninvasive transcutaneous ultrasound scans with devices such as the Dermascan and the TUPS (tissue ultrasound palpation system) as well as with very simple noninvasive negative molding or three-dimensional imaging.[94] These methods compare the thickness of the traumatized dermal tissue with the dermal tissue of adjacent normal skin at regular intervals for comparison difference measurement. Different devices are used for color analysis of scars, including pigment and vascular changes such as the Minolta Chromameter, Labscan, and Micro Color as well as narrowband simple reflectance meters such as the DermaSpectrometer and the Mexameter.[94] Computerized video camera images can objectively assess the color of scars quantitatively by analyzing images using a custom-written computer program such as the Image Tool system.[95] Skin pliability, extensibility, and tension can be assessed objectively using cicatrometers, pneumatonometers, or modified tonometers or by using other dedicated systems such as the Cutometer, Dermaflex, or Dermal Torque Meter.[94] More complex laser-based instruments currently being used to assess both live blood flow as well as objective color assessment include the laser-Doppler flowmeter (LDF), laser-Doppler imaging (LDI), and laser speckle imaging (LSPI).[94,98] These devices use a combination of red or near-infrared wavelengths and digital image-processing techniques to provide detailed blood flow assessment in real time processing. There are a number of new methods currently in development for scar assessment that combine a number of one or more high tech instruments, including combining standardized digital imaging (SDI) and spectral modeling (SpM) to objectively assess the scar digitally.[98] Additionally, techniques to assess discreet physiological processes during the scar maturation process have been undertaken, including transcutaneous oxygen tension measurement via skin electrodes; transepidermal water loss (TEWL) assessment using the Dermalab, Tewameter, or VapoMeter; and hydration of the skin surface (stratum corneum) via electrical conductance meters such as the CorneoMeter or Skicon-200.[94,99]

Superficial burn wounds heal by re-epithelialization, and deep wounds, like any other deep wound, heal by forming scar. Scar is defined as the fibrous tissue replacing normal tissues destroyed by injury or disease. Burn scars, if not managed appropriately, can become thick and elevated, resulting in what is known as scar hypertrophy, and have a prevalence of more than 65% in burn injury.[100] Factors that

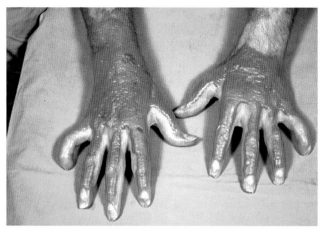

Fig. 82.35 Bilateral hands showing immature hypertrophic scarring. Note the inability of the patient to fully extend both small fingers at the interphalangeal joints.

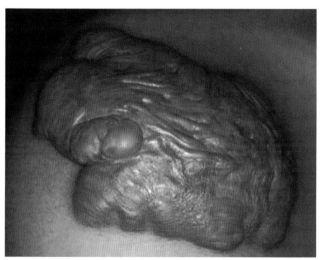

Fig. 82.36 Keloid scar on the anterior shoulder. Note the puffier and less restrictive appearance of this scar.

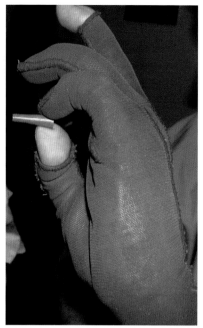

Fig. 82.37 Custom-measured compression garment. Note the open tips on some digits to allow for sensory input and facilitate fine motor dexterity.

can contribute to the development of hypertrophic scars include the presence of wound infection, the patient's genetic makeup, repeatedly harvested donor sites, the patient's age, chronic inflammatory process, location of the injury, and skin tension.[37] These types of scars are characterized as hypertrophic or keloid, and both are considered dermatoproliferative disorders of the skin.[101]

Hypertrophic scar is typically characterized as raised, red, rigid, painful, and pruritic, which often limits or restricts skin extensibility and ROM and remains within the confines of the burn[102] (Fig. 82.35). Keloid scarring shares some of the same basic characteristics as hypertrophic scar; however, keloid scars extend outside of the margin of the original injury, advance into the surrounding soft tissue, and are somewhat less contractile in form[102] (Fig. 82.36). The therapist must understand the unique underlying scar morphology to effectively manage each type of scar. Hypertrophic scars are not cosmetically appealing, and if they cross any joints, they can restrict function or distract joint position, especially over articular or highly mobile skin surfaces.[37] As the burn wound progresses toward healing or after skin grafting operations take place, scars begin to form. Generally, the deeper the burn injury and the longer the inflammatory wound process, the higher the potential is for the formation of hypertrophic

scar.[103] Also, the longer a wound remains open and not fully healed, the higher the potential is for the development of hypertrophic scar tissue. As the wound begins the healing process, collagen fibers develop to bridge the wound, forming an immature (active) scar, which appears as a red, raised, and rigid mass.[104] Extensive study with well-defined randomized controlled trials is lacking in understanding hypertrophic scar development because of the limited consensus on an adequate animal model of abnormal scarring.[101] However, progress continues to be made in understanding and potentially unlocking the scar development cascade, including the signal mediator transforming growth factor–β, the overproduction of extracellular matrix, and keratinocyte signal expression research.[101,104]

SCAR TREATMENT

The management of burns scars involves many treatment options throughout the burn injury timeline. Wound closure and minimization of the inflammatory process are crucial to close the breached skin surface and promote effective healing and minimize the appearance of the scar. Because of the imbalance in skin hydration, moisturizers also play a key role in the early management of scars, and the application of these moisturizers should be frequent to support damaged sebaceous gland functions and to mitigate the pruritic effect of the dry skin surface.

Clients usually receive custom compression garments to manage scarring during the long-term rehabilitation phase. Pressure therapy during the scar maturation phase can contribute to a more linear, softer, and a more devascularized scar (Fig. 82.37). Patients with burn wounds that heal within 7 to 14 (superficial partial-thickness burn wounds) days do not need pressure therapy.[103] Patients whose wounds heal within 14 to 21 days are closely monitored, and pressure therapy can be initiated prophylactically. In general, a burn wound that heals after 21 days requires the use of pressure garments and pressure mediated modalities.[103,105] The correct amount of pressure in suppressing the hypertrophic scar has not yet been determined.[103] Pressure of as

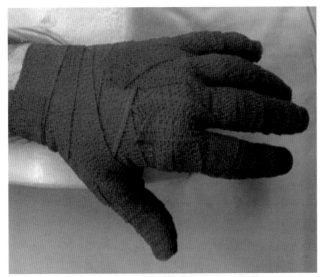

Fig. 82.38 A self-adherent wrap of the hand will exert gentle pressures of 10 to 12 mm Hg to manage immature hypertrophic burn scars. Note the full coverage of the hand, which provides uniform compression while allowing for full mobility of the hand.

little as 10 mm Hg can be effective in remodeling the scar tissue over time (Fig. 82.38). High pressures in excess of about 40 mm Hg can be destructive to tissues and cause paresthesia. Burn scars can take up to 2 years or longer to mature. Scars can begin to become thick and raised at approximately 8 to 12 weeks after the burn wounds close.[37] Clinically, custom therapeutic pressure for the prevention, control, and correction of scar hypertrophy averages 24 to 28 mm Hg, which is approximately equal and opposing to the capillary pressure (25 mm Hg). At this pressure level, many researchers believe that scars can be altered.[105] For pressure therapy to be effective, pressure garments need to be worn at all times, day and night. They should only be removed for bathing and on occasion during exercise because they should not interfere with movement.

Silicone gel sheeting has been a mainstay of burn scar management since the early 1980s[37] (Fig. 82.39). To date, the mechanism of how silicone affects the burn scar is still not known.[106] The most recent developments have pointed to a cascade of action in the epidermal signaling mechanism in which occlusion causes a decrease in TEWL and normalizes the hydration state of keratinocytes, which then signal dermal fibroblasts to downregulate extracellular matrix production.[100,107] Clinically, silicone has been observed to hydrate the burn scar, depress the height of hypertrophic scars, prevent shrinking of fresh skin grafts, and increase the pliability of a scar, thus allowing for increases in the ROM of affected joints[105,108] (Fig. 82.40). When the burn scars have matured enough to tolerate sheering forces, massage can be incorporated into the scar management regimen. Scar massage is an effective modality for maintaining joint mobility, and in the case of contractures, it helps to lengthen scar bands. Even though the benefits of scar massage are yet to be scientifically demonstrated, the general belief of those who use burn scar massage is that massage helps to soften or remodel scar tissues by freeing adhering fibrous bands and allowing the scars to become more elastic, thus improving joint mobility.[105] Intralesional corticosteroid injection can be of some limited benefit in the treatment of hypertrophic burn scar. The use of pulsed-dye laser in the treatment of hypertrophic scars is controversial and is not yet routine in most burn centers in North America.[101] Some early preclinical evidence supports the effect of interferon-α as a promising treatment for hypertrophic burn scars, but larger human studies have yet to be performed.[104]

Burn Scar Contracture: Prevention, Correction, and Challenges
Wound Healing Time: Preventing Contractures

The mere presence of a hand burn does not predict the development of BSC, impairment, or functional difficulties.[109,110] What is important is not that a hand burn has occurred but how long it takes for the burn injury to heal.[48] In response to today's burn therapy challenges, Hunter and Brand have indicated that the problem with preventing and correcting contractures is "time." Hunter[40] reported that "healing time" is critical for preventing contractures, and the seminal work of Brand demonstrates the importance of "chronic time" in managing and correcting contractures.

More than 50 years ago, Hunter[40] addressed the issue of time dependency in the context of burn injury, stating, "The prognosis of the burned hand is directly related to wound healing time." Hunter[40] further stated that the primary goal in the management of a severely burned hand is the prevention and correction of contractures and deformity. During the acute phase of burn rehabilitation, the prognosis improves with preventing contractures and hypertrophic scarring if the rate of healing time is less than 3 weeks for the burn wound and graft take including healing of graft boundaries.[8,31,33,37,48] Shichinohe and coworkers[48] revealed that burned fingers treated with skin grafting that healed within 19 days had normal ROM with TAM greater than 220 degrees, and fingers requiring 20 to 43 days to heal had abnormal ROM with TAM less than 219 degrees. After this acute healing phase, the process of preventing and correcting BSC requires considerable doses of persistence, fortitude, and chronic time to minimize deformity and hypertrophic scarring.

Time-Dependent Behavior: Correcting Contractures

All viscoelastic tissues of the body are time dependent.[14] This means that the duration of time that a force is applied to a tissue is important. In applying tension to treat contractures, Brand[17] states, "The problem is time." Therefore, an understanding of the time-dependent perspective and behavior of skin and scar requires a commitment to using a prolonged period of time to prevent and correct BSC and deformity throughout acute, intermediate, and long-term rehabilitation. The biophysical principles of skin and scar tissue should be observed together with a patient focused biopsychosocial perspective to encourage the burned person to respond optimally to the physical, physiological and psychosocial stressors of burn injury throughout acute, intermediate, and long-term rehabilitation.

Burn scar contracture is a common complication of burn injury and can be defined as "an impairment caused by replacement of skin with pathologic scar tissue of insufficient extensibility and length, resulting in a loss of motion or tissue alignment of an associated joint or anatomic structure."[1] Throughout recovery, the therapist evaluates the severity of the burn wound as it relates to risks for BSC, deformity, hypertrophic scarring, and functional limitations. Management of a severely burned hand is a scar tissue issue in which the position of comfort will become the position of contracture[111] (Fig. 82.41). BSCs can occur because of the effect of myofibroblasts and free actin in the scar.[112] Contractures are either intrinsic (loss of tissue in the injured area with subsequent distortion of the involved anatomic part) or extrinsic (loss of tissue is at a distance from the affected area, but the distorted structures are not injured themselves). Basic research on the biomechanical effects of stretch is difficult to translate into clinical practice because small forces observed in the in vitro setting suggest that stretching can increase the risk of contracture, but this has yet to be proven clinically.[113] The

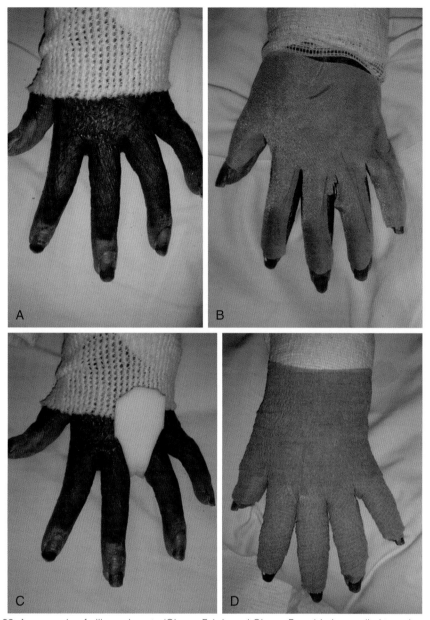

Fig. 82.39 An example of silicone inserts (Oleeva Fabric and Oleeva Foam) being applied to a dorsal-based hypertrophic scar (**A**). The inserts can be applied either to the dorsal surface (**B**) or in between the digits (**C**), and the self-adherent wrap is used to support a combination of silicone and pressure modulation (**D**).

physical manifestations of BSC, hypertrophic scarring, and overall long-term functioning are often directly attributable to how severely an individual is burned. The development and number of BSCs have been directly related to the extent of TBSA burned and can be quantified and segmented into CFUs, which relate to expectations of functional recovery required and potential for the development of skin and scar contracture (Fig. 82.42).[114] If less than 20% TBSA is burned, an individual is expected to do well unless severe burn injury occurs to the hands, in which case the potential for impaired functional outcomes increases considerably because of the multiple functional articular joint surfaces of the hand.

A burn patient tends to prefer a "position of comfort," folding joints into a flexed posture, and it is this position which can influence the new collagen fibers to fuse together in a shortened length, becoming a solid mass of collagen.[37] Prolonged immobility and the shortened, fused collagen across a joint crease can decrease ROM and

result in contracture formation.[115] The development of restrictions from burn scar occur within 5 to 7 days. Therefore, an ongoing effective problem list requires frequent updating and can be used to communicate to the burn team the location and severity of any foreseen or ongoing BSCs and deformities. For example, the therapist should frequently assess areas at risk for BSC and update the problem list to include losses in ROM (e.g., "loss of 10 degrees, from 55 to 45 degrees, in small finger MP joint flexion from November 3–10, 2019, caused by contracting dorsal ulnar hand BSC"). This documentation makes it clear that the patient is at very severe risk for right small finger MP joint hyperextension and PIP–DIP joint flexion contracture. With such losses in ROM, the exercise program and orthosis and strapping methods should be reassessed to ensure effective exercises and correct positioning of the hand within the burn hand orthosis (see Fig. 82.23). Additionally, after obtaining consent, photographic documentation is highly recommended, especially serial imaging of

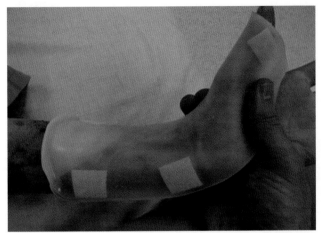

Fig. 82.40 Fabrication of a radial-based thumb spica orthosis with a silicone-lined thermoplastic (Silon-LTS). Note that this orthosis is fabricated directly onto the scar so that the silicone is directly in contact with the immature hypertrophic scar (blanching shows optimal stretch to scar).

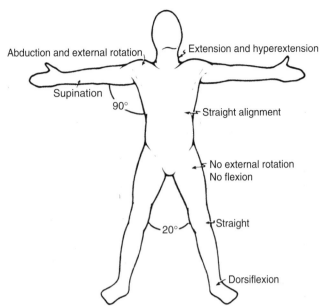

Fig. 82.41 General body positioning for prevention of burn scar contractures. (From Apfel LM, Irwin CP, Staley MJ, et al: Approaches to positioning the burn patient. In Richard RL, Staley MJ [ed]: *Burn Care and Rehabilitation Principles and Practice*, Philadelphia, FA Davis, 1994, pp 221-241; with permission.)

areas at risk for BSC and deformity. It is of utmost importance to meticulously collect and maintain dates regarding healing time and measurements of ROM for joints at risk for contracture. When an active contracture of a joint is occurring and not responding to rehabilitative efforts with exercise and orthoses, it is important to record and maintain a history of these ROM deficits over time. Documentation early in recovery of these undesirable changes can be valuable information when discussing with the surgeon the possible need for temporary joint fixation by percutaneous pinning to obtain directional control of forces of an impending burn scar and joint contracture. Furthermore, it is important to assess, monitor, and clearly document changes over time. After documenting measurements of what is presently known, how the client has occupied his or her time in the recent past should be described along with how she or he plans to occupy it in the immediate and near future. BSC and deformity evolve quickly within a short window of time. It is important to know how the client is occupying his or her time with regards to exercise, activity, and positioning on a 24-hour schedule. In turn, it is important to describe how the client is making changes in her or his daily routine on a 24-hour basis with respect to preventing or minimizing risk for BSC and deformity.

Burn scar contractures are labeled opposite of the motion that is restricted. For example, if a patient cannot fully extend the elbow, the contracture is called an elbow flexion contracture.[1] Larger TBSA is associated with a greater number of contractures, and contractures are more likely to occur with a full-thickness burn.[3,116] A contracture can develop in any skin crease overlying a joint, but the most common locations are the shoulder, hand, elbow, and knee[117] (Fig. 82.43). Scar contracture can continue to form throughout the scar remodeling phase. Orthoses, positioning, serial casting, and ROM exercises are necessary to combat this relentless process until maturation is achieved.[37] Contracture can still occur despite proper therapeutic interventions and surgical releases can be necessary in which additional orthosis use and dedicated mobilization of the joint will be required to counteract the potential redevelopment of hypertrophic scar contracture.[101,115]

Morbidity

According to the ABA's National Burn Awareness Fact Sheet for 2018, "Today, 96.7% of those treated in burn centers will survive. Unfortunately, many of those survivors will sustain serious scarring, life-long physical disabilities, and adjustment difficulties."[49] Although mortality rates have decreased, subsequent morbidity rates appear to have stagnated or possibly even worsened, especially with more and more patients surviving extensive burn injury. Richard and associates[2] expound on these current outcomes and difficulties, asserting, "The rehabilitation outcome of patients with severe burns is less than optimal and appears to have leveled off." Kowalske and coworkers[110] speak to the decreasing mortality rate and increasing morbidity rate being partly attributable to patients surviving with more complications from deep hand burns with exposed tendon or bone.

The therapist is encouraged to respond to the severity of these challenges by knowing the anatomy of the hand, upper extremity, and skin and the biomechanical and biorheological principles that govern the "science" of burn rehabilitation. Understanding and enacting the "art" of how to best establish the correct vision and goals at the correct time while implementing an efficient and effective burn therapy plan of care can be extremely difficult. Although the therapist's problem list and plan of care is straightforward, scar tissue of the hand and upper extremity often contract persistently and relentlessly. For this reason, the therapist must remain keenly aware of ensuing contractures and be vigilant in implementing and updating a creative plan of care that requires continuous time management as the scar tissue forms, remodels, and matures. Contractures are not prevented and managed well with a mere 30-minute daily treatment session and an orthosis. Typically, an effective treatment plan involves extensive and ongoing patient education and encouragement, anticontracture exercise techniques, or positioning techniques as well as orthoses for at least 6 to 8 hours per day and effective positioning and orthosis use at night. If the plan of care is implemented carefully, efficiently, and effectively, the therapist can make a profound and sustaining impact on the burn survivor's functional restoration and quality of life. With respect to the "art" of burn therapy, the overarching goal is to get recovering burn patients to do what they do not want to do so they can achieve the things they want and need to do to become

Dorsal View (Total)
(CFU 60000)

Palmar View (Total)
(CFU 100000)

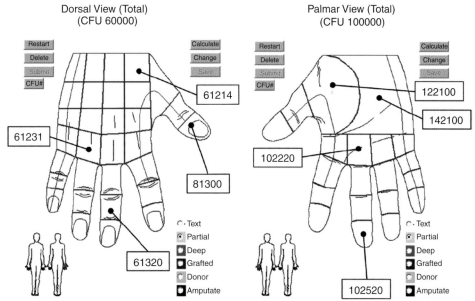

Fig. 82.42 Expanded view of the right hand surface area graphic evaluation/cutaneous functional units (SAGE/ CFU) diagrams with the examples of the CFU-numbering scheme. (From Richard R, Jones JA, Parshley P. Hierarchical decomposition of burn body diagram based on cutaneous functional units and its utility. *J Burn Care Res.* 2015;36[1];36; with permission.)

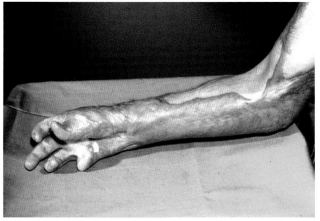

Fig. 82.43 Elbow flexion contracture and concomitant cupping deformity of the palm. Note the extensive scar spanning from the medial arm to the palm of the hand, which severely restricts elbow and hand extension.

functional. In that seemingly contradictory statement, the therapist must be able to earn the trust of the patient while remaining truly committed to using persistent yet gentle discomforting stress followed by prolonged positioning and compression to manage BSC and hypertrophic scar.

In managing skin and scar areas at risks for BSC of the hand and upper extremity, it is especially important for the therapist to help the team facilitate the burned patient's biorheological growth and psychological posttraumatic growth (PTG) throughout acute, intermediate, and long-term rehabilitation.[118,119] The therapist should be able to promote wound healing using protective orthoses and assist with wound care and dressing changes while preventing contractures, all by applying the biomechanical and biorheological principles of skin and scar. In turn, sustained and recovered motion should improve function and could lessen the problems associated with posttraumatic stress and encourage the client to experience physical and psychological PTG.[118,119]

SUMMARY

Rehabilitation management of the burned hand and upper extremity can be an overwhelming task, especially in association with other severely injured areas of the body. Therapist commitment throughout the acute, intermediate, and long-term phases of rehabilitation along with a team approach, including the physician, nurse, and family, is absolutely necessary to achieve optimal outcomes. The therapist must have a comprehensive understanding of upper extremity anatomy, edema prevention, scar formation and maturation, the use of orthoses, and the targeted use of therapeutic interventions, such as exercise, low-load prolonged-duration tension, and strengthening, to efficiently and effectively manage hand and upper extremity burns. Armed with this knowledge, an appropriate treatment plan can be developed to return the patient to a more independent and meaningful level of function. Nursing staff must be educated and encouraged to help reinforce rehabilitation goals. Most important, the family and patient must be involved in therapy and understand the goals of treatment. Patient adherence to established therapy routines and support from their loved ones are critical for an optimal outcome.

REFERENCES

1. Richard RL, Baryza M, Carr JA, et al. Burn rehabilitation and research: Proceedings from a consensus summit. *J Burn Care Res.* 2009;30(4):543–573.
2. Richard RL, Hedman T, Quick CD, et al. A clarion to recommit and reaffirm burn rehabilitation. *J Burn Care Res.* 2008;29:425–432.
3. Esselman PC, Thombs DB, Magyar-Russell G, et al. Burn rehabilitation: state of science. *Am J Phys Med Rehabil.* 2006;85:383–413.

SKIN ANATOMY AND FUNCTION

4. Falkel JE. Anatomy and physiology of the skin. In: Richard RL, Staley MJ, eds. *Burn Care and Rehabilitation Principles and Practice.* Philadelphia: FA Davis; 1994:10–28.

5. Marieb EN, Hoehn K. The integumentary system. In: Marieb EN, Hoehn K, eds. *Human Anatomy & Physiology*. 7th ed. San Francisco: Pearson Education Inc; 2007:151–174.

6. Brody G. The biomechanical properties of tissue. In: Rudolph R, ed. *Problems in Aesthetic Surgery: Biological Causes and Clinical Solutions*. St. Louis: The C.V. Mosby Company; 1986:49–64.

7. Sussman C. Assessment of the skin and wound. In: Sussman C, Bates-Jensen BM, eds. *Wound Care: A Collaborative Practice Manual for Health Professionals*. 3rd ed. Philadelphia: Lippincott Williams & Wilkins; 2007:85–122.

8. Germann G, Hrabowski H. Burned hand. In: Wolfe SW, Hotchkiss RN, Pederson WC, Kozin SH, Cohen MS, eds. *Green's Operative Hand Surgery*. 7th ed. Philadelphia: Elsevier; 2017:1926–1957.

9. Gilbert SF. The emergence of the ectoderm: the central nervous system and the epidermis. In: Gilbert SF, ed. *Developmental Biology*. 7th ed. Sunderland: Sinauer Associates Inc; 2003:391–425.

10. Greenhalgh DG, Staley MJ. Burn wound healing. In: Richard RL, Staley MJ, eds. *Burn Care and Rehabilitation Principles and Practice*. Philadelphia: FA Davis; 1994:70–102.

11. Howell JW. Management of the burned hand. In: Richard RL, Staley MJ, eds. *Burn Care and Rehabilitation Principles and Practice*. Philadelphia: FA Davis; 1994:531–575.

BIOMECHANICS OF SKIN AND SCAR

12. Pham TN, Cancio LC, Gibran NS. American Burn Association practice guidelines burn shock resuscitation. *J Burn Care Res*. 2008;29(1):257–266.

13. Hedman TL, Quick CD, Richard RL, et al. Rehabilitation of burn casualties. In: Lenhart MK, Pasquina PF, Cooper RA, eds. *Textbooks of Military Medicine: Care of the Combat Amputee, Falls Church (VA): Office of the Surgeon General*. Department of the Army; 2009:277–379.

14. Richard RL, Staley MJ. Biophysical aspects of normal skin and burn scar. In: Richard RL, Staley MJ, eds. *Burn Care and Rehabilitation Principles and Practice*. Philadelphia: FA Davis; 1994:49–69.

15. Weber E, Davis J. Rehabilitation following hand surgery. *Orthop Clin North Am*. 1978;92:529–542.

16. Brand PW, Hollister AM, Thompson DE. Chapter 7: mechanical resistance. In: *Brand PW & Hollister: Clinical Mechanics of the Hand*. 3rd ed. St. Louis: Mosby Inc; 1999:184–214.

17. Brand PW, Hollister AM, Giurintano DE, et al. Chapter 9: external stress: forces that affect joint action. In: *Brand PW & Hollister: Clinical Mechanics of the Hand*. 3rd ed. St. Louis: Mosby Inc; 1999:233–246.

18. Fess EE. Mechanical principles. In: Fess E, Gettle K, Philips C, Janson J, eds. *Hand and Upper Extremity Splinting: Principles & Methods*. 3rd ed. Philadelphia: Mosby; 2005:161–183.

19. Brand PW. Chapter 5: drag. In: Brand PW, ed. *Clinical Mechanics of the Hand*. St. Louis: C.V. Mosby Company; 1985:61–87.

20. Dunn MG, Silver FH, Swann DA. Mechanical analysis of hypertrophic scar tissue: structural basis for apparent increased rigidity. *J Invest Dermatol*. 1985;84:9–13.

21. Bell-Krotoski J. Tissue remodeling. In: Fess E, Gettle K, Philips C, Janson J, eds. *Hand and Upper Extremity Splinting: Principles & Methods*. 3rd ed. Philadelphia: Mosby; 2005:103–112.

22. Bell-Krotoski JA. Tissue remodeling and contracture correction using serial plaster casting and orthotic positioning. In: Skirven TM, Osterman AE, Fedorczyk JM, Amadio PC, eds. *Rehabilitation of the Hand and Upper Extremity*. 6th ed. Philadelphia: Mosby Inc; 2011:1597–1609.

23. Copley AL, Seaman GVF. The meaning of the terms rheology, biorheology and hemorheology. *Clin Hemorheol*. 1981;1:117–119.

24. Wilhelmi BJ, Blackwell SJ, Mancoll JS, Phillips LG. Creep vs Stretch: a review of the viscoelastic properties of skin. *Ann Plast Surg*. 1998;41:215–219.

25. Jacobs K. Dictionary of terms. In: Jacobs K, ed. *Quick Reference Dictionary for Occupational Therapy*. 2nd ed. 1999:55. Thorofare, NJ.

BURN WOUNDS

26. American Burn Association. Burn center referral criteria. Available at: http://ameriburn.org/wp-content/uploads/2017/05/burncenterreferralcriteria.pdf.

27. Lewis GM, Heimbach DM, Gibran NS. Evaluation of the burn wound: management decisions. In: Herndon DN. *Total Burn Care*. 4th ed. Philadelphia: Elsevier Inc; 2012:125–130.

28. Johnson C. Pathologic manifestations of burn injury. In: Richard RL, Staley MJ, eds. *Burn Care and Rehabilitation Principles and Practice*. Philadelphia: FA Davis; 1994:29–48.

29. Devgan L, Bhat S, Aylward S, Spence RJ. Modalities for the assessment of burn wound depth. *J Burns Wounds*. 2006;5:e2.

30. Richard R. Assessment and diagnosis of burn wounds. *Adv Wound Care*. 1999;12:468–471.

31. Deitch EA, Wheelaham TM, Rose MP. Hypertrophic burn scars: analysis of variables. *J Trauma*. 1983;23:895–898.

32. Holmes JH, Heimbach DM. Burns/inhalation injury. In: Peitzman AB, Rhodes M, Schwab CW, Yealy DM, Fabian TC, eds. *The Trauma Manual: Trauma and Acute Care Surgery*. 3rd ed. Philadelphia: Lippincott, Williams & Wilkins; 2007:387–492.

33. Saffle JR, Schnebly WA. Burn wound care. In: Richard RL, Staley MJ, eds. *Burn Care and Rehabilitation: Principles and Practice*. Philadelphia: FA Davis; 1994:119–176.

34. Hunt JL, Sato RM. Early excision of full-thickness hand and digit burns: factors affecting morbidity. *J Trauma*. 1982;22(5):414–419.

35. Staley M, Richard R, Warden GD, et al. Functional outcomes for the patient with burn injuries. *J Burn Care Rehabil*. 1996;7(4):362–368.

36. Richard RL, Dewey WS, Anyan WR, et al. Increased burn rehabilitation treatment time improves patient outcome. *J Burn Care Res*. 2014;35(3):S100.

37. Staley MJ, Richard RL. Scar management. In: Richard RL, Staley MJ, eds. *Burn Care and Rehabilitation Principles and Practice*. Philadelphia: FA Davis; 1994:380–418.

38. Ward S. Management of scar. In: Sussman C, Bates-Jensen BM, eds. *Wound Care: A Collaborative Practice Manual for Health Professionals*. 3rd ed. Philadelphia: Lippincott Williams & Wilkins; 2007:309–318.

EDEMA MANAGEMENT

39. Demling RH. The burn edema process: current concepts. *J Burn Care Rehabil*. 2005;26(3):207–227.

40. Hunter JM. Salvage of the burned hand. *Surg Clin North Am*. 1967;47:1059–1075.

41. Dewey WS, Hedman TL, Chapman TT, et al. The reliability and concurrent validity of the figure-of-eight method of measuring hand edema in patients with burns. *J Burn Care Res*. 2007;28:157–162.

42. Salisbury RE, Dingeldein GP. The burned hand and upper extremity. In: Green DP, ed. *Green's Operative Hand Surgery*. 3rd ed. Philadelphia: Elsevier Churchill Livingstone; 1993:2007–2031.

43. Villeco JP, Mackin EJ, Hunter JM. Edema: therapist's management. In: Hunter JM, Mackin EJ, Callahan AD, eds. *Rehabilitation of the Hand and Upper Extremity*. 5th ed. Philadelphia; 2002:183–193.

44. Lavelle K, Stanton DB. Measurement of edema in the hand clinic. In: MacDermid J, Solomon G, Valdes K, eds. *Clinical Assessment Recommendations: Impairment-Based Conditions*. 3rd ed. New Jersey: American Society of Hand Therapist; 2015:35–46.

45. Maihafer G, Llewellyn MA, Piller Jr WJ, et al. A comparison of the figure-of-eight method and water volumetry in measurement of hand and wrist size. *J Hand Ther*. 2003;16:305–310.

46. Kramer G, Lund T, Herndon D. Pathophysiology of burn shock and burn edema. In: Herndon DN, ed. *Total Burn Care*. 2nd ed. New York: W.B. Saunders; 2002:78–87.

POSITIONING THE UPPER EXTREMITY

47. Buescher TM, Pruitt BA. Burn scar contracture: prevention and treatment. *Probl Gen Surg.* 1994;11(4):804–815.
48. Shichinohe R, Yamamoto Y, Kawashima K, et al. Factors that affected functional outcome after a delayed excision and split-thickness skin graft on the dorsal side of burned hands. *J Burn Care Res.* 2017;38:e851–e858.
49. American Burn Association. National burn awareness week, February 4-10, 2018, burn injury fact sheet. Available at: https://ameriburn.org/wp-content/uploads/2017/12/nbaw-factsheet_121417-1.pdf.
50. Dewey WS, Richard RL, Parry IS. Positioning, splinting, and contracture management. *Phys Med Rehabil Clin N Am.* 2011;22:229–247.
51. Lester ME, Hazelton J, Dewey WS, et al. Influence of upper extremity positioning on pain, paresthesia, and tolerance: advancing current practice. *J Burn Care Res.* 2013;34:e324–e350.
52. Serghiou MA, Niszczak J, Parry I, et al. Clinical practice recommendations for positioning of the burn patient. *Burns.* 2016;42:267–275.
53. Serghiou MA, Ott S,C, Cowan A, et al. Burn rehabilitation along the continuum of care. In: Herndon DN, ed. *Total Burn Care.* 5th ed. Philadelphia: Elsevier Inc; 2018:476–508.
54. Richard RL, Hedman TL, Chapman TT, et al. Atlas of burn scar contractures: a patient education tool. *J Burn Care Res.* 2007;28:S152.

ORTHOTICS AND SERIAL CASTING

55. Fess EE. A history of splinting: to understand the present, view the past. In: Fess E, Gettle K, Philips C, Janson J, eds. *Hand and Upper Extremity Splinting: Principles & Methods.* 3rd ed. Philadelphia: Mosby; 2005:3–40.
56. Daugherty MB, Carr-Collins JA. Splinting techniques for the burn patient. In: Richard RL, Staley MJ, eds. *Burn Care and Rehabilitation: Principles and Practice.* Philadelphia: FA Davis Co; 1994:242–323.
57. Richard R, Chapman T, Dougherty M, et al. *An Atlas and Compendium of Burn Splints.* San Antonio, TX: Reg Richard, Inc; 2005.
58. Malick MH, Carr JA. *Manual on Management of the Burn Patient: Including Splinting, Mold and Pressure Techniques.* Pittsburgh: Harmarville Rehabilitation Center Educational Resource Division; 1982.
59. Vehmeyer-Heeman M, Lommers B, Van den Kerckhove E, et al. Axillary burns: extended grafting and early splinting prevents contractures. *J Burn Care Rehabil.* 2005;26(6):539–542.
60. Kolmus AM, Holland AE, Byrne MJ, et al. The effects of splinting on shoulder function in adult burns. *Burns.* 2012;38(5):638–644.
61. Richard RL. Use of the Dynasplint to correct elbow flexion contracture: a case report. *J Burn Care Rehabil.* 1986;7:151–152.
62. Grigsby-deLinde L, Knothe B. Therapist's management of the burned hand. In: Hunter JM, Mackin EJ, Callahan AD, eds. *Rehabilitation of the Hand and Upper Extremity.* 5th ed. Philadelphia: Mosby; 2002:1492–1526.
63. Colditz JC. The biomechanics of a thumb carpometacarpal immobilization orthosis: design and fitting. *J Hand Ther.* 2000;13(3):228–235.
64. Choi JS, Mun JH, Lee JY, et al. Effects of modified dynamic metacarpophalangeal joint flexion orthoses after hand burn. *Ann Rehabil Med.* 2011;35(6):880–886.
65. Wilton JC. Splinting to address the fingers. In: Wilton JC, ed. *Hand Splinting: Principles of Design and Fabrication.* London: WB Saunders; 1997:45–53.
66. Hooper RM, North ER. Dynamic interphalangeal extension splint design. *Am J Occup Ther.* 1982;36(4):257–258.
67. VanStraten O, Sagi A. "Supersplint": a new dynamic combination orthosis for the burned hand. *J Burn Care Rehabil.* 2000;21:71–73.
68. Callahan A, McEntee P. Splinting proximal interphalangeal joint flexion contractures: a new design. *Am J Occup Ther.* 1986;40(6):409–413.
69. Stack HG. A modified splint for mallet fingers. *J Hand Surg.* 1986;11:263.
70. Ward RS, Schnebly WA. Have you tried the sandwich orthosis? A method of preventing hand deformities in children. *J Burn Care Rehabil.* 1989;10(1):83–85.
71. Brand PW. The reconstruction of the hand in leprosy. *Ann Royal Coll Surg Engl.* 1952;11:350.
72. Bennett GB, Helm P, Purdue GF, et al. Serial casting: a method for treating contractures. *J Burn Care Rehabil.* 1989;10(6):543–545.
73. Serghiou MA, Ott SC, Cowan A, Kemp-Offenberg J, Suman OE. Burn rehabilitation along the continuum of care. In: Herndon DN, ed. *Total Burn Care.* 5th ed. Philadelphia: Elsevier Inc; 2018:476–508.
74. Staley M, Serghiou M. Casting guidelines, tips, and techniques: Proceedings from the 1997 American Burn Association PT/OT casting workshop. *J Burn Care Rehab.* 1998;19(3):254–260.

RANGE-OF-MOTION

75. Seftchick JL, Detullio LM, Fedorczyk JM, et al. Clinical examination of the hand. In: Skirven TM, Osterman AE, Fedorczyk JM, Amadio PC, eds. *Rehabilitation of the Hand and Upper Extremity.* 6th ed. Philadelphia: Mosby Inc; 2011:55–71f.
76. Korp K, Richard R, Hawkins D. Refining the idiom "functional range of motion" related to burn injury. *J Burn Care Res.* 2015;36:e136–e145.
77. Edgar D, Finlay V, Wu A, et al. Goniometry and linear assessments to monitor movement outcomes: are they reliable tools in burn survivors. *Burns.* 2009;35(1):58–62.
78. Holavanahalli RK, Helm PA, Gorman AR, et al. Outcomes after deep full thickness hand burns. *Arch Phys Med Rehabil.* 2007;88(12 suppl 2):S30–S35.
79. Richard R, Parry IS, Santos A, et al. Burn hand or finger goniometric measurements: sum of the isolated parts and the composite whole. *J Burn Care Res.* 2017;38:e960–e965.
80. Tuden-Neugerbauer C, Serghiou M, Herndon DN, et al. Effects of a 12-week rehabilitation program with music & exercise groups on range of motion in young children with severe burns. *J Burn Care Res.* 2008;29:939–948.
81. Foster K, Leonhard V, Ray R, et al. The impact of early autografting on functional range of motion of the hand. *J Burn Care Res.* 2018;39:S142.

STRENGTH, CONDITIONING AND ACTIVITIES OF DAILY LIVING (ADLs)

82. Rivas E, Herndon DN, Cambiaso-Daniel J, et al. Quantification of an exercise rehabilitation program for severely burned children: the standard of care at Shriners Hospitals for Children-Galveston. *J Burn Care Res.* 2018;39(6):889–896.
83. Cronan T, Hammond J, Ward CG. The value of isokinetic exercise and testing in burn rehabilitation and determination of back-to-work status. *J Burn Care Rehab.* 1990;11:224–227.
84. Covey MH, Dutcher K, Marvin JA, et al. Efficacy of continuous passive motion (CPM) devices with hand burns. *J Burn Care Rehab.* 1988;9:397–400.
85. Ibebunjo C, Martyn JAJ. Muscle dysfunction after burn and immobilization: a comparison. *J Burn Care Rehab.* 1998;19:S236.
86. Yasuhara S, Kanakubo E, Perez ME, et al. The 1999 Moyer Award: burn injury induces skeletal muscle apoptosis and activation of caspase pathways in rats. *J Burn Care Rehab.* 1999;20:462–467.

PAIN MANAGEMENT

87. Wiechman Askay S, Patterson DR. What are the psychiatric sequelae of burn pain? *Curr Pain Headache Rep.* 2008;12(2):94–97.
88. Low AJ, Dyster-Aas J, Kildal M, et al. The presence of nightmares as a screening tool for symptoms of posttraumatic stress disorder in burn survivors. *J Burn Care Res.* 2006;27(5):727–733.

SENSATION

89. Ward RS, Tuckett RP. Quantitative changes in cutaneous sensation of patients with burns. *J Burn Care Rehabil.* 1991;12:569–575.

90. Holavanahalli RK, Helm PA, Kowalske KJ. Long-term outcomes in patients surviving large burns: the skin. *J Burn Care Res*. 2010;41:631–639.

91. Mazzetto- Betti KC, Amancio AC, Farina Jr JA, et al. High-voltage electrical burn injuries: functional upper extremity assessment. *Burns*. 2009;35:707–713.

92. Weinstein S. Fifty years of somatosensory research: from the Semmes-Weinstein monofilaments to Weinstein enhanced sensory test. *J Hand Ther*. 1993;G:11.

93. Dellon AL, ed. *Evaluation of Sensibility and Re-education of Sensation in the Hand*. Baltimore: Lucas; 1988.

SCAR MANAGEMENT

Scar Assessment

94. Brusselaers N, Pirayesh A, Hoeksema H, et al. Burn scar assessment: a systematic review of objective scar assessment tools. *Burns*. 2010;36(8):1157–1164.

95. Parry IS, Walker K, Niszczak J, et al. Methods and tools used for the measurement of burn scar contracture. *J Burn Care Res*. 2010;31(6):888–903.

96. Nedelec B, Correa JA, Rachelska G, et al. Quantitative measurement of hypertrophic scar: interrater reliability and concurrent validity. *J Burn Care Res*. 2008;29(3):501–511.

97. Tyack Z, Simons M, Spinks A, et al. A systematic review of the quality of burn scar rating scales for clinical and research use. *Burns*. 2012;38(1):6–18.

98. Kaartinen IS, Välisuo PO, Alander JT, et al. Objective scar assessment—a new method using standardized digital imaging and spectral modelling. *Burns*. 2011;37(1):74–81.

99. Anthonissen M, Daly D, Fieuws S, et al. Measurement of elasticity and transepidermal water loss rate of burn scars with the Dermalab burns. 39(3):420–428.

100. Bloeman MCT, van der Veer W, Ulrich MMW, et al. Prevention and curative management of hypertrophic scar formation. *Burns*. 2009;35(4):463–475.

101. Gabriel V, Holavanahalli R. Burn rehabilitation. In: Braddom RL, ed. *Physical Medicine and Rehabilitation*. 4th ed. Philadelphia: Elsevier Inc; 2011:256–298.

102. Van der Veer WM, Bloemen MCT, Ulrich MMW, et al. Potential cellular and molecular causes of hypertrophic scar formation. *Burns*. 2009;35(1):15–29.

103. Engrav LH, Heimbach DM, Rivara FP, et al. 12-Year within-wound study of the effectiveness of custom pressure garment therapy. *Burns*. 2010;36(7):975–998.

104. Tredget E, Wang J, Jiao H, et al. Decreased fibrocytes in post-burn hypertrophic scar after treatment with interferon alpha-2b. *Wound Repair Regen*. 2008;16(2):126.

SCAR TREATMENT

105. Serghiou MA, Ott S, Whitehead C, et al. Comprehensive rehabilitation of the burn patient. In: Herndon DN, ed. *Total Burn Care*. 4th ed. Philadelphia: Elsevier Inc; 2012:517–549.

106. O'Brien L, Pandit A. Silicon gel sheeting for preventing and treating hypertrophic and keloid scars. *Cochrane Database Sys Rev*. 2006;25(1):CD003826.

107. Mustoe TA. Evolution of silicone therapy and mechanism of action in scar management. *Aesth Plast Surg*. 2008;32:82–92.

108. Van den Kerckhove E, Stappaerts K, Boeckx W, et al. Silicones in the rehabilitation of burns: a review and overview. *Burns*. 2001;27(3):205–214.

BURN SCAR CONTRACTURE

109. Chapman TT, Richard RL, Hedman TL, et al. Military return to duty and civilian return to work factors following burns with focus on the hand and literature review. *J Burn Care Res*. 2008;29:756–762.

110. Kowalske KJ, Greenhalgh DG, Ward SR. Hand burns. *J Burn Care Res*. 2007;28(4):607–610.

111. Apfel LM, Irwin CP, Staley MJ, et al. Approaches to positioning the burn patient. In: Richard RL, Staley MJ, eds. *Burn Care and Rehabilitation Principles and Practice*. Philadelphia: FA Davis; 1994:221–241.

112. Junker JPE, Kratz C, Tollback A, et al. Mechanical tension stimulates the transdifferentiation of fibroblasts into myofibroblasts in human burn scars. *Burns*. 2008;34(7):942–946.

113. Richard R, Dewey S, Parry IS, et al. Letter to the editor. *Burns*. 2013;39(3):539–541.

114. Richard R, Jones JA, Parshley P. Hierarchical decomposition of burn body diagram based on cutaneous functional units and its utility. *J Burn Care Res*. 2015;36(1):33–43.

115. Hawkins H, Finnerty CC. Pathophysiology of burn scar. In: Herndon DN, ed. *Total Burn Care*. 4th ed. Philadelphia: Elsevier Inc; 2012:507–514.

116. Kraemer MD, Jones T, Deitch EA. Burn contractures: Incidence, predisposing factors, and results of surgical therapy. *J Burn Care Rehabil*. 1988;9:261–265.

117. Schneider JC, Holavanahalli R, Heim P, et al. Contractures in burn injury: defining the problem. *J Burn Care Res*. 2006;27(4):508–514.

118. Martin L, Byrnes M, McGarry S, et al. Posttraumatic growth after burn in adults: an integrative literature review. *Burns*. 2017;43:459–470.

119. Martin L, Byrnes M, Bulsara MK, et al. Quality of life and posttraumatic growth after adult burn: a prospective, longitudinal study. *Burns*. 2017;43:1400–1410.

83

Psychosocial Issues After a Traumatic Upper Extremity Injury: Facilitating Adjustment

Susan D. Hannah, Michael K. Cheng

OUTLINE

CRITICAL POINTS

- Hands are integral in defining us as human beings. Given their importance in all aspects of life, individuals may experience significant physical, psychological, and social consequences after a hand injury. These issues can interfere with physical recovery and the resumption of activities and roles.
- Adjustment improves when the complex interplay among physical, psychological, and social elements is recognized and valued goals are integrated into the treatment plan.
- Given the intensive course of therapy after a traumatic injury, hand therapists can play a central role in facilitating physical and psychosocial adjustment.
- Ongoing assessment using brief and easily administered screening tools is important to facilitate referral for psychological intervention. Three months is a good time to identify patients in need of psychological support and counseling.
- Ongoing evaluation of coping strategies can help identify maladaptive coping behaviors and assist patients in developing more effective strategies.
- Facilitating functional goals that are meaningful to patients enhances engagement and physical and emotional recovery.
- The resumption of valued roles (e.g., spouse, caregiver, friend, worker) is critical to identity, self-worth, and recovery.
- Motivational interviewing is a structured approach that can be used to facilitate positive patient change. Motivational interviewing principles and techniques are summarized in this chapter.

INTRODUCTION

Hands are integral in defining us as human beings. They are highly specialized parts of the body and have many functions, including physical, psychological, and social.[1] They provide us with independence in work, leisure, self-care, and social interactions.[2] Hands are symbolic in communication[3] and expression[4] and are used in greetings, prayer, intimacy, and protection.[3]

Given their importance in all aspects of life, individuals may experience significant physical, psychological, and social consequences after a hand injury.[2,3,5–8] The meaning that individuals ascribe to hands are shaped by personal, family, and cultural factors. These "meanings" affect how people perceive the injury, which in turn influences adjustment and recovery.[9] This process is unique to each person and changes over time. The treatment of complex hand injuries involves long-term, one-to-one, intensive therapy. The hand therapist thereby has a unique opportunity to play a central role in facilitating physical and psychosocial adjustment. Therapists are highly specialized in physical care but also have the training and knowledge to address psychosocial issues. Psychosocial issues can create barriers to successful adjustment and should therefore be addressed in conjunction with the physical recovery of a hand injury.[9] Adjustment improves when the complex interplay among physical, psychological, and social elements is recognized and valued goals are integrated into the treatment plan.[2,10,11] This requires ongoing enquiry and assessment over the course of therapy to facilitate and provide appropriate and timely interventions. When hand therapists treat the whole person and collaboratively develop patient-centered goals, outcomes improve.[8]

Although this chapter is divided into sections, the dynamic interrelationship of a physical injury on the psychological and social aspects of each person's life requires a biopsychosocial lens rather than a biomedical and impairment approach to facilitate adjustment. This chapter describes (1) the psychosocial consequences of a serious hand and upper extremity injury, (2) setting the therapeutic stage including use of motivational interviewing (MI), (3) the importance of adopting an interdisciplinary approach to assessment and treatment planning, and (4) hand therapy–specific assessment and treatment interventions related to psychological and social issues after a traumatic hand and upper extremity injury.

SETTING THE THERAPEUTIC STAGE: TRUST, RESPECT, COMMUNICATION, AND RELATIONSHIP

Vranceanu and Ring[12] have stated: "The health provider–patient relationship is one of the most important predictors of patient satisfaction, adherence to (medical) treatment, and overall treatment success."

At some point in time, most people have either personally experienced or observed an interaction whereby a health care provider did not allow a patient to fully explain her or his symptoms, concerns, or the situational factors leading up to a particular health event. The health care provider interrupted the patient, never made eye contact, and then abruptly told the patient the cause of the problem and the solution. Interactions such as these leave patients feeling disempowered, that their concerns have not been heard, understood, or in some cases believed. Ultimately, the patient may never return for follow-up and seeks care elsewhere. The clinician may have exceptional technical and evidence-based skills, but without trust, rapport, respect, empathy, effective communication, and a safe therapeutic relationship, the patient will never benefit from this knowledge and expertise. Using the first clinical visit to develop rapport, particularly in situations in which patients are distrustful, angry, or fearful, may be more beneficial for future interactions than providing a complete and rushed evaluation and intervention.[12] Normalizing the person's experience, providing choices, asking permission to perform the physical examination, and legitimizing concerns all help to decrease anxiety.

> Mrs. Horvat fell on her left, nondominant hand 6 months ago. She developed chronic regional pain syndrome (CRPS), and it was recommended by her family physician that she seek treatment by a Certified Hand Therapist. Early on in the assessment, she mentioned that she was a two-time cancer survivor and that she had posttraumatic stress disorder. She was highly anxious and had read as much as she could about CRPS on the internet.

Mrs. Horvat had noticeable sympathetic changes in her left hand in addition to decreased motion of her fingers, thumb, and wrist; however, she was using her left hand to communicate and pick up small objects. Her pain was well controlled with medication, and she was seeing a counsellor for posttraumatic stress disorder (PTSD). The hand therapist spent time answering questions and reassuring Mrs. Horvat that she was "on the right track" because she was using her left hand for activities at home and at work. The hand therapist explained the benefits, from a cortical and emotional perspective, of integrating valued and pleasurable activities into her life to balance and distract from the pain and subsequent anxiety. Mrs. Horvat had not been provided with a comprehensive home exercise program and was unsure what she could be doing to improve the function of her hand. Given that her pain was well controlled, her hand therapist discussed the importance of working on range of motion and desensitization throughout the day in a graduated fashion. The therapist outlined her plan to perform a detailed physical evaluation during their first visit but that they would collaboratively create a treatment plan during the second visit that would address impairment needs with the goal of returning her to valued activities such as yoga. At the end of the first session, Mrs. Horvat said, "This has been the most helpful information that I have received to date. Thank you so much." This shared decision process is dynamic and complex but results in greater patient satisfaction, improved outcomes, and acceptance and adherence to recommended treatment strategies.[12]

INTERDISCIPLINARY ASSESSMENT AND PLANNING

Because of a high co-occurrence between hand injuries and disruptions in the psychological, social, and functional domain, hand treatment should use an interdisciplinary assessment approach. Brief and easily administered psychological measures can be used to assess pain, depression, anxiety, and posttraumatic stress over time and can help with referral and treatment decisions.

Information from the clinical assessment and psychological measures can then be integrated into an interdisciplinary plan. Planning should not be based on the severity of the physical injury alone because this has been found to be a poor predictor of adjustment and outcome.[2] It is important for the treatment team to have an understanding of the injury, its likely course, and the indicated interventions. Team membership is dependent on the nature of the setting and program resources. In many cases, a surgeon and hand therapist will be the core elements of a team. When indicated by assessment results, clinical judgment, or the course of recovery, the surgeon and hand therapist should collaboratively consider the potential benefits of referral to other disciplines. In some cases, the surgeon will be best positioned to facilitate a pain or surgical consultation. In other cases, the hand therapist may have a more comprehensive understanding of possible barriers to rehabilitation and recovery whereby referral to psychology may be beneficial. In either case, collaborative and consistent communication with the patient will help support engagement and effective treatment planning. This sharing of profession-specific perspectives can help each team member to integrate relevant goals into their treatment programs. For example, the hand therapist can assist the team psychologist to understand the physical aspects of the case to help assess the accuracy of the hand patient's perceptions, promote accurate and adaptive thinking, and support engagement in healthy activities that have been collaboratively identified by the team. Such a plan may involve reducing pain inputs through activity modification or challenging pain perceptions through graduated exposure and stress reduction.

Effective interdisciplinary planning integrates information related to physical, personal, social, and system factors to sequence treatment goals, reduce barriers, promote collaborative and consistent goal setting, and reduce the potential for conflict between the patient and team members and among team members. Failure to do this may result in patient resistance and limited progress, both physically and psychologically.

PSYCHOLOGICAL RESPONSES AFTER A TRAUMATIC HAND INJURY

Individuals who experience serious hand injuries face constant reminders of unwanted loss. Reminders can include posttraumatic reexperiencing, situational anxiety, neuropathic pain, increases in pain with activity, reductions in dexterity and strength, reductions in abilities to achieve important goals, and the social appraisal of others. They may develop into more rigid, intense, persistent, and pervasive problems when challenges continue to overwhelm available coping responses and supports. Development of clinical psychopathology may depend on personal factors (e.g., anxiety, high identification with lost ability), social responses (e.g., partner or peer rejection), and the availability of suitable work or retraining opportunities.

Hand injuries can be particularly stressful because of how the hand was injured and in many cases mutilated. Individuals can experience intense emotions (anxiety, guilt, fear, sadness, anger) immediately after their injury, during subsequent surgical and therapy treatments, and throughout their ongoing evaluation of its impact on their lives.[2,13] Hand therapists can educate patients about these normal responses to trauma, which may give them peace of mind.[2]

There is a wide response to a hand injury, from an individual with a minor fingertip amputation who no longer goes out in public to the person with a mangling punch press injury and resultant finger amputations who plays guitar professionally. It is important to keep in mind that the severity of a hand injury does not predict adaptation and resiliency.[2,6] However, from a hand therapy perspective, disproportionate or disabling stress responses benefit from prompt identification and referral for appropriate intervention.[6,8]

Grunert and coworkers[13] studied psychological symptoms after severe, work-related injuries and categorized them into four domains: (1) cognitive, (2) affective, (3) physiological, and (4) behavioral. They examined the incidence of these symptoms over time and documented which symptoms persisted. In the cognitive domain, individuals experienced *flashbacks* (80.6%), *nightmares* (70%), and had *concentration/attention difficulties* (13.5%) immediately after their injuries.[13] *Nightmares* and *concentration/attention* difficulties decreased significantly after 3 months, but *flashbacks* persisted in 39.4% of the sample at 18 months.[13]

The type of flashback (*replay, appraisal, projected*) experienced and its relationship to return to work have been studied.[6,13] In a *replay* flashback, the individual experiences the entire accident again, often in great detail.[6] *Replay* flashbacks respond to early treatment and are more amenable to early return to work.[6,13] An *appraisal* flashback occurs when the individual sees his or her hand in snapshot form immediately after the injury.[6] A *projected* flashback occurs when the individual sees scenes that never actually occur.[6] A combined *appraisal and projected* flashback emphasizes the individual's feeling of little or no control over the incident, thereby enhancing his or her belief of the workplace as dangerous.[13] This belief impedes successful return to work.[6]

Symptoms in the affective domain include anxiety, depression, disgust, irritability, hostility, and concerns about cosmesis.[13] Anxiety, specifically related to concern regarding reinjury, was present in 50% of the sample but declined steadily over 18 months.[13] Personal acceptance of the cosmetic effect of the hand injury was initially high (51.2%) but decreased (14.1%) by 18 months.[13] Concerns regarding *social acceptability* were still relatively high (31.8%) at 18 months.[13] Overall, emotional reactions were frequent and contributed to ongoing adjustment issues for approximately 30% of clients in the study.[13]

Symptoms in the physiological domain (startle reaction, phantom sensations, sexual dysfunction) decreased over 18 months; however, sexual dysfunction was not identified as an issue initially but was noted in 34.1% of the responses at month 3 and persisted in 12.4% of the cases at month 18.[13] This is seen clinically when patients are focused on the immediate physical aspects of their hand injury such as wound care, loss of range of motion (ROM), and pain. They may not have the opportunity to experience limitations regarding sexuality until issues such as wound healing, functional loss, and pain have been addressed.

In the behavioral domain, symptoms include *avoidance, denial, gaze aversion, alcohol or drug abuse,* and *marital distress.*[13] Of interest to hand therapists is that marital distress is not identified immediately after injury but rises to 19.4% at month 3 and persists at 18 months (14.7%).[13] This finding is observed clinically as the long-term impacts of a hand injury (physical, emotional, financial) stress significant relationships. During therapy, patients may share relationship issues with their hand therapists. Depending on the comfort level and clinical experience of the therapist involved, specific strategies related to communication, relaxation, and stress management may be aspects of hand therapy care. Referrals to family physicians, social workers, or psychologists are appropriate therapeutic options.

Also in the behavioral domain, *gaze aversion* is high initially (43.5%) but decreases to 2.9% by 18 months.[13] Long-term gaze aversion related to the hand or wound and negative reactions such as vomiting are "associated with trauma-related distress and mood disorders."

Careful observation of how a client reacts to the sight of the hand over time can help identify those in need of psychological support.[14]

PSYCHOLOGICAL ISSUES: HAND THERAPY INTERVENTION

Monitoring emotions and psychological symptoms during regular therapy sessions is an important aspect of ongoing assessment and treatment. Many psychological symptoms will decrease over time. If gaze aversion or pain-avoidance behaviors persist, there is likely an adjustment problem.[14] Does the patient take ownership of his wound care, scar management, and exercise program, or does he allow his spouse to "do" the therapy for him?

Patients should be encouraged to take control of their hand therapy program because this improves adherence. Active participation provides valuable feedback to the patient regarding sensations that are helpful, such as a stretch during passive ROM exercises, which helps them overcome the faulty assumption that all pain is harmful.

Because the best outcomes rely on regular exercises outside of the clinic situation, a clear understanding of the concept of hurt versus harm is critical. Most important, participation increases the individual's feelings of control and self-efficacy, which have been altered by the injury itself. This discussion may also need to include family members so that a clear understanding of therapy expectations and the benefits from this approach is understood.[9]

Incorporating questions related to sleep patterns, mood changes, and behavioral and physical changes can highlight persistent psychological symptoms that should be addressed.[8] Hand therapists can facilitate referrals to a family physician, psychologist, psychiatrist, or hand injury support group.

Regarding the timing of these referrals, Gustafsson and Ahlstrom[7] followed patients for 1 year after a severe hand injury and investigated changes in physical and psychological issues over time, the frequency of persisting issues, and their impact on work and life situations.[7] Problems identified immediately after injury, such as functional impairment, pain, trauma-related distress, mood disorders, and negative reactions to the sight of the hand, decreased during the first 3 months but tended to remain unchanged during the remainder of the first year. Persistent behaviors such as gaze aversion, pain-avoidance behaviors, flashback, nightmares, startle reactions, and hypervigilance are red flags. Three months is therefore a good time to identify patients in need of psychological support and counseling and to make the appropriate referrals.[7,13] It is important to note that some issues, such as marital stress and sexual concerns, may not surface until a later date and should also be monitored over time.

Standardized assessments (Table 83.1) can be used immediately after injury and at regular intervals during treatment to identify stress-related issues and changes that occur over the course of treatment. These can be an important starting point for discussions between patients and therapists when collaboratively developing a plan to address identified issues. Although people can present as coping well, they may be experiencing stress-related symptoms that should be addressed early to help prevent prolongation of maladaptive symptoms such as flashbacks, nightmares, and avoidance of accident reminders.[8,14]

Patients are often hesitant to discuss their psychological issues because of the perceived stigma associated with stress behaviors and feelings and often say, "I don't want people to think that I'm crazy." This creates tremendous stress for patients and their families, who often notice behavior changes, such as increased irritability and anger. When discussing referral to other health professionals, it is important to convey that this is part of the overall treatment program[2] because many patients

TABLE 83.1	**Psychological Measures**
Pain	Pain Catastrophizing Scale (PCS)[15,16]
	McGill Pain Questionnaire(MPQ)[17,18]
Depression	Pain Health Questionnaire 9 (PHQ-9)[19,20]
	Quick Inventory of Depressive Symptoms Self-Report 16 (QIDS-SR16)[21,22]
	Beck Depression Inventory 2 (BDI-II)[23,24]
Anxiety	Generalized Anxiety Disorder 7 (GAD-7)[19,20]
	Beck Anxiety Inventory (BAI)[24,25]
Trauma	Posttraumatic Stress Disorder Checklist for DSM-5 (PCL-5)[26,27]
	Impact of Event Scale–Revised (IES-R)[28,29]

express concern about the potential stigma of counseling. Patients need to be reassured that stress responses are normal responses to trauma but that prolonged symptoms can impede progress and adjustment, hence the addition of other treatment resources such as counseling.[9]

MENTAL HEALTH ASSESSMENT

Although individuals who have experienced serious hand injuries commonly experience psychological symptoms, rigid, intense, persistent, and pervasive problems causing significant distress or functional impairment should be assessed further by a psychologist or psychiatrist. In some cases, clinical psychopathology may arise directly and immediately from the accident itself. In other cases, overuse of limited or maladaptive coping responses or prolonged exposure to postaccident stress may result in more psychopathological processes, including depression, as a result of learned helplessness, generalized anxiety (including panic and poorly controlled worry), and development of somatoform or substance use disorders.

Many psychological approaches that have been found to be effective fall under the general framework of cognitive behavioral therapy. Newer approaches, including acceptance and commitment therapy,[30] aim not only to reduce symptoms but to recognize the importance of supporting an individual's specific values and goals and promoting increased flexibility after experiencing unwanted change.

There are excellent guidelines for the psychological and psychiatric treatment of patients with depression, anxiety, posttraumatic stress, somatoform, substance, and personality disorders that are beyond the scope of this chapter to review.[31–34]

COPING STRATEGIES

Evaluation Over Time

People experience strong emotional responses after hand injuries. Although specific symptoms of anxiety, depression, or PTSD may or may not be present, mood fluctuations are likely to occur as each person adapts to changes in her or his life.[1,35] Coping is complex and incorporates emotional, psychological, and behavioral responses to an injury and the subsequent impact of this injury on the person's life. Identifying both effective and maladaptive coping early and throughout the treatment process may therefore improve the individual's overall adjustment after his or her hand injury.[1]

Coping can be defined as cognitive and behavioral efforts to manage psychological stress and is used to manage problems that cause stress (problem-focused coping) and to regulate emotions caused by the problems (emotion-focused coping).[2,5,36] Problem-focused coping, such as modifying equipment or seeking counseling, is more common when stressful conditions are viewed as controllable through action.[37] Emotion-focused coping, such as distancing and distracting attention from the event, dominates when situations are assessed as being impossible

to change.[37] Coping strategies are evaluated as effective if they are used at the appropriate time and fit the situational and life context of that person.[37] People use several coping strategies at the same time; however, there is often a dominant strategy used at any one time.[36]

Meyer[2] divides coping strategies into engaging and disengaging strategies. Engaging strategies are associated with more positive adjustment and include determining positive meaning from the event, active problem solving, and perceiving personal control.[2] Disengaging strategies include a perception of helplessness, lack of control, catastrophizing (thinking and believing the worst), and emotional and behavioral avoidance.[2]

Emotional distress in the first weeks after a hand injury results from functional and financial loss, dependency, uncertainty about the future, disfigurement, the trauma experience itself, and pain.[36,37] In some circumstances, such as replantation, emotional distress can be delayed because the patient's primary focus is on reattachment of the fingers or hand. The functional ramifications of the hand injury have not yet been evaluated by the patient. Strategies such as avoidance and distancing, which are commonly used initially after a traumatic hand injury, can become maladaptive if used long term or in isolation.

How people respond to a hand injury depends on how they evaluate the impact of this event on their lives[37] and the coping strategies that they use vary based on this ongoing self-assessment.[36] This evaluation process occurs continuously and is influenced by personal (past and present), cultural, and situational factors.[37] Coping strategies evolve over time depending on the problem, the situation, and the personality of the individual[36] and are often subconsciously used.[1] It is important for hand therapists to recognize and assess the coping strategies used by patients and how they can affect adaptation and resiliency, either positively or negatively. Multiple coping scales can be used for this purpose.[38] Given the long-term therapeutic relationship that often develops, hand therapists have a unique opportunity to assess coping over time and assist patients in finding the most effective coping strategies for them.[1]

Hand Therapy Intervention

> Ms. Nair a 26-year-old, right-handed recent immigrant, was offered temporary work at the factory where her mother-in-law worked. Her right arm was caught in a machine for 30 minutes, resulting in a crush, avulsion injury to her volar forearm. Her coworkers were talking among themselves while waiting for the fire department and ambulance to arrive. Ms. Nair reports that no one, including her mother-in-law, came to comfort her while her forearm was caught in the machine.

From a hand therapy perspective, it is important to identify which strategies are used by the individual during each stage of recovery and determine if these strategies are assisting or hindering adjustment.

Ms. Nair initially used distancing as a strategy to avoid social situations and minimize discussion of her hand injury. However, she continued to use this as her primary coping strategy 1 year after her injury, Ms. Nair told her hand therapist that her sister-in-law was coming from India to visit. Previous conversations with Ms. Nair illustrated how close she was to her sister-in-law; however, Ms. Nair indicated that she was not going to see her during this particular visit, stating, "I don't want to see my pain on her face. I don't want her sympathy." Her hand therapist struggled with this situation, wondering if she should discuss this further and how to do so respectfully. The next day, her hand therapist asked Ms. Nair how she would feel if she did not see her sister-in-law. Ms. Nair replied that she would feel very upset if this occurred. Her hand therapist asked Ms. Nair if she would feel comfortable discussing her feelings with her sister-in-law and if this would help to "clear the air" so that they could talk about other topics and not her hand injury specifically. The following week, Ms. Nair told her therapist that she had spoken with her sister-in-law and had attended the family reunion over the weekend.

This situation highlights self-appraisal by the hand therapist regarding boundaries, roles, and possible interventions. The use of open-ended questions such as, "How would you feel if…" can be helpful in facilitating new thinking about a situation and change a potentially negative outcome to one that will ultimately benefit the injured person. In this particular situation, by avoiding social functions, Ms. Nair would have lost the potential benefits of being with family, including redefining roles, engaging in meaningful activities, and receiving relational support.

The observation of physical postures (hand-hiding), interactions with family members and listening to patients' descriptions of their daily activities can help highlight coping strategies, both behavioral and emotional, that are no longer helpful for long-term adjustment. Coping strategies, change over time and therefore should be evaluated longitudinally over the course of treatment.[1] Individualized intervention can then be initiated, with the patient being central to this process. This involves ongoing enquiry by the hand therapist to monitor change over time with a realization that adjustment is unpredictable and specific to each individual. This can be frustrating for both the patient and therapist and requires trust, mutual respect, and ongoing problem solving to be successful.

SOCIAL ISSUES AFTER A HAND INJURY

Christiansen[39] points out that "if our identities are crafted by what we do and how we do it, then it follows that any threat to our ability to engage in occupations and present ourselves as competent people becomes a threat to our identity." Because we are social beings, identity change "influences our life and the lives of others."[4]

Multiple social changes take place after a hand injury. These include reassessing life goals, reintegrating an altered body image, dealing with dependence, heightened emotions, role failures and modifications, and coping with social stigma.[2,4,40] Disfigurement can negatively affect self-image,[1] thereby affecting social interactions and relationships. One patient reported that his wife "can't stand to have me touch her anymore." A visible hand injury can discourage prospective employers from hiring individuals who are viewed as less productive. This is particularly true during difficult economic times.

Hand therapists are in a position to ask enquiring questions throughout the physical and emotional recovery phase to evaluate preinjury routines, goals, and valued roles. By asking questions and actively listening to patients as they share their stories, hopes, and aspirations, hand therapists can help to identify maladaptive coping strategies and behavior changes, such as social isolation, sleeping during the day, reliance on medication, weight gain, irritability, and anger, and assist patients in recognizing the potentially negative impact of these behaviors on recovery and adjustment.

THE IMPACT OF ROLE CHANGE: SPOUSE, CAREGIVER, FRIEND, AND WORKER

Hand injuries affect how people perform their roles as spouse, caregiver, friend, and worker.[4] Participants in a study by Shier and Chan[4] said that they experienced profound changes in their ability to perform their preinjury life roles. With respect to spousal relationships, patients reported increased dependence on their spouses, both physically and emotionally, thereby altering their spouses' lives as well as "the relationship as a whole."[4] There may be a change in intimacy because of the role that hands play in conveying feelings, emotions, and sexuality.[4] Hand injuries can jeopardize family income, status, and participation in family activities, such as sports, travel, and other shared activities. Bankruptcy and subsequent loss of a home can create significant personal and relational stress. Financial stresses may require that the role of "breadwinner" be adopted by another family member.[4,10] As discussed in the psychological section, marital distress or relationship breakdowns were reported at 3 months postinjury.[4,13] This is multifaceted and can be the result of physical intimacy issues, a breakdown

in communication, role change, psychological distress such as increased irritability and anger, dependency, and depression.

An inability to care for young children or aging parents, with resulting dependency on a child, friends or family, can significantly change the parent or caregiver role. When adults require assistance from a child to perform intimate self-care tasks such as bathing or shaving, relationships are altered by this role reversal. There are often accompanying feelings of guilt, anger, and frustration, from both the child and parent, which can further stress relationships.

Isolation from friends after a hand injury is common, particularly after the acute stage of recovery. People report that they no longer socialize with friends because they have no new experiences to share, and conversation tends to focus solely on their injury. Because their regular routines and roles have been interrupted or lost, they have minimal to no contact with coworkers. Participation in shared activities such as sports may be limited or curtailed because of their hand injury. Life goals are placed on hold, resulting in an ongoing cycle of isolation and decreased social confidence. This in turn can lead to depression, irritability, anger, and further stress on family and friends.

Work is a major source of personal satisfaction and social interaction, so a temporary or permanent loss of the worker role can have a significant impact on self-esteem.[10,13] Facilitation of early, meaningful return to work is therefore important, and depending on the situation, the hand therapist can positively impact this process.[8] Hand therapists are often required to complete reports that impact return-to-work decisions. Interventions such as work modifications, addressing fears related to reinjury and PTSD triggers, establishing safe return to work recommendations, and maximizing both impairments and work skills are elements of a comprehensive hand therapy role.

HAND THERAPY INTERVENTION: RESTORING VALUED ROLES AND PATIENT-CENTERED ASSESSMENT

Restoring Valued Roles

Christiansen[39] has stated: "Therapy becomes identity building when therapists provide environments that help persons explore possible selves and achieve success in tasks that are instrumental to identities they strive to achieve, and when it enables them to validate the identities that they have worked hard to achieve in the past."

Role change and functional loss can negatively affect self-image, leaving patients with a sense of inadequacy and loss of identity.[5,6,37] Traditionally, hand therapy has focused on impairment; however, it is important to identify and incorporate functional goals into our treatment programs that are meaningful to the patient. This enhances engagement and physical and emotional recovery. If appropriate from a cultural perspective, assisting patients in becoming independent in self-care as soon as possible is critical in the recovery process. This independence positively affects self-esteem and restores valued roles.[37] Facilitating participation in meaningful activities through adaptive equipment, activity modification, compensatory strategies, and training ensures that important roles are preserved.[41]

Mr. Smith, a 35-year-old mechanic, and father of three, sustained an amputation of his left dominant small and ring fingers after a small scratch at work and subsequent infection. The infection resulted from necrotizing fasciitis secondary to prednisone use for a preexisting medical condition. He was found unconscious by his wife and rushed to the hospital. He was the sole financial supporter of his family and stated during his initial assessment that his primary goal was to return to work as a mechanic.

Mr. Smith's treating hand therapist worked diligently with Mr. Smith to address wound care issues, scar management, desensitization, positioning, and ROM using static, serial static, and static progressive orthoses in addition to incorporating progressive strengthening and functional tasks into his treatment program. However, the hand therapist struggled with Mr. Smith's insistence that he wanted to return to work after the amputation of his left dominant small and ring fingers and his near-death experience. Through self-reflection, she realized that she held a personal belief that Mr. Smith would never return to his job as a mechanic and that this belief was interfering with her ability to provide patient-centered care. She realized that her role as therapist was to facilitate Mr. Smith's goal to the best of her ability and to incorporate his return to work goal into her treatment plan for physical, motivational, and role identity purposes. When impairment gains had plateaued, Mr. Smith's hand therapist facilitated a referral to a worker rehabilitation and work conditioning program at another facility. After 8 weeks of a progressive work simulation and conditioning program, Mr. Smith was discharged back to work as a mechanic at the light to medium physical demand classification with work modifications such as assistance with heavier tasks and a shift to include training as part of his regular duties. At discharge Mr. Smith said, "I couldn't have done this without you."

Michael sustained a severe roller crush injury of his right dominant hand and arm. His hand therapist worked with him to improve his ROM, strength, and hypersensitivity. Five months after this injury, Michael told his therapist that his 7-year-old son was devastated that he could no longer play street hockey with him. His hand therapist asked Michael to bring in his hockey stick, and they collaboratively developed a thermoplastic handle so that he could grasp his hockey stick. After playing hockey with his son, Michael said, "It was awesome. You should have seen the smile on my son's face. I don't know how many times he came over to hug me." Patient-centered modifications such as the one described have significant benefits on quality of life, restoring valued roles and relationships.

PATIENT-CENTERED ASSESSMENT

Patient-centered assessments allow hand therapists to focus on relevant and important patient issues during therapy.[42] They help build strong therapeutic relationships by giving the opportunity for the patient and therapist to identify meaningful and achievable goals together. Impairment goals, such as ROM and strength, should be integrated into activities that are valued by the patient, thus improving motivation and therapy engagement[4,41] in addition to improving outcomes.[43] Collaborative problem solving between the patient and hand therapist ensures that issues are addressed in the context of that individual's life.[41]

Mrs. Lee, a 45 year-old woman, worked at a dry cleaning business. Both of her hands were caught in the press, resulting in burn, crush amputations to all digits bilaterally. Her hand therapist addressed wound care issues, hypersensitivity, ROM, and strength; however, Mrs. Lee continued to cover her fingertips and was not using her hands functionally. The hand therapist used a patient-centered assessment to help identify which tasks and activities were most important to Mrs. Lee and incorporated them into Mrs. Lee's therapy program. She brought a keyboard to the therapy department so that Mrs. Lee could practice playing music, a passion of hers before her injury. Over time, her hand therapist noticed that Mrs. Lee started to use her hands functionally, and she was no longer hiding them in her pockets. Additionally, playing the keyboard addressed ongoing impairment issues such as hypersensitivity and ROM with the added social benefits of interaction with other patients in the treatment area.

Two evaluations can be used to identify goals that are meaningful to patients and measure change in patient perception of performance over time. These are the Canadian Occupational Performance Measure (COPM)[44] and the Patient-Specific Functional Scale (PSFS).[45]

The COPM is designed to measure patient-identified issues in self-care, productivity, and leisure with a variety of patient populations.[44] Issues are rated in terms of importance to the patient, and scores are obtained for activity performance and satisfaction with performance.[41,42]

The PSFS is a self-report measure used to identify functional limitations that are relevant to each patient.[45,46] Similar to the COPM, the goal is to measure change in individual patients rather than to compare disability among a group of individuals. Both the COPM and the PSFS are useful tools to guide patient-centered practice and monitor patient-identified goals.[46,47]

THE IMPACT OF SOCIAL STIGMA AND HAND THERAPY INTERVENTION

Social stigma and cosmetic concerns have been found to have pronounced effects on long-term social acceptability and can interfere with overall adjustment.[10] Because of the visible nature of the hand, patients become acutely aware of how others view their hands.[48] This type of feedback is coined "social body image" and is obtained from people in the patient's environment.[48] Because hands are easily viewed by others, they invoke the public curiosity and questions.[48] Initially, questions from family members may be helpful because they convey a sense of concern; however, continued questioning by family, friends, and strangers can interfere with a patient's willingness to pursue relationships and participate in social events.[2] Patients may begin to avoid activities and events, resulting in social isolation. This change in behavior should be monitored and collaborative strategies developed to address this issue. For example, patients may require help establishing boundaries with family and friends regarding their hand injury in order to feel comfortable in social situations. Progressive exposure to social situations such as a get-together with a close work colleague or friend may be one way to assist in decreasing isolation and helping patients to reestablish their support network. Assessment and provision of an aesthetic prosthesis may assist an individual with amputations or a mutilating hand injury go out in public and attend large social events such as weddings or work events. Patients must be carefully assessed for readiness psychologically before these interventions are initiated. How the individual goes about interpreting and addressing social stigma will depend on personal, family, and cultural norms.

THE IMPACT OF CULTURE AND HAND THERAPY INTERVENTION

Culture is described as a "blueprint for human behavior"[49] and contributes to how one thinks, feels, and behaves.[50] Culture operates at different levels—at the regional, community, family, and individual levels.[51] Culture is dynamic and contributes to our present diversity of "health beliefs and practices."[52] This influx of multiple health perspectives means that hand therapists need to adapt their practices to meet diverse needs.[53]

Many commonly used hand therapy assessments have a cultural bias. For example, standard questions related to utensil use ignore the fact that people in many cultures use their hands to eat. Therefore, there is a need to use evaluations such as the COPM and the PSFS to ensure that identified problems and goals are culturally relevant to each person. When goals have been established, direct observation of performance and activity analysis is critical to highlight unique ways of performing activities. This information can be used to tailor hand therapy so that activities reflect culturally important patient goals.[9]

It is important to examine personal biases, such as assumptions about the beliefs and behaviors of various cultural groups, as well as the biases and assumptions embedded in Western health care systems. These assumptions can affect whether or not an intervention is accepted by the patient and ultimately successful.[54,55] For example, the importance of "independence" is rooted in the cultural context of Western medicine and reflective of the sociocultural norms of a white middle-class population.[56] A patient may be labeled as noncompliant with treatment such as the provision of adaptive equipment to improve her independence in activities of daily living when in fact the individual believes that it is her family's responsibility to take care of her after her injury. Family values such as responsibility and role expectations supersede independence in this example.[9]

MOTIVATIONAL INTERVIEWING: IMPROVING MOTIVATION AND FACILITATING CHANGE

Motivational interviewing[57] is a structured approach to facilitate positive patient change. Motivational interviewing recognizes the central role of the patient in his or her own care and the importance of the therapy relationship in either entrenching unhealthy coping behaviors or supporting positive change.

Motivational interviewing encourages clinicians to assess a patient's readiness to accept information and to recognize when their attempts to educate or convince instead result in resistance or disengagement. When this occurs, MI supports positive change through five core principles: (1) expression of empathy, (2) development of discrepancies, (3) use of change talk, (4) acceptance of resistance and setbacks, and (5) supporting self-efficacy (Table 83.2).

Expression of empathy is intended not only to communicate respect but also to support the increased exchange of information so that the clinician can understand how unhealthy behaviors are maintained. For example, a hand patient may overuse pain medication to maintain important caregiving activities for her child rather than pursuing pain relief.

When a patient's current motivations are better understood, a clinician can promote change by increasing the patient's awareness of discrepancies between his unhealthy behaviors and his values or likely outcomes. For example, a hand patient who overuses pain medication so that he can perform important caregiving activities can be encouraged to develop a pros and cons list. Such a list can increase the patient's awareness of how overuse of medication can impair his ability to engage in these important activities safely.

Motivational interviewing also supports healthy change through the use of "change talk." Clinicians can encourage patients to imagine the long-term consequences of unhealthy and healthy behaviors. For example, a hand patient with a disfigurement injury may withdraw from her child to protect the child from temporary anxiety. The patient can be asked to imagine how their relationship will develop over years. The patient can then be asked to imagine a time in the future when her child has become accustomed to the injury and to develop a plan to achieve that goal.

Motivational interviewing encourages clinicians to remain aware and accepting of temporary conflicts and problems and to "roll with resistance." Clinicians should also be aware of their own reactions and behaviors so that their drive to help the patient (referred to as "the righting instinct") does not become expressed as irritability, judgment, dismissiveness, or disengagement.

Finally, MI recognizes that positive patient change is best maintained through the patient's own actions and community. Clinicians may encourage patients to bring family members to the therapy setting or ask patients for permission to work with trusted people, including their family physician or spiritual advisor. For example, overprotective family members may be invited to participate in hurt-versus-harm education. Just as valuable, family members may identify important barriers to activity engagement and propose creative solutions to support healthy change.

SUMMARY: ACHIEVING BETTER OUTCOMES

Adjustment after a traumatic hand and upper extremity injury improves when the complex interplay among physical, psychological, and social elements is recognized and incorporated into hand therapy treatment. Patients often share their concerns, whether they are financial, relational, or social. It is important to acknowledge these concerns and support patients as they work through the impact of a traumatic injury on their lives. Impairment goals can be integrated and matched with activities that are valued by the patient, thus improving motivation and engagement in the therapy process. When goals are collaboratively established, are culturally relevant and meaningful to *that* person engagement improves as does outcomes. Hand therapists have the skills, tools, and opportunities to play a central role in facilitating adjustment.

ACKNOWLEDGMENT

Portions of this chapter are reprinted from *The Journal of Hand Therapy*, Volume 24(2), Hannah SD. Psychosocial issues after a traumatic hand injury: facilitating adjustment, pp 95-103 (2011).

TABLE 83.2 **Motivational Interviewing Principles and Techniques**	
Increase engagement between the clinician and patient	• Identification and validation of patient-specific needs, values, and preferences
Clarify pros and cons of different coping strategies	• Development of decisional balance related to current behaviors
	• Development of decisional balance related to proposed or alternative behaviors
Use change talk	• Emphasizing the temporary nature of problems or deficits
	• Imagined consequences of continuation of current behaviors
	• Imagined consequences of proposed or alternative behaviors
Accept resistance and setbacks	• Attunement to passive withdrawal
	• Acceptance of anger, frustration, and setbacks
Elicit patient and community resources	• Accessing community resources

REFERENCES

1. Bates E, Mason R. Coping strategies used by people with a major hand injury: a review of the literature. *Br J Occup Ther.* 2014;77(6):289–182.

2. Meyer TM. Psychological aspects of mutilating hand injuries. *Hand Clin.* 2003;19:41–44.

3. Haese JB. Psychological aspects of hand injuries their treatment and rehabilitation. *J Hand Surg (British and European Volume).* 1985;10(3):283–287.

4. Schier J, Chan J. Changes in life roles after hand injury. *J Hand Ther.* 2007;20:57–69.

5. Carlsson IK, Edberg AK, Wann-Hansson C. Hand-injured patients' experiences of cold sensitivity and the consequences and adaptation for daily life: a qualitative study. *J Hand Ther.* 2010;23:53–62.

6. Grunert BK, Smith CJ, Devine CA, Fehring BA, Matloub HS, Sanger JR. Early psychological aspects of severe hand injury. *J Hand Surg.* 1988;13B(2):177–180.

7. Gustafsson M, Ahlstrom G. Problems experienced during the first year of an acute traumatic hand injury – a prospective study. *J Clin Nurs.* 2004;13:986–995.

8. Hennigar C, Saunders D, Efendov A. The injured workers survey: development and clinical use of a psychosocial screening tool for patients with hand injuries. *J Hand Ther.* 2001;14:122–127.

9. Hannah SD. Psychosocial issues after a traumatic hand injury: facilitating adjustment. *J Hand Ther.* 2011;24(2):95–103.

10. Grob M, Papadopulos NA, Zimmermann A, Biemer E, Kovacs L. The psychological impact of severe hand injury. *J Hand Surg (European Volume).* 2008;33E(3):358–362.

11. Vranceanu AM, Ring D. Value of psychological evaluation of the hand surgical patient. *J Hand Surg.* 2008;33A:985–987.

12. Vranceanu AM, Ring D. Psychosocial aspects of arm illness. In: *Rehabilitation of the Hand and Upper Extremity.* 6th ed. Mosby; 2011:1754–1765.

13. Grunert BK, Devine CA, Matloub HS, et al. Psychological adjustment following work-related hand injury: 18-month follow-up. *Ann Plast Surg.* 1992;29(6):537–542.

14. Gustafsson M, Amilon A, Ahlstrom G. Trauma-related distress and mood disorders in the early stage of an acute traumatic hand injury. *J Hand Surg (British and European Volume).* 2003;28B(4):332–338.

15. Sullivan MJL. *Pain Catastrophizing Scale User Manual.* Montreal, Quebec: McGill; 1995.

16. Pain catastrophizing scale. Available at: http://sullivan-painresearch.mcgill.ca/pdf/pcs/PCSManual_English.pdf.

17. Melzack R. McGill pain questionnaire: major properties and scoring methods. *Pain.* 1975;1:277–299.

18. McGill Pain questionnaire. Available at: https://www.google.ca/url?sa=t&rct=j&q=&esrc=s&source=web&cd=1&cad=rja&uact=8&ved=0ahUKEwioqM-UtdLXAhWB5IMKHS6ZAIwQFggrMAA&url=https%3A%2F%2Fwww.gem-beta.org%2Fpublic%2FDownloadMeasure.aspx%3Fmid%3D1348&usg=AOvVaw2rZixTLAcjspGMb5hZ-5wam.

19. Spitzer RL, Williams JBW, Kroenke K, Linzer M, deGruy FV, Hahn SR, et al. Utility of a new procedure for diagnosing mental disorders in primary care. The PRIME-MD 1000 study. *JAMA.* 1994;272:1749–1756.

20. Patient health questionnaire-9 and generalized anxiety disorder. Available at: http://www.phqscreeners.com/select-screener.

21. Rush AJ, Trivedi MH, Ibrahim HM, Carmody TJ, Arnow B, Klein DN, et al. The 16-item Quick Inventory of Depressive Symptomatology (QIDS), clinician rating (QIDS-C) and self-report (QIDS-SR): a psychometric evaluation in patients with chronic major depression. *Biol Psychiatry.* 2003;54(5):573–583.

22. Quick Inventory of depressive symptoms self-report 16. Available at: http://www.ids-qids.org/.

23. Beck AT, Epstein N, Brown G, Steer RA. An inventory for measuring clinical anxiety: psychometric properties. *J Consult Clin Psychol.* 1988;56:893–897.

24. Beck Depression Inventory – II and Beck Anxiety Inventory. Available at: https://www.pearsonclinical.ca – not an open source.

25. Beck AT, Epstein N, Brown G, Steer RA. An inventory for measuring clinical anxiety: psychometric properties. *J Consult Clin Psychol.* 1988;56:893–897.

26. Weathers FW, Litz BT, Keane TM, Palmieri PA, Marx BP, Schnurr PP. *The PTSD Checklist for DSM-5 (PCL-5).* Washington, DC: National Center for PTSD; 2013.

27. Posttraumatic stress disorder checklist for DSM-5. Available at: https://www.ptsd.va.gov/professional/assessment/adult-sr/ptsd-checklist.asp.

28. Weiss DS, Marmar CR. The impact of event scale – revised. In: Wilson J, Keane TM, eds. *Assessing Psychological Trauma and PTSD.* New York: Guilford; 1996:399–411.

29. Impact of Event Scale – Revised. Available at: https://www.ptsd.va.gov/professional/assessment/adult-sr/ies-r.asp.

30. Hayes SC. Acceptance and commitment therapy, relational frame therapy, and the third wave of behavioral and cognitive therapies. *Behavior Ther.* 2004;35(4):639–665.

31. American Psychological Association. *Clinical Practice Guideline for the Treatment of PTSD;* 2017.

32. International Society for Treatment of Stress Studies. *Effective treatments for PTSD.* 2nd ed. 2009.

33. Canadian Network for Mood and Anxiety Treatments. *Clinical Guidelines for the Management of Adults with Major Depressive Disorder;* 2016.

34. Canadian Psychiatric Association. *Clinical Practice Guidelines: Management of Anxiety Disorders;* 2006.

35. Koestler AJ. Psychological perspective on hand injury and pain. *J Hand Ther.* 2010;23(2):199–210.

36. Gustafsson M, Persson L, Amilon A. A qualitative study of coping in the early stage of acute traumatic hand injury. *J Clin Nurs.* 2002;11:594–602.

37. Gustafsson M, Ahlstrom G. Emotional distress and coping in the early stage of recovery following acute traumatic hand injury: a questionnaire survey. *Int J Nurs Stud.* 2006;43:557–565.

38. Kato T. Frequently used coping scales: a meta-analysis. *Stress Health.* 2015;31(4):315–323.

39. Christiansen CH. Defining lives: occupation as identity: an essay on competence, coherence, and the creation of meaning. *Am J Occup Ther.* 1999;53(6):547–558.

40. Richmond TS, Thompson HJ, Deatrick JA, Kauder DR. Journey towards recovery following physical trauma. *J Adv Nurs.* 2000;32(6):1341–1347.

41. Jack J, Estes R. Documenting progress: hand therapy treatment shift from biomechanical to occupational adaptation. *Am J Occup Ther.* 2010;64(1):82–87.

42. Jolles BM, Buchbinder R, Beaton DE. A study compared nine patient-specific indices for musculoskeletal disorders. *J Clin Epidemiol.* 2005;58:791–801.

43. Chan J, Spencer J. Adaptation to hand injury: an evolving experience. *Am J Occup Ther.* 2004;58(2):128–138.

44. Carswell A, McColl MA, Baptiste S, Polatajko H, Pollock N. The Canadian Occupational Performance Measure: a research and clinical literature review. *Can J Occup Ther.* 2004;71(4):210–222.

45. Stratford P, Gill C, Westaway M, Binkley J. Assessing disability and change on individual patients: a report of a patient specific measure. *Physiother Can.* 1995;47:258–263.

46. Gross DP, Battie MC, Asant AK. The patient-specific functional scale: validity in workers' compensation claimants. *Arch Phys Med Rehabil.* 2008;89:1294–1299.

47. Dedding D, Cardol M, Eyssen I, Dekker J, Beelen A. Validity of the Canadian Occupational Performance Measure: a client-centered outcome measurement. *Clin Rehabil.* 2004;18:660–667.

48. Grunert BK, Maksud-Sagrillo DP. Psychological adjustment to hand injuries: nursing management. *Plast Surg Nurs.* 1998;18(3):163–167.

49. Leininger M. *Transcultural Nursing: Concepts, Theories and Practices.* New York: John Wiley and Sons; 1978:80.

50. Paul S. Culture and its influence on occupational therapy evaluation. *Can J Occup Ther.* 1995;62(3):154–161.

51. Awaad T. Culture, cultural competency and occupational therapy: a review of the literature. *Br J Occup Ther.* 2000;66:196–199.

52. Brathewaite AC, Majumdar B. Evaluation of a cultural competence educational programme. *J Adv Nurs*. 2006;53(4):470–479.

53. Whiteford GE, Wilcock AA. Cultural relativism: occupation and independence reconsidered. *Can J Occup Ther*. 2000;67(5):324–336.

54. Campinha-Bacote J. The quest for cultural competence in nursing care. *Nurs Forum*. 1995;30(4):19–25.

55. Campinha-Bacote J. A model and instrument for addressing cultural competence in health care. *J Nurs Educ*. 1999;38(5):203–207.

56. Jungersen K. Culture, theory and the practice of occupational therapy in New Zealand/Aotearoa. *Am J Occup Ther*. 1992;46(8):745–750.

57. Miller WR, Rollnick S. *Motivational Interviewing: Preparing People for Change*. New York: Guilford; 1991.

84

Pathomechanics of Deformities of the Arthritic Hand and Wrist

Kevin C. Chung, Phillip Ross

OUTLINE

CRITICAL POINTS

- Synovial proliferation and inflammation in rheumatoid arthritis cause destruction of surrounding cartilage, bone, ligament, and tendon.
- Various pathologic mechanical forces are created as diseased synovium affects different aspects of the musculoskeletal system.
- Rheumatoid synovitis and inflammation cause cartilage, tendons, and ligaments to lose their abilities to withstand deforming forces.
- Tendon ruptures are common and may result from attrition, ischemia, or direct tissue invasion.

- Wrist deformity follows predictable patterns of collapse and degeneration often with volar migration and supination of the carpus and ulnar head prominence.
- The metacarpophalangeal joint is susceptible to ulnar and volar forces, leading to ulnar drift and zig-zag deformities.
- Boutonnière and swan-neck deformities may develop from pathology at numerous places in the rheumatoid fingers and thumb.

Rheumatoid arthritis (RA) is a chronic inflammatory condition that targets synovial joints. The inflammation and diseased synovium in RA affect all parts of the musculoskeletal system, including bone, cartilage, tendon, and muscle. Selective tissue destruction leads to altered mechanics that give rise to deformities characteristic of the disease.

SYNOVIUM

The primary hallmark of RA is synovial inflammation, and nearly all deformity in arthritic hands and wrists can be traced back to this central pathology. Normal synovium encapsulates the joint and consists of an intimal layer and a sublining, predominantly composed of type A and type B synovial cells. Type A cells are macrophage-like cells with antigen-presenting functions and are from a bone marrow lineage. Type B cells are similar to fibroblasts; these cells produce synovial fluid. Healthy synovium is only one or two cells thick, and type A and type B cells are present in roughly equal numbers.[1]

Rheumatoid Synovium

Synovial Pathology

Diseased synovium in RA contains several elements that contribute to its pathology. There is occlusion of the microvasculature, which leads to swelling of the endothelial lining. The entire structure becomes hypervascular and hypertrophic, up to 10 times the cellular thickness as normal synovial tissue. There is an invasion of lymphocytes; CD4+ T cells constitute up to half of the cells in rheumatoid synovium. Natural killer cells, synovial B cells, and dendritic cells are also seen in increased numbers.[1]

This proliferation of cells produces many chemical factors that contribute to disease development. Synoviocytes secrete increased levels of interleukin (IL)-1, IL-6, and others to increase inflammation. Transforming growth factor–β (TGF-β), IL-8, and other chemotactic factors, such as C5a and leukotriene B4, are increased to attract polymorphonuclear cells (PMNs) to the joint. Although neutrophils are relatively rare in the synovial tissue itself, they accumulate in abundance in synovial fluid.[1] In addition to chemotactic and proinflammatory factors, synovial fibroblasts and endothelial cells also produce high levels of matrix metalloproteinases (MMP), especially MMP-1, -2, -8, and -13. These enzymes are present in both the proliferated synovial tissue and synovial fluid; they target and destroy local normal tissue.[2]

Effect on Cartilage

Aggressive synoviocytes at sites of pannus overgrowth, cytokine-activated chondrocytes, and PMNs are all responsible for destruction of the cartilage in RA. IL-1, tumor necrosis factor (TNF)–α, and TGF-β from synoviocytes stimulate cartilage matrix degrading enzymes and interfere with cartilage remodeling.[3] PMNs produce MMPs, serine proteases, and cathepsins; collagenase-3 in particular cleaves type 2 collagen, which is an important step in cartilage destruction.[4] Severed collagen proteins and depleted proteoglycans decrease the ability of cartilage to absorb impacts, which leads to mechanical defects.[1]

Effect on Bone

The hypertrophic synovium in RA forms a pannus that extends over subchondral bone and cartilage. Intracellular adhesion molecules allow the pannus to remain fixed on the tissues,[4] and when there, activated osteoclasts and giant cells erode the bone.[1] TNF-α aids in stimulating progenitor cells into mature osteoclasts[3] and increases the osteoclast response to RANKL (receptor activator of nuclear factor κ-B ligand).[5] Other chemofactors, such as IL-1, increase the osteoclast bone-resorbing activity. Bone loss can range from thinned cortices and absent medullary cancellous bone to severe bone resorption such as seen in arthritis mutilans.[3]

Effect on Ligament

There is a dual mechanism of destruction for ligaments. Direct pannus infiltration can compromise ligament integrity. Secreted MMPs cleave the collagen essential for tissue strength.[2] Joint distention from increased diseased synovial fluid also stretches the ligaments intimately adjacent to the capsule.[6]

Effect on Tendons

Synovium in RA has been found to either encapsulate or directly invade tendons. Encapsulating synovium creates pressure, which occludes the vincula and disrupts blood flow.[7] Direct invasion causes destruction with MMPs and can be seen in almost 50% of cases.[2]

Effect on Muscle

Muscle is less commonly invaded by synovial pannus but is affected by the perivascular inflammation that accompanies disease development. This inflammation and blood vessel disruption can lead to muscle tightness, most commonly in the intrinsic hand muscles.[8]

TENDON RUPTURES

Extensor Tendons

One of the most frequent clinical manifestations of RA in the hands and wrist is extensor tendon ruptures. Three distinct mechanisms contribute to ruptures: attrition, ischemia, and direct tenosynovial invasion.

The process that disposes the extensor tendons to attritional ruptures stems from the synovial disease. Cellular destruction erodes the bone unevenly to create sharp edges. As the tendon moves over the rough surface, it gradually whittles down its substance until rupture occurs. Lister tubercle is the most common edge to provoke a rupture, and the small finger extensor and extensor carpi ulnaris (ECU) rubbing on the distal ulna are common, too.[9,10] Often a sequence of extensor tendon rupture is seen over time starting from the small finger and progressing to the index finger[9] (Fig. 84.1).

Ischemic extensor tendon ruptures develop as dorsal wrist synovitis compresses the tendons and weakens their blood supply, preventing the tendon from repairing itself (Fig. 84.2). Frequently, extensor pollicis longus (EPL) rupture is a combination of ischemia and attrition.[11]

Direct invasion of diseased synovium is another method by which tendons are damaged. MMPs produced by synoviocytes, particularly ones that cleave collagen-1, progressively thin the collagen fibrils that compose tendons until eventual rupture.[2] In contrast to attritional and ischemia ruptures, direct invasion by inflamed tenosynovium causes symptoms before failure, such as painful and limited motion, tendon fullness, and crepitus.[7]

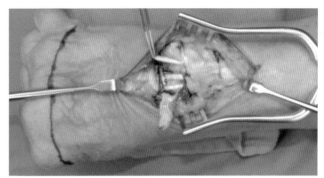

Fig. 84.1 Rupture of the extensor digiti quinti minimi (EDQM), but the extensor digitorum communis of the small finger is intact. This is an attritional rupture of the EDQM over the prominent ulnar head.

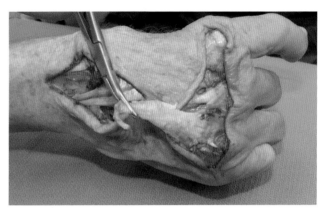

Fig. 84.2 Rupture of the ring and little extensor digitorum communis (EDC) at midcarpal level.

Flexor Tendons

Although less common than extensor tendon ruptures, flexor tendons may rupture by similar mechanisms. The wrist is the most common location, contributing to two thirds of these attritional ruptures.[7] Tendons degrade from rubbing over carpal bone spurs that pierce the floor of the carpal tunnel.[12] The scaphoid is the most frequent bone responsible, although ruptures are also seen over the trapezium, radius, lunate, ulna, and hamate. The flexor pollicis longus (FPL) is often the most frequently ruptured, which is the so-called "Mannerfelt lesion." Next affected are the index and long finger flexor digitorum superficialis (FDS) and flexor digitorum profundus (FDP) tendons. This progression from radial to ulnar is in contrast to the usual sequence of extensor tendon ruptures.[12]

Ruptures of flexor tendons in the palm and digit are less common but are still seen. Infiltrating tenosynovitis is usually the mechanism of tendon damage in these further distal locations.[7] The FPL, however, may still rub over an eroded sesamoid to cause an attritional rupture.[13] Therapeutic steroid injections may also weaken tendon structure and contribute to rupture by other mechanisms.[12]

THE WRIST

Zig-Zag Deformities

Deformities in the arthritic wrist follow predictable patters, which result from the interaction of diseased tissue and extrinsic forces. A common deformity seen is a zig-zag shape resulting from two joints inappropriately aligned in opposite directions. The wrist consists of

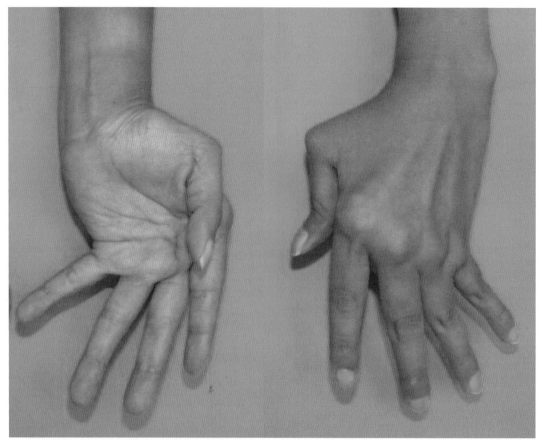

Fig. 84.3 Clinical photographs demonstrating a carpal–metacarpal–phalangeal zig-zag deformity in a 41-year-old woman with rheumatoid arthritis.

a multiarticular system, with the radiocarpal, intercarpal, and carpometacarpal (CMC) joints. There are long extensors and flexors on either side with no attachments to the intercalated bones.[14] Without proper stability from ligaments or a third muscle, terminal flexion of the proximal joint will cause the distal joint to move into extension because of increased pull from the long extensors. With extension of the proximal joint, the opposite occurs, and the distal joint is pulled into flexion. In either direction, the system falls into a zig-zag deformity[9] (Fig. 84.3).

Carpal Joint Destruction

Radiocarpal Joint

In the wrist, the zig-zag deformity starts with destruction of the wrist ligaments. Direct pannus destruction and stretching from joint effusion weaken the radioscaphocapitate (RSC) ligament volarly. With the loss of the supportive sling that the RSC provides, the scaphoid is able to rotate vertically.[6]

Scapholunate Joint

Synovitis continues to weaken the intrinsic ligaments of the wrist, next attacking the scapholunate (SL) ligament. Loss of this restraint along with the RSC renders the scaphoid unstable and allows it to flex volarly. Radial deviation of the carpus on the radius gives the extrinsic muscles shorter moment arms, and there is a loss of force balance between the intrinsic and extrinsic muscles. The increased compressive force from the extrinsic muscles causes the scaphoid to further flex and the entire system is compressed, leading to a loss of carpal height[6] (Fig. 84.4).

Midcarpal Joint

In contrast, the midcarpal joint has relatively few intrinsic ligaments. As a result, there is minimal pannus formation or synovial destruction at this level. Although the radiocarpal and SL deformities continue to progress, midcarpal motion stays well preserved (Fig. 84.5). Much of the remaining motion in unstable wrists in RA comes from the midcarpal joint.[15]

Subluxation of the Carpus

The normal wrist should have the radius, lunate, capitate, and metacarpals align in the coronal and sagittal planes. During power grip, the second metacarpal and radius stay aligned with the carpus stabilized, if not slightly ulnar, so the thumb may align closer to the forearm. The rheumatoid wrist may subluxate in multiple directions during grip, leading to substantial loss of power.[16]

This process begins at the ulnar styloid and ulnar head. Synovitis in the ulnocarpal and distal radioulnar (DRU) joints stretches the ECU sheath and ulnocarpal ligaments.[9] The ECU subluxates volarly without restraint from its sheath and loses its function as a wrist extensor and ulnar-sided stabilizer. It occasionally stops firing altogether.[16] Without dorsal–ulnar support from ligaments and the ECU, the carpus slides volarly and supinates (Fig. 84.6). This shift makes the ulna head more prominent and converts the ECU to more of a wrist flexor.[6]

With no opposition on the ulnar side of the wrist, the extensor carpi radialis longus and brevis (ECRL and ECRB) tendons create an imbalance that pulls the carpus and metacarpals to deviate radially during grip (Fig. 84.7). In addition to rotating the metacarpals radially, the pull of the radial extensors creates a compressive force

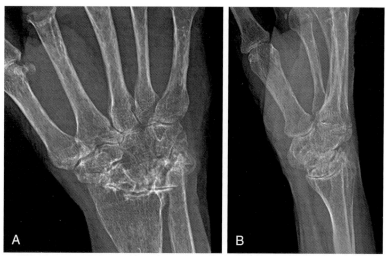

Fig. 84.4 Carpal arthritis, with ulnar subluxation. Anteroposterior (**A**) and lateral (**B**) radiographs illustrating severe radiocarpal arthritis with loss of carpal height in a 62-year-old patient with longstanding rheumatoid arthritis.

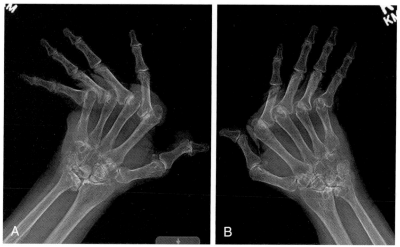

Fig. 84.5 Wrist and finger deformity. **A** and **B,** Anteroposterior radiographs showing bilateral metacarpophalangeal joint dislocations and radiocarpal and distal radioulnar joint arthritis with ulnar subluxation of the carpus. Note that the midcarpal joints are relatively spared.

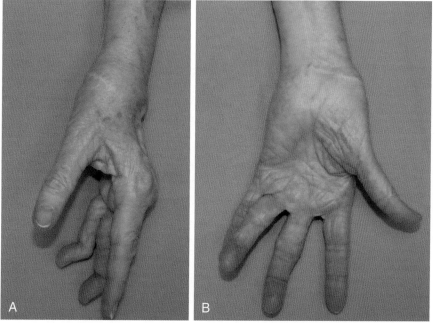

Fig. 84.6 Volarly subluxated carpus. This patient has volar subluxation (**A**) and supination (**B**) of the carpus. Also note the swan-neck deformities of the patient's middle and ring fingers.

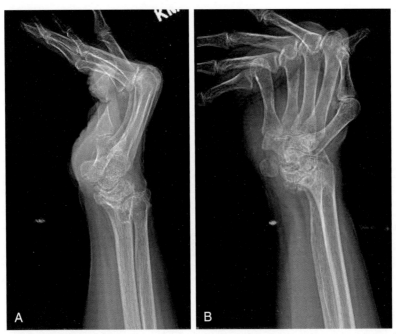

Fig. 84.7 Volar wrist. Lateral (**A**) and oblique (**B**) radiographs demonstrating volar subluxation and supination of the carpus in rheumatoid arthritis. Note that the ulnar head becomes prominent, and the metacarpals deviate radially as this change occurs.

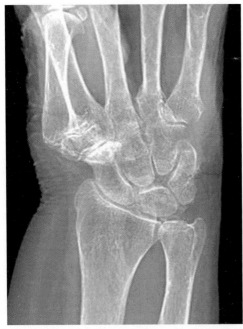

Fig. 84.8 Ulnar subluxation of the carpus seen in rheumatoid arthritis.

on the proximal carpal bones. This vector is slightly ulnar, down the inclination of the radius. In some rheumatoid wrists, the attenuated radiocarpal ligaments cannot restrain this force, and thus the carpus translocates ulnarly in addition to volarly (Fig. 84.8). In these cases, the radial styloid becomes prominent.[17] Either radial deviation of the metacarpals and ulnar translocation of the proximal carpus can contribute to the loss of grip power. These deformities also exacerbate forces causing ulnar deviation at the metacarpophalangeal joints.[16]

Distal Radioulnar Joint

A classic pattern of rheumatoid wrist deformity is that of the "caput ulna syndrome."[18] This phenomenon arises not from enlargement of the ulnar head but from movement of the wrist. When the carpus subluxates volarly and supinates, the ulnar head becomes prominent (Fig. 84.9). Synovitis in the DRU joint and destruction of the dorsal and volar radioulnar ligaments lead to DRU joint instability. Distention and synovial invasion destroy the retinaculum of the ECU. Supination of the carpus pulls the ECU into a position volar to the ulnar head to eliminate its extension moment and convert it to a deforming flexor force.[17] Destruction of the ulnar corner of the distal radius is also seen, enabling it to subluxate volarly. This change manifests clinically as an apparent dorsal migration of the ulna. Both the change in wrist position and loss of the ECU function lead to limited wrist extension. The prominence of the ulnar head serves as an abnormal contact point, leading to attritional extensor tendon ruptures.[18]

End-Stage Deformity

When the disease is allowed to progress uninterrupted, the final deformity results in a volar wrist dislocation. In time, synovitis destroys the remaining wrist ligaments. The long finger flexors pull the wrist down without restraint or opposition. The carpus dislocates volarly, and there is complete dissociation of the DRU joint. Continued dislocation leads to arthrosis and destruction of the joint. Complete fibrosis of the joint may eventually occur.[6]

Radiographic Changes

Bone erosion is a hallmark of rheumatoid changes that may be visible on radiographs, and the amount of erosion is proportional to the degree of synovitis. Changes may be seen often where ligaments insert, such as the RSC, the ulnocarpal ligaments, and the prestyloid recess.[6] Grooving of the midscaphoid and SL dissociation indicates involvement of radiocarpal ligaments and loss of support.[19]

Other common sites of radiographic erosions are the ulnar triquetrum and ulnar head. In juvenile RA, the entire carpus is often involved.[6]

Classification Systems

Classification systems of rheumatoid disease in the wrist have been developed based on both clinical and radiographic parameters. Clinically, classification follows progression of the joint destruction (Table 84.1). In stage 1, there are only synovitis and osteopenia. Stage 2 presents with limited motion and some joint erosions. Extensive deformities characterize stage 3. Patients with stage 4 have ankylosis of the wrist.[6]

Radiographic classification was developed by Larsen and coworkers[20] based on standard reference films and applies to all joints (Table 84.2). Grade I consists of slight joint abnormalities, such as swelling and osteoporosis. Grade II has definite early changes. Narrowing and erosions in all joints define grade III. In grade IV, there is severe destruction, and grade V consists of mutilating changes, with gross bone deformation and no remaining articular surfaces.

METACARPOPHALANGEAL JOINT DEFORMITIES

The metacarpophalangeal (MCP) joint is the most important articulation for finger function. There is freedom in two planes, and it has a large arc of motion, making it vulnerable to surrounding deforming forces. The classic deformity at the MCP joint is an ulnar drift with volar subluxation or dislocation[21] (Fig. 84.10).

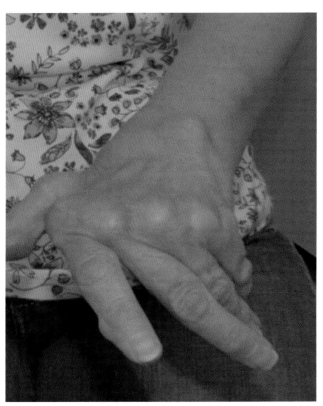

Fig. 84.9 Caput ulnae. Prominent ulnar head along with severe ulnar and volar deviation of the digits at the metacarpophalangeal joints in a 59-year-old woman with rheumatoid arthritis.

TABLE 84.1 Clinical Stages of Wrist Arthritis[6]

Stage	Characteristics
1	Synovitis, osteopenia
2	Limited range of motion; some periarticular erosions
3	Extensive joint deformities and destruction
4	Joint ankylosis

TABLE 84.2 Larsen Radiographic Grades of Arthritis[20]

Grade	Radiographic Findings
I	Osteoporosis with slight joint changes
II	Definite early degenerative changes
III	Erosions and narrowing in all joints
IV	Severe destruction
V	Mutilating changes

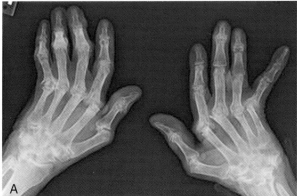
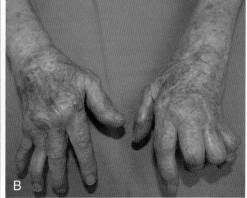

Fig. 84.10 Ulnarly subluxated metacarpophalangeal joints. Anteroposterior radiographs of bilateral hands (**A**) and clinical images (**B**) of a 77-year-old patient with rheumatoid arthritis showing severe erosion and ulnar deviation at the metacarpophalangeal joints. The patient also has significant degeneration in the carpal joints.

Factors Affecting Metacarpophalangeal Joint Deformity

Metacarpophalangeal Joint Synovitis

Synovitis of the MCP joint begins the process of deformity. Cellular proliferation and joint effusion stretch the capsule and ligamentous structures.[22] Often this starts between the metacarpal head and the collateral ligament attachment where erosions form.[21] As synovitis erodes the ligament attachments, the collateral ligaments fail, allowing the proximal phalanx to rotate ulnarly.[22]

Intrinsic Muscle Imbalance

Synovitis weakens the sagittal bands, which loosens the relationship between the base of the proximal phalanx and the extensor apparatus. The phalanx sags slightly volarly to create shorter excursion distances for the intrinsic muscles. Less tension on the intrinsic tendons combines with perivascular inflammation to cause the muscles to contract.[8] Hypoxia may also increase contraction of the ulnar sided interossei.[24] Tight intrinsic muscles result in increased, unbalanced flexion forces, which cause further volar phalanx subluxation.[25]

Wrist Deformity

Subluxation of the wrist with resultant radial deviation of the metacarpals creates another ulnar-directed force at the MCP joints. Collapse of the wrist leaves the extrinsic tendons at a length suboptimal for proper function, leaving a relative intrinsic plus imbalance.[26] In patients with increased radial inclination, the carpus may also migrate ulnarly, which further shortens the working length of the tendons.[27]

Extensor Tendon Forces

As the metacarpals deviate radially, the long finger extensor tendons migrate to the ulnar side (Fig. 84.11), pulling the phalanges with them and producing a zig-zag pattern between the wrist and the MCP joints. As the radial sagittal bands become attenuated further by direct disease invasion and synovial proliferation, the check rein against ulnar translation on the extensor tendons is eliminated.[9]

Flexor Tendon Forces

The finger flexor tendons produce a strong volar force during pinch,[28] which is transmitted to the base of the proximal phalanx by the A2 pulley. As the collateral ligaments and sagittal bands stretch out, the pulley is allowed to migrate further volar and ulnar[29] (Fig. 84.12).

Pinch and Grip

Use of the hand and fingers for normal activities of daily living puts continual tension on the ligaments and repeats the pathologic forces. For example, turning a key, lifting a mug, and cutting with a knife all apply an ulnar force to the fingers.[30] Additionally, power grip causes compression across the collapsed wrist and creates an ulnarly directed force.[31]

FINGER DEFORMITIES

Boutonnière Deformity

The boutonnière deformity is a zig-zag pattern pathology consisting of flexion at the proximal interphalangeal (PIP) joint and hyperextension at the distal interphalangeal (DIP) joint (Fig. 84.13). It is common in RA but not unique to the disease.

This deformity originates with PIP joint flexion. Proliferative synovitis and pannus stretch the overlying dorsal joint capsule and extensor mechanisms. The central slip of the extensor tendon become deficient and creates an extensor lag at the PIP joint (Fig. 84.14). Early in development, PIP flexion is passively correctable. As the deformity progresses, however, the joint becomes fixed.

In addition to the central slip, synovitis also attenuates the triangular ligament, weakening its function as a stabilizer of the lateral bands. Without a check rein, the lateral bands displace volarly, and their force changes from an extensor to a PIP joint flexor. The pathologic lateral band pull combines with the long finger tendons to create an unbalanced flexion force at the PIP joint and unbalanced extension force at the DIP joint. Eventually, the head of the proximal phalanx can prolapse through the attenuated central slip in a button-hole fashion.[32]

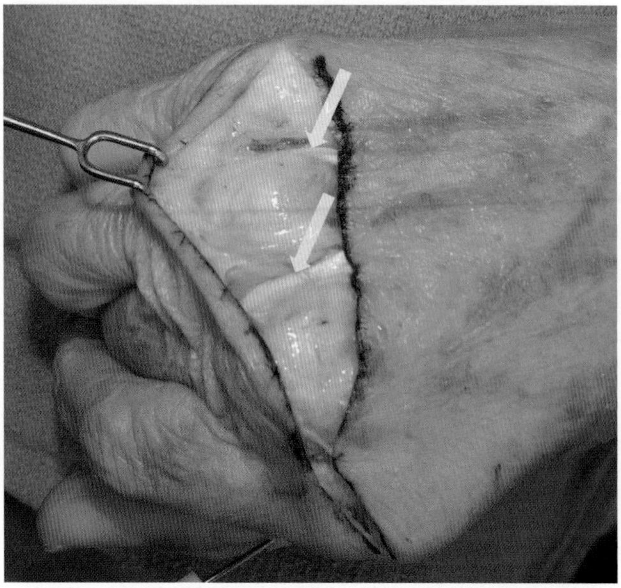

Fig. 84.11 Ulnarly subluxated extensor digitorum communis tendons. Intraoperative photograph demonstrating the subluxation of the extensor tendons at the metacarpophalangeal joints in a patient with ulnar drift.

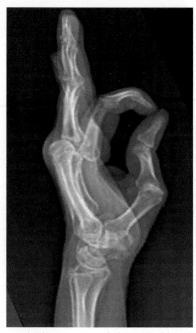

Fig. 84.12 Ulnar and volar metacarpophalangeal subluxation. Lateral radiograph demonstrating volar subluxation of the metacarpophalangeal joints.

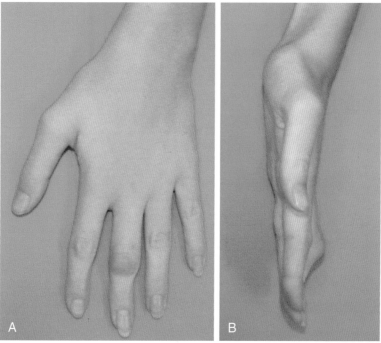

Fig. 84.13 **A** and **B,** Middle finger boutonnière: boutonnière deformity of the middle finger.

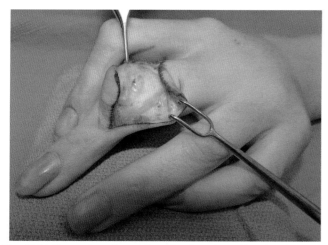

Fig. 84.14 Separation of central tendon from lateral band and removal of synovitis. Intraoperative photograph revealing synovitis and central slip attenuation leading to a boutonnière deformity.

Contracture of the oblique retinacular ligament also contributes to the deformity. As the PIP joint remains in flexion, the ligament shortening causes obligatory extension of the DIP joint. To compensate for deformity at the distal two joints, the MCP joint often becomes hyperextended as well.[33]

Boutonnière deformities are staged based on the PIP deformity (Table 84.3). Stage 1 deformities are mild with PIP flexion of 10 to 15 degrees. Usually there is full passive PIP extension. In stage 2, the PIP joint is flexed 30 to 40 degrees. Early stage 2 is passively correctable, whereas severe stage 2 is fixed. When the PIP joint flexion contracture is fixed and there is joint space destruction on radiographs, it is considered stage 3.[33]

Swan-Neck Deformity

The swan-neck deformity is another finger deformity not unique to RA. It consists of PIP joint hyperextension and DIP joint flexion.

TABLE 84.3 Stages of Boutonnière Deformity[33]

Stage	Findings
1 (mild)	PIP flexion to 10–15 degrees
2 (moderate)	PIP flexion to 30–40 degrees
3 (severe)	Fixed PIP joint contracture and joint destruction

PIP, Proximal interphalangeal.

In contrast to the boutonnière deformity, a swan-neck deformity may originate at the MCP, PIP, or DIP joints[34] (Fig. 84.15).

Metacarpophalangeal Joint

Swan-neck deformities that arise from the MCP joint are often secondary to intrinsic inbalance.[25] Synovial inflammation weakens the capsular support around the joint, and the proximal phalanx subluxates volarly on the metacarpal head as intrinsic muscles contract and lose their length. Intrinsic function then becomes concentrated on the central slip and lateral bands, producing an extension force at the PIP joint. Initially, the PIP joint stays supple, but as the intrinsic muscles contract further, PIP motion is only possible with the MCP joint flexed, which relieves tension on the intrinsic muscles. It is at this point that results on Bunnell's test for intrinsic tightness will be positive.[35] Synovitis erodes the tissue holding the lateral bands in place, and they migrate dorsally under the constant pull of the intrinsic muscles. Eventually, the dorsal skin, collateral ligaments, and dorsal capsule contract, which fixes the PIP deformity and prevents flexion. With the PIP joint hyperextended, the FDP tendon pulls the DIP joint into flexion.[25]

Proximal Interphalangeal Joint

Synovitis and pannus originating in the PIP joint cause laxity in the volar plate and joint capsule. Transverse fibers of the oblique retinacular ligament also stretch. Both factors combine to enable the PIP joint to hyperextend primarily. As this happens, the lateral bands displace dorsally and accentuate the deformity with additional extension

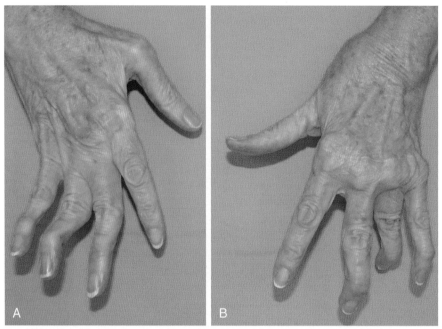

Fig. 84.15 A and **B,** Swan-neck deformity. Swan-neck deformities of the right middle and ring fingers and left middle, ring, and small fingers, with hyperextension at the proximal interphalangeal joint and flexion of the distal interphalangeal joint. Also note the ulnar deviation at the metacarpophalangeal (MCP) joints on the right and volar subluxation of the MCP joints on the left.

force.[35] Adhesions may develop between the dorsal joint and the extensor tendon, preventing excursion during flexion and between the subluxated conjoint lateral bands.[36] Constant PIP joint hyperextension relaxes tension on the terminal tendon, allowing the DIP joint to fall into flexion. Stretching or rupture of the FDS tendon, which is common in RA, and intrinsic tightness may also exacerbate the PIP joint deformity.[25]

Distal Interphalangeal Joint

Swan-neck deformity may also begin at the DIP joint. Rupture or attenuation of the terminal extensor tendon creates an extensor lag at the DIP joint, resulting in a mallet finger. Without tension on the terminal tendon, extensor forces concentrate at the PIP joint through the central slip. Constant force imbalance there leads to a gradual hyperextension and eventual permanence of the zig-zag deformity.[25]

Snapping Swan-Neck Deformity

Some swan-neck deformities may be actively overcome with flexion of the fingers. As flexion of the fingers starts, the intrinsic muscles contract to flex the MCP joints. This pull exaggerates the extension force at the PIP joint. Eventually, the long finger flexors overcome the lumbricals and interossei and force the PIP joint into flexion. As this happens, reduction of the lateral bands creates a distinct snap as they quickly move from a dorsally subluxated position back to their anatomic location.[35]

Classification

Classification for swan-neck deformities is based on motion at the PIP joint (Table 84.4). A type 1 deformity has a PIP joint that is mobile in all positions. In type 2, the flexion of the PIP joint is only achieved when the MCP joint is held flexed. When PIP joint flexion is limited in all finger positions, it is classified as type 3.[37] Type 4 deformities show severe arthritic changes.[25]

TABLE 84.4   Classification of Swan-Neck Deformity [25]

Type	Characteristics
1	PIP joint mobile in all positions (no intrinsic tightness)
2	PIP flexion only if MCP joint flexed (tight intrinsics)
3	PIP flexion limited in all positions
4	Severe arthritic changes

MCP, Metacarpophalangeal; *PIP,* proximal interphalangeal.

THUMB DEFORMITIES

Boutonnière Deformity of the Thumb

Consisting of MCP joint flexion and interphalangeal (IP) joint extension, the boutonnière deformity is the most common deformity of arthritic thumbs (Fig. 84.16). It is occasionally referred to as the "intrinsic-plus" deformity[38] and may originate at the MCP or IP joint.

Metacarpophalangeal Joint

To begin at the MCP joint, synovitis first degrades the dorsal capsule and extensor pollicis brevis (EPB) insertion. The extensor hood and EPL also stretch to give a weak extensor force. Often this synovitis manifests as dorsal bulging at the MCP joint. Flexion forces are able to dominate, and the EPL displaces volar and ulnar. Without sufficient force from the EPB, the proximal phalanx also displaces volarly on the metacarpal head. With the MCP joint unstable and flexed, the FPL can no longer exert a flexion moment on the IP joint, and the intrinsic and EPL pull it into extension. The thumb metacarpal adducts to compensate for MCP joint flexion (Fig. 84.17). Pinch accentuates the MCP joint flexion and IP joint extension, creating a cycle of pathologic loading. MCP and IP joint deformities mirror each other under the extrinsic forces, and eventually opposite 90 degree-90 degree deformities develop. Initially, the joints are passively correctible. With time,

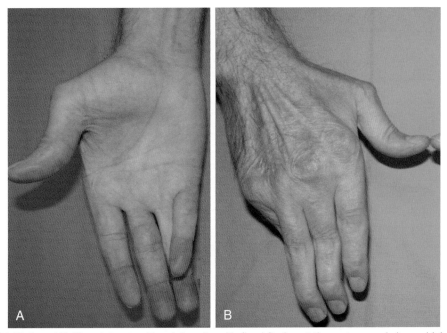

Fig. 84.16 A and **B,** Thumb boutonnière deformity with fixed flexion at the metacarpophalangeal joint and interphalangeal joint extension. There is also an abduction contracture.

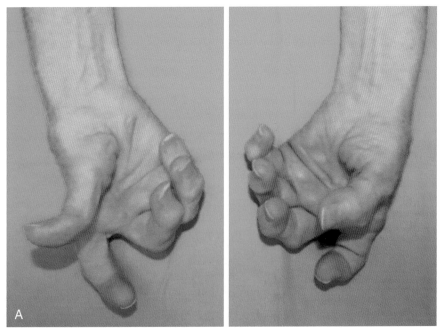

Fig. 84.17 Thumb adduction. Clinical image (**A**) and anteroposterior radiograph (**B**) of bilateral thumb adduction contractures. Also note the patient's degeneration at the radiocarpal and metacarpophalangeal joints, as well as the prior distal ulna resections.

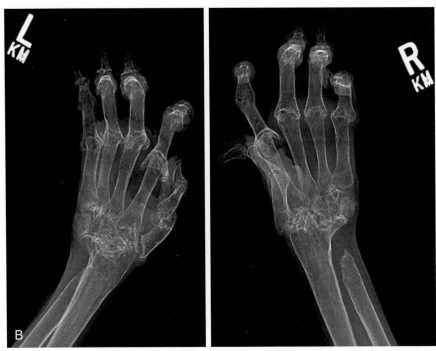

Fig. 84.17 Cont'd

degeneration and tissue contracture cause first the MCP joint and then the IP joint to become fixed in contracture.[39]

Interphalangeal Joint

The classic boutonnière deformity of the thumb originates at the MCP joint. If synovitis first causes attenuation of the IP joint volar plate and collateral ligaments, however, a boutonnière deformity may also stem from IP joint pathology. As the volar restraints become lax, the IP joint hyperextends. Rupture of the FPL tendon, often in the carpal tunnel, leaves the extension force unopposed at the IP joint and may aggravate this position. IP hyperextension causes increased tension on the intrinsic tendons of the thumb. To relieve it, the MCP joint is forced into flexion. In this scenario, IP hyperextension is typically greater then MCP joint flexion.[25]

Swan-Neck Deformity of the Thumb

The swan-neck is the second most common thumb deformity in RA. The IP joint goes into flexion whereas the MCP joint hyperextends. As in the thumb boutonnière deformity, the metacarpal is often adducted.[40]

Carpometacarpal Joint

A swan-neck deformity in the thumb may begin at the CMC joint. Pannus and inflammation erode away the capsule and articular surface, permitting dorsal and radial subluxation of the thumb metacarpal base.[25] In response, the metacarpal shaft adducts and flexes, likely from pain or adductor muscle spasm. Muscle itself is not involved, but the overlying fascia and adductor aponeurosis contract. As the disease progresses, the adduction contracture may become fixed. When the patient attempts to open the thumb, there is increased force at the MCP joint, and with time, it is stretched into hyperextension. With a strong adduction contracture resisting powerful forces to open the thumb, MCP joint dislocations are sometimes seen. Because the FPL

tendon must travel farther over the hyperextended MCP joint, it pulls the IP joint into flexion.[38]

Metacarpophalangeal Joint

Occasionally, the initial pathology of a swan-neck deformity is at the MCP joint of the thumb. Diseased synovitis stretches the volar plate, causing primary hyperextension of the proximal phalanx on the metacarpal (Fig. 84.18). Tension on the FPL as it runs over the MCP joint causes the IP joint into flexion. In these cases, the metacarpal does not necessarily develop an adduction contracture.[25]

Gamekeeper's Thumb

The gamekeeper's thumb, or radial deviation of the proximal phalanx at the MCP joint, occurs in RA. Synovitis erodes the ulnar collateral ligament, which is essential for phalanx stability on the metacarpal head. Pinch between the fingers and thumb creates a radially directed force that tests the collateral ligament competency. When insufficient, the phalanx begins to deviate. As this happens, the patient compensates for lack of thumb stability with greater adduction forces. Often a contracture then develops with the thumb metacarpal in adduction.[25]

Carpometacarpal Arthritis and Instability

Thumb stability is critical for pinch and grip functions in the hand. Both the CMC and MCP joints may become unstable in patients with RA. Synovitis generally causes cartilage destruction there, leading it to become the earliest joint affected. Fortunately, progression is slower than in other areas such as the MCP joints.[41] Although radiographic signs of arthritis are common, gross instability at CMC joint and frank dislocation are relatively rare.[40]

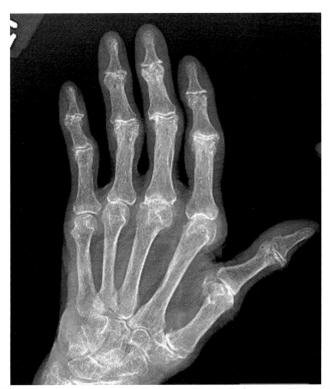

Fig. 84.18 Thumb metacarpophalangeal (MCP) dislocation, with distal radioulnar joint arthritis. The patient has thumb MCP joint subluxation and hyperextension. The patient also has erosions and severe joint space narrowing involving multiple MCP joints with volar subluxations and erosions of the proximal interphalangeal and distal interphalangeal joints with ulnar subluxations.

Combination Deformities

Described thumb deformities may occur in isolation or in combination. Boutonnière deformities have been seen with CMC dislocations.[25] Adduction contractures of the thumb metacarpal occur frequently with swan-neck deformities and gamekeeper's thumbs. Thumb instability may present with all types of deformities.[38]

SUMMARY

Although the deformities seen in the hands and wrists in RA are numerous, the primary common generator of pathology stems from synovial inflammation and pannus formation, which often compromise normal support structures. Depending on the location of disease and instability, altered anatomic forces create characteristic joint deformities commonly seen in RA.

REFERENCES

1. Firestein GS. Etiology and pathogenesis of rheumatoid arthritis. In: Harris ED, et al., ed. *Kelly's Textbook of Rheumatology*. 7th ed. Philadelphia: WB Saunders; 2005:996–1043.
2. Jain A, Brennan F, Troeberg L, et al. The role of matrix metalloproteinases in rheumatoid tendon disease. *J Hand Surg*. 2002;27A:1059–1064.
3. Goldring SR. Pathogenesis of bone and cartilage destruction in rheumatoid arthritis. *Rheumatology*. 2003;42(suppl 2):ii11–ii16.
4. Muller-Ladner U, Gay RE, Gay S. Molecular biology of cartilage and bone destruction. *Curr Opin Rheumatol*. 1998;10:212–212.
5. O'Gradaigh D, Ireland D, Bord S, et al. Joint erosion in rheumatoid arthritis: interactions between tumour necrosis factor alpha, interleukin 1, and receptor activator of nuclear factor kappa B ligand (RANKL) regulate osteoclasts. *Ann Rheum Dis*. 2004;63:354–359.
6. Taleisnik J. *The Wrist*. New York: Churchill Livingstone; 1985.
7. Ertel AN, Millender LH, Nalebuff E, et al. Flexor tendon ruptures in patients with rheumatoid arthritis. *J Hand Surg*. 1988;13A:860–866.
8. Magyar E, Talerman A, Mohácsy J, et al. Muscle changes in rheumatoid arthritis: a review of the literature with a study of 100 cases. *Virchows Arch A Pathol Anat Histol*. 1977;373:267–278.
9. Vaughan-Jackson OJ. Rheumatoid hand deformities considered in the light of tendon imbalance. *J Bone Joint Surg*. 1962;44B:764–775.
10. Stack HG, Vaughan-Jackson OJ. The zigzag deformity in the rheumatoid hand. *Hand*. 1971;3:62–67.
11. Ehrlich GE, Peterson LT, Sokoloff L, et al. Pathogenesis of rupture of extensor tendons at the wrist in rheumatoid arthritis. *Arth Rheum*. 1959;2:332–346.
12. Mannerfelt LG, Norman O. Attrition ruptures of flexor tendons in rheumatoid arthritis caused by bony spurs in the carpal tunnel: a clinical and radiological study. *J Bone Joint Surg*. 1969;51B:270–277.
13. Walker LG. Flexor pollicis longus rupture in rheumatoid arthritis secondary to attrition on a sesamoid. *J Hand Surg*. 1993;18A:990–991.
14. Landsmeer JM. Studies in the anatomy of articulation. 1. The equilibrium of the "interrelated" bone. *Acta Morphol Neerl Scand*. 1961;3:287–303.
15. Arimitsu S, Sugamoto K, Hashimoto J, et al. Analysis of radiocarpal and midcarpal motion in stable and unstable rheumatoid wrists using 3-dimensional computed tomography. *J Hand Surg*. 2008;33(2):189–197.
16. Shapiro JS, Heijna W, Nasatir S, et al. The relationship of wrist motion to ulnar phalangeal drift in the rheumatoid patient. *Hand*. 1971;3(1):68–75.
17. Hastings DE, Evans JA. Rheumatoid wrist deformities and their relation to ulnar drift. *J Bone Joint Surg*. 1975;57A:930–934.
18. Backdahl M. The caput ulnae syndrome in rheumatoid arthritis: a study of the morphology, abnormal anatomy, and clinical picture. *Acta Rheumatol Scand*. 1963;5:26–49.
19. Taleisnik J. Rheumatoid synovitis of the volar compartment of the wrist joint: its radiological signs and its contribution to wrist and hand deformity. *J Hand Surg*. 1979;4(6):526–535.
20. Larsen A, Dale K, Eek M. Radiographic evaluation of rheumatoid arthritis and related conditions by standard reference films. *Acta Radiologica Diagnosis*. 1977;18:481–491.
21. Wilson RL, Carlblom ER. The rheumatoid metacarpophalangeal joint. *Hand Clin*. 1989;5:223–237.
22. Morco S, Bowden A. Ulnar drift in rheumatoid arthritis: a review of biomechanical etiology. *J Biomech*. 2015;48(4):725–728.
23. Hakstian RW, Tubiana R. Ulnar deviation of the fingers. The role of joint structure and function. *J Bone Joint Surg*. 1967;49:299–316.
24. Akhavani MA, Paleolog EM, Kang N. Muscle hypoxia in rheumatoid hands: does it play a role in ulnar drift? *J Hand Surg*. 2011;36:677–685.
25. Feldon P, Terrono AL, Nalebuff EA, et al. Rheumatoid arthritis and other connective tissue diseases. In: Wolfe SW, Hotchkiss R, Pederson W, Kozin S, eds. *Green's Operative Hand Surgery*. 6th ed. Philadelphia: Elsevier Churchill Livingstone; 2011:1993–2066.
26. Shapiro JS. The etiology of ulnar drift: a new factor. *Clin Orthop Relat Res*. 1970;68:32–43.
27. DiBenedetto MR, Lubbers LM, Coleman CR. Relationship between radial inclination angle and ulnar deviation of the fingers. *J Hand Surg*. 1991;16(1):36–39.
28. Smith EM, Juvinall RC, Bender LF, et al. Flexor forces and rheumatoid metacarpophalangeal deformities. Clinical implications. *JAMA*. 1966;198:130–134.
29. Flatt AE. Some pathomechanics of ulnar drift. *Plast Reconstr Surg*. 1966;37:295–303.
30. Bielefeld T, Neumann D. The unstable metacarpophalangeal joint in rheumatoid arthritis: anatomy, pathomechanics, and physical rehabilitation considerations. *J Orthop Sports Phys Ther*. 2005;35(8):502–520.
31. Backhouse KM. The mechanics of normal digital control in the hand and an analysis of the ulnar drift of rheumatoid arthritis. *Ann R Coll Surg Engl*. 1968;43(3):154–173.
32. Sebastin SJ, Chung KC. Reconstruction of digital deformities in rheumatoid arthritis. *Hand Clin*. 2011;27(1):87–104.
33. Williams K, Terrono AL. Treatment of boutonniere finger deformity in rheumatoid arthritis. *J Hand Surg*. 2011;36(8):1388–1393.

34. Nalebuff EA. The rheumatoid swan-neck deformity. *Hand Clin.* 1989;5(2):203–214.

35. Welsh RP, Hastings DE. Swan neck deformity in rheumatoid arthritis of the hand. *Hand.* 1977;9(2):109–116.

36. Heywood AW. The pathogenesis of the rheumatoid swan neck deformity. *Hand.* 1979;11(2):176–183.

37. Nalebuff EA, Millender JH. Surgical treatment of the swan-neck deformity in rheumatoid arthritis. *Orthop Clin North Am.* 1975;6(3):733–752.

38. Kessler I. Aetiology and management of adduction contracture of the thumb in rheumatoid arthritis. *Hand.* 1973;5:170–174.

39. Terrono A, Millender L, Nalebuff E. Boutonniere rheumatoid thumb deformity. *J Hand Surg.* 1990;15(6):999–1003.

40. Ratliff AH. Deformities of the thumb in rheumatoid arthritis. *Hand.* 1971;3(2):138–143.

41. Leak RS, Rayan GM, Arthur RE. Longitudinal radiographic analysis of rheumatoid arthritis in the hand and wrist. *J Hand Surg.* 2003;28A(3):427–434.

85

The Arthritic Hand: Conservative Management

Jeanine Beasley, Dianna Lunsford

CRITICAL POINTS

- Arthritis is the leading cause of disability in adults.[1]
- Conservative management requires an understanding of the disease process, specific conditions, potential deformities, and the patient's individual needs.
- A comprehensive examination assists the therapist in appropriate goal setting and treatment planning.

- The goals of therapy are to reduce inflammation, decrease trauma to the joints, decrease pain, facilitate proper joint alignment, improve performance of daily living tasks, facilitate successful adjustments in lifestyle, and prevent losses of function.[2]

Nearly one in four adults, 54.4 million individuals, in the United States report that they have arthritis, and by 2040, that number is projected to increase 49% to 78.4 million.[3,4] Arthritis continues to be the leading cause of disability in adults, affecting 8.6 million people.[1] There are many different conditions that make up these rheumatic and musculoskeletal disorders. The conditions that more commonly affect the hand include rheumatoid arthritis (RA); juvenile idiopathic arthritis (JIA); osteoarthritis (OA); systemic lupus erythematosus (SLE); psoriatic arthritis (PsA); and scleroderma, or systemic sclerosis (SS) (see Chapter 92). It is clear that with this level of prevalence, therapists need to understand the disease process, how it can affect activities of daily living (ADLs), identify what is effective in the best available evidence, and implement those interventions into current practice for these individuals.

CONDITIONS

Rheumatoid Arthritis

Rheumatoid arthritis is the most common inflammatory disease of the joints.[5] This incidence appears to be rising from the previously reported 1.3 million to an estimated 1.5 million adults in the United States.[6] It is a chronic, systemic disease characterized by synovial inflammation and proliferation, which leads to loss of the articular cartilage and bone.[7] Hand involvement may be an early clinical sign and can include joint swelling and inflammation of the proximal interphalangeal (PIP) joints, metacarpophalangeal (MCP) joints, and wrists (Fig. 85.1).[7] Although current medications have altered the course of this disease, providing a substantial clinical benefit, it is important to note that these medications are not a cure.[8] Most patients will continue to have a progression of the disease, eventually resulting in cartilage breakdown, bone erosions, joint destruction, and instability, leading to functional impairment.[8] In 2010, the American College of Rheumatology/European League Against Rheumatism Collaborative Initiative developed a new RA Classification Criteria to assist with early diagnosis.[7] The scoring system (Table 85.1) involves several criteria with a score of 6 indicating a definitive presence of RA.[7]

Juvenile Idiopathic Arthritis

Approximately 30 to 100 in 100,000 children have JIA, which is made up of several disorders.[9] These are defined by the International League Against Rheumatism, and include systemic onset (Still's disease), enthesitis-related (ERA), psoriatic, oligoarticular, polyarticular seropositive, polyarticular seronegative, and undifferentiated.[10] The diagnosis is made clinically when a child younger than 16 years of age presents with persistent synovitis in any one joint for more than 6 weeks.[10] Obtaining a diagnosis is often a frustrating experience for parents seeking answers to their child's pain because there are no specific diagnostic laboratory tests. The wrist and hand involvement varies greatly in these children depending on the type of JIA. In a study by Selvaag and coworkers,[11] half of the patients demonstrated radiographic damage in the hands and wrists. Carpal involvement is more common than MCP or PIP joint involvement.[12] With carpal involvement, wrist flexion with wrist ulnar deviation is a common pattern of deformity.[12] Interestingly, some of these children may demonstrate MCP joint radial deviation with wrist ulnar deviation, which is opposite that of the more common MCP joint ulnar deviation seen in adult RA.[13] Other children may demonstrate similar deformities to those with adult-onset RA. Care must be taken to consider all potential deformities when treating these children.

Osteoarthritis

In the United States, OA is the most common joint disorder, with 27 million individuals with clinical OA.[14-16] It is a degenerative and chronic disease, with an estimated hand radiologic prevalence of approximately 6.8% overall and 54% to 67% of the adult population

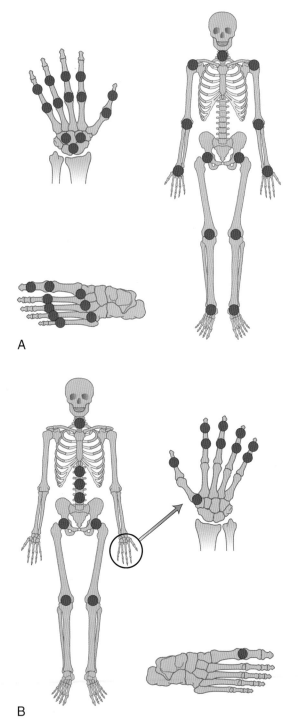

Fig. 85.1 The typical distribution of joint involvements with rheumatoid arthritis (RA) and osteoarthritis (OA). (A) Hand involvement in RA may be an early clinical sign and can include joint swelling and inflammation of the proximal interphalangeal joints, metacarpophalangeal joints, and wrists.[7] (B) In an upper extremity with OA, the joints that are most symptomatic are the distal interphalangeal joints and the first carpometacarpal joint.[21] (Redrawn from O'Dell JR, Imboden JB, Miller LD. Rheumatoid arthritis. In: Imboden JB, Hellman DB, Stone JH, eds. *Rheumatology: Current Diagnosis & Treatment.* 3rd edition. New York: McGraw Hill Medical; 2013:187-197).

TABLE 85.1 Rheumatoid Arthritis Classification Criteria to Assist with Early Diagnosis: American College of Rheumatology/European League Against Rheumatism Collaborative Initiative[7]	
Target population: patients who have at least one joint with clinical synovitis and with the synovitis not better explained by another disease	
A. Joint Involvement (Tender or Swollen)	**Score**
1 large joint	0
2–10 large joints	1
1–3 small joints (± involvement of large joints)	2
4–10 small joints (± involvement of large joints)	3
>10 joints (≥1 small joint)	5
B. Serology	
Negative RF and ACPA	0
Low-positive RF and low-positive ACPA	2
	3
C. Acute-Phase Reactants	
Normal CRP and ESR	0
Abnormal CRP and ESR	1
D. Duration of Symptoms	
<6 wk	0
≥6 wk	1
Add score of categories A–D: ≥6/10 = definite RA	**Total:**

ACPA, Anticitrullinated protein antibodies; *CRP,* C-reactive protein; *ESR,* erythrocyte sedimentation rate; *RA,* rheumatoid arthritis; *RF,* rheumatoid factor.

research demonstrates that the breakdown in the articular cartilage is caused by mechanical, biochemical, and cellular factors.[19] There is a genetic susceptibility, and OA occurs more frequently and with greater severity in women of postmenopausal age, suggesting a hormonal component.[15,20] In the upper extremity, the joints that are most symptomatic are the distal interphalangeal (DIP) joints and the first carpometacarpal (CMC) joint (see Fig. 85. 1).[21] In the lower extremities, the knees and less commonly the hips are affected.[14–16] If the patient needs to use a walker or crutches because of lower extremity pain, this activity can place additional stress on the hands. Please refer to Chapter 88 for more information on OA and the CMC joint.

Systemic Lupus Erythematosus

Systemic lupus erythematosus is one of the autoimmune connective tissue diseases resulting from complex interactions among genes, the environment, hormones, smoking, infections, drugs, and abnormalities of the adaptive immune system.[22] There is a high variability of clinical symptoms ranging from joint, skin, and organ involvement, which can be life threatening.[23] In the United States, it is estimated that between 0.5 million and 1.5 million Americans have SLE, and it is more common in women, African Americans, Asians, and Hispanics.[24] Patients with SLE exhibit a characteristic rash, which can occur on the face (butterfly rash), between the interphalangeal (IP) joints of the digits, the trunk, and the upper extremities.[23,25] There is also a tendency toward Raynaud's phenomenon.[26] Arthritis and arthralgia affects 95% of the cases, frequently involving the small joints of the hand and the wrists.[23] Swan-neck deformities are evident in many cases but are passively correctable because of ligamentous laxity.[23] The connective tissue involvement resembles RA in that it is symmetrical, with 10% developing nonerosive MCP joint ulnar deviation of the digits.[27]

55 years of age and older.[17,18] When symptomatic hand OA is combined with radiologic evidence, 26% of women and 13% of men older than the age of 70 years are affected.[17] This prevalence is expected to rise in the coming decades with the aging population.[16] OA is often called the wear-and-tear disease, increasing in prevalence with age, but

The combination of these deformities has been referred to as Jaccoud's arthropathy, including passively correctable or "reversible" joint deformities such as swan-neck, thumb subluxation, ulnar deviation, and boutonnière with an absence of articular erosions.[27]

Psoriatic Arthritis

Psoriatic arthritis is an inflammatory musculoskeletal disease associated with psoriasis.[28] PsA has been rising over 30 years with an incidence of 7.2 cases (9.1 for men and 5.4 for women) per 100,000.[29] Clinically, PsA may resemble RA, but psoriatic skin lesions, nail changes, and DIP joint involvement assist in making the diagnosis.[28] Approximately 30% (range, 6%–41%) of patients with psoriasis will develop PsA.[30] Nail changes can include pitting, oil spots, crumbling, linear pitting, splinter hemorrhages, or discoloration.[28,31] Pain from nail psoriasis can result in decreased functional ability and is often associated with DIP joint involvement.[32] Several classifications have been proposed but none has been universally accepted because it has been found that disease patterns change over time.[29,31] Some patients report a delay in obtaining a diagnosis that connects their psoriasis to PsA.

Scleroderma, or Systemic Sclerosis

Systemic sclerosis is a chronic connective tissue disease characterized by vascular, immunologic, and fibrotic changes that affect multiple internal organs, muscles, joints, tendons, blood vessels, and the skin.[33,34] It is a rare disorder, with an annual incidence in the United States of about 20 to 240 cases per 1 million adults.[35,36] The first sign of progressive skin hardening or thickening is often noted at the digits.[33] Ulcers can be evident at the PIP joints and at the tips of the digits.[34] Hand deformities can progress to MCP joint extension with PIP and DIP joint flexion. Changes to the nail folds may include dilated capillary loops or small hemorrhages.[36] Raynaud's phenomenon is present in most patients with SS.[33,37] Readers are referred to Chapters 91 and 92 for more complete information on this topic.

EXAMINATION

Examination includes inspection for the effects of the disease process on the arthritic hand and wrist with particular note made of joint deformities, skin condition, inflammation, and nodules and nodes. Also included is palpation to localize areas of tenderness and pain and to identify grating or crepitus, as well as an assessment of joint stability, range of motion (ROM), and strength. Equally important is the assessment of how the arthritic condition has affected the individual's occupational functioning. It is important to look at the client holistically and not just the hand in isolation when completing the examination with the use of a validated patient functional outcome measure (see Table 85.3).

Palpation and Skin Observation

Palpation of the joint and surrounding tissue and observation of the skin are important components of the evaluation. Grating or crepitus evident with joint compression can be indicative of damaged cartilage. For example, the grind test at the CMC joint involves compressing the joint while gently rotating the base of the metacarpal on the trapezium (Fig. 85.2).[38] Pain or crepitus at the CMC joint is generally considered a positive finding. Grating or crepitus during active range of motion (AROM) may be palpated or heard as a crunching or popping sound.[38] Volar palpation of the flexor tendons at the A1 pulley while the patient flexes and extends the digits (Fig. 85.3) may reveal tendon thickening, triggering, or periodic locking of the digit in flexion, which is indicative of flexor tenosynovitis. Examination of the skin's condition should include color, temperature, and areas of swelling.

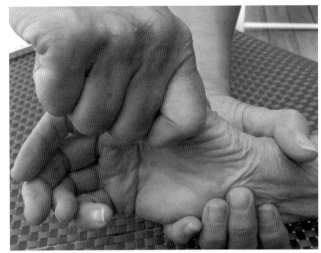

Fig. 85.2 The grind test as described by Swanson[38] for crepitus at the first carpometacarpal (CMC) joint involves compressing the joint while gently rotating the metacarpal on the trapezium at the CMC joint.

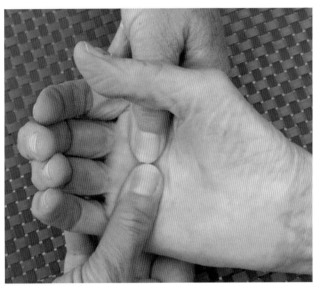

Fig. 85.3 A thickening of the flexor tendons can be palpated in the palm at the A1 pulley as the patient flexes and extends the digits.

Nodules and Nodes

Rheumatoid nodules develop in many patients with RA and most commonly may be seen at the joints or along the tendons.[39] The nodules may or may not be painful and are often largest near the elbow joint (Fig. 85.4). Some patients report an abrupt appearance of nodules, whereas others have a more gradual onset. Rheumatoid nodules can be painful when palpated and should be noted in the evaluation because they may affect orthosis design or strap placement. These nodules should not be confused with nodes, which are seen in OA caused by a bony proliferation called osteophytes. This osteophyte formation at the DIP joint is called a Heberden's node (Fig. 85.5), and at the PIP joint, it is called a Bouchard's node.[40] Patients can have RA in combination with degenerative joint disease, which explains the presence of these nodes in the RA population.

Deformities

The presence of deformities should be documented and a notation made of whether the deformity is fixed or flexible and whether the deformity is accentuated during the performance of simple activities

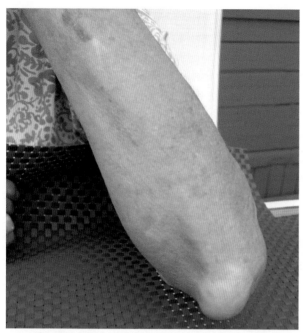

Fig. 85.4 Rheumatoid nodules near the elbow joint.

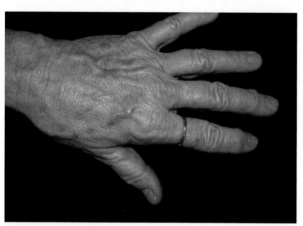

Fig. 85.5 The joints that are most symptomatic in osteoarthritis in the upper extremity are the distal interphalangeal (DIP) joints and the first carpometacarpal joint. This patient is also demonstrating Heberden's nodes at the index and middle DIP joints. (Courtesy of Dr. Donald Condit.)

or whether the deformity prevents the activity. Readers are encouraged to review a detailed description of common hand and wrist deformities in RA (see Chapter 86), OA CMC joint (see Chapter 88), and SS (see Chapter 92).

Pain

Pain is most frequently measured using the Numeric Pain Rating Scale (NPRS) or the Visual Analog Scale (VAS) in practice. The NPRS provides the patient (either verbally or on paper) an 11-point scale from 0 to 10 to choose from. On this scale, 0 is no pain, and 10 is the worst pain possible.[41,42] This scale is a valid and reliable tool that is easy to use and quick to administer. A decrease of 2 points is found to be clinically significant.[41] Another commonly used tool is the VAS, which is a 10-cm VAS, with one end being no pain and the other end being severe pain, allowing the patient to create a vertical hash mark on the scale to identify the current pain level. This can be scored again after treatment and then measured to obtain the numerical score. A difference of 2 cm or more is found to be clinically significant. This is also a valid and

reliable tool, which is quick and easy to administer.[42] These scales can be used to determine pain both at rest and with activities. Pain early in the disease process is usually greater than it is later as the disease progresses. Pain from a nerve compression caused by synovitis also may be evident. Compression of the median nerve, or carpal tunnel syndrome, is one of the most commonly seen conditions at the wrist. The ulnar nerve can also be compressed at Guyon's canal and at the cubital tunnel (see Chapters 10, 51, 53, and 55).

Range of Motion

Active range of motion measurements of the arthritic hand can vary throughout the day. Increased stiffness or gelling, which is defined as difficulty in initiating joint motion after a period of inactivity, is often noted in the morning.[39] Measurement of hand AROM has been shown to have poor reliability because measurements may vary by as much as 10 degrees with RA patients.[43] Measurement of composite digital flexion, active digital extension, and thumb opposition often give more functional information. Passive range of motion (PROM) measurements using overpressure at the end of the available ROM are not recommended, especially if there is a lack of joint stability. However, it is important to note significant discrepancies between AROM and PROM at a joint or joints, which may indicate a tendon rupture or impending rupture.

Tendon ruptures cause loss of AROM in flexion or extension and occur secondary to attrition of the tendon as it glides over roughened and irregular bone areas.[44] For example, in RA, the extensor pollicis longus (EPL) and the extensor digitorum communis (EDC) tendons of the third, fourth, and fifth digits as well as the extensor digiti quinti (EDQ) are vulnerable to attritional rupture at the wrist level.[45] The EPL can rupture at Lister's tubercle on the dorsal aspect of the distal radius, and the EDC and EDQ can rupture over the distal end of the ulna. Vaughan-Jackson syndrome refers to disruption of the digital extensor tendons, beginning on the ulnar side of the hand and, if untreated, progressing radially.[46] To test the EPL, the patient attempts to extend the thumb at all joints in forearm pronation; an inability to fully extend the thumb through the available PROM may indicate a rupture or impending rupture of the EPL. To test the EDQ, the therapist should hold the MCP joints of the index, middle, and ring fingers in flexion and have the patient attempt isolated extension of the small finger.[44,47] An inability to extend the small digit independently with no significant restriction in passive small finger extension may indicate a rupture of the EDQ. The patient often is unaware of this condition, but it should be brought to the attention of the hand surgeon.

The ROM of thumb pinch patterns should be evaluated and noted. Some patients are only able to complete a lateral pinch because of a pronation deformity of the index finger.[48] Measurement of the degree of ulnar deviation at the MCP joints can provide helpful information on the progression of this joint deformity. MCP joint ulnar deviation varies based on the MCP joint position (flexion or extension), and therefore the position of the MCP joint should be reported in combination with the ulnar drift measurement.[43] These authors recommend measuring ulnar deviation in the maximum available active MCP joint extension because this is the position commonly used in nighttime orthoses positioning.

Digit and thumb abduction should also be measured and can be especially limited in patients with SS. One method of measuring thumb and digit abduction is to trace the hand on a piece of paper with thumb and digits maximally abducted.[49]

Joint Stability

The stability of the MCP and IP joints of the digits is frequently compromised by the arthritic disease process. Stability of the IP joints is tested

TABLE 85.2	**Product Information**
Products	**Manufacturer**
Oval-8 Splint	3-Point Products: http://www.
P.O.P. Splint	3pointproducts.com
Court'R Force Brace	North Coast Medical: https://
	www.ncmedical.com
SIRIS Splint	Silver Ring Splint Company:
	http://www.silverringsplint.com
Coban, Co-Wrap, Polyform, Neoprene,	Performance Health: https://
Seam Tape, Velcro, and Aquaplast	www.performancehealth.com

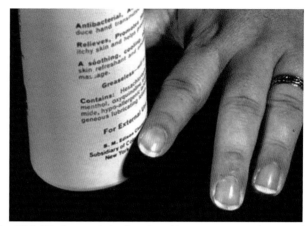

Fig. 85.6 Weakness of the first dorsal interosseous can be tested by having the patient attempt to abduct the index digit actively or against a light object to determine the appropriate muscle grade.

by stabilizing proximally and then attempting to tilt or glide the joint laterally. Instability is apparent by excessive lateral play. Testing of MCP joint stability requires that the joint be positioned in flexion during lateral stress testing because in this position, the collateral ligaments are tightened, and normally, there should be little lateral play. Instability of the MCP joints in RA often results in palmar subluxation and ulnar deviation. Thumb stability is further evaluated by having the patient attempt a tip pinch. If the thumb MCP and IP joints are unable to maintain a near-neutral position during pinch, ligament stability is questioned.

Hypermobility can be evident in just one joint (because of ligamentous or soft tissue disruption) or more generalized such as evident in hypermobility syndrome. A screen for hypermobility syndrome (Beighton test or score) has been described by Uul-Kristensen and associates.[50]

Strength and Exercise

Philips reports that a grip of 20 lb is necessary for most daily activities.[47] The standard Jamar hydraulic hand dynamometer (Performance Health; see Table 85.2) has good reliability and is the most mentioned in the literature but is often painful for the rheumatoid hand.[51] Sphygmomanometers are more comfortable for these patients, but they measure grip pressure that is affected by the amount of contact surface area, and these results can be influenced by hand size.[52] Interestingly, a study by Agnew[53] has determined correlations between the two instruments. Pinch strength can be obtained with a pinch meter; however, some patients are unable to complete a tip pinch or a three-jaw chuck pinch because of a pronation deformity of the index digit and therefore perform many daily tasks with a key or lateral pinch.[48] Joint instability, rather than weakness, can be more problematic during ADLs. Even with good muscle strength, patients are unable to maintain a grip on an object if their joints collapse into deformities. Another problem in RA and OA is weakness of the first dorsal interosseous muscle. This is tested by having the patient abduct the index digit actively against resistance (Fig. 85.6).

Activities of Daily Living and Hand Function

Examination of the patient's functional level begins as soon as the patient enters the therapy clinic. The speed with which the patient ambulates can give information about the level of pain and the extent of lower extremity involvement. Observation as the patient unbuttons and removes a coat and sits at a table can be invaluable in understanding his or her ability to maintain an upright posture, pinch and grasp, complete simple functional activities, and use the hand for mobility (e.g., using crutches or propelling a wheelchair). It is important to gain an understanding of the patient's home situation and support system when planning the treatment program and potential orthosis designs. For example, if the patient is unable to don an orthosis independently, a caregiver must be available to assist. The patient's goals for therapy need to be evaluated carefully and collaboratively to ensure that they

are realistic. The evaluation of ADL tasks should include home, work, and avocational activities. Many patients seek treatment when meaningful work and avocational activities are threatened or limited. Several functional assessments are helpful in the evaluation of these clients and are listed in Table 85.3.[54–75]

TREATMENT PLANNING

The therapist's management of arthritis is individualized and specific to the patient's condition, deformity or potential deformity, and ADL needs. The patient's personal goals should also be considered in determining the treatment plan. Patient education about the disease and treatment options is critical in the treatment process. The goals of therapy are to maintain and improve upper limb function through joint protection and energy conservation, hand exercises, assistive devices and orthoses, physical agents, fatigue and stress management, ADL training, environmental modifications, and community resources.[76]

Orthoses

Orthotic positioning is supported by the evidence and commonly used in arthritic conditions to decrease inflammation and pain, to improve function, and to minimize deformity.[77–79] In severe flexion deformities, night orthoses may be used to gently position the digits in comfortable extension, which can facilitate morning hand hygiene. Simple stretch gloves have been found to be helpful in decreasing morning stiffness and pain.[80] Wrist or digit orthoses may be used to enhance joint stability during ADLs and thus improve function.[81]

When passively correctable, the orthosis should gently support the joint(s) in a position opposite of the deformity, thereby reducing pain, improving function, and maintaining soft tissue length and balance. Of course, any attempt to realign the joints should be done gently. Orthotic positioning for common arthritic wrist and hand deformities is discussed later. Readers are referred to Chapter 84 for a detailed description of the pathoanatomy and pathomechanics of these deformities.

Swan-Neck Deformity

A swan-neck deformity is characterized by flexion of the DIP joint and hyperextension of the PIP joint (Fig. 85.7) and can be seen in RA and SLE. The swan-neck deformity can originate from abnormalities at the DIP, PIP, or the MCP joints (see Chapter 84).[82] Positioning techniques that prevent PIP joint hyperextension yet allow flexion are often very effective. These orthoses are needed for the long term and therefore should be durable. It has been reported that there is greater acceptance

TABLE 85.3   Arthritis Assessments

Assessment	Description	Scoring	Change in Outcome
Arthritis Hand Function Test[60]	11-item performance-based test designed to measure hand strength and dexterity in persons with arthritis	No summative total score; 4 subscales: grip and pinch strength, dexterity, applied dexterity and applied strength	Not established
The Arthritis Helplessness Index (AHI)[61]	Assesses self-perception of helplessness across 15 items related to managing arthritis	A higher score indicates greater perceived helplessness	Responsiveness: the 6-mo retesting indicated changes over time, and these were more strongly related to changes in pain and depression than were changes in the full AHI[61]
The Arthritis Impact Measurement Scales II (AIMS2)[62]	A standardized outcome for arthritis that includes subscales for mood, tension, and pain	A summative raw score from 5–25; a higher score indicates poorer health	Responsiveness: standardized response means that changes in AIMS2-SF scores over 3 months range from 0.36 (small) to 0.8 (high)[62,63]
Arthritis Self-Efficacy Scale [64]	Developed to measure patients' arthritis-specific self-efficacy or patients' beliefs that they could perform specific tasks or behaviors to cope with the consequences of arthritis	Range is 10–100 on each of three subscales: Self-efficacy Pain, Self-efficacy Function, and Self-efficacy Other Symptoms	Unknown
AUSCAN The Australian/ Canadian Osteoarthritis Hand Index[65]	A self-administered questionnaire that assessment pain, joint stiffness, and disability in the OA hand with 15 questions	Three scales: pain, stiffness, and function assessed at rest and during activities	Each 1-unit increase in the function subscale was associated with a clinically relevant decrease in hand strength[66]
Cochin Hand Function Scale[67]	Self-report scale of 18 tasks to measure functional ability in the hand	7-point scale from 0 (without difficulty) to 5 (impossible)	Discriminated between those who improved and those who deteriorated[68]
COPM Canadian Occupational Performance Measure[69]	Detects change in a patient's self-perception of occupational performance (self-care, productivity, and leisure)	Patients identify their most important occupational performance issues and rate their level of satisfaction and performance on a scale of 1–10	Defined as an increase in 2.0 points[69]
Health Assessment Questionnaire (HAQ) Disability Index (DI)[70]	A standardized, self-administered, written questionnaire developed to assess a patient's functional ability	The highest score for each category is added (range, 0–24) and divided by 8 to yield a continuous score (0–3)	Defined as a decrease of 0.2 points[71]
McGill Pain Questionnaire[72]	A self-reported measure of pain	0 (no pain) to 78 (severe pain)	Not established
Michigan Hand Outcomes Questionnaire[73]	Measures perception of the hands in terms of function, appearance, pain, and satisfaction	Six subscales: overall hand function, ADLs, pain, work performance, aesthetics, and patient satisfaction with hand function	Patients with RA; MCIDs were identified for the pain (3), function (11), and ADL subscales (13)[74]
Patient Specific Functional Scale[75]	Used to assess functional ability to complete specific activities	Patients rate their ability to complete an activity on a 11-point scale; 0 represents unable to perform, and 10 represents the ability to perform at prior level	Musculoskeletal MCID = 1.2 points[75]
Quick Disabilities of Arm, Shoulder & Hand[76]	11 items to measure physical function and symptoms in people with any or multiple musculoskeletal disorders of the upper limb	0–100 (most severe disability)	MCID = 9.0–11.3 for upper extremity musculoskeletal disorders[77]
Sickness Impact Profile-68 (SIP-68)[78]	A 68-question objective measure designed to assess quality of life and level of dysfunction that results from disability or illness; designed to provide a valid and sensitive assessment of outcomes that result from health care–related services	A general measure of generic health status; 0 identifies the best health to 68, which indicates the worst health	Less is known about the sensitivity of the SIP-68; results indicate that the SIP-136 has high specificity to detect change in health status; the SIP-136 total score had high specificity to detect a 3-point change in self-rated function[79]
Stanford Hand and Assessment Questionnaire[80]	Designed to measure disability in arthritis and asks patients to rate degree of difficulty in performing 24 everyday activities	The assessment generates a score on an ordinal scale from 0 (minimum disability) to 3 (maximum)	A change in score by 0.48 points or more for 95% confidence to reflects significant change (0.31 for 80% confidence)[81,83]

ADL, Activity of daily living; *MCID*, minimal clinically important difference; *OA*, osteoarthritis; *RA*, rheumatoid arthritis.

and tolerance with prefabricated orthoses (Fig. 85.8) over custom-made orthoses.[79] Many of the low-temperature plastic orthoses can wear out and need to be replaced frequently. A high-temperature plastic option, the Oval-8 splint, is available in a variety of sizes and can be obtained from 3-Point Products (Annapolis, MD) (see Fig. 85.8). A metal custom-sized orthosis, the SIRIS splint (Fig. 85.9), is available from the Silver Ring Splint Company (Charlottesville, VA). These orthoses are well tolerated by patients because they allow most ADLs and do not need to be removed for hand washing. Several studies have found that these orthoses improve dexterity in patients with RA.[78,79]

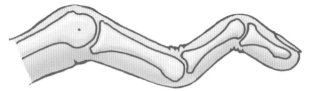

Fig. 85.7 Proximal interphalangeal (PIP) joint swan-neck deformity with PIP joint hyperextension and distal interphalangeal joint flexion.

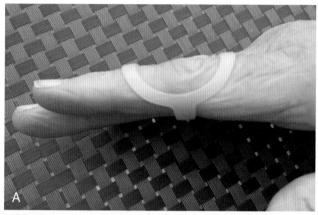

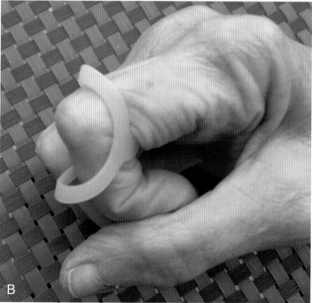

Fig. 85.8 A, Orthosis that prevents proximal interphalangeal (PIP) joint hyperextension with a swan-neck deformity. **B,** The Oval-8 splint allows PIP joint flexion during daily activities. (Orthosis courtesy of 3-Point Products, http://www.3pointproducts.com.)

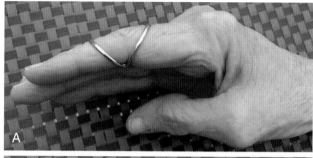

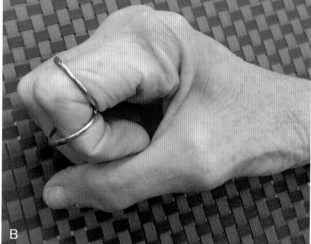

Fig. 85.9 A, Custom-sized ring orthosis, the SIRIS splint, which prevents proximal interphalangeal (PIP) joint hyperextension. **B,** The SIRIS splint allows PIP joint flexion. (Orthosis courtesy the Silver Ring Splint Company, Charlottesville, VA, http://www.silverringsplint.com.)

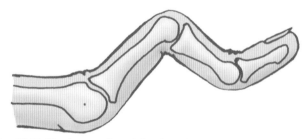

Fig. 85.10 The boutonnière deformity with proximal interphalangeal joint flexion and distal interphalangeal joint hyperextension.

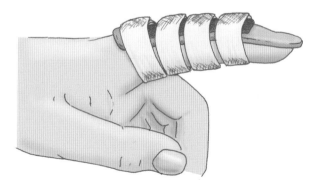

Fig. 85.11 Orthotic positioning of a boutonnière deformity when passively correctable includes proximal interphalangeal joint extension and slight distal interphalangeal joint flexion.

Boutonnière Deformity

The boutonnière deformity in RA is characterized by a posture of PIP joint flexion and DIP joint hyperextension (Fig. 85.10). In patients demonstrating good passive extension, positioning the PIP joint in extension with a DIP extension block may be used (Fig. 85.11). When the orthosis is worn consistently, this method may help to maintain passive PIP extension and prevent the deformity from becoming fixed. One study found improvements in grip strength when wearing the orthosis for 6 weeks.[83] Many patients reject this orthosis during ADLs because it limits the ability to flex the PIP joint. These patients may prefer and better tolerate nighttime positioning in this type of orthosis.

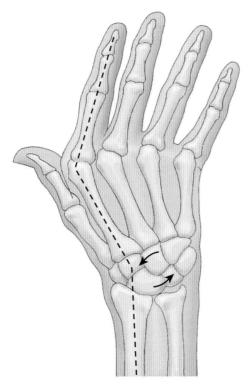

Fig. 85.12 The zigzag deformity with wrist radial deviation and metacarpophalangeal joint ulnar deviation. (Redrawn with permission from Melvin JL. *Rheumatic Disease: Occupational Therapy and Rehabilitation.* 2nd ed. Philadelphia: FA Davis; 1982.)

Metacarpophalangeal Joint Ulnar Deviation and Palmar Subluxation

Ulnar deviation of the MCP joints is the most common deformity seen in RA. It can also be seen in SLE. Factors that can contribute to the development of the ulnar deviation deformity, in the presence of weakened and diseased joint ligaments and capsules, include anatomic susceptibility, as well as ulnar and volar forces that occur during the performance of ADLs.[82] Lateral pinch activities, gripping an object, writing, and even gravity tend to place ulnar and volar forces on the MCP joints. The deformity often includes radial deviation of the wrist (Fig. 85.12).[84] Positioning the MCP joints in radial alignment requires consideration of MCP palmar subluxation and wrist radial deviation deformities. The therapist should carefully avoid forcing the digits into alignment in an orthosis that leaves the wrist position unchecked and that aggravates the wrist radial deviation deformity.[84,85] To prevent further deviation of the wrist, it is also important to provide wrist ulnar alignment with appropriate strapping (Fig. 85.13).[84] Night orthoses for this deformity should include a volar component to gently glide the subluxed proximal phalanx into alignment. According to Brand, it is important to avoid the use of the long lever arm of the digit to position the MCP joint.[86] If the proximal phalanx tilts rather than glides into position, it can wear away at the dorsal lip of the phalanx. This results in an orthosis that actually increases pain and absorption of the joint surface (Fig. 85.14). Patients who are fitted with night orthoses should be made aware of proper application techniques to avoid this joint tilting, and the orthosis should be properly formed, allowing the joint to glide into position. At later stages of RA, functional orthoses can be used to give stability to the joint during ADL performance. Day orthoses are tolerated by the patient if they allow some degree of function for ADLs, are comfortable, and are not bulky. Hand-based orthoses, such as those made of soft materials (Fig. 85.15), help with joint stability during activities. A Cochrane review of 38 studies reported these orthoses in the treatment of RA can decrease pain and improve the strength of one's grip, but may decrease hand movement.[87]

Volar Subluxation of the Carpus on the Radius

Ligament laxity resulting from chronic synovitis at the wrist and the natural volar tilt of the distal articular surface of the radius can result in volar subluxation of the carpus on the radius (Fig. 85.16).[88] The wrist, as stated by Swanson,[82] is the key joint for proper hand function, and instability at the wrist affects grip and pinch activities. Colditz[88] recommends positioning the wrist with a volar reinforcement orthosis to support the carpal area. Many patients with this deformity prefer soft or fabric orthoses with a volar rigid bar for ADLs.[89] The soft orthosis also has some flexibility, which facilitates grasping objects. D-rings for Velcro closures make it easier to don and doff the orthosis when the hand has limited mobility (Fig. 85.17). A study by Pagnotta and colleagues[81] found that static wrist orthoses decreased pain without decreasing work performance in patients with RA.

Distal Ulnar Dorsal Subluxation

Patients with RA commonly demonstrate instability of the distal ulna. The distal ulna normally is less prominent in supination and more prominent in pronation. The arthritic process often weakens the ligamentous structures, causing dorsal prominence of the distal ulna, pain, or crepitation with pronation and supination.[82] Providing stability to the dorsally subluxed distal ulna, by means of gentle ulnar-head depression, often can decrease pain and increase stability during forearm rotation activities. Positioning of a soft orthosis (see Chapter 110) with padding to depress the distal ulna on the dorsal surface, with counterforce volarly on the radius, can be accomplished using a variety of techniques (Fig. 85.18). Materials that have an elastic component can maintain a more constant pressure, increasing the stability of the ulna during rotation.

Thumb Deformities

Classification and treatment of the arthritic thumb and common patterns of thumb deformity are covered in greater detail in Chapters 87 and 88. A stable, pain-free thumb is vital to the hand because it provides a post to which the digits can grip and pinch effectively for daily functioning. Thumb IP joint instability can be seen in arthritis mutilans and RA. This instability can result in decreased pinch strength during ADLs. A solution to this situation is an orthosis to the IP joint that provides joint stability yet allows IP flexion (Fig. 85.19). The orthosis should provide durable long-term support that can be worn full time. A durable plastic option is the Oval-8 splint from 3-Point Products (http://www.3pointproducts.com). Another durable option is an orthosis from the Silver Ring Splint Company (http://www.silverringsplint.com).

Distal Interphalangeal Joint

In OA, DIP joint pain can be troublesome during periods of inflammation. Orthotic positioning can be helpful in decreasing pain during this time (Fig. 85.20). In the presence of Heberden's nodes and joint swelling, orthoses for the DIP joints need to conform well and provide even pressure distribution. Thin, or "light," orthotic positioning material is recommended, and the material should have excellent drape characteristics. This can include Polyform light or thin perforated materials such as Aquaplast. These orthoses are usually made on the dorsal surface to allow for tactile input on the volar surface for activities such as computer work or grasping objects. To hold these orthoses in place, a

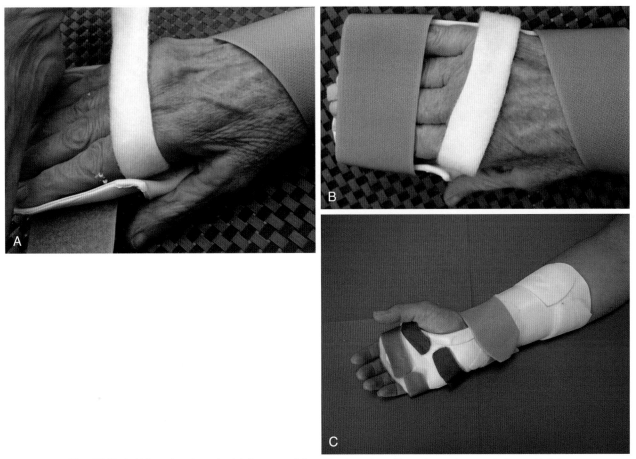

Fig. 85.13 A, When the therapist fabricates a night orthosis and positions the metacarpophalangeal joints in a position opposite that of ulnar deviation, it is important to be aware of the wrist's orientation. The therapist should carefully avoid forcing the digits into alignment with an orthosis that leaves the wrist position unchecked and could aggravate the wrist radial deviation deformity. This can be addressed with an inside out strap that gently places the wrist in neutral alignment avoiding wrist radial deviation. **B,** This night orthosis helps guide the wrist into gentle wrist ulnar alignment and the metacarpophalangeal joints into radial alignment. **C,** In some cases, the interphalangeal joints can be left free in the night orthosis to allow the patient to manage bedding. (Part B from Boozer JA. Splinting the arthritic hand. *J Hand Ther.* 1993;6:46.)

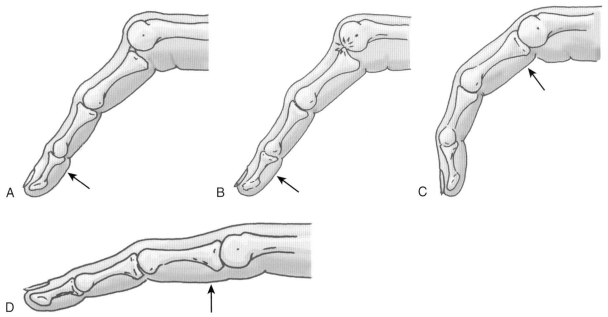

Fig. 85.14 A, When positioning the hand with rheumatoid arthritis with palmar subluxation at the metacarpophalangeal joint, if the proximal phalanx tilts rather than glides into position, it can wear away at the dorsal lip of the proximal phalanx. **B,** This results in an orthosis that actually increases pain and absorption of the joint surface. The orthosis should provide gentle force at the base of the phalanx (**C**) to gently glide the joint into position (**D**). (Redrawn from Brand P. *Clinical Mechanics of the Hand.* St. Louis: Mosby; 1985.)

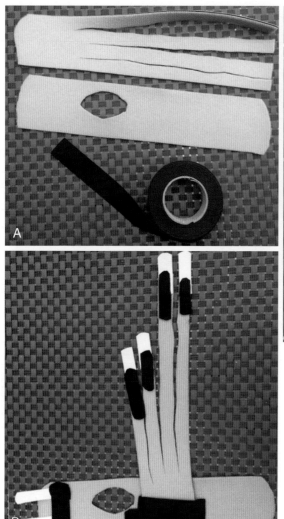

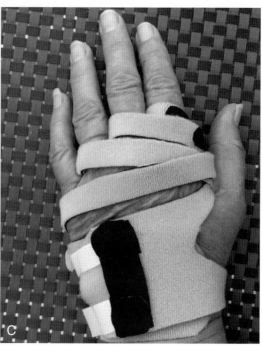

Fig. 85.15 A, A neoprene hand-based metacarpophalangeal joint alignment orthosis can be made from neoprene orthosis strapping. **B,** Velcro is secured with iron on seam tape. **C,** The orthosis allows for proper metacarpophalangeal joint alignment during daily activities.

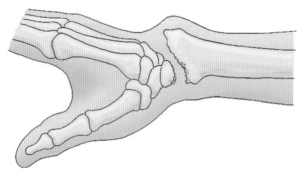

Fig. 85.16 Ligament laxity resulting from chronic synovitis at the wrist, and the natural volar tilt of the radius can result in volar subluxation of the carpus on the radius. (Redrawn with permission from Melvin JL. *Rheumatic Disease: Occupational Therapy and Rehabilitation.* 2nd ed. Philadelphia: FA Davis; 1982.)

nonadhesive wrap such as Coban is recommended to avoid slippage (see Table 85.2). Orthoses applied to DIP joints with OA have been reported to decrease pain.[90,91]

Joint Protection Principles and Adaptive Equipment

Joint protection principles are ideally initiated early in the disease process in an effort to decrease and prevent further stress on the involved joints. Current research indicates strong evidence for the efficacy of joint protection instruction in decreasing pain and promoting ADL performance for the patient with RA and OA.[92–97] A systematic review by the European League Against Rheumatism reported that education concerning joint protection with an exercise regimen is recommended for all patients with hand OA.[97] Instruction in joint protection principles can be facilitated with a stepwise approach that allows an individualized application of the six general joint protection principles to meet the needs of the client.[98] Using the chart included in this chapter (Fig. 85.21), the therapist would introduce the principle such as "respect pain" and then apply under that heading the items that relate to the individual patient. This should be implemented with an educational–behavioral joint protection approach that involves skill practice, goal setting, and home programs. These programs have been found to be more effective than short instruction or information booklets as demonstrated by fewer deformities, less morning stiffness, improved ADL scores, and joint protection technique adherence.[99] In addition, instruction in energy conservation with cognitive-behavioral strategies

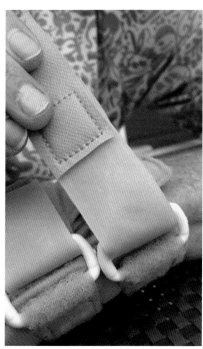

Fig. 85.17 D-rings for Velcro closures can make it easier for the patient with arthritis to don and doff the orthoses.

may decrease pain and fatigue and increase physical activity in patients with RA.[100] Although these programs can be time intensive, a randomized controlled trial of patients with early RA demonstrated that 8-hour instruction in joint protection can decrease pain, morning stiffness, and doctor visits, as well as improve grip strength, self-efficacy, and maintain function, indicating their effectiveness.[101] One systematic review found "gold" level evidence that instruction in joint protection can help people with RA to do daily activities with less pain.[92]

With the thumb, joint protection principles focus on decreasing the amount of force to the CMC joint during pinching activities. The goal is to avoid forces that could sublux the metacarpal from its position on the trapezium. Adaptive equipment that can help to increase leverage and also distribute pressure in the hand includes larger-diameter handle tools, pens, Dycem (or other nonskid materials to increase force), angled knives, book holders, broad key holders, large plastic tabs on medicine bottles, and car door openers.[95] The patient should also be instructed in using a relaxed pinch as opposed to a tight three-jaw chuck pinch when writing. There is moderate evidence to support joint protection education and adaptive equipment for increased hand function and pain reduction in patients with OA.[93] In a 7-year prospective study by Berggren and associates[102] that included joint protection, adaptive equipment, and soft orthoses for the CMC joint, after 7 months, 23 of 33 (70%) did not want an operation to the CMC joint. A joint protection approach for the patient with OA is most effective with a multimodal approach that also includes orthoses, exercise, adaptive equipment, and modalities.[103]

Joint protection principles for patients with MCP joint ulnar deviation from RA include avoiding specific activities that aggravate the deformity.[44,47,98] Examples include activities that place or push the digits into MCP joint ulnar deviation; flexion forces that contribute to palmar subluxation; lateral pinch, which can aggravate ulnar deviation of the index digit; and the pull of gravity with the hands in sustained postures.

In patients demonstrating a swan-neck deformity, joint protection principles should stress avoiding the intrinsic-plus hand grasp during ADL, which may aggravate this deformity (Fig. 85.22). In patients demonstrating a boutonnière deformity, joint protection should include avoiding activities that have prolonged and forceful PIP flexion, such as a tight, three-jaw chuck pinch when writing. Moving objects out of the hand (e.g., using a shoulder-strap tote bag instead of a handled brief case) can be helpful, and plastic grocery bags held by the handle should also be replaced with bags that can be carried closer to the body.

It is important to look at all aspects of the patient when treating symptoms of the arthritic hand. Patients often place strong forces on the hands when lifting themselves from one position to another. In some cases, adaptive equipment can also reduce the effort on the lower extremities (e.g., a lift chair, a shower chair, elevated toilet seat) and may also help to reduce the stress placed on the hands.

In addition, the therapist should take into consideration the patient's sociocultural context. The patient may or may not have insurance coverage or resources for adaptive equipment or orthoses. Options should be carefully discussed with the patient and weighed in terms of cost versus value in meeting specific needs. It has been reported in one study that 91% of the recommended kitchen adaptive equipment continued to be used 12 months later.[104] The therapist should be aware of low- or no-cost resources in the community that may assist patients in obtaining specific adaptive equipment (e.g., grab bars, elevated toilet seats) if the equipment's cost exceeds the patient's available funds. Civic, community, or religious organizations may also offer helpful resources.

Modalities

Thermal agents, such as heat and cold, are commonly used in the treatment of arthritic conditions. There is evidence supporting paraffin baths to decrease pain and stiffness in patient with RA.[105] Superficial heat has also been found to decrease pain in patients with OA.[93] During periods of acute inflammation, when joint temperatures are elevated, heat is contraindicated. Cryotherapy, which lowers joint temperatures, reduces pain, and decreases inflammation, is more applicable during the acute phase. Cold should not be used for patients with Raynaud's phenomenon, which is often seen in cases of RA and SS. In regards to electrical modalities, transcutaneous electrical nerve stimulation has been found to help decrease pain and morning stiffness in patients with RA.[106] Neuromuscular electrical nerve stimulation has been reported to improve hand function when used with the first dorsal interosseous muscle in patients with RA.[107] Ultrasound has been reported in one study to decrease pain, improve wrist extension, and improve the quality of life (using the Health Assessment Questionnaire) in patients with RA.[108] See Chapter 101 for further information on these and other physical agents.

Exercise

General principles of upper extremity exercise include avoiding painful AROM and PROM and the importance of working within the patient's comfort level. Exercise has been found to be effective in decreasing arthritis-related pain, increasing blood flow, and improving cartilage health.[95,109] General AROM exercises for the hand include wrist flexion and extension, gentle digit flexion and extension, and thumb opposition. Shoulder and elbow AROM in the supine position is also beneficial for preventing stiffness. Patients often obtain increased shoulder motion in the supine position as a result of lessening the effects of gravity during the exercise. ROM exercises should be kept pain free to prevent overstretching of joint structures, and the number of repetitions should be controlled to avoid overstressing vulnerable tissues. Hand function was reported to be increased when combining joint protection and pain-free hand home exercises.[110] Generalized conditioning for the patient with

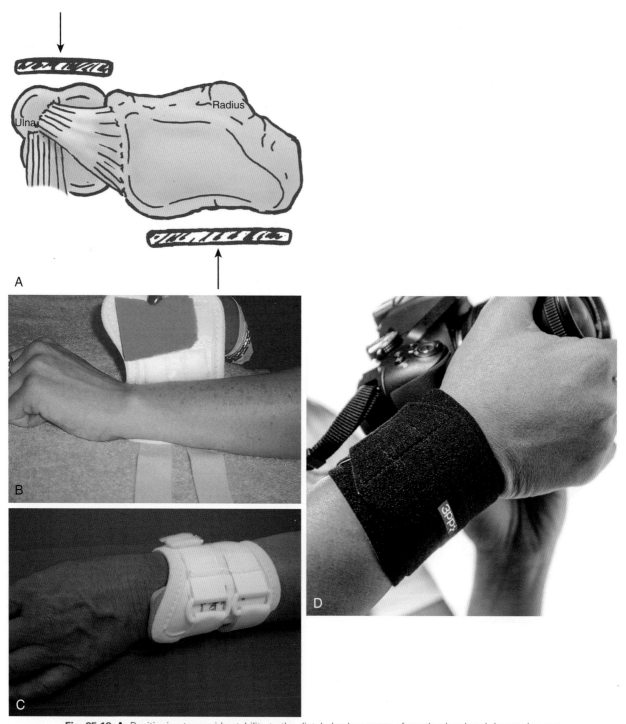

Fig. 85.18 A, Positioning to provide stability to the distal ulna by means of gentle ulnar-head depression can often decrease pain. **B,** The foam insert depresses the distal ulna dorsally and the distal radius volarly. **C,** The orthosis allows wrist motion but supports the distal ulna. **D.** A neoprene option, the 3pp Wrist P.O.P Splint from 3-Point Products. (Part A concept courtesy Judy Leonard, OTR, CHT; redrawn from Melvin JL. *Rheumatic Disease: Occupational Therapy and Rehabilitation.* 2nd ed. Philadelphia: FA Davis. 1982. Part B from Count'R-Force brace from Medical Sports, Arlington, VA. Part D used with permission from 3-Point Products.)

RA has been found to improve stamina and muscle strength.[111] Low-impact general conditioning increased the aerobic capacity and decreased depression and anxiety in patients with arthritis.[112]

More specific guidelines for exercise depend on the involved and vulnerable structures identified during the initial examination. For example, intrinsic tightness can lead to a swan-neck deformity and can be addressed with appropriate intrinsic stretching and lengthening exercises (see Fig. 85.22B). With an unstable distal radioulnar joint and dorsally subluxed ulnar head, repetitive wrist ROM exercises or, even worse, isotonic wrist curls with free weights can lead to fraying and attritional rupture of the finger extensor tendons and must be avoided. With finger flexor tenosynovitis, repetitive finger flexion exercises could exacerbate symptoms. There is moderate evidence to support hand exercises in OA for increasing grip strength, improving function, improving ROM, and pain reduction.[93] The Dynamic Stability approach has been helpful with the treatment of the patient with OA

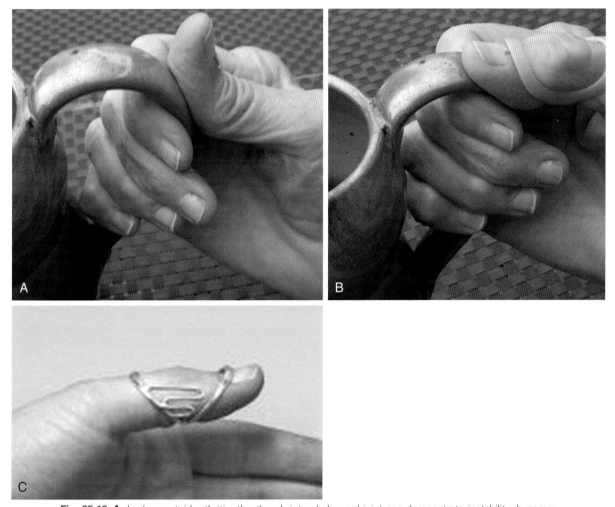

Fig. 85.19 A, In rheumatoid arthritis, the thumb interphalangeal joint can demonstrate instability, hyperextending during functional tasks. **B,** An orthosis (e.g., an Oval-8) can provide stability to the interphalangeal joint during pinch and grasping activities while allowing flexion (3-Point Products, Annapolis, MD). **C,** Custom-sized lateral alignment SIRIS splint gives thumb interphalangeal joint stability and lateral alignment during grasp and pinch activities. (Part C courtesy of the Silver Ring Splint Company, Charlottesville, VA; with permission.)

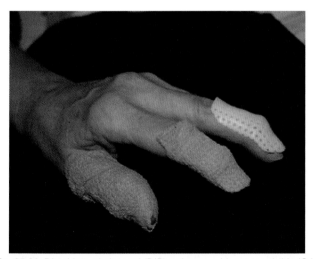

Fig. 85.20 Distal interphalangeal (DIP) orthoses with osteoarthritis (OA). Orthotic positioning can be helpful in decreasing pain during periods of inflammation. Thin, or "light," orthotic material is recommended and applied on the dorsal surface to allow for tactile input on the volar surface for activities. To hold these orthoses in place, a nonadhesive wrap such as Coban is recommended to avoid slippage (see Table 85.3). Orthoses applied to DIP joints with OA have been reported to decrease pain.[90,91]

in decreasing pain and improving CMC joint alignment (see Chapter 88).[113] Strengthening programs for the arthritic hand should be used with caution to avoid aggravation of deformities. For example, with OA and RA, even light putty-pinching exercises impart large forces to an unstable CMC joint and might aggravate a potential deformity.[86] Stability must not be sacrificed for a possible increase in strength. A stable, pain-free thumb provides a post, against which the digits can grip and pinch effectively. Grip strengthening is a common example of an exercise that can aggravate inflamed flexor tendons. A digit that is triggering or locking is not improved with grip-strengthening exercises because strengthening usually increases these symptoms. Therapy exercises should never create deforming forces or cause pain in an arthritic patient. There is moderate evidence to support carefully prescribed resistive hand exercises to improve grip strength in patients with OA. The studies avoided pain and included resistive hand exercises alone,[114] resistive hand exercises with general strengthening,[115] and hand exercises (AROM and resistive) with joint protection.[94,95,116] For the patient with RA, one study, the SARAH (Stretching And strengthening for Rheumatoid Arthritis of the Hand) trial, used carefully prescribed resistive hand exercises that resulted in increased strength, dexterity, and hand function.[117] The exercises were progressed when the patient perceived exertion (based on the Borg scale) was reported as moderate, but not higher than a level 6, and only if pain did not increase.

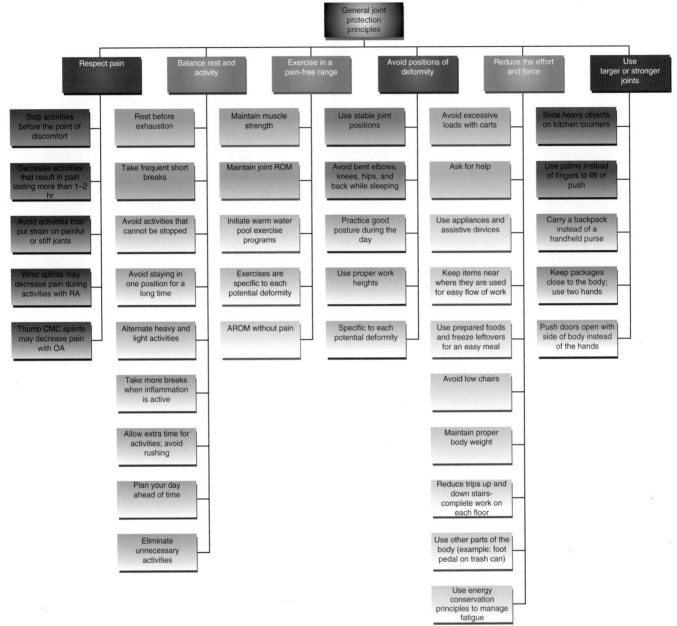

Fig. 85.21 Joint protection principles.[98] Using this chart, the therapist would introduce the principle such as "respect pain" and then apply under that heading the items that relate to the individual patient. This should be implemented with an educational–behavioral joint protection approach that involves skill practice, goal setting, and home programs. These programs have been found to be more effective than short instruction or information booklets as demonstrated by fewer deformities, less morning stiffness, improved activity of daily living scores, and joint protection technique adherence.[99] In addition, instruction in energy conservation with cognitive-behavioral strategies may decrease pain and fatigue and increase physical activity in patients with rheumatoid arthritis.[100] *AROM,* Active range of motion; *CMC,* carpometacarpal; *OA,* osteoarthritis; *RA,* rheumatoid arthritis; *ROM,* range of motion. (From Beasley J. Osteoarthritis and rheumatoid arthritis. *J Hand Ther.* 2012;25:163-172; with permission.)

Community Support

Many patients report benefits from exercise programs performed in a swimming pool. These are good for general conditioning, and they reduce strain on the weight-bearing joints. The temperature of the pool should be comfortably warm to avoid muscle guarding and joint stiffness, which can increase pain. The psychological benefits of social interaction and the informal support group this type of exercise provides should not be underestimated. A study that evaluated

interventions such as disease education, joint protection and energy conservation, psychosocial techniques, and pain management found improvements in coping with pain, managing fatigue, and maintaining a positive effect.[118] In an effort to prevent disability with arthritis, one study found that employed patients with RA can benefit from interventions such as education, self-advocacy, workplace rights and responsibilities, ergonomic reviews, reasonable accommodations, posture advice, pacing, ADLs, stress management, assertiveness, and

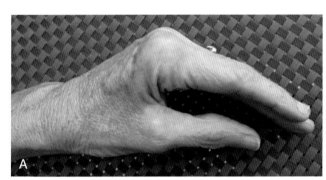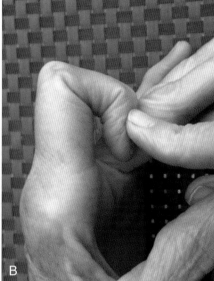

Fig. 85.22 A, Intrinsic-plus finger position. Patients developing a swan-neck deformity should avoid activities that place the digits in an intrinsic-plus position. This can include activities such as holding a book, cards, or a tray. Card holders, bookstands, and carts on wheels can reduce the need for the intrinsic-plus position. **B,** Gentle stretching to prevent intrinsic contractures in patients with early swan-neck deformity.

sleep posture and hygiene.[119] The Arthritis Foundation is a national provider of several community programs and is an excellent resource for patients and health care providers (see www.arthritis.org).

SUMMARY

Conservative management of arthritis requires an understanding of the disease process, specific conditions, potential deformities, and the patient's individual needs. A comprehensive holistic evaluation assists the therapist in appropriate goal setting and treatment planning.

Further research is needed to quantify the benefits that are clinically observed in conservative management.

REFERENCES

1. CDC. Prevalence and most common causes of disability among adults—United States, 2005. *MMWR Morb Mortal Wkly Rep.* 2009;58:421–426.
2. Hammond A, Young A, Kidao R. EULAR recommendations for patient education for people with inflammatory arthritis. *Ann Rheum Dis.* 2004;63:23–30. https://doi.org/10.1136/ard.2002.001511.
3. Hootman JM, Helmick CG, Barbour KE, Theis KA, Boring MA. Updated projected prevalence of self-reported doctor-diagnosed arthritis and arthritis-attributable activity limitation among US adults, 2015-2040. *Arthritis Rheumatol.* 2016;68(7):1582–1587. https://doi.org/10.1002/art.39692.
4. Barbour KE, Helmick CG, Boring M, Brady TJ. Vital signs: prevalence of doctor-diagnosed arthritis and arthritis-attributable activity limitation—United States, 2013-2015. *MMWR Morb Mortal Wkly Rep.* 2017;66:246–253.
5. Combe B, Landewe R, Lukas C, et al. EULAR evidence recommendations for the management of early arthritis. Report of a task force of the European Standing Committee for International Clinical Studies Including Therapeutics. *Ann Rheum Dis.* 2007;66:34–45.
6. Myasoedova E, Crowson CS, Kremers HM, Therneau TM, Gabriel SE. Is the incidence of rheumatoid arthritis rising? Results from Olmsted County, Minnesota, 1955-2007. *Arthritis Rheum.* 2010;62(6):1576–1582. https://doi.org/10.1002/art.27425.
7. Aletaha D, Neogi T, Silman AJ, et al. 2010 Rheumatoid arthritis classification criteria an American College of Rheumatology/European League Against Rheumatism Collaborative Initiative. *Arthritis Rheum.* 2010;62(9):2569–2581. https://doi.org/10.1002/art.27584.
8. Combe B. Progression in early rheumatoid arthritis. Best practice & research. *Clin Rheum.* 2009;23(1):59–69.
9. Eisenstein EM, Berkun Y. Diagnosis and classification of juvenile idiopathic arthritis. *J Autoimun.* 2014;48:31–33.
10. Turner JK, Schlesinger P. Approach to the adolescent with arthritis. In: Imboden JB, Hellman DB, Stone JH, eds. *Rheumatology: Current Diagnosis & Treatment.* 3rd ed. New York: Mc Graw Hill Medical; 2013:36–40.
11. Selvaag AM, Kirkhus E, Tornqvist L, Lilleby V, Aulie HA, Flato B. Radiographic damage in hands and wrists of patients with juvenile idiopathic arthritis after 29 years of disease duration. *Ped Rheum.* 2017;15(1):20. https://doi.org.ezproxy.gvsu.edu/10.1186/s12969-017-0151-7.
12. Giancane G, Pederzoli S, Norambuena X, Ioseliani M, Sato J, Gallo MC, et al. Frequency of radiographic damage and progression in individual joints in children with juvenile idiopathic arthritis. *Arthritis Care Res (Hoboken).* 2014;66:27–33.
13. Mier RJ, Wright FV, Bolding DJ. Juvenile rheumatoid arthritis. In: Melvin JL, Wright FV, eds. *Pediatric Rheumatic Diseases.* Bethesda, MD: The American Occupational Therapy Association; 2000:1–43.
14. Felson DT, Lawrence RC, Dieppe PA, et al. Osteoarthritis: new insights. Part 1: the disease and its risk factors. *Ann Intern Med.* 2000;133(8):635–646.
15. Zhang Y, Jordan JM. Epidemiology of osteoarthritis. *Clin Geriatr Med.* 2010;26:355–369.
16. Lawrence RC, Felson DT, Helmick CG, et al. Estimates of the prevalence of arthritis and other rheumatic conditions in the United States. Part II. National Arthritis Data Workgroup. *Arthritis Rheum.* 2008;58(1):26–35.
17. Zhang Y, Niu J, Kelly-Hayes M, Chaisson CE, Aliabadi P, Felson DT. Prevalence of symptomatic hand osteoarthritis and its impact on functional status among the elderly: the Framingham study. *Am J Epid.* 2002;156(11):1021–1027.
18. Dahaghin S, Bierma-Zeinstra SMA, Ginai AZ, Pols HAP, Hazes JMW, Koes BW. Prevalence and pattern of radiographic hand osteoarthritis and association with pain and disability (the Rotterdam study). *Ann Rheum Dis.* 2005;64(5):682–687. https://doi.org/10.1136/ard.2004.023564.
19. Feelisch M. The chemical biology of nitric oxide — an outsider's reflections about its role in osteoarthritis. *Osteoarthritis Cartilage.* 2008;16(2):S3–S13.
20. Srikanth VK, Fryer JL, Zhai G, Winzenberg TM, Hosmer D, Jones G. A meta-analysis of sex differences prevalence, incidence and severity of osteoarthritis. *Osteo Cart.* 2005;13(9):769–781.

21. Botha-Scheepers S, Riyazi N, Watt I, Rosendaal FR, Slagboom E, Bellamy N, et al. Progression of hand osteoarthritis over 2 years: a clinical and radiological follow up study. *Ann Rheum Dis.* 2009;68(8):1260–1264.

22. Frieri M. Mechanisms of disease for the clinician: systemic lupus erythematosus. *Ann Allergy Asthma Immunol.* 2013;110(4):228–232.

23. Dall'Era M. Systemic lupus erythematosus. In: Imboden JB, Hellman DB, Stone JH, eds. *Rheumatology: Current Diagnosis & Treatment.* 3rd ed. New York: Mc Graw Hill Medical; 2013:187–197.

24. Manzi S. Epidemiology of systemic lupus erythematosus. *Am J Manag Care.* 2001;7:s474–s479.

25. Lai JS, Beaumont JL, Jensen SE, Kaiser K, Van Brunt DL, Kao AH, et al. An evaluation of health-related quality of life in patients with systemic lupus erythematosus using PROMIS and Neuro-QoL. *Clin Rheum.* 2017;36(3):555–562.

26. Herrick AL. Pathogenesis of Raynaud's phenomenon. *Rheum (Ox).* 2005;44(5):587–596.

27. Santiago MB. Jaccoud's arthropathy. *Best Pract & Res Clin Rheum.* 2011;25(5):715–725.

28. Ogdie A, Weiss P. The epidemiology of psoriatic arthritis. *Rheum Dis Clin North Am.* 2015;41:545–568.

29. Wilson FC, Icen M, Crowson CS, McEvoy MT, Gabriel SE, Kremers HM. Time trends in epidemiology and characteristics of psoriatic arthritis over 3 decades: a population-based study. *J Rheumatol.* 2009;36(2):361–367.

30. Rachakonda TD, Schupp CW, Armstrong AW. Psoriasis prevalence among adults in the United States. *J Am Acad Dermatol.* 2014;70(3): 512–516.

31. Scarpa R, Cuocolo A, Peluso R, et al. Early psoriatic arthritis: the clinical spectrum. *J Rheumatol.* 2008;35(1):137–141.

32. Dalbeth N, Pui K, Lobo M, et al. Nail disease in psoriatic arthritis: distal phalangeal bone edema detected by magnetic resonance imaging predicts development of onycholysis and hyperkeratosis. *J Rheumatol.* 2012;39(4):841–843.

33. van den Hoogen F, Khanna D, Fransen J, Johnson SR, Baron M, Tyndall A, et al. 2013 classification criteria for systemic sclerosis: an American College of Rheumatology/European League Against Rheumatism collaborative initiative. *Ann Rheum Dis.* 2013;72:1747–1755. https://doi.org/10.1136/annrheumdis-2013-204424.

34. Mayes MD, Lacey Jr JV, Beebe-Dimmer J, et al. Prevalence, incidence, survival, and disease characteristics of systemic sclerosis in a large US population. *Arthritis Rheum.* 2003;48:2246–2255.

35. Mayes MD. Scleroderma epidemiology. *Rheum Dis Clin North Am.* 2003;29:239–254.

36. Boin F, Wigley F. Systemic sclerosis. In: Bartlett SJ, ed. *Clinical Care of the Rheumatic Diseases.* 3rd ed. Atlanta: Association of Rheumatology Health Professionals; 2006:193–198.

37. Park JS, Park MC, Song JJ, Park YB, Lee SK, Lee SW. Application of the 2013 ACR/EULAR classification criteria for systemic sclerosis to patients with Raynaud's phenomenon. *Arthritis Res Ther.* 2015;17(1):77. https://doi.org/10.1186/s13075-015-0594-5.

38. Swanson A. Disabling arthritis at the base of the thumb: treatment by resection of the trapezium and flexible (silicon) implant arthroplasty. *J Bone Joint Surg.* 1972;54A:456–471.

39. Anderson RJ. Rheumatoid arthritis: clinical and laboratory features. In: Klippel JH, Weyand CM, Wortmann RL, eds. *Primer on Rheumatic Diseases.* 11th ed. Atlanta: Arthritis Foundation; 1997:218–225.

40. Berenbaum F. Osteoarthritis A. Epidemiology, pathology, and pathogenesis. In: Kippel JH, Crofford LJ, Stone JH, Weyand CM, eds. *Primer on the Rheumatic Diseases.* 12th ed. Atlanta: Arthritis Foundation; 2001:285–288.

41. Farrar JT, Young JP, LaMoreaux L, Werth JL, Poole RM. Clinical importance of changes in chronic pain intensity measured on an 11-point numerical pain rating scale. *Pain.* 2001;94:149–158.

42. Grilo RM, Treves R, Preux PM. Clinically relevant VAS pain score change in patients with acute rheumatic conditions. *Joint Bone Spine.* 2007;74(4):358–361. https://doi.org/10.1016/j.jbspin.2006.06.019.

43. Hasselkus BR, Kshepakaran KK, Houge JC, Plautz KA. Rheumatoid arthritis: a two-axis goniometer to measure metacarpophalangeal laxity. *Arch Phys Med Rehabil.* 1981;62:137–139.

44. Siverman S, Wolfe T. Rheumatoid arthritis. In: Melvin JL, Ferrel KM, eds. *Adult Rheumatic Disease.* Bethesda MD: The American Occupational Therapy Association; 2000;(2):259–278.

45. Brooks P. Extensor mechanism ruptures. *Ortho.* 2009;32(9):683–684.

46. Vaughan-Jackson OJ. Rupture of extensor tendons by attrition at the inferior radio-ulnar joint. Report of two cases. *J Bone Joint Surg Br.* 1948;30B(3):528–530.

47. Philips CA. The management of patients with rheumatoid arthritis. In: Hunter JM, Schneider LH, Mackin EJ, Callahan AD, eds. *Rehabilitation of the Hand: Surgery and Therapy.* 3rd ed. Philadelphia: CV Mosby; 1990:903–907.

48. Swanson AB, Swanson GG, Winfield DL. The pronated index finger deformity in the rheumatoid hand. *Bull Hosp Jt Dis Orthop Inst.* 1984;44(2):498–510. Fall.

49. Melvin JL, LeRoy EC, Elrod CS. Systemic sclerosis. In: Melvin JL, Ferrel KM, eds. *Adult Rheumatic Diseases.* Bethesda, MD: The American Occupational Therapy Association; 2000:259–278. 2.

50. Juul-Kristensen B, Røgind H, Jensen DV, Remvig L. Inter-examiner reproducibility of tests and criteria for generalized joint hypermobility and benign joint hypermobility syndrome. *Rheumatol (Ox).* 2007;46(12):1835–1841. https://doi.org/10.1093/rheumatology/kem290.

51. Shiratori AP, da Rosa lop R, Junior NGB, Domenech SC, Gevaerd MdS. Evaluation protocols of hand grip strength in individuals with rheumatoid arthritis: a systematic review. *Revista Brasil de Reumatol (Eng Ed).* 2014;54(2):140–147.

52. Roberts HC, Denison HJ, Martin HJ, Patel HP, Syddall H, Cooper C, et al. A review of the measurement of grip strength in clinical and epidemiological studies: towards a standardized approach. *Age Ageing.* 2011;40:423–429.

53. Agnew PJ. Jamar dynamometer and adapted sphygmomanometer for measuring grip strength in patients with rheumatoid arthritis. *Occup Ther J Res.* 1991;11(5):259–270.

54. Backman C, Mackie H, Harris J. Arthritis hand function test: development of a standardized assessment tool. *Occup Ther J Res.* 1991;11:246–256.

55. Stein MJ, Wallston KA, Nicassio PM, Castner CM. Correlates of a clinical classification schema for the arthritis helplessness subscale. *Arthritis Rheum.* 1988;31:876–881.

56. Meenan RF, Mason JH, Anderson JJ, Guccione AA, Kazis LE. AIMS2: the content and properties of a revised and expanded Arthritis Impact Measurement Scales health status questionnaire. *Arthritis Rheum.* 1992;35:1–10.

57. Liang MH, Fossel AH, Larson MG. Comparisons of five health status instruments for orthopaedic evaluation. *Med Care.* 1990;28:632–642.

58. Brady TJ. Measures of self-efficacy, helplessness, mastery, and control. *Arthritis Rheum.* 2003;49(5S):S147–S164. https://doi.org/10.1002/art.11413B.

59. Bellamy N, Campbell J, Haraoui B, Buchbinder R, Hobby K, Roth JH, MacDermid JC. Dimensionality and clinical importance of pain and disability in hand osteoarthritis: development of the Australian/Canadian (AUSCAN) Osteoarthritis Hand Index. *Osteoarthritis Cartilage.* 2002;10(11):855–862.

60. Allen KD, Jordan JM, Renner JB, Kraus VB. Validity, factor structure, and clinical relevance of the AUSCAN Osteoarthritis Hand Index. *Arthritis Rheum.* 2006;54:551–556.

61. Duruoz MT, Poiraudeau S, Fermanian J, Menkes C, Amor B, Dougados M, et al. Development and validation of a rheumatoid hand functional disability scale that Poole JL. Measures of Hand Function. *Arthr Care & Res.* 2011;63(S11):S189–S199. https://doi.org/10.1002/acr.2063.

62. Poiraudeau S, Chevalier X, Conrozier T, Flippo RM, Liote F, Lefevre-Colau MM, et al. Reliability, validity, and sensitivity to change of the Cochin Hand Functional Disability Scale in hand osteoarthritis. *Osteo Cart.* 2001;9:570–577.

63. Law M, Baptiste S, Carswell S, McColl M, Polatajko H, Pol-lock N. *Canadian Occupational Performance Measure.* 3rd ed. Ottawa: CAOT; 1998.

64. Fries J, Spitz P, Kraines R, Holman H. Measurement of patient outcome in arthritis. *Arthritis Rheum.* 1980;23:137–145.

65. Goekoop-Ruiterman YP, de Vries-Bouwstra JK, Allaart CF, van Zeben D, Kerstens PJ, Hazes JM, et al. Clinical and radio-graphic outcomes

of four different treatment strategies in patients with early rheumatoid arthritis (the BeSt study): a randomized, controlled trial. *Arthritis Rheum.* 2005;52:338–339.

66. Burckhardt CS. The use of the McGill Pain Questionnaire in assessing arthritis pain. *Pain.* 1984;19(3):305–314.

67. Chung KC, Pillsbury MS, Walers MR, Hayward RA. Reliability and validity testing of the Michigan Hand Outcomes Questionnaire. *J Hand Surg.* 1998;23A:575–587.

68. Shauver MJ, Chung KC. The minimal clinically important difference of the Michigan Hand Questionnaire. *J Hand Surg.* 2009;34A:509–514.

69. Hefford C, Abbott JH, Arnold R, Baxter GD. The patient-specific functional scale: validity, reliability, and responsiveness in patients with upper extremity musculoskeletal problems. *J Orthop Sports Phys Ther.* 2012;42(2):56–65.

70. Hudak P, Amadio PC, Bombardier C. Upper extremity collaborative group development of an upper extremity outcome measure: the DASH (Disabilities of the Arm, Shoulder, and Hand). *Amer J Ind Med.* 1996;29:602–608.

71. Polson KD, ReidD, McNair PJ, Larmer P. Responsiveness, minimal importance difference and minimal detectable change scores of the shortened disability arm shoulder hand (QuickDASH) questionnaire. *Man Ther.* 2010;15(4):404–407.

72. Lillegraven S, Kvien TK. Measuring disability and quality of life in established rheumatoid arthritis. *Best Pract Res Clin Rheumatol.* 2007;21:827–840.

73. Deyo RA, Inui TS. Toward clinical applications of health status measures: sensitivity of scales to clinically important changes. *Health Serv Res.* 1984;19:275–289.

74. Greenwood MC, Doyle DV, Ensor M. Does the Stanford Health Assessment Questionnaire have potential as a monitoring tool for subjects with rheumatoid arthritis? *Ann Rheum Dis.* 2001;60:344–348.

75. Hawley D, Wolfe F. Sensitivity to change of the Health Assessment Questionnaire (HAQ) and other clinical and health status measures in rheumatoid arthritis. *Arthritis Care Res.* 1992;5:130–136.

76. Deighton C, O'Mahony R, Tosh J, Turner C, Rudolf M. Management of rheumatoid arthritis: summary of NICE guidance. *BMJ.* 2009;338:b702.

77. Kjeken I, Smedslund G, Moe RH, Slatkowsky-Christensen B, Uhlig T, Hagen KB. Systematic review of design and effects of splints and exercise programs in hand osteoarthritis. *Arthritis Care Res.* 2011;63:834–848. https://doi.org/10.1002/acr.20427.

78. Spicka C, Macleod C, Adams J, Metcalf C. Effect of silver ring splint on hand dexterity and grip strength in patients with rheumatoid arthritis: an observational pilot study. *Hand Ther.* 2009;14(2):53–57.

79. Tar Schegget M, Knipping A. A study comparing use and effects of custom-made versus prefabricated splints for swan neck deformity in patients with rheumatoid arthritis. *Brit J Hand Ther.* 2000;5(4):101–107.

80. Swezey RL, Spiegel TM, Cretin S, Clements P. Arthritic hand response to pressure gradient gloves. *Arch Phys Med Rehabil.* 1979;60(8):375–377.

81. Pagnotta A, Korner-Bitensky N, Mazer G, et al. Static wrist splint use in the performance of daily activities by individuals with rheumatoid arthritis. *J Rheumatol.* 2005;32:36–43.

82. Swanson AB. Pathomechanics of deformities in hand and wrist. In: Hunter JM, et al., ed. *Rehabilitation of the Hand: Surgery and Therapy.* 3rd ed. Philadelphia: Mosby; 1990:891–902.

83. Palchik NS, Mitchell DM, Gilbert NL, Schulz AJ, Dedrick RF, Palella TD. Nonsurgical management of the boutonniere deformity. *Arthritis Care Res.* 1990;3(4):227–232.

84. Boozer JA. Splinting the arthritic hand. *J Hand Ther.* 1993;6:46–48.

85. Flatt A. *Care of the Arthritic Hand.* 4th ed. St. Louis: Mosby; 1983.

86. Brand P. *Clinical Mechanics of the Hand.* St. Louis: Mosby; 1985.

87. Egan M, Brosseau L, Farmer M, Ouimet MA, Rees S, Tugwell P, et al. Splints and Orthosis for treating rheumatoid arthritis. *Cochrane Data Syst Rev.* 2001;4:Art. No. CD004018. https://doi.org/10.1002/14651858.CD004018.

88. Colditz JC. Arthritis. In: Pittsburgh, Malick MH, Kasch MC, eds. *Manual on Management of Specific Hand Problems.* AREN Publications; 1984:111–136.

89. Callinan NJ, Mathiowetz V. Soft versus hard resting hand splints in RA: pain relief preference and compliance. *Am J Occup Ther.* 1996;50:347–353.

90. Ikeda M, Ishii T, Kobayashi Y, Mochida J, Saito I, Oka Y. Custom-made splint treatment for osteoarthritis of the distal interphalangeal joints. *J Hand Surg.* 2010;35(4):589–593.

91. Watt F, Kennedy D, Carlisle K, et al. Night-time immobilization of the distal interphalangeal joint reduces pain and extension deformity in hand osteoarthritis. *Rheum.* 2014;53(6):1142–1149. https://doi.org/10.1093/rheumatology/ket455.

92. Steultjens EEMJ, Dekker JJ, Bouter LM, Schaardenburg DD, Kuyk MAMAH, Van den Ende ECHM. Occupational therapy for rheumatoid arthritis. *Cochrane Data Syst Rev.* 2004;1. https://doi.org/10.1002/14651858.CD003114.pub2.

93. Valdes K, Marik T. A systemic review of conservative interventions for osteoarthritis of the hand. *J Hand Ther.* 2010;23(4):334–349.

94. Dziedzic K, Nicholls E, Hammond A, Handy J, Thomas E, Hay E. Self-management approaches for osteoarthritis in the hand: A 2x2 factorial randomized trial. *Ann Rheum Dis.* 2013;74(1):108–118.

95. Stamm T, Machold K, Smolen J, et al. Joint protection and home hand exercises improve hand function in patients with hand osteoarthritis: a randomized controlled trial. *Arthritis Rheum.* 2002;47(1):44–49.

96. Christie A, Jamtvedt G, Thuve Dahm K, Moe RH, Haavardsholm EA, Birger Hagen K. Effect of nonpharmacological and nonsurgical interventions for patients with rheumatoid arthritis: an overview of systematic reviews. *Phys Ther.* 2007;87(12):1697–1715.

97. Zhang W, Doherty M, Leeb BF, et al. EULAR evidence based recommendations for the management of hand osteoarthritis: Report of a Task Force of the EULAR Standing Committee for International Clinical Studies Including Therapeutics (ESCISIT). *Ann Rheum Dis.* 2007;66(3):377–388. https://doi.org/10.1136/ard.2006.062091.

98. Beasley J. Osteoarthritis and rheumatoid arthritis. *J Hand Ther.* 2012;25:163–172.

99. Hammond A, Young A, Kidao R. A randomized controlled trial of occupational therapy for people with early rheumatoid arthritis. *Ann Rheum Dis.* 2004;63:23.

100. Furst GP, Gerber LH, Smith CC, Fisher S. A program for improving energy conservation behaviors in adults with rheumatoid arthritis. *Am J Occup Therapy.* 1987;41(2):102–111.

101. Wessel J. The effectiveness of hand exercises for persons with rheumatoid arthritis: a systematic review. *J Hand Ther.* 2004;17(2):174–180.

102. Berggren M, Joost-Davidsson A, Lindstrand J, et al. Reduction in the need for operation after conservative treatment of osteoarthritis of the first carpometacarpal joint: a seven-year prospective study. *Scand J Plast Reconstr Surg Hand Surg.* 2001;35:415–417.

103. Aebischer B, Elsig S, Taeymans J. Effectiveness of physical an occupational therapy on pain, function and quality of life in patients with trapeziometacarpal osteoarthritis: a systematic review and meta-analysis. *Hand Ther.* 2016;21(1):5–15.

104. Nordenskiöld U. Daily activities in women with rheumatoid arthritis. Aspects of patient education, assistive devices and methods for disability and impairment assessment. *Scand J Rehabil Med Suppl.* 1997;37:1.

105. Welch V, Brosseau L, Casimiro L, Judd M, Shea B, Tugwell P, et al. Thermotherapy for treating rheumatoid arthritis. *Cochrane Database Syst Rev.* 2002;2:CD002826. https://doi.org/10.1002/14651858.CD002826.

106. Brosseau L, Yonge KA, Welch V, Marchand S, Judd M, Wells GA, Tugwell P. Transcutaneous electrical nerve stimulation (TENS) for the treatment of rheumatoid arthritis in the hand. *Cochrane Database Syst Rev.* 2003;2. https://doi.org/10.1002/14651858.CD004377.

107. Oldman JA, Stanley JK. Rehabilitation of atrophied muscle in the rheumatoid arthritic hand: a comparison of two methods of electrical stimulation. *J Hand Surg (Eur).* 1989;14(3):294–297.

108. Király M, Varga Z, Szanyó F, Kiss R, Hodosi K, Bender T. Effects of underwater ultrasound therapy on pain, inflammation, hand function and quality of life in patients with rheumatoid arthritis – a randomized controlled trial. *Brazil J Phys Ther.* 2017;21(3):199–205. https://doi.org/10.1016/j.bjpt.2017.04.002.

109. Westby MD, Minor MM. Exercise and physical activity. In: Bartlett SJ, ed. *Clinical Care of the Rheumatic Diseases.* 3rd ed. Atlanta: Association of Rheumatology Health Professionals; 2006:211–220.

110. Boustedt C, Nordenskiöld U, Lundgren Nilsson A. Effects of a protection programme with an addition of splinting and exercise: one year follow-up. *Clin Rheumatol.* 2009;28(7):793–799. Epub 2009 Mar 18.

111. Hurkmans E, van der Giesen FJ, Vliet Vlieland TPM, Schoones J, Van den Ende ECHM. Dynamic exercise programs (aerobic capacity and/or muscle strength training) in patients with rheumatoid arthritis. *Cochrane Database Syst Rev.* 2009;4:Art. No. CD006853. https://doi.org/10.1002/14651858.CD006853.pub2.

112. Minor MA, Hewett JE, Webel RR, Anderson SK, Kay DR. Efficacy of physical conditioning exercise in patients with rheumatoid arthritis and osteoarthritis. *Arthritis Rheum.* 1989;32:1396–1405.

113. O'Brien VH, Russell Giveanu M. Effects of a dynamic stability approach in conservative intervention of the carpometacarpal joint of the thumb: a retrospective study. *J Hand Ther.* 2013;26:44–52.

114. Lefler C, Armstrong W. Exercise in the treatment of osteoarthritis in the hands of the elderly. *Clin Kinesiology: J American Kinesiotherapy Association.* 2004;58(2):13–17.

115. Rogers M, Wilder F. The effects of strength training among persons with hand osteoarthritis: a two-year follow-up study. *J Hand Ther.* 2007;20(3):244–250. https://doi.org/10.1197/j.jht.2007.04.005.

116. Hennig T, Hæhre L, Hornburg V, Mowinckel P, Norli E, Kjeken I. Effect of home-based hand exercises in women with hand osteoarthritis: a randomised controlled trial. *Ann Rheum Dis.* 2015;74(8):1501–1508. https://doi.org/10.1136/annrheumdis-2013-204808.

117. Heine PJ, Williams MA, Williamson E, Bridle C, Adams J, O'Brien, et al. Development and delivery of an exercise intervention for rheumatoid arthritis: Strengthening and stretching for rheumatoid arthritis of the hand (SARAH) trial. *Physiotherapy.* 2012:121–130.

118. Carandang K, Pyatak EA, Cheryl LP, Vigen CLP. Systematic review of educational interventions for rheumatoid arthritis. *Am J Occup Ther.* 2016;70(6):7006290020p1- 7006290020p12. https://doi.org/10.5014/ajot.2016.021386.

119. Macedo AM, Oakley SP, Panayi GS, Kirkham BW. Functional and work outcomes improve in patients with rheumatoid arthritis who receive targeted, comprehensive occupational therapy. *Arthritis Rheum.* 2009;61(11):1522–1530.

86

Surgery and Therapy for the Rheumatoid Hand and Wrist

Abdo Bachoura, Katie Pisano, Terri Wolfe, John D. Lubahn

OUTLINE

CRITICAL POINTS

- The goals of management are joint stability, pain-relief, and improved function rather than improved range of motion.
- Surgeon–therapist–patient cooperation is essential for successful outcomes.
- Meticulous surgical technique and therapy are both necessary.
- In the patient with rheumatoid arthritis, tendon ruptures are relatively common in the hand and wrist. Tendon transfer is most often the treatment of choice for tendon ruptures in the rheumatoid hand.
- Motion preserving wrist and small joint arthroplasty are preferred for end stage arthritis; however, arthrodesis remains a reasonable option in many patients.

INTRODUCTION

Surgery of the hand in patients with rheumatoid arthritis (RA) has changed dramatically since the first edition of *Rehabilitation of the Hand and Upper Extremity* was published in 1978. The introduction of disease-modifying antirheumatic drugs (DMARDs) and biologic medications has been extremely effective in minimizing and in some cases completely eliminating the disease in the musculoskeletal system, including, of course, the hand and upper extremity.[1,2] With diarthrodial (synovial lined) joints being spared the ravages of the disease, surgical indications, and resultant pathology have changed as well. Occasionally, one or two joints in the upper extremity will still be affected by RA despite otherwise effective medical therapy. Occasionally, joints will be affected before initiation of medical therapy. Some patients are unable to tolerate DMARDs or biologics and present to hand surgeons with complaints and findings similar to those in patients before DMARD therapy (Fig. 86.1). Other patients are not eligible for DMARDs or biologic medication treatment because of a lack of insurance coverage, or, in some patients, the disease goes undiagnosed and untreated until they present to a hand surgeon.

Principles of Treatment

A complete history and physical examination should be performed and all medications and other systemic effects of the disease noted. When symptoms of potential instability are noted in the cervical spine, a thorough neurologic examination and radiographs of the cervical spine (anteroposterior, flexion–extension lateral, and two oblique) should be performed. The combination of physical findings such as clonus and radiographic findings of instability should prompt a referral to a spine surgeon.[3] Patients with RA should be screened for cardiovascular, pulmonary, hematologic, hepatic, and other gastrointestinal conditions.

The history and examination should also address the lower extremity. If hip or knee replacement is required or surgery on the foot or ankle, this should precede surgery on the upper extremity to avoid weight bearing on a delicate upper extremity procedure. Because rehabilitation after many rheumatoid hand procedures requires prolonged therapy and orthotic positioning, pertinent social data (e.g., support at home for meal preparation and self-care postoperatively) and individual support systems are all important to consider during the preoperative evaluation.

A complete upper extremity exam should include range of motion (ROM) of the shoulder and elbow with evaluation of muscular strength. Wrist and hand function should receive similar attention with a focus on intrinsic muscle function and tightness commonly seen in association with ulnar deviation of the metacarpophalangeal (MCP) joint and ulnar subluxation of the dorsal apparatus at the MCP joint level. A description of the effects of the disease process on the upper extremity should be included, with special note of the presence of any deformities and joint contractures. A thorough neurosensory examination is critical because patients with RA are prone to carpal tunnel syndrome (CTS) from proliferative synovium causing pressure on the median nerve in the carpal tunnel. Referral for preoperative assessment by an occupational or physical therapist may be beneficial to determine patient goals and activity of daily living (ADL) needs postoperatively.

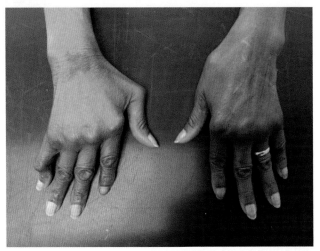

Fig. 86.1 A 70-year old woman with untreated rheumatoid arthritis. The right hand appears to be more severely affected and reveals multiple deformities, including swollen and prominent metacarpophalangeal joints, ulnar drift, and boutonnière deformities of the right small finger and thumb.

Hand surgeons should be aware of the various families of medications used in RA such as nonsteroidal antiinflammatory drugs (NSAIDs), corticosteroids, DMARDs (e.g., methotrexate, sulfasalazine), and biologics (e.g., tumor necrosis factor–α [TNF-α] inhibitors) (Table 86.1).[4] Some medications may have to be discontinued perioperatively to minimize the risk of infection and delayed wound healing.[5] On the other hand, stopping and restarting some RA medications may predispose patients to flare reactions. The latter may delay rehabilitation and negatively influence outcomes. These decisions should be made in collaboration with the patient's rheumatologist. In general, continuation of NSAIDs, methotrexate, and low-dose steroids is considered safe, whereas biologics such as TNF-α inhibitors and interleukin-1 receptor antagonists are stopped 3 to 5 half-lives before surgery and restarted approximately 2 weeks postoperatively or when the wound has healed (see Table 86.1).[4,5]

THE WRIST

Disease activity at the level of wrist may lead to various manifestations dictated by the severity of the autoimmune process and the tissue involved. RA leads to formation of a destructive synovial pannus.

TABLE 86.1	Perioperative Recommendations for Rheumatoid Medications			
Name	**Trade Name**	**Mechanism of Action**	**Half-Life**	**Perioperative Management**
NSAIDs				
Ibuprofen	Advil, Motrin	Nonselective COX inhibitor	2 hr	Continue if bleeding risk low
Naproxen	Aleve, Naprosyn	Nonselective COX inhibitor	12–24 hr	Continue if bleeding risk low
Celecoxib	Celebrex	Selective COX-2 inhibitor	11 hr	Continue
DMARDs				
Methotrexate	Rheumatrex, Trexall	Inhibits dihydrofolate reductase	3–15 hr	Continue
Sulfasalazine	Azulfidine	Suppression of IL-1, TNF-α, triggers apoptosis of inflammatory cells	5–10 hr	Insufficient data
Azathioprine	Azasan, Imuran	Purine synthesis inhibitor	3 hr	Insufficient data
Cyclophosphamide	Cytoxan	DNA crosslinking and cell death	3–12 hr	Insufficient data
Cyclosporine	Gengraf, Neoral, Sandimmune, Sangcya	Calcineurin inhibitor	~24 hr	Discontinue ~3–4 half-lives before surgery; continue after wounds healed
Hydroxychloroquine	Plaquenil, Quineprox	Suppression of interleukin-1, TNF-α, triggers apoptosis of inflammatory cells	1–2 mo	Discontinue ~3–4 half-lives before surgery; continue after wounds healed
Penicillamine	Cuprimine, Depen	Decreases rheumatoid factor levels, inhibits T cells	1 hr	Discontinue ~3–4 half-lives before surgery; continue after wounds healed
Leflunomide	Arava	Pyrimidine synthesis inhibitor	2 wk	Insufficient data
Biologic Agents				
Infliximab	Remicade	TNF-α inhibitor	10 days	Insufficient data
Etanercept	Enbrel	TNF-α inhibitor	4.3 days	Insufficient data
Adalimumab	Humira	TNF-α inhibitor	10–20 days	Insufficient data
Glucocorticoids				
Hydrocortisone	Solu-Cortef	Upregulates genes that inhibit inflammation	8 hr	Continue
Prednisone	Deltacortril, Hostacortin, Wysolone	Upregulates genes that inhibit inflammation	18–36 hr	Continue
Methylprednisolone	Solu-Medrol	Upregulates genes that inhibit inflammation	18–40 hr	Continue
Dexamethasone	Decadron	Upregulates genes that inhibit inflammation	36–54 hr	Continue

COX, Cyclooxygenase; *DMARD*, disease-modifying antirheumatic drug; *IL-1*, interleukin-1; *NSAID*, nonsteroidal antiinflammatory drug; *TNF*, tumor necrosis factor.
Data from Thorsness RJ, Hammert WC. Perioperative management of rheumatoid medications. *J Hand Surg Am.* 2012;37:1928-1931.

Synovium is found in all diarthrodial joints. It also lines the flexor tendons, deep volar carpal ligament, annular pulley system, extensor tendons, and extensor retinaculum. Synovial inflammation and hypertrophy often result in pain, swelling, flexor or extensor tendon ruptures, tendon imbalances, and CTS. Involvement of the articular surfaces of the wrist may present as radiocarpal disease with radial deviation of the radiocarpal joint and relative sparing of the midcarpal joint until later stages of the disease. The distal radioulnar (DRU) joint is also frequently involved and may be symptomatic because of articular destruction or instability and its sequela.

Wrist Synovitis

Removal of diseased synovium is performed in most procedures that involve the rheumatoid hand and wrist. Synovectomy decreases disease burden and removes the source of inflammation. Traditionally, early surgical intervention has been advocated to limit attritional extensor tendon rupture and articular destruction. Hsueh and associates[6] found that disease duration for more than 8 years and persistent tenosynovitis for more than 1 year were associated with spontaneous extensor tendon rupture in the rheumatoid wrist. Open synovectomy through a dorsal wrist approach is preferred when concomitant extensor tendon transfers, distal ulna procedures, limited wrist arthrodesis, total wrist arthrodesis, or total wrist arthroplasty (TWA) are performed.[7] Although isolated synovectomy has narrow indications in the hand, especially since the introduction of DMARDs and biologics, wrist synovectomy may be indicated for joints that have been refractory to medical management for more than 6 months and do not have evidence of substantial joint destruction.[8,9] Arthroscopic synovectomy has recently been advocated because it may provide pain relief and functional improvements while allowing for earlier rehabilitation because of its less invasive nature.[8,9]

Tendon Rupture

Tendon rupture in patients with RA is relatively common, particularly in uncontrolled, advanced disease. Three theories have been proposed to explain the pathophysiology of tendon rupture:

1. Proliferative tenosynovitis on the dorsal or volar surfaces of the hand grows into the substance of the tendon tissue, destroying it locally with proteolytic enzymes, such as collagenase, to the extent that the tendon weakens and eventually ruptures.
2. The tendon is mechanically abraded by rough bone or a sharp spike of bone.
3. Tendon rupture occurs secondary to ischemia of the tendon.

Tendon rupture occurs insidiously and is rarely associated with pain. Initially, the patient may note inability to extend the small finger or perhaps the small and ring fingers. When rupture is at the DRU joint (Vaughn-Jackson syndrome),[10] the diagnosis may be difficult because the extensor tendons at the level of the MCP joint may have subluxed ulnarward secondary to attenuation of the sagittal fibers on the radial side of the dorsal apparatus of the extensor mechanism between the central tendon and the palmar plate.

Direct tendon repair is rarely possible because of frequent delays in treatment and the condition of the tendon after rupture. Tendon transfer therefore becomes the treatment of choice, and the general principles of tendon transfer are applicable to patients with RA. The disease should be well controlled medically, and the soft tissues through which the tendon transfer must pass should be relatively free of disease. Perivascular inflammation, boggy synovium, and intrinsic muscle contractures are all relative contraindications to tendon transfer in the hand, as are skin ulceration or attenuation caused by vasculitis or chronic glucocorticoid and other immunosuppressive therapy. Tendon transfers to restore finger extension and flexion or to increase thumb mobility

may significantly improve function. Moreover, tendon transfers may improve the appearance of the hand and yield a high degree of patient satisfaction. Although tendon transfer may prove more palliative than curative, the opportunity to improve function in a patient with RA is not an opportunity to be squandered, and patients with successful outcomes are often satisfied.

FINGER EXTENSOR TENDON RUPTURES

One of the most common sites of extensor tendon rupture occurs at the DRU joint. Since the classic *Journal of Bone and Joint Surgery* article in 1948, this condition has been referred to as *caput ulnae* or *Vaughan-Jackson syndrome*.[10] Traditional teaching is that tendon rupture is the result of excursion over an osteophyte on the joint, but with rupture of the DRU joint capsule, the tendons are exposed directly to synovial fluid containing collagenase and other proteolytic enzymes, which may also play a role in tendon rupture. Sudden loss of extension of the long, ring, and small fingers or any combination of thumb and index fingers usually requires relatively prompt treatment. The tenodesis test is useful to rule out posterior interosseous nerve palsy, which may occur secondary to radiohumeral arthritis and synovitis. Occasionally, patients may compensate for loss of one or two finger extensors; however, loss of extension of more than one or two digits can cause significant functional disability. Chung and coworkers[11] reported that the duration of untreated rupture correlates with the MCP joint extension lag after reconstructive surgery ($R^2 = 0.233$; $P <.001$), and patient satisfaction negatively correlated with MCP joint extension lag ($R^2 = 0.384$; $P <.001$). Furthermore, patients who had surgery to one or two fingers had less extensor lag and higher satisfaction scores than those with surgery to three fingers. Therefore, early treatment is recommended after a digital extensor tendon rupture has been identified.[11]

Lack of extension of the MCP joint of the small finger may indicate complete rupture of the extensor digitorum communis (EDC) or extensor digiti quinti (EDQ). The EDQ commonly has two slips; sometimes only one may rupture, preserving function. Transfer is usually end to side, weaving the distal stump of the EDQ through the adjacent common extensor of the ring finger. Both tendon grafting and tendon transfer are reliable reconstruction methods for ruptured finger extensor tendons.[11]

Ruptures of the ring and small finger extensors may occasionally occur together. Under these circumstances, successful transfer of the distal stump of the small finger to the adjacent ring finger and suture of the ring finger to the long finger may result in excess abduction of the ring and small fingers, particularly the small finger. Furthermore, adequate force may not be exerted through this double side-to-side transfer to allow sufficient extension of the small finger and may exert more of an ulnar deviation force instead. Therefore, tendon transfer of the extensor indicis proprius (EIP) to the EDQ, EDC, or both is preferable if the EIP is available. The EIP may be used to motor both the ring and small fingers. When the EIP is unavailable, the flexor carpi ulnaris (FCU) may be used; however, it is an extremely strong wrist flexor, and it does not match the excursion of the finger extensors well. Similarly, the flexor carpi radialis (FCR) could be considered, but neither wrist flexor is long enough to reach the distal stumps of the finger extensors and would need to be prolonged with a graft. A better option may be the extensor carpi radialis longus (ECRL) or extensor carpi radialis brevis (ECRB). Both insert on the dorsum of the wrist, not far from the distal finger extensors and are expendable if partial or complete wrist fusion is being performed.

When all four finger extensors have ruptured, including the EDQ and EIP, weaving all four distal tendon stumps through the radial wrist extensor provides reasonably good wrist extension (Fig. 86.2).

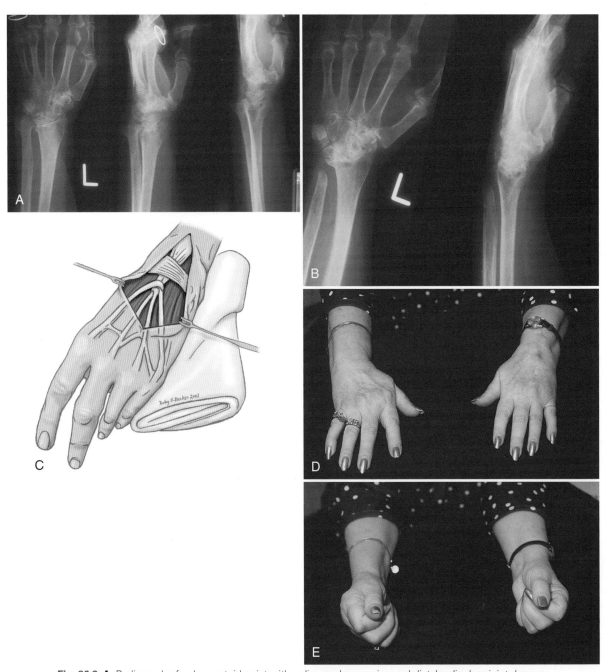

Fig. 86.2 A, Radiograph of a rheumatoid wrist with radiocarpal narrowing and distal radioulnar joint degeneration and osteophyte formation. **B,** The same wrist after radiocarpal fusion and resection of the distal ulna. **C,** Extensor carpi radialis longus to extensor digitorum communis (EDC) transfer. **D** and **E,** Postoperative flexion and extension 6 months after extensor carpi radialis longus to EDC transfer.

Alternatively, tendon transfer of the flexor digitorum superficialis (FDS) tendons to the long and ring fingers may be used to restore finger extension (Fig. 86.3). Bunnell and Boyes[12] originally described this transfer executed through the interosseous membrane. When scarring is present in the interosseous membrane or if the surgeon prefers, the FDS tendon to the long finger may be brought around the radial side of the forearm to restore extension to the index and long fingers. The FDS tendon to the ring finger is brought around the ulnar border of the forearm, restoring extension to the ring and small fingers. A Pulvertaft-type weave is used when possible to increase the strength of the transfer, weaving auAthe smaller extensor tendons that have already ruptured through the larger FDS

tendon to the long and ring fingers, respectively. Another option is to treat ruptures of multiple extensor tendons at wrist level by a free loop tendon graft using the palmaris longus or fourth toe extensor tendon.[13]

In general, rupture of multiple extensor tendons can seriously compromise hand function and even the best of transfers in the most experienced surgeon's hands, yields only fair results. Extensor tendon lag is common, and patients with severe RA are better treated with early aggressive synovectomy of the DRU joint to prevent tendon ruptures.[11] In patients with multiple extensor tendon ruptures and advanced radiocarpal arthritis, the surgeon should seriously consider wrist arthrodesis. This not only stabilizes the carpus, but it also makes an

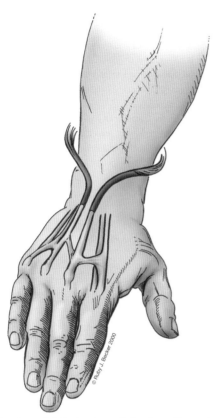

Fig. 86.3 The superficialis tendon of the long finger is transferred around the radial side of the forearm and sutured end to end to the extensor communis to the long finger. If sufficient distal tendon is present, a weave, as seen in Figure 86.4, may be used. The superficialis tendon of the ring finger is shown passing around the ulnar border of the forearm and sutured to the distal extensor communis to the ring finger.

additional five tendons potentially available for use as transfers (ECRL, ECRB, extensor carpi ulnaris [ECU], FCR, and FCU). Referral to therapy should include a list of tendon transfers, desired motion, and precautions for overstretching.

THUMB EXTENSOR TENDON RUPTURE

Rupture of the extensor pollicis longus EPL is also common and probably occurs secondary to the relatively small tunnel through which it passes at Lister's tubercle, resulting in physical change to the tendon; local synovitis and exposure to proteolytic enzymes; the acute angle rounding the tubercle as it passes from the forearm to the tip of the thumb, resulting in wear on the tendon; and finally vascular compromise.

Hypothetically, EPL rupture can be seen and treated early with end-to-end repair. In reality, the tendon ends are in no condition for end-to-end repair and better treated with intercalated grafting with a slip of EDQ or palmaris longus. Short extensors from the foot or a strip of the FCR also may be considered. Tendon transfer using the EIP is a popular treatment among many hand surgeons. Based on principles of tendon transfer, it is ideal, having similar amplitude and excursion, innervation, and force vector as the EPL. The EDQ or ECRL may also be considered.

The EIP tendon usually inserts on the ulnar side of the MCP joint of the index finger but rarely may insert radial to the index EDC.[14] When performing the transfer, the EIP is freed from distal to proximal

to the level of the extensor retinaculum and transferred subcutaneously to the distal stump of the EPL and secured to the EPL using a Pulvertaft weave. Tension is adjusted such that, with passive wrist flexion, full extension of the interphalangeal (IP) joint occurs and with passive wrist extension, slight IP joint flexion occurs.

FLEXOR TENDONS

On the palmar surface of the wrist, the flexor pollicis longus (FPL) and flexor digitorum profundus (FDP) to the index and long fingers may be abraded by a spur on the scaphoid or by spur formation at the level of the scaphotrapezial joint. The eponym for tendon ruptures at this level is Mannerfelt syndrome.[15] This must be differentiated clinically from anterior interosseous nerve (AIN) palsy, which also can be seen with RA. Rheumatoid cyst formation from the elbow joint may cause compression of the AIN and secondary loss of IP joint flexion in the thumb, as well as distal IP joint flexion in the index finger. These are the same digits affected by tendon rupture in Mannerfelt syndrome.

Careful clinical and radiologic examination of the MCP and IP joints is required in planning surgical reconstruction of the flexor tendons. Restoration of IP joint motion is particularly important in cases of previous MCP joint fusion. In the case of rupture of the FPL or FDP to the index or long finger, interposition tendon graft to the FPL may be the best option to restore thumb flexion. The palmaris longus or one of the usual two slips of the EDQ may be used for interposition tendon grafting. Tendon transfer should be considered when the patient is seen more than 6 months after the rupture and the proximal muscle of the FPL or FDP has become contracted and is no longer capable of serving as a motor unit. Transfer options include the FDS of the long or ring finger to the stump of the distal FPL. The brachioradialis (BR) is also an excellent muscle to restore flexion power to the thumb if the distal FPL is long enough to reach the BR. If not, a small intercalated tendon graft can be used. The combination of transfer of the BR to the FPL with transfer of the ECRL or ECRB to the FDP of the index and long fingers, as used for high median nerve palsy, may be a good choice for tendon rupture as well. Side-to-side tendon transfer of the FDP of the index or long finger to the FDP of the ring and small fingers is yet another choice to restore flexion to the radial two fingers.

Postoperative Management After Tendon Transfers

To treat individuals after a tendon reconstructive procedure, the therapist must be aware of the nature of the rupture and the quality of the ttendon repair. Additional care should be taken when progressing through the phases of rehabilitation with respect to the potential fragility of the involved tendons, and the focus of treatment should be on whole-body functioning.

Literature supporting any one program for post-operative management after tendon transfers in patients with RA is lacking.[16] Current trends in treatment include the following: (1) edema reduction techniques; (2) custom orthotic fabrication for protection of the transfer during healing; (3) tendon transfer training exercises; (4) functional electrical stimulation, if needed to coax a transfer through scar adhesions; and (5) functional retraining.

The goal of tendon transfer is to redistribute power to improve function. Communication with the physician and the establishment of realistic goals for the patient are important. The patient will benefit from a realistic understanding that the tendon transfer does not return joint motion to normal but rather improves current function.

General Guidelines

Protective Phase: Weeks 1 to 3

The focus of therapy is protection of the transfer while healing occurs, to prevent rupture or elongation at the tendon juncture, through the use of a custom-fabricated orthosis. The joints included in the orthosis are those that the tendon transfer either acts on or crosses. The orthosis is positioned so that any possible tension on the transfer is minimized. Other goals of therapy at this stage include reduction of postoperative edema, maintenance of ROM of uninvolved joints, and promotion of independence in ADLs.

Mobilization Period: Weeks 3 to 6

Depending on the surgeon's level of comfort with the strength of the suture line between the donor and recipient tendons, active motion of the tendon transfer may be started as early as 3.5 weeks after surgery.

During attempts to actively use the transfer, the patient should focus on the original function of the transferred muscle–tendon unit. For example, if the EIP has been transferred to the EPL, the patient should think about index finger extension while attempting to extend the thumb. Biofeedback and functional electrical stimulation are helpful to enhance the patient's efforts. Orthoses are continued but are removed during exercise sessions and for bathing. Scar massage is begun to help decrease adherence of incision scars if this is a problem. Typically, patients require at least two supervised therapy sessions weekly. Equally important is a detailed home program, with a focus on active function of the transfer.

Mobilization Period: Weeks 6 to 8

At this stage, tendon transfer training continues, as does scar massage. Gentle passive range of motion (PROM) may potentially begin at this time if needed, but caution must be observed to avoid overly zealous passive stretching exercise in a direction opposite that of the tendon transfer. For example, if thumb extension is the goal of the tendon transfer, aggressive passive thumb flexion should be avoided. Therapist and surgeon communication regarding the goals and progression of rehabilitation is essential.

After the incisions are well healed and the tendon junctures are secure, purposeful activity may be incorporated into the home program. Patients do extremely well in identifying and using their tendon transfers if they are involved in purposeful functional activities. To use the tendon transfer, the patient may perform light ADLs, such as brushing teeth and folding clothes. Patients adapt surprisingly well to the new way of using the hand. At this stage, orthoses are used at night and for protection during all but light ADLs.

Mobilization Period: 8 to 12 Weeks

Strengthening exercises may begin at this stage if needed, with resistance upgraded gradually and as tolerated, with the emphasis kept on the level of strength needed for functional activities. All other exercises are continued as needed. Orthosis use is gradually decreased during the day but may continue at night for up to 6 months, depending on the function of the transfer.

REHABILITATION GUIDELINES FOR SPECIFIC TRANSFERS

Extensor Indicis Proprius to Extensor Pollicis Longus

Rehabilitation after transfer of the EIP to the EPL to restore thumb extension usually begins 3 to 3.5 weeks after surgery. A low-temperature thermoplastic orthosis is fabricated by the therapist at the first visit to maintain the wrist in 30 to 40 degrees of wrist extension, with the thumb in palmar abduction and the MCP and IP joints in neutral to slight extension. The orthosis position may vary slightly, depending on the preference of the referring surgeon and factors specific to each individual case. Patients are instructed to use the orthosis at all times except for bathing and exercise. In some cases, the patient may be referred for the custom postoperative thermoplastic orthosis within a few days after surgery, in which case the orthosis would be worn at all times until active exercise is begun, usually 3 to 3.5 weeks after surgery.

Active tendon transfer training involves the patient's active attempts to extend the thumb. Patients who have difficulty activating the transfer may be helped by thinking about index finger extension while attempting thumb extension. Given the similar angle of pull of the original and the donor tendon in this case, most patients will benefit from functional grasp activities incorporated into ADL tasks and may not require prolonged therapy courses. Frequently, motion opposite the direction of the transfer (i.e., thumb and wrist flexion) may be limited at this early stage because of tension or adherence of the transfer. The patient is instructed to perform only gentle active wrist flexion and thumb flexion and opposition within a comfortable range. The patient is not permitted to perform passive stretching of the thumb and wrist into flexion or simultaneous thumb and wrist flexion to avoid stretching the transfer. Occasionally, adherence of the transfer may be apparent and massage along the path of the transferred tendon and the incision scar is helpful.

In addition to supervised therapy sessions, the patient is instructed in a home program of exercises to be performed three to four times a day. The EIP-to-EPL transfer would be expected to function well. Usually, 6 weeks after surgery, active range of motion (AROM) has become functional and gentle resistive exercises may begin if needed. Orthosis use is gradually decreased to use at night only. With the transferred EIP woven three times through the recipient tendon and two to three sutures placed at each weave, there is little risk of rupture. However, if the transfer has only one or two stable weaves because of a more distal rupture, or in the case of poor tendon tissue distally, the surgeon must communicate this concern to the therapist, and mobilization may be delayed until the sixth postoperative week.

Side-to-Side Transfer to Restore Finger Extension

A side-to-side tendon transfer to restore finger extension typically is protected for 3 to 3.5 weeks in a cast or custom-made thermoplastic orthosis. The position of immobilization is with the wrist in extension and the MCP joints supported in neutral extension or slight flexion, depending on the positions at which the wrist and MCP joints were tensioned during surgery. Gentle active movement of the proximal and distal IP joints may be started when pain and swelling are controlled; however, a more conservative approach would be to delay IP joint motion until 3.5 weeks postoperatively. The surgeon may delay the initiation of active tendon transfer training until 6 weeks, depending on the strength of the transfer.

Tendon transfer training involves the patient's active attempts to extend the digits with the orthosis removed. The retraining process may begin with place-and-hold exercises. For example, the digits are gently positioned in full extension, and the patient is asked to actively hold the position. The patient is then asked to initiate active finger extension from a resting position. Using the tenodesis effect created by wrist flexion facilitates this process. For example, as the wrist flexes, the fingers extend, and the patient's active efforts are enhanced. The next step is to have the patient place the hand over the edge of a table or thick book and actively extend the digits. The most difficult exercise is to have the patient place the hand on a flat surface and attempt to actively lift each digit. Adherence of the incision scar and the tendon transfer may be apparent, and scar massage is helpful to decrease adherence and facilitate excursion of the transfer. If significant extensor lag is present, a dynamic MCP joint extension assist orthosis may be helpful to support the digits and facilitate the patient's efforts.

Overzealous finger and wrist flexion and grip exercises should be avoided, especially during the early weeks of therapy to avoid overstretching the transfer.

When the patient has mastered control of the transfer, therapeutic activity, such as the use of a pegboard, and light ADLs are helpful.

Flexor Digitorum Superficialis to Extensor Digitorum Communis Transfer for Finger Extension

Transfer of the FDS to the EDC to restore finger extension typically is protected for 3 to 3.5 weeks in a cast or thermoplastic orthosis custom fabricated by the hand therapist, with the wrist in extension and the MCP joints of the digits supported in neutral. Gentle active movement of the proximal and distal IP joints is started when pain and swelling are controlled; however, a more conservative approach would be to delay IP joint motion until 3.5 weeks postoperatively. Training of this transfer can be difficult because although the FDS performs a function that is in phase with wrist extension, it is antagonistic to that of the EDC. Active retraining begins at 3.5 to 6 weeks, depending on the security of the tendon transfer suture line as determined by the surgeon. When active motion is begun, the patient is asked to place the involved hand on a table with the fingers over the edge and then to actively flex the finger from which the transfer was taken, at the proximal IP joint. This should result in extension of the digit. Demonstrating FDS activity on the opposite hand can be helpful. Blocking exercises to specifically demonstrate the function of the FDS will help as well. If the FDS is routed around the radius or ulna, gentle forearm rotation may enhance the transfer. If the transfer is through the interosseous membrane, flexion and extension of the wrist may enhance the patient's efforts.

Tendon Transfer for Flexor Pollicis Longus or Flexor Digitorum Profundus Rupture (Mannerfelt Syndrome)

The timing of rehabilitation depends on the integrity and strength of the tendon transfer suture line. Positioning after these procedures to restore flexion of the thumb or digits is typically with a dorsal block orthosis custom fabricated by the hand therapist, with the wrist flexed and the thumb or digits blocked from full extension at the MCP joints for the digits and at the carpometacarpal (CMC) and MCP joints for the thumb. Passive motion of the thumb or digits within the limits of the orthosis may begin soon after surgery, as with primary flexor tendon repair. At 3.5 weeks, gentle AROM is begun, and in the case of the graft, no reeducation is necessary because the original muscle is used. More specific retraining is needed in the case of tendon transfer. For example, with a BR transfer to the FPL, flexion of the elbow will help the patient learn to activate the transfer and achieve thumb flexion. The orthosis may be removed at 3 to 3.5 weeks to perform active exercises, with care taken to avoid simultaneous wrist and finger and thumb extension or passive stretching into extension to prevent rupture or stretching out of the transfer or graft. At 6 weeks, gentle resistance may be started, and at 12 weeks, orthosis use may be discontinued.

Summary

Tendon transfers in the hand and upper extremity are among the most rewarding procedures for a hand surgeon and hand therapist to manage. Tendon transfers involve the restoration of a function that has been completely lost and, as seen in this chapter, may involve the use of a tendon graft or, in some instances, a direct end-to-end repair. Close communication between the surgeon and the therapist is critical, especially regarding hands with RA. The therapist must know whether a stable weave has been obtained surgically; if so, motion may be started as early as 3.5 weeks. The ability of a therapist

or surgeon to teach a patient to use a transfer is a true art form. It involves educating the patient to activate the donor tendon to restore function to the recipient tendon. Modalities such as electrical stimulation may help; however, if the surgeon has adhered to the basic principles of tendon transfer, that is, trying to obtain a donor tendon with comparable amplitude, direction of pull, and excursion to the recipient tendon, the task of retraining should be relatively easy. More difficult transfers, such as the ECRB or ECRL to finger extensors, may take time to retrain, but when these are the only donors available, the time and effort should prove worthwhile to the surgeon; the therapist; and, most important, the patient.

CARPAL TUNNEL SYNDROME

Carpal tunnel syndrome is the most common compressive neuropathy of the upper extremity. Traditionally, RA has been considered a risk factor for the development of CTS.[17] Based on moderate levels of evidence, the most recent American Academy of Orthopaedic Surgeons (AAOS) Clinical Practice Guidelines reaffirm RA as a risk factor for the development of CTS.[18] This could be explained in part by the synovial inflammation and hypertrophy within the carpal tunnel leading to compression of the median nerve. It should be noted, however, that a recent study showed similar incidence of CTS in patients with RA and the general population (0.3–5.0 per 1000 person-years).[19] This trend may reflect the increased use of DMARDs and biologics for disease control.[19]

After the diagnosis has been made, treatment of early CTS in patients with RA is similar to treatment in the general population, beginning first with oral steroidal or nonsteroidal antiinflammatory medications or corticosteroid injections. Referral to therapy may be indicated for sensory evaluation, orthotic management, postural assessment, and a home exercise program (HEP). Relative to idiopathic CTS, patients with RA may respond better to corticosteroid injections because of the inflammatory nature of the disease process.[20] If signs and symptoms reflect advanced median nerve compression or the patient does not respond to nonsurgical treatment, operative treatment is recommended. The major difference between carpal tunnel release in a patient with RA and in a patient with idiopathic CTS is the requirement for concomitant synovectomy in patients with RA. An extended open carpal tunnel incision offers adequate exposure to accomplish this task.

WRIST ARTHRITIS

Limited Fusion

Rheumatoid arthritis of the wrist may disrupt the intercarpal ligaments and preferentially destroy the radiocarpal joint, with relative sparing of the midcarpal joint.[21] Therefore, limited wrist fusion alone or in combination with other bony and soft tissue procedures has been used to effectively treat patients with RA. Limited wrist fusions attempt to retain enough motion to enable the use of the wrist in a functional manner (Fig. 86.4). The functional ROM of the wrist has been defined by Palmer and coworkers[22] as 5 degrees of flexion, 30 degrees of extension, 10 degrees of radial deviation, and 15 degrees of ulnar deviation. Indications for limited wrist fusions include wrist pain resistant to medical treatment; wrist deformity with carpal instability, including ulnar translocation; end-stage arthritis of the radiolunate or the radiocarpal joint; and more active patients who desire to retain some wrist motion. Contraindications include severe mutilating deformities of the radiocarpal joint and midcarpal arthritis. The complications typically associated with limited wrist fusions include nonunion and progressive adjacent joint disease. Arthrodesis may be performed

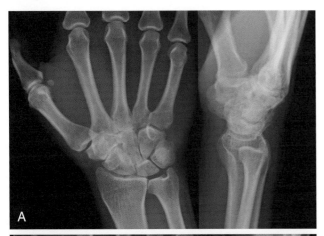

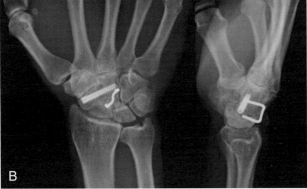

Fig. 86.4 A 36-year old carpenter with rheumatoid arthritis affecting his midcarpal articulation. **A,** Posteroanterior and lateral radiographs demonstrate arthritic changes in the scaphocapitate articulation. **B,** Subsequent fusion of this articulation with a screw and staple.

using various fixation devices, including Kirschner wires (K-wires), screws, or staples.

Motomiya and coworkers[23] retrospectively reviewed the outcomes of radiolunate arthrodesis, combined with a Darrach procedure to treat concomitant DRU joint pathology, and obtained autograft for the fusion. At the time of surgery and at final follow-up, these 22 patients were all receiving a combination of prednisolone, DMARDs, methotrexate, or biologics. At an average follow-up period of 7 years, the authors noted improved Mayo wrist scores, which assess pain, function, ROM, and grip strength. The scores improved from 37 to 72 (*P* <.001). The wrist flexion–extension arc was functional according to the range defined by Palmer and coworkers.[22] It should be noted, however, that adjacent joint disease involving the scapholunate and midcarpal joints continued to progress, as would be expected after limited fusion.

When the radioscaphoid and the radiolunate joints are affected, radioscapholunate arthrodesis may be a useful procedure to control symptoms, treat instability, and maintain a functional wrist ROM.[24] Although some patients may require further midcarpal arthrodesis, most patients seem to respond well to treatment. In a retrospective series of 23 patients treated with either radiolunate or radioscapholunate fusion, Raven and coworkers noted mean Disability of the Arm Shoulder and Hand (DASH) scores of 41.0 and a 64 degrees of flexion–extension arc of motion at a mean of 11.3 years after surgery.[24] Complications included persistent pain requiring midcarpal fusion, nonunion, and hardware penetration into the midcarpal joint requiring revision.

Total Wrist Fusion

Total wrist fusion is often the final salvage procedure for patients with end-stage wrist arthritis. Many of these patients may have had prior surgeries aimed at preserving some motion, such as limited carpal fusion. The pain control afforded by arthrodesis may be substantial but comes at the cost of no wrist motion and compromised function. A number of fusion techniques have been described, including the use of a dorsal compression plate or the use of an intramedullary pin or rush rod, also known as the "Mannerfelt technique."[25] The optimal position of the fusion is still the subject of ongoing debate. Although some authors consider slight extension and ulnar deviation the optimal position, a shared decision with the patient based on her or his activities and vocations may guide the optimal fusion position.[25] Immobilizing the wrist preoperatively for a trial period to simulate the angle of flexion or extension can be helpful to assess needs for ADLs. With dorsal compression plating, radiocarpal fusion is reliably achieved in a very high percentage of patients, but potential complications include screw fracture, plate loosening, and plate fracture as well as nonunion of the long finger CMC joint.[26] Intramedullary rush rod fusion is achieved by passing the rod through the third metacarpal and then back through the capitate and the prepared carpus in retrograde fashion through the medullary canal of the radius. Additional staples may be used to stabilize and compress the fusion.[27] Advantages include the less prominent hardware, lack of fusion of the CMC joint, and easy soft tissue coverage. In a series of 34 wrists in 25 patients, a 94% union rate was achieved as well as substantial pain relief with intramedullary fusion.[25] All patients who rated their satisfaction as excellent were fixed between 14 degrees of flexion and 10 degrees of extension.[25]

Total Wrist Arthroplasty

Rheumatoid patients may be ideally suited for joint replacement arthroplasty of the wrist, especially if they have polyarticular involvement (e.g., wrist, hand, finger, elbow, shoulder) in which preservation of motion at the wrist is important. Until relatively recently, TWA has been fraught with complications, including instability, soft tissue imbalance, and carpal component loosening.[28] Over the past 2 decades, improvements in design and technique have led to encouraging outcomes.[29] Surgeons must remember, however, that operative intervention in rheumatoid patients is palliative, and although beneficial to the patient, joint replacement arthroplasty is not a cure. The surgeon and therapist should counsel patients in advance to ensure that patients have a thorough understanding of what is involved in joint replacement and the rehabilitation program. They should be advised that close follow-up will be necessary after surgery. The patient must also adhere to an ongoing program of joint protection, both preoperatively and postoperatively, to ensure that the replacement will last as long as possible. Furthermore, patients should be made aware of lifetime restrictions on lifting more than 10 lb. The optimal candidate for wrist replacement has pancarpal arthritis and relatively normal bone stock. The patient must have a compelling need for replacement rather than fusion, limited fusion, or a "shelf procedure." Clinically, this usually is a patient with severe bilateral disease that affects both elbows and shoulders. Contraindications include active infection and the need to bear weight through the wrist with a handheld device such as a walker or cane. Distal carpal bone loss due to disease activity may limit fixation and is also a relative contraindication for TWA. In patients with significant osteopenia or erosive arthritis of the wrist, silicone implant arthroplasty remains an option (Fig. 86.5).

Ward and coworkers[28] assessed the 5- to 10-year outcomes of 19 wrists in 15 rheumatoid patients who underwent TWA using a

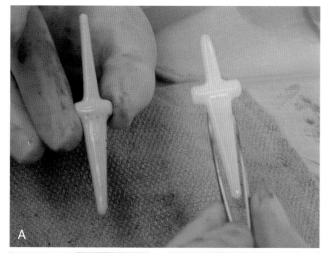

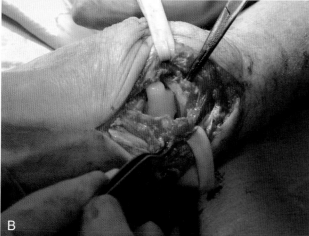

Fig. 86.5 A, Swanson monobloc trial (hand held) and silicon wrist implant (handled with forceps). **B,** After preparation of the distal radius and the carpus, the silicon prosthesis has been implanted.

cemented Universal wrist prosthesis (KMI, Carlsbad, CA) and noted that 50% of implants had failed by the time of the latest follow-up. Carpal component failure was the most commonly encountered complication. Patients who did not have a failure were able to maintain a functional ROM both flexion–extension and radioulnar deviation.[28] More recent studies assessing the medium- and long-term outcomes of TWA using biologic fixation have been more encouraging because survival rates have improved, and complications appear to have decreased in frequency.[29,30] Gil and coworkers[29] assessed outcomes of 39 patients, 31 of whom had RA using a press-fit Universal 2 TWA implant (Integra Life Sciences, Plainsboro, NJ; previously manufactured by KMI, Inc.). The mean follow-up duration was 9 years. Pain on a 0 to 10 verbal pain scale improved from 8.6 preoperatively to 0.4 postoperatively, whereas the mean flexion and extension were 37 and 29 degrees, respectively. The cumulative probability of remaining free from revision was 78% (95% confidence interval [CI], 62%–91%) at 15 years. Complications included implant loosening in three patients (7.7%). Two underwent surgical revision with an uncemented carpal component and one with revision of the carpal and radial components.

Badge and coworkers[30] assessed the outcomes of 85 uncemented Universal 2 TWA Universal in 75 patients, at a mean follow-up duration of 53 months. Pain on the visual analog scale (VAS) improved from 8.1 preoperatively to 5.4 postoperatively. ROM was preserved and remained functional with a mean extension of 29 degrees and flexion

of 21 degrees. Similarly, grip strength improved from 4.8 kg preoperatively to 10 kg at final follow-up, and the QuickDASH score improved from 61 to 46. The Kaplan-Meier probability of survival defining removal of the components as the endpoint was 91% at 7.8 years. Major complications occurred in six patients (7%); three required revision arthroplasty, and three required arthrodesis.[30]

Silicon Interposition Arthroplasty

In the 1970s, Swanson[31] introduced silicone implant arthroplasty. The monobloc silicone joint had a proximal stem that was inserted into the radius, a flexible hinge, and a distal stem that was inserted through the capitate into the long finger metacarpal. In low-demand patients and patients with vocational or avocational activities that require wrist motion, this implant remains a reasonable treatment option. In some patients with RA, bone stock may be so deficient that successful fusion or metal-on-plastic TWA is unlikely. Silicone replacement of the radiocarpal joint then becomes the preferred treatment of choice (see Fig. 86.5). The material properties of silicone are closer to that of bone; therefore, the silicone joint and stem are less likely to subside into the metacarpal distally or the radius proximally. Indications for silicone wrist replacement include pain with attempted wrist motion, decreased motion, instability, and deformity. Radiographs should reveal pancarpal arthritis with enough remaining bone stock to support the implant, specifically, an intact distal radius cortex and similar residual bone stock in the long finger metacarpal to support the implant. In a series of 23 patients who underwent 26 Swanson radiocarpal replacements, Davis, Weiland, and Volenec-Dowling[32] noted that patients had significant functional improvement in activities that require wrist extension. No improvement was seen in activities requiring strength or fine-motor control. Concomitant capsular reconstruction and tendon transfer to balance the wrist were important in the success of the arthroplasty.[32] Despite more compatible material properties with bone, silicone wrist implants also fail with time. This may lead to recurrent deformity and possibly silicone synovitis.[33]

Distal Radioulnar Joint Arthroplasty

In addition to a diseased radiocarpal joint, the DRU joint may be severely affected, leading to pain and instability, or caput ulnae syndrome, which is a constellation of palmar subluxation, supination, and ulnar translation of the carpus; palmar subluxation of the ECU; and the appearance of a prominent ulna head.[34] In turn, this may result in extensor tendon rupture, or Vaughn-Jackson syndrome. Traditional surgical treatment consisted of a Darrach procedure (associated with painful radioulnar convergence and ulnar translocations of the carpus, instability), Sauve-Kapandji procedure, or ulnar head prosthetic replacement. Wrist stability, however, may be compromised by the synovitis and ligamentous laxity. As a consequence, total DRU joint arthroplasty was developed (APTIS Medical LLC, Louisville, KY). This is a constrained prosthesis that consists of a polyethylene ulnar head replacement that articulates with a socket within a metallic radial plate (Fig. 86.6). Galvis and coworkers[34] assessed the results of 19 rheumatoid wrists that underwent total DRU joint replacement, at a mean follow-up of 39 months. The average patient age was 57 years. The authors found improvements of the pain VAS from 7.3 to 2.2, improvements in pronation and supination, and DASH scores of 24 at final follow-up. Complications included revision surgery in two patients; one patient developed implant loosening, and another patient underwent tenolysis of the ECU tendon. Furthermore, at final review, six patients had undergone radiocarpal arthrodesis.[34]

Wrist Arthroplasty: Postoperative Management
0 to 4 Weeks

At 24 to 48 hours, the dressing is changed, and the drain is removed. At this time, the patient is placed in a volar wrist support orthosis. The

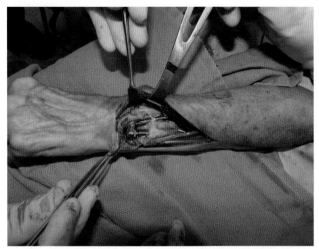

Fig. 86.6 Total distal radioulnar (DRU) joint arthroplasty (APTIS Medical LLC, Louisville, KY) used to treat DRU joint arthritis in this rheumatoid patient.

sutures are removed between 1 and 2 weeks. Depending on the stability of the prosthesis, gentle AROM for the wrist may be started as early as 2 weeks postoperatively. The surgeon and therapist need to discuss and review factors that influence the timing of initiation of wrist ROM, such as poor bone stock or weakened or frayed tendons, as well as the specific procedure and expected outcome. Under ideal circumstances, a 40- to 60-degree arc of total active flexion and extension of the wrist may be obtained. Supervised outpatient hand therapy sessions at this time are scheduled as needed. The patient should have an established home program and should be provided with information regarding joint protection. Care should be taken to address the patient's shoulder, elbow, and neck to maintain ROM and function and to avoid undue stress on the contralateral extremity.

During the first 4 weeks, techniques to promote healing of the incision and to manage postoperative swelling are reviewed. Joint protection techniques are reinforced by demonstration and practice and via use of adaptive equipment. The patient must understand that she or he cannot bear weight through the involved wrist, especially if she or he uses a device such as a cane to ambulate, and alternate arrangements (e.g., platform crutch or walker) should be made. The patient wears the volar wrist support orthosis the majority of the day and at night, removing it for bathing and exercises. The orthosis positions the wrist at 10 to 20 degrees of extension and allows for full flexion and extension of the digits and opposition of the thumb to the small finger. If the extensor tendons are repaired, the MCP joints are supported in the wrist orthosis in a neutral position to protect the tendons for 3 weeks or more postoperatively. Initiation of wrist motion may be delayed. After 3 weeks, if an extensor lag develops or persists, use of the orthosis for another 1 to 2 weeks is recommended.

4 to 8 Weeks

Gentle active motion of the wrist continues with care to avoid overexercise and to monitor for extensor lag of the digits. Edema control and scar management are part of the program, as are modalities to help with swelling, stiffness, and pain. Light grip activities, such as the weight well with no resistance and limited repetitions, can help facilitate increased ROM.

8 to 10 Weeks

By 8 to 10 weeks postoperatively, a light strengthening program may be initiated. This should begin with isometric exercise followed by progressive resistive exercise with a 1-lb (0.4-kg) weight and with education of the patient on biomechanically sound joint protection principles. A wrist orthosis, either custom made or prefabricated, may be used for heavy activities, such as gardening, or during extended use. Long-term outcomes are improved with a permanent lifting restriction of 10 lb (4 kg) after TWA.

THE METACARPOPHALANGEAL JOINT

At the level of the MCP joint, rheumatoid patients may experience triggering, soft tissue imbalances leading to ulnar drift, or frank joint destruction. The diagnosis, surgical treatment, and rehabilitation of the various disease entities are discussed in this section.

Trigger Finger

Although trigger finger in rheumatoid patients presents in a similar fashion as in nonrheumatoid patients, it has a distinct pathophysiology and a different surgical treatment. Tenosynovial ingrowth may occur anywhere tenosynovium is found, such as the flexor tendons, or dorsum of the wrist proximal or distal to the extensor retinaculum. Although this has the potential to cause tendon rupture, this synovial ingrowth more often results in limited tendon excursion as the tendon swells and no longer passes easily beneath the annular pulley system on the flexor surface of the finger. If aggressive medical treatment that includes corticosteroid injections is unsuccessful, tenosynovectomy with reduction tenoplasty or resection of one slip of the FDS is the treatment of choice, with reasonable long-term results. Release of the A1 pulley should be avoided because it increases the moment of force of the FDP tendon at the MCP joint level in an ulnar direction and may lead to premature ulnar deviation at the MCP joint in the involved digits. RA appears to be associated with an increased risk of revision trigger finger surgery (odds ratio, 1.4 [1.1–1.7, 95% CI]), as well as postoperative digital stiffness (OR, 1.7 [1.5–2.0, 95% CI]).[35]

Ulnar Drift

Metacarpophalangeal joint deformity in RA is characterized by flexion, volar subluxation, and ulnar deviation of the proximal phalanges relative to the metacarpal heads. The digital flexors deviate the fingers in an ulnar direction, whereas the metacarpals and carpus deviate radially. Patients typically complain of loss of dexterity and difficulty with pinch. Although no consensus has been reached to explain the pathophysiology, it is thought that ulnar drift develops secondary to a variety of factors, including intrinsic muscle ischemia and secondary contracture,[36] incompetence of collateral ligaments, or increased intraarticular pressure.[37]

In the early stages of the deformity, when the MCP joints are passively correctable and no volar subluxation exists, reconstruction involves synovectomy, centralization of the extrinsic extensor tendons, division of the ulnar intrinsics, and tightening of the dorsal and radial structures.[38] Crossed intrinsic transfer has been shown to have acceptable outcomes more predictable when the disease is controlled medically. In this transfer, the ulnar intrinsic tendon of the index, long, and ring fingers is transferred to the radial side of the adjacent digit. It is sutured to the oblique fibers of the radial extensor expansion. Release of the abductor digiti minimi and replacement of the first dorsal interosseous muscle to its normal position is also performed.[38]

Extensor indicis proprius tenodesis has also been described for the correction ulnar deviation in the rheumatoid hand. Monreal[39] reported the short-term outcomes of EIP tenodesis to correct ulnar drift deformity in patients with RA. The EIP tendon is divided at the musculotendinous junction, while its insertion is preserved. It is passed transversely from the radial to the ulnar side, deep to the sagittal bands at the level of the metacarpal necks and passed back radially and eventually tenodesed to the radial collateral ligament. Postoperative therapy management included immobilizing the MCP joints in extension and 10 to 15 degrees of radial deviation with the wrist and IP joints free for 6 weeks. Active and passive motion began at 6 weeks, with a night MCP joint extension orthosis for an additional 6 weeks.[39] Follow-up of 10 hands in 5 patients at 8 to 12 months demonstrated some recurrence of the ulnar deviation deformity; however, this was still favorable relative to the preoperative state.[39]

In the late stages, when the MCP joint deformity becomes fixed, MCP joint arthroplasty is the usual treatment option, and both silicon and resurfacing implants have been successfully used. Treatment of combined ulnar deviation and extensor lag has been successfully managed with silicon arthroplasty, with patients reporting decreased pain, improved function, and cosmetic appearance.[40] Chung and coworkers compared the objective and patient-rated outcomes of 33 patients with less than 100 degrees of combined deformity versus 37 patients with more severe deformity (≥100 degrees) combined MCP joint ulnar deviation and extensor lag.[40] The authors found that the severe hand deformity group attained similar functional outcomes compared with the less severe group based on the Michigan Hand Questionnaire. The group with more severe deformities, however, had statistically and clinically more significant deformities after reconstruction. The authors therefore noted that it is much easier to correct the deformities and restore the patients' hand posture when the deformities are less severe.[40]

In general, postoperative therapy management for extensor tendon realignment surgery to correct ulnar drift should involve a hand-based orthosis that provides support to align the MCP joints in neutral or slight radial deviation with straps or thermoplastic dividers. When beginning AROM, emphasizing radial-finger walking may be beneficial. Education is provided to prevent lateral stresses to the MCP joint into ulnar deviation during activities such as lifting a coffee cup. Index finger lateral pinch may need to be restricted by an orthosis to allow for additional healing time. Some individuals may require up to 12 weeks of orthotic management, especially at night time.

Metacarpophalangeal Joint Arthroplasty

Replacement of the MCP joint is typically reserved for patients with severe RA with joint destruction, late stages of ulnar drift, volar subluxation, or intrinsic tightness. There are currently two major categories of prosthetic replacements for the MCP joint: silicone interposition arthroplasty and surface replacement arthroplasty.

Silicone Arthroplasty

The Swanson silicone MCP joint arthroplasty has a long track record in the rheumatoid hand and has been used for more than 50 years.[41] This monobloc implant has a dorsal hinge that enables the implant to flex and depends less on ligamentous support for stability. The modulus of elasticity of silicone implants is less than cortical bone and suitable for the poor bone quality characteristic of advanced rheumatoid disease. Therefore, when joints are chronically dislocated and have evidence of cortical bone loss or poor bone stock, silicone implants should be used as opposed to resurfacing prostheses. The outcomes of silicone MCP joint arthroplasty were recently assessed in a multicenter study that prospectively compared patients who elected to undergo silicone MCP joint arthroplasty while continuing medical management versus patients who elected to have medical treatment only.[42] The benefits of the procedure included improvements in function, ulnar drift, extensor lag, and aesthetics, which were maintained at 7 years. The authors found that nonoperatively treated patients were also able to maintain baseline function at 7 years. When the operative and nonoperative

cohorts were compared, however, the adjusted difference showed significant benefits of the silicone arthroplasty based on the Michigan Hand Questionnaire function, satisfaction, and aesthetic components. On the other hand, grip and pinch strength did not improve after silicone MCP joint arthroplasty.[42]

Implant fractures may occur but do not always require revision unless there is clinical suspicion of silicone synovitis or instability or if alignment of the joint is compromised. Furthermore, the treatment of surface replacement dislocation with revision to a silicone MCP joint implant appears to hold the most promise in achieving a stable joint after an acute prosthetic dislocation (Fig. 86.7).[43]

Silicone synovitis, clinically characterized by swelling and pain, is a well-documented complication of silicone implants. Radiographically, silicone synovitis is demonstrated by cystic changes and osteolysis. Histologically, the pathology is characterized by a giant cell reaction and evidence of silicone fragmentation.[44] Silicone synovitis tends to occur when the prosthesis is loaded in compression and fractures and fragments. This is more commonly seen when the prostheses are used in joints that are subjected to higher loading forces, such as the radial head, trapezium, scaphoid, or lunate. Surgical treatment in the form of synovial debridement and removal of the fractured implant is effective in relieving symptoms.[44] Silicone synovitis and granuloma formation have been reported but are uncommon (0.1%) at the MCP and proximal interphalangeal (PIP) joints.[45]

Although ideally suited to last 10 years or more in low-demand patients, silicone MCP joints fail eventually, as will all other nonbiologic implants. They may remain well aligned, stable, and relatively painless in the early period after fracture but are almost certain to require revision in higher demand patients. However, they also may result in synovitis and ulnar deviation. Surgery in symptomatic patients usually is performed through the original incision. The dorsal apparatus is again identified and usually retracted in an ulnar direction. It must be carefully protected to remain functional and centralized at the close of the procedure. Occasionally, the prosthesis may fail and deviate radially. In such instances, the joint is exposed through the opposite side. The capsule is opened, and tissue is obtained for culture and pathology. Culture and biopsy of failed implants should be the norm, and the patient should be watched closely for signs of systemic infection. If the implant is broken, care must be taken to remove the entire implant. Fragments can be found in soft tissue and could later affect motion in the new joint. The metacarpal and proximal phalanx are inspected to be certain no sharp edges exist. Both are then reamed, using standard hand-powered reamers, to either the same size or one size larger. If bone stock is extremely poor, a soft tissue arthroplasty may be performed. After impacted in place, the joint is checked for stability. If stable, the extensor tendon is repositioned over the implant, the wound is closed carefully over a small rubber drain, and the fingers are immobilized.

Surface Replacement Arthroplasty

Surface replacement prostheses of the MCP joints are semiconstrained and consist of two components. They were designed primarily for MCP joints affected by osteoarthritis (OA) or posttraumatic OA; however, they can be used in patients with RA. These implants attempt to reproduce the normal kinematics of the MCP joint and rely on soft tissue constraint and good bone quality for fixation, which may be difficult to achieve in patients with advanced RA. In these patients, the surgeon needs to remember that soft tissue balance is critical to the success or failure of these implants. Patients with severe ulnar deviation and volar subluxation may be better served with standard silicone implants. In younger patients, however, and in patients who the surgeon feels comfortable with joint stability postoperatively (or even preoperatively), surface replacement arthroplasty (SRA) may be considered and may

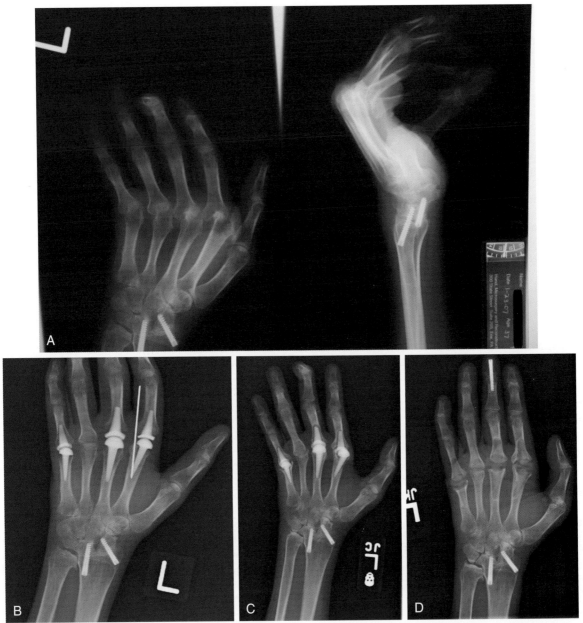

Fig. 86.7 A, 37-year old female rheumatoid patient with substantial ulnar drift and metacarpophalangeal (MCP) joint subluxation. Also note, prior radioscapholunate arthrodesis. **B,** The patient's index, long, and small digits were treated with MCP joint pyrocarbon arthroplasty. **C,** Over the next few years, the pyrocarbon implants became loose. **D,** The pyrocarbon implants were subsequently revised to Swanson-type silicone implants.

in fact serve the patient better in the long term by not failing mechanically. The surgical approach is basically the same for these implants, with the main difference between these and a standard silicone implant being that the surface replacement implants consist of two separate proximal and distal components instead of the single component. The proximal component in each replaces the metacarpal head, and the distal component replaces the base of the proximal phalanx. Intramedullary stems stabilize both proximal and distal components, and both proximal and distal components are stabilized, usually using a press-fit technique. Guided osteotomies unique to each prosthesis are used first on the metacarpal head and then on the proximal phalanx. The medullary canals are then broached to the desired size. The proximal phalanx is generally broached first because it determines the size of

the implant. The metacarpal is then broached to the appropriate size as well as remembering a chamfer cut on the volar surface of the distal metacarpal. Trial implants are placed and checked for stability, and if stable and satisfactory, the final implants are impacted in place. In our experience, preservation of the radial and ulnar collateral ligaments is key to preventing ulnar and volar subluxation in either the long or short term.

The Ascension pyrocarbon MCP joint prosthesis (Ascension Orthopaedics, Austin, TX) has been used in patients with RA (see Fig. 86.7B and C).[46] Outcomes have been reported to be successful, with reasonable survivorship statistics when the implants are used in patients with minimal deformity.[46] This resurfacing prosthesis relies on press-fit fixation and has a pyrocarbon coated graphite core. The use of pyrocarbon is desirable because it is considered inert, has excellent wear characteristics, and has an elastic modulus is similar to cortical bone.[46–48] Recent outcome studies on MCP joint resurfacing arthroplasty have been lacking, and most literature available on pyrocarbon small joint arthroplasty describes the results of PIP joint arthroplasty in patients with OA. Medium-term outcomes have blunted the enthusiasm for these implants because of concerns that bone ongrowth does not reliably occur (see Fig. 86.7B and C). These medium-term studies have revealed high revision rates, implant subsidence, loosening, squeaking, and implant fractures.[47–49] Because of concerns about relatively high revision rates and progressive loosening, most hand surgeons in the United States are reluctant to use these implants in rheumatoid patients and prefer the silicone implant instead.

The SR MCP joint implant (Stryker, Kalamazoo, MI; formerly Small Bone Innovations) is designed with separate proximal and distal components that require ligamentous stability for success. The implant is a metal-on-polyethylene design, and implant fixation may be achieved either with the use of bone cement or press-fit fixation. Similar to the pyrocarbon MCP joint implants, limited recent outcome studies exist in patients with RA.

Metacarpophalangeal Joint Fusion and Salvage Options

Arthroplasty is a better option for MCP joint arthritis affecting the fingers than arthrodesis.[50] However, in certain patients, arthrodesis, particularly of the index finger, may more reliably increase stability in pinch and prevent ulnar deviation by the ulnar deforming forces. PIP and distal interphalangeal (DIP) joint function should be normal when considering index MCP joint fusion. Salvage procedures after failed implants with loss of bone or infection include various modifications of soft tissue arthroplasty.[51,52] When reasonable bone stock remains, Fowler arthroplasty is recommended,[53] in which the metacarpal is cut in the shape of a chevron and intercalated in a V-shaped cut in the base of the proximal phalanx. Leonard Goldner has stated that the best results from soft tissue arthroplasty exceed the best results from silicone replacement, but the latter yields more consistent results.

Therapy After Metacarpophalangeal Joint Arthroplasty

Because rehabilitation after MCP joint replacement requires prolonged therapy and orthotic positioning for 3 to 6 months, pertinent social data (i.e., support at home for meal preparation and self-care postoperatively) and insurance benefits are important to consider during the preoperative evaluation. The goal of the therapy program must be patient focused on pain relief, improvement of cosmesis, restoration of a functional arc of motion, and satisfactory alignment of the joint. Patients and their insurance carriers need to realize that at least weekly visits are necessary to achieve this goal.

Postoperative Management After Metacarpophalangeal Joint Arthroplasty

Hand function and patient satisfaction after MCP joint implant arthroplasty are based on a goal-oriented and structured postoperative therapy program, along with a HEP, usually lasting 3 to 6 months. In general, it is important for the therapist to appreciate that the index and long fingers require less flexion at the MCP joint than the ring and small fingers for most ADLs.[54] Considering the individual patient's unique goals as the treatment program is developed is important for a successful outcome. An experienced hand therapist who is skilled in patient education, joint protection training, dynamic orthotic positioning, and use of adaptive equipment must direct the rehabilitation program.

General Overview of Postoperative Therapy

General therapy goals following MCP joint implant arthroplasty include the following:

1. Optimal wound healing
2. Prevention of scar adherence
3. Control of postoperative swelling
4. Neutral alignment and the desired degree of ROM at the reconstructed MCP joints
5. Optimal performance of ADLs and vocational and avocational pursuits
6. AROM of the shoulder, elbow, and remaining nonoperative joints
7. Functional skills with solid joint protection principles

There has been a recent shift in postoperative management after MCP joint arthroplasty away from the use of a dynamic extension assist orthosis and toward use of a short-arc motion (SAM) protocol.[55] Close communication among the patient, surgeon, and therapist is essential to select the most beneficial treatment regimen. The most effective postoperative protocol is one that is based on the patient's tissue response to the exercises and orthotic positioning program instituted by the therapist. It is important to know the type and design of implant used because this information may guide treatment. The desired result after MCP joint arthroplasty is an arc of motion that is functional for the patient. In addition, patients are generally satisfied if their pain has been relieved and the deformity improved.

Weeks 1 to 2. The patient, therapist, and surgeon will decide on the most appropriate postoperative plan, either with use of a (1) static orthosis and SAM program or (2) a dynamic extension orthosis program (see Fig. 86.8A–C). Both are described next:

Static Orthosis and Short-Arc Motion Program. Two orthoses are fabricated within the first 1 to 2 postoperative weeks. For nighttime, a static, forearm-based resting orthosis is used with the wrist in slight extension and ulnar deviation, the MCP joints in extension and in neutral alignment, and the PIP joints in a resting position. The daytime orthosis will also be forearm based but will leave the IP joints free. Both orthoses should have either a thermoplastic insert between each finger or Velcro straps to prevent ulnar drift. Another option is to fabricate the daytime orthosis and create a separate component to add to the orthosis for night that extends to include the IP joints. Satisfactory results have also been obtained with use of one resting orthosis only, with the MCP joints held in 40 degrees of flexion and IP joints in slight (10–20 degrees) of flexion.[56]

Therapy during this time includes orthosis management, edema control, initiation of a HEP, scar management, ADL instruction, and joint protection principles as necessary.

Exercise: Immediate Active Motion. Escott and coworkers[56] describe a postoperative management program that initiates active flexion and extension at the level of the MCP joint within the first week after surgery, as well as PROM at the level of the wrist and IP joints. Chim and coworkers[55] provide a protocol after MCP joint arthroplasty that describes the advancement of allowable motion at the new joint, starting at 0 to 30 degrees during week 1 and increasing by 10 degrees each week (Box 86.1). At this time, the patient should continue to be immobilized in an orthosis at all times except for exercise. Education should be provided to prevent lateral stresses to the MCP joint.

Dynamic Orthosis Program. Another approach to MCP joint arthroplasty postoperative management involves immediate postoperative orthotic positioning with a dorsal MCP joint extension outrigger fabricated at the first visit, which should be scheduled no later than 1 week after the surgery date. Therapy consists of AROM and gentle PROM of the reconstructed MCP joints, with care to control alignment, care of the incision, and skin inspection. Edema control and

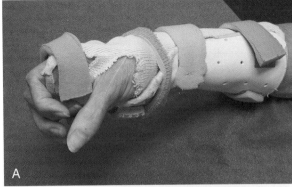

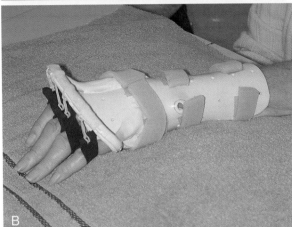

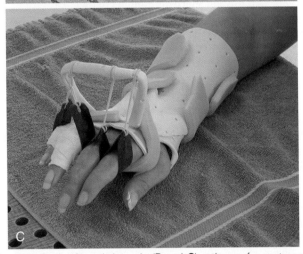

Fig. 86.8 Static (**A**) and dynamic (**B** and **C**) orthoses for metacarpophalangeal joint replacement. Although both are acceptable, the static orthosis is preferable when stability is marginal. Both should allow proximal interphalangeal and distal interphalangeal joint motion. Note cylinder casting for boutonnière deformities in the ring and small fingers.

BOX 86.1 Short-Arc Motion Protocol After Metacarpophalangeal Joint Arthroplasty[55]

Time After Surgery (wk)	Exercise
1–2	May perform IP flexion–extension only (hourly). Begin 0–30 degrees of MCP motion (consider template).
3	Advance MCP motion 0–40 degrees if no extension lag is present.
4	Advance MCP motion 0–50 degrees if no extension lag is present.
5	Advance MCP motion 0–60 degrees if no extension lag is present. Light prehensile activities may begin in therapy.
6	Consider buddy taping as needed. May initiate ADLs. Consider NMES if extensor tendon gliding is poor.

ADLs, Activities of daily living; *IP,* interphalangeal; *MCP,* metacarpophalangeal; *NMES,* neuromuscular electrical nerve stimulation.

for MCP joint alignment is fabricated. This orthosis should provide not only an extension assist but also a radial pull to the reconstructed MCP joints. Additionally, the outrigger component is helpful in correcting any pronation–supination deformities at the level of the MCP joints. AROM and light PROM exercises for MCP joint flexion and extension are begun within the orthosis, with careful monitoring to ensure control of alignment and rotation. Edema control techniques such as compression bandages and Coban for finger edema are implemented at this time. Care must be taken to avoid traction on the skin in an ulnar direction by the compression bandages. A static orthosis with MCP joints supported in neutral or radial alignment also may be fabricated for night use.

Orthosis Specifications. The purpose of the dynamic orthosis (Fig. 86.9) is to control the position and alignment of the reconstructed MCP joints and at the same time to allow guided ROM. In supporting the fingers in a neutral position (MCP joints at 0 degrees) while allowing movement of the reconstructed joint, the orthosis helps influence the encapsulation process and maintain capsular length throughout the period of scar remodeling.[57] The orthosis also is necessary to guide the motion of the joint in flexion and extension and prevent recurrence of the ulnar deviation deformity.

The dynamic orthosis may be worn during the day while a static forearm-based wrist orthosis with MCP support in neutral is worn at night, depending on individual considerations. A static night orthosis (Fig. 86.10) should have either an ulnar border with a trough or Velcro straps (Velcro USA, Manchester, NH) to prevent ulnar drift. The dynamic orthosis is based dorsally with an extension outrigger. Finger slings with elastic traction, which attach to the outrigger, support the MCP joints in extension while avoiding hyperextension. They are placed at the proximal end of the proximal phalanges to guide motion and alignment of the digits. A 90-degree angle of pull from the proximal phalanx to the outrigger, maintaining the reconstructed MCP joints in a neutral position of extension when at rest, must be achieved. In addition, the pull should be in a radial direction to prevent recurrence of ulnar drift and to prevent lateral and medial instability by decreasing stress on the lateral capsular structure. Additional outriggers (Fig. 86.11) may be required to act as a force couple to correct pronation–supination rotation deformities, especially at the index finger. The traction device (rubber bands or springs) should be relaxed enough to allow for approximately 70 degrees of active MCP joint flexion.[58] The force magnitude must be kept low enough to prevent pain and swelling.

ADL training using joint protection principles are included. A home program of AROM within the orthosis and elevation to control edema is critical. Variations to the program are made based on problems identified throughout the postoperative course of therapy (Table 86.2).

Because of the nature and chronicity of RA, ROM exercises are emphasized for the neck, shoulders, elbows, wrists, hips, and knees. Specific details for postoperative therapy for MCP joint replacement are as follows.

3 to 5 Days to 2 Weeks. The bulky dressing is removed, and a light compressive dressing is applied. The dressing is changed at each office visit until suture removal at 10 to 14 days postoperatively. At the initial therapy visit, a dynamic MCPJ extension assist orthosis with control

TABLE 86.2 Postoperative Management of Metacarpophalangeal Joint Arthroplasties

Problems Identified in Therapy Program	Solutions and Interventions
Edema and postoperative pain	Leave patient in postoperative cast for longer period (1–3 wk) in proper position. Use resting hand orthosis at night and outrigger during the day. Fabricate postoperative orthosis before surgery, understanding that adjustments will be needed.
Fragile skin	Use silicone "second skin" padding under dorsal hand portion of outrigger.
Lack of MCP joint flexion at 3 wk	Use removable cylinder casts for PIP joint extension or volar PIP joint extension orthoses to focus effort at the MCP joint in a lumbrical-plus position. Wear volar-based dynamic MCP joint flexion outrigger for stretching joint capsule.
Lack of MCP joint extension	Increase time in the dynamic-extension outrigger; limit flexion activities, particularly of the index and long fingers.
Rotation of index finger	Use supination outrigger on dynamic-extension orthosis.
Difficulty with applying orthosis straps because of weak pinch from arthritis and uninvolved hand	Use larger straps, all ulnar to radial direction, and a D-ring sewn on strap for ease and loss of pinch strength.
Tendency for ulnar deviation	Use a functional ulnar deviation orthosis.
Orthosis slippage (rotates on the forearm)	Use a neoprene strap around wrist to anchor the orthosis in place.
Lack of extension	Position at night with the MCP joints supported in extension; duration of use varies up to 6 mo to 1 yr; wear daytime functional orthosis with support and protection of MCP joint to protect against lateral stresses and support in extension.

MCP, Metacarpophalangeal; *PIP,* proximal interphalangeal.

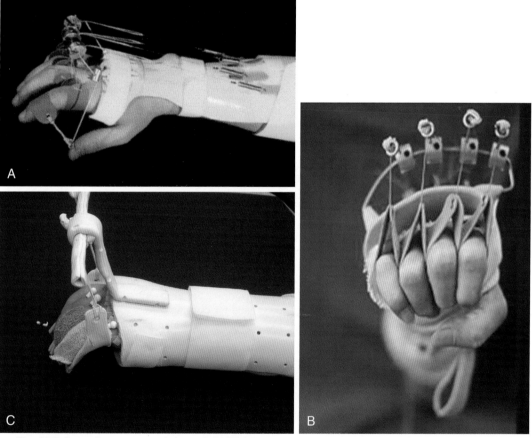

Fig. 86.9 Dynamic metacarpophalangeal (MCP) joint extension orthoses can vary in design. **A,** Dynamic orthosis with rubber bands pulling to a dorsal outrigger to maintain MCP joint extension. Rubber bands may be pulled in a radial direction to avoid recurrence of ulnar deviation. **B,** This orthosis uses a Phoenix Outrigger Kit to achieve the same goal. **C,** This higher profile orthosis design, although also using rubber band traction, requires less force to initiate and maintain motion.

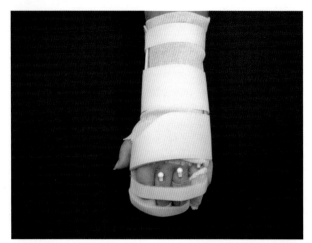

Fig. 86.10 This static night extension orthosis uses Velcro straps to position the fingers in optimal alignment and prevent ulnar drift.

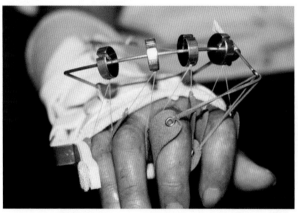

Fig. 86.11 This orthosis has an additional outrigger that allows for the creation of a force couple (i.e., two equal and opposite forces that act along parallel lines by the combined pull of the two slings). A force couple is used to control rotation of the involved digit and produces a corrective rotational torque in either supination or pronation on the digit without interfering with flexion and extension.

Boozer and coworkers[59] compared the forces involved in high-profile positioning versus low-profile dynamic positioning. They found that even though the low-profile orthosis is easier to apply and more acceptable to the patient, the high-profile orthosis requires less force to initiate and maintain motion, and the high-profile force couple design provides greater index-digit supination during ROM. When fabricating low-profile orthoses, it is imperative to keep the force as low as possible. This study demonstrated that 40% more force was required to move the low-profile sling versus the high-profile sling.[59]

Within the dynamic orthosis, the wrist is held in neutral to 20 degrees of extension and 10 to 20 degrees of ulnar deviation. The thumb may be included in the orthosis if it has been reconstructed, or to limit lateral pinch.

A static orthosis may be provided for the patient to wear while sleeping. The night orthosis is made with support of the wrist and of the MCP joints in neutral extension with control of alignment. The night orthosis is worn for 3 to 6 months after surgery or longer as determined by joint alignment and the presence of extensor lag. It is critical to have patients demonstrate the ability to remove and apply their orthosis using proper techniques to avoid inappropriate stress to the reconstructed MCP joints when applying the orthosis, which is especially important during the initial postoperative period.

Exercise. The encapsulation process around the MCP joint begins during the first week. During this time, the emphasis is on edema reduction with AROM and gentle PROM performed within the orthosis. The shelf (or tabletop) position is emphasized. The MCP joint is flexed and then the fingers curl from this intrinsic-plus position, slowly flexing into the palm. The focus is on the ROM of the MCP joint. If needed, PIP joint extension orthoses can be used to activate the EDC in the intrinsic-plus position.[53]

Occasionally, the index finger may show a tendency toward supination or pronation, and an additional outrigger may be needed (see Fig. 86.11). This outrigger allows creation of a force couple (i.e., two equal and opposite forces that act along parallel lines by the combined pull of the two slings). This coupling produces a torque in the required direction on the digit without interfering with flexion and extension or exercise performance.

During the second week after surgery, collagen formation increases around the implant. The reconstructed joints become more stable during the second and third postoperative week. This may be perceived by the patient and therapist as increased stiffness of the reconstructed joints. It is important to monitor the ROM of the MCP joints during this time to ensure that the desired degree of motion is maintained during this phase of scar production and early scar maturation.

Because the small finger may tend to have weak flexor power resulting from chronic subluxation at the MCP joint, it should be closely monitored to ensure that the desired degree of flexion is achieved. Often this is difficult for the patient to observe, and mirrors may be helpful to demonstrate MCP joint flexion during AROM exercises. Buddy taping the small finger at the proximal phalanx level to the ring finger may assist with small finger MCP joint flexion.

Weeks 3 to 4. The implant is clinically stable at 21 days, and out-of-orthosis exercises may be added (dynamic program) or continued (SAM program) with monitoring and control of alignment during exercises. Radial finger walking is encouraged to prevent ulnar drift. Passive flexion cuffs or rubber-band traction can be used if MCP joint flexion is not at the desired range. The frequency and duration of orthotic positioning and therapy are determined by objective measurements of AROM and PROM. If active MCP flexion is improving but MCP joint extension is limited, more emphasis is placed on active extension and EDC gliding exercises, and more time may be spent in the static MCP extension orthosis.

In the late fibroblastic stage (4 weeks), coordination and balancing exercises to maintain flexion and extension may be initiated. Joint protection principles are constantly reviewed to modify and correct the patient's behaviors and habits.

Week 5. At 5 weeks, light ADLs and functional activities are permitted with joint protection principles observed. Avoiding deforming postures, respecting pain, using the forearm instead of the hand for carrying objects such as a grocery bag, and avoiding static positions for prolonged periods can be helpful. Therapy continues with ROM exercises and light functional strengthening. The dynamic orthosis may be continued if needed to control alignment and to provide an extension assist if an extensor lag is present.

Weeks 6 to 8. At 6 weeks, the implant is encapsulated, and the daytime dynamic orthosis may be discontinued. It may be beneficial for some patients to use a small hand-based orthosis during activities (Fig. 86.12) to protect the reconstructed joints from undesirable forces imparted during activities. Return to light or supervisory work is allowed. The therapist must reinforce to the patient the importance of performing gentle, tolerable exercise while respecting pain and to avoid lateral stress to the MCP joints during ADLs and carrying tasks.

At 8 weeks, the scar remodeling and maturation phase is well under way, and functional strengthening as well as night positioning is continued if a persistent extension lag or tendency toward flexion

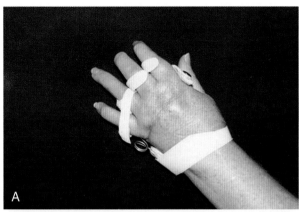

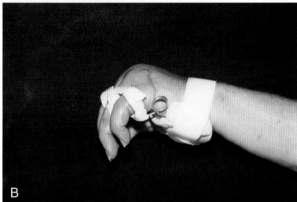

Fig. 86.12 A and **B,** This hand-based orthosis is spring-loaded to maintain the metacarpophalangeal joints in extension yet allow for flexion during functional activities. It also maintains the digits in neutral alignment, preventing ulnar drift.

contracture or deviation of digits exists. Wear of the night orthosis can continue for 3 months to 1 year.[55,56]

Outcomes

Improved appearance, improved function, and decreased pain are all important motivators for individuals to undergo MCP joint arthroplasty.[60] Patient satisfaction after 1 year has been reported to be high in all three of these domains as reported in a randomized, controlled trial of 33 patients who received both Swanson and NeuFlex implants.[60] An average of a 42-degree arc of motion at MCP joint has been reported after Swanson implant arthroplasty.[56]

Postoperative Therapy for Pyrolytic Carbon Implants for Rheumatoid Arthritis (Metacarpophalangeal Joint)

Beckenbaugh and Lund[61] have developed specific guidelines for postoperative management for patients with RA after MCP joint arthroplasty with pyrolytic carbon implants and separate guidelines for patients with OA and trauma.[62] These guidelines are summarized in Box 86.2.

THE PROXIMAL INTERPHALANGEAL JOINT

Proximal Interphalangeal Joint Arthroplasty

Indications for PIP joint replacement include a history and physical findings of pain, stiffness, and loss of motion. These should be coupled with the radiographic findings of loss of 50% or more of the articular surface of the PIP joint, bone stock loss, hypertrophic spurs, and subluxation or angulation. In general, PIP joint

arthroplasties are reserved for the central digits; however, in certain unique instances, the index or small finger PIP joint may be better served by arthroplasty than arthrodesis. In these patients, the collateral ligaments and dorsal apparatus must be protected with a small custom-molded finger orthosis in as close to full extension as possible. Some surgeons prefer to avoid replacement of the index finger PIP joint because the relatively high forces with grip and pinch predispose the joint to early failure.[63] Fusion of the painful and unstable PIP joint in the index finger is the procedure of choice, particularly in younger patients.

Volar, dorsal, or lateral approaches may be used.[64,65] In a long-term study of surface replacement prostheses, Murray and coworkers[66] reported that PIP joint prostheses implanted through a volar approach failed more often than those implanted via a dorsal approach (relative risk, 6.59; $P = .004$). It should be noted, however, that other surgeons have reported satisfactory outcomes with the volar approach.[65] The authors prefer to use a dorsal curvilinear or straight incision. The central slip may be split centrally or the Chamay approach may be used to gain access to the joint (Fig. 86.13 and Video 86.1).[64]

Similar to the MCP joint, currently three basic implant types are : available for PIP joint arthroplasty in the United States: silicone, pyrocarbon, and metal-on-polyethylene. If a resurfacing implant is selected, the collateral ligaments should be preserved.

The silicone implant is a Swanson-type dynamic spacer that remains popular for low-demand, usually older, patients, often with osteoporosis. The Swanson-type silicone implants used to treat the PIP joint are identical to those used in the MCP joint. The literature shows high patient satisfaction with significant pain relief.[67,68] Over time, stress and wear may lead to mechanical failure and degradation and may result in implant fracture in up to 30% of cases.[63,67,68] Full PIP joint ROM after Silastic implant arthroplasty is not expected.[68] Joint stability is achieved through reconstruction of ligamentous and musculotendinous systems. Postoperative management depends on the soft tissue reconstruction performed.

Surface replacement pyrocarbon and metal-on-polyethylene arthroplasty are designed to mimic normal mechanics of the PIP joint by using a virtual axis as opposed to a fixed axis as seen with the silicone joints. Furthermore, they have more desirable wear properties than silicone implants. Similar to the SR MCP prosthesis, the SR PIP implant is composed of a cobalt–chromium proximal phalanx stem and an ultra-high-molecular-weight polyethylene articular surface (see Fig. 86.13A). Fixation may be achieved with or without bone cement. Contraindications for use of this implant include acute or chronic infection, loss of the extensor mechanism or flexor tendon function, an inadequate soft tissue envelope, and incompetent collateral ligaments or volar plate of the PIP joint. Relative contraindications include the presence of static swan-neck or boutonnière deformities.[66,69] Murray and coworkers[66] found that the cumulative 5-year incidence of implant failure occurred more frequently in patients with RA than those with OA (20% vs 8%, $P = .17$). Implant failure was salvaged with arthro desis, revision arthroplasty, or amputation. Jennings and Livingstone[69] retrospectively reviewed 39 SR PIP arthroplasties used to treat OA and RA at a mean of 9.3 years postoperatively. Although an average PIP arc of 56 degrees of motion was maintained, results were poor in the two patients with RA because one of these patients developed a progressive boutonnière deformity, and the other had a revision to a silicon arthroplasty secondary to persistent pain.[69]

As for the pyrolytic PIP joint implants, medium-term outcomes have blunted enthusiasm for their use. Sweets and Stern[47] presented the results of 31 osteoarthritic PIP joints treated with pyrocarbon arthroplasty (Ascension Orthopedics, Inc., Austin, TX). At a mean follow-up duration of 55 months, PIP joint ROM was 31 degrees.

Postoperative Therapy for Pyrolytic Carbon Implants (MCP Joint)

For patients with rheumatoid arthritis (RA), the postoperative protocol includes an immediate postoperative dressing that is well padded and includes a dorsal or volar plaster orthosis with the wrist in 10 to 15 degrees of dorsiflexion. In contrast to the "safe position," in which the metacarpophalangeal (MCP) joints are flexed and the proximal interphalangeal (PIP) joints are extended, after pyrocarbon implant, the MCP joints are held in extension to achieve more stability while the PIP joints are held in slight (5–10 degrees) flexion. On the fourth postoperative day, the bulky dressing is changed, and a second postoperative orthosis is applied that may be less bulky but now maintains the wrist in neutral to slight dorsiflexion and slight ulnar deviation to counter the tendency of rheumatoid wrists to collapse in radial deviation while the MCP joints are still held in full extension and the PIP joints in slight flexion. This position is maintained for the next 3 weeks, maintaining MCP joint extension while allowing PIP joint flexion and extension in the orthosis. Beckenbaugh and coworkers[62] recommend a radiograph in the orthosis to confirm satisfactory position of the implants. Postoperative edema is managed by light compressive bandages, being careful not to apply too much tension or torque to the skin, which could result in blister formation and potential skin loss. Retrograde massage of the fingers may be initiated at this time as well. While the PIP joints are allowed active and passive motion, care must be taken to avoid rotation, compression, or distraction of the PIP joints.

At 3 weeks, the plaster orthosis is removed and a light dressing applied. A dynamic MCP joint extension orthosis is fabricated with Orthoplast (WisdomKing.com, Inc., Oceanside, CA) and an outrigger for daytime use and to guide the patient during active exercise. As with the postoperative plaster, the wrist is again positioned in neutral with 10 to 15 degrees of ulnar deviation. The MCP joints are at 0 degrees, also with slight radial deviation, and the PIP joints are left free for active motion. Radial outriggers can be added to prevent ulnar drift at the proximal phalanx and derotational slings as needed to correct index finger pronation or supination. Evaluation of MCP joint resting position is critical. If the MCP joints tend to hyperextend, the tension on the dynamic extension in the outrigger must be decreased and in some cases discontinued, applying a static orthosis to hold the MCP joints in neutral position. The Mayo protocol recommends that a resting orthosis be worn at night, which is usually more comfortable for the patient. The resting orthosis holds the wrist at 0 to 10 degrees of dorsiflexion with slight ulnar deviation. The MCP joints are at 0 degrees with finger dividers or Velcro (Velcro USA, Manchester, NH) straps to maintain slight radial deviation. The PIP joints are in a "relaxed position," allowing active flexion, and the thumb is excluded from the orthosis unless the MCP joint of the thumb has been fused or replaced, in which case it is incorporated in the orthosis.

If intrinsic tightness is present or there is significant IP joint stiffness, a third orthosis may prove helpful. This orthosis is applied to the volar surface of the forearm and extends to the PIP joints, allowing full PIP joint flexion. The orthosis holds the MCP joint in 10 degrees of extension with slight ulnar deviation of the wrist. A radiograph in the orthosis may prove helpful to demonstrate good position of the implants.

A unique therapeutic feature of this implant is the restriction of flexion at the MCP joint for the first 3 to 6 weeks. Although some flexion of up to 45 degrees may be safe and maintain stability of the joint, the therapist is advised to err on the side of being conservative unless the surgeon communicates directly that for one reason or another, early flexion is desirable. Exercise is confined to the dynamic orthosis during this time frame, with the motion allowed to be between 0 and 45 degrees of flexion. If more aggressive motion is started, the therapist and surgeon run the risk of recurrent ulnar deviation or an extensor lag, or both. For certain patients, an exercise template may be helpful to limit motion. As in the management of silicone implants, all exercise should be carried out in a slow, deliberate, pain-free manner, allowing PIP joint and distal interphalangeal (DIP) joint flexion, radial finger walking, and gentle tip-to-tip pinch with opposition to the thumb with MCP joint flexion that does not exceed 45 degrees. Exercise should be done hourly throughout the day with repetitions of 10 to 15 cycles. In this 2- to 6-week postoperative interval, sound joint protection principles are also important to reinforce good alignment of the implant and the remainder of the finger. Resistive exercises are deferred until 6 weeks to prevent subluxation of the implant, and activities of

daily living (ADLs) such as using a toothbrush may be modified by using a built-up handle on the brush. This same handle modification can be applied to a hairbrush or a razor. At between 4 and 6 weeks, light functional activities are encouraged while the patient is still wearing the orthosis, and a follow-up radiograph is encouraged to be certain the implants have remained in a stable position. At 6 weeks, dynamic flexion can be increased in the orthosis to 60 degrees, and under the supervision of a therapist, some active flexion without resistance can be initiated out of the orthosis, incorporating active flexion and extension of the PIP and DIP joints as well as the MCP joint. Shoulder, neck, elbow, and wrist motion are also encouraged at this time with light activities.

12 Weeks

Beckenbaugh[62,63] recommends not flexing the MCP joint beyond 60 degrees for the first year. This requires careful monitoring on the part of the patient and the therapist to avoid undue stress on the implant. Good joint protection principles are equally important and must be incorporated into the patient's day-to-day existence. Therapy visits are decreased when the patient can maintain alignment of the implant during active range of motion (AROM) without evidence of ulnar drift or hyperextension. The dynamic orthosis is discontinued and the static orthosis is used at night for a minimum of 1 year. The Mayo protocol recommends wearing the static night orthosis indefinitely to maintain the digits in full extension and neutral deviation.

Management of Metacarpophalangeal Joint Replacements in Osteoarthritis and Posttraumatic Osteoarthritis (Mayo Approach)

The main difference in the care and management of patients undergoing joint replacement of osteoarthritis (OA) or posttraumatic OA is that the soft tissues are generally healthier than soft tissues in patients with RA. This may be less of a consideration as disease-modifying drugs such as adalimumab (Humira; Abbott Laboratories, Abbott Park, IL) become more commonplace and tissues better preserved; nevertheless, when disease-modifying drugs are used, patients are at greater risk for infection, and soft tissues are still less forgiving, although they are healthier in appearance. At 2 to 4 days postoperative, the bulky orthosis applied in the operating room for MCP joint replacement in the OA or posttraumatic OA patient is removed, the dynamic orthosis is fabricated for daytime use, and exercises are begun in the orthosis; a resting static orthosis is used only at night. Good communication with the surgeon is important to be sure that the surgeon has no concerns regarding the stability of the implant. If only the central digits, such as the long or ring finger, have been replaced, buddy taping to the adjacent uninvolved digit may be all that is required, and a dynamic orthosis may not be necessary. Under these circumstances, a protective static orthosis is still recommended for the patient to wear during the day, when not exercising.

1 Week Postoperative

Active flexion continues but is limited to 60 degrees during the first 2 weeks to protect the extensor tendon. Exercises are performed in the same slow, deliberate pain-free manner, in the dynamic orthosis or buddy tape, to assure that no rotation or ulnar deviation occurs throughout the arc of flexion. Exercises include AROM of the MCP joint between 0 to 45 and 0 to 60 degrees, opposition of each fingertip to the thumb, tip to tip only (no lateral pinch), with a focus on maintaining full MCP joint extension.

4 to 6 Weeks

Light ADLs without the orthosis are initiated, observing joint protection principles and maintaining neutral alignment. Flexion of the MCP joint to 60 degrees is allowed, but night orthotic positioning is continued. If there is stiffness and 60 degrees flexion is not achieved by this time, a dynamic flexion orthosis may be required.

6 Weeks

At 6 weeks, the orthosis can be removed during the day for most activities, with the therapy program focused on ADLs and avocational activities, as well as on maintaining good alignment of the implant in flexion and extension. In general, by 12 weeks, all activities are permitted, with the exception of some extreme activities such as operating air-driven power tools and using a sledge hammer.

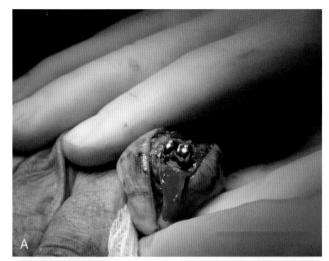

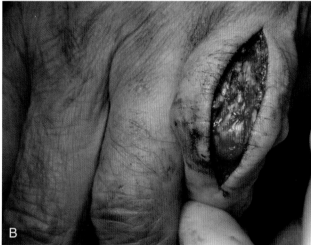

Fig. 86.13 A, The Chamay approach to the proximal interphalangeal joint was used in this patient to place a surface replacement implant. **B,** Subsequent repair of the extensor mechanism.

TABLE 86.3 Treatment Options for Boutonnière Deformity Based on Classification

Stage	PIP Joint	DIP Joint
1. Mild	Splinting	Extensor tenotomy
• Passively correctable	Injection or	
• Normal articular surface	tenosynovectomy	
2. Moderate	Treat as stage 1	Extensor tenotomy
• Passively correctable	± Extensor	
• Normal articular surface	reconstruction	
2. Moderate	Treat as stage 1	Extensor tenotomy
• Partially passively correctable	Convert to correctable	
• Normal articular surface	Extensor reconstruction	
2. Moderate to severe	Treat as above	Extensor tenotomy
• Fixed	If correctable →extensor reconstruction	
• Normal articular surface	If not correctable → salvage	
3. Joint destruction	Arthrodesis or arthroplasty	Extensor tenotomy

DIP, Distal interphalangeal; *PIP,* proximal interphalangeal.
Data from Williams K, Terrono AL. Treatment of boutonniere finger deformity in rheumatoid arthritis. *J Hand Surg Am.* 2011;36:1388-1393.

addition, the one patient with considerable migration of the implant also had RA. Again, these results demonstrate that patients with RA may have less successful outcomes after pyrocarbon arthroplasty even when hemiarthroplasty is used.

Postoperative Management of Proximal Interphalangeal Joint Arthroplasty

To plan an appropriate treatment program after PIP joint replacement, the therapist must first know which implant was used and what surgical approach or procedure was performed. It is helpful for the therapist to be aware that a functional hand has an index finger PIP joint that can flex to 45 degrees, a long finger PIP joint that can flex to 60 degrees, and a ring and small finger PIP joint that can flex to 70 degrees.[54]

Swanson Silicone Implant

A systematic literature review reports that the average PIP joint arc of motion achieved with the Swanson implant is 44 degrees.[77] Over time, stress and wear may lead to mechanical failure and degradation and may result in implant fracture or dislocation, silicone synovitis, infection, pain recurrence, stiffness, or deformity.[45] Full PIP joint ROM after Silastic implant arthroplasty is not expected. In fact, more than 90 degrees of PIP flexion may lead to implant fracture.[78] The Swanson silicone implant is a flexible hinge that acts as a dynamic spacer to maintain internal alignment and spacing of the reconstructed joint and as an internal mold that supports the healing capsuloligamentous system while early motion begins.[79] The implant becomes stabilized by the encapsulation process.[41,79,80] Joint stability is achieved through reconstruction of ligamentous and musculotendinous systems. Postoperative management depends on the soft tissue reconstruction performed.

Three surgical approaches may used: volar, dorsal, or lateral. A variety of surgical techniques have been described in association with these approaches. Table 86.4 describes these techniques along with the structures that are released or repaired and will require protection, the structures left intact, and general treatment guidelines. Therapists must

However, 12 of 31 implants in the proximal phalanx subsided more than 2 mm, and 5 of 31 implants in the middle phalanx subsided more than 2 mm. In some cases, implant subluxation lead to implant dislocation. Other complications included implant fracture, and almost 50% of implants were loose by radiographic criteria. In addition, 35% of patients reported squeaking in their joints at some point postoperatively.[47] Long-term outcome studies have corroborated high revision rates, usually secondary to implant loosening or instability.[48] Although some authors have recently reported low complication rates and long-term survivorship in patients with OA,[70] most hand surgeons in the United States are reluctant to use pyrocarbon implants in rheumatoid patients.

Because of the generally poor results of PIP pyrocarbon arthroplasty, some authors have attempted PIP joint hemiarthroplasty instead.[71] Compared with total joint arthroplasty, proximal phalanx hemiarthroplasty is technically simpler and preserves more bone stock. Prerequisites to this procedure are intact collateral ligaments and adequate bone stock and bone quality of the distal aspect of the proximal phalanx. Based on an average follow-up period of 4.6 years, these implants demonstrated improvements in pain and clinically important improvements in function based on the DASH score. PIP joint ROM, grip strength, and pinch strength were preserved. In the series by Pettersson and coworkers,[71] 20% of RA patients had treatment failures. In

TABLE 86.4		Surgical Techniques Common to Proximal Interphalangeal Joint Arthroplasty		
Procedure[a]	Approach	Released or Repaired Structures Requiring Protection	Structures Left Intact	Postoperative Treatment
Central slip sparing technique	Dorsal	Collateral ligaments and palmar plate; joint is dislocated volarly	Extensors, allowing immediate AROM	Buddy taping to radial digit for exercise; forearm trough or hand based static extension orthosis
Palmar approach[92]	Volar	Flexor sheath insertion; palmar plate; and UCL; joint is dorsally dislocated	Extensors and flexors, allowing early mobilization	Pulley ring; 30-degree extension block for 4 wk; night static extension orthosis
Lateral approach[93]	Lateral	Collateral ligaments and volar plate; joint is opened like a book	Extensors and flexors, allowing early mobilization	Buddy tapes or dynamic splint; night static extension splint
Central slip splitting technique[94]	Dorsal	Central slip is longitudinally split and detached; palmar plate is possibly disrupted	Collateral ligaments, increasing joint stability	Mobilization is delayed 2–4 wk; night extension orthosis; daily dynamic extension orthosis
Dorsal Chamay repair[95]	Dorsal	Triangular flap is dissected from extensor apparatus and lifted up	Central tendon, allowing early AROM	Extension orthotic positioning for PIP joint; flexion may progress quickly

[a]The central slip sparing technique, the lateral approach, the palmar approach, and the central slip splitting technique are commonly used with the Swanson implant. The central slip splitting technique is also commonly used with the pyrocarbon implant as well as the dorsal Chamay procedure.[57,80,86]

AROM, Active range of motion; *PIP,* proximal interphalangeal; *UCL,* ulnar collateral ligament.
Reprinted with permission from Feldscher SB. Postoperative management for PIP joint pyrocarbon arthroplasty. *J Hand Ther.* 2010;23(3):315-322.

understand what structures require protection with each procedure to better understand postoperative needs with regard to exercise and protective orthotic positioning. As new procedures and implants are introduced, we must consider what structures are disrupted and what type of postoperative protection will be required.

Surface Replacement Arthroplasty

Surface replacement arthroplasty has recently gained popularity in an effort to improve joint biomechanics. SRA is a technically demanding procedure that requires an experienced hand therapist who is able to provide diligent monitoring, clinical reasoning, and a problem-solving approach to treatment. Direct communication between the surgeon and therapist is essential. Potential complications must be recognized early, and treatment modified. Each patient and each joint are unique and may require a variety of treatment solutions. Two implants commonly used with SRA are the Ascension PIP joint implant and the Stryker implant (SR PIP).

Ascension Proximal Interphalangeal Joint Implant

Pyrocarbon is a strong, fatigue- and wear-resistant, ceramic-like material made of pyrolytic carbon.[81] The Ascension PIP joint implant is a two-component, bicondylar, semiconstrained prosthesis designed to replace the articulating surfaces of the PIP joint and accommodate maximum anatomic ROM.[82] The proximal component has a dorsal groove to allow central tendon tracking.[82] Final implant fixation stabilization occurs 6 to 24 months postoperatively.[83]

Ascension has published a therapy protocol (Ascension protocol) for a PyroCarbon PIP Total Joint as a guideline for patients with OA or traumatic arthritis (http://www.smith-nephew.com).[84] To apply this protocol to individuals with RA, it is important to assess each individual case by case and make modifications as needed. Up to 3 weeks of immobilization may be indicated in the case of RA to provide soft tissue stabilization before initiating active motion at the PIP joint. AROM is dictated by extensor tendon status and surgical technique.

In general, after arthroplasty using a PyroCarbon PIP implant with a dorsal approach in an individual with RA, postoperative management begins at 1 to 2 weeks postsurgery with the fabrication of a dorsal, static finger orthosis, with the PIP joint blocked at 15 to 20 degrees

of flexion.[84] This orthosis may be used for up to 3 months postsurgery. A SAM protocol is initiated 3 weeks postsurgery, beginning with fabrication of an exercise orthosis which allows for 30 to 45 degrees of PIP joint flexion.[85] Avoiding hyperextension is crucial during this period.[85] PIP joint flexion is advanced based on the ability to maintain active extension vs stiffness. If a PIP joint active extensor lag is present, then the progression of flexion is delayed, whereas if stiffness is present, SAM is increased.[54] When appropriate, light ADL activities are incorporated into the program. The patient is educated about joint protection techniques and the importance of avoiding lateral and rotational forces at the PIP joint and not overstressing the new joint.

Several precautions require discussion. Lateral stress to the PIP joint must be avoided for a minimum of 12 weeks. Index fingers must be closely monitored because of lateral forces applied during pinch. Flexion must not be regained at the expense of extension. If an extension lag develops, flexion increments should be more modest, and extension orthotic positioning and exercises emphasized. PIP joint hyperextension must be avoided. If hyperextension is noted, a dorsal block orthosis should be fabricated for full-time use with the PIP joint at 30 degrees of flexion, allowing for a 30- to 60-degree arc of motion. When joint stability is regained, the orthosis can be weaned and ROM progressed.

Table 86.5 compares the Swanson implant to the Ascension pyrocarbon implant.[37–39,41,42,48–53,64,68,69] Most important, note that the Swanson implant has one component, and the Ascension implant has two components.

In the recent past, dynamic orthoses were primarily used to manage the PyroCarbon implant postoperatively and may still be beneficial in the hands of a skilled surgeon and therapist. These approaches are described in detail elsewhere.[86] When dynamic orthoses after PIP joint arthroplasty are applied, the goals are to prevent recurrent deformity and guide motion of the PIP joint during healing to influence the orientation of the healing capsular structures so as to obtain desired mobility, stability, and alignment. When therapists apply a dynamic orthosis to an Ascension implant, force is applied to only one half of the implant (Fig. 86.14). If the soft tissue stabilization is not adequate or the force is too great, implant migration may occur. It is vital that all orthoses are checked with radiographs

TABLE 86.5 Comparison of the Swanson Implant with the Ascension Pyrocarbon Implant

	Swanson Implant	Ascension Implant
Number of components	One	Two
Fixation	Noncement	Noncement
Joint stability	Achieved through reconstruction of ligamentous and musculotendinous systems. Encapsulation process. Osseous ingrowth	Attained from surrounding capsuloligamentous structures. Press fit stabilized by insertion into medullary canals followed by appositional bone growth
Implant stabilization	Occurs when released ligaments and scar have healed	Final implant fixation stabilization occurs 6–24 mo postoperatively
Surgery	Volar, dorsal, or lateral approach	Dorsal approach using a Chamay or extensor tendon splitting technique
Postoperative management	Depends on surgical technique and structures repaired	Based on repair of extensor tendon
ROM goals	Long finger, 0/45; ring finger, 0/60; small finger, 0/70. Not recommended for use in index fingers	0/75. Believed safe for use in index fingers
Stress level	Unable to withstand full ROM and functional stress	Designed to accommodate maximum anatomic ROM
Uses	Sedentary low-demand patients	A better option for younger active patients
Isolated disability	Yes	No

ROM, Range of motion.
Reprinted with permission from Feldscher SB. Postoperative management for PIP joint pyrocarbon arthroplasty. *J Hand Ther.* 2010;23(3):315-322.

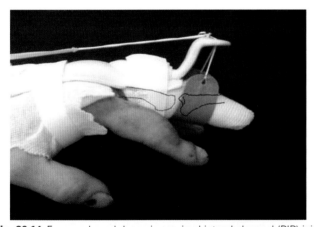

Fig. 86.14 Forearm-based dynamic proximal interphalangeal (PIP) joint extension orthosis with a two-component implant drawn in position. Note that the force is applied to only one half of the implant. The proximal component is held stable in the orthosis, while the force is applied distally. If the soft tissue stabilization is not adequate or the force is too great, implant migration could occur. It is vital that all orthoses are checked with radiographs to ensure proper joint alignment. Poor alignment will not necessarily be visible to the naked eye. (Reprinted with permission from Feldscher SB. Postoperative management for PIP joint pyrocarbon arthroplasty. *J Hand Ther.* 2010; 23[3]:315-322.)

(as recommended by the manufacturer) to ensure proper joint alignment. Poor alignment may not be visible to the naked eye, especially in an edematous finger.

Stryker SR PIP Implant

The SR PIP implant has two components: a distal component that combines a titanium alloy stem (which has an external surface to allow bone growth) with an ultra-high-molecular-weight-polyethylene articulating surface and a proximal component consisting of a cobalt–chromium–molybdenum articulating surface. The components articulate on each other to form a semiconstrained prosthetic replacement for the PIP joint.[76] The kinematics of this implant have been found to closely mimic those of a normal joint with well-preserved soft tissues.[87] The implant is designed to allow a 90-degree arc of flexion–extension; however, a stable pain-free 60-degree PIP joint arc of motion is considered a good result.[76] A dorsal or volar surgical approach can be used. Postoperative guidelines are similar to those previously described for these approaches. Specific treatment guidelines are available at www.stryker.com.

Postoperative Management of Proximal Interphalangeal Joint Hemiarthroplasty

There is limited research regarding optimal postoperative programs for individuals with RA undergoing PIP joint hemiarthroplasty. Pettersson and coworkers[71] described a postoperative program, with results that suggested that patients with RA may have less successful outcomes. The program included immobilization in PIP joint extension for 3 to 7 days in a resting orthosis, while a separate orthosis was fabricated allowing 30 degrees of flexion.[71] The latter orthosis was modified over 4 to 8 weeks, progressively allowing up to 90 degrees of flexion.[71] Strengthening and unrestricted activity was permitted after 2 to 3 months.[71] The author also emphasized the need to avoid PIP hyperextension using a PIP extension block orthosis if required.[71]

Boutonnière Deformity

The digital extensor mechanism is intricate and complex as it interconnects the MCP, PIP, and DIP joints through the combined action of the intrinsic and extrinsic tendons. The intrinsic muscles (the interossei and lumbricals) link the MCP and PIP joints, whereas the oblique retinacular ligament links the PIP and DIP joints. The development of pathology at one joint may subsequently lead to pathology at an adjacent joint. This is demonstrated in both boutonnière and swan-neck deformities. The boutonnière deformity is characterized by hyperflexion of the PIP joint in addition to hyperextension of the DIP joint. Whereas the pathologic process of a swan-neck deformity may be initiated at the MCP, PIP, or DIP joint, the cause of deformity in a boutonnière digit is most often related to pathology of the central slip. Stretching of the PIP joint attenuates the central slip, leading to inability to completely extend the PIP joint. Over time, the lateral bands migrate volarly and volar to the axis of rotation at the PIP joint.[72] As a result, they contribute to flexion of the PIP joint. The lateral bands course distal to the PIP joint and unite at the terminal tendon, contributing to the hyperextension seen in the deformity. Over time, the deformity may become fixed as the lateral bands become adherent to the transverse retinacular ligament volarly. Similarly, the collateral ligaments and volar plate of the PIP joint becomes stiff, and the FDS tendon contracts. Patients with a boutonnière deformity often complain of inability to flex the DIP joint because this may limit grasp. The patients attempt to compensate by hyperextending the MCP joint. In rheumatoid patients, as in those with nonrheumatoid boutonnière deformity, treatment is based on whether the PIP joint deformity is passively correctable, the severity of the deformity, and the status of the articular surfaces of the PIP joint (Table 86.3).[72] When the articular surface of the PIP joint is intact, nonoperative treatment is the first line of treatment. The application of serial casting to the PIP joint with the DIP joint free is usually effective in improving PIP joint extension and often converts a fixed deformity to a flexible deformity. Prescribing DIP joint blocking exercises while the PIP is immobilized can be helpful to lengthen the oblique retinacular ligament and to realign the lateral bands. Terminal extensor tendon tenotomy may be performed when the deformity is flexible. This is a relatively simple procedure and restores the patient's ability to flex the DIP joint. Patients should be informed that an extensor lag at the DIP joint may develop. This is usually well tolerated, however. Central slip reconstruction may be an option for patients with a substantial yet passively correctable deformity and an intact PIP joint surface, although historically, outcomes have been unpredictable.[73] Various techniques are available, including central slip reconstruction with local tissue and lateral band dorsal realignment or reconstruction, in conjunction with a terminal tendon tenotomy. If the articular surface of the PIP joint is arthritic or the fixed contracture is severe, arthrodesis of the PIP joint is effective at positioning the digit in a more functionally tolerable position. Because of the forces imparted on the index digit during pinch, arthrodesis offers a reliable treatment option. PIP joint arthroplasty may be offered for mild deformity of the ulnar sided digits in combination with extensor tendon reconstruction.

Swan-Neck Deformity

The swan-neck deformity is characterized by PIP joint hyperextension and DIP joint flexion. In patients with RA, synovial inflammation of the MCP, IP, joints and tendons is responsible for the observed deformities. When assessing a patient with a swan-neck deformity, it is important to consider the status of both the PIP joint and intrinsic muscle flexibility because these factors influence treatment. The PIP joint may be fixed or supple, arthritic or nonarthritic, or fixed and nonarthritic.

Although nonoperative treatment is not as effective as it is in a boutonnière deformity, therapy plays a role in the correction of intrinsic tightness. Additionally, oval-8 orthoses or Silver Ring Splints that prevent PIP joint hyperextension can improve joint stability and functional grasp. Nalebuff[74] classified the rheumatoid swan-neck into one of four types based on the PIP joint mobility and integrity and offered several treatment recommendations:

- Type 1: swan-neck with a flexible PIP joint. This may be treated by DIP joint fusion, dermodesis, flexor tenodesis, or retinacular ligament reconstruction.
- Type 2: swan-neck with tight intrinsics. This may be treated with an intrinsic release.
- Type 3: swan-neck with fixed deformity and an intact articular surface of the PIP joint. This type may be treated by PIP joint manipulation, skin release and lateral band mobilization.
- Type 4: swan-neck with a stiff and arthritic PIP joint. This is best treated with fusion or arthroplasty of the PIP joint.

Postoperative Management of Boutonniere and Swan-Neck Deformities

Postoperative management of the PIP joint depends on the type of deformity present before surgery in addition to the surgical procedure performed. One must take into consideration the needs of a stiff PIP joint versus a laterally deviated PIP joint versus one having a boutonnière or swan-neck deformity.[54] In the case of a preoperatively stiff PIP joint, AROM and dynamic flexion splinting may need to be initiated earlier in the rehabilitation process.[54] When PIP joint lateral deviation is present, an orthosis may need to be applied laterally to better align the joint and AROM may be delayed, allowing for adequate tissue healing.[54] With a boutonnière deformity, an orthosis is typically applied with the PIP joint in full extension, and AROM may

be delayed to allow for adequate tissue healing.[54] Finally, in the case of a swan-neck deformity, a PIP joint dorsal block orthosis is usually applied in 20 to 30 degrees of flexion, and AROM may be delayed to allow for adequate tissue healing.[54] In general, night orthosis use may continue for up to 3 months.[54] Joint protection education on avoiding lateral stresses during ADLs is imperative, and buddy straps may be required to maintain good joint alignment.[54] Overall, the goal of therapy is to slowly advance PIP joint flexion without sacrificing extension.

Proximal Interphalangeal Joint Arthrodesis

Fusion of the PIP joint is the treatment of choice when the deformity is severe and the joint is arthritic. Furthermore, fusion may be selected as a salvage option after failed PIP joint arthroplasty. Although motion is eliminated, this procedure may offer predictable pain relief, joint correction, and stability. The index finger in particular does well with fusion because it is subjected to greater forces with pinch. Fusion of the PIP joint in 25 to 40 degrees offers pain relief and improved function, provided that the procedure is without complications. Fusion of the PIP joint may be achieved with either single or dual column small plate fixation, intramedullary pins or screw, or K-wires and a tension band construct.[75,76] Patient age, activity level, bone stock, bone quality, and soft tissue quality should all be considered when deciding on the most appropriate fixation construct. Plate fixation and intramedullary linked screw arthrodesis tends to result in stiffer fixation constructs and may be more desirable in younger, more active patients because these methods allow early motion of the MCP and DIP joints.[76]

Postoperative Management of Proximal Interphalangeal Joint Arthrodesis

Rehabilitation consists of immobilization of the involved joint for 6 to 12 weeks or until bony healing occurs. When deemed safe, it is essential to begin to incorporate ADL and function-based activities because the patient will have learned to bypass the involved digit.

THE DISTAL INTERPHALANGEAL JOINT

Replacement of the DIP joint, although technically feasible, rarely is performed. In most patients, DIP joint fusion is a far more satisfactory procedure (see Fig. 86.7C and D). Although not allowing motion, arthrodesis provides pain relief and correction of deformity, leaving the joint in a functional position and allowing for early mobilization of the finger. As with the PIP joint, replacement of the DIP joint of the index or small finger is relatively contraindicated because of the high forces across the joint in pinch and grip; therefore, because of the high probability of failure in a short time in high-demand, younger patients, replacement of these joints is reserved for more sedentary individuals. For central digits or for patients in whom replacement of the DIP joint in a border digit is selected, the technique is similar to that used for the PIP and MCP joints. We prefer an H-shaped incision with the transverse component of the incision over the DIP joint. The incision extends in a palmar direction to the midaxial line on both the radial and ulnar sides of the joint before extending proximally and distally for ideal exposure and release of the collateral ligaments. To preserve stability and extension of the DIP joint postoperatively, the terminal tendon to the dorsal apparatus is left intact whenever possible. The terminal tendon can be safely reflected in a radial or ulnar direction and exposure of the joint achieved through the ulnar collateral ligament. Some surgeons also consider dividing the terminal tendon. The distal surface of the middle phalanx is removed with an oscillating saw and the proximal surface of the distal phalanx debrided and flattened with a rongeur. A trial fit is performed using a single-axis type of implant, and the final prosthesis is impacted into place. After

TABLE 86.6 Nalebuff[87] Classification of Rheumatoid Thumb Deformities

Type	CMC Joint	MCP Joint	IP Joint
I (boutonnière)	Not involved	Flexed	Hyperextended
II (uncommon)	CMC flexed and adducted	Flexed	Hyperextended
III (swan neck)	CMC subluxed, flexed, and adducted	Hyperextended	Flexed
IV (gamekeeper's)	CMC not subluxed; flexed and adducted	Hyperextended, UCL unstable	Not involved
V	May or may not be involved	Volar plate unstable	Not involved
VI (arthritis mutilans)	Bone loss at any level	Bone loss at any level	Bone loss at any level

CMC, Carpometacarpal; *IP*, interphalangeal; *MCP*, metacarpophalangeal; *UCL*, ulnar collateral ligament.

wound closure and repair of the terminal tendon, the DIP joint is positioned in extension for 6 weeks. Often a cylinder cast is the best way to maintain DIP joint extension. Sutures are left in place for 7 to 10 days. At 6 weeks, a gentle ROM program begins, but orthotic positioning is continued for a total of 12 weeks.

THE THUMB

The authors would like to acknowledge Andrew L. Terrono, MD; Edward A. Nalebuff, MD; and Cynthia A. Philips, MA, OTR/L, CHT, for their contributions to the chapter on the rheumatoid thumb in the sixth edition of *Rehabilitation of the Hand and Upper Extremity*, much of which has been incorporated into this section. Readers are urged to refer to the aforementioned chapter for a more detailed description of the rheumatoid thumb.

Rheumatoid arthritis often involves the thumb. Pain and disruption of the normal thumb biomechanics often lead to substantial loss of the patient's ability to carry out ADLs. Evaluation of the thumb should be placed in the context of global hand function.

The deformities encountered in the rheumatoid thumb are the result of ligamentous instability and imbalances of the intrinsic and extrinsic muscles and tendons of the thumb. Nalebuff classified the rheumatoid thumb into six types based on deformities to the thumb CMC, MCP, and IP joints (Table 86.6).[87] These six thumb deformities, unfortunately, do not exhaust the range of deformities one encounters in RA.[88]

Nonoperative and operative treatment are aimed at preventing and correcting the various thumb deformities and restoring function. When deformities are passively correctable, hand therapy helps to maintain joint mobility and joint protection through the use of orthoses and activity modification. These interventions, along with medical treatment, may afford patients considerable relief and may slow the progression of deformity. When nonoperative measures have been expended, surgery may be useful to correct the deformity, provide stability, and relieve pain. Surgical procedures used to treat the rheumatoid thumb are guided more by the joint involved than by the specific type of deformity.

Fusion of the thumb IP joint should be considered in patients in whom the IP joint is grossly unstable, with or without intact extrinsic tendons. Arthrodesis of the IP joint of the thumb does not cause significant functional loss and in fact improves the patient's ability to pinch objects with force.[88] Fusion at this level often makes it possible to correct rotational deformities by positioning the IP joint in

a slightly flexed and pronated position. In patients with the collapse type of deformity, the use of supplemental bone grafting is useful to achieve fusion and to restore length. Several techniques may be used to achieve arthrodesis, including K-wires, tension band constructs, single retrograde compression screws, or plates. Arthroplasty for IP joint involvement in the rheumatoid thumb is rarely indicated because it does not provide good lateral stability.[88] Refer to the Tendon Rupture section for the management of FPL and EPL tendon ruptures.

The surgical procedures found useful to treat the MCP joint in rheumatoid patients include synovectomy, EPL tendon transfer, arthrodesis, arthroplasty, capsulodesis, and sesamoidesis. Tendon transfer has a role in treating the early stages of type I thumb deformity (boutonnière thumb). If both the IP and MCP joints have satisfactory passive motion, tendon transfer of the EPL one joint proximal to insert at the base of the proximal phalanx is an excellent treatment for this condition, correcting the deformities at both joints (Fig. 86.15). For an MCP joint that is grossly unstable or in which the articular cartilage has been destroyed, arthrodesis or arthroplasty may be useful. The ideal position of a thumb MCP joint fusion is 15 degrees of flexion. If the CMC joint has limited motion, 5 degrees of adduction and 20 degrees of pronation may be needed to allow the thumb to oppose to the index finger.[88] Arthroplasty with a Swanson-type implant is useful for patients with a flexion deformity.[88] This procedure is usually supplemented by reinforcing or shortening the extensor mechanism. Patients undergoing arthroplasty at this level are usually not started on early motion because of concerns about instability. In hyperextension deformities of the MCP joint, arthrodesis of the joint in a slightly flexed position is advisable. Some authors are reluctant to insert a flexible implant in patients with a hyperextension deformity of the thumb MCP joint because of the lack of volar stability. However, if arthroplasty is selected, it is advisable to repair or reconstruct the volar plate.[88]

At the CMC joint, the surgical procedures performed include various types of arthroplasties and, in specific instances, arthrodesis. Because RA commonly affects multiple joints, it is ordinarily not advisable to fuse the CMC joint. Subsequent involvement at the MCP joint level requiring fusion would leave the patient with very little mobility.[88]

Postoperative Therapy After Operative Procedures of the Rheumatoid Thumb

Synovectomy

The goal of therapy after synovectomy is to mobilize the flexor tendon, with respect to tendon integrity. Because a synovectomy may be performed by dissecting the tendon as opposed to A1 pulley release, overly aggressive programs risk rupturing the debrided tendon and require diligent management. Close communication between surgeon and therapist is critical.[89] Education of the patient regarding the complexity of the procedure and activity restrictions is an important part of the therapy plan.

Metacarpophalangeal and Interphalangeal Joint Arthrodesis

Rehabilitation consists of immobilization of the involved joint for 6 to 12 weeks or until bony healing occurs. When deemed safe, it is essential to begin to incorporate ADL and function-based activities because the patient will have learned to bypass the thumb during this time period.

Therapy Guidelines for Multiple Procedures

When patients have one or more procedures at the same time, protecting one while mobilizing another can be difficult. The Saunders chart (Table 86.7)[86] can help with staging the positioning and the therapy plan.

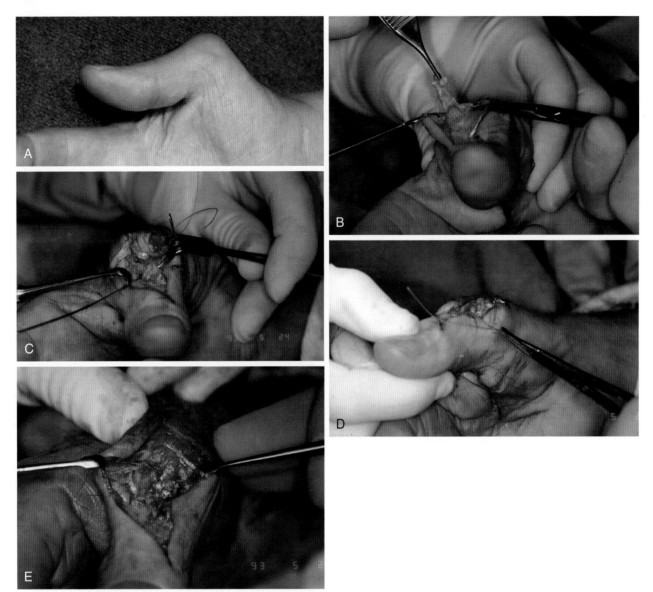

Fig. 86.15 A, Boutonnière deformity of the thumb (Nalebuff type I). **B** and **C,** Tendon transfer of the extensor pollicis longus proximally to the site of insertion of the extensor pollicis brevis, allowing the hyperextended interphalangeal joint to drop into a more flexed position and active extension of the metacarpophalangeal joint. **D** and **E,** The extensor pollicis longus anchored to bone at the base of the proximal phalanx.

TABLE 86.7	Rehabilitation Management After Multiple Procedures: Sandy Saunders Matrix[86]			
Therapeutic Management	**Wrist**	**MCP Joint**	**Thumb**	**PIP Joint**
Surgery	Darrach	MCP joint arthroplasty Swanson	MCP joint fusion	IP joint fusion
Protection	4–6 wk Volar wrist orthosis	5–6 wk Dorsal extension outrigger	MCP joint—no motion 6–8 wk Thumb spica orthosis	PIP joint 6–8 wk Gutter extension orthosis
Movement	Wrist extension–flexion Supination–pronation when comfortable	MCP joint, extension–flexion dynamic orthosis, wrist extension–flexion	IP joint, CMC joint, wrist	MCP joint, DIP joint wrist

CMC, Carpometacarpal; *DIP,* distal interphalangeal; *IP,* interphalangeal; *MCP,* metacarpophalangeal; *PIP,* proximal interphalangeal.

This approach can also help with surgeon and patient communication with simple visual feedback. For example, if a patient with OA has a basal joint arthroplasty, carpal tunnel release, and PIP joint arthroplasty of the ring finger all scheduled for the same time, the thumb must be protected in a thumb spica orthosis, wrist in neutral position, and ring finger PIP joint in extension with the ability to mobilize in 2 to 3 days. Charting what needs to be stabilized and what needs to mobilized and at what intervals makes clear the type of orthosis and therapy program required.

ACKNOWLEDGMENT

The authors would like to acknowledge Sheri Feldscher, OT, CHT, for her contributions to the chapter "Joint Replacement in the Hand and Wrist: Surgery and Therapy" in the sixth edition of *Rehabilitation of the Hand and Upper Extremity*, much of which has been incorporated into this chapter.

REFERENCES

1. Gogna R, Cheung G, Arundell M, et al. Rheumatoid hand surgery: is there a decline? A 22-year population-based study. *Hand (N Y)*. 2015;10:272–278.
2. Dafydd M, Whitaker IS, Murison MS, et al. Change in operative workload for rheumatoid disease of the hand: 1,109 procedures over 13 years. *J Plast Reconstr Aesthet Surg*. 2012;65:800–803.
3. Dreyer SJ, Boden SD. Natural history of rheumatoid arthritis of the cervical spine. *Clin Orthop Relat Res*. 1999;366:98–106.
4. Thorsness RJ, Hammert WC. Perioperative management of rheumatoid medications. *J Hand Surg Am*. 2012;37:1928–1931.
5. Barnard AR, Regan M, Burke FD, et al. Wound healing with medications for rheumatoid arthritis in hand surgery. *ISRN Rheumatol*. 2012;2012:251962.
6. Hsueh JH, Liu WC, Yang KC, et al. Spontaneous extensor tendon rupture in the rheumatoid wrist: Risk factors and preventive role of extended tenosynovectomy. *Ann Plast Surg*. 2016;76(suppl 1):S41–47.
7. Tubiana R. Technique of dorsal synovectomy on the rheumatoid wrist. *Ann Chir Main Memb Super*. 1990;9:138–145.
8. Lee HI, Lee KH, Koh KH, et al. Long-term results of arthroscopic wrist synovectomy in rheumatoid arthritis. *J Hand Surg Am*. 2014;39:1295–1300.
9. Shim JW, Park MJ. Arthroscopic synovectomy of wrist in rheumatoid arthritis. *Hand Clin*. 2017;33:779–785.
10. Vaughan-Jackson OJ. Rupture of extensor tendons by attrition at the inferior radio-ulnar joint: report of two cases. *J Bone Joint Surg Br*. 1948;30:528–530.
11. Chung US, Kim JH, Seo WS, et al. Tendon transfer or tendon graft for ruptured finger extensor tendons in rheumatoid hands. *J Hand Surg Eur*. 2010;35:279–282.
12. Bunnell S, Boyes JH, eds. *Bunnell's Surgery of the Hand*. 5th ed. Philadelphia: JB Lippincott; 1970.
13. Bora Jr FW, Osterman AL, Thomas VJ, et al. The treatment of ruptures of multiple extensor tendons at wrist level by a free tendon graft in the rheumatoid patient. *J Hand Surg Am*. 1987;12:1038–1040.
14. Yamaguchi S, Viegas SF. Extensor indicis proprius tendon: case report of a rare anatomic variation. *Clin Anat*. 2000;13:63–65.
15. Mannerfelt L, Norman O. Attrition ruptures of flexor tendons in rheumatoid arthritis caused by bony spurs in the carpal tunnel: a clinical and radiological study. *J Bone Joint Surg Br*. 1969;51:270–277.
16. O'Sullivan MB, Singh H, Wolf JM. Tendon transfers in the rheumatoid hand for reconstruction. *Hand Clin*. 2016;32:407–416.
17. Geoghegan JM, Clark DI, Bainbridge LC, et al. Risk factors in carpal tunnel syndrome. *J Hand Surg Br*. 2004;29:315–320.
18. American Academy of Orthopaedic Surgeons. Management of carpal tunnel syndrome evidence-based clinical practice guideline. www.aaos.org/ctsguideline.
19. Lee KH, Lee CH, Lee BG, et al. The incidence of carpal tunnel syndrome in patients with rheumatoid arthritis. *Int J Rheum Dis*. 2015;18:52–57.
20. Evers S, Bryan AJ, Sanders TL, et al. Corticosteroid injections for carpal tunnel syndrome: long-term follow-up in a population-based cohort. *Plast Reconstr Surg*. 2017;140:338–347.
21. Hindley CJ, Stanley JK. The rheumatoid wrist: patterns of disease progression. A review of 50 wrists. *J Hand Surg Br*. 1991;16:275–279.
22. Palmer AK, Werner FW, Murphy D, et al. Functional wrist motion: a biomechanical study. *J Hand Surg Am*. 1985;10:39–46.
23. Motomiya M, Iwasaki N, Minami A, et al. Clinical and radiological results of radiolunate arthrodesis for rheumatoid arthritis: 22 wrists followed for an average of 7 years. *J Hand Surg Am*. 2013;38:1484–1491.
24. Raven EE, Ottink KD, Doets KC. Radiolunate and radioscapholunate arthrodeses as treatments for rheumatoid and psoriatic arthritis: long-term follow-up. *J Hand Surg Am*. 2012;37:55–62.
25. Lautenbach M, Millrose M, Langner I, et al. Results of Mannerfelt wrist arthrodesis for rheumatoid arthritis in relation to the position of the fused wrist. *Int Orthop*. 2013;37:2409–2413.
26. Berling SE, Kiefhaber TR, Stern PJ. Hardware-related complications following radiocarpal arthrodesis using a dorsal plate. *J Wrist Surg*. 2015;4:56–60.
27. Kluge S, Schindele S, Henkel T, et al. The modified Clayton-Mannerfelt arthrodesis of the wrist in rheumatoid arthritis: operative technique and report on 93 cases. *J Hand Surg Am*. 2013;38:999–1005.
28. Ward CM, Kuhl T, Adams BD. Five to ten-year outcomes of the universal total wrist arthroplasty in patients with rheumatoid arthritis. *J Bone Joint Surg Am*. 2011;93:914–919.
29. Gil JA, Kamal RN, Cone E, et al. High survivorship and few complications with cementless total wrist arthroplasty at a mean followup of 9 Years. *Clin Orthop Relat Res*. 2017;475:3082–3087.
30. Badge R, Kailash K, Dickson DR, et al. Medium-term outcomes of the Universal-2 total wrist arthroplasty in patients with rheumatoid arthritis. *Bone Joint J*. 2016;98-B:1642–1647.
31. Swanson AB. Flexible implant arthroplasty for arthritic finger joints: rationale, technique, and results of treatment. *J Bone Joint Surg Am*. 1972;54:435–455.
32. Davis RF, Weiland AJ, Dowling SV. Swanson implant arthroplasty of the wrist in rheumatoid arthritis. *Clin Orthop Relat Res*. 1982;166:132–137.
33. Jolly SL, Ferlic DC, Clayton ML, et al. Swanson silicone arthroplasty of the wrist in rheumatoid arthritis: a long-term follow-up. *J Hand Surg Am*. 1992;17:142–149.
34. Galvis EJ, Pessa J, Scheker LR. Total joint arthroplasty of the distal radioulnar joint for rheumatoid arthritis. *J Hand Surg Am*. 2014;39:1699–1704.
35. Werner BC, Boatright JD, Chhabra AB, et al. Trigger digit release: rates of surgery and complications as indicated by a United States Medicare database. *J Hand Surg Eur*. 2016;41:970–976.
36. Akhavani MA, Paleolog EM, Kang N. Muscle hypoxia in rheumatoid hands: does it play a role in ulnar drift? *J Hand Surg Am*. 2011;36:677–685.
37. Morco S, Bowden A. Ulnar drift in rheumatoid arthritis: a review of biomechanical etiology. *J Biomech*. 2015;48:725–728.
38. Ellison MR, Flatt AE, Kelly KJ. Ulnar drift of the fingers in rheumatoid disease. Treatment by crossed intrinsic tendon transfer. *J Bone Joint Surg Am*. 1971;53:1061–1082.
39. Monreal R. Extensor Indicis proprius tenodesis to correct finger ulnar drift deformity in rheumatoid arthritis. *Hand (N Y)*. 2016;11:336–340.
40. Chung KC, Burke FD, Wilgis EF, et al. A prospective study comparing outcomes after reconstruction in rheumatoid arthritis patients with severe ulnar drift deformities. *Plast Reconstr Surg*. 2009;123:1769–1777.
41. Swanson AB. Silicone rubber implants for replacement of arthritis or destroyed joints in the hand. *Surg Clin North Am*. 1968;48:1113–1127.
42. Chung KC, Kotsis SV, Burns PB, et al. Seven-year outcomes of the silicone arthroplasty in rheumatoid arthritis prospective cohort study. *Arthritis Care Res (Hoboken)*. 2017;69:973–981.

43. Wanderman N, Wagner E, Moran S, et al. Outcomes following acute metacarpophalangeal joint arthroplasty dislocation: an analysis of 37 cases. *J Hand Surg Am.* 2018;43:289.e1–289.e6.

44. Pugliese D, Bush D, Harrington T. Silicone synovitis: longer term outcome data and review of the literature. *J Clin Rheumatol.* 2009;15:8–11.

45. Foliart DE. Swanson silicone finger joint implants: a review of the literature regarding long-term complications. *J Hand Surg Am.* 1995;20:445–449.

46. Cook SD, Beckenbaugh RD, Redondo J, et al. Long-term follow-up of pyrolytic carbon metacarpophalangeal implants. *J Bone Joint Surg Am.* 1999;81:635–648.

47. Sweets TM, Stern PJ. Pyrolytic carbon resurfacing arthroplasty for osteoarthritis of the proximal interphalangeal joint of the finger. *J Bone Joint Surg Am.* 2011;93:1417–1425.

48. Dickson DR, Nuttall D, Watts AC, et al. Pyrocarbon proximal interphalangeal joint arthroplasty: minimum five-year follow-up. *J Hand Surg Am.* 2015;40:2142–2148.e4.

49. Petscavage JM, Ha AS, Chew FS. Arthroplasty of the hand: radiographic outcomes of pyrolytic carbon proximal interphalangeal and metacarpophalangeal joint replacements. *AJR Am J Roentgenol.* 2011;197:1177–1181.

50. Rizzo M. Metacarpophalangeal joint arthritis. *J Hand Surg Am.* 2011;36:345–353.

51. Vainio K. Vainio arthroplasty of the metacarpophalangeal joints in rheumatoid arthritis. *J Hand Surg Am.* 1989;14:367–368.

52. Weilby A. Resection arthroplasty of the metacarpophalangeal joint a.m. Tupper using interposition of the volar plate. *Scand J Plast Reconstr Surg.* 1977;11:239–242.

53. Fowler SB. Arthroplasty of the metacarpophalangeal joint in rheumatoid arthritis. *J Bone Joint Surg.* 1962;44A:1037.

54. Beasley J. American society of hand therapists (ASHT) webinar, Postoperative Management of PIP IRA.

55. Chim HW, Reese SK, Toomey SN, et al. Update on the surgical treatment for rheumatoid arthritis of the wrist and hand. *J Hand Ther.* 2014;27:134–141; quiz 142.

56. Escott BG, Ronald K, Judd MG, et al. NeuFlex and Swanson metacarpophalangeal implants for rheumatoid arthritis: prospective randomized, controlled clinical trial. *J Hand Surg Am.* 2010;35:44–51.

57. Robinson S, Rosenblum N, eds. *Concepts in Hand Rehabilitation.* New York: Churchill-Livingstone; 1986.

58. Hunter JM, et al., ed. *Rehabilitation of the Hand.* 3rd ed. St. Louis: Mosby; 1990.

59. Boozer JA, Sanson MS, Soutas-Little RW, et al. Comparison of the biomedical motions and forces involved in high-profile versus low-profile dynamic splinting. *J Hand Ther.* 1994;7:171–182.

60. Bogoch ER, Escott BG, Ronald K. Hand appearance as a patient motivation for surgery and a determinant of satisfaction with metacarpophalangeal joint arthroplasty for rheumatoid arthritis. *J Hand Surg Am.* 2011;36:1007–1014: e1–4.

61. Beckenbaugh RD, Lund A. *ICL 01 Advances in the Treatment of Rheumatoid Hand and Wrist.* San Antonio, TX: Joint Annual Meeting ASSH & ASHT; 2006.

62. Beckenbaugh RD. *Arthroplasty of the MP/PIP Joint, Postop Management.* Beverly Hills, CA: AAHS 38th Annual Meeting; 2008.

63. Herren DB, Keuchel T, Marks M, et al. Revision arthroplasty for failed silicone proximal interphalangeal joint arthroplasty: indications and 8-year results. *J Hand Surg Am.* 2014;39:462–466.

64. Cheah AE, Yao J. Surgical approaches to the proximal interphalangeal joint. *J Hand Surg Am.* 2016;41:294–305.

65. Duncan SFM, Smith AA, Renfree KJ, et al. Results of the volar approach in proximal interphalangeal joint arthroplasty. *J Hand Surg Asian Pac.* 2018;23:26–32.

66. Murray PM, Linscheid RL, Cooney 3rd WP, et al. Long-term outcomes of proximal interphalangeal joint surface replacement arthroplasty. *J Bone Joint Surg Am.* 2012;94:1120–1128.

67. Mares O, Clairemidi A, Wavreille G, et al. Swanson-type silastic arthroplasties of the PIP joint for rheumatoid arthritis. Results of 19 implants at 5.3 years of follow-up. *Chir Main.* 2010;29:242–248.

68. Takigawa S, Meletiou S, Sauerbier M, et al. Long-term assessment of Swanson implant arthroplasty in the proximal interphalangeal joint of the hand. *J Hand Surg Am.* 2004;29:785–795.

69. Jennings CD, Livingstone DP. Surface replacement arthroplasty of the proximal interphalangeal joint using the SR PIP implant: long-term results. *J Hand Surg Am.* 2015;40:469–473.e6.

70. Storey PA, Goddard M, Clegg C, et al. Pyrocarbon proximal interphalangeal joint arthroplasty: a medium to long term follow-up of a single surgeon series. *J Hand Surg Eur.* 2015;40:952–956.

71. Pettersson K, Amilon A, Rizzo M. Pyrolytic carbon hemiarthroplasty in the management of proximal interphalangeal joint arthritis. *J Hand Surg Am.* 2015;40:462–468.

72. Williams K, Terrono AL. Treatment of boutonniere finger deformity in rheumatoid arthritis. *J Hand Surg Am.* 2011;36:1388–1393.

73. Kiefhaber TR, Strickland JW. Soft tissue reconstruction for rheumatoid swan-neck and boutonniere deformities: long-term results. *J Hand Surg Am.* 1993;18:984–989.

74. Nalebuff EA. The rheumatoid swan-neck deformity. *Hand Clin.* 1989;5:203–214.

75. Mikolyzk DK, Stern PJ. Steinmann pin arthrodesis for salvage of failed small joint arthroplasty. *J Hand Surg Am.* 2011;36:1383–1387.

76. Capo JT, Melamed E, Shamian B, et al. Biomechanical evaluation of 5 fixation devices for proximal interphalangeal joint arthrodesis. *J Hand Surg Am.* 2014;39:1971–1977.

77. Squitieri L, Chung KC. A systematic review of outcomes and complications of vascularized toe joint transfer, silicone arthroplasty, and PyroCarbon arthroplasty for posttraumatic joint reconstruction of the finger. *Plast Reconstr Surg.* 2008;121:1697–1707.

78. Melvin JL. Therapist's management of osteoarthritis in the hand. In: Mackin EJ, Callahan AD, Skirven TM, et al., eds. *Rehabilitation of the Hand and Upper Extremity.* 5th ed. St. Louis: Mosby; 2002.

79. Swanson AB, de Groot Swanson G. Flexible implant resection arthroplasty of the proximal interphalangeal joint. *Hand Clin.* 1994;10:261–266.

80. Swanson AB, Swanson GD, Leonard J. Postoperative rehabilitation programs in flexible implant arthroplasty of the digits. In: Hunter JM, Mackin EJ, Callahan AD, eds. *Rehabilitation of the Hand: Surgery and Therapy.* 4th ed. St. Louis: Mosby; 1995.

81. Herren DB, Schindele S, Goldhahn J, et al. Problematic bone fixation with pyrocarbon implants in proximal interphalangeal joint replacement: short-term results. *J Hand Surg Br.* 2006;31:643–651.

82. U.S. Food & Drug Administration. Summary of safety and probable benefit, ascension PIP; HDE # H010005. Available at: https://www.accessdata.fda.gov/scripts/cdrh/cfdocs/cfhde/hde.cfm?ID=H010005.

83. Beckenbaugh RD, Klawitter J, Cook S. Osseointegration and mechanical stability of pyrocarbon and titanium hand implants in a load-bearing in vivo model for small joint arthroplasty. *J Hand Surg Am.* 2006;31:1240–1241. author reply 1241–1242.

84. Ascension Orthopedics Inc. *Ascension PIP PyroCarbon Total Joint Arthroplasty Post-Operative Therapy Protocol.* Integra LifeSciences Corporation; 2017. Available at: https://www.integralife.com/file/general/1524246421.pdf.

85. Feldscher SB. Postoperative management for PIP joint pyrocarbon arthroplasty. *J Hand Ther.* 2010;23:315–322.

86. Lubahn JD, Wolfe TL, Feldscher SB. Joint replacement in the hand and wrist: surgery and therapy. In: Skirven TM, Osterman AL, Fedorczyk J, et al., eds. *Rehabilitation of the Hand and Upper Extremity.* 6th ed. Philadelphia: Elsevier Mosby; 2011:1376–1398.

87. Nalebuff EA. Diagnosis, classification and management of rheumatoid thumb deformities. *Bull Hosp Joint Dis.* 1968;29:119–137.

88. Terrono AL, Nalebuff EA, Philips CA. The rheumatoid thumb. In: Skirven TM, Osterman AL, Fedorczyk JM, et al., eds. *Rehabilitation of the Hand and Upper Extremity.* 6th ed. Philadelphia: Elsevier Mosby; 2011:1344–1355.

89. Schindele SF, Herren DB, Simmen BR. Tendon reconstruction for the rheumatoid hand. *Hand Clin.* 2011;27:105–113.

90. Schneider LH. Proximal interphalangeal joint arthroplasty: the volar approach. *Semin Arthroplasty.* 1991; 2(2):139–147.

91. Lipscomb PR. Synovectomy of the distal two joints of the thumb and fingers in rheumatoid arthritis. *J Bone Joint Surg Am.* 1967;49(6):1135–1140.

92. Swanson AB, Maupin BK, Gajjar NV, Swanson GD. Flexible implant arthroplasty in the proximal interphalangeal joint of the hand. *J Hand Surg Am.* 1985;10(6 Pt 1):796-805.

93. Chamay A. A distally based dorsal and triangular tendinous flap for direct access to the proximal interphalangeal joint.. *Ann Chir Main.* 1988;7(2):179–183.

87

Surgery Management of the Osteoarthritic Thumb Carpometacarpal Joint

Michael B. Gottschalk, Sanjeev Kakar

OUTLINE

CRITICAL POINTS

- Thumb carpometacarpal (CMC) arthritis is the second most common cause of arthritis in the hand with patients complaining of pain with pinch and grasp. Patients are tender at the CMC joint with plain radiographs being used as an adjunct to the clinical exam.

- Conservative options should be trialed first and may include hand therapy, orthosis, antiinflammatory medications, and joint injections.
- A combination of trapezial-sparing and trapezial-sacrificing procedures exist that should be considered and discussed with the patient in detail.

INTRODUCTION

The trapeziometacarpal (TM) joint of the thumb is a common source of pain secondary to degenerative changes. It is more common in postmenopausal women, although older men are also subject to developing symptoms.[1-3] Because of evolutionary changes, the human thumb is unique in that it allows oppositional pinch. This complex interplay of movement accounts for the thumb providing 40% of hand function.[4] The bony anatomy allows for range of motion (ROM) along multiple planes, thereby permitting thumb circumduction. There is minimal bony support with the majority of stability being afforded by static and dynamic restraints.[5] The two most important include the volar oblique and dorsal radial ligament.[6] Strauch and coworkers[6] performed a biomechanical study on 38 thumbs and serially sectioned the ligaments about the carpometacarpal (CMC) joint. The authors found the dorsal radial ligament to be the primary restraining force to dorsal dislocation.

During key pinch, there is a 12-fold increase in pressure seen at the thumb CMC joint. Given that the thumb accounts for 40% of hand function and with this repetitive loading, it is prone to degenerative changes.[4,7,8] Conservative measures can be effective and range from therapy, orthoses, and corticosteroid injections. For patients who fail conservative measures, several surgical options are widely available, including both trapezial-sparing and trapezial-sacrificing procedures. Surgical treatment is often decided based on patient characteristics, radiographic findings (e.g., involvement of the scaphotrapeziotrapezoid [STT] joint), and surgeon preference. Nonoperative treatment is covered in Chapters 85 and 88.

PATHOPHYSIOLOGY

Several theories have been postulated regarding the pathophysiology of thumb CMC arthritis. Attenuation of the volar anterior oblique ligament (ligamentous laxity theory) was first believed to be the primary cause of CMC osteoarthritis (OA) secondary to dorsal radial subluxation of the TM joint.[9,10] Eaton and Littler[11] described a theory whereby the flexion-adduction forces created by key pinch caused impingement and dorsal subluxation of the CMC base. More recently, the role of gender has been considered because there is an increase prevalence in women, leading some to believe there is a difference in bony morphology as well as hormonal differences.[12] The hormonal theory describes a causal relationship with higher levels of estrogen and relaxin in women that may result in a higher incidence in CMC instability.[12-14] Posttraumatic arthritis can also ensue after injuries such as a Bennett's or Rolando fracture.[15]

ASSESSMENT AND DIAGNOSIS

Patients often present with pain located over the palmar or dorsal aspect of the base of the thumb TM joint that is exacerbated with activities such as key pinch or opening a jar. The history should focus on the timing of onset, exacerbating factors or activities, recent trauma, and previous treatments. Many patients may have concomitant carpal tunnel syndrome.[16]

Clinically, patients are tender at the thumb CMC joint. This can be elucidated by a myriad of tests, including the grind test, metacarpophalangeal (MCP) extension test, lever test, or a combination of gentle distraction and dorsal to volar pressure of the base of the thumb metacarpal that reduces the subluxated TM joint.[17,18] Gelberman and colleagues[19] have shown that the extension and metacarpal adduction maneuvers have more specificity than tenderness to palpation over the CMC joint and have more sensitivity then the grind test. The examiner should palpate for tenderness at the STT joint,[20] as well as other causes of radial-sided wrist pain, including de Quervain's tenosynovitis, Wartenberg's syndrome, and scaphoid pathology. It is important

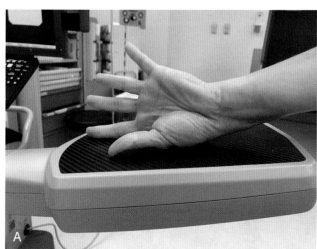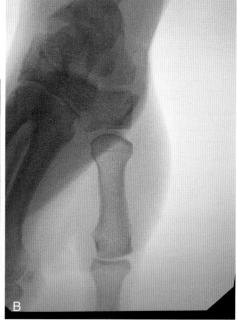

Fig. 87.1 A, Photograph of the correct position for a Roberts anteroposterior view of the thumb. The hand is hyperpronated against the cassette or image intensifier as shown. **B,** The fluoroscopic view of the hand shown in A demonstrating visualization of the carpometacarpal joint in addition to the scaphotrapeziotrapezoid joint.

to note that both trigger thumb and de Quervain's tenosynovitis can occur with CMC arthritis and may make it more difficult to discern the root cause of the patient's pain.[21]

With advanced thumb CMC arthritis, the thumb may assume a Z deformity with thumb metacarpal adduction and compensatory MCP joint hyperextension. The hyperextension of the thumb MCP is secondary to the deforming force by the extensor pollicis brevis and is a compensatory mechanism to allow grasp given that the arthritic CMC joint limits motion.[22]

Standard radiographs include posteroanterior, lateral, and oblique views. Other views, such as the Roberts and pinch lateral views, may be helpful in examining the extent of CMC joint degeneration in addition to concomitant adjacent joint disease.[23] The Roberts view (Fig. 87.1) allows one to appreciate the disease in a coronal plane at the CMC and STT joint and is especially useful when considering trapezial-preserving procedures such as TM arthrodesis or prosthetic arthroplasty. It can also assist with examining index and thumb metacarpal impingement. Stress radiographs of bilateral thumb CMC joints may be helpful for eliciting early signs of CMC instability and OA (Fig. 87.2). Concomitant radiographic findings that may affect the treatment include adjacent OA of the MCP or interphalangeal joint.

The most common radiographic classification used for thumb CMC arthritis was described by Eaton and Littler[11] (Table 87.1). It is a four-stage classification system that evaluates both the CMC and STT joints. Despite its widespread use, the inter- and intraobserver reliability and its ability to guide treatment can be variable.

SURGICAL MANAGEMENT: TRAPEZIAL-SPARING PROCEDURES

Several surgical options are available in the treatment of patients with CMC OA. In younger patients in whom the STT joint maybe spared, trapezial-sparing procedures may be considered. These include denervation, metacarpal extension osteotomy, arthroscopy, prosthetic arthroplasty, and arthrodesis.

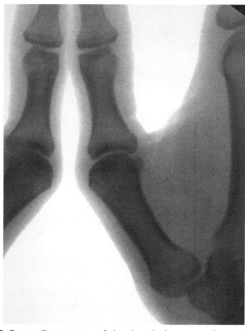

Fig. 87.2 Stress fluoroscopy of the thumb demonstrating extrusion of the base of the thumb consistent with early carpometacarpal osteoarthritis.

Carpometacarpal Denervation

Trapeziometacarpal denervation includes the removal of sensory nerve endings that innervate the CMC joint. There are several proposed benefits, including pain relief with minimal postoperative rehabilitation, all while maintaining the column of the thumb and possibly strength. The procedure addresses innervation from the superficial branch of the radial nerve, lateral antebrachial cutaneous nerve, median nerve, and the deep motor branch of the ulnar nerve. Mixed results have been

TABLE 87.1 Eaton and Littler Classification of Thumb Trapeziometacarpal Osteoarthritis

Stage	Characteristics
I	Subtle CMC joint space widening caused by effusion and ligamentous laxity Normal articular contours No significant osteophytes
II	CMC joint space narrowing with sclerosis Osteophytes or loose bodies <2 mm Partial joint subluxation
III	Significant CMC joint space narrowing with sclerosis; cyst formation Osteophytes >2 mm Joint subluxation
IV	Advanced CMC degeneration with significant subluxation Minimal joint space with moderate cystic changes and osteophytes Scaphotrapezial involvement

CMC, Carpometacarpal.

TABLE 87.2 Badia Arthroscopic Classification of Thumb Trapeziometacarpal Osteoarthritis

Stage	Arthroscopic Changes
I	Intact articular cartilage; disruption of the dorsoradial ligament and diffuse synovial hypertrophy; inconsistent attenuation of the AOL
II	Frank eburnation of the articular cartilage on the ulnar third of the base of first metacarpal and central third of the distal surface of the trapezium; disruption of the dorsoradial ligament and more intense synovial hypertrophy; constant attenuation of the AOL
III	Widespread, full-thickness cartilage loss with or without a peripheral rim on both articular surfaces; less severe synovitis; frayed volar ligaments with laxity

AOL, Anterior oblique ligament.

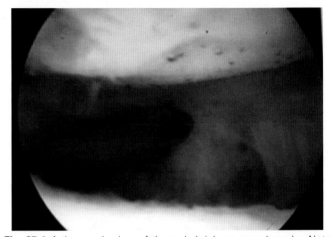

Fig. 87.4 Arthroscopic view of thermal shrinkage capsulorraphy. Note the prominent volar oblique ligament.

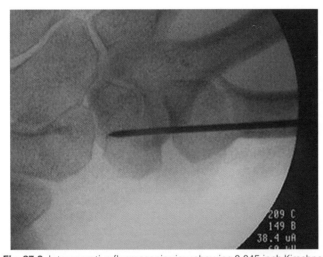

Fig. 87.3 Intraoperative fluoroscopic view showing 0.045-inch Kirschner wire placement for stabilization of metacarpal base osteotomy. Note extension posture of metacarpal and the centralization of metacarpal base on trapezium also maintained with same-wire fixation.

reported in the literature. Lorea and colleagues[24,25] used a two-incision technique and noted that of 43 patients with a mean of 60 years of age, the majority were satisfied and demonstrated improved Kapandji scores and key pinch. None of the patients developed a Charcot joint. Reported complications include paresthesias, hypertrophic scarring, and hypoesthesia.[26]

Extension Metacarpal Osteotomy

First metacarpal extension osteotomy may be useful in patients with early CMC OA (Fig. 87.3). The osteotomy redirects the joint forces dorsally, thereby unloading the diseased volar aspect of the metacarpal articular surface. Tomaino[27] prospectively performed an extraarticular 30-degree extension osteotomy in 12 patients. At an average follow-up of 2.1 years, patients demonstrated increased grip and pinch strength with union occurring at an average of 7 weeks. Parker and coworkers[28] noted that at an average of 9 years, patients may continue to have improvement in their pain and function even in more moderate CMC OA.

Carpometacarpal Arthroscopy

Advantages of basilar thumb joint arthroscopy include its relatively minimally invasive approach and speed of recovery with decreased morbidity. Badia[29] described an arthroscopic staging system for CMC OA (Table 87.2). In the early stages of disease, patients may have synovitis without frank subluxation and are amenable to arthroscopic synovectomy with or without radiofrequency shrinkage capsulorrhaphy (Fig. 87.4). Furia[30] reported results with arthroscopic synovectomy in patients with Eaton stage I and II arthritis and found an improvement in Disability of the Arm, Shoulder and Hand (DASH) scores and pinch strength with an 83% satisfaction rate.

Arthroscopic hemitrapeziectomy with or without interposition may be advocated with advanced CMC joint involvement, in which the STT joint is spared (Fig. 87.5). Menon[31] reported results with arthroscopic hemitrapeziectomy and the use of autogenous tissue, allograft fascia lata, or Gore-Tex (WL Gore, Elkton, MD) in 33 thumbs and reported an 87.8% success rate in relieving pain. Patient pinch strength averaged 11 lb.

Adams and coworkers[32] have described their results with using acellular dermal matrix allograft (Graftjacket; Wright Medical Technology, Inc., Arlington, TN). In patients with Eaton stage II and III arthritis, 94% of patients were either partially or completely satisfied by an arthroscopic hemitrapeziectomy with interposition. More than 70% of patients had minimal to no difficulty in activities of daily living with an average grip strength of 18.5 kg and an average pinch strength of 3.9 kg.

Carpometacarpal Arthrodesis

Thumb TM arthrodesis has traditionally been used for the treatment of young, active male laborers and those with posttraumatic arthritis after a Bennett's fracture. Several methods have been reported, including headless compression screws, plates, Kirschner wires, and tension band constructs. The proposed position of the thumb basal joint is one that allows for key pinch and has been described as 10 to 20 degrees of radial abduction, 30 to 40 degrees of palmar abduction, and slight extension.[5]

Hartigan and coworkers[33] and Goldfarb and Stern[34] reviewed their outcomes of CMC fusion to excisional arthroplasty in 141 patients with 10 years of follow-up. Patients who underwent arthrodesis had stronger pinch strength, whereas those that underwent excisional arthroplasty had better ROM. The arthrodesis group had a higher complication rate with nonunion being the most common. Rizzo and colleagues[35] have reviewed their long-term results after CMC arthrodesis and noted similar improvements in pain, pinch, and grip strength. Thirty-nine of 126 patients developed radiographic evidence of STT OA, with 8 being symptomatic.

Vermeulen and associates[36] performed a randomized controlled trial comparing CMC arthrodesis with ligament reconstruction with tendon interposition (LRTI). The study was prematurely stopped because the CMC arthrodesis cohort had a significantly higher complication rate of 71%. The complications included 6 mild complications (scar tenderness and sensory disturbances), 6 moderate complications

(neuromas, delayed union, and type I complex regional pain syndrome [CRPS]) and 3 severe complications (2 nonunions requiring additional surgery and type 1 CRPS). The authors concluded that they do not routinely recommend CMC arthrodesis for patients older than 40 years of age with stage II or III CMC OA.

Implant Arthroplasty: Hemiarthroplasty and Total Joint Arthroplasty

Purported advantages of prosthetic arthroplasty include the maintenance of the thumb column with perceived improved strength and cosmesis. Swanson[37] reported the outcomes of silicone CMC arthroplasty at 5 years postoperatively in 46 patients. Despite an improvement in pain and grip strength, 17.4% of the patients developed instability complications. Sollerman and coworkers[38] reported their results of 33 patients with 39 silastic replacements, and despite early promising results, at 12 years, more than half had implant wear and dislocations, resulting in diminished thumb strength and function. Minami and coworkers[39] noted that at an average of 15 years, more than 70% of implants subsided or fractured. Given these high complication rates, the prosthesis has mostly been abandoned.

With improvements in material technology, prosthetic hemiarthroplasty has gained some popularity. Martinez de Aragon and associates[40] reported 80% survival of 54 pyrolytic carbon arthroplasty at a mean of 22 months. Most patients reported a 90% increase in strength compared with the contralateral side with 15 requiring secondary procedures. Vitale and associates[41] compared trapeziectomy and APL suspension arthroplasty with pyrolytic carbon and found that the former cohort had a significantly lower risk of complications (72.8%), reoperations (87.7%), and revision surgery (87.2%) when controlling for age and sex.

To guard against the risk of prosthetic wear on the trapezium, total joint arthroplasties have been used to treat CMC joint arthritis. Johnston and colleagues[42] have demonstrated an 86% survivability at 26 years. In a similar case series, Cootjans and coworkers[43] reviewed 166 patients at 80 month follow-up with more than 96% survivorship. Despite these results, caution needs to be paid to the generalizability of prosthetic arthroplasty given that it is a technically demanding procedure, and the outcomes, in general, do not supersede trapeziectomy and suspension arthroplasty.

SURGICAL MANAGEMENT: TRAPEZIAL-SACRIFICING PROCEDURES

Excision Arthroplasty

Gervis and Wells[44] popularized trapeziectomy as a treatment for basilar thumb joint arthritis with excellent results. Given this, others have

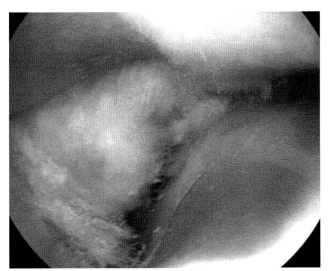

Fig. 87.5 Arthroscopic view of Badia stage III trapeziometacarpal arthritis. Note the nearly complete loss of cartilage on trapezium, metacarpal cartilage deterioration, and poor integrity of the capsule.

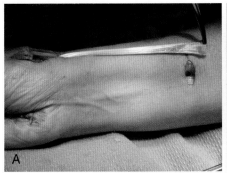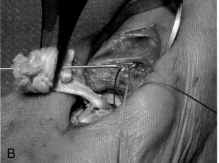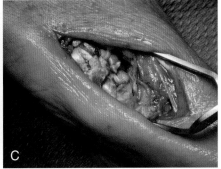

Fig. 87.6 Diagram illustrating Tomaino's technique for trapezial excisional arthroplasty with entire flexor carpi radialis used for ligament reconstruction and tendon interposition. (**A**) Flexor carpi radialis harvest demonstrating retrieval from the distal incision. (**B**) Technique for performing the anchovie technique for interposition arthroplasty. (**C**) Completion of the ligament reconstruction with tendon interposition.

adopted the technique with modifications. Meals and associates[45] described hematoma distraction arthroplasty (HDA) whereby the metacarpal is temporarily suspended with a Kirschner wire, allowing the trapezial space to fill in with scar tissue. In a prospective case series of 26 patients at 2-year follow-up, the authors noted improved motion, pain relief, and strength. Gray and Meals[46] reviewed their results at 6.5 years after surgery and found that nearly 82% of their patients were pain free, with average increases in grip and key pinch of 21% and 11%, respectively.

Corain and coworkers[47] reported their prospective randomized study of 64 patients undergoing LRTI compared with 56 patients undergoing HAD for stage 3 or 4 OA. The results were similar between the two groups, including DASH scores, grip strength, trapezial height, and ROM. The authors reported a 15% complication rate in the LRTI group and concluded that HDA was more favorable in terms of difficulty, time, and recovery. One of the concerns with HDA is the proximal subsidence of the thumb metacarpal, especially in younger patients.

Ligament Reconstruction and Tendon Interposition

To guard against proximal migration of the thumb metacarpal, Burton and Pellegrini[48] combined trapeziectomy with ligament reconstruction using a distally based flexor carpi radialis tendon (FCR). The authors reported their results of 25 procedures at an average follow-up period of 2 years. The study reported metacarpal migration of 11% in the LRTI cohort versus 50% in the silicone cohort. Excellent results were reported in 92% of LRTI patients with improved pinch and grip strength. The authors concluded that trapeziectomy with LRTI had become their preferred method of the treatment of CMC OA. As of 2012, a survey performed by Wolf and Delaronde[49] polling members of the American Society for Surgery of the Hand demonstrated that 62% of the responding physicians use trapeziectomy with LRTI as their method of surgical treatment for stage III arthritis. Davis and colleagues[50] conducted a prospective randomized clinical trial comparing trapeziectomy, LRTI, or tendon interposition in 76 patients. After 1-year follow-up, it was noted that pain relief, hand function, and thumb strength were similar among cohorts.

To build off this concept of suspension arthroplasty, many adaptations have been described. The Weilby procedure uses a distally based strip of the FCR weaved around the abductor pollicis longus (APL) and remaining FCR[51] to suspend the thumb metacarpal after trapeziectomy. Others have used a strip of the APL to suspend the thumb metacarpal.[52] Sammer and Amadio[52] modified the APL weave to incorporate the extensor carpi radialis longus (ECRL) for further stabilization and have reported improved strength with this technique.

Despite many other types of tendon weaves, the FCR has been the most popularized given its location and ease in which it can be harvested and used to suspend the thumb metacarpal (Fig. 87.6). In cases in which the FCR is attenuated or injured, Jones and colleagues[53] have outlined other options for reconstruction, including hematoma distraction arthroplasty or using a strip of the ECRL to restore stability.

In more advanced disease, a zig-zag deformity may be present with adduction of the thumb metacarpal and MCP joint hyperextension (Fig. 87.7). In treating the TM arthritis, should the MCP joint be concomitantly addressed to improve the posture and pinch biomechanics of the thumb? Brogan and coworkers[54,55] compared the results of 203 patients who underwent either a trapeziectomy and suspension arthroplasty (LRTI or Weilby procedure) with or without MCP joint hyperextension. The authors found that patients with mild, untreated MCP hyperextension (<30 degrees) had no statistical difference in outcomes compared with those without any MCP hyperextension.

Poulter and Davis[56] reviewed the results of 297 thumbs that underwent CMC arthroplasty and demonstrated that patients with untreated MCP hyperextension of less than 30 degrees did not significantly influence their outcomes. However, when comparing the results of those patients to the patients with greater than 35 degrees of MCP hyperextension, the authors recommended MCP capsulodesis or fusion.

Suture Suspension Arthroplasty

Given the encouraging results of ligament suspension arthroplasty procedures, suture suspension has gained recent popularity. Yao and associates[57] reported their 5-year results in 16 thumbs after undergoing arthroscopic hemitrapeziectomy and suture suspensionplasty. The authors demonstrated maintenance of the trapezial space by 71%, a decrease of QuickDASH scores of 58.2 points, and increases in ROM. Complications of this technique may include hardware irritation, iatrogenic metacarpal fracture, and impingement of the first and second metacarpal from overtightening.

To guard against thumb and index finger impingement, Endress and Kakar and colleagues[58] advocated the use of a double-suture

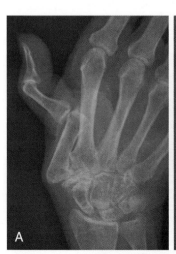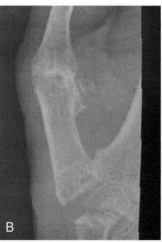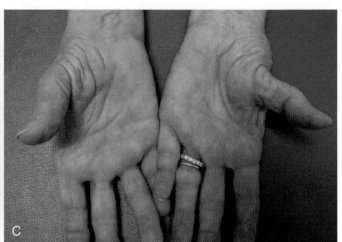

Fig. 87.7 Preoperative (**A**) and postoperative (**B**) radiographs and clinical photograph (**C**) showing a patient with severe Z-deformity caused by advanced trapeziometacarpal joint collapse and good clinical outcome after trapezial resection, ligament reconstruction tendon interposition with abductor pollicis longus tendon, and metacarpophalangeal joint fusion. Note clinical improvement compared with the untreated, contralateral thumb.

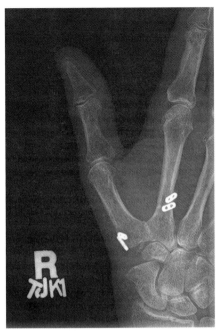

Fig. 87.8 Radiograph demonstrating double-suture suspensionplasty as described by Kakar.[67]

suspensionplasty with FCR to APL tendon imbrication (Fig. 87.8). The authors demonstrated improvement in strength, trapezial height, and pain at an average of 17 months. Biomechanical testing has shown that double-suture suspension maintains trapezial height and resists metacarpal load more favorably than single suture suspension or LRTI, thereby possibly allowing early rehabilitation.[59]

More recently, DeGeorge and colleagues[60] investigated the functional, radiographic outcomes, and complications of trapeziectomy and FCR to APL suspension with or without suture-button suspensionplasty for thumb basilar joint arthritis in 70 patients. After a follow up averaging 2 years, there was no difference in functional outcomes between the patients although those that had a suture suspension had less thumb metacarpal subsidence.

SUMMARY

Thumb CMC arthritis is a common cause of hand disability; as such, having a structured method of treatment is important for patient satisfaction. Initial nonoperative treatment should combine a multifaceted approach, including hand therapy, analgesia, and splinting with selective injections. After patients fail nonoperative treatment, surgical interventions are tailored along a trapezial-preserving or trapezial-sacrificing approach.

REFERENCES

1. Armstrong AL, Hunter JB, Davis TR. The prevalence of degenerative arthritis of the base of the thumb in post-menopausal women. *J Hand Surg.* 1994;19(3):340–341.
2. Sodha S, Ring D, Zurakowski D, Jupiter JB. Prevalence of osteoarthrosis of the trapeziometacarpal joint. *J Bone Joint Surg Am.* 2005;87(12):2614–2618.
3. Sonne-Holm S, Jacobsen S. Osteoarthritis of the first carpometacarpal joint: a study of radiology and clinical epidemiology. Results from the Copenhagen osteoarthritis study. *Osteoarthritis Cartilage.* 2006;14(5):496–500.
4. Moran SL, Berger RA. Biomechanics and hand trauma: what you need. *Hand Clin.* 2003;19(1):17–31.
5. Van Heest AE, Kallemeier P. Thumb carpal metacarpal arthritis. *J Am Acad Orthop Surg.* 2008;16(3):140–151.
6. Strauch RJ, Behrman MJ, Rosenwasser MP. Acute dislocation of the carpometacarpal joint of the thumb: an anatomic and cadaver study. *J Hand Surg.* 1994;19(1):93–98.
7. Yuan BJ, Moran SL, Tay SC, Berger RA. Trapeziectomy and carpal collapse. *The J Hand Surg.* 2009;34(2):219–227.
8. Cooney 3rd WP, Chao EY. Biomechanical analysis of static forces in the thumb during hand function. *J Bone Joint Surg Am.* 1977;59(1):27–36.
9. Pellegrini Jr VD. Osteoarthritis of the trapeziometacarpal joint: the pathophysiology of articular cartilage degeneration. I. Anatomy and pathology of the aging joint. *J Hand Surg.* 1991;16(6):967–974.
10. Pellegrini Jr VD, Olcott CW, Hollenberg G. Contact patterns in the trapeziometacarpal joint: the role of the palmar beak ligament. *J Hand Surg.* 1993;18(2):238–244.
11. Eaton RG, Littler JW. A study of the basal joint of the thumb. Treatment of its disabilities by fusion. *J Bone Joint Surg Am.* 1969;51(4):661–668.
12. Ladd AL, Weiss AP, Crisco JJ, et al. The thumb carpometacarpal joint: anatomy, hormones, and biomechanics. *Instr Course Lect.* 2013;62:165–179.
13. Ateshian GA, Rosenwasser MP, Mow VC. Curvature characteristics and congruence of the thumb carpometacarpal joint: differences between female and male joints. *J Biomech.* 1992;25(6):591–607.
14. Wolf JM, Scher DL, Etchill EW, et al. Relationship of relaxin hormone and thumb carpometacarpal joint arthritis. *Clin Orthop Relat Res.* 2014;472(4):1130–1137.
15. McQuillan TJ, Kenney D, Crisco JJ, Weiss AP, Ladd AL. Weaker functional pinch strength is associated with early thumb carpometacarpal osteoarthritis. *Clin Orthop Relat Res.* 2016;474(2):557–561.
16. Florack TM, Miller RJ, Pellegrini VD, Burton RI, Dunn MG. The prevalence of carpal tunnel syndrome in patients with basal joint arthritis of the thumb. *J Hand Surg.* 1992;17(4):624–630.
17. Model Z, Liu AY, Kang L, Wolfe SW, Burket JC, Lee SK. Evaluation of physical examination tests for thumb basal joint osteoarthritis. *Hand (N Y).* 2016;11(1):108–112.
18. Choa RM, Parvizi N, Giele HP. A prospective case-control study to compare the sensitivity and specificity of the grind and traction-shift (subluxation-relocation) clinical tests in osteoarthritis of the thumb carpometacarpal joint. *J Hand Surg Eur Vol.* 2014;39(3):282–285.
19. Gelberman RH, Boone S, Osei DA, Cherney S, Calfee RP. Trapeziometacarpal arthritis: a prospective clinical evaluation of the thumb adduction and extension provocative tests. *J Hand Surg.* 2015;40(7):1285–1291.
20. Barron OA, Glickel SZ, Eaton RG. Basal joint arthritis of the thumb. *J Am Acad Orthop Surg.* 2000;8(5):314–323.
21. Li YK, White CP. Five things to know about...carpometacarpal osteoarthritis of the thumb. *CMAJ.* 2013;185(2):149.
22. Baker RH, Al-Shukri J, Davis TR. Evidence-based medicine: thumb basal joint arthritis. *Plast Reconstr Surg.* 2017;139(1):256e–266e.
23. Melville DM, Taljanovic MS, Scalcione LR, et al. Imaging and management of thumb carpometacarpal joint osteoarthritis. *Skeletal Radiol.* 2015;44(2):165–177.
24. Lorea P, Dury M, Marin Braun F, Dekkai T, De Mey A, Foucher G. Trapeziometacarpal denervation. Description of surgical technique and preliminary results from a prospective series of 14 cases. *Chir Main.* 2002;21(4):209–217.
25. Lorea P, Ezzedine R, Marchesi S. Denervation of the proximal interphalangeal joint: a realistic and simple procedure. *Tech Hand Up Extrem Surg.* 2004;8(4):262–265.
26. Arenas-Prat JM. Wagner approach for first carpometacarpal joint denervation. *Tech Hand Up Extrem Surg.* 2012;16(2):107–109.
27. Tomaino MM. Treatment of Eaton stage I trapeziometacarpal disease with thumb metacarpal extension osteotomy. *J Hand Surg.* 2000;25(6):1100–1106.
28. Parker WL, Linscheid RL, Amadio PC. Long-term outcomes of first metacarpal extension osteotomy in the treatment of carpal-metacarpal osteoarthritis. *J Hand Surg.* 2008;33(10):1737–1743.
29. Badia A. Trapeziometacarpal arthroscopy: a classification and treatment algorithm. *Hand Clin.* 2006;22(2):153–163.

30. Furia JP. Arthroscopic debridement and synovectomy for treating basal joint arthritis. *Arthroscopy.* 2010;26(1):34–40.

31. Menon J. Arthroscopic management of trapeziometacarpal joint arthritis of the thumb. *Arthroscopy.* 1996;12(5):581–587.

32. Adams JE, Merten SM, Steinmann SP. Arthroscopic interposition arthroplasty of the first carpometacarpal joint. *J Hand Surg Eur.* 2007;32(3):268–274.

33. Hartigan BJ, Stern PJ, Kiefhaber TR. Thumb carpometacarpal osteoarthritis: arthrodesis compared with ligament reconstruction and tendon interposition. *J Bone Joint Surg Am.* 2001;83-A(10):1470–1478.

34. Goldfarb CA, Stern PJ. Indications and techniques for thumb carpometacarpal arthrodesis. *Tech Hand Up Extrem Surg.* 2002;6(4):178–184.

35. Rizzo M, Moran SL, Shin AY. Long-term outcomes of trapeziometacarpal arthrodesis in the management of trapeziometacarpal arthritis. *J Hand Surg.* 2009;34(1):20–26.

36. Vermeulen GM, Brink SM, Slijper H, et al. Trapeziometacarpal arthrodesis or trapeziectomy with ligament reconstruction in primary trapeziometacarpal osteoarthritis: a randomized controlled trial. *J Bone Joint Surg Am.* 2014;96(9):726–733.

37. Swanson AB. Disabling arthritis at the base of the thumb: treatment by resection of the trapezium and flexible (silicone) implant arthroplasty. *J Bone Joint Surg Am.* 1972;54(3):456–471.

38. Sollerman C, Herrlin K, Abrahamsson SO, Lindholm A. Silastic replacement of the trapezium for arthrosis—a twelve year follow-up study. *J Hand Surg.* 1988;13(4):426–429.

39. Minami A, Iwasaki N, Kutsumi K, Suenaga N, Yasuda K. A long-term follow-up of silicone-rubber interposition arthroplasty for osteoarthritis of the thumb carpometacarpal joint. *Hand Surg.* 2005;10(1):77–82.

40. Martinez de Aragon JS, Moran SL, Rizzo M, Reggin KB, Beckenbaugh RD. Early outcomes of pyrolytic carbon hemiarthroplasty for the treatment of trapezial-metacarpal arthritis. *J Hand Surg.* 2009;34(2):205–212.

41. Vitale MA, Hsu CC, Rizzo M, Moran SL. Pyrolytic carbon arthroplasty versus suspensionplasty for trapezial-metacarpal arthritis. *J Wrist Surg.* 2017;6(2):134–143.

42. Johnston P, Getgood A, Larson D, Chojnowski AJ, Chakrabarti AJ, Chapman PG. De la Caffiniere thumb trapeziometacarpal joint arthroplasty: 16-26 year follow-up. *J Hand Surg, Eur.* 2012;37(7):621–624.

43. Cootjans K, Vanhaecke J, Dezillie M, Barth J, Pottel H, Stockmans F. Joint survival analysis and clinical outcome of total joint arthroplasties with the ARPE implant in the treatment of trapeziometacarpal osteoarthritis with a minimal follow-up of 5 years. *J Hand Surg.* 2017;42(8):630–638.

44. Gervis WH, Wells T. A review of excision of the trapezium for osteoarthritis of the trapezio-metacarpal joint after twenty-five years. *J Bone Joint Surg Br.* 1973;55(1):56–57.

45. Kuhns CA, Emerson ET, Meals RA. Hematoma and distraction arthroplasty for thumb basal joint osteoarthritis: a prospective, single-surgeon study including outcomes measures. *J Hand Surg Am.* 2003;28(3):381–389.

46. Gray KV, Meals RA. Hematoma and distraction arthroplasty for thumb basal joint osteoarthritis: minimum 6.5-year follow-up evaluation. *J Hand Surg Am.* 2007;32(1):23–29.

47. Corain M, Zampieri N, Mugnai R, Adani R. Interposition arthroplasty versus hematoma and distraction for the treatment of osteoarthritis of the trapeziometacarpal joint. *J Hand Surg Asian Pac.* 2016;21(1):85–91.

48. Burton RI, Pellegrini Jr VD. Surgical management of basal joint arthritis of the thumb. Part II. Ligament reconstruction with tendon interposition arthroplasty. *J Hand Surg.* 1986;11(3):324–332.

49. Wolf JM, Delaronde S. Current trends in nonoperative and operative treatment of trapeziometacarpal osteoarthritis: a survey of US hand surgeons. *J Hand Surg.* 2012;37(1):77–82.

50. Davis TR, Brady O, Barton NJ, et al. Trapeziectomy alone, with tendon interposition or with ligament reconstruction? *J Hand Surg Br.* 1997;22(6):689–694.

51. Weilby A. Tendon interposition arthroplasty of the first carpo-metacarpal joint. *J Hand Surg.* 1988;13(4):421–425.

52. Sammer DM, Amadio PC. Description and outcomes of a new technique for thumb Basal joint arthroplasty. *J Hand Surg.* 2010;35(7):1198–1205.

53. Jones Jr DB, Rhee PC, Shin AY, Kakar S. Salvage options for flexor carpi radialis tendon disruption during ligament reconstruction and tendon interposition or suspension arthroplasty of the trapeziometacarpal joint. *J Hand Surg.* 2013;38(9):1806–1811.

54. Brogan DM, Kakar S. Metacarpophalangeal joint hyperextension and the treatment of thumb basilar joint arthritis. *J Hand Surg.* 2012;37(4):837–838.

55. Brogan DM, van Hogezand RM, Babovic N, Carlsen B, Kakar S. The effect of metacarpophalangeal joint hyperextension on outcomes in the surgical treatment of carpometacarpal joint arthritis. *J Wrist Surg.* 2017;6(3):188–193.

56. Poulter RJ, Davis TR. Management of hyperextension of the metacarpophalangeal joint in association with trapeziometacarpal joint osteoarthritis. *J Hand Surg, Eur.* 2011;36(4):280–284.

57. Yao J, Cheah AE. Mean 5-Year Follow-up for suture button suspensionplasty in the treatment of thumb carpometacarpal joint osteoarthritis. *J Hand Surg.* 2017;42(7):569 e561-569 e511.

58. Endress RD, Kakar S. Double tightrope for basilar thumb arthritis. *J Hand Surg.* 2014;39(12):2512–2516.

59. Hooke AW, Parry JA, Kakar S. Mini tightrope fixation versus ligament reconstruction - tendon interposition for maintenance of post-trapeziectomy space height: a biomechanical study. *J Hand Surg.* 2016;41(3):399–403.

60. DeGeorge Jr BR, Chawla SS, Elhassan BT, Kakar S. Basilar thumb arthritis: the utility of suture-button suspensionplasty. *Hand (NY).* 2019;14(1):66–72.

88

Therapist's Management of the Thumb Carpometacarpal Joint with Osteoarthritis

Kristin Valdes, Lori Algar, Corey Weston McGee

OUTLINE

CRITICAL POINTS

- Anatomically the carpometacarpal (CMC) joint of the thumb presents with instability inclining the joint to articular wear.
- Ligamentous laxity, muscle forces, contact forces, and lack of neuromuscular control are four mechanisms by which thumb CMC osteoarthritis (OA) is believed to occur.
- Conservative therapeutic management of thumb CMC OA includes use of an orthosis, dynamic stability exercises, joint mobilizations, modalities, and multimodal interventions.

- Assessment of outcomes in therapy should include evaluation of body functions (range of motion via the Kapandji index and intermetacarpal distance, pinch and grip strength, and pain) and patient function or activity and participation.
- Postsurgical management depends on the specific structures involved, the intentions of the surgery, and specifics related to the patient but includes a progression from protective phase to active motion to strengthening.

Osteoarthritis (OA) at the carpometacarpal (CMC) joint of the thumb is a common diagnosis among older individuals and involves symptoms that impact function and occupational performance.[1-3] It has been found that approximately 26.2% of women and 13.4% of men age 71 to 100 years old have symptomatic thumb CMC joint OA.[3] In addition, arthritis at the base of the thumb was found to be responsible for hand pain in 70% of individuals examined with radiographs,[4] and it has been suggested that this particular disease may be underdiagnosed.[5]

The most common symptoms specific to thumb CMC OA include thumb pain during activity,[2] pain at rest, decreased grip and pinch strength,[3] decreased motion,[6] and thumb deformity. These symptoms impact function, including writing, fingering small objects, and carrying a 10-lb bundle.[3] In addition, individuals with hand OA in general have been found to have difficulty with household management, functional mobility, personal care, active recreation, wringing cloths, opening containers,[7] caring for grandchildren, and using cell phones.[8] The functional concerns associated with thumb CMC joint OA necessitate the role of hand therapy for treatment of patients with this condition. A survey of hand therapists suggests that more than half of hand therapists have a caseload in which approximately one quarter is composed of individuals with thumb pain.[9]

ANATOMICAL CONSIDERATIONS

Joint Classification

The thumb CMC is one of three saddle joints in the human body; the others are the sternoclavicular joint and the incudomalleolar joint of the inner ear. Saddle joints are biaxial, allowing movement in the sagittal and frontal planes. This biaxial movement is available because of reciprocal concavity and convexity of the two articulating bones. In the thumb CMC joint, the articular surface of the trapezium is generally convex in

an ulnoradial direction and concave from a palmar-dorsal direction, and the surface of the first metacarpal (MC) is the reverse (Fig. 88.1).

Motions

The saddlelike architecture of the trapeziometacarpal joint allows the thumb CMC to produce flexion, extension, adduction, abduction, and combinations of such (i.e., opposition and reposition). The thumb CMC's primary motions are palmar abduction and adduction, which predominantly occur in the sagittal plane and flexion and extension, which occur predominantly in the frontal plane. Opposition and reposition are secondary movement patterns derived from these primary biaxial movements.

Abduction and adduction occur when the convex articular surface of the thumb MC moves on the fixed concave (dorsovolar) surface of the trapezium (Fig. 88.2). During abduction, the convex articular surface of the MC rolls palmarly almost 45 degrees and slides dorsally on the concave surface of the trapezium. Full abduction at the CMC joint elongates the adductor pollicis muscle and most ligaments at the CMC joint, especially those embedded within the posterior aspect of the joint capsule.[10] Full abduction opens the webspace of the thumb, forming a wide curvature useful for grasping large and cylindrical objects.

Flexion and extension occur when the concave articular surface of the MC moves across the convex (radioulnar) trapezial surface (Fig. 88.3). When moving from full extension into flexion, the concave surface of MC rolls about 45 to 50 degrees[11] and simultaneously slides in an ulnar direction and pronates slightly.[10,12]

Opposition is produced by combining the biaxial motions, abduction and flexion, which results in the addition of out-of-plane motion, namely MC pronation[13] (Fig. 88.4). The prime mover responsible for opposition, the opponens pollicis (OP), flexes and pronates the thumb MC and is facilitated by a groove on the transverse surface of

PALMAR VIEW

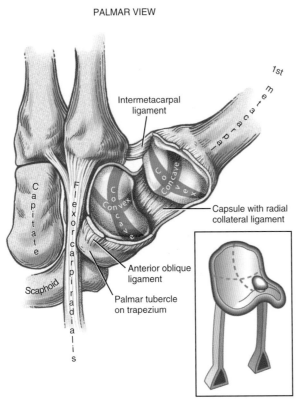

Fig. 88.1 The carpometacarpal saddle joint.

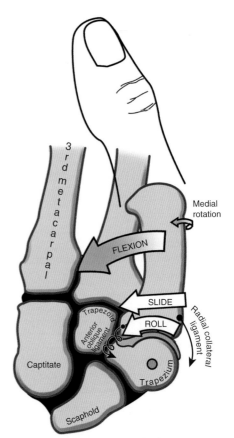

Fig. 88.3 Thumb flexion.

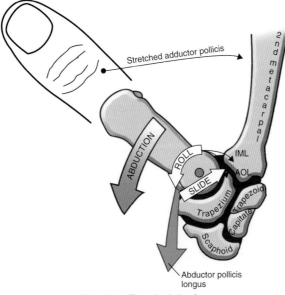

Fig. 88.2 Thumb abduction.

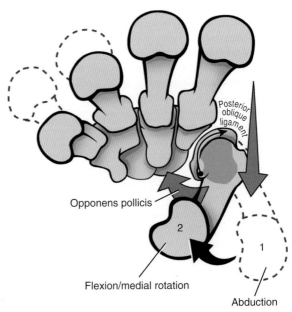

Fig. 88.4 Thumb opposition.

the trapezium. In addition to MC pronation, trapezial movement augments opposition. During opposition, fluoroscopic study has revealed trapezial twisting relative to the scaphoid and trapezoid.[14] Full opposition is considered the thumb CMC's most stable position (i.e., closed-pack).[15] Opposition is stabilized by making several dorsal capsular ligaments taut and by activating the supporting musculature. It should be noted that although the joint is most congruent in full opposition, only about half of the surface area of the joint is load bearing. Considering the large and frequent loads (forces) that cross this joint, the relatively small contact area may naturally predispose the joint to large and potentially damaging stress.[16] Opposition allows the thumb tip to

make pulp-to-pulp contact with opposing fingers and enables various prehensile and grasp patterns. Achieving precision tip and three-point pinch or gross spherical and cylindrical grasps is made possible when the thumb opposes and generates forces opposite to the fingers.

The final out-of-plane motion, reposition, occurs when the thumb returns from opposition back into the anatomic position. This motion combines adduction with extension and supination of the MC.[13] Reposition allows for the hand to rest on or weight bear onto flat surfaces and prepositions the thumb for grasping large-diameter objects.

TABLE 88.1   Primary Actions of Muscles Crossing the Thumb Carpometacarpal Joint

Primary Action	Muscle(s)
Flexion	Adductor pollicis, flexor pollicis brevis, flexor pollicis longus, opponens pollicis
Extension	Extensor pollicis brevis, extensor pollicis longus, abductor pollicis longus
Abduction	Abductor pollicis brevis, abductor pollicis longus
Adduction	Adductor pollicis, extensor pollicis longus
Opposition	Opponens pollicis, flexor pollicis brevis, abductor pollicis brevis, flexor pollicis longus, abductor pollicis longus
Reposition	Extensor pollicis longus, extensor pollicis brevis

Muscles

Cooney and Chao[17] report there to be eight muscles that act on the CMC joint; however, recent evidence suggests that in addition, the first dorsal interosseous (FDI) muscle, the "lateral thenar muscle," may also have a role in control of the thumb CMC joint.[18,19] Table 88.1 lists the primary actions performed by the eight muscles that cross the CMC joint of the thumb.[17] By necessity, these actions are associated with relatively large joint forces, potentially 10 to 18 times greater than the resistive (external) force applied to the distal end of the digit.[17] The large joint forces ultimately reflect that these thumb muscles must generate higher forces to match the demands of the task given that the leverage available to them (based on moment arm length) is much smaller than the leverage available to the external forces (Torque = Force × Lever arm). In theory, even when performing daily activities with presumably lower force demands (e.g., turning a key, flossing teeth, or handwriting), significant muscular-based loads are likely acting on the thumb CMC joint. Recent evidence supports that in a less innocuous activity, opening of a sealed jar, high loads likely act upon the thumb CMC joint over time. Depending on how one approaches jar opening, the act of attempting to open a sealed jar is expected to result in anywhere between 82.6 and 206.0 lb*seconds of load to the thumb CMC across the duration of the act.[20]

The naturally strongest motions of the thumb typically involve a combination of flexion and adduction of the CMC joint, usually associated with a strong lateral pinch. Fig. 88.5 shows the relative torque potential and actions of seven thumb muscles that cross the CMC joint based on data from cadaver specimens. In this diagram, the orientation of the solid lines is indicative of muscle line of pull and the relative length of the solid line represents the individual muscle's (or it's individual heads') torque-generating capacity. The lines with tic marks, however, illustrate the maximal torque generating capacity of the combined prime movers into the flexion–extension and adduction–abduction planes. For example, the adductor pollicis (oblique head) is shown producing a combined adduction and flexion torque across the CMC joint (solid line), whereas the maximum flexion torque is about 50% greater than the maximum adduction torque (line with tic marks). It should be noted that the oblique head of the adductor pollicis is theoretically capable of producing the greatest torque of all the thumb muscles that cross the CMC joint.

In the next section, we will explore the theories that intend to explain the development of thumb CMC OA, two of which directly relate to the topic of thumb musculature. One theory relates more to aforementioned evidence on the deleterious effect of generating repetitive and large thumb CMC pinch forces on supporting ligamentous stabilizers and articular surfaces. Another theory is that poor thumb neuromuscular control results in inadequate help from muscular stabilizers and maladaptive compensatory strategies to produce the desired motions (i.e., use of the extensor pollicis longus [EPL] to produce CMC extension while also loading the thumb

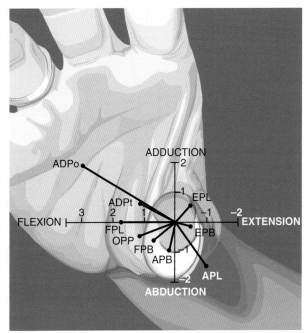

Fig. 88.5 The relative torque potential and actions of seven thumb muscles that cross the carpometacarpal joint. *ADPo,* Oblique head of the adductor pollicis; *ADPt,* transverse head of the adductor pollicis; *APB,* abductor pollicis brevis; *APL,* abductor pollicis longus; *EPB,* extensor pollicis brevis; *EPL,* extensor pollicis longus; *FPB,* flexor pollicis brevis; *FPL,* flexor pollicis longus; *OPP,* opponens pollicis.

metacarpophalangeal [MCP] and generating a CMC adduction force). Whether or not this is a symptom of weakness, just a lack of responsiveness by muscles that are believed to be dynamic stabilizers of the thumb CMC or both is not yet known; however, this theory has recently led to a paradigm shift in hand therapy. This shift in thinking is grounded in early work of Paul Brand and Hollister[21] and Poole and Pelligrini[22] and is now supported by some basic scientific evidence that the strength of the FDI significantly predicts its ability to reduce an induced MC subluxation in vivo[19] and that the OP and FDI distract and ulnarly approximate the base of the thumb MC relative to the trapezium in vitro.[18] Further evidence in support of a neuromuscular cause and effect of thumb CMC OA is that the thumb ligamentous mechanoreceptors accountable for the responsiveness of muscular stabilizers are less prominent in the ligaments of the osteoarthritic thumb CMC than they are in healthy thumb CMC joints.[23] In summary, the muscles surrounding the CMC afford it mobility and stability but are also likely sources of instability and articular wear.

Ligaments

The bony architecture of the thumb CMC is notably shallow and thus possesses little intrinsic stability; the intrinsic stability of this joint is primarily achieved by its ligaments.[24] More specifically, the thumb CMC ligaments have four specific functions: (1) controlling the extent and direction of joint motion, (2) maintaining normal alignment of the joint, (3) controlling forces, and (4) dissipating forces produced by activated muscles.[15,24,25] As few as 3 and as many as 16 ligaments have been identified. Volar and dorsal ligaments have been named as primary stabilizers of the CMC joint.[13] For the purposes of this chapter, 5 primary ligaments will be described, 3 dorsal and 2 volar. The 3 dorsal ligaments are the dorsal radial ligament (DRL), dorsal central ligament (DCL), and posterior oblique ligament (POL), and the 2 volar are the anterior or volar (beak) oblique ligament (AOL) and ulnar collateral ligament (UCL) (Fig. 88.6). Table 88.2 describes the origins and insertions of these 5 ligaments. Given the large arc of motion native to the thumb CMC, the ligaments of the thumb CMC joint are, out of necessity, fundamentally loose fitting

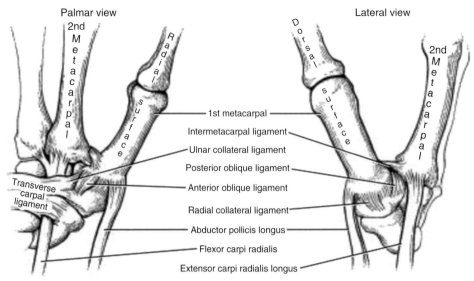

Fig. 88.6 Thumb ligaments.

TABLE 88.2	**Primary Thumb Carpometacarpal Ligaments[15,24,26]**			
	Name	**Insert**	**Origin**	**Function**
Volar ligaments	Anterior oblique ligament (AOL)[a]	Articular margins of the trapezium and first metacarpal	Ulnar to the volar styloid process at the base of the first metacarpal	Taut in extension and adduction; shortened during flexion, abduction, and opposition; secondary restraint to posterior shear, translation, and dislocation
	Ulnar collateral ligament (UCL)	Superficial and ulnar to the AOL on the palmar–ulnar tubercle of the first metacarpal	Distal margin of the transverse carpal ligament and ulnar to the insertion of the TCL onto the trapezial ridge	Taut in abduction and pronation; shortened during supination and adduction; secondary restraint to posterior shear, translation, and dislocation
Dorsal ligaments (i.e., deltoid ligament)	Dorsal central ligament (DCL)	Dorsal edge of the base of the thumb metacarpal	Dorsoradial tubercle of the trapezium; travels ulnar to the DRL and deep to the EPB tendon	Taut during flexion, abduction, and opposition; shortened during extension and adduction; primary restraint to posterior shear, translation, and dislocation
	Dorsal radial ligament (DRL)	Dorsal edge of the base of the thumb metacarpal	Dorsoradial tubercle of the trapezium	Taut during flexion, abduction, and opposition; shortened during extension and adduction; primary restraint to posterior shear, translation, and dislocation
	Posterior oblique (POL)	Dorsoulnar aspect of the thumb metacarpal and the palmar–ulnar tubercle along with the IML	Dorsoulnar side of the trapezium immediately adjacent to the DRL	Taut during flexion, abduction, and opposition; shortened during extension and adduction; primary restraint to posterior shear, translation, and dislocation

[a]Described as two heads: superficial and deep ("beak") fibers.
EPB, Extensor pollicis brevis; *IML,* intermetacarpal ligament; *TCL,* transverse carpal ligament.

yet are critical in resisting the CMC's tendency to subluxate with pinch and gripping. Failure of the ligaments to perform these functions can make the joint susceptible to excessive play and degeneration.[26]

In general, extension, abduction, and opposition elongate most of the ligaments of the CMC joint of the thumb. New evidence counters early literature[27,28] that describes the AOL as being the primary dynamic stabilizer of the thumb CMC. More recently, several authors have illustrated that the DRL prevents radial subluxation,[29–31] has

more dense and organized collagen bundles, and is better innervated with mechanoreceptors than is the AOL.[15] Early research emphasized changes in the volar ligaments but did not report on dorsal ligamentous changes with CMC OA, whereas more recently, there is emerging evidence to suggest that there are mechanoreceptor innervation density changes in the DRL of arthritic thumbs.[32,33] The histology and the pathohistology of this ligament reinforce biomechanical findings and beckon additional research on the role of proprioceptive interventions.

The volar beak ligament (anterior oblique ligament) is completely lax during the screw-home-torque phase of opposition in power pinch and power grasp and therefore plays no part in prevention of dorsal subluxation during power pinch or power grip.[34]

BIOMECHANICAL AND NEUROMUSCULAR CONSIDERATIONS

Numerous mechanisms for thumb CMC OA development have been proposed, all of which are strongly grounded in cadaveric and biomechanical research. Ligamentous laxity, muscle forces, contact forces, and lack of neuromuscular control are four mechanisms by which thumb CMC OA is believed to occur. The etiology, however, is likely not explained by any one particular theory but rather is likely explained by the interaction between all. This multifaceted etiology is explained by factors intrinsic to the individual and the demands placed on the hand. Any part of the "synovial organ," whether it is the joint, ligament, periarticular muscles, or joint innervation, may be involved in the development of joint OA.[35]

Ligamentous Laxity

According to this theory, ligaments that normally stabilize the CMC joint are lax or become weak or partially ruptured because of overuse and are less able to resist the radial-directed forces that naturally accompany lateral pinch. As a result, the base of the first MC slides or migrates radially, or radial dorsally, relative to the trapezium.[16] Potentially damaging shear forces may concentrate near the palmar aspect of the trapezium, adjacent to the attachments of the anterior oblique ligament.[16] The literature suggests that hypermobility of the thumb CMC is strongly linked to the presence of OA in young patients with Ehlers-Danlos syndrome[36] or just the general population of persons with joint hypermobility.[37] A presumed precursor to OA development, dorsoradial MC subluxation, is also significantly related to an objective measure of generalized joint laxity.[38,39]

Another point of consideration is the impact of distal joint hypermobility on the thumb CMC joint. Basic science research demonstrates that when the thumb MCP postures in 30 degrees of flexion, the MC exerts loads onto the trapezium in a centrally distributed fashion, whereas when it postures in hyperextension, the MC's load shifts onto the more volar aspect of the trapezium in a manner more consistent with that that occurs with radial subluxation.[40] Whether or not this phenomenon is compensatory so as to increase the available thumb working space after the formation of an adduction contracture or if this is a mechanism by which arthritis develops is unknown.[41]

Muscle Forces

According to this theory, thumb CMC OA develops as a result of repetitive and large loads on the CMC, muscle strength imbalance[42] and higher force generating capacity.[43] The strength of the adductor pollicis, when compared with the weaker opposing thenar intrinsic and extrinsic extensors and abductors, is suggested to contribute to the collapsed CMC deformity. Additionally, a subluxated CMC joint affects the moment arms of the muscles that cross the region, which may further bias the MC into radial subluxation.[44]

Recent evidence[45] contradicts early theory of the abductor pollicis longus (APL) having a stabilizing effect.[22] According to Mobargha and associates,[45] the APL and EPL produce large compressive forces and do not approximate the thumb MC. The strength of the adductor pollicis, when compared with the weaker opposing thenar intrinsic and extrinsic extensors and abductors, is suggested to contribute to the collapsed CMC deformity. Additionally, a subluxated CMC joint affects the moment arms of the muscles that cross the region, which may further bias the MC into radial subluxation.[45]

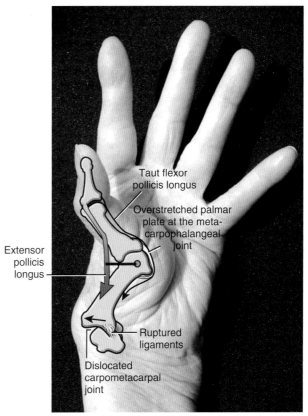

Fig. 88.7 Zig-zag deformity of the thumb.

Conversely, the authors report that the FDI provides the strongest distraction of the joint. The early theory that the APL's occasional insertion onto the trapezium may have a stabilizing effect on the trapezium is also no longer supported in the literature.[46] When the MC collapses in adduction, the APL likely has no useful moment arms to effect CMC extension.

When thumb MCP hyperextension is present, the altered line of pull of the extensor pollicis brevis (EPB) can further contribute to the collapse deformity related to the EPB's insertion on the thumb proximal phalanx.[47] Therapists should consider this when attempting to regain CMC extension and should place the thumb's MCP and interphalangeal (IP) joints in flexion so as to avoid encouraging the MCP hyperextension deformity.

This MCP hyperextension deformity also results in other biomechanical changes in the thumb. The EPL loses its mechanical advantage and ability to act on the IP and further contributes to the MCP extension deformity. Moreover, the flexor pollicis longus (FPL) becomes shortened and loses its ability to act on the IP joint. Given this inefficient IP joint flexion, the force required for pinch is transmitted to the MC head instead of the tip of the distal phalanx (Fig. 88.7).

Contact Forces

A foundational study in the understanding of thumb CMC mechanics performed by Cooney and Chao[17] reports CMC joint compression forces up to 12 times larger than the contact forces applied at the distal end of the thumb during lateral pinch. Others have reported that depending on the posture of the thumb, trapezial loads were as large as 6 to 24 times the applied load.[48] Giurintano and coworkers[48] reported loads acting on the CMC joint to be 24 times the applied loads when grasping a screwdriver and 18 times the applied load during a key grasp. Maximal-effort lateral pinch can concentrate very large joint forces across a relatively small part of the joint's articular cartilage.[16] The relatively limited area of this force can create large and potentially damaging intraarticular stress within this region of the joint.

Additionally, research suggests that women appear to have more variance in trapezial contact force and area than do men and also trend toward having increased CMC contact forces and peak pressure.[49] Given that there are no apparent gender differences in the kinematics of the MC relative to the trapezium in healthy joints,[50] these findings support the theory that other factors such as trapezial geometry or the protective or deleterious effects of estrogen and relaxin are at play.[13]

Lack of Neuromuscular Control

The healthy thumb CMC joint depends on a refined integration of sensory input from muscles, ligaments, and skin and motor output—that is, neuromuscular control.[32] Evidence describes the reduced presence of mechanoreceptors in the ligaments supporting the arthritic thumb CMC joint compared with healthy thumb CMC joints, suggesting a neuromuscular component to thumb CMC joint OA.[32] The reflexive proprioceptive responsiveness of thumb CMC joint mechanoreceptors is described by Mobargha.[51] In this study, electrostimulus was provided to the DRL in healthy-handed individuals while the thumb was placed into stable (i.e., tip) and unstable (i.e., lateral) pinches. When unstable, stimulus to the DRL resulted in reflexive activity in the stabilizing intrinsic and extrinsic musculature, whereas when in a stable posture, there was an inhibitory effect on such. To date, this experiment has not yet been carried out in persons with arthritic thumb CMC joints; however, given the aforementioned reduced mechanoreceptor density, one would anticipate a reduced reflexive responsiveness of stabilizing musculature. Other sensorimotor disturbances are already documented when arthritis is located elsewhere in the hand,[52] so such impairments might also be expected when OA is localized to the thumb CMC. Whether or not this reduction in receptor density is a response to or predictor of joint disease remains unknown. However, experts describe that joints with ligamentous injuries may remain stable as long as the neuromuscular control of the joint remains intact through adequate proprioceptive input.[53] Beyond this, the experience of pain during thumb use could explain altered neuromuscular control and could subsequently explain motor learning, or lack thereof, during rehabilitation. Further study in this area is needed, but this evidence appears to have sparked a paradigm shift in our approach to hand therapy for persons with predispositions to proprioceptive changes.

THERAPY INTERVENTIONS

Orthoses

One common treatment intervention to decrease the symptoms associated with OA at the thumb CMC joint is an orthosis. Studies have suggested that 70% to 88% of therapists recommend an orthosis when working with an individual with CMC arthrosis.[9,54] An orthosis is generally recommended for this diagnosis to provide stability to the joint for ligamentous laxity, assist with preventing or deterring dorsal–radial subluxation of the MC on the trapezium, provide proprioceptive input into the thumb, provide rest to an inflamed joint, or discourage use of the thumb in a position of deformity. The goal of providing an orthosis to an individual with thumb CMC joint OA is to assist with increasing function and decreasing pain.

There are a large number of possible options for the orthosis design, including static immobilization (Fig. 88.8) or neoprene support orthoses (Fig. 88.9), custom or prefabricated designs, and

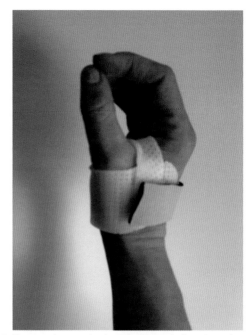

Fig. 88.8 Custom thermoplastic orthosis excluding the wrist and metacarpophalangeal joint and positioning the carpometacarpal joint in palmar abduction, slight flexion, and medial rotation of the metacarpal.

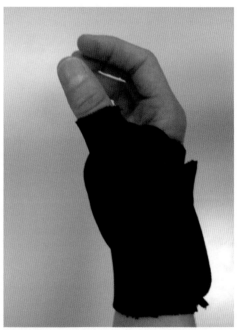

Fig. 88.9 Prefabricated neoprene carpometacarpal orthosis.

patterns that include or exclude the wrist and thumb MCP joint. Generally speaking, orthoses for thumb CMC joint OA position the thumb into palmar abduction, slight flexion, and medial rotation of the MC. This position of the thumb is clinically believed to promote natural stability at the base of the thumb by increasing the congruity of the joint surfaces.[55,56] This position also assists with maintenance of the webspace, which is often shortened with deformity related to this diagnosis.

An orthosis has been shown via research studies and systematic reviews[57–62] to decrease pain for individuals with OA at the base of the thumb. The available research studies, however, do not identify one specific orthosis design that is superior in decreasing pain and increasing function.[57-59] The selection of an orthosis, therefore, should be an evidence-based decision considering the therapist's experience and comfort in fabrication, the patient's preferences and needs, and the available research evidence. Hand therapists may opt to provide the support necessary for good or improved pinch mechanics and the support needed to decrease pain with pinching. For example, an individual presenting with symptomatic arthritis at the base of the thumb with MCP joint hyperextension may be a candidate for inclusion of the MCP joint in the orthosis in flexion. MCP joint hyperextension and the change in muscle leverage because of the MCP joint hyperextension can impact the stability of the CMC joint and encourage dorsal–radial subluxation of the MC.[63] A cadaveric study[61] has suggested that 30 degrees of flexion at the MCP joint shifts pressure in the CMC joint dorsally. Another study[64] evaluated differences in outcomes for individuals with and without inclusion of the thumb MCP joint in an orthosis and found no differences; however, individuals with MCP joint hyperextension were excluded, and this population has not been exclusively studied. As another example, an individual with symptomatic thumb CMC joint OA who is required to wear gloves daily for work may be an appropriate candidate for a low-profile custom or prefabricated orthosis including only the CMC joint as long as this provides the support needed for greater stability and decreased pain. As further discussion related to selection of the most appropriate orthosis for each individual, research studies suggest a patient preference for prefabricated neoprene orthoses compared with custom thermoplastic orthoses.[65-67] Additionally, another study[68] has suggested that the greater the stability provided by an orthosis, the greater the impact on functionality of the involved hand, meaning less restrictive orthoses allow greater functional use of the involved hand.

It is important to note that because individuals with mild to moderate OA are considered better candidates for conservative treatment than those with severe OA, the studies on using an orthosis for thumb CMC OA generally involve participants with milder cases of OA. Sound clinical judgment should be used when treating referrals with severe CMC joint OA. For example, an orthosis may not be appropriate when there is a subluxed MC that is not easily reducible. Additional high-quality studies are needed to assist with identifying the most appropriate orthoses for different clinical presentations, including severe joint destruction, MCP joint hyperextension, and so on.

Related to the frequency and duration of wear of an orthosis for symptomatic thumb CMC joint OA, it is common to recommend use during the daytime to reduce pain with functional use of the hand or at night during sleep to rest the joint in a stable position. One randomized controlled trial (RCT)[69] with individuals with varying degrees of arthritis at the base of the thumb evaluated the use of a prefabricated long opponens orthosis including the wrist and thumb MCP joint during sleep only. They concluded that this orthosis worn only at night during sleep did decrease pain in the long term (at 1-year follow-up) but not in the short term.[69] More often, research studies evaluate the effectiveness of using an orthosis for thumb CMC arthritis during functional use of the hand. It has been found that wear of an orthosis during function allows decreased pain within the first 4 weeks of wear[70,71] and that pain continues to decrease with continued wear.[72] The duration of orthosis wear can be individualized and may be long term or as needed during flareup of symptoms. Research studies have found no thenar muscle atrophy[71] to occur and no decrease in grip or pinch strength[73] after prolonged use of an orthosis for CMC joint arthritis at the thumb.

Dynamic Stability Exercises

The dynamic stability approach,[74] originally called this by the late Jan Albrecht, OTR/L, CHT, in 2000, is grounded in the early biomechanical

work and experiences of Poole and Pelligrini,[22] who described that strengthening of the thenar muscles and APL would assist in stabilizing the thumb CMC; Boutan,[75] who reports that the OP and FDI were coordinated in their effort to stabilize the CMC; Taylor,[76] who advocated for the restoration of the first webspace; and Brand and Hollister,[21] who were the first to describe the CMC stabilizing effects of the FDI. The retrospective therapy outcomes of the dynamic stability approach were first reported by O'Brien and Giveans,[77] who found clinically significantly improved pain and disability according to the Quick Disability of the Arm, Shoulder and Hand (DASH) after an average of two skilled therapy visits.[77] In addition, Wouters[78] prospectively explored the benefits of the dynamic stability approach compared to an orthosis only "standard of care" group and reported significantly better pain reduction in the dynamic stability group at 3 months. The authors also explored what intrinsic factors explained patient responsiveness to the program and reported that when the dominant hand was treated and when greater thumb MCP flexion was available, pain at rest and pain during loading were lower, respectively.[78]

The objectives of the dynamic stability approach are to preserve the CMC joint, minimize dependence on orthoses, and reduce pain. This is accomplished through a multimodal and staged approach that includes manual release of the adductor and any overactive muscle, joint mobilization to reduce the subluxated MC and realign the CMC joint, neuromuscular reeducation and strengthening, use of adaptive tools and joint protection techniques, and orthoses as needed with a goal of gradual weaning.

Throughout each stage of the approach, the client is taught to respect pain. The approach takes pain into consideration so as to reduce risk of flare up but also to ensure that optimal neuromuscular facilitation can occur. As was indicated earlier in the chapter, motor learning can be impaired when pain is present, and like other sources of chronic pain, cortical changes are likely already present and need to be changed and not perpetuated. Although no evidence currently exists on cortical changes when living with thumb CMC OA, recent research supports that, like in clients with type 1 chronic regional pain syndrome,[79] there appears to be the presence of limb disregard. This approach takes a neuromuscular reeducation approach by focusing heavily on relearning patterns of muscle activity that best maintain the "stable C" positioning during prehension. The "stable C" position involves the closed-pack posture of the CMC where the dorsal ligaments are taut and the joint most congruent. This is accomplished through opposing the first MC to the second and third metacarpals, achieving a MCP joint posture of about 30 degrees of flexion, and maintaining a well-opened (i.e., noncollapsed) first webspace (Fig. 88.10).

Phase 1 of the dynamic stability approach is to work to release the adductor pollicis through manual release (Fig. 88.11). Release of this muscle is done to increase the potential range of motion (ROM) of the thumb often lost because of webspace contracture and is a precursor to begin achieving congruency of the thumb CMC joint. This release may also be achieved through use of a chip-bag clip via placing pressure on the adductor pollicis to promote relaxation. The release techniques are performed for a duration of 30 seconds several times daily. After achieving improved adductor extensibility, additional manual approaches are used to centralize the MC on the trapezium, assist in production of synovial fluid to aid in joint nutrition, and reduce pain. Several forms of grade I mobilizations were described by O'Brien and Giveans,[77] including CMC traction to open the joint space (Fig. 88.12), an ulnar glide to reduce the dorsoradially subluxated MC, and rolling the MC into reposition. These mobilization techniques are held for 1 to 3 minutes and performed twice daily.

After these two manual approaches to better seat the MC on the trapezium, neuromuscular reeducation is undertaken to help maintain

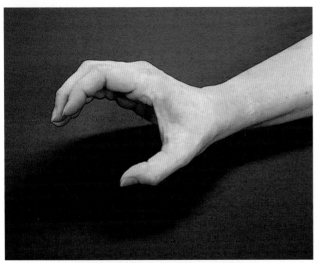

Fig. 88.10 The "stable C" position.

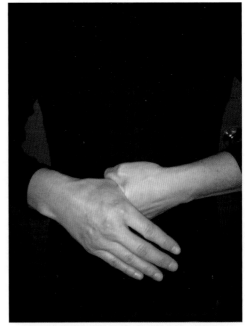

Fig. 88.12 Carpometacarpal joint traction.

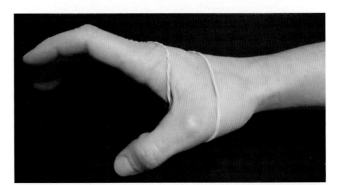

Fig. 88.13 The abductor pollicis brevis is selectively targeted to open up the webspace.

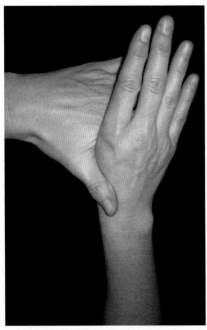

Fig. 88.11 Release of the adductor pollicis through manual release.

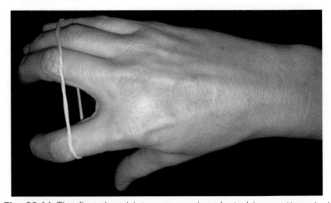

Fig. 88.14 The first dorsal interosseous is selected in an attempt at maintaining the metacarpal out of the radially subluxated posture.

the gains made through manual techniques. Neuromuscular training first comes in the form of selected pain-free active motion without resistance, progressing to light isometric and later adding isotonic exercises. Retraining without resistance and then isometrically occurs three times daily for 10 to 15 repetitions depending on the tolerance of the client. When progressing into maximal resistances, the frequency and intensity reduce to once a day for 8 to 10 repetitions. The target muscles and rationales for their training are as follows:

- The **abductor pollicis brevis** is selectively targeted to open up the webspace (Fig. 88.13).
- The **OP** is targeted to restore the pronation often lost with adductor pollicis tightness.
- The **FDI** is selected in an attempt at maintaining the MC out of the radially subluxated posture (Fig. 88.14).
- The reeducation of **EPB** is emphasized to break the pattern of an EPL-dominant thumb initiating CMC extension and should be performed with the MCP and IP joints posturing in flexion to minimize

recruitment of the dominant EPL and mitigate the potential of the EPB and EPL to hyperextend the MCP joint.

- The **flexor pollicis brevis** (**FPB**) is emphasized with the intent of maintaining MCP flexion during prehension and preventing the MCP hyperextension collapse.

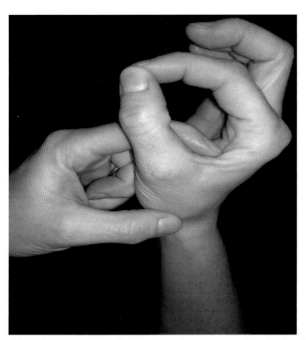

Fig. 88.15 Providing manual support to the metacarpal in the "stable C" position.

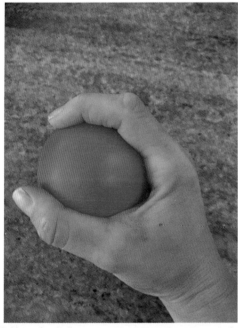

Fig. 88.16 Use of a ball to promote appropriate posture for dynamic stability exercise for the thumb carpometacarpal joint, including thumb opposition and first dorsal interossei contraction though index abduction.

The program as presented by O'Brien and Giveans[77] recommends neuromuscular reeducation of the APL as well; however, given recent evidence of the compressive loading effect of the APL,[46] we recommend deemphasizing this muscle. For a patient with an unstable CMC, doing FDI neuromuscular reeducation may be painful initially. In this case, providing manual support of the MC while in the "C" position while co-contracting the OP, EPB, and FPB may be helpful (Figs. 88.15 and 88.16).

The dynamic stability approach is multimodal and also includes early incorporation of joint protection training with emphasis on preventing the collapse deformity and key pinch, a CMC or CMC/MCP stabilization orthosis for wear during dynamic activities but working toward weaning to avoid disuse of newly reeducated motor programs, modalities to enhance pain management and prepare for stretching, elastic taping techniques to facilitate reeducation, and the use of prescribed therapeutic occupations to facilitate motor training and work toward translating exercise into real-world scenarios.

Joint Mobilization

Manual therapy techniques for joint mobilization of a symptomatic CMC joint of the thumb can include joint distraction or mobilization with movement (MWM). Joint distraction to the CMC joint is a gentle mobilization technique in which the therapist grasps the patient's thumb and gently distracts or "pulls" on the CMC joint space to open the space to decrease pain. MWM is a manual technique that is applied to a joint to promote restoration of normal joint alignment and arthrokinematics rather than the stretching of the joint capsule.[80] The technique includes sustained manual correction of subtle joint malalignment, with active movement immediately superimposed on the corrected joint position.[81] The active movement chosen is one that produced pain previously but, when performed with manual correction of joint alignment, occurs pain free.[82] For example, the therapist centralizes the first MC in the joint space and then asks the patient to perform active thumb abduction. Both joint distraction and MWM are performed to reduce pain and improve hand function. A case study found that a combined program of MWM and application of elastic tape reduced pain, increased ROM, and increased tip pinch strength in a patient with severe functional impairment related to dominant CMC OA.[83] A systematic review on the conservative management of CMC OA found moderate-quality evidence that manual therapy (Kaltenborn technique, posterior–anterior gliding with distraction, grade 3 of CMC joint for 3 minutes with a 1-minute pause) improves pain at a short-term follow-up. They found no significant improvement in hand strength at short-term follow-up when comparing manual therapy with a control group.[84]

Modalities

Superficial heat and cold modalities commonly used for treating OA of the CMC joint of the thumb include hot packs, paraffin baths, warm baths, fluidotherapy, cold packs, ice baths, and ice massage. The goals of these thermal modalities are to reduce pain, decrease inflammation, improve function, and increase or maintain ROM. As a general rule, cold modalities are used for acute inflammation and heat for joint stiffness. Paraffin in particular is commonly used in the treatment of hand OA. According to in vivo studies, paraffin treatment can increase temperature in the joint capsule by 7.5°C and 4.5°C in the muscle,[85] allowing increased lymph flow and absorption of exudates.[86] An RCT has found that compared with a control, paraffin treatments decreased pain at rest and pain with performance of activities of daily living and increased ROM for individuals with hand OA.[87]

Other modalities are considered in the treatment of OA at the base of the thumb preoperatively to assist with addressing the chronic inflammation that may be present and destructive to the joint via weakening ligaments and cartilage. A systematic review[84] reported that laser treatment did not produce a meaningful effect on pain, function, hand strength, ROM, or stiffness. The review reported that evidence is scarce for ultrasound, electrotherapy, or acupuncture.

Multimodal Interventions

Multimodal interventions can be defined as performing multiple interventions (e.g., joint protection education, orthosis provision, therapeutic exercises, joint mobilization) in hand therapy to improve hand function and decrease pain. In clinical practice, interventions are not often performed in isolation. A systematic review and meta-analysis on the effect of conservative intervention on CMC OA reported on the effects of manual therapy and therapeutic exercise.[84] They found moderate quality evidence for the provision of manual therapy and therapeutic exercise for the improvement of pain in thumb CMC OA at short- and intermediate-term follow-up.[84] They also reported that therapeutic exercise combined with manual therapy improved grip strength at the short-term follow up and at an intermediate-term follow-up.[84] Another systematic review found that multimodal interventions are more effective in decreasing pain compared with single interventions.[88] They report that single interventions seem not to be effective.[88] The systematic review by Villafane and associates[84] also reported on one study that provided an orthosis combined with therapeutic exercise and education program. Outcomes assessed were pain, hand strength, function, ROM and stiffness. The evidence found that a program of orthosis provision, exercise, and education provides no significant improvement in pain, hand strength, function, ROM, or stiffness at a long-term follow-up.[84]

OCCUPATION-BASED INTERVENTIONS

Conducting an occupational profile is imperative for clients with thumb CMC OA. The profile will reveal patterns of hand use and the demands of the client's occupations, including those that most aggravate symptomology. Understanding these factors will enable the therapist to better plan joint protection with targeted interventions (e.g., simulating and modifying occupations), make education relative to the needs of the client (e.g., "When you micropipette like this, huge pressures are placed on your painful thumb joint, whereas if you tried this…"), and build in home programming into the clients' existing habits and routines. Making joint protection interventions relevant to occupational demands will likely support lifestyle modification. Adherence to therapy recommendations will be supported by exploring how they can be incorporated into existing routines (e.g., "practicing dynamic stability exercises during your morning bus-ride commute"). Last, the use of activity could be used in place of some exercises (e.g., reinforcing activation of the FPB during card playing to prevent MCP collapse and then grading up to slightly more resistive activities such as handwriting or brushing teeth). Recent evidence supports that the use of occupations results in better improvement in strength,[89,90] motion, and discomfort than rote activity in a hand therapy context; however, more evidence specific to this is needed. Keeping our interventions occupation based may improve compliance, carry-over, and effectiveness, including better motor performance of the targeted stabilizing muscles.

MEASURING OUTCOMES

In clinical practice, it is important to measure body functions using a variety of validated and reproducible measures, including grip and pinch strength (Fig. 88.17), pain, and ROM.[91] The Kapandji Index is a useful and reliable tool for measuring thumb ROM in persons with CMC OA[92] and has been found to be a more psychometrically sound method of assessing ROM at the thumb than goniometric measurement[93] (Table 88.3). Assessment of palmar abduction at the thumb is indicated when treating individuals with thumb CMC joint OA and has routinely been assessed with a goniometer; however, evidence supports that the intermetacarpal distance method (Fig. 88.18) to measuring thumb abduction has the most optimal psychometrics in healthy and arthritic thumb CMC joints.[94] For more specificity and sensitivity in strength measurements, an instrument such as the Rotterdam Intrinsic Hand Myometer, a handheld myometer, can be used to gather objective

and responsive measurements of CMC palmar abduction and opposition, thumb MCP flexion, and index finger abduction strength.[95]

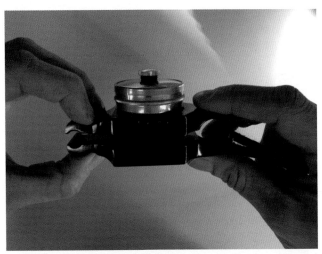

Fig. 88.17 Assessment of the body function of palmar or three-point pinch using a pinch gauge.

TABLE 88.3	**The Kapandji Index**
Score	**Location Achieved**
1	Radial side of the proximal phalanx of the index finger
2	Radial side of the middle phalanx of the index finger
3	Tip of the index finger
4	Tip of the long finger
5	Tip of the ring finger
6	Tip of the small finger
7	Distal interphalangeal joint crease of the small finger
8	Proximal interphalangeal joint crease of the small finger
9	Metacarpophalangeal joint crease of the small finger
10	Distal palmar crease below small finger

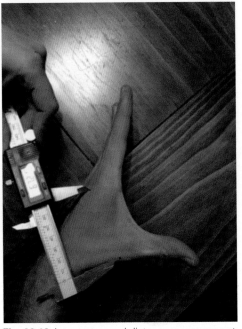

Fig. 88.18 intermetacarpal distance measurement.

In addition to assessing body functions, it is important to measure patient function or activity and participation using a validated outcome measure. Villafane and coworkers[84] found that a number of outcome measures were used to determine the effectiveness of interventions in the conservative management of CMC OA. Some of these outcome measures are specific to hand OA, and others are more global. The measures found by Villafane and coworkers[84] included the Australian/Canadian Hand Osteoarthritis Index (AUSCAN), DASH, Global Assessment of Change, Short Form 36 (SF-36), Canadian Occupation Performance Measure (COPM), and Cochin Hand Functional Scale.[84] Based on the findings from a systematic review, outcome measures used with individuals with thumb CMC OA emphasize body functions and activity and participation.[96] Some of the difficulties experienced by individuals with CMC OA, such as caring for grandchildren, wringing out washcloths, and using cell phones,[8] are not addressed by the available outcome measures and additional measures may need to be developed that capture more OA-specific issues.[97] Perhaps using more than one outcome measure can better capture all aspects of the symptoms and functional deficits of patients with CMC OA. See Chapter 14 for additional information on self-report measures and their clinical utility. The International Classification of Functioning, Disability and Health provides a comprehensive guide to understanding the experience of a hand injury, so it can be used as a reference during evaluation of an individual with thumb CMC OA to ensure consideration of environmental factors, personal factors, and activity and participation in compliment of body function.

POSTSURGICAL MANAGEMENT

Carpometacarpal OA may result in reduced cartilage thickness, increased ligament laxity with resultant instability, and subluxation of the base of the MC on the trapezium, which in turn results in a first MC adduction contracture and decreased thumb webspace. The severity of symptoms does not necessarily correspond with the radiographic stage of the disease; instead, the main indications for surgery are pain and loss of function.[98] Surgeons often tell patients to tell them when they are ready for the surgery rather than the surgeon making the decision to proceed to surgery.

Generally speaking, hand rehabilitation after surgery for arthritis at the base of the thumb is guided by the specific structures involved, the intentions of the surgery, and specifics related to the patient. Repair of ligament for stability, need for bone consolidation, intention of using scar formation for stability, and poor healing are reasons to progress

slowly or immobilize for a longer period of time following surgery, whereas variables such as stable fixation or lack of soft tissue repair are reasons to progress more quickly to ROM and strengthening. Ultimately, the focus of hand therapy after thumb CMC joint surgery is to support a functional, pain-free, stable thumb.

A systematic review[99] was conducted on the role of postoperative management of CMC OA. Unfortunately, the majority of the studies identified in the review focused on descriptions or comparisons of surgical techniques, and the authors were unable to draw definite conclusions regarding optimal postoperative immobilization, therapy protocols, and the best time to release patients to unrestricted activity after surgery for basal joint arthritis.[99] As with any hand injury, sound clinical reasoning is therefore needed when treating individuals postoperatively for a CMC joint procedure.

Surgical procedures most frequently comprise trapeziectomy with or without ligament reconstruction and tendon interposition (LRTI). Trapeziectomy with LRTI has been found to be the only surgery performed by 93% of surgeons for basal joint arthritis in one study on this topic.[100] Trapeziometacarpal arthrodesis is another option for surgical intervention for arthritis at the base of the thumb. Arthrodesis was at one time considered to be only appropriate for severe cases of CMC OA because of loss of ROM of the CMC joint. A recent study[101] found that participants who underwent joint arthrodesis had 25% better pinch strength and comparable ROM to the group that underwent an LRTI procedure. In addition, surgical options have included a variety of joint implant options and denervation of the thumb CMC joint. Hypermobility of the thumb MCP joint (>30 degrees of hyperextension in particular)[102] may also necessitate a volar plate arthroplasty or joint capsulodesis or MCP joint arthrodesis in conjunction with the basal joint surgery (Fig. 88.19). See Chapter 87 for a full description of the procedures.

There are three main phases of the postoperative care of a patient after surgery for thumb CMC joint arthritis. Table 88.4 outlines a typical postoperative therapy program. Because this program will vary considerably across clinical settings, it is meant only as a general guide. The phases include immobilization, initiation of ROM exercises, and finally the initiation of strengthening exercises. In the immobilization phase, the thumb and wrist are immobilized in a cast or an orthotic device for a period of 2[99] to 6 weeks[103] (Fig. 88.20).

Phase 2 is the initiation of ROM exercises. A systematic review[99] found that postoperative thumb exercise protocols were quite variable across the studies included in the review. Some patients simply

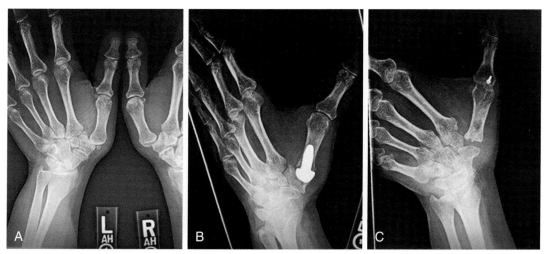

Fig. 88.19 A, Symptomatic osteoarthritis at the base of the left thumb. **B,** Stablyx implant. **C,** Excision implant and arthrodesis.

TABLE 88.4   Hand Therapy Management After a Surgery for Basal Joint Arthritis at the Thumb

Phase	Hand Therapy Guidelines After a Surgical Procedure for Basal Joint Arthritis at the Thumb[a]
I: Immobilization	• Thumb spica cast or splint is applied postoperatively and is worn full time for up to the first 4 postoperative weeks. Time frames will vary because of physician preference and the procedure performed. • Treatment focus at this time is on edema control, using ice and elevation and AROM of the uninvolved digits and thumb IP joint
II: AROM	• The cast is removed, and a thumb spica orthosis fabricated (if it has not already been done) and worn at all times except during exercise. • AROM may be now be performed at the digits and wrist. • AROM is initiated at the thumb as dictated by the surgical procedure. Each procedure has its own precautions. For example, after LRTI, flexion and adduction must be avoided early on to protect the surgically incised dorsal side of the capsule. A second example is that no abduction and circumduction are performed after a CMC arthrodesis. • By week 6–8, the protective orthosis may be weaned to a soft or neoprene orthotic to continue to provide protection yet allow for increased mobility and function.
III: Strengthening	• Start with isometric exercises and progress to strengthening exercises as tolerated. • Strengthening exercises may be performed for the wrist, grip strengthening, or pinch strengthening depending on presenting deficits and functional needs. Monitor the thumb MCP joint for hyperextension and avoid resistive activities that contribute to poor positioning of the MCP joint. • Use an orthosis as directed by therapist or physician to protect tissues during resistive activities. • Return to work and normal activities at weeks 8–12, but this will vary depending on the procedure performed and the patient's occupational demands.

[a]Time frames vary.

AROM, Active range of motion; *CMC,* carpometacarpal; *IP,* interphalangeal; *LRTI,* ligament reconstruction tendon interposition; *MCP,* metacarpophalangeal.

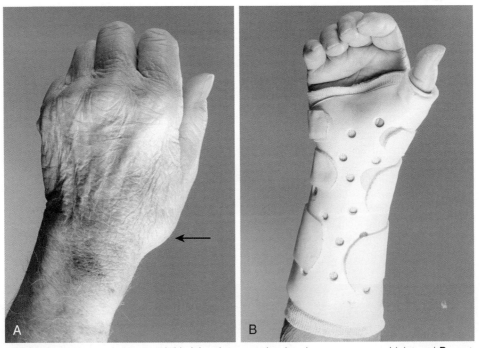

Fig. 88.20 A, Arrow is pointing at arthritic joint change at the thumb carpometacarpal joint and **B,** custom thumb spica orthosis.

were shown exercises after the immobilization was discontinued, other patients were referred to a therapist after the period of immobilization, and some patients were only referred to a therapist if it was thought they were not making satisfactory progress during follow-up visits. A small powered study[103] looked at the differences between patients who received a home program only with patients who received occupational therapy once weekly. They found no significant differences between the home program group (*n* = 5) and the occupational therapy group (*n* = 4). However, they found an increase in grip and pinch strength only in the occupational therapy group and decreased strength in the home program group.[103] Some researchers do not describe the exercise program performed in therapy. Generally, thumb ROM exercises include opposition exercises that gradually progress from aiming to the tip of the small finger to reaching the base of the small finger.[104] Another author described performing AROM exercises for CMC and MCP joints supervised by a therapist, with no CMC flexion or adduction exercises allowed to protect surgical reconstruction when there was soft tissue reconstruction.[105]

Finally, phase 3 involves strengthening and returning the patient to unrestricted activity. One author reported starting isometric thumb strengthening exercises on postoperative day 18.[106] In another study, Vermeulen and associates[107] did not specify the resistive exercises performed at 4 weeks after surgery but indicated that standardized hand therapy was performed, and it focused on regaining functionality by increasing strength. The systematic review mentioned earlier found that the time for return to full unrestricted activity was only mentioned in 5 of the 19 studies, and the range for time to return to full activity was 5 to 12 weeks in those 5 studies.[99]

Postoperative management necessitates that the thumb be immobilized in a thumb spica cast or orthosis with the CMC and MCP joints stabilized while the IP joint is left unrestricted. Horlock and coworkers[108] observed loss of movement at the MCP and IP joints after surgery and were concerned that this may have resulted from postoperative immobilization. They studied the effects of immobilization on the results of simple excision of the trapezium by comparing mobilization at 1 week and at 4 weeks after surgery.[108] The patients in the early mobilization group were instructed to remove their splints during the day to allow light use of the hand and were taught active exercises for the thumb.[108] The early mobilization group wore their orthoses for heavy activities and protection at night for 6 weeks.[108] The late mobilization group received custom-made orthoses at 2 weeks that were worn continuously until 4 weeks when they

were removed for gentle use and mobilization.[108] They discontinued the orthoses at 6 weeks or except when performing heavy tasks or at the discretion of the patient.[108] They found that the early mobilization group experienced more convenience than the late mobilization group. Furthermore, they found decreased MCP joint ROM in the late mobilization group. However, complications were observed in 15% of the participants in the early group compared with 5% in the semirigid group.[108]

There are a number of surgical procedures that address the CMC joint that are discussed in Chapter 87. See Table Table 88.5 for the impact of some surgical procedures on the rehabilitation program.

CONCLUSION

In summary, hand therapists commonly treat individuals with symptomatic OA at the thumb CMC joint, which has a high prevalence of occurrence because of biomechanical and neuromuscular concerns, including ligament laxity, muscle forces across the joint, contact forces to the articular surface, and lack of neuromuscular control. Conservative hand therapy treatment of this diagnosis includes evidence-based interventions designed to provide increased function and decreased pain. If surgical intervention is required at the thumb CMC joint, specifics on soft tissue involvement will assist in guiding the treatment progression as intended to restore ROM and function while maintaining the stability gained through surgical intervention.

TABLE 88.5	Impact of Carpometacarpal Surgical Procedures on the Rehabilitation Program		
Surgical Procedure	**Information to Note**	**Impact on Hand Therapy**	**Relevant Research**
Trapeziectomy	Can be performed with or without temporary K-wire and casting to allow scarring	ROM and functional use of the hand begin earlier after surgery when no K-wire or immobilization is used. Typically, proximal migration of the metacarpal is expected, and is greater without the allowance for scarring and without tendon interposition.[109]	A significant correlation has been found between remaining trapezial height and key pinch force,[109] but this is not consistently reported.[110]
Trapeziectomy with LRTI	Ligament reconstruction is completed after soft tissue interposition.	Requires protection of the healing ligament reconstruction	Often studied, but there is no one consistent or accepted postoperative rehabilitation protocol.[99]
Trapeziometacarpal arthrodesis using K-wire until consolidation occurs	K-wire and immobilization usually needed until consolidation is noted	Hand therapy referral for orthotic fabrication for immobilization and protection to accommodate K-wires and allow ROM at the uninvolved joints until consolidation is noted on radiographs at which time formal therapy may begin.	Perfect bone union was not needed for a good postsurgical outcome.[111]
Trapeziometacarpal arthrodesis using internal bone bridging	Can be performed with a plate and screw construct, power staple, and tension band wiring (with or without K-wire)	Stable fixation from the hardware allows decreased immobilization time and quicker return to function.	Function and motion were found to be similar to LRTI, and pinch strength was found to be 25% greater.[112]
Suture-button suspensionplasty or tightrope procedure	Uses hardware through the base of the first and second metacarpals after removal of the trapezium	Requires no soft tissue healing, therefore allowing an accelerated recovery.[113]	Mean time of 64-month follow-up suggests improvement in ROM and strength and pain relief,[113] although product rupture has been reported.[114]
Stablyx joint replacement	Saddle-shaped prosthesis with a portion to replace the distal trapezium and the proximal metacarpal. Said to have inherent stability because of the design and fit of the components	Can use stabilization with the flexor carpi radialis tendon and can occur with ligament repair, so it may require a period of immobilization for this soft tissue healing	Research findings not available at this time

TABLE 88.5   Impact of Carpometacarpal Surgical Procedures on the Rehabilitation Program—cont'd

Surgical Procedure	Information to Note	Impact on Hand Therapy	Relevant Research
PyroDisk	Designed to resurface the thumb CMC joint, is stabilized by the flexor carpi radialis tendon (which is passed through the implant)	Will likely require healing time for the soft tissue stabilization	No superiority found over trapeziectomy with or without LRTI, and 5-year survival of the prosthesis was 90%[115] Study has suggested a 20% decrease in strength postoperatively[116]
Thumb CMC joint denervation	Nerve resection to denervate the CMC joint to decrease pain	Requires short immobilization period after surgery and allows quick return to functional use[117]	Has not been compared with other surgical procedures Found to reduce pain and improve key pinch but seems to be a better option for earlier stage OA[117]
Thumb CMC joint procedure with volar plate arthroplasty of the thumb MCP joint	Usually tightening of the volar plate to decrease or eliminate thumb MCP joint hyperextension and related instability	May require dorsal blocking of the thumb MCP joint until the volar plate heals	Therapy protocol in one study allowed thumb MCP joint motion at 6 weeks after surgery but required use of an orthosis for the MCP joint until at least 16 weeks after surgery.[118]
Thumb CMC joint procedure with thumb MCP arthrodesis	Fusion of the thumb MCP joint to address MCP joint hypermobility and thumb instability	May require immobilization of the MCP joint until bony consolidation occurs	Typically found to be indicated (or a volar plate arthroplasty) when MCP hyperextension is >30 degrees[102]

CMC, Carpometacarpal; *LRTI*, ligament reconstruction and tendon interposition; *OA*, osteoarthritis *ROM*, range of motion.

REFERENCES

1. Lee HJ, Paik N, Lim J, Kim KW, Gong HS. The impact of digit-related radiographic osteoarthritis of the hand on grip strength and upper extremity disability. *Clin Orthop*. 2012;470:2202–2208.
2. Marshall M, van der Windt D, Nicholls E, Myers H, Dziedzic K. Radiographic thumb osteoarthritis: frequency, patterns, and associations with pain and clinical assessment findings in a community-dwelling population. *Rheumatol*. 2011;50:735–739.
3. Zhang Y, Niu J, Kelley-Hayes M, Chaisson CE, Aliabadi P, Felson D. Prevalence of symptomatic hand osteoarthritis and its impact on functional status among the elderly: the Framingham study. *Am J Epidemiol*. 2002;156:1021–1027.
4. Eaton RG, Glickel SZ. Trapeziometacarpal osteoarthritis: staging as a rationale for treatment. *Hand Clinics*. 1987;3:455–469.
5. Haara MM, Heliovaara M, Kroger H, et al. Osteoarthritis in the carpometacarpal joint of the thumb: prevalence and associations with disability and mortality. *J Bone Joint Surg*. 2004;86-A:1452–1457.
6. Gehrmann SV, Tang J, Li ZM, Goitz RJ, Windolf J, Kaufmann RA. Motion deficit of the thumb in CMC joint arthritis. *J Hand Surg*. 2010;35A:1449–1453.
7. Kjeken I, Dagfinrud H, Slatkowsky-Christensen B, et al. Activity limitations and participation restrictions in women with hand osteoarthritis: patients' descriptions and associations between dimensions of functioning. *Ann Rheum Dis*. 2005;64:1633–1638.
8. Stamm T, van der Giesen F, Thorstensson CA, et al. Patient perspective of hand osteoarthritis in relation to concepts covered by instruments measuring functioning: a qualitative European multi-centre study. *Ann Rheum Dis*. 2009;68:1453–1460.
9. O'Brien VH, McGaha JL. Current practice patterns in conservative thumb CMC joint care: survey results. *J Hand Ther*. 2014;27:14–22.
10. Imaeda T, Niebur G, Cooney WP, et al. Kinematics of the normal trapeziometacarpal joint. *J Orthop Res*. 1994;12:197–204.
11. Cooney WP, Lucca MJ, Chao EY, et al. The kinesiology of the thumb trapeziometacarpal joint. *J Bone Joint Surg*. 1981;63A:1371–1381.
12. Crisco J, Halilaj E, Moore D, Patel T, Weiss A, Ladd A. In vivo kineobarghaatics of the trapeziometacarpal joint during thumb extension-flexion and abduction-adduction. *J Hand Surg*. 2015;40:289–296.
13. Ladd A, Weiss A, Crisco J, Hagert E, Wolf J, Glickel S, et al. The thumb carpometacarpal joint: anatomy, hormones, and biomechanics. *AAOS Instr Course Lect*. 2013;62:165–179.
14. Zancolli EA, Ziadenberg C, Zancolli Jr E. Biomechanics of the trapeziometacarpal joint. *Clin Orthop Relat Res*. 1987;220:14–26.
15. Ladd AL, Lee J, Hagert E. Macroscopic and microscopic analysis of the thumb carpometacarpal ligaments: a cadaveric study of ligament anatomy and history. *J Bone Joint Surg Am*. 2012;94:1468–1477.
16. Pellegrini Jr VD. Osteoarthritis of the trapeziometacarpal joint: the pathophysiology of articular cartilage degeneration. I. Anatomy and pathology of the aging joint. *J Hand Surg*. 1991;16A:967–974.
17. Cooney III WP, Chao EYS. Biomechanical analysis of static forces in the thumb during hand function. *J Bone Joint Surg*. 1977;59:27–36.
18. Adams J, O'Brien V, Magnusson E, Rosenstein B, Nuckley D. *Radiographic Analysis of Simulated First Dorsal Interosseous and Opponens Pollicis Loading upon Thumb CMC Joint Subluxation: a Cadaver Study*. New York: Hand; 2017. 1558944717691132.
19. McGee C, O'Brien V, Van Nortwick S, Adams J, Van Heest A. First dorsal interosseous muscle contraction results in radiographic reduction of healthy thumb carpometacarpal joint. *J Hand Ther*. 2015;28:375–380.
20. McGee C, Mathiowetz V. Evaluation of hand forces during a joint-protection strategy for women with hand osteoarthritis. *AJOT*. 2017;71: 7101190020p1-7101190020 p8.
21. Brand PW, Hollister A. *Mechanics of Individual Muscles at Individual Joints. Clinical Mechanics of the Hand*. 2nd ed. St. Louis: Mosby; 1993:254.
22. Poole JU, Pellegrini VD. Arthritis of the thumb basal joint complex. *J Hand Ther*. 2000;13:91–107.
23. Ludwig C, Mobargha N, Okogbaa J, Hagert E, Ladd A. Altered innervation pattern in ligaments of patients with basal thumb arthritis. *J Wrist Surg*. 2015;4:284–291.
24. Bettinger PC, Linscheid RL, Berger RA, Cooney WP, An K. An anatomical study of the stabilizing ligaments of the trapezium and trapeziometacarpal joint. *J Hand Surg [Am]*. 1999;24:786–797.
25. Lee J, Ladd A, Hagert E. Immunofluorescent triple-staining technique to identify sensory nerve endings in human thumb ligaments. *Cells Tissues Organs*. 2012;195:456–464.

26. Zhang A, Van Nortwick S, Hagert E, Yao J, Ladd A. Thumb carpometacarpal ligaments inside and out: a comparative study of arthroscopic and gross anatomy from the Robert A. Chase Hand and Upper Limb Center at Stanford University. *J Wrist Surg.* 2013;2:55–62.

27. Eaton RG, Littler JW. Ligament reconstruction for the painful thumb carpometacarpal joint. *J Bone Joint Surg Am.* 1973;55:1655–1666.

28. Pellegrini Jr VD, Olcott CW, Hollenberg G. Contact patterns in the trapeziometacarpal joint: the role of the palmar beak ligament. *J Hand Surg Am.* 1993;18:238–244.

29. Colman M, Mass DP, Draganich LF. Effects of the deep anterior oblique and dorsoradial ligaments on trapeziometacarpal joint stability. *J Hand Surg Am.* 2007;32:310–317.

30. Strauch RJ, Behrman MJ, Rosenwasser MP. Acute dislocation of the carpometacarpal joint of the thumb: an anatomic and cadaver study. *J Hand Surg Am.* 1994;19:93–98.

31. Van Brenk B, Richards RR, Mackay MB, Boynton EL. A biomechanical assessment of ligaments preventing dorsoradial subluxation of the trapeziometacarpal joint. *J Hand Surg Am.* 1998;23:607–611.

32. Mobargha N, Ludwig C, Ladd A, Hagert E. Ultrastructure and innervation of thumb carpometacarpal ligaments in surgical patients with osteoarthritis. *Clin Orthop Relat Res.* 2014;472:1146–1154.

33. Ludwig CA, Mobargha N, Okogbaa J, Hagert E, Ladd A. Altered innervation pattern in ligaments of patients with basal thumb arthritis. *J Wrist Surg.* 2015;4:284–291.

34. Edmunds JO. Traumatic dislocations and instability of the trapeziometacarpal joint of the thumb. *Hand Clinics.* 2006;22:365–392.

35. Brandt KD, Dieppe P, Radin E. Etiopathogenesis of osteoarthritis. *Med Clin North Am.* 2009;93:1–24.

36. Gamble JG, Mochizuki C, Rinsky LA. Trapeziometacarpal abnormalities in Ehlers-Danlos syndrome. *J Hand Surg Am.* 1989;14:89–94.

37. Jónsson H, Valtýsdóttir ST, Kjartansson O, Brekkan A. Hypermobility associated with osteoarthritis of the thumb base: a clinical and radiological subset of hand osteoarthritis. *Ann Rheum Dis.* 1996;55:540–543.

38. Beighton P, Solomon L, Soskolne CL. Articular mobility in an African population. *Ann Rheum Dis.* 1973;32:413–418.

39. Wolf JM, Schreier S, Tomsick S, Williams A, Petersen B. Radiographic laxity of the trapeziometacarpal joint is correlated with generalized joint hypermobility. *J Hand Surg Am.* 2011;36:1165–1169.

40. Moulton MJ, Parentis MA, Kelly MJ, et al. Influence of metacarpophalangeal joint position on basal joint-loading in the thumb. *J Bone Joint Surg Am.* 2001;83:709–716.

41. Poulter RJ, Davis TR. Management of hyperextension of the metacarpophalangeal joint in association with trapeziometacarpal joint osteoarthritis. *J Hand Surg Eur.* 2011;36:280–284.

42. Brandt KD, Radin EL, Dieppe PA, van de Putte L. Yet more evidence that osteoarthritis is not a cartilage disease. *Ann Rheum Dis.* 2006;65:1261–1264.

43. Chaisson C, Zhang Y, Sharma L, Kannel W, Felson D. Grip strength and the risk of developing radiographic hand osteoarthritis: results from the Framingham Study. *Arthritis Rheum.* 1999;42:33–38.

44. Belt E, Kaarela K, Lehtinen J, et al. When does subluxation of the first carpometacarpal joint cause swan-neck deformity of the thumb in rheumatoid arthritis: a 20-year follow-up study. *Clin Rheumatol.* 1998;17:135–138.

45. Mobargha N, Esplugas M, Garcia-Elias M, Lluch A, Megerle K, Hagert E. The effect of individual isometric muscle loading on the alignment of the base of the thumb metacarpal: a cadaveric study. *J Hand Surg EUR.* 2016;41:374–379.

46. Schulz CU, Anetzberger H, Pfahler M, Maier M, Refior HJ. The relation between primary osteoarthritis of the trapeziometacarpal joint and supernumerary slips of the abductor pollicis longus tendon. *J Hand Surg Br.* 2002;27:238–241.

47. Poulter RJ, Davis TR. Management of hyperextension of the metacarpophalangeal joint in association with trapeziometacarpal joint osteoarthritis. *J Hand Surg Eur Vol.* 2011;36:280–284.

48. Giurintano DJ, Hollister AM, Buford WL, Thompson DE, Myers LM. A virtual five-link model of the thumb. *Med Eng Phys.* 1995;17:297–303.

49. Qi Zheng. *The Etiology of Thumb Carpometacarpal Osteoarthritis: Early Indications from In Vivo Joint Contact Mechanics.* Unpublished Master's Thesis. University of Kansas; 2014.

50. Halilaj E, Rainbow M, Got J, et al. In vivo kinematics of the thumb carpometacarpal joint during three isometric functional tasks. *Clin Ortho Relat Res.* 2014;472:1114–1122.

51. Mobargha N. *The Proprioception and Neuromuscular Stability of the Basal Thumb Joint.* Unpublished Doctoral Thesis. Stockholm, Sweden: Karolinska Institutet; 2015.

52. Magni NE, McNair P, Rice D. Sensorimotor performance and function in people with osteoarthritis of the hand: a case-control comparison. *Semin Arthritis Rheum.* doi.org/10.1016/j.semarthrit.2017.09.008

53. Tan AL, Toumi H, Benjamin M, et al. Combined high-resolution magnetic resonance imaging and histological examination to explore the role of ligaments and tendons in the phenotypic expression of early hand osteoarthritis. *Ann Rheum Dis.* 2006;65:1267–1272.

54. Davenport BJ. An investigation into therapists' management of osteoarthritis of the carpometacarpal joint of the thumb in the UK. *Hand Ther.* 2009;14:2–9.

55. Standring S. *Gray's Anatomy: The Anatomical Basis of Clinical Practice.* 39th ed. St Louis: Elsevier; 2005.

56. Flatt AE. *The Care of the Rheumatoid Hand.* 4th ed. St. Louis: CV Mosby; 1983.

57. Egan MY, Brousseau L. Splinting for osteoarthritis of the carpometacarpal joint: a review of the evidence. *Am J of Occup Ther.* 2007;61:70–78.

58. Valdes K, Marik T. A systematic review of conservative interventions for osteoarthritis of the hand. *J Hand Ther.* 2010;23:334–351.

59. Kjeken I, Smedslund G, Moe RH, Slatkowsky-Christensen B, Unlig T, Hagen KB. Systematic review of design and effects of splints and exercise programs in hand osteoarthritis. *Arthritis Care Res.* 2011;63:834–848.

60. Bertozzi L, Valdes K, Vanti C, Negrini S, Pillastrini P, Villafane JH. Investigation of the effect of conservative interventions in thumb carpometacarpal osteoarthritis: systematic review and meta-analysis. *Disabil Rehabil.* 2015;37:2025–2043.

61. Spaans AJ, van Minnen P, Kon M, Schuurman AH, Schreuders AR, Vermeulen GM. Conservative treatment of thumb base osteoarthritis: a systematic review. *J Hand Surg.* 2015;40:16–21.

62. Aebischer B, Elsig S. Taeymans J Effectiveness of physical and occupational therapy on pain, function and quality of life in patients with trapeziometacarpal osteoarthritis- a systematic review and meta-analysis. *Hand Ther.* 2016;21:5–15.

63. Omokawa S, Ryu J, Tang JB, Han J, Kish VL. Trapeziometacarpal joint instability affects the moment arms of thumb motor tendons. *Clin Orthop.* 2000;372:262–271.

64. Moulton MJ, Parentis MA, Kelly MJ, et al. Influence of metacarpophalangeal joint position on basal joint-loading in the thumb. *J Bone Joint Surg.* 2001;83A:709–716.

65. Cantero-Tellez R, Villafane JH, Valdes K, Berjano P. Effect of immobilization of metacarpophalangeal joint in thumb carpometacarpal osteoarthritis on pain and function. A quasi-experimental trial. *J Hand Ther.* 2018;31(1):68–73.

66. Weiss S, LaStayo P, Mills A, Bramlet D. Splinting the degenerative basal joint: custom-made or prefabricated neoprene? *J Hand Ther.* 2004;17:401–406.

67. Sillem H, Backman CL, Miller WC, Li LC. Comparison of two carpometacarpal stabilizing splints for individuals with thumb osteoarthritis. *J Hand Ther.* 2011;24:216–226.

68. Becker SJ, Bot AG, Curley SE, Jupiter JB, Ring D. A prospective randomized comparison of neoprene vs thermoplast hand-based thumb spica splinting for trapeziometacarpal arthrosis. *Osteoarthritis Cartilage.* 2013;21:668–675.

69. Hamann N, Heidemann J, Heinrich k, et al. Stabilization effectiveness and functionality of different thumb orthoses in female patients with firth carpometacarpal joint osteoarthritis. *Clin Biomech.* 2014;29:1170–1176.

70. Rannou F, Dimet J, Boutron I, et al. Splint for base-of-thumb osteoarthritis: a randomized trial. *Ann Intern Med.* 2009;150:661–670.

71. Bani MA, Arazpour M, Kashani RV, Mousavi ME, Maleki M, Hutchins SW. The effect of custom-made splints in patients with the first carpometacarpal joint osteoarthritis. *Prosthet Orthot Int.* 2012;37: 139–144.

72. Arazpour M, Soflaei M, Bani MA, et al. The effect of thumb splinting on thenar muscle atrophy, pain, and function in subjects with thumb carpometacarpal joint osteoarthritis. *Prosthet Orthot Int.* 2017;41:379–386.

73. Gomes Carreira AC, Jones A, Natour J. Assessment of the effectiveness of a functional splint for osteoarthritis of the trapeziometacarpal joint of the dominant hand: a randomized controlled study. *J Rehabil Med.* 2010;42:469–474.

74. Albrecht JE. *Caring for the Painful Thumb: More than a Splint.* 2nd ed. North Mankato, MN: Jan Albrecht; 2015.

75. Boutan M. Role du couple opposant-1er interosseux dorsal dans la stabilite de l'articulation trapezo=metacarpienne. *Ann Kinesither.* 2000;27:316–324.

76. Taylor J. Restoration of dynamic stability in early osteoarthritis of the carpometacarpal joint of the thumb. *Br J Hand Ther.* 2000;5:37–41.

77. O'Brien V, Giveans MR. Effects of a dynamic stability approach in conservative intervention of the carpometacarpal joint of the thumb: a retrospective study. *J Hand Ther.* 2013;26:44–51.

78. Wouters RM. *The Effect of an Exercise Program in Patients with Thumb base Osteoarthritis: a Prospective Cohort Study with Propensity Score Matching* [Unpublished Master's Thesis]. Utrecht, The Netherlands: Utrecht, University; 2016.

79. Schwenkreis P, Janssen F, Rommel O, et al. Bilateral motor cortex disinhibition in complex regional pain syndrome (CRPS) type I of the hand. *Neurology.* 2003;61:515–519.

80. Backstrom KM. Mobilization with movement as an adjunct intervention in a patient with complicated de Quervain's tenosynovitis: a case report. *J Orthop Sports Phys Ther.* 2002;32:86–94.

81. Vicenzino B, Paungmali A, Teys P. Mulligan's mobilization-with-movement, positional faults and pain relief: current concepts from a critical review of literature. *Man Ther.* 2007;12:98–108.

82. Exelby L. Peripheral mobilisations with movement. *Man Ther.* 1996;1:118–126.

83. Villafane JH, Langford D, Alguacil-Diego IM, et al. Management of trapeziometacarpal osteoarthritis pain and dysfunction using mobilization with movement technique in combination with kinesiology tape: a case report. *J Chiropr Med.* 2013;12:79–86.

84. Villafane JH, Valdes K, Vanti C, et al. Investigation of the effect of conservative interventions in thumb carpometacarpal osteoarthritis: systematic review and meta-analysis. *Disabil Rehabil.* 37(22):2025–2043.

85. Borrell RM, Parker R, Henley EJ, Masley D, Repinecz M. Comparison of in vivo temperatures produced by hydrotherapy, paraffin wax treatment and fluidotherapy. *Phys Ther.* 1980;60:1273–1276.

86. Stimson CW, Rose GB, Nelson PA. Paraffin bath as thermotherapy: an evaluation. *Arch Phys Med Rehabil.* 1958;39:219–227.

87. Dilek B, Gozum M, Sahin E, et al. Efficacy of paraffin bath treatment in hand osteoarthritis: a single-blinded randomized controlled trial. *Arch Phys Med Rehabil.* 2013;94:642–649.

88. Aebisher B, Elsig S, Taeymans J. Effectiveness of physical and occupational therapy on pain, function and quality of life in patients with trapeziometacarpal osteoarthritis – a systematic review and meta-analysis. *Hand Ther.* 2016;21:5–15.

89. Guzelkucuk U, Duman I, Taskaynatan M, Dincer K. Comparison of therapeutic activities with therapeutic exercises in the rehabilitation of young adult patients with hand injuries. *J Hand Surg.* 2007;32:1429–1435.

90. Che Daud A, Yau M, Barnett F, Judd J, Jones R, Muhammad Nawawi R. Integration of occupation based intervention in hand injury rehabilitation: a randomized controlled trial. *J Hand Ther.* 2016;29: 30–40.

91. Gelberman R, Boone S, Osei D, Cherney S, Calfee R. Trapeziometacarpal arthritis: a prospective clinical evaluation of the thumb adduction and extension provocative tests. *J Hand Surg.* 2015;40:1285–1291.

92. Jha B. Measuring thumb range of motion in first carpometacarpal joint arthritis: the inter-rater reliability of the Kapandji Index versus goniometry. *Hand Ther.* 2016;21:45–53.

93. McGee C, Carlson K, Koethe A, Mathiowetz V. Inter-rater and inter-instrument reliability of goniometric thumb active and passive flexion range of motion measurements in healthy hands. *Hand Ther.* 2017;22:110–117.

94. De Kraker M, Selles R, Schreuders T, Stam H, Hovius S. Palmar abduction: reliability of 6 measurement methods in healthy adults. *J Hand Surg.* 2009;34:523–530.

95. McGee C. Measuring intrinsic hand strength in healthy adults: the accuracy intrarater and inter-rater reliability of the Rotterdam intrinsic hand myometer. *J Hand Ther.* https://10.1016/j.jht.2017.03.002.

96. Valdes K, Naughton N, Algar L. Linking ICF components to outcome measures for orthotic intervention for CMC OA: a systematic review. *J Hand Ther.* 2016;29:396–404.

97. Stamm T, van der Giesen F, Thorstensson CA, et al. Patient perspective of hand osteoarthritis in relation to concepts covered by instruments measuring functioning: a qualitative European multi-centre study. *Ann Rheum Dis.* 2009;68:1453–1460.

98. Glickel SZ. Clinical assessment of the thumb trapeziometacarpal joint. *Hand Clin.* 2001;17:185–195.

99. Wolfe T, Chu JY, Woods T, et al. A systematic review of postoperative hand therapy management of basal joint arthritis. *Clin Orthop Relat Res.* 2014;472:1190–1197.

100. Yuan F, Aliu O, Chung KC, Mahmoudi E. Evidence-based practice in the surgical treatment of thumb carpometacarpal joint arthritis. *J Hand Surg.* 2017;42. 104.e1-112.e1.

101. Davis TR, Brady O, Dias JJ. Excision of the trapezium for osteoarthritis of the trapeziometacarpal joint: a study of the benefit of ligament reconstruction or tendon interposition. *J Hand Surg Am.* 2004;29:1069–1077. https://doi.org/10.1016/j.jhsa.2004.06.017.

102. Brogan DM, van Hogezand RM, Babovic N, Carlsen B, Kakar S. The effect of metacarpophalangeal joint hyperextension on outcomes in the surgical treatment of carpometacarpal joint arthritis. *J Wrist Surg.* 2017;6:188–193.

103. Poole JL, Walenta MH, Alonzo V, et al. A pilot study comparing of two therapy regimens following carpometacarpal joint arthroplasty. *Phys Occup Ther Geriatr.* 2011;29:327–336.

104. Rocchi L, Merolli A, Cotroneo C, et al. Abductor pollicis longus hemitendon looping around the first intermetacarpal ligament as interposition following trapeziectomy: a one-year follow-up study. *Orthop Traumatol Surg Res.* 2011;97:726–733.

105. Ataker Y, Gudemez E, Ece SC, et al. A. Rehabilitation protocol after suspension arthroplasty of thumb carpometacarpal joint osteoarthritis. *J Hand Ther.* 2012;25:374–382.

106. Yao J, Lashgari D. Thumb basal joint: Utilizing new technology for the treatment of a common problem. *Jn Hand Ther.* 2014;27:127–132.

107. Vermeulen GM, Spekreijse KR, Slijper H, Feitz R, Hovius SER, Selles RW. Comparison of arthroplasties with or without bone tunnel creation for thumb basal joint arthritis: a randomized controlled trial. *J Hand Surg Am.* 2014;39(9):1692–1698.

108. Horlock N, Belcher HJ. Early versus late mobilisation after simple excision of the trapezium. *J Bone Joint Surg Br.* 2002;84:1111–1115.

109. Smet LD, Sioen W, Spaepen D, van Ransbeeck H. Treatment of basal joint arthritis of the thumb: trapeziectomy with or without tendon. *Hand Surg.* 2004;9:5–9.

110. Downing ND, Davis TR. Trapezial space height after trapeziectomy: mechanism of formation and benefits. *J Hand Surg.* 2001;26:862–868.

111. Smeraglia F, Soldati A, Orabona G, Ivone A, Balato G, Pacelli M. Trapeziometacarpal arthrodesis: is bone union necessary for a good outcome? *J Hand Surg (Eur).* 2015;40:356–361.

112. Kazmers N, Hippensteel K, Calfee R, et al. Locking plate arthrodesis compares favorably with LRTI for thumb trapeziometacarpal arthrosis: early outcomes from a longitudinal cohort study. *HSS Journal.* 2017;13:54–60.

113. Yao J, Cheah E. Mean 5-year follow-up for suture button suspensionplasty in the treatment of thumb carpometacarpal joint osteoarthritis. *J Hand Surg.* 2017;42:569.e1–569.e11.

114. Sonoda LA, Jones NF. Failed suture button suspensionplasty of the thumb carpometacarpal joint salvaged using pyrocarbon arthroplasty. *J Hand Surg.* 2017;42:665.e1–665.e4.

115. Barrera-Ochoa S, Vidal-Tarrason N, Correa-Vazquez E, Reverte-Vinaixa MM, Font-Segura J, Mir-Bullo X. Pyrocarbon interposition (PyroDisk) implant for trapeziometacarpal osteoarthritis: minimum 5-year follow-up. *J Hand Surg Am.* 2014;39:2150–2160.

116. Odella S, Querenghi AM, Sartore RA, DeFelice A, Dacatra U. Trapeziometacarpal osteoarthritis: pyrocarbon interposition implants. *Joints.* 2014;2:154–158.

117. Giesen T, Klein HJ, Franchi A, Medina JA, Elliot D. Thumb carpometacarpal joint denervation for primary osteoarthritis: a prospective study of 31 thumbs. *Hand Surg Rehabil.* 2017;36:192–197.

118. Qadir R, Duncan SF, Smith AA, Merritt MV, Ivy CC, Iba K. Volar capsulodesis of the thumb metacarpophalangeal joint at the time of basal joint arthroplasty: a surgical technique using suture anchors. *J Hand Sur.* 2014;39:1999–2004.

89

Surgical and Postoperative Management of Shoulder Arthritis

Wayne W. Chan, Surena Namdari, Brian G. Leggin, Martin J. Kelley, Joseph R. Kearns, Gerald R. Williams, Jr.

OUTLINE

CRITICAL POINTS

- Types of shoulder arthritis include osteoarthritis, inflammatory arthritis such as rheumatoid arthritis, and the other arthritides such as gout and pseudogout.
- Common to all forms of shoulder arthritis is shoulder pain that has worsened over time as well as stiffness, weakness, grinding, or clicking with movement and functional limitation of the affected arm.
- Nonoperative management strategies should be exhausted before choosing surgical options.

- Surgical options include arthroscopic shoulder debridement with or without capsular release, humeral hemiarthroplasty with or without glenoid reaming, total shoulder arthroplasty, and reverse shoulder arthroplasty.
- Rehabilitation is a standard component of postoperative management and varies according to the specific procedure performed.

Arthritis is a general term used to describe a wide range of pathologic conditions that result in loss of cartilage at the joint surfaces. The shoulder (i.e., glenohumeral joint) is the third most commonly affected large joint, after the hip and knee. There are many etiologies of glenohumeral arthritis, but in some cases, the exact cause remains unclear. In general, arthritis can be thought of in the following broad categories: osteoarthritis (OA), inflammatory arthritis, and other arthritides (Box 89.1).

Osteoarthritis can be divided into primary and secondary types. Primary OA is without an identifiable cause. Examples of secondary OA include posttraumatic (i.e., instability or intraarticular fracture) and postsurgical (i.e., capsulorrhaphy) arthritis. Inflammatory arthritides are systemic diseases in which rheumatoid arthritis (RA) represents the most common form. Arthritis from inflammatory bowel disease, ankylosing spondylitis, and psoriatic arthritis are also in the family of inflammatory arthritides.

The category of other arthritides encompasses a wide range of diagnoses. Crystal deposition diseases, such as gout and pseudogout, can involve the shoulder. Additional types of glenohumeral arthritis include arthritis associated with acromegaly, glenohumeral dysplasia, neuropathic arthropathy, and septic arthropathy. Atraumatic osteonecrosis or avascular necrosis (AVN) can result in humeral head subchondral bone collapse and may be secondary to systemic corticosteroid use, alcoholism, Gaucher's disease, sickle cell disease, or irradiation. Rotator cuff tear arthropathy (RCTA) is a unique form of arthritis with well-known pathoanatomy but poorly understood etiology.

Although shoulder arthritis entails a broad range of etiologies, the focus of this chapter is to discuss the surgical management of the more common conditions: OA, RA, and RCTA. Many of the surgical principles discussed are also applicable to other causes of glenohumeral arthritis.

DIAGNOSIS

The majority of cases of glenohumeral arthritis can be diagnosed based on history, physical examination, and plain radiographs. Consideration should be given to the list of differential diagnoses, which includes cervical spine disease, cardiac or pulmonary etiologies, diaphragmatic irritation, Charcot's arthropathy, tumors, and acute trauma.

Specific clinical features of shoulder arthritis presenting in a particular individual are dependent on the type of arthritis. However, in general, there is a predominant symptom of shoulder pain that has worsened over time. Initially, the pain occurs with use of the joint and is relieved by rest. With disease progression, the pain and discomfort can be brought on by minimal activity and may even occur at rest and at nighttime. In addition to the pain, other symptoms usually include stiffness, weakness, grinding, and clicking with movement and functional limitation of the affected arm. Patients with inflammatory arthritis may specifically report morning stiffness that improves throughout the day and swelling around the shoulder.

BOX 89.1 Types of Glenohumeral Arthritis

Osteoarthritis
Primary
Secondary
  Posttraumatic
  Postsurgical
  Instability
  Hypoplastic glenoid

Systemic Inflammatory Diseases
Rheumatoid arthritis
Ankylosing spondylitis
Psoriatic arthritis
Inflammatory bowel disease

Other Arthritides
Rotator cuff tear arthropathy
Crystalline arthropathy
  Gout
  Pseudogout
  Osteonecrosis
  Idiopathic
  Corticosteroid induced
  Alcoholism
  Post-traumatic
  Gaucher's disease
  Postirradiation necrosis
  Hemoglobinopathies: sickle cell disease, hemophilia, hemochromatosis
Neuropathic arthropathy
  Syringomyelia
  Peripheral neuropathy
Infectious
  Septic arthritis
  Lyme arthritis
Arthritis associated with acromegaly

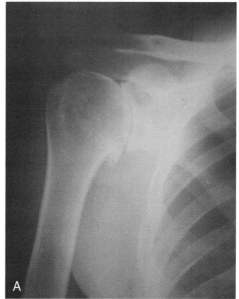

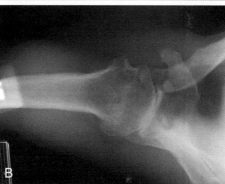

Fig. 89.1 Radiographs of a patient with glenohumeral osteoarthritis. **A,** The anteroposterior view shows joint space narrowing, subchondral sclerosis, and osteophytes on the inferior aspect of the humeral head and neck. **B,** The axillary view is better for evaluating glenohumeral joint space narrowing. (Courtesy of Virak Tan, MD.)

In all patients with glenohumeral arthritis, physical examination will demonstrate decreased motion (active and passive) and crepitus, and there may be generalized atrophy of the shoulder girdle muscles secondary to disuse. Other physical findings are more specific to the disease process.

The basic minimal radiographs for shoulder arthritis should include an anteroposterior (AP) view in the scapular plane in both internal and external rotation (ER) and an axillary view.[1] The major indication for using computed tomography (CT) is to quantitate posterior glenoid erosion and version for operative planning. CT can also assist in evaluating glenoid bone stock, central erosion, and rotator cuff muscle quality.[2]

At present, magnetic resonance imaging (MRI) is the preferred imaging method in the setting of inflammatory arthritis. It is accurate and noninvasive and may provide additional information regarding intraarticular pathology. Moreover, MRI is helpful in quantifying cuff tear size, retraction, muscle atrophy, and fatty degeneration,[3] which may be helpful in preoperative planning.

SPECIFIC ARTHRITIDES AFFECTING THE SHOULDER

Osteoarthritis

Osteoarthritis is the most common ailment affecting human joints. In general, patients with OA of the shoulder joint are younger and more active than patients with lower extremity arthritis. This is particularly

true when the arthritis is related to instability or trauma. Although much has been published regarding the epidemiology of OA, there is a dearth of data related specifically to the glenohumeral joint.

When searching for causes of OA, two major hypotheses surface.[4,5] One emphasizes the role of physical forces causing failure of articular cartilage. The other hypothesis implicates a failure of the regulation between degradation and repair of articular cartilage. The common pathway is eventual cartilage breakdown. Other well-documented factors that have been associated with the development of OA include aging, trauma, and genetic factors. Primary OA of the shoulder is likely to have a similar etiology and pathogenesis as other joints in the body. Although not typically a weight-bearing joint, the muscles about the shoulder can generate significant forces across the joint.

Physical examination of patients with OA reveals a symmetrical restriction of both active and passive motions, with a greater loss of ER compared with internal rotation (IR) secondary to anterior soft tissue contractures. There may be a slight prominence of the coracoid process and loss of normal shoulder contour caused by a posteriorly subluxated humeral head in the setting of posterior glenoid wear. Localized posterior joint line tenderness is also common.[6]

The cardinal radiographic features of glenohumeral OA (Fig. 89.1) are asymmetrical joint space narrowing, subchondral sclerosis, subchondral cyst formation, and osteophyte formation.[7] Osteophyte formation is commonly seen on the inferior aspect of the humeral head and neck but is also present circumferentially. The axillary view is better than the AP view for evaluating glenohumeral joint space narrowing and can often show humeral head flattening that is not always appreciated on the AP view. The axillary view can also give a rough estimate of posterior glenoid wear, humeral head subluxation, and glenoid version. Barring contraindications (relative or absolute), total shoulder arthroplasty (TSA) is generally the standard surgical treatment for glenohumeral arthritis.[8]

Rheumatoid Arthritis

Rheumatoid arthritis is a chronic, progressive inflammatory disease that affects multiple organ systems, including the musculoskeletal system. Although its etiology is not clearly defined, there are data to suggest an antigen-driven mechanism, which results in activation of immune pathways to cause tissue destruction, especially in and around synovial joints. Multiple stimuli can trigger the cascades of inflammatory response, some of which may be infectious, cross-reactivity, and autoimmunity. This constellation may help explain the wide variations in clinical presentation and the severity of involvement of the disease in different individuals.

The incidence of RA has been reported to be between 20 and 40 per 100,000 white adults, with a prevalence rate of 0.5% to 2%.[9] There is a two- to fourfold higher frequency in women.[10–12] The disease prevalence also increases with age. It is believed that there is a genetic predisposition to the development of RA because there is an increased frequency of the disease among first-degree relatives. The prevalence of RA in a sibling of someone who has RA is four to eight times higher than the prevalence in the general population.[13,14]

The clinical hallmark of RA is morning joint stiffness and polyarticular arthritis. The shoulders are not commonly symptomatic early in the inflammatory disease process, with only 4% of rheumatoid patients initially presenting with shoulder symptoms.[15] However, with progression of the disease, as many as 91% of patients report shoulder symptoms.[16] When the glenohumeral joint is involved, it is often bilateral and is usually associated with deformities of the hand and elbow.[17] The rheumatoid process may affect the entire shoulder girdle, including the bursae, tendons, and all four articulations of the shoulder.

Examination of a rheumatoid shoulder is likely to reveal boggy synovitis, generalized atrophy, and decreased active and passive range of motion (AROM and PROM). In contrast to OA, the loss of active motion in RA is often greater than the loss of passive motion. Because of a higher prevalence of dysfunctional or torn rotator cuffs, there may also be weakness and atrophy.

The radiographic features of a rheumatoid shoulder parallel those of any joint affected by RA.[18] There are regional osteopenia, symmetrical joint space narrowing, and juxtaarticular erosions. These erosions are best seen at the synovial reflection on the superior aspect of the humeral head. Osteophytes are not a prominent feature but may be present. Central glenoid erosion may also be present on the AP view, seen as medialization of the glenoid joint surface. Additionally, in the case of rotator cuff insufficiency, the AP view will help determine superior migration of the humerus, which contributes to superior glenoid erosion. The axillary view is the best way to estimate joint space narrowing as well as medial erosion of the glenoid surface with respect to the coracoid process (Fig. 89.2A). The extent of humeral head deformity associated with juxtaarticular erosions is best evaluated with the axillary view and can be verified on MRI (Fig. 89.2B).

Surgical management of a rheumatoid shoulder depends on the stage of disease. For early disease, patients may benefit from joint debridement, bursectomy, and synovectomy. When glenoid bone stock is adequate and the humeral head can be centered on the glenoid by

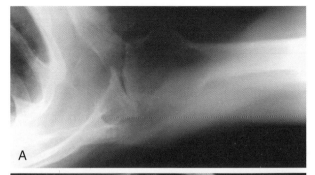

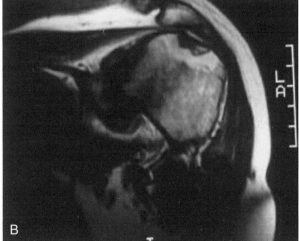

Fig. 89.2 Axillary radiographs of a patient with rheumatoid arthritis of the shoulder. **A,** There are marginal erosions of the humeral head and medialization of the glenoid joint surface beyond the base of the coracoid process. **B,** Magnetic resonance imaging confirms the severe joint destruction with juxta-articular erosions in addition to thinning of the superior cuff. (Courtesy of Gerald R. Williams, Jr., MD.)

a functional cuff, TSA provides pain relief superior to hemiarthroplasty.[19,20] In the setting of advanced disease, reverse total shoulder arthroplasty (RTSA) is often indicated because of significant bone loss or proximal humeral migration associated with rotator cuff dysfunction.[21,22]

Rotator Cuff Tear Arthropathy

The clinical features of RCTA have been described in the literature since the 19th century; however, its pathogenesis remains elusive. Two main theories have been proposed to explain this distinct clinical entity of severe glenohumeral joint destruction that occurs in association with a chronic massive rotator cuff defect. One theory points to mechanical and nutritional factors as being causative, and the other implicates crystal deposition as the inciting factor.

In 1981, McCarty and colleagues[23] introduced the term *Milwaukee shoulder* to describe four patients with glenohumeral degenerative joint disease and rotator cuff defects whose joint fluid contained active collagenase, neutral proteinase, and hydroxyapatite crystals. These authors postulated that the syndrome begins with capsular, synovial, or cartilage damage, which in turn precipitates hydroxyapatite crystal deposition. The crystals are then phagocytized by macrophage-like synoviocytes. Phagocytosis of the crystals stimulates the synoviocytes to release collagenase and protease that attack all the periarticular tissues, including articular cartilage, the rotator cuff, and adjacent soft tissues. The tissue damage leads to further crystal deposition and perpetuates the cycle of joint destruction. In a more recent study, Antoniou and colleagues[24] demonstrated a significant relationship between the presence of crystals

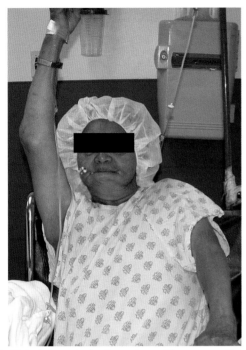

Fig. 89.3 Clinical photograph of a patient with rotator cuff arthropathy of the left shoulder. She essentially has no active elevation of the arm because of chronic rotator cuff insufficiency and superior migration of the humeral head. (Courtesy of Virak Tan, MD.)

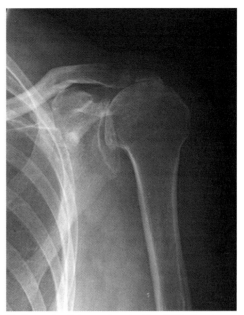

Fig. 89.4 Radiograph of the patient in Fig. 89.3 showing osteopenia, proximal humeral head migration, narrowing of the acromiohumeral space, acromion erosions, and superior glenoid bone loss. (Courtesy of Virak Tan, MD.)

and glenohumeral arthritis with massive rotator cuff tears. However, it is not clear which developed first: the massive cuff defect and abnormal joint mechanics that cause the crystals to appear in the synovial fluid or the deposition of apatite crystals that generate cytokines and lead to a massive tear. Regardless of the sequence, the presence of apatite crystals in synovial fluid leads to the production of inflammatory mediators, which is detrimental to the glenohumeral joint.

In 1983, Neer and colleagues[25] put forth the concept that mechanical and nutritional factors lead to RCTA. They postulated that a small percentage of untreated, chronic, full-thickness cuff tears progress to RCTA. The mechanical factors cited are gross instability of the humeral head, proximal migration against the coracoacromial arch, and rupture or dislocation of the long head of the biceps, resulting in further impingement and instability. Nutritional factors include decreased perfusion of nutrients into the articular cartilage because of leakage of synovial fluid from the joint. In addition, disuse of the joint alters water and glycosaminoglycan concentration of the articular cartilage causing softening and collapse. These authors believed that the combination of instability, inactivity and disuse, proximal humeral migration, and poor nutrition ultimately lead to subchondral bone collapse on both the humeral head and glenoid.

Regardless of the exact pathogenesis, RCTA is characterized by rotator cuff insufficiency, degenerative changes of the glenohumeral joint, superior migration of the humeral head, and recurrent (often hemorrhagic) effusions. The most significant physical finding in RTCA is the lack of or limited active elevation of the shoulder (Fig. 89.3). This loss of motion is not only related to the rotator cuff deficiency but also to the glenohumeral incongruity that resulted from the high-riding humeral head. There is marked atrophy of the supra- and infraspinatus muscles, and patients may also have recurrent swelling (i.e., Codman's "fluid sign"). In the setting of an incompetent coracoacromial arch as a static humeral head restraint, patients will have superior escape of the humeral head and "pseudoparalysis" of the arm.

Typically, radiographs show osteopenia, proximal humeral head migration, narrowing or obliteration of the acromiohumeral space, acromial erosions, and superior glenoid bone loss (Fig. 89.4). Humeral head collapse, osteophytes, cyst formation, and subchondral sclerosis may also be seen. According to Neer, humeral head collapse is a hallmark of RCTA. The axillary view is useful for evaluating glenoid erosion and medial migration. In addition, anterior subluxation on the axillary view suggests anterosuperior escape.

Whereas hemiarthroplasty with an anatomic, slightly oversized or hooded humeral component was a historic treatment option for RCTA, the reverse shoulder arthroplasty has emerged as the procedure of choice with reasonable outcomes at long-term follow-up.[26,27]

MANAGEMENT OF SHOULDER ARTHRITIDES

After all nonoperative management strategies have been exhausted, several surgical options are available to patients with glenohumeral arthritis. In general, the surgical armamentarium includes arthroscopic joint debridement[28–31] with or without capsular release, humeral hemiarthroplasty[32–34] with or without glenoid reaming, TSA,[8,35,36] and reverse shoulder arthroplasty.[21,37–41] Arthrodesis has a limited role in the treatment of glenohumeral OA; however, discussion of this topic is beyond the focus of this chapter.

DEBRIDEMENT AND CAPSULAR RELEASE

In active, high-demand, young patients (usually younger than 40 years of age) with mild to moderate glenohumeral arthritis, arthroscopic joint debridement and capsular release can be a useful procedure for pain relief and restoration of motion. A nonconcentric or incongruent joint is a relative contraindication to debridement because the results have been poor.[31,42] Although the debridement can be done by open technique, most are performed arthroscopically. Furthermore, arthroscopy can be both diagnostic and therapeutic for early-stage arthritis, especially in cases in which there are small focal lesions that are not easily seen by imaging studies.

Surgical Technique

Shoulder arthroscopy is performed in the beach-chair or lateral position. Standard posterior viewing and anterior working portals are used. After diagnostic arthroscopy, chondral lesions are debrided of loose fragments until a stable edge is obtained. Any degenerative or frayed labrum is also debrided to a stable rim with a shaver. In the presence of substantial stiffness and the absence of severe bone deformity, capsular release may increase postoperative range of motion (ROM). Release of the rotator interval and anterior capsule down to the 4 o'clock position is achieved with an electrocautery probe. This is an important step to gain ER. Further release of the axillary pouch and posterior capsule can also be done with an arthroscopic punch, depending on the restriction in preoperative motion. Tendinopathy of the long head of the biceps tendon can be addressed with a tenotomy or a tenodesis. Loose bodies that are encountered in the axillary pouch and small inferior osteophytes off the humeral head can be removed to alleviate mechanical symptoms. At the completion of debridement of the glenohumeral joint, the arthroscope is removed, and manipulation of the shoulder may be performed to ensure that adequate capsular releases have been achieved. The arthroscope is then inserted into the subacromial space through the posterior portal. A bursectomy is performed to assess the rotator cuff. As clinically warranted, subacromial decompression, distal clavicle resection, or both can be done accordingly. In cases of inflammatory arthritis, a thorough synovectomy and bursectomy are essential for pain relief.

Postoperative Rehabilitation

Rehabilitation begins with passive shoulder ROM on the first postoperative day. The sling is discontinued within 2 to 3 days as tolerated. Active shoulder motion is started according to pain tolerance, and patients are allowed to return to their regular recreational activities after 4 to 6 weeks.

Results

In 1986, Ogilvie-Harris and Wiley[30] reported on 54 patients undergoing arthroscopic shoulder debridement for degenerative arthritis. Nearly two thirds of their patients with mild disease achieved a successful result, whereas only 30% of those with moderate to severe disease had a good result. Weinstein and colleagues[31] noted good to excellent outcomes in 80% of patients undergoing arthroscopic debridement for early glenohumeral OA. The average age of the group was 46 years, and all patients reported at least some improvement in pain. At final follow-up (12–63 months), only two patients had reported return of pain to preoperative levels. There was a trend toward increasing severity of articular cartilage damage and unfavorable results. In 2002, Cameron and colleagues[28] reported on arthroscopic debridement of grade 4 glenohumeral articular lesions and noted pain relief for at least 28 months in their patients. They found that chondral lesions larger than 2 cm^2 were predictive of ultimate failure of the debridement. Similarly, Kerr and McCarty[29] concluded that the grade of the chondral lesion did not influence outcome scores, but patients with bipolar changes had lower scores.

More recently, debridement and capsular release has led to mixed results. In 2015, Skelley and associates[43] examined 33 patients with a mean age of 55 years and grade II to IV chondral changes. Patients' pain and preoperative pain scores returned to baseline at 3.8 months, with 61% of the patients reporting dissatisfaction with the outcome. Subsequently, 42% of the patients underwent a TSA at an average of 8.8 months. The remaining patients had similar preoperative and postoperative American Shoulder and Elbow Surgeons Shoulder and visual analog scale scores. In contrast, Mitchell and colleagues[44] described a more durable outcome at 5 years, with 77% of the 49 shoulders avoiding

TSA. The procedure they described included chondroplasty, capsular release synovectomy, humeral osteoplasty, axillary nerve neurolysis, subacromial decompression, loose body removal, microfracture, and biceps tenodesis.

SHOULDER HEMIARTHROPLASTY

Although the procedure of choice for most patients with glenohumeral arthritis is a TSA, there are several scenarios when replacing only the humeral side of the joint (i.e., hemiarthroplasty) is indicated. First, in a young patient who has isolated humeral head arthrosis (i.e., uninvolved glenoid) and an intact rotator cuff (such as in AVN or posttraumatic arthropathy), hemiarthroplasty is a reasonable option because it preserves glenoid bone stock. In certain instances, even when there is arthritic involvement of the glenoid, a hemiarthroplasty with concentric glenoid reaming has the additional benefit of eliminating the risk of glenoid loosening (Fig. 89.5). The ream-and-run arthroplasty, as developed by Matsen and colleagues,[45] restores a concentric glenoid surface and stimulates fibrocartilage ingrowth. Saltzman and colleagues[46] evaluated the ream-and-run procedure in patients younger than 55 years of age and found significant functional and pain improvement. A more recent study[47] focusing on ream-and-run arthroplasty in patients with biconcave glenoids yielded similar results but found that younger patients and early postoperative stiffness were associated with worse outcomes.

Another indication for shoulder hemiarthroplasty is when the arthritis occurs in the setting of an irreparable rotator cuff tear, proximal humeral head migration, and preserved preoperative active overhead elevation. Typically, this can be seen with RCTA, OA, or RA. The use of a prosthetic glenoid component under these circumstances has been associated with premature glenoid loosening; therefore, hemiarthroplasty, or more commonly RTSA, is a better choice. Inadequate glenoid bone stock to accept a prosthesis is yet another reason to select hemiarthroplasty over TSA.

Results

In 2006, Wirth and colleagues[34] reported the results of 64 hemiarthroplasties done for primary or secondary glenohumeral arthritis. Fifty shoulders were followed for a minimum of 5 years (mean, 7.5 years), and the average age of the patients was 63 years. The authors included patients with nonconcentric glenoids as long as concentricity could be achieved with reaming and patients with humeral head subluxation that was correctable by soft tissue balancing. Postoperatively, these patients were found to have improvement in the pain score and the shoulder ROM. Kaplan-Meier analysis estimated a 98.4% survival rate at 8 years. The authors concluded that in carefully selected patients, shoulder hemiarthroplasty provided good to excellent pain relief and functional improvement that was sustained at 5 to 10 years postoperatively.

In a prospective study, Lynch and colleagues[33] reported on 37 consecutive patients (38 shoulders) who underwent uncemented humeral hemiarthroplasty combined with reaming of the glenoid to a diameter 2 mm larger than the prosthetic head. Of the 35 shoulders that were followed for 2 years or longer, 26 had primary and 4 secondary OA, and 5 had capsulorrhaphy arthrosis. According to patient self-assessment ratings, 32 shoulders demonstrated improved comfort and function, 1 demonstrated no change from the preoperative level, and 2 had worse function postoperatively. Long-term follow-up in patients younger than 50 years of age undergoing hemiarthroplasty revealed lasting pain relief, improved ROM, and survivorship of 75.6%.[48] Modest results were also achieved in the treatment of patients with a biconcave glenoid, with 75% survivorship with a mean follow-up of 3.7 years.[47]

Several authors[32,49] presented their results of biological glenoid resurfacing and humeral head replacement as an alternative to total

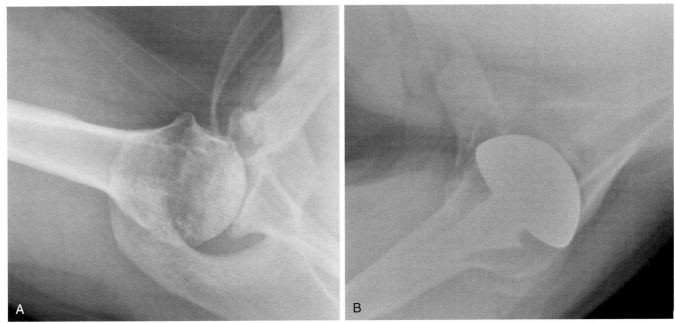

Fig. 89.5 Hemiarthroplasty with concentric glenoid reaming ("ream and run"). **A,** Preoperative axillary radiograph showing Walch B2 (biconcave) glenoid. **B,** Postoperative axillary radiograph with no posterior subluxation. (Courtesy of Gerald R. Williams, Jr., MD.)

shoulder replacement. Krishnan and colleagues[32] reported on 36 shoulders in which they concluded that biological resurfacing of the glenoid can provide pain relief similar to TSA and recommended Achilles tendon allograft as their material of choice for this procedure. Nicholson and colleagues[49] concluded that glenoid resurfacing with lateral meniscus allograft was not perfect but did provide significant pain relief, increased ROM, and patient satisfaction in the short term. Namdari and colleagues[42] performed a systematic review of seven studies using a variety of tissue sources and uncovered modest improvements in outcomes scores; a reoperation rate of 26%; and a complication rate of 13%, including infection, stiffness, and brachial neuritis. Puskas and associates[50] investigated their own prospective cohort using capsular interposition, meniscal allograft, or human dermal allograft combined with either a resurfacing or stemmed hemiarthroplasty. At a follow-up period ranging from 16 months to 34 months, 4 of the 6 patients undergoing capsular interposition, 3 of the 5 receiving meniscal allograft, and 5 of the 6 patients implanted with human dermal allograft underwent a revision surgery, with a combined 10 of the 17 patients undergoing conversion to either an anatomic or RTSA. Based on these more recent studies demonstrating poor results, this technique has largely fallen out of favor.

TOTAL SHOULDER ARTHROPLASTY

When deciding whether to use a glenoid component in shoulder arthroplasty for arthritis, the surgeon must individualize each case and weigh the risks and benefits of possible improved pain relief versus early glenoid loosening. Unconstrained humeral and glenoid prostheses are the treatment of choice for glenohumeral arthritis with an intact (or reparable), functional rotator cuff. Most arthroplasty systems use a stemmed humeral component in conjunction with a polyethylene glenoid component. However, humeral head resurfacing without an intramedullary stem has proponents, particularly when the glenoid is not being resurfaced.[51–54] In addition, there are a variety of options for glenoid replacement, including all-polyethylene designs, metal-backed designs, and hybrid designs with metal peg sleeves but no metal

backing. Recently, posteriorly augmented glenoid components have become available to address patients with severe posterior glenoid wear and the preliminary results at a 2-year minimum follow-up are comparable to a standard polyethylene implant.[55] There are also options with regard to articular conformity and constraint in which less conforming radii of curvature yield more physiologic translations and exhibit lower loosening scores than conforming designs.[56,57] In general, most surgeons use modular humeral components with humeral head offset options and an all-polyethylene cemented glenoid component with some degree of articular mismatch.

Surgical Technique

There are general principles that are applicable to all types of arthritides when arthroplasty is performed for the glenohumeral joint. Some principles are more relevant to specific pathologies seen in the particular form of the arthritis. For example, because of the associated incidence of proximal humeral migration and irreparable rotator cuff insufficiency, coracoacromial arch preservation is more germane in cases of RA and RCTA than in primary OA. The most important principle of patient positioning is to provide adequate access to the humeral shaft during reaming and humeral stem insertion while balancing appropriate glenoid exposure. This requires that the patient be in the beach-chair position with the thorax and pelvis laterally on the operating table so the entire shoulder and arm are unsupported by the table. The arm may then be maximally adducted, extended, and externally rotated to provide unobstructed instrumentation of the intramedullary canal.

Exposure

An extended deltopectoral approach is used whether the procedure is a hemiarthroplasty or TSA. The skin incision begins at the coracoid process and extends inferolaterally toward the deltoid tuberosity. The interval between the deltoid and pectoralis major is identified and dissected superiorly to the clavicle and inferiorly to the inferior margin of the pectoralis major tendon. The cephalic vein is preserved and may be taken laterally with the deltoid or medially with the pectoralis major. Because the majority of contributing branches arise from the deltoid, lateral retraction is most common. The upper 1.0 to 1.5 cm of the pectoralis major tendon may be released from the humerus for added exposure or correction of severe IR contractures.

The conjoined tendon of the coracobrachialis and short head of the biceps brachii is identified deep to the deltopectoral groove. The clavipectoral fascia is incised lateral to the conjoined tendon. This incision is extended proximally to the coracoacromial ligament, which can be preserved in all cases. The rotator cuff is then inspected. If a full-thickness rotator cuff tear is identified, the surgeon needs to assess whether it is reparable. In most cases of primary or posttraumatic OA, the cuff is intact or can be repaired. In all cases of RCTA and many cases of RA, rotator cuff integrity cannot be restored adequately. Retracting the conjoined tendon medially exposes the subscapularis tendon. The musculocutaneous nerve may enter the posterior surface of the conjoined tendon as close as 1.5 to 2.0 cm distal to the tip of the coracoid. Under these circumstances, excessive traction on the conjoined tendon should be avoided. The anterior humeral circumflex vessels are coagulated or ligated, and the axillary nerve is identified and protected throughout the remainder of the case. Next, the long head of the biceps is identified within the groove and tenodesed to the upper border of the pectoralis major tendon.

The method of managing the subscapularis tendon depends on the extent of subscapularis and anterior capsular contracture. If preoperative passive ER with the arm at the side is greater than 10 degrees, the subscapularis is incised 1.5 to 2.0 cm medial to its insertion on the lesser tuberosity. A lesser tuberosity osteotomy continues to gain favor because of the theoretical advantage of bone-to-bone healing. Alternatively, if the bone–tendon junction appears compromised, a subscapularis peel is performed by elevating the subscapularis insertion off the lesser tuberosity. After appropriate capsular release, the subscapularis may be repaired anatomically, either tendon to tendon or via suture osteosynthesis of the lesser tuberosity osteotomy. When preoperative passive ER is between 10 degrees and −30 degrees, additional subscapularis length is needed for ER. In most cases, complete release of the subscapularis provides adequate excursion of the tendon without lengthening. Alternatively, the subscapularis can be released directly from its insertion on the lesser tuberosity to ensure maximal length. At the time of closure, the subscapularis is reinserted at the level of the humeral osteotomy site. Every 1 cm of medial advancement yields approximately 20 to 30 degrees of ER. In the rare case of severe IR contractures (i.e., passive external of less than −30 degrees), subscapularis Z-lengthening may be required. This can be accomplished by direct release of the subscapularis from the lesser tuberosity followed by separation of the subscapularis from the underlying anterior capsule. After separating these two structures, the anterior capsule is then released from the glenoid, thereby creating a medially based subscapularis flap and a laterally based capsular flap that can be sutured in a lengthened position at the time of closure. Subscapularis Z-lengthening is difficult and may compromise the strength of the subscapularis repair; with modern techniques of subscapularis release, this is rarely needed.

Humeral Preparation

After taking down the subscapularis and capsule, the humeral head is dislocated by simultaneously adducting, extending, and externally rotating the arm. Humeral osteophytes are removed to define the anatomic neck. The humeral osteotomy can be performed in one of two ways. In the first method, the native boundary of the humeral anatomic neck guides the osteotomy. Theoretically, this technique ensures that the humeral cut reproduces the native humeral retroversion and neck-shaft angle for that particular patient. However, identification of the native anatomic neck can be difficult when the humeral head is deformed and obscured by significant osteophytes. The second method

uses a mechanical cutting guide at a predetermined "average" neck-shaft angle. These guides can be intramedullary or extramedullary. Retroversion can be determined using the known average relationship between the distal humeral epicondylar axis and the plane of the articular surface (i.e., 30 degrees of retroversion). The goal of the osteotomy is to permit anatomic placement of the prosthetic head on the cut surface of the humerus.

After the humeral osteotomy has been performed, the resected head is used for sizing on the back table. In addition, trial humeral heads can be placed on the cut surface of the metaphysis to aid in humeral head sizing. The humeral canal is reamed using sequentially larger reamers. In the presence of hard, necrotic bone within the humeral metaphysis (i.e., AVN), initial passage of the reamer can be difficult. In this instance, it is advisable to first drill a hole in the metaphysis as large as the initial reamer to minimize hoop stress on the proximal humeral metaphysis. After adequate drilling, sequential reamers can be passed as usual. An appropriately sized broach is then used to prepare the proximal metaphysis by cutting out channels for the fins of the prosthesis. The broach is left in place to protect the humeral metaphysis during posterior retraction that is required for glenoid exposure. Alternatively, the glenoid can be prepared after the humeral osteotomy but before humeral intramedullary preparation.

A retractor is placed between the humerus and the glenoid to posteriorly displace the humeral metaphysis. The glenoid is inspected, and a decision is made with regard to concentric glenoid reaming or resurfacing. If the native glenoid is preserved and hemiarthroplasty is the choice procedure, the need for concentric glenoid reaming is assessed. After the glenoid has been concentrically reamed, the next step is soft tissue balancing and trialing of the humeral head component (see the following).

Ream-and-Run Arthroplasty

In patients who demand a high level of physical activity, a ream-and-run arthroplasty eliminates the concern for glenoid component failure. It is a surgical option that requires careful patient selection, a high level of technical expertise, and dedication from the patient to consistent postoperative rehabilitation. After adequate glenoid exposure, a capsular release is performed while preserving the labrum. If preoperative films indicate posterior subluxation, capsular release stops at the inferior glenoid. If the patient is stiff without posterior subluxation, a 360-degree release is performed. Any residual cartilage is curetted from the surface of the glenoid. In patients with a notable biconcavity, a burr is used to smooth down the ridge before reaming the glenoid concentrically. A 2-mm mismatch in the glenoid reamer is used to optimize the load transfer. The goal of reaming is to achieve a concentric glenoid articulation while prioritizing preserving glenoid bone stock over normalizing glenoid version.

Glenoid Preparation

If adequate bone is available, the rotator cuff is intact and functional, and the patient's age and activity level are appropriate, glenoid resurfacing with a polyethylene component is preferred. To prepare for the glenoid component, the labrum is circumferentially excised, including the biceps anchor. In cases of greater than 25% posterior subluxation, release of the posterior capsule should be avoided.

The glenoid is prepared with a motorized reamer, correcting the glenoid version to neutral position (perpendicular to the plane of the scapula) as needed by eccentric reaming. The asymmetrical glenoid reaming limit is 0.5 to 1.0 cm. Beyond this degree of reaming, the remaining glenoid bone may be insufficient to safely anchor glenoid component. Therefore, the preoperative CT scan should be reviewed carefully to determine the degree of correction that is possible with reaming alone. If complete correction does not seem possible, a decision must be made to either accept incomplete correction or bone graft the glenoid. The advent of augmented glenoid components[58-60] gives the surgeon an additional option for addressing eccentric glenoid wear. The glenoid surface is then prepared to accept either a pegged or keeled component, and the component is placed.

Soft Tissue Balancing and Trialing

Regardless of whether a glenoid component is implanted, soft tissue balancing is a step in shoulder arthroplasty. Appropriate tension in the capsule and rotator cuff ensures maximal ROM and stability. Soft tissue tension is assessed by placing a humeral head on the broach or the trial stem. A humeral head is selected that approximates the size of the resected native humeral head. With the humeral head reduced, subluxation of approximately 50% of the humeral head diameter indicates appropriate soft tissue balance. In addition, the subscapularis should reach the proposed repair[58] site with enough laxity to allow a minimum of 30 to 40 degrees of ER. This may require circumferential release of the subscapularis and excision of the anterior capsule. If the posterior capsule is too lax, a larger humeral head can be placed. However, if the larger head compromises subscapularis length, a posterior capsular shift is performed, and the smaller head size is used. This capsulorraphy can be accomplished from the anterior approach "through the joint" with the trial prosthetic humeral head removed. After a humeral head size has been selected, the trial implant is removed. The final humeral component can be secured to the humerus using either cemented or press-fit techniques.

Closure

The technique of subscapularis repair depends on how the subscapularis was taken down. If the tendon was incised medial to its insertion, anatomic tendon-to-tendon repair of the subscapularis is performed. Our preference is a lesser tuberosity osteotomy, and this can be repaired anatomically with interfragmentary sutures in addition to rotator interval closure and a suture passed from the neck of the prosthesis through the bone–tendon junction. If the tendon was released directly from the lesser tuberosity, it is reattached through drill holes at the osteotomy site. If Z-lengthening of the subscapularis is planned, then the medially based subscapularis flap is sutured to the laterally based capsular flap in a lengthened position. The subcutaneous tissue and skin are closed in standard fashion.

Postoperative Rehabilitation

The rehabilitation program after a shoulder arthroplasty should be individualized according to the patient's goals, motivation, and physical ability. Patients with good preoperative rotator cuff function and bone quality can enroll in the standard program, whereas patients with poor preoperative rotator cuff function are placed in a limited goals program. A general scheme of postoperative rehabilitation is outlined in the following.

Phase I

Rehabilitation begins the first postoperative day with patient education, when they are informed to expect swelling and discoloration and instructed in the use of ice and modalities for edema control. Patients can use their extremity for waist-level activities and bring the hand to the mouth with the arm adducted but are to avoid lifting, carrying, pushing, pulling, and leaning on the operated side. Pendulum exercises, supine passive forward elevation, and ER in the scapular plane are initiated (Fig. 89.6). Patients in the limited goals category

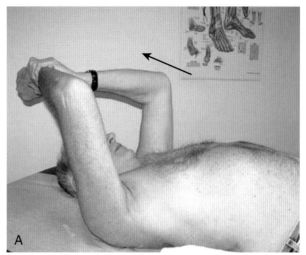

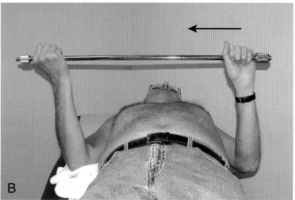

Fig. 89.6 Phase I stretching exercises. **A,** Passive supine forward flexion is achieved by using the power of the opposite arm (in this case, the left) to move the right shoulder into flexion . **B,** Passive supine external rotation with the aid of a stick. (Courtesy of Virak Tan, MD.)

can achieve forward flexion by the table slide technique, typically after a period of immobilization or rest. The exercises are performed four to six times daily and are continued until full passive ROM is achieved.

Postoperative treatment, at this stage, is dependent on the subscapularis tendon repair technique. Protection of the subscapularis is critical for a successful outcome because of the importance of this muscle in shoulder function and stability.[61]

Phase II

At 6 weeks after surgery, patients should be able to perform many of their waist-level activities of daily living (ADLs). Patients then progress to phase II ROM exercises. These exercises include extension, cross-body adduction, and IR behind the back. An effective stretch for the inferior capsule is having the patient supine with the hands behind the head and the shoulders abducted and externally rotated.

Also at this point, phase I strengthening exercises with elastic bands can be instituted (Fig. 89.7). Patients are instructed to begin with the band that provides the least resistance. They are asked to work up to 3 sets of 10 repetitions as tolerated and progress to the next level of resistance thereafter. When strength is achieved at the highest resistance band with the arm at the side, phase II strengthening exercises can begin with shoulder abduction to 45 degrees, forward elevation to slightly below shoulder level, and ER at 45 degrees of abduction in the supported position. In addition, shoulder shrugs and scapular retraction exercises can begin.

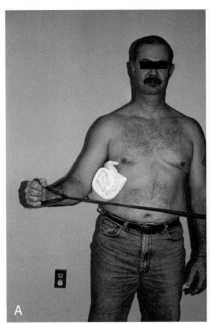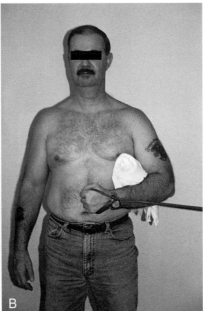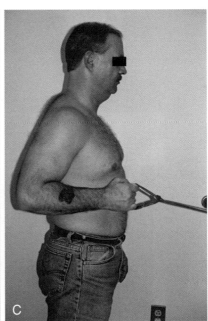

Fig. 89.7 Phase I strengthening exercises with elastic bands. External rotation (**A**), internal rotation (**B**), and extension (**C**) with the arm at the side. (Courtesy of Gerald R. Williams, Jr., MD.)

Patients in the limited goals category begin the phase II stretching exercises at 6 weeks postoperatively. They may also initiate submaximal rotator cuff isometrics and scapular strengthening at this time.

Phase III

At 8 to 12 weeks after surgery, the patient should have full and pain-free passive ROM as well as good rotator cuff strength. Phase II strengthening exercises with the elastic band can usually be started if they have not already. Progression of resistance for shoulder shrugs, scapular retraction, biceps curls, and triceps extension is accomplished. Patients with limited goals should have adequate soft tissue healing and stability of the glenohumeral components and can begin strengthening exercises with the arm at the side.

Phase IV

The patient will be progressed to this phase at 12 to 24 weeks after surgery. This phase includes work- or sport-specific training as well as suggestions for modification of work, sport, or functional activities. Patients are discouraged from participating in heavy work or recreational activities that result in high loads and forces to the glenohumeral joint.[62] Golf, swimming, bicycling, aerobics, and running activities are acceptable activities for patients after shoulder arthroplasty.

Patients in the limited goals category should be able to perform normal daily activities with modifications to use lower shelves and a stepstool for higher shelves.

Results

The results of shoulder arthroplasty are generally favorable. TSA in glenohumeral OA has been successful in relieving pain, increasing ROM, and improving ADLs. Pain relief is more predictable in TSA than in hemiarthroplasty. Pain relief and improved function can be expected in approximately 90% of patients with a survivorship of more than 90% at 10 years and more than 80% at 20 years.[36]

As in OA, shoulder arthroplasty in RA reliably achieves relief of pain. Improved function, however, is dependent on the preoperative status of the rotator cuff, deltoid, and other periarticular soft tissues. Boyd and colleagues[63] reported the results of TSA and hemiarthroplasty

with the intent of more clearly outlining the indications for glenoid resurfacing. They concluded that TSA and hemiarthroplasty demonstrated similar functional improvements. However, in the patients with RA, pain relief, ROM, and patient satisfaction were greater in those receiving a TSA than a hemiarthroplasty.

In 2004, Sperling and colleagues[36] reported on shoulder arthroplasty for RA in 247 patients. Follow-up averaged 11.6 years, and the postoperative results showed significant long-term pain relief and better active abduction and ER with both hemiarthroplasty and TSA. There was not a significant difference in pain and ROM between the two procedures for patients with a thin or torn rotator cuff. However, among patients with an intact rotator cuff, improvement in pain and abduction were significantly greater, and the risk of revision was significantly lower, for TSA.

In 2011, Zarkadas and associates[64] reported outcomes for patients on average 9 years after TSA or hemiarthroplasty. Patients who received TSA reported significantly better ROM and strength compared with patients who received hemiarthroplasty but only slightly superior functional results. Results demonstrate that patients who underwent TSA were equally as active as patients with hemiarthroplasty.

REVERSE TOTAL SHOULDER ARTHROPLASTY

The "reversed shoulder" is a ball-and-socket design in which the ball is on the glenoid side and the socket is on the humeral side (Fig. 89.8). Current designs use a medialized center of rotation to decrease torque on the glenoid anchoring points and to increase the deltoid lever arm.[65] However, the degree of medialization differs among implants, and the optimal amount is not known. Although only made available in the United States since 2004, the reversed shoulder has been in use in Europe for 2 decades.[40] The collective experience suggests that in the setting of shoulder arthritis, the reverse shoulder arthroplasty is best for patients with end-stage severe cuff arthropathy who are older and low demand with active elevation less than 90 degrees. In addition, the deltoid must be functional, and there should be sufficient bone on the glenoid side to allow for secure screw fixation of the component.

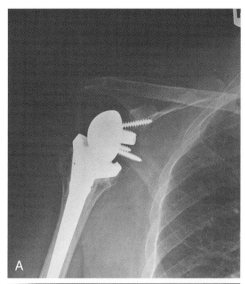

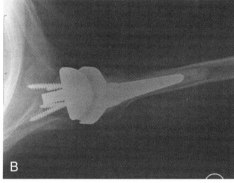

Fig. 89.8 Radiographs of a reverse shoulder prosthesis. Anteroposterior (**A**) and axillary (**B**) views. (Courtesy of Virak Tan, MD.)

Surgical Technique

The patient is placed in the standard beach-chair position after induction of anesthesia. The prosthesis can be placed using the superior deltoid-splitting or the deltopectoral approach. The superior approach is more difficult in patients with anterior soft tissue contracture or inferior humeral osteophytes, and inferior glenoid sphere placement is more challenging than with the deltopectoral approach. In addition, the superior approach has the added disadvantage of potential postoperative deltoid detachment. For this reason, some surgeons prefer the deltopectoral approach in all cases. However, the rate of postoperative dislocation may be higher with the deltopectoral approach, particularly if the subscapularis is not repaired. Because the deltopectoral approach is described in the surgical technique section for shoulder arthroplasty, a description of the superior approach is provided in the following.

A skin incision is made perpendicular to Langer's lines about the lateral aspect of the shoulder. Alternatively, the incision can be made in Langer's lines, and medial and lateral skin flaps can be raised to expose the deltoid. After the subcutaneous dissection, the anterior deltoid is sharply released from the distal clavicle and acromion and extended distally in line with the muscle fibers between the anterior and medial deltoid. Care should be exercised to limit the dissection to within 3 to 4 cm of the lateral margin of the acromion to avoid injury to the axillary nerve. The coracoacromial ligament is released with the anterior deltoid, and bursectomy and acromioplasty are performed as needed for exposure of the humeral head. If the biceps is present, it should be released or tenodesed in the bicipital groove. Any intact anterior and posterior cuff tendon should be retained.

The humeral head is dislocated superiorly and through the wound by extension of the arm, ER, and pushing up at the elbow. Large humeral osteophytes are difficult to remove through a superior approach. However, small osteophytes are removed with a rongeur, and an initial humeral cut is made through the head with the intramedullary guide in place. The humeral head osteotomy is done at 0 or 10 degrees of retroversion and is completed after removal of the resection guide. Appropriate head resection is achieved when the top of the humeral osteotomy lines up with the inferior half of the glenoid with downward traction of the arm. This ensures clear visualization for instrumentation of the glenoid surface.

The glenoid is exposed by placing a retractor inferiorly under the scapular neck and levering down the humerus. The labrum is excised, and a complete capsulotomy or capsulectomy is performed to allow palpation of the inferior scapular neck. Reaming of the glenoid is determined in part by the existing anatomy and should allow the glenoid base plate to sit with its inferior border aligned with the inferior border of the native glenoid. This has been shown to decrease contact of the humerus with the inferior scapula and potentially decrease inferior scapular notching. Inferior tilting of the glenoid base plate has not been definitively shown to decrease inferior humeral–scapular contact and requires substantial inferior reaming that may compromise the subchondral bone of the glenoid. Preservation of the subchondral bone allows better support of the prosthesis. When reaming is completed, the appropriate size base plate is implanted and secured to the glenoid with screws. It is important to align the superior and inferior screw holes so that the superior and inferior locking screws can be placed in the base of the coracoid and the lateral scapular border, respectively.

Preparation of the humeral side is done by delivering the osteotomy surface through the wound. Reaming of the canal and metaphysis is done sequentially using hand or power reamers. If power is used, the reamer should be held loosely so that if the reamer binds on the humerus, the reamer spins in the surgeon's hand rather than cracking the humerus. Reaming is continued until the flange of the reamer is at the level of the osteotomy and in contact with the cortical bone at the metaphysis. The epiphysis is then reamed, usually using an intramedullary guide. A trial humeral stem is seated down the canal, and a trial cup is placed onto the stem. The joint is reduced and taken through the ROM. Appropriate soft tissue tensioning is achieved when there is no toggling or impingement of the components. The joint should remain stable and fully engaged throughout the ROM. Any mismatch must be addressed at this time by trialing different components or removing overhanging bone.

After the correct-size implants are selected, the prosthetic humeral stem is cemented in place and the glenosphere attached to the base plate. The definitive polyethylene humeral cup is impacted onto the stem, and the joint is reduced. Final assessment of stability and ROM is performed. After thorough irrigation, the deltoid is repaired in a side-to-side manner and back to the acromion with transosseous nonabsorbable sutures. Closure of the skin is done in the standard fashion.

Postoperative Rehabilitation

Rehabilitation after a reverse shoulder arthroplasty is not standardized but dependent on surgeon preference and the quality of the glenoid fixation. Some authors report initiating no postoperative rehabilitation and allowing patients to use their arm freely for functional activities after the initial healing process. Others have advocated immobilization for as long as 4 to 6 weeks after surgery.[39] Still others have initiated passive ROM on the first postoperative day with limits of 90 degrees of passive elevation and 0 degrees of ER for the first 6 weeks and active movement allowed after 6 weeks.[21]

TABLE 89.1	Published Series for Reverse Shoulder Arthroplasty for Rotator Cuff Tear Arthropathy					
Reference	No. of Shoulders	Follow-up (mo)	Active Elevation (Pre-/Postoperative)	Constant Score (Pre-/Postoperative)	Complication Rate (%)	Reoperation and Revision Rate (%)
Baulot et al[69] (1995)	16	27	NA	14/69	NA	13
Sirveaux et al[41] (2004)	80	44	73/138	22.6/65.6	15	5
Boileau et al[38] (2006)	21	40	53/123	18/66	19	5
Frankle et al[39] (2005)	60	33	55/105	34/68 (ASES score)	17	12
Al-Hadithy et al[72] (2014)	41	20–101 (mean, 60)	55/108	24/60	10	2
Levy et al[68] (2014)	166	24	62/120	37/72 (ASES score)	NA	NA

ASES, American Shoulder and Elbow Surgeons; *NA*, not available.

Our approach to rehabilitation depends on the patient's preoperative deltoid function and postoperative stiffness. Patients with good deltoid function are allowed to use their arms for waist-level activities for the first 6 postoperative weeks. Thereafter, they are allowed unrestricted use of their arms. Patients with postoperative stiffness begin PROM exercises within the first 7 to 10 days postoperatively. Exercises are restricted to supine passive forward elevation. ER ROM is restricted to 0 degrees. Patients may also perform pulleys and chair stretch to help improve passive forward elevation. Beyond 6 weeks from surgery, these patients are progressed to AROM and strengthening.

Patients with poor deltoid function begin strengthening and functional training at 6 weeks. Deltoid strengthening is emphasized with a supine elevation progression. Gravity is virtually eliminated, and the patient can practice raising the arm past 90 degrees while strengthening the deltoid. The patient begins with the elbow bent to 90 degrees to decrease the lever arm and weight of the extremity. When the patient can comfortably perform 30 repetitions in this position, he or she gradually extends the elbow to increase the weight of the extremity until he or she can perform 30 repetitions with the elbow fully extended. Next the head is slightly elevated to gradually add the weight of gravity to the exercise. This sequence continues until the patient is able to raise the arm while standing upright. This exercise can be enhanced with the use of weighted balls, dumbbells, or elastic resistance.

Boudreau and associates[66] described a four-phase rehabilitation program guided by three postoperative concepts—joint protection, deltoid function, and establishing appropriate ROM and functional expectations. The goals of the first phase are to maintain the integrity of the replaced joint while restoring PROM. In the first 3 weeks, flexion and scapular plane elevation are gradually increased to 90 degrees as tolerated, and ER should be progressed to 20 to 30 degrees in the scapular plane. After the first 3 weeks, passive elevation can be advanced to patient tolerance, typically up to 140 degrees.[66] Rehabilitation in patients who have required reverse shoulder arthroplasty for a revision of failed anatomic TSA needs to be managed on case-by-case basis and generally requires a longer period of immobilization.

At 6 weeks, active assisted range of motion (AAROM) and AROM as well as initiation of gentle strengthening can be started. The primary goal is restoring dynamic shoulder stability and enhanced mechanics. An elevation progression program is used, and periscapular strengthening begins as well.[66] Phase 3 begins at 12 weeks when the patient is able to isotonically activate each deltoid head and periscapular muscles. The patient can start upper extremity strengthening to improve functional independence. Phase 4 commences at about 4 months postsurgery when the patient is able to demonstrate functional pain-free

shoulder AROM and is independent with an appropriate strengthening program.[66]

In 2016, Liu and coworkers[67] looked retrospectively at return to sports after shoulder arthroplasty, comparing outcomes after hemiarthroplasty and RTSA. Included were patients with contraindication for anatomic TSA and indications for hemiarthroplasty or RTSA. A similar postoperative rehabilitation protocol was followed that included 4 weeks in a sling, PROM at 2 weeks, AROM at 6 weeks, and strengthening at 3 months.[67]

Although no literature was identified that compared rehabilitative programs with self-directed home programs, Levy and colleagues[68] described treatment of self-directed stretching and strengthening. Patients were immobilized in a sling for 6 weeks and encouraged to initiate pendulum exercises. At 6 weeks, patients were instructed in supine AAROM and were encouraged to use the extremity for light ADLs with a 2-lb weight restriction. After 3 months, patients were encouraged to continue self-directed stretching and strengthening and were allowed to return to activities within comfort levels.[68]

All reverse prostheses have a limitation of ROM compared with an anatomic joint, especially with respect to IR. Moreover, the complication rate, including dislocations and acromial stress fractures, is higher with reversed implants. Therefore, the decision to institute a formal therapy program should be made carefully. In general, less therapy for reverse implants than for anatomic implants is wise.

Results

The clinical outcome of reverse shoulder arthroplasty for RCTA is generally more favorable than when done for other diagnoses (e.g., failed prosthetic arthroplasty or fracture). Several series have been published with short- to midterm results showing overall improvement in pain, constant scores of 55 to 65, and active forward flexion from 105 to 140 degrees (Table 89.1). Active ER is not improved if the posterior cuff is deficient.[38,39,41,69] Bacle and colleagues[70] followed up on their initial midterm outcome study looking at long-term outcomes (minimum 10-year follow-up). Although the overall prosthetic survival was excellent (93%), patients showed deteriorating functional outcomes and high rates of scapular notching (73%) and complications (29%). Despite the cautious optimism with the reversed shoulder, there are relatively high complication and reoperation rates.

Furthermore, there are unsolved problems with these prostheses. First, deltoid tension is difficult to assess intraoperatively. Undertensioning can lead to instability, and overtensioning can limit ROM and may cause an acromial stress fracture.[71] Second, inferior scapular notching has been noted in a majority of cases with the Grammont design. Although the clinical significance of this finding is unclear, there is a concern that it could lead to loosening of the glenoid component. The trade-off is to have the glenosphere be more laterally offset, thereby minimizing impingement of polyethylene humeral cup on the scapular neck. However, this design results in a shorter deltoid lever arm and has the theoretical disadvantage of increased shear stresses at the glenoid component–bone interface.

Al-Hadithy and associates[72] evaluated outcomes of reverse shoulder arthroplasty. Constant scores improved from 34 points to 71 points, and shoulder forward flexion improved from 55 degrees to 110 degrees over an average follow-up period of 5 years. Scapular notching was present in 68% of shoulders, but there was no observed association with deterioration of Constant score at 24 months and final follow-up.[72] RTSA has been shown to improve pain and function in patients with RCTA, with a low complication rate.[72]

Levy and coworkers[68] concluded rapid improvement of pain in patients treated with TSA and reverse shoulder arthroplasty, although those treated with TSA can expect a more consistent and effective recovery of pain, function, and shoulder elevation. Patients receiving anatomic TSA were found to have a more predictable postoperative course of recovery, whereas patients undergoing reverse shoulder arthroplasty can expect a variable length of recovery with greater improvements of shoulder flexion ROM.[68]

SUMMARY

Although multiple types of glenohumeral arthritis exist, the most common are OA, RA, and RCTA. The pathogenesis of all types of glenohumeral arthritis is poorly understood. The clinical presentation, prognosis, and recommended treatment are largely dependent on the arthritis type. When nonoperative measures fail, surgical management includes several options. Debridement and capsular releases may have a role for active, high-demand, young patients with mild to moderate arthritis. The most commonly performed procedure for end-stage glenohumeral arthritis is prosthetic shoulder replacement. Indications for hemiarthroplasty continue to be refined and in the future may become the procedure of choice for end-stage shoulder arthritis in younger, active patients. At present, TSA is preferred in patients older than 50 years of age with an intact and functional rotator cuff and adequate glenoid bone stock to accept a glenoid component. Reverse shoulder arthroplasty is most commonly used for low-demand, older adult patients with glenohumeral arthritis in the setting of a massive, irreparable rotator cuff defect.

REFERENCES

1. Green A, Norris TR. Imaging techniques for glenohumeral arthritis and glenohumeral arthroplasty. *Clin Orthop Relat Res.* 1994;(307):7–17.
2. Friedman RJ, Hawthorne KB, Genez BM. The use of computerized tomography in the measurement of glenoid version. *J Bone Joint Surg Am.* 1992;74(7):1032–1037.
3. Iannotti JP, et al. Magnetic resonance imaging of the shoulder. Sensitivity, specificity, and predictive value. *J Bone Joint Surg Am.* 1991;73(1):17–29.
4. Kumar V, Cotran RS, Robbins SL. Osteoarthritis. In: RS Kumar V, ed. *Basic Pathology.* Philadelphia: W.B. Saunders; 1992:693.
5. Howell DS, TB, Trippel SB. Etiopathogenesis of osteoarthritis. In: HD Moskowitz R, Goldberg V, Mankin H, eds. *Osteoarthritis: Diagnosis and Medical/Surgical Management.* Philadelphia: W.B. Saunders; 1992:233.
6. DN C. In: WG Iannotti J, ed. *Disorders of the Shoulder: Diagnosis and Management.* Philadelphia: Lippincott, Williams & Wilkins; 2007:563–632.
7. Neer 2nd CS. Replacement arthroplasty for glenohumeral osteoarthritis. *J Bone Joint Surg Am.* 1974;56(1):1–13.
8. Williams GRJ,IJ. Unconstrained prosthetic arthroplasty for glenohumeral arthritis with an intact or repairable rotator cuff: indications, technique, and results. In: WG Iannotti J, ed. *Disorders of the Shoulder: Diagnosis and Management.* Philadelphia: Lippincott, Williams & Wilkins; 2007:697–726.
9. Rheumatoid EH. *Arthritis.* Philadelphia: WB Saunders; 1997.
10. Silman A,HM. *Epidemiology of the Rheumatic Diseases.* Oxford: Oxford University Press; 1993.
11. Chan KW, et al. Incidence of rheumatoid arthritis in central Massachusetts. *Arthritis Rheum.* 1993;36(12):1691–1696.
12. Hochberg MC. Adult and juvenile rheumatoid arthritis: current epidemiologic concepts. *Epidemiol Rev.* 1981;3:27–44.
13. JC B. The etiology of rheumatoid arthritis. In: HE Kelley W, Ruddy S, Sledge C, eds. *Textbook of Rheumatology.* Philadelphia: W.B. Saunders; 1985:879.
14. Kumar V, CR, Robbins SL. Rheumatoid arthritis. In: RS Kumar V, ed. *Basic Pathology.* Philadelphia: W.B. Saunders; 1992:145.
15. Haskard D,GR. Management of chronic inflammatory arthropathy. In: Watsons M, ed. *Surgical Disorders of the Shoulder.* New York: Churchill-Livingstone; 1991.
16. C P. Painful shoulders in patients with rheumatoid arthritis. Prevalence, clinical and radiological features. *Scand J Rheumatol.* 1986;15:275–279.
17. Bennett WF,GC. Operative treatment of the rheumatoid shoulder. *Curr Opin Rheumatol.* 1994;6:177–182.
18. Larson A, DK, Eek M. Radiographic evaluation of rheumatoid arthritis and related conditions by standard reference film. *Acta Radiol Diagn.* 1977;18:481–491.
19. Tan V, LB, Williams GRJ. Complications of shoulder arthroplasty. In: WG Iannotti J, ed. *Disorders of the Shoulder: Diagnosis and Management.* Philadelphia: Lippincott, Williams, & Wilkins; 1999:1608–1623.
20. Sperling JW, et al. Total shoulder arthroplasty versus hemiarthroplasty for rheumatoid arthritis of the shoulder: results of 303 consecutive cases. *J Shoulder Elbow Surg.* 2007;16(6):683–690.
21. Rittmeister M, Kerschbaumer F. Grammont reverse total shoulder arthroplasty in patients with rheumatoid arthritis and nonreconstructible rotator cuff lesions. *J Shoulder Elbow Surg.* 2001;10(1):17–22.
22. Holcomb JO, et al. Reverse shoulder arthroplasty in patients with rheumatoid arthritis. *J Shoulder Elbow Surg.* 2010;19(7):1076–1084.
23. McCarty DJ, et al. "Milwaukee shoulder"--association of microspheroids containing hydroxyapatite crystals, active collagenase, and neutral protease with rotator cuff defects. I. Clinical aspects. *Arthritis Rheum.* 1981;24(3):464–473.
24. Antoniou J, et al. Milwaukee shoulder: correlating possible etiologic variables. *Clin Orthop Relat Res.* 2003;407:79–85.
25. Neer 2nd CS, Craig EV, Fukuda H. Cuff-tear arthropathy. *J Bone Joint Surg Am.* 1983;65(9):1232–1244.
26. Favard L, et al. Reverse prostheses in arthropathies with cuff tear: are survivorship and function maintained over time? *Clin Orthop Relat Res.* 2011;469(9):2469–2475.
27. Ek ET, et al. Reverse total shoulder arthroplasty for massive irreparable rotator cuff tears in patients younger than 65 years old: results after five to fifteen years. *J Shoulder Elbow Surg.* 2013;22(9):1199–1208.
28. Cameron BD, et al. Non-prosthetic management of grade IV osteochondral lesions of the glenohumeral joint. *J Shoulder Elbow Surg.* 2002;11(1):25–32.
29. Kerr BJ, McCarty EC. Outcome of arthroscopic debridement is worse for patients with glenohumeral arthritis of both sides of the joint. *Clin Orthop Relat Res.* 2008;466(3):634–638.
30. Ogilvie-Harris DJ, Wiley AM. Arthroscopic surgery of the shoulder. A general appraisal. *J Bone Joint Surg Br.* 1986;68(2):201–207.
31. Weinstein DM, et al. Arthroscopic debridement of the shoulder for osteoarthritis. *Arthroscopy.* 2000;16(5):471–476.
32. Krishnan SG, et al. Humeral hemiarthroplasty with biologic resurfacing of the glenoid for glenohumeral arthritis. Two to fifteen-year outcomes. *J Bone Joint Surg Am.* 2007;89(4):727–734.
33. Lynch JR, et al. Self-assessed outcome at two to four years after shoulder hemiarthroplasty with concentric glenoid reaming. *J Bone Joint Surg Am.* 2007;89(6):1284–1292.
34. Wirth MA, et al. Treatment of glenohumeral arthritis with a hemiarthroplasty: a minimum five-year follow-up outcome study. *J Bone Joint Surg Am.* 2006;88(5):964–973.
35. Orfaly RM, et al. Shoulder arthroplasty in cases with avascular necrosis of the humeral head. *J Shoulder Elbow Surg.* 2007;16(suppl 3):S27–S32.

36. Sperling JW, Cofield RH, Rowland CM. Minimum fifteen-year follow-up of Neer hemiarthroplasty and total shoulder arthroplasty in patients aged fifty years or younger. *J Shoulder Elbow Surg.* 2004;13(6):604–613.

37. Safran O, SL. Iannotti JP. Cuff deficiency: unconstrained and constrained shoulder arthroplasty. In: WG Iannotti J, ed. *Disorders of the Shoulder: Diagnosis and Management.* Lippincott, Williams & Wilkins; 2007:727–751.

38. Boileau P, et al. Neer Award 2005: the Grammont reverse shoulder prosthesis: results in cuff tear arthritis, fracture sequelae, and revision arthroplasty. *J Shoulder Elbow Surg.* 2006;15(5):527–540.

39. Frankle M, et al. The Reverse Shoulder Prosthesis for glenohumeral arthritis associated with severe rotator cuff deficiency. A minimum two-year follow-up study of sixty patients. *J Bone Joint Surg Am.* 2005;87(8):1697–1705.

40. Seebauer L. Total reverse shoulder arthroplasty: European lessons and future trends. *Am J Orthop (Belle Mead NJ).* 2007;36(12 suppl 1):22–28.

41. Sirveaux F, et al. Grammont inverted total shoulder arthroplasty in the treatment of glenohumeral osteoarthritis with massive rupture of the cuff. Results of a multicentre study of 80 shoulders. *J Bone Joint Surg Br.* 2004;86(3):388–395.

42. Namdari S, et al. What is the role of arthroscopic debridement for glenohumeral arthritis? A critical examination of the literature. *Arthroscopy.* 2013;29(8):1392–1398.

43. Skelley NW, et al. Arthroscopic debridement and capsular release for the treatment of shoulder osteoarthritis. *Arthroscopy.* 2015;31(3):494–500.

44. Mitchell JJ, et al. Survivorship and patient-reported outcomes after comprehensive arthroscopic management of glenohumeral osteoarthritis: minimum 5-Year Follow-up. *Am J Sports Med.* 2016;44(12):3206–3213.

45. Weldon 3rd EJ, et al. Optimizing the glenoid contribution to the stability of a humeral hemiarthroplasty without a prosthetic glenoid. *J Bone Joint Surg Am.* 2004;86-A(9):2022–2029.

46. Saltzman MD, et al. Shoulder hemiarthroplasty with concentric glenoid reaming in patients 55 years old or less. *J Shoulder Elbow Surg.* 2011;20(4):609–615.

47. Getz CL, et al. Survivorship of hemiarthroplasty with concentric glenoid reaming for glenohumeral arthritis in young, active patients with a biconcave glenoid. *J Am Acad Orthop Surg.* 2017;25(10):715–723.

48. Schoch B, et al. Shoulder arthroplasty in patients younger than 50 years: minimum 20-year follow-up. *J Shoulder Elbow Surg.* 2015;24(5):705–710.

49. Nicholson GP, et al. Lateral meniscus allograft biologic glenoid arthroplasty in total shoulder arthroplasty for young shoulders with degenerative joint disease. *J Shoulder Elbow Surg.* 2007;16(suppl):S261–S266.

50. Puskas GJ, et al. Unacceptable failure of hemiarthroplasty combined with biological glenoid resurfacing in the treatment of glenohumeral arthritis in the young. *J Shoulder Elbow Surg.* 2015;24(12):1900–1907.

51. Alund M, et al. Outcome after cup hemiarthroplasty in the rheumatoid shoulder: a retrospective evaluation of 39 patients followed for 2-6 years. *Acta Orthop Scand.* 2000;71(2):180–184.

52. Fink B, et al. Surface replacement of the humeral head in rheumatoid arthritis. *Arch Orthop Trauma Surg.* 2004;124(6):366–373.

53. Levy O, Copeland SA. Cementless surface replacement arthroplasty (Copeland CSRA) for osteoarthritis of the shoulder. *J Shoulder Elbow Surg.* 2004;13(3):266–271.

54. Levy O, et al. Copeland surface replacement arthroplasty of the shoulder in rheumatoid arthritis. *J Bone Joint Surg Am.* 2004;86-A(3):512–518.

55. Wright TW, et al. Preliminary results of a posterior augmented glenoid compared to an all polyethylene standard glenoid in anatomic total shoulder arthroplasty. *Bull Hosp Jt Dis (2013).* 2015;73(suppl 1):S79–S85.

56. Karduna AR, et al. Joint stability after total shoulder arthroplasty in a cadaver model. *J Shoulder Elbow Surg.* 1997;6(6):506–511.

57. Walch G, et al. The influence of glenohumeral prosthetic mismatch on glenoid radiolucent lines: results of a multicenter study. *J Bone Joint Surg Am.* 2002;84-A(12):2186–2191.

58. Knowles NK, Ferreira LM, Athwal GS. Augmented glenoid component designs for type B2 erosions: a computational comparison by volume of bone removal and quality of remaining bone. *J Shoulder Elbow Surg.* 2015;24(8):1218–1226.

59. Cil A, Sperling JW, Cofield RH. Nonstandard glenoid components for bone deficiencies in shoulder arthroplasty. *J Shoulder Elbow Surg.* 2014;23(7):e149–e157.

60. Sabesan V, et al. Correction of acquired glenoid bone loss in osteoarthritis with a standard versus an augmented glenoid component. *J Shoulder Elbow Surg.* 2014;23(7):964–973.

61. Kuhn JE,DR, Desir W. Shoulder replacement. In: BS Di Giacomomo G, ed. *Shoulder Surgery and Rehabilitation.* Basel, Switzerland: Spring; 2016:67–92.

62. Williams GRJ,IJ. Diagnostic tests and surgical techniques. In: CW. Kelley M, ed. *Orthopedic Therapy of the Shoulder.* Philadelphia: JB Lippincott; 1994:158–224.

63. Boyd Jr AD, et al. Total shoulder arthroplasty versus hemiarthroplasty. Indications for glenoid resurfacing. *J Arthroplasty.* 1990;5(4):329–336.

64. Zarkadas PC, et al. Patient reported activities after shoulder replacement: total and hemiarthroplasty. *J Shoulder Elbow Surg.* 2011;20(2):273–280.

65. De Wilde LF, Audenaert EA, Berghs BM. Shoulder prostheses treating cuff tear arthropathy: a comparative biomechanical study. *J Orthop Res.* 2004;22(6):1222–1230.

66. Boudreau S, et al. Rehabilitation following reverse total shoulder arthroplasty. *J Orthop Sports Phys Ther.* 2007;37(12):734–743.

67. Liu JN, et al. Sports after shoulder arthroplasty: a comparative analysis of hemiarthroplasty and reverse total shoulder replacement. *J Shoulder Elbow Surg.* 2016;25(6):920–926.

68. Levy JC, et al. Speed of recovery after shoulder arthroplasty: a comparison of reverse and anatomic total shoulder arthroplasty. *J Shoulder Elbow Surg.* 2014;23(12):1872–1881.

69. Baulot E, Garron E, Grammont PM. Grammont prosthesis in humeral head osteonecrosis. Indications--results. *Acta Orthop Belg.* 1999;65(suppl 1):109–115.

70. Bacle G, et al. Long-term outcomes of reverse total shoulder arthroplasty: a follow-up of a previous study. *J Bone Joint Surg Am.* 2017;99(6):454–461.

71. Wong MT, et al. Implant positioning in reverse shoulder arthroplasty has an impact on acromial stresses. *J Shoulder Elbow Surg.* 2016;25(11):1889–1895.

72. Al-Hadithy N, et al. Reverse shoulder arthroplasty in 41 patients with cuff tear arthropathy with a mean follow-up period of 5 years. *J Shoulder Elbow Surg.* 2014;23(11):1662–1668.

90

Surgical and Postoperative Management of Elbow Arthritis

Dafang Zhang, Neal C. Chen

OUTLINE

CRITICAL POINTS

Indications

- Surgical treatment of elbow arthritis is indicated after failing conservative measures.
- Open or arthroscopic debridement procedures are indicated for the early stages of osteoarthritis or posttraumatic arthritis.
- Open or arthroscopic synovectomy is indicated for the early stages of rheumatoid arthritis.
- Interposition arthroplasty is a temporizing option in the young, active patient who would not otherwise be a candidate for total elbow arthroplasty.
- Total elbow arthroplasty is the mainstay of surgical treatment for severe elbow arthritis but should be used judiciously.

Pitfalls

- Semiconstrained and unlinked total elbow arthroplasty have better survivorship than fixed-hinge total elbow arthroplasty.
- Common causes of revision of total elbow arthroplasty include aseptic loosening, instability, and infection.
- Common causes of reoperation with implant retention after total elbow arthroplasty include infection, triceps rupture, and periprosthetic fracture.
- Ulnar neuropathy is a prevalent nonoperative complication after total elbow arthroplasty.

INTRODUCTION TO ELBOW ARTHRITIS

Various pathologies lead toward cartilage destruction of the elbow, commonly described as elbow arthritis. Clinically, patients manifest with pain, decreased range of motion (ROM), and diminished elbow function. Radiographic features may include osteophytes, intraarticular loose bodies, subchondral cysts or erosions, and joint space narrowing. Common etiologies of elbow arthritis include inflammatory arthritis, posttraumatic arthritis, and osteoarthritis (OA). Hemophilic arthropathy, neurogenic arthropathy, and septic arthritis are also less common types of arthritis.

Options for nonoperative treatment of elbow arthritis includes oral nonsteroidal antiinflammatory drugs, occasional intraarticular corticosteroid injections, and therapy to maintain joint mobility. Disease-modifying antirheumatic drugs (DMARDs) have revolutionized the treatment of rheumatoid arthritis (RA). Today, surgical intervention for the rheumatoid elbow is less frequent than in the era before DMARDs.[1] Orthotic use has a role in symptomatic management of arthritic flares, but the duration of immobilization must be limited and balanced against the risk of stiffness.

Surgical treatments can be categorized as nonarthroplasty and arthroplasty options. Nonarthroplasty options usually consist of treatments aimed at removing geometric blocks to motion. Total elbow arthroplasty is an option for advanced elbow arthritis; however, because of finite survival of elbow prostheses, total elbow arthroplasty has limited utility in younger or active patients.

JOINT-PRESERVING SURGICAL OPTIONS

Most joint-preserving surgical options focus on the removal of intraarticular loose bodies and geometric blocks to motion. In RA, arthroscopy may be performed to debulk synovitis and intraarticular disease burden. Joint-preserving surgeries may be performed via an open or arthroscopic approach. The choice as to which technique is most appropriate for the individual patient is determined by the severity of the disease and the experience and comfort level of the surgeon.

Outerbridge-Kashiwagi Procedure and Ulnohumeral Arthroplasty

Primary OA of the elbow classically affects middle-aged male laborers, resulting from heavy loading and repetitive use of the affected elbow. Elbow OA is characterized by osteophytes that impinge and limit motion. Kashiwagi[2] described an open elbow debridement procedure that he named the Outerbridge-Kashiwagi procedure, consisting of removal of loose bodies, the thickened olecranon fossa membrane, and osteophytes in the anterior and posterior elbow compartments by creating a window through the olecranon fossa. Morrey[3] described ulnohumeral arthroplasty, in which the posterior compartment is debrided by elevating rather than splitting the triceps and a bone trephine is used to debride encroaching osteophytes around the olecranon and coronoid fossae.

We perform open debridement with the patient supine and the operative arm placed across the chest over a bump. An extensile posterior skin incision is used. The triceps is elevated from its medial or lateral margin. The ulnar nerve is usually released and mobilized to protect it during this procedure. Loose bodies, osteophytes, and the thickened membrane in the olecranon fossa are excised. The floor of the olecranon fossa is then opened with a bone trephine, the size of which is determined by the diameter of the olecranon fossa, to gain access to the anterior compartment of the elbow. Care must be taken to center the window in the olecranon fossa. Fenestration too distal risks injury to the trochlea and deviation too medial or lateral can result in fracture of the distal humerus. Usually, a trephine 10 to 16 mm in diameter is appropriate.

If necessary, the anterior compartment is entered by elevating the anterior compartment off the lateral supracondylar ridge and splitting the common extensor distally. The medial compartment can be entered in a similar fashion as needed. Flexion and extension of the elbow delivers the coronoid into view and allows for excision of osteophytes about the coronoid process. At the conclusion of the procedure, the elbow is irrigated and closed over a suction drain, which can be safely removed within 24 hours. The elbow is placed in a soft dressing for early mobilization.

Postoperative Rehabilitation

This procedure is performed usually as an outpatient, but if performed as an inpatient, patients are generally discharged from the hospital after the closed-suction drain is removed. Patients are encouraged to perform progressive passive and active flexion and extension elbow ROM exercises at home and with supervision by a therapist. At 10 to 14 days postoperatively, patients are assessed in the office and continued on a formal therapy regimen for ROM. Strengthening may proceed as the patient tolerates beginning between 4 to 6 weeks after surgery, depending on whether the collateral ligaments were detached during surgery.

Morrey[3] describes using an indwelling brachial plexus nerve catheter starting in the recovery room for 3 days and continuous passive motion for 6 days. Patients are discharged with a hinged elbow orthosis with instructions for progressive active flexion and extension exercises.

Results of Surgery

The Outerbridge-Kashiwagi procedure and ulnohumeral arthroplasty alleviates pain and improves motion, but results may deteriorate over time. Morrey[3] reported good pain relief in 14 of 15 elbows that underwent ulnohumeral arthroplasty with minimum 2-year follow-up. Longer term studies demonstrate deterioration of results. Minami and coworkers[4] reported good pain relief in 27 of 44 elbows at 10 years.

Motion is reliably restored after this operation; however, the long-term gains are generally more modest than those seen intraoperatively, particularly in extension. Flexion is reported to improve by an average of 10 to 20 degrees at final follow-up and extension by an average of 6 to 11 degrees[3–6] Antuña and coworkers[5] reported improvement in mean Mayo Elbow Performance Score (MEPS) from 55 preoperatively to 83 postoperatively at mean 80-month follow-up. Similarly, Phillips and coworkers[6] reported good or excellent functional results in 65% of patients using the MEPS and 85% of patients using the Disabilities of the Arm, Shoulder and Hand (DASH) score at mean 75-month follow-up.

Ulnar neuropathy is encountered in over 15% of cases.[5] Antuña and coworkers[5] recommend prophylactic decompression or translocation of the ulnar nerve in elbows with preoperative flexion arc less than 100 degrees. Radiographic recurrence of olecranon and coronoid osteophytes occurs in more than 50% of elbows at medium-term follow-up[4–5]; however, radiographic recurrence of osteophytes does not correlate with functional outcome measures or elbow ROM.[6]

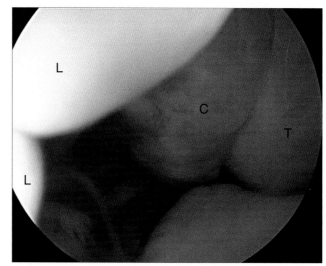

Fig. 90.1 Arthroscopic visualization of the coronoid process *(C)*, trochlea *(T)*, and multiple loose bodies *(L)* from the anterolateral viewing portal.

Elbow Arthroscopy

Arthroscopic elbow debridement is an alternative to open debridement. Elbow arthroscopy may be useful for an array of indications, ranging from simple loose body removal to ulnohumeral arthroplasty and capsular release. These procedures can be technically demanding. Elbow arthroscopy is potentially hazardous because of the close proximity of major upper extremity nerves to the entry portals and joint capsule.

The procedure is performed in the supine, prone, or lateral position. Surface anatomy is marked, and the elbow joint is insufflated with saline through the posterolateral soft spot. An anterolateral viewing portal is established, and then an anteromedial working portal is established using an inside-out technique. Loose bodies are removed, and osteophytes on the coronoid process and coronoid fossa are debrided (Fig. 90.1). The portals are switched so the camera is introduced medially and the working portal is switched laterally. If the patient has limitations in extension, the thickened anterior capsule may be released with an arthroscopic shaver or a biter. The radial nerve is in close proximity to the anterior joint capsule.

The camera is placed in the posterolateral viewing portal, and a straight posterior working portal through the triceps is established. Loose bodies in the posterior elbow are removed, and osteophytes on the olecranon process and olecranon fossa are debrided. If the patient has limitations in flexion, the posterior capsule may be released arthroscopically. The medial and lateral gutters are examined because they can house loose bodies. Large loose bodies in the lateral gutter can be excised using a small mini-open incision. Care should be taken around the medial gutter because of the proximity of the ulnar nerve.

A small joint arthroscope can be introduced into the lateral gutter through a soft spot portal. A lateral working portal can also be introduced to remove loose bodies or to debride the capitellum.

In patients with preoperative flexion limited to 90 degrees, it is appropriate to consider prophylactic release and transposition of the ulnar nerve to prevent secondary neuropathy with increased postoperative flexion. If the nerve subluxates after release, a subcutaneous transposition may be performed, although this may preclude further arthroscopic surgery.

Postoperative Rehabilitation

Patients are generally discharged from the recovery unit on the day of surgery. Patients are encouraged to perform progressive active flexion and extension elbow ROM exercises at home. Formal therapy begins on postoperative day 1. Strengthening begins as the patient tolerates.

Krishnan and coworkers[7] use an in-hospital stay overnight and continuous passive motion for 1 week. Patients who lack motion compared with the intraoperative gains at 1 week are started on dynamic flexion–extension orthoses for 6 weeks.

The critical element to consider with rehabilitation is whether ulnar nerve release has been performed in the setting of the arthroscopy. If an in situ release has been performed and the nerve is stable, then ROM as tolerated is recommended. However, if the ulnar nerve subluxates but was not transposed, then the arc of motion should be restricted to avoid higher degrees of flexion for the first 3 to 4 weeks to try to allow the ulnar nerve to stay in the groove.

Results of Surgery

Similar to open debridement, arthroscopic elbow debridement for primary OA alleviates pain and improves motion. Removal of loose bodies appears to provide the most reliable benefit, whereas patients with severe arthritis tend to benefit the least.[8–10] Dominant arm involvement is associated with better postoperative function.[11]

In the short term, Krishnan and coworkers[7] reported good or excellent MEPS in 11 elbows. Adams and coworkers[12] reported 81% excellent or good function in 42 elbows. Midterm results are similar: Galle and coworkers[13] reported improvement in mean MEPS from 57 to 87. MacLean and coworkers[8] reported improvement in DASH score from 34.0 to 12.7.

Flexion is reported to improve by an average of 9 to 40 degrees at final follow-up and extension by an average of 7 to 33 degrees.[7,11–14] Greater preoperative flexion–extension arc of motion is associated with greater postoperative flexion–extension arc of motion and function.[11] Subgroup analysis found that continuous passive motion devices had inferior MEPS and ROM compared with use of dynamic orthoses.[12]

Synovectomy

Although DMARDs have been very successful, in refractory cases of inflammatory arthritis, surgical intervention can be beneficial. Synovectomy is the surgical treatment of choice in mild RA of the elbow (Larsen grade I or II). This procedure may be performed open or arthroscopically. Although traditionally performed with concurrent radial head resection, routine resection of the radial head has fallen out of favor because of concerns that it concentrates forces at the lateral edge of the ulnohumeral joint and leads to accelerated deterioration.[15] Our current practice is to resect the radial head only in cases in which we believe that there is a high probability that resection of the radial head will improve pain.

Open synovectomy is performed with the patient supine, with careful control of the cervical spine, with the operative arm placed across the chest with a bump. An extensile lateral approach is used to access the elbow joint. The extensor carpi radialis longus and brachioradialis are elevated off the lateral supracondylar ridge, and the capsule is identified deep to the brachialis. The common extensor origin is split. The capsular tissue is incised without violating the lateral collateral ligament. This approach allows synovectomy as well as radial head resection if desired. The triceps can be elevated posteriorly to address the posterior compartment.

Arthroscopic synovectomy is performed similar to the prior description of arthroscopic elbow debridement. Arthroscopy is particularly dangerous because the capsule may be thinned and attenuated. The brachialis may be atrophic. In addition, synovitis can make visualization very difficult. Magnetic resonance imaging may be valuable to characterize synovitis preoperatively. Steroid injections prior to surgery may help attenuate synovitis before surgery.

Postoperative Rehabilitation

Patients are generally discharged from the recovery unit on the day of surgery. Patients are encouraged to perform progressive active flexion and extension elbow ROM exercises at home. For more extensive synovectomies, patients are initiated on a formal therapy for progressive ROM on postoperative day 1; otherwise, at 7 to 10 days postoperatively, patients are assessed in the office and initiated on a formal therapy regimen for ROM. At 6 weeks postoperatively, patients are advanced to progressive strengthening exercises.

Lee and Morrey[16] use an indwelling brachial plexus nerve catheter starting in the recovery room for 2 days, during which continuous passive motion is used. We do not use an indwelling catheter in these cases.

Results of Surgery

Although open synovectomy with radial head resection is an effective option for pain relief for patients with early stage RA in the short term, long-term follow-up shows that these results deteriorate.[15,17] Gendi and coworkers[18] suggest that patients with primarily limitations of forearm rotation benefit more from synovectomy and radial head resection than patients with limitations of flexion–extension. There is a current trend to avoid radial head resection if possible. The results of arthroscopic synovectomy similarly deteriorate over time. Functional outcomes significantly improve after surgery but decline to a middle ground within 2 years.[16,19] Although there are a few reports suggesting good long-term outcomes of synovectomy,[20] this surgical tactic is used more sparingly now than in the past. Results after synovectomy are generally less favorable with Larsen grade IV disease compared with Larsen grade I or grade II disease.[19]

Interposition Arthroplasty

Interposition arthroplasty was a more common method of treatment for arthritis before the development of modern total elbow prostheses. Today, interposition arthroplasty may be an option in younger, more active patients who are not be candidates for total elbow arthroplasty. Usually autologous fascia lata or Achilles tendon allograft is interposed between the articular surfaces of the elbow.

The procedure is performed with the patient supine, with the operative arm placed across the chest with a bump. An extensile posterior skin incision is used, and medial and lateral flaps are developed. The ulnar nerve is identified and protected. The anterior soft tissues are reflected off the lateral supracondylar ridge, and the extensor mass is split to access the lateral side. The radial head is resected. The medial elbow is accessed by similarly reflecting the anterior soft tissues and capsule from the medial supracondylar ridge. The remaining bony surfaces are prepared with a burr.

Hotchkiss[20a] describes a technique in which the medial collateral ligament and lateral collateral ligament are preserved, and the interposition tissue is drawn through the joint after preparation of the bony surfaces. The interposition material is then secured using either drill holes through the bone or suture anchors.

If the collateral ligaments are not intact, an internal hinge or an external fixator may be applied. Usually this consists of placing an axis pin through the ulnohumeral joint and then applying the internal hinge or external fixator relative to the axis pin. If possible, the joint articulation is distracted by 3 to 4 mm to unload the shear forces on the graft.

Postoperative Rehabilitation

Usually, patients have a single shot intrascalene block or an indwelling interscalene nerve catheter and begin supervised ROM exercises on postoperative day 1. If an external fixator is present, this is maintained about 6 to 8 weeks after the initial surgery; however, they may be removed earlier if there are pin site problems. Rehabilitation should be expected to take about 1 year before reaching durable results. The elbow should avoid positions of varus or valgus stress, and axial loading is not permitted for the first 3 months after surgery.

Results of Surgery

Interposition arthroplasty has fair results in the short-term for pain relief and functional improvement. MEPS improved postoperatively for the majority of patients, whether a fascia lata autograft or an Achilles tendon allograft was used. MEPS improved in the cohort of patients who did not have a distraction external fixator applied for various reasons. Almost all patients were able to delay total elbow arthroplasty in the short term.[21–24]

Larson and coworkers[24] reported mean flexion–extension arc improvement from 51 to 97 degrees and mean pronation–supination arc improvement from 85 to 123 degrees in their cohort. Nolla and coworkers[24] reported mean flexion–extension arc improvement from 48 to 110 degrees.

Instability is a commonly encountered complication of this operation, occurring in up to 31% of cases.[24] Preoperative instability is predictive of poor postoperative functional outcomes[23] and patient satisfaction.[22] Substantial bone loss, such as loss of one column of the distal humerus in a posttraumatic scenario, is also predictive of postoperative instability.[24]

The survival of interposition arthroplasty free of revision has been reported to be 88% at 5 years.[23] Major reasons for reoperation are instability, infection, and conversion to total elbow arthroplasty. The role of interposition arthroplasty is debated. It is an option for young patients with debilitating ulnohumeral arthrosis; however, it is an option that should be used judiciously.

JOINT-REPLACING SURGICAL OPTIONS

Total elbow arthroplasty has evolved from a basic hinge, to an unconstrained design, and then to a more complex semiconstrained design. The elbow joint undergoes multiple different forces that lead to failure. As a result, elbow arthroplasty is less durable than hip or knee arthroplasty. Modern total elbow arthroplasty consists of prosthetic replacement of the humeral and ulnar articulations and resection of the radial head. The most common modes of failure for total elbow arthroplasty are aseptic loosening, instability, and infection. Thoughtful patient selection and surgical decision making are the keys to a durable outcome.

Total Elbow Arthroplasty

Total elbow arthroplasty is the mainstay of surgical treatment for end-stage elbow arthritis. Total elbow arthroplasty was first reported by Dee[25] in the early 1970s. Early total elbow arthroplasty designs were a fixed hinge at the ulnohumeral articulation. Although they provide good pain relief, these hinges loosened relatively rapidly. Because the hinge is highly constrained, forces are primarily absorbed at the interface between the prosthesis and cement. The typical pattern of aseptic loosening observed is anterior migration of the proximal tip of the humeral stem and posterior migration of the axis of the hinged implant. This loosening pattern results from the posteriorly directed forces on the elbow prosthesis with cyclic flexion and extension.

Modern total elbow prostheses are either linked or unlinked. Some convertible implants provide surgeons the ability to insert the implant as linked or unlinked at the time of surgery, depending on intraoperative findings.

Unlinked total elbow prostheses are unconstrained implants, meaning that the humeral component is not directly attached to the ulnar component. Their development are a response to the failures of the original fixed hinge design. In unlinked total elbow arthroplasty, the soft tissues around the elbow maintain stability of the prosthetic elbow joint. Stability of the unlinked total elbow arthroplasty depends on adequate bone stock and competent soft tissue restraints. In theory, an unlinked design results in less loading of the cement–implant interface and less aseptic loosening. However, unlinked prostheses are difficult to implant properly and are problematic if the elbow is unstable.

The majority of modern linked total elbow prostheses are semiconstrained implants. They represent a middle ground in design between the fixed hinge and unlinked implants. Semiconstrained implants consist of a humeral and ulnar component with an articulation that allows for a limited amount motion between the humeral and ulnar components (Fig. 90.2). This loose articulation maintains more freedom of motion in the prosthetic articulation than the fixed hinge and therefore decreases loading of the cement–implant interface. In contrast to unlinked prostheses, semiconstrained prostheses can be used in patients with incompetent collateral ligaments.

A retrospective review of a comprehensive Medicare patient population database by Triplet and coworkers[1] showed that total elbow arthroplasty utilization is unchanged despite a growing Medicare population. Despite increases in office visits, total elbow arthroplasty utilization remains constant, likely secondary to improved medical management with DMARDs and surgeons' comfort with fracture fixation options.

Total elbow arthroplasty is primarily used for inflammatory arthritis, followed by posttraumatic arthritis and OA.[26,27] Functional outcomes at long-term follow-up are significantly better in patients with RA compared with patients with posttraumatic arthritis.[27] Moreover, total elbow arthroplasties performed for posttraumatic arthritis have substantially higher rates of implant revision than those performed for inflammatory arthritis, 57% compared with 27% at 6-year follow-up in a series by Perretta and coworkers.[28] Implant longevity is to a large degree a reflection on the demands placed on the prosthesis by the patient. Patients with inflammatory arthritis, in general, have lower functional demands than patients with posttraumatic arthritis, and this is reflected in their satisfaction, function, and implant survival.

The preferred candidate for total elbow arthroplasty is an older adult patient, generally older than 70 years of age, with inflammatory arthritis and low functional demands. Some surgeons have advocated total elbow arthroplasty for other indications. Chronologically young but physiologically older adult patients with end-stage arthritis and low functional demands or patients with irreparable periarticular elbow fractures may be considered for total elbow arthroplasty. Celli and coworkers[29] reported a series of 55 elbows in 49 patients age 40 years or younger who underwent total elbow arthroplasty with long-term follow-up. Overall implant survival rates were 95.2% at 8 years and 89.5% at 15 years. Patients with inflammatory arthritis had better functional outcomes and lower reoperation rates than those with posttraumatic arthritis. Currently, total elbow arthroplasty is being used less frequently for these less conventional indications.

Revision total elbow arthroplasty is challenging because of the lack of bone stock, the poor quality of soft tissues, and scarring of the ulnar nerve. The rate of adverse events is similar in primary and revision total elbow arthroplasties[30]; however, revision total elbow arthroplasty has poorer functional outcome and final ROM.[27]

Surgical Technique

There are various ways to approach the elbow for total elbow arthroplasty. In general, the procedure is performed under tourniquet control in the lateral position, with the arm supported by a bump or arm holder. An extensile posterior skin incision is used. The ulnar nerve is identified and decompressed. At the end of the case, the ulnar nerve is either transposed or left in situ per surgeon discretion. Exposure of the joint is accomplished by cutting and repairing, splitting, or elevating the triceps. Synovectomy is performed, and the radial head is resected. Bony resection is performed using cutting jigs specific to the implant

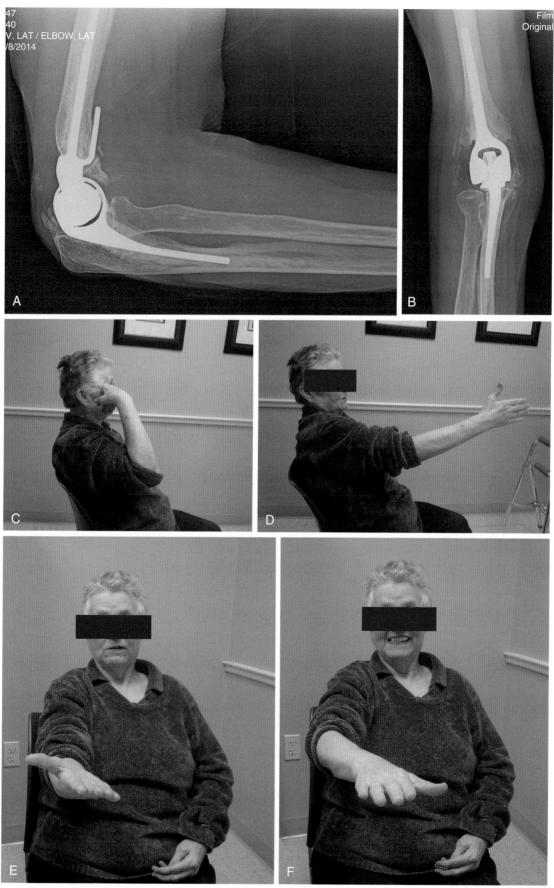

Fig. 90.2 Postoperative anteroposterior (**A**) and lateral (**B**) plain radiographs of a semiconstrained total elbow arthroplasty performed for posttraumatic arthritis with acceptable postoperative flexion (**C**), extension (**D**), pronation (**E**), and supination (**F**).

design. After the distal humerus is cut, the shaft of the humerus is prepared with intramedullary reamers and rasps. The proximal ulna is prepared in a similar fashion, usually with a large reamer to remove the chondral surface of the olecranon and then with progressive reamers to open the metaphyseal ulna and the proximal ulnar canal.

The components are trialed to ensure ease of implantation and to check that there is no impingement between the humeral and ulnar sides of the joint. Impingement places the elbow at risk of loosening, and in cases of unlinked prostheses, dislocation. The elbow is cycled to help with adjustments in alignment. After the final implant is inserted, it is crucial to reconstruct the triceps mechanism firmly before closure.

Postoperative Rehabilitation

Patients are placed in a posterior plaster orthosis at the conclusion of the surgery. Postoperative rehabilitation after total elbow arthroplasty is dictated by the quality of the soft tissue, the status of the ulnar nerve, the status of the triceps mechanism, and the type of implant used. In cases of poor soft tissue quality, the elbow is immobilized for 2 weeks to allow for soft tissue healing. Emphasis during this time is placed on edema control and distal ROM exercises. Nerve-gliding exercises can be performed, especially if there has been substantial surgery around the ulnar nerve. While in an orthosis, the position of the shoulder, elbow, and wrist can be altered to elicit ulnar nerve excursion. At 2 weeks postoperatively, patients are assessed in the office and initiated on a formal therapy regimen for ROM.

In the early postoperative period, triceps management is the most important consideration. If the triceps mechanism has been reattached or is of poor quality, a safe arc of motion should be identified intraoperatively. Passive ROM exercises may be performed within the safe arc initially. This is gradually progressed depending on the quality of triceps repair. In general, elbow ROM can be advanced more rapidly after about 4 to 6 weeks. Some patients who have had multiple revisions do not have an intact triceps mechanism, and in these cases, patients will rely on gravity to extend the elbow.

If the elbow is unlinked, it is important to take note of the quality of the collateral ligaments. Varus and valgus stresses on the implant are avoided depending on which ligament is at risk. In general, after about 6 weeks, the precautions are lifted. At 6 weeks postoperatively, patients are advanced to progressive strengthening exercises. For long-term management, it is important to work in coordination with the rehabilitation team and be clear about loading limits for the patient. These limits vary among practices and should be defined early with the rehabilitation team.

Results of Surgery

Unlinked total elbow arthroplasty reliably alleviates pain, improves ROM, and restores function; however, there are concerns about long-term survivorship. Ewald and coworkers[31] reported on 202 elbows in 172 patients who underwent unlinked capitellocondylar total elbow arthroplasty for RA. Patients had excellent functional improvement with mean 24-degree improvement in flexion–extension arc of motion. However, the complication rate of capitellocondylar total elbow arthroplasty is relatively high, ranging from 15% to 57% in the literature.[31–35] Ikavalko and coworkers[36] reported on 525 elbows in 406 patients who underwent unlinked Souter-Strathclyde total elbow arthroplasty with mean 5-year follow-up period. Average flexion was improved; however, of the 525 cases, 108 further operations were performed in 82 patients, including 33 operations for aseptic loosening and 30 operations for dislocation. A disproportionate, specific mode of failure of the unlinked total elbow arthroplasty is instability, although other modes of failure, including aseptic loosening and infection, are also observed.[37–39]

Semiconstrained total elbow arthroplasty is comparably effective at pain relief and functional restoration. Long-term survivorship appears to vary among studies. Gill and Morrey[40] reported on 78 elbows in 69 patients that underwent semiconstrained Coonrad-Morrey total elbow arthroplasty for RA with minimum 10-year follow-up. Good or excellent functional results were seen in 86% of patients using the MEPS. ROM was improved, and the overall survival rates of the implant were 94.4% at 5 years and 92.4% at 10 years. Gschwend and coworkers[41] reported on 36 elbows in 32 patients who underwent semiconstrained GSB III total elbow arthroplasty for RA or posttraumatic arthritis with a minimum 10-year follow-up period. Mean flexion–extension arc of motion improved 37 degrees in patients with RA and 67 degrees in patients with posttraumatic arthritis. The overall survival rate of the implant was 87.7% at 10 years. The predominant mode of failure for linked total elbow arthroplasty is aseptic loosening, followed by infection.[40–42]

Comparative studies between types of total elbow arthroplasty are limited. Little and coworkers[43] compared outcomes of consecutive series of 33 Souter-Strathclyde, Kudo, and Coonrad-Morrey arthroplasties. Although pain relief and ROM were similar among the implants, survival of the implant at 5 years, assessed by revision surgery and radiographic signs of loosening as endpoints, respectively, were 85% and 81% for the Souter-Strathclyde, 93% and 82% for the Kudo, and 90% and 85% for the Coonrad-Morrey prostheses. Plaschke and coworkers[44] reviewed 324 elbows in 234 patients who underwent primary total elbow arthroplasty for various diagnoses using the Danish National Patient Register and found that unlinked total elbow arthroplasty had a higher risk of revision surgery than linked total elbow arthroplasty.

Patients who undergo total elbow arthroplasty for inflammatory arthritis generally have better outcomes than patients with posttraumatic arthritis.[27,45] This has been attributed to lower functional demands of patients with inflammatory arthritis because of limitations of multiple joints. Moreover, patients with total elbow arthroplasties for posttraumatic arthritis are more likely to undergo reoperation or implant revision than patients with RA.[28,44]

In a systematic review by Little and coworkers[46] of 3618 implantations in 86 articles, the complication rates of total elbow arthroplasties ranged from 14% to 80%, with a median rate of 33%. Aseptic loosening was reported in 9% of cases, with asymptomatic radiolucencies in 14%. The wound complication rate was 9%, not associated with postoperative immobilization, and the deep infection rate was 5%. In a review by Lovy and coworkers[30] using the National Surgical Quality Improvement Program database, adverse events after total elbow arthroplasty were found to be associated with smoking, dependent functional status, hypertension, and OA (versus RA). Perretta and coworkers[28] reported the rate of reoperation after total elbow arthroplasty to be 41%, with the most common indication for reoperation being component loosening. In a review by Jenkins and coworkers[26] of 1146 primary total elbow arthroplasties for various diagnoses using the Scottish Morbidity Record, implant survivorship was found to be higher for surgeons who performed at least 10 total elbow arthroplasties per year.

Revision Arthroplasty

Common reasons for revision total elbow arthroplasty are aseptic loosening, infection, and periprosthetic fracture. Revision total elbow arthroplasty often presents challenges of lack of bone stock, poor quality of soft tissues, and scarring of the ulnar nerve. Although adverse event rates are similar in primary and revision total elbow arthroplasties,[30] revision total elbow arthroplasties have poorer functional outcome and final ROM.[27] Careful preoperative planning is crucial to a successful outcome.

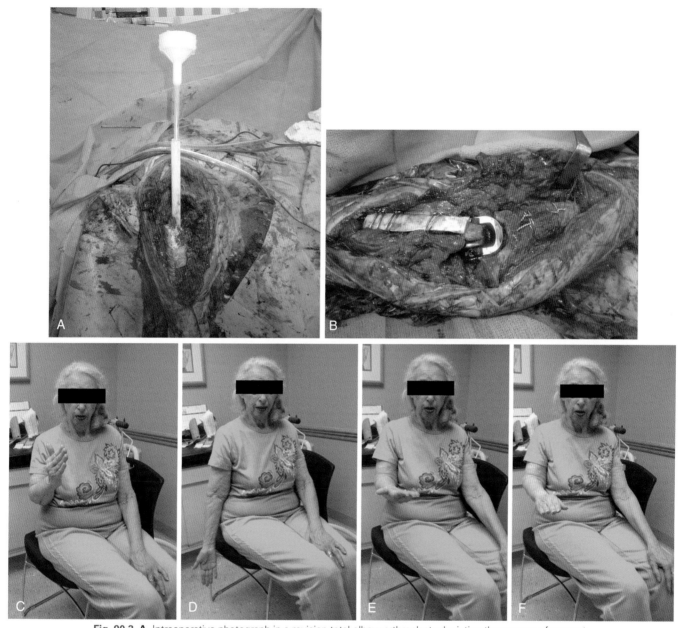

Fig. 90.3 A, Intraoperative photograph in a revision total elbow arthroplasty depicting the process of cementing the ulnar canal after the use of a fibular allograft strut and impaction grafting to reconstruct deficient bone stock. **B,** Intraoperative photograph depicting the fibular allograft strut reconstruction of deficient ulna *(left)* and cerclage wiring of the distal humerus *(right)*, with a semiconstrained implant in place *(center)*. Postoperative clinical assessment showing acceptable postoperative **C,** flexion, **D,** extension, **E,** supination, and **F,** pronation.

Infected total elbow arthroplasty may be treated by irrigation and debridement and polyethylene exchange, one-stage revision, two-stage revision, or resection of the arthroplasty. In two-stage treatment, the prosthesis is removed followed by a prolonged course of intravenous antibiotics, usually for at least 6 weeks. This is followed by a period when the elbow is left without an arthroplasty and the patient is off antibiotics. It is theorized that this period allows any residual infection to re-present itself. After a new infectious workup, if there is no evidence of infection recurrence, then the elbow may be reimplanted.

Periprosthetic fractures are particularly difficult to manage. The Mayo Classification categorizes type I fractures as periarticular, type II fractures as adjacent to the stem of the prosthesis, and type III fracture as well beyond the tip of the stem.[47] The location of the periprosthetic fracture dictates the appropriate surgical approach. Bone grafting,

including strut allografts, may be useful in cases of deficient bone stock (Fig. 90.3). Negative-pressure wound therapy has an increasing role in minimizing edema in a traumatized wound bed. Rehabilitation is generally similar to that for primary total elbow arthroplasty but may be affected by the quality of the soft tissue, remaining bone support, and the stability of the prosthesis.

SUMMARY

Elbow arthritis is the sequela of one of a number of joint destructive processes, including RA, posttraumatic arthritis, and OA. A variety of surgical options are available when nonoperative management is unsuccessful. These surgical options range from joint-preserving to joint-reconstructing to joint-replacing procedures. Choice of the optimal procedure is based on the etiology and severity of the arthritis, the experience and training of the surgeon, and the profile and demands of the patient. Rehabilitation is a routine and necessary aspect of postoperative management and varies according to the specific procedure performed, expectations for functional restoration, and preferences of the treating surgeon.

REFERENCES

1. Triplet JJ, Kurowicki J, Momoh E, et al. Trends in total elbow arthroplasty in the Medicare population: a nationwide study of records from 2005 to 2012. *J Shoulder Elbow Surg.* 2016;25(11):1848–1853.

2. Kashiwagi D. Outerbridge Kashiwagi arthroplasty for osteoarthritis of the elbow. In: Kashiwagi D, ed. *Proceedings of the International Congress.* Kobi, Japan, Amsterdam: Excerpta Medica; 1986.

3. Morrey BF. Primary degenerative arthritis of the elbow. Treatment by ulnohumeral arthroplasty. *J Bone Joint Surg Br.* 1992;74(3):409–413.

4. Minami M, Kato S, Kashiwagi D. Outerbridge-Kashiwagi's method for arthroplasty of osteoarthritis of the elbow: 44 elbows followed for 8-16 years. *J Orthop Sci.* 1996;1:11–16.

5. Antuña SA, Morrey BF, Adams RA, et al. Ulnohumeral arthroplasty for primary degenerative arthritis of the elbow: long-term outcomes and complications. *J Bone Joint Surg Am.* 2002;84-A(12):2168–2173.

6. Phillips NJ, Ali A, Stanley D. Treatment of primary degenerative arthritis of the elbow by ulnohumeral arthroplasty. A long-term follow-up. *J Bone Joint Surg Br.* 2003;85(3):347–350.

7. Krishnan SG, Harkins DC, Pennington SG, et al. Arthroscopic ulnohumeral arthroplasty for degenerative arthritis of the elbow in patients under fifty years of age. *J Shoulder Elbow Surg.* 2007;16(4):443–448.

8. MacLean SB, Oni T, Crawford LA, et al. Medium-term results of arthroscopic debridement and capsulectomy for the treatment of elbow osteoarthritis. *J Shoulder Elbow Surg.* 2013;22(5):653–657.

9. Ogilvie-Harris DJ, Schemitsch E. Arthroscopy of the elbow for removal of loose bodies. *Arthroscopy.* 1993;9:5–8.

10. Rupp S, Tempelhof S. Arthroscopic surgery of the elbow. Therapeutic benefits and hazards. *Clin Orthop Relat Res.* 1995;313:140–145.

11. Lim TK, Koh KH, Lee HI, et al. Arthroscopic débridement for primary osteoarthritis of the elbow: analysis of preoperative factors affecting outcome. *J Shoulder Elbow Surg.* 2014;23(9):1381–1387.

12. Adams JE, Wolff LH, Merton SM, et al. Osteoarthritis of the elbow: results of arthroscopic osteophyte resection and capsulectomy. *J Shoulder Elbow Surg.* 2008;17(1):126–131.

13. Galle SE, Beck JD, Burchette RJ, et al. Outcomes of elbow arthroscopic osteocapsular arthroplasty. *J Hand Surg Am.* 2016;41(2):184–191.

14. Miyake J, Shimada K, Oka K, et al. Arthroscopic debridement in the treatment of patients with osteoarthritis of the elbow, based on computer simulation. *Bone Joint J.* 2014;96-B(2):237–241.

15. Rymaszewski LA, Mackay I, Amiss AA, et al. Long-term effects of excision of the radial head in rheumatoid arthritis. *J Bone Joint Surg Am.* 1984;66(1):109–113.

16. Lee BP, Morrey BF. Arthroscopic synovectomy of the elbow for rheumatoid arthritis. A prospective study. *J Bone Joint Surg Am.* 1997;79B:770–772.

17. Summers GD, Taylor AR, Webley M. Elbow synovectomy and excision of the radial head in rheumatoid arthritis: a short term palliative procedure. *J Rheumatol.* 1988;15(4):566–569.

18. Gendi NST, Axon JMC, Carr AJ, et al. Synovectomy of the elbow and radial head excision in rheumatoid arthritis. Predictive factors and long-term outcome. *J Bone Joint Surg Br.* 1997;79(6):918–923.

19. Horiuchi K, Momohara S, Tomatsu T, et al. Arthroscopic synovectomy of the elbow in rheumatoid arthritis. *J Bone Joint Surg Am.* 2002;84-A(3):342–347.

20. Ishii K, Inaba Y, Mochida Y, et al. Good long-term outcome of synovectomy in advanced stages of the rheumatoid elbow. *Acta Orthop.* 2012;83(4):374–378.

20a. Tan V, Daluiski A, Capo J, Hotchkiss R. Hinged elbow external fixators: indications and uses. *J Am Acad Orthop Surg.* 2005;13(8):503–514.

21. Ljung P, Jonsson K, Larsson K, et al. Interposition arthroplasty of the elbow with rheumatoid arthritis. *J Shoulder Elbow Surg.* 1996;5(2 Pt 1):81–85.

22. Cheng SL, Morrey BF. Treatment of the mobile, painful arthritic elbow by distraction interposition arthroplasty. *J Bone Joint Surg Br.* 2000;82(2):233–238.

23. Larson AN, Morrey BF, et al. Interposition arthroplasty with an Achilles tendon allograft as a salvage procedure for the elbow. *J Bone Joint Surg Am.* 2008;90(12):2714–2723.

24. Nolla J, Ring D, Lozano-Calderon S, et al. Interposition arthroplasty of the elbow with hinged external fixation for post-traumatic arthritis. *J Shoulder Elbow Surg.* 2008;17(3):459–464.

25. Dee R. Total replacement arthroplasty of the elbow for rheumatoid arthritis. *J Bone Joint Surg Br.* 1972;54(1):88–95.

26. Jenkins PJ, Watts AC, Norwood T, et al. Total elbow replacement: outcome of 1,146 arthroplasties from the Scottish Arthroplasty Project. *Acta Orthop.* 2013;84(2):119–123.

27. Plaschke HC, Thillemann TM, Brorson S, et al. Outcome after total elbow arthroplasty: a retrospective study of 167 procedures performed from 1981 to 2008. *J Shoulder Elbow Surg.* 2015;24(12):1982–1990.

28. Perretta D, van Leeuwen WF, Dyer G, et al. Risk factors for reoperation after total elbow arthroplasty. *J Shoulder Elbow Surg.* 2017;26(5):824–829.

29. Celli A, Morrey BF, et al. Total elbow arthroplasty in patients forty years of age or less. *J Bone Joint Surg Am.* 2009;91(6):1414–1418.

30. Lovy AJ, Keswani A, Dowdell J, et al. Outcomes, complications, utilization trends, and risk factors for primary and revision total elbow replacement. *J Shoulder Elbow Surg.* 2016;25(6):1020–1026.

31. Ewald FC, Simmons Jr ED, Sullivan JA, et al. Capitellocondylar total elbow replacement in rheumatoid arthritis. Long-term results. *J Bone Joint Surg Am.* 1993;75(4):498–507.

32. Ovesen J, Olsen BS, Johannsen HV, et al. Capitellocondylar total elbow replacement in late-stage rheumatoid arthritis. *J Shoulder Elbow Surg.* 2005;14(4):414–420.

33. Trancik T, Wilde AH, Borden LS. Capitellocondylar total elbow arthroplasty. Two-to eight-year experience. *Clin Orthop Relat Res.* 1987;223:175–180.

34. Dennis DA, Clayton ML, Ferlic DC, et al. Capitello-Condylar total elbow arthroplasty for rheumatoid arthritis. *J Arthroplasty.* 1990;(suppl 5):S83–S88.

35. Ruth JT, Wilde AH. Capitellocondylar total elbow replacement. A long-term follow-up study. *J Bone Joint Surg Am.* 1992;74(1):95–100.

36. Ikavalko M, Lehuto MUK, Repo A, et al. The Souter-Strathclyde elbow arthroplasty: a clinical and radiological study of 525 consecutive cases. *J Bone Joint Surg Br.* 2002;84(1):77–82.

37. Landor I, Vavrik P, Jahoda D, et al. Total elbow replacement with the Souter-Strathclyde prosthesis in rheumatoid arthritis. Long-term follow-up. *J Bone Joint Surg Br.* 2006;88(11):1460–1463.

38. Kodama A, Mizuseki T, Adachi N. Kudo type-5 total elbow arthroplasty for patients with rheumatoid arthritis: a minimum ten-year follow-up study. *Bone Joint J.* 2017;99-B(6):818–823.

39. Qureshi F, Draviaraj KP, Stanley D. The Kudo 5 total elbow replacement in the treatment of the rheumatoid elbow: results at a minimum of ten years. *J Bone Joint Surg Br.* 2010;92(10):1416–1421.

40. Gill DR, Morrey BF. The Coonrad-Morrey total elbow arthroplasty in patients with rheumatoid arthritis. A ten to fifteen year follow-up. *J Bone Joint Surg Am.* 1998;80A:1327–1335.

41. Gschwend N, Scheier NH, Baeher AR. Long term results of the GSB III elbow arthroplasty. *J Bone Joint Surg Br.* 1999;81(6):1005–1012.

42. Schneeberger AG, Adams R, Morrey BF. Semiconstrained total elbow replacement for the treatment of post-traumatic osteoarthrosis. *J Bone Joint Surg Am*. 1997;79(8):1211–1222.

43. Little CP, Graham AJ, Karatzas G, et al. Outcomes of total elbow arthroplasty for rheumatoid arthritis: comparative study of three implants. *J Bone Joint Surg Am*. 2005;87(11):2439–2448.

44. Plaschke HC, Thillemann TM, Brorson S, et al. Implant survival after total elbow arthroplasty: a retrospective study of 324 procedures performed from 1980 to 2008. *J Shoulder Elbow Surg*. 2014;23(6):829–836.

45. Toulemonde J, Ancelin D, Azoulay V, et al. Complications and revisions after semi-constrained total elbow arthroplasty: a mono-centre analysis of one hundred cases. *Int Orthop*. 2016;40(1):73–80.

46. Little CP, Graham AJ, Carr AJ. Total elbow arthroplasty: a systematic review of the literature in the English language until the end of 2003. *J Bone Joint Surg Br*. 2005;87-B:437–444.

47. O'Driscoll SW, Morrey BF. Periprosthetic fractures about the elbow. *Orthop Clin North Am*. 1999;30(2):319–325.

91

Scleroderma: Surgery

A. Lee Osterman, Meredith Osterman

CRITICAL POINTS

- Scleroderma is a systemic disease that manifests challenging hand problems for patients.
- Factor in the overall health of the patient, current medications, vascular problems, and activity goals when addressing hand pathology.
- Digital ischemia, calcinosis, joint contractures, and skin changes are the primary manifestations of scleroderma in the hand.
- CREST syndrome includes calcinosis, Raynaud's phenomenon, esophageal dysmotility, scleroderma, and telangiectasias.

- Botox shows promising results for digital ischemia.
- Calcinosis can lead to nerve compression, skin ulcerations, joint contractures, and pain.
- Recommended surgical treatment for the radiocarpal joint is fusion and for the small joints of the hand include arthroplasties for the metacarpophalangeal joints and fusions for the proximal interphalangeal and distal interphalangeal joints.

HISTORY AND PATHOGENESIS

Hippocrates described the clinical findings associated with scleroderma, including thickened skin, in his writings from 460 BC. The first detailed description of the condition came from Dr. Carlo Curzio in Naples in 1752 when he saw a patient with woodlike hardened skin. His patient was a 17-year-old girl who was assigned to him upon her admission to the hospital. He chronicled her symptoms and her treatment in his monograph. These symptoms included tightness around the mouth and hardness of the skin in different areas of the body and around the neck. Treatments used at that time included baths in vapor and warm milk, bleeding from the foot, and small therapeutic doses of quicksilver. Robert Goetz was the first to develop a detailed description of scleroderma as a systemic disease and to document the progressive nature of the disease in 1945.[1]

Scleroderma is derived from the Greek words *skleros*, meaning hard or indurated, and *derma*, skin. Systemic sclerosis (SSc) is an autoimmune disease characterized by skin induration and thickening as well as tissue fibrosis of visceral organs and alterations in immunity. Cutaneous systemic sclerosis can be limited (limited cutaneous systemic sclerosis [lcSSc]) and confined to the distal extremities or diffuse (diffuse cutaneous systemic sclerosis [dcSSc]), involving the trunk and proximal extremities as well. The American College of Rheumatology has developed diagnostic criteria for SSc, with a diagnosis that requires the presence of one major criterion or two minor criteria.[2]

Major criteria include symmetrical thickening, tightening, and induration of the skin of the fingers and proximal to the metacarpophalangeal

(MCP) joints. The involvement may extend even further proximally to include the entire upper extremity, face, neck, and trunk.

Minor criteria include sclerodactyly limited only to the fingers, pitting scars of the digits or ischemic loss of the substance of the pads of the digits, and bibasilar pulmonary fibrosis.

CREST is the acronym used to describe the clinical features of *c*alcinosis, *R*aynaud's phenomenon, *e*sophageal dysfunction, *s*clerodactyly, and *t*elangiectasia. This constellation of symptoms is seen in lcSSc. dcSSc is characterized by involvement of multiple visceral organs leading to pulmonary fibrosis and pulmonary hypertension, renal insufficiency, renal crisis, and CREST. The findings of sclerodactyly and digital ulceration are seen with equal frequency in both the limited and diffuse forms of the disease (Table 91.1).

The pathogenesis at the cellular level involves the T cells, fibroblasts, and cytokines. T cells are seen in the skin biopsies of patients with SSc. Both the T cells and cytokines act on the fibroblasts to induce collagen deposition. The obliterative vascular pathology occurs from both diffuse intimal hyperplasia and adventitial fibrosis leading to ischemic digital ulcers and systemic arterial pathology with pulmonary hypertension.[3] Antibodies commonly tested for in SSc include antinuclear, anticentromere, topoisomerase I, ribonucleic acid polymerase, and U3/ribonucleoprotein. Peripheral ischemia is associated with anticentromere antibodies as well as anti–Scl-70 antibodies.[4]

The estimated prevalence of the disease is 1 case per 4000 population.[5] The risk of SSc is higher in blacks and in women, with women four times greater than men. The peak onset is between 30 and 50 years of age.

TABLE 91.1 Comparison of Diffuse versus Limited Scleroderma

Parameter	Diffuse Scleroderma	Limited Scleroderma or CREST
Frequency	30%–40%	60%–65%
Skin involvement	Proximal trunk and extremities	Fingers, feet, face
Raynaud's phenomenon	Concomitant with disease onset	May precede other features by years
Telangiectasia	May be present	Often extensive, florid
Renal disease	30%–40%	None
Pulmonary fibrosis	30%–40%	10%–20%
Pulmonary hypertension	20%, usually with interstitial lung disease	Late, 20%–50%
Digital ulcers	Common	Common
Anesthesia risk	Increased	
Sclerodactyly	Same	Same

CREST, Calcinosis, Raynaud's phenomenon, esophageal dysfunction, sclerodactyly, and telangiectasia.

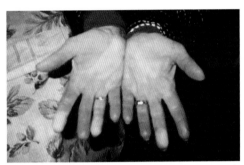

Fig. 91.1 Raynaud's phenomenon in a patient with systemic sclerosis. Note the significant pallor of the long finger.

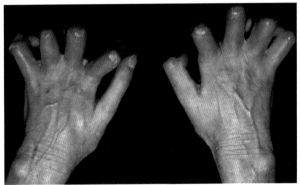

Fig. 91.2 Note the severe flexion deformities at the level of the proximal interphalangeal joints, the tightened and shortened skin, and hyperextension deformities present at the metacarpophalangeal joints. Thumb adduction contractures are present bilaterally.

CLINICAL FINDINGS

Digital ischemia, calcinosis, joint contractures, and skin changes are the primary manifestations of scleroderma in the hand. Physical examination findings include changes in the pigmentation of the skin to alternating areas of hyperpigmentation and hypopigmentation, a so-called salt-and-pepper appearance. Dilated telangiectatic small vessels just beneath the skin may be visible. Edematous skin progressing eventually to tight and shiny hardened skin with loss of folds, loss of sweating, and hair loss is also characteristic. These changes usually start distally in the fingers and progress proximally over time. Digital ulcers, necrotic lesions, and cutaneous calcinosis are common, especially in the digits. Flexion contractures of the joints may eventually occur as well as bony resorption of the distal phalanx. Raynaud's phenomenon (Fig. 91.1), seen in 90% and often early in the disease, is distinguished by episodes during which the fingers turn white, then blue, and then finally red and is the result of intermittent digital vasospasm. This vasospasm is often the initial presenting symptom of scleroderma and is brought on by cold or stress. This is in contrast to Raynaud's disease where the vasospastic changes are unrelated to underlying sclerosis. There can be some overlap with findings seen in other similar disorders such as lupus, rheumatoid arthritis (RA), and dermatomyositis; this is known as *overlap syndrome.*[6]

Digital deformity follows a rather predictable pattern with time in these patients (Fig. 91.2) Flexion contractures develop in the proximal interphalangeal (PIP) joints.[7-11] These begin with loss of the ability to extend the PIP joints with the resultant development of stiffness and contracture. These can become quite severe with time. The skin located over the dorsum of the joints may blanch because of the severe flexion deformity coupled with the hardened skin. Thinning of the extensor mechanism may eventually result in rupture. The skin may eventually break down with progressive increase in severity of the deformity. The underlying PIP joint may then become exposed, predisposing the patient to infection of the joint or bone.

With the increasing PIP flexion deformity comes the compensatory hyperextension deformity at the MCP joints. With longstanding hyperextension deformities, the soft tissue structures, including the collateral ligaments and capsular tissues, contract, resulting in stiffness at the MCP joint level as well.

Rarely, a hyperextension deformity at the PIP joint occurs as a result of subluxation at the MCP joint level.

Relative to the thumb, a contracture typically develops in the first webspace. This limits the patient's ability to grasp objects, especially larger things (Fig. 91.3). This is a result of the tightening of the skin and underlying deeper soft tissue structures in this area.

A study by Herrick and associates[12] looked at the functional ability of scleroderma patients in 140 patients, using an 11-item functional questionnaire, found that functional limitations were largely related to contractures and decreased range of motion (ROM), especially in the hand. Another study by Poole and associates[13] followed 60 patients with scleroderma who were administered assessments of grip and pinch strength, joint ROM, and pain and were observed for the presence of digital ulcers, digital scars, calcium deposits, puffy fingers, and tendon friction rubs over a 5-year span. They concluded that hand impairment persisted over time, and functional ability decreased.

Soft tissue calcinosis is also commonly seen in these patients (Fig. 91.4). This can be especially problematic when it develops over the

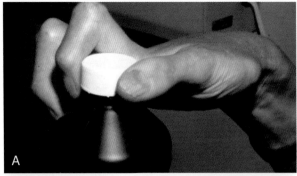

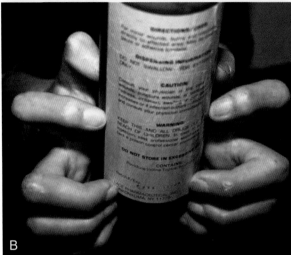

Fig. 91.3 A, Note the thumb adduction contracture, making it difficult for the patient to grasp objects, particularly larger ones. **B,** The patient is forced to use both hands as demonstrated.

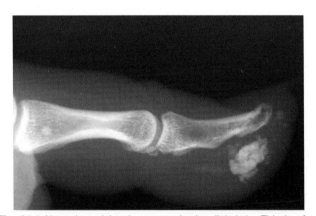

Fig. 91.4 Note the calcinosis present in the digital tip. This is often symptomatic, requiring debulking or excision.

already compromised skin over the dorsal aspect of the flexed PIP joints and can result in skin breakdown and difficulty in healing.

Treatment

Treatment of patients with sclerosis is multidisciplinary with hand surgeons, rheumatologists, and hand therapists working in conjunction. Pharmaceutical treatments, avoidance of vasospastic stimulators, wound care, and therapy[14–17] are the initial mainstays of treatment. Surgical intervention is reserved as a last resort given the increased risks of delayed wound healing, infection, vascular damage and ischemia.

SURGICAL TREATMENT

For many reasons, surgical treatment can be very challenging in patients with scleroderma. There is potential difficulty with healing of surgical incisions postoperatively due to poor skin quality and impaired vascularity as a result of the disease. There is also a high risk of recurrence of the deformities because of the underlying disease process. Surgical treatment is therefore undertaken after a course of conservative management, including therapy and orthotic positioning . Preoperative evaluation is critical to assess pulmonary and renal function, which may increase the risk of general anesthesia. Local or regional anesthetic is a reasonable alternative surgical option.

Surgical treatment in patients with scleroderma is aimed at the predictable problems that develop, including calcinosis in the soft tissues, joint contractures, and digital ischemia with ulcerations.

Calcinosis

Calcinosis cutis is the collection of interstitial calcific masses, most commonly in the subcutaneous tissues and fascia of the hand and is present in 8.9% to 73.1% of patients with SSc and is part of the CREST constellation of findings.[9,11,18,19] It can also be found in other rheumatologic conditions such as dermatomyositis and systemic lupus erythematosus. It results from hydroxyapatite calcium phosphate deposition in soft tissue.[20] Calcinosis can be found in a single digit or widespread throughout the hand and can cause pain, decreased function, and occasional ulceration with calcium exudation. It occurs frequently in the pulp surfaces, over bony prominences, and at points of stress as a result of mechanical stress in addition to the underlying systemic process. It is often found over the dorsal aspect of PIP joints affected by flexion deformity and along the radial portion of the digits that oppose the thumb during pinch, mainly the index and long fingers. Occasionally, the soft tissue calcifications can become symptomatic, especially when they form in the distal tips of the digits. Patients may complain of pain or may develop recurrent trauma to the skin over the area, resulting in skin breakdown and difficulty healing, predisposing the patient to infection. If the skin does break down, white chalky-appearing drainage may be seen.

In 2011, Reiter and coworkers[23] performed an extensive review of the medical treatment options. The results showed that no single proposed treatment has been successful in resolving or preventing the calcinosis or decreasing complications associated with digital calcinosis.

Surgical debridement to debulk the calcific mass has provided reasonable pain relief and improvement in function. Care must be taken to minimize exposure because of the increased risk of vascular compromise and flap necrosis. We prefer a limited surgical exposure using a curette or high-speed burr. Warm saline irrigation helps leach the calcium from the fibrous pulp septae. Often the deposit encompasses the digital nerve, which requires appropriate protective care. Often complete resection is not necessary, and simple debulking of the calcinosis can be very helpful in relieving symptoms. Residual scar tenderness and recurrent calcification are common. The outcome literature[11,18,20,24] for debulking has shown variable results and is compromised by retrospective design, small study size, short follow-up, lack of functional evaluations, and patient heterogenicity.

Proximal Interphalangeal Joint Contracture

The largest functional limitations were the result of contractures and decreased ROM in the hands. Therefore, surgically addressing and improving the contractures in the hands of a patient with scleroderma can result in significant functional improvement. Surgical treatment of the PIP joints consists of soft tissue procedures, joint arthrodesis, or joint arthroplasty.

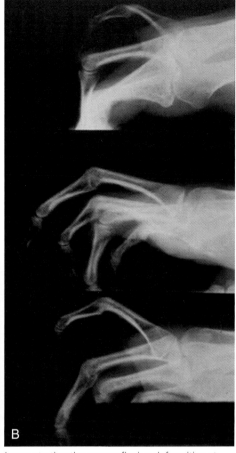

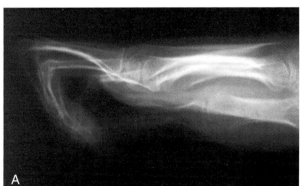

Fig. 91.5 Preoperative (**A**) and (**B**) postoperative radiographs demonstrating the severe flexion deformities at the proximal interphalangeal joint level treated with arthrodesis resulting in solid fusion and better functional positions of the digits.

Reconstructive soft tissue procedures should usually be reserved for younger patients with less severe joint deformities. The risk of the development of recurrent deformities is high if soft tissue procedures are performed, but they can provide improvement in function for a period of time. Surgical treatment consists of releasing or excising the volar plate and collateral ligaments at the level of the PIP joints to correct the flexion deformity. Skin coverage will probably be necessary for the palmar aspect of the joint, and most often this is done with full-thickness skin grafting. A midaxial or palmar incision is recommended in this setting. Anandacoomarasamy and coworkers[10] found that the tight volar skin was the structure contributing most to the flexion deformity at the PIP joint. The tight volar plate and collateral ligaments do contribute but to a lesser degree to the overall deformity. The patients treated surgically with soft tissue procedures do tend to maintain the improved position of the joints, but the joints often become stiff again with progression of the disease.

Arthrodesis is the more common surgical treatment for the joint at the level of the PIP joint. It can be undertaken using tension band fixation or other methods based on the preferences of the operating surgeon (Fig. 91.5). Often the dorsal soft tissue deficiency requires a percutaneous pin technique or full intramedullary fixation with a screw. Lipscomb and coworkers[25] found that interphalangeal (IP) joint arthrodesis attempts in patients with scleroderma resulted in solid bony fusion in all of the patients treated. In addition, time to ultimate fusion was found to be shorter than in cases in which arthrodesis is attempted for other conditions. Judicious shortening of the bony elements is necessary for correction of the deformity and to minimize stress on the vascular structures. The standard accepted positions of

arthrodesis are applicable in patients with scleroderma. However, because of the associated vascular insufficiency that is often present, the digits may not tolerate the desired amount of straightening, and fusion in a slightly more flexed position may be required to maintain vascularity of the digit. This should be assessed intraoperatively after arthrodesis at the PIP joint level, and the position of the digit should be adjusted to maintain viability of the digit.

Arthroplasty at the level of the PIP joint has been performed in patients with scleroderma. Norris and Brown[26] reported on their results following 20 replacement arthroplasties at the PIP joints in six patients. These patients had improved hand function and appearance postoperatively, but no long-term results have been published.

Metacarpophalangeal Joint Contracture

The characteristic extension and hyperextension deformities that result at the MCP joint level can also be treated surgically with good results. Both soft tissue reconstruction and joint arthroplasty have been performed.[1,8,10,11,27–30]

At the MCP joint level, the dorsal capsule contributes most to the overall contracture seen compared to the PIP joint with its pan tissue involvement Anandacoomarasamy and associates[10] described a soft tissue procedure to address this. Adhesions are present between the extensor apparatus and the capsule, further contributing to stiffness. Through a single transverse dorsal incision, these adhesions can be cleared and a capsulectomy can address the thickened dorsal capsule. The collateral ligaments and volar plate are also released, and the joints are pinned in the intrinsic-plus position for 3 weeks postoperatively. Full-thickness skin graft is often required to address the resultant

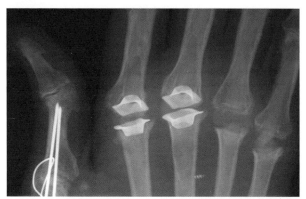

Fig. 91.6 With a preserved arc of motion of at least 50 degrees, patients can successfully be treated for involvement at the metacarpophalangeal joint level with implant arthroplasties with good results.

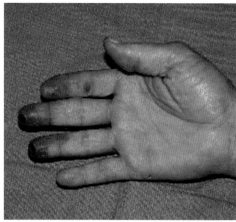

Fig. 91.7 Digital ischemia can result in chronic painful nonhealing digital ulcerations in patients with systemic sclerosis.

defect over the dorsal aspect of the joints. Over time the deformity does recur, although to a lesser degree.

Joint arthroplasty is the more commonly performed and widely accepted surgical treatment for deformity at the MCP joint (Fig. 91.6). Although both excisional and implant replacement arthroplasties have been performed, Nalebuff[27] notes that implant replacements are not as successful in patients with SSc as they are in patients with other types of arthritis, including degenerative and RA at the same level. Gilbart and coworkers[28] reported good functional results with the surgical combination of PIP joint fusion and excisional arthroplasty at the MCP joint level for correction of the severe "finger-in-palm" deformity commonly seen in severe late disease. Melone and coworkers[29] reported results following a large series of 70 patients treated with 211 IP joint arthrodeses including the PIP and DIP joint levels, in addition to 28 implant arthroplasties performed at the MCP joint level. In follow-up ranging from 1 to 15 years, the average arc of motion at the replaced MCP joint level was 50 degrees. Given these results, there appears to be no clear consensus regarding the use of excisional versus implant replacement arthroplasties at the MCP joint level for patients with scleroderma, and both treatments seem to show reasonable and acceptable results. It is recommended that patients have at least 50 degrees of motion preoperatively before undergoing an implant replacement arthroplasty at the MCP joint level.

Thumb Adduction Contracture

An adduction contracture of the first webspace is also typical in patients with scleroderma. The contracture comes from the skin as well as the underlying muscles and deeper soft tissue structures. Surgical release of the first webspace is often helpful in restoring grasp and pinch. A soft tissue release of the contracted adductor attachment as well as a Z-plasty lengthening of the skin of the first webspace is the generally accepted treatment for this problem. Skin grafts may be needed for the webspace along with the soft tissue release. In addition, an arthrodesis at the MCP joint or IP joint may be needed to improve thumb-to-index pinch if deformity in these joints is seen.[25,29,30] Excision of the trapezium as well as reconstruction of the ligaments at the basilar thumb joint may also be required if symptoms and radiographic changes are present.

Digital Ulceration and Vascular Insufficiency

Impaired digital blood flow in patients with SSc can be compounded by the coexistence of Raynaud's phenomenon present in up to 95% of individuals. The resultant vascular insufficiency can lead to digital ulceration, infection, and eventual amputation in some cases (Fig. 91.7). Bogoch and Gross[18] found that recurrent digital ulceration is present in up to 70% of patients with scleroderma. They reported that nearly 30% of these patients can go on to develop gangrene.

BOX 91.1 Drugs Used to Treat Raynaud's Phenomenon and Digital Ulcerations

Direct Vasodilators
Calcium channel blockers
α-Adrenergic inhibitors
Nitrate patches or nitroglycerin ointment
Angiotensin-converting enzyme inhibitors
Angiotensin receptor blockers
Prostacyclin analogues
Phosphodiesterase type 5 inhibitors
Botox

Endothelial Integrity and Vascular Health
Endothelin receptor blockers
Fish oils, vitamin E, vitamin C
Probucol, other statins
Low-dose aspirin
Anticoagulants

Perfusion-Enhancing and Thermoregulatory Agents
Serotonin inhibitors
Serotonin reuptake inhibitors
Calcitonin gene-related peptide
Pentoxifylline, cilostazol

A recent study[31] confirmed the relationship between angiogenic vascular biomarkers and the occurrence of digital ulceration. Endoglin and vascular endothelial growth factor (VEGF) serum levels are potential risk factors, and VEGF has a predictive value for the occurrence of new digital ulceration.

Nonsurgical management of digital ulcerations that are not acutely infected should be attempted initially. This consists of cessation of smoking, avoidance of exposure of the digits to cold, and biofeedback. Medications such as β-blockers, α-blockers, vasodilators, and calcium channel blockers have also been used (Box 91.1). In a double-blind, randomized trial,[32] tadalafil (Cialis; Eli Lilly, Indianapolis, IN) was found to improve symptoms in patients with resistant Raynaud phenomenon, heal digital ulcers, and improve quality of life outcomes. Tadalafil is a phosphodiesterase type 5 enzyme inhibitor for use in erectile dysfunction and pulmonary arterial hypertension. Phosphodiesterase inhibitors promote nitric oxide release in blood vessels, allow for smooth muscle relaxation, and ultimately increase blood flow. Patel and Nagle[33] reported a case of digital ulcer healing in a medically compromised patient with scleroderma with a daily dose of 5 mg of tadalafil and the application of a wound vac. Sequential nerve blockade has shown some success in some individuals.

Neumeister and coworkers[34,35] reported an exciting development, the use of Botox injection for ischemic digits. After injection of 50 to 100 units of Botox around each neurovascular bundle, 16 of 19 patients (84%) had pain reduction at rest; 13 felt immediate relief, 3 had gradual pain reduction over 1 to 2 months, and 3 had no or minimal pain relief. Tissue perfusion results demonstrated a marked increase in blood flow (8.15% to 425%) to the digits. All patients with chronic finger ulcers healed within 60 days. As important, 63% of patients remained pain-free (13–59 months) with a single injections, while 21% required repeated injections because of recurrent pain. However, Bello and coworkers[36] looked at blood flow after Botox injections in patients with scleroderma using laser doppler imaging and found no statistically significant improvement in blood flow at 4-month follow-up.

Surgical management includes debridement, excision of prominent areas of calcinosis, repositioning of the digits to avoid stretching and pressure in areas of already tight skin, and sympathectomy. Ward and Van Moore[37] looked at nonsurgical versus surgical management of digital ulcerations in 12 patients with scleroderma and digital ulcerations involving 15 hands. Nonsurgical management was successful in obtaining healing in 6 patients in an average of 6 weeks. The remaining nine hands were treated with palmar digital sympathectomy as described by Flatt[38] for treatment of Raynaud's phenomenon. In this technique, 2 cm of adventitial stripping of the proper and common digital arteries, often including the superficial transverse arch, is performed under magnification. Sympathectomy resulted in healing in all patients in an average of 3.7 weeks. Three sympathectomy patients did develop recurrent ulcerations at 6, 9, and 11 months postoperatively. The remaining sympathectomy patients remained free of ulcerations at last follow-up of 51 months. Preoperative digital brachial indices were 1.03 and improved to 1.11 postoperatively. This was not a significant improvement. It is thought that the sympathectomy does not improve actual pressures in the digit but does improve low-velocity flow to the digit improving nutrition and perfusion. Three of the surgically treated patients did report continued pain in the digits despite resolution of ulceration. Preoperative arteriography demonstrated complete unreconstructible ulnar artery occlusion at the level of the midforearm in all patients. If a short-segment reconstructible occlusion is identified, then vein graft reconstruction and palmar sympathectomy are recommended. If no reconstructible occlusion is found, then palmar sympathectomy alone is performed.[17]

Ruch and associates[39] reported on 22 patients (29 hands) with a diagnosis of scleroderma and a history of nonhealing painful digital ulcers. All were unresponsive to conservative treatment modalities. All were treated with periarterial sympathectomy, including circumferentially stripping 1 cm of adventitia from the radial and ulnar arteries at the wrist, the superficial palmar arch, and the common digital arteries. Preoperative and postoperative isolated cold stress testing and cutaneous perfusion as measured by laser Doppler were performed. Eighty-two percent of patients reported improvement in pain, subjective ulcer healing, and reduction in occurrence of ulcerations postoperatively. Cutaneous perfusion showed statistically significant improvements during isolated cold stress testing over 2 years postoperatively. However, digital temperatures were not significantly improved with sympathectomy. The authors note that the search for a reconstructible arterial lesion using preoperative arteriography is imperative (Fig. 91.8). If a short-segment reconstructible occlusion is identified, then vein graft reconstruction and palmar sympathectomy are recommended. If no reconstructible occlusion is found, then palmar sympathectomy alone is performed.

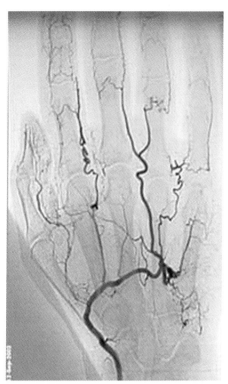

Fig. 91.8 Preoperative arteriography demonstrating complete occlusion of the ulnar artery proximal to the wrist. Note the "corkscrew"-appearing collateral vessels often seen in patients with systemic sclerosis.

Nerve Compression in Scleroderma

Carpal tunnel syndrome has long been observed in patients with scleroderma[40] and is thought to be caused by fibrosis and edema of the surrounding soft tissues. Ko and coworkers[41] described a case report in which a thickened palmaris longus and distal antebrachial fascia were noted to be the causes of compression of the median nerve proximal to the carpal tunnel. Based on this experience and others, it is recommended that patients with scleroderma and carpal tunnel symptoms have these structures examined and released, if needed, as well as the carpal tunnel itself. Ulnar nerve compression at Guyon's canal secondary to calcinosis has also been documented.[42]

Wrist Arthrosis

Wrist arthritis with accompanying pain and stiffness can also be seen in patients with SSc, especially in the face of the diagnosis of *overlap syndrome* as previously discussed. Radiographic changes mimic those seen in other inflammatory arthritides such as RA.[43] One treatment option is wrist arthrodesis by the standard means, with good results and solid bony fusion. Total wrist arthroplasty maintains ROM at the wrist joint and can be used with good success in some individuals (Fig. 91.9). Most comparative studies indicate that patients prefer wrist arthroplasty over arthrodesis in general.

THE CHANGING PARADIGM OF SURGERY IN SCLERODERMA

Paul Klee (1879–1940), a Swiss painter, developed systemic scleroderma from which he died. His tombstone reads: "I belong not only to this life. I live well with the dead, as with those not born. Nearer to the heart of creation than others, but still too far."[44] The fundamental solutions to scleroderma remain elusive, but progress in the treatment of the musculoskeletal deformities has progressed.

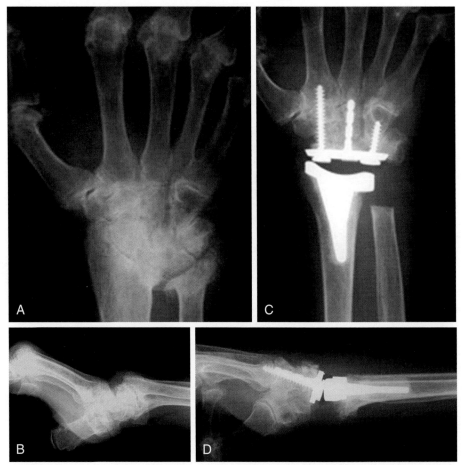

Fig. 91.9 Preoperative (**A** and **B**) and postoperative (**C** and **D**) radiographs of a patient with systemic sclerosis and rheumatoid arthritis diagnoses, the so-called overlap syndrome. Eight years after total wrist arthroplasty, the patient maintained functional range of wrist motion and pain relief.

REFERENCES

1. Handley B. The History of Scleroderma. *Scleroderma News*. 2017;47(2).
2. Van den Hoogen F, Khanna D, Fransen J, et al. Classification criteria for systemic sclerosis. *Arthritis Rheum*. 2013;65(11):2737–2747.
3. Gu YS, Kong J, Cheema GS, Keen CL, Wick G, Gershwin ME. The immunobiology of systemic sclerosis. *Semin Arthritis Rheum*. 2008;38(2):132–160.
4. Herrick AL, Heaney M, Hollis S, Jayson MI. Anticardiolipin, anticentromere and anti-scl-70 antibodies in patients with systemic sclerosis and severe digital ischaemia. *Ann Rheum Dis*. 1994;53(8):540.
5. Mayes MD. Scleroderma epidemiology. *Rheum Dis Clin North Am*. 2003;29:239–254.
6. Iaccarino L, Gatto M, Bettio S, Caso F, Rampudda M, Zen M, et al. Overlap connective tissue disease syndromes. *Autoimmun Rev*. 2013;12(3):363–737.
7. Pope JE. Musculoskeletal involvement in scleroderma. *Rheum Dis Clin N Am*. 2003;29:391–408.
8. Jakubietz MG, Jakubietz RG, Gruenert JG. Scleroderma of the hand. *J Soc Surg Am. Hand*. 2005;5:42–47.
9. Choo AD, Middleton G, Wilson RL. Nonrheumatoid inflammatory arthroses of the hand and wrist. *J Hand Surg Am*. 2015;40(12):2477–2487.
10. Anandacoomarasamy A, Manolios N, Kirkham S. Reconstructive hand surgery for scleroderma joint contractures. *J Hand Surg*. 2007;32A:1107–1112.
11. Fox P, Chung L, Chang J. Management of the hand in systemic sclerosis. *J Hand Surg Am*. 2013;38:1012–1016.
12. Herrick A, Rooney B, Finn J, Silman A. Lack of relationship between functional ability and skin score in patients with systemic sclerosis. *J Rheumatol*. 2001;28:292–295.
13. Poole JL, Watzlaf VJ, D'amico F. A five-year followup of hand function and activities of daily living in systemic sclerosis (scleroderma). *J Hand Ther*. 2004;17(4):407–411.
14. Askew LJ, Beckett VL, An K, Chao EYS. Objective evaluation of hand function in scleroderma patients to assess effectiveness of physical therapy. *Br J Rheum*. 1983;22:224–232.
15. Mouthon L, Poole JL. Physical and occupational therapy. In: Varga J, Denton C, Wigley F, eds. *Scleroderma: From Pathogenesis to Comprehensive Management*. New York: Springer; 2012:629–639.
16. Poole JL. Musculoskeletal rehabilitation in the person with scleroderma. *Curr Opin Rheumatol*. 2010;22(2):205–212.
17. Maddali Bongi S, Del Rosso A, Galluccio F, Tai G, Sigismondi F, Passalacqua M, et al. Efficacy of a tailored rehabilitation program for systemic sclerosis. *Clin Exp Rheumatol*. 2009;27(3 suppl 54):44–50.
18. Bogoch ER, Gross DK. Surgery of the hand in patients with systemic sclerosis: outcomes and considerations. *J Rheumatol*. 2005;32(4):642–648.
19. Schlenker JD, Clark DD, Weckesser EC. Calcinosis circumscripta of the hand in scleroderma. *J Bone Joint Surg Am*. 1973;55(5):1051–1056.
20. Mendelson BC, Linscheid RL, Dobyns JH, Muller SA. Surgical treatment of calcinosis cutis in the upper extremity. *J Hand Surg Am*. 1977;2(4):318–324.
21. Deleted in review.
22. Deleted in review.

23. Reiter N, El-Shabrawi L, Leinweber B, Berghold A, Aberer E. Calcinosis cutis: part II. Treatment options. *J Am Acad Dermatol.* 2011;65(1):15–22.

24. Lapner MA, Goetz TJ. High-speed burr debulking of digital calcinosis cutis in scleroderma patients. *J Hand Surg Am.* 2014;39(3):503–510.

25. Lipscomb P, Simons G, Winkelmann R. Surgery for sclerodactylia of the hand: experience with six cases. *J Bone Joint Surg.* 1969;51:1112–1117.

26. Norris RW, Brown HG. The proximal interphalangeal joint in systemic sclerosis and its surgical management. *Br J Plastic Surg.* 1985;38(4):526–531.

27. Nalebuff E. Surgery in patients with systemic sclerosis of the hand. *Clin Orthop Rel Res.* 1999;366:91–97.

28. Gilbart MK, Jolles BM, Lee P, Bogoch ER. Surgery of the hand in severe systemic sclerosis. *Inl Hand Surg Br.* 2004;29(6):599–603.

29. Melone CP, McLoughlin JC, Beidner S. Surgical management of the hand in scleroderma. *Curr Opin Rheum.* 1999;11:514–520.

30. Jones NF, Imbriglia JE, Steen VD, Medsger TA. Surgery for scleroderma of the hand. *J Hand Surg.* 1987;12A:391–400.

31. Silva I, Almeida C, Teixeira A, Oliveira J, Vasconcelos C. Impaired angiogenesis as a feature of digital ulcers in systemic sclerosis. *Clin Rheumatol.* 2016;35(7):1743–1751.

32. Shenoy PD, Kumar S, Jha LK, Choudhary SK, Singh U, Misra R, et al. Efficacy of tadalafil in secondary Raynaud's phenomenon resistant to vasodilator therapy: a double-blind randomized cross-over trial. *Rheumatology.* 2010;4912:2420–2428.

33. Patel RM, Nagle DJ. Nonoperative management of scleroderma of the hand with tadalafil and subatmospheric pressure wound therapy: case report. *J Hand Surg.* 2012;37A:803–806.

34. Neumeister MW, Chambers CB, Herron MS, et al. Botox for ischemic digits. *Plast Reconstr Surg.* 2009;124:191–200.

35. Neumeister MW. Botulinum toxin Type A in the treatment of Raynaud's phenomenon. *J Hand Surg.* 2010;35A:2085–2092.

36. Bello Rj, Cooney CM, Melamed E, Follimar KE, Wigley FJ, Lifchez SD. A randomized, double-blinded, placebo controlled clinical trial assessing the therapeutic efficacy of botulinum toxin in treating scleroderma-associated Raynaud's phenomenon: level 1 evidence. *J Hand Surg.* 2016;41(9):S2.

37. Ward WA, Van Moore A. Management of finger ulcers in scleroderma. *J Hand Surg.* 1995;20A:868–872.

38. Flatt AE. Digital artery sympathectomy. *J Hand Surg.* 1980;5:550–556.

39. Ruch DS, Holden M, Paterson Smith B, et al. Periarterial sympathectomy in scleroderma patients: intermediate- term follow-up. *J Hand Surg.* 2002;27A:258–264.

40. Barr WG, Blair SJ. Carpal tunnel syndrome as the initial manifestation of scleroderma. *J Hand Surg.* 1988;13A:378–380.

41. Ko CY, Jones NF, Steen VD. Compression of the median nerve proximal to the carpal tunnel in scleroderma. *J Hand Surg.* 1996;21A:363–365.

42. Thurman RT, Jindal P, Wolff TW. Ulnar nerve compression in Guyon's canal caused by calcinosis in scleroderma. *J Hand Surg.* 1991;16A:739–741.

43. Allali F, Tahiri L, Senjari A. Erosive arthropathy in systemic sclerosis. *BMC Public Health.* 2007;7:260.

44. Friedewald P, Paul Klee. *Life and Work.* New York: Prestel Publishing; 2011.

92

Scleroderma: Therapy

Janet L. Poole, Carole Dodge

CRITICAL POINTS

- Early intervention is the key to improved outcomes.
- Every effort must be made to preserve hand function by focusing on improving joint motion and mobility of the skin.
- Use heat before passive stretching.
- Stretching should focus on maintaining metacarpophalangeal joint flexion, interphalangeal joint extension, thumb and digit abduction, wrist motion, and lateral pinch.

- Ulcerations are an emergent situation because they can quickly lead to decreased joint motion and permanent loss of motion.
- Avoid cold and teach behavior strategies to manage Raynaud's phenomenon.
- Few studies have been conducted that address the efficacy of orthotic intervention for systemic scleroderma.

Scleroderma refers to a group of disorders that includes sclerosis of the skin as a predominant feature (Box 92.1).[1,2] Systemic sclerosis or systemic scleroderma (SSc) refers to the autoimmune connective tissue disease characterized by vascular disease and fibrosis of the skin and internal organs.[3,4] SSc is a generalized disease often seen in rheumatic disease and hand clinics because of severe hand impairment and corresponding functional disability.[4,5]

EPIDEMIOLOGY, PATHOGENESIS, AND CLASSIFICATION

Systemic sclerosis is considered a rare disease because the prevalence is fewer than 1 in 2000.[6] However, SSc is found across all racial groups and all ages. The prevalence is slightly higher in African Americans, who also tend to have an earlier onset and more severe disease.[7] SSc affects women three to four times more often than men, and the peak age of onset is in the childbearing years.[7] SSc is rare in children. It is more common to see localized or linear scleroderma in children.[8]

BOX 92.1 Classification of Scleroderma

Scleroderma
- Localized Scleroderma
  - Morphea
  - Linear
- Systemic scleroderma/Systemic sclerosis
  - Limited Scleroderma (CREST)
  - Diffuse Scleroderma

The cause of SSc is not known, but it is thought that the autoimmune processes result in abnormal collagen buildup.[9] Collagen is the major part of connective tissue that is found in skin, tendons, joints, ligaments, and organs, such as the kidneys, lungs, and heart. Collagen is the basic component of scar tissue, which is essential for repair after injury. However, an overproduction of collagen interrupts vital systems by replacing functioning cells with "scars." When this process happens in the lungs, for example, it results in pulmonary fibrosis (scarring in the lungs), which causes problems with breathing. Although the cause of scleroderma is unknown, when there is a specific genetic background and a potential trigger, the immune system may be activated.[9] This results in damage to the blood vessels and causes the cells to make too much collagen in the skin and other internal organs.[10]

There are two major subtypes of adult SSc, *limited cutaneous* and *diffuse cutaneous* (Box 92.1). It is essential for clinicians to understand the clinical features of each subtype.

Limited Cutaneous Systemic Sclerosis

In limited cutaneous systemic sclerosis (lcSSc) the skin manifestations are limited to the distal extremities (distal to the elbows and knees) and face.[10–12] The skin changes are stable or slowly progressive, and hand motion may remain nearly normal. Raynaud's phenomenon is usually present for a long period before skin thickening occurs. Patients with lcSSc are more prone to digital ulcers, ischemia, and gangrene. There is a prominence of telangiectasis (dilated capillaries) and subcutaneous calcinosis, although the latter may be microscopic or occur late; and the serum is positive for anticentromere antibody (ANA) in 70% to 80% of patients.[10–12] People with this subtype rarely develop myocardial or renal disease but are prone to late (after 10-plus years) appearance of primary pulmonary arterial hypertension, interstitial lung disease, and gastrointestinal (GI) involvement, including intestinal malabsorption and biliary cirrhosis.[10–12]

Limited SSc used to be referred to as CREST syndrome, the acronym referring to the symptoms of calcinosis, Raynaud's phenomenon, esophageal dysfunction, sclerodactyly (scleroderma of the digits), and telangiectasias.[10–12]

Diffuse Cutaneous Systemic Sclerosis

The second subtype of SSc is diffuse cutaneous systemic sclerosis (dcSSc).[10–12] In dcSSc, there is often rapid progression of skin thickening, beginning distally in the extremities and progressing proximally to include the trunk. Raynaud's phenomenon usually occurs within 1 year of onset of skin changes. Tendon friction rubs (TFRs) are palpable, polyarthritis is common, and the serum is positive for antibody Scl-70.[11,13] These patients are at a higher risk for developing early and often severe internal involvement in the first 2 years of the disease, such as renal crisis, myocardial failure, interstitial lung disease, and GI complications.[14] dcSSc produces the most severe hand deformities early in the disease course as the fibrosis affects all of the soft tissue: skin, fat, fascia, muscle, tendon sheath, ligament, and joint capsule.[15]

Diagnostic Tests and Epidemiology

A definitive diagnosis and classification of disease subtypes can be determined using the 2013 European League Against Rheumatism classification.[1,16] Although the cause is unknown and genetic predisposition is still uncertain, significant strides have been made in early detection and prediction of who will develop SSc.[10,12,17] Young and Khanna[12] state that the presence of Raynaud's phenomenon, puffy fingers, and positive ANA are suggestive of SSc because 90% have Raynaud's phenomenon, 95% have sclerodactyly, and 95% have a positive ANA. There are two diagnostic procedures that should be done to make a definitive diagnosis[12]: the nail fold capillary microscopy to detect characteristic capillary dilation or avascular areas in the nail fold and the presences of serum antinuclear antibody determinations of anticentromere and antinucleolar antibodies. Antibody testing is important to predict organ involvement and disease progression.[1,18] Knowing one's antibodies can help patients, and physicians be alert for the potential for severe sclerosis and organ failure before irreversible scarring occurs. Prognosis is determined by the degree of internal organ involvement. Optimal patient care includes an integrated, multispecialty medical management to promptly and effectively recognize, evaluate, and manage complications and limit end-organ dysfunction.[19]

Localized Form of Scleroderma

There is also a localized form of scleroderma in which fibrotic lesions occur in a single patch (morphea), multiple hypopigmented or depigmented patches (guttate morphea), confluent patches (generalized morphea), or linear bands.[8,20] There is no associated systemic or visceral involvement.[20] Localized scleroderma primarily occurs in children and young adults, mostly female. Morphea begins with an area of erythematous or violaceous discoloration of the skin, progressing to a waxy or ivory-colored sclerotic patch surrounded by an inflammatory border. The lesions often soften after a few months or years.

In children, morphea affects the associated soft tissue and can retard bone growth. Linear scleroderma that crosses a joint may lead to a severe contracture and fibrotic distortion of the nearby neurovascular compartment. When this occurs in the hand, usually only one or two digits are involved. Hand therapy can be designed according to the program outlined later in this chapter for dcSSc, except that the precautions for Raynaud's phenomenon, swelling, associated conditions, and hand deformity patterns do not apply.

MEDICAL MANAGEMENT

There are three major components of SSc that can be addressed with medications: vascular damage (e.g., renal crisis, pulmonary arterial hypertension), immune cell activation, and fibrogenesis. The current medical philosophy in rheumatology is a combination strategy treating all three processes because this is more likely to control the disease than single-agent therapy.[10] In addition, most patients receive medications to manage associated symptoms such as gastroesophageal reflux disease, Raynaud's phenomenon, and joint inflammation.

Vascular Damage

Treatment of vascular disease is critical to control SSc. The most effective interventions are the calcium channel blockers (nifedipine).[10] Until the 1990s, renal disease was a major cause of death.[21] The risk of renal damage from scleroderma renal crisis has been reduced by early detection, prompt initiation of angiotensin-converting enzyme inhibitor therapy (ACE), and avoidance of high-dose corticosteroids. Short-acting ACE inhibitors (e.g., Captopril) are now used to control blood pressure. If these are not effective, then calcium channel blockers may be initiated.[10] This approach improved the 10-year survival rate from 54% to 66% from 1972 to 2002.[21] Currently, pulmonary fibrosis and pulmonary hypertension are the leading causes of death in SSc.[21] Patients with pulmonary arterial hypertension are treated with endothelin-1 receptor blockers and phosphodiesterase-5 (PDE5) inhibitors.[22,23]

Immune Cell Activation

Cyclophosphamide (Cytoxan) and methotrexate or mycophenolate have been proven to be effective immunosuppressive drugs to treat skin involvement.[10] Autologous stem cell transplantation was shown to increase overall survival in one randomized controlled trial comparing hematopoietic stem cell therapy with month-pulse cyclophosphamide in persons with dSSc.[24] However, patient selection and screening are crucial because of deaths associated with severe cardiac disease.[24] One study examined hand function in five patients who received autologous stem cell transplantation. Over a 12-month period, hand function improved, skin softened, and tenosynovitis resolved.[25] Both hand length (less contracture) and digit abduction improved. In this study, loss of finger abduction was a more sensitive measure of finger clawing than loss of hand length.[25]

Fibrogenesis

New strategies against fibrosis based on advanced understanding of the molecular biology of SSc hold promise. Cyclophosphamide is now recommended for treating severe skin disease and interstitial lung disease in SSc.[26,27]

QUALITY OF LIFE AND HAND FUNCTION

Comprehensive disability outcome assessments of patients with SSc focused attention on the physical and functional limitations that can impair quality of life. Hand dysfunction, such as decreased strength, joint contractures, Raynaud's phenomenon, pain, and digital ulcers, has been shown to be associated with decreased performance and poorer quality of life.[28–31] Therapeutic measures that can minimize patient functional impairment include preventing contractures of small and large joints, softening the skin, relieving joint pain and swelling, strengthening weak muscles, reducing fatigue associated with systemic inflammation, and managing ischemic hand ulcers (see the Associated Hand Conditions section). In particular, the striking effect of hand dysfunction, reflected by reduced ability to make a fist and reduced hand spread, suggests that a major goal of treatment should be to lessen hand dysfunction.[32]

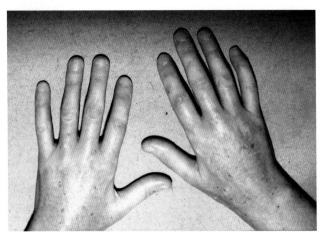

Fig. 92.1 This patient has early-stage systemic scleroderma with diffuse swelling and telangiectasias over the fingers and dorsum of the hand.

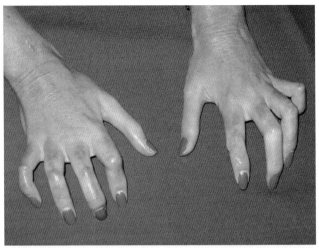

Fig. 92.2 Classic severe hand deformities seen in diffuse cutaneous systemic sclerosis, with loss of metacarpophalangeal joint flexion and proximal interphalangeal (PIP) joint extension. Note the tight skin, pigment changes, and healed ulcers (scars) over the PIP joints of the left middle and fifth fingers.

HAND INVOLVEMENT IN SYSTEMIC SCLEROSIS

Early Signs and Symptoms

In the early stages, patients with lcSSc and dcSSc appear very similar, but with time, patients with dcSSc develop more severe limitations in the hand, and patients with lcSSc often have more limitations distal to the metacarpophalangeal (MCP) joints. Typically, the first symptoms are *swelling* (nonpitting edema) and *tightness* in the hands, feet, and possibly the face. People with lcSSc typically have Raynaud's phenomenon for years before symptoms appear. Those with dcSSc develop Raynaud's phenomenon shortly before or within 1 year of onset of the skin changes.[10]

Initially, some patients have no other symptoms beyond the swelling and feeling of tightness in their fingers (sclerodactyly or acrosclerosis) (Fig. 92.1). Others develop arthralgias or inflammatory arthritis with associated malaise, joint pain, and fatigue.[3,33] In the hand, joint swelling associated with arthritis may be masked by the diffuse edema, especially in dcSSc.[33] The only obvious symptoms may be pain and aching in the joints and limited joint motion. Although the synovitis may be mild, it is a serious problem because it prevents joint motion and increases the risk of contractures. Synovitis may be associated with pulmonary arterial hypertension.[3,34] Some people with dcSSc develop severe hand limitations in a matter of weeks, but others with lcSSc may maintain near-full joint motion for 10 to 20-plus years. Each patient must be assessed and treated individually. Assessments that include measurements of joint motion and questions about changes in hand mobility over the previous 1-month, 6-month, and 1-year periods are helpful for evaluating the progression and disease activity for rehabilitation purposes.[35]

In very mild cases, the skin can be the primary or only tissue involved. In most cases, however, joint limitations result from fibrosis of all the soft tissues: skin, fascia, muscle, tendon, and joint capsule.[3,36] Rheumatologists monitor skin changes in SSc using the Modified Rodnan Skin (thickness) Score (MRSS): 0 = normal skin; 1 = mild; 2 = moderate; 3 = severe thickening.[37] However, in clinical practice, it is helpful to understand the three stages of skin involvement: early, classic, and late.[38,39] In the *edematous stage* (see Fig. 92.1), the hands, feet, and possibly the face are puffy, especially in the morning. This evolves into a taut pitting or nonpitting edema in the fingers, hands, forearms, toes, and feet. The epidermis and epidermal appendages (e.g., hair, nails, and sweat and mammary glands) remain intact. In the *indurative stage* (Fig. 92.2), the edema subsides and is replaced by tight, hidebound skin that feels dry and coarse and often itches. This can happen quickly in dSSc, whereas in lSSc, the induration can occur much more slowly. Areas of hypopigmentation or hyperpigmentation are common. The epidermis becomes shiny, thin, and adherent to the underlying subcutis or hypodermis.[38,39] The skin thickening is less severe in lSSc; however, telangiectasias are much more prominent. Hair disappears or becomes coarser, and sweating is noticeably impaired. These changes are considered diagnostic. The *atrophic stage* occurs several years after the beginning of the classic skin changes. The skin softens and becomes more pliable, but epidermal atrophy and "tethering" of the dermis to underlying tissues occur. Skin may look "normal" but feels taut and adherent. This may be part of a total remission or can occur while other symptoms (e.g., finger ulcers) continue to be active.[38,39]

Deformity Patterns

Diffuse Cutaneous Systemic Sclerosis

The typical deformity seen in the hands of patients with dSSc consists of loss of MCP joint flexion, proximal interphalangeal (PIP) joint extension, distal interphalangeal (DIP) motion, thumb and digit abduction, opposition, flexion, and wrist motion in all planes (see Fig. 92.2).[15,40] About 12% to 65% of people with SSc have joint involvement, swelling, stiffness, and inflamation.[33] Sclerosis of the skin, collateral ligaments, joint capsules, and flexor tendon sheaths results in attenuation of the central slip and palmer displacement of the lateral bands, causing flexion contractures of the PIP joints.[33] MCP joint hyperextension results when patients attempt to compensate for limitations at the PIP joints and contractures develop when there is sclerosis of the soft tissue between the extensor tendons and joint capsules.[33] At the DIP joint, the distal phalanx may be shortened from resorption, or there may be joint erosion or narrowing in the DIP joint.[34] Other biomechanical considerations are tightening of the first webspace in adduction, loss of the palmer arches of the hand, and loss of intrinsic muscle function. These biomechanical changes along with pain resulting from Raynaud's phenomenon, calcium deposits, digital ulcers, or swelling contribute to diminished hand use and muscular guarding.

Consequently, to counteract deforming forces, therapy must focus on preserving MCP joint flexion, thumb carpometacarpal (CMC) abduction, and PIP joint extension. From a functional standpoint, preserving lateral pinch is the most critical goal.

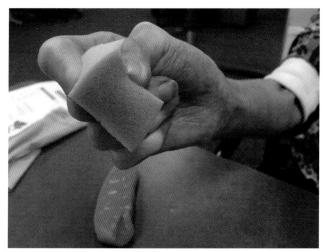

Fig. 92.3 This patient has had diffuse cutaneous systemic sclerosis for 2 years. She can barely pinch and is unable to do a true lateral pinch. Therapy that would increase index metacarpophalangeal joint flexion 15 to 20 degrees would significantly improve her ability for pinch and hand function.

Thumb function represents about 45% of all hand function. As sclerosis progresses, tip-to-tip pinch and then palmar pinch are lost. Lateral pinch, which is the last function lost, is the most important because it is the power pinch. Loss of lateral pinch represents a tremendous loss of hand function, and its restoration either conservatively or surgically should be a prime goal in the treatment of patients with SSc (Fig. 92.3).

Limited Cutaneous Systemic Sclerosis

Patients with lSSc also may have arthralgias. They may maintain full or near-full joint range of motion (ROM) for years with function limited more by ischemic fingertip ulcers, Raynaud's phenomenon, and calcinosis. The most common scenario is that sclerodactyly results in mild to moderate PIP joint flexion and extension contractures and stiff DIP joints in slight flexion.[40] The MCP joints often have good mobility, but PIP joint flexion contractures encourage MCP joint extension, which can result in loss of MCP joint flexion.[40] The primary therapeutic goal is to maintain PIP joint extension and MCP joint flexion and digit span. There is generally very little that can be done for the DIP joints. If therapy time is limited, the focus should be on maintaining MCP joint and thumb function because the PIP and DIP joints are limited more by vascular disease rather than soft tissue restriction. Maintaining thumb abduction is important. Lateral pinch is also important but is usually maintained naturally because MCP joint flexion is present.

Associated Hand Conditions

Raynaud's Phenomenon

Raynaud's phenomenon is defined as an episodic ischemia characterized by blanching (vasospasm), cyanosis, and suffusion or hyperemia erythema as the blood returns. Raynaud's phenomenon occurs in up to 95% of people with SSc and is the first symptom in 70% of patients.[41] Raynaud's phenomenon occurs in the fingers, toes, nose, ears, and tip of the tongue. Raynaud's phenomenon can be caused by vasospastic stimuli such as cold or stress, nicotine, or vasoconstrictive medications, but it may occur without any perceivable trigger. Raynaud's phenomenon in patients with SSc is thought to be caused by an abnormal balance between regulation of vasoconstriction and vasodilation of the cutaneous blood vessels.[42] Patients should use a range of behavioral methods to help control the symptoms of vasospasm (Box 92.2). Pharmacologic management such as calcium channel blockers (nifedipine)

BOX 92.2 Behavioral Methods Patients Can Use to Reduce the Symptoms of Raynaud's Phenomenon

- Avoid nicotine and caffeine.
- Avoid cold temperatures and prepare in advance for exposure to the cold.
- Dress warmly and wear layers of clothing, keeping the core warm to increase the temperature of the arms and legs (e.g., a warm vest such as a fleece vest).
- New lightweight, high-tech fabric clothes and undergarments specifically designed to retain heat are available in camping-goods stores or catalogues.
- Wear hats and scarves outside in the cold to retain body heat.
- Have an emergency kit available (always bring a sweater, mittens or gloves, and a blanket in the car).
- Avoid air conditioning because cold exacerbates Raynaud's phenomenon. Take gloves and sweaters to indoor air-conditioned indoor events.
- Use chemical hand warmers.
- Warm up the car on cold days using an automatic car starter or heated seats or covers and close vents when possible to avoid drafts.
- Insulate hands from strong detergents, irritating chemicals, and bacteria (wear gloves).
- Take care of skin; keep skin moist.
- Avoid carrying bags by the handles and holding objects such as cell phones too tightly, which impairs circulation to the fingers.
- Use an electric blanket or sheet to warm the bed before getting in. If you do not like sleeping with an electric blanket, use it only to prewarm the bed.

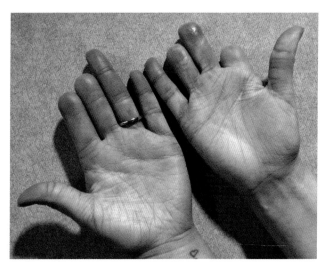

Fig. 92.4 Color changes with Raynaud's phenomenon and amputations from unhealed ulcers.

may be used if nonpharmacological interventions do not work.[43] Complications of Raynaud's phenomenon are irreversible tissue injury and digital ulcers in the fingers and loss of or amputations of the fingers (Fig. 92.4).[42]

Digital Ischemic Ulcers

Digital ischemic ulcers can cause significant pain and inhibit the ability to manipulate objects and perform daily activities.[44] The most common ulcers are *small ulcers over the fingertips or palmar surface,* often the size of a pinhead or smaller. These ulcers are caused by cutaneous ischemia from Raynaud's phenomenon and are very painful.[45] As the ulcer scars in, the ratio of viable tissue to the available blood supply comes into balance, the ulcer appears healed, and the pain stops. Unfortunately, new ulcers tend to appear, and patients usually have several at one time. Furthermore, ulcers can take many months to heal[45] and can lead to complications, including osteomyelitis, digital infarction, tissue loss, and amputations.[45] In hand therapy, digital ischemic ulcers are a major problem because they are painful and limit the patient's ability to exercise, stretch the finger joints, and manipulate objects. Determining the effect of these ulcers on function and the need for specific adaptive measures is therefore part of the hand assessment.[35] The focus of treatment is to improve function by using adaptive equipment and techniques to reduce pain, protect the ulcers during activities, reduce the occurrence of Raynaud's phenomenon, and reduce muscular guarding elicited by the fear of hurting the hands during activities.[35] Specific instructions are provided later in the chapter.

Another type of digital ischemic ulcer occurs over the dorsum of the PIP joints. The PIP joints are vulnerable to trauma and thus prone to these ulcers, because of the flexion contractures that stretch the taut skin over the dorsum of the joint (see Fig. 92.2).[45] Active flexion reduces the blood supply to this area, as evidenced by dorsal blanching during grip and flexion exercises, and impedes wound healing and closure. These ulcers are a result of fibrosis and mechanical pressure as opposed to arterial occlusion or full digital ischemia. In the early stages, the ulcer appears as a demarcated, tender area (see Fig. 92.2). The ulcer may remain like this for a long time or develop an open, necrotic center. Some ulcers stay open; others develop thick scabs.

Ulcers can also occur on the sides of the hand or ends of the fingers as a result of a more generalized ischemia to the digit secondary to Raynaud's phenomenon, fibrosis, or thrombosis of the digital arteries. Fortunately, these are less common than the first two types of ulcers. These ulcers can progress to gangrene. Often, the digit is allowed to auto amputate to preserve the maximal amount of digit length possible; otherwise, surgical amputation may be indicated.[46]

Nonpharmacologic interventions were reviewed by Moran[47] and are discussed later in this chapter. However, pharmacologic interventions have been shown to be effective in preventing and healing of digital ischemic ulcers. These medications prevent vascular spasm and induce vasodilation such as calcium channel blockers and PDE5 inhibitors (sildenafil, tadalafil, bosentan, and intravenous prostacyclins).[4] Some medications may cause serious cardiac, GI, and psychological side effects, and many patients cannot tolerate them. Some people need to take the medications only in the winter season.

For all open ulcers, meticulous wound and skin care is important. This includes keeping the wound clean and moist, using antibacterial soap, avoiding exposure to dirt, and using antibiotic ointment as prescribed. These patients are vulnerable to developing staphylococcal infections and can quickly progress to osteomyelitis. All patients should be taught to recognize the signs of infection and promptly report them to their health professionals.

Telangiectasias

Telangiectasias are lesions formed by dilated capillaries that appear as dark red spots in the skin or just beneath the surface (see Fig. 92.1). They are commonly found in the face and hands and generally are not painful. However, those on the fingerpads may be tender to touch and need the same protection as palmar ulcers.

Calcium Deposits

Accumulation of calcium salts (*calcinosis cutis*) under the skin is a common symptom of SSc. Calcinosis is found in about 15% of patients with dcSSc and 25% of patients with lcSSc.[48] In the hand, subcutaneous deposits tend to be localized (*circumscripta*) and may feel like a pebble or stone under the skin (Fig. 92.5). In the upper extremity, deposits

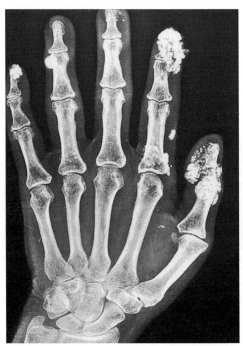

Fig. 92.5 Radiograph showing calcium deposits (calcinosis) in a patient with systemic scleroderma.

tend to occur over functional pressure areas such as the volar aspect of the thumb interphalangeal (IP) joint, heel of the hand, lateral surface of the index finger, medial aspect of the palm or ulna, and the elbow.[49] Calcium deposits in the hands and fingers results in sensitivity of the overlying skin and subcutaneous tissues with pressure and can significantly impair function.

The skin can break down over the deposits, allowing white chalky calcium to extrude. The breakdown can lead to ulcers, infection, and decreased function. Patients often mistake the calcium for pus. Unless there are obvious signs of infection, such as heat, redness, pain, or thick green-yellow discharge, this is a noninfectious process. However, any skin breakdown should be cleaned three times a day with a bactericidal agent and kept protected and clean. Treatment for Raynaud's phenomenon and digital ulcers is important in the prevention of calcinosis.[48] Corticosteroid injections may decrease the inflammation.[48] Medical and nonmedical interventions are reviewed and summarized by Valenzuela and Chung.[48]

Particularly troublesome deposits can be surgically removed, but because they recur frequently, this is done only in selected cases. Therapy includes placing pressure-relieving, doughnut-type pads over the deposit or padding equipment and utensils to reduce pressure over the deposit.[45]

Resorption

Resorption of the distal tuft of the distal phalanx (acro-osteolysis) occurs in 20% to 25% of patients with SSc.[4] The result is shortening of the digit, with the tip becoming sharpened.[3,50] Depending on the severity, overall shortening of the finger(s) can occur (Fig. 92.6). Resorption is detected by comparing digit length between both hands. The cause is not known but could be because of ischemic digital ischemia or retractile pressure from thickened skin.[3]

Tendon Friction Rubs

Tendon friction rubs are a form of crepitation noticed with passive or active motion of a joint.[36] Assessment consists of palpation of the tendon during passive or active joint motion and is positive

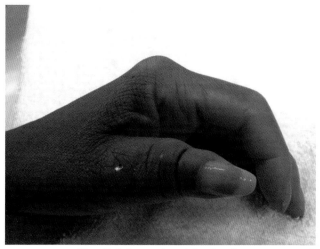

Fig. 92.6 Resorption of the thumb.

BOX 92.3 Hand Therapy Goals

- Every effort must be made to preserve hand function.
- Loss of hand function is the most limiting factor when performing ADLs and is what reminds patients most of their disease.
- Maintain wrist and forearm motion for participation in ADLs.
- Maintain motion in the hand.
- Prevent loss of MCP joint flexion.
- Prevent loss of PIP joint extension.
- Prevent loss of digit abduction, with emphasis on the thumb CMC joint.
- Maintain lateral pinch.
- Mobilize the skin in all directions.
- Manage Raynaud's phenomenon.
- Encourage engagement in ADLs.

ADL, Activity of daily living; *CMC,* carpometacarpal; *MCP,* metacarpophalangeal; *PIP,* proximal interphalangeal.

---

if a leathery, rubbing, or crepitus sensation is noted.[51] TFRs result from fibrinous deposits within the tendon sheaths and overlying fascia[36] and often occur in the flexor and extensor tendons of the fingers but are also common over tendons of the wrists, elbows, knees, and ankles. TFRs are highly associated with the dcSSc subtype, more severe skin thickening, joint contractures, and organ involvement, particularly of the heart, kidneys, and GI systems.[52] They are often noticeable with motion and may or may not be painful. Treatment usually consists of nonsteroidal antiinflammatory drugs or low-dose corticosteroids.[36,52]

HAND REHABILITATION

Philosophy and Approach

Hand rehabilitation should start as soon as a patient is diagnosed with SSc, and patients should be referred *before* there is any apparent loss of motion or functional deficit because early intervention is the key to improved outcomes. Emphasis should be placed on self-management and self-monitoring strategies. The overall goals of hand therapy are to improve hand function and quality of life. (See Box 92.3 for hand therapy goals.) General guidelines to follow are listed below.

- Intervention and home programs should focus on improving joint motion, decreasing soft tissue tightness of the extrinsic and intrinsic muscles of the hand, and mobilizing the skin.

- Teach patients how to perform their exercises independently and how to regularly monitor their own joint motion to evaluate whether the exercises are preventing loss of motion.
- Patients need to recognize that significant time must be devoted to performing their home program as long as their disease is active.
- Instruct patients in skin care and inspection with aggressive attention and intervention to prevent digital ulcers that might lead to permanent loss of joint motion.

Specific goals are to:
1. Maintain wrist and forearm motion.
2. Maintain motion in the hand.
    a. Prevent loss of MCP joint flexion.
    b. Prevent loss of PIP joint extension.
    c. Prevent loss of digit abduction, with emphasis on the thumb CMC joint.
3. Maintain lateral pinch.
4. Mobilize the skin in all directions.
5. Manage Raynaud's phenomenon.
6. Encourage engagement in activities of daily living (ADLs).

Even with early intervention and prevention strategies, it is often not possible to prevent all deformities. Deformities occur when there is active disease and fibrosis that cannot be controlled with pharmacologic treatment. Pain, illness, and ulcers that prevent adequate ability to perform ROM exercises also contribute to the likelihood of deformities developing over time.

In general, studies examining the effectiveness of current rehabilitation techniques, including paraffin, stretching, massage, joint mobilization, strengthening, and orthotics, show positive results. However, these studies are few in number and have small sample sizes, and some have flaws in study design. For reviews, see Mouthon and Poole,[5] Poole,[53] and Willems and associates.[54]

ASSESSMENT

Range of Motion

Goniometric measurements should be performed to evaluate active and passive ROM at the initiation of therapy to obtain accurate baseline data and repeated at regular intervals as long as the disease is active. Measurements should be performed and recorded in accordance with the American Society of Hand Therapists' (ASHT's) Clinical Assessment Recommendations.[55]

Patients should be shown how to monitor their own joint motion. The fingertip to proximal palmar crease distance can be recorded in centimeters both in the clinic and as part of home monitoring. Hand tracings on paper can be made in the clinic and are an effective method for patients to use to self-monitor loss of IP extension and loss of abduction of the digits, including abduction and extension of the thumb (Fig. 92.7). For thumb abduction and to stretch the webspace, patients can find the largest cylindrical object (e.g., a water bottle, soup can, spice jar, tomato paste can) that will fit tightly in the webspace without a gap (Fig. 92.8). To monitor MCP joint flexion, patients can place an index card with the angle cut out over the MCP joints when making a composite fist (Fig. 92.9). Using a smartphone for pictures of the hands is also an excellent way to document change.

Although goniometry is the gold standard to measure joint motion, there are other assessments that evaluate functional joint motion and have been found to be reliable and valid in persons with SSc: the Hand Mobility in Scleroderma (HAMIS) Test, the Hand Function Index (HFI), and the Kapandji Index (see Chapter 88; also see Mouthon and Poole[5] for a review and description of the assessments). The HAMIS was developed specifically for persons with SSc.[56,57] The assessment includes nine items: finger flexion, extension, and abduction; thumb abduction; pincer grip; wrist flexion and extension; and forearm

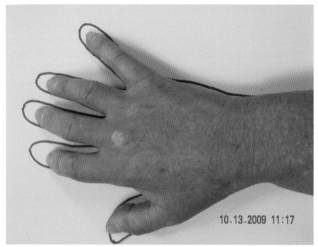

Fig. 92.7 Tracing outline of hand to document thumb and digit abduction. This is a helpful self-monitoring tool for both home and clinic.

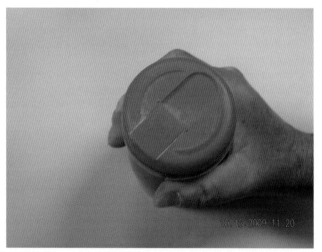

Fig. 92.8 Placing the largest cylindrical object that will fit tightly into the webspace without a gap can be used to both stretch and monitor thumb web span and abduction.

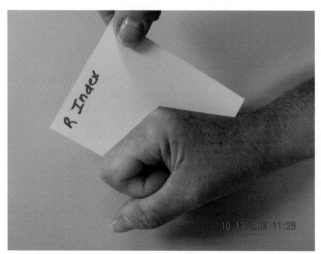

Fig. 92.9 Self-assessment of range of motion is easier using a template with the desired amount of degrees cut out. The template can be made out of cardboard or thermoplastic scraps.

pronation and supination.[56,57] Items are scored from 0 (can perform item fully) to 3 (cannot do item). A modified version of the HAMIS, the mHAMIS, consists of 4 of the 9 items: finger flexion, finger extension, finger abduction, and dorsal extension.[58]

Strength

Grip and pinch strength should also be assessed at baseline and at regular intervals to help monitor any functional loss and highlight the need for modifications to the treatment plan. Grip strength should be measured with the Jamar Dynamometer. The second handle position should be used and the procedure should follow the guidelines in the ASHT Clinical Assessment Recommendations.[59] A pinch gauge is the most common tool used to measure maximal isometric strength of lateral, tip, and three-point or tripod pinch. The procedure should follow the ASHT Clinical Assessment Recommendations.[59]

Coordination, Dexterity, and Hand Function

Coordination can be assessed with the 9-Hole Peg Test[60] at the initiation of treatment and again at regular intervals. Fibrosis of the skin results in loss of excursion of both the intrinsic and extrinsic muscles of the hand contributing to a loss of overall mobility of the hand. Observing the patient perform various functional hand tasks that tend to be limited by SSc will aid in the development of the treatment plan. Examples include using different prehension patterns and performing dexterity tasks such as picking up coins from a table, manipulating the coins without dropping them, holding tools and utensils for feeding and grooming, and manipulating fasteners on clothes.

The Arthritis Hand Function Test (AHFT), an 11-item performance based test designed to measure grip and pinch strength and dexterity, has been shown to be valid in people with SSc.[61] The dexterity items include the 9-Hole Peg Test, applied dexterity tasks (buttoning, handling coins, opening/closing safety pins, tying a shoe, cutting putty), and applied strength tasks (pouring water, lifting a tray of cans).

Self-Care and Activities of Daily Living

Participation in ADLs may be compromised when there are contractures, calcinosis, digital ulcers, or extensive cardiopulmonary or GI systemic involvement. Self-reports of ability and hand function during ADL performance, which have been shown to be reliable and valid in persons with scleroderma, are listed below.

- The Michigan Hand Questionnaire (MHQ) is a 37-item self-report with six subscales: overall hand function, ADLs, pain, work performance, aesthetics, and patient satisfaction with hand function.[62] Items are scored on a 5-point Likert scale from 1 (very good, not at all difficult, always, very mild, and very satisfied) to 5 (very poor, very difficult, never, severe, and very dissatisfied). Raw scores are converted to a scale from 0 to 100 according to a scoring algorithm.
- The Scleroderma Health Assessment Questionnaire (SHAQ) consists of the eight categories on the HAQ: dressing and grooming, eating, rising, walking, hygiene, reach, grip, and outside activity.[63] Items are scored form 0 (no difficulty) to 3 (unable to do). The SHAQ also includes visual analog scales (VASs) for pain, patient global assessment, vascular, digital ulcers, lung involvement, and GI involvement.
- The Cochin Hand Function Scale (CHFS) (also known as the Duruoz Hand Index) is a self-report of hand function, containing 18 items related to daily activities (kitchen, dressing, hygiene, office, and other).[64,65] Items are scored on a scale from 0 (no difficulty) to 5 (impossible to do).
- The McMaster-Toronto Arthritis Patient Preference Disability Questionnaire (MACTAR) covers broad areas such as domestic care, self-care, professional activities, leisure activities, social interaction, and roles.[65,66] Patients identify 10 activities they have difficulties with

BOX 92.4   Resources for Patients and Clinicians

Institutional Names and Addresses

1. Scleroderma Foundation
300 Rosewood Drive, Suite 105, Danvers, MA 01923 (800-722-HOPE)
www.scleroderma.org
The Scleroderma Foundation has brochures and educational materials for patients, caregivers, and health professionals. There is also information regarding support groups, discussion boards, and the annual conferences. Downloadable Brochure: Stretching Exercises for the Hand and Face , 2019 by Janet L. Poole https://www.scleroderma.org/site/DocServer/Form_16c_low_res.pdf?docID=19809&AddInterest=1281 Video version: http://www.youtube.com/sclerodermaUS

2. The Scleroderma Research Foundation
220 Montgomery Street, Suite 484, San Francisco, CA 94104 (800-441-CURE)
www.srfcure.org
The Scleroderma Research Foundation has information for patients and health professionals and information about research trials. The foundation sponsors free webinar series

3. International Scleroderma Network
7455 France Avenue South, No. 266, Edina, MN 55435-4702 (800-564-7099; direct line, 952-831-30913)
https://sclero.org/
Educational information on caregiving, disability, medications, equipment, Medicare, and medical services.

4. The Arthritis Foundation
1355 Peachtree St NE, Suite 600, Atlanta, GA 30309 (800-283-7800)
www.arthritis.org
Free consumer education booklets on systemic scleroderma, self-management methods and medications, and information about treatment resources.

5. The Arthritis Society (National Office)
41 King William St., Suite 203, Hamilton, Ontario L8R 1A2, Canada (866-279-0632)
www.scleroderma.ca/
Email: info@scleroderma.ca/
Offers specialized patient care programs, consumer education materials, and an annual conference.

6. Scleroderma & Raynaud's UK (SRUK) Society (United Kingdom)
18-20 Bride Lane, London, UK (+020-7000-1925)
www.sruk.co.uk/scleroderma
E-mail: info@sruk.co.uk
Offers educational and resources for patients and families.

7. Sjögren's Syndrome Foundation 6707 Democracy Boulevard, Suite 325, Bethesda, MD 20817 (800-475-6473)
www.sjorgens.org

Books for Patients from Amazon.com
The First Year: Scleroderma: An Essential Guide for the Newly Diagnosed (The First Year Series), 2004, by Karen Gottesman and Daniel E. Furst.
If You Have to Wear an Ugly Dress, Learn to Accessorize: Guidance, Inspiration, and Hope for Women with Lupus, Scleroderma, and Other Autoimmune Illnesses, 2013, by Linda McNamara and Karen Kemper
Scleroderma Coping Strategies, 2011, by B. Bianca Podesta
Internet Self-management Program: Taking Charge of Systemic Sclerosis (TOSS) https://www.selfmanagescleroderma.com.

Adaptive Equipment and Clothing Resources
Damart Catalogue (thermal undergarments)
See international website: www.damartusa.com

Adapted from Melvin JL: Scleroderma (Systemic Sclerosis): Treatment of the Hand. In: Skirven TM, Osterman AL, Fedorczyk JM, Amadio PM (eds). *Rehabilitation of the Hand and Upper Extremity.* 6th ed, Philadelphia: Elsevier; 2011:1434-1448.

and then rank the activities from 1 (most important) to 10 (least important). Each item is also rated on the degree of difficulty in performing the activity from 0 (not difficult) to 10 (very difficult).

- The QuickDASH (Disability of the Arm, Shoulder and Hand)[67] and Patient Rated Wrist Hand Evaluation (PRWE)[68] can be completed in the hand clinic at initial assessment, and at regular intervals. However, only the DASH has been shown to be valid with SSc.[69]

Skin

- Note the presence of Raynaud's phenomenon and any color changes in the skin, including biphasic color changes and blanching. Ask the patient to indicate the triggers for Raynaud's phenomenon and what the patient does to prevent occurrences of Raynaud's phenomenon.
- Pictures are beneficial to document areas of skin thickening; the presence calcium deposits; and evidence of any open, closed, or old healed ulcers.
- Edema of the wrist, distal palmar crease, and proximal phalanx of the digits can be assessed with a volumeter or with circumferential measurements in centimeters. Observe the hands and forearms for loss of skin mobility with absence of wrist and digit creases.
- Fingerprints may also disappear with the tightening of the skin decreasing the ability to pick up and manipulate small objects.
- Severity of skin thickening is assessed with the Modified Rodnan Skin Score.[37] Skin areas are graded on a scale from 0 to 3, with 0 indicating no involvement, 1 indicating mild, 2 indicating moderate, and 3 indicating severe thickening. This is usually performed by the rheumatologist.

Pain

- Pain can be assessed using a self-report numeric reporting 10-point scale, a VAS, or with the Faces Pain Scale.[70]
- The 10-point Pain VAS from the HAQ can be used to evaluate pain and is reliable and valid in persons with SSc.[63]
- The Brief Pain Inventory (BPI) is a standardized pain inventory that evaluates pain across different time frames and includes a pain related interference subscale applicable to chronic musculoskeletal conditions.[71]
- The McGill Pain Questionnaire (Short Form) can also be used in SSc and has been shown to be valid.[72]

INTERVENTIONS

When a therapist first encounters a patient with SSc, the current musculoskeletal condition guides the approach of the treatment intervention for either prevention or early- or late-stage contracture rehabilitation.

Education

Education should begin upon initial presentation and referral to therapy. Patients must be educated regarding the disease characteristics, how changes in the skin are related to the underlying anatomy, how to live with a chronic autoimmune disease, and the importance of advocating for oneself in the management of a rare chronic disease. Gauging level of acceptance of the disease and pain and fatigue levels can play an important role in the ability of the individual to participate in self-management strategies. (See Box 92.4 for resources for patients and clinicians.)

Pain

Raynaud's phenomenon is one of the most common symptoms of SSc and often the first to be exhibited. Patients should be instructed in the self-management techniques listed next to decrease triggers because it is temperature change, rather than the cold itself, that is likely to trigger a Raynaud's phenomenon episode.[73] Box 92.2 and the website from the Raynaud's and Scleroderma Association (http://www.raynauds.org.uk/component/content/article/138) provide other helpful hints on Raynaud's phenomenon and managing digital ulcers.

Thermal biofeedback has been recommended for patients with Raynaud's phenomenon, but a systematic review of complementary and alternative medicine for Raynaud's phenomenon found that biofeedback was no better than sham biofeedback.[74] Since that review, a recent study comparing biofeedback, deep oscillation, and no treatment found that biofeedback resulted in a significant improvement of Raynaud's phenomenon compared with control patients, whereas deep oscillations reached significance. However, the sample size was very small, and the two interventions were not compared with each other.[75]

Range of Motion

When possible, ROM and stretching should be initiated before any visible deformity appears. As previously stated, careful attention should be paid to maintaining MCP joint flexion, IP joint extension, thumb and digit abduction, lateral pinch, and active and passive motion of the wrist. Although deformities may not be completely preventable, the goals are to minimize the occurrence and delay the development of contractures for as long as possible. Because stretching programs are a major component of management of the hands in persons with SSc, specific stretching exercises for both early- and late-stage contractures are discussed in a separate section later in this chapter.

Skin Management

Proactively monitoring the skin for changes in thickness, color, and ulcers is imperative for maintaining skin mobility. Signs that the skin is becoming tighter include blanching or darkening of the skin or increasing redness over the joints.[39] Skin should be inspected daily, and when digital ulcers become visible, appropriate treatment must be initiated. Ulcers are extremely painful and can lead to permanent joint contractures if not dealt with on a timely basis. Small silicone digit pads can be used over the IP joints for protection and comfort when needed.

Applying techniques such as myofascial release, manual edema massage,[76] and negative-pressure therapy[77] can assist in maintaining skin mobility, decrease swelling, soften the skin texture, and relieve pain. Studies have shown that manual edema massage is effective in the early edematous phase of SSc and that connective tissue massage in conjunction with joint mobilization and hand exercises did improve fist closure and hand function.[78]

Strength

Signs of decreasing strength may be dropping objects or difficulty opening jars and containers of various sizes and shapes. Lifting and carrying may also be affected because of the overall level of fatigue associated with SSc. It is important that patients move their extremities throughout the available range against resistance to remain strong. This can be accomplished through exercises and many household tasks such as when pulling clothes out of a washer, cleaning mirrors or counters, or doing yardwork.

Coordination

Manipulating small objects with individual fingers and the thumb is something most people take for granted, but this simple activity can be very difficult when the intrinsic muscles of the hand are tight. It is important to prevent adduction tightness and to maintain webspaces

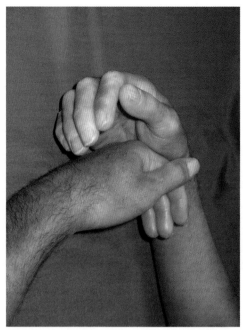

Fig. 92.10 The heel of the hand can push down on the proximal phalanges of the other hand to stretch metacarpophalangeal joints into flexion.

between the digits. Lacing the finger together is a way patients can monitor webspace tightness. Manipulating small objects in the hands can also help maintain dexterity.

Activities of Daily Living

Daily participation in ADLs is crucial to maintain hand function as well as monitor any gradual loss of impairment. Having difficulty grasping utensils or pulling tickets from a parking machine or dropping change should be recognized as signs that joint motion and strength are declining. This is a red flag indicating that the patient needs to emphasize or return to performing exercises to halt the loss of hand function that could further compromise ADL participation.

Strategies for Management of Early- and Late-Stage Contractures

Intervention for contractures is dependent on the disease severity and whether the contractures are recently occurring or longstanding. Intervention for early stage contractures focuses on stretching to prevent any further loss of motion, whereas intervention for late-stage contractures emphasizes preserving joint mobility for gross grasp and pinch and using assistive devices. The next section describes specific strategies to manage both early- and late-state contractures.

Early-Stage Contractures

In SSc, losses in motion can be gradual. Patients may not recognize immediately that ROM has been compromised. In fact, we recommend that stretching exercises commence before any noticeable tightness or beginning contractures are observed. A thorough, individualized stretching program must be designed, and stretching exercises should be done to achieve full passive joint motion to all involved joints.

Helpful Hints

- Use heat to warm up tissues before performing stretching exercises, particularly hand stretches.
- Ensure that the stretching program focuses on these motions: flexion of the MCP joints to counteract tightening of the skin on the dorsum of the hand (Fig. 92.10), extension of the PIP and DIP (Fig. 92.11),

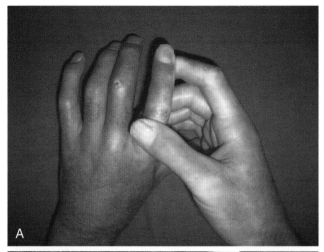

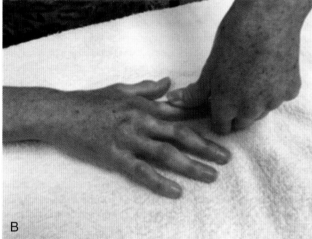

Fig. 92.11 A and **B,** The proximal interphalangeal (PIP) joints can be stretched by stabilizing the metacarpophalangeal joints and extending the PIP joint.

joints, abduction of the thumb (see Fig. 92.8) and digits (Fig. 92.12), and flexion and extension of the wrists (Figs. 92.13 and 92.14).

- Exercises should be performed once or twice a day. Each exercise should held for 5 to 10 seconds and repeated 5 to 10 times depending on tightness.
- Use objective ROM measures to monitor joint motion on a weekly basis as long as disease is active. Telemonitoring may be a promising way to monitor home programs.[79]

Teaching effective stretching programs must be individualized and can be time consuming. Many patients who already have contractures may have difficulty holding or positioning the joints of the opposite hand to achieve the needed passive stretch. In addition, pain and the presence of digital ulcers may limit tolerance to passive stretch.

Passive stretching should be followed with active digit and wrist ROM exercises and functional activities to maximize the effects from stretching. Tendon-gliding and -blocking exercises can be performed with an emphasis on involved joints. Putty exercises are an effective modality for strengthening the extrinsic and intrinsic muscles of the hand and can also be used for resistance to add a passive stretch to the IP joints and hand.

Using a variety of functional activities such as practicing opening and closing various sized containers with different types of closures (e.g., jars, packages, zip lock bags), working on pinch with foam cubes, grasping and releasing large beans or cubes for composite grasp, and adapting tools and utensils with cylindrical foam for improved performance with ADLs should be part of daily treatment intervention. Working on patient-identified goals combined with stretching exercises was shown to improve hand function.[80]

Late-Stage Contractures

Factors that contribute to the development of deformities are active and aggressive disease, late referral to therapy, lack of financial resources, lack of availability of experienced clinicians, pain, ulcers that prevent ROM, and severity of organ involvement.

Passive stretching to the digits and wrist is still indicated, especially on the less affected joints, to prevent further loss of motion and to maintain

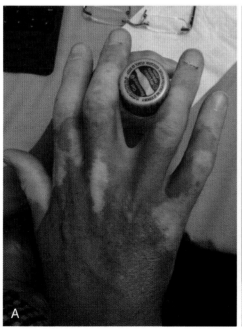

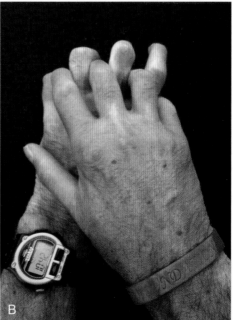

Fig. 92.12 A, Wedging the top of a bottle between the fingers provides an effective stretch of the webspace. It is well tolerated and can be done innocuously. **B,** Clasping the hands deeply is an easy, effective way to stretch the webspaces. It is well tolerated and cannot hurt the skin. This also can be done in warm water.

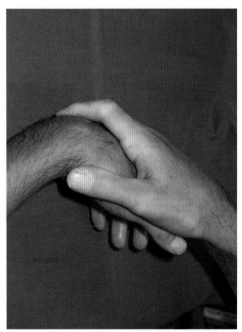

Fig. 92.13 For wrist flexion, the patient can flex the wrist for active motion and then gently push on the dorsum of the hand for a passive wrist flexion stretch. (Courtesy of The Scleroderma Foundation. Stretching exercises for the hand and face. http://www.scleroderma.org/site/DocServer/Form_16c_low_res.pdf?docID=19809&AddInterest=1281.)

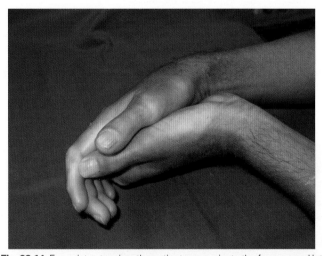

Fig. 92.14 For wrist extension, the patient can supinate the forearm and let the wrist extend actively. Then the palm of one hand can be used to press on the palm of the other hand for a passive stretch for wrist extension.

mobility for gross grasp and lateral pinch needed for ADLs. Patients should be taught to use adaptive techniques and assistive devices. Learning to grasp between the palms of both hands or supporting a weight on the forearms improves lifting and carrying of larger objects. Adaptive equipment, such as cylindrical foam on utensils and tools, button hooks, zipper pulls, jar and bottle openers, and elastic shoelaces, makes grasp and manipulation tasks less frustrating. Every effort should be made toward maintaining ADL independence and engagement in meaningful activity.[80]

Specific Exercises for Both Early- and Late-Stage Contractures

The importance of daily home exercises for the upper extremities, with an emphasis on the hands, must be stressed. As stated earlier, loss of motion can be gradual and go unnoticed by the patient until there is significant and irreversible loss of motion. Pictures of the hands in different positions, which can be replicated over time, are an excellent way to monitor motion improvement or loss. The goal is for the patient to be able to perform the exercises independently. Working with patients to develop the best technique to get the most from the exercises requires experimenting with different holding patterns because there is usually bilateral hand involvement. It is often helpful to instruct a family member or friend to assist with the exercises if the patient has difficulty. Compliance with the daily home exercise program will have the greatest effect on long-term outcome. Exercises may be uncomfortable, but it is essential to achieve maximum range in all motions. Changes in skin color such as blanching or increased redness are expected while patients are performing the exercises. See Mouthon and Poole,[5] Poole,[53] and Willems and coworkers[54] for reviews of evidence to support hand exercises and stretching in people with SSc.

Passive Exercises

Sustained passive ROM exercises should be performed to all joints in all planes of motion to maintain mobility. As stated earlier, emphasis should be placed on the thumb webspace and lateral pinch, MCP joint flexion, PIP joint extension, and abduction of the digits; wrist flexion and extension; radial and ulnar deviation; circumduction; and forearm supination and pronation. The therapist should work with the patient to identify key exercises that *must* be performed, especially if multiple joints in the upper extremities are involved.

Usually doing 5 to 10 repetitions, and holding each stretch for 5 and 10 seconds can be tolerated initially and increased gradually to patient tolerance. For some patients, it is more beneficial to do fewer repetitions of exercise throughout the day than attempting to perform too many at one time, which may exacerbate pain. The goal is to reduce stiffness throughout the day for successful participation in ADLs.

Active Exercises

Tendon-gliding exercises help to maintain tendon excursion and joint mobility. Prevention of PIP joint contractures is dependent on facilitating gliding of the dorsal hood, lumbrical muscles, lateral bands, and central slip. Blocking and reverse blocking exercises can be effective in targeting specific PIP joint limitations to prevent tightness of the collateral ligaments that are at risk. Digit abduction is crucial to maintain webspaces and prevent tightening of the MCP joint capsule and collateral ligaments. Finger adduction and abduction exercises help to reduce swelling by stimulating the muscle pump action around the MCP joints. Exercise putty can be used for many self-stretching activities. Flattening the hand on the table with the added resistance of the putty along with additional assist from opposite hand can facilitate IP joint extension, decrease intrinsic tightness, and maintain the width and length of the hand. Rolling putty from the wrist to fingertips helps to stretch the palm and extend the digits (Fig. 92.15), which will allow patients to don gloves and place their hands in their pockets. Composite grasp will prevent MCP joint hyperextension and facilitate ability to touch the fingertips to the palm for holding and manipulation of tools, utensils, and small objects.

Putty can be used to maintain lateral pinch by using a long, rolled piece between the thumb and index digit as if holding a key and squeezing repeatedly the length of the putty. Mobilization of the lumbricals and dorsal expansion can be performed by looping putty or a rubber band over the middle phalanges in an intrinsic-plus position (MCP joints flexed and IP joints straight) and spreading the fingers apart (Fig. 92.16)

Foam cubes can be used to maintain lateral pinch, mobilize the hand, and facilitate grasp for self-care activities. Exercises using a gyro ball, flex

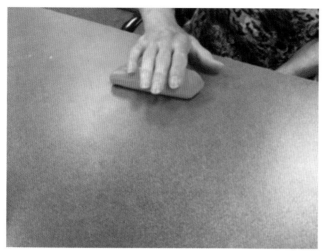

Fig. 92.15 Rolling putty from the wrist to the fingertips helps to stretch the palm and extend the digits.

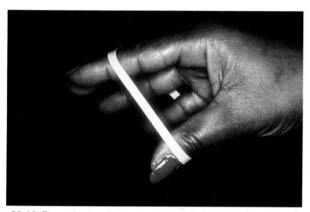

Fig. 92.16 For patients with severe, classic limitations, this rubber band exercise is useful for strengthening and mobilizing the extensor communis and thumb abductor muscles.

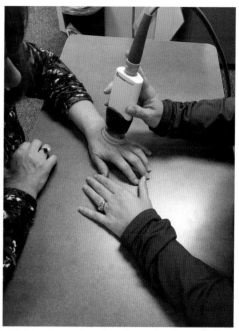

Fig. 92.17 Lymphatouch to the skin on the dorsum of the hand.

bar, wrist roller, Velcro board, and hammer are examples of active activities that patients can use to facilitate and improve these motions. Wrist exercises should include flexion and extension (see Figs. 92.13 and 92.14),

Modalities

Thermal modalities should be included as part of the intervention plan during all phases of treatment. Microvascular destruction of circulatory vessels is responsible for compromised circulation and should not be exacerbated. Thus, precautions must be observed before application of any thermal modalities because 90% of patients have presence of Raynaud's phenomenon[12,41] or temperature sensitivity. Cold must be avoided secondary to the adverse effects on the circulation.

Paraffin wax has been effective, along with stretching exercises, in improving hand motion in patients with SSc.[5,53,54] The moist heat provides warmth to increase tissue extensibility before passive stretching, decreases pain, and adds needed moisture to the skin. Temperature should be between 120°F and 130°F and tested regularly with a candy or meat thermometer because most paraffin units do not have an external temperature gauge. The amount of dips will vary with patient tolerance; dips can be as few as three or as many as eight. The wax should be left on for a period of 15 to 20 minutes for maximum effectiveness. Home paraffin units are easily purchased in stores and online.

If there are any digital ulcers, paraffin may still be used by donning examination gloves and taping closed at the wrists before dipping in the wax.

Commercially available heated mitts, hot packs, and heating pads may also be used if there are enough protective layers between the heat source and the skin; the heat can be applied for a maximum of 20 minutes. If swelling is present, heat should be applied with the extremity in elevation.[81]

The Lymphatouch (previously known as PhysioTouch) is a device designed to mobilize fibrotic tissue and improve tissue health by providing three-dimensional fascial release, changing the collagen matrix.[82] The Lymphatouch's negative-pressure lift of the dermis or collagen provides selective stimulation to mechanoreceptors (Fig. 92.17). Benefits include improved lymphatic flow, decreased inflammation, and reduced pain.[77] More information can be found at https://www.youtube.com/user/lymphatouch.

Orthotic Intervention and Scleroderma

With many rheumatic diseases, custom-fabricated orthoses may be included as part of the intervention plan to prevent deformities, provide support, or rest joints. Current evidence for the use of hand orthoses for patients with scleroderma is lacking.[33,53,83] A 1987 study of the efficacy of a dynamic orthosis in reducing PIP joint contractures in patients with SSc found that only 8 of the 19 participants completed the study and that in the participants who dropped out, the orthosis exacerbated symptoms such as Raynaud's phenomenon. In the 8 participants who completed the study, PIP joint extension extension did not improve.[84] It is important to note that orthotic interventions and designs (e.g., serial static or static progressive orthoses) for contracture correction have advanced since 1987, but there are no reported studies assessing their efficacy for patients with SSc. A recent study included static and dynamic orthoses as part of a comprehensive intervention.[85] However, while the study did not report any increases in digital ulcers from the orthoses, the actual effectiveness of the orthoses could not be determined.[85] Clinical experience by one of the authors (CD) suggests that fibrotic tissue is resistant to orthotic intervention. If a therapist decides to use a static or static progressive orthosis to increase joint motion, the patient's hand must be carefully monitored for compromised vascularity (Fig. 92.18).

Orthotic intervention for comfort and protection for patients with SSc with hand involvement is clearly indicated. Microvascular destruction of circulatory vessels is responsible for compromised circulation and should not be exacerbated. Trauma to ulcers on the PIP joint or pressure to ulcers on the fingertips can be excruciatingly

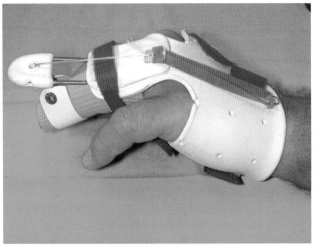

Fig. 92.18 Dynamic proximal interphalangeal joint extension orthosis.

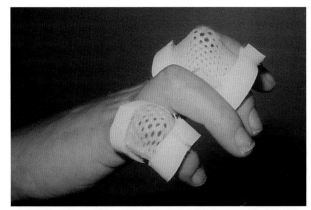

Fig. 92.20 These proximal interphalangeal (PIP) joint cylinder orthoses are bivalved and "bubbled" over dorsal PIP joint ulcers. The goals of this orthosis are to immobilize the PIP joint and protect against trauma to encourage dorsal PIP joint ulcers to heal. These orthoses can dramatically improve function by allowing the patient to use the hands without fear of injury. They are made from $\frac{1}{16}$-inch perforated Aquaplast.

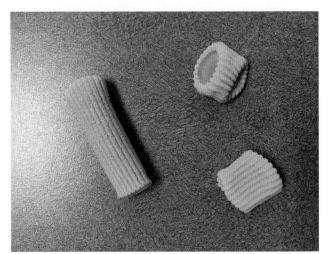

Fig. 92.19 Silipos antibacterial digit pads and digital caps can be worn over the proximal interphalangeal joints to cushion and over the fingertips for protection.

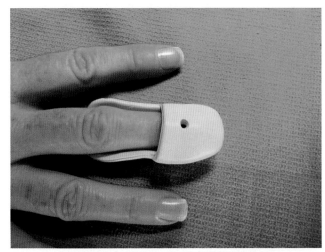

Fig. 92.21 Protective orthosis for digital ulcer.

painful. Without protection of ulcers, patients are reluctant to use their hands and digits, which can further compromise functional ROM and strength.

Silipos antibacterial digit pads and digital caps can be worn over the PIP joints to cushion and over the fingertips for protection. These pads contain an antimicrobial and are latex free and hypoallergenic, and the mineral oil in the pads helps to moisturize the skin (Fig. 92.19). (See https://www.silipos.com/products/antibacterial-digital-pads.)

If patients need greater protection over the dorsal PIP joints or fingertips, custom thermoplastic PIP orthoses and digit-tip protectors can be fabricated by the therapist (Figs. 92.20 and 92.21). Examples include low-temperature protective orthoses; protective padding (e.g., self-adherent foam or gauze wrap, e.g. Mepilex, AG Coban [3M, St. Paul, MN], neoprene sleeves, gloves with only the essential finger sleeves, i.e., with the others cut off) over the ulcer, if possible; and adaptive padding of equipment and handles. When there are diffuse, multiple ulcers, wearing thin cotton laboratory gloves can help protect the hands and keep them warm.

SURGERY

In general, surgery may be indicated for pain, ulcers, severe contractures. or circulation issues.[33,86,87] The PIP joint may be fused in a position of optimal function; however, wound healing is a concern because of the compromised vascular system.[33,86] Digital sympathectomy involving removing the adventitia (outer covering of the digital arteries) has been somewhat successful in optimizing circulation in a digit.[33,42] A detailed discussion of surgery for the hand in patients with SSc is given in Chapter 91.

SUMMARY

Systemic sclerosis is an autoimmune connective tissue disease that results in severe deformities in the hands. The contractures along with digital ulcers, Raynaud's phenomenon, and calcium deposits compromise hand function needed to participate in meaningful occupations. Patients should be referred to hand therapy upon initial diagnosis. Exercises to maintain the mobility of the joints of the hand and wrist should be started before there is any noticeable decreases in joint motion. Interventions should focus on mobilizing tissue; ROM exercises to increase MCP joint flexion, PIP joint extension, and abduction of the thumb and digits; strengthening exercises for all upper extremity muscles and preservation of lateral pinch; and provision of education regarding methods to prevent Raynaud's phenomenon and reduce the effects of ulcers on function. A self-monitoring system should be included so patients can know for sure that they are maintaining their ROM.

REFERENCES

1. van den Hoogen F, Khanna D, Fransen J, et al. classification criteria for systemic sclerosis: an American College of Rheumatology/European League against Rheumatism collaborative initiative. *Arthritis Rheum.* 2013;65(11):2737–2747.
2. Wollheim FA. Classification of systemic sclerosis. Visions and reality. *Rheumatology (Oxford).* 2005;44(10):1212–1216.
3. Morrisroe KB, Nikpour M, Proudman SM, et al. Musculoskeletal manifestations of systemic sclerosis. *Rheum Dis Clin North Am.* 2015;41(3):507–518.
4. Young A, Namas R, Dodge C, et al. Hand impairment in systemic sclerosis: various manifestations and currently available treatment. *Curr Treatm Opt Rheumatol.* 2016;2:252–269.
5. Mouthon L, Poole JL. Physical and Occupational Therapy. In: Varga J, Denton C, Wigley F, Kuwana M, Allanore Y, eds. *Scleroderma: From Pathogenesis to Comprehensive Management.* 2nd ed. New York: Springer; 2017:603–613.
6. Orphanet. The Portal for Rare Diseases and Orphan Drugs. Available at: http://www.orpha.net/consor/cgi-bin/Education_AboutRareDiseases.php?lng=EN.
7. Barnes JK, Mouthon L, Mayes MD. Epidemiology, environmental, and infectious risk factors. In: Varga J, Denton CP, Wigley FM, Allanore Y, Kuwana M, eds. *Scleroderma: From Pathogenesis to Comprehensive Management.* 2nd ed. New York: Springer; 2017:11–24.
8. Zulian F, Cuffaro G, Sperotto F. Scleroderma in children: an update. *Curr Opin Rheumatol.* 2013;25(5):643–650.
9. Desbois AC, Cacoub P. Systemic sclerosis: an update in 2016. *Autoimmun Rev.* 2016;15:417–426.
10. Denton CP, Khanna D. Systemic sclerosis. *Lancet.* 2017;390:1685–1699.
11. Sims R. Assessment and management of progressive skin involvement in diffuse scleroderma. In: Varga J, Denton CP, Wigley FM, Allanore Y, Kuwana M, eds. *Scleroderma: From Pathogenesis to Comprehensive Management.* 2nd ed. New York: Springer; 2017:489–498.
12. Young A, Khanna D. Systemic sclerosis: a systematic review on therapeutic management from 2011 to 2014. *Curr Opin Rheumatol.* 2015;27(3):241–248.
13. Hachulla E, Launay D. Diagnosis and classification of systemic sclerosis. *Clin Rev Allergy Immunol.* 2011;40(2):78–83.
14. Domsic RT, Rodriguez-Reyna T, Lucas M, Fertig N, Medsger Jr TA, et al. Skin thickness progression rate: a predictor of mortality and early internal organ involvement in diffuse scleroderma. *Ann Rheum Dis.* 2011;70(1):104–109.
15. Bálint Z, Farkas H, Farkas N, et al. A three-year follow-up study of the development of joint contractures in 131 patients with systemic sclerosis. *Clin Exp Rheumatol.* 2014;32(6 suppl 86):S68–S74.
16. Jordan S, Maurer B, Toniolo M, Michel B, et al. Distler O. Performance of the new ACR/EULAR classification criteria for systemic sclerosis in clinical practice. *Rheumatology (Oxford).* 2015;54(8):1454–1458.
17. Nihtyanova SI, Tang EC, Coghlan JG, Wells AU, Black CM, Denton CP, et al. Improved survival in systemic sclerosis is associated with better ascertainment of internal organ disease: a retrospective cohort study. *QJM.* 2010;103(2):109–115.
18. Steen VD. Autoantibodies in systemic sclerosis. *Semin Arthritis Rheum.* 2005;35(1):35–42.
19. Hinchcliff M, Varga J. Systemic sclerosis/scleroderma: a treatable multisystem disease. *Am Fam Physician.* 2008;78(8):961–968.
20. Zulian F, et al. Systemic sclerosis and localized scleroderma in childhood. *Rheum Dis Clin North Am.* 2008;34(1):239–255.
21. Steen VD, Medsger TA. Changes in causes of death in systemic sclerosis, 1972-2002. *Ann Rheum Dis.* 2007;66(7):940–944.
22. Nagaraja V, Denton CP, Khanna D, et al. Old medications and new targeted therapies in systemic sclerosis. *Rheumatology (Oxford).* 2015;54(11):1944–1953.
23. Rao V, Khanna D, et al. Scleroderma and fibrosing disorders: advances in management. *Int J Adv Rheumatol.* 2010;8(2):53–62.
24. Khanna D, Georges GE, Couriel DR, et al. Autologous hematopoietic stem cell therapy in severe systemic sclerosis ready for clinical practice. *JAMA.* 2014;311(24):2485–2487.
25. Englert H, Kirkham S, Moore J, et al. Autologous stem cell transplantation in diffuse scleroderma. impact on hand structure and function. *Intern Med J.* 2008;38(9):692–696.
26. Charles C, Clements P, Furst DE, et al. Systemic sclerosis: hypothesis-driven treatment strategies. *Lancet.* 2006;367(9523):1683–1691.
27. Quillinan NP, Denton CP, et al. Disease-modifying treatment in systemic sclerosis: current status. *Curr Opin Rheumatol.* 2009;6:636–641.
28. Poole JL, Steen V. The use of the Health Assessment Questionnaire (HAQ) to determine physical disability in systemic sclerosis. *Arthritis Care Res.* 1991;4:27–31.
29. Poole JL, Watzlaf V, D'Amico F, et al. Hand risk factors for the development of disability in systemic sclerosis (scleroderma). *J Hand Ther.* 2004;17:407–411.
30. Mouthon L, Mestre-Stanislas C, Bérezné A, Rannou F, Guilpain P, Revel M, et al. Impact of digital ulcers on disability and health-related quality of life in systemic sclerosis. *Ann Rheum Dis.* 2010;69(1):214–217.
31. M, Hudson M, Taillefer SS, Schier O, Baron M, Thombs BD. Frequency and impact of symptoms experienced by patients with systemic sclerosis: results from a Canadian National Survey. *Rheumatology (Oxford).* 2011;50(4):762–767.
32. Clements PJ, Wong WK, Hurwitz EL, et al. Correlates of the disability index of the health assessment questionnaire: a measure of functional impairment in systemic sclerosis. *Arthritis Rheum.* 1999;42:2372–2380.
33. Jakubietz MG, Jakubietz RG, Gruenert JG. Scleroderma of the hand. *J Hand Surg Am.* 2005;5(1):42–47.
34. Avouac J, Walker U, Tyndall A, Kahan A, Matucci-Cerinic M, Allanore Y, et al. Characteristics of joint involvement and relationships with systemic inflammation in systemic sclerosis: results from the EULAR Scleroderma Trial and Research Group (EUSTAR) database. *J Rheumatol.* 2010;37:1488–14501.
35. Melvin JL. Scleroderma (Systemic Sclerosis): treatment of the Hand. In: Skirven TM, Osterman AL, Fedorczyk JM, Amadio PM, eds. *Rehabilitation of the Hand and Upper Extremity.* 6th ed. Philadelphia: Elsevier; 2011:1434–1448.
36. Avouac J, Clements PJ, Khanna D, et al. Articular involvement in systemic sclerosis. *Rheumatology.* 2012;51:1347–1356.
37. Clements P, Lachenbruch P, Siebold J, et al. Inter- and intra-observer variability of total skin thickness score (modified Rodnan TSS) in systemic sclerosis. *J Rheumatol.* 1995;22(7):1281–1285.
38. Clements PJ, Medsger Jr TA, Feghali CA. Cutaneous involvement in systemic sclerosis. In: Clements PJ, Furst DE, eds. *Systemic Sclerosis.* 2nd ed. New York: Lippincott Williams & Wilkins; 2004:129–150.
39. Sherber NS, Wigley FM. Evaluation and management of skin disease. In: Varga J, Denton CP, Wigley FM, Allanore Y, Kuwana M, eds. *Scleroderma: From Pathogenesis to Comprehensive Management.* 2nd ed. New York: Springer; 2017:473–488.
40. Palmer DG, Hale GM, Grennan DM, Pollock M, et al. Bowed fingers. A helpful sign in the early diagnosis of systemic sclerosis. *J Rheumatol.* 1981;(2):266–272.
41. Meier FM, Frommer KW, Dinser R, et al. Update on the profile of the EUSTAR cohort: an analysis of the EULAR Scleroderma Trials and Research group database. *Ann Rheum Dis.* 2012;71(8):1355–1360.
42. Herrick AL, Wigley FM, Matucci-Cerinic M. Raynaud's phenomenon, digital ulcers and nailfold capillaroscopy. In: Varga J, Denton CP, Wigley FM, Allanore Y, Kuwana M, eds. *Scleroderma: From Pathogenesis to Comprehensive Management.* 2nd ed. New York: Springer; 2017:297–316.
43. Thompson AE, Pope JE, et al. Calcium channel blockers for primary Raynaud's phenomenon: a meta-analysis. *Rheumatology (Oxford).* 2005;44(2):145–150.
44. Mouthon L, Carpentier PH, Lok C, Clerson P, Gressin V, Hachulla E, et al. Ischemic digital ulcers affect hand disability and pain in systemic sclerosis. *J Rheumatol.* 2014;41(7):1317–1323.
45. Spence RJ. Managing complicated digital ulcers. In: Varga J, Denton CP, Wigley FM, Allanore Y, Kuwana M, eds. *Scleroderma: From Pathogenesis to Comprehensive Management.* 2nd ed. New York: Springer; 2017:723–730.
46. Jones MF. Surgical treatment of the hand in systemic sclerosis. In: Clements P, Furst D eds. *Systemic Sclerosis.* 2nd ed. Philadelphia: Lea & Febiger; 269–277.

47. Moran ME. Scleroderma and evidence based non-pharmaceutical treatment modalities for digital ulcers: a systematic review. *J Wound Care.* 2014;23(10):510–516.

48. Valenzuela A, Chung L. Calcinosis. In: Varga J, Denton CP, Wigley FM, Allanore Y, Kuwana M, eds. *Scleroderma: From Pathogenesis to Comprehensive Management.* 2nd ed. New York: Springer; 2017:461–471.

49. Avouac J, Guerini H, Wipff J, et al. Radiological hand involvement in systemic sclerosis. *Ann Rheum Dis.* 2006;65(8):1088–1092.

50. Johnstone EM1, Hutchinson CE, Vail A, Chevance A, Herrick AL, et al. Acro-osteolysis in systemic sclerosis is associated with digital ischaemia and severe calcinosis. *Rheumatology (Oxford).* 2012;51(12):2234–2238.

51. Steen VD, Medsger Jr TA, et al. The palpable tendon friction rub: an important physical examination finding in patients with systemic sclerosis. *Arthritis Rheum.* 1997;40(6):1146–1151.

52. Doré A, Lucas M, Ivanco D, Medsger Jr TA, Domsic RT, et al. Significance of palpable tendon friction rubs in early diffuse cutaneous systemic sclerosis. *Arthritis Care Res.* 2013;65(8):1385–1389.

53. Poole J. Musculoskeletal Rehabilitation in the Person with Scleroderma. *Curr Opin Rheumatol.* 2010;22:205–212.

54. Willems LM, Vriezekolk JE, Schouffoer AA, Poole JL, Stamm TA, Bostrom C, et al. Effectiveness of non-pharmacological interventions in systemic sclerosis: a systemic review. *Arthritis Care Res.* 2015;67:1426–1439.

55. Gibson G. Goniometry. In: ASHT, ed. *Clinical Assessment Recommendations.* 3rd ed. USA; 2015:71–80.

56. Sandqvist G, Eklund M, et al. Hand Mobility in Scleroderma (HAMIS) test: the reliability of a novel hand function test. *Arthritis Care Res.* 2000;13(6):369–374.

57. Sandqvist G, Eklund M, et al. Validity of HAMIS: a test of hand mobility in scleroderma. *Arthritis Care Res.* 2000;13(6):382–387.

58. Sandqvist G, Nilsson JÅ, Wuttge DM, Hesselstrand R, et al. Development of a modified Hand Mobility in Scleroderma (HAMIS) test and its potential as an outcome measure in systemic sclerosis. *J Rheumatol.* 2014;41:2186–2192.

59. Schectman O, Sindu B. Grip Assessment. In: ASHT, ed. *Clinical Assessment Recommendations.* 3rd ed. USA; 2015:1–8.

60. Mathiowetz V, Weber K, Kashman N, Volland G, et al. Adult norms for the Nine-Hole Peg Test of finger dexterity. *Occup Ther J Res.* 1985;5:24–38.

61. Poole JL, Gallegos M, O'Linc S. Reliability and validity of the arthritis hand function test in women with scleroderma. *Arthritis Care Res.* 2000;13:69–73.

62. Schouffoer AA, van der Giesen FJ, Beaart-van de Voorde LJ, Wolterbeek R, Huizinga TW, et al. Validity and responsiveness of the Michigan Hand Questionnaire in patients with systemic sclerosis. *Rheumatology (Oxford).* 2016;55(8):1386–1393.

63. Steen VD, Medsger Jr TA. The value of the Health Assessment Questionnaire and special patient-generated scales to demonstrate change in systemic sclerosis patients over time. *Arthritis Rheum.* 1997;40:1984–1991.

64. Brower LM, Poole JL. Reliability and validity of the Duruöz Hand Index in persons with systemic sclerosis. *Arthritis Care Res.* 2004;51:805–809.

65. Rannou F, Poiraudeau S, Berezné A, Baubet T, Le-Guern V, Cabane J, et al. Assessing disability and quality of life in systemic sclerosis: construct validities of the Cochin hand function scale, health assessment questionnaire (HAQ), systemic sclerosis HAQ, and MOS SF-36. *Arthritis Rheum.* 2007;57(1):94–102.

66. Mouthon L, Rannou F, Berezne A, Pagnoux C, Guilpain P, Goldwasser F, et al. Patient preference disability questionnaire in systemic sclerosis: a cross-sectional survey. *Arthritis Rheum.* 2008;59(7):968–973.

67. Gummesson C, Ward MM, Atrosi I. The shortened Disabilities of the Arm, Shoulder and Hand questionnaire (QuickDASH): validity and reliability based on responses within the full-length DASH. *BMC Musculoskelet Disord.* 2006;18:1–7.

68. MacDermid JC, Turgeon T, Richards RS, et al. Patient rating of wrist pain and disability. a reliable and valid measurement tool. *J Ortho Trauma.* 1998;12(8):577–586.

69. Varju C, Balint Z, Solyom AI, Farkas H, Karpati E, Berta B, et al. Cross-cultural adaptation of the Disabilities of the Arm, Shoulder, and Hand (DASH) questionnaire into Hungarian and investigation of its validity in patients with systemic sclerosis. *Clin Exp Rheumatol.* 2008;26(5):776–783.

70. Stuppy DJ. The faces of pain scale: reliability and validity with mature adults. *App Nurs Res.* 1998;11:84–89.

71. Tan G, Jensen MP, Thornby JI, Shanti BF. Validation of the brief pain inventory for chronic nonmalignant pain. *J Pain.* 2004;5:133–137.

72. El-Baalbaki G, Lober J, Hudson M, Baron M, Thombs BD, et al. Measuring pain in systemic sclerosis: comparison of the short-form McGill Pain Questionnaire versus a single-item measure of pain. *J Rheumatol.* 2011;38(12):2581–2587.

73. Groundry B, Bell L, Langtree M, Moorthy A. Diagnosis and management of Raynaud's phenomenon. *BMJ.* 2012;344:e289.

74. Malenfant D, Catton M, Pope JE, et al. The efficacy of complementary and alternative medicine in the treatment of Raynaud's phenomenon: a literature review and meta-analysis. *Rheumatology (Oxford).* 2009;48(7):791–795.

75. Sporbeck B, Mathiske-Schmidt K, Jahr S, et al. Effect of biofeedback and deep oscillation on Raynaud's phenomenon secondary to systemic sclerosis: results of a controlled prospective randomized clinical trial. *Rheumatol Int.* 2012;32:1469–1473.

76. Bongi SM, Del Rosso A, Passalacqua M, et al. Manual lymph drainage improving upper extremity edema and hand function in patients with systemic sclerosis in edematous phase. *Arthritis Care Res.* 2011;63:1134–1141.

77. Murphy SL, Barber M, Homer K, Dodge C, Khanna D. Occupational therapy treatment to improve upper extremity function in individuals with early systemic sclerosis: A pilot study. *Arthritis Care Res.* 2018;70:1653–1660.

78. Maddali-Bongi S, Landi G, Galluccio F, Del Rosso A, Miniati I, Conforti ML, et al. The rehabilitation of facial involvement in systemic sclerosis: efficacy of the combination of connective tissue massage, Kabat's technique and kinesiotherapy: a randomized controlled trial. *Rheumatol Int.* 2010;31(7):895–901.

79. Piga M, Tradori I, Pani D, et al. Telemedicine applied to kinesiotherapy for hand dysfunction in patients with systemic sclerosis and rheumatoid arthritis: recovery of movement and telemonitoring technology. *J Rheumatol.* 2014;41:1324–1333.

80. Stefanantoni K, Sciarra I, Iannace N, et al. Occupational therapy integrated with a self-administered stretching program on systemic sclerosis patients with hand involvement. *Clin Exp Rheumatol.* 2016;34:157–161.

81. Fedorczyk JM. The use of physical agents in hand rehabilitation. In: Skirven TM, Osterman AL, Fedorczyk JM, Amadio PC, eds. *Rehabilitation of the Hand and Upper Extremity.* 6th ed. Philadelphia: Elsevier; 2011:495–1511.

82. Iivarinen JT, Korhonen RK, Jurvelin JS. Modeling of interstitial fluid movement in soft tissue under negative pressure - relevance to treatment of tissue swelling. *Comput Methods Biomech Biomed Engin.* 2016;19:1089–1098.

83. Casale R, Buonocore M, Matucci-cerinic M. Systemic Sclerosis (Scleroderma): an Integrated Challenge in Rehabilitation. *Arch Phys Med Rehabil.* 1997;78:767–773.

84. Seeger MW, Furst DE. Effects of splinting in the treatment of hand contractures in progressive systemic sclerosis. *Am J Occup Ther.* 1987;41(2):118–121.

85. Rannou F, Boutron I, Mouthon L, et al. Personalized physical therapy versus usual care for patients with systemic sclerosis: a randomized controlled trial. *Arthritis Care Res.* 2017;69:1050–1059.

86. Anandacoomarasamy A, Englert H, Manolios N, et al. Reconstructive hand surgery for scleroderma joint contractures. *J Hand Surg Am.* 2007;32(7):1107–1112.

87. Avouac J, Buch MH, Allanore Y. Tendons, joints, and bone. In: Varga J, Denton CP, Wigley FM, Allanore Y, Kuwana M, eds. *Scleroderma: From Pathogenesis to Comprehensive Management.* 2nd ed. New York: Springer; 2017:11–24.

93

Understanding Pain Mechanisms: The Basis of Clinical Decision Making for Pain Modulation

Melanie B. Elliott, Mary F. Barbe

OUTLINE

CRITICAL POINTS

Forms of Pain and Hypersensitivity

- Acute pain is a normal response of nociceptors to noxious stimuli.
- Allodynia is a painful response to a normally nonpainful stimulus, such as light touch.
- Hyperalgesia is a heightened painful response to a noxious stimulus.

- Persistent pain is chronic pain. It is a heightened painful response to a painful stimulus.
- Spontaneous pain is the presence of pain symptoms despite a lack of stimuli.

INTRODUCTION: ACUTE VERSUS PERSISTENT PAIN

Noxious stimulation of tissues with high-intensity heat, cold, mechanical, and chemical stimuli induce acute pain. *Acute pain* is typically defined as pain of rapid or sudden onset, described as being sharp and localized, and serves to warn the organism of impending tissue damage. This type of pain has also been termed *nociceptor pain* because nociception is the physiological sensory process of encoding and signaling of noxious stimuli to the central nervous system (CNS) after activation of nociceptor endings.[1]

However, alterations in peripheral or central pain pathways elicited by inflammation or tissue or nerve damage can induce *hypersensitivity*. Various types of altered pain perceptions to stimuli include *allodynia* (a painful response to a normally nonpainful stimulus, such as light touch) and *hyperalgesia* (a heightened painful response to a noxious stimulus) (see Table 93.1 for detailed definitions of various terms used to describe pain). For example, pain occurring as a result of inflammatory responses (e.g., inflammatory cytokine release from injured tissues or tissues affected by inflammatory disorders or diseases) can induce hypersensitivity to both painful and nonpainful stimuli. Such *inflammatory pain* may improve as inflammation resolves,[2–4] although an individual with a chronic inflammatory condition may have perpetuated pain symptoms even with remission of inflammatory signs.[1]

There are also several types of stimulus-independent pain, such as *spontaneous pain* (the presence of pain symptoms despite a lack of stimuli).

Pain symptoms are considered *persistent* or *chronic* when they persist despite no obvious sign of non-neural tissue injury. Persistent (chronic) pain after tissue or nerve injury or chemotherapy or in association with a metabolic disorders (e.g., diabetes and viral infections), cancer, or arthritis is associated with chronic neuroinflammation, dysfunction, or pathological changes in nociceptor signaling or other aspects of the peripheral nervous system, or pathological neuroplasticity in the CNS. *Neuropathic pain* is a form of persistent pain that has been recently redefined by the International Association for the Study of Pain (IASP) as pain caused by a lesion or disease of the peripheral or central somatosensory nervous system.[5] Although controversial,[6] the IASP in 2016 proposed the adoption of a new term, *nociplastic pain*, to capture the type of persistent pain conditions with no clear medial explanation (as in *idiopathic pain*), as in no clear evidence of actual or threatened tissue damage that might cause activation of peripheral nociceptors and no evidence of disease or lesion of the somatosensory system circuitry (see Table 93.1).

Whatever the term used, most agree that persistent and neuropathic pain conditions are linked to physiological attributes other than traditional neuronal transmission. These are debilitating conditions with

TABLE 93.1	Pain Terminology
Pain Term	**Description**
Acute pain	Pain of rapid or sudden onset; described as being sharp and localized
Allodynia	Perception of pain produced by stimuli that are not normally painful, such as stroking of skin, light pinch, or movement of joint
Central sensitization	Increased responses to painful or innocuous stimuli in central nervous system circuitry, e.g., dorsal horns and at supraspinal sites, after remodeling of said circuitry
Hyperalgesia	A heightened response to noxious (painful) stimuli
Inflammatory pain	Pain occurring from inflammation, e.g., inflammatory cytokine and mediator release, from injured tissues or tissues affected by inflammatory disorders or diseases
Neuralgia	Severe pain typically of a stabbing or burning sensation caused by infection or an irritated or damaged nerve (e.g., trigeminal neuralgia or postherpetic neuralgia caused by shingles)
Neuropathic pain	Pain caused by a lesion or disease of the somatosensory nervous system
Nociceptor pain	Pain that arises from actual or threatened damage to non-neural tissue and is due to the activation of nociceptors; a term used to describe pain occurring with a normally functional nervous system
Nociplastic pain	Pain that arises from altered nociception despite no clear evidence of actual or threatened tissue damage that might cause activation of peripheral nociceptors or evidence of disease or lesion of the somatosensory system
Pain of unknown origin (idiopathic pain)	Pain of unknown causes and origin; pain that cannot be classified as neuropathic, nociceptive, or nociplastic pain
Peripheral sensitization	Increased responses to painful or innocuous stimuli by primary afferents in the periphery
Persistent or chronic pain	Pain of long duration with a slower, gradual onset; described as dull, diffuse, and poorly localized
Recurrent pain	Recurring or episodic; pain that accompanies a reinjury, or it may be a painful episode associated with a disease process such as rheumatoid arthritis
Spontaneous pain	The presence of pain symptoms despite a lack of stimuli

high morbidity and impact on an individual's quality of life, particularly because these conditions are resistant to standard analgesics.[7,8] A review of epidemiologic studies estimates the prevalence of pain with neuropathic characteristics is between 6.9% and 10%.[9] A better understanding of their etiology is key for improving the treatment of patients with such pain.[2]

NEUROANATOMICAL BASIS OF SOMATIC PAIN: PERIPHERAL MECHANISMS

The Nociceptor: Transducers of Acute Pain

Nociception is the physiological neural response initiated by noxious or potentially tissue-damaging stimuli. It is also the mechanism of acute pain generation. This response is mediated by peripheral afferent nerve fibers called nociceptors located in the skin, muscle, joints, periosteum, and viscera. Nociceptor endings in the tissues are unencapsulated ("free") and are associated with thinly myelinated axons of medium diameter (Aδ fibers) or unmyelinated, small-sized axons (C fibers). The three main functional classes of nociceptors (mechanical, thermal, and polymodal) are widely distributed throughout their target tissues (albeit at varying degrees of density to allow for differential sensory ability in the fingertips versus the back, for example,[10] and often work in unison). The specific properties of the nociceptors are determined by membrane-bound ion channels on the peripheral terminal that cause depolarization of these first-order primary afferent neurons. Upon activation, these ion channel receptors transduce an external stimulus into a change in the membrane potential via the opening of a sodium–calcium or transient receptor potential (TRP) channel or the closing of a potassium (K+) channel. One example of this process is proton (H+) activation of acid-sensing ion channels (ASIC) as part of the inflammatory soup activation of nociceptors (Fig. 93.1).[11] Detection of increased lactic acid in muscles, for example, is one cause of

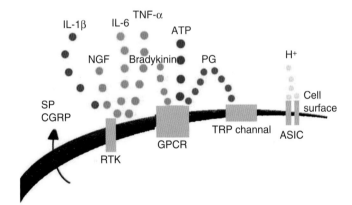

Fig. 93.1 Peripheral mediators of inflammation. The inflammatory mediators released by the nociceptors or non-neuronal cells inflamed area bind to receptors on the membrane surface of peripheral nociceptors, lowering the threshold of the nociceptors. One or more inflammatory mediators may bind to the same receptor. Likewise, a receptor can interact with one or more inflammatory mediators. *ASIC*, Acid-sensitive ion channel, receptors for extracellular protons; *ATP*, adenosine triphosphate; *CGRP*, calcitonin gene-related peptide; *GPCR*, G protein–coupled receptor; *H*, hydrogen ions; *IL*, interleukin; *NGF*, nerve growth factor; *PG*, prostaglandin; *RTK*, receptor tyrosine kinase; *SP*, substance P; *TNF*, tumor necrosis factor. (Adapted from Yan YY, Li CY, Zhou L, et al. Research progress of mechanisms and drug therapy for neuropathic pain. *Life Sci.* 2017;190:68-77.)

muscle soreness after exercise. If the membrane potential is of sufficient magnitude to reach the activation threshold for voltage-gated sodium (Na+) channels (NaV), an action potential be generated followed by its propagation along the axon of an afferent neuron centrally to the spinal cord.

TABLE 93.2 Types of Nociceptors

Type	Respond to Stimuli	Diameter (µm)	Conduction Velocity, Mean Range (m/sec)	Response
Aδ type I (myelinated)	Thermal, extreme heat (>50°C)	1–5	6.9 ± 6.17 (3.5–31)	Painful hot as burning
Aδ type II/A-HTMR (myelinated)	High-intensity mechanical: noxious skin pinch, penetration and probing by sharp object, squeezing	1–5	6.9 ± 6.17 (3.5–31)	Sharp, pricking sensation
C-HTMR (unmyelinated)	High-intensity mechanical: noxious skin pinch, penetration and probing by sharp object, squeezing	0.2–1.5	1.0 ± 0.20 (0.5–1.9)	Sharp, pricking sensation
C polymodal (unmyelinated)	Polymodal, firm stroking, chemical, heat (38°–60°C), and cold (10°–21°C) stimuli	0.2–1.5	0.7 ± 0.04 (0.2–1.5)	Burning, dull, aching; long lasting
C nociceptor (unmyelinated)	Thermal, extreme heat (>45°C), and extreme cold (<5°C)	0.2–1.5	0.7 ± 0.04 (0.2–1.5)	Painful hot or cold as burning or aching; freezing pain as stinging

HTMR, High-threshold mechanoreceptors.

Types of Nociceptors and Their Functionality

Nociceptors have varied thresholds and sensitivities to external and internal stimuli with which they are able to adapt or maladapt to their microenvironment.[12] Different subsets are also sensitive to different ranges of stimuli, with most being defined as polymodal based on anatomical and in vivo and in vitro electrophysiological data.[13] However, anatomical and electrophysiological data have also shown that some nociceptors respond to narrower ranges of stimuli.[11] Also, some recent studies using genetically encoded Ca^{2+}-indicators technology in transgenic mice have found that under control conditions, most sensory neurons are modality specific rather than polymodal, that is, they response to mechanical pinch but not noxious hot or cold.[14,15] More studies using additional techniques are needed to elucidate this topic.

Many of the Aδ nociceptors mentioned earlier are mechanical nociceptors activated by intensive pressure, such as a noxious skin pinch, probing the skin with sharp objects, and squeezing. These nerves are moderate in diameter (1–5 µm), thinly to moderately myelinated, and have a broad range of conduction velocities from slow to moderately fast (Table 93.2).[16,17] The Aδ nociceptors can be further divided into two subtypes: a high-heat threshold type I (responds >50°C) and a low-heat threshold type II that also responds to high-intensity mechanical stimuli and thus considered an A-HTMR (myelinated high-threshold mechanoreceptor). The type of pain typically perceived after activation of A-HTMR is a sharp, pricking sensation with an exact location. These large and fast mechanical nociceptors are the sensory neurons underlying "fast pain/first pain."[13,16]

The Aδ nociceptors differ from Aβ mechanoreceptors both morphologically and functionally. Aβ mechanoreceptors have larger axonal diameters (6-12 µm) and are moderately myelinated. They respond to innocuous stimuli, such as light touch, and are commonly associated with the experience of pleasure.[17]

C nociceptors or C fibers are extremely prevalent in number and make up 80% of the total fibers in cutaneous nerves. These nociceptors have axons with small diameters (0.2–1.5 µm) and can be divided into two main groups: those that respond to mechanical stimulation but not to thermal stimuli (C-HTMR [unmyelinated high-threshold mechanoreceptor]) and those that respond to thermal as well as other noxious stimuli (C-polymodal), as shown in Table 93.2. The C-HTMR nociceptors are high-threshold afferents with slow conduction velocities that respond to intensive pressure, such as a noxious skin pinch, probing the skin with sharp objects, and squeezing. The C-polymodal nociceptors are unmyelinated and are activated by firm stroking of the skin, chemical stimuli, and high temperatures (38°–60°C) or cold temperatures (10°–21°C).[17] This subset of C nociceptors is also called group IV afferents because they have unmyelinated, very small-diameter axons (<1 mm) that conduct very slowly. Mechanically insensitive cutaneous nociceptors have also been identified that respond only to heat and are thus called thermal receptors (see Table 93.2). C nociceptors also are located within joints, muscles, and viscera. As a component of visceral nerves, C nociceptors are thought to transmit unpleasant sensations associated with distention of the bowel and bladder, chemical secretions, and inflammation of the visceral structures. Hypersensitivity in these nociceptors is one cause of "functional" visceral pain disorders, such as irritable bowel syndrome or bladder pain syndrome. Pain processing from C nociceptors is slow, and the injury is poorly localized; thus, they are considered the sensory neurons underlying "slow pain."[13,16,17] Pain associated with activation of the C fibers is burning, dull, aching, and long-lasting in nature (see Table 93.2). Several categories of C fibers also respond to chemical stimuli and can produce sensation consistent with itching.[18] Yet not all nociceptors are responsive under typical conditions to noninjurious stimuli. The term *silent nociceptors* has been used to describe high-threshold C fibers that have little or no spontaneous activity and that are activated only by intense physical stimuli.

C nociceptors can also be divided into peptidergic or nonpeptidergic subsets.[17] The peptidergic C subdivision release a variety of peptides, including substance P and calcitonin gene-related peptide (CGRP), and express tropomyosin receptor kinase A (trkA) receptors that bind nerve growth factor (NGF), as shown in Fig. 93.1.[19] The nonpeptidergic C subset expresses fluoride-resistant acid phosphatase and c-Ret neurotrophin receptors (the receptor for the glial cell line–derived family of neurotrophic factors), also termed IB4 nociceptors because they bind IB4 lectin.[16,20–22] Receptor differences between these two subsets lead to differential responsiveness to chemical mediators released and contribute to varied levels of pain modulation at the site of injury.

It is important to also realize that afferents also have efferent properties. For example, peptidergic nociceptors have the ability to release substances from their peripheral terminals, such as substance P (see Fig. 93.1).[12,23,24] This peripheral release of substances from nociceptors plays roles in normal tissue remodeling, tissue healing by inducing of collagen production from fibroblasts and tenocytes (via release of

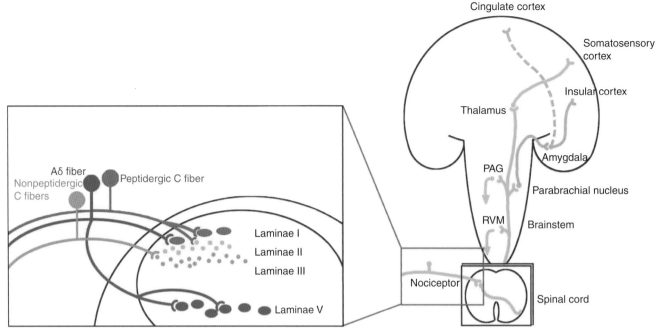

Fig. 93.2 Anatomy of pain pathways. *Left,* The site of laminar termination of afferent fibers within the dorsal horn. Peptidergic C fibers terminate on neurons (*red* and *green*) located in laminae I and II. Nonpeptidergic C fibers terminate on interneurons *(blue)* in laminae II. Aδ fibers terminate on neurons both in the superficial laminae I, laminae II, and deep laminae V. *Right,* Pain messages ascend (transmit) to the cerebral cortex (somatosensory cortex, cingulate cortex, and insular cortex) via the ascending pathways (through the brainstem, parabrachial nucleus [PB], amygdala, or the thalamus). The cerebral cortical areas process transmitted nociceptive information for localization and type of stimuli and for emotional context. There are also a descending feedback system (including periaqueductal gray [PAG] area and rostral ventral medulla [RVM]) and various neurotransmitters that modulate pain, leading to pain relief or hypersensitivity. (Adapted from Yan YY, Li CY, Zhou L, et al. Research progress of mechanisms and drug therapy for neuropathic pain. *Life Sci.* 2017;190:68-77.)

substance P), and vasodilation and plasma extravasation when CGRP and substance P are released after tissue injury.[12,24] The latter events are essential for injury-induced inflammatory processes yet also help drive the pain associated with inflammation.[12]

Projection of Nociceptors Into the Spinal Cord

Because nociceptors are sensory neurons, they, like other peripheral sensory neurons, are pseudounipolar in shape, with two axons branching from a main axon of the cell body (Fig. 93.2). The cell body is located in the dorsal root ganglia or sensory cranial nerve ganglia, similar to other types of sensory neurons. A peripherally projecting axon carries impulses from the nociceptor terminal located in the skin, joints, or viscera from the peripheral site centrally to the spinal cord (see Fig. 93.2). A centrally projecting axon projects into the spinal cord, where it terminates in the dorsal horn and releases excitatory neurotransmitters, such as glutamate and substance P, onto second-order projection neurons and interneurons.[3,12,25] However, first, these centrally projecting nociceptive axons ascend or descend for several spinal segments in a small pathway called Lissauer's tract (located in the posterolateral sulcus at the tip of the dorsal horn) before terminating in the dorsal horn gray matter.[26] Subsets of the afferent collaterals express the transient receptor potential vanilloid 1 (TRPV1), which transduces a nociceptive response to capsaicin.[26] These TRPV1-expressing nociceptors send collaterals to neurons located in the ventral horn of the spinal cord to modulate locomotor central pattern generators to ensure a rapid withdrawal from aversive stimuli, for example.

That said, key synapses of the C-nociceptor and A-nociceptor axons are in laminae within the dorsal horn. Most nociceptive fibers terminate in laminae I and II, with a few connections to deeper laminae.[10,17] Lamina II is most commonly referred to as the *substantia gelatinosa.* The A-nociceptor fibers terminate primarily in laminae I, II, and V, laminae containing many wide dynamic range (WDR) neurons. In contrast, most somatic C-nociceptors terminate primarily in lamina I and II, which contains both excitatory and inhibitory interneurons that respond to both noxious and non-noxious stimuli (see Fig. 93.2).[10,17] Within lamina I, for example, approximately 80% of the cells expression the neurokinin 1 receptor, the main receptor for substance P. Second-order neurons in lamina I project primarily to the thalamus, periaqueductal gray (PAG) area of the midbrain, parabrachial nucleus, and rostroventromedial medulla (RVM) nucleus in the medulla, indicating that they play roles in both transmission of ascending pain information to supraspinal centers and in descending pain modulation originating from these same centers (Figs. 93.2 and 93.3). Interestingly, neurons in laminae VII and VIII receive bilateral input from polymodal nociceptors and project to neurons of the brainstem reticular formation bilaterally; therefore, these latter laminae contribute to diffuse pain sensations.[27]

NEUROANATOMICAL BASIS OF PAIN IN THE HEAD AND NECK: PERIPHERAL MECHANISMS

Head and neck pain may be generated from signaling received by the trigeminal nerve, which is the fifth cranial nerve and a widely distributed nerve in the head. The trigeminal nerve has three branches, the ophthalmic, maxillary, and mandibular, responsible for translating sensory input from the face, scalp, oral cavity, periosteum, calvarium,

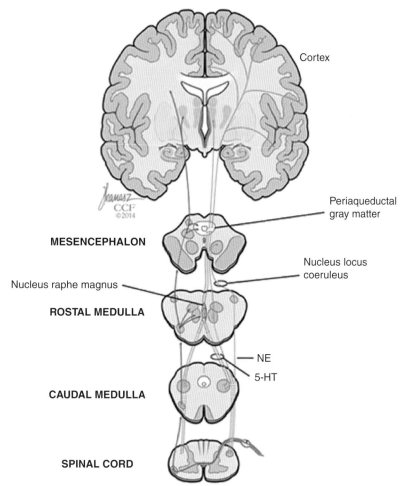

Fig. 93.3 Descending modulation of afferent input into the dorsal horn. Several sites in the descending pain system serve to modulate the ascending pain signal from the dorsal horn, including the periaqueductal grey (PAG) area, dorsolateral pontine tegmentum, and rostroventral medulla (RVM). The PAG region controls pain signaling by sending projections descending to synapse in the dorsal horn and to the nucleus raphe magnus located in the RVM, which release serotonin (5-HT). Descending modulation also includes the noradrenergic input from the locus coeruleus to the dorsal horn. (Adapted from Bourne S, Machado AG, Nagel SJ. Basic anatomy and physiology of pain pathways. *Neurosurg Clin North Am.* 2014;25(4):629-638.)

and meningeal vessels to the brain. Common trigeminal pain disorders include migraine, tension-type headache, and posttraumatic headache, whereas less common disorders such as trigeminal neuralgia also exist. Migraine is the predominant headache phenotype after concussion or traumatic brain injury prevalent in 49% to 90% of military service and nonmilitary patients.[28–30] Posttraumatic headache and migraine commonly share features, including sensitivity to light and sound (photophobia and phonophobia), nausea and vomiting, unilateral headache, pulsate quality, moderate to severe intensity, and headache that is aggravated by routine physical activity.[28,31–34] In addition, cutaneous hypersensitivity to a mechanical stimulus, mechanical allodynia, is a painful response commonly reported in patients with migraine and posttraumatic headache.[35–37] Testing for trigeminal or facial allodynia, light sensitivity, and spontaneous pain behaviors has been used in animals to study the mechanisms of migraine and posttraumatic headache.[37–41]

A migraine attack is elicited by the activation of the trigeminal pain pathway in which the sensitization of the peripheral trigeminal pain neurons, central trigeminal pain neurons, or both has been proposed (peripheral or central sensitization).[42] Similarly, altered nociceptive signaling in the trigeminal pain pathway was shown in association

with headache behaviors (facial allodynia and light sensitivity) after cortical contusion injury in rodents[38,39,41] and acute concussion or closed head injury models, expanding on the understanding of the mechanisms of these disorders.[43–48] As a result of concussion or other types of brain injury, inflammation of the meningeal tissues and particularly the dura will trigger the activation and sensitization of the meningeal nociceptors.[49–52] Periosteal inflammation is an additional sensitizer and activator of the trigeminal ganglia neurons after head injury.[44,53] Extracranial structures, such as those in the skin, meninges, periosteum, and cranium, are innervated by the trigeminal ganglia, or adjacent area such as the neck have ganglia that converge in the trigeminal pathway; these structures are also potential sources of inflammation after concussion in addition to the intracranial structures of the trigeminal pathway. Inflammation-induced sensitization of trigeminal pain neurons remain a predominant mechanism underlying the persistence of posttraumatic headache whether localized to the trigeminal ganglia or centrally either in the caudal brain stem trigeminal nucleus caudalis, thalamic relay ventral posterior medialis nucleus, or sensory cortex.[38,39,43,44] Concussions, as with other types of traumatic brain injury, are heterogeneous injuries whereby the parameters affecting injury (e.g., location, impact force, history of concussion, age, gender, and genetic factors) have an impact on the central pain nuclei in the trigeminal system.

Release of inflammatory mediators, such as cytokines, prostaglandins, nitric oxide, bradykinins, and histamine, sensitize nociceptors (see Fig. 93.1), and central trigeminal pain neurons in the injured brain contribute to the development of headache.[38,39,42–44,54] Inflammatory mediators lower the threshold for activation of meningeal nociceptors and consequently increase the release of excitatory nociceptive neuropeptides such as CGRP in response to an even smaller degree of vessel dilation or other stimulus.[54,55] CGRP, nitric oxide, and nitric oxide synthase (NOS) are essential pain signaling molecules in the development of migraine and posttraumatic headache pathophysiology.[38,56–58] Increases in CGRP and the inducible isoform of NOS in the trigeminal pain pathway are associated with headache behaviors in models of cortical contusion[38,39,59] and postconcussion headache.[48] Triggers postulated to cause the release of CGRP that may play a role in posttraumatic headache continue to be strong areas of interest for their role in eliciting algesia and nociception. Anandamide, an endogenous cannabinoid, is released on demand after injury and is also a ligand of the TRPV1.[60] When activated, TRPV1 releases CGRP. To date, a majority of studies indicate that meningeal or periosteal inflammation sensitizes the trigeminal nociceptors after head injury. However, evidence shows additional mechanisms in other central pain regions may also contribute to posttraumatic headache.[59,61–65]

PERIPHERAL SENSITIZATION: MECHANISMS

The term *neuroplasticity*, a phenomenon that occurs in the peripheral nervous system and CNS, is broadly defined as altered functioning of the nervous system in response to different environmental conditions. Plasticity underlies the pathophysiologic states involved in chronic pain conditions. When nociceptive pathways are suddenly activated by stimuli that are normally not painful (allodynia), when symptoms of pain are heightened or exaggerated in response to the inducing stimulus, or when pain symptoms are present in the absence of any stimulus, sensitization has occurred.

Peripheral sensitization involves altered nociceptor function by which there is a reduced threshold of activation and enhanced responsiveness.[8] This results from both direct and indirect mechanisms, such as (1) increased numbers of immune cells that secrete proinflammatory cytokines; (2) an increase in mediators in general in the inflammatory soup that maintain enhanced activation of the afferent terminals; (3) alterations or dysregulation of the expression or ion channels in the peripheral afferent terminals; (4) increased spontaneous or ectopic activity in the afferent neuron; and (5) even alterations in surrounding cells, such as in epidermal cells, that maintain the enhanced activity.[1,8,10–12,17,66]

With regard to the inflammatory soup, a variety of chemical mediators are released from injured cells and infiltrating immune cells into the local injured site that then sensitize the peripheral end terminals of the nociceptors. As introduced earlier, inflammatory cytokines, CGRP and substance P, and NGF, as well as norepinephrine (NE), capsaicin, histamine, serotonin (5-HT), bradykinin, and prostaglandin E_2, are among the chemical mediators that affect the threshold of nociceptors (see Fig. 93.1).[10,12,17] Other mediators, including proteases, additional growth factors, chemokines and damage-associated molecular patterns (DAMPs), continue to be identified.[17,67,68] These mediators have a variety of cellular origins. Cellular sources of inflammatory cytokines include damaged tissue cells, damaged axons and cells within the nerve (axons, Schwann cells, intraneural fibroblasts, satellite glial cells), and infiltrating immune cells (mast cells, neutrophils, lymphocytes, and macrophages).[68,69] These inflammatory

mediators form an "inflammatory soup" and act both directly and indirectly on nociceptor terminals in peripheral tissues.[17,68,69] Sensory afferent terminals expression receptors for nearly every component of the inflammatory soup so that such exposure decreases the stimulation threshold or increases responsiveness during inflammation.[1,17] Under conditions of inflammation, non-nociceptive Aβ/δ mechanoreceptors elicit enhanced responses to pressure and movement, high-threshold Aδ and C nociceptors respond to less intense stimuli such as light pressure, and silent nociceptors become responsive to mechanical stimulation. The magnitude and duration of the mechanical hypersensitivity appear to be related to the severity of the nerve or tissue inflammation.

Nerve injury, or repeated or prolonged activation of nociceptors, can lead to altered gene expression within these neurons so that the density, distribution, and even expression type of ion channels on the neuronal membrane change. For example, repeated exposure to inflammatory mediators or nerve injury can lead to increased density of voltage-gated sodium channels and voltage-gated calcium channels on the nociceptor terminals. This change results in a dramatic increase in abnormal action potentials and subsequent neuropathic pain.[12,17] A massive aggregation of various ion channels on the neuronal membrane can also contribute to spontaneous nerve activity, discussed later. Neural growth factors, such as NGF, when upregulated in cells and tissues surrounding peptidergic C fibers, signal through TrakA and p75 receptors to increase gene expression of neuropeptides, such as substance P, leading to enhanced pain as well.

With regard to increased spontaneous activity, which has also been termed *ectopic discharge*, "silent nociceptors" can become spontaneously active after exposure to inflammatory mediators.[12,70] There is also a decrease in threshold to depolarization also that they can be elicited by non-noxious stimuli, analogous to an allodynic state so that they fire in response to moderate stimuli such as touch rather than intense stimuli.[12] Such maladaptive neuroplasticity may be the common mechanism of pain associated with inflammatory diagnoses (i.e., diagnoses that end in "-itis").[1] There are studies showing increased levels of tumor necrosis factor–α at midaxonal level, and tissue inflammation around an axon increased firing activity of a nociceptor axon (termed *ectopic discharge*). For example, as a result of peripheral sensitization, presynaptic changes of the afferent neurons increase the release of neurotransmitters from their central terminals within the spinal cord dorsal horns. According to several investigators, this afferent barrage of excitatory transmitters into the dorsal horn is the presynaptic component of central sensitization, to be discussed later in this chapter.

In summary, peripheral sensitization is a function of chemically induced nociceptor hyperactivity that leads to a state of increased sensitivity to normally nonpainful stimuli (allodynia) or increased responsiveness to noxious stimuli (hyperalgesia) that is perceived with exaggerated or prolonged pain and may develop into chronic pain.

PHYSIOLOGIC BASIS OF PAIN: CENTRAL MECHANISMS

Ascending Pathways of Pain Transmission

Ascending pain impulses are carried from the spinal cord via multiple pathways, including the spinothalamic, spinoreticular, spinomesencephalic, and spinohypothalamic–limbic pathways (Table 93.3; see also Fig. 93.3).[71,72] Collectively, these pathways, as well as a few others not listed here, are known as the *anterolateral system*. This system includes not only pain and temperature sensibilities but also crude tactile and pressure modalities from innocuous mechanoreceptors with large receptive fields.

TABLE 93.3 Components of the Anterolateral System, the Ascending Pathways of Pain Transmission

Pathway	Origin in Spinal Cord	Supraspinal Termination Site	Mode of Ascension	Function
Spinothalamic	Laminae I, IV–VII	Thalamus: VPL, CL	Contralateral	Carries information of type and location of noxious stimuli for relay to cortex; VPL to SI cortex for specific location and type perception; POm to limbic cortices for emotional response; CL to widespread cortical areas
Spinoreticular (spinoreticular-thalamic)	Laminae VII, VIII	Reticular formation in medulla and pons that projects to CL and intralaminar thalamic nuclei	Most contralateral, some ipsilateral	For modulation of pain and perception of pain
Spinomesencephalic	Laminae I, V–VII	Reticular formation in the mesencephalon, PAG area, and colliculi	Predominantly contralateral, but a large ipsilateral subset	For modulation of pain
Spinobrachial (subset of spinomesencephalic)	Laminae I, V–VII	Parabrachial nuclei and amygdala (a limbic structure)	Bilateral	Emotional aspect of pain
Spinohypothalamic	Laminae I, V, VIII	Hypothalamus (center of autonomic nervous system control)		Pain's effects on neuroendocrine and cardiovascular systems

CL, Centrolateral nucleus; *PAG,* periaqueductal grey; *SI,* somatosensory cortex area 1; *VPL,* ventral posterior lateral nucleus of the thalamus.

The *spinothalamic tract* is the primary nociceptive pathway and is also the most studied of the known pathways (see Table 93.3).[71] It consists of axons of nociceptive-specific and WDR neurons from laminae I, IV, V, VI, and VII. Although there is a small ipsilateral projection, most of the axons decussate in the ventral white commissure of the spinal cord before ascending contralaterally in the anterolateral white matter to the ventroposterolateral (VPL) nucleus, medial nucleus of posterior complex (POm), and central lateral (CL) nuclei of the thalamus. Noxious and non-noxious impulses such as pain, crude touch, and temperature are transmitted.[71] The primary function of this tract is to carry the discriminatory features of type and location of the noxious stimulus via relays through the VPL nucleus to the primary somatosensory cortex (see Fig. 93.3). However, there are also spinothalamic connections to the CL nucleus, a nucleus with projections to widespread cortical areas, and to the POm, a nucleus involved in the nondiscriminative, affective component of pain. These additional connections expand the roles of the spinothalamic tract to include the emotional response to pain and the perception of pain.[73] The latter includes pain quality (e.g., burning, sharp, dull), cardiovascular changes (e.g., increased heart rate), and neuroendocrine effects (e.g., nausea).

The *spinoreticular tract* (see Table 93.3) consists primarily of fibers from nociceptive neurons in laminae VII and VIII.[71] Note that a few of the neurons contributing to this tract are either inhibited or excited by innocuous cutaneous sensation. The spinoreticular tract consists primarily of axons from the cervical cord and ascends in the anterolateral quadrant of the spinal cord along with the spinothalamic tract. However, not all the fibers in this tract cross the midline and ascend on the contralateral side. A small percentage of ipsilateral projections exist. Fibers of this tract project to various nuclei in the reticular formation of the medulla and pons. These reticular nuclei project to medial thalamic nuclei such as CL and other intralaminar nuclei, forming a *spinoreticular–thalamic–cortical circuit*. The polysynaptic nature of this circuitry allows for modulation of the pain signals through numerous brainstem and supraspinal afferents and efferents. In addition, the projections through intralaminar nuclei connect with many cortical areas, including the limbic prefrontal cortex. Consequently, this pathway

serves as an important route for pain perception rather than the location of the noxious stimulus.

A smaller group of nociceptive neurons located in laminae I and V to VII contribute to the *spinomesencephalic tract*, in which fibers project to the mesencephalic reticular formation, the PAG region, and superior colliculus, as well as a few collaterals to the thalamus (see Table 93.3).[71] Most of the axons ascend to the contralateral midbrain, but a prominent group from the upper cervical cord ascends ipsilaterally. Axons terminating in the PAG region contribute to pain modulation via the descending pain pathways.[74] The *spinoparabrachial tract* is a component of the spinomesencephalic tract. Fibers of this latter tract project to the parabrachial nuclei and then to the amygdala, a limbic structure serving as the center of emotion. Thus, the spinoparabrachial tract contributes to the emotional and affective component of pain.

Another pain pathway, the *spinohypothalamic–limbic tract*, arises from neurons in laminae I, V, and VIII.[71] This tract projects to the hypothalamus, the center of supraspinal autonomic control. This pathway is one mechanism through which pain affects neuroendocrine and cardiovascular outputs (see Table 93.3).

Descending Pathways of the Central Nervous System: Their Role in Pain Modulation

Basic research has identified and substantiated the central mechanisms of pain control implicating an even more potent control of nociception than the gate-control theory proposed by Melzack and Wall in the mid-1960s. Supraspinal modulation controls nociception predominantly via the midbrain and medullary structures. Higher brain centers send input to the PAG region and then continues onto the RVM, which can both facilitate or inhibit descending pain.[27] The descending pathway of pain control consists of excitatory connections that originate from the PAG region and synapse in the medulla within the nucleus raphe magnus[71,72] (see Figs. 93.2 and 93.3). Additional excitatory connections project from the PAG region to the nucleus reticularis paragigantocellularis and the lateral tegmental nucleus located in the medulla. Descending serotonergic neurons from the nucleus raphe magnus, as well as noradrenergic neurons from the lateral tegmental nucleus, have excitatory connections on the spinal interneurons in the dorsal horns.

Noradrenergic projections from the locus coeruleus also communicate with the RVM and PAG.[27,71] These spinal interneurons contain endogenous opiates and GABA (γ-aminobutyric acid), both inhibitory neuropeptides.[71] When activated, these interneurons play a role in suppressing nociceptive activity of the incoming A and C nociceptors.

Endogenous opiates such as enkephalins and endorphins have been discovered by several investigators.[74,75] Cell bodies containing enkephalin and dynorphin have been located at multiple sites. β-Endorphins have been located primarily within neurons of the hypothalamus that send axons to the PAG and RVM regions to exert analgesia via opioid receptors.[27] These enkephalin-containing neurons in the superficial dorsal horn inhibit the neurons that form the spinothalamic tract and, when activated, inhibit the transmission of nociceptive information to the higher centers of the brain. The endogenous opioids also may inhibit the sensations carried by the A and C nociceptors through both presynaptic and postsynaptic actions on the WDR and nociceptor-specific neurons.

Many of the components of endogenous cannabinoid (eCB) system have been studied for their role in pain responses and modulation. The eCB includes endogenously produced cannabinoids, their receptors, and proteins involved in their synthesis and degradation.[76,77] The contribution of the eCB to pain is indicated by the abundant distribution of CB receptors within multiple pain processing sites, including the dorsal root ganglia, spinal cord dorsal horn, brainstem, and the cortex.[78] Pain studies have focused on the presence of CB1, eCBs, and degrading enzymes within the PAG-RVM circuit, whereby analgesia is produced via PAG glutamatergic-projecting neurons and RVM ON/OFF cell signaling.[78] Cannabinoids injected centrally into the descending pain pathway at locations known to induce opioid-mediated analgesia such as the dorsolateral PAG, dorsal raphe nucleus, or RVM have been shown to produce antinociceptive effects.[79] Although the three identified CB receptors (CB1, CB2, and GPR55) contribute to nociceptive signaling and pain, they differ from one another in their potential for exerting psychotropic effects and immunomodulatory actions. The CB1 receptor binds the primary psychoactive constituent in *Cannabis* sativa, (-)-Δ^9-tetrahydrocannabinol (Δ^9-THC), which has known analgesic properties.[80,81] CB1 receptor is constituently expressed in high levels in the CNS, whereas the CB2 receptor expression is limited but upregulates after injury or during inflammation.[82,83] Systemic administration of CB2 receptor agonists elicited short-term antinociception in a model of migraine[84] inhibited pain behaviors after cortical contusion in mice and in models of peripheral inflammatory and neuropathic pain. The G protein–coupled receptor 55 (GPR55) has a wide distribution in the CNS, including expression in hippocampus, thalamus, and regions of the midbrain.[85] Although CB ligands activate the GPR55, there is responsiveness to a lysophospholipid, non-CB ligand, L-α-lysophosphatidylinositol (LPI).[86] Microinjection of the GPR55 ligand LPI in the PAG region is pronociceptive,[87] in which blockade exerts antinociception actions.

Higher Cortical Centers: Their Role in the Affective Dimension of Pain

As discussed previously, there is an unpleasant, emotional aspect to pain, a psychological phenomenon termed *secondary affect*.[73,88] Multiple mechanisms contribute to this affect. First, as discussed previously, parallel-serial spinal projections carrying pain information to lower brainstem and limbic structures contribute to activation of arousal, autonomic, and somatomotor systems.[27,71,88] Second, there are parallel serial spinal projections to thalamic nuclei with both specific and widespread cortical projections. The medial thalamic nuclei, such as intralaminar and CL nuclei, project pain signals to prefrontal, insular, anterior cingulate, and posterior parietal cortices, whereas lateral thalamic nuclei, such as VPL nuclei, project predominantly to the primary

and secondary somatosensory (SI and SII) cortices.[71] Third, many cortical regions receive direct or indirect input from the numerous pain pathways. Fourth, research has revealed a global and bilateral integration of the brain regions mediating pain processing. For example, SI and SII, cortices highly involved in the localization and discrimination of pain, project to limbic cortical and subcortical regions (corticolimbic pathway), including many of the same regions that receive input directly from the ascending spinal pain pathways.[89] Neuroimaging studies of brain regions in combination with psychophysical assessment of pain revealed that the perception of stimulus intensity involves diverse cortices such as those important in somatosensory processing (SI, SII, and the posterior insular cortex), motor processing (including the cerebellum, basal ganglia, supplementary motor cortex, and anterior cingulate cortex), affective and autonomic processing (the anterior cingulate and insular cortices), and attentional processing so as to assign response priorities (the anterior cingulate, SI, and premotor cortex).[89–93] Many of these brain regions are activated bilaterally by nociceptive stimuli.[93,94] Even the expectation of pain seems to have an effect on the processing of nonpainful somatosensory stimulation in many of these cortical regions. In summary, localization of pain, unpleasantness from the intensity of the pain, and the psychological and emotional aspects of pain are linked through numerous somatosensory, motor, and limbic cortical and subcortical centers. The involvement of the motor cortices in these global circuits and the potential for an impact on motor processing should be of interest to clinicians.

CENTRAL SENSITIZATION: MECHANISMS

The phenomenon of central sensitization is defined as adaptations within the CNS to external or internal stimuli that are characterized by (1) abnormal pain responses such as hyperalgesia or allodynia; (2) diverse biochemical and cellular adjustments, including altered neurotransmitter, receptor, or ion channel expression; or (3) changes in the structure and functional properties of neurons.[95] Changes in the synaptic network involving the afferent nociceptor neurons and second-order transmission neurons are signs of persistent CNS changes that lead to sensitization.[96] Two distinct forms of central sensitization have been described: activity dependent and transcription dependent.[66,95] The activity-dependent form is a rapid central response induced by afferent nociceptor input that produces short-lasting synaptic changes, in turn enhancing synaptic transmission in the spinal cord.[66,97] Such changes may be an immediate response to activity-induced excitatory facilitation and diminished inhibition.[98] The transcription-dependent form refers to a slow induction of central changes in synaptic transmission distinguished by prolonged effects in which neuroplasticity may outlast the initial input or require low-threshold peripheral drive.[66,98]

Among the proposed mechanisms of central sensitization accounting for persistent pain are changes in calcium permeability, receptor overexpression, and synapse location[67,99] but also disrupted circuitry and transmitter imbalances within descending facilitation and inhibition (Fig. 93.4).[99] Cortical and subcortical maladaptive plasticity has also been proposed to underlie central sensitization.[99] Altered synaptic spine density, or axonal degeneration or regeneration and aberrant connectivity, along with changes in glial function affect nociceptive molecular signaling and in turn contribute to the persistence of pain.[98] A good deal of progress has been made over the past decade into providing evidence for the presence of central sensitization and identifying postulated cellular and molecular mechanisms responsible for such neuroplasticity.[100] With steadfast progress into the examination of underlying pathophysiologic mechanisms of central sensitization, clinical and basic science research will ultimately lead to improved pharmacologic interventions for chronic pain.

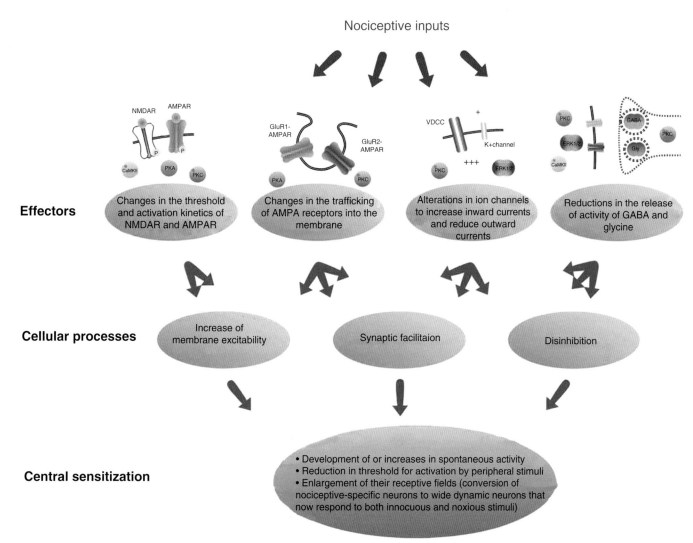

Fig. 93.4 Multiple cellular processes lead to central sensitization. Central sensitization is not defined by activation of a single molecular pathway but rather represents the altered functional status of nociceptive neurons. During central sensitization, these neurons display one or all of the following: i, development of or an increase in spontaneous activity; ii, reduction in threshold for activation; and iii, enlargement of nociceptive neuron receptive fields. These characteristics can be produced by several different cellular processes, including increases in membrane excitability, a facilitation of synaptic strength, and decreases in inhibitory transmission (disinhibition). Similarly, these mechanisms can be driven by different molecular effectors, including protein kinase A (PKA), protein kinase C (PKC), calcium/calmodulin dependent protein kinase II (CaMKII), and extracellular signal related kinase 1 and 2 (ERK1/2). These kinases participate in changes in the threshold and activation kinetics of N-methyl-D-aspartate receptor (NMDA) and α-amino-3-hydroxy-5-methyl-4-isoxazolepropionic acid receptor (AMPAR), and in their trafficking to the membrane, cause alterations in ion channels that increase inward currents and reduce outward currents and reduce the release or activity of GABA (γ-aminobutyric acid) and glycine. (Adapted from Latremoliere A, Woolf CJ. Central sensitization: a generator of pain hypersensitivity by central neural plasticity. *J Pain.* 2009;10(9):895-926.r)

SUMMARY

The information provided in this chapter regarding nociception, the transmission of nociceptive input, and the mechanisms involved in pain modulation should serves as a basis for clinical decision making. Further investigations into the neuroscience of pain are required to uncover additional information regarding pain pathways and control mechanisms. Clinicians must consider the source of pain mediation, the clinical assessment of pain, and the proposed mechanism of pain modulation when selecting an intervention and establishing a plan of care. The clinician should then form a hypothesis regarding the nature of the pain, the related symptoms, and the expected outcome of treatment.

REFERENCES

1. Woller SA, Eddinger KA, Corr M, Yaksh TL. An overview of pathways encoding nociception. *Clin Exp Rheumatol.* 2017;35 suppl 107(5):40–46.

2. Taneja A, Della Pasqua O, Danhof M. Challenges in translational drug research in neuropathic and inflammatory pain: the prerequisites for a new paradigm. *Eur J Clin Pharmacol.* 2017;73(10):1219–1236.

3. Xin DL, Hadrevi J, Elliott ME, et al. Effectiveness of conservative interventions for sickness and pain behaviors induced by a high repetition high force upper extremity task. *BMC Neurosci.* 2017;18(1):36.

4. Jain NX, Barr-Gillespie AE, Clark BD, et al. Bone loss from high repetitive high force loading is prevented by ibuprofen treatment. *J Musculoskelet Neuronal Interact.* 2014;14(1):78–94.

5. Kosek E, Cohen M, Baron R, et al. Do we need a third mechanistic descriptor for chronic pain states? *Pain.* 2016;157(7):1382–1386.

6. Granan LP. We do not need a third mechanistic descriptor for chronic pain states! Not yet. *Pain.* 2017;158(1):179.

7. Sindrup SH, Holbech J, Demant D, Finnerup NB, Bach FW, Jensen TS. Impact of etiology and duration of pain on pharmacological treatment effects in painful polyneuropathy. *Eur J Pain.* 2017;21(8):1443–1450.

8. Spiegel DR, Pattison A, Lyons A, et al. The role and treatment implications of peripheral and central processing of pain, pruritus, and nausea in heightened somatic awareness: a review. *Innov Clin Neurosci.* 2017;14(5-6):11–20.

9. van Hecke O, Austin SK, Khan RA, Smith BH, Torrance N. Neuropathic pain in the general population: a systematic review of epidemiological studies. *Pain.* 2014;155(4):654–662.

10. Voscopoulos C, Lema M. When does acute pain become chronic? *Br J Anaesth.* 2010;105(suppl 1):i69–i85.

11. St John Smith E. Advances in understanding nociception and neuropathic pain. *J Neurol.* 2017.

12. Gold MS, Gebhart GF. Nociceptor sensitization in pain pathogenesis. *Nat Med.* 2010;16(11):1248–1257.

13. Dubin AE, Patapoutian A. Nociceptors: the sensors of the pain pathway. *J Clin Invest.* 2010;120(11):3760–3772.

14. Benard J, Bettan-Renaud L, Gavoille A, et al. In vitro chemical eradication of small cell lung cancer: application in autologous bone marrow transplantation. *Eur J Cancer Clin Oncol.* 1988;24(10):1561–1566.

15. Emery EC, Luiz AP, Sikandar S, Magnusdottir R, Dong X, Wood JN. In vivo characterization of distinct modality-specific subsets of somatosensory neurons using GCaMP. *Sci Adv.* 2016;2(11):e1600990.

16. Basbaum AI, Bautista DM, Scherrer G, Julius D. Cellular and molecular mechanisms of pain. *Cell.* 2009;139(2):267–284.

17. Yan YY, Li CY, Zhou L, Ao LY, Fang WR, Li YM. Research progress of mechanisms and drug therapy for neuropathic pain. *Life Sci.* 2017;190:68–77.

18. Hassan I, Haji ML. Understanding itch: an update on mediators and mechanisms of pruritus. *Indian J Dermatol Venereol Leprol.* 2014;80(2):106–114.

19. Chandran V, Coppola G, Nawabi H, et al. A systems-level analysis of the peripheral nerve intrinsic axonal growth program. *Neuron.* 2016;89(5):956–970.

20. Chandran GT, Li X, Ogata A, Penner RM. Electrically transduced sensors based on nanomaterials (2012-2016). *Anal Chem.* 2017;89(1):249–275.

21. Lewin GR, Lechner SG, Smith ES. Nerve growth factor and nociception: from experimental embryology to new analgesic therapy. *Handb Exp Pharmacol.* 2014;220:251–282.

22. Lewin GR, Nykjaer A. Pro-neurotrophins, sortilin, and nociception. *Eur J Neurosci.* 2014;39(3):363–374.

23. Fedorczyk JM, Barr AE, Rani S, et al. Exposure-dependent increases in IL-1beta, substance P, CTGF, and tendinosis in flexor digitorum tendons with upper extremity repetitive strain injury. *J Orthop Res.* 2010;28(3):298–307.

24. Frara N, Fisher PW, Zhao Y, et al. Substance P increases CCN2 dependent on TGF-beta yet Collagen Type I via TGF-beta1 dependent and independent pathways in tenocytes. *Connect Tissue Res.* 2017:1–15.

25. Elliott MB, Barr AE, Clark BD, Wade CK, Barbe MF. Performance of a repetitive task by aged rats leads to median neuropathy and spinal cord inflammation with associated sensorimotor declines. *Neuroscience.* 2010;170(3):929–941.

26. Mandadi S, Hong P, Tran MA, et al. Identification of multisegmental nociceptive afferents that modulate locomotor circuits in the neonatal mouse spinal cord. *J Comp Neurol.* 2013;521(12):2870–2887.

27. Ossipov MH, Morimura K, Porreca F. Descending pain modulation and chronification of pain. *Curr Opin Support Palliat Care.* 2014;8(2):143–151.

28. Lucas S, Hoffman JM, Bell KR, Dikmen S. A prospective study of prevalence and characterization of headache following mild traumatic brain injury. *Cephalalgia Int J Headache.* 2013.

29. Theeler B, Lucas S, Riechers 2nd RG, Ruff RL. Post-traumatic headaches in civilians and military personnel: a comparative, clinical review. *Headache.* 2013;53(6):881–900.

30. Theeler BJ, Flynn FG, Erickson JC. Headaches after concussion in US soldiers returning from Iraq or Afghanistan. *Headache.* 2010;50(8):1262–1272.

31. Hoffman JM, Lucas S, Dikmen S, et al. Natural history of headache after traumatic brain injury. *J Neurotrauma.* 2011;28(9):1719–1725.

32. Lucas S. Headache management in concussion and mild traumatic brain injury. *PM R J Inj Funct Rehabil.* 2011;3(10 suppl 2):S406–S412.

33. Seifert TD. Sports concussion and associated post-traumatic headache. *Headache.* 2013;53(5):726–736.

34. Headache Classification Committee of the International Headache S. The International Classification of Headache Disorders, 3rd edition (beta version). *Cephalalgia Int J Headache.* 2013;33(9):629–808.

35. Ofek H, Defrin R. The characteristics of chronic central pain after traumatic brain injury. *Pain.* 2007;131(3):330–340.

36. Burstein R, Yarnitsky D, Goor-Aryeh I, Ransil BJ, Bajwa ZH. An association between migraine and cutaneous allodynia. *Ann Neurol.* 2000;47(5):614–624.

37. Burstein R, Jakubowski M, Garcia-Nicas E, et al. Thalamic sensitization transforms localized pain into widespread allodynia. *Ann Neurol.* 2010;68(1):81–91.

38. Elliott MB, Oshinsky ML, Amenta PS, Awe OO, Jallo JI. Nociceptive neuropeptide increases and periorbital allodynia in a model of traumatic brain injury. *Headache.* 2012;52(6):966–984.

39. Macolino CM, Daiutolo BV, Alberston BK, Elliott MB. Mechanical allodynia induced by traumatic brain injury is independent of restraint stress. *J Neurosci Methods.* 2014.

40. Recober A, Kuburas A, Zhang Z, Wemmie JA, Anderson MG, Russo AF. Role of calcitonin gene-related peptide in light-aversive behavior: implications for migraine. *J Neurosci.* 2009;29(27):8798–8804.

41. Daiutolo BV, Tyburski A, Clark SW, Elliott MB. Trigeminal pain molecules, allodynia, and photosensitivity are pharmacologically and genetically modulated in a model of traumatic brain injury. *J Neurotrauma.* 2016;33(8):748–760.

42. Bernstein C, Burstein R. Sensitization of the trigeminovascular pathway: perspective and implications to migraine pathophysiology. *J Clin Neurol.* 2012;8(2):89–99.

43. Benromano T, Defrin R, Ahn AH, Zhao J, Pick CG, Levy D. Mild closed head injury promotes a selective trigeminal hypernociception: implications for the acute emergence of post-traumatic headache. *Eur J Pain.* 2015;19(5):621–628.

44. Feliciano DP, Sahbaie P, Shi X, Klukinov M, Clark JD, Yeomans DC. Nociceptive sensitization and BDNF up-regulation in a rat model of traumatic brain injury. *Neurosci Lett.* 2014;583:55–59.

45. Mustafa G, Hou J, Tsuda S, et al. Trigeminal neuroplasticity underlies allodynia in a preclinical model of mild closed head traumatic brain injury (cTBI). *Neuropharmacology.* 2016;107:27–39.

46. Levy D, Edut S, Baraz-Goldstein R, et al. Responses of dural mast cells in concussive and blast models of mild traumatic brain injury in mice: potential implications for post-traumatic headache. *Cephalalgia Int J Headache.* 2016;36(10):915–923.

47. Bree D, Levy D. Development of CGRP-dependent pain and headache related behaviours in a rat model of concussion: implications for mechanisms of post-traumatic headache. *Cephalalgia Int J Headache.* 2016.

48. Tyburski A, Cheng L, Assari S, Darvish K, Elliott M. Frequent mild head injury promotes trigeminal sensitivity concomitant with microglial proliferation, astrocytosis, and increased neuropeptide levels in the trigeminal pain system. *J Headache Pain.* 2017. [in press].

49. Woolf CJ, Salter MW. Neuronal plasticity: increasing the gain in pain. *Science.* 2000;288(5472):1765–1769.

50. Amenta PS, Jallo JI, Tuma RF, Elliott MB. A cannabinoid type 2 receptor agonist attenuates blood-brain barrier damage and neurodegeneration in a murine model of traumatic brain injury. *J Neurosci Res.* 2012.

51. Amenta PS, Jallo JI, Tuma RF, Hooper DC, Elliott MB. Cannabinoid receptor type-2 stimulation, blockade, and deletion alters the vascular inflammatory responses to traumatic brain injury. *J Neuroinflamm.* 2014;11(1):191.

52. Woolf CJ, Ma Q. Nociceptors--noxious stimulus detectors. *Neuron.* 2007;55(3):353–364.

53. Benromano T, Defrin R, Ahn AH, Zhao J, Pick CG, Levy D. Mild closed head injury promotes a selective trigeminal hypernociception: implications for the acute emergence of post-traumatic headache. *Eur J Pain.* 2014.

54. Levy D, Kainz V, Burstein R, Strassman AM. Mast cell degranulation distinctly activates trigemino-cervical and lumbosacral pain pathways and elicits widespread tactile pain hypersensitivity. *Brain Behav Immun.* 2012;26(2):311–317.

55. Levy D, Burstein R. The vascular theory of migraine: leave it or love it? *Ann Neurol.* 2011;69(4):600–601.

56. Goadsby PJ, Edvinsson L, Ekman R. Vasoactive peptide release in the extracerebral circulation of humans during migraine headache. *Ann Neurol.* 1990;28(2):183–187.

57. Recober A, Goadsby PJ. Calcitonin gene-related peptide: a molecular link between obesity and migraine? *Drug News Perspect.* 2010;23(2):112–117.

58. Edvinsson L, Mulder H, Goadsby PJ, Uddman R. Calcitonin gene-related peptide and nitric oxide in the trigeminal ganglion: cerebral vasodilatation from trigeminal nerve stimulation involves mainly calcitonin gene-related peptide. *J Auton Nerv Syst.* 1998;70(1-2):15–22.

59. Hazra A, Macolino C, Elliott MB, Chin J. Delayed thalamic astrocytosis and disrupted sleep-wake patterns in a preclinical model of traumatic brain injury. *J Neurosci Res.* 2014. [in press].

60. Akerman S, Kaube H, Goadsby PJ. Vanilloid type 1 receptors (VR1) on trigeminal sensory nerve fibres play a minor role in neurogenic dural vasodilatation, and are involved in capsaicin-induced dural dilation. *Br J Pharmacol.* 2003;140(4):718–724.

61. Meents JE, Neeb L, Reuter U. TRPV1 in migraine pathophysiology. *Trends Mol Med.* 2010;16(4):153–159.

62. Tyburski AL, Cheng L, Assari S, Darvish K, Elliott MB. Frequent mild head injury promotes trigeminal sensitivity concomitant with microglial proliferation, astrocytosis, and increased neuropeptide levels in the trigeminal pain system. *J Headache Pain.* 2017;18(1):16.

63. Onyszchuk G, LeVine SM, Brooks WM, Berman NE. Post-acute pathological changes in the thalamus and internal capsule in aged mice following controlled cortical impact injury: a magnetic resonance imaging, iron histochemical, and glial immunohistochemical study. *Neurosci Lett.* 2009;452(2):204–208.

64. Hall ED, Bryant YD, Cho W, Sullivan PG. Evolution of post-traumatic neurodegeneration after controlled cortical impact traumatic brain injury in mice and rats as assessed by the de Olmos silver and fluorojade staining methods. *J Neurotrauma.* 2008;25(3):235–247.

65. Hall KD, Lifshitz J. Diffuse traumatic brain injury initially attenuates and later expands activation of the rat somatosensory whisker circuit concomitant with neuroplastic responses. *Brain Res.* 2010;1323: 161–173.

66. Latremoliere A, Woolf CJ. Central sensitization: a generator of pain hypersensitivity by central neural plasticity. *J Pain.* 2009;10(9):895–926.

67. Lacagnina MJ, Watkins LR, Grace PM. Toll-like receptors and their role in persistent pain. *Pharmacol Ther.* 2017.

68. Kiguchi N, Kobayashi D, Saika F, Matsuzaki S, Kishioka S. Pharmacological regulation of neuropathic pain driven by inflammatory macrophages. *Int J Mol Sci.* 2017;18(11).

69. Al-Shatti T, Barr AE, Safadi FF, Amin M, Barbe MF. Increase in inflammatory cytokines in median nerves in a rat model of repetitive motion injury. *J Neuroimmunol.* 2005;167(1-2):13–22.

70. Feng B, Gebhart GF. Characterization of silent afferents in the pelvic and splanchnic innervations of the mouse colorectum. *Am J Physiol Gastrointest Liver Physiol.* 2011;300(1):G170–G180.

71. Bourne S, Machado AG, Nagel SJ. Basic anatomy and physiology of pain pathways. *Neurosurg Clin N Am.* 2014;25(4):629–638.

72. Boadas-Vaello P, Castany S, Homs J, Alvarez-Perez B, Deulofeu M, Verdu E. Neuroplasticity of ascending and descending pathways after somatosensory system injury: reviewing knowledge to identify neuropathic pain therapeutic targets. *Spinal Cord.* 2016;54(5):330–340.

73. Garland EL. Pain processing in the human nervous system: a selective review of nociceptive and biobehavioral pathways. *Prim Care.* 2012;39(3):561–571.

74. Lau BK, Vaughan CW. Descending modulation of pain: the GABA disinhibition hypothesis of analgesia. *Curr Opin Neurobiol.* 2014;29:159–164.

75. Agarwal N, Pacher P, Tegeder I, et al. Cannabinoids mediate analgesia largely via peripheral type 1 cannabinoid receptors in nociceptors. *Nat Neurosci.* 2007;10(7):870–879.

76. Zogopoulos P, Vasileiou I, Patsouris E, Theocharis SE. The role of endocannabinoids in pain modulation. *Fundam Clin Pharmacol.* 2013;27(1):64–80.

77. Mechoulam R. Endocannabinoids and psychiatric disorders: the road ahead. *Rev Bras Psiquiatr.* 2010;32(suppl 1):S5–S6.

78. Palazzo E, Luongo L, Novellis V, Rossi F, Maione S. The role of cannabinoid receptors in the descending modulation of pain. *Pharmaceuticals (Basel).* 2010;3(8):2661–2673.

79. Mendiguren A, Aostri E, Pineda J. Regulation of noradrenergic and serotonergic systems by cannabinoids: relevance to cannabinoid-induced effects. *Life Sci.* 2017.

80. Mechoulam R, Hanus LO, Pertwee R, Howlett AC. Early phytocannabinoid chemistry to endocannabinoids and beyond. *Nat Rev Neurosci.* 2014;15(11):757–764.

81. Turcotte D, Le Dorze JA, Esfahani F, Frost E, Gomori A, Namaka M. Examining the roles of cannabinoids in pain and other therapeutic indications: a review. *Expert Opin Pharmacother.* 2010;11(1):17–31.

82. Ashton JC. The use of knockout mice to test the specificity of antibodies for cannabinoid receptors. *Hippocampus.* 2011.

83. Atwood BK, Mackie K. CB2: a cannabinoid receptor with an identity crisis. *Br J Pharmacol.* 2010;160(3):467–479.

84. Greco R, Mangione AS, Sandrini G, Nappi G, Tassorelli C. Activation of CB2 receptors as a potential therapeutic target for migraine: evaluation in an animal model. *J Headache Pain.* 2014;15:14.

85. Henstridge CM. Off-target cannabinoid effects mediated by GPR55. *Pharmacology.* 2012;89(3-4):179–187.

86. Kotsikorou E, Sharir H, Shore DM, et al. Identification of the GPR55 antagonist binding site using a novel set of high-potency GPR55 selective ligands. *Biochemistry.* 2013;52(52):9456–9469.

87. Deliu E, Sperow M, Console-Bram L, et al. The Lysophosphatidylinositol Receptor GPR55 Modulates Pain Perception in the Periaqueductal Gray. *Molecul Pharmacol.* 2015;88(2):265–272.

88. Villemure C, Schweinhardt P. Supraspinal pain processing: distinct roles of emotion and attention. *Neuroscientist.* 2010;16(3):276–284.

89. Quintero GC. Advances in cortical modulation of pain. *J Pain Res.* 2013;6:713–725.

90. Bogdanov VB, Vigano A, Noirhomme Q, et al. Cerebral responses and role of the prefrontal cortex in conditioned pain modulation: an fMRI study in healthy subjects. *Behav Brain Res.* 2015;281:187–198.

91. Xie YF, Huo FQ, Tang JS. Cerebral cortex modulation of pain. *Acta Pharmacol Sin.* 2009;30(1):31–41.

92. Becker S, Gandhi W, Schweinhardt P. Cerebral interactions of pain and reward and their relevance for chronic pain. *Neurosci Lett.* 2012;520(2):182–187.

93. Alomar S, Bakhaidar M. Neuroimaging of neuropathic pain: review of current status and future directions. *Neurosurg Rev.* 2016.

94. Oertel BG, Preibisch C, Martin T, et al. Separating brain processing of pain from that of stimulus intensity. *Hum Brain Mapp.* 2012;33(4):883–894.

95. Woolf CJ. Central sensitization: implications for the diagnosis and treatment of pain. *Pain.* 2011;152(suppl 3):S2–S15.

96. Woolf CJ. What is this thing called pain? *J Clin Invest.* 2010;120(11):3742–3744.

97. Woolf CJ. Central sensitization: uncovering the relation between pain and plasticity. *Anesthesiology.* 2007;106(4):864–867.

98. Kuner R. Central mechanisms of pathological pain. *Nat Med.* 2010;16(11):1258–1266.

99. Meacham K, Shepherd A, Mohapatra DP, Haroutounian S. Neuropathic pain: central vs. peripheral mechanisms. *Curr Pain Headache Rep.* 2017;21(6):28.

100. Roussel NA, Nijs J, Meeus M, Mylius V, Fayt C, Oostendorp R. Central sensitization and altered central pain processing in chronic low back pain: fact or myth? *Clin J Pain.* 2013;29(7):625–638.

94

Pain Assessment

Kenneth A. Taylor, Jane M. Fedorczyk

OUTLINE

CRITICAL POINTS

- Pain is multidimensional; more than one test or measure may be needed in the examination.
- Pain may be the cause or the result of other musculoskeletal impairments, so both examination and plan of care should address these relationships.
- Identifying the predominant pain mechanism assists the therapists in developing an appropriate plan of care.

- Psychosocial factors have a significant association with pain intensity and outcomes in overall musculoskeletal pain, as well as in upper extremity rehabilitation–specific populations.
- High pain intensity at initial onset is predictive of developing persistent pain and complex regional pain syndrome.

The International Association for the Study of Pain (IASP) defines pain as "an unpleasant sensory and emotional experience associated with actual or potential tissue damage, or described in terms of such damage."[1] This definition originated in 1979[2] and rightfully places emphasis on pain as an experience that is influenced by both sensory and affective processes. However, a significant amount of research on pain has been done since the inception of the IASP's definition of pain, and many researchers have proposed revisions to this definition, citing that it should include cognitive and social components.[3] Furthermore, some proponents of a more updated definition argue an embodied view of pain, defining pain in terms of action rather than perception—"an experience that, as part of a protective strategy, attempts to defend one's *self* in the presence of inferred threat."[4]

Pain is the primary reason that patients seek medical attention. The underlying mechanisms that lead to pain are complex and multidimensional; for a review of these mechanisms, refer to Chapter 93. This complex interplay between environmental, biological, psychological, sociological, and evolutionary drivers results in different individual experiences for each patient who may have had a similar injury or surgery. Additionally, understanding that pain is a multidimensional experience and not solely driven by tissue damage or nociception (even in cases when nociception may be the dominant driver) should help clinicians to reconcile wild variations in objective clinical observations and patient self-report. Appreciating that the experience of pain is highly variable, it is often necessary to collect more than one test or measure regarding pain.

Pain is a common complaint encountered by rehabilitation professionals across all settings and specialties. Although pain is often related to neuromusculoskeletal dysfunction, ruling out signs and symptoms of more sinister pathology is of utmost importance. Individuals presenting with complaints of pain may have underlying pathology related to the neuromuscular, pulmonary, cardiovascular, integumentary,

metabolic, or endocrine systems. Furthermore, the presence of pain at any stage of chronicity or healing may result in significant changes in muscle performance, range of motion (ROM), overall quality of motion, edema, or sensory discrimination. Because of these changes, individuals with pain may experience an altered ability to perform activities of daily living and work-related activities and participate in sports or leisure activities. In turn, these limitations may adversely impact the individual's overall quality of life. Because pain is a highly individual and multifactorial experience that can significantly impede quality of life and overall function and, in some cases, be related to serious and sinister pathology, pain assessment should always be included in a comprehensive regional examination along with appropriate medical screening. Appropriate assessment of pain will help direct interventions for pain management or alleviation, targeted at the underlying dominant mechanism(s).

CLINICAL ASSESSMENT OF PAIN

Despite pain typically being an unpleasant experience for the individual, it serves as an evolutionary, adaptive mechanism to protect the individual and ideally results in a modification of behavior that will be helpful in recovery from or prevention of injury or pathology. Although most aches and pains seen by clinicians in a rehabilitation setting are likely to be neuromusculoskeletal in nature, the initial goal of pain assessment should be to rule out the likelihood of pain from more sinister or serious pathology.

Referred pain is pain that occurs at a site remote from the source of disease or injury. The onset, duration, and perception of pain largely depend on the primary cause.[5] Referred pain from pathology or injury to visceral structures occurs as a result of convergence of visceral and peripheral nociception on the same common nerve root of the spinal cord (Fig. 94.1).[6,7] In the upper limb, referred pain is generally

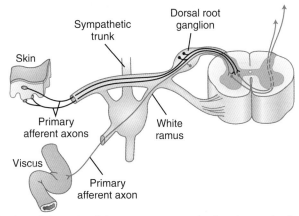

Fig. 94.1 Schematic of the convergence-projection theory of referred pain.

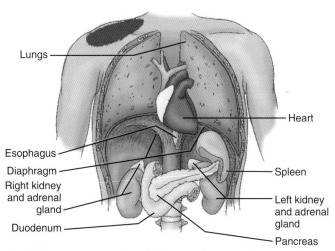

Fig. 94.2 Direct pressure from inflamed, infected, or obstructed organs near the diaphragm can refer pain to the ipsilateral shoulder. (From Goodman CC, Snyder TEK, eds. *Differential Diagnosis for Physical Therapists: Screening for Referral.* 4th ed. St. Louis: Saunders Elsevier; 2007.)

limited by visceral structures to the shoulder girdle region (Fig. 94.2). An inflamed, infected, ischemic, or obstructed heart, lungs, spleen, pancreas, or gallbladder may apply direct pressure to the diaphragm and refer pain to the shoulder. The gallbladder is on the right side of the diaphragm and may refer pain to the right shoulder. The heart and spleen may refer pain the left shoulder. The location of the pancreas allows it to refer pain to either shoulder. The connection here is that the diaphragm is innervated by the phrenic nerve, which is composed of cervical nerve roots C3 to C5. The shoulder cutaneous area is also innervated by nerve roots C4 and C5.[6] Recording vital signs and asking appropriate screening questions regarding the cardiovascular, pulmonary, endocrine, and gastrointestinal systems should be included at a minimum to rule out the likelihood of non-neuromusculoskeletal dysfunction that may be presenting in a neuromusculoskeletal fashion.

Additionally, pain in the upper limb may be referred because of an inflammatory or compressive insult to the cervical nerve roots. The cervical nerve roots C4, C5, C6, C7, and C8 may refer pain to the shoulder, elbow, forearm, or hand on the ipsilateral side.[6,8] This is further discussed in the section on peripheral neuropathic pain.

Traditional Classification of Pain

In classifying pain, clinicians traditionally have used a temporal-based classification system based on assumed tissue healing over time. Readers will be familiar with this process of identifying pain as acute, subacute, or chronic. Within this traditional taxonomy, *acute* pain is pain that lasts from days to weeks. Pain that lasts from more than 1 week up to 3 months may be classified as *subacute*, and pain lasting longer than 3 to 6 months is considered *chronic*. However, this specific taxonomy for classifying pain carries forward the outdated Cartesian idea of pain being an input from peripheral tissue, placing an emphasis on the healing of that tissue as the driver of pain rather than approaching pain as a multidimensional-dependent output of an individual's nervous system. This view is problematic in evidence-based health care because the nociception is not necessary for pain to be experienced, nor is it sufficient in and of itself to produce a pain experience.[9,10] Pain is not a good indicator of tissue status. Furthermore, the assumption with the traditional tissue-based temporal classification of pain is that acute pain is assumed to be driven by peripheral tissue status to protect the local tissue and chronic pain is assumed driven by maladaptive processing with almost mutual exclusivity. There is evidence to challenge this belief that maladaptive processing and acute pain are mutually exclusive and that individuals who have traditionally been classified as having acute pain have a much more heterogeneous presentation than is implied by the use of this traditional classification for musculoskeletal pain.[11] Central neurophysiological mechanisms drive the pain state for a subgroup of individuals with acute pain, such as those with acute or subacute whiplash,[12,13] osteoarthritis,[14,15] rheumatoid arthritis,[14,16] and other diagnoses. If these central mechanisms are the dominant driver of an individual's pain state, then interventions that are traditionally used for acute-type pain are unlikely to be effective or will have notably less efficacy. The classification of pain as acute, subacute, or chronic may not help clinicians in the selection of successful interventions to relieve or manage pain. Although this traditional classification remains a useful descriptor for summarizing temporal aspects of pain, an alternate taxonomy or classification of pain will be presented based on identifying the dominant driver of the individual's pain state, which is more likely to help clinicians select appropriate interventions, regardless of time since pain onset.

Mechanism-Based Classification of Pain

A mechanism-based classification approach has been proposed by several different authors[17–24] as an alternative to the traditional temporal-based classification to better inform pain management interventions (see Chapter 96). As the name implies, this approach to classifying pain focuses on identifying the dominant neurophysiological mechanism that is driving the individual's pain experience. Within this framework, there are three predominant mechanisms: nociception dominant, peripheral neuropathic dominant, and nociplastic dominant (sometimes referred to as central sensitization dominant).[18–20,25]

Nociception-Dominant Pain

A nociception-dominant pain state implies that the patient's presentation is driven by peripheral nociception. This type of pain state is typically what clinicians may think of when considering acute pain in the temporal-based taxonomy of pain. However, it is important to point out that although many acute pain states may be dominated by nociception, many people who are traditionally considered to have a chronic pain state may also have a nociception-dominant pain state as well. Box 94.1 lists signs and symptoms that can be used to identify nociception-dominant pain and signs and symptoms that are typically absent when nociception is the driving mechanism behind the individual's pain.[20]

BOX 94.1 Signs and Symptoms of Nociception-Dominant Pain

Characterized by:

Pain is localized to the area of injury or dysfunction

There is a clear proportionate mechanical or anatomical nature to aggravating and easing factors

Usually intermittent and sharp with movement or mechanical provocation and may be more of a constant dull ache or throb at rest

Typically, an absence of:

Pain in association with other dysesthesias

Night pain or disturbed sleep

Antalgic postures or movement patterns

Pain variously described as burning, shooting, sharp, or electric-like

Data from Smart KM, Blake C, Staines A, Thacker M, Doody C. Mechanisms-based classifications of musculoskeletal pain: part 3 of 3: symptoms and signs of nociceptive pain in patients with low back (+/- leg) pain. *Man Ther.* 2012;17(4):352-357.

From the typically absent signs and symptoms for nociception-dominant pain, it is important to point out that night pain, disturbed sleep, and antalgic movements may still be present in this group, especially in those with upper extremity nociception-dominant pain. For example, individuals with shoulder pain often complain of pain waking them at night that may be related to position changes or sleeping position preference.

Peripheral Neuropathic–Dominant Pain

Overall population prevalence of pain with neuropathic characteristics is estimated to be between 6.9% and 10%.[26] In 2011, the IASP altered its definition of neuropathic pain,[27] which can be seen in Table 94.1. Along with this new definition, neuropathic pain was originally clarified to contrast with nociceptive pain. This dichotomy between nociceptive pain and neuropathic pain was criticized for being too narrow and ill-fitting for patients who may not fit in either category but have a very real pain experience.[25] In 2016, an IASP task force published its recommendations[25] for changes to mechanistic descriptors of pain to avoid this dichotomy and include a third descriptor (see next section). These recommendations were adopted by the IASP in 2017.[28] Signs and symptoms of peripheral neuropathic–dominant pain are listed in Box 94.2.[19,27]

When considering the common signs and symptoms of peripheral neuropathic–dominant pain, there are a few caveats to keep in mind. Although neuroanatomically logical *pain* is typically defined as pain being referred in a dermatomal or cutaneous distribution, is important to point out that neuroanatomically logical pain from cervical nerve roots may be outside of traditionally identified dermatomes. Slipman and colleagues[8] used fluoroscopy to mechanically stimulate the cervical nerve roots of C4 to C8 and demonstrated a significant difference between dermatomal maps that most clinicians will be familiar with and what Slipman and colleagues referred to as dynatomal maps—maps of where pain was recorded during their study when mechanically stimulating each nerve root. The implication of these findings is that neuroanatomically logical *pain* should be considered pain that is referred in a dermatomal, cutaneous, or dynatomal distributions. These dynatomal maps are depicted in Figure 94.3 and are specific to pain, not sensory dysesthesias.

Nociplastic-Dominant Pain

Central sensitization is a naturally occurring phenomenon that results in significant abnormal processing in the central nervous system (CNS)

TABLE 94.1 International Association for the Study of Pain (IASP) Taxonomy

IASP TAXONOMY	
Term	**IASP Definition**
Nociception	The neural process of encoding noxious stimuli
Nociceptive pain	Pain that arises from actual or threatened damage to non-neural tissue and is caused by the activation of nociceptors
Neuropathy	A disturbance of function or pathological change in a nerve: in one nerve, mononeuropathy; in several nerves, mononeuropathy multiplex; if diffuse and bilateral, polyneuropathy
Neuropathic pain	Pain caused by a lesion or disease of the somatosensory nervous system
Central sensitization	Increased responsiveness of nociceptive neurons in the CNS to their normal or subthreshold afferent input
Nociplastic pain	Pain that arises from altered nociception despite no clear evidence of actual or threatened tissue damage causing the activation of peripheral nociceptors or evidence for disease or lesion of the somatosensory system causing the pain
Allodynia	Pain caused by a stimulus that does not normally provoke pain
Hyperalgesia	Increased pain from a stimulus that normally provokes pain

CNS, Central nervous system.

Data from IASP Taxonomy—IASP. https://www.iasp-pain.org/Taxonomy?navItemNumber=576.

BOX 94.2 Signs and Symptoms of Peripheral Neuropathic–Dominant Pain

Characterized by:

Pain that is neuroanatomically logical

Sensory dysfunction that is neuroanatomically logical

History of nerve injury, pathology, or mechanical compromise or other medical cause

Pain or symptom provocation with mechanical or movement tests (e.g., active or passive motion, neurodynamic tests) that move, load, or compress neural tissue

Pain may be described as shooting, burning, or pricking

Data from Smart KM, Blake C, Staines A, Thacker M, Doody C. Mechanisms-based classifications of musculoskeletal pain: part 2 of 3: symptoms and signs of peripheral neuropathic pain in patients with low back (+/- leg) pain. *Man Ther.* 2012;17(4):345-351.

of somatosensory input from the peripheral nervous system. As previously mentioned, the IASP recently introduced the term *nociplastic* as a descriptor to replace central sensitization. Nociplastic pain is the result of altered nociception in the absence of clear evidence of actual or threatened tissue damage (nociceptive-dominant pain) or insult or disease of the somatosensory system (neuropathic-dominant pain) related to the pain.[24] This phenomenon is associated with expansion of the receptive fields, hyperalgesia, allodynia, and prolonged pain after stimuli have been removed.[29,30] This can be a protective mechanism in acute injuries that should resolve over time. However, this altered processing may persist beyond the expected time relative to the inciting stimulus,

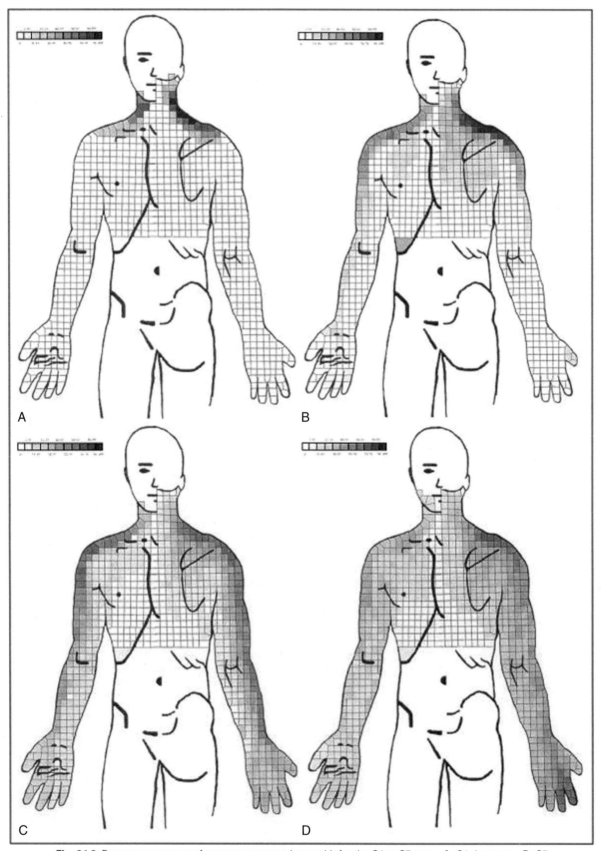

Fig. 94.3 Percent occurrence of symptom provocation per bit for the C4 to C7 roots. **A,** C4 dynatome. **B,** C5 dynatome. **C,** C6 dynatome. **D,** C7 dynatome. (From Slipman CW, Plastaras CT, Palmitier RA, Huston CW, Sterenfeld EB. Symptom provocation of fluoroscopically guided cervical nerve root stimulation. Are dynatomal maps identical to dermatomal maps? *Spine [Phila Pa 1976].* 1998;23[20]:2235-2242.)

BOX 94.3 Signs and Symptoms of Nociplastic-Dominant Pain

Characterized by:

Disproportionate, nonmechanical, unpredictable pattern of pain provocation in response to multiple or nonspecific aggravating and easing factors

Pain disproportionate to the nature and extent of injury or pathology

Strong association with maladaptive psychosocial factors (e.g., negative emotions, poor self-efficacy, maladaptive beliefs, and pain behaviors)

Diffuse or nonanatomical areas of pain or tenderness on palpation

Pain may be described as shooting, burning, or pricking

Data from Smart KM, Blake C, Staines A, Thacker M, Doody C. Mechanisms-based classifications of musculoskeletal pain: part 1 of 3: symptoms and signs of central sensitisation in patients with low back (+/- leg) pain. *Man Ther.* 2012;17(4):336-344.

resulting in ongoing neuroplastic and nociplastic changes that maintain the patient's pain experience. As time from injury or inciting stimulus increases and pain remains, the likelihood of nociplastic changes, such as central sensitization, as the predominant driver of the individual's pain state increases. However, it is of paramount importance that the reader understands that nociplastic-dominant pain is not synonymous with chronic pain and should not be regarded as such. Patients traditionally classified as having chronic pain may have a nociception-dominant or peripheral neuropathic–dominant pain state rather than a nociplastic-dominant pain state.[18,20,22] To further complicate things, it is possible for individuals to present without one clear dominant driver—more of a mixed-driver presentation.[31] Although there remains no agreed upon gold standard test for the identification of nociplastic or central sensitization–dominant pain, the Delphi-derived clinical signs and symptoms[32] that have been shown to be most predictive of central sensitization– or nociplastic-dominant pain are listed in Box 94.3.[18]

Nijs and colleagues[11] have identified additional characteristics of central sensitization: hypersensitivity to bright light, touch, noise, pesticides, mechanical pressure, medication, or temperature (high and low). Additionally there are some symptoms that might be related but are not necessarily characteristics of the presence of central sensitization that clinicians should assess: fatigue, sleep disturbances, unrefreshing sleep, concentration difficulties, feelings of swollenness in the affected body part, tingling, and numbness.[11]

The presence of central sensitization has been shown to be predictive of pain duration and intensity after surgery in those undergoing procedures for shoulder impingement syndrome[33] and spinal fusion.[34] The presence of central sensitization mediates treatment effect in individuals with chronic whiplash[35] and chronic lateral epicondylalgia[36] as well. Furthermore, the presence of central sensitization explains 40% of variance in upper limb function 1.5 years after surgery among breast cancer survivors.[37] Therefore, to provide optimal treatment, it is important to understand the dominant driver behind the patient's pain state.

Nociplastic mechanisms have been identified as being characteristic of several common diagnoses, including chronic whiplash-associated disorders, fibromyalgia, and chronic fatigue syndrome.[11] These mechanisms may be present in at least a subgroup of individuals with a particular diagnosis even if that particular diagnosis is not characterized by nociplastic mechanisms. These diagnoses with subgroups of individuals having nociplastic mechanisms as the dominant driver of their pain include osteoarthritis,[14,15] rheumatoid arthritis,[14,16] subacromial impingement syndrome,[33] myofascial pain syndrome,[14,30,38,39] chronic shoulder pain,[40] chronic lateral elbow pain,[36] nontraumatic neck pain,[41,42] postcancer pain,[37,43,44] acute and subacute whiplash,[12,13] and athletic overuse injuries.[45,46]

Although the traditional, temporal-based framework of acute, subacute, and chronic classifies patients based on time since pain onset, understanding the timeline of an individual's pain alone does not adequately inform the best approaches for treatment interventions. Clinicians should attempt to identify the dominant mechanism(s) driving the individual's pain state regardless of which temporal-based category the individual falls within to inform treatment.

IDENTIFYING THE DOMINANT DRIVER

Figure 94.4 shows an algorithm for clinical decision making when trying to assess and identify the dominant mechanism driving the individual's pain experience. If the clinician is concerned about the potential presence of sinister pathology based on the individual's subjective complaints and other objective findings, then referral to the appropriate provider for follow-up is necessary. If the individual's pain appears to be neuromusculoskeletal in nature, then the first step is ruling out peripheral neuropathic mechanisms as the dominant driver of the individual's pain state. Using the criteria described previously and in Box 94.2, the clinician should be able to differentiate whether the patient's pain fits this presentation or not. Physician providers will have additional options at their disposal to further identify peripheral neuropathic–dominant based pain that rehabilitation providers may not.[27]

If peripheral neuropathic–dominant pain has been ruled out, then the clinician can follow the algorithm further to help aide in identifying the presence of central sensitization (nociplastic pain) as the dominant driver of the individual's pain state. One tool that can be used after peripheral neuropathic–dominant pain has been ruled out is the Central Sensitization Inventory (CSI)[47] (Fig. 94.5). The CSI is a self-report measure that may be administered to identify symptoms of central sensitization. The tool has been shown to be a valid, reliable, and consistent measure and may also be used as a responsive treatment outcome measure.[48] A cutoff score of 40 points or greater on Part A of the CSI has been identified as indicative of potential presence of central sensitization as a dominant driver of the individual's pain state.[49] A score of 0 to 100 is obtained in Part A of the CSI by assigning a score of 0, 1, 2, 3, and 4 points to the individual's selection of never, rarely, sometimes, often, and always, for each of the 25 items, respectively. Part B of the CSI helps the clinician identify if the individual has been previously diagnosed by a physician with disorders specifically within the family of central sensitivity syndrome, as well as anxiety and depression (which may co-occur in those with central sensitization).[47,50] If an individual selects yes on one or more of the items in Part B, the presence of central sensitization should be considered, especially if the individual surpasses the cutoff score for Part A and signs and symptoms from Box 94.3 are present.[47] Identifying the dominant driver of the individual's predominant pain mechanism can help inform the interventions for that specific individual (see Chapter 96).

Tests and Measures for the Clinical Assessment of Pain

When dealing with pain, it is impossible to separate an individual's pain experience from the person her- or himself. Any attempt to collect clinical examination information will always involve a concomitant need for subjective response from the individual being examined. This makes quantifying pain much more difficult than ROM or strength, for example. As previously discussed, pain is a multidimensional experience. Thus, multiple different types of information regarding the individual's pain experience are needed. The selection of the appropriate measure for pain assessment depends on the aspect of pain the therapist is trying to capture. Table 94.2 associates commonly used pain measures with the appropriate dimension of pain. Many of the tools described subsequently may assess only one dimension of pain. Multidimensional tools may be more helpful because they integrate pain and other symptoms with function.

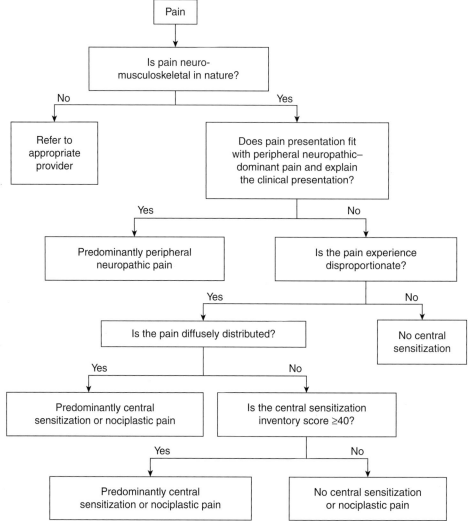

Fig. 94.4 Clinical decision-making algorithm for differentiating peripheral neuropathic-dominant pain from central sensitization—dominant pain. (Adapted Nijs J, Goubert D, Ickmans K. Recognition and treatment of central sensitization in chronic pain patients: not limited to specialized care. *J Orthop Sports Phys Ther.* 2016;46[12]:1024-1028.)

Subjective Interview Information

The therapist may ask a series of questions regarding the patient's pain experience as part of the subjective portion of the clinical examination.[51] Questions should elicit information regarding the intensity, quality, temporal, physical, and descriptive characteristics of pain and pain-related beliefs. Intensity usually is described in terms of the severity of the pain. The quality of the pain may be described as a burning, sharp, stabbing, dull, and so on. The temporal aspects of pain include whether the pain is constant or intermittent, time since initial onset of pain, and how the pain behaves over a typical 24-hour period. They also may include the time of day that the pain is better or worse and what activities seem to exacerbate or alleviate the pain. The physical characteristics of pain refer to the location of the pain and whether the pain is radiating, localized, or diffuse. When conducting the interview, the therapist needs to be careful not to ask leading questions regarding pain. Likewise, broad-based questions (e.g., "Do you have pain at all times?") also should be avoided. Box 94.4 reviews commonly asked questions during a pain interview. Additional questions or outcome measures that may lead to insight about potential maladaptive beliefs about pain should be used as well. It is important to include questions that assess patient cognitions because it has been well established that pain experience and cognitions regarding pain are interrelated.[18,52–56] Information gathered from the subjective interview will aid the clinician in formulating an initial hypothesis regarding the dominant driver of the patient's pain state.

Assessing Sleep Quality in Relation to Pain

Sleep has been identified as an important variable when considering the likelihood of a pain state persisting in chronicity. Among those patients with chronic pain disorders, sleep complaints are present in 67% to 88%.[57,58] Furthermore, of individuals diagnosed with insomnia, at least 50% also have chronic pain.[59] Of note, results of multiple prospective studies indicate sleep disturbance increases the risk of incident cases of chronic pain in individuals who are pain free, worsens the long-term prognosis of existing persistent musculoskeletal pain, and influences daily fluctuations in pain.[60] Although many clinicians tend to assume that pain leads to poorer sleep, the literature on the relationship between sleep and pain indicates that poor sleep quality and decreased total sleep may have a stronger effect on persistent pain experience than the effect of pain on these dimensions of

Central Sensitization Inventory: Part A

Please circle the best response to the right of each statement.						
1	I feel unrefreshed when I wake up in the morning.	Never	Rarely	Sometimes	Often	Always
2	My muscles feel stiff and achy.	Never	Rarely	Sometimes	Often	Always
3	I have anxiety attacks.	Never	Rarely	Sometimes	Often	Always
4	I grind or clench my teeth.	Never	Rarely	Sometimes	Often	Always
5	I have problems with diarrhea and/or constipation.	Never	Rarely	Sometimes	Often	Always
6	I need help in performing my daily activities.	Never	Rarely	Sometimes	Often	Always
7	I am sensitive to bright lights.	Never	Rarely	Sometimes	Often	Always
8	I get tired very easily when I am physically active.	Never	Rarely	Sometimes	Often	Always
9	I feel pain all over my body.	Never	Rarely	Sometimes	Often	Always
10	I have headaches.	Never	Rarely	Sometimes	Often	Always
11	I feel discomfort in my bladder and/or burning when I urinate.	Never	Rarely	Sometimes	Often	Always
12	I do not sleep well.	Never	Rarely	Sometimes	Often	Always
13	I have difficulty concentrating.	Never	Rarely	Sometimes	Often	Always
14	I have skin problems such as dryness, itchiness or rashes.	Never	Rarely	Sometimes	Often	Always
15	Stress makes my physical symptoms get worse.	Never	Rarely	Sometimes	Often	Always
16	I feel sad or depressed.	Never	Rarely	Sometimes	Often	Always
17	I have low energy.	Never	Rarely	Sometimes	Often	Always
18	I have muscle tension in my neck and shoulders.	Never	Rarely	Sometimes	Often	Always
19	I have pain in my jaw.	Never	Rarely	Sometimes	Often	Always
20	Certain smells, such as perfumes, make me feel dizzy and nauseated.	Never	Rarely	Sometimes	Often	Always
21	I have to urinate frequently.	Never	Rarely	Sometimes	Often	Always
22	My legs feel uncomfortable and restless when I am trying to go to sleep at night.	Never	Rarely	Sometimes	Often	Always
23	I have difficulty remembering things.	Never	Rarely	Sometimes	Often	Always
24	I suffered trauma as a child.	Never	Rarely	Sometimes	Often	Always
25	I have pain in my pelvic area.	Never	Rarely	Sometimes	Often	Always
					Total=	

Fig. 94.5 A, Central Sensitization Inventory (CSI), Part A. **B,** Central Sensitization Inventory (CSI), Part B. (From Mayer TG, Neblett R, Cohen H, et al. The development and psychometric validation of the central sensitization inventory. *Pain Pract.* 2012;12[4]:276-285.)

Central Sensitization Inventory: Part B

	Have you been diagnosed by a doctor with any of the following disorders? Please check the box to the right for each diagnosis and write the year of the diagnosis.	NO	YES	Year Diagnosed
1	Restless Leg Syndrome			
2	Chronic Fatigue Syndrome			
3	Fibromyalgia			
4	Temporomandibular Joint Disorder (TMJ)			
5	Migraine or tension headaches			
6	Irritable Bowel Syndrome			
7	Multiple Chemical Sensitivities			
8	Neck Injury (including whiplash)			
9	Anxiety or Panic Attacks			
10	Depression			

Fig. 94.5, cont'd

TABLE 94.2 Pain Measure Applied to the Dimension of Pain

Dimension of Pain	Pain Measure(s) Used
Spatial (location)	Pain drawings, body diagrams, or verbal descriptions
Intensity (how much)	Verbal or visual rating scales
Quality or nature	Patient interviews or self-report questionnaires
Temporal	Rating scales of worst, best, and average pain over a given time period, time since initial onset, pain behavior across a 24-hour period
Functional impairment	Self-report or specific outcome questionnaires

sleep.[60] Human and animal studies have both shown that inadequate or interrupted sleep dampens pain inhibition mehanisms.[61-63] Furthermore, restoration of good sleep increases the likelihood that persistent pain will resolve over time.[60] Aberrant glial activation from sleep disturbance resulting in glial long-term potentiation and a subsequent low-grade neuroinflammatory state has been proposed by experts as a major underlying mechanism to explain the relationship between poor sleep and the development of persistent pain states.[64]

Assessing the sleep quality and quantity of individuals in pain is important at all stages of pain assessment. Individuals with recent-onset pain may be at higher risk of developing a persistent pain state if their sleep is poor, and those who already have persistent pain states have a higher likelihood of persistent pain remission if prevalent sleep problems are addressed adequately.[60] From a clinical perspective, it is important to get a good idea of how the individual's sleep habits were before symptom onset and how they may have changed since onset. Clinicians should assess the patient's typical habits in the hours leading up to bedtime, as well as delineating how much time is spent

in bed compared with how much of the time in bed is spent sleeping. Gathering this information helps clinicians understand both the individual's sleep hygiene (habits surrounding the bedroom, sleep, and evening rituals) and his or her overall sleep efficiency (duration spent sleeping divided by the time spent in bed). The increasing prevalence of wearable technology that tracks an individual's sleep habits throughout the night may help in providing more objective assessment of these values if the individual regularly uses such technology. Using a sleep log may also aid the clinician in quantifying current sleep quality and duration and changes over the course of treatment if wearable technology is not available. The Pittsburgh Sleep Quality Index (PSQI) may be used to quantify perceived sleep quality, sleep efficiency, and daily disturbances.[65,66] The PSQI is a valid and reliable tool for screening for sleep dysfunction in clinical and nonclinical samples.[67] Strategies for improving sleep hygiene and sleep efficiency are presented in Chapter 96.

Rating Scales

Many rating scales have been suggested in the literature to measure the intensity of a patient's pain.[51,68] These rating scales are relatively quick and easy to administer. They can be presented in a verbal or visual format. Rating scales can be used as part of the initial assessment of pain as well as before, during, or after subsequent treatment sessions or procedures. However, when the dominant driver of the individual's pain experience is nociplastic in nature, constant cues from clinicians for pain attention may facilitate the maintenance of pain hypervigilance and communicate the message that the pain output is important or should be strongly monitored (which may not be the case in individuals with nociplastic-dominant pain). Facilitating pain hypervigilance may hinder rehabilitation progress and only help to maintain the abnormal processing of stimuli within the nervous system.

The information obtained from the rating scales has been criticized as being one dimensional[51] and not providing a true representation of the individual's total pain experience. The information gained from the

BOX 94.4 Commonly Asked Questions Regarding Pain During the Patient Interview

Location of Pain

Where do you feel pain? (patient may point to painful areas)

Is your pain deep (within a joint) or superficial?

Nature of Pain

Is your pain constant or intermittent?

If constant, does it vary in intensity?

If intermittent, when do you have pain?

How long does your pain last?

What is the frequency of the pain? (frequent, occasional)

How long have you had this pain?

Have you ever had pain like this before? (prior history)

Do you have pain now? (during interview)

Beliefs or Cognitions About Pain

What do you think is happening when you feel the pain?

What do you think will make your pain better?

What do you think will keep your pain from getting better?

What are your expectations regarding your recovery?

Does the pain make you afraid to move?

Behavior of Pain

Describe your pain (e.g., throbbing, aching, burning, sharp, dull).

Does the pain move or spread to other areas?

Is the pain aggravated by movement?

Is the pain aggravated by certain positions?

Can you demonstrate the movement or positions that cause pain?

Do you have stiffness associated with pain?

Describe how your pain behaves over a typical 24-hour period.

Do you have pain at rest?

Do you have pain at night or in the morning?

Does the pain wake you from sleep?

Do you have pain during activity?

Do you have pain after activity, and if so, how long after activity does it take to appear or resolve?

What makes your pain worse?

What helps to ease your pain?

What do you do to relieve the pain?

Indicate the position on the line which best describes:

	No pain	Pain as bad as it could be
How you feel right now:	⊢————————————⊣	
When you feel the best:	⊢————————————⊣	
When you feel the worst:	⊢————————————⊣	
The worst pain ever felt:	⊢————————————⊣	

Fig. 94.6 Visual analog scales from Schultz upper extremity pain assessment form. (Copyright 1993, Karen Schultz-Johnson.)

rating scales is momentary and therefore may provide the clinician with limited information regarding the effectiveness of an applied intervention in short- and long-term variations or changes in pain intensity. To administer a numerical pain rating scale (NPRS), the therapist generally asks the patient to assign a number to his or her pain intensity or to "rate the pain" on a scale of 0 to 10, with 0 referring to no pain, and 10 being the worst pain imaginable. The visual analog scale (VAS) has several modifications (Fig. 94.6). Commonly, it includes a 10-cm horizontal or vertical line that represents a range of pain intensity. The line may have no marks or descriptive words except at the ends of the line, which represent no pain at one end and the worst pain imaginable at the opposite end. Other visual scales may place more word descriptors along the continuum. The patient places a mark on the line to indicate her or his level of pain. A problem that may occur when using the rating scales is that the patient may initially start on the scale near or at the end of the scale, indicating the worst pain, and then the patient's pain experience becomes worse. In this case, the patient's response on the scale may exceed the upper limit. Additionally, patients often rate their pain on what they perceive as an average pain scale for other people, giving a much higher rating. In this case, the clinician may ask the patient to rate on her or his own 0 to 10 scale without thinking of other people's experiences.

Using rating scales, clinicians can garner information regarding the individual's pain at worst, pain at best, and pain on average over a given period (days, weeks, months). This scale can also be used to determine pain with specific activities, which may aide clinicians in identifying pain threshold or pain tolerance of the individual. Pain threshold is defined as the minimum stimulus intensity that results in pain. Pain threshold is highly reproducible in different individuals within clinical pain experiments and in the same individual at different time periods. Conversely, pain tolerance is highly variable and correlates well with the affective and cognitive components of pain. Tolerance implies a question about how much pain an individual is willing to accept in a given situation.[1] Pain tolerance may be affected by fatigue, lack of control, stress, environment, and anxiety. During examination, therapists should determine whether any of the variables that modulate pain tolerance are present.

Body Diagrams and Pain Drawings

The patient or the therapist can fill out a diagram of the human body with both front and back views. For individuals with pain specific to only the hands, an enlarged diagram of the upper quarter (Fig. 94.7) may be an appropriate alternative to a full-body diagram. This would allow more detailed information regarding the location, intensity, and quality of the pain to be illustrated specifically in the upper quarter. However, when examining a patient with longstanding pain, it may be preferable to use a full-body diagram to determine all potential pain complaints. As previously mentioned, individuals with nociplastic pain typically report diffuse, spreading pain or secondary hyperalgesia, so using a full-body diagram may allow for assessment of underlying pain

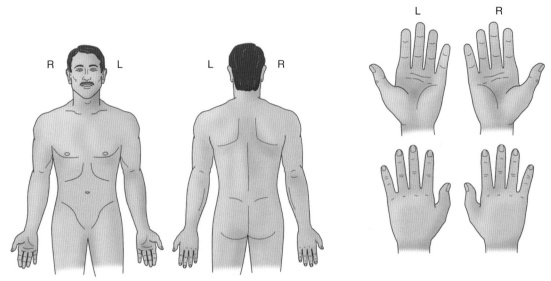

Fig. 94.7 Body diagram specifically for upper quarter pain from Schultz upper extremity pain assessment form. *L*, Left; *R*, right. (Copyright 1993, Karen Schultz-Johnson.)

mechanisms. Colored pencils, degrees of shading, or symbols can be used to represent the intensity and the quality of the pain. Numbness and other paresthesias associated with the pathologic conditions can be included in this format by using different identification markings such as dotted areas for paresthesias and cross hatches for areas of numbness. Letters such as "E" and "I" can be used to identify the pain as being located externally or internally. These would indicate that the pain is perceived as superficial or deep, respectively. Numbers may be used to give a numerical rating to the different areas of pain located on the diagram.

The McGill Pain Questionnaire

The McGill Pain Questionnaire (Fig. 94.e1) provides a comprehensive look at the multidimensional aspects of pain. A short form and a long form have been suggested for clinical use. The long form consists of four parts. One part of the questionnaire involves word descriptors that are categorized and ranked regarding quality and intensity. The patient selects only one word from each group of words. A group of words may be omitted if it does not match the patient's perception of pain. Another part includes a rating scale that could be a modified VAS or a present pain index; this consists of a numerical value being assigned to a descriptive word. The remaining parts include a body diagram and a questionnaire regarding the previously described temporal aspects of pain.[68,69]

Pressure Pain Threshold

Numerous authors have reported the reliable use of a pressure algometer (Fig. 94.8) to quantify the amount of pressure necessary to produce point tenderness as reported by the patient's report of pain with pressure.[70–73] Lower algometer scores would indicate increased point tenderness or pain sensitivity. Higher pressure tolerance scores would indicate less sensitivity. The pressure algometer may be used to measure hyperalgesia (see Table 94.1) to mechanical stimuli. Primary hyperalgesia such as point tenderness would be examined at the site of injury, and secondary hyperalgesia is examined away from the site of injury. Primary hyperalgesia is related to nociception-dominant or peripheral neuropathic–dominant pain states through peripheral sensitization of the nervous system. Secondary hyperalgesia is a sign of nociplastic

changes within the CNS that may be dominating the individual's pain state. Nociplastic mechanisms (central sensitization) have been identified in the literature using pressure algometry in individuals with carpal tunnel syndrome (CTS),[70] but the presence of secondary hyperalgesia alone does not exclude the role of other pain mechanisms.[74]

Monofilaments (Von Frey or Semmes-Weinstein) may be used to examine and map allodynia (see Table 94.1), which may be indicative of nociplastic-dominant pain. Mapping allodynia may be useful as an outcome measure during reassessment. Allodynia may be seen postoperatively along surgical scars and is commonly referred to as a hypersensitive scar; in early post-operative cases of allodynia, nociplastic changes (central sensitization) may be present as an underlying mechanism even when it is not the predominant mechanism behind the individual's pain state. Allodynia is a common symptom of complex regional pain syndrome (CRPS; for a full review of CRPS, see Chapter 97) but is often present without CRPS. The monofilaments may be applied in a graded manner just as they are used for sensibility testing. However, the response with allodynia will be painful rather than just a positive response to light touch.

Assessing Thermal Hyperalgesia

Thermal sensitivity may result from both peripheral sensitization and central sensitization after injury. Peripheral nociceptor sensitization (as within nociception-dominant pain states) often results in heat hyperalgesia, and peripheral nerve injury (peripheral neuropathic–dominant pain) is often accompanied by cold hyperalgesia over the local area of injury.[75,76] A common example of heat hyperalgesia is the case of a sunburn (nociception-dominant pain state). When a person is sunburnt, a hot shower becomes very uncomfortable and even painful depending on the water's temperature over the area of the sunburn (local to the area of tissue injury). Thermal hyperalgesia and sensitivity over the local area of injury may indicate peripheral nociceptor or nerve sensitization; however, thermal hyperalgesia and sensitivity in *uninjured* areas may indicate a nociplastic-dominant pain state (either heat or cold). Bilateral thermal hyperalgesia can be been found in some individuals with strictly unilateral CTS, and thermal pain sensitivity has been found as an important predictive factor for success in management of CTS.[77,78] Cold hyperalgesia in individuals with unilateral lateral epicondylalgia also distinguishes between individuals with more severe

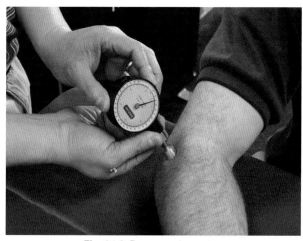

Fig. 94.8 Pressure algometer.

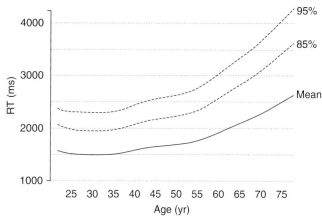

Fig. 94.9 Mean response times (RTs) for age groups with 85% and 95% cutoffs for abnormal performance when assessing left–right discrimination at the shoulders. (From Breckenridge JD, McAuley JH, Butler DS, Stewart H, Moseley GL, Ginn KA. The development of a shoulder specific left/right judgement task: validity & reliability. *Musculoskelet Sci Pract.* 2017;28[suppl C]:39-45.)

pain and disability.[79] Although studies have used expensive laboratory equipment to precisely deliver the thermal stimulus, a clinical ice pain test for cold hyperalgesia has been shown to correlate with quantitative laboratory measures.[80] Placing ice against the individual's skin for 10 seconds, a pain intensity rating of more than 5 of 10 indicated 90% likelihood of cold hyperalgesia in individuals with neck pain.[81] Although this test demonstrates promising initial utility, the use of this "low-tech" alternative test to assess cold hyperalgesia in individuals with upper extremity pain has yet to be studied at the time of writing.

Assessing Left–Right Discrimination

Because of CNS neuroplasticity in response to pain, individuals with upper extremity pain may have a distorted somatosensory homuncular representation of the painful limb, leading to decreased ability to discriminate between left and right caused by altered processing. These changes have been shown to occur in individuals with CRPS,[82–85] phantom pain,[86–89] CTS,[90,91] brachial plexus injuries,[92] focal dystonia,[93] and osteoarthritis of the hand.[94] Assessment of left–right discrimination can be done through use of card-based systems or through computer, tablet, or phone applications that measure side-to-side differences in accuracy and speed. The presence of altered left–right discrimination may indicate nociplastic changes as at least one mechanism at play in the individual's pain, if not the predominate pain mechanism. Age-appropriate cutoffs for individuals specifically for left–right discrimination of the shoulder have been reported and are depicted in Figs. 94.9 and 94.10.[95] Accuracy and reaction time averages by trial and separate days among 50 healthy individuals in a narrow age range have been reported that are specific to left–right discrimination of the hand using both card-based (average reaction time, 1.56 sec for day 1 and 1.35 sec for day 2; average accuracy, 96.2% for day 1 and 96.1% for day 2) and tablet-based (average reaction time ,1.55 sec; average accuracy, 92.5%) testing methods.[96]

Self-Report Questionnaires

Numerous self-report questionnaires have been described in the literature over the past couple of decades. These include quality of life questionnaires such as the Short Form 36[97]; region-specific questionnaires such as the Disabilities of the Arm, Shoulder and Hand (DASH)[98] and Patient-Rated Wrist Evaluation (PRWE)[99]; and disease-specific questionnaires such as the Carpal Tunnel Instrument,[100] Patient-Rated Tennis Elbow Evaluation (PRTEE),[101] and Patient Rated Ulnar Nerve

Evaluation (PRUNE).[102] These examples of self-report outcome measures allow correlation between pain complaints and functional performance. The Michigan Hand Outcomes Questionnaire may be used to determine how the patient feels about his or her pain and function.[68,103] Descriptions of many types of questionnaires specific to the upper extremity are presented elsewhere.[68,104] Pain assessment scales within these questionnaires may be more valuable than independent pain assessment tools in determining the outcome of therapy intervention depending on the patient's underlying dominant pain mechanism. To learn more about the use of these measures, see Chapter 14.

Pain Mechanism and Pain Belief– or Cognition-Specific Questionnaires

Self-report questionnaires such as the CSI (as previously described), Pain Catastrophizing Scale (PCS),[105] Psychological Inflexibility in Pain Scale (PIPS),[106] Pain Vigilance and Awareness Questionnaire (PVAQ),[107] Injustice Experience Questionnaire (IEQ),[108] and Brief Illness Perception Questionnaire (B-IPQ)[109] can be useful in collecting information specific to underlying pain mechanisms or pain-related cognitions and beliefs. The painDETECT questionnaire (PD-Q)[110] is a validated screening tool that may be used to screen for the presence of neuropathic mechanisms that might be driving the individual's pain state.[111] Additionally, the Revised Neurophysiology of Pain Questionnaire[112] may be used to gain an understanding of the individual's working knowledge of pain overall. This information can be important to gather, even in recent-onset pain states. For example, among individuals with CTS, misinterpreting nociception and depression was significantly associated with pain intensity, whereas sex, age, and electrophysiological measures did not have a significant correlation with pain intensity.[113] Research also indicates that pain in individuals with trigger finger has moderate correlation with psychological factors (predominantly pain catastrophizing).[114] Additionally, pain intensity 10 to 14 days after minor hand surgery correlates significantly with presurgery pain catastrophizing, pain anxiety, self-efficacy, and depression.[115] Pain catastrophizing among individuals with persistent pain was found to be predictive of pain intensity, disability, and psychological distress independent of the level of impairment.[115] The information gathered from these questionnaires can be helpful in tailoring specific

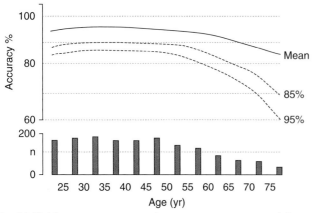

Fig. 94.10 Mean accuracy scores (percent correct responses) for age groups with 85% and 95% cutoffs for abnormal performance when assessing left–right discrimination at the shoulders. (From Breckenridge JD, McAuley JH, Butler DS, Stewart H, Moseley GL, Ginn KA. The development of a shoulder specific left/right judgement task: validity & reliability. *Musculoskelet Sci Pract.* 2017;28[suppl C]:39-45.)

educational interventions to address identified maladaptive beliefs, cognitions, and behaviors related to pain (e.g., with pain neuroscience education), which can in turn improve the individual's pain experience.[116] This information can also help the clinician understand more about the patient's pain experience up to that point in time.

ASSESSING RISK FOR DEVELOPMENT OF PERSISTENT PAIN

Several potential factors have been identified that may contribute to the development of persistent pain states (chronic pain). Although they fit into three different categories, they remain interrelated. Physiological factors that have been identified as contributing to development of persistent pain states include poor sleep (as mentioned previously), advancing age, and low physical activity.[74] Psychological factors that contribute to development of persistent pain states include depression, anxiety, anger or hostility, self-esteem, and general emotional functioning.[74,117] Social factors outside of advancing age include recent divorce, separation, or death of a spouse; low education levels and low family income; and tenuous housing and employment status, history of physical or sexual abuse, and being a recent immigrant or nonwhite; these factors may all contribute to predisposing someone to developing a persistent pain state.[74]

Among individuals with distal radius fractures, a baseline pain intensity score (>35 or 50 on the PRWE pain subscale) was found to be a strong predictor of developing a persistent pain state 12 months after the fracture.[118] Likewise, among individuals with wrist fractures, pain greater than or equal to 5 out of 10 on a NPRS in the first week after fracture when asked, "What is your average pain over the past 2 days?" was predictive of developing CRPS.[119] This finding of higher pain severity at baseline has also been found to be predictive of poor outcome (persistent pain) among individuals with shoulder or neck pain, elbow pain, and general musculoskeletal pain.[120] As previously mentioned, multiple psychosocial factors are predictive of pain intensity at all stages of chronicity. Therefore, it is imperative that health care providers deliver appropriate treatment that is specific to the individual's pain state quickly as well as address the pain from an evidence-informed and biopsychosocial perspective to decrease the likelihood of complex and persistent pain state development by addressing modifiable risk factors.

REFERENCES

1. IASP Terminology - IASP. https://www.iasp-pain.org/terminology?navItemNumber=576. Accessed August 12, 2019.
2. Pain terms: a list with definitions and notes on usage. Recommended by the IASP subcommittee on taxonomy. *Pain.* 1979;6(3):249.
3. Nicholas MK, Ashton-James C. Embodied pain: grasping a thorny problem? *Pain.* 2017;158(6):993–994.
4. Tabor A, Keogh E, Eccleston C. Embodied pain-negotiating the boundaries of possible action. *Pain.* 2017;158(6):1007–1011.
5. Weisberg J. Pain. In: Hecox B, Andemicael Mehreteab T, Weisberg J, eds. *Physical Agents : A Comprehensive Text for Physical Therapists.* Norwalk, CT: Appleton & Lange; 1994:473, xv.
6. Goodman CC, Snyder TEK. Pain types and viscerogenic pain patterns. In: Goodman CC, Snyder TEK, eds. *Differential Diagnosis for Physical Therapists : Screening for Referral.* 4th ed. St. Louis: Saunders/Elsevier; 2007:110–112.
7. Basbayn AU, Jessell TM. The perception of pain. In: 4th ed. Kandel ER, Schwartz JH, Jessell TM, eds. *Principles of Neural Science.* New York: McGraw-Hill, Health Professions Division; 2000:1414, xli.
8. Slipman CW, Plastaras CT, Palmitier RA, Huston CW, Sterenfeld EB. Symptom provocation of fluoroscopically guided cervical nerve root stimulation. Are dynatomal maps identical to dermatomal maps? *Spine (Phila Pa 1976).* 1998;23(20):2235–2242.
9. Moseley GL, Vlaeyen JW. Beyond nociception: the imprecision hypothesis of chronic pain. *Pain.* 2015;156(1):35–38.
10. Mischkowski D, Palacios-Barrios EE, Banker L, Dildine TC, Atlas LY. Pain or nociception? Subjective experience mediates the effects of acute noxious heat on autonomic responses. *Pain.* 2018;159(4):699–711.
11. Nijs J, Van Houdenhove B, Oostendorp RA. Recognition of central sensitization in patients with musculoskeletal pain: application of pain neurophysiology in manual therapy practice. *Man Ther.* 2010;15(2):135–141.
12. Sterling M, Jull G, Vicenzino B, Kenardy J. Sensory hypersensitivity occurs soon after whiplash injury and is associated with poor recovery. *Pain.* 2003;104(3):509–517.
13. Sterling M, Jull G, Kenardy J. Physical and psychological factors maintain long-term predictive capacity post-whiplash injury. *Pain.* 2006;122(1-2):102–108.
14. Yunus MB. Role of central sensitization in symptoms beyond muscle pain, and the evaluation of a patient with widespread pain. *Best Pract Res Clin Rheumatol.* 2007;21(3):481–497.
15. Lluch E, Torres R, Nijs J, Van Oosterwijck J. Evidence for central sensitization in patients with osteoarthritis pain: a systematic literature review. *Eur J Pain.* 2014;18(10):1367–1375.
16. Morris VH, Cruwys SC, Kidd BL. Characterisation of capsaicin-induced mechanical hyperalgesia as a marker for altered nociceptive processing in patients with rheumatoid arthritis. *Pain.* 1997;71(2):179–186.
17. Vardeh D, Mannion RJ, Woolf CJ. Toward a mechanism-based approach to pain diagnosis. *J Pain.* 2016;17(suppl 9):T50–69.
18. Smart KM, Blake C, Staines A, Thacker M, Doody C. Mechanisms-based classifications of musculoskeletal pain: part 1 of 3: symptoms and signs of central sensitisation in patients with low back (+/- leg) pain. *Man Ther.* 2012;17(4):336–344.
19. Smart KM, Blake C, Staines A, Thacker M, Doody C. Mechanisms-based classifications of musculoskeletal pain: part 2 of 3: symptoms and signs of peripheral neuropathic pain in patients with low back (+/- leg) pain. *Man Ther.* 2012;17(4):345–351.
20. Smart KM, Blake C, Staines A, Thacker M, Doody C. Mechanisms-based classifications of musculoskeletal pain: part 3 of 3: symptoms and signs of nociceptive pain in patients with low back (+/- leg) pain. *Man Ther.* 2012;17(4):352–357.
21. Malfait AM, Schnitzer TJ. Towards a mechanism-based approach to pain management in osteoarthritis. *Nat Rev Rheumatol.* 2013;9(11):654–664.
22. Smart KM, Blake C, Staines A, Doody C. The Discriminative validity of "nociceptive," "peripheral neuropathic," and "central sensitization" as mechanisms-based classifications of musculoskeletal pain. *Clin J Pain.* 2011;27(8):655–663.

23. Gierthmuhlen J, Binder A, Baron R. Mechanism-based treatment in complex regional pain syndromes. *Nat Rev Neurol.* 2014;10(9):518–528.

24. Chimenti RL, Frey-Law LA, Sluka KA. A mechanism-based approach to physical therapist management of pain. *Phys Ther.* 2018;98(5):302–314.

25. Kosek E, Cohen M, Baron R, et al. Do we need a third mechanistic descriptor for chronic pain states? *Pain.* 2016;157(7):1382–1386.

26. van Hecke O, Austin SK, Khan RA, Smith BH, Torrance N. Neuropathic pain in the general population: a systematic review of epidemiological studies. *Pain.* 2014;155(4):654–662.

27. Haanpaa M, Attal N, Backonja M, et al. NeuPSIG guidelines on neuropathic pain assessment. *Pain.* 2011;152(1):14–27.

28. IASP. IASP Council. Adopts task force recommendation for third mechanistic descriptor of pain. http://www.iasp-pain.org/Publications-News/NewsDetail.aspx?ItemNumber=6862; 2017. Accessed October 2, 2018.

29. Woolf CJ. Central sensitization: implications for the diagnosis and treatment of pain. *Pain.* 2011;152(suppl 3):S2–15.

30. Yunus MB. Central sensitivity syndromes: a unified concept for fibromyalgia and other similar maladies. *J Indian Rheumatol Assoc.* 2000;8:27–33.

31. Nijs J, Goubert D, Ickmans K. Recognition and treatment of central sensitization in chronic pain patients: not limited to specialized care. *J Orthop Sports Phys Ther.* 2016;46(12):1024–1028.

32. Smart KM, Blake C, Staines A, Doody C. Clinical indicators of 'nociceptive', 'peripheral neuropathic' and 'central' mechanisms of musculoskeletal pain. A Delphi survey of expert clinicians. *Man Ther.* 2010;15(1):80–87.

33. Gwilym SE, Oag HC, Tracey I, Carr AJ. Evidence that central sensitisation is present in patients with shoulder impingement syndrome and influences the outcome after surgery. *J Bone Joint Surg Br.* 2011;93(4):498–502.

34. Bennett EE, Walsh KM, Thompson NR, Krishnaney AA. Central sensitization inventory as a predictor of worse quality of life measures and increased length of stay following spinal fusion. *World Neurosurg.* 2017;104:594–600.

35. Jull G, Sterling M, Kenardy J, Beller E. Does the presence of sensory hypersensitivity influence outcomes of physical rehabilitation for chronic whiplash? A preliminary. *RCT. Pain.* 2007;129(1-2):28–34.

36. Coombes BK, Bisset L, Vicenzino B. Cold hyperalgesia associated with poorer prognosis in lateral epicondylalgia: a 1-year prognostic study of physical and psychological factors. *Clin J Pain.* 2015;31(1):30–35.

37. De Groef A, Meeus M, De Vrieze T, et al. Pain characteristics as important contributing factors to upper limb dysfunctions in breast cancer survivors at long term. *Musculoskelet Sci Pract.* 2017;29:52–59.

38. Vierck Jr CJ. Mechanisms underlying development of spatially distributed chronic pain (fibromyalgia). *Pain.* 2006;124(3):242–263.

39. Yunus MB. Fibromyalgia and overlapping disorders: the unifying concept of central sensitivity syndromes. *Semin Arthritis Rheum.* 2007;36(6):339–356.

40. Kuppens K, Hans G, Roussel N, et al. Sensory processing and central pain modulation in patients with chronic shoulder pain: a case-control study. *Scand J Med Sci Sports.* 2017.

41. Malfliet A, Kregel J, Cagnie B, et al. Lack of evidence for central sensitization in idiopathic, non-traumatic neck pain: a systematic review. *Pain Physician.* 2015;18(3):223–236.

42. Scott D, Jull G, Sterling M. Widespread sensory hypersensitivity is a feature of chronic whiplash-associated disorder but not chronic idiopathic neck pain. *Clin J Pain.* 2005;21(2):175–181.

43. Fernández-Lao C, Cantarero-Villanueva I, Fernández-de-las-Peñas C, Del-Moral-Ávila R, Menjón-Beltrán S, Arroyo-Morales M. Widespread mechanical pain hypersensitivity as a sign of central sensitization after breast cancer surgery: comparison between mastectomy and lumpectomy. *Pain Med.* 2011;12(1):72–78.

44. Schmidt BL, Hamamoto DT, Simone DA, Wilcox GL. Mechanism of cancer pain. *Mol Interv.* 2010;10(3):164–178.

45. Bahr R. No injuries, but plenty of pain? On the methodology for recording overuse symptoms in sports. *Br J Sports Med.* 2009;43(13):966–972.

46. van Wilgen CP, Keizer D. Neuropathic pain mechanisms in patients with chronic sports injuries: a diagnostic model useful in sports medicine? *Pain Medicine.* 2011;12(1):110–117.

47. Mayer TG, Neblett R, Cohen H, et al. The development and psychometric validation of the central sensitization inventory. *Pain Pract.* 2012;12(4):276–285.

48. Scerbo T, Colasurdo J, Dunn S, Unger J, Nijs J, Cook C. Measurement properties of the central sensitization inventory: a systematic review. *Pain Pract.* 2017.

49. Neblett R, Cohen H, Choi Y, et al. The Central Sensitization Inventory (CSI): establishing clinically significant values for identifying central sensitivity syndromes in an outpatient chronic pain sample. *J Pain.* 2013;14(5):438–445.

50. Aggarwal VR, McBeth J, Zakrzewska JM, Lunt M, Macfarlane GJ. The epidemiology of chronic syndromes that are frequently unexplained: do they have common associated factors? *Int J Epidemiol.* 2006;35(2):468–476.

51. Breivik H, Borchgrevink PC, Allen SM, et al. Assessment of pain. *Br J Anaesth.* 2008;101(1):17–24.

52. Van Oosterwijck J, Nijs J, Meeus M, et al. Pain neurophysiology education improves cognitions, pain thresholds, and movement performance in people with chronic whiplash: a pilot study. *J Rehabil Res Dev.* 2011;48(1):43–58.

53. Wakaizumi K, Yamada K, Oka H, et al. Fear-avoidance beliefs are independently associated with the prevalence of chronic pain in Japanese workers. *J Anesth.* 2017;31(2):255–262.

54. Yoshida T, Molton IR, Jensen MP, et al. Cognitions, metacognitions, and chronic pain. *Rehabil Psychol.* 2012;57(3):207–213.

55. Jensen MP, Sole E, Castarlenas E, et al. Behavioral inhibition, maladaptive pain cognitions, and function in patients with chronic pain. *Scand J Pain.* 2017;17:41–48.

56. Taylor SS, Davis MC, Yeung EW, Zautra AJ, Tennen HA. Relations between adaptive and maladaptive pain cognitions and within-day pain exacerbations in individuals with fibromyalgia. *J Behav Med.* 2017;40(3):458–467.

57. Morin CM, LeBlanc M, Daley M, Gregoire JP, Merette C. Epidemiology of insomnia: prevalence, self-help treatments, consultations, and determinants of help-seeking behaviors. *Sleep Med.* 2006;7(2):123–130.

58. Smith MT, Haythornthwaite JA. How do sleep disturbance and chronic pain inter-relate? Insights from the longitudinal and cognitive-behavioral clinical trials literature. *Sleep Med Rev.* 2004;8(2):119–132.

59. Taylor DJ, Mallory LJ, Lichstein KL, Durrence HH, Riedel BW, Bush AJ. Comorbidity of chronic insomnia with medical problems. *Sleep.* 2007;30(2):213–218.

60. Finan PH, Goodin BR, Smith MT. The association of sleep and pain: an update and a path forward. *J Pain.* 2013;14(12):1539–1552.

61. Bjurstrom MF, Irwin MR. Polysomnographic characteristics in nonmalignant chronic pain populations: a review of controlled studies. *Sleep Med Rev.* 2016;26:74–86.

62. Palermo TM, Wilson AC, Lewandowski AS, Toliver-Sokol M, Murray CB. Behavioral and psychosocial factors associated with insomnia in adolescents with chronic pain. *Pain.* 2011;152(1):89–94.

63. Mason P. Deconstructing endogenous pain modulations. *J Neurophysiol.* 2005;94(3):1659–1663.

64. Nijs J, Loggia ML, Polli A, et al. Sleep disturbances and severe stress as glial activators: key targets for treating central sensitization in chronic pain patients? *Expert Opin Ther Targets.* 2017;21(8):817–826.

65. Cole JC, Motivala SJ, Buysse DJ, Oxman MN, Levin MJ, Irwin MR. Validation of a 3-factor scoring model for the Pittsburgh Sleep Quality Index in older adults. *Sleep.* 2006;29(1):112–116.

66. Tomfohr LM, Schweizer CA, Dimsdale JE, Loredo JS. Psychometric characteristics of the Pittsburgh Sleep Quality Index in English speaking non-Hispanic whites and English and Spanish speaking Hispanics of Mexican descent. *J Clin Sleep Med.* 2013;9(1):61–66.

67. Mollayeva T, Thurairajah P, Burton K, Mollayeva S, Shapiro CM, Colantonio A. The Pittsburgh Sleep Quality Index as a screening tool for sleep dysfunction in clinical and non-clinical samples: a systematic review and meta-analysis. *Sleep Med Rev.* 2016;25:52–73.

68. Scudds RA. Pain outcome measures. *J Hand Ther.* 2001;14(2):86–90.

69. Melzack R. The McGill Pain Questionnaire: major properties and scoring methods. *Pain.* 1975;1(3):277–299.

70. Courtney CA, Kavchak AE, Lowry CD, O'Hearn MA. Interpreting joint pain: quantitative sensory testing in musculoskeletal management. *J Orthop Sports Phys Ther.* 2010;40(12):818–825.

71. Fischer AA. Pressure threshold meter: its use for quantification of tender spots. *Arch Phys Med Rehabil.* 1986;67(11):836–838.

72. Fischer AA. Pressure algometry over normal muscles. Standard values, validity and reproducibility of pressure threshold. *Pain.* 1987;30(1):115–126.

73. Nirschl RP. Elbow tendinosis/tennis elbow. *Clin Sports Med.* 1992;11(4):851–870.

74. Courtney CA, Fernandez-de-Las-Penas C, Bond S. Mechanisms of chronic pain - key considerations for appropriate physical therapy management. *J Man Manip Ther.* 2017;25(3):118–127.

75. de Medinaceli L, Hurpeau J, Merle M, Begorre H. Cold and post-traumatic pain: modeling of the peripheral nerve message. *Biosystems.* 1997;43(3):145–167.

76. Raja SN, Campbell JN, Meyer RA. Evidence for different mechanisms of primary and secondary hyperalgesia following heat injury to the glabrous skin. *Brain.* 1984;107(Pt 4):1179–1188.

77. de la Llave-Rincon AI, Fernandez-de-las-Penas C, Fernandez-Carnero J, Padua L, Arendt-Nielsen L, Pareja JA. Bilateral hand/wrist heat and cold hyperalgesia, but not hypoesthesia, in unilateral carpal tunnel syndrome. *Exp Brain Res.* 2009;198(4):455–463.

78. Fernandez-de-Las-Penas C, Fernandez-Munoz JJ, Navarro-Pardo E, da-Silva-Pocinho RF, Ambite-Quesada S, Pareja JA. Identification of subgroups of women with carpal tunnel syndrome with central sensitization. *Pain Med.* 2016;17(9):1749–1756.

79. Coombes BK, Bisset L, Vicenzino B. Thermal hyperalgesia distinguishes those with severe pain and disability in unilateral lateral epicondylalgia. *Clin J Pain.* 2012;28(7):595–601.

80. Rebbeck T, Moloney N, Azoory R, et al. Clinical ratings of pain sensitivity correlate with quantitative measures in people with chronic neck pain and healthy controls: cross-sectional study. *Phys Ther.* 2015;95(11):1536–1546.

81. Maxwell S, Sterling M. An investigation of the use of a numeric pain rating scale with ice application to the neck to determine cold hyperalgesia. *Man Ther.* 2013;18(2):172–174.

82. Moseley GL. Why do people with complex regional pain syndrome take longer to recognize their affected hand? *Neurology.* 2004;62(12):2182–2186.

83. Maihofner C, Handwerker HO, Neundorfer B, Birklein F. Patterns of cortical reorganization in complex regional pain syndrome. *Neurology.* 2003;61(12):1707–1715.

84. Schwoebel J, Friedman R, Duda N, Coslett HB. Pain and the body schema: evidence for peripheral effects on mental representations of movement. *Brain.* 2001;124(Pt 10):2098–2104.

85. Schwoebel J, Coslett HB, Bradt J, Friedman R, Dileo C. Pain and the body schema: effects of pain severity on mental representations of movement. *Neurology.* 2002;59(5):775–777.

86. Flor H, Elbert T, Knecht S, et al. Phantom-limb pain as a perceptual correlate of cortical reorganization following arm amputation. *Nature.* 1995;375(6531):482–484.

87. MacIver K, Lloyd DM, Kelly S, Roberts N, Nurmikko T. Phantom limb pain, cortical reorganization and the therapeutic effect of mental imagery. *Brain.* 2008;131(Pt 8):2181–2191.

88. Nico D, Daprati E, Rigal F, Parsons L, Sirigu A. Left and right hand recognition in upper limb amputees. *Brain.* 2004;127(Pt 1):120–132.

89. Flor H, Devor M, Jensen T. Phantom limb pain: causes and cures. In: Dostrovsky JO, Carr DB, Kolzenburg M, eds. *Progress in Pain Research and Management.* Vol. 24. Seattle: IASP Press; 2003.

90. Schmid AB, Soon BT, Wasner G, Coppieters MW. Can widespread hypersensitivity in carpal tunnel syndrome be substantiated if neck and arm pain are absent? *Eur J Pain.* 2012;16(2):217–228.

91. Schmid AB, Coppieters MW. Left/right judgment of body parts is selectively impaired in patients with unilateral carpal tunnel syndrome. *Clin J Pain.* 2012;28(7):615–622.

92. Moseley GL. Graded motor imagery for pathologic pain: a randomized controlled trial. *Neurology.* 2006;67(12):2129–2134.

93. Fiorio M, Tinazzi M, Aglioti SM. Selective impairment of hand mental rotation in patients with focal hand dystonia. *Brain.* 2006;129(Pt 1):47–54.

94. Gilpin HR, Moseley GL, Stanton TR, Newport R. Evidence for distorted mental representation of the hand in osteoarthritis. *Rheumatology (Oxford).* 2015;54(4):678–682.

95. Breckenridge JD, McAuley JH, Butler DS, Stewart H, Moseley GL, Ginn KA. The development of a shoulder specific left/right judgement task: validity & reliability. *Musculoskelet Sci Pract.* 2017;28(suppl C):39–45.

96. Zimney KJ, Wassinger CA, Goranson J, Kingsbury T, Kuhn T, Morgan S. The reliability of card-based and tablet-based left/right judgment measurements. *Musculoskelet Sci Pract.* 2017.

97. Brazier JE, Harper R, Jones NM, et al. Validating the SF-36 health survey questionnaire: new outcome measure for primary care. *BMJ.* 1992;305(6846):160–164.

98. Hudak PL, Amadio PC, Bombardier C. Development of an upper extremity outcome measure: the DASH (disabilities of the arm, shoulder and hand) [corrected]. The Upper Extremity Collaborative Group (UECG). *Am J Ind Med.* 1996;29(6):602–608.

99. Mulders MAM, Kleipool SC, Dingemans SA, et al. Normative data for the patient-rated wrist evaluation questionnaire. *J Hand Ther.* 2017.

100. Levine DW, Simmons BP, Koris MJ, et al. A self-administered questionnaire for the assessment of severity of symptoms and functional status in carpal tunnel syndrome. *J Bone Joint Surg Am.* 1993;75(11):1585–1592.

101. Rompe JD, Overend TJ, MacDermid JC. Validation of the patient-rated tennis elbow evaluation questionnaire. *J Hand Ther.* 2007;20(1):3–10. quiz 11.

102. MacDermid JC, Grewal R. Development and validation of the patient-rated ulnar nerve evaluation. *BMC Musculoskelet Disord.* 2013;14:146.

103. Chung KC, Pillsbury MS, Walters MR, Hayward RA. Reliability and validity testing of the Michigan Hand Outcomes Questionnaire. *J Hand Surg Am.* 1998;23(4):575–587.

104. Amadio PC. Outcome assessment in hand surgery and hand therapy: an update. *J Hand Ther.* 2001;14(2):63–67.

105. Osman A, Barrios FX, Gutierrez PM, Kopper BA, Merrifield T, Grittmann L. The pain catastrophizing scale: further psychometric evaluation with adult samples. *J Behav Med.* 2000;23(4):351–365.

106. Barke A, Riecke J, Rief W, Glombiewski JA. The Psychological Inflexibility in Pain Scale (PIPS) - validation, factor structure and comparison to the Chronic Pain Acceptance Questionnaire (CPAQ) and other validated measures in German chronic back pain patients. *BMC Musculoskelet Disord.* 2015;16:171.

107. Roelofs J, Peters ML, McCracken L, Vlaeyen JW. The Pain Vigilance and Awareness Questionnaire (PVAQ): further psychometric evaluation in fibromyalgia and other chronic pain syndromes. *Pain.* 2003;101(3):299–306.

108. Rodero B, Luciano JV, Montero-Marin J, et al. Perceived injustice in fibromyalgia: psychometric characteristics of the Injustice Experience Questionnaire and relationship with pain catastrophising and pain acceptance. *J Psychosom Res.* 2012;73(2):86–91.

109. Broadbent E, Wilkes C, Koschwanez H, Weinman J, Norton S, Petrie KJ. A systematic review and meta-analysis of the brief illness perception questionnaire. *Psychol Health.* 2015;30(11):1361–1385.

110. Freynhagen R, Baron R, Gockel U, Tolle TR. painDETECT: a new screening questionnaire to identify neuropathic components in patients with back pain. *Curr Med Res Opin.* 2006;22(10):1911–1920.

111. Freynhagen R, Tolle TR, Gockel U, Baron R. The painDETECT project - far more than a screening tool on neuropathic pain. *Curr Med Res Opin.* 2016;32(6):1033–1057.

112. Catley MJ, O'Connell NE, Moseley GL. How good is the neurophysiology of pain questionnaire? A Rasch analysis of psychometric properties. *J Pain.* 2013;14(8):818–827.

113. Nunez F, Vranceanu AM, Ring D. Determinants of pain in patients with carpal tunnel syndrome. *Clin Orthop Relat Res.* 2010;468(12):3328–3332.

114. Kennedy SA, Vranceanu AM, Nunez F, Ring D. Association between psychosocial factors and pain in patients with trigger finger. *J Hand Microsurg.* 2010;2(1):18–23.

115. Vranceanu AM, Jupiter JB, Mudgal CS, Ring D. Predictors of pain intensity and disability after minor hand surgery. *J Hand Surg Am.* 2010;35(6):956–960.

116. Louw A, Diener I, Butler DS, Puentedura EJ. The effect of neuroscience education on pain, disability, anxiety, and stress in chronic musculoskeletal pain. *Arch Phys Med Rehabil.* 2011;92(12):2041–2056.

117. Burke AL, Mathias JL, Denson LA. Psychological functioning of people living with chronic pain: a meta-analytic review. *Br J Clin Psychol.* 2015;54(3):345–360.

118. Mehta SP, MacDermid JC, Richardson J, MacIntyre NJ, Grewal R. Baseline pain intensity is a predictor of chronic pain in individuals with distal radius fracture. *J Orthop Sports Phys Ther.* 2015;45(2):119–127.

119. Moseley GL, Herbert RD, Parsons T, Lucas S, Van Hilten JJ, Marinus J. Intense pain soon after wrist fracture strongly predicts who will develop complex regional pain syndrome: prospective cohort study. *J Pain.* 2014;15(1):16–23.

120. Mallen CD, Peat G, Thomas E, Dunn KM, Croft PR. Prognostic factors for musculoskeletal pain in primary care: a systematic review. *Br J Gen Pract.* 2007;57(541):655–661.

95

Medical Management for Pain

Peter P. Pham, Michael P. Gaspar, Patrick M. Kane

CRITICAL POINTS

- Pain can be classified in functional terms or by its temporal pattern. These classifications are helpful for devising medical treatment regimens.
- Nociceptive pain arises from actual or threatened damage to non-neural tissue and is caused by the activation of nociceptors. Treatment options include opioids, antiinflammatory agents, and acetaminophen.
- Neuropathic pain arises as a direct consequence of a lesion or disease affecting the somatosensory system. These conditions tend to respond favorably to "atypical" pain medications, including anticonvulsants and antidepressants. The use of opioids for treatment of neuropathic pain is controversial.

- Acute pain typically has a distinct onset after a specific bodily insult, and it tends to improve or resolve when the underlying injury has been treated. In most cases, acute pain is a physiologic response. This category includes postsurgical pain and is often managed with combination therapy that may include opioids.
- Chronic pain is typically defined as pain that lasts for at least 3 months. Characteristics may vary, but chronic pain is generally considered a maladaptive response to an injury or condition. Opioid use for treatment of chronic nonmalignant pain is generally not advised because of potential negative sequelae of prolonged use, including tolerance and dependence.

Pain is a ubiquitous phenomenon common to the human experience, yet it remains incompletely understood and difficult to define. Nevertheless, our understanding of pain has progressed dramatically over time, and with this knowledge, medical treatment options for pain have similarly evolved. Because pain is often the motivating factor for patients with upper limb disorders to seek care with a hand surgeon or hand therapist, tertiary care providers should possess a well-versed understanding of different types of pain, including the medical treatment options that specifically target each type. This chapter outlines the most common medical treatments for hand and upper extremity pain of which hand surgeons and therapists should be aware.

HISTORICAL PERSPECTIVE ON MEDICAL PAIN MANAGEMENT

The word "pain" is derived from the Latin *poena* with origins in both Greek and Roman mythology. *Poena* was the Roman spirit of punishment while *Poine* was the Greek goddess of revenge, who sent by the gods when they had been angered.[1] As the title of these mythological characters might suggest, pain was perceived as a form of punishment inflicted by the gods, a view that persisted for thousands of years. Based on these misconceptions, early unsuccessful attempts at "treating" pain included religious offerings and animal sacrifices, among other rituals aimed at appeasing the gods. However, early evidence of success with medical pain management can also be traced as far back as 4000 BC

when Assyrians documented their use of willow leaves (genus *Salix*), which contain a form of salicylic acid, for treatment of inflammatory rheumatic pain.[2] Centuries later, the ancient Greek physician Hippocrates prescribed willow bark as an effective analgesic for mothers undergoing childbirth.[2]

Opium shares a similar historical chronology as salicylic acid, as the Sumerians first documented their use of opium in 4000 BC.[3] The Sumerians were so fascinated with its euphoric effects that they referred to opium simply as "joy," and its source, the poppy plant, as the "plant of joy."[3] In the early 19th century, German pharmacist Friedrich Wilhelm Serturner isolated the active ingredient found in opium and named it morphine after the Greek god of dreams, Morpheus.[3] As the analgesic effects of opioids became more widely touted, their medicinal use grew exponentially, and by the start of the 20th century, opioids were the predominant agent used for medical analgesia. However, issues with opioid dependence led to an exploration of alternatives to opioid analgesics, an area of medicine that remains of utmost importance today.

PAIN CLASSIFICATIONS

Pain can be classified both in functional terms and based on the temporal pattern of its onset and duration. These classifications are helpful for devising treatment plans, but it should be noted that these categories are not necessarily mutually exclusive, and medical treatment regimens should always be explored on a case-by-case basis.

FUNCTIONAL CLASSIFICATION

Nociceptive Pain

Nociceptive pain refers to pain that arises from actual or threatened damage to non-neural tissue.[4] This type is the broader of the two main functional categories of pain and includes pain secondary to traumatic injury or surgery itself. Nociceptive pain involves peripheral inflammation secondary to the release of inflammatory mediators. Prostaglandin-E_2 (PGE_2), which is synthesized by cyclooxygenase-2 (COX-2) from arachidonic acid (AA), is responsible for nociceptor sensitization.[5] After being sensitized, activated nociceptors release additional peptides, including substance P, which in turn stimulates the release of histamine and serotonin (5-HT) from mast cells and platelets, respectively.[5]

Neuropathic Pain

Neuropathic pain was most recently defined by the International Association for the Study of Pain (IASP) Special Interest Group on Neuropathic Pain (NeuPSIG) as "pain arising as a direct consequence of a lesion or disease affecting the somatosensory system."[4,6,7]

Mixed Pain

As the name suggests, *mixed pain* shares traits of both nociceptive and neuropathic pain and is a relatively new functional category. Recent work suggests that patients with mixed pain have greater clinical complexity and are less likely to respond to medical management compared with those with either nociceptive or neuropathic pain alone.[8]

TEMPORAL CLASSIFICATIONS

Acute Pain

Acute pain typically has a distinct onset that generally follows an identifiable traumatic event or surgical procedure.[9] It is usually limited in duration and tends to improve or resolve when the underlying injury has been treated. For the most part, acute pain is considered a normal physiologic response and is thus a protective mechanism.[9]

Chronic Pain

Chronic pain is typically defined as pain that lasts for at least 3 months, and although it may arise from a specific injury, it often has an unclear etiology.[10] In contrast to acute pain, chronic pain is generally considered as a maladaptive response to an injury or other cause.[11]

TYPES OF MEDICATIONS FOR PAIN MANAGEMENT

Opioids

Opioids are inhibitory neuromodulators that function to inhibit pain by acting on specific opioid receptors.[12,13] The pertinent opioid receptors are divided into mu-1 (μ1), μ2, kappa (κ) and delta (δ) receptors,[12,14,15] whose functions can be summarized as follows:

μ1: analgesia, physical dependence
μ2: euphoria, respiratory depression, and inhibition of gut mobility
κ: spinal analgesia, meiosis, and sedation
δ: analgesia, respiratory depression, and physical dependence

The clinical effects of a specific opioid depend on several of its inherent properties, which can also be used to classify them. For example, receptor affinity can be categorized as agonist, partial agonists, agonist–antagonist, or antagonist, whereas the intrinsic activity at a given receptor can be described as weak or strong.[12-15] Opioids can also be classified based on their derivation as natural, synthetic, or semisynthetic.[12,13]

Despite their widespread use as analgesics after acute injury or surgery, consensus opioid postoperative prescribing guidelines do not exist. As a result, clinicians often rely on their experience and best clinical judgment in determining a proper opioid regimen, although certain key principles should guide opioid prescribing behavior. Significant variation in patients' pain tolerance, history of opioid use, and underlying genetics and physiology may necessitate differing dosages or dosing intervals even when the underlying injury or condition is identical.[16,17] Opioid doses should be titrated to a response and tapered as pain improves. Many practitioners now suggest that opioids should be avoided in patients with chronic nonmalignant pain because of the risk of tolerance and dependence,[17,18] and opioids are also not recommended as first-line therapy for neuropathic pain.[19,20] In addition, opioids should be used with extreme caution in patients with obstructive sleep apnea because of their depressive effects on the respiratory system.[21]

Nonopioids

Nonsteroidal Antiinflammatory Drugs

Nonsteroidal antiinflammatory drugs (NSAIDs) can be classified based on their activity against the COX enzymes as nonspecific NSAIDs (ns-NSAIDs) or COX-2–specific inhibitors (COXibs). Of note, whereas COX-2 is upregulated in the setting of inflammation, COX-1 is responsible for the conversion of AA to various prostaglandins necessary for homeostatic functions that regulate renal blood flow and gastroprotective mechanisms.[5] As a consequence of such mechanisms of action, ns-NSAIDs increase the risk of renal failure and are less preferred than COXibs.[22] Although COXibs have also been scrutinized for their potential cardiotoxic effects, recent evidence has challenged this opinion, with newer studies claiming that COXibs may in fact be cardioprotective.[23]

Acetaminophen

Acetaminophen is currently one of the most widely recognized and widely used pain medications in the world. Despite its ubiquity, the mechanism by which it exerts its analgesic effects remains poorly understood. Unlike NSAIDs, acetaminophen is thought to have little effect on COX-1 and COX-2 and thus little antiinflammatory effect. Rather, acetaminophen is thought to act through central nervous system (CNS) pathways because of its ability to cross the blood–brain barrier and may provide relief by elevating the pain threshold.[24,25] This selective permeability within the CNS provides evidence for acetaminophen's role as an antipyretic agent that modulates the heat-regulating center of the hypothalamus.[24,25]

The main limitation of acetaminophen use is its documented renal and hepatotoxicity. However, these adverse effects are minimal in healthy patients with absent to mild preexisting kidney liver disease who adhere to the maximum daily dosing guidelines.[26] Because of its comparatively mild side effect profile, acetaminophen is not only an effective stand-alone first-line treatment option for pain but is also a useful component in combination medications with opioids and NSAIDs.[24,25]

Gabapentinoids

Gabapentin and pregabalin are two antiepileptic medications that have proven efficacy in treating patients with peripheral neuropathic pain; some authors recommend these agents as first-line treatment of upper limb neuropathic pain.[27-29] Because of their potential sedative effects, these medications are particularly useful in patients with neuropathic pain and concomitant sleep disturbance, a presentation commonly seen in carpal tunnel syndrome.[30-32]

Antidepressants

Because chronic pain is often correlated with psychological disorders such as depression and anxiety,[33] treatment regimens for pain should also take into consideration these underlying disorders. The complex interplay between psychosocial factors and upper limb pain is discussed in greater detail in Chapter 118. Antidepressants, including tricyclic antidepressants and serotonin norepinephrine reuptake inhibitors (SNRIs), have proven efficacy against neuropathic pain in numerous controlled trials.[34,35] In fact, recent studies have shown that duloxetine (an SNRI) demonstrates equivalent efficacy as pregabalin for treatment of diabetic neuropathic pain.[36] Although the exact mechanism by which antidepressants treat neuropathic pain is somewhat unclear, animal models suggest that norepinephrine plays an important role in the inhibition of neuropathic pain. Thus, inhibition of norepinephrine reuptake promotes increased activity, leading to greater inhibition of neuropathic pain.[34]

CURRENT CONCEPTS AND CONTROVERSIES IN MEDICAL MANAGEMENT

Over the past decade, opioid abuse has become the focus of fierce public debate because of the ongoing public health crisis that continues to plague the United States.[37] Recent studies specific to upper extremity surgery report that surgeons regularly overprescribe opioids postoperatively in light of the fact that patients typically only use one third of their prescribed amount.[38,39] Despite efforts to curb this growing public health concern, opioids remain an important modality for treating moderate to severe pain when prescribed and used responsibly. A survey of 5703 patients who underwent outpatient surgery found that 30% reported moderate to severe pain despite use of prescribed analgesia 24 hours postoperatively.[40] Notably, upper limb surgeries were among those most frequently identified as causing the highest levels of pain.[40] Other studies have found that as many as 70% of patients believe that their postoperative pain management is inadequate.[41,42] On the other hand, recent findings demonstrate that even short-term postoperative opioid use is a risk factor for developing chronic use problems in opioid-naïve patients.[38,43-45] Thus, tertiary care providers, hand surgeons in particular, are faced with the difficult task of optimizing pain control while minimizing risks associated with opioid use.[46] This challenge underscores the importance of multimodal pain management regimens that include nonopioids as well as interdisciplinary pain management interventions coordinated by hand therapists, which will be discussed in the next chapter.

REFERENCES

1. Smith W, et al. *A Dictionary of Greek and Roman Antiquities*. London: William Wayte, GE. Marindin.; 1890.
2. Jack DB. One hundred years of aspirin. *Lancet*. 1997;350(9075):437–439.
3. Brownstein MJ. A brief history of opiates, opioid peptides, and opioid receptors. *Proc Natl Acad Sci U S A*. 1993;90(12):5391–5393.
4. Loeser JD, Treede RD. The Kyoto protocol of IASP basic pain terminology. *Pain*. 2008;137:473–477.
5. Ricciotti E, FitzGerald GA. Prostaglandins and inflammation. *Arterioscler Thromb Vasc Biol*. 2011;31(5):986–1000.
6. Treede RD, Jensen TS, Campbell JN, et al. Neuropathic pain: redefinition and a grading system for clinical and research purposes. *Neurology*. 2008;70:1630–1635.
7. Finnerup NB, Haroutounian S, Kamerman P, et al. Neuropathic pain: an updated grading system for research and clinical practice. *Pain*. 2016;157(8):1599–1606.
8. Ibor PJ, Sánchez-Magro I, Villoria J, Leal A, Esquivias A. Mixed pain can be discerned in the primary care and orthopedics settings in Spain: a large cross-sectional study. *Clin J Pain*. 2017;33(12):1100–1108.
9. Kent ML, Tighe PJ, Belfer I, et al. The ACTTION-APS-AAPM pain taxonomy (AAAPT) multidimensional approach to classifying acute pain conditions. *J Pain*. 2017;18(5):479–489.
10. Dworkin RH, Bruehl S, Fillingim RB, Loeser JD, Terman GW, Turk DC. Multidimensional diagnostic criteria for chronic pain: introduction to the ACTTION-American Pain Society Pain Taxonomy (AAPT). *J Pain*. 2016;17(suppl 9):T1–T9.
11. Kim W, Kim SK, Nabekura J. Functional and structural plasticity in the primary somatosensory cortex associated with chronic pain. *J Neurochem*. 2017;141(4):499–506.
12. Argoff CE. Clinical implications of opioid pharmacogenetics. *Clin J Pain*. 2010;26(suppl 10):S16–S20.
13. Owusu Obeng A, Hamadeh I, Smith M. Review of opioid pharmacogenetics and considerations for pain management. *Pharmacotherapy*. 2017;37(9):1105–1121.
14. Lutz PE, Kieffer BL. The multiple facets of opioid receptor function: implications for addiction. *Curr Opin Neurobiol*. 2013;23(4):473–479.
15. Feng Y, He X, Yang Y, Chao D, Lazarus LH, Xia Y. Current research on opioid receptor function. *Curr Drug Targets*. 2012;13(2):230–246.
16. Solhaug V, Molden E. Individual variability in clinical effect and tolerability of opioid analgesics - Importance of drug interactions and pharmacogenetics. *Scand J Pain*. 2017;17:193–200.
17. Webster LR. Risk factors for opioid-use disorder and overdose. *Anesth Analg*. 2017;125(5):1741–1748.
18. Volkow ND, McLellan AT. Opioid abuse in chronic pain—misconceptions and mitigation strategies. *N Engl J Med*. 2016;374(13):1253–1263.
19. Gaskell H, Derry S, Stannard C, Moore RA. Oxycodone for neuropathic pain in adults. *Cochrane Database Syst Rev*. 2016;7:CD010692.
20. Cooper TE, Chen J, Wiffen PJ, et al. Morphine for chronic neuropathic pain in adults. *Cochrane Database Syst Rev*. 2017;5:CD011669.
21. Gaspar MP, Kane PM, Jacoby SM, Gaspar PS, Osterman AL. Evaluation and management of sleep disorders in the hand surgery patient. *J Hand Surg Am*. 2016;41(10):1019–1026.
22. van Walsem A, Pandhi S, Nixon RM, Guyot P, Karabis A, Moore RA. Relative benefit-risk comparing diclofenac to other traditional non-steroidal anti-inflammatory drugs and cyclooxygenase-2 inhibitors in patients with osteoarthritis or rheumatoid arthritis: a network meta-analysis. *Arthritis Res Ther*. 2015;17:66.
23. Zingler G, Hermann B, Fischer T, Herdegen T. Cardiovascular adverse events by non-steroidal anti-inflammatory drugs: when the benefits outweigh the risks. *Expert Rev Clin Pharmacol*. 2016;9(11):1479–1492.
24. Candido KD, Perozo OJ, Knezevic NN. Pharmacology of acetaminophen, nonsteroidal antiinflammatory drugs, and steroid medications: implications for anesthesia or unique associated risks. *Anesthesiol Clin*. 2017;35(2):e145–e162.
25. Myers SH, LaPorte DM. Acetaminophen: safe use and associated risks. *J Hand Surg Am*. 2009;34(6):1137–1139.
26. Ramachandran A, Jaeschke H. Acetaminophen toxicity novel insights into mechanisms and future perspectives. *Gene Expr*. 2017;20.
27. Duman I, Aydemir K, Ozgul A, Kalyon TA. Assessment of the efficacy of gabapentin in carpal tunnel syndrome. *J Clin Rheumatol*. 2008;14(3):175–177.
28. van Seventer R, Bach FW, Toth CC, Serpell M, Temple J, Murphy TK, et al. Pregabalin in the treatment of post-traumatic peripheral neuropathic pain: a randomized double-blind trial. *Eur J Neurol*. 2010;17:1082–1089.
29. Brunton L, Laporte D. Use of gabapentin and pregabalin for hand surgery patients. *J Hand Surg Am*. 2012;37(7):e1486–e1488.
30. Roth T, Lankford DA, Bhadra P, Whalen E, Resnick EM. Effect of pregabalin on sleep in patients with fibromyalgia and sleep maintenance disturbance: a randomized, placebo-controlled, 2-way crossover polysomnography study. *Arthritis Care Res (Hoboken)*. 2012;64(4):e597–e606.
31. Roth T, Bhadra-Brown P, Pitman VW, Resnick EM. Pregabalin improves fibromyalgia-related sleep disturbance. *Clin J Pain*. 2016;32(4):e308–e312.
32. Roth T, van Seventer R, Murphy TK. The effect of pregabalin on pain-related sleep interference in diabetic peripheral neuropathy or postherpetic neuralgia: a review of nine clinical trials. *Curr Med Res Opin*. 2010;26(10):2411–2419.
33. Bair MJ, Robinson RL, Katon W, et al. Depression and pain comorbidity: a literature review. *Arch Intern Med*. 2003;163(20):2433–2445.

34. Obata H. Analgesic mechanisms of antidepressants for neuropathic pain. *Int J Mol Sci.* 2017;18(11). pii:E2483. https://doi.org/10.3390/ijms18112483. Review.

35. Aiyer R, Barkin RL, Bhatia A. Treatment of neuropathic pain with venlafaxine: a systematic review. *Pain Med.* 2012;18(10):1999.

36. Roy MK, Kuriakose AS, Varma SK, Jacob LA, Beegum NJ. A study on comparative efficacy and cost effectiveness of pregabalin and duloxetine used in diabetic neuropathic pain. *Diabetes Metab Syndr.* 2017;11(1):31–35.

37. Soelberg CD, Brown Jr RE, Du Vivier D, Meyer JE, Ramachandran BK. The US Opioid Crisis: current federal and state legal issues. *Anesth Analg.* 2017;125(5):1675–1681.

38. Waljee JF, Zhong L, Hou H, Sears E, Brummett C, Chung KC. The use of opioid analgesics following common upper extremity surgical procedures: a national, population-based study. *Plast Reconstr Surg.* 2016;137(2):355e–364e.

39. Rodgers J, Cunningham K, Fitzgerald K, Finnerty E. Opioid consumption following outpatient upper extremity surgery. *J Hand Surg.* 2012;37(4):645–650.

40. McGrath B, Elgendy H, Chung F, Kamming D, Curti B, King S. Thirty percent of patients have moderate to severe pain 24 hours after ambulatory surgery: a survey of 5703 patients. *Can J Anaesth.* 2004;51:886–891.

41. Apfelbaum JL, Chen C, Mehta SS, Gan TJ. Postoperative pain experience: results from a national survey suggest postoperative pain continues to be undermanaged. *Anesth Analg.* 2003;97:534–540.

42. Wu CL, Raja SN. Treatment of acute postoperative pain. *Lancet.* 2011;377:2215–2225.

43. Brummett CM, Waljee JF, Goesling J, et al. New persistent opioid use after minor and major surgical procedures in us adults. *JAMA Surg.* 2017;152(6):e170504.

44. Johnson SP, Chung KC, Zhong L, et al. Risk of prolonged opioid use among opioid-naïve patients following common hand surgery procedures. *J Hand Surg Am.* 2016;41(10):947–957.e3.

45. Shah A, Hayes CJ, Martin BC. Characteristics of initial prescription episodes and likelihood of long-term opioid use - United States, 2006–2015. *MMWR Morb Mortal Wkly Rep.* 2017;66(10):265–269.

46. Cheatle MD. Prescription opioid misuse, abuse, morbidity, and mortality: balancing effective pain management and safety. *Pain Med.* 2015;16(suppl 1):S3–S8.

96

Pain Management: Principles of Therapist's Interventions

Patti Carrillo, Kenneth A. Taylor, Jane M. Fedorczyk

OUTLINE

CRITICAL POINTS

- Pain is a highly personal experience, so each treatment plan needs to be unique and individualized to best meet patient expectations and needs.
- Identification of the primary pain mechanism will assist in selecting appropriate evidence-informed treatment interventions.

- Evidence consistently suggests implementation of multimodal treatment strategies for best outcomes, with significant support for use of exercise as a primary intervention for treatment of pain.
- Function is an objectively measurable outcome of therapy intervention and should be the primary goal in hand therapy treatment planning.

INTRODUCTION: CHALLENGES OF PAIN TREATMENT

Pain is defined as an unpleasant sensory and emotional experience associated with actual or potential tissue damage.[1] Pain is a universal subjective experience and as such is as complex and varied as the individuals who experience it. The pathway from nociception to pain is not straightforward, and nuances make each patient's experience and perception unique. The complex pain phenomenon begins with nociception processed by the nervous system, which is then filtered and shaped by each individual's biological, psychological, and socioeconomic factors. These factors include, but are not limited to, medical comorbidities, emotional disposition, understanding of the pain episode, perceptions about disability, coping mechanisms, and access to care.[2] Because the pain experience is unique to the individual, the treatment of pain has always been challenging to health care providers.

As challenging as it may be to treat pain, it is a common, symptom, diagnosis, or condition. Clinicians worldwide have witnessed dramatic increases in numbers of patients seeking treatment for pain. Twenty years ago, it was estimated that roughly one in seven Americans experienced persistent pain.[3] The prevalence of pain has increased dramatically in the intervening decades with current figures suggesting that pain impacts one in four or more than 100 million individuals in the United States.[3] This represents an impact greater than the incidence of diabetes, heart disease, and cancer combined.[4] With the escalation of pain conditions, pain is now cited as the primary reason that individuals access the health care system in the United States.[4] Frequently, entry into the health care system with complaints of pain will result in a typical biomedical intervention—prescription of pain medication.[4] This common treatment practice combined with escalating numbers of patients in pain has resulted in what the Centers for

Disease Control and Prevention (CDC) is now referring to as a prescription pain medication crisis. Although there is moderate evidence in the literature suggesting that nonsteroidal antiinflammatory drugs and opioids demonstrate some efficacy in the treatment of short-term pain (<12 weeks), these options are not without potential for significant adverse effects.[5] The CDC recognizes overdose and opioid use disorder as among the most serious risks associated with opioid use.[6] Alarmingly, the CDC reports that in the 15 years from 1999 to 2014, more than 165,000 individuals died from overdoses related to the use of prescribed opioid medication.[6] In addition, more than 1000 individuals in the United States are treated in emergency departments every day for misuse or overdose of prescribed opioid medications.[7] It is clear that other pain treatment options are needed, and rehabilitation professionals should embrace their role in pain management.

Historically, treatment of pain in rehabilitation was derived from pain models that were almost entirely biomedical in their approach. Dysfunctions resulted in departure from normal physical and biomechanical structure and function. When these "abnormalities" were corrected using therapeutic interventions, the pain drivers were eliminated, and patients returned "back to normal." Discrepancies between biomedical model predictions and the realities observed with patients in pain treatment settings were at times frustrating to therapists. Patients were expected to feel better and to be better when tissue healed. Led by pain neuroscience researchers, therapists have begun to adopt more comprehensive models of pain management. These new pain treatment models acknowledge the overlap and connections among biological, psychological, and social factors.[8] At the same time, strides have been made in understanding the nervous system's processing of pain, as discussed in Chapters 93 and 94, and researchers are beginning to develop a body of evidence supporting the use of a variety of traditional as well as emerging therapy interventions.

INTERVENTIONS FOR PAIN MANAGEMENT

After a thorough pain assessment and classification as described in Chapter 94, the therapist is tasked with selection and implementation of pain-modulating interventions. Evidence-informed approaches are influencing treatment choices and infusing treatment with a level of scientific authority, which in some instances had previously been lacking. However, even with expanding evidence, there are still gaps in the research, and there are areas of therapy intervention on which the research base remains silent. In the clinical setting, treating therapists are daily translating research into clinical practice, and even where evidence is less than compelling, therapists must use sound decision making to ensure that quality patient care is rendered to achieve the best patient outcome. The integration of evidence into practice emphasizes that a lack of evidence is not always synonymous with a lack of effect and that although randomized controlled trials and systematic reviews offer high-quality evidence, as clinicians, we are tasked with implementation of best available evidence, which consists of less than perfect research. In the pursuit of research evidence, we cannot as hand therapists abandon the opinions and advice of experienced clinicians, and we must also remain sensitive to the desires and preferences of our patients.[9]

Physical Agents for Pain Modulation

Traditional therapy intervention for pain management has been rooted for decades in the application of pain-relieving thermal and electrotherapeutic modalities. Physical agents have been valued and used for their analgesic effects and for their contributions to edema management and tissue healing. When contemplating the use of physical agents in a treatment plan, the hand therapist should consider the physiologic rationale, biophysical properties, proposed mechanisms of pain modulation, and precautions or contraindications for each physical agent to ensure safe and effective use on the hand-injured patient. Selection of a particular modality will depend on the source of pain mediation and other contributing factors such as edema, inflammation, and muscle guarding. In addition, selection may be made through the consideration of potential contraindications or precautions with the injured hand.[10,11] Chapter 101 provides information on the use of physical agents in hand therapy, including pain modulation.

Superficial heat and cold application typically take form as hot packs, cold packs, paraffin treatments, ice massage, or fluidotherapy. Although the mode of delivery varies, the mechanism of pain modulation in this group of agents is primarily accomplished by reducing the activation of nociceptors in the periphery.[12] Other short-term physiological changes have also been described in association with these modalities, including changes in nerve conduction and blood flow, as well as changes in tissue extensibility and tone.[12] Thermal modalities are therefore often used as an adjunct to stretching programs to enhance benefit and promote comfort and can be successfully used before other manual therapies such as soft tissue or joint mobilizations.

Other traditional physical agents are used to modify pain through a variety of delivery mechanisms and theoretical pain inhibition mechanisms. Therapeutic ultrasound delivers mechanical energy to the target tissue, where depending on the specific parameters selected, either thermal or nonthermal effects are produced. Thermal effects are similar to those attributed to superficial heating agents but occurring in deeper tissue. Nonthermal effects are thought to facilitate cellular function and metabolic activity, therefore aiding in deep tissue healing.[12] Electrical stimulation in the form of transcutaneous nerve stimulation (TENS) delivered by pulsed or alternating (interferential) current applies low- to medium-frequency electrical current to the skin via self-adhering electrodes. A number of parameters, including,

frequency, duration, and amplitude, can be manipulated to alter the pain-relieving benefits of this treatment. Electroanalgesia is thought to alleviate pain through two mechanisms: the gate control theory of pain and through the release of endogenous opioids.[13] Therapists may use ultrasound and electrical stimulation as methods of transdermal drug delivery to resolve pain and inflammation.[10,11] Iontophoresis and phonophoresis deliver analgesics and antiinflammatory agents transdermally. These methods are typically used to treat the painful target tissue, such as tendon that is readily palpable in a symptomatic tendinopathy. However, current information related to tendon pathologies suggests that tissue inflammation may not consistently play as great a role in mediating pain as previously thought.[14]

Low-level laser therapy (LLLT) is another agent used to alleviate pain in part by accelerating tissue healing. LLLT treatment consists of the application of red and near-infrared light to the skin over the involved area. The mechanism of action is thought to be through the production of nonthermal or photochemical reactions in the cells.[12] Laser is thought to produce inhibitory effects on the peripheral nervous system as well.[12]

The efficacy of physical agents has long been debated. Several Cochrane reviews and other systematic reviews all point to the limited efficacy of commonly used physical agents in hand therapy.[5,15-17] In large part, this is because of limitations in the literature: studies are poorly designed, small and underpowered, and heterogeneic. Effects are found to be short term and often no better than placebo. Knowing this, the hand therapist can still capitalize on their treatment effects. Patients experiencing long-term pain often welcome even brief periods of relief. Physical agents can be used before or after performance of exercises or other therapeutic interventions to allow for greater participation by the patient. Thermal agents and some electroanalgesic agents (TENS or interferential current) can also rather easily be transferred to home administration by the patient, providing needed relief within the patient's own control at any time. Therapists also need to acknowledge that patients arrive at the clinic with expectations of what their treatment may include, especially if the patient has received prior care, which is often the case among patients with chronic or multisite pain. Early establishment of patient rapport and therapeutic alliance may necessitate the inclusion of some physical agents to establish patient "buy in" for the overall treatment plan. The plan of care should include a range of interventions designed to move the patient from passive dependent treatment to more functional, independent, and movement-based interventions.

Psychosocial Treatment Model

Historically, pain treatment within the biomedical model considered pain to be a symptom. Within this model, the goal was to identify the underlying pathomechanical or pathophysiological problem and treat it. When the underlying physical issues were resolved, the pain symptom would also be resolved.[18] This model often worked, especially in acute injury cases, but there were patients whose pain did not respond and resolve as expected.

In recent years, there has been a departure from the biomedical model, instead offering a more holistic treatment model that recognized the contributions of emotional stress and psychosocial factors in the treatment of illnesses, particularly chronic illnesses and pain.[19] This newer model attempted to address both disease, the physical state, and illness, which was viewed as a more complex interaction of biological, psychological, and social factors. Holistic approaches applying the biopsychosocial model to the treatment of pain offer patients more comprehensive care in dealing with the physical, emotional, and social aspects of pain, especially when it is chronic. Interdisciplinary pain treatment programs are equipped with teams of professionals to deal with all aspects of pain, but access remains difficult for many patients.

Even without the benefits of an interdisciplinary team, therapists can and should use holistic concepts when treating patients with pain. Evidence has demonstrated that psychosocial interventions, when combined with other treatment options, provide additional benefit for musculoskeletal pain conditions.[5]

Cognitive Behavioral Treatment Concepts

One way for hand therapists to incorporate psychosocial interventions is with cognitive behavioral techniques. Cognitive behavioral treatment or therapy[20] (CBT) can be conceptualized as a series of feedback loops including the individual's thoughts, feelings, and behaviors (Fig. 96.1). Each aspect of the individual influences the others and can be used to create positive (or negative) changes. How we think about things influences how we feel and what we choose to do. Conversely, feedback from actions or behaviors can similarly change how we feel and therefore what we think. For hand therapists, this is particularly empowering because our typical work on functional behaviors has the potential to impact our patients' thoughts and emotions related to their pain experiences. The primary goal of CBT is to identify and modify or replace maladaptive cognitions, emotions, and behaviors with more adaptive ones, thereby improving coping and functioning by the patient.[20] Specific techniques vary among clinicians, but the components of CBT remain constant. These components are education, skill acquisition, skill consolidation, and generalization and maintenance.[18] It is important to state that clinicians should always practice within their level of skill and training as well as within their local practice credential. By incorporating CBT into treatment, hand therapists are not conducting

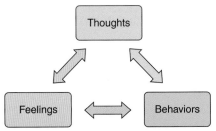

Fig. 96.1 Cognitive Behavioral Theory feedback loops depicted here provide the foundation for change within the CBT treatment model. Each domain can impact the others resulting in positive or negative change.

"psychotherapy" but rather acknowledging the psychosocial aspects of the patient and incorporating an additional dimension into existing treatment techniques for the purpose of greater treatment effect. Some patients may not be responsive to the subtle incorporation of CBT into their treatment plan, and they may benefit from referral to behavioral health professionals.

Cognitive Behavioral Interventions in Hand Therapy

Pain Neuroscience Education. Education is one of the cornerstones of CBT. The ability to impact thinking has the ability to impact emotions and behaviors. In a nutshell, this is how patients change and improve. Patients are often provided with information about their injury, tissue damage, and structural abnormalities. Rather than helping patients cope with their pain, this information may actually increase their concerns, fears, and anxieties, resulting in increased rather than decreased pain. Pain neuroscience education is a newer approach, which is increasing in use among rehabilitation professionals, and has been demonstrating the ability to positively impact pain, stress, anxiety, and disability in patients with musculoskeletal pain.[21]

Rather than emphasizing injury and tissue damage or degeneration, pain neuroscience education provides patients with more information about pain. Patients are taught about nociception and the neural pathways that lead to the brain producing pain. At the same time, information is provided about how neurologic signals are transmitted and how they can be regulated. The key message of pain neuroscience education is that nociception and pain are not the same. There is also an emphasis on the ability of the nervous system to change and reinterpret these signals, leaving patients with a hopeful message that pain is part of a larger system that can be influenced by many different inputs. Current evidence suggests that pain neuroscience education is best provided in direct one-on-one communication in sessions as brief as 30 to 45 minutes and accompanied by a variety of teaching tools such as graphics, examples, and worksheets. Pain neuroscience education has also been demonstrated to be most effective when applied in combination with other therapy interventions such as manual therapy and exercise.[21]

Cognitive Restructuring. All humans are subject to their own "preconceived notions," or automatic thoughts, and this applies to thoughts about pain as well. CBT, as one of its pillars, examines the fallacies that can commonly occur in cognition and processes those errors or distortions with patients, offering alternative ways to think about pain situations. Common cognitive distortions as they relate to pain can be found in Table 96.1 along with cognitive reframing,

TABLE 96.1	**Reframing Common Cognitive Distortions**	
Cognitive Distortion	**Example of Cognitive Distortion**	**Example of Reframing**
Polarized thinking: all or nothing; right or wrong	"Exercise is bad because it makes me hurt. I'd better stop moving; it's making me worse."	"Movement is good. Gradual exercise will make my body stronger."
Overgeneralization: overgeneralizing based on one event	"I can't go grocery shopping. Last time I went, I couldn't get out of bed for 2 days."	"If I pace myself and make a short shopping list, it won't be so bad. I just overdid it last time."
Catastrophizing: everyday problems = disasters	"Another muscle spasm. I must have reinjured myself. I'm pretty sure I'll need that surgery."	"I'm having a spasm; maybe I should apply the cold pack and do some stretches like my therapist suggested."
Overly responsible: takes on too much; "just say no"	"We are having a party for 50 people, and I have to make all of the food because that is what everyone expects."	"We could always cater the party or ask everyone to bring a dish and focus on enjoying each other's company."
Emotional reasoning: can't distinguish feelings from facts	"I am in so much pain that I can't believe how bad I feel. I can't even tie my own shoes let alone provide for my family. I feel like I'm no good to anyone."	"I'm going to follow my routine using strategies I learned in therapy. After I shower and get dressed, I will feel a little better, and I'll do my home exercises."
Filtering: focusing only on the negative	"I'm having pain. I'm back to square one."	"Actually, my pain is not as intense as it used to be, and it's been a week since I had a major pain episode. I'm making progress."

Data from Vranceanu A, Safren S. Cognitive-behavioral therapy for hand and arm pain. *J Hand Ther.* 2011;2:124-130, and from personal communication with J Carrillo, PhD, cognitive behavioral clinical psychologist.

which can be offered as an alternative way for patients to interpret their thoughts about pain in a more positive way.[20] The process of trying to relearn the way one thinks about and interprets pain is difficult and takes time. It is important to reinforce these concepts during treatment sessions but also to assist the patient in developing self-monitoring skills. One way to accomplish this is through the use of a *thought* journal in which patients record their thoughts about pain as they emerge in daily life. Then patients can record their moods, make an assessment of their cognitive distortions, and record alternative reframed thoughts. Over time, this process becomes more automatic, and it is hoped that patients may learn new ways to process thoughts about pain. Ultimately, this becomes a tool whereby patients realize a greater degree of control over their thoughts, feelings, and actions related to their pain responses.[20]

Skills Acquisition and Consolidation. In addition to recognizing and altering thoughts about pain, it is also important to equip patients with new pain management behaviors to assist in dealing with their pain. A primary tenant of CBT is that each component—thoughts, emotions, and behaviors—has the ability to influence each other. Changing behaviors as they relate to pain can simultaneously alter thoughts and feelings about pain as well. In assisting patients to gain new pain management skills, the emphasis is placed on the development of self-efficacy and independence, not on the particular skill because patients respond differently to different methods.[18]

Relaxation Training. It is common for patients with pain, especially those with chronic pain, to experience stress along with comorbid anxiety, anger, and depression.[19] These can predate the pain but nonetheless are capable of heightening the pain experience. Conversely affective disorders can also emerge after pain events, especially when pain is prolonged.[19] Physiological stress responses occur in reaction to fear or perceived threats to safety.[22] Epinephrine, norepinephrine, and cortisol are released, and when this happens repeatedly or when levels remain elevated for prolonged periods, the body develops a sensitized physiological stress response, which is easily triggered. This leads to prolonged elevation of cortisol, systemic inflammation, and increased pain. The stress–cortisol–pain cycle becomes self-perpetuating. The ability to break the cycle and invoke a relaxation response may help to reduce both stress and pain. Two widely used relaxation techniques are diaphragmatic breathing and progressive muscle relaxation. Diaphragmatic breathing trains patients to breathe slowly and deeply, engaging the diaphragm in abdominal excursion, the diaphragm in abdominal excursion rather than shallow, rapid chest breathing, which uses smaller accessory muscles. Diaphragmatic breathing has been demonstrated to impact emotions by decreasing negative cognitions and has also been shown to decrease cortisol levels and thus directly impacts the stress cycle.[23]

Progressive muscle relaxation is a whole-body relaxation technique in which participants alternately tense and relax muscle groups and regions of the body. It is thought that over time, with prolonged states of stress, the body "learns" to be tense. This state of muscle tension is often so persistent that it becomes "normal." Through progressive muscle relaxation exercise, patients are able to feel the difference between tense and relaxed states, and it is thought that over time, muscle relaxation can be relearned.[20]

Both diaphragmatic breathing and progressive muscle relaxation fall within the scope of therapist's practice expertise and can be performed in the clinic and issued as part of a home exercise program. Numerous online resources can be found to assist patients with home practice of these techniques. It is always prudent for therapists to curate a list of reliable digital and online resources to guide patients in their independent practice of these techniques at home.

Activity Modification and Pacing. Another important and helpful technique when implementing CBT strategies is the concept of activity modification and pacing. Therapists often encounter pain patients who are at either extreme of the activity spectrum. At one extreme, patients are afraid to move and are not engaging in much activity at all. At the other extreme, patients try to do everything, and in the course of doing so, they exacerbate pain symptoms and at times even risk disrupting healing tissue. Activity modification and pacing techniques are helpful skills for patients to learn regardless of where they fall on the activity spectrum and across many diagnoses regardless of the mechanism of pain generation.

Activity modifications or accommodations are described as a group of strategies that allow patients to perform daily activities with greater ease and less pain. Some examples include assistive devices, adaptations to tools, equipment or work surfaces, and stopping or avoiding certain activities or ways of performing activities.[24] Activity pacing is a specific strategy used to help patients manage their pain by thoughtfully planning and performing activities with alternate periods of activity and rest or by segmenting tasks into multiple shorter time blocks or by simultaneously slowing down. In activity pacing, the individual's pain tolerance is not exceeded. Research has shown that the ability to perform valued activities plays an important role in overall health and emotional well-being, and conversely, the inability to engage in desired activities reduces quality of life and increases risk for the development of depression.[24] Therefore, preservation of valued activities is an important facet of an overall hand therapy treatment program.

To begin the process of implementing activity pacing and activity modification strategies, patients first need to realize that activities impact their pain. Activity logs or journals can be helpful in allowing patients to reflect on their actions and make connections about how their actions affect pain levels.[25] Patients can then begin the process of collaborating with their hand therapist to devise strategies that both build the patient's confidence and foster self-efficacy associated with function. Therapists may wish to develop materials for patients, including examples of adaptive devices, sources to obtain devices, and simple cost-effective strategies, as well as ideas from other patients regarding tips they found to be helpful while navigating this same process.[24] Ultimately, the therapist's goal is to provide a "toolbox of ideas" so that patients can become effective problem solvers on their own behalf.[25]

Patient Advice, Education, and Self-Management

Although certainly similar to and in some instances overlapping with pain neuroscience education (PNE), patient advice, education, and self-management instruction are to be differentiated. PNE is a discrete program of education specifically using cognitive behavioral approaches to engage patients in the management of their own pain with the goals of reducing fear and anxiety about pain, "rethinking" pain, and practicing and implementing new behaviors to cope with pain. There is a growing literature base supporting PNE as an effective treatment intervention for pain management, especially related to chronic pain and when implemented in combination with other therapy interventions.[5] Patient advice, education, and self-management information includes "everything else" hand therapists typically share with patients to facilitate their understanding and participation in their own care. The evidence supporting the use of self-management advice and education is derived primarily from expert opinion as contained in treatment guidelines developed by consensus panels. There is weak support based on low to moderate-quality studies for this collection of interventions.[5] Despite limited evidence, there are still strong recommendations for the inclusion of patient education within a broader treatment plan.

Home Exercise Program

Therapists should take the time to explain their hypothesis of why the patient has a chief symptom of pain, including the source of pain mediation. When the patient gains an understanding of his or her pain condition, the therapist is likely to see a reduction in anxiety about the rehabilitation process. Patients need to understand that therapy, especially exercise, is not going to cause more pain or tissue damage. Education should also empower the patient to be an active participant in the plan of care. This may need to be continually emphasized with some patients. If the patient is an active participant, compliance with therapy visits and home programs should be evident. It is important to provide patients with written instructions with pictures or videos for home programs because pain may distract their ability to remember the entire program.

In our current technology-driven era, it is also possible more than ever for hand therapists to use computer-and smartphone-based activities to enhance patient home exercise programs. Several digital and online home exercise generating programs allow therapists to email programs directly to patients complete with pictures, customized instructions, and even video clips. To further customize exercise programs or home instructions, it has been suggested that the therapist may take pictures or video clips on the patient's own smartphone with the patient receiving instruction or performing exercises in the clinic.[26] These simple tools can be invaluable in reminding the patient of correct technique, therefore improving safety and compliance. In addition, numerous smartphone gaming and puzzle apps have been suggested as potential enhancements to therapy programs as they can engage a variety of fine-motor and proprioceptive skills.[26] Use of a smartphone as an adjunct to certain aspects of the therapy plan of care is convenient, low cost, and motivating.

Posture

Including instruction and advice about posture is also an important part of the information that can be offered by hand therapists. Initially, posture retraining may focus on determining a position of comfort (i.e., a position that results in tolerable or minimized pain). Therapists may need to instruct patients in appropriate positions for sleeping, driving, or working. Patients who report sleep difficulty secondary to pain will benefit from education about sleeping postures. Extra pillows for upper limb support in the supine or sidelying position may improve the patient's ability to sleep. If the patient can improve his or her hours of sleep, pain tolerance may improve because the inability to sleep is one of the variables that affects pain tolerance. A patient's workstation should be evaluated to determine whether any positions or activities may exacerbate his or her pain. Modifications should be made if awkward postures or limb movements are evident. This is particularly true in patients with sedentary jobs, such as those who primarily use a computer for their work activities.

Posture assessment may reveal common postural faults in patients with upper quarter pain, such as forward head and rounded shoulders. Imbalances between muscle groups may exist as well. Flexibility exercises should be given to stretch tight muscles, and strengthening exercises should be performed to strengthen weak muscles.[27] Exercises to promote trunk and scapular stability will reduce postural faults and enhance functional performance of the upper limbs. The exercises need to be integrated to match the patient's source of pain mediation and tolerance for exercise. The exercises should not aggravate the patient's pain.

Rest, Active Rest, and Pain-free Movement

Therapists need to be thorough in instruction to patients regarding activity. These instructions will vary widely depending on the diagnosis, chronicity, and mechanism of pain. The instructions will evolve as the patient response and progress warrant. Patients should be instructed to avoid motions or functional activities that aggravate their pain. This intervention is an essential component to all patients, regardless of the source of pain mediation. It may not be possible to avoid all activities, especially activities of daily living; therefore, instruction on how to modify these activities may minimize pain. Patients must have a good understanding that constant rest or complete immobilization are detrimental to healing musculoskeletal tissues. Orthoses or limb positioning should be used to offer intermittent rest to painful or injured tissues, but pain-free, controlled range of motion (ROM) exercises should be performed throughout the day.

In cases of acute peripheral nociceptive pain, patients may experience some discomfort during exercise, but it should subside quickly after exercise. Patients and therapists can gauge the vigor of the therapeutic exercise program by observing tissue reactivity. Pain associated with exercise should subside within 30 minutes, edema should not increase, and there should not be a loss of motion if the vigor of exercise is appropriate. If pain, edema, and stiffness increase for a persistent time after exercise, the therapeutic exercise program should be reassessed and downgraded.

Lifestyle Changes

Finally, specific global tactics may be used to promote musculoskeletal tissue healing as well as decrease pain (Table 96.2). These lifestyle changes may be beneficial for all sources of pain mediation and tissue healing. The nervous system is highly vascularized and metabolically demanding; therefore, nerves depend on good blood flow to maintain function and health.[28] The global tactics focus on lifestyle changes that promote increased blood flow, increased oxygen, and stress-free use of the hand and upper extremity. Pain, especially chronic pain, is often associated with inactivity and can in fact be both a cause and an effect of inactivity. There are additional lifestyle practices that have also been associated with musculoskeletal pain, including smoking, poor diet, poor weight management, altered sleep habits, and high levels of stress.[29]

Most would agree that smoking is harmful to health in numerous ways. In relation to the musculoskeletal system, smoking directly impacts exercise capacity, has been shown to delay healing, increases complication rates after surgery and trauma, is associated with increased systemic inflammation, and is linked to reports of increased pain.[29] Tobacco users have demonstrated slowed collagen production and weaker scar tissue formation, leading to increased risk for recurrent injury.[30] Smoking is also reported to impact local inflammation in conditions such as lateral elbow tendinopathy and has been reported to be an independent risk factor for this upper extremity condition.[29] Conversely, smoking cessation has been shown over time to reverse all of the negative impacts mentioned. Since 2012 the American Physical Therapy Association has advocated that physical therapists should take an active role in helping patients to stop smoking, a position that seems generalizable to all rehabilitation professionals. Research has shown that most smokers do contemplate smoking cessation but are more than twice as likely to take action if two or more health care providers

TABLE 96.2	Lifestyle Changes to Enhance Nerve and Tissue Healing	
Increase Blood Flow	**Increase Oxygen**	**Reduce Stress**
Reduce caffeine	Hydration	Joint protection
Smoking cessation	Focused breathing	Activity modification
Exercise	Exercise	Mindfulness

discuss it with them. At the same time, more than 60% of adult smokers never receive any information from medical providers regarding their smoking habit.[30] Therapists in general are in a unique position to have input given the number of interactions during which patients are contacted.[30] Materials to assist patients with smoking cessation have been created by the US Department of Health and Human Services and are available online.[31]

Unhealthy diet and excess weight are other modifiable lifestyle behaviors that can impact pain. An optimal diet provides nutrients needed for tissue repair, may decrease systemic inflammation, and improves overall energy levels.[29] These in turn can over time reduce body mass to a healthy level, which facilitates activity by easing joint loading and energy expenditure.

Lifestyle modification advice typically offered for management of chronic conditions and illnesses such as cardiovascular disease and diabetes is similarly warranted in musculoskeletal care, especially in the management of chronic pain. A novel concept has been proposed in the literature suggesting a longitudinal approach to care in chronic musculoskeletal conditions given that we know behavioral modification occurs slowly and is subject to relapse.[32] Current treatment models across the board subscribe to relatively brief episodes of rehabilitation care carried out at fairly high frequency (e.g., two to three visits per week for 1 to 2 months). Researchers are proposing a model that better matches the natural history of chronic musculoskeletal conditions in which contact with the therapist makes sense over a longer time frame but with less frequent contacts. This allows patients to internalize behavioral change concepts, allows support through potential symptom flare-ups, and fosters progressive independence on the part of the patient. Although this proposed treatment concept makes sense to therapists, referral sources and third-party insurers may not embrace the concept with enthusiasm. As therapist practice evolves toward greater autonomy and with technologies such as telehealth, this type of strategy may gain traction in the near future.[32]

Addressing Sleep Disturbance and Insomnia in Individuals with Pain

The importance of sleep as it relates to pain is discussed in Chapter 94. If poor sleep quality or duration is present, then pain inhibition mechanisms in the body are less effective.[33–35] Addressing sleep disturbances and overall sleep quality and quantity has notable potential to improve homeostatic mechanisms related to overall pain fluctuations from day to day.[36] Additionally, sleep deprivation has been shown to have significant adverse effect on tissue healing in rat models.[37] Therefore, addressing altered sleep has notable potential for improving rehabilitation outcomes with regard to tissue healing and overall pain.

Exercise to improve sleep quality is one of the most readily available interventions; however, it is not universally effective in dealing with altered sleep or insomnia. Current best evidence for nonpharmacologic management of chronic insomnia and decreased sleep quality supports the use of cognitive behavioral therapy for insomnia (CBT-i).[38,39] Although most upper extremity and hand rehabilitation professionals are unlikely to be trained as a cognitive behavioral therapists, clinicians can still apply components of this intervention approach through patient education aimed at behavior change to improve multiple measures of sleep. CBT-i is typically described in five components: cognitive therapy, stimulus control, sleep restriction, sleep hygiene, and relaxation. Because most therapists are not psychologists or psychiatrists, a description of the cognitive therapy component will not be described here. It is important to point out that although some components may be more effective than others delivered in isolation, rehabilitation professionals are encouraged to use the approaches described next in tandem with exercise for compounding effect.

TABLE 96.3 Stimulus Control and Sleep Hygiene General Recommendations

Stimulus control	Go to bed only when sleepy
	When unable to sleep, leave the bedroom for 15–20 minutes and return only when sleepy
	Avoid nonsleep activities in the bedroom (e.g., reading, watching television, video games)
Sleep hygiene	Go to bed at the same time each night
	Wake up at the same time each morning
	Avoid daytime napping longer than 20 minutes
	Avoid visual access to a clock
	Limit use of caffeine, nicotine, and alcohol, especially around bedtime
	Avoid ingesting large volumes of water before bed
	Keep the bedroom at a cool temperature and dark
	Avoid bright lights or electronic screens within the hour before bedtime

Stimulus Control

The concept of stimulus control is based on facilitating associations between the individual's presence in bed and sleep while preventing learned associations between being in bed and any other activity outside of sleep or sex.[38,39] Examples of general recommendations for stimulus control are listed in Table 96.3.

Sleep Hygiene

Sleep hygiene revolves around leveraging multiple different factors (e.g., physiological, behavioral, environmental) to facilitate higher quality sleep.[38,39] Examples of general recommendations for sleep hygiene are listed in Table 96.3.

Sleep Restriction

Sleep restriction is an intervention that can be used to directly attempt to increase sleep efficiency

$$\left(\frac{\text{average 1-2 week total sleep time (minutes)}}{\text{average 1-2 week total time in bed (minutes)}} \times 100 \right),$$

resulting in decreased time spent awake in bed and increased drive for sleep.[33,38] Current literature on sleep restriction indicates this is the most effective component for addressing fragmented or overall decreased sleep.[38] Although sleep restriction is effective, reporting of parameters used for sleep restriction in clinical trials is variable and often omitted[40]; however, general recommendations for sleep restriction are presented in Table 96.4. Sleep restriction should be used with caution in patients with comorbid diagnoses of epilepsy or bipolar disorder because of the potential to cause adverse effects.[38]

Relaxation

Relaxation involves whatever relaxation technique is effective for the individual to promote sleep through reduced muscle tension and decreased cognitive activity or arousal.[38,39] This may include mindfulness, mediation, guided imagery, focused breathing, or progressive muscle relaxation.[38,39,41]

Manual Therapy

Manual therapy as an intervention can take many forms and can involve many different tissue types. Soft tissue can be mobilized via

TABLE 96.4 General Recommendations for Sleep Restriction[a]

Sleep window	Adjusted based on TST from 1- to 2-week sleep log
	Sleep window positioned based on patient preference
	Minimum TIB of 5 hours to limit adverse effects
Sleep efficiency criterion:	
≥85% over 5 days	Increase TIB by 15 min
80%–85% over 5 days	No change in TIB
<80% over 5 days	Decrease TIB by 15 min unless TIB is already at the minimum

[a]General recommendations based on a combination of original recommendations described by Spielman and associates[42] and the most commonly used protocols in intervention trials.[40]
TIB, Time in bed; TST, total sleep time.

massage or scar tissue mobilization, with either therapists' hands or the use of instruments. Joints can be mobilized or manipulated with low-amplitude, high-velocity thrust application, and neural tissue can be mobilized through application of specific tensioning and gliding forces. Research has begun to shed more light on the mechanisms through which these techniques modify pain responses in individuals.

Massage and Soft Tissue Mobilization

Massage and soft tissue mobilization are often well tolerated by patients, perhaps too well tolerated at times. Hand therapists should carefully evaluate the role these interventions may play in the treatment plan and consider the goals they are attempting to achieve through their use. Passive treatments can habituate patients to patterns of inactivity that are likely counter to the ultimate therapy goal of return to function. However, there are desirable benefits of soft tissue work, especially when it can be used as a segue to more active interventions.

Research has demonstrated numerous mechanisms by which pain is altered by soft tissue mobilization. A general response to massage is relaxation, which in turn can decrease levels of the stress hormone cortisol. The benefits of cortisol reduction have been discussed previously. Massage also alters the release of neurotransmitters in the central nervous system (CNS), increasing inhibition through descending control pathways. In the periphery, healing is promoted by reduction of inflammation, which is accomplished by altered gene expression in the tissue. Massage has been shown to reduce mechanical and chemical irritants, which results in decreased activation of nociceptors.[43] However, in the literature, the effects of massage and soft tissue mobilization are very limited. The benefits are often found to be short term, at times no better than sham treatments, and most successful when used as a limited part of a multimodal treatment plan.

A popular form of soft tissue work in current use is instrument assisted soft tissue mobilization. In this type of massage technique, hard instruments, either plastic or metal, are used to apply scraping type strokes to the treatment area. This can result in posttreatment soreness, swelling, and bruising. The benefit is stated to be the remodeling of scar tissue in the treatment area. Preclinical research to support these claims is very limited at this time.[44] A small pilot study conducted on patients with carpal tunnel syndrome compared instrument-assisted techniques with soft tissue manipulation with clinician's hands. The results showed that both groups improved, but there were no significant between group differences.[45] Because of potential adverse effects of posttreatment soreness, swelling, and ecchymosis, it is recommended that before using this intervention, therapists should be adequately trained in proper use of the various instruments and should adequately describe the treatment and potential side effects to the patient before treatment execution.

Joint Mobilization and Manipulation

Joint mobilizations and manipulations include a wide variety of passive movement techniques applied by therapists to affect joint position, joint mobility, and pain. Chapter 104 provides a detailed overview of manual therapy along with specific application criteria. Joint mobilizations and manipulations have been shown in the literature to produce short-duration pain-relieving effects by increasing pain thresholds and decreasing motor neuron excitability.[43] There have also been a number of studies demonstrating regional effects.[46–48] Thoracic and cervical spinal manipulations have demonstrated effects on the shoulder and elbow, respectively, and elbow mobilizations have been shown to improve shoulder ROM. A systematic review examining effective treatment options for musculoskeletal pain determined that manual therapy effects in the literature were mostly for nonacute pain and were mostly studied in combination with other interventions.[5] In this same review, the quality of evidence was determined to be moderate to high, and pooled estimates of effectiveness were considered significant. Effects were short term, ranging from immediate to 6 weeks.

In another systematic review,[47] it was noted that most evidence on manual therapy in the upper extremity was related to the shoulder. Evidence related to the elbow was all in patient populations presenting with lateral elbow pain. The most favorable mobilization for treatment of lateral elbow pain is Mulligan's mobilization with movement, which consistently was found to decrease pain and improve pain-free function, particularly gripping.

The evidence for use of manual therapy for the wrist and hand is extremely limited.[48] A very low number of studies have examined the use of mobilizations at the wrist. There is not a strong consensus on the best techniques. All mobilizations have been found to reduce pain, and in some instances, ROM has improved a bit earlier than comparison groups. One study compared a carpal tunnel surgery group with a manual therapy group.[49] A novel approach was taken in manual therapy, treating the entire pathway of the median nerve from the cervical spine to the wrist. This treatment methodology was based on theory and evidence that although a peripheral neuropathy, carpal tunnel syndrome may in fact be more complex manifesting sensitization of the CNS as well.[50] In both studies, the therapists performed cervical mobilizations along with upper extremity soft tissue mobilization at known common compression sites for the median nerve along with specific median nerve–gliding maneuvers.[49,50] In these studies, the manual therapy group demonstrated greater improvement in pain and function at initial follow-up (3 months). The two groups were found to have similar outcomes at long-term follow-up (6 months and 1 year). The significance here is that conservative treatment by hand therapists is able to achieve similar outcomes as surgery regarding the studied outcome measures but with significantly less risk to the patient.

Because of the low number of studies dedicated to the hand combined with the high number of articulations in the hand, resulting in high variability, little clinically relevant data exist at this time regarding application of joint mobilizations in the hand.[48] So although the entirety of the existing evidence is supportive of the use of joint mobilization and manipulation as part of a multimodal treatment approach for short-term effects at the shoulder and elbow, there is a need to develop more studies related to the distal upper extremity to further understand how manual therapy may help hand therapy patients in regards to pain relief and improvement of function.

Neural Mobilization

Neural mobilizations are interventions performed manually by hand therapists and adapted into exercises for patient independent performance when appropriate. Neurodynamic mobilization is particularly effective in patients presenting with peripheral neurogenic pain. The purpose of neurodynamic mobilization is to restore normal functioning to the nervous system by moving nerves or surrounding tissue.

Studies have shown that neural mobilization can have significant physiological impact after nerve injury and can play a role in returning the nerve and surrounding structures to homeostasis.[51] Additional information on nerve mobilization is available in Chapter 103.

Current evidence suggests that in the upper extremity, neurodynamic strategies are helpful in the treatment of carpal tunnel syndrome and lateral elbow pain, but evidence for benefit in ulnar nerve compressions is lacking.[51] Numerous studies have evaluated neurodynamic techniques in carpal tunnel syndrome, and the findings indicate that greatest benefit is derived from median nerve–sliding techniques. Sliding techniques produced improvements in pain and function and resulted in decreased intraneural edema.[51] Nerve gliding has also been found to improve nerve conduction, whereas tensioning maneuvers have been found to negatively affect nerve conduction.[52,53] Lateral elbow pain has been positively affected by use of cervical lateral gliding techniques.[51]

Neurodynamic movements can successfully improve symptoms and function in patients with nerve compression syndromes of the upper extremity when applied manually by the hand therapist in the clinic and when performed as exercises by the patient. Based on current evidence, therapists should take care to select appropriate movement patterns to emphasize nerve sliding while limiting nerve tensioning in the involved structures. Patients should also be counselled on the impact that daily activity can have on neural dynamics so that they have awareness of potential undesired forces created in postures and movements during functional activity.

Exercise

The therapy intervention with the strongest evidence for its effective treatment of musculoskeletal pain is exercise.[5] Exercise improves pain, function, and quality of life with medium to large effect sizes and this occurs with a wide variety of exercise types applied to all musculoskeletal areas of pain and all mechanisms of pain generation.[5] This is not entirely surprising because we know that exercise has been shown to be helpful for management of all types of chronic health conditions and illnesses from diabetes[54] to cardiovascular disease,[55] and exercise is also an essential component in healthy weight maintenance.[56] In the rehabilitation setting, graded exercise provides a pathway for returning to function. Patients are normally cautious during early healing stages, in part because of the nature of the pain they experience and also because of their understanding or lack of understanding about tissue healing. It is vital that hand therapists explain concepts of tissue healing in ways that will not cause patients to be fearful of moving. By understanding the concept of mechanotherapy or mechanotransduction, therapists can convey to patients the process by which the body heals itself from a cellular level.[57] Movement in and of itself is a healing force and not to be feared. Movement, even gentle movement, produces mechanical loading of tissue. This mechanical loading causes physical perturbation at the cellular level, which results in an array of chemical signaling within and between cells. Cell-to-cell communication triggers a cascade of molecular activities extending far beyond the original location of mechanical input and results in tissue healing. Therapeutic exercise is therefore a catalyst in promoting the repair and remodeling of injured tissue.[57] Therapists can conceptualize graded therapeutic exercise in all of its forms as a means of managing tissue loading. Too little mechanical loading will result in an insufficient stimulus to heal or cause tissue changes; too much loading, and the forces may overwhelm the tissue resulting in pain and possible tissue degradation. Administered skillfully, movement and exercise are key components of tissue healing and pain relief. Although the global effects of exercise are well established in the literature, many of the specifics related to type of exercise and dosing continue to emerge.

Exercise for Central Sensitization Pain

Patients referred to therapy with central sensitization pain present with a cluster of signs and symptoms that is recognizable. According to Smart and coworkers,[58] these signs and symptoms are disproportionate, nonmechanical, unpredictable patterns of pain with nonspecific aggravating and easing factors; pain that is disproportionate to the injury or pathology; maladaptive psychosocial factors; and diffuse nonanatomic pain and tenderness with palpation. Patients with central sensitization pain often report that they are apprehensive about exercise because activity has flared up their symptoms in the past. This group of patients typically has habituated to greater and greater levels of inactivity over time because of their negative pain responses to exercise attempts. Although exercise typically induces hypoalgesia by activating descending inhibitory pain mechanisms, this is not always the case in individuals with central sensitization.[58] In fact, the opposite can happen, and exercise that is too aggressive can trigger sensitized peripheral nociceptors and cause significant increases in pain for prolonged periods of time.[58] A key concept in prescribing exercise with this patient group is to appropriately match patient symptom levels and symptom irritability with exercise intensity. In the centrally sensitized patient, lower exercise intensities are capable of inducing exercise hypoalgesia, which in turn will reinforce exercise performance.

In the literature, the exercise most associated with pain relief in patients with chronic pain and central sensitization is aerobic exercise. Aerobic exercise is known to activate descending pain modulation and as such can be a contributor to overall pain relief. Any form of aerobic activity will produce beneficial effects, and the exercise does not have to directly engage the painful areas. The therapist should start with brief, low-intensity activity, progressing in a graded manner. Walking programs are an ideal way to accomplish this goal with upper extremity patients.

Another form of exercise noted in the literature as beneficial for treatment of central sensitization is strengthening exercise, in particular isometric strength training. Isometric exercise has been noted as having analgesic effects especially when performed at lower intensity of contraction between 25% and 50% of maximum voluntary contraction, for longer duration holds, upward to 90 seconds.[59] Other studies have indicated that light resistance exercises performed for higher repetitions are beneficial for this population in part because of their conditioning effects.[8] Finally, there is evidence to suggest that complementary exercises such as yoga, tai chi, and Pilates demonstrate some efficacy with centrally sensitized pain populations.[59] This may in part be because of the generally gentle, noncompetitive, self-paced nature of these practices along with their focus on breathing and relaxation of muscle tension.

Exercise for Peripheral Neuropathic Pain

Patients presenting to therapy with peripheral neuropathic pain presentations will, according to Smart and associates,[60] display a unique pattern of signs and symptoms. These include pain referred in a dermatomal or cutaneous distribution; history of nerve injury, pathology, or mechanical compromise; and pain or symptom provocation with mechanical or movement tests such as neurodynamic tests that move, load, or compress neural tissue.[60] Treatment of peripheral neuropathic pain consists primarily of the application of neurodynamic mobilization both in the form of therapist generated mobilizations as discussed in the previous section on manual therapy and through patient performance of neurodynamic exercises. These exercises are described in more detail in Chapter 102.

Accurate performance of nerve mobilization exercises is very important so that the proper force be imparted to the desired tissue. Step-by-step instructions with pictures, cell phone photos, or short narrated cell phone videos are very helpful to aid in proper performance and compliance with neurodynamic exercises. Improper performance of exercises can lead to significant aggravation of the symptom pattern. Dosing is also an extremely important component of neurodynamic exercises, although there is no consensus in the literature to give clinicians guidance. In general, nerve mobilization exercises should be selected based on irritability of the nerve as noted during upper limb neurodynamic testing. Highly symptomatic conditions initially respond better to gliding or sliding techniques that promote greater excursion of the nerve while keeping tension levels low. The exercises may induce mild stretching sensations but should not reproduce the pattern of nerve pain. Exercises should be performed in low numbers of repetitions with higher frequency throughout the day. It is crucial to educate the patient about not exceeding prescribed dosing and about monitoring their exercise responses because flare-ups of pain may be (and usually are) latent. Patients should be instructed in how to manage aggravation of symptoms with techniques such as application of thermal modalities, decreasing intensity of exercises, decreasing frequency of exercise, use of prescribed antiinflammatory drugs as directed, and positioning for comfort. As the symptom presentation improves, neurodynamic exercises can be increased gradually by modifying intensity and frequency, adding progressive tensioning maneuvers, and evaluating surrounding soft tissue for mobility impairments. It is common, for example, that proximal muscles such as the upper trapezius, pectoral muscles, and scalenes may be limited in flexibility because of the adoption of accommodating postures over time to alleviate neural stress and pain.

Exercise for Nociceptive Pain

Patients presenting to therapy with nociceptive pain present with a cluster of clinical criteria predictive of nociceptive pain, including pain localized to the area of pain or dysfunction; clear, proportionate mechanical or anatomical nature to aggravating and easing factors; usually intermittent and sharp with movement or mechanical provocation; may be a more constant dull ache or throb at rest; the absence of pain in association with other dysesthesias; night pain with disturbed sleep; antalgic postures or movement patterns; and pain variously described as burning, shooting, sharp, or electric shock–like.[61] In most outpatient hand therapy settings, this will likely represent a large portion of the patients treated. Therapeutic exercise interventions for patients with nociceptive pain are in large part based on the physical impairments noted on the evaluation. Typical impairments may include edema, limited ROM, and strength and endurance deficits as well as neuromuscular deficits in coordination or proprioception.

Depending on the acuity of the pain and associated diagnosis (e.g., trauma, fracture, surgery, "itis," "osis," or "opathy"), initial exercise intervention may be focused on promoting circulation, alleviating swelling, and promoting tissue healing. ROM exercises can be used to activate muscle pumping action, which in turn stimulates circulation and helps to alleviate stiffness and joint limitations caused by edema. For wider spread swelling, exercise concepts such as those used as part of a more comprehensive edema decongestion or mobilization program can be helpful. Edema mobilization techniques generally include a series of exercises that aim to decrease limb swelling through repeated muscle contraction. Such routines begin with core or proximal clearing exercises such as diaphragmatic breathing or core muscle activation. Exercises then proceed from proximal to distal, which is proposed to decongest and clear more proximal swelling first, thus allowing distal edema to drain. It is important to

state that although studies report patient satisfaction with these techniques, accompanied by subjective reports of improvement, the small amount of evidence available does not demonstrate statistical significance.[62] Additional information about edema mobilization for orthopedic patients can be found in Chapter 57. As tissue healing occurs, patients will progress through ROM exercises to stretching, in which more stress is placed on involved tissue to restore tissue length and joint mobility. A limited pool of evidence supports implementation of stretching programs for pain relief.[63] However, greater pain relief is noted when stretching exercise is combined with strengthening exercise.[63] Strengthening exercise, as discussed in a previous section, has been demonstrated to produce pain-relieving effects.[8,58] In addition, exercise can improve function, thereby decreasing disability, and can help prevent development of chronic pain.[58] Even with multiple known benefits of exercise, research on specifics of load, intensity, duration, total volume of activity, and variation based on tissue type is only beginning to emerge regarding specific exercise prescription. There are several specific areas of upper extremity rehabilitation that have growing bodies of research supporting the implementation of exercise in the treatment plan.

Treatment of painful conditions at the shoulder, variously called shoulder impingement, impingement syndrome, subacromial pain syndrome, or rotator cuff tendinopathy, have been found in numerous studies and systematic reviews to benefit from exercise interventions.[64–68] In summary, these studies concluded that exercise is effective in decreasing shoulder pain and improving function. The addition of manual therapy techniques to a therapeutic exercise regimen enhanced the benefit above that of exercise alone.[68,69] Specific, progressive, moderately painful exercises including both concentric and eccentric resistive exercises for the scapular stabilizers and rotator cuff were found to be more effective than pain-free general ROM and stretching exercises for the shoulder region.[64] This information may be valuable when considering how to structure exercise programs to treat peripheral nociceptive pain. Peripheral nociceptive pain responds to more intense and more specific exercises compared with the exercises recommended for central sensitization pain, which are more global in their scope, are lower intensity, and are recommended to be pain free. Additional studies comparing the effectiveness of therapeutic exercise versus surgery for shoulder impingement concluded that exercise can be as effective as surgery.[66–68] The authors admit to low- and moderate-quality evidence; however, they still conclude that the effects of exercise on pain and function are equal to surgery outcomes and that given the significant discrepancy between the interventions in terms of risk and cost, exercise is recommended as a first-line intervention to improve pain and function.

Lateral elbow tendinopathy is another painful upper extremity condition frequently treated with exercise. Although there are limitations in the quality of the literature, evidence suggests that exercise is effective in reducing pain and disability over time.[69] There is little consensus, however, on the type of exercise or dosing of exercise for optimum benefit. Eccentric exercise is popular and has been studied frequently in recent years, but the literature stops short of advocating eccentric exercise over other forms of strengthening. There is some evidence to support concentric and isometric exercises along with eccentric strengthening.[69–71] Unfortunately, there is no clear guidance on how to determine appropriate resistance intensity or exercise duration.[69] In addition to a variety of strengthening methods for the wrist extensor group, some researchers have found that scapular stabilizers as well as rotator cuff muscles have been found to be impaired in groups with lateral elbow tendinopathy.[71] Although causation has not been established, it is suggested that these muscle groups warrant evaluation and appropriate strengthening if indicated.[72]

The final painful upper extremity condition for which exercise is often prescribed by hand therapists is thumb carpometacarpal (CMC) osteoarthritis. The research advocating this has not progressed as far as it needs to. Principles and programs currently in use are widely based on biomechanical analysis of the thumb CMC joint with the intended goal to stabilize the painful hypermobile joint; others are based on physiologic ROM of the thumb combined with resistive exercise in functional gripping and pinching positions.[72,73] A small number of clinical trials do point to benefit from multimodal treatment for thumb CMC osteoarthritis.[74,75] In all experimental treatment plans, exercise was used; however, there is not a clear consensus on the combination of components best used within the multimodal treatment plan. So although there is still much that needs further study, it does appear that exercise is widely used and beneficial to patients with thumb CMC osteoarthritis.

Other Treatments: Emerging and Complementary

There are other interventions that are increasingly used in the treatment of patients with painful conditions of the upper extremity. Although some are newer such as elastic tape and dry needling, others are ancient practices such as cupping therapy that have found new popularity as favorites among elite athletes and on social media. Elastic taping is discussed at length in Chapter 103, and readers are referred there for additional information.

Dry needling is an intervention that has been performed for more than 20 years, but it began to gain popularity over the past decade. The intervention primarily consists of insertion of needle monofilaments (acupuncture needles) into myofascial trigger points for the purpose of pain reduction and normalization of muscle function.

There are numerous variations and schools of thought currently taught involving different needle placement, target tissue, and combination of dry needling with electrical stimulation in which the needle acts as an internal electrode in the muscle (Fig. 96.2). As with any emerging intervention, the body of evidence regarding dry needling is not without problems and is small but is growing rapidly. Current systematic reviews, including one that looked at the evidence for the upper quarter, indicate that dry needling can be an effective part of multimodal treatment of pain.[76-78] A case study using dry needling along with manual therapy for lateral elbow tendinopathy reported that the patient experienced rapid improvement in pressure pain threshold and pain-free grip over eight treatment sessions in 4 weeks. The results were sustained at 4-month follow-up, and in fact, pain-free grip was even greater than at the conclusion of treatment.[79] Dry needling has been reported as effective in both acute and chronic conditions. The pain-relieving underpinnings of dry needling are thought to be many, including the activation of opioid- and nonopioid-based pain reduction mechanisms, normalization of nociceptive channels, and reversal of hyperalgesia. A number of synergistic mechanisms are proposed to mediate analgesia via biochemical and mechanical processes in neural, connective, and muscle tissue.[80] Dry needling is an invasive technique, and although the overall risks are considered very low, any therapist desiring to offer this intervention should undertake adequate training. In addition, dry needling is not universally included in all state therapy practice acts, and contact with local professional associations and state licensure boards would be prudent before undertaking training in dry needling.

Cupping captured the world's attention when elite athletes were seen at the Olympic Games with telltale circular bruising on their backs and shoulders. Cupping has been practiced as an indigenous therapy in many cultures for thousands of years. The intervention consists of placing a round vessel on the skin in the treatment area and using one of a few methods to create negative pressure within the cup, thus creating a suctioning effect that anchors the rim of the vessel to the skin and draws the soft tissue upward into the vacuum. The method typically used in clinical setting today consists of hard plastic bell-like cups that are activated using a manual pump to create negative pressure inside the cups. After being set, the cups are left in place for 5 to 20 minutes or alternatively moved around over the surface of the skin, creating a deep massaging effect (Fig. 96.3). Other than short-term pain reduction, the most typically noted after effects are local erythema, possible mild edema, and immediate or latent ecchymosis.[81] Although it is clear by observation that cupping does impart tensile and mechanical stresses to superficial somatic structures, there are no reliable data to date clarifying the mechanisms responsible for any therapeutic effects derived from this intervention.[81] One theory proposes that increased circulation facilitates the body's elimination of chemical irritants in

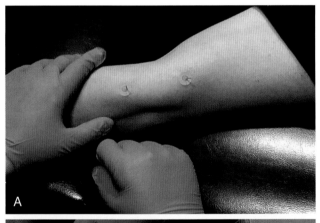
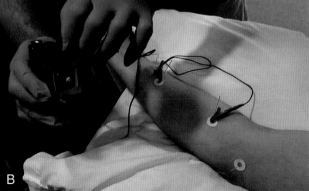

Fig. 96.2 **A,** Dry needling treatment setup for lateral elbow pain. **B,** Dry needling combined with electrical stimulation for medial forearm and elbow pain associated with ulnar nerve compression.

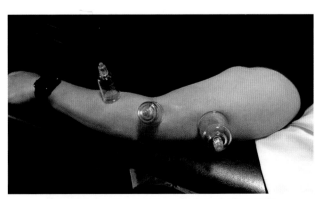

Fig. 96.3 Cupping treatment for lateral elbow pain

the local tissue. Other theories pull from traditional Chinese medicine, suggesting that cupping stimulates acupuncture or acupressure sites and in doing so activates similar neural mechanisms to block pain signals. Others suggest that by manipulating the skin and fascia, the inhibitory receptive fields of dorsal horn neurons are activated, resulting in noxious inhibitory control.[81] Finally, it is suggested that the procedure induces deep relaxation, which imparts all of the benefits previously discussed in this chapter regarding stress reduction and stress management. Research related to cupping is limited and generally poor quality because of small study size and significant study bias.[82] The decision to include cupping into a treatment plan, like many other treatment modalities, depends on the training of the clinician, the proposed rationale for using the intervention, and the patient's desire to receive the intervention. Currently, there is no strong evidence base in favor of cupping, and there is no consensus on the mechanism of action by which any benefits may be derived. Therefore, when used, cupping may most effectively be seen as an adjunct intervention in a larger treatment strategy.

CHOOSING THE BEST INTERVENTIONS FOR YOUR PATIENT

Given the wide variety of treatment options available, how does a hand therapist best select interventions for individual patients? There are a number of guiding principles that may be helpful in the clinical decision-making process.

Evidence Informed

Hand therapists are committed to rendering care that is based on current best evidence. The evidence often lacks the clarity that clinicians want; however, it is possible to translate the existing evidence into daily practice with great benefit to the patient. Figure 96.4 depicts the current best evidence for effective treatment options for musculoskeletal pain. The literature currently offers strongest support to the use of exercise as an intervention for pain.[12] Moderate evidence exists for the incorporation of manual therapy techniques and psychosocial strategies.[12] Other treatment techniques and interventions are currently supported by weak or scant evidence in the

literature.[12] This does not mean that these interventions are not to be used, but as evidence-informed practitioners, we do need to be aware of the potential limitations of certain interventions and plan treatment accordingly. When existing literature presents gaps instead of guidance, clinicians must remember that evidence-informed practice is a continuum that includes randomized controlled trials as well as expert opinion. Patient preference also plays a role in creatively adapting the treatment plan to the patient's individual needs and can also provide motivation and increased patient "buy in" to the overall treatment plan and can improve compliance with clinic appointments and self-management strategies.

Mechanism of Pain Generation

As our knowledge about pain and its underlying mechanisms grows, hand therapists can begin to match treatment interventions based on the pain drivers and the mechanisms of pain relief in individual interventions. Table 96.5 summarizes the classification of pain using a mechanism-based nomenclature and then links each classification to typical associated diagnoses, patterns of presentation in the clinic, and evidence-based treatment interventions.

Regional Involvement

We have seen in the exercise and manual therapy literature that patient treatment may often benefit from a broader perspective. Manual therapy procedures performed on a particular joint are found to impact a distant area of pain such as a cervical mobilization impacting the more distal upper extremity. Similarly, strengthening of the proximal muscle groups has been known to impact muscle and joint function more distally in the extremity as well. The musculoskeletal system is interconnected in ways we do not always understand such that "seemingly unrelated impairments in a remote anatomical region may contribute to, or be associated with, the patient's primary complaint."[83] This concept is known as regional interdependence and is separate from referred pain. In upper extremity referred pain, the pain generator is proximal, usually within the cervical spine. In this instance, treatment of the cervical spine will greatly impact pain, whereas treatment of the distal location of pain referral will not. In regional interdependence models, after referred pain has been ruled out as the primary pain

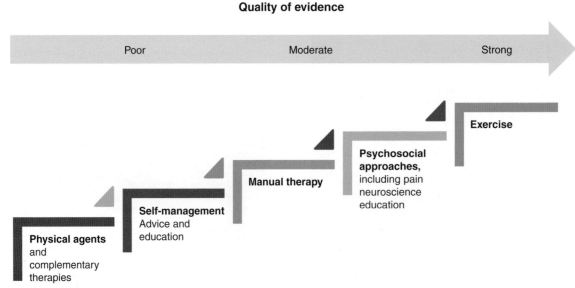

Quality of evidence

Poor   Moderate   Strong

Exercise

Psychosocial approaches, including pain neuroscience education

Manual therapy

Self-management Advice and education

Physical agents and complementary therapies

Fig. 96.4 Strength of evidence support for common therapy interventions. (Adapted from Baxter GD, Basford JR. Overview of other electrophysical agents including thermal agents. In: Sluka KA, ed. *Mechanisms and Management of Pain for the Physical Therapist.* 2nd ed. Philadelphia: Wolters Kluwer Health; 2016:225-236.)

TABLE 96.5   Summary of Evidence-Informed Therapy Interventions for Pain

Mechanism-Based Classification of Pain	Associated Diagnoses	Description and Presenting Symptoms	Evidence-Informed Therapy Interventions
Nociception dominant (peripheral sensitization)	Local MSK strain or sprain Trauma Surgery Tendinitis Tendinosis Tendinopathy	Localized, discrete pain pattern Pain proportionate to corresponding injury Related to inflammation Protective mechanism Heat hyperalgesia	• Physical agents • Manual therapy • Activity modification • Orthoses • Postural education • Graded exercise
Peripheral neuropathic dominant	Radiculopathy Peripheral nerve compression Adherent nerve root Diabetic peripheral neuropathy	Radiating pain Burning pain Numbness or tingling Cold hyperalgesia Hypoesthesia[5]	• Unloading (traction) • Neurodynamic mobilization • Stretching of adverse neural tension

Central sensitization dominant (nociplastic)	Primary presentation in these diagnoses:
	• Fibromyalgia
	• Chronic fatigue syndrome
	• Irritable bowel syndrome
	• Chronic whiplash
	Accompanying presentation in these diagnoses:
	• Chronic low back pain
	• TMJ dysfunctions
	• RA
	• Chronic HA
		• Amplification of nociceptive signaling to the CNS
		• Impaired central pain inhibition mechanisms
		• Widespread, nonanatomical, nonmechanical, persistent pain.
		• Often unresponsive to pharmacologic and surgical interventions
		• Pain characterized as severe, constant; easily aggravated; accompanied by burning, coldness, crawling, nondermatomal, nonmyotomal
		• Pain at rest
		• Spontaneous pain
		• Presence of "top-down" sensitizers (depression, anxiety)
		• Presence of "bottom-up" sensitizers (inflammation)
			• Exercise
			  • Aerobic
			  • Strengthening
			  • Stabilization
			  • Isometric
			• Posture education
			• Relaxation
			• Breathing
			• Sleep hygiene
			• Manual therapy
			• Physical agents
			• Cupping
			• Dry needling
			• Pain neuroscience education

CNS, Central nervous system; *HA,* headache; *MSK,* musculoskeletal; *RA,* rheumatoid arthritis; *TMJ,* temporomandibular joint.

generator, what is suggested is that the area proximal to and distal to the primary pain location be evaluated and then treated based on the findings of the examination. So, for example, in lateral elbow pain, the therapist would also evaluate the shoulder, scapula, and wrist. Findings might then indicate a need for scapula and rotator cuff strengthening as well as wrist mobility exercises.

Multimodal Treatment

Consistently, the literature indicates benefit of an intervention when used in combination with other interventions. Although separately interventions may not demonstrate significant clinical benefit, when used in combination with other interventions, the effects are often greater. A plan of care that incorporates a variety of treatment interventions may better address different facets of each individual's pain. Use of a multimodal treatment concept also prompts therapists to be cognizant of their own treatment biases and encourages therapists to cultivate and maintain skill in a broad range of treatment tools.

Focus on Function

Although patients often state a desire for alleviation of pain, they also desire to be able to return to function doing all the things they need to and want to be able to do. Use of outcome measures allows therapists to quickly identify areas of functional deficit, which can be used to structure both treatment goals and interventions. Focusing on function can also be a strong motivator to patients, engaging them in all aspects of their care.

SUMMARY

Pain is complex in nature; therefore, there are no simple "one size fits all" treatment plans. As in other areas of rehabilitation, planning an intervention strategy begins with thorough patient assessment and development of a therapy problem list. Therapist–patient collaboration and creativity can then be used to develop the best treatment plan for the individual patient. Options begin with those interventions available within the clinic and within the therapist's skill set. It goes without saying that therapists must always treat within their personal level of preparation and skill level and within the scope of practice for their discipline as well as their local professional practice act. Treatment interventions should be evidence based, and when no clear evidence exists, then options should be "evidence informed," remembering that evidence is a continuum, and we are charged with implementation of the *best available evidence.* Treatment should also be consistent with patient preferences because patient engagement will assist with compliance both in self-management as well as attendance at appointments. Finally, the focus of the intervention plan should be function with the ultimate goal of improving the patient's functional ability and independence.

REFERENCES

1. IASP Terminology: pain. Available at: https://www.iasp-pain.org/terminology?navItemNumber=576#Pain. Accessed on November 8, 2017.
2. Gatchel R, McGeary D, McGeary C. Interdisciplinary chronic pain management. *Am Psychol.* 2014;69:119–130.

3. Pain as a public health Challenge. In: *Institute of Medicine: Relieving Pain in America: A Blueprint for Transforming Prevention, Care, Education, and Research*. Washington DC: National Academies Press; 2011:55–112.

4. National Institutes of Health. Fact Sheet - pain management. Available at: https://report.nih.gov/nihfactsheets/viewfactsheet.aspx?csid=57. Accessed on November 4, 2017.

5. Babatunde O, Jordan J, Van der Windt D, et al. Effective treatment options for musculoskeletal pain in primary care: a systematic overview of current evidence. *PLoS One*. 12(6): e0178621. https://doi.org/10.1371/journal.pone.0178621

6. Dowell D, Haegerich T, Chou R. CDC guideline for prescribing opioids for chronic pain — United States, 2016. *MMWR Recomm Rep (Morb Mortal Wkly Rep)*. 2016;65(No. 1):1–49.

7. Opioid Overdose. Available at: https://www.cdc.gov/drugoverdose/index.html Accessed on October 23, 2017.

8. Louw A, Puentedura E, Zimney K, et al. Know pain; know gain? A perspective on pain neuroscience education in physical therapy. *J Orthop Sports Phys Ther*. 2016;46:131–134.

9. MacDermid JC. Evidence-based practice. In: Skirven TM, Osterman AL, Fedorczyk JM, Amadio PC, eds. *Rehabilitation of the Hand and Upper Extremity*. 6th ed. St. Louis: Mosby; 2011.

10. Fedorczyk JM. The role of physical agents in modulating pain. *J Hand Ther*. 1997;10:110–121.

11. Fedorczyk JM, Michlovitz SL. Pain and limited motion. In: Michlovitz SL, Nolan, eds. *TP. Modalities for Therapeutic Intervention*. 4th ed. Philadelphia: FA Davis; 2005:185–206.

12. Baxter GD, Basford JR. Overview of other electrophysical agents including thermal agents. In: Sluka KA, ed. *Mechanisms and Management of Pain for the Physical Therapist*. 2nd ed. Philadelphia: Wolters Kluwer Health; 2016:225–236.

13. Sluka KA, Walsh DM. Transcutaneous electrical nerve stimulation and interferential therapy. In: Sluka KA, ed. *Mechanisms and Management of Pain for the Physical Therapist*. 2nd ed. Philadelphia: Wolters Kluwer Health; 2016:203–224.

14. Fedorczyk JM. Tendinopathies of the elbow, wrist, and hand: histopathology and clinical considerations. *J Hand Ther*. 2012;25:191–201.

15. Rankin IA, Sargent H, Rehman H, Gurusamy KS. Low-level laser therapy for carpal tunnel syndrome. *Cochrane Database Syst Rev*. 2017;(8).

16. Page MJ, O'Conner D, Pitt V, Massy-Westropp N. Therapeutic ultrasound for carpal tunnel syndrome. *Cochrane Database Syst Rev*. 2013;(3).

17. Page MJ, Green S, Mrocki MA, et al. Electrotherapy modalities for rotator cuff disease. *Cochrane Database Syst Rev*. 2016;(6).

18. Sluka KA. Introduction: definitions, concepts, and models of pain. In: Sluka KA, ed. *Mechanisms and Management of Pain for the Physical Therapist*. 2nd ed. Philadelphia: Wolters Kluwer Health; 2016:3–16.

19. Gatchel R, Peng YB, Fuchs P, et al. The biopsychosocial approach to chronic pain: scientific advances and future directions. *Psychol Bull*. 2007;133:581–624.

20. Vranceanu A, Safren S. Cognitive-behavioral therapy for hand and arm pain. *J Hand Ther*. 2011;2:124–130.

21. Louw A, Diener I, Butler DS, et al. The effect of neuroscience education on pain, disability, anxiety, and stress in chronic musculoskeletal pain. *Am J Phys Med Rehabil*. 2011;92:2041–2056.

22. Hannibal K, Bishop M. Chronic stress, cortisol dysfunction, and pain: a psychoneuroendocrine rationale for stress management in pain rehabilitation. *Phys Ther*. 2014;94:1816–1825.

23. Ma X, Yue Z, Gong Z, et al. The effect of diaphragmatic breathing on attention, negative affect and stress in healthy adults. *Front Psychol*. 2017;8:1–12.

24. Kjeken I, Darre S, Latowkowsy-Christensen B, et al. Self-management strategies to support performance of daily activities in hand osteoarthritis. *Scand J Occup Ther*. 2013;20:29–36.

25. Scott-Dempster C, Toye F, Truman J, et al. Physiotherapists' experiences of activity pacing with people with chronic musculoskeletal pain: an interpretative phenomenological analysis. *Physiother Theory Pract*. 2014;30:319–328.

26. Algar L, Valdes K. Using smartphone applications as hand therapy interventions. *J Hand Ther*. 2014;27:254–257.

27. Novak CB, Mackinnon SE. Repetitive use and static postures: a source of compression and pain. *J Hand Ther*. 1997;10:151–159.

28. Weisburg J. Pain. In: Heacox B, Weisberg J, Andemicael-Mehreteab T, eds. *Integrating Physical Agents in Rehabilitation*. 2nd ed. Pearson; 2006.

29. Dean E, Soderlund A. What is the role or lifestyle behavior change associated with non-communicable disease risk in managing musculoskeletal health conditions with special reference to chronic pain? *BMC Musculoskeletal Dis*. 2015;16:1.

30. Pignataro R, Ohtake P, Swisher A, Dino G. The role of physical therapists in smoking cessation: opportunities for improving treatment outcomes. *Phys Ther*. 2012;92:757–766.

31. Smokefree.gov. Available at: www.smokefree.gov. Accessed on April 12, 2019.

32. Beattie P, Silfies S, Jordon M. The evolving role of physical therapists in the long-term management of chronic low back pain: longitudinal care using assisted self-management strategies. *Braz J Phys Ther*. 2016;20(6):580–591.

33. Bjurstrom MF, Irwin MR. Polysomnographic characteristics in nonmalignant chronic pain populations: a review of controlled studies. *Sleep Med Rev*. 2016;26:74–86.

34. Palermo TM, Wilson AC, Lewandowski AS, Toliver-Sokol M, Murray CB. Behavioral and psychosocial factors associated with insomnia in adolescents with chronic pain. *Pain*. 2011;152(1):89–94.

35. Mason P. Deconstructing endogenous pain modulations. *J Neurophysiol*. 2005;94(3):1659–1663.

36. Finan PH, Goodin BR, Smith MT. The association of sleep and pain: an update and a path forward. *J Pain*. 2013;14(12):1539–1552.

37. Gumustekin K, Seven B, Karabulut N, et al. Effects of sleep deprivation, nicotine, and selenium on wound healing in rats. *Int J Neurosci*. 2004;114(11):1433–1442.

38. Kay-Stacey M, Attarian H. Advances in the management of chronic insomnia. *BMJ*. 2016;354:i2123.

39. Trauer JM, Qian MY, Doyle JS, Rajaratnam SM, Cunnington D. Cognitive behavioral therapy for chronic insomnia: a systematic review and meta-analysis. *Ann Intern Med*. 2015;163(3):191–204.

40. Kyle SD, Aquino MRJ, Miller CB, et al. Towards standardisation and improved understanding of sleep restriction therapy for insomnia disorder: a systematic examination of CBT-I trial content. *Sleep Med Rev*. 2015;23(suppl C):83–88.

41. Mansel JK, Carey EC. Nonpharmacologic approach to sleep disorders. *Cancer J*. 2014;20(5):345–351.

42. Spielman AJ, Saskin P, Thorpy MJ. Treatment of chronic insomnia by restriction of time in bed. *Sleep*. 1933.87;10(1):45–56.

43. Sluka KA, Milosavljevic S. Manual therapy. In: Sluka KA, ed. *Mechanisms and Management of Pain for the Physical Therapist*. 2nd ed. Philadelphia: Wolters Kluwer Health; 2016:237–250.

44. Loghmani M, Bane S. Instrument-assisted soft tissue manipulation: evidence for its emerging efficacy. *J Nov Physiother Phys Rehabil*. 2016;S3:012.

45. Burke J, Buchberger D, Carey-Loghmani T, et al. A pilot study comparing two manual therapy interventions for carpal tunnel syndrome. *J Manip Physiol Ther*. 2007;30:50–61.

46. Fernandez-De-La-Penas C, Perez-Dr-Heredia M, Brea-Rivera M, Miangolarra-Page J. Immediate effects on pressure pain threshold following a single cervical spine manipulation in healthy subjects. *J Orthop Sports Phys Ther*. 2007;37(6):325–329.

47. Boyles R, Ritland B, Miracle B, et al. The short-term effects of thoracic thrust manipulation on patients with shoulder impingement syndrome. *Man Ther*. 2009;14:375–380.

48. Heiser R, O'Brien V, Schwartz D. The use of joint mobilization to improve clinical outcomes in hand therapy: a systematic review of the literature. *J Hand Ther*. 2013;26:297–311.

49. Fernandez-De-La-Penas C, Cleland J, Palacios-Cena M. The effectiveness of manual therapy versus surgery on self-reported function, cervical of motion, and pinch grip force in carpal tunnel syndrome: a randomized clinical trial. *J Orthop Sports Phys Ther*. 2017;47:151–161.

50. Fernandez-De-La-Penas C, Ortega-Santiago R, de la Llave-Rincon A, et al. Manual physical therapy versus surgery for carpal tunnel syndrome: a randomized parallel-group trial. *J Pain*. 2015;16(11):1087–1094.

51. Basson A, Olivier B, Ellis R, et al. The effectiveness of neural mobilization for neuromusculoskeletal conditions: a systematic review and meta-analysis. *J Orthop Sports Phys Ther*. 2017;47(9):593–615.

52. Goyal M, Mehta S, Rana N, et al. Motor nerve conduction velocity and function in carpal tunnel syndrome following neural mobilization: a randomized clinical trial. *Int J Health Allied Sci.* 2016;5(2):104–110.

53. Ginanneschi F, Cioncoloni D, Bigliazzi J, et al. Sensory axons excitability changes in carpal tunnel syndrome after neural mobilization. *Neurol Sci.* 2015;36:1611–1615.

54. Colberg SR, Sigal RJ, Yardley JE, et al. Physical activity/exercise and diabetes. A position statement of the American Diabetes Association. *Diabetes Care.* 2016;39:2065–2079.

55. Myers J. Exercise and cardiovascular health. *Circulation.* 2003;107:e2–e5.

56. Miller WC, Koceja DM, Hamilton EJ. A meta-analysis of the past 25 years of weight loss research using diet, exercise, or diet plus exercise intervention. *Int J Obes.* 1997;21:941–947.

57. Khan K, Scott A. Mechanotherapy: how physical therapists' prescription of exercise promotes tissue repair. *Br J Sports Med.* 2009;43:247–251.

58. Smart K, Blake C, Staines A, Thacker M, Doody C. Mechanisms-based classifications of musculoskeletal pain: Part 1 of 3: symptoms and signs of central sensitization in patients with low back (+/- leg) pain. *Man Ther.* 2012;17:336–344.

59. Bement MH, Sluka KA. Exercise-induced hypoalgesia – an evidence-based review. In: Sluka KA, ed. *Mechanisms and Management of Pain for the Physical Therapist.* 2nd ed. Philadelphia: Wolters Kluwer Health; 2016:117–202.

60. Smart K, Blake C, Staines A, Thacker M, Doody C. Mechanisms-based classifications of musculoskeletal pain: Part 2 of 3: symptoms and signs of peripheral neuropathic pain in patients with low back (+/- leg) pain. *Man Ther.* 2012;17:345–351.

61. Smart K, Blake C, Staines A, Thacker M, Doody C. Mechanisms-based classifications of musculoskeletal pain: Part 3 of 3: symptoms and signs of nociceptive pain in patients with low back (+/- leg) pain. *Man Ther.* 2012;17:352–357.

62. Knygsand-Roenhoej K, Maribo T. A randomized clinical controlled study comparing the effect of modified manual edema mobilization treatment with traditional edema technique in patients with a fracture of the distal radius. *J Hand Ther.* 2011;24:184–193.

63. Mata Diz J, Miranda de Souza J, Oliveira Leopoldino A, Oliveira V. Exercise, especially combined stretching and strengthening exercise, reduces myofascial pain: a systematic review. *J Physiother.* 2017;63:17–22.

64. Marinkko L, Chacko J, Dalton D, Chacko C. The effectiveness of therapeutic exercise for painful shoulder conditions: a meta-analysis. *J Shoulder Elbow Surg.* 2011;20:1351–1359.

65. Hallgren H, Holmgren T, Oberg B, et al. A specific exercise strategy reduced the need for surgery in subacromial pain patients. *Br J Sports Med.* 2014;48:1431–1436.

66. Saltychev M, Aarimaa V, Virolainen P, Laimi K. Conservative treatment or surgery for shoulder impingement: systematic review and meta-analysis. *Disabil Rehabil.* 2015;37(1):1–8.

67. Haik M, Alburquerque-Sendin F, Moreira R, et al. Effectiveness of physical therapy treatment of clearly defined subacromial pain: a systematic review of randomized controlled trials. *Br J Sports Med.* 2016;50:1124–1134.

68. Steuri R, Sattelmayer M, Elsig S, et al. Effectiveness of conservative interventions including exercise, manual therapy, and medical management in adults with shoulder impingement: a systematic review and meta-analysis of RCTs. *Br J Sports Med.* 2017;0:1–10.

69. Raman J, MacDermid J, Grewal R. Effectiveness of different methods of resistance exercises in lateral epicondylosis – a systematic review. *J Hand Ther.* 2012;25:5–26.

70. Heijnders I, Chung-Wei C. The effect of eccentric exercise in improving function or reducing pain in lateral epicondylitis is unclear. *Br J Sports Med.* 2015;49(16):1087–1088.

71. Stasinopoulos D, Stasinopoulos I. Comparison of effects of eccentric training, eccentric-concentric training, and eccentric-concentric training combined with isometric contraction in the treatment of lateral elbow tendinopathy. *J Hand Ther.* 2017;30:13–19.

72. Day J, Bush H, Nitz A, Uhl T. Scapular muscle performance in Individuals with lateral epicondylalgia. *J Orthop Sports Phys Ther.* 2015;45(5):414–424.

73. Valdes K, von der Heyde R. An exercise program for carpometacarpal osteoarthritis based on biomechanical principles. *J Hand Ther.* 2012;25:251–263.

74. Villafane J, Cleland J, Fernandez-De-Las-Penas C. The effectiveness of a manual therapy and exercise protocol in patients with thumb carpometacarpal osteoarthritis: a randomized controlled trial. *J Orthop Sports Phys Ther.* 2013;43(4):204–213.

75. Shankland B, Beaton D, Ahmed S, Nedlec B. Effects of client-centered multimodal treatment on impairment, function, and satisfaction of people with thumb carpometacarpal osteoarthritis. *J Hand Ther.* 2017;30:307–313.

76. Furlan A, van Tulder M, Cerkin D, et al. Acupuncture and dry needling for low back pain. *Cochrane Database Syst Rev.* 2005;1. Art. No.:CD001351.

77. Kalichman L, Vulfsons S. Dry needling in the management of musculoskeletal pain. *J Am Board Fam Med.* 2010;23:640–646.

78. Kietrys D, Palombaro K, Azaretto E, et al. Effectiveness of dry needling for upper-quarter myofascial pain: a systematic review and meta-analysis. *J Orthop Sports Phys Ther.* 2013;43(9):620–634.

79. Fernandez-Carnero J, Fernandez-de-las-Penas C, Cleland J. Mulligan's mobilization with movement and muscle trigger point dry needling for the management of chronic lateral epicondylalgia: a case report. *J Musculoskelet Pain.* 2009;17(4):409–415.

80. Butts R, Dunning J, Perreault T, et al. Peripheral and spinal mechanisms of pain and dry needling mediated analgesia: a clinical resource guide for health care professionals. *Int J Phys Med Rehabil.* 2016;4(2):1000327.

81. Rozenfeld E, Kalichman L. New is the well-forgotten old: the use of dry cupping in musculoskeletal medicine. *J Bodyw Mov Ther.* 2016;20:173–178.

82. Cao H, Li X, Liu J. An updated review of the efficacy of cupping therapy. *PLoS One.* 2012;7(2):e31793.

83. Wainer R, Whitman J, Clelanc J, Flynn T. Regional interdependence: a musculoskeletal examination model whose time has come. *J Orthop Sports Phys Ther.* 2007;37(11):658–660.

97

Complex Regional Pain Syndromes: Types 1 and 2

L. Andrew Koman, Elizabeth Anne McBride, Beth Paterson Smith, Thomas L. Smith

CRITICAL POINTS

- Complex regional pain syndrome (CRPS) type 1 (traditional reflex sympathetic dystrophy) or type 2 (traditional causalgia) is the preferred diagnostic descriptor.
- The Budapest expert consensus recommendations provide improved diagnostic specificity and sensitivity over previous options.
- There is no pathognomonic marker for CRPS; it occurs in an extremity after a noxious event in the absence of ongoing cellular damage and must *not* be explainable by an alternative diagnosis with the exception that peripheral nerve diagnoses may coexist with CRPS type 2.
- CRPS may be sympathetically mediated or sympathetically independent; these descriptors are defined by the patient's response to a sympatholytic intervention. Traditionally, a stellate block or a continuous autonomic nerve block is the most common option.
- Three-phase bone scans (TFBSs), if positive, support a diagnosis of CRPS type 1 or 2; however, the absolute diagnostic value of these scans is low, and TFBS is not a pathognomonic marker.
- Management of CRPS is predominantly medical. Surgical correction of nociceptive or neural dysfunction is appropriate to correct ongoing pain excitation or to correct post–dystrophic deformity. In general, intra- and postoperative sympatholytic protection and modulation are recommended by using continuous blocks or parenteral or oral sympatholytics.

- Surgery is appropriate in selected cases in which pain can be controlled by sympatholytic intervention; continuous peripheral nerve catheters or epidural catheters used after surgery are usually the preferable pain control modality.
- Amputation as a treatment is relatively contraindicated because of both symptom recurrence and difficulty using a prosthesis. Amputation has a role in individuals with chronic infection and severe function impairing deformity.
- Patients with CRPS may experience another dystrophic event affecting a previously nonpainful limb.
- There is no consistent time course for CRPS.
- 10th revision of the International Statistical Classification of Diseases and Related Health Problems coding:

  CRPS Type 1
      Upper limb
          G90.511 right
          G90.512 left
          G90.513 bilateral
  CRPS Type 2
      Upper limb
          G54.42 left
          G54.43 bilateral

Chronic posttraumatic extremity pain that is out of proportion to the injury and persists in the absence of ongoing injury or cellular damage is a significant disability, interferes with function and health-related quality of life (HRQOL), and increases compensation in liability actions.[1,2] Historically, this clinical entity has been commonly termed *reflex sympathetic dystrophy* (RSD), *causalgia*, and *algodystrophy*. Currently, *complex regional pain syndrome* (CRPS) is the most accepted term used to describe this clinical entity. CRPS has no pathognomonic marker and cannot exist if an alternative diagnosis explains the clinical symptoms and signs.[3,4] CRPS is a clinical diagnosis that includes pain, autonomic dysfunction, trophic changes, and functional impairment. CRPS is divided into type 1, in which a noxious event without identifiable nerve injury is causative, and type 2, in which an identifiable nerve injury exists.

Complex regional pain syndrome is based on terminology proposed by the International Association for the Study of Pain in 1993 and refined in 2003 during a workshop in Budapest.[3,4] The validated Budapest criteria provide descriptive terminology based on clinical features, location, and specifics of the injury, without implying mechanism, cause, or sympathetic maintenance. The proposed criteria better discriminates between CRPS and non-CRPS. Although a third category, CRPS–NOS (not otherwise specified), was proposed, this category has not been included in the 10th revision of the International Statistical Classification of Diseases and Related Health Problems. The Budapest criteria requires "pain which is persistent and out of proportion to the injury", one symptom in a minimum of three of four of categories, one sign in two of four categories, and no alternative diagnosis (Box 97.1) CRPS-1 may be sympathetically mediated (SMP) or sympathetically independent (SIP); these descriptors are defined by the response to a sympatholytic intervention. Traditionally, a stellate block or a continuous autonomic nerve block is the most common option to define

BOX 97.1   Diagnostic Criteria for Type 1 Complex Regional Pain Syndrome

- One (1) **symptom** in a minimum of three of four of the following categories:
  - Sensory: hyperpathia or allodynia
  - Vasomotor: temperature asymmetry, skin color changes, or skin color asymmetry
  - Sudomotor or edema, sweating changes, or sweating asymmetry
  - Motor or trophic: decreased ROM, motor dysfunction (weakness, tremor, dystonia), or trophic changes (e.g., hair, nail, skin)
- One (1) **sign** in a minimum of two of four of the following categories:
  - Sensory: evidence of hyperalgesia (to pinprick), allodynia (e.g., to light touch, temperature), hyperpathia, or allodynia
  - Vasomotor: temperature asymmetry (>1 degree) or skin color changes or asymmetry
  - Sudomotor: evidence of edema, sweating changes, or sweating asymmetry
  - Motor or trophic: evidence of decreased ROM, motor dysfunction (weakness, tremor, dystonia), or trophic changes (e.g., hair, nail, skin)

ROM, Range of motion.

SMP versus SIP, but relief with oral sympatholytics is supportive of the diagnosis of SMP. The classic definition of SMP is based on relief from a phentolamine block.[5–9]

The term *reflex sympathetic dystrophy* used in the United States and North America and *algodystrophy* used in Europe were generic terms describing chronic extremity posttraumatic pain accompanied by dysfunction, autonomic activity, and impaired extremity function. These two terms have been replaced with the new terminology of CRPS. CRPS type 1 (traditional RSD or algodystrophy) occurs without an identifiable peripheral nerve injury; CRPS type 2, causalgia, is clinical RSD with a peripheral nerve abnormality.[10,11] Either may be SMP or SIP.

Physiologic manifestations of CRPS are normal responses to an initial noxious insult that are prolonged abnormally and persist in the absence of ongoing or impending cellular damage. Patients presenting with CRPS report incapacitating pain beyond the traumatized area and outside normal nerve distributions with associated functional compromise. In CRPS, a complex series of peripheral and central events affect peripheral autonomic control; modify central nervous system (CNS) activity; and produce pain, autonomic dysfunction, trophic changes, and functional impairment.

Pain may be nociceptive or neuropathic. The former originates from a mechanical source in the absence of an identifiable nerve injury. Neuropathic pain emanates from an injury or dysfunction of a peripheral nerve combined with trophic changes, autonomic dysfunction, and functional impairment. Thus, a localized neuroma or neuroma-in-continuity, a cause of neuropathic pain, is not per se CRPS type 2. The presence of a nociceptive focus (e.g., mechanical irritation of the wrist secondary to an unstable distal radioulnar joint or injury to a peripheral nerve) serves as a trigger to further exaggerate physiologic responses mediated through inappropriate α-adrenergic activity within the dorsal horn of the spinal cord.[12,13] After a peripheral injury, excitation and sensitization of wide-dynamic-range neurons (internuncial connections in the dorsal horn of the spinal cord) increase the conscious appreciation of pain.[13,14] SMP occurs when *receptor disease* (receptor disease refers to the concept that increased sensitivity of adrenergic receptors is responsible for CRPS) predominates and sympatholytic intervention (e.g., intravenous phentolamine or stellate ganglion block) decreases α-adrenergic tone with subsequent decreased pain, normalization of autonomic function, and increased physical capability.[6] Over time, physiologic or anatomic adaptation occurs or permanent structural damage may alter peripheral and CNS architectural structures. When this occurs, sympathetic blockade is no longer effective, and pain becomes SIP.[15]

DEMOGRAPHICS

The incidence of CRPS varies with reports from Olmsted County, Minnesota, of approximately 5.5 in 100,000 with a prevalence of 21 in 100, 000[16]; however, the incidence in the Netherlands was greater at 26.2 in 100,000.[17] The estimated female preponderance of CRPS varies from 1:1.6 to 4.5:1.[17–19] The incidence of CRPS type 1 is greater that CRPS type 2. Smokers are more frequently affected.[16,20] Age at onset is most frequently between 30 and 55 years (mean, 40 years); however, individuals of any age may be affected.[21] Although CRPS can develop in any patient, epidemiologically, white women who smoke cigarettes are affected most frequently. An identifiable nociceptive injury is diagnosed in less than 50% of cases.[22–24]

Complex regional pain syndrome is observed frequently (20%–40%) after fracture of the distal radius.[25–28] In addition, traumatic or iatrogenic injuries to the following nerves have been documented to contribute to and to precipitate CRPS: the palmar cutaneous branch of the median nerve, the median nerve at any level, the dorsal branch of the ulnar nerve, the superficial radial nerve, the ulnar nerve at the elbow, and the posterior interosseous nerve.[29] The reported incidence of CRPS after simultaneous median nerve decompression and palmar fasciectomy for Dupuytren's disease is supported in spite of previous reports to the contrary.[30–33] Familial or genetic factors have been implicated as risk factors for CRPS.[34] Patients with CRPS do not report higher pain scores or lower levels of psychological distress than do patients with back pain or local neuropathy.[35] Self-induced disorders such as factitious disorders may be confused with CRPS.[36]

DIAGNOSIS

General

The diagnosis of CRPS is based on clinical findings. In patients with CRPS, pain is initiated in the periphery by a noxious or traumatic event(s), is influenced by posttraumatic interventions and activity, is exacerbated by physiologic or anatomic variables, and is determined in part by congenital or genetic factors.[29,37–40] There are no pathognomonic tests for CRPS; early diagnosis and treatment are important for optimal recovery. However, onset is frequently delayed 2 to 12 weeks after the precipitating injury, and definitive diagnosis often is made weeks to months after injury.[15,29]

Symptoms and Signs

Pain, a prerequisite of CRPS, often is described as burning, throbbing, tearing, cutting, searing, shooting, and aching. Characteristic types of pain in CRPS include hyperalgesia, allodynia, and hyperpathia. Hyperalgesia, pain that is greater than expected for a given painful stimulus, is considered primary when it affects the immediate area surrounding the injury. Hyperalgesia is termed secondary when it causes distant discomfort in nontraumatized skin either proximal or distal to the initial injury area.[41,42] Pain secondary to normally nonpainful stimuli is called allodynia. Hyperpathia is delayed pain that typically outlasts the initiating stimulus and spreads beyond normal dermatomal borders. Vascular abnormalities and cold sensitivity (a painful response to cold exposure) are also commonly experienced by patients with CRPS.[43]

Trophic changes associated with CRPS include stiffness; edema; and atrophy of the hair, nails, and skin. Hyperkeratosis of the skin may occur. Symptoms of vasomotor or autonomic nervous system dysfunction occur in 80% of patients.[44,45] A variety of testing methods can be used to demonstrate abnormal autonomic function in most patients.[44-46]

The subjective symptoms of patients with CRPS may be quantified by the use of validated instruments that evaluate pain, cold sensitivity, and numbness. These instruments include variations of the McGill Pain Questionnaire,[47,48] the Carpal Tunnel Instrument,[49] and the McCabe Cold Sensitivity Severity Scale.[50] Extremity function may be analyzed using the Carpal Tunnel Instrument Function Scale[49] and the Disabilities of the Arm, Shoulder and Hand (DASH) form from the American Academy of Orthopaedic Surgery.[51] The RAND Short Form 36 Health Survey[52] may be used to measure the HRQOL of patients with CRPS. This survey assesses physical, social, and emotional functioning; perceived health; overall life satisfaction; perceived pain; and work performance.[53,54]

Physical Examination

The physical examination must include an assessment of the entire patient, including the cervical spine, thoracic spine, shoulder girdle, involved extremity, contralateral limb, and both lower extremities. A careful neurologic assessment is required to determine the presence or absence of discogenic or degenerative cervical disease, peripheral neuropathy, arthritis, or arthrofibrosis.[29,39] It is advisable, if possible, to observe the patient's extremity during ambulation or while the patient is seated. Note if the motion of the affected limb is restricted or "normal." Also observe the posture of the affected extremity and its activity during the movement of the "normal" extremity. Normal arm swing during gait is not a consistent finding.[29] Restricted shoulder range of motion (ROM), which may be secondary to adhesive capsulitis, is common. This condition, often called shoulder–hand syndrome, negatively impacts HRQOL and requires specific treatment modalities. Shoulder–hand problems often may be overlooked without directed examination of the shoulder. The involved extremity must be assessed for sensibility, hyperpathia, allodynia, discoloration, swelling, atrophy, vasomotor and autonomic tone, neurologic function, vascular status, grip, and pinch. In addition, any nociceptive foci should be noted. Reevaluation after or during sympatholytic treatment may reveal additional findings, facilitate the identification of trigger areas, delineate underlying inflammatory processes, and clarify any structural injury. Any mechanical–nociceptive or neuropathic abnormalities that are correctable by noninvasive or surgical means should be addressed and may have a positive impact on outcomes.[23,24,29]

Diagnostic Testing

There is no pathognomonic marker for CRPS; therefore, tests augment or quantify historical data and clinical findings. The clinical evaluation may be aided by information from validated instruments evaluating HRQOL, symptoms, and function. Combined with a standardized examination, this information provides reproducible and quantifiable data. Specific testing modalities provide an analysis of anatomic integrity, physiologic performance, and functional capacity. Categorization of the patient with CRPS using reproducible physiologic assessments guides treatment decisions and documents disease status.[29,39,55] It is often advisable to evaluate bone density and osteopenia, sudomotor performance, vasomotor and thermoregulatory control, components of blood flow, and endurance testing.[29,39,55,56] Radiographs may be used to assess the amount of regional osteopenia and abnormalities of bone microstructure, a finding observed in 70% to 80% of patients with CRPS.[27,56] The classic radiographic finding associated with CRPS is periarticular osteopenia; however, CRPS may affect both cortical and cancellous bone.[57-59] Genant and colleagues[57] described five patterns of resorption that occur in CRPS:

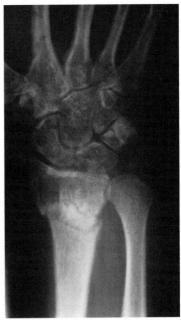

Fig. 97.1 Plain radiographic films of a patient with type 1 complex regional pain syndrome after fracture of the distal ends of the radius and ulna. The fracture line is visible. There is diffuse osteopenia in addition to juxtacortical demineralization and subchondral erosions and cysts. (From Koman LA. *Orthopaedic Manual.* Winston-Salem, NC: Orthopaedic Press; 1998.)

patchy, irregular trabecular bone, subperiosteal, intracortical, endosteal, and subchondral and juxtachondral surface erosions. However, radiographic changes often occur later in the progression of CRPS, and all imaging in patients with CRPS has poor sensitivity, reasonable specificity, a low positive predictive value, and a moderate negative predictive value[60] (Fig. 97.1).

Three-phase bone scans "should not be used as a major criterion in diagnosing reflex sympathetic dystrophy."[61] A third-phase scan with positive findings is not a prerequisite for the diagnosis of CRPS or SMP.[60-63] The diagnostic importance of abnormal phases of bone scans has been a subject of debate which is now clarified. *Three-phase bone scans are not pathognomonic; although they may support the diagnosis by themselves, they are not exclusionary.* Abnormal findings on three phase scans, in any phase, may assist in the corroboration of the diagnosis of RSD.[64,65] Although it has been stated that only a third-phase scan correlates with RSD,[66] abnormal findings in any phase of a three-phase scan document abnormal physiology of blood flow, bone turnover, or both. Unfortunately, bone scan findings do not correlate with the traditional staging criteria for RSD, do not predict recovery, do not determine the potential for response to treatment, and do not necessarily revert to normal after successful treatment.[61-66] However, the presence of positive third-phase bone scan findings provides objective corroboration for the clinical diagnosis of CRPS[29,39] (Figs. 97.2 and 97.3).

Sudomotor performance may be evaluated using resting sweat output, galvanic skin response, peripheral autonomic surface potentials, sympathetic skin response, and quantitative sudomotor axon reflex test. These tests provide an objective measure of sweat function by indirect or direct means.[67-72]

Vasomotor and thermoregulatory control can be assessed by monitoring digital pulp temperature(s), laser Doppler fluxmetry measurements of cutaneous perfusion (Fig. 97.4), or laser Doppler perfusion imaging of cutaneous perfusion profiles. These studies indirectly

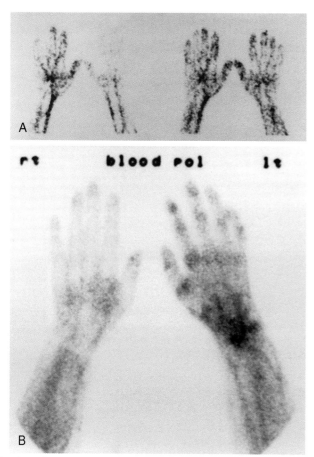

Fig. 97.2 Three-phase bone scans. **A,** Phase I, a "dynamic phase," evaluates vascular perfusion by visual or quantitative analysis or radiotracer uptake after an intravenous injection. Each image represents a 3- to 5-second interval and allows an assessment of flow dynamics. **B,** Phase II, a "blood pool" image, documents total tissue uptake of tracer during the first 3 to 5 minutes after injection. Phase III is a conventional bone scan (see Fig. 97.3). (From Koman LA. *Orthopaedic Manual.* Winston-Salem, NC: Orthopaedic Press; 1998.)

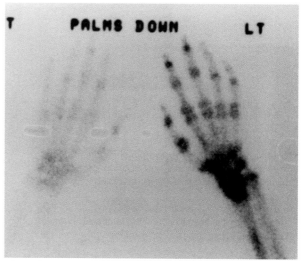

Fig. 97.3 An abnormal (phase III) bone scan demonstrating increased periarticular uptake throughout the hand. This is a scan of the patient whose x-ray film is seen in Fig. 97.1. Notice the increased radiolucency at the fracture site. (From Koman LA. *Orthopaedic Manual.* Winston-Salem, NC: Orthopaedic Press; 1998.)

evaluate cutaneous perfusion and provide reproducible profiles of physiologic capacity if combined with a physiologic stressor.[29,39,73,74]

Under normal conditions, 80% to 90% of total finger blood flow is involved in thermoregulation. However, in patients with CRPS, the percentage of blood flow involved in thermoregulatory activity may vary. Thermoregulatory flow is calculated by subtracting the nutritional flow from the total flow. Nutritional flow may be measured by using vital capillaroscopy.[74–76] This technique measures nutritional blood flow of the nail fold capillaries by direct evaluation of red blood cell flow through a single capillary loop by using an epi-illumination microscope and computerized analyses of flow (Fig. 97.5). Patients with CRPS have reduced nutritional flow and are unable to modulate flow compared with normal patients. Decreased nutritional flow occurs in patients with longstanding CRPS and may be secondary, in part, to irreversible changes in arteriovenous shunt mechanisms or arteriovenous shunt control.[38,44,45]

Endurance testing may be performed by using a variety of computerized diagnostic techniques that quantify muscle energy, strength, and endurance. Subtle abnormalities in function may be assessed only by careful analysis of these test results.[29,39]

Diagnostic blockade may be used to determine whether CRPS is SMP or SIP. The most common diagnostic blockade procedures performed are stellate ganglion block, phentolamine testing, epidural injections, and controlled trials of oral sympatholytic medications. Diagnostic blockade is performed classically with stellate ganglion block or intravenous phentolamine[77,78]; however, phentolamine currently is not used and is difficult to obtain in the United States.

Stellate ganglion block is performed by injecting the cervical sympathetic trunk with a short- to medium-acting stabilizing agent (e.g., lidocaine) (Fig. 97.6). Decreased pain after injection is presumptive evidence that pain is SMP. The inability to obtain pain reduction after or during the test suggests either an alternative diagnosis or that irreversible peripheral changes have occurred that have changed the previously SMP to SIP pain. A brief response to oral sympatholytic medications is presumptive evidence of complex regional pain that is SMP. However, the use of a continuous block is the most reliable pain management technique and may provide lasting relief.[29,39,79,80]

TREATMENT

General Principles

Prognostic data are primarily from anecdotal reports but imply that patients with CRPS treated within the first year of injury will show significant improvement in 80% of patients, and only 50% of those treated after 1 year will improve. However, patients with CRPS after distal radius fractures appear to have a poorer prognosis. Stiffness and decreased finger function in these patients at 3 months correlate with residual impairment and morbidity at 10 years.[81] Although early intervention is important, it is not always possible. Many patients are treated inadvertently before diagnosis. Thus, the natural history may be improved by medical intervention despite an incorrect or incomplete diagnosis.

Effective treatment of CRPS requires recognition and prompt intervention[18,23,24,29] and initiation of treatment. It is appropriate to stage the CRPS patient by determining (1) if the pain is SMP or SIP, (2) if total blood flow is high or low, (3) the extent of abnormal arteriovenous shunting or nutritional deprivation, (4) if permanent structural damage has occurred, and (5) if there are mechanical or neural dystrophic pain generators.[29] The degree of soft tissue contracture should be assessed because patients with significant arthrofibrosis and atrophy often have sustained irreversible trophic

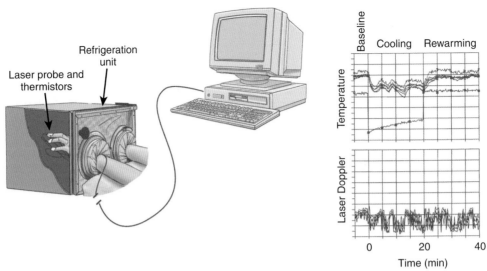

Fig. 97.4 Digital microvascular physiology can be evaluated by using an isolated cold stress test combining digital temperature and laser Doppler fluxmetry measurements. Digital temperatures are monitored with thermistors attached to each digit of both extremities. Microvascular cutaneous perfusion is assessed with a laser Doppler probe attached to one digit of each extremity. Digital temperature and laser Doppler fluxmetry measurements are sampled by using custom computer software, and the results of the test are plotted for analysis. (From Koman LA. *Orthopaedic Manual.* Winston-Salem, NC: Orthopaedic Press; 1998.)

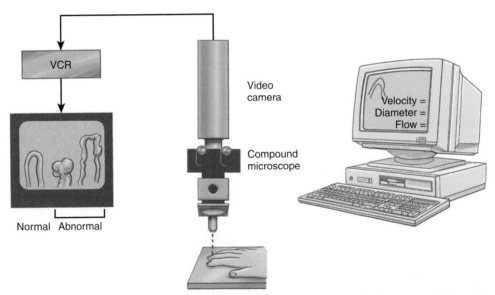

Fig. 97.5 Nutritional capillaries may be visualized directly through a compound microscope, which provides epi-illumination from the microscope. Magnification within the microscope and use of a video camera allow direct visualization of cell motion within the capillaries and permit the identification of normal or abnormal capillary morphology. Videotape analysis facilitates quantitation of the diameter of the capillaries and velocity of red blood cell flow within the ascending and descending capillary loop. Abnormal morphology diagnostic of collagen vascular disease also can be observed. (From Koman LA. *Orthopaedic Manual.* Winston-Salem, NC: Orthopaedic Press; 1998.)

changes that indicate a less favorable prognosis. Nociceptive foci should be identified and treated. Effective sympatholytic treatment often requires the use of multiple modalities.[29,82] It is important to recognize that the treatment of patients with CRPS remains largely empirical because of the paucity of randomized controlled trials (RCTs).[39,83]

Hand Therapy

Hand therapy is an important aspect of management of CRPS affecting the upper extremity. The active involvement of a hand therapist

in the management of a patient with CRPS provides an independent assessment of progress; continuity of care; and a vital feedback loop among the patient, physician, insurance carriers, and rehabilitation personnel. Pain modulation techniques used in hand therapy include contrast baths, desensitization, fluidotherapy (Chattanooga Medical, Chattanooga, TN), static orthotic positioning, electrical stimulation, and ultrasound. Edema is controlled by using manual lymphatic drainage techniques or light compression garments. ROM activity can be aided by ultrasound and paraffin baths along with dynamic orthotic positioning and continuous passive motion equipment as long as the

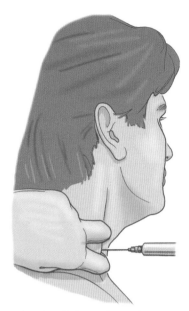

Fig. 97.6 Schematic of technique of needle placement for stellate block.

patient's pain does not increase. The Cochrane database suggests that long-term, large-scale RCTs are required for specific proof to delineate optimal therapy options in patients with CRPS.[84,85]

Pharmacologic Interventions

The use of oral, topical, and parenteral pharmacologic intervention is well documented in the management of patients with CRPS. The most commonly used drugs include antidepressants, anticonvulsants, membrane-stabilizing agents, adrenergic agents, and steroids. The use of these medications is largely empirical; however, theoretical mechanisms support their use in patients with chronic pain. Oral medications (e.g., anticonvulsants, local anesthetics) may stabilize hypersensitive membranes; may provide competitive inhibition of neurotransmitters (e.g., bretylium); may block or influence neurotransmitter activity, receptor affinity, or both; or may increase nutritional flow or decrease inappropriate arteriovenous shunting.[86]

The use of almost all these agents are unlabeled indications according to the US Food and Drug Administration (FDA). Therefore, practitioners must be familiar with the pharmacology, physiologic actions, side effects, potential complications, indications, potential drug interactions, and contraindications of all medications prescribed.

Vitamins

The use of vitamin C supplementation as a prophylactic agent to prevent CRPS is controversial, and there is no clear consensus on its use with contradictory RCTs. Meta-analyses have shown "no substantial benefit" to "high benefit."[87–94] However, the current role of vitamin C in CRPS can be summarized in the AAOS report based on level II therapeutic evaluations:

> *The number of causal/association criteria met was adequate to support the scientific premise of the effect of vitamin C in preventing CRPS after DRF. Furthermore, vitamin C administration is of relatively low cost and has few complications unless administered in large doses. Owing to sufficient epidemiological evidence availability, the American Academy of Orthopaedic Surgeons recommendation of vitamin C to prevent CRPS has practical merit.*[90]

If CRPS prophylaxis with vitamin C is elected, a dose of 500 mg/day for 50 days is appropriate.

Oral Pharmacologic Choices

Detailed recommendations for oral pharmacologic agents are beyond the scope and purview of this chapter. Antidepressants, anticonvulsants, membrane-stabilizing agents, adrenergic agents, and steroids, among others, are used for their sympatholytic properties, to decrease pain, to improve nutritional, and to ameliorate muscle hypertonia. In general, narcotics are not overly helpful in the management of patients with CRPS. Drug selection must be personalized. These powerful agents are associated with significant side effects. A few generalizations are provided for perspective to guide patient understanding, to facilitate patient support, and to augment provider understanding but not treatment.

Antidepressants are frequently used to decrease anxiety, to improve sleep, and to provide a sympatholytic effect. In general, tricyclic antidepressants are preferable to other types of antidepressants for CRPS.[86]

Anticonvulsants are commonly used because of their theoretical effect on membrane stabilization, which decreases nociceptive and neuropathic pain generation. Pregabalin and gabapentin are approved for neuropathic pain and are frequently used to treat patients with CRPS. The use of oral membrane-stabilizing agents such as mexiletine and tocainide is limited because of the numerous side effects associated with these agents.[39,86]

Steroids are used frequently as a primary oral medication. A dose pack is often used with a high initial dose that is rapidly tapered. Avascular necrosis is a concern but is rare with short-term use.

Adrenergic agents have direct effects on presynaptic and postsynaptic hypersensitivity; therefore, theoretically, they should benefit many patients with CRPS. However, these agents are used rarely.

Calcium channel blockers increase nutritional perfusion and are valuable in patients with decreased total blood flow and inappropriate arteriovenous shunting or in patients with nutritionally compromised extremities as a result of reduced blood flow.[39,86]

Parenteral Medications

Parenteral interventions include intramuscular, intravenous, and intrathecal drugs.

Intravenous Agents. Intravenous agents that have been or are used to manage CRPS include calcitonin, bisphosphonates, ketamine, immunoglobulins, guanethidine, reserpine, bretylium tosylate, steroids, lidocaine, and Marcaine.[95]

Calcitonin and Bisphosphonates

Calcitonin may be administered intranasally or intravenously and has been used frequently in Europe in patients with CRPS. Pain reduction occurs in many patients with CRPS, and "the effects of calcitonin surpass that of bisphosphonates . . . as a short term medication in more chronic stages of the illness [CRPS]."[95]

Bisphosphonates block osteoclastic activity, a possible antiinflammatory property, and appear to be more effective in early stages of CRPS when increased bone turnover is occurring.[27,96,97]

Immunoglobulins have been used in refractory patients with CRPS. However, an RCT in patients with CRPS of 1 to 5 years' duration for 6 weeks was not successful at relieving pain in patients diagnosed with moderate to severe CRPS.[98]

Guanethidine, reserpine, and bretylium tosylate were widely used but are effectively obsolete options in the management of CRPS.[83] *At this time, these drugs are not clinically relevant* based on consistent lack of support of their use in controlled studies, their side effects, and commercial unavailability.

Ketamine, an *N*-methyl-D-aspartate (NMDA) receptor antagonist, is increasingly being used by anesthesia pain management specialists in the treatment of patients with CRPS. Ketamine is an anesthetic agent and may be administered intramuscularly or intravenously administered in a controlled setting. In patients with CRPS, it is used intravenously and has been shown to decrease pain, decrease swelling, and improve ROM. The precise mechanisms of action of ketamine is incompletely understood. However, the primary mechanism is as an NMDA antagonist. Additionally, there appear to be hypnotic, antidystonic, sympatholytic, and analgesic effects. These effects are mediated by blockade of HCN1, cholinergic, aminergic, antidepressant, and opioid receptors. Ketamine's impact on chronic pain and as an antidepressant outlast the actual drug levels, which suggests mediation by secondary increases in structural synaptic connectivity and neuronal response to the ketamine-induced hyperglutamatergic state.

Intravenous ketamine has been used to manage refractory CRPS on an inpatient[99] or outpatient basis.[100] Ketamine has a selective effect on relieving pain caused by CRPS without causing prolonged sedation and respiratory depression. However, hallucinations and cognitive dissociation may occur; these effects are countered by midazolam. Physical dependency (addiction), tolerance, and constipation are not side effects associated with ketamine. A variety of doses have been used with continuous high doses used in intensive care units. Continuous lower doses are used in hospital units, and 1- to 3-hour lower dose infusions are administered in a clinic or emergency department setting. Ketamine has also been used as part of multimodal care protocols (e.g., in combination with an epidural).[101–103] The FDA-approved drug insert supports the safety of ketamine.

Continuous Blocks and Serial Stellates

Continuous autonomic (sympathetic) blockade using lidocaine hydrochloride or other similar agents is used to determine the presence and control of SMP,[39] to protect and "treat" patients preoperatively,[104,105] and to treat patients with CRPS. Similarly, single stellate blocks facilitate determining the SMP component of CRPS. Although serial blocks are still advocated by some, we prefer continuous blocks because they are more reliable and better tolerated.[106] Continuous blocks are used prophylactically.

Intrathecal Epidural Medications

Continuous epidural infusions with clonidine and other agents have been used with variable efficacy for patients with advanced refractory cases of CRPS.[107–109]

Surgical and Ablative Therapies

Sympathectomy may be achieved by cervicothoracic ablation, periarterial stripping, or neurolytic blockade. Cervicothoracic ablation provides relatively short-term efficacy that is maintained for 6 to 12 weeks. This period is followed by increased peripheral hypersensitivity secondary to receptor upregulation. Periarterial sympathectomy that is performed in the periphery does not result in receptor upregulation or increased sensitivity of a receptor to a transmitter; however, it is not documented to be effective in any controlled studies involving CRPS. The use of percutaneous cervicothoracic sympathectomy using phenol and alcohol provides ease of administration with reversibility and eliminates the potential problems of receptor upregulation. Alternative therapies include thorascopic transection of the superior cervical ganglia[110] and radiofrequency ablation.[111,112] Implantable stimulators in the spinal cord and neurosurgical instrumentation in the thalamus and gray matter, as well as cingulotomy (i.e., transection of a portion of the brain) have been performed.[113–119]

Surgical Management

Surgical management of a nociceptive or neuropathic pain generator is an important option in the management of patients with CRPS types 1 and 2. Contrary to dogma, surgery can be performed safely in patients with SMP with prophylaxis provided by regional continuous blockade. A mechanical irritant exaggerates or incites abnormal peripheral fibers with resultant secondary CNS adaptations. Sympatholytic medications or treatments may be required to reduce pain and hypersensitivity sufficiently to delineate underlying nociceptive foci. If possible, these mechanical or neural areas of irritation then should be surgically repaired under the protection of continuous autonomic blockade. In CRPS type 2, common nociceptive foci include neuroma, neuroma in continuity, compression neuropathy, irritation of the superficial radial nerve (often by a fixation pin), irritation of the median nerve, and irritation of the dorsal branch of the ulnar nerve. In CRPS type 1, stenosing tenosynovitis of the first, second, or third dorsal compartment; internal derangements of the wrist; and osteochondral fractures often are precipitating and exacerbating events.[28,120–122]

SUMMARY

Although the pathophysiology of complex regional pain remains ill defined, the use of sequential treatment modalities that decrease pain and restore function is vital for a successful outcome. Early recognition, diagnosis, and intervention in patients with complex regional pain are important; however, most patients receive partial treatment before their definitive diagnosis. CRPS is common after fractures of the distal radius and ulna and may complicate relatively "trivial" trauma with exaggerated pain responses. After surgery, CRPS can create a stormy postoperative course and should be suspected if pain seems excessive. Often, patients with an expected postsurgical course have mild CRPS that complicates recovery; these patients will respond dramatically to sympatholytic drugs, not narcotics. Treatment should be multifactorial and should be based on physiologic criteria. Treatment paradigms should decrease inappropriate autonomic function, restore appropriate arteriovenous shunting, and identify and correct underlying nociceptive foci.

REFERENCES

1. Van Velzen GA, Perez RS, van Gestel MA, et al. Health-related quality of life in 975 patients with complex regional pain syndrome type 1. *Pain*. 155(3):629–634.
2. Crick JC, Crick JC. *Jury Verdicts related to Reflex Sympathetic Dystrophy Poster #3; 26th SOA Meeting*. Florida: Amelia Island; 2009.
3. Harden RN, Bruehl S, Stanton-Hicks M, Wilson PR. Proposed new diagnostic criteria for complex regional pain syndrome. *Pain Med*. 2007;8(4):326–331.
4. Harden RN, Bruehl S, Perez RS, et al. Validation of proposed diagnostic criteria (the "Budapest Criteria") for complex regional pain syndrome. *Pain*. 2010;150(2):268–274.
5. Raja SN, Treede RD, Davis KD, Campbell JN. Systemic alpha-adrenergic blockade with phentolamine: a diagnostic test for sympathetically maintained pain. *Anesthesiology*. 1991;74:691–698.
6. Raja SN, Turnquist JL, Meleka S, Campbell JN. Monitoring adequacy of α-adrenoceptor blockade following systemic phentolamine administration. *Pain*. 1996;64:197–204.
7. Campbell JN, et al. Diagnosis and management of sympathetically maintained pain. In: Fields HL, Liebeskind JC, eds. *Progress in Pain Research and Management*. Vol. 1. Seattle: IASP Press; 1994.
8. Dotson RM. Causalgia: reflex sympathetic dystrophy—sympathetically maintained pain: myth and reality. *Muscle Nerve*. 1993;16:1049.
9. Ochoa JL, Verdugo RJ. The mythology of reflex sympathetic dystrophy and sympathetically maintained pains. *Phys Med Rehab Clin North Am*. 1993;4:151.

10. Boas RA. Complex regional pain syndromes: symptoms, signs, and differential diagnosis. In: Janig W, Stanton-Hicks M, eds. *Reflex Sympathetic Dystrophy: A Reappraisal—Progress in Pain Research and Management.* Vol. 6. Seattle: IASP Press; 1996.

11. Amadio PC, Mackinnon SE, Merritt WH, et al. Reflex sympathetic dystrophy syndrome: consensus report of an ad hoc committee of the American Association for Hand Surgery on the definition of reflex sympathetic dystrophy syndrome. *Plast Reconstr Surg.* 1991;87:371–375.

12. Campbell JN, Meyer RA, Raja SN. Is nociceptor activation by alpha-1 adrenoreceptors the culprit in sympathetically maintained pain? *Am Pain Soc J.* 1992;1:3.

13. Campbell JN, et al. Myelinated afferents signal the hyperalgesia associated with nerve injury. *Pain.* 1988;32:89.

14. Yung Chung O, Bruehl SP. Complex regional pain syndrome. *Curr Treat Options Neurol.* 2003;5(6):499–511.

15. Li Z, Smith BP, Smith TL, Koman LA. Diagnosis and management of complex regional pain syndrome complicating upper extremity recovery. *J Hand Ther.* 2005;18(2):270–276.

16. Sandroni P, Benrud-Larson LM, McClelland RL, Low PA. Complex regional pain syndrome type I: incidence and prevalence in Olmsted County, a population-based study. *Pain.* 2003;103(1-2):199–207.

17. de Mos M, de Bruijn AG, Huygen FJ, et al. The incidence of complex regional pain syndrome: a population-based study. *Pain.* 2007;129:12–20.

18. Pappagallo M, Rosenberg AD. Epidemiology, pathophysiology, and management of complex regional pain syndrome. *Pain Pract.* 2001;1(1):11.

19. Allen G, Galar BS, Schwartz L. Epidemiology of CRPS: a retrospective chart review of 134 patients. *Pain.* 1999;80:539.

20. An HS, Hawthorne KB, Jackson WT. Reflex sympathetic dystrophy and cigarette smoking. *J Hand Surg.* 1988;13A:458.

21. Wilder RT, Berde CB, Wolohan M, et al. Reflex sympathetic dystrophy in children: clinical characteristics and follow-up of seventy patients. *J Bone Joint Surg.* 1992;74A:910–919.

22. Mailis A, Wade J. Profile of Caucasian women with possible genetic predisposition to reflex sympathetic dystrophy: a pilot study. *Clin J Pain.* 1994;10:210.

23. Veldman PHJM, Reynen HM, Arntz IE, Goris RJ. Signs and symptoms of reflex sympathetic dystrophy: prospective study of 829 patients. *Lancet.* 1993;342:1012–1016.

24. Subbarao J, Stillwell GK. Reflex sympathetic dystrophy syndrome of the upper extremity: analysis of total outcome of management of 125 cases. *Arch Phys Med Rehabil.* 1988;62:549.

25. Atkins RM, Duckworth T, Kanis JA. Algodystrophy following Colles' fracture. *J Hand Surg.* 1989;14B:161.

26. Atkins RM, Duckworth T, Kanis JA. Features of algodystrophy after Colles' fracture. *J Bone Joint Surg.* 1990;72B:105.

27. Bickerstaff DR, Charlesworth D, Kanis JA. Changes in cortical and trabecular bone in algodystrophy. *Br J Rheumatol.* 1993;32:46.

28. Laulan J, Bismuth JP, Sicre G, Garaud P. The different types of algodystrophy after fracture of the distal radius: predictive criteria of outcome after 1 year. *J Hand Surg.* 1997;22B:441–447.

29. Koman LA, Poehling GG, Smith TL. Complex regional pain syndrome: reflex sympathetic dystrophy and causalgia. In: Green DP, ed. *Green's Operative Hand Surgery.* New York: Churchill Livingstone; 1999.

30. Gonzalez F, Watson HK. Simultaneous carpal tunnel release and Dupuytren's fasciectomy. *J Hand Surg.* 1991;16B:175.

31. Nissenbaum M, Kleinert HE. Treatment considerations in carpal tunnel syndrome with coexistent Dupuytren's disease. *J Hand Surg.* 1980;5:544.

32. Lilly SI, Stern PJ. Simultaneous carpal tunnel release and Dupuytren's fasciectomy. *J Hand Surg Am.* 2010;35(5):754–759.

33. Buller M, Schulz S, Kasdan M, Wilhelmi BJ. The incidence of complex regional pain syndrome in simultaneous surgical treatment of carpal tunnel syndrome and dupuytren contracture. *Hand (N Y).* 2017.

34. Griepp ME, Thomas AF. Familial occurrences of reflex sympathetic dystrophy. *Clin J Pain.* 1991;7:48.

35. Ciccone DS, Bandilla EB, Wu W. Psychological dysfunction in patients with reflex sympathetic dystrophy. *Pain.* 1997;71:323.

36. Mailis-Gagnon A, Nicholson K, Blumberger D, Zurowski M. Characteristics and period prevalence of self-induced disorder in patients referred to a pain clinic with the diagnosis of complex regional pain syndrome. *Clin J Pain.* 2008;24(2):176–185.

37. de Takats G. Sympathetic reflex dystrophy. *Med Clin North Am.* 1965;49:117.

38. de Takats G, Miller DS. Post-traumatic dystrophy of the extremities: a chronic vasodilator mechanism. *Arch Surg.* 1943;46:469.

39. Koman LA, et al. Reflex sympathetic and other dystrophies. In: Peimer C, ed. *Surgery of the Hand and Upper Extremity.* New York: McGraw-Hill; 1996.

40. Satteson ES, Harbour PW, Koman LA, Smith BP, Li Z. The risk of pain syndrome affecting a previously non-painful limb following trauma or surgery in patients with a history of complex regional pain syndrome. *Scand J Pain.* 2017.

41. Sieweke N, Birklein F, Riedl B, et al. Patterns of hyperalgesia in complex regional pain syndrome. *Pain.* 1999;80:171–177.

42. Baron R, Blumberg H, Janig W. Clinical characteristics of patients with complex regional pain syndrome in Germany with special emphasis on vasomotor function. In: Janig W, Stanton-Hicks M, eds. *Reflex Sympathetic Dystrophy: A Reappraisal—Progress in Pain Research and Management.* Vol. 6. Seattle: IASP Press; 1996.

43. Wasner G, Schattschneider J, Heckmann K, Maier C, Baron R. Vascular abnormalities in reflex sympathetic dystrophy (CRPS I): mechanisms and diagnostic value. *Brain.* 2001;124(Pt 3):587–599.

44. Koman LA. Current status of noninvasive techniques in the diagnosis of upper extremity disorders. Part I. Evaluation of vascular competency. *Instr Course Lect.* 1983;32:61–76.

45. Pollock FE, Koman LA, Smith BP, Poehling GG. Patterns of microvascular response associated with reflex sympathetic dystrophy of the hand and wrist. *J Hand Surg.* 1993;18A:847–852.

46. Schürmann M, Gradl G, Andress HJ, et al. Assessment of peripheral sympathetic nervous function for diagnosing early post-traumatic complex regional pain syndrome type I. *Pain.* 1999;80:149–159.

47. Davidoff G, Morey K, Amann M, Stamps J. Pain measurement in reflex sympathetic dystrophy syndrome. *Pain.* 1988;32:27–34.

48. Huskisson EC. Measurement of pain. *Lancet.* 1974;2:1127.

49. Levine DW, Simmons BP, Koris MJ, et al. A self-administered questionnaire for the assessment of severity of symptoms and functional status in carpal tunnel syndrome. *J Bone Joint Surg.* 1993;75A:1585–1592.

50. McCabe SJ, Mizgala C, Glickman L. The measurement of cold sensitivity of the hand. *J Hand Surg.* 1991;16A:1037.

51. American Academy of Orthopaedic Surgeons. *Council of Musculoskeletal Specialty Societies, Institute for Work and Health. Disabilities of the Arm, Shoulder, and Hand: Outcomes Data Collection Package, Version 1.1;* 1996.

52. RAND Health Sciences Program. *RAND 36-Item Health Survey 1.0.* Santa Monica, CA: RAND Corp; 1992.

53. Stewart AL, Greenfield S, Hays RD, et al. Functional status and well-being of patients with chronic conditions. *JAMA.* 1989;262:907–913.

54. Stewart AL, Ware JE, Brook RH. Advances in the measurements of functional status: construction of aggregate indexes. *Med Care.* 1981;19:473–488.

55. Sandroni P, Low PA, Ferrer T, et al. Complex regional pain syndrome I (CRPSI): prospective study and laboratory evaluation. *Clin J Pain.* 1998;14:282–289.

56. Mussawy H, Schmidt T, Rolvien T, Rüther W, Amling M. Evaluation of bone microstructure in CRPS-affected upper limbs by HR-pQCT. *Clin Cases Miner Bone Metab.* 2017;14(1):54–59.

57. Genant HK, Kozin E, Bekerman C, et al. The reflex sympathetic dystrophy syndrome. *Radiology.* 1975;117:21–32.

58. Atkins RM, Tindale W, Bickerstaff D, Kanis JA. Quantitative bone scintigraphy in reflex sympathetic dystrophy. *Br J Rheumatol.* 1993;32:41–45.

59. Otake T, Ieshima H, Ishida H, et al. Bone atrophy in complex regional pain syndrome patients measured by microdensitometry. *Can J Anaesth.* 1998;45:831–838.

60. Schürmann M, Zaspel J, Löhr P, et al. Imaging in early posttraumatic complex regional pain syndrome: a comparison of diagnostic methods. *Clin J Pain.* 2007;23(5):449–457.

61. Lee GW, Weeks PM. The role of bone scintigraphy in diagnosing reflex sympathetic dystrophy. *J Hand Surg.* 1995;20A:458.

62. Moon JY, Park SY, Kim YC, et al. Analysis of patterns of three-phase bone scintigraphy for patients with complex regional pain syndrome diagnosed using the proposed research criteria (the 'Budapest Criteria'). *Br J Anaesth.* 2012;108(4):655–661.

63. Werner R, Davidoff G, Jackson MD, Cremer S, Ventocilla C, Wolf L. Factors affecting the sensitivity and specificity of the three-phase technetium bone scan in the diagnosis of reflex sympathetic dystrophy syndrome in the upper extremity. *J Hand Surg Am.* 1989;14(3):520–523.

64. Kozin F, Ryan LM, Carerra GF, et al. The reflex sympathetic dystrophy syndrome (RSDS). III. Scintigraphic studies, further evidence for the therapeutic efficacy of systemic corticosteroids, and proposed diagnostic criteria. *Am J Med.* 1981;70:23.

65. Kozin F, Soin JS, Ryan LM, et al. Bone scintigraphy in the reflex sympathetic dystrophy syndrome. *Radiology.* 1981;138:437–443.

66. Mackinnon SE, Holder LE. The use of three-phase radionuclide bone scanning in the diagnosis of reflex sympathetic dystrophy. *J Hand Surg.* 1984;9A:556.

67. Low PA, Caskey PE, Tuck RR, et al. Quantitative sudomotor axon reflex test in normal and neuropathic subjects. *Ann Neurol.* 1983;14:573–580.

68. Poudel A, Asahina M, Fujinuma Y, Yamanaka Y, Katagiri A, Araki N, et al. Skin sympathetic function in complex regional pain syndrome type 1. *Clin Auton Res.* 2015;25(6):367–371.

69. Chelimsky TC, Low PA, Naessens JM, Wilson PR, Amadio PC, O'Brien PC. Value of autonomic testing in reflex sympathetic dystrophy. *Mayo Clin Proc.* 1995;70(11):1029–1040.

70. Knezevic W, Bajada S. Peripheral autonomic surface potential: a quantitative technique for recording autonomic neural function in man. *Clin Exp Neurol.* 1985;21:201.

71. Fagius J, Karhuvaara S, Sundlöf G. The cold pressor test: effects of sympathetic nerve activity on human muscle and skin nerve fascicles. *Acta Physiol Scand.* 1989;137:325.

72. Baron R, Maier C. Reflex sympathetic dystrophy: skin blood flow, sympathetic vasoconstrictor reflexes and pain before and after surgical sympathectomy. *Pain.* 1996;67:317.

73. Gulevich SJ, Conwell TD, Lane J, et al. Stress infrared telethermography is useful in the diagnosis of complex regional pain syndrome, type I (formerly reflex sympathetic dystrophy). *Clin J Pain.* 1997;13:50–59.

74. Koman LA, Smith BP, Smith TL. Stress testing in the evaluation of upper-extremity perfusion. *Hand Clin.* 1993;9:59.

75. Fagrell B. Microcirculation of the skin. In: Mortillaro NA, ed. *The Physiology and Pharmacology of the Microcirculation.* Vol. 2. Orlando: Academic Press; 1984.

76. Ostergren J, Fagrell B. Skin microvascular circulation in the sympathetic dystrophies evaluated by videophotometric capillaroscopy and laser Doppler fluxmetry. *Intl J Microcirc.* 1988;7:289.

77. Raja SN, Meyer RA, Campbell JN. Peripheral mechanisms of somatic pain. *Anesthesiology.* 1988;68:571.

78. Raja SN, Davis KD, Campbell JN. The adrenergic pharmacology of sympathetically-maintained pain. *J Reconstr Microsurg.* 1992;8:63.

79. Dellon AL, Andonian E, Rosson GD. CRPS of the upper or lower extremity: surgical treatment outcomes. *J Brachial Plex Peripher Nerve Inj.* 2009;4:1.

80. Hobelmann Jr CF, Dellon AL. Use of prolonged sympathetic blockade as an adjunct to surgery in the patient with sympathetic maintained pain. *Microsurgery.* 1989;10(2):151–153.

81. Field J, Warwick D, Bannister GC. Features of algodystrophy ten years after Colles' fracture. *J Hand Surg [Br].* 1992;17(3):318.

82. Viel E, Ripart J, Pelissier J, et al. Management of reflex sympathetic dystrophy. *Ann Med Intern.* 1999;150:205–210.

83. Rowbotham MC. Pharmacologic management of complex regional pain syndrome. *Clin J Pain.* 2006;22(5):425–429. Review.

84. Bengtson K. Physical modalities for complex regional pain syndrome. *Hand Clin.* 1997;13:443–483.

85. Smart KM, Wand BM, O'Connell NE. Physiotherapy for pain and disability in adults with complex regional pain syndrome (CRPS) types I and II. *Cochrane Database Syst Rev.* 2016;2:CD010853.

86. Czop C, Smith TL, Rauck R, Koman LA. The pharmacologic approach to the painful hand. *Hand Clin.* 1996;12:633–642.

87. Evaniew N, McCarthy C, Kleinlugtenbelt YV, Ghert M, Bhandari M. Vitamin C to prevent complex regional pain syndrome in patients with distal radius fractures: a meta-analysis of randomized controlled trials. *J Orthop Trauma.* 2015;29(8):e235–e241.

88. Chen S, Roffey DM, Dion CA, Arab A, Wai EK. Effect of perioperative vitamin C supplementation on postoperative pain and the incidence of chronic regional pain syndrome: a systematic review and meta-analysis. *Clin J Pain.* 2016;32(2):179–185.

89. Meena S, Sharma P, Gangary SK, Chowdhury B. Role of vitamin C in prevention of complex regional pain syndrome after distal radius fractures: a meta-analysis. *Eur J Orthop Surg Traumatol.* 2015;25(4):637–641.

90. Malay S, Chung KC. Testing the validity of preventing chronic regional pain syndrome with vitamin C after distal radius fracture. [Corrected]. *J Hand Surg Am.* 2014;39(11):2251–2257. https://doi.org/10.1016/j.jhsa.2014.08.009. Epub 2014 Sep 16. Review. Erratum in: *J Hand Surg Am.* 2014 Dec;39(12):2551.

91. Ekrol I, Duckworth AD, Ralston SH, Court-Brown CM, McQueen MM. The influence of vitamin C on the outcome of distal radial fractures: a double-blind, randomized controlled trial. *J Bone Joint Surg Am.* 2014;96(17):1451–1459.

92. Pouskoulas CD, Aeschbach A, Ruppen W. Anaesthesia and pain therapy: perioperative management of patients with complex regional pain syndrome. *Anasthesiol Intensivmed Notfallmed Schmerzther.* 2012;47(11 12):688–695.

93. Zollinger PE, Kreis RW, van der Meulen HG, van der Elst M, Breederveld RS, Tuinebreijer WE. No Higher risk of CRPS after external fixation of distal radial fractures - subgroup analysis under randomised vitamin C prophylaxis. *Open Orthop J.* 2010;4:71–75.

94. Zollinger PE, Tuinebreijer WE, Breederveld RS, Kreis RW. Can vitamin C prevent complex regional pain syndrome in patients with wrist fractures? A randomized, controlled, multicenter dose-response study. *J Bone Joint Surg Am.* 2007;89(7):1424–1431.

95. Wertli MM, Kessels AG, Perez RS, Bachmann LM, Brunner F. Rational pain management in complex regional pain syndrome 1 (CRPS 1)—a network meta-analysis. *Pain Med.* 2014;15(9):1575–1589.

96. Varenna M, Adami S, Sinigaglia L. Bisphosphonates in complex regional pain syndrome type I: how do they work? *Clin Exp Rheumatol.* 2014;32(4):451–454. Epub 2014 Jun 24. Review.

97. Kingery WS. A critical review of controlled clinical trials for peripheral neuropathic pain and complex regional pain syndromes. *Pain.* 1997;73(2):123–139. Review.

98. Satoh H, Terai T, Nakanishi H, Ono T, Shibayama F. Effect of tiapride on the activity of neuroleptics and other kinds of drugs in mice and rats. *Nihon Yakurigaku Zasshi.* 1988;91(2):71–80.

99. Correll GE, Maleki J, Gracely EJ, et al. Subanesthetic ketamine infusion therapy: a retrospective analysis of a novel therapeutic approach to CRPS. *Pain Med.* 2004;5:263–275.

100. Correll GE, Maleki J, Gracely EJ, et al. Subanesthetic ketamine infusion therapy: a retrospective analysis of a novel therapeutic approach to CRPS. *Pain Med.* 2004;5:263–275.

101. Goldberg ME, Domsky R, Scaringe D, et al. Multi-day low dose ketamine infusion for the treatment of CRPS. *Pain Physician.* 2005;8:175–179.

102. Lavand'homme P, DeKock M, Waterloos H. Intraoperative epidural analgesia combined with ketamine provides effective preventative analgesia in patients undergoing major digestive surgery. *Anesthesiology.* 2005;103:813–820.

103. Puchalski P, Zyluk A. Results of the treatment of chronic, refractory CRPS with ketamine infusions: a preliminary report. *Handchir Mikrochir Plast Chir.* 2016;48(3):143–147.

104. Kiefer RT, Rohr P, Ploppa A, et al. Efficacy of ketamine in anesthetic dosage for the treatment of refractory complex regional pain syndrome: an open-label phase II study. *Pain Med.* 2008;9(8):1173–1201.

105. Hobelmann Jr CF, Dellon AL. Use of prolonged sympathetic blockade as an adjunct to surgery in the patient with sympathetic maintained pain. *Microsurgery.* 1989;10(2):151–153.

106. Ducic I, Maloney Jr CJ, Barrett SL, Dellon AL. Perioperative epidural blockade in the management of post-traumatic complex pain syndrome of the lower extremity. *Orthopedics*. 2003;26(6):641–644.

107. Hord AH, Rooks MD, Stephens BO, et al. Intravenous regional bretylium and lidocaine for treatment of reflex sympathetic dystrophy: a randomized, double-blind study. *Anesth Analg*. 1992;74:818–821.

108. Eisenach JC, Rauck RL, Buzzanell C, Lysak SZ. Epidural clonidine analgesia for intractable cancer pain: phase I. *Anaesthesiology*. 1989;71:647–652.

109. Rauck RL, Eisenach JC, Jackson K, et al. Epidural clonidine treatment for refractory reflex sympathetic dystrophy. *Anesthesiology*. 1993;79:1163–1169.

110. Eisenberg E, Geller R, Brill S. Pharmacotherapy options for complex regional pain syndrome. *Expert Rev Neurother*. 2007;7(5):521.

111. Sharony R, Saute M, Uretzky G. Video assisted thoracic surgery: our experience with patients. *J Cardiovasc Surg*. 1994;35:173.

112. Wilkinson HA. Percutaneous radiofrequency upper thoracic sympathectomy: a new technique. *Neurosurg*. 1984;15:811.

113. Wilkinson HA. Radiofrequency percutaneous upper-thoracic sympathectomy: technique and review of indications. *N Engl J Med*. 1984;311:34.

114. Barolat G, Schwartzmann R, Woo R. Epidural spinal cord stimulation in the management of reflex sympathetic dystrophy. *Appl Neurophysiol*. 1987;50:442.

115. Calvillo O, Didie J, Smith K. Neuroaugmentation in the treatment of complex regional pain syndrome of the upper extremity. *Acta Orthop Belg*. 1998;64:58.

116. Hassenbusch SJ, Stanton-Hicks M, Schoppa D, et al. Long-term results of peripheral nerve stimulation for reflex sympathetic dystrophy. *J Neurosurg*. 1996;84:415–423.

117. Hosobuchi Y. Subcortical electrical stimulation for control of intractable pain in humans: report of 122 cases, 1970-1984. *J Neurosurg*. 1986;64:543.

118. Robaina FJ, Dominguez M, Díaz M, et al. Spinal cord stimulation for relief of chronic pain in vasospastic disorders of the upper limbs. *Neurosurgery*. 1989;24:63–67.

119. Santo JL, Arias LM, Barolat G, et al. Bilateral cingulumotomy in the treatment of reflex sympathetic dystrophy. *Pain*. 1990;41:55–59.

120. Walker AE, Nulson F. Electrical stimulation of the upper thoracic portion of the sympathetic chain in man. *Arch Neurol Psychiatry*. 1948;59:559.

121. Jupiter JB, Seiler 3rd JG, Zienowicz R. Sympathetic maintained pain (causalgia) associated with a demonstrable peripheral-nerve lesion. Operative treatment. *J Bone Joint Surg Am*. 1994;76(9):1376–1384.

122. Cheung K, Klausmeyer MA, Jupiter JB. Abductor digiti minimi flap for vascularized coverage in the surgical management of complex regional pain syndrome following carpal tunnel release. *Hand (N Y)*. 2017;12(6):546–550.

98

Therapists' Management of Complex Regional Pain Syndrome

Tara L. Packham, Janet Holly

OUTLINE

CRITICAL POINTS

- Early recognition is critical for better outcomes.
- Comprehensive pain and symptom management includes both "top-down" and "bottom-up" approaches.
- Using contemporary knowledge of neuroplasticity, most treatments focus on avoiding provocation of pathological pain and retraining the nervous system with comfortable sensory inputs.
- The ultimate aim is return the patient to participation in meaningful roles, not eliminate impairments.

Complex regional pain syndrome (CRPS) is a predictably unpredictable management challenge in hand therapy. Careful collaboration and regular communication between the patient and his or her health care team, including therapist(s), surgeon, family physician, and pain specialists, will support maximal recovery and best functional outcomes.[1] For a thorough discussion of the diagnostic criteria, pathophysiology, prognosis, and medical management, please refer to Chapter 97. Early diagnosis and skilled rehabilitation have been supported by multiple clinical practice guidelines as critical for maximizing functional return[2-4]; however there is emerging evidence that early hand therapy intervention may also prevent the development of CRPS after distal radius fractures.[5,6]

Before progressing to practical recommendations for assessment and treatment, it is helpful to first lay a theoretical foundation for our conceptualizations of pain and sensory processing and for the associated general rehabilitation approaches. Melzack and Wall[7] postulated that pain should be understood as a multidimensional experience, including a complex combination of sensory-discriminative, affective–motivational, and cognitive components. The contemporary definition of pain from the International Association for the Study of Pain reflects this combination of sensory and emotional elements (Box 98.1).[8]

Woolf[9] has proposed a neurobiological classification of pain, closely linked to stimulus thresholds, responses and related behaviors. *Nociceptive pain* is a protective behavioral response to a high threshold, intense stimulus; *inflammatory pain* is also an adaptive protective response triggered by immune system activation from tissue damage or infection. Inflammatory pain creates tenderness, in which less intense stimuli trigger a protective response at lower thresholds. The third category is *pathological pain*; this category includes both *neuropathic pain* and *nociplastic pain*[8] and frequently includes features of central sensitization. Pathological pain is associated with disproportionate and escalating responses to subthreshold stimuli or even in the absence of any appreciable stimulus. Clinically, this may be seen as dynamic tactile allodynia, hyperalgesia, and spatial summation (refer to Box 98.2 for definitions).[9] However, it is important to note that these three categories are not mutually exclusive but may coexist (e.g., in postoperative pain after carpal tunnel release). Furthermore, the type of stimuli that elicit or increase pain may be multisensory. Melzack and Wall[7] relate a story from Livingston's work with causalgia (CRPS II) in a United States naval hospital in the early 1940s, when special orders from Washington were given to prevent airplanes from passing over the hospital because the sound provoked so much pain. Indeed, this phenomenon of hyperacusis in CRPS was described by de Klaver and associates,[10] who reported it in more than one third of their sample presenting with severe CRPS. Although hypersensitivities to light and sound are accepted as common features of altered sensory processing in migraine, so multisensory sensitivity can be present in persons with CRPS, reflecting the abnormal processing of the central nervous system (CNS) across multiple innocuous inputs.[10]

A final theoretical keystone for pain management is the overall paradigm of the practitioner. Some therapists use a "bottom-up" approach, that is, starting with a focus on impairments or activity components and building toward meaningful functional activities and overall participation and role performance. Indeed, this approach is often necessary in hand rehabilitation, in which recovery protocols are designed around tissue healing parameters, and the initial focus is on restoring function by maximizing the recovery of injured structures.[11] Evaluation is thus focused on measuring impairments in the target components. "Top-down" approaches start with an evaluation of the individual's overall participation, and the focus may be remediation or adaptation to improve role engagement, minimize environmental challenges, provide equipment for alternative approaches to tasks, and prioritize meaningful activities as both a means and end for interventions. In pain management, the terms "bottom-up" and "top-down" are also

---

BOX 98.1   International Association for the Study of Pain Definition of Pain

Defining Pain

"An unpleasant sensory and emotional experience associated with actual or potential tissue damage, or described in terms of such damage" (International Association for the Study of Pain. http://www.iasp-org/Taxonomy).

BOX 98.2   Definitions for Pain Features

Defining Pain

"An unpleasant sensory and emotional experience associated with actual or potential tissue damage, or described in terms of such damage" (International Association for the Study of Pain (http://www.iasp-org/Taxonomy).

Pain Features

Allodynia: pain caused by a stimulus that does not normally provoke pain; may be seen related to different types of somatosensory stimuli (touch, pressure, thermal; moving or static).

Hyperalgesia: increased pain from a stimulus that normally provokes pain (e.g., pinprick).

Summation: increasing response with repeated application of a stimulus; can be spatial (e.g., pain from pinprick is perceived over a larger and larger area of the skin) or temporal, in which the sensation continues for an increasing duration after removal of the stimulus.

Dysesthesia: an abnormal and unpleasant sensation; may be spontaneous or evoked by a particular stimulus.[8]

BOX 98.3   COMPACT Domains for CRPS

Domain	Outcome Measure
Pain	Pain intensity
	Short Form McGill Pain Questionnaire (version 2)
	PROMIS 29 Profile (version 2)
	EuroQoL-5D-5L
Disease severity	CRPS Severity Score
	CRPS symptom questions
Participation and function	PROMIS 29 Profile (version 2)
	EuroQoL-5D-5L
Emotional and psychological function	PROMIS 29 Profile (version 2)
	PROMIS suicidal ideation question
	EuroQoL-5D-5L
Catastrophizing	Pain Catastrophizing Scale
Self-efficacy	Pain Self-Efficacy Questionnaire
Person's global impression of change	Global Impression of Change (for follow-up visits)

Adapted from Grieve S, Perez RS, Birklein F, et al. Recommendations for a first Core Outcome Measurement set for Complex regional PAin syndrome Clinical sTudies (COMPACT). *Pain.* 2017;158(6):1083-1090.

---

used, with slightly different but complementary meanings. Bottom-up approaches focus on peripheral contributions to pain signaling via the stimuli, nerve transmission, and facilitation or inhibition outside of the CNS (e.g., application of ice or topical pain relievers, acupuncture, transcutaneous electrical nerve stimulation [TENS]). Top-down approaches focus on changing the perception and response to pain stimuli in the CNS by addressing pain-related fear, maladaptive movement patterns, or communication patterns between the somatosensory and motor cortices. For CRPS, we advocate that a thoughtful combination of these approaches is the optimal rehabilitation strategy.[12]

EVALUATIONS TO INFORM DIAGNOSIS

Early recognition is a key part of therapists' management for CRPS. In this pursuit, several standardized assessments have been developed with clear ties to the Budapest clinical criteria, which may assist in evaluation. The 16-item CRPS severity scale (CSS) has been widely used and continues to be validated in clinical practice and research.[13] An alternate 14-item standardized assessment of CRPS signs for clinicians has been proposed using a 4-point scale (none, mild, moderate, or severe) and continues to be developed.[14] Applying Woolf's categorization to CRPS, we can begin to understand that early CRPS features may present as inflammatory pain but will have additional features such as vasomotor instability that will align with the Budapest criteria. Type 2 CRPS is by definition a form of neuropathic pain and thus falls in the pathological category. Although type 1 CRPS is not widely accepted as a form of neuropathic pain, the syndrome also fits the categorization of pathological pain and sometimes nociplastic pain. This shared quality of pathological pain, coupled with the equivalence of the clinical presentation, may explain why many clinicians do not find the type 1 or type 2 differentiation particularly useful.

Although the Budapest criteria are the current diagnostic standard, the pursuit of clinical evaluations to inform diagnosis continues. Skin surface temperature asymmetry of greater than 1°C between affected and unaffected hands has been proposed as a diagnostic indicator,[15] but methods lack utility and reproducibility. Preliminary work reported the safety, reliability, and diagnostic sensitivity estimates for a cold pressor test combined with infrared thermometric measures of skin surface temperature using standardized evaluation points related to peripheral innervation[16,17]; this provides a rationale for continuing to pursue further validation of this method. Beyond diagnosis, however, thorough assessment of the individual constellation of presenting signs and symptoms is invaluable for formulating client-centered treatment goals, selecting the appropriate approaches and individual interventions, and predicting treatment response and overall recovery trajectories.

Examination

Examination of the person with symptoms of or a confirmed diagnosis of CRPS should incorporate both top-down and bottom-up lenses. This approach is reflected in the recent development of a core measurement set for all clinical studies of CRPS, known as Core Outcome Measurement set for complex regional PAin syndrome Clinical sTudies (COMPACT). COMPACT advocates for evaluation of seven key areas, each linked to a specific evaluation (Box 98.3).

Peripheral examination may include testing for allodynia, skin temperature asymmetry, edema, and other clinical signs of CRPS. The overarching principle is understanding and documenting the elements of the Budapest criteria: persistent pain that is disproportionate and cannot be explained by any other diagnosis. Symptoms often extend regionally beyond the territory of the original insult, and consideration of the entire limb is important; comparison with the contralateral limb is also critical (Fig. 98.1). Although there are a lack of validated condition-specific assessments,[18] the following summary of clinical assessment techniques applied in a standardized fashion can inform diagnostic evaluation and treatment planning. Assessment may also include consideration of potential nociceptive foci (e.g., addressing an adherent scar contributing to evoked pain with movement); however, it is important to maintain clear communication with the client: this is not searching for the "cause" of the pain but simply identifying

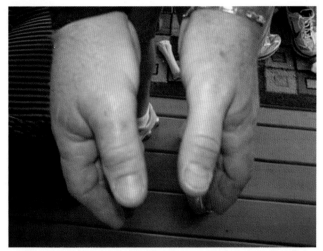

Fig. 98.1 Comparing affected and nonaffected limbs for symptom presentation. Note the swelling, shiny skin, and color changes suggesting vasodilation.

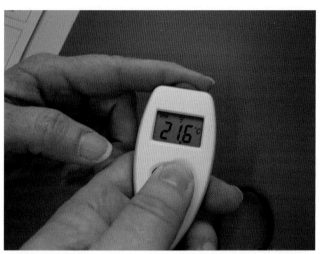

Fig. 98.2 Infrared skin surface thermometer. Note the small aperture suitable for measuring a fingertip and the temperature reading (in degrees Celsius) indicating skin surface, not body core temperature.

modifiable factors that can be contributors to the overall pain experience. A final yet critical point regarding assessment must be stated explicitly: the need for objective documentation of impairments should not supersede the cultivation of the therapeutic alliance with the person. Completing baseline measures of active range of motion (ROM) or grip strength may not be appropriate, and informed consent to explain the benefits and risks of completing formal evaluations is paramount. It should be carefully weighed if the information gained will substantially influence the nature of your *initial* treatment plan versus the risk to trust, rapport, and client autonomy.

Allodynia

This painful response to a non-noxious stimuli can be evoked with many different modalities or types of stimuli. Descriptions of clinical evaluations include testing for (1) dynamic mechanical allodynia by light stroking with a feather or cotton ball; (2) static mechanical allodynia by firm pressure applied to a joint using algometers, or use of calibrated monofilaments; or (3) cold allodynia by touching with an ice cube or an ice water test tube.

Autonomic and Vasomotor Changes

Edema should be measured using standardized procedures and noting qualities such as pitting or brawniness. In the absence of measurable edema, persons with CRPS may nonetheless report that their hand feels swollen; this should alert the therapist to also consider body perception disturbance. Changes in limb color and temperature should also be noted: increased temperature and redness indicates vasodilation, whereas skin that is blue and cool to the touch indicates vasoconstriction.[19] The client should also be asked if this is a consistent pattern or if it fluctuates between the two and what triggers for this change have been noted. It is not unusual for clients to use cell phone cameras to document fluctuations in color and edema, and observations made from these images can be described as subjective assessment findings.

Infrared thermometers that measure the temperature of the skin surface can be used to quantify skin temperature asymmetry.[16,20] Both the size and range of the temperature sensor should be considered when purchasing equipment to optimize utility for measurements on the hand; it also is worth noting if the measure is for skin surface temperature or an estimate of body core temperature (Fig. 98.2). Surface moisture must be removed from the hand, particularly in the presence of hyperhidrosis, before taking thermometric measures.

Joint Range of Motion

Goniometric assessment of active and passive joint motion can identify contractures and patterns of weakness. However, caution is needed when interpreting ROM measures because the inherent variability of the condition is reflected in poor measurement reliability.[21]

Motor Function

The same variability that challenges measurement reliability in measuring active movement also contributes to the instability seen in dynamometry measures of grip strength.[22] Incoordination may be documented using common observational tools such as bilateral rapid alternating pronation and supination or the "finger-to-nose" evaluation using the affected limb. Dystonias (sustained abnormal limb postures associated with more severe and chronic disease) should also be noted.

Sudomotor and Trophic Changes

Changes in the quality and growth patterns of the hair and nails should be noted. Skin color, texture, and moisture should also be noted, with abnormal patterns of sweating (both increased and decreased are possible) also recorded. In individuals with dystonia or motor extinction, there is also a risk of skin breakdown between the digits, creating a risk of infection. On rare occasions, we have also observed a pattern of fine blisters in the cutaneous territory reported as being the most painful. Sepsis associated with CRPS has been reported as leading to amputation.[4]

Self-Reported Measures Validated for Complex Regional Pain Syndrome

Global or "top-down" evaluations of CRPS should include evaluations of daily activities and role participation, not just impairments. This is often best achieved by validated self-report questionnaires. A systematic review of the measurement tools validated for the CRPS population reported six evaluations specifically targeting the upper extremity[18]; none of the three self-reported tools were in the English language. Other evaluations not specific to the upper extremity focused only on pain qualities and did not address activities or function. Neither the Disabilities of the Arm, Shoulder and Hand (DASH)[23] nor the Patient-Rated Wrist/Hand Evaluation (PRW/HE)[24] have been explicitly validated with the CRPS population, although both have been used in CRPS trials. The COMPACT battery proposes use of the Patient-Reported Outcomes Measurement Information System®, 29

Item version (PROMIS 29) item evaluation of general health and Euro-Qual 5D-5L as global evaluations,[25] and validation of these choices is underway. Also in development is the Hamilton Inventory for CRPS (HI-CRPS), which includes a 40-item self-reported component addressing symptoms, daily activities, and participation.[26] The Bath Body Perception scale was developed at a CRPS research center in the United Kingdom to describe neuroplastic changes to the body schema but has not undergone formal psychometric testing.[27] Building on this tool, a small study described preliminary use of a digital medium that allowed persons with CRPS to create a virtual representation of their perceived body schema, including qualitative reports of the value of a means of expressing these altered perceptions.[28] Therapists may find the novel tools described here useful for communication but should not rely on the results as measures of treatment outcome.

Pain Assessment

Pain assessment is addressed in detail in Chapter 94; however, we will explore some issues specific to CRPS here. Consensus guidelines suggest that comprehensive assessment of pain outcomes should include measures of pain intensity, physical and emotional functioning, symptoms and adverse events related to treatment, patient impression of improvement and satisfaction with treatment, and adherence.[29] Other important elements include spatial mapping of where the pain is perceived and temporal aspects of pain. The CRPS-specific recommendations from COMPACT mirror these guidelines but also recommend assessment of pain qualities.[25] Although agreement does not exist on whether both types 1 and 2 are neuropathic in nature, the pain quality experienced by persons with CRPS is concordant with neuropathic pain. Birklein and associates[30] reported the most common pain qualities reported from the McGill Pain Questionnaire (German version) in a cohort of 145 persons with CRPS were tearing (31%), burning (18%), and stinging (18%). The 78 pain descriptors included in the McGill Pain Questionnaire support a nuanced description of CRPS pain[31] but require strong language and comprehension skills. Self-reported evaluations of pain qualities that do not exclusively focus on screening for neuropathic pain can be helpful for patients to communicate their pain experience.

Short Form of the McGill Pain Questionnaire, Version 2. This evaluation includes six items (hot-burning, cold-freezing, itching, pain from light touch, numbness, and tingling or pins-and-needles) addressing neuropathic qualities; other subscales address continuous pain, intermittent pain, and affective qualities for a total of 22 items.[32]

painDETECT Questionnaire. The painDETECT Questionnaire (PDQ) was developed for neuropathic pain screening but also demonstrates the potential to be used as an outcome measure.[33] It has seven pain quality items (burning, tingling, light touch, numbness, light pressure, and hot–cold sensitivity), a temporal pattern item, and a radiating item. Although not included in the scoring, the PDQ also includes a three numeric rating scale for current pain, worst pain, and average pain intensity, as well as a body diagram for noting pain sites.[34]

Pain-QuILT. This online interactive tool allows visual mapping of 16 different pain qualities onto a body map and records intensity ratings for each quality.[35] Users can save files in a password-protected account for repeated measures and have the option to link their account to their clinicians (see https://app.painquilt.com).

Brief Pain Inventory. The Brief Pain Inventory (BPI) is a self-administered questionnaire that has been translated and validated in 14 languages. It not only quantitatively measures pain as present, worst, least and average but also measures its impact on daily function. The BPI provides 15 qualitative descriptors for pain, as well as a body diagram. It is widely used in the clinical environment.[36]

Examination tools using a standardized stimulus and subjective ratings of perceived responses are also known as psychophysical evaluations. Several novel psychophysical evaluations have been proposed for CRPS and other forms of painful somatosensory disorders.

Radboud Evaluation of Sensitivity, English Version. The original Radboud Evaluation of Sensitivity (RES) had eight items self-rated using a 100-mm visual analog scale (VAS); six of these use a standardized sensory stimulus. Preliminary psychometric evaluation of the English translation supported the reliability of this tool in a hand injury population, including persons with CRPS.[37]

Allodynography and the Rainbow Pain Scale. These complementary clinical examination techniques from the somatosensory rehabilitation method[38] use calibrated monofilaments from the Semmes-Weinstein set to evaluate static mechanical allodynia. In this context, allodynia is defined as a painful response (3 of 10 on a numeric rating scale or 30 mm on a 100-mm VAS) to a single touch with a 15-g (#5.18) monofilament. Allodynography uses this definition to map the borders of the territory of allodynic skin; this is useful to direct sensory reeducation efforts[39] and to avoid evoked pain, which may sustain the allodynic response.[40] The Rainbow Pain Scale uses seven different sizes of monofilaments (starting with the #2.44 filament) to generate a categorical rating of the allodynia threshold, or the minimum amount of pressure required to stimulate a painful response in the center of the allodynic territory.[41] Initial estimates of test–retest reliability, interrater reliability, and validity are promising, but ongoing validation of the techniques is required.[42]

Somatosensory Examination

Somatosensory deficits in patients with CRPS may present as sensory loss (painful numbness), dysesthesia and mislocalization, or sensory gain (allodynia, hyperesthesia, summation), with sensory losses presenting more frequently.[43] For a thorough discussion of sensory evaluation techniques, refer to Chapter 10. Special considerations for persons with CRPS should include (1) the tendency for sensory abnormalities in type 1 CRPS to present regionally, often without following a clear pattern of nerve distribution or dermatomes; (2) the potential for persons with CRPS type 2 to present with both localized (related to the known nerve injury) and regional symptoms (resulting from the syndrome); (3) the risk of temporal and spatial summation adding variability to results, especially with repeated stimuli or multiple tests; and (4) the potentially heightened impact of the environment (light, sound, temperature) and limb positioning on the observed results.

Other Assessments to Consider for Comprehensive Evaluation

A recent review of assessments used in CRPS research[44] highlights the broad spectrum of outcome measures reported in clinical trials. The COMPACT recommendations for CRPS seek to focus this to key domains, including self-reported evaluations for concepts such as pain-related fears, beliefs, and (mis)perceptions. Relevant evaluations of these domains include the following.

Pain Catastrophizing Scale

This 13-item self-reported scale evaluates elements of catastrophic thinking, including rumination, magnification, and helplessness.[45] A score of 30 of 52 indicates potentially catastrophic thought patterns.[45] This has been associated with poorer outcomes in hand surgery and rehabilitation and higher levels of pain and disability in CRPS.[46]

Pain Self Efficacy Questionnaire

This is a 10-item questionnaire intended to measure beliefs about the ability to manage activities despite pain and cope despite adversity.[47]

This strength-based lens is therefore negatively correlated with catastrophic thinking and pain disability but remains unrelated to pain intensity.

Tampa Scale for Kinesiophobia

Also available in several shorter versions, the original Tampa Scale for Kinesiophobia (TSK) has 17 items evaluating fear of movement and reinjury, with normative data in several languages.[48] A study of persons recently diagnosed with CRPS reported high baseline scores on the TSK-11 significantly predicted higher levels of disability at 1 year after diagnosis.[46]

Although the concepts of catastrophic thinking and fear of movement have added to our understanding of pain behavior, we caution therapists to refrain from labeling clients as "catastrophizers" or "kinesiophobic." When faced with evoked pain and spontaneous exacerbations, persons with CRPS may have adaptively altered their movement patterns to allow them to continue to function or may need to exercise vigilance by attending to pain triggers. It may be important to help them reframe these behaviors as unhelpful in the long term, but it is equally important to recognize that they may have effectively served as adaptive coping strategies in the short term. Failure to acknowledge the person's attempts to adaptively manage his or her condition by the negative connotations sometimes assigned to catastrophic thinking and guarding may counter self-efficacy. For further reflections on these concepts, readers are directed to Chapter 96 for a discussion of pain management principles and Chapters 83 and 118 for advice on facilitating psychosocial adjustment after injury.

EVIDENCE-INFORMED REHABILITATION INTERVENTIONS FOR COMPLEX REGIONAL PAIN SYNDROME

In the past decade, there has been a proliferation of studies evaluating rehabilitation strategies for CRPS. Despite this upsurge, there is an ongoing need for high-quality trials of interventions recruiting sufficient participants and using robust outcome measures to increase the confidence in the resultant estimates of effectiveness. Notwithstanding the existing gaps in the literature, current clinical practice guidelines for CRPS management strongly endorse rehabilitation interventions offered by allied health professionals (physical therapy, occupational therapy, and psychology) as first-line treatments.[2,3] A recent Cochrane review of physiotherapy interventions for CRPS[49] concluded that there was not sufficient high-quality evidence to endorse any treatments for the reduction of pain and disability; however, existing evidence suggested there may be benefit for graded motor imagery or mirror therapy.[49] However, with the emergence of international collaborations to support research (http://www.crpsconsortium.org) and advancing technologies generating both new understandings of the neurophysiology and targeted treatment options, the evidence should continue to evolve.

Given a lack of clear direction from the current state of the evidence, theoretical frameworks can be used to guide decision making. We earlier introduced the idea of selecting a combination of "bottom-up" and "top-down" approaches. In our experience, the clinical presentation of peripheral manifestations of pain such as persistent inflammation and vasomotor changes can be matched to bottom-up management strategies. Similarly, top-down approaches can address the impact of maladaptive neuroplasticity and central sensitization, with a broader focus on increasing functional use and participation in valued life roles. Accordingly, we have organized the following discussion of treatment options into general considerations and bottom-up and top-down approaches to CRPS management.

General Considerations

Comprehensive care of patients with CRPS is best realized by a multidisciplinary health care team. In the hand therapy setting, this may include the family doctor, orthopedic or plastic surgeon, pain specialist, psychologist, and hand therapist(s). Although this team may not be physically located in the same space, consistent communication about treatment goals and strategies can greatly reduce patient anxiety and increase adherence to treatment in all its forms. Addressing psychological health in this population has been described as ". . . crucial to successful treatment."[3] Ongoing formal and informal evaluation of mental health concerns will help the hand therapist to identify the need for psychological consultation and support. As with many other pain conditions, mental health issues were historically thought to predispose to the development of the syndrome. However, this view has been challenged by controlled prospective studies and evidence synthesis.[50] Nonetheless, persons with CRPS, especially those with intense pain or longstanding symptoms, may present with anxiety, depression, and thoughts of self-harm[51]; recent work also suggests a higher prevalence of posttraumatic stress disorder in persons with CRPS attending a pain center.[52] These concerns must be addressed to achieve progress in rehabilitation and recovery.

Other historical perspectives challenged by more recent evidence include the "no pain, no gain" approaches to exercise and desensitization. The current paradigm centers on grading of activity based on the overall level of challenge to the nervous system, (e.g., contributions of environment and context) and not just the physical movement or exercise, treatment task, or activity. Function in the real-world environment is the priority, not completing a prescribed therapy program. This demands careful consideration of work and life demands as important contributors to the grading of neuromatrix inputs: high salience inputs are more likely to provoke signs and symptoms. For example, a professional violinist after distal radius fracture who is having difficulties with activities because of intense pain that involve movements of prehension and radial deviation may be thinking about the need for that movement to hold a bow and as such is unconsciously weighting these inputs with greater salience.[53] Explaining the cognitive process and the unconscious assignment of greater salience or threat secondary to financial risk and possible loss of vocation may assist with moving forward by providing the person with an explanation for the greater magnitude of signs and symptoms during specific movements. Therefore, soliciting and valuing the feedback of the person with pain to guide treatment planning for every session will greatly assist outcomes. The need for ongoing evaluation was summarized very clearly by the previous author of this chapter in the sixth edition of *Rehabilitation of the Hand*:

> *Through the examination, the therapist can determine the irritability of the patient's involved tissues and formulate a treatment plan. If the therapist fails to make an accurate assessment of the patient's signs and symptoms, in many instances he or she becomes the "pain terrorist." . . . Treatment program development requires clinical reasoning, frequent if not daily observation of the patient, assessment of the patient's response to previous treatments, and assessment of the patient's level of [tissue and system] irritability. The therapist must clinically decide at each visit the vasomotor state of the patient's extremity. There is no support in the literature to suggest an appropriate dosage or duration for treatment. It is only through this ongoing evaluation process that these parameters can be determined and modified.*

Mark Walsh

Bottom-Up Approaches: Address the Signs and Symptoms

Inflammation

A hot, red, swollen hand is typical of 'warm' CRPS, and is a clear treatment target for the hand therapist (see Fig. 98.1). However, evidence specific to CRPS is currently of generally low quality, derived from small studies. A randomized controlled trial (RCT) reported manual lymph drainage techniques using a home program of self-massage and therapist hands-on treatment reported only short-term benefit without increasing pain.[54] Low-level laser was superior to usual care using interferential current when used twice daily for 10 days in acute-onset CRPS (3–5 weeks after symptom onset), but persistent effects were not reported.[55] A recent study added neuromuscular electrical stimulation or 30-minute warm whirlpool baths to daily physiotherapy and found similar improvements in both groups for ROM but favored whirlpool baths for swelling.[56] Although the evidence for contrast baths lacks clarity in other populations because of heterogeneity[57] and lacks evidence for this population, we continue to use this modality selectively for both inflammation and graded thermal sensory reeducation.

Prevention of Vasoconstriction and Hypoxia

There has been a proliferation of trials investigating the antioxidant influence of vitamin C for the prevention of CRPS after fracture.[58] The evidence suggests a protective effect for immediately commencing a 500 mg daily dose for 50 days. From a rehabilitation lens, Gillespie and associates[5] describe how implementation of a multimodal strategy including early motion at adjacent joints, careful monitoring of casting, and healthy eating recommendations for patients after distal radius fracture dramatically reduced the incidence of CRPS in this population.

Pain and Painful Somatosensory Disturbances

By definition, pain is a cardinal feature of CRPS. It is therefore not surprising that meaningful pain reduction is a valued indicator of outcome for persons with CRPS.[59] Although there is a lack of consensus on the minimum clinically important difference in pain trials, a study of meaningful pain reduction in CRPS reported a 3-cm change on a 10-cm VAS or a 50% reduction of pain intensity was related to patient perception of treatment success.[60]

Several modalities have been posited to reduce pain in CRPS. Korpan and coworkers[61] investigated acupuncture for pain reduction to facilitate participation in a physical rehabilitation program, but was unable to demonstrate a direct benefit. TENS applied proximally to an area of allodynia in a study by Ryan and coworkers[62] (*n* = 8) of persons with CRPS in one upper limb failed to achieve target enrollment to generate estimates of effect. Scrambler therapy purports to use cutaneous electrostimulation to disrupt peripheral afferent signaling and thus provide long-term pain relief in persons with refractory CRPS when used daily over a 1- 2-week period[63]; however, these claims have not yet been supported by robust evidence in this population.

Other therapeutic interventions for addressing painful somatosensation in upper limb CRPS have also been proposed. Moseley and coworkersl[64] described a tactile discrimination training program (*n* = 13) using therapist or helper stimulation of the painful area with two different sizes of probe (2- and 11-mm wine corks). Participants were asked to simultaneously discriminate between the size of the probe and the location of the stimulation. In short-term follow-up, participants reported both a reduction in pain and improvements in two-point discrimination.[64] A subsequent study combined tactile discrimination with mirror visual feedback and reported the combination to be more effective than tactile discrimination alone in a small study

(*n* = 10) on same-day comparisons and 2 days later; participants were not evaluated for lasting benefits.[65] Somatosensory rehabilitation is a formal program for the evaluation and treatment of the painful consequences of altered nerve function, including both painful numbness and allodynia.[38,66] Packham and colleagues[41] reported the effectiveness of this method for addressing allodynia in an uncontrolled retrospective cohort of persons with CRPS of one upper limb (*n* = 48). Resolution of the allodynia was reported after an average of 81 days of a supervised home program, with associated reduction of pain of more than 50% as reported by the French version of the McGill Pain Questionnaire. Techniques of sensory–motor reeducation for persons with CRPS were also described by Lewis and coworkers[39] and illustrated with a small case series (*n* = 4).

Desensitization is a concept frequently listed in management protocols for CRPS but seldom described or evaluated; one of the few effectiveness studies of desensitization for upper limb injuries excluded persons with CRPS.[67] Pleger and coworkers presented a brief but detailed report on a graded approach to tactile desensitization matched to current pain experience in a case series of six persons with CRPS of one upper limb.[68] They reported parallel gains in two-point discrimination, decreased pain intensity, and normalization of somatosensory maps on functional magnetic resonance imaging; however, desensitization was only one component of their graded rehabilitation program. Furthermore, dosage and duration of treatment were highly variable.[68] Lewis and coworkers[39] also described a personalized, graded approach to sensory retraining, which they termed *desensitization*; however, it is important to note that stimulation was not applied directly to the painful area but to areas adjacent to the pain but still lacking normal sensory function. In our experience, direct desensitization may be helpful for persons with peripheral sensitization evidenced by numbness or dysesthesias but should be avoided in persons in whom allodynia and summation are suggestive of central sensitization.

Stiffness

Passive range of motion (PROM) is most appropriately used only after the person's signs and symptoms are stabilized and as a means to improve functional use of the hand, not merely in pursuit of premorbid joint range. Included in passive motion techniques are joint mobilization procedures to increase ROM and decrease pain and static progressive orthoses for joint contractures or soft tissue limitations with functional implications.[69] Careful consideration of the value of PROM weighed against the potential of evoked pain or temporal summation effects is warranted. There are no data supporting aggressive PROM after medical intervention such as regional or stellate ganglion blocks. Anecdotally, the authors have seen a carefully selected subset of patients with sympathetically maintained pain benefit from a collaborative approach of tailored therapy intensity in relation to pain blocks.

There are multiple effective options for providing superficial heat for preconditioning before passive stretch.[70] However, the use of heat may be contraindicated in persons with thermal allodynia or may need careful titration and monitoring to minimize pain evocation that would counter any therapeutic benefits. The combined effect of warmth, active movement, and tactile stimulation provided by a whirlpool bath or fluidotherapy can be helpful or may create a sensory overload; again, carefully graded introduction of the individual components is important to find the "just-right" balance of comfort and challenge. Similarly, use of static progressive orthoses with prolonged and uniform gentle pressure may be better tolerated by this population than short-term dynamic orthosis use or PROM. In the absence of literature directly addressing use of these strategies in CRPS, therapists are encouraged to weigh the evidence for other conditions against the symptom presentation of the individual client and use a combination of clinical reasoning and careful monitoring to

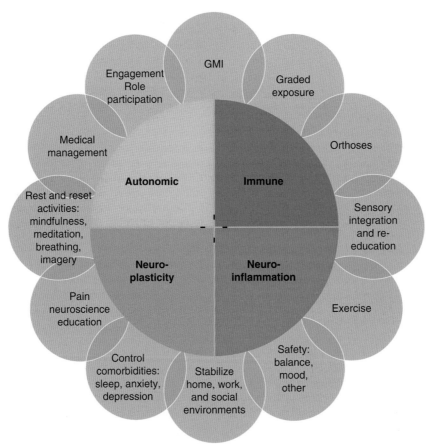

Fig. 98.3 Holistic treatment of complex regional pain syndrome. The center of the diagram illustrates the mechanisms, and management approaches form the outer ring. *GMI,* graded motor imagery.

inform treatment planning. Thoughtfully combining bottom-up strategies to manage signs and symptoms with top-down strategies to address overall participation and function is the key to holistic management (Fig. 98.3).

Top-Down Approaches: Address the Person and Systems

Therapists caring for persons with CRPS must maintain a holistic view of the person. Hand therapists often see this population early and may continue to follow the person if the condition persists. Clinical practice guidelines emphasize the goals of care are to "…reduce pain, preserve or restore function, and enable patients to manage their condition and improve their quality of life."[2] These goals can be achieved by a tailored approach of intervention strategies addressing the evidence of maladaptive neuroplasticity and its functional consequences.

Sensorimotor Incongruence

Since publication of the first RCT on graded motor imagery (GMI),[71] it has become one of the gold standards of CRPS rehabilitation. The principles underpinning GMI as an effective intervention for CRPS were progressively illustrated by (1) an initial RCT of GMI,[71] (2) a second trial illustrating sequential activation of the cortical networks involved in sensory and motor processing was the key component of GMI for correcting sensorimotor incongruence in chronic CRPS rather than sustained attention,[72] and (3) a trial with longer follow-up illustrated one of three patients with either CRPS or phantom limb pain still had benefits 6 months later.[73] Despite these findings, a subsequent study did not determine efficacy for CRPS in the naturalistic setting of a clinic.[74] Although the original GMI protocol instructs participants to practice the various components every waking hour, the multisite trial by Johnson and coworkers[74] could not achieve compliance at the same treatment intensity. Furthermore, they

found that participants were not ready to progress through all GMI stages after only 2 weeks. Subsequently, the original research protocol has now been modified to be progressed only when the person has achieved a stable level of proficiency over the course of a week[75] instead of following a steady progression based on a temporal standard. See Chapter 100 for a more in-depth description of GMI in diverse populations. Box 98.4 summarizes clinical pearls for using GMI for persons with CRPS.

Laterality Discrimination

Because some persons with CRPS feel pain when even thinking about movement,[76] it is important to start with laterality discrimination. The key principles in early studies was for the participant to be able to discriminate between left and right hand or shoulder by viewing images of the part of the body affected by CRPS. Clinically, it is important to determine the appropriate baselines for a client to perform this task. This may be 1 image or 40 depending on the individual person's capacity to perform the activity without excessive aggravation of all signs and symptoms. For success with this technique, it is crucial that the clinician determine what a true baseline is for each individual. To progress to the next level, there should be consistency of ability to perform the task for at least 1 week. Observations by the therapist are essential; it is not sufficient to give a quick demonstration and commence a home program, or autonomic reactions many be missed, and the person may abandon the program because this was not anticipated and addressed.

Motor Imagery: Imagined Movements

If the person can complete laterality recognition without signs and symptom aggravation over a period of a week, it is time to start imagined movements. They should imagine using the limb without actually

BOX 98.4 Clinical Pearls for Using Graded Motor Imagery in Patients with Complex Regional Pain Syndrome

Laterality

Determine an appropriate baseline (signs and symptoms).

- Sweating responses from the autonomic nervous system (ANS) during this activity may be found on another part of the body (e.g., upper lip, back).
- Clients may also experience vertigo or nausea-like symptoms from strong ANS responses they may not believe are activity related. These need to be respected as part of the client baseline.

Establish a relaxation technique for sign or symptom control **before** starting the task. This empowers the person by being able to reduce the signs or symptoms during the task.

Ensure client is aware that the task is the **process of participating** and not necessarily completion.

During the task, observe the person carefully for increasing vigilance and reactions to images. These give insights to areas of greater body perception disruption (e.g., Is D1 more difficult than D5?).

In the game of concentration, the patient may try to match the dorsal image of a hand in a certain position with a palmar image in the same positions.

Initially remove more threatening images from the game. These are the images that draw out negative comments (e.g., "It looks like a claw") or actual physical recoil responses to the images.

Start with images oriented toward the patient and change orientation to make more difficult.

In the beginning, it may be necessary to use laterality recognition images of the elbow or shoulder if the person is unable to tolerate the images of the hand

Tools for Laterality

NOIgroup cards, photographs, or magazines

Apps

- NOI Recognise (>80% accuracy, 2.0 sec +/– 0.5 sec hands and shoulders)
- Orientate

Use Google Images to find a variety of pictures and postures

Create a PowerPoint slide show to use in the clinic and at home.

Activities with children: The patient gets to participate in play assisting in fulfilling his or her life role as a parent or grandparent.

- Paint or draw hand pictures.
- Trace outlines of hands.

Observe sculptures at a museum or park, determining the left and right limbs (added bonus of getting people out of the house improving overall activity level and decreasing social isolation).

Barriers to Progress in Laterality

Sleep dysfunction (new learning is consolidated during sleep)

Not really looking at the images but focusing purely on the thumb to determine left and right and complete the task.

Posttraumatic stress disorder (PTSD)[52]

- Difficulties looking at specific limb images because of previous traumatic exposures involving limb dismemberment (car accident victims, first responders, military).
- The addition of a psychologist to surmount this barrier will likely be required.

Motor Imagery

Determine an appropriate baseline (signs and symptoms).

Use relaxation technique for sign and symptom control throughout the task to maximize repetitions.

Remind the client that the goal is the process of participating and not necessarily task completion.

Watch the person carefully for signs of increasing vigilance.

Start off with visual imagery using the seven senses as a relaxation exercise to decrease the vigilance level of the ANS. Then incorporate the imagined movement into the imagery location.

If the shoulder is involved, imagine movements below 90 degrees of elevation or internal rotation at 0 degrees of abduction first and then progress to external rotation and elevation above 90 degrees.

As imagined movements become easier, imagine the movement with light loads, progressing them slowly to imagining heavier loads.

Barriers to Progress in Motor Imagery

Difficulties focusing on tasks

Kinesiophobia: Patients may need to think about someone else moving first.

Mirror Visual Feedback

Determine appropriate baselines for signs and symptoms.

Remind client to use relaxation technique throughout mirror therapy for control of ANS "fight-or-flight" responses to maximize treatment intensity.

Start with laterality recognition tasks first as a warm-up to facilitate success with mirror therapy.

Add picking up small objects, particularly related to functional tasks:

- Toothbrush, hairbrush, coins
- Empty plastic cup

Progress to bigger and heavier objects:

- Apple, banana, orange
- Glass or mug

Add tactile sensory (touch, thermal, gentle pressure, vibration, proprioception) inputs on both hands at same time.

Adding smells or noise may also assist (bell, rattle, scented lotion).

Practice in various emotional states (happy, sad, stressed, anxious).

Tools for Mirror Visual Feedback

Mirror box

Sensory input objects:

- Paint brush
- Cold spoon or warm spoon (or test tubes)
- Eraser or wine cork for pressure
- Tuning forks (use the same frequency for each side)

Barriers to Progress in Mirror Visual Feedback

Other body perception disorders such as anorexia or intolerances to mirrors

PTSD: Scars or the lack of scar reflected in the mirror may triggers memories of traumatic events.

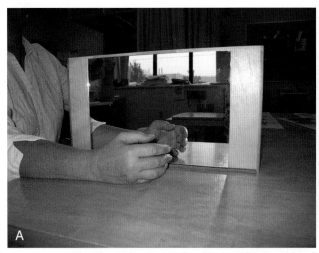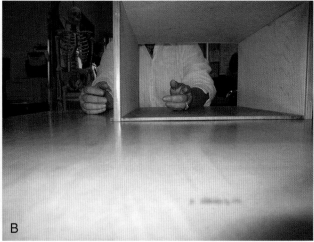

Fig. 98.4 Using a mirror box for visual feedback. Ideally, the box should be positioned where the mirror image is easily viewed (**A**) and large enough (**B**) for the person to be comfortable moving his or her limb inside.

moving, thus activating the supplementary motor area in the brain[77] but without producing muscle contraction in the limb (see Box 98.4).

Mirror Therapy

Mirror therapy is a process to "trick the brain" that the affected limb is moving without eliciting CRPS signs and symptoms. The concept involves first watching the unaffected limb moving and then progressing to bilateral movements. Treatment is most effective when the mirror is well positioned to support the visual illusion, fooling the brain into believing the limb it sees reflected in the mirror is indeed the affected limb (Fig. 98.4). Movements are to be made in a slow and smooth manner and progress from simple to complex to fine-motor dexterity tasks.[75]

When mirror therapy is no longer difficult, the client should progress to typical strengthening and flexibility exercises in a paced, graded manner, respecting load baselines and activity tolerances versus a traditional exercise prescription model.

Beyond GMI, other approaches to addressing sensorimotor incongruence have been proposed. Schmid and coworkers[78] described pain reduction in a small prospective cohort ($n = 10$) provided with an intensive 2-week home program based on principles of sensorimotor retraining. Participants with upper limb CRPS were provided with a series of discs containing raised dots (inspired by Braille) and a variety of perceptual training exercises, focusing on bimanual hand use, speed, and memory training.[78] Anecdotally, this is an approach we have also used in practice as a way of using tactile discrimination principles[64] but allowing the client to have control and removing the need to have a therapist or partner administer sensory stimuli. The key is providing activities that can be done without vision: raised characters can be easily made using puff paint or glitter glue on stiff cardboard. An alternate media is to mount Braille-like patterns starting with large dried beans (e.g., fava) and reducing to smaller forms such as dried peas or tapioca pearls. Other activities can include identifying shapes made of Lego blocks, sponge, or craft foam with vision occluded or discriminating between different forms of textiles such as velvet, flannel, and satin. Size discrimination of identical shapes is another task variation or sorting a mixture of coins, safety pins, or dried beans by size.

Body Perception Disturbances

Body perception disturbances do not refer to the emotional percept of body image but rather to disruption or alteration of the cortical representation of the body or body schema used for sensory integration and

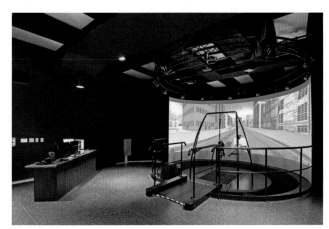

Fig. 98.5 Example of a CAREN virtual reality laboratory. (Used with permission of the Ottawa Hospital.)

motor planning (although the person experiencing a disrupted schema may also experience changes in body image).[79] Much of the foundational work in this area is experimental in focus, exploring the nature of body representation and its relationship to pain,[80,81] and has not yet been translated into clinical interventions. However, several reports describe the longitudinal effects of interventions targeting body representations. Sensorimotor reeducation using tactile stimulation of areas of cutaneous dysesthesias immediately adjacent to painful skin areas was related to modest improvements in body perception disturbance in a case described by Lewis and coworkers.[39] Prism glasses were used to improve body perception in a case study reported by Bultitude and Rafal[82] and in a small cohort study ($n = 7$) by Christophe and coworkers[83] to correct "pseudo-neglect," or spatial alterations in visual attention. The cohort used the glasses twice daily for 4 days and reported both immediate and sustained (2-week follow-up) improvements in pain.

Virtual reality (VR) has grown out of the world of gaming and is now being explored as a treatment medium for a range of health conditions. VR uses the alteration of multimodal stimuli to create an actual presence or immersion in a virtual world. VR modalities can vary from MIRAGE illusion boxes to head-mount VR systems to fully immersive CAREN (Fig. 98.5) and CAVE VR laboratories. There is a body of work looking at VR as distraction therapy in the management of acute pain, particularly during burn debridement techniques.[84] VR has also been examined for increasing ROM in chronic pain.[85] A Cochrane review of stroke interventions reported improvements in arm function, as well as activity of daily living (ADL) function with the use of VR.[86] Embodiment in the VR world has already been examined for the treatment of eating disorders, in which the person has schematic misperceptions about body size.[87]

Given the capacity to alter the body in the virtual world and the body perception and embodiment dysfunctions also seen in persons with CRPS, this technology has generated pilot studies to explore the potential for improving outcome in this population. Early work by Sato and coworkers[88] looked at nonimmersive VR mirror feedback therapy in a pilot study of five persons with CRPS. Four of the five participants achieved a 50% reduction in pain, with qualitative reports of increased use of the affected arm as pain reduced. Three of five participants were able to reduce their medications after participating in the study.[88] In a pediatric CRPS study of four participants using head-mount VR, a representational avatar was used in immersive sessions to complete game tasks.[89] The participants were provided stereoscopic images, audio feedback, and haptic feedback through floor vibration to enhance the virtual world to assist with the feeling of embodiment.

In 2015, Lewis and coworkers[90] conducted an RCT using a MIRAGE-augmented VR box. They made virtual adjustments to the size and shape of the viewed limb and reported improved ownership of the affected limb in persons with CRPS. Mouraux and coworkers[91] used three-dimensional glasses and a Kinect camera to create a virtual form of mirror therapy for persons with persistent neuropathic pain, including CRPS. They reported improvements in pain after a single session, with cumulative effects across multiple sessions. Another study by Lewis and coworkers[92] showed that the MIRAGE system and visual illusions can modulate pain in patients with chronic CRPS. Given the outcome of these early studies and the ability to modulate a multimodal spatial environment in a controlled manner, VR may be a promising future treatment for CRPS.

Kinesiophobia and Learned Nonuse

Stress loading was first described in a retrospective case series ($n = 52$) 30 years ago,[93] but replication of the results using more robust study designs has not been reported in the ensuing decades. The program consisted of a sequential and graded program of compression loading through the painful limb (scrubbing) and distraction loading (carrying) with increasing frequency and duration. Secondary increases in pain and swelling were reported to resolve within several days, allowing for continued participation and progression of program. Beyond the low quality of the supporting evidence,[94] there are several other caveats to this approach. First, the theoretical mechanism of action was related to decreasing sympathetic overactivity, which has now been abandoned as a causal mechanism in CRPS, particularly in persons with a longer duration of symptoms. The justification for continued loading despite symptom flare is not concordant with our current understandings of pain mechanisms and is difficult to reconcile with any pain neuroscience education (PNE) the client may have already received. Second, given the contemporary emphasis on early identification and intervention, the core weight-bearing and traction elements of stress loading may not be appropriate until after healing of the initial or precipitating event (e.g., a hand fracture or tendon repair).

Graded exposure in vivo for reducing pain-related fear of movement in CRPS was described in a small single case experimental design study ($n = 8$) by de Jong and coworkers.[95] They targeted persons with CRPS symptoms lasting at least 6 months and reporting high levels of kinesiophobia on the Tampa Scale. A standardized test using pictures of daily activities was used to grade the perceived level of threat associated with specific activities, and the treatment program was customized using this hierarchy. They reported that the graded exposure program

improved function and decreased both pain intensity and pain-related fear.[95] A later cross-sectional study of persons with CRPS suggested that both pain-related fear and pain intensity were important predictors of disability,[96] confirming the importance of targeting pain-related fears in comprehensive rehabilitation. This provided justification for a larger study using graded exposure by den Hollander and coworkers[97] to reduce kinesiophobia in persons with CRPS. They conducted an RCT ($n = 46$), comparing graded exposure to potentially painful activities with traditional physiotherapy in which activities were titrated to avoid producing pain. In the population studied (persons with moderate kinesiophobia but without anxiety or depression), a 4-month graded exposure program reduced pain and improved function.[97]

A proposed alternative to graded pain exposure is the pain-exposure physical therapy or PEPT program. This method was tested in persons who did not have a high level of fear of movement but excluded persons with mood disorders. Intensity of stimulation was not graded; instead, they exposed all participants to functional activities and discontinued all forms of pain control, including medications and orthoses.[98] A pilot study of 20 persons with CRPS was first undertaken to ensure the safety of the method; they reported the only adverse effects to be (1) a temporary increase in edema in 2 participants and (2) a temporary increase in pain in 5 participants.[99] A second larger trial reported benefits for those who completed the program as prescribed, but the overall intention-to-treat analysis did not find PEPT to be better than a traditional physiotherapy program.[98]

Pain-Related Disability

One of the largest studies of rehabilitation of persons with CRPS was conducted by Oerlemans and coworkers, which was an RCT with 135 participants.[100] They compared outcomes for individually tailored therapy consisting of physical therapy (focused on movement, pain, and other symptoms), occupational therapy (focusing on management of inflammation, sensory reeducation, and functional activity), or social work (general education on pain and coping). Participants who received the "active" programs of physical or occupational therapy saw greater improvements than those in the social work "passive" control group. A more recent retrospective cohort ($n = 60$) compared persons who had received just physiotherapy with those receiving both physical and occupational therapy for CRPS after upper limb injury.[101] Although both groups improved with treatment, those with the multidisciplinary management reported higher participation in daily activities.

Pain Neurophysiology Education

The purpose of PNE is to provide persons with a sound understanding of the neurophysiology of pain. This may be particularly important for this client group, who often feel they have not been given adequate information about CRPS.[102] PNE has been found to be an effective treatment tool in other chronic pain conditions, with lasting benefits for participants.[103,104] Research looking at the effectiveness of PNE with CRPS has not been conducted but is merited.[102,105] See Box 98.5 for a quick reference guide to PNE.

In CRPS, the constant stimulation of nociceptors in the peripheral nervous system results in central sensitization and a greater salience to CNS inputs. Work done by Bruehl and Chung[106] also highlighted the role of psychological and behavioral factors in exacerbating pain and potentially helping to maintain the condition in some clients. As such, a context-specific PNE session can assist persons with CRPS with both understanding their condition and improving self-management.

The principle behind PNE is to explain the physiology of pain rather than focusing on tissue damage. Persons with pain are taught how central sensitization can create nociplastic pain even when threat no longer exists to their tissues.[8] With this understanding in place, it removes a substantial barrier to increasing their engagement in ADLs and physical activity.

BOX 98.5   Quick Reference for Pain Neurophysiology Education

Key Components of Pain Neurophysiology Education

1. When people know why they hurt, they generally hurt less.
2. Pain is normal and always real. It is dependent on how your brain is processing information from many sources (peripheral and central) to determine threats.
3. We do not have pain receptors but rather other receptors that signal potential danger.
4. Pain can exist without tissue damage, and tissue damage can exist without pain.
5. The nervous system balances factors that *may* threaten the body and those that promote safety.
6. Pain relies on contexts, including your *thoughts, memories, beliefs,* and *current situation.*
7. The nervous system can adapt and become overprotective (hypervigilant), protecting us when there is no immediate threat to tissue. However, it can also adapt to become less protective.[110]

Teaching Resources for PNE

Explain Pain or *Explain Pain Supercharged* (Noigroup Publications)

Painful Yarns and Metaphors and Stories to Help Understand the Biology of Pain (Noigroup Publications)

Therapeutic Neuroscience Education: Teaching Patients About Pain (International Spine and Pain Institute)

How Does Your Brain Respond To Pain? https://www.youtube.com/watch?v=I7wfDenj6CQ

TEDxAdelaide: Lorimer Moseley. Why Things Hurt, https://www.youtube.com/watch?v=gwd-wLdlHjs&list=PLMXXJ4hJ3GhkkBR9EY2p-dt8QUPCodqj7i&index=3

Brainman Chooses: Pain Treatment. https://www.youtube.com/watch?v=jl-wn9rC3rOl

Understanding Pain and What To Do About It. https://www.youtube.com/watch?v=cLWntMDgFcs

Understanding Pain in Less Than 5 Minutes. https://www.youtube.com/watch?v=5KrUL8tOaQs

Why Things Hurt. https://www.youtube.com/watch?v=gwd-wLdlHjs

PNE also provides the person with tools to promote self-management of pain.[107] Oral instruction followed by written pain neurophysiology education has been found to be more effective than just written or oral.[107] Use of metaphors or examples that are specific to your client will assist with her or his understanding.[108] PNE needs to be reinforced during therapy activities to ensure consolidation of the information and optimize outcomes.[109]

Adult learning principles are an important foundation for pain neuroscience teaching. Adults enter a learning experience to create change in (1) skills, (2) behavior, (3) knowledge level, or (4) their attitudes. Adults also learn through visual, auditory, kinesthetic, and experiential learning styles. A mixed format of presenting the material may be necessary for success.

Readiness to learning is a key principle in being successful with PNE[111] because participants come with preconceived thoughts and emotions. Readiness can be identified through a frank discussion or by using the Pain Stages of Change Questionnaire.[112] Biases need to be determined in advance[111] by exploring beliefs around CRPS to break down any barriers to learning. PNE is best offered and reinforced in teachable moments rather than formal sessions. Using in-the-moment strategies throughout treatment will assist the person to applying this learning in future everyday life situations. A good example of this is using a past "bad day" strategy to plan for addressing bad days in the future, fostering self-appraisal of what worked, and exploring what could be changed.[111] Moving PNE from knowledge to application is critical to foster self-management.

Breathing and Relaxation Techniques for Control of Autonomic Nervous System Fight-or-Flight Response

Persons with CRPS frequently present with autonomic signs and symptoms, and these symptoms may be exacerbated by treatment.[1] Rehabilitation therapies have not targeted these areas in the past, often leaving these concerns to be addressed by medical management. However, with evolving literature in other areas of rehabilitation, there are opportunities to translate the self-management strategies to address autonomic symptoms to this population.

Relaxation techniques have been used to mediate pain and distress in fibromyalgia,[113] acute pain,[114] and chronic low back pain.[115] Mindfulness has also been used in the treatment of chronic pain. A 2017 systematic review by Hilton and coworkers[116] found that low-quality evidence mindfulness offers a small decrease in pain compared with

BOX 98.6   Summary of Relaxation Activities

Relaxation Activities

Imagery[117]	Picture in your mind a place that gives you joy and you feel safe. Use all your senses to explore it in your mind.	Quick and easy and needs little training to achieve a result; suitable to use during other treatment techniques for control of signs and symptoms
Autogenic (box) breathing	Breathe in for a count of 4. Hold for a count of 4. Breathe out for a count of 4. Hold empty for a count of 4.	Easy to use in any situation and needs little training to achieve a result.
Progressive relaxation[113]	Tense the muscles and notice what it feels like to have tense muscles. Then release the muscles and notice what it feels like to relax them. With practice, the patient can then be able to identify tense muscles by scanning and then consciously relaxing them.	May cause pain by firing mechanoreceptors in some individuals; requires some practice
Meditation[113]	Many forms	Requires training
Mindfulness[116]	Be attentive to the moment without judging your thoughts or feelings.	Requires training to be proficient
Respiration control	Slow the breathing rate below normal.	Requires brief training to be proficient in stressful situations
Qigong[120,119]	Use breathing and meditation during what is described as internal movement.[120]	A very portable technique but requires training

control participants. A recent uncontrolled cohort study found support for the use of breathing interventions and guided imagery for pain reduction in persons with chronic pain.[117] A wide variety of relaxation techniques exist, from those that are useful for in-the-moment control to those that require greater practice for proficiency. Box 98.6 provides an overview of options for relaxation practice.

Breathing relaxation techniques have been shown to directly impact autonomic nervous system sympathetic activity.[118] Breathing relaxation techniques decrease heart rate and perceived stress and improve performance even in times of severely increased stress such as combat training. The effect is postulated to result from sympathetic inhibition achieved by slow deep breathing; this inhibition occurs during the second half of the inspiratory process and the start of the expiration process. The opposite is true of rapid shallow breathing, which upregulates the sympathetic nervous system.[118] However, only Qigong, a form of movement and meditation, has been studied for its effects on the signs and symptoms of chronic CRPS. Wu[119] demonstrated a change in pain but no other signs and symptoms in chronic CRPS, but a second study failed to demonstrate effectiveness.[120]

SUMMARY

By definition, CRPS is a complex condition with multiple contributing factors for the development and maintenance of pain and other symptoms.[3,46] Because it is more commonly seen in the upper limb than the lower limb, hand therapists will undoubtedly encounter this clinical management challenge. Critical skills for successful management of CRPS include (1) early recognition, (2) client-centered and comprehensive evaluation and intervention, (3) application of contemporary understandings of neuroplasticity for selecting and tailoring treatments and patient education, and (4) an overarching goal of assisting patients to maximize their participation in meaningful life roles. Although rehabilitation is considered the cornerstone of CRPS management, the evidence for conservative interventions is continuing to evolve. At present, evidence-informed therapist management should consider a combination of bottom-up modalities to modulate pain and other clinical signs and symptoms and top-down approaches to support patients to participate in meaningful activities and roles within their physical and social environments. Self-management strategies are integral to achieve this goal. Communication and collaboration with other health care team members for comprehensive care of the psychological consequences of this syndrome are also keys to success.

REFERENCES

1. Birklein F, O'Neill D, Schlereth T. Complex regional pain syndrome: an optimistic perspective. *Neurology.* 2015;84(1):89–96.
2. Goebel A, Barker C, Turner-Stokes L, et al. *Complex Regional Pain Syndrome in Adults: UK Guidelines for Diagnosis , Referral and Management in Primary and Secondary Care.* London: Royal College of Physicians; 2012.
3. Harden RN, Oaklander AL, Burton AW, et al. Complex regional pain syndrome: practical diagnostic and treatment guidelines. *Pain Med.* 2013;14:180–229.
4. Perez RSGM, Zollinger PE, Dijkstra PU, et al. Evidence based guidelines for complex regional pain syndrome type 1. *BMC Neurol.* 2010;10(20). Available at: https://bmcneurol.biomedcentral.com/articles/10.1186/1471-2377-10-20. Accessed November 29, 2017.
5. Gillespie S, Cowell F, Cheung G, Brown D. Can we reduce the incidence of complex regional pain syndrome type I in distal radius fractures? The Liverpool experience. *Hand Ther.* 2016;21(4):123–130.
6. Dilek B, Ayhan C, Yagci G, Yakut Y. Effectiveness of the graded motor imagery to improve hand function in patients with distal radius fracture: a randomized controlled trial. *J Hand Ther.* 2018;31(1):2–9.e1. https://doi.org/10.1016/j.jht.2017.09.004.
7. Melzack R, Wall PD. *The Challenge of Pain.* New York: Basic Books Inc; 1983.
8. International Association for the Study of Pain. *Taxonomy.* Available at http://www.iasp-pain.org/Taxonomy. Accessed November 18, 2017.
9. Woolf CJ. Review series introduction What is this thing called pain ? *J Clin Invest.* 2010;120(11):10–12.
10. de Klaver MJM, van Rijn MA, Marinus J, Soede W, de Laat JAPM, van Hilten JJ. Hyperacusis in patients with complex regional pain syndrome related dystonia. *J Neurol Neurosurg Psychiatry.* 2007;78(12):1310–1313.
11. Winthrop Rose B, Kasch MC, Aaron DH, Stegink-Jansen CW. Does hand therapy literature incorporate the holistic view of health and function promoted by the world health organization? *J Hand Ther.* 2011;24(2):84–88.
12. Packham TL, Holly J. Mechanism-specific rehabilitation management of CRPS: proposed recommendations from evidence synthesis. *J Hand Ther.* 2018;31(2):238–249. https://doi;/10.1016/j.jht.2018.01.007
13. Harden RN, Maihofner C, Abousaad E, et al. A prospective, multisite, international validation of the complex regional pain syndrome severity score. *Pain.* 2017;158(8):1430–1436.
14. Packham T, MacDermid JC, Henry J, Bain JR. The Hamilton Inventory for complex regional pain syndrome: a cognitive debriefing study of the clinician-based component. *J Hand Ther.* 2012;25(1):97–112.
15. Cho CW, Nahm FS, Choi E, et al. Multicenter study on the asymmetry of skin temperature in complex regional pain syndrome. *Medicine (Baltimore).* 2016;95(52):e5548. Available from: http://journals.lww.com/md-journal/Fulltext/2016/12300/Multicenter_study_on_the_asymmetry_of_skin.9.aspx. Accessed November 29, 2017.
16. Packham TL, Fok D, Frederiksen K, Thabane L, Buckley N. Reliability of infrared thermometric measurements of skin temperature in the hand. *J Hand Ther.* 2012;25(4):358–362.
17. Packham T, MacDermid JC, Bain J, Buckley DN. Cold-pressor stimulated skin temperature asymmetries for the identification of CRPS. *Canadian Can J Pain.* 2018;2(1). https://doi.org/10.1080/24740527.2018.1504283
18. Packham T, MacDermid JC, Henry J, Bain J. A systematic review of psychometric evaluations of outcome assessments for complex regional pain syndrome. *Disabil Rehabil.* 2012;34(13):1059–1069.
19. Wasner G. Vasomotor disturbances in complex regional pain syndrome-A review. *Pain Med (United States).* 2010;11(8):1267–1273.
20. Burnham RS, McKinley RS, Vincent DD. Three types of skin-surface thermometers: a comparison of reliability, validity, and responsiveness. *Am J Phys Med Rehabil.* 2006;85(7):553–558.
21. Geertzen JH, Dijkstra PU, Stewart RE, Groothoff JW, Ten Duis HJ, Eisma WH. Variation in measurements of range of motion: a study in reflex sympathetic dystrophy patients. *Clin Rehabil.* 1998;12(3):254–264.
22. Geertzen JHB, Dijkstra PU, Stewart RE, Groothoff JW, Ten Duis HJ, Eisma WH. Variation in measurements of grip strength. A study in reflex sympathetic dystrophy patients. *Acta Orthop Scand Suppl.* 1998;69(279):4–11.
23. Hudak PL, Amadio P, Bombardier C, Collaborative Group UE. Development of an upper extremity outcome measure: the DASH (Disabilities of the Arm, Shoulder, and Hand). *Am J Ind Med.* 1996;29:602–608.
24. Mehta SP, MacDermid JC, Richardson J, MacIntyre NJ, Grewal R. A systematic review of the measurement properties of the patient-rated wrist evaluation. *J Orthop Sport Phys Ther.* 2015;45(4):289–298.
25. Grieve S, Perez RS, Birklein F, et al. Recommendations for a first Core Outcome Measurement set for complex regional PAin syndrome Clinical sTudies (COMPACT). *Pain.* 2017;158(6):1083–1090.
26. Packham TL, MacDermid JC, Michlovitz SL, Buckley DN. Content validity of the patient-reported Hamilton Inventory for CRPS. *Can J Occup Ther.* 2018;85(2):99–105. https://doi.org/10.1177/0008417417734562.
27. Lewis J, McCabe C. Correcting the body in mind: body perception disturbances in complex regional pain syndrome (CRPS) and rehabilitation approaches. *Pr Pain Manag.* 2010. April:60–66.
28. Turton AJ, Palmer M, Grieve S, Moss TP, Lewis J, McCabe CS. Evaluation of a prototype tool for communicating body perception disturbances in complex regional pain syndrome. *Front Hum Neurosci.* 2013;7:517.
29. Turk DC, Dworkin RH, Allen RR, et al. Core outcome domains for chronic pain clinical trials: IMMPACT recommendations. *Pain.* 2003;106(3):337–345.

30. Birklein F, Riedl B, Sieweke N, Weber M, Neundorfer B. Neurological findings in complex regional pain syndromes - analysis of 145 cases. *Acta Neurol Scand*. 2000;101(4):262–269.

31. Melzack R. The McGill Pain Questionnaire: from description to measurement. *Anesthesiology*. 2005;103(1):199–202.

32. Lovejoy TI, Turk DC, Morasco BJ. Evaluation of the psychometric properties of the revised short-form McGill Pain Questionnaire. *J Pain*. 2012;13(12):1250–1257.

33. Packham TL, Cappelleri JC, Sadosky A, Macdermid JC, Brunner F. Measurement properties of painDETECT: Rasch analysis of responses from community-dwelling adult with neuropathic pain. *BMC Neurol*. 2017;17(1):48. Available from: https://bmcneurol.biomedcentral.com/articles/10.1186/s12883-017-0825-2. Accessed March 4, 2017.

34. Freynhagen R, Baron R, Gockel U, Tölle TR. painDETECT: a new screening questionnaire to identify neuropathic components in patients with back pain. *Curr Med Res Opin*. 2006;22(10):1911–1920.

35. Lalloo C, Kumbhare D, Stinson JN, Henry JL. Pain-QuILT: clinical feasibility of a web-based visual pain assessment tool in adults with chronic pain. *J Med Internet Res*. 2014;16(5):e127. Available from: https://www.jmir.org/2014/5/e127. Accessed November 29, 2017.

36. Keller S, Bann CM, Dodd SL, Schein J, Mendoza TR, Cleeland CS. Validity of the brief pain inventory for use in documenting the outcomes of patients with noncancer pain. *Clin J Pain*. 2004;20(5):309–318.

37. Packham TL, MacDermid JC, Michlovitz S, Cup E, Van de Ven-Stevens L. Cross cultural adaptation and refinement of an English version of a Dutch patient-reported questionnaire for hand sensitivity: the Radboud evaluation of sensitivity. *J Hand Ther*. 2018;31(3):371–380. https://doi.org/10.1016/j.jht.2017.03.003.

38. Spicher C, Quintal I, Vittaz M. *Reeducation Sensitive Des Douleurs Neuropathiques*. 3rd ed. Montpellier, France: Sauramps Medical; 2015.

39. Lewis JS, Coales K, Hall J, McCabe CS. "Now you see it, now you do not": sensory-motor re-education in complex regional pain syndrome. *Hand Ther*. 2011;16(2):29–38.

40. Bennett GJ. What is spontaneous pain and who has it? *J Pain*. 2012;13(10):921–929.

41. Packham TL, Spicher CJ, MacDermid JC, Michlovitz S, Buckley DN. Somatosensory rehabilitation for allodynia in complex regional pain syndrome of the upper limb: a retrospective cohort study. *J Hand Ther*. 2018;31(1):10–19. https://doi.org/10.1016/j.jht.2017.02.007.

42. Packham TL, Spicher CJ, MacDermid JC. Research poster abstracts. Evaluating a sensitive issue: reliability and validity of allodynia measures used in the somatosensory rehabilitation method. *Can J Pain*. 2017;1(1):A158. Available from: http://www.tandfonline.com/doi/full/10.1080/24740527.2017.1329323. Accessed November 29, 2017.

43. Borchers AT, Gershwin ME. Complex regional pain syndrome: a comprehensive and critical review. *Autoimmun Rev*. 2014;13(3):242–265.

44. Grieve S, Jones L, Walsh N, McCabe C. What outcome measures are commonly used for complex regional pain syndrome clinical trials? A systematic review of the literature. *Eur J Pain*. 2016;20(3):331–340.

45. Sullivan M. *The Pain Catastrophizing Scale User Manual*. Montreal: McGill University; 2009.

46. Bean DJ, Johnson MH, Heiss-Dunlop W, Lee AC, Kydd RR. Do psychological factors influence recovery from complex regional pain syndrome type-1? A prospective study. *Pain*. 2015;156(11):2310–2318.

47. Nicholas MK. The pain self-efficacy questionnaire: taking pain into account. *Eur J Pain*. 2007;11(2):153–163.

48. Roelofs J, Van Breukelen G, Sluiter J, et al. Norming of the Tampa scale for kinesiophobia across pain diagnoses and various countries. *Pain*. 2011;152(5):1090–1095.

49. Smart KM, Wand BM, O'Connell NE. Physiotherapy for pain and disability in adults with complex regional pain syndrome (CRPS) types I and II. *Cochrane Database Syst Rev*. 2016;2016(2):CD010853. Available from: http://onlinelibrary.wiley.com/doi/10.1002/14651858.CD010853.pub2/full. Accessed November 29, 2017.

50. Beerthuizen A, Stronks DL, Huygen FJPM, Passchier J, Klein J, Spijker AVT. The association between psychological factors and the development of complex regional pain syndrome type 1 (CRPS1) - A prospective multicenter study. *Eur J Pain*. 2011;15(9):971–975.

51. Lee D-H, Noh EC, Kim YC, et al. Risk factors for suicidal ideation among patients with complex regional pain syndrome. *Psychiatry Investig*. 2014;11(1):32.

52. Speck V, Schlereth T, Birklein F. Increased prevalence of posttraumatic stress disorder in CRPS. *Eur J Pain*. 2017;21:466–473.

53. Borsook D, Edwards R, Elman I, Becerra L, Levine JD. Pain and analgesia: the value of salience circuits. *Prog Neurobiol*. 2013;104:93–105.

54. Duman I, Ozdemir A, Tan AK, Dincer K. The efficacy of manual lymphatic drainage therapy in the management of limb edema secondary to reflex sympathetic dystrophy. *Rheumatol Int*. 2009;29(7):759–763.

55. Kocic M, Lazovic M, Dimitrijevic I, Mancic D, Stankovic A. Procena terapijskog efekta lasera male snage i interferentnih struja kod bolesnika sa kompleksnim regionalnim bolnim sindromom primenom infracrvene termovizijske kamere. *Vojnosanit Pregl*. 2010;67(9):755–760.

56. Devrimsel G, Turkyilmaz AK, Yildirim M, Beyaza MS. The Effects of Whirlpool bath and Neuromuscular Electrical Stimulation on Complex Regional Pain Syndrome. *J Phys Ther Sci*. 2015;27(1):27–30.

57. Breger Stanton DE, Lazaro R, MacDermid JC. A systematic review of the effectiveness of contrast baths. *J Hand Ther*. 2009;22(1):57–70.

58. Aïm F, Klouche S, Frison A, Bauer T, Hardy P. Efficacy of vitamin C in preventing complex regional pain syndrome after wrist fracture: a systematic review and meta-analysis. *Orthop Traumatol Surg Res*. 2017;103(3):465–470.

59. Llewellyn A, McCabe CS, Hibberd Y, et al. Are you better? A multi-centre study of patient-defined recovery from complex regional pain syndrome. *Eur J Pain*. 2018;22(3):551–564. https://doi.org/10.1002/ejp.1138.

60. Forouzanfar T, Weber WE, Kemler M, van Kleef M. What is a meaningful pain reduction in patients with complex regional pain syndrome type 1? *Clin J Pain*. 2003;19(5):281–285.

61. Korpan MI, Dezu Y, Schneider B, Leitha T, Fialka-Moser V. Acupuncture in the treatment of posttraumatic pain syndrome. *Acta Orthop Belg*. 1999;65(2):197–201.

62. Ryan CG, King R, Robinson V, et al. Transcutaneous electrical nerve stimulation using an LTP-like repetitive stimulation protocol for patients with upper limb complex regional pain syndrome : a feasibility study. *Hand Ther*. 2016;22(2):52–63.

63. Raucci U, Tomasello C, Marri M, Salzano M, Gasparini A, Conicella E. Scrambler Therapy MC-5A for complex regional pain syndrome: case reports. *Pain Pract*. 2016;16(7):103–109.

64. Moseley GL, Zalucki NM, Wiech K. Tactile discrimination, but not tactile stimulation alone , reduces chronic limb pain. *Pain*. 2008;137:600–608.

65. Moseley GL, Wiech K. The effect of tactile discrimination training is enhanced when patients watch the reflected image of their unaffected limb during training. *Pain*. 2009;144(3):314–319.

66. Spicher CJ. *Handbook for Somatosensory Rehabilitation*. Montpellier, France: Sauramps Medical; 2006.

67. Goransson I, Cederlund R. A study of the effect of desensitization on hyperaesthesia in the hand and upper extremity after injury or surgery. *Hand Ther*. 2010;16(1):12–18.

68. Pleger B, Tegenthoff M, Ragert P, et al. Sensorimotor returning in complex regional pain syndrome parallels pain reduction. *Ann Neurol*. 2005;57(3):425–429.

69. Li Z, Smith BP, Smith TL, Koman LA. Diagnosis and management of complex regional pain syndrome complicating upper extremity recovery. *J Hand Ther*. 2005;18(2):270–276.

70. Szekeres M, MacDermid JC, Grewal R, Birmingham T. The short-term effects of hot packs vs therapeutic whirlpool on active wrist range of motion for patients with distal radius fracture: a randomized controlled trial. *J Hand Ther*. 2018;31(3):276–281.

71. Moseley GL. Graded motor imagery is effective for long-standing complex regional pain syndrome: a randomised controlled trial. *Pain*. 2004;108(1–2):192–198.

72. Moseley GL. Is successful rehabilitation of complex regional pain syndrome due to sustained attention to the affected limb? A randomised clinical trial. *Pain*. 2005;114(1–2):54–61.

73. Moseley GL. Graded motor imagery for pathologic pain: a randomized controlled trial. *Neurology*. 2006;67(12):2129–2134.

74. Johnson S, Hall J, Barnet S, et al. Using graded motor imagery for complex regional pain syndrome in clinical practice: failure to improve pain. *Eur J Pain*. 2012;16:550–561.

75. Moseley GL, Butler DS, Beames TB, Giles TJ. *The Graded Motor Imagery Handbook*. Adelaide, Australia: Noigroup Publications; 2012.

76. Moseley GL, Zalucki N, Birklein F, Marinus J, van Hilten JJ, Luomajoki H. Thinking about movement hurts: the effect of motor imagery on pain and swelling in people with chronic arm pain. *Arthritis Rheum*. 2008;59(5):623–631.

77. Park I, Chang W, Lee M, et al. Which motor cortical region best predicts imagined movement? *Neuroimage*. 2015;113:101–110.

78. Schmid A-C, Schwarz A, Gustin SM, Greenspan JD, Hummel FC, Birbaumer N. Pain reduction due to novel sensory-motor training in complex regional pain syndrome I – A pilot study. *Scand J Pain*. 2017;15:30–37.

79. Lewis JS, Kersten P, McPherson KM, et al. Wherever is my arm? Impaired upper limb position accuracy in complex regional pain syndrome. *Pain*. 2010;149(3):463–469.

80. Bultitude JH, Walker I, Spence C. Space-based bias of covert visual attention in complex regional pain syndrome. *Brain*. 2017;140(9):2306–2321.

81. Boesch E, Bellan V, Moseley GL, Stanton TR. The effect of bodily illusions on clinical pain. *Pain*. 2016;157(3):516–529.

82. Bultitude JH, Rafal RD. Derangement of body representation in complex regional pain syndrome: report of a case treated with mirror and prisms. *Exp Brain Res*. 2010;204:409–418.

83. Christophe L, Chabanat E, Delporte L, et al. Prisms to shift pain away: pathophysiological and therapeutic exploration of CRPS with prism adaptation. *Neural Plast*. 2016;2016:ID1694256. Available from: https://www.hindawi.com/journals/np/2016/1694256. Accessed November 29, 2017.

84. Hoffman HG, Chambers GT, Meyer WJ, et al. Virtual reality as an adjunctive non-pharmacologic analgesic for acute burn pain during medical procedures. *Ann Behav Med*. 2011;41(2):183–191.

85. Li A, Montaño Z, Chen VJ, Gold JI. Virtual reality and pain management: current trends and future directions. *Pain Manag*. 2011;1(2):147–157. https://doi.org/10.2217/pmt.10.15.

86. Laver KE, Lang B, George S, et al. Virtual reality for stroke rehabilitation. *Cochrane Syst Rev*. 2017. Issue 11. Art. No.: CD008349. Available from: http://onlinelibrary.wiley.com/doi/10.1002/14651858.CD008349.pub4/full.

87. Keizer A, Van Elburg A, Helms R, Dijkerman HC. A virtual reality full body illusion improves body image disturbance in anorexia nervosa. *PLoS One*. 2016;11(10):1–21.

88. Sato K, Fukumori S, Matsusaki T, et al. Nonimmersive virtual reality mirror visual feedback therapy and its application for the treatment of complex regional pain syndrome: an open-label pilot study. *Pain Med*. 2010;11(4):622–629.

89. Won A, Tataru C, CM C, et al. Two virtual reality pilot studies for the treatment of pediatric CRPS. *Pain Med*. 2015;16(8):1644–1647.

90. Lewis JS, Newport R, McCabe CS. Changing appearance using visual illusions improves ownership of the painful hand in complex regional pain syndrome. In: *European Pain Federation EFIC*. Vienna, Austria; 2015.

91. Mouraux D, Brassinne E, Sobczak S, et al. 3D augmented reality mirror visual feedback therapy applied to the treatment of persistent, unilateral upper extremity neuropathic pain: a preliminary study. *J Man Manip Ther*. 2017;25(3):137–143. https://doi.org/10.1080/10669817.2016.1176726.

92. Lewis J, Newport R, McCabe CS. Changing hand appearance using visual illusion modulates hand pain in longstanding complex regional pain syndrome. In: *CRPS Cork 2017*. Cork. Ireland: International Association for the Study of Pain; 2017.

93. Watson HK, Carlson L. Treatment of reflex sympathetic dystrophy of the hand with an active "stress loading" program. *J Hand Surg Am*. 1987;12(5 Pt 1):779–785.

94. Daly AE, Bialocerkowski AE. Does evidence support physiotherapy management of adult complex regional pain syndrome type I? A systematic review. *Eur J Pain*. 2009;13(4):339–353.

95. de Jong JR, Vlaeyen JWS, Onghena P, Cuypers C, Den Hollander M, Ruijgrok J. Reduction of pain-related fear in complex regional pain syndrome type I: the application of graded exposure in vivo. *Pain*. 2005;116(3):264–275.

96. de Jong JR, Vlaeyen JWS, De Gelder JM, Patijn J. Pain-related fear, perceived harmfulness of activities, and functional limitations in complex regional pain syndrome type I. *J Pain*. 2011;12(12):1209–1218.

97. den Hollander M, Goossens M, de Jong J, et al. Expose or protect? A randomized controlled trial of exposure in vivo vs pain-contingent treatment as usual in patients with complex regional pain syndrome type 1. *Pain*. 2016;157(10):2318–2329.

98. Barnhoorn KJ, van de Meent H, van Dongen RTM, et al. Pain exposure physical therapy (PEPT) compared to conventional treatment in complex regional pain syndrome type 1: a randomised controlled trial. *BMJ Open*. 2015;5(12):e008283. Available from: http://bmjopen.bmj.com/content/5/12/e008283. Accessed on November 29, 2017.

99. Van De Meent H, Oerlemans M, Bruggeman A, et al. Safety of "pain exposure" physical therapy in patients with complex regional pain syndrome type 1. *Pain*. 2011;152(6):1431–1438.

100. Oerlemans HM, Oostendorp RA, de Boo T, Goris RJ. Pain and reduced mobility in complex regional pain syndrome I: outcome of a prospective randomised controlled clinical trial of adjuvant physical therapy versus occupational therapy. *Pain*. 1999;83(1):77–83.

101. Rome L. The place of occupational therapy in rehabilitation strategies of complex regional pain syndrome: comparative study of 60 cases. *Hand Surg Rehabil*. 2016;35(5):355–362.

102. Grieve S, Adams J, McCabe C. "What I Really Needed Was the Truth". Exploring the information needs of people with complex regional pain syndrome. *Musculoskeletal Care*. 2016;14(1):15–25.

103. Nijs J, Meeus M, Cagnie B, et al. A modern neuroscience approach to chronic spinal pain: combining pain neuroscience education with cognition-targeted motor control training. *Phys Ther*. 2014;94(5):730–738.

104. Louw A, Diener I, Landers MR, Zimney K, Puentedura EJ. Three-year follow-up of a randomized controlled trial comparing preoperative neuroscience education for patients undergoing surgery for lumbar radiculopathy. *J Spine Surg*. 2016;2(4):289–298.

105. Louw A, Zimney K, Cox T, O'Hotto C, Wassinger CA. The experiences and beliefs of patients with complex regional pain syndrome: an exploratory survey study. *Chronic Illn*. 2018;14(2):104–118. https://doi.org/10.1177/1742395317709329.

106. Bruehl S, Chung OY. Psychological and behavioral aspects of complex regional pain syndrome management. *Clin J Pain*. 2006;22(5):430–437.

107. Nijs J, Paul van Wilgen C, Van Oosterwijck J, van Ittersum M, Meeus M. How to explain central sensitization to patients with "unexplained" chronic musculoskeletal pain: practice guidelines. *Man Ther*. 2011;16(5):413–418.

108. Gallagher L, McAuley J, Moseley GL. A randomized-controlled trial of using a book of metaphors to reconceptualize pain and decrease catastrophizing in people with chronic pain. *Clin J Pain*. 2013;29(1):20–25.

109. Nijs J, Torres-Cueco R, van Wilgen CP, et al. Applying modern pain neuroscience in clinical practice: criteria for the classification of central sensitization pain. *Pain Physician*. 2014;17(12):447–457.

110. Moseley GL, Butler DS. *Explain Pain Supercharged: The Clinician's Handbook*. Adelaide, Australia: Noigroup Publications; 2017.

111. Russell SS. An Overview of adult-learning processes. *Urol Nurs*. 2006;26(5):349–352.

112. Carr JL, Moffett JA, Sharp DM, Haines DR. Is the Pain Stages of Change Questionnaire (PSOCQ) a useful tool for predicting participation in a self-management programme? Further evidence of validity, on a sample of UK pain clinic patients. *BMC Musculoskelet Disord*. 2006;7:101. Available from: https://bmcmusculoskeletdisord.biomedcentral.com/articles/10.1186/1471-2474-7-101. Accessed on November 29, 2017.

113. Hassett A, Gevirtz R. Nonpharmacologic treatment for fibromyalgia: patient education, cognitive-behavioral therapy, relaxation techniques, and complementary and alternative medicine. *Rheum Dis Clin North Am*. 2009;35(2):393–407.

114. Seers K, Carroll D. Relaxation techniques for acute pain management: a systematic review. *J Adv Nurs.* 1998;27(3):466–475.

115. Carroll D, Seers K. Relaxation for the relief of chronic pain: a systematic review. *J Adv Nurs.* 1998;27(3):476–487.

116. Hilton L, Hempel S, Ewing BA, et al. Mindfulness meditation for chronic pain: systematic review and meta-analysis. *Ann Behav Med.* 2017;51(2):199–213.

117. Khan N, Khatri S. Immediate effectiveness of relaxation in management of chronic low back pain. *Rom J Phys Ther.* 2016;22(37):23–29.

118. Jerath R, Crawford MW, Barnes VA, Harden K. Self-regulation of breathing as a primary treatment for anxiety. *Appl Psychophysiol Biofeedback.* 2015;40(2):107–115.

119. Wu W. Controlled trial shows complex regional pain syndrome responding to Qigong training. *Heal Essent Inf Altern Heal Care.* 1999;5(1):5.

120. Kattapong V. Qigong for complex regional pain syndrome. *Relias.* 2001;4:56–58.

Proprioception in Hand Rehabilitation

Elisabet Hagert, Christos Karagiannopoulos, Susanne Rein

CRITICAL POINTS

- A healthy and maintained innervation of a joint is essential for both normal joint homeostasis and functioning joint proprioception. Denervation procedures should therefore only be advocated in patients with chronic joint pain who have either failed to respond to other treatments or have underlying chronic joint pathology (e.g., degenerative arthritis).

- *Cross-education* is a neural adaptation that is defined as the increase in strength or functional performance of the untrained injured limb after unilateral training of the opposite (uninjured) limb. In patients with wrist injuries (e.g., distal radius fracture), training of the uninjured hand during the period of casting or immobilization will improve the clinical outcome of the injured hand.

- The early rehabilitation phase should emphasize techniques for the control of inflammation, early active ROM, sensory reeducation, and restoration of the proprioceptive senses that control joint position and kinesthesia. Improvement in all of these areas is a prerequisite for restoring the body's unconscious or anticipatory neuromuscular function toward proper wrist joint dynamic stability and control.

- The late rehabilitation phase should emphasize strengthening techniques with proper progressions through isometric, isotonic,

and perturbation exercises that aim to restore the body's unconscious neuromuscular function toward proper joint dynamic stability. Closed- or open-chain perturbation exercises should be selected based on patient-specific rehabilitation goals.

- Scapholunate joint instability benefits from dynamic stabilization exercises that are directed toward the extensor carpi radialis longus and brevis, abductor pollicis longus, flexor carpi ulnaris, and flexor carpi radialis (FCR) muscles while avoiding the activation of the extensor carpi ulnaris (ECU). The recommended position for these exercises is with the forearm in pronation. Lunotriquetral instability requires dynamic stabilization exercises focused on the ECU and gradually progress to include both the ECU and FCR muscles. The recommended position for these exercises is with the forearm in supination.

- Wrist fractures may lead to various concomitant impairments such as excessive edema, pain, joint stiffness, sensibility deficits, and ligamentous instabilities. Therapeutic progression should follow the aforementioned early and late rehabilitation criteria. Timely identification of concomitant ligamentous instabilities is of critical importance in order to customize a rehabilitation approach toward proper joint-protective dynamic stabilization exercises.

INTRODUCTION

The experience of hands is tactile. . . . They live in the land of feeling where touch is everything. And where the mystery of touch is the bridge between nerve and soul.

Harry Martinsson, Human Hands, 1971[1]

Martinsson's poem of the human hand[1] and its intimate role in bridging the outer world with our innermost perceptions is an eloquent description of the role of proprioception in allowing us a conscious and unconscious interaction with the world around us. Although *tactility* in this poem pertains to the sensory role of the skin, this sensory function originates from fine nerve endings and mechanoreceptors located

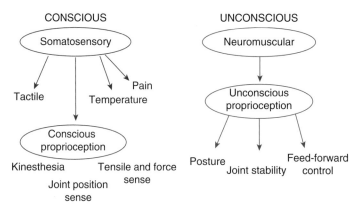

Fig. 99.1 A schematic presentation of the different proprioception senses. The somatosensory senses are conscious appreciations of proprioception, whereas the neuromuscular senses reflect the unconscious control in joint proprioception.[20]

primarily in the pulp of the fingertips. As such, the delicate sensation in our fingers becomes part of a greater sensory–motor system known as "proprioception."

The term *proprioception* is derived from Latin, *proprius*, belonging to one's own, and *-ception*, to perceive. The term was first introduced by the 1932 Nobel laureate in physiology or medicine, Sir Charles Scott Sherrington,[2] who, in 1906, defined proprioception as sensations arising in the deep areas of the body, contributing to conscious sensations ("muscle sense"), total posture ("postural equilibrium"), and segmental posture ("joint stability").

The proprioceptive sensations may be divided into unconscious neuromuscular and conscious somatosensory senses, as shown in Figure 99.1. The latter include kinesthesia, the sense of joint position and the sense of force. The neuromuscular senses include postural control, joint stability, and feed-forward control.

Conscious Proprioception Senses

The conscious joint senses—kinesthesia and joint position sense (JPS)—were first recognized by Henry Charlton Bastian in the 19th century.[3] The term *force sense* was defined by Ernst Heinrich Weber.[4] Although these senses are of great importance in our conscious appreciations of joint motion and position, thorough investigations have concluded that these senses are primarily influenced by the action of muscle spindles,[5] with some afference from skin receptors[6] and minor from joint receptors.[7] Skin receptors are primarily of importance in the kinesthesia of finger joints[8] because the muscles controlling the fingers are located at a distance, in the forearm and hand. Joint receptors are similarly thought to be of importance whenever a muscle traverses more than one major joint, thus limiting the sensitivity of the muscle spindle in detecting motion[9] or under circumstances in which input from muscle and skin is not available.[10]

In the human hand, the dependency on cutaneous sensation for finger kinesthesia and JPS is readily appreciated in patients with sensory loss after nerve injury.[11] Similarly, the kinesthesia and JPS of the wrist is primarily influenced by muscle receptors and not joint sensation. This has been recently described in studies on patients who have undergone partial wrist denervation, in whom the conscious joint senses remained intact despite the surgical removal or desensitization of the anterior or posterior interosseous nerves.[12]

Unconscious Proprioception Senses

The unconscious proprioception sense is equivalent to joint neuromuscular sense. This sense includes the anticipatory control of muscles around a joint through so-called feed-forward control, as well as the ability to unconsciously maintain joint stability and equilibrium.[13] The

neuromuscular sense is greatly influenced by spinal reflexes for immediate joint control, as well as integrations in the cerebellum for planning, anticipating, and executing joint control. Hence, although the neuromuscular control of a joint is the hardest to objectively quantify or assess, it is likely of greatest importance in maintaining joint stability.

Conscious assessment techniques (e.g., JPS) used to measure conscious proprioception cannot be applied to the unconscious proprioception sense. Rather, this sense demands techniques assessing reflex muscle activation,[14] for instance, through the use of electromyography (EMG)[15] or sensory nerve activation potential (SNAP), in determining muscle control.[16]

MECHANORECEPTORS

Joint stability relies on fine interactions of mechanical and dynamic components. Although static joint stability is constituted by osseous and ligamentous integrity, the dynamic elements of joint stability concern proprioceptive control of the compressive and directional muscular forces acting on the joint.[17] The core of joint stability is best described with the concept of "tensegrity," which entails stability through a synergy of ligament tensile and joint compressive forces.[18,19]

Ligaments are not only passive structures for stabilizing and limiting joint movement; they also have viscoelastic behavior facilitating joint homeostasis and, more important, are regarded as proprioceptive sensory organs.[17,20] The innervation of ligaments is characterized by specific sensory nerve endings, which can be classified because of their typical morphological and neurophysiological properties into four groups according to Freeman and Wyke[21] (Fig. 99.2 and Table 99.1). Sensory nerve endings, so-called mechanoreceptors, are able to detect mechanical stimuli (e.g., changes in joint position and velocity), transform them into neural excitations, and signal this information from the joint via afferent nerves and dorsal root ganglia to the spinal cord. Sensory nerve endings are found mostly close to ligament insertions into bone as well as in the epiligamentous region of ligaments,[22,23] where they can act as monitors of tension and force applied to the ligament.[24]

Ruffini Endings

Ruffini endings (type I, synonym: dendritic or spray endings) were discovered by the Italian histologist Angelo Ruffini at the end of the 19th century.[25] Ruffini endings are oval corpuscles with a thin collagenous capsule containing terminal branches of an afferent axon (see Fig. 99.2A). They capture the direction and speed of motion as slow-adapting mechanoreceptors and are therefore important for joint position and kinesthesia. They react on intraarticular and atmospheric pressure changes, the direction, the amplitude, and the speed of active and passive joint movement. They respond to axial load and tension but not to

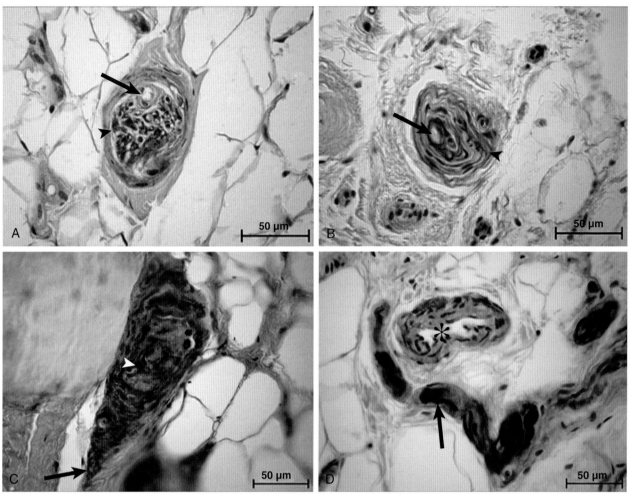

Fig. 99.2 Immunohistochemical staining of sensory nerve endings using low-affinity nerve growth factor receptor p75 (p75) (magnification ×400). **A,** A Ruffini ending characterized by p75 immunoreactive (IR) dendritic nerve endings *(arrowhead)*, a clearly visible central axon without IR *(arrow)*, and a thin and at times partial encapsulation of the corpuscle. **B,** In contrast, the Pacini corpuscle has an onion-layered p75 IR capsule *(arrowhead)* and central axon *(arrow)*. **C,** The Golgi-like ending is larger with an afferent nerve fascicle *(arrow)* coursing to the center of the corpuscle. Typically smaller corpuscles within the Golgi-like ending are seen *(arrowhead)*. **D,** Finally, free nerve endings *(arrow)* are p75 IR and often located close to vessels *(star)*.

vertical compressive joint forces, highlighting their importance in specifying joint position and rotation.[23] The Ruffini endings are the most commonly found nerve endings in the wrist and basal thumb ligaments.

Pacini Corpuscles

Although Pacini corpuscles were first described by Johannes Gottlieb Lehmann[26] in his doctoral thesis in 1741 and in the same year by the German anatomist and botanist Abraham Vater,[27] this discovery fell into oblivion for a while.[28] Only when the Italian anatomist Filippo Pacini rediscovered this corpuscle in 1835 did this corpuscle and its synonym, Vater-Pacini-corpuscles, also appear in literature.[29] Pacini corpuscles, type II, have an elongated, conical body with a thick lamellar capsule and a central afferent nerve ending running from the base to the tip (see Fig. 99.2B). These mechanoreceptors adapt very fast, perceiving vibrations and de- and acceleration of joints. They are even able to detect mechanical disturbances at a certain distance.[30] These receptors are nonreactive in immobile joints. Contrary to Ruffini endings, Pacini corpuscles are sensitive to compressive forces but not to tensile forces.[23]

Golgi-like Endings

The Golgi-like endings, type III, are named after the Italian anatomist and Nobel laureate for physiology or medicine (1906) Camillo Golgi,[31] who initially discovered this sensory nerve endings as the "Golgi tendon organ" in the myotendinous junction in 1878. To express that ligaments are not containing the Golgi tendon organ of the myotendinous junction, these ligamentous receptors are described as "Golgi-like endings."[23,32] They are the largest sensory end organs in the ligamentous tissue. They consist of a thin fusiform capsule enclosing many tightly branching terminal nerve filaments of a large axon (see Fig. 99.2C). These slowly adapting mechanoreceptors respond to extreme joint movement.[23]

Free Nerve Endings

Free nerve endings, type IV, have no fibrous capsule (see Fig. 99.2D). These are specific nociceptors that do not adapt and detect noxious mechanical, chemical, or inflammatory stimuli.[32]

Unclassifiable Corpuscles

Corpuscles that cannot be classified as Ruffini, Pacini, Golgi-like endings, or free nerve endings are regarded as unclassifiable corpuscles, type V, according to Hagert.[33]

According to the classification of Erlanger and Gasser (1937) as well as Lloyd and Hunt for afferent and efferent nerve fibers (Table 99.2), the afferents of Ruffini endings and Pacini corpuscles are myelinated

TABLE 99.1 Classification of Mechanoreceptors in Ligaments

Type	Corpuscles	Morphology	Neurophysiology	Joint Function
I	Ruffini ending	Coil shaped, partial encapsulation, arborizing nerve branches with bulbous terminals, 50–120 μm	Slowly adapting Low threshold	Static joint position changes in velocity and amplitude
II	Pacini corpuscle	Rounded, ovular corpuscle, thick lamellar or onion-like capsule, 20–50 μm	Rapidly adapting Low threshold	Joint acceleration and deceleration
III	Golgi-like ending	Large, spherical, partial encapsulation groups of arborizing and terminal nerve endings >150 μm	Rapidly adapting High threshold	Extreme ranges of joint motion
IV	Free nerve ending	Various appearances, often close to blood vessels	A-δ: fast C fibers: slow	Noxious, chemical, nociceptive, inflammatory
V	Unclassifiable	Variable in size, appearance, and degree of encapsulation	Unknown	Unknown

Based on Freeman MA, Wyke B. The innervation of the knee joint. An anatomical and histological study in the cat. *J Anat.* Jun 1967;101:505-532. Modified by Hagert. *Outlining the Morphology and Function of the Various Sensory Nerve Endings Found in the Human Hand.* Reprinted from Hagert E. *Wrist Ligaments—Innervation Patterns and Ligamento-Muscular Reflexes.* PhD thesis, Karolinska Institutet, 2008, p. 24.

TABLE 99.2 Two Classification Systems of the Nerve Fiber Groups[a]

Diameter (μm)	Conduction Velocity (m/sec)	Myelin Sheath	ERLANGER AND GASSER[33a]		LLOYD[33b] AND HUNT[33c]	
			Fiber Type	Afference or Efference	Fiber Type	Afference
10–20	60–120	Yes (thick)	A-α	α-Motoneuron skeletal muscle (extrafusal)	I a	Muscle spindle
					I b	Golgi-tendon organ
7–15	40–90	Yes	A-β		II	Ruffini, Pacini, Golgi-like endings
4–8	20–50	Yes	A-γ	γ-Motoneuron Skeletal muscle (intrafusal)		
2–5	10–30	Yes (thin)	A-δ		III	Free nerve endings
1–3	5–20	Yes (thin)	B	Sympathetic preganglionic		
0.5–1.5	0.5–2.0	No	C	Sympathetic postganglionic	IV	Free nerve endings

[a]According to Erlanger and Gasser as well as Lloyd and Hunt. The first system, described by Erlanger and Gasser, applies to both, sensory (afferent), and motor (efferent) nerve fibers, whereas the second system, described by Lloyd and Hunt, applies only to sensory (afferent) nerve fibers.

group II and Aβ fibers with nerve conduction velocities of 36 to 72 m/sec. Golgi-like endings of the periarticular tissue belong to group II, whereas the originally described Golgi tendon organ of the myotendinous junction are Ib fibers. The afferents of free nerve endings are either thin myelinated group III and Aδ fibers with a conduction velocity between 4 to 36 m/sec or unmyelinated group IV and C fibers with conduction velocity of 0.4 to 2 m/sec.[34,35]

INNERVATION OF JOINTS IN THE HUMAN HAND

Wrist

The innervation of wrist ligaments has been intensively studied.[32,36] Its pattern was found to vary distinctly, with a pronounced innervation in the dorsal ligaments and in the entire scapholunate interosseous ligament (SLIL),[36] an intermediate innervation in the volar triquetral ligaments, and only limited to occasional innervation of the volar radial ligaments.[32,37] Based on this, the dorsal ligaments and the SLIL are considered sensory important ligaments in wrist proprioception, with the Ruffini ending being the predominant mechanoreceptor type.

Free nerve endings are the predominant receptor type in the triangular fibrocartilage complex (TFCC) with its seven different parts, namely, the subsheath of the extensor carpi ulnaris tendon sheath, the ulnocarpal meniscoid, the articular disk, as well as the dorsal and volar radioulnar, ulnolunate, and ulnotriquetral ligaments.[38,39] The articular disk

and ulnolunate ligament are rarely innervated, indicating a primarily mechanical function. Both radioulnar ligaments are richly innervated by all types of sensory nerve endings, and the volar radioulnar ligament has the highest amount of Ruffini endings, mediating JPS (see Fig. 99.2A). The ulnotriquetral ligament, the subsheath of the extensor carpi ulnaris tendon sheath, and the ulnocarpal meniscoid have all types of sensory nerve endings and therefore distinct proprioceptive qualities.[39]

Finger Joints

Ruffini endings and Pacini corpuscles have been identified in the distal interphalangeal joint (DIP), with a greater density of innervation in the proximal region compared with midsubstance/distal region.[40] In addition, Ruffini endings have been mainly found in the proximal volar plate, where they are particularly able to monitor joint position changes. Pacini corpuscles, on the other hand, were primarily seen in association with the C1 pulley, suggesting that they sense acceleration and deceleration of the finger.[40] The density of free nerve endings and Pacini corpuscles was consistently greater in palmar areas than in dorsal or lateral parts of the proximal interphalangeal (PIP) and metacarpophalangeal joint capsules.[41]

Basal Thumb Joint

The dorsal ligaments of the basal thumb (carpometacarpal [CMC]-1) joint have an abundance of sensory nerve endings mainly close to the metacarpal insertion, whereas the ulnar collateral show little and the anterior oblique ligament no innervation. As with the wrist ligaments, Ruffini endings are the predominant receptor type in the CMC-1, indicating a function in providing information regarding thumb position and velocity.[22] In contrast, unclassifiable corpuscles predominate in CMC-1 joint osteoarthritis, suggesting an alteration of the mechanoreceptor population and distribution that accompanies the development of osteoarthritis.[42]

SUPRASPINAL CONTROL

The unconscious and conscious proprioceptive information is mediated by afferent nerve fibers to the spinal cord (Fig. 99.3). The spinal ganglion cells of the conscious proprioception, together with their epicritic afferents, form the posterior funiculus, which extends to the gracilis and cuneatus nuclei in the medulla oblongata. There is the synapse to the second neuron, which crosses to the contralateral side and ends as the medial lemniscus in the ventral posterolateral nucleus of the thalamus. The axons of the third neuron in the thalamus project to the primary somatosensory cortex.

The unconscious proprioceptive information of the lower half of the body is transmitted via the anterior and posterior spinocerebellar tractus, and those of the upper half of the body are transmitted via the cuneocerebellar fibers to the cerebellum. There are also connections to the thalamus and the cortex and thus to the conscious perception of proprioception.[43] Proprioceptive information is processed on three hierarchically arranged levels of the spinal cord, brainstem, and motor cortex.[44]

The spinal cord integrates proprioceptive information from all parts of the body.[45] Neural connections between proprioceptors and motor neurons are flexibly connected via a network of interneurons,[46] which are responsible for the intrinsic functions of the spinal cord, and are called the propriospinal apparatus.[35] Reflexes are regenerated at the level of the spinal cord (e.g., direct automatic motor responses to proprioceptive afferents). The motor neurons in the anterior horn of the spinal cord are controlled via interneurons by ascending and descending influences.[44] The convergence results in a summation of excitatory and inhibitory influences.[35]

The brainstem integrates proprioceptive, vestibular, and visual information. The centers of the brainstem influence the network of motor neurons and interneurons via descending pathways. The brainstem is thus not only a stopover from the cortex to the spinal cord but also has a direct influence on the postural control and the performance of automated and stereotyped movements (see Fig. 99.3).[45]

Cortical projections of proprioceptive afferents lead to conscious perception of joint position, kinesthesia, and strength.[47] Complex voluntary movements are initiated and controlled in the somatotopically arranged areas of the motor cortex. The descending corticospinalis tractus directly influences the activity of motor neurons and thus controls motor functions. The cortex indirectly influences the motor neurons via the brainstem.

In addition to these major centers of motor control, the cerebellum and basal ganglia are also involved in motor control. The spinocerebellum receives unconscious proprioceptive information from the spinocerebellar tract, such as extremity position, joint angle, and muscle tension and length. This uses the cerebellum along with other sensory and central information for the modification of motor activities.[45] With the help of proprioceptive information, the cerebellum calculates the body's position in space and establishes maintenance of postural control as well as planning and performing movements.[43] Furthermore, the sensory afferents to the spinocerebellum, in the sense of a feedback mechanism, contribute to the regulation of muscle tone

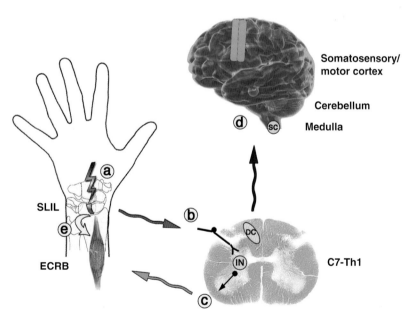

Fig. 99.3 The principles of wrist proprioceptive pathways. Stimuli elicited by mechanoreceptors in intraarticular ligaments *(a)* convey afferent information to the dorsal horn of the spinal cord *(b)*, where a fast monosynaptic effect on the α-motoneuron takes place *(c)* for immediate control of the muscles around the wrist joint. The afferent information is, furthermore, conveyed to the cerebellum and cortex *(d)* for a higher supraspinal control of wrist stability. Some research also advocated the presence of local fusiform reflexes, where afferent information form mechanoreceptors is believed to stimulate the γ-motoneurons directly through local reflex arcs *(e)*. *DC,* Dorsal column of spinal cord; *ECRB,* extensor carpi radialis brevis; *IN,* interneuron; *SC,* spinocerebellar pathway; *SLIL,* scapholunate interosseous ligament. (Reprinted from Hagert E *Wrist Ligaments—Innervation Patterns and Ligamento-Muscular Reflexes.* PhD thesis, Karolinska Institutet, 2008, p.15.[33])

via the regulation of γ-motoneurons.[45] The basal ganglia are connected with afferents and efferents via the thalamus to the cortex and participate in the tuning of higher order cognitive motor processes. They also influence spinal motor function via descending connections to the brainstem.[43,48]

LIGAMENTOMUSCULAR REFLEXES

Background

According to Freeman and Wyke's[49] reflex theory, a polysynaptic reflex arc originates from the ligamentous and capsular mechanoreceptors. This influences the activity of the joint-stabilizing musculature via γ-motoneurons and thus coordinates the muscle tone to maintain joint stability in rest position and movement.[50] Solomonow[20] supports the theory that excitatory and inhibitory reflex arcs originating from the ligamentous receptors modulate the activity of joint-stabilizing muscles. These finely tuned interactions between ligamentous structures and muscles protect the ligaments from overload and potential damage.

In 1958, Ivar Palmer was the first to demonstrate the existence of reflexes between the medial collateral ligament of the knee and its periarticular muscles acting on that joint.[51] Since then, the existence of such ligamentomuscular reflexes has been studied by stimulation of ligaments at the knee joint,[52] ankle joint,[53] shoulder joint,[54] wrist,[15] and CMC-1.[55] Different opinions exist in literature about the connection and the importance of ligamentomuscular reflex arcs. Some studies observed muscular responses with very short latencies (between 20 and 40 msec), postulating a direct influence of the joint stabilizing muscles via α-motoneurons as a protective reflex.[15,56] However, the majority of studies on this topic yielded significantly longer latencies (between 60 and 500 msec) for muscular responses after ligamentous or capsular stimulation of different joints, suggesting a polysynaptic reflex.[52,54,57] The different latencies for different joints depend on the distance to the spinal cord.[56]

The current state of research suggests an indirect regulation of muscle activity via γ-motoneurons rather than a direct monosynaptic ligamentomuscular reflex via α-motoneurons.[48,58] Thus, ligamentous mechanoreceptors, along with other proprioceptive afferents and descending neuronal influences, activate γ motoneurons of the spinal cord, which affect the sensitivity of muscle spindles (see Fig. 99.3). These in turn modulate the excitability of α-motoneurons and thus muscle stiffness via autogenous and heterogeneous reflex arcs.[48] In turn, increasing muscle stiffness results in functional enhanced joint stability.[48,59]

In addition, ligamentous and capsular mechanoreceptors play an important role in supraspinal sensorimotor control of dynamic joint stability. An animal study has shown that impairment of these proprioceptive afferents leads to changes in voluntary motor function and even in the processing of visual and vestibular influences on postural control.[49] In humans, an influence of ligamentous receptors on higher motor centers is assumed.[48,53]

Wrist Reflexes

Studies on in vivo wrist joint proprioception using EMG[15] and SNAP[60] have shown that the wrist has distinct patterns of reflex activation following disturbance of the SLIL. Within 20 msec of joint perturbation, antagonist muscles are activated, indicating fast joint protective reflexes through monosynaptic spinal control.[15] Deafferentation of the SLIL by anesthetizing the posterior interosseous nerve (PIN) results in significant loss of these joint protective reflexes.[61] Similarly, sectioning of the SLIL significantly reduces the afferent signals through primarily the median and radial nerves.[60] These findings show that denervation of the anterior interosseous nerve (AIN), PIN, or both, although

resulting in no alteration of conscious wrist proprioception,[12,62] has adverse effects on the unconscious neuromuscular control of the wrist joint. Hence, denervation procedures should only be carefully advocated in wrists in which the proprioceptive function may already be considered inferior (e.g., advanced wrist osteoarthritis) and not as a routine in minor procedures (e.g., removal of ganglion cysts) because these patients may develop disturbances in their joint proprioceptive functions.

PROPRIOCEPTION REHABILITATION: THEORY AND PRACTICE

Background

Historically, a dearth of research evidence has limited the rehabilitation of wrist and hand proprioception deficits to only certain methods that have derived from basic science knowledge and clinical research from other joints such as the shoulder,[63] knee,[64] and ankle.[65] Because recent research initiatives have led to the discovery that significant sensorimotor control impairment prevails for up to 3 months after wrist trauma,[66,67] strong clinical interest has emerged on the implementation of innovative rehabilitation paradigms toward wrist and hand proprioceptive deficits.[68] Furthermore, emerging evidence has coined the importance of timely implementation of sensorimotor control training strategies after injury to restore proper conscious and unconscious proprioceptive senses of the upper extremity as a whole.[48]

It has been recognized that one of the initial therapy objectives should be to enhance the body's joint position and motion senses.[14,69] Consequently, training methods should advance into eliciting centrally driven involuntary neuromuscular control responses toward optimal functional recovery.[14] This section's aim is to provide an evidence-based guideline, outlining the most current proprioceptive rehabilitation principles and strategies after common wrist trauma.

Both high- and low-energy trauma pathomechanics can lead to various types of wrist fractures[70] and ligamentous injuries,[71] causing significant physical and functional impairments.[72] Specifically, the initial 3-month period after these injuries has been determined to be critical for both the recovery of physical impairments (i.e., wrist pain, edema, sensibility, active range of motion [ROM], muscle strength, and proprioception)[66,73] and restoration of function.[73] Distal radius fracture (DRF) is considered the most common type of wrist trauma, which leads to significant wrist sensorimotor control impairment and functional disablement during this period.[73] Wrist sensorimotor control impairment after DRFs has been linked to clinically meaningful deficits of pain, sensibility, joint positions sense, muscle strength, and muscle endurance.[66] The exact cause of wrist sensorimotor control deficit after DRF has yet to be clearly determined. A plethora of potential etiologic factors such as pain, acute edema, and injury to peripheral neuroreceptors after disruptive trauma may be legitimate primary causes of sensorimotor control impairment that necessitate further investigation.[69] Central neuroplastic brain changes caused by chronic pain[74] have been proposed as a possible mechanism of wrist JPS impairment after DRF.[66,67] Similarly, capsuloligamentous injury at the wrist joint may lead to significant sensorimotor control impairment because it disrupts vital rapid ligament-to-muscle proprioceptive reflex pathways that mediate proper wrist neuromuscular control.[75] Thus, a comprehensive rehabilitation program (Table 99.3) that focuses on restoring proper function of both the wrist conscious and unconscious proprioceptive pathways is critical for improving the aforementioned physical impairments and reestablishing proper wrist joint dynamic control.

TABLE 99.3 Rehabilitation Strategies and Treatment Plan in Wrist Proprioception Reeducation

Stages of Proprioception Rehabilitation	Rehabilitation Plan	Purpose	Techniques	Assessment of Outcome
1	Basic rehabilitation	Edema and pain control, promote motion	Basic hand therapy techniques	VAS, degree of joint motion (ROM)
2	Proprioception awareness	Promote conscious joint control	Mirror therapy	VAS and ROM
3	Joint position sense	Ability to replicate a predetermined joint angle	Blinded passive and active reproduction of joint angle	Accuracy of joint motion, measured with goniometer or exercise machine
4	Kinesthesia (TTDPM)	Ability to sense joint motion without audiovisual cues	Motion detection using an exercise machine (preferable) or manual passive motion	Degree of joint angle at which motion was sensed, measured with goniometer or exercise machine
5	Conscious neuromuscular rehabilitation	Strengthening of specific muscles to enhance joint stability	Isometric training Eccentric training Isokinetic training Coactivation	Evaluation of specific muscle strength, wrist stability during coactivations, joint stability during isometric exercises
6	Unconscious neuromuscular rehabilitation	Reactive muscle activation	Powerball exercises Plyometric training	Muscle activation patterns using EMG

EMG, Electromyography; *ROM,* range of motion; *TTDPM,* threshold to detection of passive motion; *VAS,* visual analogue scale.
Reprinted with permission from Hagert E. Proprioception of the wrist joint: a review of current concepts and possible implications on the rehabilitation of the wrist. *J Hand Ther.* 2010;23:2-17.

The Conscious Proprioception Senses

The conscious proprioception senses are the easiest to comprehend, quantify, and appreciate and are therefore frequently used in proprioception reeducation strategies. These include JPS, kinesthesia, and tensile and force sensation.[14]

Joint position sense is defined as the ability to accurately reproduce a specific joint angle, ideally without visual or auditory aid. *Kinesthesia,* on the other hand, is the ability to sense the motion of the joint, and is frequently measured as the smallest change in joint angle needed to elicit a conscious awareness of joint motion, as related to time ($\Delta°$/sec).[48] *Tensile and force sensation* is the ability to consciously appreciate the change in joint torque and the force involved in torque generation. Principally, this relates to the proprioception generated from muscle spindles and Golgi-tendon organs in muscle tendons rather than joint proprioception per se.

It is important, however, to also recognize that other somatosensory modalities can contribute to the conscious sensation of a joint. These include tactile, nociceptive, and vibratory senses, which may all enhance or mimic the sensation of joint motion. Vibrations applied over tendons have, for instance, been shown to elicit illusory joint motions, and cutaneous mechanoreceptors have similarly been shown to be of importance in the kinesthesia of finger joints.[8]

Joint Position Sense and Kinesthesia

The two conscious modalities of proprioception, JPS and kinesthesia, are well suited for the earliest stages of proprioception reeducation because they can be used in all stages of wrist rehabilitation without the risk of inducing harm.[63] Both JPS and kinesthesia can be tested using a number of tools, from a standard manual goniometer to more advanced testing equipment, such an Upper Limb Exerciser (Biometrics Ltd, Ladysmith, VA) or a Biodex Dynamometer (Biodex Medical Systems Inc, Shirley, NY) for isokinetic exercises. The important thing to realize is that any hand therapist with access to a goniometer can assess proprioception and provide proprioception reeducation.

Joint position sense is, as mentioned earlier, the ability to accurately replicate a given joint angle. This can be done either passively

or actively, with visual cues or blinded. Passive JPS is when the therapist moves the wrist and the patient signals when the target position is reached. Active JPS is when the patient moves the wrist actively to the predetermined target position. It is advisable to start JPS training with visual cues and progress to blindfolded exercises when the patient feels comfortable in the experimental setting. The results of JPS exercises are easily assessed using a goniometer to determine the accuracy of reproducing a specific joint angle.

Kinesthesia is defined as the ability to sense changes in joint angle and should thus be recorded as the degree of joint motion needed before the patient is consciously aware of the wrist being moved, so-called *threshold to detection of passive motion* (TTDPM). The difficulty in assessing TTDPM is the large influence of other sensory modalities in appreciating joint motion. Hence, to adequately test kinesthesia, all auditory and visual cues should be removed.

Ultimately, wrist proprioceptive rehabilitation should progress through an early and late phase (Fig. 99.4), aiming to gradually enhance functional recovery after a disruptive osseous or ligamentous wrist or hand injury.[14,69]

EARLY REHABILITATION PHASE (HAGERT STAGES 1–4)

Basic Hand Therapy: Pain Control

Depending on injury type, severity level, and comorbidity incidence (e.g., nerve injury, increased edema, hand and wrist stiffness, fracture nonunions or malunions),[76] the early rehabilitation phase should encompass methods directed toward the management of various physical impairments. This should include inflammation control (i.e., pain, edema, and sensibility loss) and active ROM and conscious proprioception (i.e., JPS and kinesthesia) restoration.[14,69] This early phase is clinically applicable to acute type of injuries (e.g., DRFs, carpal bone fractures, extrinsic or intrinsic wrist ligamentous disruption). Thus, its primary aim is to allow for proper physiologic tissue healing time while preventing functional overload during the initial 8 weeks after injury.

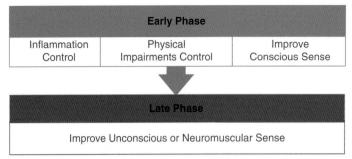

Fig. 99.4 Proprioceptive rehabilitation classification system with early and late phases. (From Karagiannopoulos C, Michlovitz S. Rehabilitation strategies for wrist sensorimotor control impairment: from theory to practice. *J Hand Ther.* 2016;29:154-165.)

During this phase, proper inflammation control improves localized edema and pain, enabling peripheral wrist receptors to produce sensory feedback more effectively for conscious proprioception.[75] Efficacious posttraumatic pain management methods would also reverse the possible development of central neuroplastic changes within sensorimotor cortex centers that have been associated with possible JPS and kinesthesia deficits.[77,78] Emphasis on early techniques of active ROM, sensory reeducation, and submaximal isometrics could restore vital conscious sensorimotor pathways and lead to an improved sense of wrist joint position and motion.[14]

Proprioception Awareness

Depending on symptom presentation and pain severity, effective pain control during the early phase can be achieved via various therapeutic interventions. These interventions may include physical and thermal modalities (e.g., cold pack, moist heat, and electrical stimulation)[79]; patient education for proper body mechanics to reduce wrist joint overloading[80]; activity modifications to prevent reinjury[81]; and regional desensitization methods of the wrist and the hand, incorporating closed-chain active range of motion (AROM) techniques[82] as well as various forms of tactile and vibration stimuli[83] that enhance the injured body area receptors' ability to elicit normal proprioceptive sensory feedback for restoration of the normal sense of joint motion and position. An example of an effective closed chain wrist AROM technique is rolling a weighted ball forward or back on a table (Fig. 99.5). This is a safe stress-loading technique, which improves recognition of joint motion and position, enhances active wrist flexion and extension active motions, and improves pain.[84] The patient can slowly advance this exercise by moving the wrist toward the end range of its physiological AROM. This method can also be progressed to wall towel wipes, promoting functional AROM improvements of the whole upper extremity kinetic chain (Fig. 99.6). Examples of therapeutic activities that use tactile or vibration stimuli for wrist and hand desensitization include an upper extremity whirlpool; manual or instrument assisted soft tissue mobilization techniques; grasping or manipulating rice, marbles, and small objects of different textures; and the application of a low-frequency vibration stimulus with a mini vibrator over hypersensitive skin or scar regions. Tactile stimulation and vibration techniques are used to enhance wrist and hand kinesthetic and JPS perception by improving the sensory function of cutaneous and musculotendinous receptors (i.e., better muscle spindle activation),[14] potentially leading to improved dexterity and wrist joint neuromuscular control for functional activities.

Implementing early wrist AROM methods is clinically important for developing proper proprioceptive awareness and allowing for faster return to function.[85] Early functional ROM exercises restore proper awareness for joint position and kinetic control that is required for a

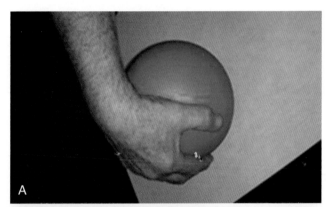

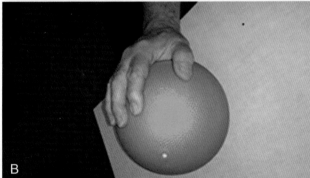

Fig. 99.5 A and **B,** Closed-chain active range of motion exercise via rolling a ball on a table.

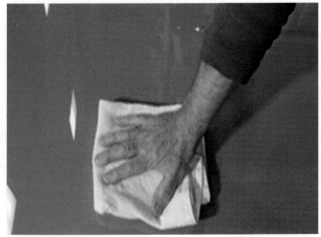

Fig. 99.6 Wall towel slides for range of motion and tactile sensory reeducation.

multitude of body functions.[14] This could become more urgent when the nondominant side is involved. Often, the nondominant side is perceived as less important by patients, thus requiring a longer rehabilitation time for functional recovery after wrist trauma.[86] Examples of wrist and hand ROM functional tasks that a patient can readily incorporate in a daily home program consist of grasping a light cylindrical stick, turning a small hammer, grasping and placing marbles in a bucket, rolling a ball on a table, simulating dart-throwing motion (DTM) with the wrist, turning book pages, turning a bottle cap, wiping a table or a wall with a towel, and practicing typing and writing skills. All of these functional exercises promote active wrist ROM by training both conscious and unconscious proprioceptive pathways at the wrist and hand. Performance of these therapeutic activities can produce an influx of visual and tactile sensory feedback from cutaneous and muscle peripheral receptors, which enhance wrist joint position and motion awareness. Improved conscious proprioception senses is considered a precursor for retraining proper neuromuscular joint function, which relies on rapid feed-forward control reflexes.[14] Restoring neuromuscular joint control leads to proper anticipatory wrist motor patterns, which are required to produce precise wrist AROM during function.[75]

Early functional wrist ROM exercises could also be used for the contralateral uninjured side during periods of protection or immobilization of the injured side. This exercise approach is supported by current research evidence, which has pointed to a possible clinical benefit of exercising the noninvolved side in an effort to induce motor control gains at the injured side.[87] Contralateral wrist exercises could produce up to a 31% increase of neuromuscular control and strength of the immobilized wrist.[87] Similar contralateral strengthening effects have been reported at the lower extremity after gastrocnemius strengthening.[88] Although the neurophysiologic mechanism of this outcome is not fully understood, it is attributed to a central cross-over training effect in the brain. Excitation of the contralateral primary sensorimotor cortex produces a central laterality effect that enhances the sensorimotor control function of the injured side.[87,88]

Mirror Therapy

Mirror therapy can also contribute to a patient's early sensory reeducation process via a similar cross-over training effect, deriving from visual stimuli to the brain.[14,89] Mirror therapy has been advocated as an effective intervention for pain control and functional ROM gains after wrist trauma,[90] hemiplegia,[91] and phantom limb pain after amputations.[92] Ultimately, mirror therapy could enhance conscious wrist proprioception through illusionary visual feedback from the reflected image of the uninjured side, which is placed in front of the mirror.[14] Visual stimulation from the uninjured arm is believed to promote cortical reorganization, leading to decreased pain and improved cortical representation of the injured side.[89] Mirror therapy exercises may range from simple wrist AROM to more functional tasks of grasping or manipulating objects (Fig. 99.7). (For more information, refer to Chapter 100 on graded motor imagery.)

Joint Position Sense

Early training of wrist JPS can be enhanced by manual training techniques.[14] One manual method entails passive placement of the involved wrist in specific wrist positions (flexion, neutral, or extension angles) with the patient's eyes closed. The patient is to memorize each position for 3 seconds and then actively move away from that position. The patient is then asked to reproduce the memorized position as accurately as possible with the eyes closed.[69] A wrist universal goniometer can be used to initially guide wrist passive positioning and assess the patient's accuracy to reproduce the memorized angle (Fig. 99.8). This exercise

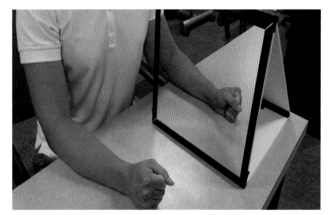

Fig. 99.7 Mirror therapy exercise with hand active range of motion.

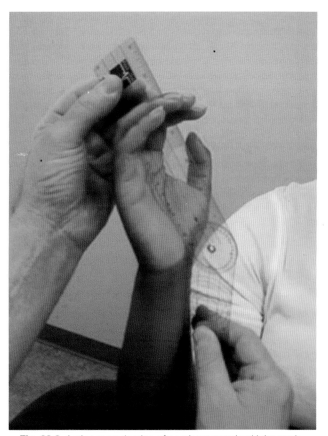

Fig. 99.8 Active reproduction of a wrist memorized joint angle.

can also incorporate the uninvolved side, requiring the patient to perform contralateral angle matching. In this case, passive wrist positioning and memorization takes place at the noninvolved side followed by reproduction of the memorized wrist position by the involved or ipsilateral wrist.[93] Another manual method to enhance early wrist JPS and neuromuscular joint dynamic control is the use of submaximal muscle isometrics at various wrist joint positions.[14] This type of activity should only be performed in nonprovocative wrist positions within the available ROM when proper tissue healing has been achieved after wrist trauma. The amount of submaximum force and the number of repetitions should be determined based on patient's tolerance and symptoms.[69] Controlled nonpainful muscle effort is believed to elicit sensory input from muscle receptors (i.e., muscle spindles and Golgi tendon organs) that are responsible for mediating important kinesthetic and JPS wrist senses.[94]

As previously stated, isometric muscle exercises can also be applied at the noninjured wrist, inducing an important central cross-education effect and potentially increase muscle recruitment at the injured wrist.[87] The neurophysiologic basis of these manual rehabilitation methods can only be supported by benchmark scientific knowledge and expert opinions.[95] Further research is needed to determine their clinical efficacy.

LATE REHABILITATION PHASE (HAGERT STAGES 5 AND 6)

The late sensorimotor control rehabilitation phase should be initiated after the initial 8 weeks or when adequate healing of the implicated wrist osseous or ligamentous tissues has been reached.[69] Depending on the type of intervention, tissue quality, and surgeon's preference, this phase may be delayed after surgical repairs (e.g., complex wrist fractures or ligament injury) that require longer postoperative protection periods. In such cases, this strengthening phase can be postponed for an additional 2 to 4 weeks, depending on the healing requirements of the injured tissue and recovery of tensile strength.[96] This late phase aims to restore the body's unconscious or anticipatory neuromuscular function required for proper wrist joint dynamic stability and control. Thus, it mainly encompasses muscle strengthening techniques, intending to restore proper reactive motor control patterns that enhance essential wrist synergistic and reciprocal muscle activation patterns that are needed for proper upper extremity function.[14]

Conscious Neuromuscular Control

During this phase, advanced isometric and isotonic strengthening exercises are initiated to instill proper wrist conscious and unconscious neuromuscular control. These strengthening exercises should be directed at selected wrist agonist and antagonist muscle groups that regulate wrist joint dynamic control during upper extremity activity.[97] Isometric exercises should precede isotonic exercises. Contrary to the early phase, isometric exercises are now applied with optimum force based on a patient's muscle strength and endurance deficits.[69] Their primary purpose is to safely enhance greater joint dynamic stability and neuromuscular recruitment at different training-specific wrist angles.[98] Angle-specific joint control enhances the patient's conscious awareness of joint position and motion during function. As adequate dynamic joint-specific motor control is established, isotonic (i.e., concentric and eccentric contraction) resistance exercises are then applied to improve joint neuromuscular control throughout the patient's available wrist ROM. Besides improving muscle strength, isotonic exercises also restore conscious and unconscious central proprioceptive neuropathways (i.e., sensory feedback input and descending feed-forward motor control) that regulate normal wrist joint reciprocal and recurrent neuromuscular performance during functional tasks.[14]

Wrist isotonic exercises typically encompass free hand weight or elastic band resistance[99] that can be readily applied both in a clinical setting and home exercise programs.[100] Resisted wrist flexion and extension with handheld free-weight exercises isolate the wrist flexor and extensor groups while recruiting the hand digital flexor muscles for concurrent grasp control.[101] The aim of these exercises is to improve wrist reciprocal neuromuscular control. Resisted wrist ulnar and radial deviation (RD) can also be performed with the elbow extended in a standing position.[99] These exercises enhance the neuromuscular function of the wrist ulnar and radial deviator muscle groups that depend on recurrent motor recruitment patterns.[14] Isometric and isotonic exercise intensity and duration parameters should be adjusted based on each individual patient's muscle strength and endurance levels after an injury. Gradual increase of resistance should aim to improve muscle neuromuscular recruitment and strength, and gradual increase in the

duration of isometric contraction and the number of isotonic repetitions should aim to improve muscle endurance.[102] Decreased muscle endurance during prolonged hand-grip isometric efforts has been linked to significant wrist JPS and neuromuscular control impairments after DRF.[66] Increased postexercise fatigue has also been found to induce significant elbow JPS deficit among healthy individuals.[103] Further research is needed to fully determine the adverse effects of muscle fatigue on wrist sensorimotor control.

Unconscious Neuromuscular Control

The late rehabilitation phase is finally advanced to perturbation or reactive exercises that are purported to improve the sensorimotor control, unconscious or anticipatory, of the involved limb.[14] Acquiring adequate conscious neuromuscular control for all the implicated muscles is an important prerequisite before initiating these types of exercises. The ultimate goal of these exercises is to improve global joint stability for the whole upper extremity because it represents a continuous kinetic-chain unit.[69] This type of exercise depends on the activation of complex neurophysiological sensorimotor control pathways that entail the excitation of rapid ligament-to-muscle joint reflexes that are regulated by the spinal cord as well as automatic descending feedback input, which is prestored, generated, and centrally regulated by cortical and cerebellar centers.[14] Perturbation exercises require the rapid activation or co-contraction of multiple muscle groups that need to optimally function synergistically to produce global dynamic joint stability.[104] These exercises are reserved for the final proprioception rehabilitation stages[14,69] because they embody the highest level of functional training before allowing a patient to return to full unrestricted activity.

Upper extremity perturbation exercises can be performed via both closed- and open-kinetic chain strategies that use various commercially available exercise devices and equipment.[69] Common exercise equipment that is used in the clinic for perturbation exercises may include a weighted ball, Swiss ball, BOSU ball, and handheld perturbation devices (e.g., flexbar, body-blade, gyroscope).[105] Use of this equipment induces reactive muscle activations while focusing on various functional movement patterns. Perturbations should initially be applied in more predictable directions and gradually advance into more random and unpredictable motion patterns. Perturbation exercises should also progress from shorter to longer time durations, aiming to improve functional muscle endurance.[69]

The clinical selection of either closed- or open-chain exercise should solely depend on the patient's specific rehabilitation program. Thus, both closed- and open-chain exercise strategies can contribute to functional improvements, depending on the patient's functional goals.[69] An example of upper extremity closed-chain perturbation exercise is a weighted or swiss ball wall rolling in clockwise or counterclockwise directions while applying axial loading to the whole upper extremity. This exercise can be advanced by pressing the ball against the wall and adding therapist-directed perturbations to the ball in multiple directions (Fig. 99.9). Having a patient's vision blocked could make these exercises even more challenging. Closed-chain exercises may be advanced further by positioning the patient to work harder against the influence of gravity. For example, swiss ball push-ups can be initiated against the wall and progress to the floor. Closed-chain proprioceptive exercises may also incorporate a foam pad or BOSU ball, progressing from double- to single-arm support positions (Fig. 99.10).[106]

Open-chain perturbation exercises typically entail the involved upper extremity being challenged by an external handheld oscillating device. Examples of these exercises may include oscillation of a handheld flexbar, body-blade, or a gyroscope in various directions (Fig. 99.11).[107] Typically, a flexbar presents less challenge than using a body-blade or a gyroscope, and it can be performed during the early or late rehabilitation phases.[108]

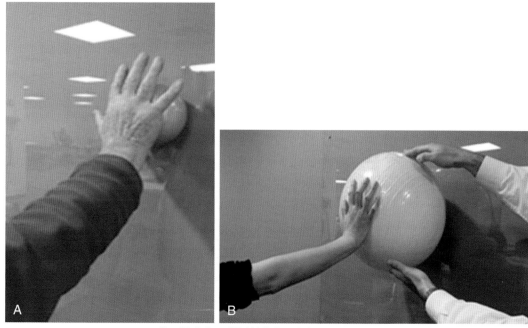

Fig. 99.9 **A** and **B**, Wall closed-chain exercises.

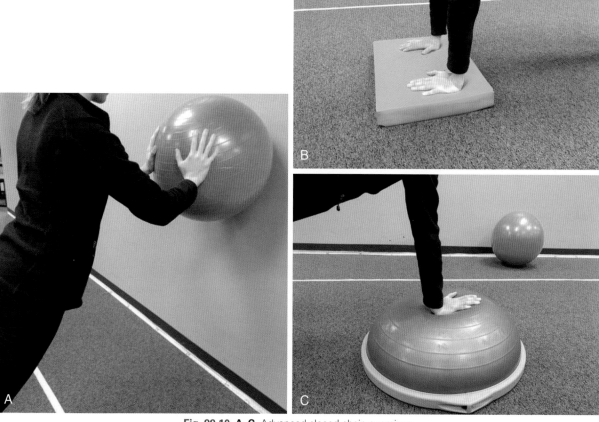

Fig. 99.10 **A–C**, Advanced closed-chain exercises.

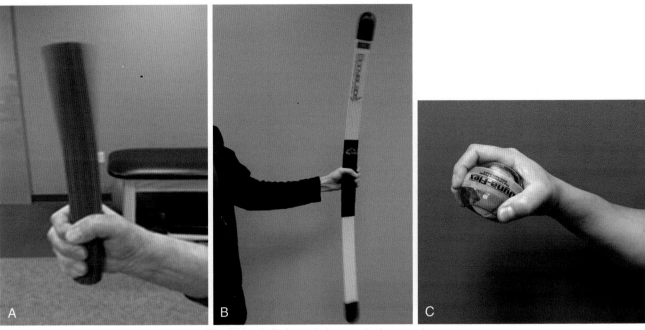

Fig. 99.11 A–C, Open-chain perturbation exercises.

Flexbar exercises can be advanced by using its commercially available colors that offer variable elastic resistance. Body-blade and gyroscope exercises are more demanding because of the increased force requirements to maintain proper arm and trunk stability and coordination during these instrument-generated perturbations. Open-chain proprioceptive exercises should be performed with the upper extremity in different positions, aiming to elicit muscle coactivation patterns based on the specific rehabilitation program.[69] Arm position also determines the degree of exercise difficulty. The further the arm is abducted away from the body's midline, the greater the expected exercise loads. Conversely, using double-hand grasp, having the elbow flexed, and maintaining the arm closer to the body's midline decrease the exercise challenge.[107] This might be a position of choice for patients with lower strength capacity or when open-chain perturbation exercises are first introduced.

NEUROMUSCULAR REEDUCATION APPLIED IN PRACTICE

Background

Regardless of injury type (i.e., soft tissue, ligamentous instability, fracture) or medical intervention (i.e., operative or nonoperative), initial injury treatment typically encompasses some form of protection or immobilization to allow for proper tissue healing.[93] Thereafter, therapy should progress based on the aforementioned rehabilitation guidelines that initially focus on improving physical impairments (i.e., edema, sensibility, active ROM, and conscious proprioception).[14,69] Improving these physical impairments is considered a clinically important prerequisite for restoring proper wrist sensorimotor function.[67] One distinguishing element of wrist sensorimotor control rehabilitation is the focus on specific dynamic stabilization strategies. Physiologically, normal biomechanical function of the wrist joint requires the presence of intact capsuloligamentous tissue and highly responsive muscular function that provides proper neuromuscular control throughout its ROM.[14,75,109] Thus, application of specific dynamic stabilization techniques should be incorporated as soon as proper tissue healing has been attained after the early rehabilitation phase.[69]

The application of dynamic stabilization exercises should be based on a thorough knowledge of wrist anatomy and biomechanics. Unarguably, wrist dynamic support derives from the surrounding muscles at specific anatomic positions. In cadaveric testing of the role of muscles on the stability of the carpus, it has been found that the forearm muscles, in addition to providing motion in the sagittal and frontal planes, act in a transverse plane to provide wrist joint stability by either supinating or pronating the carpus.[109,110] Using physiological joint loads on the forearm muscles while monitoring carpal alignment through the use of an electromagnetic motion tracking device,[109] the extensor carpi radialis longus and brevis (ECRL/B), abductor pollicis longus (APL), and flexor carpi ulnaris (FCU) muscles were all found to be carpal supinators. In contrast, the extensor carpi ulnaris (ECU) is considered to induce carpus pronation.[110] Dissimilar to these muscles, the flexor carpi radialis (FCR) muscle is known for its dual role in wrist stability, promoting both supination and pronation of the scaphoid and triquetral carpal bones, respectively.[109,110] Given no ligamentous injury, these muscles work synergistically to provide global dynamic support throughout wrist kinetic function.[75,110] However, upon specific wrist ligamentous injury, these muscles may have a more specialized action. The biomechanical function of carpus supinator muscles directly favors the stability of the scapholunate (SL) articulation, whereas it can be detrimental to an unstable lunotriquetral (LT) joint. The concomitant function of the ECU and the FCR, which both induce pronation of the triquetrum, provides critical dynamic support at the LT joint.[109] When the ECU muscle becomes isolated, it can further destabilize an injured SL articulation.[110] Finally, the ECU and pronator quadratus (PQ) muscle synergistic actions offer critical dynamic stability at the distal radioulnar (DRU) joint.[18,109] All of these muscle biomechanical relationships should be considered before establishing a dynamic stabilization program (Table 99.4). Thus, exercise prescription after wrist ligamentous injuries (e.g., scapholunate, LT, and DRU joint instabilities) should be exclusively directed toward muscle groups that play a designated supportive role for the recovery of each given injured joint. The following sections of this chapter outline specific neuromuscular retraining exercise strategies that are indicated for patients with common wrist traumatic conditions.

TABLE 99.4 Wrist Neuromuscular Retraining Recommendations Targeting Specific Joint Protective Muscle Groups[109,110]

Types of Instability	Dynamic Stabilizers	Avoid
SL	ECRL, ECRB, APL, FCU (carpal supinators) FCR (scaphoid supinator)	ECU (carpal pronator)
LT	ECU (carpal pronator), FCR (triquetrum pronator)	ECRL, ERCB, APL, FCU (carpal supinators)
Midcarpal	ECU, FCU, FCR	
DRU joint	ECU and PQ	

APL, Abductor pollicis longus; *DRU,* distal radioulnar; *ECRB,* extensor carpi radialis brevis; *ECRL,* extensor carpi radialis longus; *ECU,* extensor carpi ulnaris; *FCR,* flexor carpi radialis; *FCU,* flexor carpi ulnaris; *LT,* lunotriquetral; *PQ,* pronator quadratus; *SL,* scapholunate.

SCAPHOLUNATE INSTABILITY

Patients with SL joint instability benefit from dynamic stabilization exercises that are directed toward the carpus supinator muscles.[109] The synergistic action of the ECRL, ECRB, APL, FCU, and FCR muscles support the congruency of the SL joint while allowing for proper healing of the SL interosseous ligament (SLIL). Exercises that promote the action of the ECU tendon should be avoided.[110] ECU muscle loading results in pronation of the scaphoid, which can potentially widen the SL joint and subject the SLIL in tensile stresses that could compromise its healing potential.[75,110] The recommended position for wrist flexion or extension neuromuscular reeducation exercises is with the forearm in pronation. In this position, the ECU tendon is located more ulnarly as it crosses the wrist in a straight line toward its insertion at the base of the fifth metacarpal. In pronation, the ECU tendon has weaker biomechanical advantage as a wrist extensor and carpus pronator.[109,110] Thus, wrist flexion and extension strengthening exercises (i.e., isometrics and isotonics) in pronation can maximize an ECRL, ECRB, FCU, and FCR carpus supination effect while minimizing any ECU adverse influence against SL joint stability.[110] Such exercises can be completed via either free weights or elastic resistance strategies (Fig. 99.12).[111,112]

A strengthening program can be further enhanced by incorporating a DTM pattern,[110,111] which occurs at near 45 degrees between the wrist sagittal and transverse planes of motion.[113] DTM consists of coupled motions that combine wrist flexion with ulnar deviation (UD) and wrist extension with RD. It is considered the wrist's functional motion pattern that naturally occurs during most manual activities.[111] Wrist DTM is known to produce a protective effect to the SL joint stability because it enhances the biomechanical advantage of the carpus supination muscles. Thus, wrist extension and flexion neuromuscular reeducation exercises should be initially performed in a DTM pattern of motion within the unconstrained available ROM.[111] DTM exercises should be performed with caution after an acute SL injury or surgical repair of the SL ligament.[111] Early exercising through excessive wrist flexion and UD could induce increased SL interval gapping.[114] In these cases, early DTM should be modified, avoiding wrist flexion and UD beyond wrist neutral.[110,111]

In light of currently known wrist kinematics,[110,114] resistive exercises in straight planes of wrist RD and UD should be used with caution because of increased shearing stress at the SL interval.[110] Carpal instability dissociative at the SL joint predisposes the scaphoid to palmar flex away from a dorsiflexed lunate and triquetrum bones.[115] This

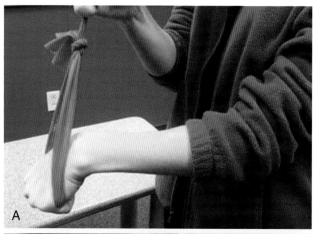
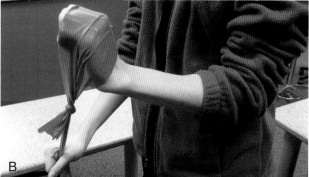

Fig. 99.12 A and **B,** Elastic resistance exercises for scapholunate instability.

faulty position could be further exaggerated by straight plane RD and UD motions that naturally force the proximal carpal row to palmar- and dorsiflex, respectively.[110] Wrist UD and RD resistive exercises should be incorporated during later rehabilitation phases when adequate SL interval capsule–ligamentous tissue tensile strength has been attained.

LUNOTRIQUETRAL INSTABILITY

Patients with LT joint instability benefit from dynamic stabilization exercises that promote triquetral pronation. Exercises that promote carpus supination muscle action should be avoided to allow for proper LT joint capsuloligamentous healing.[109,110] Early LT instability rehabilitation stages should focus primarily on the ECU muscle and gradually progress to inducing the combined actions of both the ECU and FCR muscles toward the dynamic stability of the LT joint. Co-contraction of both muscles is known to pronate the triquetrum.[116] However, isolated FCR contraction promotes scaphoid and lunate flexion, which could potentially be harmful before LT interval healing. Thus, FCR muscle activation is reserved for later rehabilitation stages when proper LT joint tissue healing levels are attained.[110] Proper dynamic stabilization exercises for LT instability should be performed in supination. In this position, the ECRL, ECRB, APL, and FCU muscles lose their mechanical advantage to act as strong carpus supinators. Conversely, the ECU tendon becomes a powerful wrist extensor and carpus pronator, contributing to maximum LT joint stability. This occurs as the ECU tendon shifts radially over the ulna and angulates ulnarly toward its distal insertion, causing its moment arm to increase.[110]

Dynamic stabilization exercises for LT instability should encompass both isometric and isotonic strategies of the ECU muscle.[117] Submaximum wrist extension isometric exercises should be initiated first with

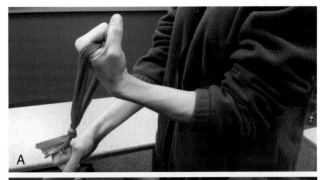
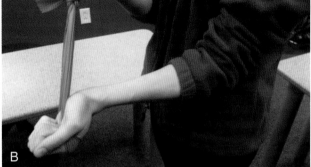

Fig. 99.13 **A** and **B,** Elastic resistance exercises for lunotriquetral instability.

the wrist in neutral or supinated position based on a patient's available ROM. ECU muscle retraining should progress via isotonic exercises. Wrist flexion isometric or isotonic exercises should be introduced during the later rehabilitation stage after adequate LT ligamentous healing has occurred. Isotonic exercises encompass both elastic or free-weight resistance strategies and should be done in supination for maximum LT joint stability (Fig. 99.13).[110] Similar to the SL interval injury, wrist UD and RD isotonic exercises should be introduced once adequate healing has been reached because of increased potential for shearing forces at the LT interval. Rhythmic stabilization into wrist flexion and extension would also be an effective proprioception retraining strategy[68] during the late rehabilitation as coactivation of the FCR and ECU muscles could contribute to restoring proper LT joint dynamic neuromuscular control.[109]

MIDCARPAL INSTABILITY

Midcarpal instability is classified as a carpal instability nondissociative disruption between the proximal and distal carpal rows.[115,118] Patients with midcarpal instability benefit from dynamic stabilization exercises that prioritize both ECU and FCR muscle retraining.[76,109,110] The ECU combined effects of powerful wrist extension and carpus pronation moments promote congruency and stability of the midcarpal articulation[110] and control the palmarly directed carpal sag deformity that develops at the ulnar wrist side.[118] The FCR additionally complements the ECU action as activation of the FCR leads to further pronation of the ulnar carpus.[116] Neuromuscular training for midcarpal instability should be done with the forearm supinated because this position maximizes the desired ECU and FCR muscle carpus pronation effects.[110] Rhythmic stabilization of the FCR and ECU via alternating wrist flexion and extension isometrics[68] or using a reverse DTM isotonic pattern should be the core exercise strategy for a midcarpal instability dynamic stabilization program. During reverse DTM motion, the supinated wrist reciprocates from a flexion–radial to extension–UD plane of motion.[75,110] UD isometrics could also complement the aforementioned exercises with the arm supinated. UD isometrics elicit a

simultaneous activation of the ECU and FCU tendons,[14] contributing further to midcarpal joint stability as they cross the dorsal and volar aspects of the ulnar wrist.[110] This exercise could progress to various positions of forearm rotation, emphasizing a strong UD moment throughout the entire available supination–pronation functional range.

DISTAL RADIOULNAR JOINT INSTABILITY

Dynamic stabilization exercises for DRU joint instability should prioritize the PQ and ECU muscles.[18,110] Contraction of the PQ, which connects the distal radius and ulna, increases DRU joint congruency. Additionally, the ECU, which directly connects to the ulnocarpal ligament and TFCC via its fibrous sheath, crosses the ulnar–carpal joint before its distal attachment at the base of the fifth metacarpal.[119] Essentially, both the PQ and ECU tendons offer valuable dynamic proprioceptive support at the DRU joint and TFCC structure during forearm rotation.[14,18] When ECU tendon isometric or isotonic exercises are used for DRU joint and TFCC instability, the forearm should be placed in slight supination. In this position, the DRU joint gains congruency while the ECU still retains its strong wrist extension and UD biomechanical advantage.[110] Neuromuscular retraining of the PQ muscle should also progress via isometric and isotonic exercises at midranges of forearm rotation using either free weights or elastic resistance. Early ECU and PQ strengthening exercises should avoid moving the forearm into full pronation as the DRU joint becomes vulnerable to dorsal subluxation at this position.[18]

WRIST FRACTURES

Upper extremity trauma may result in various types of wrist fractures that may implicate the distal radius and carpal bones. DRF is the most frequent fracture of the upper extremity and can result in significant osseous deformity and ligamentous instabilities[96] that impair proper wrist neuromuscular control.[66] Dorsal angulation and shortening of the distal radius or proximal carpus collapse after ligamentous disruption can alter the length–tension relationships of the long wrist flexor and extensor muscles that cross the radiocarpal joint, leading to significant muscle weakness.[120] Concomitant SL, LT, and DRU joint instabilities, which are frequently associated with DRF, can lead to significant wrist dynamic control impairment. All these wrist trauma cases require proper neuromuscular retraining irrespective of postfracture medical management.

Thorough dynamic stabilization exercises after wrist fractures should aim to restore neuromuscular control for all the implicated muscles for ultimate kinetic stability and function.[14,48,69] Specific focus should be directed to weakened wrist extensors, preventing a faulty hand substitution with the digital extensors that is observed during wrist extension.[72] Restoring proper neuromuscular function between the wrist extensors and the intrinsic and extrinsic digital flexors should also be prioritized. These muscles work synergistically to allow for proper hand-grasping mechanics.[101] Joint-specific dynamic stabilization exercises, based on the previous guidelines, should apply for SL, LT, midcarpal, and DRU joint instabilities after wrist fractures.[110] Dynamic stabilization methods should progress through isometric and isotonic exercises toward optimal functional recovery.[14,69] Gentle midrange isometrics could be safely initiated at the end of the early rehabilitation phase based on an appropriate healing status of the underlying osseous or ligamentous tissues.[69] These exercises help to instill proper wrist kinesthetic awareness of motion and position.[14] Isometrics should be progressed by increasing the applied force and varying the application angle[98] before advancing into more demanding isotonic (i.e., concentric, eccentric) and perturbation strengthening strategies, which ultimately help to improve anticipatory neuromuscular control toward optimal wrist joint dynamic stability.[69]

REFERENCES

1. Martinsson H. Människans händer [Man's hands]. *Dikter Om Ljus Och Mörker* [Poems of light and darkness]. Sweden: Bonnier; 1971;(1):41
2. Sherrington CS. *The Integrative Action of the Nervous System*. New Haven, CT: Yale University Press; 1906.
3. Bastian HC. The "muscular sense"; its nature and cortical localisation. *Brain*. 1888;10:1–137.
4. Weber EH. In: Wagner R, ed. *Der Tastsinn und das Gemeingefühl. Handwörterbuch der Physiologie*. Leipzig: W. Engelmann; 1905.
5. Proske U. Kinesthesia: the role of muscle receptors. *Muscle Nerve*. 2006;34:545–558.
6. Luu BL, Day BL, Cole JD, Fitzpatrick RC. The fusimotor and reafferent origin of the sense of force and weight. *J. Physiol*. 2011;589:3135–3147.
7. Burke D, Gandevia SC, Macefield G. Responses to passive movement of receptors in joint, skin and muscle of the human hand. *J Physiol*. 1988;402:347–361.
8. Collins DF, Refshauge KM, Todd G, Gandevia SC. Cutaneous receptors contribute to kinesthesia at the index finger, elbow, and knee. *J Neurophysiol*. 2005;94:1699–1706.
9. Sturnieks DL, Wright JR, Fitzpatrick RC. Detection of simultaneous movement at two human arm joints. *J Physiol*. 2007;585:833–842.
10. Ferrell BYWR, Gandevia SC, Mccloskey DI. The role of joint receptors in human kinaesthesia when intramuscular receptors cannot contribute. *J Physiol*. 1987;386:63–71.
11. Moberg E. The role of cutaneous afferents in position sense, kinaesthesia, and motor function of the hand. *Brain*. 1983;106(Pt 1):1–19.
12. Patterson RW, Van Niel M, Shimko P, Pace C, Seitz Jr WH. Proprioception of the wrist following posterior interosseous sensory neurectomy. *J Hand Surg Am*. 2010;35:52–56.
13. Sjolander P, Johansson H, Djupsjobacka M. Spinal and supraspinal effects of activity in ligament afferents. *J Electromyogr Kinesiol*. 2002;12:167–176.
14. Hagert E. Proprioception of the wrist joint: a review of current concepts and possible implications on the rehabilitation of the wrist. *J Hand Ther*. 2010;23:2–17.
15. Hagert E, Persson JK, Werner M, Ljung BO. Evidence of wrist proprioceptive reflexes elicited after stimulation of the scapholunate interosseous ligament. *J Hand Surg*. 2009;34A:642–651.
16. Bergquist ER, Hammert WC. Timing and appropriate use of electrodiagnostic studies. *Hand Clinics*. 2013;29:363–370.
17. Frank CB. Ligament structure, physiology and function. *J Musculoskelet Neuronal Interact*. 2004;4:199–201.
18. Hagert E, Hagert CG. Understanding stability of the distal radioulnar joint through an understanding of its anatomy. *Hand Clin*. 2010;26:459–466.
19. Ingber DE. The architecture of life. *Sci Am*. 1998;278:48–57.
20. Solomonow M. Sensory-motor control of ligaments and associated neuromuscular disorders. *J Electromyogr Kinesiol*. 2006;16:549–567.
21. Freeman MA, Wyke B. The innervation of the knee joint. An anatomical and histological study in the cat. *J Anat*. 1967;101:505–532.
22. Hagert E, Lee J, Ladd AL. Innervation patterns of thumb trapeziometacarpal joint ligaments. *J Hand Surg Am*. 2012;37:706–714. e701.
23. Rein S, Hagert E, Hanisch U, Lwowski S, Fieguth A, Zwipp H. Immunohistochemical analysis of sensory nerve endings in ankle ligaments: a cadaver study. *Cells Tissues Organs*. 2012;197:64–76.
24. Takebayashi T, Yamashita T, Minaki Y, Ishii S. Mechanosensitive afferent units in the lateral ligament of the ankle. *J Bone Joint Surg Br*. 1997;79:490–493.
25. Ruffini A. Sur un novel organe nerveux terminal et sur la présence des corpuscles Golgi-Mazzoni dans le conjunctiv sous-cutané de la pulpe des doigts de l'homme. *Arch Ital Biol*. 1894;21:249–265.
26. Lehmann JG. Dissertatio inauguralis medica de consensu partium corporis humani occasione spasmi singularis in manu ejusque digitis ex hernia observati; exposito simul nervorum barchialium et cruralium coalitu peculiari atque papillarum nervearum in digitis dispositio. *Wittenberg*. 1741.
27. Vater A. Dissertatio de consensu partium corporis humani occasione spasmi singularis in manu eiusque digitis ex hernia observati exposito simul nervorum brachialium et cruralium coalitu peculiari atque papil-
larum nervearum in digitis dispositione. In: Haller A, ed. *Disputationum Anatomicarum Selectarum. Göttingen: Vandenhoeck*. 1741:953–972.
28. Bentivoglio M, Pacini P. Filippo Pacini: a determined observer. *Brain Res Bull*. 1995;38:161–165.
29. Pacini F. Sopra un particolare genere di piccoli corpi globosi scoperti nel corpo umano da Filippo Pacini, Alunno interno degli Spedali riuniti di Pistoia. *Letter to the Accademia Medico-Fisica di Firenze*; 1835.
30. Macefield VG. Physiological characteristics of low-threshold mechanoreceptors in joints, muscle and skin in human subjects. *Clin Exp Pharmacol Physiol*. 2005;32:135–144.
31. Golgi C. *Della Terminazione Dei Nervi Nei Tendini E Di Un Nuovo Apparato Nervoso Terminale Muscolo-Tendineo*. Milano: Atti della Settima Riunione Staordinaria della Societa Italiana di Scienze Naturali in Varese, Tipografia G. Bernardoni; 1878
32. Hagert E, Forsgren S, Ljung BO. Differences in the presence of mechanoreceptors and nerve structures between wrist ligaments may imply differential roles in wrist stabilization. *J Orthop Res*. 2005;23:757–763.
33. Hagert E. *Wrist Ligaments- Innervation Patterns and Ligamento-Muscular Reflexes*; 2008.
33a. Erlanger J, Gasser HS. *Electrical Signs of Gassernervous Activity*. Oxford: Univ Penn Press. 1937.
33b. Lloyd D. Neuron patterns controlling transmission of ipsilateral hind limb reflexes in cat. *J Neurophysiol*. 1943;6(4):293–315.
33c. Hunt CC . Relation of function to diameter in afferent fibers of muscle nerves. *J Gen Physiol*. 1954;38(1):117–131.
34. Gilman S. Joint position sense and vibration sense: anatomical organisation and assessment. *J Neurol Neurosurg Psychiatry*. 2002;73:473–477.
35. Costanzo LS. *Physiology*, 6th ed. Philadelphia: Elsevier. 2018:74.
36. Mataliotakis G, Doukas M, Kostas I, Lykissas M, Batistatou A, Beris A. Sensory innervation of the subregions of the scapholunate interosseous ligament in relation to their structural composition. *J Hand Surg*. 2009;34A:1413–1421.
37. Hagert E, Garcia-Elias M, Forsgren S, Ljung BO. Immunohistochemical analysis of wrist ligament innervation in relation to their structural composition. *J Hand Surg*. 2007;32A:30–36.
38. Hagert E, Chim H, Moran SL. Anatomy of the distal radioulnar joint and ulnocarpal complex. In: Greenberg JA, ed. *Ulnar-Sided Wrist Pain: A Master Skills Publication*. Chicago: American Society for Surgery of the Hand; 2013:11–21.
39. Rein S, Semisch M, Garcia-Elias M, Lluch A, Zwipp H, Hagert E. Immunohistochemical mapping of sensory nerve endings in the human triangular fibrocartilage complex. *Clin Orthop Relat Res*. 2015;473:3245–3253.
40. Chikenji T, Berger Ra, Fujimiya M, Suzuki D, Tsubota S, An KN. Distribution of nerve endings in human distal interphalangeal joint and surrounding structures. *J Hand Surg Am*. 2011;36:406–412.
41. Chen YG, McClinton MA, DaSilva MF, Wilgis S. Innervation of the metacarpophalangeal and interphalangeal joints: a microanatomic and histologic study of the nerve endings. *J Hand Surg Am*. 2000;25:128–133.
42. Ludwig A, Mobargha N, Okogbaa J, Hagert E, Ladd L. Altered innervation pattern in ligaments of patients with basal thumb arthritis. *J Wrist Surg*. 2015;4:284–291.
43. Johnson EO, Babis GC, Soultanis KC, Soucacos PN. Functional neuroanatomy of proprioception. *J Surg Orthop Adv*. 2008;17:159–164. Fall.
44. Ghez C. The control of movement. *Principles of Neural Science*. 1991:533–646.
45. Riemann BL, Lephart SM. The sensorimotor system, part I: the physiologic basis of functional joint stability. *J Athl Train*. 2002;37:71–79.
46. Jankowska E. Interneuronal relay in spinal pathways from proprioceptors. *Progress in Neurobiology*. 1992;38:335–378.
47. Matthews PBC. Where does Sherrington's "muscular sense" originate? Muscles, joints corollary discharges? *Neuroscience*. 1982:189–218.
48. Riemann BL, Lephart SM. The sensorimotor system, part II: the role of proprioception in motor control and functional joint stability. *J Athl Train*. 2002;37:80–84.
49. Ma Freeman, Wyke B. Articular contributions to limb muscle reflexes. The effects of partial neurectomy of the knee-joint on postural reflexes. *Br J Surg*. 1966;53:61–68.

50. Freeman MA, Wyke B. Articular reflexes at the ankle joint: an electromyographic study of normal and abnormal influences of ankle-joint mechanoreceptors upon reflex activity in the leg muscles. *Br J Surg.* 1967;54:990–1001.

51. Palmer I. Pathophysiology of the medial ligament of the knee joint. *Acta Chir Scand.* 1958;115:312–318.

52. Dyhre-Poulsen P, Krogsgaard MR. Muscular reflexes elicited by electrical stimulation of the anterior cruciate ligament in humans. *J Appl Physiol.* 2000;89:2191–2195.

53. Sterling-Hauf T. *Nachweis propriozeptiver Reflexe des menschlichen Sprunggelenkes nach Stimulation des Ligamentum fibulotalare anterius.* Dresden, Germany: Medical Faculty, Technical University of Dresden; 2016.

54. Diederichsen LP, Norregaard J, Krogsgaard M, Fischer-Rasmussen T, Dyhre-Poulsen P. Reflexes in the shoulder muscles elicited from the human coracoacromial ligament. *J Orthop Res.* 2004;22:976–983.

55. Mobargha N. *The Proprioception and Neuromuscular Stability of the Basal Thumb Joint.* Stockholm, Sweden: Dept of Clinical Science and Education, Karolinska Institutet; 2015.

56. Solomonow M, Lewis J. Reflex from the ankle ligaments of the feline. *J Electromyogr Kinesiol.* 2002;12:193–198.

57. Jerosch J, Steinbeck J, Schröder M, Westhues M, Reer R. Intraoperative EMG response of the musculature after stimulation of the glenohumeral joint capsule. *Acta Orthop Belg.* 1997;63:8–14.

58. Sojka P, Johansson Hk, Sjölander P, Lorentzon R, Djupsjöbacka M. Fusimotor neurones can be reflexy influenced by activity in receptor afferents from the posterior cruciate ligament. *Brain Research.* 1989;483:177–183

59. Louie JK, Mote CD. Contribution of the musculature to rotatory laxity and torsional stiffness at the knee. *J Biomech.* 1987;20:281–300.

60. Vekris MD, Mataliotakis GI, Beris AE. The scapholunate interosseous ligament afferent proprioceptive pathway: a human in vivo experimental study. *J Hand Surg.* 2011;36A:37–46.

61. Hagert E, Persson JK. Desensitizing the posterior interosseous nerve alters wrist proprioceptive reflexes. *J Hand Surg.* 2010;35A:1059–1066.

62. Gay A, Harbst K, Hansen DK, Laskowski ER, Berger RA, Kaufman KR. Effect of partial wrist denervation on wrist kinesthesia: wrist denervation does not impair proprioception. *J Hand Surg Am.* 2011;36:1774–1779.

63. Myers JB, Lephart SM. The role of the sensorimotor system in the athletic shoulder. *J Athl Train.* 2000;35:351–363.

64. Swanik CB, Lephart SM, Giannantonio FP, Fu FH. Reestablishing proprioception and neuromuscular control in the ACL-injured athlete. *J Sport Rehabil.* 1997;6:182–206.

65. Hoffman M, Payne VG. The effects of proprioceptive ankle disk training on healthy subjects. *J Orthop Sports Phys Ther.* 1995;21:90–93.

66. Karagiannopoulos C, Sitler M, Michlovitz S, Tierney R. A descriptive study on wrist and hand sensori-motor impairment and function following distal radius fracture intervention. *J Hand Ther.* 2013;26:204–214. quiz 215.

67. Karagiannopoulos C, Sitler M, Michlovitz S, Tucker C, Tierney R. Responsiveness of the active wrist joint position sense test after distal radius fracture intervention. *J Hand Ther.* 2016;29:474–482.

68. Valdes K, Naughton N, Algar L. Sensorimotor interventions and assessments for the hand and wrist: a scoping review. *J Hand Ther.* 2014;27:272–285. quiz 286.

69. Karagiannopoulos C, Michlovitz S. Rehabilitation strategies for wrist sensorimotor control impairment: from theory to practice. *J Hand Ther.* 2016;29:154–165.

70. Chen NC, Jupiter JB. Management of distal radial fractures. *J Bone Joint Surg Am.* 2007;89:2051–2062.

71. Forward DP, Lindau TR, Melsom DS. Intercarpal ligament injuries associated with fractures of the distal part of the radius. *J Bone Joint Surg Am.* 2007;89:2334–2340.

72. Diaz-Garcia RJ, Oda T, Shauver MJ, Chung KC. A systematic review of outcomes and complications of treating unstable distal radius fractures in the elderly. *J Hand Surg Am.* 2011;36:824–835. e822.

73. MacDermid JC, Richards RS, Roth JH. Distal radius fracture: a prospective outcome study of 275 patients. *J Hand Ther.* 2001;14:154–169.

74. May A. Chronic pain may change the structure of the brain. *Pain.* 2008;137:7–15.

75. Hagert E, Lluch A, Rein S. The role of proprioception and neuromuscular stability in carpal instabilities. *J Hand Surg Eur Vol.* 2016;41:94–101.

76. McKay SD, MacDermid JC, Roth JH, Richards RS. Assessment of complications of distal radius fractures and development of a complication checklist. *J Hand Surg Am.* 2001;26:916–922.

77. Sharma L, Pai YC. Impaired proprioception and osteoarthritis. *Curr Opin Rheumatol.* 1997;9:253–258.

78. Flor H, Nikolajsen L, Staehelin Jensen T. Phantom limb pain: a case of maladaptive CNS plasticity? *Nat Rev Neurosci.* 2006;7:873–881.

79. Minor MA, Sanford MK. The role of physical therapy and physical modalities in pain management. *Rheum Dis Clin North Am.* 1999;25:233–248. viii.

80. Valdes K, Marik T. A systematic review of conservative interventions for osteoarthritis of the hand. *J Hand Ther.* 2010;23:334–350; quiz 351.

81. Stamm TA, Machold KP, Smolen JS, et al. Joint protection and home hand exercises improve hand function in patients with hand osteoarthritis: a randomized controlled trial. *Arthritis Rheum.* 2002;47:44–49.

82. Mesplie G, Grelet V, Leger O, Lemoine S, Ricarrere D, Geoffroy C. Rehabilitation of distal radioulnar joint instability. *Hand Surg Rehabil.* 2017;36:314–321.

83. Watson J, Gonzalez M, Romero A, Kerns J. Neuromas of the hand and upper extremity. *J Hand Surg Am.* 2010;35:499–510.

84. Watson HK, Carlson L. Treatment of reflex sympathetic dystrophy of the hand with an active "stress loading" program. *J Hand Surg Am.* 1987;12:779–785.

85. Valdes K. A retrospective pilot study comparing the number of therapy visits required to regain functional wrist and forearm range of motion following volar plating of a distal radius fracture. *J Hand Ther.* 2009;22:312–318. quiz 319.

86. Harris JE, Eng JJ. Individuals with the dominant hand affected following stroke demonstrate less impairment than those with the nondominant hand affected. *Neurorehabil Neural Repair.* 2006;20:380–389.

87. Lee M, Gandevia SC, Carroll TJ. Unilateral strength training increases voluntary activation of the opposite untrained limb. *Clin Neurophysiol.* 18 2009.

88. Fimland MS, Helgerud J, Solstad GM, Iversen VM, Leivseth G, Hoff J. Neural adaptations underlying cross-education after unilateral strength training. *Eur J Appl Physiol.* 2009;107:723–730.

89. Naito E, Roland PE, Ehrsson HH. I feel my hand moving: a new role of the primary motor cortex in somatic perception of limb movement. *Neuron.* 2002;36:979–988.

90. Altschuler EL, Hu J. Mirror therapy in a patient with a fractured wrist and no active wrist extension. *Scand J Plast Reconstr Surg Hand Surg.* 2008;42:110–111.

91. Yavuzer G, Selles R, Sezer N, et al. Mirror therapy improves hand function in subacute stroke: a randomized controlled trial. *Arch Phys Med Rehabil.* 2008;89:393–398.

92. Grünert-Plüss N, Hufscmid U, Santschi L, Grünert J. Mirror therapy in hand rehabilitation: a review of the literature, the St Gallen Protocol for mirror therapy and evaluation of a case series of 52 patients. *Hand Ther.* 2008;13:4–11.

93. Hincapie OL, Elkins JS, Vasquez-Welsh L. Proprioception retraining for a patient with chronic wrist pain secondary to ligament injury with no structural instability. *J Hand Ther.* 2016;29:183–190.

94. Smith JL, Crawford M, Proske U, Taylor JL, Gandevia SC. Signals of motor command bias joint position sense in the presence of feedback from proprioceptors. *J Appl Physiol (1985).* 2009;106:950–958.

95. Carroll TJ, Herbert RD, Munn J, Lee M, Gandevia SC. Contralateral effects of unilateral strength training: evidence and possible mechanisms. *J Appl Physiol (1985).* 2006;101:1514–1522.

96. Handoll HH, Elliott J. Rehabilitation for distal radial fractures in adults. *Cochrane Database Syst Rev.* 2015;25:CD003324.

97. Bawa P, Chalmers GR, Jones KE, Sogaard K, Walsh ML. Control of the wrist joint in humans. *Eur J Appl Physiol.* 2000;83:116–127.

98. Folland JP, Hawker K, Leach B, Little T, Jones DA. Strength training: isometric training at a range of joint angles versus dynamic training. *J Sports Sci.* 2005;23:817–824.

99. Szymanski DJ, Szymanski JM, Molloy JM, Pascoe DD. Effect of 12 weeks of wrist and forearm training on high school baseball players. *J Strength Cond Res.* 2004;18:432–440.

100. Bruder AM, Taylor NF, Dodd KJ, Shields N. Physiotherapy intervention practice patterns used in rehabilitation after distal radial fracture. *Physiotherapy.* 2013;99:233–240.

101. Mitsukane M, Sekiya N, Himei S, Oyama K. Immediate effects of repetitive wrist extension on grip strength in patients with distal radial fracture. *Arch Phys Med Rehabil.* 2015;96:862–868.

102. Dudley GA, Fleck SJ. Strength and endurance training. Are they mutually exclusive? *Sports Med.* 1987;4:79–85.

103. Allen TJ, Ansems GE, Proske U. Effects of muscle conditioning on position sense at the human forearm during loading or fatigue of elbow flexors and the role of the sense of effort. *J Physiol.* 2007;580:423–434.

104. Fitzgerald GK, Axe MJ, Snyder-Mackler L. The efficacy of perturbation training in nonoperative anterior cruciate ligament rehabilitation programs for physical active individuals. *Physical therapy.* 2000;80:128–140.

105. Escamilla RF, Yamashiro K, Dunning R, Mikla T, Grover M, Kenniston M, et al. An electromyographic analysis of the shoulder complex musculature while performing exercises using the Bodyblade classic and Bodyblade pro. *Int J Sports Phys Ther.* 2016;11:175–189.

106. Behm D, Colado JC. The effectiveness of resistance training using unstable surfaces and devices for rehabilitation. *Int J Sports Phys Ther.* 2012;7:226–241.

107. Arora S, Button DC, Basset FA, Behm DG. The effect of double versus single oscillating exercise devices on trunk and limb muscle activation. *Int J Sports Phys Ther.* 2013;8:370–380.

108. Vasiliadis AV, Lampridis V, Georgiannos D, Bisbinas IG. Rehabilitation exercise program after surgical treatment of pectoralis major rupture. A case report. *Phys Ther Sport.* 2016;20:32–39.

109. Salva-Coll G, Garcia-Elias M, Leon-Lopez MT, Llusa-Perez M, Rodriguez-Baeza A. Effects of forearm muscles on carpal stability. *J Hand Surg Eur Vol.* 2011;36:553–559.

110. Esplugas M, Garcia-Elias M, Lluch A, Llusa Perez M. Role of muscles in the stabilization of ligament-deficient wrists. *J Hand Ther.* 2016;29:166–174.

111. Wolff AL, Wolfe SW. Rehabilitation for scapholunate injury: Application of scientific and clinical evidence to practice. *J Hand Ther.* 2016;29:146–153.

112. Holmes MK, Taylor S, Miller C, Brewster MBS. Early outcomes of 'The Birmingham Wrist Instability Programme': a pragmatic intervention for stage one scapholunate instability. *Hand Ther.* 2017;22:90–100.

113. Crisco JJ, Coburn JC, Moore DC, Akelman E, Weiss AP, Wolfe SW. In vivo radiocarpal kinematics and the dart thrower's motion. *J Bone Joint Surg Am.* 2005;87:2729–2740.

114. Garcia-Elias M, Alomar Serrallach X, Monill Serra J. Dart-throwing motion in patients with scapholunate instability: a dynamic four-dimensional computed tomography study. *J Hand Surg Eur Vol.* 2014;39:346–352.

115. Garcia-Elias M. The treatment of wrist instability. *J Bone Joint Surg Br.* 1997;79:684–690.

116. Salva-Coll G, Garcia-Elias M, Llusa-Perez M, Rodriguez-Baeza A. The role of the flexor carpi radialis muscle in scapholunate instability. *J Hand Surg Am.* 2011;36:31–36.

117. Leon-Lopez MM, Salva-Coll G, Garcia-Elias M, Lluch-Bergada A, Llusa-Perez M. Role of the extensor carpi ulnaris in the stabilization of the lunotriquetral joint. An experimental study. *J Hand Ther.* 2013;26:312–317; quiz 317.

118. Niacaris T, Ming BW, Lichtman DM. Midcarpal Instability: a comprehensive review and update. *Hand Clin.* 2015;31:487–493.

119. Moritomo H. Anatomy and clinical relevance of the ulnocarpal ligament. *J Wrist Surg.* 2013;2:186–189.

120. Tang JB, Ryu J, Kish V, Wearden S. Effect of radial shortening on muscle length and moment arms of the wrist flexors and extensors. *J Orthop Res.* 1997;15:324–330.

Graded Motor Imagery

Susan Watkins Stralka

CRITICAL POINTS

- Graded motor imagery (GMI) is a sequential program and should be tailored for each patient.
- GMI should be part of a comprehensive therapeutic treatment plan.
- Patients with both musculoskeletal and neurologic conditions who cannot move or are afraid of movement may benefit from GMI.
- More evidence is needed to support the benefits of GMI.

BACKGROUND

Graded motor imagery (GMI) is a technique of rehabilitation described by Moseley and Butler[1] as a way to sequentially train the brain. Recent neuroscience research using advanced and improved technologies such as functional magnetic resonance imaging (fMRI) and transcranial magnetic stimulation (TMS) demonstrate brain reorganization after the use of rehabilitation techniques such as GMI.[2,3] GMI has been shown to sequentially activate distinctly ordered stages of brain function[2] using positron emission tomography (PET), which reveals brain activation through blood flow measurements. There is a large body of literature on the differences in central nervous system (CNS) organization and function between patients with persistent or chronic pain compared with healthy control participants.[4–6] Change in cerebral organization in patients with complex regional pain syndrome (CRPS) with reorganization in central cortical somatosensory and motor networks results in altered processing of tactile and nociceptive stimuli.[7] Moseley's interest in GMI came about after reviewing a research report of delayed reaction time in a left–right hand discrimination task that occurred in people with hand pain.[4,8] In this report, the body schema, which is a real-time cortical representation of the body in space generated by proprioceptive, somatosensory, vestibular, and other sensory inputs, was examined to see if pain had an effect on this representation, which it did.[4,8] This report stimulated Moseley's interest in studying how a therapist can provide treatment that is less threatening than imagined movements. Other research reports found that patients with chronic unilateral pain required a longer response time (RT) with a left–right discrimination task.[9] Lundborg,[10] Merzenich and Charms,[11] and Byl and Merzenich[12] reported that the brain has the ability to reorganize, to change its input and output throughout lifetime, and this is called *neuroplasticity*.

These research studies provided evidence that cortical representation is subject to change. Flor and Moseley's[13,14] investigation of the mechanism of phantom limb pain, which is caused by a body part that no longer exists, has largely contributed to our understanding of the development and maintenance of pain perceptions. These studies have shown that the brain itself plays a major role in chronic pain when it reacts to past experiences and reorganizes itself after amputation and persistent pain.[15] Mirror neurons are brain cells that fire when one acts as well as when one observes the same action performed by another; they have recently been identified as being involved in central sensitization (i.e., the development and maintenance of chronic pain).[16] These mirror neurons fire through both observation and imagining, as well as with execution of movement. Fadiga and coworkers[17] provided evidence that mirror neurons in humans fired after the observation of a movement and resulted in actual motor facilitation in brain studies. This same study demonstrated that mirror neurons fire not only when a person performs an activity but also when observing another person performing the same activity, which may assist in functional recovery. Evidence from research on limb amputation confirmed that there were changes in cortical representation from pre- to postamputation.[18] It has been noted that the somatosensory cortex that formerly received input from the amputated limb with phantom limb pain reorganizes and receives input from neighboring regions. Reorganization changes occurred only in amputees with phantom limb pain after amputation but not in amputees without pain. Ramachandran's[15] research studies also suggested that phantom limb and phantom sensations that occurred when certain areas of the face of amputees were stimulated were linked to cortical reorganization after injury and amputation. This author suggested that this phenomenon may be maintained in some amputees because of input from peripheral nerves that were damaged and continued to send random signals to the brain.[15] These studies with amputees support past knowledge that the human brain is malleable or plastic and that "top-down training" such as mirror therapy or GMI may be helpful in dealing with phantom limb sensations or pain. Ramachandran's research was embraced by many, and interest in the investigation and use of mirror therapy for phantom limb pain developed. Investigators asserted that phantom pain results from a mismatch between motor output and visual feedback. While observing the reflected image of the uninvolved limb in a mirror placed on the involved side, the brain is "tricked" into thinking that the amputated limb is restored, thus reestablishing the visual feedback that would overrule this mismatch.[16] According to Rock and Victor[19,20] in 1964, the brain has been shown to prioritize visual input over proprioceptive input, so when the unaffected limb moves in front of the mirror, it appears as though the affected limb is functioning normally when watching the image in the mirror. Flor[13] and Moseley and Butler's[1] research findings demonstrated through fMRI that the duration and extent of injury correlated with remapping of the brain after chronic pain, stroke, dystonia, phantom limb pain, and CRPS involving specific sensory and motor cortical networks.[13] Ramachandran and Moseley reported that the changes in the cortical map are thought to be part of "maladaptive neuroplasticity " that develops after injury.[1,18] A number of studies have emphasized the importance of correct left–right identification, which reflects an intact body schema. Central abnormalities include disruption of sensory and motor cortical processing and disrupted body schema causing sensory disturbances, dysfunctional motor control, and spreading of symptoms.[21,22] With recent neuroscience advances in the understanding of brain activity and its relationship to clinical symptoms, a new roadmap for treating patients with persistent pain symptoms and loss of motor control has evolved. The importance of identifying and treating both "bottom-up" or peripheral symptoms and "top-down" symptoms (i.e., brain training) has opened a new avenue for consideration with therapy patients. GMI is called a "brain-based treatment" or a "top-down treatment" because the intervention has been shown to turn on specific brain areas or sequentially activate cortical premotor and motor networks in a graded manner.[1] It has been termed a *graded exposure* process with pacing to avoid trigging a protective response such as pain. Graded exposure requires appropriate patient education regarding pain and activity and allows for a reduction of pain with gradual improvement toward movement.

GRADED MOTOR IMAGERY PHASES

Phase 1: Laterality Training or Left–Right Identification

The first stage of the GMI training is laterality or left–right recognition; the difference between identifying left from right is dependent on an intact body schema. Laterality identification assesses how quickly and accurately the patient identifies whether an image of a hand, arm, or other body part is the left or right. Laterality cards are commercially available flash cards, each containing a photo of a left or right hand or arm. The patient is asked to quickly identify whether the image is of a left or right hand or arm (Fig. 100.1). This identification is done first in the clinic, and then the patient is sent home with pictures or magazines to use for home training. Cards may be purchased or fabricated. Laterality training is progressed by increasing the number of cards, improving the time or increasing the difficulty of the pictures.[23] Laterality training is the first phase in the GMI training because it is thought that until the patient has an accurate cortical representation of her or his body, it is counterproductive to move forward with cortical retraining.[23] The average RT of identifying the hand cards is greater than 80% accuracy and less than 2 ± 0.05 seconds[1] (Table 100.1). The patient should perform left–right training multiple times a day and for short periods at a time. According to Moseley and Acerra,[24] by disengaging the primary motor cortex, it promotes inhibition and helps with desmudging in the sensory cortex. Laterality training activates premotor cortices and reestablishes left and right concepts in the brain, which helps to decrease the firing of painful neurotags.[25] (Neurotags are formed by neurons that have learned to link with each other in the interpretation of a single input.) Phase I of GMI is usually performed at home by the patient for at least a 2-week period but varies from patient to patient. Additional timeframes are discussed later in the chapter.

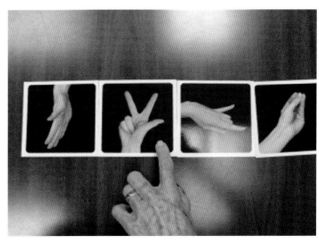

Fig. 100.1 Laterality training is the first phase in the graded motor imagery program and is used to develop an accurate cortical representation of the body.

TABLE 100.1 General Guidelines for Left–Right Discrimination
Accuracy of ≥80%
A time of 1.6–2.5 sec variable with body part
A response time of 2.0–2.05 sec
Accuracy and response times should be reasonably equal for the left and right
Often the involved limb takes more time to identify in the acute phase

Adapted from Mosely GL, Butler DS, Beames TB, Giles TJ. *The Graded Motor Imagery Handbook.* Adelaide, Australia: NOI Group; 2012.

Left–right identification cards include the hands, feet, knees, backs, and shoulders. There are computer-driven laterality recognition software programs called Recognize and Orientate.

Phase 2: Motor Imagery or Mental Imagery Rehearsal

Motor imagery has been around for many years, and it was a common practice with athletes before performing their sports (Fig. 100.2). During the past decade, there has been a rapid growth in the use of motor imagery in rehabilitation and psychology.[26,27] With motor imagery, the patient imagines his or her involved limb in a certain position. The patient is asked to imagine pain-free movement of that limb without increasing symptoms. Imagined hand movements are thought to activate the cortex in a similar manner to executed movements. Parsons[28] has shown that a motor imagery program, performed sequentially, activates cortical mechanisms associated with movement without evoking pain. When there is no pain, the patient then imagines the limb moving or imagines performing an activity with the limb. It is important to pace this phase by first having the patient imagine a static position before imagining movement of the limb. This phase of imagined movement is self-generated and activates areas of the brain similar to those of actual movement.[2] Other methods of using motor imagery involve having the patient view pictures of limb motions on the television or on video clips and then imagine performance of the observed motion(s) without pain. This is a conscious access to neurosignatures or movement memories representing intention, preparation, carrying out, and eventual movement, an approach that has been used in sports with healthy people.[27] The rationale for imagined movements is based on the findings that people with ongoing arm pain may experience pain just by thinking about movement. A Cochrane review on mental imagery revealed that mental imagery and physical practice more effectively improved upper extremity function than physical activity alone.[29] Even

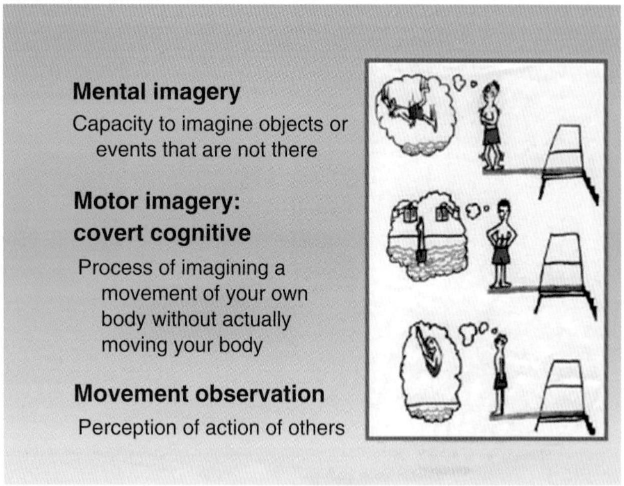

Mental imagery
Capacity to imagine objects or
events that are not there

Motor imagery:
covert cognitive
Process of imagining a
movement of your own
body without actually
moving your body

Movement observation
Perception of action of others

Fig. 100.2 Motor imagery involves imagined movements that are thought to activate the cortex similar to executed movements and are thought to be helpful in retraining the involved limb.

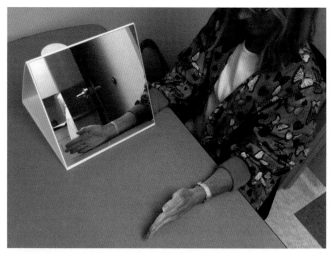

Fig. 100.3 Mirror therapy involves looking into a mirror and seeing the reflected image of the uninvolved limb in the mirror.

though information from several research studies suggests that mental imagery may be very helpful and is a promising technique, more studies are needed to confirm its efficacy.

Phase 3: Mirror Therapy or Mirror Visual Feedback

Mirror therapy involves looking into a mirror and seeing the reflected image of the uninvolved limb in the mirror, which has been placed on the involved side, in front of the involved limb. The reflected image appears to be that of the involved limb (Fig. 100.3). The first step is to have the patient look at the image in the mirror and see the illusion of the involved hand. This creates the illusion that the injured hand is now without pain. It is important for the patient to be comfortable, with both hands relaxed. The patient is then asked what hand he or she sees in the mirror. When the reflected image in the mirror has been identified by the patient as the involved hand, movement of the uninvolved hand in front of the mirror can begin. If there are no increased symptoms while looking at the image of movement in the mirror, then bimanual movement may begin. The patient should move both hands in a bilateral synchronous manner to feel the movement at the same time as she or he is observing the reflection of the normal limb movement.[30] According to McCabe and coworkers,[30] mirror therapy is thought to provide strong positive sensory feedback to the motor cortex that not all movements need to be painful. Another theory notes that mirror therapy may work because of increased attention to the limb, causing improved ownership[25]; however, the exact mechanisms of mirror therapy are still not fully understood. McCabe and coworkers[30] reported using mirror therapy alone in treating patients with CRPS; this treatment was effective in patients with early CRPS. Others report use of all three phases of GMI because this is a sequential order that does not overwhelm the sensitized nervous system and exacerbate symptoms. Moseley and Butler[1] suggest that the entire three-phase approach be performed sequentially. This is a graded approach to cortical activation using techniques that activate cortical regions affiliated with movement preparation (priming) and then slowly staging movement execution of sight.[29] Laqueux and associates[31] reported on seven patients with CRPS who were treated with a modified GMI program and who had lessened pain as reflected on the short form McGill pain Questionnaire ($P = .046$), grip force improvement ($P = .042$), and global impression of change ($P = .015$) but not improved function on the DASH (Disabilities of the Arm, Shoulder and Hand) questionnaire.

All three phases of GMI use the principle of graded exposure; some studies have demonstrated that premature exposure to sensory or motor stimuli in patients with CRPS and limb pain leads to activation of painful neurotags.[1] The phasing in from left–right identification to motor imagery and then followed by mirror therapy follows the principles of graded exposure and is less likely to set off a painful neurotag or central sensitization. The goal in pain management with GMI is to achieve movement with decreased pain without causing increased symptoms. There is research backing the graded exposure theory that reveals improvement in cortical representation or reorganization in the brains neural network.[1,13,17] Moseley and Butler[1] stated that GMI helps prevent adverse responses by avoiding nonproductive neural pathways and reinforcing the development of productive pathways. Many have just looked at mirror therapy rather than all three phases of GMI,[30] and other studies have looked at the entire GMI process.[1] It is important to emphasize that GMI is just one part of treating patients with persistent chronic pain and should be combined with other therapies.

PAIN AND GRADED MOTOR IMAGERY

Within the past 2 decades, progress has been made in the understanding of the changes in the CNS when there is persistent pain. According to Melzack's[32] neuromatrix theory published in 1996, a combination of cortical mechanisms, when activated, produces danger for the brain and pain.

The brain considers multiple inputs when interpreting whether the incoming stimuli are dangerous to the body. The brain then evaluates all inputs and decides if protective action is needed, which determines the response. Researchers have determined that pain disrupts the body schema and the internal cortical representation of the involved limb in the homunculus, thus causing proprioceptive and sensorimotor dysfunctions, such as dystonia. Melzack[32] states that pain is produced by the brain after a neural signature has been activated and the brain concludes that the body is in danger.[1,31] Thus, a neurotag is formed by neurons that have learned to link with each other in the interpretation of a single input and therefore produce a programmed output. With GMI, we want to turn off painful neurotags and turn on painless neurotags. GMI works on the underlying mechanism that neural networks, which are normally involved in movement planning and execution, are also equally active during perception, perceptual reorganization, and imagined movements.[27] In recent years, it has become increasingly clear that pain includes both peripheral and central features.[23] The management of hands and upper extremities after musculoskeletal injuries has traditionally focused on the tissue, joint or bone involvement, and the signs and symptoms originating from the physiological impairments. The peripheral identification of symptoms works for acute injuries, but when pain persists and symptoms increase, the therapist should consider that there is CNS plastic reorganization.[33] This involvement of the CNS is called *central sensitization (central sensitivity)* and, after acute injury or immobilization, should be addressed at the initial visit. This amplification of neural signaling within the CNS elicits pain and hypersensitivity and is considered a form of maladaptive plasticity.[11,34]

The early indications for the use of GMI as described by Moseley[34] were for CRPS, phantom limb, and stroke. These three conditions involve cortical abnormalities or changes, and Moseley suggested that sequential cortical organization treatment without setting off a painful neurotag was necessary. In previous research, Moseley found that early movement of the involved limb in patients with CRPS evoked intolerable pain, and activating neural networks first, without movement, would reduce pain and swelling in patients with CRPS.[1,24] Moseley's research with 13 patients with chronic CRPS compared a motor imagery program with ongoing therapy without GMI. The GMI program consisted of 2 weeks each of hand laterality recognition tasks or left–right identification and imagined hand movements for another 2 weeks followed by mirror therapy. The results showed that not starting with limb movement but instead starting with left–right recognition is effective for patients with CRPS.[25]

A 1995 research study by Flor and associates[6] proved that there is neuronal activation in the somatosensory cortical area representing the amputated limb during the patient's experience of phantom pain. Flor and associates[6] proposed that mirror therapy would reverse the cortical reorganization seen in patients with phantom limb pain and would alleviate the pain; this theory was supported through brain imaging. There is a relationship between the cortical reorganization and pain: as the cortical changes reverse and return to normal, the pain reduces, correlating with the maladaptive reorganization.[6,13] This illustrates that pain is a complex and dynamic process that is unique to each patient with pain. Therefore, incorporating GMI (i.e., retraining the brain) is necessary when treating patients with persistent pain.

Stroke and Graded Motor Imagery

Recovery after stroke depends on the remaining cortical sensorimotor networks for functional recovery and the reorganization processes. Neural reorganization depends on the information provided by sensorimotor efferent–afferent feedback loops.[35] When a functional area or system of the brain is completely damaged, recovery is achieved by other areas of the brain that are recruited to take over the functions of the area damaged by stroke.[36–38] Priming, as described by Stoykov and Madhaan,[39] is a change in behavior based on previous stimuli. The general theory about priming is that the brain that has been primed by prior activation is generally more responsive to accompanying or subsequent training. It has been suggested that GMI may be a priming technique. Studies on brain mapping have investigated motor priming as a tool for inducing neuroplasticity and enhancing the effects of rehabilitation. Other research has studied priming as a way to facilitate motor learning. In a 2011 article, Pomeroy and coworkers[40] categorized priming as a restorative intervention that reduces impairment by targeting underlying neural mechanisms in neurologic disorders such as stroke. Evidence has shown that GMI, as a targeted intervention designed to improve sensorimotor recovery in upper and lower extremities, to increase the functional use of the extremities, and to work in conjunction with conventional therapies directly influences brain changes or brain reorganization. However, current evidence has also shown that motor imagery may provide additional benefits to conventional therapies for neurologic injuries. More randomized studies are needed to assess the benefits of motor imagery for cortical insults in both acute

and chronic conditions. Further information on this subject is beyond the scope of this chapter and can be reviewed in an article by Muratori and coworkers[41] in the *Journal of Hand Therapy*. GMI seems to be a feasible tool to consider when used with conventional stroke therapies.[39]

Implications for Upper Extremity and Hand Rehabilitation

Symptoms after injury to the hand and upper extremity most often are related to acute musculoskeletal consequences and can be addressed by determining the tissue involved and developing the appropriate treatment strategies. After soft tissue, nerve, and bone injury of the hand, neuroscientific evidence over the years has shown that the primary sensory and motor areas of the cortex can change as a consequence of injury. In a 2017 randomized controlled study after distal radius fractures, 36 participants were randomly selected for the GMI ($n = 17$) or the control group ($n = 19$). The GMI group received traditional therapy with GMI, and the control group received traditional therapy for 8 weeks. The GMI group had improved range of motion as well as improved function on the DASH outcome measure with less pain.[42] Patients who have been immobilized may develop persistent pain and abnormal sensations such as allodynia and hyperalgesia. Allodynia and hyperalgesia are symptoms of CNS involvement called *central sensitization*.[34] Treating these symptoms by only addressing the peripheral changes is not always adequate. Strategies targeting brain changes are necessary, and the use of GMI is indicated. Individual case studies and a few small sample population studies reveal improvement in sensorimotor recovery after stroke using mirror therapy alone or using GMI. Polli and coworkers[43] used GMI in a nonrandomized controlled study of the clinical effect of GMI in 28 stroke patients (14 experimental and 14 control participants). The Wolf Motor Function Test and the 66-point motor section of the Fugl-Meyer Assessment were used to assess the outcomes of treatment for both groups. The experimental group treated with GMI had better outcome scores than the control group treated with conventional therapy.[43]

CONCLUSION

The cortical representation of the body and the cortical reorganization that occurs after injury and immobilization and the functional consequences should be considered in all patients.[33] GMI is not a preset program but a guideline for progressing patients starting with non-movement and progressing into movement therapies as the symptoms decline. As with other therapy treatments, GMI must be individually tailored for each patient and should not be used as a single treatment choice but incorporated into the overall treatment program. GMI is one of the treatments to arise from the paradigm shift in neuroplasticity.[35] Moseley and Butler[1] in their 2012 *Graded Motor Imagery Handbook* stress the importance of educating the patient in the updated neuroscience of pain before starting GMI. This knowledge allows the patient to be in control and not a passive recipient of treatment. For GMI to be successful, the therapist must use clinical reasoning regarding the timing and progression of GMI. At this time, few studies exist that identify the parameters of GMI, such as time frames and frequency. In general, brief sessions offered throughout the day are recommended (e.g., 15 minutes at a time for at least five to eight sessions daily).

In summary, GMI can be useful for upper extremity injuries in patients who have pain or do not want to move, patients who have kinesophobia (i.e., fear of movement), and patients who lack sensory motor control. Further research is needed to define parameters for the use of GMI for specific diagnostic groups. Although this treatment technique is in need of further research support, evidence is mounting advocating its benefits.

REFERENCES

1. Moseley LG, Butler DS, Beames TB, Giles TJ. *The Graded Motor Imagery Handbook*. Adelaide, Australia: NOIi Group Publication; 2012.
2. Flor H. Cortical Reorganization and Chronic Pain: implication for rehabilitation. *J Rehabil Med Suppl*. 2003;41:66–72.
3. Flor H. The modification of cortical reorganization and chronic pain by sensory feedback. *Appl Psychophysiol Biofeedback*. 2012;27(3):215–227.
4. Harris AJ. Cortical origin of pathological pain. *Lancet*. 1999;354:464–466.
5. Cacchio A, De Blasis E, DeBlasis V, et al. Mirror therapy in complex regional pain syndrome type 1 of the upper limb in stroke patients. *Neurorehabil Neural Repair*. 2009;23:792–799.
6. Flor H, Denke C, Shaefer M, Grusser S. Effects of sensory discrimination training on cortical reorganization. *Lancet*. 2001;352:1763–1764.
7. Maihofner C, Handwerker H, Neundorfer B, et al. Patterns of cortical reorganization in complex regional pain syndrome. *Neurology*. 2003;61:1707–1715.
8. Schwoebel J, Friedman R, Duda N, et al. Pain and the body schema-evidence for peripheral effects on mental representation of movement. *Brain*. 2001;124:2098–2104.
9. Hudson M, McCormick K, Zalucki N, et al. Expectation of pain replicates the effect of pain in a hand laterality task: bias in information processing toward the painful side? *Eur J Pain*. 2006;10:219–224.
10. Lundborg G. Peripheral Nerve Injuries: pathophysiology and strategies for treatment. *J Hand Ther*. 1993.
11. Merzenich M, de Charms C. Neural representations experience and change. In: Llinass R, Churchland P, eds. *The Mind Brain Continuum*. 1996:61–81.
12. Byl N, Merzenich M. The neural consequences of repetitions; clinical implications of a learned hypothesis. *J Hand Ther*. 197;10:160–174
13. Flor H, Elbert T, Knecht S, et al. Phantom limb pain as a perpetual correlate of cortica reorganization following arm amputation. *Nature*. 1995;375:482–484.
14. Moseley L, Gallace A, Spence C. Bodily illusions in health and disease: physiological and clinical perspectives and the concept and the concept of a cortical body matrix. *Neurosci Biobehav Rev*. 2012;36:34–46.
15. Ramachandran VS. Phantom limbs, neglect syndromes, repressed memories, and Freudian psychology. *Int Re Neurobio*. 1994;37:291–333.
16. Rizzolatti G, Singalia C. The mirror neuron system. *Annal Re Neurosci*. 27:169–191.
17. Fadiga L, Di Pellegrino G, Singalia C, et al. Understanding motor events, a neurophysiological study. *Exp Brain Res*. 1992;91:176.
18. Ramachandran V, Rodgers-Rmachandran D. Synaesthesia in phantom limb induced with mirrors. *Prac Bio Sci*. 1996;263:3377–3386.
19. Rock I, Victor J. Vision and Touch: an experimental created conflict between the two senses. *Science*. 1964;143:594–596.
20. Pain syndrome and phantom limb pain. *Neurosci Letters*. 2010;486(3):240–245.
21. Reinersmann A, Haameyer G, Blankenburg M, et al. Left is where the L is right. Significantly delayed reaction time in limb laterality recognition in both complex regional pain syndrome and phantom limb pain. *Neurosci Letters*. 2010;486(3):240–245.
22. Moseley LG, Bray H. Disrupted working body schema of the trunk in people with back pain. *Br J Sports Med*. 45:168–173
23. Priganc V, Stralka S. Graded motor imagery. *J Hand Ther*. 2011;24:164–169.
24. Moseley G, Acerra N. Complex regional pain syndrome is associated with distorted body schema of the affected part. *Neuro Sci*. 2005;238:5501–5505.
25. Moseley G. Is successful treatment of complex regional pain syndrome due to sustained attention to the affected. *Limb*. 2006;114:5461.
26. Guilliot A, Moschberger K, Collet C. Coupling movement with imagery as a new perspective for motor imagery practice. *Behav Brain Funct*. 2013;9:9081–9089.
27. Lotze M, Halsband U. Motor imagery. *J Physiol Paris*. 2006;99:386–395.
28. Parsons LM. Integrating cognitive psychology, neurology and neuroimaging. *Acta Psychol (Amst)*. 2001;107:155–181.
29. Wang J, Fritzsch C, Bernarding J, et al. A comparison of neural mechanisms in mirror therapy and movement observation therapy. *J Rehabil Med*. 2013;45:410–413.
30. McCabe CS, Haigh RC, Ring EFJ, et al. A controlled pilot study of the utility of mirror visual feedback in the treatment of complex regional pain syndrome. *Rheumatology*. 2003;42:97–101.
31. Laqueux E, Charest J, Caron EL, et al. Modified graded motor imagery for complex regional syndrome type 1 of the upper extremity in the acute phase: a patient series. *Int J Rehab Res*. 2012;35:138–145.
32. Melzack R. Evolution of the Neuromatrix Theory of Pain. The Prithvi Raj Lecture: presented at the Third World Congress of World Institute of Pain, Barcelona 2004. At 2005 World Institute of Pain. *Reprinted Pain Practice*. 2005;5(2):85–94.
33. Neblett R. The central sensitization inventory (CSI) establishing clinically significant values for identifying central sensitization in out patients. *J Pain*. 2013;14(5):428–445.
34. Moseley GL. Graded motor imagery for pathologic pain: a randomized controlled trial. *Neurology*. 2006;67. 2139–2134.
35. Najiha A, Jagatheesan A, Rathod VJ. Mirror therapy: a review of evidences. *Int J Physio and Res*. 2015;3(3):1086–1090.
36. Seniow J, Bilik M, Lesniak M, et al. Transmagnetic stimulation combined with physiotherapy in rehabilitation of poststroke hemiparesis: a randomized double-blind, placebo-controlled study. *Neurorehabil Neural Repair*. 2012;26(9):1072–1079.
37. Kopp B, Kunkel W, Muhlnickel K, et al. Plasticity in the motor system related to therapy-induced improvement after stroke. *Neuroreport*. 10;(199):807–810.
38. Carey L, Seitz R. Functional neuroimaging in stroke recovery and neurorehabilitation: conceptual issues and perspectives. *Int J Stroke*. 2007;2(4):245–264.
39. Stoykov M, Madhaan S. Motor priming in neurorehabilitation. *J Neuro Phy Thr*. 2015;39:33–39.
40. Pomeroy VN, Ward NS, Johansen-Berg H, et al. Clinical efficacy of functional strength training for upper limb motor recovery early after stroke: neural correlates and prognostic indicators. *Int J Stroke*. 2014;9(2):240–245.
41. Muratori LM, Lamberg EM, Quinn L, Duff SV. Applying principles of motor learning and control to upper extremity rehabilitation. 2013;26(2):94–102.
42. Dilek B, Ayhan C, Yagci, Yakut Y. Effectiveness of GMI to improve hand function in pts with distal radius fractures: a randomized controlled trial. *J Hand Ther*. 2017.
43. Polli A, Mosely GL, Gioia E, et al. Graded motor imagery for patients with stroke: a non-randomized controlled trial of a new approach. *Eur J Phys Rehabil Med*. 2017;53:14–23.

101

The Use of Physical Agents in Hand Rehabilitation

Jane M. Fedorczyk, Christina M. Read

OUTLINE

CRITICAL POINTS

- Physical agents should be incorporated into the plan of care with other therapy interventions.
- Signs of cold sensitivity should be monitored for when using cryotherapy.
- The use of thermal agents should be avoided if the sympathetic autonomic efferents are not functioning because of nerve injury or vessel repair.
- Neuromuscular electrical nerve stimulator treatments should be monitored by the therapist to ensure quality contractions.
- More evidence is needed to support the use of physical agents in hand therapy practice.

Physical agents are included in the plan of care for hand and upper extremity patients to decrease pain, increase range of motion (ROM), increase muscle strength, and facilitate tissue healing. To use physical agents in a safe and judicious manner, therapists should have a strong foundation of the biophysical properties, clinical indications, precautions, and contraindications. Therapists need to perform a comprehensive clinical examination to determine whether the use of a physical agent is warranted and to determine treatment effectiveness. It is beyond the scope of this chapter to cover all aspects of the use of physical agents to the depth that they would be covered in an entry-level therapy course. Key texts are available for readers who desire additional information.[1,2] In recent years, several states have adjusted practice act requirements; therefore, readers are advised to investigate state licensure laws to determine individual professional limitations or requirements before applying physical agents in the clinic.

In the first part of this chapter, the theory and principles of each group of physical agents commonly used in hand therapy are discussed. In the second part of this chapter, the clinical application of physical agents to address impairments common to patients with hand and upper extremity injuries is discussed.

THERMAL AGENTS

Thermal agents rely on several methods of heat transfer to alter the temperature of the target tissue. Table 101.1 reviews the different methods of heat transfer and the associated thermal agents. Thermotherapy consists of superficial and deep heating agents that increase tissue temperature at different levels of penetration. Cryotherapy techniques reduce tissue temperature by removing heat from the tissues in direct contact with the cold agent. Thermal agents should always be used as adjuncts to other

therapeutic interventions that will help achieve the established therapy goals. Therapists should understand the biophysical principles, clinical indications, precautions, and contraindications for safe and effective use of thermal agents. Box 101.1 outlines the precautions and contraindications for the use of thermal agents; in particular, impaired sensation or circulation will limit the use of thermal agents because of diminished temperature regulation capabilities. The vasa nervosum and nervi vasorum control vasomotor response in arteries (Fig. 101.e1). If the nerve is injured or impaired, these sympathetic autonomic efferents may not be able to communicate with the nearby artery to signal the appropriate vasomotor response to an environmental temperature change, and tissue damage may occur.[3] Information on treatment parameters and application techniques for ultrasound, superficial heating agents, and cryotherapy are outlined in Table 101.e1.

Superficial Heating Agents

Superficial heating agents include hydrocollator packs, air-activated heat wraps, paraffin, heating pads, and Fluidotherapy (DJO Global, Dallas, TX). These agents can increase tissue temperature as much as 2 cm in depth; therefore, they work well in the hand and wrist. The depth of penetration will depend on (1) the physical agent used, (2) the composition of the target tissue, (3) the duration of treatment, (4) the initial temperature difference, and (5) how long the agent stays hot.

Tissue temperatures must be elevated between 40° and 45°C (104°–113°F) to achieve therapeutic benefit.[4] Above this range, there is the potential for tissue injury, and below this range, the therapeutic benefits may not be achieved because the heating is considered to be mild. The proposed benefits of therapeutic heating include vasodilation or increased blood flow, decreased pain, increased tissue extensibility, and decreased muscle tension.

TABLE 101.1   Methods of Heat Transfer for Agents Commonly Used in Hand Therapy

Method	Definition	Associated Thermal Agent(s)
Conduction	Transfer of thermal energy by direct contact between two surfaces	Hot packs Paraffin Commercial cold packs Ice bags Ice massage
Convection	Transfer of thermal energy by fluid movement from one place to another	Fluidotherapy
Conversion	The transition of one form of energy to another (e.g., mechanical energy to kinetic energy)	Ultrasound

BOX 101.1   Precautions and Contraindications for Physical Agents

Heat Contraindications
1. Decreased sensation to thermal or painful stimuli
2. Vascular compromise or disease
3. Recent or potential hemorrhage

Heat Precautions
1. Area of malignancy
2. Area of untreated infection; okay 24 hours after antibiotic therapy started
3. Acute inflammation or injury (wait at least 48 hours)
4. Corn allergy (Fluidotherapy)
5. Not advised to use in combination with liniments, heat rubs, and herbal packs

Cold Contraindications
1. Identified cold-sensitive conditions
    a. Cold urticaria
    b. Cryoglobulinemia
    c. Paroxysmal cold hemoglobinuria
    d. Raynaud's phenomenon or disease
2. Decreased sensation to thermal or painful stimuli
3. Vascular compromise or disease
4. Over open wounds

Cold Precautions
1. Hypertension
2. Aversion to cold therapy
3. Thermoregulatory disorders
4. Prolonged exposure to cold

Ultrasound Contraindications
1. Include heat contraindications listed
2. Should not be performed over the eyes, heart, or reproductive organs
3. Should not be performed over a pregnant uterus
4. Should not be used within a known malignant area
5. Should not be used with patients with cardiac pacemakers
6. Caution and selective use over epiphyseal plates of children

Ultrasound Precautions
Lower intensity may be needed due to refractory effects with

1. Metal plates, screws, pins, external fixators
2. Joint replacement components

Electrotherapy Contraindications
1. Unshielded cardiac pacemakers or other implanted electrical devices (may interfere with normal operation)
2. Should not be performed over a pregnant uterus
3. Should not be performed over carotid sinus
4. Should not be performed over thoracic region of body
5. Should not be used within area of deep venous thrombosis; risk of thrombus or embolism

Electrotherapy Precautions
1. Pain serving a protective function
2. Area of infection, malignancy, or peripheral vascular disease; FDA does not directly state, but increases in circulation may exacerbate these conditions
3. Excessive adipose tissue may require higher current amplitudes
4. Decreased sensation to thermal or painful stimuli (direct current)
5. Damaged or fragile skin or open skin surface
6. Contraindications, allergies, or previous adverse reactions associated with medications or substances used in iontophoresis
7. Adverse skin reactions at electrode interface
    a. Irritation
    b. Allergic reaction to adhesive polymer electrodes
    c. Direct current, especially from cathode
    d. Unbalanced biphasic pulsed-current waveforms

Patient-Specific Precautions
1. Age
2. Altered cardiorespiratory status (e.g., acute myocardial infarction, congestive heart failure, high blood pressure, low blood pressure, chronic obstructive pulmonary disease)
3. Patients unable to provide feedback or follow directions
    a. Infants or small children
    b. Cognitive ability
    c. Language barriers

FDA, Food and Drug Administration.

The increase in blood flow is limited primarily to the skin located beneath the heat source. Vasodilation occurs in response to the heat to regulate tissue temperature to prevent a burn. There is a secondary vasodilation response in coordination with a spinal cord reflex that is stimulated by the heating of cutaneous afferents. No change in skeletal muscle blood flow is expected. Along with the increased blood flow, metabolic rate (cellular activity) and oxygen saturation within the local tissue increase.[5] Although these effects are only observed while the tissue temperature is elevated, these hemodynamic and metabolic effects may facilitate tissue healing.

Elevation of tissue temperature creates some temporary neuromuscular effects that may reduce pain and muscle tension. These changes only occur when the tissue temperature is elevated and maintained. As tissue temperature decreases, the neuromuscular effects reverse. Sensory nerve conduction velocity increases with elevated temperature.[6,7] Because the increase in temperature is temporary, the therapeutic benefit is unclear, but it may contribute to a reduction in pain. Elevation of muscle temperature decreases the firing rate of the muscle spindle afferents (type II afferents) and increases the firing rate of the type Ib afferents from the Golgi tendon organs.[4,8] These changes in firing rates lead to a decrease in alpha motor neuron activity and thus a reduction in muscle (extrafusal fiber) activity. Superficial heat may not sufficiently increase muscle temperature to achieve these neuromuscular effects, but the heating of skin does decrease gamma efferent firing, which elicits a similar response.[9] Basically, skeletal muscles heated to at least 42°C (107.6°F) relax and become more flexible. The therapeutic benefits may be decreased pain and increased ROM, especially if muscle guarding or spasm is present.

There are several proposed mechanisms for pain modulation with heat modalities. The counterirritant theory suggests that thermal receptors in the target tissue are activated and conduct impulses about temperature increases in the tissue environment more quickly than impulses from pain fibers.[10] This physiologic response is related to the gating mechanism of pain.[11] Increases in tissue temperature also increase the activation threshold of pain fibers (nociceptors), which may reduce the number of pain signals sent to the spinal cord. The elevated threshold of nociceptors may also be related to a decrease in chemical mediators within the target tissue that either activate or sensitize nociceptors. The increased blood flow associated with temperature elevation may remove these chemical mediators and decrease nociceptor activity in the local tissue.

Tissue extensibility also increases with temperature increases.[12,13] The viscosity of ground substance in collagen connective tissues such as joint capsule, ligaments, and tendons decreases. Because of the neuromuscular effects, there is increased muscle flexibility. Although these effects are seen only while the tissue temperature is elevated, the decreased perception of joint stiffness allows the patient to participate in ROM exercises.

Ultrasound

Ultrasound is considered a deep heating agent. It is probably the most widely used physical agent in hand therapy practice. Treatments are likely to be ineffective if the (1) ultrasound treatment is not focused on the correct structure, (2) dosing parameters are incorrect, and (3) the transducer is moved too quickly. Electrical energy is converted into mechanical energy (sound propagation) via the piezoelectric effect. A ceramic or quartz piezoelectric crystal located within the transducer expands and contracts from the applied electrical current (Fig. 101.1). The crystal creates an electric voltage potential that replicates the sound wave pattern determined by the selected frequency. The sound waves are initially propagated longitudinally into the target tissue and then transversely at bone or metal interfaces. These sound waves leave the transducer as a collimated focused beam similar to a flashlight. The larger the sound head, the more collimated the beam. Molecules and cells within the target tissue expand and contract to produce vibration (Fig. 101.2). The vibration increases kinetic energy of the molecules, which increases tissue temperature, provided the ultrasound was delivered in the continuous mode with sufficient intensity.[14]

Frequency determines the depth of penetration within the target tissue. The collimated beam is more divergent with the 1-MHz transducer, which will transmit sound waves through the superficial tissue layers so that the ultrasound energy will be absorbed in deeper tissues

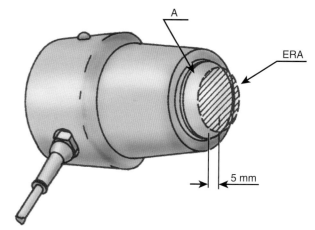

Fig. 101.1 The *shaded area* is the piezoelectric crystal (transducer) mounted in the ultrasound applicator. The effective radiating area (ERA) of the transducer is noted. (Used with permission of Henley International, Sugar Land, TX.)

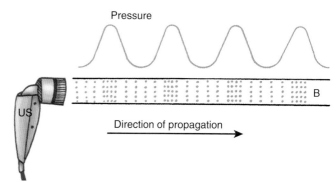

Fig. 101.2 Diagram of a collimated ultrasound beam *(B)* coming from an ultrasound *(US)* applicator. The associated pressure wave is diagrammed above. Areas of increased molecular concentration (:::) are condensations. Areas of decreased molecular concentration are rarefactions (:.:). (From Ziskin MC, McDiarmid T, Michlovitz SL. Therapeutic ultrasound. In: Michlovitz SL, ed. *Thermal Agents in Rehabilitation.* 2nd ed. Philadelphia: FA Davis; 1990.)

at 2 to 5 cm. Energy is absorbed in the superficial tissue layers up to 2 cm with the 3-Hz sound head. Ultrasound is absorbed within tissues with a high protein content (e.g., collagen); thus, collagen-rich connective tissues such as tendon, ligament, and joint capsule absorb sound waves well.[14]

Acoustic impedance occurs at tissue interfaces such as bone. Sound waves are reflected away from the bone either in the opposite direction or transversely. Standing waves may occur if the longitudinal incident waves are superimposed on reflected sound waves. Standing waves are known as "hot spots" and have the potential to cause tissue damage. Excessive heating of the periosteum at the bone interface may also cause pain because of standing waves. If this occurs during treatment, the patient usually pulls away from the transducer and reports pain. This is a clinical sign of standing wave formation, and treatment should be modified or discontinued for that session. Standing waves can be avoided if the transducer is kept moving, if the 3-MHz frequency is selected, and if the intensity is not too high.[14]

The effective radiating area (ERA) is the portion of the transducer that actually produces and emits sound waves. The beam nonuniform ratio (BNR) compares the maximum point intensity on the transducer

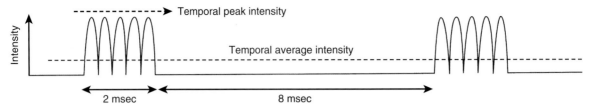

Fig. 101.3 A typical pulsing pattern. The total pulse period is 10 msec. The pulse duration is 2 msec. The duty cycle is 0.20 (20%). (From Ziskin MC, McDiarmid T, Michlovitz SL. Therapeutic ultrasound. In: Michlovitz SL, ed. *Thermal Agents in Rehabilitation.* 2nd ed. Philadelphia: FA Davis; 1990.)

(spatial peak intensity) with the average spatial intensity across the sound head (spatial average intensity). The lower the BNR is, the more evenly distributed the energy from the transducer. Optimally, the BNR should be 1:1, but manufacturing guidelines require the BNR to be 6:1 or lower. Most units on the market today have an ERA equal to the size of the transducer face plate with the perimeter emitting less energy than the center of the face plate and a BNR of 6:1. The manufacturer specifications or equipment manuals supply this information. A variety of sizes of applicators are available for use, ranging from 0.5 to 5.0 cm^2.

Ultrasound waves markedly attenuate in air. Therefore, air between the applicator face and body surface must be eliminated or minimized. A coupling medium such as a commercially available water-soluble gel is spread in a layer between the applicator and skin surface. If a small irregular area is to be treated with ultrasound, a small applicator with a gel pad interface can be used.[15] Coupling through a water bath[16] or water-filled balloon[15] is less efficient.

Therapists have the option to select continuous or pulsed-wave ultrasound treatments. With pulsed-wave ultrasound, the intensity is periodically interrupted so that no ultrasound energy is being produced during the off time in the duty cycle. Continuous-wave ultrasound produces thermal and nonthermal effects, whereas pulsed-wave ultrasound emphasizes the nonthermal effects of ultrasound because heat does not really accumulate. This is a result of the dissipation of heat by conduction during the off time of the pulse period. Duty cycles may be calculated by dividing the duration of the pulse (on time) by the pulse period (on time + off time). Therefore, if the pulse is 2 seconds of a 10-second pulse period, the duty cycle would be 20%.[14] Figure 101.3 shows a typical pulsed-wave ultrasound pattern. The physiologic effects of a particular duty cycle are unclear. Low-duty cycles of 10% or 20% have been studied in chronic wound healing, but no other work has been demonstrated at high-duty cycles.

Spatial average intensity is the rate at which ultrasound energy (in watts) is delivered and averaged over the area of the transducer (in square centimeters).[14] Intensity is the strength of the ultrasound treatment. All factors held constant, the greater the intensity is, the greater the tissue temperature elevation with continuous ultrasound. Most units display spatial average intensity. When using pulsed-wave ultrasound, the temporal average intensity can be calculated by multiplying the duty cycle by the spatial average intensity. For example, if the spatial average intensity selected was 2.0 W/cm^2 and the duty cycle is 20%, the temporal average intensity is 0.4 W/cm^2. Although the temporal average intensity over the pulse period is low, it is still 2.0 W/cm^2 during the pulse period, which may be too high for some target tissues in the upper extremity. There are no clear-cut guidelines on how to select a treatment intensity, but the World Health Organization does set an upper limit of 3.0 W/cm^2 ultrasound units. The correct intensity will achieve the desired goal and do no harm.

Selecting continuous- or pulsed-wave mode determines whether the thermal or nonthermal effects will predominate during the ultrasound treatment. Thermal effects are related to temperature elevation and are the same as those for the superficial heating agents discussed

TABLE 101.2 Comparisons of Physiologic Effects of Heat Versus Cold		
Cryotherapy		**Thermotherapy**
↓	Pain	↓
↓	Blood flow and metabolic activity	↑
↓	Nerve conduction velocity	↑
↓	Muscle spasm	↓
↓	Muscle and tissue elasticity and extensibility	↑
↑	Tissue healing	↑
↑	Heart rate	↑
↑	Blood pressure	↓

previously. The two primary nonthermal effects are cavitation and acoustic streaming.[14] Cavitation is the formation of gas bubbles within the cells in response to the vibration within the target tissue. Stable cavitation may enhance cellular diffusion, but unstable cavitation may result in cell implosion and tissue damage.[4] Unstable cavitation can be avoided by selecting the pulsed-wave mode and using lower treatment intensities in the continuous-wave mode. Acoustic streaming is the movement of fluids and gas bubbles within cells in response to vibration. Acoustic streaming is theorized to facilitate cell membrane permeability and ion exchange, which have potential tissue healing benefits.[17]

Ultrasound has all the same clinical indications as the superficial heating agents discussed previously, but it focuses on smaller treatment areas and may target structures greater than 2 cm in depth. Most structures in the wrist and hand can be sufficiently heated to elevate tissue temperature to a therapeutic level, but ultrasound as a deep heating agent is needed for similar indications at the forearm, elbow, and shoulder. Ultrasound may promote tissue healing first by increasing blood flow and oxygenation caused by thermal effects and second as a result of the nonthermal effects. Studies of delayed-healing wounds have demonstrated that low-intensity pulsed-wave ultrasound, which emphasizes nonthermal effects, releases growth factors from macrophages, increases angiogenesis, and facilitates collagen production.[17] These benefits promote the fibroplasia phase of tissue healing. During remodeling, tensile strength may increase when thermal ultrasound is combined with controlled stress exercises. Increased tissue extensibility will facilitate collagen reorganization and gains in tensile strength.

Cryotherapy

The physiologic effects of cold are for the most part the exact opposite of those associated with thermotherapy. Table 101.2 reviews these comparisons. Cold is primarily used after acute injury or surgery to control pain and edema. The normal patient response to cold in terms of sensory changes is the feeling of cold followed by burning, pain or discomfort, tingling, and numbness.[18] Although the timing is not standardized among patients, the order of these sensory changes is

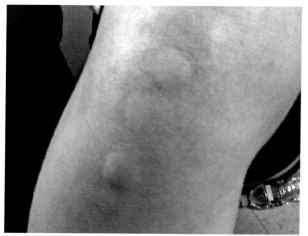

Fig. 101.4 Wheal formation, or local cold urticaria, after ice massage to the knee.

consistent. It is this author's experience that patients do not tolerate ice bags or ice baths applied directly to the hand but do find ice applied directly to the shoulder or elbow tolerable. Commercial cold packs are more commonly used at the hand and wrist.

The application of cold results in decreased blood flow and vasoconstriction in response to decreases in tissue temperature.[19,20] Vasoconstriction is an immediate response to attempt to regulate temperature. There is a decrease in blood viscosity, which further reduces blood flow. Prolonged cold exposure such as in an ice bath below 10°C (50°F) may result in a reflex vasodilation called the hunting response.[20] This response is usually observed in the skin, but it may occur in deeper tissues as well.

There may also be a decrease in the inflammatory response if cold is applied immediately after injury.[19–22] Because of the decrease in blood flow, the chemical mediators associated with inflammation such as histamine and prostaglandins may not be able to circulate and promote vasodilation. Decreased blood flow also reduces metabolic activity, including the synthesis of prostaglandins that mediate inflammation. There is also a decrease in oxygen uptake within cells caused by reduced metabolic demand. With prolonged cold exposure, this may result in hypoxia and tissue damage, as observed in frostbite and peripheral nerve palsy.[20,21]

The mechanisms of pain modulation are similar to those with heat based on the gating mechanism and counterirritant theory.[10,11] In addition, decreased blood flow may lessen the inflammatory response and further modulate pain. Reduced edema means that there will be less tissue distention and therefore less pain. A decrease in the circulating chemical mediators that promote inflammation and activate or sensitize nociceptors will also modulate pain.

The patient may report an increase in joint stiffness or at least the perception of increased stiffness after the application of cold. The viscosity of the ground substance will increase with decreases in tissue temperature. Although muscle tension will decrease in response to cold, which may reduce muscle spasm, guarding, or spasticity, the muscles will be less flexible to movement.[23–25] With cold exposure, decreased nerve conduction velocity[26] and muscle spindle and Golgi tendon organ activity may also contribute to decreases in pain.

Several cold sensitivity symptoms and conditions need to be addressed before applying cold to hand and upper extremity patients. It is normal for the skin underlying the cold source to become red during cryotherapy because of hyperemia or vasodilation of skin blood vessels. The entire area should be red. However, if wheals or hives develop as a result of a histamine reaction, this is an allergic reaction to cold. It is called local cold urticaria, and the wheals are raised with red borders and blanching in the center[20,21] (Fig. 101.4). This is the most common

cold sensitivity condition observed, and the cold treatment should cease if a wheal develops.

Systemic urticaria is a systemic allergic reaction that results in flushing of the face, increased heart rate, and a sharp decrease in blood pressure that can lead to syncope or lightheadedness.[20] Raynaud's disease or phenomenon is a vasospastic disorder that occurs in response to cold. It usually affects the fingers, and in response to cold, the fingers blanch (pallor), become blue or purple (cyanosis), turn bright red (rubor), and then return to normal color. This cyclic response is associated with autoimmune disorders such as lupus erythematosus and rheumatoid arthritis. It has also been associated with nerve compression syndromes and trauma.[20] Patients likely know whether they have ever had any of these responses to cold, so be sure to ask about them when obtaining your patient's history during the clinical examination.

Cryoglobulinemia is associated with autoimmune conditions, chronic liver disease, multiple melanoma, and infections. In response to cold exposure, an abnormal blood protein forms a gel, decreasing blood flow and resulting in ischemia and eventually gangrene.[20] Paroxysmal cold hemoglobinuria[20] is a condition in which hemoglobin is released and lysed red blood cells can be identified in urine, although the urine is not red. Anemia develops in the patient, which may be mild or severe. Although neither of these cold sensitivity problems is common, therapists should ask patients about these conditions when obtaining their history and monitor the patients' response to cryotherapy carefully because the sequelae can be severe.

ELECTROTHERAPY

Devices and Electrodes

Electrotherapy may be used for pain modulation, for muscle reeducation, and to facilitate tissue healing. Electrotherapeutic currents are delivered across the skin using surface electrodes to disperse the current within the target tissues. A variety of electromedical devices on the market offer one or more therapeutic currents, current modulators, and channels. There are both clinical line-powered and battery-powered portable units. Portable units may be used in the clinic but also by patients at home if they have appropriate durable medical equipment coverage with their insurance plan. Many electromedical device manufacturers and distributors have consolidated or ceased operations. Therapists may recommend that patients rent or purchase devices from online sources if there is not a local vendor in their practice area. Portable units are more convenient to use during functional activity. They also may be used for pain modulation while the patient performs "controlled" therapeutic exercises or activities or to augment motor learning during functional activities such as reaching.

Electrodes are available in a variety of sizes, shapes, and materials. The success of electrotherapy begins with appropriate electrode selection, preparation, and placement. Electrodes for the hand and upper limb need to be able to conform to the target area and serve as an efficient conductor of the electrotherapeutic current. Some electrode materials are better conductors of electricity and have less resistance to current flow at the skin–electrode interface.

Metal and flexible carbon or rubber electrodes are not commonly used in therapy There are a variety of commercially available electrodes for single or multiple use that have been developed. These electrodes are coated with an adhesive polymer and come in a variety of shapes and sizes. Most have a pigtail coming from the electrode so that the lead wire from the electrotherapy unit can easily be secured to the electrode. Reusable electrodes may be used for multiple applications provided that adequate skin preparation and electrode cleansing are performed. Single-use electrodes have an adhesive quality similar to that of an adhesive bandage, which is a more appropriate choice for patients with sensitive skin and those who experienced an adverse reaction to another electrode. They are meant to be used once and thrown away. The adhesive polymers typically have some resistance to current flow, but their ease of application enhances patient compliance, and they also conform well to the hand. Patients may have an allergic reaction to the adhesive polymer. If this occurs, the electrodes should be replaced with another type, and the reaction should be reported to the electrode vendor.

Skin preparation in the area where the electrodes will be placed is essential to promote decreased skin resistance to current flow. It should make the treatment more comfortable because less current should be needed to achieve the desired clinical response. The skin should be cleansed with soap and water or rubbing alcohol to remove dirt, dry skin cells, oils, and lotions. This is important for all types of electrotherapy, but it is considered essential when performing iontophoresis. The alcohol swab is often packaged with the iontophoresis electrodes. If the skin is hairy and the electrodes cannot make uniform contact, the hair should be clipped or shaved. This author prefers trimming the hair with scissors rather than shaving. Shaving creates skin irritability, which may be exacerbated by the electrotherapeutic current.

Therapeutic Currents

There are three types of therapeutic currents: direct, alternating, and pulsed. The therapeutic current is not determined by the power source of the electromedical device. Oscillators and potentiometers within the electromedical device create the type of therapeutic current to be used for the treatment.

Direct Current

Direct current (DC) is defined as the unidirectional flow of charged particles that continues when the circuit is closed and stops when the circuit is opened.[27] The direction of flow is determined by the polarity selected. DC current is used for iontophoresis in hand therapy, but it may also be used for wound healing and to stimulate denervated muscle. The recognition of polarity is important when a treatment method requires a specific polarity such as iontophoresis. The negative electrode, termed the *cathode*, attracts positive ions from the tissue, and the *anode*, or positive electrode, attracts negative ions from the tissue.

An alkaline reaction will build up under the cathode, and an acidic reaction will build up under the anode; both may cause a skin reaction under the electrodes. The typical skin reaction is redness termed *hyperemia*, but a full-thickness burn is always a potential. The most common adverse reaction is blister formation under the electrode, especially the cathode, because the alkaline reaction is more caustic to human skin. The commercial electrodes used for iontophoresis contain buffering agents to minimize the pH changes under the electrodes and minimize the risk of skin irritation or burn.

The size of the electrode will also reduce the risk of skin irritation or burn. The electrode should be large enough to cover the target tissue and disperse the current evenly. If the electrode is too small (≤1 cm in diameter), the current cannot be dispersed and irritation or a burn is more likely. In the United States, the Food and Drug Administration (FDA) approves all electrodes. Therapists should avoid making "homemade" electrodes when using any type of electrotherapy, especially with DC, because they are not regulated by the FDA.

Alternating Current

Alternating current (AC) is the bidirectional flow of charged particles.[27] It is typically represented as a sinusoidal waveform, but it can be symmetrical or asymmetrical. A common example of a stimulator using AC is interferential current (IFC). IFC is typically used for pain modulation. IFC uses a high carrier frequency to overcome skin resistance to current flow, so it is usually considered a comfortable form of electrotherapy.

AC may be modulated and acts in a fashion similar to a biphasic pulsed current. Burst-modulated AC current or "Russian" stimulation is used for muscle strengthening. Bursting of current results in phases of current delivery that act similarly to individual pulses, but the current density is higher than with most pulsed (see next section) currents. Although commonly used for larger muscle groups such as the quadriceps and hamstrings, this type of current may be used for neuromuscular reeducation in the hand and upper extremity.

Most electrotherapy units that have IFC will also have the burst-modulated AC for muscle strengthening. This may be confusing to therapists but is an easy way to remember that IFC is used for pain modulation, so there is no way to establish on/off time ratios for muscle contractions with the IFC controls.

Pulsed Current

Pulsed current is the flow of charged particles, unidirectional or bidirectional, that is delivered in finite periods of time (microseconds), before the next electrical event. The time between electrical events or pulses does not equate to on or off time cycles. Pulsed currents are primarily used for pain modulation or neuromuscular reeducation. On an oscilloscope, the visual representation of the pulse is called a waveform.[27]

Waveforms can be monophasic or biphasic, depending on the direction of current flow. With monophasic waveforms, polarity does not change; current flow is unidirectional. In biphasic waveforms, each pulse has two phases that cross the isoelectric line of polarity; current flow is bidirectional. Biphasic pulses may be symmetrical or asymmetrical in shape (Fig. 101.5). Symmetrical biphasic waveforms are balanced; the area within each phase is equal but opposite polarity. The phases look like mirror images. Asymmetrical biphasic waveforms can be balanced or unbalanced.[27] Therapists want to use only balanced asymmetrical biphasic waveforms in clinical practice. The manufacturer's specifications located on either a product information sheet or in the user's manual will indicate that an asymmetrical biphasic waveform is balanced with the phrase "zero net DC effect." This just means that even though the phases may not look equal, the total electrical charge in each direction is the same. In an unbalanced waveform, this is not the case, so the sensation under one stimulation electrode will be more intense than under the counterpart electrode.

Measurable Characteristics of Waveforms and the Stimulus Parameters

Amplitude

Amplitude is another term for *intensity*. Both terms are used interchangeably in the peer-reviewed literature, on devices, and among clinicians. The therapist or the patient has full adjustability of the amplitude controls on any device. When the intensity of one phase is measured, the highest point of the phase is called the *peak amplitude*. When intensity measurements are taken for biphasic pulses, the distance from the isoelectric line of one phase to its peak and the distance between the isoelectric line of the other phase to its peak are combined for a *peak-to-peak amplitude*. The device manual will provide information on whether you are setting *peak* or *peak-to-peak amplitude* (Fig. 101.6).

Pulse and Phase Duration

Phase duration is the time that elapses from the beginning of the phase to the end of the phase. If the waveform is biphasic, then the two phases, the lead and decay phases, would constitute the pulse. Pulse duration is the time that elapses from the beginning of the pulse to the end of

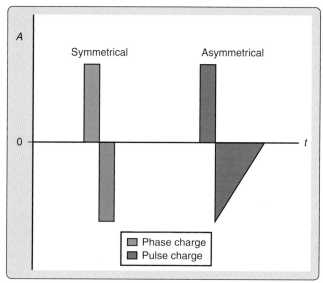

Fig 101.5 Biphasic pulses can be symmetrical or asymmetrical in shape. Pulse charge combines both phases of the pulse and phase charge keeps the phases separate. In a symmetrical biphasic pulse, the pulse charge is the same in each phase. *A,* Current amplitude in milliamps; *t,* time in microseconds; *0,* the zero point, or isoelectric line.

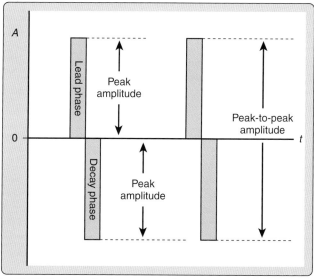

Fig. 101.6 Peak amplitude versus peak-to-peak amplitude. *A,* Current amplitude in milliamps; *t,* time in microseconds; *0,* the zero point, or isoelectric line.

the pulse. Pulse duration is also known as pulse width, but because the unit of measure is in microseconds (time), duration is the more appropriate term. Phase or pulse duration exists only for pulsed current units, and it is either preset or fully adjustable within the unit (Fig. 101.7). For clinical applications, a device with a fully adjustable pulse duration is preferred. Check the device manual to determine whether you are setting the phase or pulse duration because this varies among units. Muscle stimulators with a biphasic pulse have the therapist set the phase duration.

Other Time-Dependent Characteristics

There may be intervals of time between phases called interphase intervals. An interpulse interval is the time between pulses. As the frequency of pulses increases, the time between pulses will need to decrease to

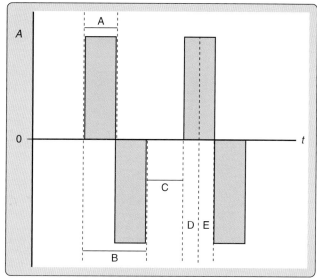

Fig. 101.7 Time-dependent characteristics of a pulse or waveform. *A,* phase duration; *B,* pulse duration; *C,* interpulse interval; *D,* rise time; *E,* fall time. *A,* Current amplitude in milliamps; *t,* time in microseconds; *0,* the zero point, or isoelectric line.

accommodate the increase in pulses. The time that it takes the leading edge of a phase to go from the isoelectric line to peak amplitude is known as the rise time, and the time that it takes the phase to return to the isoelectric line is called the decay of fall time (see Fig. 101.7).

Pulse Charge and Frequency

Pulse charge is both amplitude and time dependent. It is considered the "power of the waveform." In other words, there is a certain level of amplitude and pulse duration that must be achieved to produce the desired clinical response in addition to frequency. Some electromedical devices allow the therapist to determine the pulse charge in microcoulombs (see Fig. 101.7).

Frequency is also known as pulse rate on pulsed-current generators and as beat frequency on IFC units. Essentially, frequency is the number of pulses (pulsed current), beats (IFC), and cycles (AC) that are delivered in 1 second. If the frequency is set at 5 pulses per second (pps), then the interpulse interval times are longer than if the frequency was set at 100 pps.

Pulse charge is determined by pulse duration and amplitude. Thus, frequency, pulse duration, and amplitude are the three primary parameters that need to be manipulated to produce one of three clinical responses: (1) perceptible tingling, (2) muscle twitching, and (3) tetanizing muscle contractions. Devices that to not deliver pulsed current like IFC will rely on frequency and amplitude to achieve the clinical response to treatment.

Current Modulators

Many electrotherapy devices have a built-in ramp-up to gradually increase to peak amplitude or clinical response. This prevents a startle response in the patient and typically makes the treatment more comfortable. Some muscle stimulators have controls to allow the therapist to establish the appropriate ramp-up and ramp-down to ease in and out of tetanized muscle contractions.

Other current modulators modify amplitude, pulse or phase duration, and frequency during continuous sensory-level stimulation (perceptible tingling) to prevent sensory receptor accommodation. If the tingling response is held constant, eventually the sensory receptors in the target tissue will perceive the unchanged stimulus and will no longer fire in response to the electrical stimulus. Current modulators minimize the risk of this occurring during a treatment session

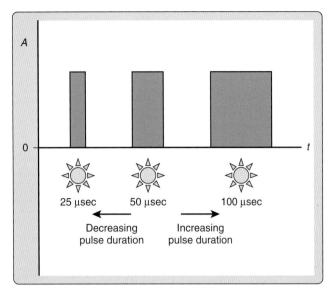

Fig. 101.8 Pulse duration modulation. *A*, Current amplitude in milliamps; *t*, time in microseconds; *0*, the zero point, or isoelectric line.

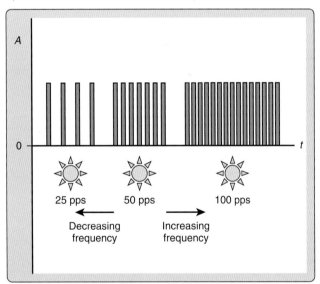

Fig. 101.9 Frequency modulation. *A*, Current amplitude in milliamps; *t*, time in microseconds; *0*, the zero point, or isoelectric line.

for pain modulation. Portable pulsed-current generators, commonly called transcutaneous electrical nerve stimulation (TENS) units, have several current modulators that may work alone or in conjunction with another. IFC units also have current modulators called scan, which is amplitude modulation, and sweep, which is frequency modulation. Current modulators never increase the parameters established by the therapist; they only modify the parameters by decreasing from the selected levels (Figs. 101.8 and 101.9).

In many applications of therapeutic current, it is desirable to alternate periods of electrical stimulation with periods of no stimulation. Many electrotherapy units allow the therapist to establish on and off time cycles. This is a requirement for neuromuscular electrical stimulation. A typical cycling for muscle stimulation for strengthening is 10 seconds of stimulation followed by 50 seconds of rest. This rest period is to minimize muscle fatigue.

Precautions and Contraindications

Therapists should carefully review the patient's history to determine that it is safe to use electrotherapy. Box 101.1 outlines the precautions

and contraindications for the use of electrotherapy. Adverse reactions to electrodes are the most common problem, so the patient's skin should be carefully inspected before and after treatment.

Electroanalgesia

Electroanalgesia is a general term to describe the outcome of using electrical stimulation for pain modulation. TENS has been commonly used to describe pain suppression with electrotherapy since Melzack and Wall[11] proposed the gate-control theory in 1965. Three modes of stimulation have been described to promote electroanalgesia: sensory, motor, and noxious.[27] Sensory and motor are commonly used in hand rehabilitation, but noxious level is not. Table 101.3 reviews parameters used for each of the levels and the theoretical level of pain modulation The parameters for each level of electroanalgesia are established based on the likelihood of stimulating specific nerve fibers: sensory, motor, and pain consistent with the strength duration curve[28,29] (Fig. 101.10).

Sensory- and Motor-Level Stimulation

Sensory- and motor-level stimulation are commonly used to modulate peripheral nociceptive- or neurogenic-mediated pain.[28] Electrode placements are on or near the site of the painful tissue. Sensory-level stimulation, also known as high rate or conventional TENS, creates a clinical response of perceptible tingling. Motor-level stimulation, also known as low-rate or "acupuncture-like" TENS, creates a clinical response of muscle twitching. At low current amplitudes, motor-level and sensory-level stimulation are very similar. The underlying mechanism for reducing pain is that the electrical current will stimulate large primary sensory afferents that may block or "gate" impulses from primary nociceptive (Ad and C) fibers. Patients typically have an immediate response to the stimulation and maintain the analgesic effect during the treatment and for a short time thereafter.[28,29]

Motor-level stimulation may be used at higher current amplitudes to cause muscle twitching. In this situation, electrodes are typically placed over motor points, peripheral nerves, or segmental nerve roots that correlate with the site of pain. A motor point is where the motor nerve branch pierces the muscle belly for innervation. Muscle twitching may be uncomfortable, so it is not recommended for acutely painful, irritable conditions. This author finds it most beneficial for pain of muscular origin. Higher amplitude motor-level stimulation may activate central mechanisms of pain modulation, including the release of endogenous opiates.[28,29]

Treatment duration in the clinic for both motor- and sensory-level electroanalgesia is usually 20 minutes; however, if used at home, electroanalgesia may be used as much as is needed to control pain. Patients may use it more or less depending on the carryover between breaks from stimulation and the pain intensity. There is little residual analgesic effect, but this may be condition and patient dependent. Sensory-level stimulation may be incorporated into a controlled exercise program as demonstrated by Rizk and coworkers[30] and Cannon[31] with patients with shoulder adhesive capsulitis and flexor tenolysis, respectively. The twitching muscle contractions used in motor-level stimulation are not conducive to being combined with controlled exercise.

Pulsed-current generators called TENS units and IFC units are commonly used for pain modulation. Both have current modulators to prevent accommodation to prolonged sensory-level stimulation. The high volt pulse current stimulator may also be used for acute or postoperative pain modulation. It does not have the current modulators found on the IFC or the pulsed-current generators, so it is not recommended for long-term pain control.

TABLE 101.3	Common Parameters of Electrical Stimulation Used for Pain Modulation		
Type	**Suggested Stimulation Parameters**	**Indications**	**Theoretic Level of Control**
Sensory-level stimulation	Pulse duration: 50–100 µsec Frequency: 80–100 pps Amplitude: tingling Treatment duration: variable Pain relief: mainly during treatment	Nociceptive pain Peripheral neurogenic pain	Local control based on gate-control theory
Motor-level stimulation	Pulse duration: 200–300 µsec Frequency: 2–10 pps Amplitude: visible muscle twitch Treatment duration: 30–45 min Pain relief: 2–6 hr after treatment	Nociceptive pain Peripheral neurogenic pain Central pain	Local control or central mechanisms
Noxious-level stimulation	Original: Pulse duration: <1 sec Frequency: 1–5 pps or >100 pps Amplitude: painful or noxious No motor response Treatment duration: brief; 2–3 sec of probe application total treatment in a few minutes Pain relief: several hours to days Current: Similar to original but delivered by electrodes not a probe Amplitude: painful or noxious No motor response Treatment duration: variable Pain relief: Several hours to days	Central pain Complex regional pain syndromes	Central mechanisms

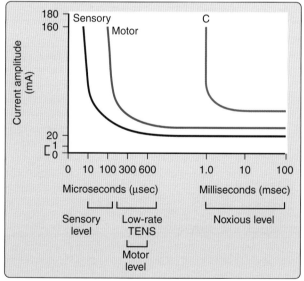

Fig. 101.10 Strength duration curves for sensory, motor, and pain fibers (*C*).

Noxious-Level Stimulation

Noxious-level stimulation, also known as electroacupuncture, and brief intense TENS are used when other methods of pain modulation have failed. The underlying mechanism for using this form of electroanalgesia is to apply a painful stimulus to target the release of endogenous opiates.[28,29] The painful stimulation is produced by creating a strong sensory response without a motor response. A burning sensation may be perceived by the patient (Fig. 101.11). This was previously performed with a specialized unit and probe.

A recent study[32] used self-adhesive gel electrodes and details are available in (Table 101.4).

Neuromuscular Electrical Stimulation

The primary clinical indication for neuromuscular electrical stimulation (NMES) is to augment muscle strength by stimulating the intact peripheral nerve to achieve a muscle contraction.[27] As a result of increasing strength, active range of motion (AROM) increases; disuse atrophy decreases; and, if present, edema may decrease. The term *functional electrical stimulation* may be used if NMES is being combined with functional training, such as orthosis substitution at the shoulder, where NMES reduces a shoulder subluxation instead of a sling or brace. NMES selectively stimulates large muscle fibers, or the fast-twitch fibers, first. This is in contrast to volitional or active exercise, which first recruits the small muscle fibers, or slow-twitch type II fibers. With postsurgical immobilization, the large fibers quickly atrophy, and NMES can selectively recruit these fibers for stimulation.[33] This makes NMES a valuable tool as an adjunct to active exercise for atrophy reduction and to increase strength.

Electrically elicited contractions are more forceful than volitional contractions because of the fiber recruitment order and the synchronous firing of motor units (motor neuron + muscle fibers that it innervates). As a result, they also produce more fatigue.[33] Patients are not able to complete as many electrically elicited contractions during an NMES session compared with volitional exercise. Higher frequencies also increase fatigue because of the increased firing rate of the motor units.

Neuromuscular Electrical Stimulation Parameters

Pulsed or burst-modulated AC may be used for NMES.[27,33,34] There are no studies that indicate that one type of electrotherapeutic current is better than another for hand and upper extremity muscles. Therapist preference and equipment availability are the likely decision-making factors. The waveforms used with pulsed-current generators may be monophasic or biphasic (asymmetrical or symmetrical, respectively). Some vendors indicate that monophasic and asymmetrical biphasic

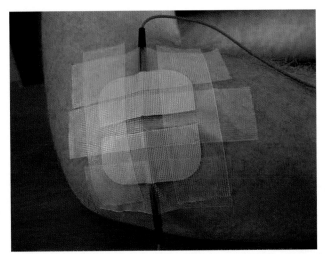

Fig. 101.11 Noxious-level stimulation electrode placement for tennis elbow. After proper skin preparation to the target area, small electrodes are placed over the focal area of pain parallel to the direction of the musculotendinous unit (common extensor tendon). As a precaution, electrodes are secured with tape to prevent migration if the patient moves or the surrounding muscle contracts.

pulsed-current waveforms are more effective for small muscles in the hand and forearm. In this author's experience, the type of current has not had much of an impact on treatment outcome.

Frequency needs to be set within the range of 30 to 80 pps to achieve a tetanic contraction.[27,33,34] Typical frequencies used for the upper extremity muscles are 35 to 55 pps. It is important to establish ramp-up and ramp-down times to create a smooth tetanic muscle contraction. Typically, a 2-second ramp up is sufficient followed by a 1-second ramp down. In patients with spasticity or high tone, longer ramp times, up and down, are recommended.[33] On most units, this ramp time is included in the on time or contraction time of the muscle, so therapists may need to increase the on time to account for the ramp times to allow sufficient contraction time at peak amplitude.

The current amplitude needs to be set high enough to allow a strong tetanic contraction.[27,33,34] The limiting factors are the patient's tolerance and fatigue. The patient needs to be informed that the strongest contractions produce the greatest strength gains. Ideally, the patient should perform 10 strong quality contractions; therefore, depending on muscle fatigue, the on/off time cycle ratios need to be between 1:3 and 1:12.[34] Therapists should look for units with the greatest range of customization to allow appropriate rest between contractions.

On a pulsed-current unit, ideally, there should be a fully adjustable pulse duration setting. The variable pulse duration allows for some fine tuning of motor unit recruitment, so as pulse duration is increased, more motor units may be recruited, and fewer are recruited as pulse duration is decreased. The latter is important to prevent current overflow into adjacent muscles. The variable pulse duration feature is particularly useful when stimulating reinnervated muscles after peripheral

TABLE 101.4	**Evidence for Using Physical Agents**			
Author (Year)	**Patient Population**	**Intervention**	**Results**	**Conclusions**
ULTRASOUND				
Desmeules et al[75] (2015)	Systematic review and meta-analysis • 11 studies included	• 2 studies compared effectiveness of therapeutic US with a placebo or control group • 8 studies compared therapeutic US with other interventions • 1 study compared two different therapeutic US dosages	• No significant benefit of including therapeutic US with an exercise program but also unable to exclude the possibility of benefit • Hyperthermia with US therapy found to be superior to therapeutic heat for overall pain and function at 10 wk	Minimal evidence to suggest US is not superior to a placebo for pain and self-reported function Minimal evidence that addition of US to an exercise program is not superior to an exercise program alone for pain and function More high-quality evidence needed to determine efficacy
NEUROMUSCULAR ELECTRICAL STIMULATION (NMES)				
Gorgey et al[76] (2009)	7 healthy individuals (6 males, 1 female)	4 NMES protocols (MVIT): 1. Standard (100-Hz, 450-μs pulses, amplitude to evoke 75% MVIT) 2. Short pulse duration (100-Hz, 150-μs pulses, amplitude to evoke 75% MVIT) 3. Low-frequency (25-Hz, 450-μs pulses, amplitude to evoke 75% MVIT) 4. Low-amplitude (100-Hz, 450-μs pulses, amplitude set to evoke 45% MVIT)	Peak torque measured before and after treatment and percent fatigue calculated: • Low-frequency protocol resulted in less fatigue than the other 3 protocols • No change in muscle fatigue when amplitude and pulse duration were decreased	Change in muscle fatigue with decreased frequency but not with a change in amplitude or pulse duration only implies correlation, not causation

Continued

TABLE 101.4 Evidence for Using Physical Agents—cont'd

TRANSCUTANEOUS ELECTRICAL STIMULATION (TENS)

Pantaleão et al[77] (2011)	56 healthy individuals (28 males, 28 females) who were TENS naïve Mean age, 22 yr (range, 18–36 yr)	4 groups (n =14 for each group): 1. Control 2. Placebo TENS 3. Fixed pulse amplitude TENS 4. Adjusted pulse amplitude TENS Treatment time, 40 minutes	• PPTs measured in dominant hand and forearm before, during, and after treatment • PPTs increased in adjusted pulse amplitude TENS group compared with all other groups in both the hand and forearm	Pulse amplitude in this shoulder should be adjusted during TENS to achieve maximal analgesic effect
Moran et al[78] (2011)	130 health individuals (65 males, 65 females) who were TENS naïve Age range, 18–64 yr	5 groups (n = 26 per group): 1. Strong nonpainful TENS 2. Sensory threshold TENS 3. Below sensory threshold TENS 4. No current placebo TENS 5. Transient placebo TENS Active TENS (80 Hz) applied for 30 min; transient placebo TENS applied for 42 sec and then automatically reset to 0mA	• PPT measured at two points in the hand and forearm before and after treatment • PPT at the forearm: significant difference between strong nonpainful TENS group compared with below sensory threshold TENS, no-current placebo TENS, and transient placebo TENS groups • PPT at the hand: significant difference between the strong nonpainful TENS group compared with the transient placebo TENS and no-current TENS • No significant difference between strong nonpainful TENS and sensory threshold TENS	TENS should be delivered at the highest intensity tolerated to produce greatest hypoalgesia
Desmeules et al[79] (2016)	Systematic review; included six studies	• TENS vs US • TENS vs corticosteroid injections • TENS vs heat	TENS vs ultrasound • TENS greater for pain relief at 3 wk • No significant difference at 4 wk • 1 study showed improved ROM in US group • 1 study showed no significant difference in ROM in either group TENS vs corticosteroid injections • Improved pain at rest, at night, and during movement with injection vs TENS TENS vs heat therapy • No significant differences between groups	No conclusions could be made on the use of TENS for the treatment of rotator cuff tendinopathy; further research needed

TABLE 101.4 Evidence for Using Physical Agents—cont'd

TRANSCUTANEOUS ELECTRICAL STIMULATION (TENS)

Macedo et al[80] (2015)	112 healthy women	7 groups (n = 16): 1. Control 2. Placebo TENS 3. Conventional TENS 4. Burst TENS 5. Cryotherapy 6. Cryotherapy and burst TENS 7. Cryotherapy and conventional TENS Interventions lasted 25 min	Pain threshold and tolerance measured with pressure algometer at lateral epicondyle before and after intervention: • Pain threshold declined in control and placebo groups • Pain threshold increased for burst TENS, cryotherapy, and cryotherapy with burst TENS groups • No change in conventional TENS and cryotherapy with conventional TENS groups • Similar results for pain tolerance • Increase in pain tolerance for cryotherapy with burst TENS significantly higher than other groups ($P < .001$)	The combination of cryotherapy and burst TENS can be effective in the reduction of pressure-induced pain

INTERFERENTIAL CURRENT (IFC)

Fuentes et al[81] (2010)	Systematic review and meta-analysis; 20 studies involving IFC included	• 7 studies: use of IFC on joint pain • 9 studies: use of IFC on muscle pain • 3 studies: use of IFC on soft tissue shoulder pain • 1 study: use of IFC on postoperative pain	• Opposing results for 2 studies focusing on IFC alone vs placebo group on pain intensity at discharge • 2 studies found IFC was not significantly better than manual therapy, traction, or massage • 3 studies found IFC used as a co-intervention was favorable compared with the control group	IFC alone was not superior to placebo or other therapy at discharge or follow-up Minimal evidence to suggest IFC used as an adjunct treatment relieves musculoskeletal pain compared with no treatment or placebo

NOXIOUS-LEVEL STIMULATION

Stackhouse et al[32] (2016)	40 asymptomatic volunteers (21 females, 19 males) between 18 and 60 yr Only 39 completed follow-up testing	3 intervention groups: 1. Cycling (n = 13) (60–70 W for 20 min) 2. Eccentric exercise (n = 14) (4 × 15 eccentric plantarflexion with full body weight on dominant leg) 3. NES (n = 13) (self-adhesive gel electrodes placed on either side of Achilles tendon on dominant leg) • 10 minutes of high-frequency electrical stimulation with the parameters: 150 pps, 10-sec on time, 2-sec ramp-up, 10-sec off time, symmetrical biphasic waveform, pulse duration of 400 µs • 10 minutes of low-frequency electric stimulation with the parameters: 2 pps, applied continuously, symmetrical biphasic waveform, pulse duration of 400 µs	Main outcome measure was PPT: • Immediately posttreatment: increased PPT with to baseline for NES and eccentric exercise groups • Morning-after treatment: only eccentric group maintained higher PPT	Some evidence that a single session of NES and eccentric exercise can result in immediate decreases in pain sensitivity for asymptomatic individuals More research is needed for clinical populations and to demonstrate effects of repeated intervention

Continued

TABLE 101.4 Evidence for Using Physical Agents—cont'd

		LOW-LEVEL LASER THERAPY (LLLT)		
Bjordal et al[44] (2008)	Systematic review (18 RCTs) and meta-analysis (13 RCTs; 730 patients with lateral elbow tendinopathy)	LLLT wavelengths: 632–1064 nm Placement on treatment: tendon insertion, acupuncture points, or trigger points Control groups (placebo or other nonlaser treatments) with at least 10 individuals per group	• Trials that targeted acupuncture points reported negative results • Trials with the following wavelengths reported negative results: 820, 830, and 1064 nm • Trials of 904- and 632-nm wavelengths demonstrated a greater weighted mean difference for pain relief on a 100-mm VAS vs placebo	Some evidence that LLLT at 904-nm wavelength offers short-term pain relief in lateral elbow tendinopathy both alone and with an exercise program but unable to have firm conclusion Minimal evidence for success with 632-nm wavelengths These findings conflict with prior reviews
		US, TENS, AND LLLT		
Page et al[82] (2016)	Cochrane systematic review • 47 trials (2388 participants; 67% women; average age, 53 yr) • 43 trials included participants without calcification	• 16 trials studied the effect of an electrotherapy modality delivered in isolation • Electrotherapy was delivered for an average of 3 wk	• US produced no clinically important additional benefits when used with other therapy interventions • 2 placebo-controlled trials showed favorable results with LLLT up to 3 wk • 10 trials found combining LLLT with other interventions had few additional benefits • No adverse effects reported by participants for US, LLLT, or TENS	Low-quality evidence that US may have short-term benefits for patients with calcific tendinitis over placebo Individuals with rotator cuff disease may get short-term benefits over placebo from LLLT It is uncertain whether TENS is superior to placebo for pain and function

MVIT, Maximal voluntary isometric torque; *NES*, noxious electrical stimulation; *PPT*, pressure pain threshold; *RCT*, randomized controlled trial; *ROM*, range of motion; *US*, ultrasound; *VAS*, visual analog scale.

nerve injuries. The units with fixed pulse durations of 250 to 300 μsec may not have sufficient pulse duration for the reinnervating muscles.

Neuromuscular electrical stimulation devices should have two channels to allow reciprocal motion on each channel.[27,34] There should also be an interrupt switch if the patient needs to stop the treatment immediately. For functional training, it is nice to have external triggers such as a heel or hand switch. These external triggers override on/off time cycles. The heel switch is particularly useful during gait training, even for the upper extremity if trying to restore arm swing.

Electrode Preparation and Placement

Electrode preparation and placement are essential to achieving the desired muscle contraction. Because NMES can be uncomfortable, it is recommended that high-quality, low-impedance electrodes be used. The clinic should also be stocked with a variety of sizes to accommodate the size range of the upper extremity muscles. The electrodes and configuration should "fit" the muscle, and the electrodes should be on or near the motor point of the desired muscle A bipolar electrode configuration, two electrodes over the target muscle, is suitable for larger muscles of the proximal upper extremity and superficial muscles in the forearm such as the wrist extensors (Fig. 101.e2). With biphasic pulsed currents, it may be necessary to apply electrodes of different sizes to the area stimulated, thus increasing current density under the smaller electrode and thereby obtaining a stronger tissue response. A monopolar configuration is recommended when several muscles are located close together as in the forearm and hand. A probe electrode works best for a monopolar electrode setup, especially during the initial application, because the probe makes it easier to locate small muscles. The electrode

to complete the circuit is placed away from the target tissue, proximally on the upper extremity[34] (Fig. 101.e3).

The authors believe that NMES should be an "attended" treatment by the therapist to establish appropriate parameters, modify parameters as needed, and achieve a good treatment outcome. After the parameters and electrode placement have been established, the therapist should monitor for 10 strong quality muscle contractions. Fibrillation or poor-quality contractions are a sign of fatigue. This author recommends that if fatigue occurs after seven or eight contractions, the treatment for that session should be discontinued and the parameters for the next session adjusted. However, if fatigue occurs in the first five contractions, then stop the treatment and adjust the on/off time cycle to increase off time. You may be able to decrease the on time, but it will depend on the initial setting. If the on time is set for 10 seconds and you have 3 seconds allotted for ramp, you really cannot reduce the on time. If the on time is greater than 7 seconds at peak amplitude, decrease it to 7 seconds. If you used an on/off ratio of 1:5, increase the off time to a 1:8 or 1:10 ratio. Frequency may be lowered, but it must remain at a level to achieve tetany, at least 35 pps.

IONTOPHORESIS AND PHONOPHORESIS

Iontophoresis delivers ionizable substances through the skin using DC. The polar effects of DC create electrostatic repulsion of like charges (likes repel; opposites attract).[35] Phonophoresis is the use of ultrasound to enhance the delivery of topically applied medications.[36] The potential benefits to transdermal delivery include direct application to the target tissue, resulting in higher concentrations of medication in the target tissue, and gastrointestinal absorption or liver metabolism factors are eliminated. Injections produce higher concentrations of medication to the target tissue, but this is an invasive procedure with a potential risk of injury, and the injections are frequently painful to the recipient.[36]

Iontophoresis is commonly used to reduce pain associated with tendinopathies, calcific tendinitis, and painful scar. Treatment outcome may be influenced by current amplitude, treatment duration, pH changes under the electrodes, correct polarity, drug concentration, and using more than one substance within the delivery electrode.

The typical treatment is to deliver a current dose of 40 mA/min.[35] Portable DC current generators (Fig. 101.12) commonly used 5 to 10 years ago have now been replaced by wireless battery-driven patches (Fig. 101.13). The instructions on the patch packaging instruct the patient to leave the patch on for 4 to 6 hours. Dosage delivery is typically complete in 4 hours for the average patient. It is the author's experience that this method of delivery tends to be more comfortable for the patient, but it is difficult to say whether or not it is superior in the terms of desired effect.

Dexamethasone sodium phosphate (4 mg/mL), a common antiinflammatory medication in injectable form, is commonly used for the treatment of tendinopathies. It is not clear whether this is an appropriate concentration for iontophoresis. The cathode is used to deliver the dexamethasone sodium phosphate.[28] Studies are limited regarding the appropriate parameters of iontophoresis, especially as related to the ionizable substances or medications delivered.

Less is known about the effective parameters for phonophoresis. Transmission quality of the ultrasound is affected by the coupling medium used with the drug.[37] Therapists should follow application guidelines used for ultrasound treatments. Byl[36] completed an extensive review of phonophoresis that may be useful for additional reading. Reviews indicate that phonophoresis is not a superior treatment to iontophoresis[38] or ultrasound alone.[39]

LOW-LEVEL LASER THERAPY

LASER is an acronym for light amplification by stimulated emission of radiation. Low-level laser therapy (LLLT) received FDA approval in the United States in 2002 for the treatment of pain associated with carpal tunnel syndrome and in 2004 for iliotibial band syndrome. The infrared lamp on LLLT units was approved for the management of minor muscle and joint pain in 2003.[40] LLLT generates light of a single wavelength that is coherent (travels in a straight line), monochromatic, and polarized (concentrated beam). It produces the proposed physiologic changes by creating photochemical reactions within cells. It does not produce a thermal or sensory effect.[40,41]

It is theorized that the light applied to the target tissue is absorbed by chromophores within cellular organs, especially mitochondria. A chromophore is part of a molecule responsible for color. Hemoglobin, lycopene, and beta-carotene are chromophores. The proposed physiologic effects of LLLT include (1) increased adenosine triphosphate production, (2) increased oxygen consumption, (3) decreased prostaglandin synthesis, (4) decreased edema, (5) decreased cell membrane permeability of neurons, (6) increased levels of serotonin and endorphins, (7) increased lymphatic flow, and (8) increased skin circulation. Therefore, the clinical indications are to reduce pain and inflammation and promote tissue healing associated with musculoskeletal conditions such as carpal tunnel syndrome and tennis elbow.[40–44] Box 101.e1 provides information on treatment, documentation, and contraindications with use of LLLT. For the safety of both the patient and therapist, it is recommended that both parties wear goggles during treatment.

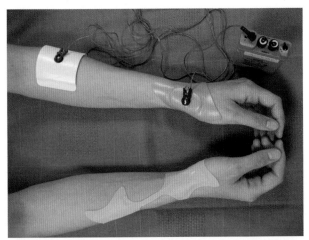

Fig. 101.12 Iontophoresis setup for de Quervain's tenosynovitis on the left wrist and transdermal patch without direct current on the right wrist.

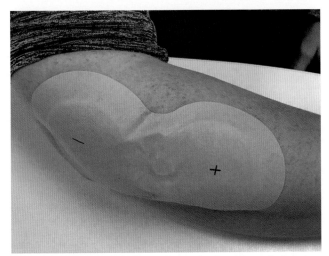

Fig. 101.13 IontoPatch STAT (http://www.iontopatch.com) placed over the lateral elbow to for treatment of lateral elbow tendinopathy.

CLINICAL APPLICATIONS FOR PHYSICAL AGENTS

This section focuses on the application of physical agents in clinical practice. The decision to use a physical agent to treat impairments identified during the examination process is influenced by patient factors (other than the impairments), clinic factors, and administrative considerations. The components of clinical reasoning to reach a determination about the use of a physical agent include the following.

What are the results of the patient examination? The results of the examination will indicate the list of patient impairments that may be treated with physical agents. The tests and measures performed will serve as baseline values to determine treatment effectiveness and outcome. Most important, examination results should reveal any comorbidities and other patient conditions that may make the use of a physical agent unsafe or suggest that the physical agent should be used with caution. Finally, the therapist will develop a hypothesis as to the source(s) of the present impairment(s). Using sound clinical reasoning and experience, the therapist can determine the physiologic appropriateness of physical agent use.

What is the expected duration of this episode of care (visits per week, number of weeks)? Insurance copayments are on the rise for therapy visits, so many patients want to reduce their number of clinic visits to save money. If the patient is not going to be seen more than once weekly and if only followed for a short duration, the use of a physical agent in the clinic may not be suitable to achieve goals. In this case, emphasis should be placed on physical agents that may be used at home.

What physical agent equipment is available to me? As will be discussed later, there is a paucity of evidence to support the use of physical agents, so clinics are less likely to stock all options. Most clinics probably limit the selection of equipment to therapist preference. If considering a unit for home use, the therapist needs to determine whether it is appropriate to use the agent at home, and if so, he or she needs to find out whether the patient has the means to cover the cost of the home device if it is not covered by insurance.

What other treatments do I plan to incorporate into my plan of care? Some physical agents may be used to treat more than one impairment, so agents that have multiple indications may be best suited for patients with more than one impairment. Other therapeutic interventions may be combined with the use of a physical agent such as "heat and stretch."

Decreasing Pain, Edema, and Inflammation

The use of physical agents for pain modulation is the most common indication in hand therapy practice. Every physical agent presented in this chapter has the ability to reduce pain, including NMES to reduce shoulder subluxations.[45] Figure 101.14 is a clinical decision-making tree that puts the information presented in the previous section into practical use. After a comprehensive assessment of pain, the therapist can determine the source of pain mediation[28,46] (see Chapter 94). Physical agents appear to work best on peripheral nociceptive or neurogenic pain of short duration and appear to be less effective on complex pain syndromes.[46-51]

As previously mentioned, the selection of the physical agent will depend on a review of the precautions and contraindications. In the case of peripheral nerve injury, thermal agents may need to be avoided or used with caution.

Associated impairments may determine the selection. This is particularly true for pain associated with edema and inflammation. Cryotherapy techniques or low-intensity, pulsed-wave ultrasound may be the most beneficial[22,28] (Fig. 101.e4). Interstitial edema can contribute to pain caused by increased pressure on mechanoreceptors or through chemical mediators located within the inflammatory exudate that sensitize or activate nociceptors.[52] Cold, compression, elevation, active exercise, and retrograde massage have been recommended for edema management.[52-54]

There has been some experimental investigation for the use of electrical stimulation for edema control.[55,56] In a frog model, sensory-level cathodal high-voltage, pulsed-wave current, applied immediately after injury, demonstrated that edema formation could be delayed. These findings could not be reproduced in edematous hands.[56] The authors believe that the use of electrical stimulation to manage edema is not practical. Readers are referred to Chapter 57 for information regarding edema management.

Low-intensity, pulsed ultrasound (LIPUS) has been shown to facilitate wound healing in chronic dermal wounds.[17] An associated benefit may be a reduction of interstitial edema and pain. LIPUS is thought to accelerate the early stages of inflammation and enhance wound-healing rates in chronic wounds.

Range of Motion and Muscle Strength

The application of heat and controlled stress results in increased tissue extensibility during and shortly after the treatment is applied. This is caused by the viscoelastic properties of connective tissue and the response to preconditioning.[12,13] Controlled stress should be applied simultaneously with heating (Fig. 101.e5). This is an ideal preconditioning technique that allows the therapist to determine how compliant

the tissues are to controlled stress.[57] Depending on the target tissue, superficial or deep heat may be used. Both AROM and passive range of motion (PROM) benefit from preconditioning.

The application of heat may also enhance motion by decreasing pain, altering contractile properties of muscle, and increasing blood flow. Heat also decreases the perception of joint stiffness. The application of cryotherapy may enhance motion by decreasing pain and edema. Although joint stiffness may be perceived, the benefits of pain and edema reduction may improve ROM gains. Both AROM and PROM benefit from decreased pain and edema.

Neuromuscular electrical stimulation may be used to augment muscle strength to improve AROM. As previously mentioned, the stronger the contractions are, the greater the strength gains. NMES is particular useful in the presence of disuse atrophy and to promote learning after immobilization. NMES does not take the place of volitional exercise, but it can enhance the AROM gains. NMES should be discontinued when the patient is able to perform a manual muscle test against gravity with minimal resistance (F+ contraction).[32,33] The emphasis on volitional exercise will promote the normal muscle physiology in terms of recruitment order and rate coding of the motor units. This may assist coordination and proprioception during functional activities.

Other than the application of heat and controlled stress for preconditioning, physical agents are not used to resolve joint contracture. The authors believe that low-load prolonged stress in the form of orthotic intervention is the first choice to resolve joint stiffness or tendon tightness. NMES has been used in the neurologic population to contract the antagonist to a muscle with spasticity in the hopes of reducing spasticity and increasing motion.[58]

Wound Healing, Scar Management, and Tendon Repairs

Wound, scar, and tendon management are covered elsewhere (see Chapters 15, 16, 31, 33, and 82). The use of LIPUS and electrical stimulation for delayed-healing wounds is well established.[17,59] However, the incidence of delayed-healing wounds is quite low in hand therapy. Additional information on the use of physical agents, especially ultrasound, with tissue healing may be found elsewhere.[60,61]

The two primary interests for rehabilitation after tendon repair are to prevent rupture or gapping and to maximize tendon gliding. Physical agents may have a role in both by preconditioning the tissue before active exercise is performed. This will decrease the drag or work of flexion requirements on the healing tendon during gliding exercise, which may enhance gliding without increasing the risk of rupture or gapping.

There has been uncertainty about the use of ultrasound over tendon repair sites, with the notion that use during the first few weeks would attenuate or damage the repair.[62,63] Basic science studies using animal models (chickens and rabbits) have demonstrated that there are no adverse effects from the use of ultrasound.[64-66] However, it is not practical to apply ultrasound over the area of tendon repair while sutures are still in place. Since this debate began, postoperative tendon management has progressed to more vigorous controlled stress, specifically early active mobilization. The benefits of ultrasound may not be superior to the early controlled stress alone. The use of ultrasound with recently repaired tendons is likely to remain controversial, but it does warrant further research.

In postsurgical tendon repairs, NMES can be applied to the affected muscle group to aid in strong muscle contraction to assist in tendon gliding. Proper timing is extremely important. After tendon repair, application of NMES at high intensity is the equivalent of performing resistive activities. It is necessary to wait at least 6 weeks after surgical repair before applying NMES at a level to elicit strong muscle

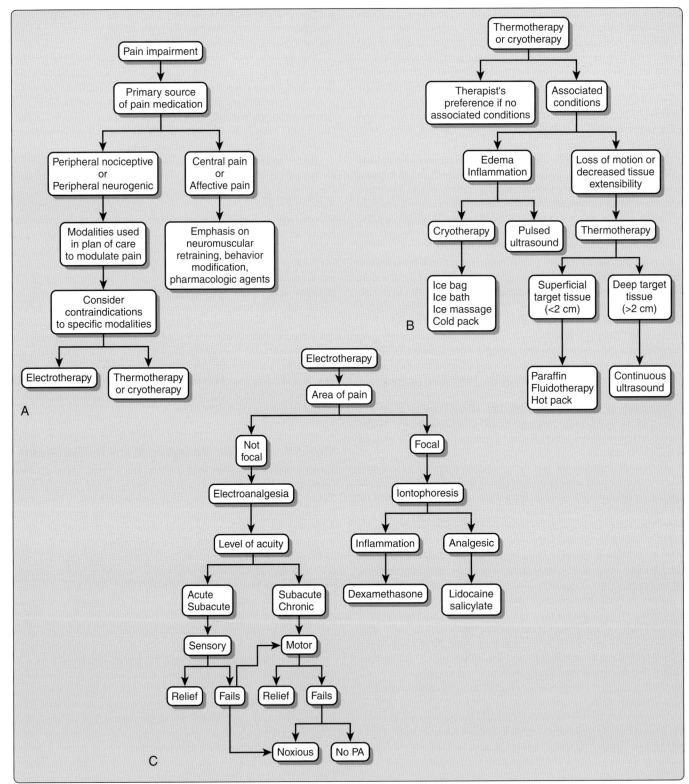

Fig. 101.14 Clinical decision-making tree for pain impairment. *PA,* Physical agents.

contraction. After tenolysis, NMES may be applied earlier, at 7 to 10 days after surgery, if tendon integrity and nutrition are considered good, but care should be taken not to overexercise the involved tendon, thereby causing an inflammatory response. If the tendons are frayed,

electrical stimulation must be avoided. It is best practice to discuss the introduction of NMES for tendon gliding with the surgeon who performed the tendon repair or tenolysis.

SUMMARY

A compelling issue in practice today is the need to support our therapeutic interventions with the best available evidence. Unfortunately, there is a lack of strong evidence to support the use of physical agents with any of the impairments covered in this chapter, especially in the hand and upper extremity patient population However, there has been an abundance of meta-analyses and systematic reviews to remind therapists that the evidence is limited (see Table 101.4).[32,39,42–44,47,51,67–82]

Several factors need to be considered in the clinical decision-making process to use a physical agent as part of the plan of care for a hand and upper extremity patient. Reviewing the results of the examination to determine how a physical agent may contribute to treatment goals and the potential contraindications or precautions will promote safe and judicious use. Although evidence is limited to support the use of physical agents, therapists can provide documentation to support their use with individual patients by collecting and reevaluating baseline tests and measures to assess treatment outcome.

REFERENCES

1. Michlovitz SL, Nolan TP. *Modalities for Therapeutic Intervention*. 4th ed. Philadelphia: FA Davis Company; 2005.
2. Cameron MH. *Physical Agents in Rehabilitation: From Research to Practice*. 3rd ed. St. Louis: W.B. Saunders Co.; 2008.
3. Sunderland S. *Nerves and Nerve Injuries*. 2nd ed. New York: Churchill Livingstone; 1978.
4. Lehmann JF, deLateur BJ. Therapeutic heat. In: Lehman JF, ed. *Therapeutic Heat and Cold*. 4th ed. Baltimore: Williams & Wilkins; 1990.
5. Abramson DI, Mitchell RE, Tuck S, et al. Changes in blood flow, oxygen uptake, and tissue temperatures produced by the topical application of wet heat. *Arch Phys Med Rehabil*. 1961;42:305–318.
6. Currier DP, Kramer JF. Sensory nerve conduction: heating effects of ultrasound and infrared. *Physiother Can*. 1982;34:241.
7. Halle JS, Scoville CR, Greathouse DG. Ultrasound's effect on the conduction latency of the superficial radial nerve in man. *Phys Ther*. 1981;61:345–350.
8. Mense S. Effects of temperature on the discharges of muscle spindles and tendon organs. *Pfleugers Archiv*. 1978;374:159–166.
9. Michlovitz SL, Rennie S. Heat therapy modalities: beyond the fake and bake. In: Michlovitz SL, Nolan TP, eds. *Modalities for Therapeutic Intervention*. 4th ed. Philadelphia: FA Davis; 2005:63–65.
10. Gammon SD, Starr I. Studies on the relief of pain by counterirritation. *J Clin Invest*. 1941;20:13–20.
11. Melzack R, Wall PD. Pain mechanisms: a new theory. *Science*. 1965;150:971–979.
12. Lehmann JF. Effect of therapeutic temperatures on tendon extensibility. *Arch Phys Med Rehabil*. 1970;51:481–487.
13. Warren GC, Lehmann JF, Koblanksi JN. Heat and stretch procedures: an elevation using rat tail tendon. *Arch Phys Med Rehabil*. 1976;57:122.
14. Sparrow KJ. Therapeutic ultrasound. In: Michlovitz SL, Nolan TP, eds. *Modalities for Therapeutic Intervention*. 4th ed. Philadelphia: FA Davis; 2005:79–86.
15. Klucinec B, Scheidler M, Denegar C, et al. Transmissivity of coupling agents used to deliver ultrasound through indirect methods. *J Orthop Sports Phys Ther*. 2000;30:263–269.
16. Draper DO, Sunderland S, Kirkendall DT, Ricard M. A comparison of temperature rise in human calf muscles following applications of underwater and topical gel ultrasound. *J Orthop Sports Phys Ther*. 1993;17:247–251.
17. Dyson M. Role of ultrasound in wound healing. In: McCulloch JM, Kloth LC, Feedar JA, eds. *Wound Healing Alternatives in Management*. 2nd ed. Philadelphia: FA Davis; 1995:318–345.
18. Bugaj R. The cooling, analgesic, and rewarming effects of ice massage on localized skin. *Phys Ther*. 1975;55:11–19.
19. Enwemeka CS, Allen C, Avila P, et al. Soft tissue thermodynamics before, during, and after cold pack therapy. *Med Sci Sports Exerc*. 2002;34(1):45–50.
20. Michlovitz SL. Heat therapy modalities: frozen peas and more. In: Michlovitz SL, Nolan TP, eds. *Modalities for Therapeutic Intervention*. 4th ed. Philadelphia: FA Davis; 2005:43–60.
21. Swenson C, Swärd L, Karlsson J. Cryotherapy in sports medicine. *Scand J Med Sci Sports*. 1996;6(4):193–200.
22. Daniel DM, Stone ML, Arendt DL. The effect of cold therapy on pain, swelling, and range of motion after anterior cruciate ligament reconstructive surgery. *Arthroscopy*. 1994;10:530–533.
23. Knuttsson E, Mattsson E. Effects of local cooling on monosynaptic reflexes in man. *Scand J Rehabil Med*. 1969;1:126–132.
24. Eldred E, Linsley DF, Buchwald JS. Effects of cooling on mammalian muscle spindles. *Exp Neurol*. 1960;2:144.
25. Newton M, Lehmkuhl D. Muscle spindle response to body heating and localized muscle cooling: implications for relief of spasticity. *J Am Phys Ther Assoc*. 1965;45:91–105.
26. Herrera E, Sandoval MC, Camargo DM, Salvini TF. Motor and sensory nerve conduction are affected differently by ice pack, ice massage, and cold water immersion. *Phys Ther*. 2010;90(4):581–591.
27. Section on Clinical Electrophysiology, American Physical Therapy Association. *Electrotherapeutic Terminology in Physical Therapy*. Alexandria, VA: APTA Publications; 1990.
28. Fedorczyk J. The role of physical agents in modulating pain. *J Hand Ther*. 1997;10:110–121.
29. Snyder-Mackler L. Electrical stimulation for pain control. In: Robinson AJ, Snyder-Mackler L, eds. *Clinical Electrophysiology: Electrotherapy and Electrophysiologic Testing*. 2nd ed. Baltimore: Williams & Wilkins; 1995:285–292.
30. Rizk TE, Christopher RP, Pinals RS, et al. Adhesive capsulitis (frozen shoulder): a new approach to its management. *Arch Phys Med*. 1983;64:29–33.
31. Cannon NM. Enhancing flexor tendon glide through tenolysis and hand therapy. *J Hand Ther*. 1989;3:122.
32. Stackhouse SK, Taylor CM, Eckenrode BJ, et al. Effects of noxious electrical stimulation and eccentric exercise on pain sensitivity in asymptomatic individuals. *PM R*. 2016;8:415–424.
33. Robinson AJ. Neuromuscular electrical stimulation for control of posture and movement. In: Robinson AJ, Snyder-Mackler L, eds. *Clinical Electrophysiology: Electrotherapy and Electrophysiologic Testing*. 2nd ed. Baltimore: Williams & Wilkins; 1995:157–210.
34. Delitto A, Snyder-Mackler L, Robinson AJ. Electrical stimulation of muscle: techniques and applications. In: Robinson AJ, Snyder-Mackler L, eds. *Clinical Electrophysiology: Electrotherapy and Electrophysiologic Testing*. Baltimore: Williams & Wilkins; 1995:123–153.
35. Ciccone CD. Iontophoresis. In: Robinson AJ, Snyder-Mackler L, eds. *Clinical Electrophysiology: Electrotherapy and Electrophysiologic Testing*. Baltimore: Williams & Wilkins; 1995:335–358.
36. Byl NN. The use of ultrasound as an enhancer for transcutaneous drug delivery: phonophoresis. *Phys Ther*. 1995;75:539.
37. Cameron MH, Monroe LG. Relative transmission of ultrasound by media customarily used for phonophoresis. *Phys Ther*. 1992;72:142–148.
38. Hoppenrath T, Ciccone CD. Is there evidence that phonophoresis is more effective than ultrasound in treating pain associated with lateral epicondylitis? *Phys Ther*. 2006;86(1):136–140.
39. Klaiman MD, Shrader JA, Danoff JV, et al. Phonophoresis versus ultrasound in the treatment of common musculoskeletal conditions. *Med Sci Sports Exerc*. 1998;30:1349–1355.
40. Enwemeka CS. Therapeutic light. *Rehab Manag*. 2004;17(1):20–25. 56–57.
41. Bukowski EL, Dellagatta EM. Electromagnetic radiation: laser, ultraviolet, and diathermy. In: Michlovitz SL, Nolan TP, eds. *Modalities for Therapeutic Intervention*. 4th ed. Philadelphia: FA Davis; 2005:141–148.
42. Enwemeka CS, Parker JC, Dowdy DS, et al. The efficacy of low-power lasers in tissue repair and pain control: a meta-analysis study. *Photomed Laser Surg*. 2004;22(4):323–329.

43. Woodruff LD, Bounkeo JM, Brannon WM, et al. The efficacy of laser therapy in wound repair: a meta-analysis of the literature. *Photomed Laser Surg.* 2004;22(3):241–247.

44. Bjordal JM, Lopes-Martins RA, Joensen J, et al. A systematic review with procedural assessments and meta-analysis of low level laser therapy in lateral elbow tendinopathy (tennis elbow). *BMC Musculoskelet Disord.* 2008;9:75.

45. Chantraine A, Baribeault A, Uebelhart D, Gremion G. Shoulder pain and dysfunction in hemiplegia: effects of functional electrical stimulation. *Arch Phys Med Rehabil.* 1999;80:328–331.

46. Fedorczyk JM, Michlovitz SL. Pain and limited motion. In: Michlovitz SL, Nolan TP, eds. *Modalities for Therapeutic Intervention.* 4th ed. Philadelphia: FA Davis; 2005:185–206.

47. Chapman CE. Can the use of physical modalities for pain control be rationalized by the research evidence? *Can J Physiol Pharmacol.* 1991;69:704–712.

48. van der Windt D, van der Heijden G, van den Berg S, et al. Ultrasound therapy for musculoskeletal disorders: a systematic review. *Pain.* 1999;81:257–271.

49. Meyler WJ, deJongste MJ, Rolf CA. Clinical evaluation of pain treatment with electrostimulation: a study of TENS in patients with different pain syndromes. *Clin J Pain.* 1994;10:22–27.

50. Carroll D, Moore RA, McQuay HJ, et al. Transcutaneous electrical nerve stimulation (TENS) for chronic pain. [Systematic Review]. *Cochrane Database Syst Rev.* 2004;2.

51. Gam AN, Johannsen F. Ultrasound therapy in musculoskeletal disorders: a meta-analysis. *Pain.* 1995;63:85–91.

52. Flowers KR. Edema: differential management based on the stages of wound healing. In: Hunter JM, Mackin EJ, Callahan AD, eds. *Rehabilitation of the Hand: Surgery and Therapy.* St. Louis: CV Mosby; 1995:87–91.

53. Sorenson MK. The edematous hand. *Phys Ther.* 1989;69:1059–1064.

54. Walsh MT, Muntzer E. Wound management. In: Stanley BG, Tribuzi SM, eds. *Concepts in Hand Rehabilitation.* Philadelphia: FA Davis; 1992:167–177.

55. Mendel FC, Fish DR. New perspectives in edema control via electrical stimulation. *J Athl Train.* 1993;28:63–74.

56. Griffin JW, Newsome LS, Stralka SW, et al. Reduction of chronic posttraumatic hand edema: a comparison of high voltage pulsed current, intermittent pneumatic compression, and placebo treatments. *Phys Ther.* 1990;70:279–286.

57. Flowers KR. A proposed decision hierarchy for splinting the stiff joint, with an emphasis on force application parameters. *J Hand Ther.* 2002;15(2):158–162.

58. Glinsky J, Harvey L. Efficacy of electrical stimulation to increase muscle strength in people with neurological conditions: a systematic review. *Physiother Res Int.* 2007;12(3):175–194.

59. Kloth LC. Electrical stimulation in tissue repair. In: McCulloch JM, Kloth LC, Feedar JA, eds. *Wound Healing Alternatives in Management.* 2nd ed. Philadelphia: FA Davis; 1995:275–314.

60. Michlovitz SL. Is there a role for ultrasound and electrical stimulation following injury to tendon and nerve? *J Hand Ther.* 2005;18(2):292–296.

61. Nussbaum E. The influence of ultrasound on healing tissues. *J Hand Ther.* 1998;11:140–147.

62. Stevenson JH, Pang CY, Lindsay WK. Functional, mechanical, and biomechanical assessment of ultrasound therapy on tendon healing in the chicken toe. *Plast Reconstr Surg.* 1986;77:965–972.

63. Enwemeka CS, Rodriquez O, Mendosa S. The biomechanical effects of low intensity ultrasound on healing tendons. *Ultrasound Med Biol.* 1990;16:801–807.

64. Enwemeka CS. The effects of therapeutic ultrasound on tendon healing: a biomechanical study. *Am J Phys Med Rehabil.* 1989;68:283–287.

65. Roberts M, Rutherford JH, Harris D. The effect of ultrasound on flexor tendon repairs in the rabbit. *J Hand Surg.* 1982;14B:17–20.

66. Turner SM, Powell ES, Ng CS. Effect of ultrasound on the healing of cockerel tendon: is collagen cross-linkage a factor? *J Hand Surg.* 1989;14B:428–433.

67. Enwemeka CS, Parker JC, Dowdy DS, et al. The efficacy of low-power lasers in tissue repair and pain control: a meta-analysis study. *Photomed Laser Surg.* 2004;4:323–329.

68. Vanderthommen M, Duchateau J. Electrical stimulation as a modality to improve performance of the neuromuscular system. *Exerc Sport Sci Rev.* 2007;35:180–185.

69. Dehail P, Duclos C, Barat M. Electrical stimulation and muscle strengthening. *Ann Readapt Med Phys.* 2008;51:441–451.

70. Speed CA. Therapeutic ultrasound in soft tissue lesions. *Rheumatology.* 2001;40:1331–1336.

71. MacAuley D. Ice therapy: how good is the evidence? *Int J Sports Med.* 2001;22:379–384.

72. Bleakley C, McDonough S, MacAuley D. The use of ice in the treatment of soft-tissue injury: a systematic review of randomized controlled trials. *Am J Sports Med.* 2004;32:251–261.

73. Andres BM, Murrell GA. Treatment of tendinopathy: what works, what does not, and what is on the horizon. *Clin Orthop Relat Res.* 2008;466:1539–1554.

74. Robertson VJ, Baker KG. A review of therapeutic ultrasound: effectiveness studies. *Phys Ther.* 2001;81:1339–1350.

75. Desmeules F, Boudreault J, Roy JS, et al. The efficacy of therapeutic ultrasound for rotator cuff tendinopathy: a systematic review and meta-analysis. *Phys Ther in Sport.* 2015;16:276–284.

76. Gorgey AS, Black CD, Elder PA, et al. Effects of electrical stimulation parameters on fatigue in skeletal muscle. *J Orthop Sports Phys Ther.* 2009;39(9):684–692.

77. Pantaleão MA, Laurino MF, Gallego NLG, et al. Adjusting pulse amplitude during transcutaneous electrical nerve stimulation (TENS) application produces greater hypoalgesia. *J Pain.* 2011;12(5):581–590.

78. Moran F, Leonard T, Hawthorne S, et al. Hypoalgesia in response to transcutaneous electrical nerve stimulation (TENS) depends on stimulation intensity. *J Pain.* 2011;12(8):929–935.

79. Desmeules F, Boudreault J, Roy JS, et al. Efficacy of transcutaneous electrical nerve stimulation for rotator cuff tendinopathy: a systematic review. *Physiotherapy.* 2016;102:41–49.

80. Macedo LB, Josué Am, Maia PHB, et al. Effect of burst TENS and conventional TENS combined with cryotherapy on pressure pain threshold: randomized, controlled, clinical trial. *Physiotherapy.* 2015;101:155–160.

81. Fuentes JP, Olivo SA, Magee DJ, et al. Effectiveness of interferential current therapy in the management of musculoskeletal pain: a systematic review and meta-analysis. *Phys Ther.* 2010;90:1219–1238.

82. Page MJ, Green S, Mrocki MA, et al. Electrotherapy modalities for rotator cuff disease. *Cochrane Database Syst Rev.* 2016;6:CD012225.

102

Neurodynamic Treatment, Examination, and Intervention with Nerve Gliding

Mark T. Walsh

OUTLINE

CRITICAL POINTS

- Neuropathic pain is often a major component of neural tension dysfunction.
- The nervous system is designed to accommodate movement via excursion and strain. Excess strain can lead to compromise of the nervous system's physiologic function and mechanical injury.
- Neuropathology manifests as alterations in neurodynamics; neurophysiology (symptoms) and mechanics (limitation of motion).

- The application of neurodynamic testing and treatment via neural intervention requires a profound respect for the sensitivity of the nervous system to excess movement, especially in the diseased state.
- Treatment requires continuous and sound clinical reasoning when applying these techniques.

NEUROPATHIC PAIN

The use of neurodynamic testing (NDT) and neurodynamic intervention (NDI) mandates that the clinician understand that the clear majority of patients with neural tension dysfunction (NTD) present with neuropathic pain (NP) as a primary feature.[1,2] The International Association for the Study of Pain now defines NP as "pain caused by a lesion or disease of the somatosensory system."[3] The reasons for the change are (1) NP is not a single disease, (2) the lesion of the somatosensory system is encompassing, and (3) current therapy for NP is not satisfactory.[3] The multiple mechanisms of NP are not fully understood as evidenced by the list of reported mechanisms compiled by Allen in Box 102.1.[4] These multiple mechanisms compound the difficulties in managing the condition. NP includes painful peripheral neuropathies and generalized polyneuropathies, leaving central pain syndromes, complex regional pain syndromes (CRPSs), and mixed pain syndromes as separate entities.[5]

In the normal pain state, afferent (nociceptor) and central nervous system (CNS) (spinal cord tracts, thalamic, and cortical) hyperexcitability occurs. The diagnosis can include negative sensory signs (deficit of perception of mechanical or vibratory stimuli) indicating injury to large afferent fibers and a loss of noxious and thermal perception, indicating small fiber afferent damage in the peripheral nervous system (PNS).[5] Patients with NP usually have abnormal sensation or hypersensitivity in the area affected. Positive symptoms can be spontaneous pain (no stimulus required) or evoked pain secondary to a mechanical or thermal stimulus causing hypersensitivity. This is usually defined by allodynia (pain perceived from a nonpainful stimulus) or hyperalgesia

(perceived increase in pain from a nociceptive stimulus).[6] Table 102.1 [6A] defines and assesses the negative and positive sensory symptoms and signs of the NP patient. An additional feature is summation in which multiple lighter stimuli summate to provoke the NP. Finally, the concept of central sensitization requires secondary allodynia and hyperalgesia in an area adjacent to the injured PNS territory and requires the involvement of the CNS.[5] This NP state leads to altered neurodynamics (pathoneurodynamics), both mechanical and physiological.[2] For successful use of NDT and NDI techniques, the therapist must appreciate the interaction between the patient's pain and the accompanying pathoneurodynamics.

Although it is beyond the scope of this chapter to discuss the potential mechanisms and the pathophysiology of NP, readers are referred to Chapters 93 and 94 on pain or the references sited for a more in-depth explanation. However, one theory to consider is the direct effect on chemical sensitization of the PNS. The chemical may be of non-neurogenic origin because of injury to connective tissue. Endogenous chemicals such as bradykinins, serotonin, histamine, prostaglandins, and leukotrienes are released and have been shown to affect nociceptive afferents. These endogenous chemicals may also be neurogenic in origin called neuropeptides and include substance P, calcitonin gene-related peptide, vasoactive intestinal peptide, and enkephalins. These chemicals are released by injured primary afferent neurons as a result of physical or chemical to peripheral nociceptive afferents.[7]

As previously noted, NP presents with a variety of symptoms that are summarized in Box 102.1.[5] Patients with NP often present with continuous and spontaneous pain that may not be related to

BOX 102.1   Potential Neuropathic Pain Mechanisms

Ectopic impulses
Neurogenic inflammation
Gene-regulated C-fos changes
Primary afferent nociceptor neuropeptide changes
Ephaptic connections
Sympathetic dysfunction
Neuronal sprouting: peripheral and central
Central sensitization
Thalamic low-threshold spike bursts
Nervi nervorum
Possible theoretical neuropathic pain mechanisms compiled by Allen[4]

BOX 102.2   Neuropathic Pain Terminology

Allodynia: nonpainful stimulus provokes pain
Hyperalgesia: increased response to painful stimulus
Hyperpathia: increased response to painful stimulus continues after it is withdrawn
Dysesthesia: unpleasant abnormal sensation (spontaneous or evoked)

any particular stimulus and may linger after the removal of an evoking stimulus (hyperpathia). The existence of spontaneous discharge has been confirmed in animal studies by Eliav and colleagues[8] in the presence of induced neurogenic inflammation. This neurogenic inflammation and increased mechanosensitivity may also be responsible for the distant projection of pain or its sometimes

TABLE 102.1   Defining and Assessing Components of Positive and Negative Symptoms of Neuropathic Pain

	Definition	Bedside Assessment	Expected Pathological Response
NEGATIVE SYMPTOMS AND SIGNS			
Hypoesthesia	Reduced sensation to nonpainful stimuli	Touch skin with painter's brush, cotton swab, or gauze	Reduced perception, numbness
Pall-hypoesthesia	Reduced sensation to vibration	Apply tuning fork on bone or joint	Reduced perception threshold
Hypoalgesia	Reduced sensation to painful stimuli	Prick skin with single pin stimulus	Reduced perception, numbness
Thermal hypoesthesia	Reduced sensation to cold or warm stimuli	Contact skin with objects of 10°C (metal roller, glass with water, coolants such as acetone); contact skin with objects of 45°C (metal roller, glass with water)	Reduced perception
SPONTANEOUS SENSATIONS OR PAIN			
Paraesthesia	Nonpainful ongoing sensation (skin crawling sensation)	Grade intensity (0–10); area in cm^2	N/A
Paroxysmal pain	Shooting electrical attacks for seconds	Number per time; grade intensity (0–10); threshold for evocation	N/A
Superficial pain	Painful ongoing sensation, often a burning sensation	Grade intensity (0–10); area in cm^2	N/A
EVOKED PAIN			
Mechanical dynamic allodynia	Pain from normally nonpainful light moving stimuli on skin	Stroke skin with painter's brush, cotton swab, or gauze	Sharp burning superficial pain; present in the primary affected zone but spreads beyond into unaffected skin areas (secondary zone)
Mechanical static hyperalgesia	Pain from normally nonpainful gentle static pressure stimuli on skin	Apply manual gentle mechanical pressure to skin	Dull pain; present in the area of affected (damaged or sensitized) primary afferent nerve endings (primary zone)
Mechanical punctate, pinprick hyperalgesia	Pain from normally stinging but nonpainful stimuli	Prick skin with a safety pin, sharp stick, or stiff von Frey hair	Sharp superficial pain; present in the primary affected zone but spreads beyond into unaffected skin areas (secondary zone)
Temporal summation	Increasing pain sensation (wind-up-like pain) from repetitive application of identical single noxious stimuli	Prick skin with safety pin at intervals of <3 sec for 30 sec	Sharp superficial pain of increasing intensity
Cold hyperalgesia	Pain from normally nonpainful cold stimuli	Contact skin with objects of 20°C (metal roller, glass with water, coolants such as acetone); control: contact skin with objects of skin temperature	Painful, often burning, temperature sensation; present in the area of affected (damaged or sensitized) primary afferent nerve endings (primary zone)
Heat hyperalgesia	Pain from normally nonpainful heat stimuli	Contact skin with objects of 40°C (metal roller, glass with water); control: contact skin with objects of skin temperature	Painful burning temperature sensation; present in the area of affected (damaged or sensitized) primary afferent nerve endings (primary zone)
Mechanical deep somatic hyperalgesia	Pain from normally nonpainful pressure on deep somatic tissues	Apply manual light pressure at joints or muscles	Deep pain at joints or muscles

Baron R. Mechanisms of Disease: Neuropathic Pain—A Clinical Perspective. *Nature Clinical Practice: Neurology.* 2006;2:95–106. (with permission).[6A]

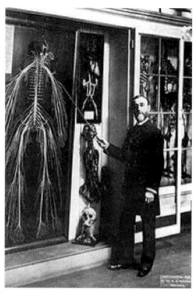

Fig. 102.1 Photograph of the dissected nervous system by Rufus Weaver, MD, titled "Harriet," demonstrating the concept of the nervous system continuum. (Courtesy of Drexel University Department of Anatomy, Philadelphia, PA.)

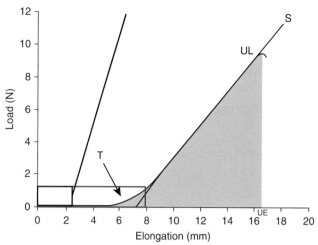

Fig. 102.2 Load deformation curve taken from the work of Grenwal and associates.[114] The *red area* represents the toe *(T)* region, where the nerve safely unfolds the undulations before tension starts to occur. The *blue area* represents the increase in stiffness of the nerve and the reduction in the toe region secondary to fibrosis that forms in the nerve connective tissue. (Adapted from Grenwal et al. *Hand Clin.* 1992;12:195-204; with permission.)

widespread nature.[6] NP may be perceived as deep (cramping, aching, throbbing) or superficial (burning, pinching, stabbing). There often is a delayed response to mechanical stimuli, which may occur after repeated stimulation.[9] Paroxysmal pain may also occur and is described as electric shock–like or shooting. Spontaneous ectopic discharge and lowered threshold mechanoreceptor function may be responsible for some of the bizarre symptoms reported by patients with NP.[6] Pain may radiate from a focal point along a continuous track or may be referred to other areas described as clusters or clumps of pain.[8,10] The specific evaluation of NP has been postulated by Galer and Jensen[11] using the Neuropathic Pain Scale (NPS). The scale is designed to measure the distinct qualities of NP. Preliminary testing shows the NPS to be discriminant and have predictive validity. More recently, additional outcome measures have been developed. Bouhassira and associates[12] developed the Neuropathic Pain Symptom Inventory (NPSI), which allows for the discrimination and quantification of five distinct clinically relevant dimensions that are sensitive to treatment. The classification system may assist in developing more specific treatment. Finally, Bennett and coworkers[13] developed an inventory that allows for identifying NP distinct from nociceptive pain.

BIOMECHANICAL AND PHYSIOLOGIC CONCEPTS

Nervous System Continuum

The nervous system is a continuum.[14] The peripheral, central, and autonomic nervous systems all combine to form one system that interacts as a unit of input and output. This continuum is achieved mechanically, electrically, and chemically. Figure 102.1 is an anatomic prosection demonstrating this concept visually prepared by Dr. Rufus Weaver and displayed in 1893 at the Columbian Exposition in Chicago. This anatomic preparation demonstrates how placing tension or strain on either the PNS or CNS could have a potential effect on the nervous system in another location. For example, the NDT of the upper extremity alters neuraxial or meningeal tension and provides the clinician with screening maneuvers to examine the irritability of the patient's nervous system and its accompanying interfacing tissues.[14]

Strain

The nervous system as a continuum requires mechanisms for compression, elongation, tension, and glide.[2] Haftek[15] investigated the effect of slow and quick stretch on albino rat tibial nerves. He reported that the initial process of elongation did not affect the nerve fiber but was physiologic in nature, described as unfolding. Progressive strain to failure demonstrated that histologic rupture of the epineurium occurred first with damage to the vascular system. Before epineural rupture, damage in the form of neurapraxia or axonotmesis occurs.[15] These strain levels are much higher than the clinician would want to impart when performing NDT or NDI. Figure 102.2 is a representation of initial unfolding *(red box)* followed by the linear sloping line, which represents the development of additional strain to the ultimate failure of the nerve.

The strain or stress that occurs along the course of the nerve because of upper extremity joint motion must also be considered. Strain is the percentage of the change in length that occurs in a nerve because of unfolding in response to extremity movement. Millesi and colleagues,[16] Wright and colleagues,[17–19] Kleinrensink and colleagues,[20] and most recently, Manvell and colleagues[21] demonstrated in cadavers that motion of the upper extremity results in stress being imparted along the entire course of the nervous system as measured by strain. Finally, the NDT for the median nerve is the most sensitive of the three major nerves and the most specific for the median nerve compared with the other NDT for the ulnar and radial nerves.[22] Research performed in animal, cadaver, and limited human models[23] verifies that the nervous system has multiple mechanisms to attenuate strain, tension, and elongation and that upper extremity and spinal motion can affect tension throughout the nervous system. These results explain structural differentiation when performing the NDT.

Tension within the nerve can also affect intraneural blood flow and nerve function. Lundborg and Rydevik[24] determined that lower limits of strain (5%–10%) demonstrated the first signs of changes in blood flow in the epineural and perineural vessels. The upper stretch limit was 11% to 18%, causing complete occlusion that resolved after relaxation of the nerve. Using rabbit sciatic nerve, Ogata and Naito[25] found that strain limits greater than 15.7% resulted in complete ablation of blood flow to the nerve. Complete ablation of blood flow also occurred when external compression was greater than 50 to 70 mm

Hg. Studying the effect of strain on rat tibial nerve function, Kwan and associates[26] reported strains of 6% or greater resulted in a 60% decrease in compound nerve action potential (CNAP) after 20 minutes. They concluded that longstanding low stress could affect the functional properties of the nerve.

In 1992, Wall and associates,[27] using rabbit tibial nerves and measuring nerve conduction, also determined that strain rates of 6% or greater resulted in a 70% decrease in CNAP after 20 minutes. Recovery occurred to within 10% of prestretch values when the load was removed. At 12% strain, there was a rapid reduction in CNAP with complete conduction block after 50 minutes. There was only a 40% recovery after the load was removed. It was their opinion that mechanical deformation contributed to decreased nerve conduction and ischemia. Wall and colleagues[27] concluded that the response to stretch might not be immediate; however, prolonged stretch may cause irreversible damage. The role of repeated versus continuous strain on nerve function was studied by Watanabe and colleagues.[28] The authors applied a continuous traction at 1, 2, 5, and 12 N of force and a repetitive traction at 60 and 120 cycles per hour to the brachial plexus of a rat. They determined that there were no changes in blood–nerve barrier permeability, functional grip strength, and electrophysiologic function, as measured by CNAP. In contrast, repetitive traction resulted in significant changes in all three measures with the higher repetitions (120 cycles per hour) causing the greatest change. The practical application of this information is that it supports that maximal strain rates using the NDT and NDI should be less than 4% to 6% (see Fig. 102.2). Repetitive applications or oscillations of NDI may result in damage to the nerve if performed in the painful ranges. The clinician must rely on the patient's response (pain or paresthesia, symptoms) to determine the amount of strain because presently it cannot be measured any other way clinically.

The nervous system's ability to accommodate tension is a product of an intraneural and extraneural anatomic design. Internally, the nerve is designed with undulations creating a tortuous nature.[29] A second mechanism that the nerve uses to tolerate elongation is intraneural gliding.[29] The unique framework of the nerve's connective tissue allows intraneural excursion between individual nerve fibers and their surrounding endoneurium and the encasing perineurium of each of the fascicles. The epineurium allows excursion to occur between it and the perineurium of each fascicle.

Excursion

Extraneural gliding provides for attenuation of tension via a gliding surface between the paraneurium and the epineurium.[16] Extraneural excursion or gliding has been demonstrated in the CNS[30] and PNS.[23,29]

Peripheral Nervous System

Neural excursion has also been demonstrated to occur in the PNS. McLellan and Swash[31] demonstrated that the median nerve underwent an excursion of 7.4 mm distally and 4.3 mm proximally with wrist and finger motion and elbow flexion–extension. In 1986, Wilgis and Murphy[32] measured excursion of the brachial plexus, median, ulnar, and radial nerves in 15 cadaver arms. The greatest excursions occurred at the brachial plexus level (15.3 mm) with movement of the shoulder, the median nerve wrist level (proximal, 14.5 mm and distal, 6.8 mm), the ulnar nerve wrist level (13.8 mm), and 6.8 mm distal excursion of the ulnar nerve with elbow extension to flexion. In vivo studies using ultrasonography confirmed the presence of nerve excursion.[23,33,34] Dilley and colleagues[33] reported total median nerve excursion of 10.4 mm in the upper arm and 4.2 mm in the forearm with elbow extension as the moving component. They also confirmed the concept of the nervous system continuum by demonstrating that the distal motion affects the nerve proximally. Passive wrist and index finger extension also result in similar median nerve excursions of up to 4.5 mm. Finally, the excursions that occur in vivo are less than those that occur in the cadaver studies previously mentioned. Dilley and colleagues[35] also studied ulnar nerve sliding during upper limb movements in healthy participants. Their finding demonstrated minimal movement of up to 4 mm in the forearm with wrist extension and little movement with shoulder abduction and elbow flexion. Ultrasound images from these data supports the concept that changing the position of the shoulder, elbow, wrist, and fingers can affect nerve excursion distally or proximally (structural tissue differentiation [STD]). These CNS and PNS studies support the continuum theory, which explains the nerve tensioning and gliding that is imparted with the NDT and NDI. Additional information will be covered during the NDI portion of the chapter.

An integral component in understanding peripheral nerve excursion is appreciating that the interfacing tissues surrounding the nerve along its entire course are also required to adapt in length in relationship to joint motion. Millesi and colleagues[36] reported that the median nerve bed must adapt by as much as 20% in length at the elbow and wrist to accommodate nerve motion. Zoech and colleagues[37] specifically investigated the difference in the length of the median nerve bed in positions of maximal flexion and extension of the upper extremity. They demonstrated that maximal extension required a 4.3% change in length, and flexion resulted in as much as a 14.9% decrease in overall length. Therefore, not only must the peripheral nerve be able to adapt to elongation and tension, but the interfacing tissues that form the nerve bed must also adapt independently to changes in length resulting from joint motion. This same adaptation of the nerve bed occurs within the CNS.[30]

Neural Vasculature and Movement

In addition to the PNS's ability to accommodate movement, its physiology and function are also dependent on its vascularity and the maintenance of a pressure gradient system. This system allows for the maintenance of vascular perfusion and physiology and is best depicted by Sunderland's[29] model as shown by the formula PA > PC > PF > PV > PT. This model requires arterial pressure (PA) to be greater than capillary pressure (PC), which is greater than fascicular pressure (PF), which exceeds venous return pressure (PV) and ultimately is greater than tunnel pressure (PT). Alterations of any one of these five pressures can effect circulation and axoplasmic flow[38,39] throughout the nerve. Alterations in PT often result in the more common peripheral nerve entrapments in the upper extremity such as cubital tunnel syndrome, ulnar tunnel syndrome, and carpal tunnel syndrome (CTS).

Pechan and Julis,[40] examining ulnar nerve pressures at the elbow, demonstrated a twofold increase in cubital tunnel pressure with cervical spine and shoulder motion and a sixfold increase with ulnar nerve provocative testing (elbow flexion, wrist extension, and the arm above the head). This study further supports the concept that remote motions can have an influence on not only neural motion and strain but also neural pressures and vascular flow. Studying the rabbit vagus nerve, Dahlin and McLean[41] examined various compressive forces verified nerve conduction blocks attributed to changes in axoplasmic flow. Nemoto and colleagues[42] clamped a dog sciatic nerve at one of two locations proximal and distal to the experimental compression site. Their work established that two low-grade compressions exceeded the expected damage caused by an isolated compression. This supports the theory of double crush (DC) described by Upton and McComas.[39] In addition to affecting vascular flow, axoplasmic flow is also altered with less external pressure than occurs with minor CTS.[38] Schmid and Coppieters[43] conducted a Delphi study in an attempt to determine if there was consensus for the causative mechanism of DC. From the panel of experts, 14 plausible mechanisms were identified with high plausibility of four: impaired axonal transport, ion channel up- or downregulation, inflammation in the dorsal root ganglia, and neuroma in continuity. Whatever the mechanism, the presence of DC remains controversial.[44]

Taken collectively, these general principles emphasize the key point —that the nervous system is designed for movement. As with any other soft tissue structure, when the nervous system is in a diseased and hyperirritable state, mechanical stresses such as compression and tension may provoke pain syndromes and movement dysfunction associated with the nervous system and its interfacing tissues. The clinician should maintain awareness that not only is direct and local tissue affected, but other tissues innervated by the involved nerves may also be the source of the patient's pain and movement dysfunction.

NEUROPATHOLOGY AND ITS MANIFESTATIONS

Neuropathology

Although it is not the intent of this chapter to discuss neural pathology in detail, the neuropathologic consequences on the mechanical, physiological, vascular flow, and axoplasmic flow properties of the nerve must be considered when using the NDT and NDI (gliding, sliding, or tensioning) techniques for examination and intervention. These factors contribute to the cause of hyperirritability of the PNS and its interfacing tissues. The vascular system may be compromised by external compression or NTD, which may be the result of adaptive shortening of the peripheral nerve secondary to scarring of the nerve (intra- or extraneural). This scarring leads to limiting the toe region of the load deformation curve and an increase in nerve stiffness as represented by the blue box and steeper slope of the nerve (see Fig. 102.2). Compromise of the nerve's vascularity can lead to a state of inflammation in or around the connective tissues of the nerve, increasing its level of irritability.[14,38,45] Vascular changes may also lead to alterations in neurovascular dynamics and intraneural fibrosis.[14,16,29] External compression can lead to compromise in axoplasmic flow. This compromise reduces the transport of neural filaments, microtubules, and neurotransmitters along the axon to its terminal ending and the return of metabolic byproducts, potentially altering the nerve's physiology. Because of this chemically mediated inflammatory process or the loss of intra- or extraneural gliding capabilities, mechanical irritability of the nerve will occur, resulting in repetitive forces being placed across the fixed (adherent) nerve segment. This loss in neural motion tolerance in one segment requires force attenuation to be achieved over a shorter segment of the nerve, exposing it to further damage or injury.

Mechanical sensitivity of the PNS is supported by animal studies. In the rat model, Bove and colleagues[46] determined that inflaming the peripheral nerve resulted in C and Aδ axons increased mechanical sensitivity. Eliav and associates[8] demonstrated in the rat that saphenous nerve perineural–induced inflammation did not damage the axon; however, it did elevate spontaneous activity and mechanosensitivity in myelinated axons. Experimental progressive compression of rat peripheral nerve resulted in local and remote immune-mediated inflammation, which could explain the widespread symptoms sometimes seen in compression or other neuropathies.[47] This was also supported by Dilley and coworkers,[10] who studied mechanical sensitivity from inflammation and its relationship to stretch and reported that "the most sensitive fibers fired at 3% stretch."

This neuropathologic process increases the nerve's vulnerability throughout the upper extremity such as in the confined space of the cubital or carpal tunnel. The interfacing tissues that surround the nerve along its course also create these spaces or tunnels. Two examples of these are the median nerve passing through the pronator muscle or the radial nerve passing through the supinator muscle. Nerves are also more vulnerable at relatively fixed points (branching or innervating locations), and motion introduced at these levels minimizes the nerve's capability of tolerating elongation forces. Finally, the nerve is vulnerable to external compression whenever it rests across a hard surface such as the radial sensory nerve as it passes across the radius.

The final consequence of peripheral neuropathology is fibrosis.[14,29,48] Occurring in two ways, intra- and extraneural fibrosis removes the nerve's inherent ability to elongate or potentiate tension within the nerve fascicles and the gliding that occurs between the connective tissue layers of the nerve and its interfacing tissues. Intraneural fibrosis causes the loss of the tortuous course of the nerve or its undulations,[29] resulting in the loss of internal glide and the unfolding capability of the nerve (see Fig. 102.2). Extraneural fibrosis limits the nerve's ability to move within its nerve bed or between the interfacing tissues, creating mechanical interference. In either scenario, the lack of nerve mobility results in increased stress or strain delivered to a shorter nerve segment as joint motion occurs.[37] This fibrosis may ultimately lead to the onset of pain and adaptive shortening of the nervous system, altering joint movement and extremity function.

Clinical Manifestations

Baron and colleagues[5] and Jensen and Finnerup[6] have described the clinical manifestations of this pathologic process. Simplified, these manifestations are pathophysiologic: symptoms reported by the patient such as paresthesia and pain and pathomechanical alterations in neural mechanics, which are limiting isolated or multi-segmented motion of the upper extremity.[1,2] Elvey[49] also described the clinical response observed through a series of clinical examination techniques. These techniques result in provocation of the patient's symptoms (pathophysiologic) and identifying motion dysfunction or limitations (pathomechanical) of the involved extremity, spinal segment, or both. Elvey[49] and Butler[14] describe a resistance encountered with NDT resulting from altered neural mechanics. Elvey[49] and Jull[50] theorize that the resistance encountered results from hyperirritability of nervous tissue, causing a protective reflexive muscle contraction. The presence of a protective muscle response was verified by van der Heide and associates[51] measuring motion and electromyography activity while performing the neural provocation tests.

NEURODYNAMIC TESTING AND NEURODYNAMIC INTERVENTION RESEARCH

Anatomic Relationships to the Neurodynamic Testing

It is often assumed that the NDT and NDI are neural tissue specific. These techniques are multisegmental and often involve mechanical deformation of other innervated structures such as arteries, fasciae, and nerve roots and accompanying meningeal tissues. To confirm that there is a relationship with neural tissue, participants with less neural extensibility have been shown to have less upper trapezius length,[52] which may be indicative of patients attempting to shorten the segment to reduce the tension on mechanically sensitive neural tissue. It is wise for the clinician to keep these multisegmental innervations in mind because they may produce a false-positive NDT result. This can be minimized via STD.[1]

Excursion

Additional cadaver studies have been conducted to examine neural excursion and its relationship to component movements of the NDT of the upper extremity.[53,54] Bay and colleagues[55] demonstrated that wrist position (extension) plays a significant role in excursion with movement of the fingers (extension–flexion). Coppieters and Alshami[54] confirmed that greater excursion occurred with a sliding technique, a two-component motion moving two joints simultaneously, than with a one-component movement (one joint), and the least amount of excursion occurred with full upper extremity tensile loading technique (NDT of the median nerve).

Strain

There is anatomic evidence supporting that the NDT and NDI also produce changes in strain in the brachial plexus and peripheral nerves.[17-20,56] Lewis and colleagues[56] studied five fresh cadavers to measure strain in the median nerve distal to the axilla with the application of the NDT. They reported a significant increase in tension with elbow and wrist extension, contralateral cervical lateral flexion, and ipsilateral straight leg raise. The importance of these findings is that remote motions can increase or decrease tension in the nerves at locations distant to the motion which is another example of STD.

Kleinrensink and colleagues[20] reported additional evidence of strain within the brachial plexus and peripheral nerves. In three cadavers, they investigated the strain of the brachial plexus and the three major nerves of the upper extremity while applying the NDT to the three major nerves and modification with cervical contralateral lateral flexion, a sensitizing and STD component. Significant increases in strain in the nerves and brachial plexus occurred in all three tests. A specific NDT for each nerve also caused strain in the brachial plexus and the other peripheral nerves. These results question the specificity of each NDT and confirm the sensitivity. They concluded that the median nerve NDT was the most sensitive. In the cadavers, Manvell and associates[21] examined the best position to isolate the radial nerve. They demonstrated that the additional component motions of shoulder abduction of 40 degrees, and extension of 25 degrees, wrist ulnar deviation, and thumb flexion significantly increase radial nerve tension and significantly differentiated between the median and ulnar nerves. These findings support earlier work that demonstrated that strain in the median nerve measured in the axilla and the proximal and distal forearm was increased even with remote joint positioning.[17-19] These two studies support the work of Lewis and colleagues[56] that remote joint motion will cause strain along the entire course of the nerve. Therefore, the clinical ability of the NDT or NDI to isolate a segment of the nerve is difficult.

Byl and colleagues[53] determined that maximum nerve strain occurred with the full tensile loading of the median nerve NDT: 8.2% ulnar nerve and 6.7% median nerve. Coppieters and Alshami[54] also demonstrated increases in median nerve strain using six different components of the median nerve NDT. Maximum tension occurred with the full median nerve tensile loading measured at the wrist (4.7%) and above the elbow (4.2%). These results contradict one another in terms of the "safe zone" of strain in the nerve (4%–6%) to avoid compromise of blood flow and conduction. Finally, Coppieters and Butler[57] determined that strain on the median nerve was significantly less when performing sliding movements compared with tension movements. All three tensioning techniques resulted in strains greater than 4%.

Normal Responses to the Neurodynamic Testing

Kenneally and colleagues[58,59] and Yaxley and Jull[60] have investigated the response of the NDT in normal participants. Recently, these responses in asymptomatic participants were reexamined. Lohkamp and Small[61] examined the NDT of the median nerve to establish normal range of motion (ROM) and sensory response with and without STD. Key sensory findings were described as stretch (58%–63%), pain (20%–27%), and paresthesia (8%–11%). Maximum contralateral cervical lateral flexion (STD) increased pain response and was located more proximally. Sensory response was present beyond the median nerve

distribution. This demonstrates that the median nerve NDT may also create strain on other nerves as well. There was a statistically significant (2-degree) difference between the dominant versus the nondominant side, but this may be clinically insignificant. There was no significance for gender.[61] Martinez and colleagues[62] examined asymptomatic participants using the NDT for the ulnar nerve. The key findings were as follows: sensory responses differed based on sex and hand dominance, the distribution of the symptoms were primarily over the ulnar nerve distribution, and the descriptive symptoms were pain and stretch.

Other authors have investigated the neural and kinetic response to the NDT. Jull[50] studied 20 asymptomatic participants using surface electromyography, elbow goniometry, and pain perception in two groups of more or less extensible neural tissues. In the less extensible group, there was greater electromyographic (EMG) activity and less elbow extension. Pain perception was not significantly different between the two groups. The result of this study is evidence of a reflexive muscle contraction tissue barrier in response to the application of the NDT and a possible correlation between the patient's perceived pain and limitation of motion measured at the elbow. Coppieters and colleagues[63] attempted to quantify the increased upper trapezius tone and limitation of motion by measuring the scapula elevation force combined with wrist–elbow motion using electrogoniometry in a pilot experiment with five asymptomatic participants. They determined that there was greater scapula elevation force with NDT tensile loading. In a further study of 35 normal participants,[64] NDT was applied in five test variations in the upper extremity. As each variant was applied, there was an increase in the patient's subjective response and a decrease in elbow ROM. Coppieters and colleagues[64] concluded that although NDT assessed non-neural and neural structures, the high level of paresthesia supports that some of the response is neurogenic in nature. The finding of reduced elbow extension also supports that the components of NDT can be used for STD.

The studies discussed were conducted using instrumentation to examine the issue of reliability. Coppieters and associates[65] studied stability and reliability in the laboratory and clinical environment in symptomatic and asymptomatic individuals. They determined that the "pain onset" and "submaximal pain" for the NDT for the median nerve can be measured reliably. ROM of elbow extension corresponds with these two pain features and can be intra and interreliably measured in the clinic. The radial and ulnar nerve NDT reliability of asymptomatic participants without the use of stabilizing equipment was studied by Petersen and colleagues.[66] They determined that the intrarater reliability was good with small measurement error. In all these studies, the authors reported a high level of intrarater reliability for the application of the NDT for the upper extremity. Because all these studies on normal participants reported subjective responses, it confirms neurogenic involvement in the patient population is more difficult and complex. Several of these studies also attempted to quantify the NDT. These results provide early evidence of the potential for objective measurement of NDT and confirms the hypothesis of altered extremity mobility as a component of a positive NDT result.

The use of high-frequency ultrasound images has demonstrated the effectiveness in assessing median nerve excursion in vivo.[33] Dilley and associates[35] examined ulnar nerve excursion during four different upper limb movements similar to components of the ulnar nerve NDT. They demonstrated that ulnar nerve excursion occurred in the forearm and to a lesser extent in the upper arm. Additionally, the amount of excursion was dependent on the wrist and shoulder position. Echigo and colleagues[67] also used ultrasonography to examine median nerve excursion during nerve gliding exercises. Their study examined the component motions of passive wrist–finger extension and active finger flexion measuring median nerve excursion in the forearm. Passive wrist and digital extension resulted in distal nerve gliding and proximal excursion occurred for active hook fist and active grasp. Coppieters and colleagues[68] confirmed the earlier cadaver findings. Using ultrasonography, they confirmed significantly more excursion occurred using the sliding technique than the tension technique.

Specificity, Sensitivity, and Reliability in Normal and Symptomatic Participants

Cadaver studies have examined the sensitivity and specificity of the NDT of the upper extremity.[20,56] Recently, the specificity of NDT has been examined using various sensory perception[69,70] and experimentally induced pain models.[71,72] Using a thermal pain sensitivity model in a quasiexperimental design in healthy participants, Beneciuk and colleagues[69] determined that the group treated with NDI (gliding) had a decrease in temporal summation, improved ROM, and a decrease in sensory descriptors rating. The NDT alters the sensory perception threshold, and there is a weak but significant effect of age, with perception leaning toward hypoesthesia.[70] In two separate studies using an experimentally induced pain model, the straight leg raise[73] and slump test[72] and the median nerve NDT[71] did not affect the experimentally induced pain, indicating that the neurodynamic test is specific to the nervous system. Boyd and associates[74] determined that mechanosensitivity was diminished in the straight-leg test in those patients with type 2 diabetes with neuropathy, which could lead to a false-negative result.

Sandmark and Nisell[75] investigated the validity of five common manual neck pain–provoking tests including the NDT. They determined that the median nerve NDT had a specificity of 94%, a sensitivity of 77%, a positive predictive value of 85%, and negative predictive value of 91% in 22 of 75 participants randomly selected with reported neck pain. Sterling and associates[76] examined the response of the brachial plexus tension test, which has the same component motions as the NDT median nerve in symptomatic patients diagnosed with whiplash injury and symptomatic controls. Participants with whiplash had significantly reduced elbow extension and increased pain sensitivity than control participants. Whiplash patients were also divided into three groups: (1) arm pain reproduced with NDT, (2) arm pain not reproduced with NDT, and (3) no arm pain. Participants in group 1 had a significant reduction in elbow motion and nonsignificant increase in pain sensitivity compared with group 2. Participants in group 1 also had significantly greater loss of motion and higher pain intensity compared with the asymptomatic side. Finally comparing group 1 with 3, group 1 had significantly greater loss of motion and higher pain intensity. The authors concluded that careful assessment is necessary when examining and treating patients with nonprovocative techniques with sensitive nerve tissue.[76] The reliability was also examined for normal participants and patients with CTS. The authors concluded that the NDT of the median nerve can be used to diagnose CTS based on significantly higher ICC's. However, I question if the difference in motion is clinically significant and the authors did not include the symptom response to the test.[77] These results are also in contrast to a systematic review conducted by Nee and associates.[78] Yeung and colleagues[79] reported a sensitivity value of 0.9 and a specificity value of 1.0; however, the exact statistical method was not elucidated.

Neurodynamic Testing Validity and Variables

Multiple authors have also investigated the presence of positive NDT results in patient populations. In a study of 60 patients with repetitive strain injury, Elvey and associates[80] found that the NDT was positive in 59 of the Repetitive Strain Injury (RSI) patients for reproduction of their symptoms. In a study of 40 patients reporting pain and paresthesia associated with a neck injury, the NDT was performed and compared with 20 normal participants. A positive test result was based on symptom

provocation.[81] The NDT was also found to be useful in identifying and having diagnostic accuracy for those patients with cervical radiculopathy. Patient symptom provocation and reduced tissue extensibility (limitation of motion) were the criteria for a positive test result.[82] Selvaratnam and colleagues[83] assessed ROM for the NDT. In one of the few control group studies, they compared three groups of participants: a group with a known brachial plexopathy, a group with sports injury, and an asymptomatic group of 25 participants. A goniometric apparatus was used to measure upper extremity joint position and cervical motion while performing the Upper Limb Neural Tension Test (ULNTT) now referred as the NDT of the upper limb. The upper extremity joints were sequentially moved until the motion elicited pain or end range was achieved based on pain onset and tolerance. The authors found a significant difference in ROM to sensory change between the brachial plexus group and the sports group with less motion and earlier onset of pain in the ROM in the brachial plexus group. Similarly, there was a significant group interaction with a greater reduction of motion in the brachial plexus group than the asymptomatic group. Trillos and coworkers[84] investigated the accuracy of the NDT for the median nerve for CTS. They reported a sensitivity of 93%, specificity of 6%, and a positive predictive value of 86.9%. Finally, in a whiplash injury population, Yeung and colleagues[79] examined limitations of knee motion with the slump test (another neurodynamic test) and symptom onset. The addition of knee extension in the slump test increased cervical pain and produced a greater limitation of knee extension.

The clinician should also be aware that there are false positives and negatives with NDT. Boyd and associates[74] determined that patients with type 2 diabetes mellitus and peripheral neuropathy may have a limited response to the NDT studying straight leg raise. They cautioned that the clinician may overstretch or harm the PN. Baselgia and associates[85] also reported on the possibility of a false-negative result using NDT with patients with entrapment neuropathies. Their recommendation was that NDT should not be used in isolation.

Based on the available clinical research, it appears that a positive response is the provocation of the patient's symptoms, not to be confused with the normal response in asymptomatic participants (normal participants). Additionally, a limitation of motion was present in those studies that compared patients with normal participants. Interrater reliability remains questionable; therefore, caution should be exercised when comparing the results of two clinicians, even in the same patient population. Although intrarater reliability was reported to be strong, the criteria used was not clearly defined. The specificity and sensitivity have been reported to be high, and recent studies appear to support this concept. The clinician is also wise to continually consider that non-neural structures are being mechanically deformed, which may lead to potential errors in specificity and sensitivity and therefore the need for STD. Finally, NDT should be applied with care and not stand alone to confirm neural tissue involvement secondary to possible false positives and negatives, which may mislead the clinician.

Examination and Treatment Concepts

Several concepts need to be emphasized regarding NDT and NDI. The first concept is the order of NDT component movement and the role it plays. Nee and associates[86] measured the effect of NDT median nerve in the forearm for strain and excursion using seven unfixed cadavers. The authors compared three movement scenarios: (1) standard test, (2) distal to proximal, and (3) proximal to distal. They determined that the pattern of excursion was significantly different when shoulder abduction was the first movement, noting minimal excursion in the forearm. Otherwise, median nerve excursion for all other individual component motion caused the median nerve to glide toward the moving joint. They also concluded that the relative strain and position of the nerve at the endpoint of the NDT did not differ. Clinically different NDT

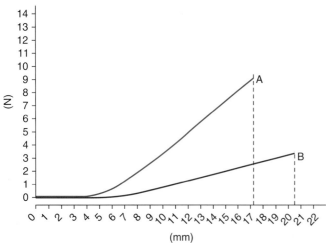

Fig. 102.3 Load deformation curve of the nerve and its relationship to the rate of application of neurodynamic testing (NDT) and neurodynamic intervention. Note that the slower application of force (blue) line results in less slope, a greater toe length, and greater length before failure of the nerve compared with the faster application of force (red) line with a shorter toe region, steeper slope, and earlier failure of the nerve. Although based on experimental data, this supports the need for the slower application of the components of the NDT upper limb for examination and treatment. A is from Kwan and coworkers[26] and is 1 cm/min. B is from Haftek,[15] 0.5 mm/min. (Data in A from Kwan M, Wall EJ, Massie J, Garfin SR. Strain, stress, and stretch of peripheral nerve: rabbit experiments in vitro and in vivo. *Acta Orthop Scand.* 1992;63:268. Data in B from Haftek J. Stretch injury of peripheral nerve: acute effects of stretching on rabbit nerve. *J Bone Joint Surg.* 1970;52[2]:355.)

sequences may still change the mechanical load to each segment where strain is applied for a longer period of a time on an individual segment or because of different ranges of motion may occur with sequences.[86]

The second concept is STD. This applies to the principle that a remote component motion alters or increases the symptoms such as cervical or scapular depression.[87] Traditional thinking would be to use this principle to determine if symptoms increased. I propose the opposite, that is, to use a remote site to decrease the symptoms considering that the nerve is already mechanically sensitive and any additional tension may cause an adverse effect.[1] Nee and Butler[87] also eluded to several other concepts: patient education, recognizing that potential non-neural structure involvement and gliding and tensile loading techniques should be nonprovoking.

Last is the concept that application rate (speed) of loading the PNS will affect the nerve's compliance ability in terms of neural elongation. Two classic studies examined this issue. Kwan and associates[26] loaded a rabbit tibial nerve at a rate of 1 cm/min and determined that the mean elongation was 38.5%, which confirmed previous reported study by Rydevik and colleagues.[88] In contrast, Haftek[15] examined the behavior of the rabbit tibial nerve, which was subjected to load at a rate of 0.5 mm/min and determined the mean elongation was 51.1% before failure. This effect is demonstrated in Figure 102.3, which is the graphic representation of Kawan and Haftek's data. What this graphic representation portrays is that slower load allows for safer accommodation to nerve movement.

Basic Science

There are basic science studies that support the use of NDI (gliding). In an unembalmed cadaver study, the authors injected a dye just beneath the epineurium of the tibial nerve, and the initial spread was measured. Repeated plantar to dorsiflexion was performed for 1 minute at the rate

of 30 repetitions, and the spread of the dye was remeasured. The results showed a significant dispersion of the dye, which possibly represents the dispersion of fluid that occurs with NDI.[89] Santos and associates[90] demonstrated in the animal model that NM and NDI provided evidence that the treatment reverses pain and suggests the involvement of glial cells and an increase in nerve growth factor (NGF) involvement. In the rat model, Santos and associates[91] used a chronic constriction injury (CCI) model and demonstrated that NDI (tensioning) facilitates pain relief using endogenous modulation. da Silva and associates[92] also studied CCI in rats and observed an increase in NGF and myelin protein zero in the NM group. Additionally, electron microscopy demonstrated high numbers of axons with myelin sheath thickness and less interaxonal fibrosis then the CCI group only.

Altered Mechanosensitivity and Neural Mechanics

The purpose of using NDI is to effect a change in the compliance (excursion and strain) of the neural tissue and to decrease its increased state of mechanosensitivity. As discussed earlier in detail, mechanosensitivity is increased in peripheral nerves in patients with NP for several reasons. Wilgis and Murphy[32] first theorized that neural excursion is compromised in patients with compression syndromes and certain diseased states. There is a growing body of literature that supports this theory of altered neural compliance. Hough and colleagues[93] studied median nerve excursion in patients with CTS and normal participants in a case-controlled study using Doppler ultrasound technique. Longitudinal median nerve excursion was significantly greater in control participants than patients with the elbow extended and flexed. An in vivo study by Greening and colleagues[94] studied two groups of patients (postwhiplash and nonspecific arm pain) compared with control participants using high-resolution ultrasonography examining median nerve movement in the forearm during inspiration–expiration. Longitudinal median nerve movement was reduced by 71% and 68%, respectively, compared with the control group. These findings may play a role in the underlying pathophysiology of these conditions.

Neurodynamic Intervention (Neural Mobilization)
Neurogenic and Neuropathic Pain

Neurodynamic intervention as a form of treatment was reported as early as 1880 by Marshall.[95] He described the use of "nerve stretching" to relieve pain. The author describes stretching and its effects on the PNS and CNS. Among the many points that Marshall discusses are some disastrous results, the importance of the rate of application, and that less force should be applied in the case of a diseased nerve. "Strong or sustained neurodynamic test typically constitute highly sensitized techniques and are often contraindicated in some asymptomatic participants, let alone patients with sensitized or compromised neural tissue."[1] Today the clinical technique for the application of NDI as a treatment approach is based on an eclectic compilation of theoretical concepts based on scientific evidence and empirical experience. There are reported clinical studies using NM for the treatment of NP. Nee and Butler[87] in a review paper discussed importance of integrating neurobiology with neurodynamics and clinical evidence for the treatment of peripheral NP. These concepts included patient education regarding the NDT and its association with the patients pain and the reason for NDI, structural tissue differentiation (STD) for identifying and confirming the presence of neural and non-neural tissue involvement, neurodynamic sequencing, and that NDI (gliding or tensile loading techniques)[87] *SHOULD NOT* provoke the patients symptoms. In a systematic review, Ellis and Hing[96] examined the use of NM in randomized controlled studies (RCTs). Their analysis concluded that limited evidence supported the use of NM and a lack of quantity and quality of research. The studies examined included multiple diagnoses and NM techniques that lacked consistency in applying NM. This further confirms the need for standardization of NM interventions.[96] A systematic review and meta-analysis of chronic nerve related musculoskeletal pain and NM by Su and associates[97] examined 20 clinical articles. They found multiple variations in NM techniques and dosage, duration, and frequency of treatment. They concluded that treatment of confirmed neural tissue involvement using NM (NDI) is superior to minimal treatment. However, this does not confirm that NM plays a positive role in treatment overall.[97] Basson and associates[98] in another systematic review and meta-analysis examined the use of NM (NDI) for neuromusculoskeletal conditions. Multiple "conditions" and NM techniques were included in the 40 studies examined. The lack of consistency of the definition of NM is problematic with most reviews. They concluded that NM was effective for lumbar- and cervical-related pain, but the evidence does not presently support NM for other conditions.[98]

More recently controlled studies have been published. Nee and associates[99] performed a randomized trial of patients with nerve-related neck and arm pain. The experimental group received education and a combination of gliding and tensile loading techniques, whereas the control group received only advice to remain active. Their conclusion was that NM provides clinically relevant benefits in comparison to advice only. Day and associates[100] examined 32 patients with nonradicular peripheral NP. The specific interventions were postural education, scapular stabilization, neural gliding, manual therapy, and proximal and distal nerve "stretching" using a specific treatment matrix. Outcome measures were the QuickDASH (Disability of the Arm, Shoulder and Hand), numeric pain rating scale, and grip strength. They concluded that a comprehensive treatment program including NM appears to be effective for reducing disability and pain.[100]

Nerve Compression Syndromes

In the study by Pinar and colleagues,[101] two groups of patients received a volar resting wrist orthosis. The experimental group performed "nerve-gliding exercises" described by Totten and Hunter[101A] (which are tensile loading techniques) that the other group did not. Each of the six exercises was performed for 10 repetitions five times per day for 10 weeks. Both groups reported significant improvement. The experimental group also reported a more rapid pain reduction and greater functional movement.[101] In a similar randomized study using orthotic positioning and nerve and tendon gliding as described by Totten and Hunter, Akalin and colleagues[102] reported significant improvement in both groups: 72% in the orthosis-only group versus 93% in the orthosis plus exercise group. However, the difference was not significant. In contrast, Brininger and colleagues[103] found no difference between the group receiving an orthosis and tendon and nerve-gliding exercises and the control group receiving an orthosis only with CTS population. A similar finding was reported by Heebner and Roddey[104] comparing two groups, one receiving standard care and the other standard care plus nerve and tendon gliding. The nerve-gliding exercise was performed for 10 repetitions with a 5-second hold three to five times per day. The nerve-gliding exercise as described was a nerve-tensioning exercise and not a sliding exercise. Bialosky and colleague[105] found no significant difference between the sham treatment and an actual NDI (gliding) treatment in participants with CTS. However, they did report that there was a reduction in temporal summation in the NDI group.

Recent RCTs have also examined NM and CTS. Horng and colleagues[106] studied the effectiveness of tendon gliding and nerve gliding using three groups. All three groups received splint and paraffin, whereas group 1 had additional tendon gliding and group 2 nerve gliding. Outcome measures were DASH, Hand Questionnaire, and the physical domain of the World Health Organization quality of Life

Questionnaire–Brief Version. The nerve gliding exercises used tensile loading exercises at the wrist and hand. There were significant improvements in symptom severity and pain scale on all three groups; however, only group 1 showed a significant change in functional status. Their conclusion was that tendon gliding was more effective than nerve gliding. It should be noted that the nerve gliding described was tensile loading, which may have affected the outcome.[106] NM was compared with ultrasound and laser in an RCT by Wolny and associates[107] using two-point discrimination as the dependent variable. Both groups improved significantly. The NM group received single joint tensioning at the elbow and wrist, which are meant to elongate the nerve bed.[107] Oskouei and associates,[108] performed a randomized study of the outcome of routine therapy and NM composed of manual techniques that widen the carpal tunnel, stretch the transverse carpal ligament, and oscillatory movement of the elbow and not the wrist. Except for distal sensory latencies, significant improvements were found in the other outcome measures: symptom severity scale, functional status scale, median nerve NDT, visual analog scale, and distal motor and sensory latencies.[108] Two recent systematic reviews concluded that there is limited evidence on the effectiveness of nerve gliding; however, they were of the opinion that nerve gliding may accelerate recovery of function in a review of 13 publications.[109] In the other review, 9 RCT studies were analyzed, concluding that the findings were inconclusive regarding the effectiveness of various NM techniques.[110] The underlying issue regarding treatment is the lack standardization of the nomenclature, of clinical application, and of the dosage and duration or frequency. Regarding its use in compression neuropathies, the above holds true, and in addition, various stages of compression were all used together rather than using mild, moderate, or severe, for example.

PRACTICAL APPROACH TO NEURODYNAMIC TESTING AND NEURODYNAMIC INTERVENTION

Neurodynamic Examination

The neurodynamic examination (NDE) of the patient requires that the therapist perform a complete upper quarter screening examination before proceeding with the NDE (see Chapter 9). In addition, a differential tissue assessment must be completed to rule out any potential tissue that may be attributed to the patient's signs and symptoms. Only after these two components are addressed should the therapist proceed with the NDE, which is composed of five components as summarized in Box 102.3.[49,87] The examination requires the presence of active motion dysfunction as the first component of the NDE. The purpose of examining for active dysfunction is to determine the patient's willingness to move and for the therapist to gain insight into the patient's limitation of motion and pain. Before initiating the examination, the therapist should observe the presenting posture of the patient for evidence of antitension posture; an example is shown in Figure 102.4. In this patient with a diagnosis of right cubital tunnel syndrome after submuscular anterior transposition, note how the patient is attempting to minimize tension in her nervous system by posturing in cervical rotation and lateral flexion to the ipsilateral side. There is increased tone in the upper trapezius, as noted by scapular elevation, and the right extremity is positioned in shoulder adduction and internal rotation, elbow flexion, pronation, and wrist flexion.

An example of the active dysfunction examination is depicted in the series of photographs in Figure 102.5 of a patient after repair of the left median nerve at the wrist. In Figure 102.5A, the initial test of the patient's willingness to move is examined by asking the patient to comfortably place his hands over his head. In the following photographs, the patient is specifically requested to perform shoulder abduction in the coronal plane within his comfort range while various components

BOX 102.3 Summary of Neuron-Orthopedic Examination

Active Dysfunction

1. Active abduction and forward flexion

Observe cervical spine and extremity joint positioning and patient's willingness to move

    Specific motions: observe joint position changes in upper quarter

    Coronal plane shoulder abduction with elbow extended

    Coronal plane shoulder abduction with proximal (cervical spine) component

        Ipsilateral rotation

            Ipsilateral lateral flexion or side bending

            Contralateral rotation - if needed

            Contralateral lateral flexion - if needed

    Coronal plane shoulder abduction with distal component

        Wrist flexion

            Wrist extension

            Variation with elbow and forearm position

2. Passive motion limitation

Neurodynamic Test: Upper Limb

3. Nerve trunk hyperalgesia

Local peripheral nerve palpation sites

    Brachial plexus

        Posterior triangle: trunks

        Axilla: cords

    Median nerve

        Medial humerus

        Medial to biceps

        Pronator

        Carpal tunnel

    Ulnar nerve

        Medial humerus

        Cubital tunnel

        Proximal

        Distal: flexor carpi ulnaris origin

        Guyon's canal: pisiform

        Hook of hamate

        Dorsal ulnar cutaneous nerve

    Radial nerve

        Spiral groove

        Radial head: anterior

        Radial tunnel

        Radial sensory: brachioradialis insertion

4. Tender spots

Local tissue tender points in tissues innervated by the peripheral nerve or cervical segment involved

5. Local dysfunction

Cervical spine segmental stiffness for the segmental levels composing the brachial plexus and/or the peripheral nerves involved

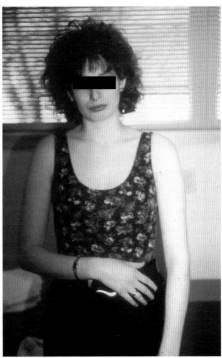

Fig. 102.4 Example of antitension posture (neural tension dysfunction). Note how the patient is attempting to minimize the tension in the right upper extremity.

The therapist must pay close attention to the presence of encountered resistance (reflexive muscle contraction)[14,49,51] and the level of irritability (patient response)[1,14,87] to avoid progressing beyond the endpoint of protective resistance and symptoms that may exacerbate the patient's symptoms. The encountered resistance (protective muscle contraction) was investigated by van der Heide and colleagues[51] by examining 20 asymptomatic participants measuring the EMG activity. They found that the onset of pain and the increase in EMG activity were highly reliable and compared favorably with the onset of muscle activity. An example of the sequence of this motion for the median nerve NDT is demonstrated in Figure 102.6. The therapist can vary the order in which each component motion is applied; however, it is recommended that the test for each nerve first be applied in a standardized manner. The final position of each joint and the patient response are recorded for baseline purposes to monitor progress.

It is recommended that the sensitizing components of scapular depression and cervical contralateral lateral flexion be applied only after the base components have been tested and only if necessary to elicit the symptoms. The subtracting of the sensitizing motions can be applied to confirm the involvement of the nervous system by eliminating the symptoms (STD) and avoiding the symptom exacerbation. The therapist should keep in mind that the NDT affects multiple aspects, including neurophysiology, blood flow, inflammation, neural mechanical sensitivity, and muscle response.[1] Each NDT should be applied slowly to avoid going beyond the encountered resistance. Although there are no clear data, it is the author's recommendation that each component be applied at a rate of 10 to 15 seconds using the work of Kwan and Haftek.[15,26] Video application of each of the three main neurodynamic tests for the upper extremity can be found on the companion website. As a reminder the purpose of STD is to eliminate the pain, not increase it. An example is scapulae elevation instead of depression or ipsilateral

are altered to determine the effect on motion and symptoms. The therapist should note how the position of the head and joints of the upper extremity changes with each movement. The active dysfunction examination is also summarized in Box 102.3.

After active motion assessment, passive motion is examined using the NDT, the second component of the NDE. The base component motions of the NDT for the three major nerves in the upper extremity are outlined in Box 102.4. As each successive sequence of motion is applied, the previous positions are maintained to successively apply low-level asymptomatic tension to the nervous system.

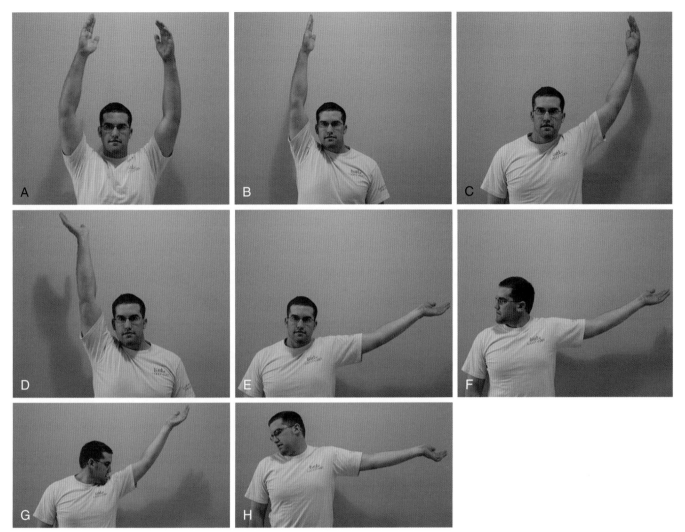

Fig. 102.5 Active motion dysfunction of a patient after median nerve repair at the wrist. **A,** Active shoulder elevation and coronal plane abduction of the uninvolved side (**B**) and involved side (**C**). Coronal plane abduction with wrist extension of the uninvolved side (**D**) and involved side (**E**). (Note the change in shoulder abduction when comparing sides.) Coronal plane abduction with cervical rotation to the contralateral side (**F**), cervical rotation to the ipsilateral side (**G**), and cervical lateral flexion to the contralateral side (**H**). (Note again the change in shoulder abduction when tension is altered using a proximal component.)

cervical rotation–lateral flexion or side bend to alleviate the pain. Any of the components of the NDT can be used in this way.

In addition to active and passive motion dysfunction, the therapist should be able to demonstrate palpable neural hyperalgesia, which is the third component of the NDE, along the course of the hypothesized nerves involved.[9,14,87] As with the NDT, the response to neural palpation is subject to the magnitude and rate of the load.[9] Repeated palpation may also preload the neural tissue, causing increased mechanosensitivity, which may lead to a false-positive result.[9] Box 102.3 includes a summary of the anatomic locations where each of the peripheral nerves can be palpated, keeping in mind that many of these locations will be an indirect palpation and the nerve itself will not be palpable. Elvey[49] described the presence of local tender points as the fourth component of NDE in tissues innervated by the hypothesized peripheral nerve or nerve root segment. The therapist should anticipate that these structures will be sensitive. Often, muscle tenderness may be confused with myofascial trigger points. Finally, there will be the presence of local dysfunction, the fifth component of NDE, within the cervical segment(s) contributing to the peripheral nerve involved.[49] This local cervical dysfunction may present as segmental hypomobility

or tenderness to palpation of the segments contributing to the involved peripheral nerve.

The interpretation of a positive NDT result will result in reproduction of the patient's symptoms and motion limitations determined by patient tolerance or encountered resistance. During the initial testing, the endpoint at which the therapist ceases continuing the motion or adding components should be the onset of patient symptoms or resistance encountered. Altering a distal or proximal component (joint) motion (STD) should result in a change in the baseline results of the NDT. For example, placing the wrist in a neutral position may increase elbow extension or cervical ipsilateral lateral flexion may improve elbow extension when performing a particular NDT.[87] These changes in motion or response are then documented for comparison with the baseline test performed. A positive test result may also be confirmed by identifying a difference in response or motion limitation by comparing the involved to the noninvolved side. It is beyond the scope of this chapter to explain in complete detail the principles of NDE and its findings. Readers are referred to the additional sources in the references and urged to pursue furthering their knowledge for a more in-depth understanding.

BOX 102.4 **Upper Extremity Neurodynamic Testing Components**

Median Nerve
Shoulder abduction
Shoulder external rotation
Forearm supination
Wrist and finger extension
Elbow extension

Sensitizing Components (only as needed; apply with care)
Shoulder depression
Cervical contralateral lateral flexion

Ulnar Nerve
Shoulder abduction
Shoulder external rotation
Pronation or supination
Wrist and small finger extension
Elbow flexion

Sensitizing Components (only as needed; apply with care)
Shoulder depression
Cervical contralateral lateral flexion

Radial Nerve
Shoulder abduction
Shoulder internal rotation
Pronation
Wrist and thumb–index flexion
Elbow extension

Sensitizing Components (only as needed; apply with care)
Shoulder depression
Cervical contralateral lateral flexion

Upper limb neurodynamic test components for the three major nerves in the upper extremity. Note that the sensitizing components are added after the primary component motion if necessary.

Guiding Principles

After the therapist has confirmed that neural tissue is the patient's problem, the development of a logical NDI approach using neural gliding (sliding), which has been shown to create better hypoalgesia effects than tensioning.[111] NDI can be guided by three basic principles. First, education of the patient and the therapist is imperative. The patient must understand the role the nervous system plays in his or her pathology, the concept of neural mechanics, and how these interact to alter movement and function. A sound comprehension of the concepts of neural tension and gliding is crucial to preventing exacerbation and assists with treatment progression. Sound clinical reasoning that formulates a working hypothesis is required. These hypotheses must include (1) the source of the symptoms or dysfunction, (2) contributing factors, (3) precautions and contraindications to examination or treatment, (4) management, and (5) prognosis.[1,87,112]

The second basic principle is NDI application and prescription. In most cases, the therapist is presented with a patient whose pathologic process has occurred over an extended period, resulting in pain and movement dysfunction. These adaptive changes may take months to alter with treatment. Although NDI techniques are used in the clinic, the restoration of movement and elimination of pain require the diligent use of a home program that is periodically adjusted based on reassessment and response to treatment. The third principle is the therapist

empowering the patient in the performance and follow-through of the exercise program. This is achieved through assisting the patient in observing and appreciating the changes in his or her symptomatology, improvements in impairments such as specific joint or multisegment motion limitations, and the ability to use his or her upper extremity for functional activities without the onset of pain.

Treatment Guidelines

As discussed earlier in the literature review, no clear-cut protocol for the development and implementation of NDI exists. A thorough working knowledge of the nervous system and the NDE components is required. The NDT components are transformed into NDI techniques and exercises for treatment and home. NDT is a dynamic process, changing daily, affecting diagnosis and treatment hypotheses. Therefore, examination, evaluation, and ongoing reevaluation should continuously guide treatment progression and implementation as the hypothesis(es) regarding the specific tissues at fault and the location becomes refined. The concepts of nerve tension (stress and strain) and glide (excursion) play a major role in treatment formulation. Tensile loading creates strain within the nerve by pulling on one or both ends of the nerve simultaneously, causing the nerve and its bed to unfold. The clinician must be especially cautious if the nerve has been preloaded because this will have a profound effect on the nerve's neurophysiology because of alterations in vascular and axoplasmic flow. In contrast, glide refers to placing tension on the nerve at one point while simultaneously releasing it at another. Coppieters and Butler[57] refer to this as a sliding technique. The overall resting tension or strain is significantly minimized with sliding.[54,57] Gliding can also occur within the nerve[16] or between the nerve and its interfacing tissue.[17–19,31,32] Figure 102.7 is an illustration of these two concepts. A clinical example of these two concepts is presented in Figure 102.8. The clinician should proceed with tensioning only if necessary and with great caution.

The presenting level of patient symptom irritability guides the use of tension or glide. In patients with highly irritable symptoms, sliding techniques may be the most appropriate approach. When using sliding techniques, the therapist needs to be aware of the tissue barriers (reflexive muscle contraction) encountered. Treatment and home exercises are performed in the pain and tension-free ROM below the stimulus threshold. It may be necessary to begin at remote sites from the hypothesized location, including the lower limb and spine, progressing toward the specific site of involvement as tolerated. Patients whose symptoms are of low irritability may be able to tolerate single-joint progressing to multijoint tension when symptoms are mild and absent at rest and recovery from any exacerbation is rapid. It may be appropriate to tension the involved nerve to the point of the tissue barrier directly or at a more remote site and progress toward the hypothesized location to elongate the tissue bed. Perhaps restoring mobility or improving tolerance to tension at a remote location may assist the nerve in attenuating tension throughout its course, thereby decreasing symptoms. As irritability decreases, the therapist can begin to work through the tissue barriers to restore movement to the extremity and increase function. At this level, there may be a transient response of paresthesia or discomfort that should quickly resolve. At no time should there be a sustained stretch.[1] Figure 102.9 is an algorithm to depict treatment progression.

The tissues hypothesized to be at fault, neural or non-neural, will also guide treatment. The treatment of non-neural tissues may initially require the nervous system be placed in a position of antitension or slack. This would allow for direct treatment of the non-neural tissues while minimizing mechanical deformation of the sensitized nerve and avoiding further risk of exacerbation. The clinician should be aware of any underlying mechanically sensitive neural tissue in the treated area. For example, if the clinician is attempting to improve glenohumeral motion, the combination of ipsilateral cervical flexion and scapular

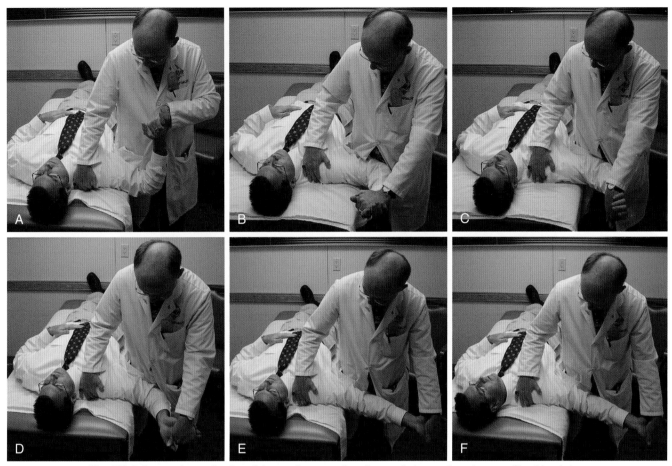

Fig. 102.6 Successive application of the median nerve (base) upper limb neural tension test. Shoulder abduction (**A**), shoulder external rotation (**B**), forearm supination (**C**), wrist–hand extension (**D**), elbow extension (**E**), additional sensitizing motions of contralateral cervical flexion, and scapular depression if needed (**F**).

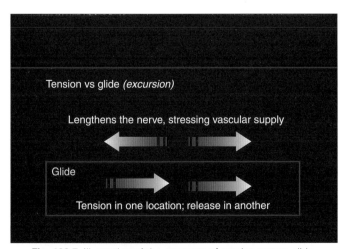

Fig. 102.7 Illustration of the concepts of tension versus glide.

elevation may minimize the additional neural tension created by glenohumeral motion. Care should always be taken not to exceed the clinical limit of the nervous system, which is determined by the patient's symptoms.

Finally, the therapist should have a working hypothesis as to the existence of any intraneural or extraneural fibrosis. If intraneural fibrosis is suspected, it may be more appropriate to attempt to increase neural compliance at a location that is remote from the hypothesized site of the lesion. It is my opinion that these therapeutic techniques are unlikely to improve the internal structure of a fibrotic nerve based on our knowledge of connective tissue. However, if it is hypothesized that the nerve's ability to glide (slide) within its tissue bed is compromised (extraneural fibrosis), treatment of the interfacing tissues at the site(s) hypothesized may be indicated. This may be performed in conjunction with glide or tension of the nerve in question, depending on the level of irritability. Box 102.5 summarizes the guidelines that the treating practitioner should consider when developing a treatment strategy.

Augmenting Neural Mobilization

Using other treatment techniques can augment NDI. Superficial and deep heating modalities may be used to precondition the tissues, keeping in mind this may alter the stimulus threshold for provoking symptoms, which could result in a delayed exacerbation response. Massage, joint mobilization, or other manual techniques can be applied to assist in restoring mobility and decreasing interfacing tissue adherence with the nerve in a slack (antitension) position. Postural education and awareness and the use of physiologic ROM exercises to improve soft tissue mobility and strength can be used in conjunction with NDI techniques. The list of combining and augmenting treatments is exhaustive if the clinical state of the nerve and its interfacing tissues is respected.

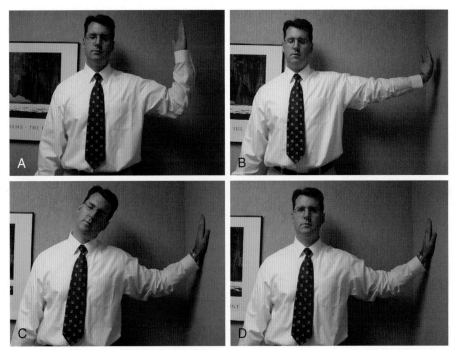

Fig. 102.8 Examples of home exercises used for neurodynamic intervention. **A** and **B,** Gliding. Note that as tensile loading is placed in one location, it is relieved in another location. **C** and **D,** Note that tension is applied using one joint only while maintaining one component in the slack position and maintaining the preload tension position of the other joints of the upper extremity. This should all be non–symptom provoking.

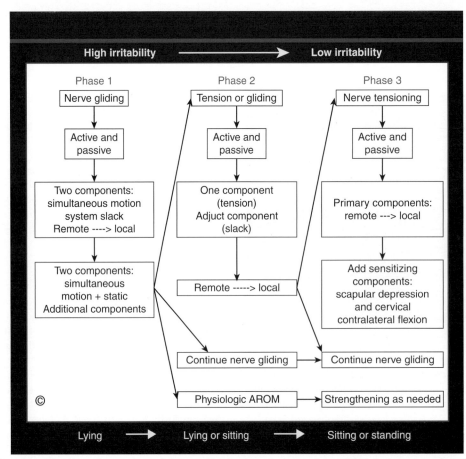

Fig. 102.9 Algorithm of neurodynamic intervention treatment progression. *AROM,* Active range of motion.

<table>
<tr><td>

BOX 102.5 Treatment Guidelines

Working Knowledge and Understanding of the Neurodynamic Test Components
Evaluation and Reevaluation
Response to treatment-changing hypothesis

Hypothesis of Location and Tissues at Fault
Tension vs Glide (Excursion)
Tension: lengthens the nerve; stresses vascular supply
Glide: tension in one location and release in another

Irritable vs Nonirritable
Irritable: gliding (tissue barriers), selected component distal to site (lower extremity or trunk), pain-free range tension free
Nonirritable: tension, (+) symptoms (mild) rapid recovery, select component or nerve directly involved

Neural vs Non-neural Components
Treat non-neural tissues directly with tension eliminated (nontension component position)
Treat non-neural tissues under tension (nonirritable)

Intraneural vs Extraneural Fibrosis
Intraneural: Attempt to increase mobility away from site
Extraneural: Treat interfacing tissue in conjunction with glide or tension

</td><td>

BOX 102.6 Precautions and Contraindications

Precautions
Irritable conditions
Spinal cord signs
Nerve root signs
Severe unremitting night pain, lacking a diagnosis
Recent paresthesia, anesthesia, or complex regional pain syndrome types I and II
Mechanical spine pain with peripheralization

Contraindications
Recently repaired peripheral nerve
Malignancy
Active inflammatory conditions
Neurologic: acute inflammatory/demyelinating diseases

</td></tr>
</table>

Progression of Neurodynamic Intervention Techniques

The progression of NDI techniques is depicted in Figure 102.9 and is dictated by the patient's response. Progression requires continual clinical reasoning to avoid further injury or exacerbation. All motions used to involve the neural system should be performed within the asymptomatic range. Only when symptoms are under control should consideration be given to challenging the tissue barriers, and only if this is necessary to improve function or range. This is an oversimplification of the concept, but the most important aspect is its consideration for the level of irritability of the tissues involved. These concepts can be applied actively by the patient, passively by the therapist, via active physiologic joint motion using individual or multiple NDT components in small- or large-amplitude movements. It is this author's recommendation that all treatments start with sliding techniques.

At present, no clear guidelines or research supports the most effective amplitude, dose, duration, or frequency necessary to achieve the desired result. The use of oscillatory movements have been suggested, keeping in mind that the rate of application plays a role in the nerves ability to tolerate elongation or excursion.[112] At no time should a tension technique be sustained for a prolonged period.[1,87] As a rule, Elvey and colleagues[113] have supported this, recommending that end-range grades should not be used, and the duration should be less than that used for joint mobilization. Therefore, sound clinical reasoning regarding these parameters is necessary to progress NDI techniques and exercises. For the present, the progression can only be based on the patient's clinical response to the treatment.

The use of additional component joint motions of the NDT will result in increased tension within the nervous system. As irritability decreases and mobility improves, additional component motions can be combined as appropriate and necessary. Working from a remote site and progressing toward the hypothesized involved site or nerve is another way to progress NDI. For example, if the ulnar nerve was involved at the level of the elbow, it may be more appropriate because of irritability to initiate nerve gliding at the shoulder, cervical spine, or

wrist before using the elbow joint for mobilizing the nerve. The adaptive changes of nerve physiology and mechanical behavior that occur over time will require patience. Therefore, these principles are best applied in conjunction with a home program with periodic visits to adjust the exercise prescription.

Contraindications and Precautions

The contraindications and precautions for the use of NDT upper limb and NDI are listed in Box 102.6. The application of the NDT or NDI techniques can easily result in significant exacerbation and prolonged recovery of the patient's symptoms when applied incorrectly. Cord and nerve root signs, especially in the presence of hard neurologic signs (reflex changes, motor weakness, and sensory changes), may indicate the presence of NTD within the CNS, necessitating that these patients be approached with caution. Unremitting night pain not associated with a mechanical cause or undiagnosed may indicate pain of visceral origin. For example, cardiac, hepatic, diaphragmatic, and upper gastrointestinal structures can refer pain to the upper quadrant. Recent sensory changes may indicate a systemic neurologic or inflammatory disease such as multiple sclerosis and rheumatoid arthritis or may be indicative of a recent CNS pathology such as nerve root compression and a peripheral lesion. CRPS may be an underlying component of the patient's pain, and aggressive handling may contribute to further exacerbation of the patient's symptoms. Pain originating from cervical spine structures may also refer pain to the upper extremity. In all these cases, the clinician must exercise caution in the application of the NDT and NDI techniques. Mechanical mobilization of the nervous system is contraindicated in the case of a recently repaired nerve, malignancy (primary or metastatic) involving a nerve or its surrounding tissues, and active neurologic or inflammatory diseases.

SUMMARY

In this chapter, I have proposed that there is a need to reexamine previous terminology and thought processes for neural system dysfunction and neuropathic and neurogenic pain. For example, I propose that STD be used to decrease the patient's symptoms with NDT to avoid the exacerbation of the patient's symptoms, which could be disastrous. This process is based on the concept of neurodynamics,[1,2] which serves to explain the PNS mechanical and physiological behavior. This concept is leading clinicians to examine and treat NP and other PNS disturbances in a different light with greater understanding. The judicious use of the NDT and NDI requires the therapist to have a sound knowledge of the nervous system's histology, vascularity, anatomy, physiology, biomechanics, and pathology. Only through the application of this knowledge is it possible to effectively examine and treat the PNS. Clinically recognizing how nervous system pathology may manifest itself is required before proceeding with the NDT and NDI. Research on this topic has centered on basic science and asymptomatic and selected patient populations. Basic science and clinical research on PNS behavior and pain theoretically supports the validity of NDT and NDI. Recently, there has been an increase in more rigorous studies and RCTs that have begun to create a better understanding. Several studies have examined the use of NDI as a treatment approach. Although the results are promising, further controlled studies are required to identify the appropriate patient population for NDI. Unfortunately, there are no studies to support an appropriate dose, duration, or frequency or application of NDT and NDI techniques, leaving it to the clinician to determine these parameters.

Treatment begins with the clinician's awareness of his or her own knowledge, clinical limitations, and the contraindications and precautions for NDI. Application of NDI is guided by the principles of clinician and patient education regarding neurodynamics and the avoidance of symptom exacerbation via examination and treatment. Clinicians are reminded that NDI as a treatment rarely stands alone and is augmented by other treatment techniques used each day for their patients. Finally, progression is based on continuous reassessment of the patient's response to the treatment strategies. NDI is an additional treatment tool available to clinicians and their patients presenting with difficult and complicated diagnoses of upper extremity NP and PNS dysfunction.

REFERENCES

1. Shacklock M. Improving application of neurodynamic (neural tension) testing and treatments: a message to researchers and clinicians. *Manual Ther.* 2005;10(3):175–179.
2. Shacklock M. 1st ed. *Clinical Neurodynamics: A New System of Musculoskeletal Treatment.* vol. 1. Philadelphia: Elsevier Butterworth Heinemann; 2005:251.
3. Jensen T, et al. A new definition of neuropathic pain. *Pain.* 2011;152:2204–2205.
4. Allen R. Neuropathic pain in the cancer patient. *Neurol Clin.* 1998;16(4):869–887.
5. Baron R, Binder A, Wasner G. Neuropathic pain: diagnosis pathophysiological mechanisms and treatment. *Lancet Neurol.* 2010;9:807–819.
6. Jensen T, Finnerup N. Allodynia and hyperalgesia in neuropathic pain: clinical manifestations and mechanisms. *Lancet Neurol.* 2014;23:924–935.
6A. Baron R. Mechanisms of Disease Neuropathic Pain—A Clinical Perspective. *Nat Clin Pract Neurol.* 2006;2:95–106.
7. Weinstein J. Neurogenic and non-neurogenic pain and inflammatory mediators. *Orthop Clin North Am.* 1991;22:235–246.
8. Eliav E, Benoliel R, Tal M. Inflammation with no axonal damage of the rat saphenous nerve trunk induces ectopic discharge and mechanosensitivity in myelinated axons. *Neurosci Letter.* 2001;311:49–52.
9. Clark E, et al. Mechanically evoked sensory and motor responses to dynamic compression of the ulnar nerve. *Muscle Nerve.* 2007;35:303–311.
10. Dilley A, Lynn B, Pang S. Pressure and stretch mechanosensitivity of peripheral nerve following local inflammation of the nerve trunk. *Pain.* 2005;117:62–472.
11. Galer B, Jensen M. Development and preliminary validation of a pain measure specific to neuropathic pain: the neuropathic pain scale. *Neurology.* 1997;48:332–338.
12. Bouhassira D, et al. Development and validation of the neuropathic pain symptom inventory. *Pain.* 2004;108:248–257.
13. Bennett M, et al. The S-LANSS score for identifying pain of predominantly neuropathic origin: validation for use in clinical and postal research. *J Pain.* 2005;6:149–158.
14. Butler D. *The Sensitive Nervous System.* Adelaide Australia: Noigroup Publications; 2000.
15. Haftek J. Stretch injury of peripheral nerve: acute effects of stretching on rabbit nerve. *J Bone Joint Surg.* 1970;52B:354–365.
16. Millesi H, Zoch G, Reihsner R. Mechanical properties of peripheral nerves. *Clin Orthop Relat Res.* 1995;314:76–83.
17. Wright T, Cowin D, Wheeler D. Radial nerve excursion and strain at the elbow and wrist associated with upper-extremity motion. *J Hand Surg.* 2005;30A:990–996.
18. Wright T, et al. Ulnar nerve excursion and strain at the elbow and wrist associated with upper extremity motion. *J Hand Surg.* 2001;26A:655–662.
19. Wright T, et al. Excursion and strain of the median nerve. *J Bone Joint Surg.* 1996;78A:1897–1903.
20. Kleinrensink G, et al. Upper limb tension tests as tools in the diagnosis of nerve and plexus lesions. *Clin Biomech.* 2000;15(1):9–14.
21. Manvell J, et al. Improving the radial nerve neurodynamic test: an observation of tension of the radial, median, and ulnar nerves during upper limb positioning. *Man Ther.* 2015;20:790–796.
22. Kleinrensink G, et al. Upper limb tension tests as tools in the diagnosis of nerve and plexus lesions: anatomical and biomechanical aspects. *Clin Biomech.* 2000;15:9–15.
23. Dilley A, et al. Quantitative in vivo studies of median nerve sliding in response to wrist, elbow, shoulder and neck movements. *Clin Biomech.* 2003;18:899–907.
24. Lundborg G, Rydevik B. Effects of stretching the tibial nerve of the rabbit. A preliminary study of the intraneural circulation and the barrier function of the perineurium. *J Bone Joint Surg.* 1973;55B:390–401.
25. Ogata K, Naito M. Blood flow of peripheral nerve effects of dissection, stretching and compression. *J Hand Surg.* 1986;11B:10–14.
26. Kwan M, et al. Strain. stress, and stretch of peripheral nerve: rabbit experiments in vitro and in vivo. *Acta Orthopedic Scandinavia.* 1992;63:267–272.
27. Wall E, et al. Experimental stretch neuropathy: changes in nerve conduction under tension. *J Bone Joint Surg.* 1992;74B:126–129.
28. Watanabe M, et al. The implication of repeated versus continuous strain on nerve function in a rat forelimb model. *J Hand Surg.* 2001;26A:663–669.
29. Sunderland S. *Nerve and Nerve Injuries.* London: Churchill and Livingston; 1978.
30. Breig A. *Adverse Mechanical Tension in the Central Nervous System.* New York: John Wiley & Sons; 1978.
31. McLellan D, Swash M. Longitudinal sliding of the median nerve during movements of the upper limb. *J Neurol Neurosurg Psychiatry.* 1976;39:566–570.
32. Wilgis E, Murphy R. The significance of longitudinal excursion in peripheral nerves. *Hand Clin.* 1986;2:761–766.
33. Dilley A, Greening J, Lynn B. The use of cross-correlation analysis between high-frequency ultrasound images to measure longitudinal median nerve movement. *Ultrasound Med Biol.* 2001;27:1211–1218.
34. Nakamichi K, Tachibana S. Transverse sliding of the median nerve beneath the flexor retinaculum. *J Hand Surg.* 1992;17B:213–216.
35. Dilley A, Summerhayes C, Lynn B. An in vivo investigation of ulnar nerve sliding during upper limb movements. *Clin Biomech.* 2007;22:774–779.
36. Millesi H, Zoch G, Rath T. The gliding apparatus of peripheral nerve and its clinical significance. *Annals Hand Upper Limb Surg.* 1990;9:87–96.
37. Zoech G, et al. Stress strain in peripheral nerves. *Neuro Orthop.* 1991;10:73–82.
38. Lundborg G. Intraneural microcirculation. *Orthop Clin North Am.* 1988;19:1–12.
39. Upton A, McComas A. The double crush in nerve entrapment syndrome. *Lancet.* 1973;2:359–362.

40. Pechan J, Julis I. The pressure measurement in the ulnar nerve. a contribution to the pathophysiology of the cubital tunnel syndrome. *J Biomech.* 1975;8:75–79.
41. Dahlin L, McLean G. Effects of graded experimental compression on slow and fast axonal transport in rabbit vagus nerve. *J Neurosci.* 1986;72:19–30.
42. Nemoto K, et al. An experimental study of the "double crush" hypothesis. *J Hand Surg.* 1987;12A:552–559.
43. Schmid A, Coppieters M. The double crush syndrome revisited - a Delphi study to reveal current expert views on mechanisms underlying dual nerve disorders. *Manual Therapy.* 2011;16:557–562.
44. Molinari W, Elfar J. The double crush syndrome. *J Hand Surg.* 2013;38A:799–801.
45. Mackinnon S, Dellon A. Experimental study of chronic nerve compression clinical implications. *Hand Clin.* 1986;2:639–650.
46. Bove G, et al. Inflammation induces ectopic mechanical sensitivity in axons of nociceptors innervating deep tissues. *J Neurophysiol.* 2003;90:1949–1955.
47. Schmid A, et al. Local and remote immune-mediated inflammation after mild peripheral nerve compression in rats. *J Neuropathol Exp Neurol.* 2013;72:662–680.
48. Lundborg G, Dahlin L. The pathophysiology of nerve compression. *Hand Clin.* 1992;8:215–227.
49. Elvey R. Physical evaluation of the peripheral nervous system in disorders of pain and dysfunction. *J Hand Ther.* 1997;10:122–129.
50. Balster S, Jull G. Upper trapezius muscle activity during the brachial plexus tension test in asymptomatic subjects. *Man Ther.* 1997;2:144–149.
51. van der Heide B, Allison G, Zusman M. Pain and muscular responses to a neural tissue provocation test in the upper limb. *Man Ther.* 2001;6:154–162.
52. Edgar D, Jull G, Sutton S. The relationship between upper trapezius muscle length and upper quadrant neural tissue extensibility. *Aust Physiother.* 1994;40:99–103.
53. Byl C, Purrlitz C, Byl N. Strain in the median and ulnar nerves during upper limb extremity positioning. *J Hand Surg.* 2002;27A:1032–1040.
54. Coppieters M, Alshami A. Longitudinal excursion and strain in the median nerve during novel nerve gliding exercises for carpal tunnel syndrome. *J Orthop Res.* 2007:972–980.
55. Bay B, Sharkey N, Sxabo R. Displacement and strain of the median nerve at the wrist. *J Hand Surg.* 1997;22A:621–627.
56. Lewis J, Ramot R, Green A. Changes in mechanical tension in the median nerve: possible implications for the upper limb tension test. *Physiotherapy.* 1998;84:254–261.
57. Coppieters M, Butler D. Do "Sliders" slide and "Tensioners" tension? an analysis of neurodynamic techniques and considerations regarding their application. *Man Ther.* 2008;13:213–221.
58. Kenneally M, Rubenach H, Elvey R. The upper limb tension test: the SLR test of the arm. In: Grant R, ed. *Physical Therapy of the Cervical and Thoracic Spine.* New York: Churchill Livingstone; 1988:67–194.
59. Kenneally M. The Upper Limb Tension Test. In *Proceedings or the Fourth Biennial Conference of the Manipulative Therapists Association of Australia.* Melbourne, Australia; 1983
60. Yaxley G, Jull G. A modified upper limb tension test: an investigation of responses in normal subjects. *Aust Physiother.* 1991;37:143–152.
61. Lohkamp M, Small K. Normal response to upper limb neurodynamic Test 1 and 2A. *Man Ther.* 2011;16:125–130.
62. Martinez M, Cubas C, Girbes E. Ulnar nerve neurodynamic test: study of the normal sensory response in asymptomatic individuals. *J Orthop Sports Phys Ther.* 2014;44:450–456.
63. Coppieters M, et al. A qualitative assessment of shoulder girdle elevation during upper limb tension Test 1. *Man Ther.* 1999;4:33–38.
64. Coppieters M, et al. Addition of test components during neurodynamic testing: effect on range of motion and sensory responses. *J Orthop Sports Phys Ther.* 2001;31(5):226–237.
65. Coppieters M, et al. Reliability of detecting "Onset Pain" and "Submaximal Pain" during neural provocation testing for the upper quadrant. *Physiother Res Int.* 2002;7(146–156).
66. Petersen S, Covill L. Reliability of the radial and ulnar nerve biased upper extremity neural tissue provocation tests. *Physiother Theory Pract.* 2010;26:476–482.
67. Echigo A, et al. The excursion of the median nerve during nerve gliding exercise: an observation with high-resolution ultrasonography. *J Hand Ther.* 2008;21:221–228.
68. Coppieters M, Hough D, Dilley A. Different nerve gliding exercises induce different magnitudes of median nerve longitudinal excursion: an in vivo study using dynamic ultrasound imaging. *J Orthop Sports Phys Ther.* 2009;39:164–171.
69. Beneciuk K, Bishop M, Beorge S. Effects of upper extremity neural mobilization on thermal pain sensitivity: a sham-controlled study in asymptomatic participants. *J Orthop Sports Phys Ther.* 2009;30:428–438.
70. Costantiini M, et al. Age and upper limb tension testing affects current perception thresholds. *J Hand Ther.* 2006;19:307–317.
71. Coppieters M, Alshami A, Hodges P. An experimental pain model to investigate the specificity of neurodynamic test for the median nerve in the differential diagnosis of hand symptoms. *Arch Phys Med Rehabil.* 2006;87:1412–1417.
72. Coppieters M, et al. The impact of neurodynamic testing on the perception of experimentally induced muscle pain. *Man Ther.* 2005;10:52–60.
73. Boyd B, et al. Mechanosensitivity of the lower extremity nervous system during straight-leg raise neurodynamic testing in healthy individuals. *J Orthop Sports Phys Ther.* 2009;39:780–790.
74. Boyd B, et al. Mechanosensitivity during lower extremity neurodynamic testing is diminished in individuals with type 2 diabetes mellitus and peripheral neuropathy: a cross sectional study. *BioMed Central Neurol.* 2010;10:1–14.
75. Sandmark H, Nisell R. Validity of five common manual neck pain provoking tests. *Scand J Rehab Med.* 1995;27:131–136.
76. Sterling M, Treleaven J, Jull G. Responses to a clinical test of mechanical provocation of nerve tissue in whiplash associated disorder. *Man Ther.* 2002;7:89–94.
77. Talebi G, Oskouei A, Shakori S. Reliability of upper limb tension test 1in normal subjects and patients with carpal tunnel syndrome. *J Back Musculoskelet Rehabil.* 2012;25:209–214.
78. R N, et al. The validity of upper-limb neurodynamic tests for detecting peripheral neuropathic pain. *J Orthop Sports Phys Ther.* 2012;42(5):413–424.
79. Yeung E, Jones M, Hall B. The response to the slump test in a group of female whiplash patients. *Aust Physiother.* 1997;43(4):245–252.
80. Elvey R, Quinter J, Thomas A. A clinical study of RSI. *Aust Fam Physician.* 1986;15:1314–1322.
81. Quintner J. A study of upper limb pain and paraesthesiae following neck injury in motor vehicle accidents: assessment of the brachial plexus tension test of Elvey. *Br J Rheumatol.* 1989;28(6):528–533.
82. Wainner R, Fritz J, Irrgang J. Reliability and diagnostic accuracy of the clinical examination and patient self-report measures for cervical radiculopathy. *Spine.* 2003;28:52–62.
83. Selvaratnam P, Matyas T, Glasgow E. Noninvasive discrimination of brachial plexus involvement in upper limb pain. *Spine.* 1994;19(1):26–33.
84. Trillos M, Soto F, Briceno-Ayala L. Upper limb neurodynamic test 1 in patients with clinical diagnosis of carpal tunnel syndrome: a diagnostic accuracy study. *J Hand Ther.* 2018;31:333–338.
85. Baselgia L, et al. Negative neurodynamic tests do not exclude neural dysfunction in patients with entrapment neuropathies. *Arch Phys Med Rehabil.* 2017;98:480–486.
86. Nee R, et al. Impact of order of movement on nerve strain and longitudinal excursion: a biomechanical study with implications for neurodynamic test sequencing. *Man Ther.* 2010;15:376–381.
87. Nee R, Butler D. Management of peripheral neuropathic pain: integrating neurobiology, neurodynamics, and clinical evidence. *Phys Ther Sport.* 2006;7:36–49.
88. Rydevik B, et al. An in vitro mechanical and histological study of acute stretching on rabbit tibial nerve. *J Orthop Res.* 1990;8(5):694–701.
89. Brown C, et al. The effects of neurodynamic mobilization on fluid dispersion within the tibial nerve at the ankle: an unembalmed cadaveric study. *J Man Manip Ther.* 2011;19:26–34.

90. Santos F, et al. Neural mobilization reverses behavioral and cellular changes that characterize neuropathic pain in rats. *Molecular Pain*. 2012;8. 1744-8069-8-57.

91. Santos F, et al. The neural mobilization technique modulates the expression of endogenous opioids in the periaqueductal gray and improves muscle strength and mobility in rats with neuropathic pain. *Behav Brain Funct*. 2014;10:1–8.

92. da Silva J, et al. Neural mobilization promotes nerve regeneration by nerve growth factor and myelin protein zero increased after sciatic nerve injury. *Growth Factors*. 2015;33:8–13.

93. Hough A, Moore A, Jones M. Reduced longitudinal excursion of the median nerve in carpal tunnel syndrome. *Arch Phys Med Rehabil*. 2007;88:569–576.

94. Greening J, Dilley A, Lynn B. In vivo study of nerve movement and mechanosensitivity of the median nerve in whiplash and non-specific arm pain patients. *Pain*. 2005;115:248–253.

95. Marshall M. Nerve stretching for the relief or cure of pain. *Lancet*. 1883:1029–1036.

96. Ellis R, Hing W. Neural mobilization: a systematic review of randomized controlled trials with an analysis of therapeutic efficacy. *J Man Ther*. 2008;16(1):8–22.

97. Su Y, Lim E. Does evidence support the use of neural tissue management to reduce pain and disability in nerve-related chronic musculoskeletal pain? A systematic review with meta-analysis. *Clin J Pain*. 2016;32(11):991–1004.

98. Basson A, et al. The effectiveness of neural mobilization for neuromusculoskeletal conditions: a systematic review and meta-analysis. *J Orthop Sports Phys Ther*. 2017;47(9):593–615.

99. Nee R, et al. Neural tissue management provides immediate clinically relevant benefits without harmful effects for patients with nerve-related neck and arm pain: a randomized trial. *J Physiother*. 2012;58: 23–31.

100. Day J, et al. Outcomes following the conservative management of patients with non-radicular peripheral neuropathic pain. *J Hand Ther*. 2014;27(3):192–200.

101. Pinar L, et al. Can we use nerve gliding exercises in women with carpal tunnel syndrome. *Adv Ther*. 2005;22:467–475.

101A. Totten P, Hunter J. Therapeutic Techniques to Enhance Nerve Gliding in Thoracic Outlet Syndrome and Carpal Tunnel Syndrome. *Hand Clin*. 1991;7:505–520.

102. Akalin E, et al. Treatment of carpal tunnel syndrome with nerve and tendon gliding exercises. *Am J Phys Med Rehabil*. 2002;81:108–113.

103. Brininger M, et al. Efficacy of a fabricated customized splint and tendon and nerve gliding exercises for the treatment of carpal tunnel syndrome: a randomized controlled trial. *Arch Phys Med Rehabil*. 2007;99:1429–1435.

104. Heebner M, Roddey T. The effects of neural mobilization in addition to standard care in persons with carpal tunnel syndrome from a community hospital. *J Hand Ther*. 2008;21:229–241.

105. Bialosky J, et al. A Randomized sham-controlled trial of a neurodynamic technique in the treatment of carpal tunnel syndrome. *J Orthop Sports Phys Ther*. 2009;39:709–723.

106. Horng Y, et al. The comparative effectiveness of tendon and nerve gliding exercises in patients with carpal tunnel syndrome: a randomized trial. *Am J Phys Med Rehabil*. 2011;90:435–442.

107. Wolny T, et al. Effect of manual therapy and neurodynamic techniques vs ultrasound and laser on 2pd in patients with CTS: a randomized controlled trial. *J Hand Ther*. 2016;29:235–245.

108. Oskouei A, et al. Effects of neuromobilization maneuver on clinical and electrophysiological measures of patients with carpal tunnel syndrome. *J Phys Ther Sci*. 2014;26:1017–1022.

109. Ballestero-Perez R, et al. Effectiveness of nerve gliding exercises on carpal tunnel syndrome: a systematic review. *J Manipulat Physiol Ther*. 2016;49:50–59.

110. Lim Y, Chee D, Girdler S. Median nerve mobilization techniques in the treatment of carpal tunnel syndrome: a systemic review. *J Hand Ther*. 2017;30:397–406.

111. Beltran-Alacreu H, et al. Comparison of hypoalgesic effects of neural stretching vs gliding: a randomized controlled trial. *J Manipulat Physiol Ther*. 2015;38:644–652.

112. Walsh M. Upper limb neural tension testing and mobilization: fact, fiction and practical approach. *J Hand Ther*. 2005;18:241–258.

113. Elvey R. Treatment of Arm pain associated with abnormal brachial plexus tension. *Austr J Physiother*. 1986;(32):225–230.

114. Grewal R, Xu J, Sotereanos D, Woo S. Biomechanical Properties of Peripheral Nerves. *Hand Clin*. 1996;12:195–204.

Taping Techniques

Tambra Marik

CRITICAL POINTS

- Therapeutic elastic tape has stretch qualities, allowing tape to move with the skin.
- Research supports short-term benefits of therapeutic elastic taping for pain relief in patients with shoulder impingement, medial epicondylitis, and lateral epicondylitis.
- The benefits of specific tension and direction of therapeutic elastic tape application require more research to fully understand therapeutic benefits.

- Therapeutic rigid tape is a nonelastic tape that is postulated to provide joint support, unload injured soft tissue structures, contribute to muscular inhibition, and facilitation and improve joint proprioception.
- Therapeutic rigid tape should be applied on top of adhesive hypoallergenic protective tape to protect the skin.

INTRODUCTION TO THERAPEUTIC TAPING

Therapeutic taping is commonly used as a rehabilitation intervention in the management of upper extremity pathology. Elastic and rigid tapes are two types of therapeutic tapes that have varying qualities. Elastic tape contains stretch qualities that are designed to mimic human skin.[1] Elastic tape is theorized to assist the body with healing or movement based on the cut of the tape and stretch tension and direction upon application to the involved structures. The rigid tape has nonstretch qualities that can provide structural support to joints.[2] Both types of tapes are proposed to enhance proprioception.[1,3] This chapter is an introduction to the background, theoretical concepts, upper extremity research evidence, basic application guidelines, and contraindications for therapeutic taping. Basic taping instructions for common clinical conditions are provided in the appendices. However, therapists are encouraged to pursue advanced training to master taping techniques to achieve safe and beneficial clinical outcomes when applying tape to a client.

ELASTIC TAPE INTRODUCTION

Dr. Kenzo Kase is considered to be the original founder of an elastic tape product and many tape application techniques that are widely used in rehabilitation clinics. Dr. Kase worked with product engineers to invent a tape that is flexible, lightweight, and hypoallergenic to avoid skin rashes.[4] The elastic tape is thought to mimic the physical characteristics off the human epidermis because of the tape's thin, lightweight quality.[1]

Dr. Kase's Kinesio Tex Tape and Kinesio-tape are common brand name tapes that have been investigated in the literature. Several manufactures market similar elastic tapes with a variety of brand names such as Kinesiology Tape, Acu or Aku-tape, Kinesio Tex, Kinesio Elastic Tape, Kinesio-Orthopaedic Tape, Athletic Tape, Rock Tape, and Neuroproprioceptive tape. This chapter refers to all elastic therapeutic tape products as "elastic tape." This chapter is an introduction to elastic taping. Therefore, specific qualities of brand name elastic tapes will not be promoted or discouraged. Therapists are encouraged to try varying brands of tapes to explore each tape's comfort and adhesive qualities for patient application.

Common characteristics of the therapeutic elastic tapes include weft angles to the right that provide the ability to longitudinally stretch approximately 35% of the tape's resting length (Fig. 103.1).[1] The stretch characteristics are hypothesized to create convolutions in the tape to permit the tape to recoil back toward the original length when applied to the skin.[5] The elastic tapes are prestretched by 15% to 25% when removing the paper backing when not applying additional mechanical stretch to the tape. Thus, tape applied to the skin without a mechanical stretch will have a 15% to 25% stretch. However, therapists can vary the amount of stretch from paper off tension (no stretch) to mechanically stretching the tape up to a recommended 75% to meet the desired therapeutic benefit. Most brand-name elastic tapes are latex free, waterproof, and made from cotton with an acrylic adhesive backing. Therapists are encouraged to read each taping manufacture's contents and guidelines before tape application because of the varying characteristics of brand-name elastic tapes. Stretch qualities can vary depending on the elastic tape manufacturer. The quality of the tape material is theorized to limit the clinical benefits.[5]

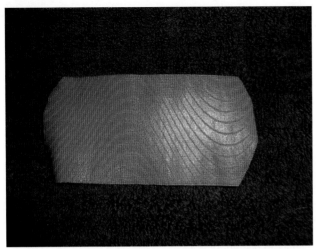

Fig. 103.1 Elastic tape longitudinal stretch qualities. (Photograph from the author's personal collection.)

THEORETICAL CLINICAL BENEFITS AND EVIDENCE FOR ELASTIC TAPE APPLICATION

Some of the proposed clinical benefits of elastic taping include pain reduction; changes in muscle recruitment activity patterns; improved blood and lymphatic circulation; and realignment of joints, muscle, or fascia.[1] Other postulated benefits of elastic taping are improvement of proprioceptive feedback.[6] The research produced during the past 15 years can provide therapists with scientific evidence that may complement proposed theoretical concepts. The research and theory can assist therapists to make sound judgments to determine the potential clinical benefits of therapeutic taping.

Theoretical Benefits of Elastic Taping for Pain Reduction

Taping application with an affixed tension to the tape combined with placing the targeted muscle in a stretched position is purported to allow convolutions in the tape to occur upon application.[1] The convolutions are theorized to lift the epidermis to reduce pressure on mechanoreceptors.[1] Thereby, nociceptive input is reduced resulting in decreased pain intensity. A second theory advocating elastic tape for pain reduction is the inhibition of nociceptive impulses.[7] The tape is thought to deform and stimulate large-fiber cutaneous mechanoreceptors that may inhibit nociceptive impulses to the spinal column and decrease pain via an ascending pathway.[7]

Research Evidence for Pain Reduction

Three randomized controlled trials (RCTs) investigated pain reduction with elastic tape application in patients with shoulder impingement.[8–10] The taping application described in the studies were based on a protocol for shoulder impingement suggested by Kase and coworkers.[1] The first strip was a Y-strip (cut down the middle, producing two tails) applied to supraspinatus from insertion to origin with no stretch to the tape. The second Y-strip was applied to the deltoid from insertion to origin with no tension to the tape. Last, a third I-strip (no cut down the middle) was applied from the coracoid process around to the posterior deltoid. A downward pressure with 50% to 75% stretch was applied to the location of pain or tenderness (Appendix 1).

The first study found a positive short-term benefit for pain reduction during range of motion (ROM) in the elastic tape intervention group compared with a sham taping technique. However, there was no difference between the groups after 6 days.[8]

The second study investigated a group receiving elastic taping combined with a movement with mobilization (MWM) technique compared with a therapeutic exercise group.[9] The authors reported a significant improvement with pain-free shoulder abduction and flexion compared with the therapeutic exercise group at 10-day follow-up.[9]

The third study investigated the short-term benefits on the reduction of pain intensity during movement, nocturnal pain, and pain-free shoulder ROM in participants with shoulder impingement.[10] The tape application to the experimental group was the same as described earlier, but the authors added a fourth Y-strip. The fourth strip was applied with 50% stretch from the thoracic spine to the medial border of the scapula. The authors did not provide a rationale for the fourth piece of tape. The elastic taping group demonstrated significant improvements with pain reduction nocturnally and pain reduction with motion immediately after tape application compared with the sham tape group.[10] However, there was no significant difference between the groups at 1-week follow-up.[10]

Chang and coworkers[11] investigated the effect of elastic tape application on baseball players with medial epicondylitis and healthy collegiate athletes. Three conditions with an interval of 1 week between conditions were applied to study participants. The conditions were (1) no tape, (2) placebo (elastic tape without right angle weft), and (3) elastic tape (right angle weft). The elastic tape application consisted of a Y-strip from insertion of wrist flexor muscles to 2 cm proximal to the medial epicondyle (see Appendix 1). The dominant arm was taped in the healthy participants, and the involved arm was taped in the medial epicondylitis group. Both taping groups improved with pressure pain tolerance.[11]

A case series examined the effect of elastic tape in individuals with lateral epicondylitis.[12] The tape was applied twice a week for 2 weeks. The tape application description was described as the "origin-to-insertion" technique. No other details were provided for tape application. A significant improvement was found with visual analog pain measures, grip strength and Patient-Rated Forearm Evaluation Questionnaire (PRFEQ) scores at 2 and 6 weeks of follow-up.[12]

Theoretical Benefits of Elastic Taping for Muscle Facilitation and Inhibition

Elastic tape application is hypothesized to enhance muscle activity when applied to a lengthened muscle by pulling on the fascia. One of the purported mechanisms to facilitate or inhibit muscle activity is by the direction of the taping application.[1,5] The proposed technique for muscle facilitation is to apply elastic tape from the muscle origin to muscle insertion. The tape application from origin to insertion is thought to enhance muscle activity by moving the fascia and skin toward the origin. Conversely, elastic tape applied from muscle insertion to origin is theorized to inhibit muscle activity by pulling the fascia toward the insertion (Fig. 103.2).[1,5] It is important to note that evidence for this proposed direction of tape application for muscle inhibition versus muscle facilitation is inconclusive as will be discussed later.

Research Evidence for Muscle Facilitation

The evidence for using elastic tape for muscle facilitation presumably to increase strength and ROM has demonstrated mixed results. Several studies have supported short-term benefits of improved strength with elastic tape with an application from muscle origin ending at the muscle insertion.[13–16] Waked and coworkers[17] studied hand strength outcomes comparing a standard therapy (positioning, orthosis, and stretching) group with a group receiving muscle facilitation taping technique combined with standard therapy. The muscle facilitation directional technique (origin to insertion) was applied to the wrist extensors combined with a functional correction technique to the digit flexors in patients

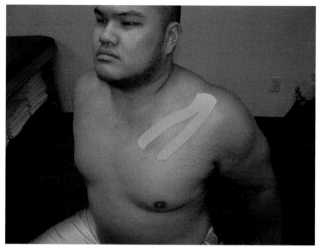

Fig. 103.2 Inhibition taping for the pectoralis minor. (Blaydes Chum photograph from the author's personal collection.)

with dorsal hand burns. The authors reported significant increases with grip strength at 2 and 4 weeks of follow-up compared with the participants in the traditional therapy without taping group.[17]

Healthy individuals were measured for their immediate biceps peak torque strength in three conditions: (1) elastic tape applied from the biceps insertion to origin with 75% tension, (2) sham elastic taping consisting of two vertical strips applied without tension at the proximal and distal biceps, and (3) no tape.[18] The authors reported significant improvements with concentric elbow torque strength in the first group.[18]

Peak torque of healthy individuals' shoulder external rotation strength was measured comparing elastic tape origin-to-insertion technique, sham tape technique, and no tape.[19] The origin-to-insertion technique was applied to the infraspinatus and teres minor with 50% tension to the muscle belly, and the placebo group received the same elastic tape application with no tension applied to the tape. The mean torque in the group with application from origin to insertion with 50% tension demonstrated increased external rotation strength but not reaching statistical significance. However, the sham taping (no tension) group demonstrated significant improvements with internal rotation ROM.[19]

A cross-over, pretest–posttest repeated measure design was performed on baseball players with shoulder impingement to measure muscle performance and scapular kinematics with elastic tape application compared with placebo tape application (3M Micropore tape) applied to the lower trapezius. The origin-to-insertion technique was applied by enveloping the lower trapezius in both groups, but the elastic tape was applied with 10% to 20% tension. The authors reported significant improvements with scapular posterior tilt when raising the arm and improvements with lower trapezius activation when lowering the arm in the elastic tape group.[20]

Van Herzeele and coworkers[21] studied scapular kinematics in healthy female handball players with taping technique speculated to provide a mechanical effect on scapular motions. The tape originated at the coracoid process anteriorly and was pulled over the upper trapezius following the muscle fibers of the lower trapezius posteriorly and ending at the thoracic spine. The authors reported immediate improvements with scapula posterior tilt and upward rotation in the taping condition compared with no taping.[21] Improvements with scapular kinematics indicate that axioscapular muscles likely improved their muscle fiber recruitment to facilitate muscle activity.

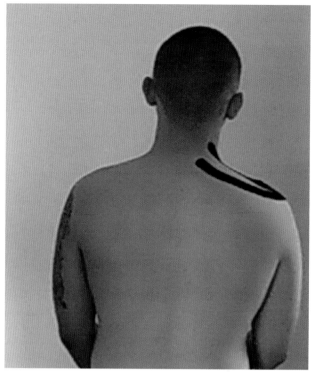

Fig. 103.3 Inhibition taping for the right upper trapezius. (John Martin photograph from the author's personal collection.)

Evidence for Muscle Inhibition

Few researchers have studied the effect of applying elastic tape from insertion to origin to inhibit muscle activity. Shaheen and coworkers found scapular kinematics improved with elastic tape muscle facilitation and muscle inhibition techniques in participants with shoulder impingement.[22] Although the study did not measure muscle activity with an electromyography receiver, one could deduce that improved scapular kinematics is likely related to improved muscle activation.

One small study with 12 participants researched the effects of elastic tape on trapezius muscle activity and typing speed. Trapezius muscle activity and typing speed were measured without tape and immediately after tape application. The elastic tape was applied from insertion to origin with 10% to 20% tension to two tape tails that enveloped the upper trapezius muscle (Fig. 103.3). The authors reported that typing speed was correlated with muscular activity of the trapezius with and without tape. However, the taping conditions resulted in decreased upper trapezius activity. This study may provide foundational evidence to support the insertion to origin taping technique to prevent overactivation of the upper trapezius muscle during typing activities.[23] However, stronger evidence is needed to determine the efficacy of elastic tape application for muscle inhibition.

Research Evidence for Elastic Tape Tension and Direction for Muscle Facilitation and Inhibition

The original recommendations for directional taping for muscle facilitation and inhibition have been a subject of controversy. For example, immediate grip strength was measured in blindfolded conditions with elastic tape application to the wrist extensor group: (1) facilitatory from muscle origin to insertion, (2) inhibitory from muscle insertion to origin, and (3) no tape. The authors found no significant difference with grip strength between the three conditions.[24]

The mechanism for improving strength (muscular facilitation) with elastic taping continues to be questioned. Fukui and coworkers[25] studied the physiological movement of skin with three-dimensional motion analysis. The authors' findings propose that skin moves according to certain physiological rules. These findings suggest that there is a sliding mechanism between superficial fascia and subcutaneous tissue. Isokinetic strength of the gluteus maximus muscle was significantly stronger when elastic tape was applied from insertion to origin compared with taping from origin to insertion and compared with a sham tape technique.[25]

The amount of stretch tension required to effect muscle activity is another area of study. Mohammadi and coworkers[15] reported short-term benefits (up to 2 hours after application) of elastic tape applied to the wrist and digit flexors and extensors with 50% tension. Lemos and coworkers[16] found short-term (up to 48 hours after application) improvements with grip strength with 25% to 35% of stretch tension during application in participants with no upper extremity pathology.

Despite the growing amount of evidence generated to support elastic tape to effect muscle activity, the amount of tape tension and direction of tape application is inconclusive. There remains unanswered questions to clearly support the therapeutic benefits of elastic taping for improved muscle activity.

THEORETICAL BENEFITS OF ELASTIC TAPE FOR IMPROVED BLOOD AND LYMPHATIC CIRCULATION

Elastic tape is purposed to improve vascular transport systems by lifting the skin and creating space between the skin and subcutaneous tissue.[1,5] The created space is considered to enhance healing by improving blood flow to injured tissues. Additionally, the space may contribute to edema reduction by propelling extracellular fluid forward toward lymphatic drains.[1,5] The elastic components of tape are proposed to lift epidermis tissue to aid in lymphatic drainage.[26]

Research Evidence for Lymphatic Circulation

Elastic tape has been found to decrease water composition in women with breast cancer–related lymphedema. Tsa and coworkers[27] compared elastic tape application with a standard pneumatic device. The authors found significant differences with a reduction of water composition in both groups but no significant difference between the groups. However, a more recent pilot trial reported a greater percentage of edema reduction in a group receiving multilayer compression (53.21% reduction) versus elastic tape (24.45% reduction) in women with breast cancer–related lymphedema.[28]

An RCT investigated the effect of elastic tape in individuals with hand edema after a stroke. The authors found a medium effect with edema reduction at the hand metacarpophalangeal and wrist joints and decreased pain scores.[29]

Elastic Taping for Positional Stimulus

Kase and coworkers[1] describe how elastic tape can create a mechanical correction by using the stretch qualities of the tape. A mechanical correction is used to provide sensory input to the nervous system to allow the body to adapt to the sensory stimulus. The sensory stimulus provided through elastic tape application can have clinical implications to promote or limit movement patterns. The theoretical mechanism of the mechanical correction is to apply elastic tape to position the tissue in the desired position. The body will adjust position to minimize the created tension from the tape, or the tape will block the action of the joint or tissue movement (Fig. 103.4).[1]

Evidence for Realignment of Joints, Fascia, and Muscle

The mechanical correction technique uses elastic tape to assist positioning of muscle, fascia tissue, or joint position.[1] There is minimal

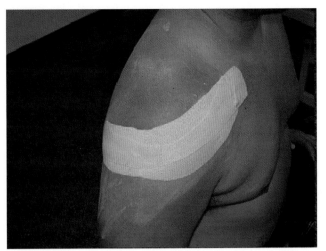

Fig. 103.4 Taping for sensory stimuli to block humeral head anterior translation. (Blaydes Chum photograph from the author's personal collection.)

research specifically measuring the effect of soft tissue realignment after application with the mechanical correction technique. Nevertheless, the technique has been part of the overall taping application in shoulder studies in which three pieces of tape were applied. The mechanical correction technique is one of the three tape applications in the previously discussed shoulder studies.[8–10] The discussed studies describe the I-strip application with 50% to 75% stretch in the anterior region of the humeral head. Theoretically, the body will adjust, or the tape will block an anterior translation of the humeral head.

Theoretical Concepts of Elastic Tape for Proprioceptive Feedback

Enhanced proprioceptive feedback is theorized to be another clinical indication for elastic taping. The elastic tape is thought to provide sensory input, allowing a person to identify the position of the a limb in space and perceive limb motion.[6]

Research Evidence for Proprioceptive Feedback

Healthy participants were measured for proprioceptive feedback magnitude in conditions with and without tape.[6] The proprioception magnitude demonstrated a moderate correlation with muscle activity of the scapular stabilizers in the taping condition. The authors suggest that the results indicate the taping condition provides proprioceptive feedback that affects muscle activity of the scapular-stabilizing muscles.[6] Presumably, muscle activity of the scapular stabilizers provides movement control during arm elevation.

Basic Elastic Tape Application Guidelines and Precautions

Specific instructions for three elastic taping techniques can be found in the appendix. There are important basic guidelines and precautions the therapist should be familiar with before applying tape to a patient. Proper application of tape requires an evaluation of the involved structures and constant reevaluation after tape application. Clients are advised to wear the tape for 3 to 5 days, providing there is a notable therapeutic benefit. There are seven important essentials for therapists to consider for tape application[1]:

1. Skin preparation
2. Tape removal
3. Removal of tape from paper backing and base application
4. Selection of elastic strip type

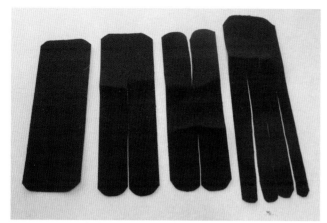

Fig. 103.5 Elastic taping "I," "Y," "X," and fans shapes listed from left to right. (Photograph from the author's personal collection.)

5. Tissue stretch
6. Tape stretch
7. Tape direction and tape removal

Skin Preparation

The client's skin should be clean, shaven, and dry to allow the tape adhesive to adhere. Spraying the skin with rubbing alcohol followed by rubbing the area with a dry towel is a helpful clinical tool for tape application. Some individuals may require a protective skin barrier to avoid skin redness or a rash. Skin barrier products such as Allkare Protective Barrier Wipes can be used to assist with protecting the client's skin. Liquid magnesium hydroxide can serve as an inexpensive over-the-counter barrier. The liquid is applied to the skin and allowed to dry before applying tape to the client.

Tape Removal

Clients should be advised to remove the tape after 3 to 5 days or if the client has skin reaction or discomfort. Tape removal should be in a rolling matter with tension applied between the skin and the tape. The skin should be pushed away from the tape rather than pulling the tape away from the skin.[1] Therapists should caution clients to avoid ripping off the tape to avoid skin irritation. Application of body oil between the tape and skin may help decrease discomfort when removing the tape.

Removal of Tape From Paper Backing

The paper backing should only be removed from its base application when beginning the taping process. Therapists should avoid tactile contact with the adhesive back of the tape to avoid losing any adhesive qualities.[1] The paper backing can gradually be removed after the base has been applied. Gradual removal of the paper backing will allow the therapist to control the desired stretch to the tape as the paper is removed. There should be no stretching of the tape at the initial base and the end application to avoid skin irritation. The desired stretch is only applied after the base application and before the end application. The paper off tension (no stretch to tape) technique results in a small amount of stretch to the tape. Therefore, there will always be some stretch with tape application. The tape should be rubbed after application to the skin to create warmth that will augment the adhesive qualities of the tape.

Selection of Elastic Strip Type

The four clinically common shapes of elastic tape are "Y," "I," "X," and a fan shape. The "Y" shape is most commonly used to surround a muscle (Fig. 103.5). The "I" strip can be used directly on a muscle or applied

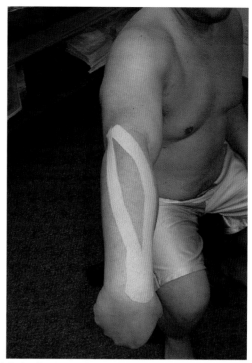

Fig. 103.6 Application to the wrist extensor group with soft tissue structures stretched. (Blaydes Chum photograph from the author's personal collection.)

over a painful area. Additionally, "I" strips can be used to help address movement patterns. "X" strips are used when a muscle origin and insertion may change with varying movement patterns.[1] Fan strips are used for lymphatic correction.[1] Rounding the edges after cutting the shapes can help prevent the edges from rolling up.

Tissue Stretch

The client's skin and muscle should be on stretch during application. Stretching the tissues along with the stretch quality of the tape aids with convolutions in the skin. Skin convolutions are thought to promote the normal flow of blood and lymphatic fluids (Fig. 103.6).[1]

Tape Stretch

Recommended tape stretch application is between paper off (stretch tension at 15%–20%) up to a strong stretch of 75%. The amount of stretch depends on the therapeutic goals. The therapist can subjectively gauge stretch application by considering the quality of elastic tape. Stretching elastic tape to its full capacity is considered 100% stretch. So, if the desired stretch is 30%, the therapist will gauge 30% of the available 100% stretch. Stretching 100% is not recommended to protect the patient from a skin reaction.

Tape Direction

There are some basic theories for tape direction. Tape application from the muscle insertion to origin is recommended when the goal is to rest the muscle and inhibit activity.[1] Tape application from the muscle origin to insertion is recommended when the goal is to increase activity of weak muscles.[1] The most effective direction of tape application remains questionable, as previously discussed.

Contraindication for Elastic Taping

In the event of a risk of a client having a skin reaction because of fragile skin or an allergic reaction or sensitivity to tape, a test patch is recommended. Some individuals can have an adverse reaction to adhesive tape because of varying causes that may be unknown to the therapist. Therapists are encouraged to perform a test patch of tape on the dorsum of the hand with 25% stretch for up to 24 hours. Stretch application of 100% is contraindicated in all individuals because of the risk of blistering, erythema, or a skin rash caused by the shearing forces of the tape.

The six conditions that are contraindicated for elastic tape application are deep vein thrombosis (DVT), kidney problems or renal failure, congestive heart failure (CHF), infections, cancers, and open wounds.[30]

Never apply elastic tape to a patient with a DVT because the tape lifts the skin, which creates space that can allow blood clots to break free and travel to vital organs (heart, lungs, or brain). The consequences could be fatal.[30]

Elastic tape should not be applied to people with kidney problems or CHF. The elastic tape improves blood circulation and promotes lymphatic drainage. Individuals with kidney problems may not be able to process body fluids. The elastic tape may cause fluid to move back to the heart in individuals with CHF, potentially causing the heart to overwork.[30]

Avoid applying elastic tape to infected tissue and patients with cellulitis. Elastic tape may encourage the spread of infected fluid to other parts of the body.

Last, elastic tape should not be applied to individuals with cancer because the tape may aid the spread of cancer cells to other parts of the body.[30]

Conclusion for Elastic Taping

Elastic tape is an adjunct to a rehabilitation therapy plan and is used with a variety of other therapeutic interventions. Therapists are encouraged to avoid tape application if there is any concern for health complications.

The benefits of therapeutic elastic taping continue to be investigated. It remains unknown whether therapeutic elastic taping is superior to other efficacious interventions for specific diagnoses to attain optimum therapeutic benefits. Many of the elastic tape investigations have been performed on healthy individuals. However, there is evidence to support short-term pain relief for individuals with shoulder impingement, medial epicondylitis, and lateral epicondylitis.

Rigid Tape Introduction

Rigid tape is a nonelastic therapeutic tape that is commonly used in upper extremity rehabilitation clinics. There are several varying types of rigid tape. Athletic trainers often use a white tape containing zinc oxide to adhere to the skin and provide joint support. Commonly investigated and used rehabilitation therapeutic rigid taping techniques originated with Jenny McConnell.[31] The unique characteristic of rehabilitation rigid tape is the amount of longitudinal fibers. Rigid tapes with 85 or more longitudinal fibers are considered high quality.[32] Therapeutic rigid tapes have a high tensile strength and are made with a rayon backing containing zinc oxide adhesive to provide support. Most investigated rehabilitative rigid tapes require the application of an underlying skin protective tape with hypoallergenic micropore fibers followed by the therapeutic rigid tape application (Figs. 103.7 and 103.8).[33] Leuko Tape and Endura Tape are two commonly used types of therapeutic rigid tape and protective tape.

Theoretical Clinical Benefits and Evidence for Therapeutic Rigid Tape Application. The proposed clinical benefits of therapeutic rigid taping include mechanical effects of tape for joint positioning, tissue deloading for pain reduction, inhibition of overactive muscles, facilitation of underactive muscles, and promotion of proprioception.[34,35] Theoretical mechanisms to support the proposed clinical benefits of rigid tape application and a review of the upper extremity literature are discussed next.

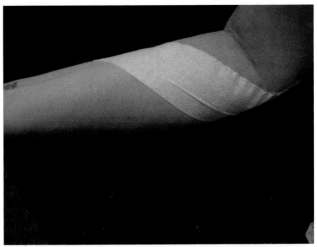

Fig. 103.7 Underlying protective tape applied to skin before applying rigid tape. (Photograph from the author's personal collection.)

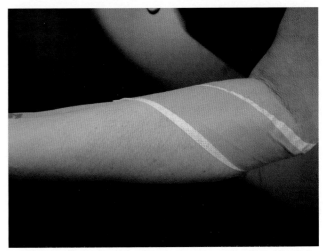

Fig. 103.8 Rigid tape applied over protective tape. (Photograph from the author's personal collection.)

Theoretical Benefits for Mechanical Effects of Rigid Tape

Rigid tape is often used as an adjunct to upper extremity rehabilitation to decrease pain. The mechanism for pain reduction via joint positioning from the tape properties is not fully understood, but it is likely related to the mechanical effects of rigid taping. The mechanical effects of rigid tape are joint support, joint realignment, and biomechanical correction.[36] Rigid tape is used for joint support and injury prevention by applying the tape to act as an external support to a joint. Additionally, rigid tape can be used as an external support to help realign a joint after injury and prevent further injury. However, therapists should use rigid tape with caution for joint support and realignment purposes. If an external support is to provide mechanical support to a ligament, it should exceed the strength of the ligament. Unfortunately, rigid tape does not exceed the strength of a ligament. The biomechanical effects of taping can be used as an adjunct after joint mobilization techniques to assist with changing the desired joint mechanics. The rigid tape is used to maintain the joint position after an application of a mobilization movement that has successfully realigned a joint.

Research Evidence for Mechanical Effects of Rigid Tape

Few studies have investigated the mechanical benefits of rigid tape application to achieve pain relief in joints of the upper extremity. One

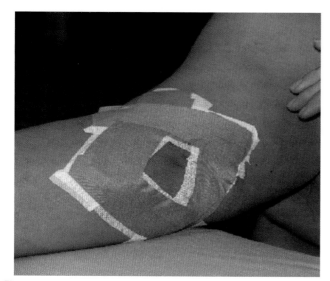

Fig. 103.9 Pain reduction via tissue unloading for lateral epicondylalgia. (Photograph from the author's personal collection.)

study compared two groups of participants with lateral epicondylitis: (1) MWM techniques to the elbow followed by rigid taping to maintain a lateral glide to the wrist extensor group and (2) a traditional therapy group in individuals with lateral epicondylitis. The authors found significant improvements with visual analog scale pain scores and functional outcomes in the group receiving MWM followed by rigid taping (Appendix 2).[37]

Theoretical Benefits of Pain Reduction via Tissue Unloading

McConnell[38] proposed the application of tape to reduce strain to inflamed tissue to allow the therapist to direct treatment to specific structures without pain. Tape may be used to unload painful structures to minimize the aggravation of the symptoms so treatment can be directed at improving the patient's function. In this case, grip strength improvements are assumed to increase function. This involves specific muscle training of the dynamically unstable segment(s) and increasing the mobility of the less flexible surrounding soft tissues.[38]

Research Evidence for Pain Reduction via Tissue Unloading

Rigid tape for tissue unloading has been investigated in individuals with lateral epicondylalgia. A randomized crossover study measured pain-free grip, and pain thresholds were measured pretreatment, immediately after treatment, and 30 minutes posttreatment. The treatment conditions were application of a diamond tape, sham tape technique, and no tape. The authors found a significant improvement with pain-free grip in the diamond tape condition compared with other taping conditions. There was a trend of decreased pain threshold in the diamond tape group, but it was not statistically significant.[39]

Shamsoddini and coworkers[40] performed pre- and posttest analysis on individuals with lateral epicondylitis, comparing no tape with the diamond tape technique. The authors reported significant improvements with grip strength and wrist extensor strength and pain reduction with up to 10 minutes after application of the diamond shape technique (Fig. 103.9).[40]

An RCT compared a diamond tape group combined with traditional therapy to a traditional therapy only group in participants with lateral epicondylitis. Pain-free grip strength was significantly improved in the diamond taping and traditional therapy group compared with the traditional therapy group at a 4-week follow-up.[39]

Last, the diamond taping technique was studied, comparing taping with Cyriax manipulation techniques in subjects with lateral epicondylitis. Both groups improved with grip, pain, and functional measures at a 1-week follow-up.[42] However, there was a significant improvement in the manipulation group with pain and function compared with the taping group.

A randomized trial compared three groups of participants with lateral epicondylitis: (1) a forearm band, (2) rigid tape applied from the volar mid forearm and spiraled around the epicondyle, and (3) a control group measuring pain-free grip and function. The forearm band group demonstrated a significant improvement with pain-free grip strength at a 4-week follow-up.[43]

Rigid Tape for Neuromuscular Benefits (Muscle Inhibition and Facilitation)

The neuromuscular effects of rigid taping to affect muscle facilitation and inhibition are not clearly understood. One proposed theory for the mechanism of muscle inhibition with tape application is to decrease myosin and actin cross-bridging. Muscle actin and myosin cross-bridging is proposed to be reduced when applied adjacent to the muscle. The theoretical basis for tape application adjacent to the muscle is that taping across the line of muscle fibers combined with compression to the overlying soft tissue reduces muscle function by bunching muscle fibers. The bunching of muscle fibers is the logic of reducing myosin and actin cross bridging.[44] An accepted rationale for muscle facilitation is the relationship between cutaneous afferents and motor unit activity. An increased stimulation of cutaneous afferent receptors when applying rigid tape directly over stretched skin is proposed to enhance muscle facilitation.[45]

Research Evidence for Neuromuscular Benefits (Muscle Inhibition and Facilitation)

Published research evidence varies as to whether rigid tape can consistently facilitate or inhibit muscles of the upper extremity. Most of the current reported research includes both healthy participants and participants with upper extremity symptoms. As a result, it is difficult to draw a conclusion to support the efficacy of rigid taping for neuromuscular benefits.

In a study comparing no tape, rigid tape (Endura Fix), and extra-rigid tape (Endura Sport) applied to the lower trapezius of healthy participants, the authors found a reduction of muscle facilitation as opposed to the expected result of muscle facilitation in the taping condition. The two types of rigid tape were aligned and gently applied to the lower trapezius. The authors concluded that a different effect may be seen with participants with pathology.[2]

The taping technique and benefits for muscle facilitation are inconclusive. Shaheen and coworkers[22] found improvements with scapular kinematics in asymptomatic individuals after rigid tape application over the lower trapezius. Improvements with the amount of scapular upward rotation, posterior tilt, and external rotation were found with the taping condition.[22] Improved scapular kinematics can logically relate to improvements with axioscapular muscle facilitation and inhibition.

Upper trapezius inhibition and lower trapezius facilitation was reported in a repeated-measure within-subjects study.[33] The authors applied tape adjacent to the upper trapezius and along the fibers of lower trapezius in participants with expected subacromial impingement syndrome (SIS) during a reaching task. These authors reported a significant difference with reduced upper trapezius activity and lower trapezius activation in taping conditions compared with no tape.[33]

In a cross-sectional laboratory-based study, Smith and coworkers investigated participants with shoulder SIS compared with age- and

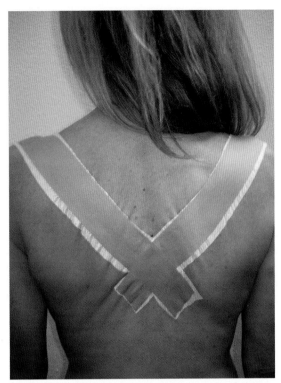

Fig. 103.10 Proprioceptive rigid taping for thoracic spinal extension. (Tambra Marik photograph from the author's personal collection.)

gender-matched asymptomatic participants.[46] Tape was applied as described in the study discussed earlier. The authors found a reduction with upper trapezius muscle activation but no difference with lower trapezius muscle activation.[46] Clinical application is limited because both of the discussed studies were performed in laboratories with no functional outcomes measured.

Scapular kinematics were measured in a laboratory study investigating the effect of elastic tape and rigid tape on participants with SIS.[41] The application of rigid tape was applied to improve posture.[47] The rigid tape was applied from the center of the spine of the scapula to T12 diagonally followed by bilateral application on the paraspinals from T1 to T12. The elastic tape was applied as follows: (1) facilitation theory (origin to insertion) to the supraspinatus, (2) inhibition theory (insertion to origin) to the deltoids, and (3) mechanical correction technique from the coracoid process to the posterior deltoid. The authors found that both types of tape improved scapular external rotation with movement in the sagittal plane. However, scapular retraction and posterior rotation improved with elastic tape application with motion in the scapular plane.

Theoretical Benefits for Enhanced Proprioception with Rigid Tape Application

Some authors postulate that rigid taping provides a form of proprioceptive biofeedback.[35] The rigid tape is applied while the joint or joints are is in the desired positions (Fig. 103.10). Tension is likely created on the skin when the joints move away from the desired positions. Proprioceptive feedback occurs from cutaneous sensory cues when the joints move in a direction outside of the parameters.[35] Therefore, rigid tape can provide feedback to the nervous system to promote movement of joints in a desired direction or limit undesired movement patterns (see Appendix 2).

The mechanical properties of rigid tape for joint support previously discussed may play a role with improved proprioception. It could be

argued that the tape provides stimulation to cutaneous receptors or joint mechanoreceptors to improve the protective reflex arc.[48] Despite varying opinions on the exact mechanism that contributes to improved proprioception, the rationale for taping is to permit optimal functional movement.

Research Evidence for Enhanced Proprioception

Improvement with thoracic extension has been reported in participants with SIS when wearing rigid posture taping compared with a placebo taping or no-tape conditions.[47] Posture taping with rigid tape has been compared with elastic taping to determine the effect of scapular kinematics.[41] The authors concluded that both taping techniques improved scapular external rotation and reduced pain in the sagittal plane of motion.[41]

Basic Rigid Tape Guidelines and Precautions

Specific instructions for three rigid taping techniques can be found in Appendix 2. There are important basic guidelines and precautions the therapist should be familiar with before applying tape to a patient. Proper application of tape requires an evaluation of the involved structures and constant reevaluation after tape application. Clients are advised to wear the tape for up to 48 hours, providing there is a notable therapeutic benefit and no skin reaction. Listed below are recommendations for therapists to consider when applying rigid tape[36]:

- Apply tape to clean, dry, and shaven skin.
- Apply the adhesive hypoallergenic protective underlay tape to the skin first (this will decrease the traction forces of the rigid tape).
- Apply the tape from distal to proximal when possible.
- Apply the anchor followed by laying the tape down on the skin. Avoid pulling the skin.
- Avoid transverse circumferential taping but apply an oblique orientation if wrapping around a limb.
- Take extra care to apply a smooth application avoiding creases or folds.
- Apply a test patch for 24 hours to monitor negative skin reactions.
- A test patch to the dorsum of the hand is recommended for individuals who may have an adverse reaction to tape.

Removal of tape should be performed slowly with one hand applying pressure to the skin while the other hand gently peels the tape back on itself. Avoid ripping the tape off from the skin. Use blunt band-aid scissors to cut the tape if needed to begin peeling tape off the skin.

Recent research has found that stretch and compression could disturb nociceptive signals and alter pain.[49] Therapists should take extra care to ensure there is no tension to the tape in painful regions.

Therapists should use caution with rigid tape application. As previously discussed in the section describing elastic tape application, some individuals may have an adverse reaction to adhesive tape. Avoid applying rigid tape to individuals with fragile and thin skin. Caution should be used when applying tape to people with peripheral vascular diseases, peripheral neuropathies, diabetes, prolonged use of steroid or anticoagulant medication, and cognitive loss.[36] Contraindications for rigid tape application are skin allergy or sensitivity to tape, open wounds, skin infections or conditions, fragile skin, circulatory conditions (bleeding or clotting disorders), and sensory loss to the area being taped.[36]

Conclusion for Rigid Tape

Rigid taping is a popular intervention in rehabilitation of the upper extremity. The majority of the existing evidence for upper extremity rigid taping focuses on the elbow and the shoulder. The exact mechanism for the clinical benefits with rigid tape application are not completely understood. However, the evidence suggests there are some short-term benefits for pain reduction and improved movement patterns in individuals with lateral epicondylitis and SIS. Upper extremity rehabilitation therapists can potentially use the rigid taping techniques as an adjunct to other interventions. However, clinicians should use caution because of the lack of long-term results. Clinicians are encouraged to use taping techniques if the tape ultimately improves functional outcomes, has a low risk of harming the patient, and is cost and time effective.

APPENDIX A: ELASTIC TAPE APPLICATION

Shoulder Taping for Subacromial Impingement (Video 103.1)[1,8]

- Use standard 2-inch elastic tape.
- The first strip is a "Y" strip. Cut a "Y" strip the length of the client's supraspinatus. Apply the base of the tape at the insertion of supraspinatus with paper off tension. Instruct the client to perform cervical side bending to the contralateral side. Surround the supraspinatus muscle with the two strips with paper off tension.
- The second strip is a "Y" strip to surround the deltoid. Cut a "Y" strip long enough to surround the client's posterior and anterior portions of their deltoid.
- Apply the base of the "Y" strip at the deltoid tuberosity with no tension. The anterior tail is applied to the anterior deltoid with light tension. Instruct the client to position the shoulder in external rotation and horizontal abduction when the anterior tail is applied. The posterior tail is a applied to the posterior deltoid with light tension. Instruct the client to horizontally adduct and internally rotate the shoulder when the posterior tail is applied.
- The third strip is an "I" strip. Cut the "I" strip to measure from the client's coracoid process to the posterior deltoid. Instruct the patient to externally rotate the shoulder with the shoulder adducted to the side before applying the "I" strip. Apply the base of the "I" to the coracoid process. Apply 50% to 75% stretch with downward pressure over the area of pain or tenderness.
- Rub the tape to enhance adhesive properties.

Forearm and Elbow Taping for Medial Epicondylitis (Video 103.2)[1,11]

- Measure a "Y" strip from 2 cm inferior to the medial epicondyle of the humerus to the wrist joint line.
- Apply the base of "Y" strip with no tension in the region of the wrist flexor insertion. Instruct the client to extend the elbow, hyperextend the wrist, and supinate the forearm when the two tails are applied. The first tail is applied with 15% to 20% stretch to the middle of the forearm. The second tail is applied with 15% to 20% stretch along the medial edge of the forearm to surround the wrist flexor muscle group.
- Rub the tape to enhance the adhesive qualities of the tape.

Forearm and Elbow Taping for Lateral Epicondylitis[5,12]

- Cut an "I" strip from the dorsal metacarpal heads to the lateral epicondyle of the humerus. Cut the "I" strip to an "X" strip. Cut one end of the "X" short to cover the length of the metacarpals. Cut the other end of the "X" to cover the wrist extensors. The middle portion of the "X" will cover the dorsal wrist.
- The patient is instructed to position in wrist flexion, forearm pronation, and elbow extension during tape application. The short tails of the "X" are applied to the metacarpals 2 and 5 with no tension. The middle portion of the "X" is applied with no tension to light tension. The long tails of the "X" are applied with 15% to 25% stretch while surrounding the wrist extensor group.
- Rub the tape to enhance the adhesive qualities of the tape.

APPENDIX B: RIGID TAPE APPLICATION

Taping for Lateral Epicondylitis Following the Movement with Mobilization Technique (Video 103.3)[37]

- Apply a hypoallergenic underlying piece of tape from the origin of extensor carpi radialis to the mid volar forearm.
- Apply a lateral glide to the extensor muscle group.
- Maintain the lateral glide with one hand while the other hand applies the rigid tape.
- Place the rigid tape on top of the hypoallergenic tape beginning at the origin of extensor carpi radialis and ending at the mid volar forearm.

Taping to Avoid Ulnar Deviation in de Quervain's Tenosynovitis (Video 103.4)

- Apply hypoallergenic underlying piece of tape from the head of metacarpal 1 to the radial forearm ending approximately 3 inches from the elbow flexion crease.
- Position the client.

Posture Taping for Improved Scapular Kinematics (Video 103.5)[47]

- Apply two adhesive hypoallergenic protective pieces of underlay tape 2 inches wide, such as Leuko Tape cover roll, on the paraspinals from T1 to T12. Apply one piece on each side of the spine. Apply to two hypoallergenic protective underlay pieces of tape 2 inches wide from the center of the spine of the scapula to T12. Apply one on each scapula.
- Instruct the client to extend the thoracic spine while fully retracing and depressing the scapula.
- Lay the rigid tape (1½ inch wide) on top of the underlay tape on each side of the spine with the client in the above posture. The length will vary depending on the client's size.
- Lay the rigid tape (1½ inch wide) on top of the underlay tape from the middle of the scapula spine to T12 with client in the above posture.

Diamond Taping for Pain Relief in Lateral Epicondylitis[39,40]

- Cut four pieces of adhesive hypoallergenic underlay tape (2 inches wide) 3 to 4 inches long. Cut four pieces of rigid tape (1½ inches wide) 3 to 4 inches long.
- Apply underlay tape distally to proximally, making a diamond around the lateral epicondyle.
- Apply the rigid tape on the underlay tape moving distal to proximal in a diamond shape. Apply a tractional force on soft tissues toward the epicondyle and perpendicular to the line of tape to give an "orange peel" appearance to the skin. The ends overlap each other and can be secured with an additional piece of tape.[39]

REFERENCES

1. Kase K, Wallis J, Kase T. *Clinical Therapeutic Applications of the Kinesio Taping Method.* Tokyo, Japan: Ken Ikai Co Ltd; 2003.
2. Alexander CM, Stynes S, Thomas A, Lewis J, Harrision PJ. Does tape facilitate or inhibit the lower fibres of trapezius? *Man Ther.* 2003;8:37–41.
3. Cools AM, Witvrouw EE, Danneels LA, Cambier DC. Does taping influence electromyographic muscle activity in the scapular rotators in healthy shoulders? *Man Ther.* 2002;7:154–162.
4. Kase K, Hashimoto T. *Changes in the Volume of the Peripheral Blood Flow;* 1998. Unpublished data www.http://kinesiotaping.com/content.asp?CustComKey=13776&CategoryKey=13777pn=Page&DomName=kinesiotaping.com.

5. Kumbrink BK. *Taping: An Illustrated Guide*. Berlin, Heidelberg, New York: Springer –Verlag Berlin Heidelberg; 2012.

6. Lin Jiu–jenq, Hung Cheng–Ju, Yang Pey–Lin. The effects of scapular taping on electromyographic muscle activity and proprioception feedback in healthy shoulders. *J Orthop Res*. 2011;29(1):53–57.

7. Montalvo Alicia M, Cara Ed Le, Myer Gregory D. Effect of kinesiology taping on pain in individuals with musculoskeletal injuries: systematic review and meta-analysis. *Phys Sportsmed*. 2014;42(2):48–57.

8. Thelen Mark D, Dauber James A, Stoneman Paul D. The clinical efficacy of kinesio tape for shoulder pain: a randomized, double-blinded, clinical trial. *J Orthop Sports Phys Ther*. 2008;38(7):389–395.

9. Djordjevic, Olivera C, et al. Mobilization with movement and kinesiotaping compared with a supervised exercise program for painful shoulder: results of a clinical trial. *J Manipulative Physiol Ther*. 2012;35(6):454–463.

10. Shakeri Hassan, et al. Clinical effectiveness of kinesiological taping on pain and pain–free shoulder range of motion in patients with shoulder impingement syndrome: a randomized, double blinded, placebo–controlled trial. *Int J Sports Phys Ther*. 2013;8(6):800.

11. Chang HY, Wang CH, Chou KY, Cheng SC. Could forearm kinesio taping improve strength, force sense, and pain in baseball pitchers with medial epicondylitis? *Clini J Sport Med*. 2012;22(4):327–333.

12. Dilek Banu, et al. Kinesio taping in patients with lateral epicondylitis. *J Back Musculoskelet Rehabil*. 2016;29(4):853–858.

13. Donec Venta, Varžaitytė Lina, Kriščiūnas Aleksandras. The effect of Kinesio Taping on maximal grip force and key pinch force. *Polish Annals Med*. 2012;19(2):98–105.

14. Lee Jung-Hoon, Yoo Won-Gyu, Lee Kyung-Soon. Effects of head-neck rotation and kinesio taping of the flexor muscles on dominant-hand grip strength. *J Phys Ther Sci*. 2010;22(3):285–289.

15. Mohammadi H, Kalantari K, Naeimi S, et al. Immediate and delayed effects of forearm kinesio taping on grip strength. *Iran Red Crescent Med. J*. 2014;16(8):e19791. https://doi.org/10.5812/ircmj.19797.

16. Lemos T, Pereira K, Protassio C, Lucas L, Matheus J. The effect of Kinesio Taping on handgrip strength. *J Phys Ther Sci*. 2015;27:567–570.

17. Waked IS, Eladi HM, Elgohary HM. Impact of kinesiology taping on handgrip strength following dorsal hand burn. *Intl J of Ther & Rehab Research*. 6;2:131–136.

18. Fratocchi Giancarlo, et al. Influence of Kinesio Taping applied over biceps brachii on isokinetic elbow peak torque. A placebo controlled study in a population of young healthy subjects. *J Sci Med Sport*. 2013;16(3):245–249.

19. Alam Sarfaraz, et al. Immediate effect of Kinesio taping on shoulder muscle strength and range of motion in healthy individuals: a randomised trial. *Hong Kong Physiother J*. 2015;33(2):80–88.

20. Hsu Yin-Hsin, et al. The effects of taping on scapular kinematics and muscle performance in baseball players with shoulder impingement syndrome. *J Electromyogr Kinesiol*. 2009;19(6):1092–1099.

21. Van Herzeele, Maarten, et al. Does the application of kinesiotape change scapular kinematics in healthy female handball players? *Int J Sports Med*. 2013;34(11):950–955.

22. Shaheen Aliah F, et al. Scapular taping alters kinematics in asymptomatic subjects. *J Electromyogr Kinesiol*. 2013;23(2):326–333.

23. Huang Tsun-Shun, Cheng Wei-Cheng, Lin Jiu-Jenq. Relationship between trapezius muscle activity and typing speed: taping effect. *Ergonomics*. 2012;55(11):1404–1411.

24. Cai C, et al. Facilitatory and inhibitory effects of Kinesio tape: fact or fad? *J sci med sport*. 2016;19(2):109–112.

25. Fukui T, Otake Y, Kondo T. The effects of new taping methods designed to increase muscle strength. *J Phys. Ther. Sci*. 2017;29:70–74.

26. Schuster E, Murray HM. *Proceedings from KinesioTape Workshop: concepts and Practical Application of the KinesioTaping Method*. Baltimore: Progressive Rehab Concepts; 2005.

27. Tsai Han-Ju, et al. Could Kinesio tape replace the bandage in decongestive lymphatic therapy for breast-cancer-related lymphedema? A pilot study. *Support Care Cancer*. 2009;17(11):1353.

28. Smykla A, et al. Effect of Kinesiology Taping on breast cancer-related lymphedema: a randomized single-blind controlled pilot study. *BioMed Research Int*. 2013.

29. Bell A, Muller M. Effects of kinesio tape to reduce hand edema in acute stroke. *Topics in Stroke Rehab*. 2013;20(3):283–288.

30. *Kinesiology Tape Info Center. When not to use KT tape or any other kinesiology tape*; 2011. Available at: http://www.kinesiologytapeinfo.com/when-not-to-use-kt-tape-or-any-other-kinesiology-tape/. Accessed October 21, 2017.

31. McConnelll Institute. Expanding orthopaedic healthcare knowledge globally. Available at: http://mcconnell-institute.com/index.html. Accessed October 26, 2017.

32. Prentice WE. *Arnheim's Principles of Athletic Training*. 13th ed. Boston: McGraw-Hill; 2009.

33. Selkowitz David M, et al. The effects of scapular taping on the surface electromyographic signal amplitude of shoulder girdle muscles during upper extremity elevation in individuals with suspected shoulder impingement syndrome. *J Orthop Sports Phys The*. 2007;37(11):694–702.

34. Host Helen H. Scapular taping in the treatment of anterior shoulder impingement. *Phys Ther*. 1995;75(9):803–812.

35. Morrissey Dylan. Proprioceptive shoulder taping. *J Bodyw Mov Ther*. 2000;4(3):189–194.

36. Constantinoou M, Brown M. Review of the principles and effects. In: *Therapeutic Taping for Musculoskeletal Conditions*. Chatsworth, Australia: Elsevier Australia; 2010:10–33.

37. Amro Akram, et al. The effects of Mulligan mobilisation with movement and taping techniques on pain, grip strength, and function in patients with lateral epicondylitis. *Hong Kong Physiother J*. 2010;28(1):19–23.

38. McConnell Jenny. A novel approach to pain relief pre-therapeutic exercise. *J Sci Med Sport*. 2000;3(3):325–334.

39. Vicenzino Bill, et al. Initial effects of elbow taping on pain-free grip strength and pressure pain threshold. *J Orthop Sports Phys Ther*. 2003;33(7):400–407.

40. Shamsoddini Alireza, Hollisaz Mohammad Taghi. Effects of taping on pain, grip strength and wrist extension force in patients with tennis elbow. *Trauma Monthly*. 2013;18(2):71.

41. Deleted in review.

42. Prabhakar Ashish J, Kage. Vijay. Comparison of Cyriax physiotherapy and taping technique in subjects with tennis elbow: a randomized clinical trial. *Romanian J Phys Ther/Revista Romana de Kinetoterapie*. 2013;19(31).

43. Kachanathu, John Shaji, et al. Forearm band versus elbow taping: as a management of lateral epicondylitis. *J Musculoskelet Res*. 2013;16(01):1350003.

44. Parkhurst Thomas M, Carolyn N. Burnett. Injury and proprioception in the lower back. *J Orthop Sports Phys Ther*. 1994;19(5):282–295.

45. MacGregor Kerren, et al. Cutaneous stimulation from patella tape causes a differential increase in vasti muscle activity in people with patellofemoral pain. *J Orthop Res*. 2005;23(2):351–358.

46. Smith Mike, et al. Upper and lower trapezius muscle activity in subjects with subacromial impingement symptoms: is there imbalance and can taping change it? *Phys Ther Sport*. 2009;10(2):45–50.

47. Lewis Jeremy S. Christine Wright, and Ann Green. Subacromial impingement syndrome: the effect of changing posture on shoulder range of movement. *J Orthop Sports Phys Ther*. 2005;35(2):72–87.

48. Heit Eric J, Lephart Scott M, Rozzi Susan L. The effect of ankle bracing and taping on joint position sense in the stable ankle. *J Sport Rehab*. 1996;5(3):206–213.

49. Chen Shu-Mei, Kai Lo Sing, Cook Jill. The effect of rigid taping with tension on mechanical displacement of the skin and change in pain perception. *J Sci Med Sport*. 2017.

104

Manual Therapy in the Management of Upper Extremity Musculoskeletal Disorders

Frank Fedorczyk

OUTLINE

CRITICAL POINTS

- Manual therapy remains a popular treatment approach in the management of upper extremity musculoskeletal disorders despite the lack of strong evidence to support its efficacy.
- Progress has been made toward understanding the mechanisms of manual therapy that relate to its effect. This may lead to better informed choices related to selection of techniques as well as the selection of the patient appropriate for this intervention.
- Efficacy has been demonstrated for the use of manual therapy in the management of select upper extremity musculoskeletal disorders, but the current best evidence is of moderate methodologic quality.

- Despite this growth, there is still much that is unknown, particularly related to the selection of manual therapy techniques.
- No formal evidence-informed guidelines are available to aid in selection.
- Strong clinical reasoning skills are required to make the best evidence-informed selection. Consider the "wise action" approach.

INTRODUCTION

The inclusion of manual therapy in the management of common musculoskeletal disorders of the upper extremity remains popular, although systematic reviews continue to find only small to moderate effect sizes and fall short of recommending these interventions over other treatment choices. Such findings continue to highlight the difficulty in designing studies that accurately reflect the manner in which this care is delivered, the complex interaction of the patient and the provider, and the multifactorial nature of the mechanisms of manual therapy. Manual therapy encompasses a disciplined clinical reasoning approach to the individual patient and her or his problem; however, study design is often limited to investigating the effect of a particular technique versus a sham technique or other intervention. Clinical and personal equipoise, placebo mechanisms, and the context in which care is delivered have been recognized as confounding factors with the potential to influence outcomes.[7,8] In clinical practice, the concept of regional interdependence is often incorporated into the treatment plan with areas remote from the site of pain or dysfunction, such as the cervical and thoracic spine, being addressed through manual techniques with greater benefit reported versus treating the painful site alone.[9–11]

Close to 30 years have passed since Rothstein's observation on the growth and maturation of manual therapy led him to state "much time has passed, and although a lot has changed, little has changed."[12] In this time, the change has been positive with manual therapy moving further away from expert opinion and anecdotal driven decision

making. Tacit assumptions regarding the mechanisms of manual therapy have not only been challenged but for the most part discarded. The utility of clinical prediction rules that after being defined, the current best evidence for the selection of treatment in select musculoskeletal disorders has been questioned after critical appraisal.[13,14] A comprehensive model related to the mechanisms of manual therapy has been described that includes proposed neurophysiological responses to the mechanical stimulus along with psychosocial influences consistent with accepted models of pain and disability.[15]

The intent of this chapter is to provide a brief review of the proposed mechanisms of manual therapy, review the relevant evidence available related to the efficacy of manual therapy in the management of upper extremity musculoskeletal disorders, and discuss the principles and clinical reasoning processes relevant to the selection of joint-based passive movement techniques commonly used for the purposes of decreasing pain and improving joint range of motion (ROM). Neurodynamic and soft tissue–based techniques are not discussed because they are covered elsewhere in this text. Although clinically important, the description and selection of manual therapy techniques directed at the cervical and thoracic spine are beyond the scope of this chapter.

MECHANISMS OF MANUAL THERAPY

In 2009, a model was proposed to account for the multiple pain inhibitory mechanisms of manual therapy. It was postulated that the mechanical stimulus from a manual therapy technique resulted in

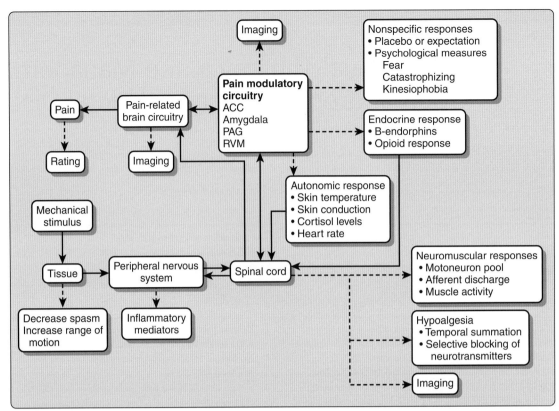

Fig. 104.1 Mechanisms of manual therapy comprehensive model. *ACC,* Anterior cingular cortex; *PAG,* periaqueductal gray; *RVM,* rostral ventromedial medulla. (From Bialosky JE, Bishop MD, Price DD, et al. The mechanisms of manual therapy in the treatment of musculoskeletal pain: a comprehensive model. *Man Ther.* 2009;14:531–538.)

neurophysiological responses within the peripheral and central nervous systems responsible for pain inhibition.[16] The described neurophysiological responses would result in the clinical outcomes associated with manual therapy (Fig. 104.1). Recognizing that the outcomes of manual therapy result from the interaction of multiple complementary mechanisms, the mode was expanded to include factors associated with the interaction between the provider and patient and to link manual therapy pain inhibition with other core outcome domains such as resting pain, emotional distress, fatigue, and satisfaction.[15] The intent of the model remains to help guide future research to assist clinicians in selecting the appropriate intervention for the clinical presentation.

The clinical relevance of this model is highlighted when considering the proposed mechanical effects of manual therapy on the joint and periarticular connective tissues. Often purported to exert an effect by means of joint repositioning,[17] the evidence suggests that any change in joint position is most likely transient and therefore unlikely to result in a lasting therapeutic outcome.[18] With respect to the ability of manual therapy to affect connective tissue or more specifically to elongate shortened tissue, one has to consider the nature of this type of problem and the effects of tensile stress on connective tissue. As with joint repositioning, any effects are most likely to be transient with increases in motion or tissue length related to the viscoelastic properties of the connective tissue.[19] It has been recommended that when true joint stiffness secondary to shortening of periarticular joint structures is the limiting factor in loss of motion, other treatment methods such as orthotic intervention may be more beneficial than passive joint mobilization. However, manual therapy may be of value in preconditioning the tissues before active exercise or orthotic intervention and allow for a greater therapeutic benefit than either alone.

EFFICACY OF MANUAL THERAPY

Reporting on the efficacy of manual therapy, DiFabio[20] stated that there was a paucity of valid research in all areas and a particular absence of controlled trials involving manual therapy applied to the peripheral joints. Since DiFabio's observation, numerous studies of variable quality and design have been published related to the use and effect of manual therapy techniques in the management of patients with select upper extremity musculoskeletal disorders. The majority of the published work has been related to the management of specific shoulder and elbow disorders with several systematic and critical reviews now available.[1-6] In a recent search, no systematic reviews could be found pertaining to the use of joint-based manual therapy specifically at the wrist or hand. However, one systematic review of therapy interventions for improving joint motion included two case series involving the use of manual therapy in the management of distal radius fractures and one prospective cohort study investigating its use for stiffness and pain after immobilization for metacarpal fracture.[21] The authors concluded that there was evidence to support the use of mobilization to increase ROM after metacarpal fracture, but the results were inconclusive with respect to management of the distal radius fractures. A limited number of studies have been published that have investigated the use of joint mobilization in the management of carpal tunnel syndrome and mobilization with movement (MVM) for de Quervain's tenosynovitis. No definitive conclusions can be drawn in terms of efficacy because these studies are of low to moderate quality.[22-24]

Systematic Reviews

A 2003 Cochrane review of physiotherapy interventions for shoulder pain found that combining mobilization with exercise resulted in additional benefit compared with exercise alone for rotator cuff disease, but not for adhesive capsulitis.[25] A 2016 update of manual therapy and exercise for rotator cuff disease identified 1 trial of 60 reviewed to be of high quality and found no clinically important differences in outcomes between a combination of exercise and manual therapy compared to placebo of inactive ultrasound.[2] A 2014 update of this review on manual therapy and exercise for adhesive capsulitis concluded that the best available data show that manual therapy and exercise may not be as effective as glucocorticoid injection in the short term.[3] The authors concluded that the overall results of their review provided little evidence to guide treatment parameters.

Another systematic review found inconsistent evidence of the effectiveness of manual therapy for various shoulder disorders compared with control interventions and no treatment.[4] Fourteen randomized controlled trials (RCTs) meeting the inclusion criteria of the review were analyzed within subgroups of adhesive capsulitis, shoulder impingement syndrome, and nonspecific shoulder pain. The authors concluded that there was no clear evidence to suggest additional benefits of manual therapy over other interventions in the management of shoulder impingement syndrome and that manual therapy was not shown to be more effective than other conservative interventions for adhesive capsulitis. They noted that the lack of clear description of techniques and treatment parameters as well as the wide range of manual therapy made it difficult to provide clear guidelines for the clinician but acknowledged that high-grade mobilizations may be more effective in improving ROM compared with low-grade mobilizations. They also acknowledged the contrasting view of an earlier published review regarding treatment efficacy for impingement syndrome that concluded the evidence for the addition of joint mobilization is moderately strong.[26,27]

Camarinos and Marinko[5] concluded in their review that the evidence suggests that the patients receiving manual therapy interventions for painful shoulder conditions, particularly high-grade or end-range mobilization, demonstrated improvements in both active and passive ROM. No definitive conclusions could be made with regard to the efficacy of treating pain. Common to the previous reviews, it was stated that the optimal form of manual therapy technique could not be identified.

Similarly, the consensus regarding the effectiveness of manual therapy in the management of tennis elbow appears to be that there is limited high-quality evidence available to guide the clinician in the selection of a particular method.[28,29] Herd and Meserve[7] reported that in terms of specific techniques, Mulligan's MWM was the most frequently studied and was shown to provide benefits such as decreased pain immediately and during short- and long-term follow-up. They cautioned that the generalizability of the studies was limited because of the design and outcome measures used. Consistent with this view are the findings of a systematic review of MWM for all peripheral joints.[30] The authors' stated purpose was to undertake a systematic review to critically evaluate the literature regarding the overall efficacy of MWM prescription and use at peripheral joints in an attempt to formulate guidelines for clinical practice. They identified 25 studies that met their inclusion criteria with 4 being true RCTs; 6 RCTs with participants as their own controls; and the remainder divided among nonexperimental designs, case studies, and case reports. Each article was assessed for methodological quality using a valid and reliable critical appraisal tool with the RCTs deemed to be of moderate methodological quality. Three of the 4 true RCTs were related to tennis elbow and 1 to the shoulder. In the 6 RCTs in which the participants were their own controls, 3 were related to tennis elbow, 2 to the ankle, and 1 to the shoulder. It was concluded that in general, the efficacy of MWM was well established with common effects including increases in strength, reduction in pain,

increases in pain pressure thresholds, and improved function. However, because of the methodological quality of the studies, the authors were unable to provide any specific guidelines for clinical practice.

Several randomized controlled trials (RCTs) of higher quality have been published demonstrating the efficacy of manual therapy in the management of painful shoulder and elbow conditions. Review of the techniques used in these trials may provide some guidance in the selection of technique process.

Yang and colleagues[31] compared the use of three mobilization techniques in the management of subjects with frozen shoulder syndrome. Inclusion criteria were having a painful stiff shoulder for at least 3 months, having limited ROM of 25% or greater compared with the noninvolved shoulder in at least two shoulder motions, and having physician consent. The techniques that were compared were described as midrange mobilization, end-range mobilization, and MWM. A multiple treatment trial design was used over a 12-week period. Improvements in mobility and functional ability were reported in all subjects. Comparing the effectiveness of the three techniques, end-range mobilization and MWM were found to be more effective than midrange mobilization. MWM was also found to improve movement strategies in terms of scapulohumeral rhythm.

Johnson and colleagues[32] compared the effectiveness of anterior and posterior glide mobilization techniques for improving shoulder external rotation ROM in patients with adhesive capsulitis. Inclusion criteria included a diagnosis of primary or idiopathic adhesive capsulitis, unilateral condition, age between 25 and 80 years, normal findings on radiographs within the previous 12 months, no previous shoulder surgery, no previous manipulation under anesthesia, and external rotation ROM that worsened with shoulder abduction. All participants received six therapy sessions consisting of ultrasound, joint mobilization, and upper body ergometer exercise. Treatment differed between groups in the direction of the mobilization technique performed. No significant difference in shoulder external rotation ROM between groups was noted at baseline. By the third treatment, individuals in the anterior mobilization group had a mean improvement in external rotation of 3 degrees. The individuals in the posterior mobilization group had a mean improvement of 31.3 degrees. Both groups were reported to have a significant decrease in pain.

Also investigating the effects of joint mobilization on ROM and disability in patients with stiff and painful shoulders, Vermeulen and colleagues[33] compared the use of high- and low-grade mobilization techniques in the management of phase II (freezing) adhesive capsulitis. The mobilization techniques included inferior glide of the head of the humerus, inferior glide in abduction–external rotation, posterior glide, anterior glide, and lateral distraction of the humerus. The high-grade group received grade III or IV mobilization, whereas the low-grade group received the same techniques as grade I or II. (See discussion of grades of movement.) Improvement was demonstrated in joint mobility and reduction of disability in both groups. Statistically significant improvement in passive abduction and active and passive external rotation was reported in the high-grade group. The authors concluded that high-grade mobilization techniques appear to be more effective in improving glenohumeral joint mobility and reducing disability than low-grade mobilization, with the overall difference between the two interventions being small. Because there was no control group not receiving mobilization, the natural history of the disorder must be considered when interpreting these results. Teys and colleagues[34] investigated the effects of a MWM technique on ROM and pressure pain threshold in individuals with limited and painful shoulder motion. Twenty-four participants meeting the inclusion criteria of inability to elevate the arm more than 100 degrees in the plane of the scapula because of the presence of anterior shoulder pain and duration of pain longer than 1 month and for less than 1 year received treatment consisting of either a MWM technique or a sham technique. A control condition was also included in which the participant was seated but without any manual contact between the therapist and participant. The MWM technique consisted of the application of a posterolateral glide to the affected shoulder. The authors reported significant and clinically meaningful improvements in both ROM and pressure pain threshold immediately after treatment in the MWM group. No follow-up was reported.

Guimaraes and colleagues[35] investigated the immediate effects of MWM versus a sham technique on ROM, strength, and function in patients with shoulder impingement syndrome. Twenty-seven participants met the inclusion criteria of pain in the shoulder lasting longer than 1 week, pain located in the anterolateral area of the shoulder, positive signs for at least one of the clinical tests to evaluate subacromial impingement syndrome (SIS) associated with painful movement during arm elevation, or pain during external rotation of the shoulder with the arm abducted to 90 degrees. The authors concluded the MWM technique was no more effective than a sham intervention in improving shoulder ROM during external rotation and abduction and function as assessed via Disability of the Arm, Shoulder and Hand (DASH) and Shoulder Pain and Disability Index (SPADI) patient self-report measures.[35]

Last, Bisset and colleagues[36] investigated the efficacy of MWM and exercise compared with corticosteroid injection or a wait-and-see approach over 1 year in patients diagnosed with tennis elbow. Physical therapy consisting of MWM and exercise was demonstrated to have a superior benefit over the wait-and-see approach in the first 6 weeks and over corticosteroid injection after 6 weeks with outcome measures of global rating of change, pain-free grip, and assessor's rating of severity. The MWM techniques included sustained lateral glide with pain-free grip and sustained lateral glide of the elbow with movement.[37]

Again, although the preceding may provide some guidance in the selection of a manual therapy technique, the generalizability is limited to the diagnoses and conditions studied. When presented with a patient not fitting these criteria, sound clinical reasoning is paramount in the decision-making process and is highlighted in the following discussion.

THE SELECTION OF TECHNIQUE

The selection of a manual therapy technique for any particular peripheral joint disorder is often based on the therapist's personal preferences, biases, and previous experiences with that technique along with a consideration of the problem being addressed. Pathoanatomic, biomechanical, and neurophysiologic principles are also influencing factors. As evident, despite the growth and maturation of manual therapy practice, standardized, evidenced-based guidelines remain unavailable to assist in this decision-making process. Limited evidence is available of specific joints and diagnoses that may aid in technique selection; however, whether this can be applied to other joints and conditions is unknown. Principles that have long guided clinicians and remain popular have been questioned in terms of their validity and efficacy, with the findings often contradictory to the stated principle.[19,38] A classic example is that the concave–convex rule, which describes a method to determine the direction of a glide, is not always correct. To increase glenohumeral external rotation, the concave–convex rule says to apply an anterior glide; however, a recent study demonstrated that greater improvement in external rotation was achieved with a posterior glide.[32]

The difficulty in developing standardized guidelines is multifactorial but at least in part is attributable to the variability often seen in the clinical presentation of individuals referred with the same diagnosis. It is common for one person to respond favorably to a particular technique but another does not. Exploring the reasons for this is beyond

the scope of this chapter, but this clinical dilemma highlights the value of a patient-centered, disciplined clinical reasoning approach when deciding which technique(s) to choose. This approach or treatment paradigm has been described in great detail elsewhere with the essence best captured by the term *wise action approach*.[39,40] When using the approach, a wise action is chosen with consideration to the best of science, the best of current therapies, and the best of the patient–therapist relationship. As evident, this is consistent with the description of evidence-based and evidence-informed practice. The following reviews the principles and processes involved in the selection of a technique that are thought to be important in allowing the clinician to arrive at this wise action. These principles have been described thoroughly by Hengeveld and Banks[41,42] and are components of what has been referred to as the Maitland-Australian approach.

General Considerations

After a thorough examination in which an assessment is made of the nature of the patient's movement-related disorder, the therapist will then decide whether treatment by passive movement is indicated and appropriate. Conditions that may preclude this type of treatment include those with an active underlying disease process, unstable fractures, severe osteoporosis, long-term steroid or anticoagulant use, surgical procedures in which the tissue must be protected, or a condition in which a strong psychosocial component is suspected. Although this list can go on, the decision is ultimately made by applying the wise action principle.

After it is determined that the patient and his or her condition are appropriate for treatment by passive movement, one must then consider the purpose or intent of the technique. The answer to this question is fairly generic at this point and may include stretching a tight or shortened tissue to relieve pain or to impart a controlled degree of stress on the tissue or joint. Next, the direction of movement should be determined, with the intent of the technique, anatomic and biomechanical considerations, and previous experience being some of the factors influencing this decision. With the intent of the technique and direction of movement selected, consideration is then given to where in the joint available ROM the technique will be applied and the manner of application. Possibilities include the beginning of range, midrange, end range, or through range, with the manner of application referring to the amplitude and rhythm of the movement.

These decisions are also influenced largely by the intent of the technique, pathoanatomic and pathobiologic considerations, and the type of disorder. The type of disorder is a phrase that is used to refer to the reason the patient is seeking treatment. This could be pain, stiffness, weakness, "giving way," and so on. After these determinations are made, the position of the patient, the position of the therapist, and the manual contacts that will best allow the technique to be performed are considered. The patient's position should be one in which he or she is comfortable and relaxed and that allows easy access to the joint being treated. The therapist's starting position should be one that allows complete control of the movement and allows forces to be applied in the direction intended and is comfortable and easy to maintain. In general, manual contacts should be as broad as possible for the technique in use to distribute the force over a larger contact area. This should allow better patient comfort as well as therapist control of the movement. When possible, the passive movement should be accomplished by movement of the body or arms of the therapist and not by pushing with the fingertips or hands (Fig. 104.2).

Grades of Movement

Grades of movement are used to denote the position in the available range at which the technique is performed and the amplitude of the movement. They are best thought of as a guide to facilitate communication between the therapist and the exact points in the range.[43] They also may allow the therapist to think in finer detail about the technique and enhance acquisition of the skill. Grades I through V have been described and are often depicted on a movement diagram (Box 104.1). Grade I is a small-amplitude movement performed at the beginning of the available range. Grade II is a large-amplitude movement performed in the resistance-free part of the range. Grade III is a large-amplitude movement performed into resistance or up to the limit of the available range. Grade IV is a small-amplitude movement performed into resistance or up to the limit of the available range. Grade V is small amplitude, high-velocity thrust performed usually, but not always, at the end of the available range. Pluses and minuses are often used, particularly with grades III and IV, to give further detail related to the vigor of the technique. For example, grade V would be performed at that part in the range where resistance to movement is first perceived, whereas grade V+ would be a more vigorous technique taken further into the resistance portion of the range. The concept of grades of movement can be applied to both passive accessory motion (glide) and passive physiologic motion. Again, it is important to emphasize that the clinical utility of grades of movement is that they provide a simple means of communicating aspects of the technique (where in the range the technique is performed, the

amplitude of the movement, and the vigor or strength used) that would otherwise require lengthy descriptions.

Options Available in the Choice of Technique

Numerous options are available when considering the type of movement to be used and the method of application. Treatment by passive movement can include the use of physiologic motions, accessory motions, or any combination of the two (Fig. 104.3). For example, if the purpose or intent of a technique is to improve external rotation at the shoulder, the choices could include external rotation, anterior or posterior glide, a combined motion of anterior glide and external rotation, or even the combined physiologic motions of external rotation and abduction. Further decisions to be made would include where in the range to perform the technique (i.e., the grade of movement, the strength of the technique, and the rhythm in which the technique is performed) (Fig. 104.4).

This decision-making process is aided by the use of the wise action approach. When considering the best of science, questions to ask could be the following. (1) Is there any evidence available to support one particular technique or movement over the other? (2) Based on anatomy, what tissues could be limiting motion, and what is the best position to stretch them? (3) Considering the pain sciences and proposed mechanisms of manual therapy, what is the dominant pain mechanism, and would one type of movement be more appropriate than another?

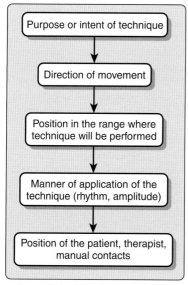

Fig. 104.2 General considerations for applying a manual joint-based technique.

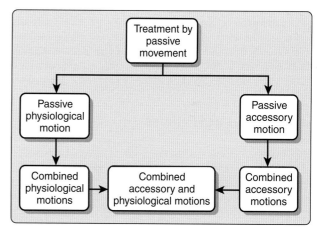

Fig. 104.3 Passive movement options for manual joint-based techniques. (Modified from Hengeveld E, Banks K. Principles of selection and progression of mobilization/manipulation techniques. In: Hengeveld E, Banks K, eds. *Maitland's Peripheral Manipulation*. 4th ed. Edinburgh: Elsevier Butterworth Heinemann; 2005:187.)

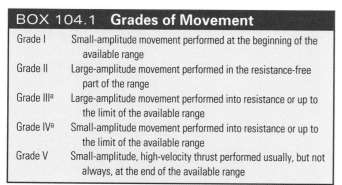

BOX 104.1	**Grades of Movement**
Grade I	Small-amplitude movement performed at the beginning of the available range
Grade II	Large-amplitude movement performed in the resistance-free part of the range
Grade III[a]	Large-amplitude movement performed into resistance or up to the limit of the available range
Grade IV[a]	Small-amplitude movement performed into resistance or up to the limit of the available range
Grade V	Small-amplitude, high-velocity thrust performed usually, but not always, at the end of the available range

[a]Pluses and minuses may be used with grades III and IV to give further detail related to the vigor of the technique.

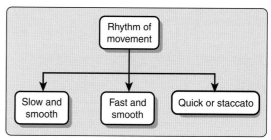

Fig. 104.4 Rhythm of movement options for manual joint-based techniques. (Modified from Hengeveld E, Banks K. Principles of selection and progression of mobilization/manipulation techniques. In: Hengeveld E, Banks K, eds. *Maitland's Peripheral Manipulation*. 4th ed. Edinburgh: Elsevier Butterworth Heinemann; 2005:185.)

Reflection on the best of current therapies may lead you to question whether one particular approach, such as Mulligan's MWM, would be more appropriate and whether there is evidence to support this.

Last, when considering the best of the patient–client interaction, attention is focused on the clinical presentation and the assessments made after the patient interview and physical examination. These assessments, which have been referred to as hypothesis categories, can include the patient's perspective on his or her experience, activity capabilities, and restrictions; the pathobiological mechanisms of the disorder; contributing factors to the development and maintenance of the problem; contraindications to and precautions of treatment; and prognosis. Taken collectively, this allows an assessment of what Maitland referred to as the SINS of the problem. SINS is an acronym for the severity, irritability, nature, and stage of the disorder. *Severity* encompasses not only the amount or intensity of a symptom, often assessed by means of a numerical pain rating, but also the degree to which the problem is restricting participation in activities relevant to the individual. *Irritability* is a construct that is used to describe the amount of activity required to bring the symptoms on, the amount of the symptom brought on, and how long it takes to settle. *Nature* refers to many aspects of the disorder, including the pathobiological mechanisms, psychosocial factors, and the medical diagnosis. *Stage* can refer to how acute or chronic the problem is, but perhaps more important, the stability of the disorder.

Thinking about the clinical presentation in such great detail can enhance the development of clinical reasoning strategies and promote pattern recognition skills. Thinking in a global sense, four distinct clinical patterns have been described along with empirically based guidelines for the selection and progression of passive movement techniques for each. The four patterns include a pain-dominant group, a stiffness-dominant group, a group with components of both pain and stiffness, and a group in which momentary pain is the dominant feature (Fig. 104.5).

Clinical Groups and Patterns

Pain Group

In the pain group, as implied, the limitation of movement is caused by pain. Stiffness cannot be assessed because pain is provoked easily and often early in the range. Pain at rest is common. If it were not for the pain, the joint may well have full ROM. These are typically highly irritable disorders, with little activity provoking much pain that takes a long time to settle. Pathobiological mechanisms may include inflammation,

peripheral sensitization with primary hyperalgesia, and centrally induced secondary hyperalgesia. The pain experience may be heightened by fear and anxiety associated with movement. Careful positioning is required with attention to finding a pain-easing position in which to perform the technique. It is also important that the joint is well supported and the manual contacts are comfortable. The patient should feel confident that the therapist will not move the joint into the painful part of the range. This can be accomplished by using the body to block motion, especially when performing passive physiologic techniques.

Often, the first choice of movement is an accessory motion performed early in the range; of small amplitude; and in a smooth, slow rhythm (Fig. 104.6 and Videos 104.1 and 104.2). As the pain eases, the amplitude of the movement can be increased with the goal being to move through as large a range as possible with the least amount of pain. Treatment can be progressed to include passive physiologic motions following the same principles. As pain eases and stiffness is encountered, small-amplitude movements just to the point of resistance can be used to provoke a controlled degree of pain. Assessment is made while performing the technique, after the technique is applied, and on follow-up at the next treatment session. If no exacerbation is experienced, the vigor and duration of the technique can be progressed.

Stiffness Group

In the stiffness group, pain is minimal and often reported only when the stiff joint is stretched vigorously. The pain eases quickly when the stretch is released, and no latent pain is experienced. Patients commonly seek treatment due to difficulty performing normal daily activities because of the loss of motion but not pain. For example, a person with a stiff elbow lacking flexion may report difficulty fastening the top button of a shirt or bringing a glass to his or her mouth. Initial treatment can include the physiologic motion that is stiff (in this case, flexion) performed in the resistance portion of the range as a small-amplitude movement or an accessory motion performed at the limit of the stiff physiologic movement (Fig. 104.7 and Video. 104.3).

As best stated by McClure and Flowers,[19] when limited ROM is thought to be caused by a structural change in the periarticular tissues, the therapist should consider which structures could potentially limit that ROM. Selection of a stretching technique should then be based on what type of maneuver will best put tension on the restricting tissue. The vigor of the technique can gradually be increased with each bout of mobilization typically lasting 1 to 2 minutes. A typical routine would include using the passive physiologic motion first followed by the accessory motion at the limit of the physiologic range and repeating this sequence three to four times. This can provoke a degree of treatment soreness that is often eased by performing the passive physiologic

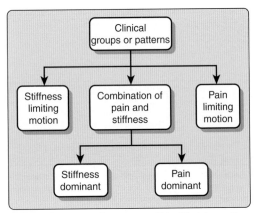

Fig. 104.5 Clinical presentation groups. (Modified from Hengeveld E, Banks K. Principles of selection and progression of mobilization/manipulation techniques. In: Hengeveld E, Banks K, eds. *Maitland's Peripheral Manipulation*. 4th ed. Edinburgh: Elsevier Butterworth Heinemann; 2005.)

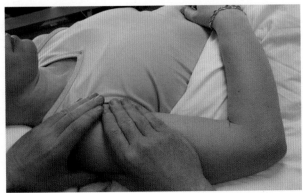

Fig. 104.6 Grade I or II posterior to anterior glide of the glenohumeral joint.

motion as a large-amplitude, through-range movement but not to the same degree of stretching.

Treatment can be progressed by performing combined physiologic and accessory motions synchronously or combining two physiologic motions performed in a synchronous manner. An example is performing external rotation with forward elevation of the shoulder (Fig. 104.8). This could also be combined with an inferior glide of the head of the humerus so that two physiologic motions and one accessory motion are performed together. The patient could be supine or sidelying. When treating the stiff joint, other options such as orthotic intervention should be kept in mind with manual therapy as an adjunctive or complementary treatment for preconditioning and pain modulation.

Pain and Stiffness Group

Most patients seeking treatment for musculoskeletal disorders of the upper extremity present with both pain and stiffness components to

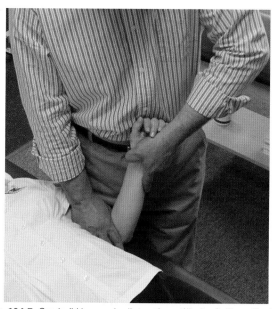

Fig. 104.7 Grade IV long-axis distraction at limit of elbow flexion.

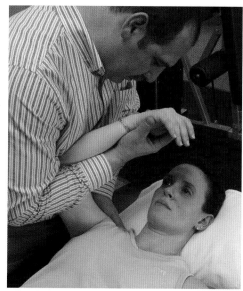

Fig. 104.8 Grade III or IV combined physiologic external rotation and flexion into resistance of available motion of the shoulder.

their problem. Determining which component is dominant can be quite a challenge, requiring greater attention to detail in the patient interview and physical examination. When pain is the greater component, guidelines similar to those for the pain group should be followed until the response to treatment, as related to the behavior of the pain, is known. Then treatment can be directed toward the stiffness component with greater confidence and less risk of exacerbation. When stiffness is the dominant component, treatment is similar to that for the stiffness group but with greater respect to the pain. Passive accessory motion can be performed in the position of the limited physiologic motion but not quite as far into the range.

Momentary Pain Group

A challenging, but often rewarding, group to treat consists of those who present with momentary pain. Frequently described as catches, twinges, or jabs of pain, the individual will state that the pain only comes on with certain movements but has difficulty identifying the painful movements. A movement may provoke the pain in an inconsistent manner. The challenge of the physical examination is to identify the offending movement, which is then often the direction first used as the treatment. A controlled degree of the familiar pain is then provoked by use of small-amplitude, end-range movements, usually an accessory motion or combined physiologic movement such as the shoulder quadrant position (Fig. 104.9 and Video 104.4). The rhythm of the movement can be a bit quicker or even staccato-like. Any treatment soreness is usually eased by larger amplitude, through-range maneuvers. Disorders of this type can be handled quite firmly, particularly when pathology such as instability or an intraarticular lesion has already been ruled out. They tend to be nonsevere, nonirritable, and very stable with minimal activity or participation restriction, involving pain that comes on quickly but can ease just as fast, and with the history revealing little to no change noted over time. The response to treatment can be fairly quick, with improvement in four to six sessions. Problems of this nature can often be underexamined and undertreated, with the value of treatment by passive movement not realized.

There are many other considerations that are relevant to the selection of the technique decision-making process that include the particular joint being treated, the medical diagnosis, the source of the symptoms, and the history and onset of the disorder, to name a few. It is beyond the scope of this chapter to review all these factors, and readers are referred elsewhere for a detailed discussion.[41,42] The intent

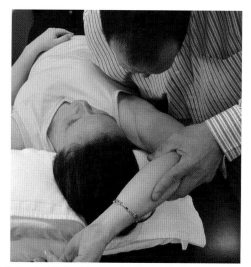

Fig. 104.9 Grade IV shoulder quadrant technique, which may be used to treat momentary pain.

of the preceding was to provide an introduction to this process, review general guidelines from one particular approach, and provoke thought, not only about the selection of a technique but also the detail required of the reasoning behind the selection.

MOBILIZATION WITH MOVEMENT

Before concluding, a brief discussion of Mulligan's MWM treatment approach is warranted because these techniques have gained popularity in both the clinical realm and research agenda. Introduced by Brian R. Mulligan, a physiotherapist from New Zealand, this approach has been summarized as follows:

> MWM is a manual therapy treatment technique in which a manual force, usually in the form of a joint glide, is applied to a motion segment and sustained while a previously impaired action is performed. The technique is indicated if, during its application, the technique enables the impaired joint to move freely without pain or impediment. The direction of the applied force (translation or rotation) is typically perpendicular to the plane of movement or impaired action and in some instances it is parallel to the treatment plane.[6]

The proposed mechanism for the clinical efficacy of MWM is based on a mechanical model that proposes that minor positional faults occur after injury or strain, resulting in movement restrictions, pain, or both. The MWM technique, or correctional mobilization, is thought to restore pain-free function by means of repositioning.[17] The positional fault theory was challenged in a critical review of the literature published up until 2003 in which the authors concluded that there was no substantive evidence that supported or refuted the hypothesis that a reversal of a positional fault was the predominant mechanism of action for MWM.[18] Although there has been some evidence of positional change after application of the technique, this was transient and could not account for any lasting benefit attributed to the technique. An alternative hypothesis was considered based on the hypoalgesic effect noted when a MWM technique (Video 104.5) was applied for tennis elbow. It was proposed that the combination of sympathoexcitation nonopioid hypoalgesia and improvement in motor function (pain-free grip strength) was an indirect sign of a possible involvement of endogenous pain-inhibition systems.[18] This mirrors the model discussed earlier, proposing that the outcomes associated with manual therapy most likely result from the interaction of complex inhibitory mechanisms at the peripheral, spinal cord, and supraspinal levels.[16] The clinical efficacy of the MWM has been demonstrated for a few select musculoskeletal disorders, as previously noted. Although there have been several RCTs investigating the effects, the level of evidence has been assessed to be of low to moderate quality. Like other manual therapy techniques and approaches, further research has been recommended to validate the proposed mechanisms and effectiveness of MWM. Continued use of MWM in clinical practice is advocated when used in the context of sound clinical reasoning strategies and can be thought of as another option falling under the category of a combined accessory glide with active or resisted physiologic motion technique.

SUMMARY

Despite critical review and limited high-quality evidence to support the efficacy and superiority over other treatment options, manual therapy has maintained its popularity in the management of upper extremity musculoskeletal disorders. The degree of uncertainty that exists surrounding the selection of the best technique(s) and complementary treatment for a particular disorder remains best managed by adopting sound clinical reasoning strategies and applying wise action principles. This approach allows for consideration of the proposed underlying mechanism in decision making without being bound to rigid dogma. Examples of the many options are demonstrated in the videos that accompany this chapter (Videos 104.6 to 104.14).

It may also be advantageous to keep in mind the concept of *the technique as the brainchild of ingenuity*. Although a standardized description of a base set of techniques is required and necessary for teaching purposes and the acquisition of skill, adaptation is encouraged to deal with the variability encountered with respect to patient size, therapist size, and the clinical presentation at hand. This also allows the development of new techniques as new evidence and knowledge emerge.

REFERENCES

1. Heiser R, O'Brien VH, Schwartz DA. The use of joint mobilization to improve clinical outcomes in hand therapy: a systematic review of the literature. *J Hand Ther.* 2013;26:297–311.
2. Page MJ, Green S, Kramer S, et al. Manual therapy and exercise in adhesive capsulitis (frozen shoulder). *Cochrane Database Syst Rev.* 2014;26(8):CD011275.
3. Page MJ, Green S, McBain B, et al. Manual therapy and exercise for rotator cuff disease. *Cochrane Database Syst Rev.* 2016;6:CD012224.
4. Westad K, Tjoestvolsen F, Hebron C. The effectiveness of Mulligan's mobilization with movement (MWM) on peripheral joint in musculoskeletal conditions: a systematic review. *Musculoskelet Sci Pract.* 2018;39:157–163.
5. Camarinos J, Marinko L. Effectiveness of manual physical therapy for painful shoulder conditions: a systematic review. *J Man Manip Ther.* 2009;17:206–215.
6. Ho CY, Sole G, Munn J. The effectiveness of manual therapy in the management of musculoskeletal disorders of the shoulder: a systematic review. *Man Ther.* 2009;14:463–474.
7. Herd CR, Meserve BB. A systematic review of the effectiveness of manipulative therapy in treating lateral epicondylalgia. *J Manip Ther.* 2008;16:225–237.
8. Cook C, Sheets C. Clinical equipoise and personal equipoise: two necessary ingredients for reducing bias in manual therapy trials. *J Man Manip Ther.* 2011;19(1):55–57.
9. Bialosky JE, Bishop MD, Penza CW. Placebo mechanisms of manual therapy: a sheep in wolf's clothing? *J Orthop Sports Phys Ther.* 2017;47(5):301–304.
10. Sueki DG, Cleland JA, Wainner RS. A regional interdependence model of musculoskeletal dysfunction: research, mechanisms, and clinical implications. *J Man Manip Ther.* 2013;21(2):90–102.
11. Bang MD, Deyle GD. Comparison of supervised exercise with and without manual therapy for patients with shoulder impingement syndrome. *J Orthop Sports Phys Ther.* 2000;30(3):126–137.
12. Wassinger CA, Rich D, Cameron N, et al. Cervical and thoracic manipulations: Acute effects upon pain pressure threshold and self-reported pain in experimentally induced shoulder pain. *Man Ther.* 2016;21:227–232.
13. Rothstein JM. Manual therapy: a special issue and a special topic. *Phys Ther.* 1992;72:839–841.
14. Haskins R, Rivett DA, Osmotherly PG. Clinical prediction rules in the physiotherapy management of low back pain: a systematic review. *Man Ther.* 2012;17:9–21.
15. Stanton TR, Hancock MJ, Maher CG, Koes BW. Critical appraisal of clinical prediction rules that aim to optimize treatment selection for musculoskeletal conditions. *Phys Ther.* 2010;90:843–854.
16. Bialosky JE, Bishop MD, Price DD, et al. The mechanisms of manual therapy in the treatment of musculoskeletal pain: a comprehensive model. *Man Ther.* 2009;14:531–538.
17. Mulligan BR. *Manual Therapy: "NAGS," "SNAGS," MWMS" etc.* 5th ed. Wellington: Plane View Services Ltd; 2004.
18. Vicenzino B, Paungmali A, Teys P. Mulligan's mobilization-with-movement, positional faults and pain relief: current concepts from a critical review of literature. *Man Ther.* 2007;12:98–108.

19. McClure PW, Flowers KR. Treatment of limited shoulder motion: a case study based on biomechanical considerations. *Phys Ther.* 1992;72:929–936.

20. DiFabio RP. Efficacy of manual therapy. *Phys Ther.* 1992;72:853–864.

21. Michlovitz SL, Harris BA, Watkins MP. Therapy interventions for improving joint range of motion: a systematic review. *J Hand Ther.* 2004;17:118–131.

22. Coyle JA, Robertson VJ. Comparison of two passive mobilizing techniques following Colles' fracture: a multi-element design. *Man Ther.* 1998;3:34–41.

23. Tal-Akabi A, Rushton A. An investigation to compare the effectiveness of carpal bone mobilisation and neurodynamic mobilisation as methods of treatment for carpal tunnel syndrome. *Man Ther.* 2000;5:214–222.

24. Handoll HH, Madhok R, Howe TE. Rehabilitation for distal radial fractures in adults. *Cochrane Database Syst Rev.* 2002;(2):D003324. Review. Update in: *Cochrane Database Syst Rev.* 2006;3:CD003324.

25. Green S, Buchbinder R, Hetrick S. Physiotherapy interventions for shoulder pain. *Cochrane Database Syst Rev.* 2003;(2):D004258.

26. Michener LA, Walsworth MK, Burnet EN. Effectiveness of rehabilitation for patients with subacromial impingement syndrome: a systematic review. *J Hand Ther.* 2004;17:152–164.

27. Desmeules F, Côté CH, Frémont P. Therapeutic exercise and orthopedic manual therapy for impingement syndrome: a systematic review. *Clin J Sport Med.* 2003;13:176–182.

28. Bisset L, Paungmali A, Vicenzino B, Beller E. A systematic review and meta-analysis of clinical trials on physical interventions for lateral epicondylalgia. *Br J Sports Med.* 2005;39:411–422.

29. Vicenzino B, Cleland JA, Bisset L. Joint manipulation in the management of lateral epicondylalgia: a clinical commentary. *J Man Manip Ther.* 2007;15:50–56.

30. Hing W, Bigelow R, Bremner T. Mulligan's mobilization with movement: a systematic review. *J Man Manip Ther.* 2009;17:E39–E66.

31. Yang JL, Chang CW, Chen SY, et al. Mobilization techniques in subjects with frozen shoulder syndrome: randomized multiple-treatment trial. *Phys Ther.* 2007;87:1307–1315.

32. Johnson AJ, Godges JJ, Zimmerman GJ, et al. The effect of anterior versus posterior glide joint mobilization on external rotation range of motion in patients with shoulder adhesive capsulitis. *J Orthop Sports Phys Ther.* 2007;37:88–99.

33. Vermeulen HM, Rozing PM, Obermann WR, et al. Comparison of high-grade and low-grade mobilization techniques in the management of adhesive capsulitis of the shoulder: randomized controlled trial. *Phys Ther.* 2006;86:355–368.

34. Teys P, Bisset L, Vicenzino B. The initial effects of a Mulligan's mobilization with movement technique on range of movement and pressure pain threshold in pain-limited shoulders. *Man Ther.* 2008;13:37–42.

35. Guimaraes JF, Salvini TF, Siqueria AL, et al. Immediate effects of mobilization with movement vs sham technique on range of motion, strength, and function in patients with shoulder impingement syndrome. *JMPT.* 2016;39(9):605–615.

36. Bisset L, Beller E, Jull G, et al. Mobilisation with movement and exercise, corticosteroid injection, or wait and see for tennis elbow: randomised trial. *Br Med J.* 2006;333(7575):939.

37. Vicenzino B. Lateral epicondylalgia: a musculoskeletal physiotherapy perspective. *Man Ther.* 2003;8:66–79.

38. Brandt C, Sole G, Krause MW, Nel M. An evidence-based review on the validity of the Kaltenborn rule as applied to the glenohumeral joint. *Man Ther.* 2007;12:3–11.

39. Jones MA, Rivett DA. Introduction to clinical reasoning. In: Jones MA, Rivett DA, eds. *Clinical Reasoning for Manual Therapists.* Edinburgh: Elsevier Butterworth Heinemann; 2004:3–24.

40. Butler DS. Clinicians and their decisions. In: Butler DS. *The Sensitive Nervous System.* Adelaide: Noigroup Publications; 2000:128–151.

41. Hengeveld E, Banks K. Principles of selection and progression of mobilization/manipulation techniques. In: Hengeveld E, Banks K, eds. *Maitland's Peripheral Manipulation.* 4th ed. Edinburgh: Elsevier Butterworth Heinemann; 2005:179–236.

42. Hengeveld E, Banks K. Principles and method of mobilization/manipulation techniques. In: Hengeveld E, Banks K, eds. *Maitland's Peripheral Manipulation.* 4th ed. Edinburgh: Elsevier Butterworth Heinemann; 2005:165–178.

43. Jones MA, Magarey ME. Clinical reasoning in the use of manual therapy techniques for the shoulder girdle. In: Tovin BJ, Greenfield BH, eds. *Evaluation and Treatment of the Shoulder: An Integration of the Guide to Physical Therapist Practice.* Philadelphia: F.A. Davis; 2001:317–346.

105

Optimizing Outcomes: Concepts of Patient Preference, Health Literacy, and Adherence to Treatment

Joy C. MacDermid

OUTLINE

CRITICAL POINTS

This SIMPLE strategy to improve adherence is:

S: Simplify.

I: Individualize.

M: Manage psychosocial barriers.

P: Promote therapeutic alliance, self-efficacy, and resiliency.

L: Limit bias.

E: Evaluate adherence and outcomes.

Strategies

- Engage patients in evidence-based shared decision making.
- Evaluate and obtain congruence with the patient with respect to goals, problem definition, and agreed-upon and useful solutions.
- Set clear expectations about your role, the therapy processes, and expected outcomes.
- Use teach back.
- Have home programs and education resources in multiple formats, including web, print, and multimedia.
- Integrate self-evaluation and adherence monitoring tools in the treatment plan.
- Use simple nontechnical language (grade 6–8 level).

- Consider culture, gender, and other social factors in how information is presented.
- Use SMART goals.
- Build partnership and trust.
- Show respect and consider the power balance.
- Provide positive role modeling.
- Provide clear and consistent feedback about progress.
- Demonstrate caring and empathy in a professional context.
- Enact needed therapist role (i.e., coach, consultant, or care provider).
- Measure adherence and discuss barriers.
- Discuss progress on standardized outcomes and expectations.
- Modify programs based on patient's lifestyle, physical abilities, and adherence profile.
- Prioritize the most essential elements of the program.
- Link home program components to the patient's daily activities.
- Use graded meaningful activities that provide performance accomplishment.

Increasingly, hand therapists are expected to deliver efficient and high-quality care in a limited number of visits. Therapy can involve exercise, instruction on safety and protection, graded return to normal activity, symptom management, and health promotion advice. The patient's enactment of these requires independent participation and ongoing adherence. This requires integrated understanding, intention, ability, and commitment. That is, patients must understand the instructions, see the information as relevant to them, adjust their decisional balance, follow the instructions correctly, and have the abilities and resources to continue the program in the face of competing demands. Thus, health literacy, adherence, fidelity, and patient centeredness are all important and interdependent aspects that influence the effectiveness of hand therapy. The World Health Organization (WHO) has stated that "increasing the effectiveness of adherence interventions may have a far greater impact on the health of the population than any improvement in specific medical treatments."[1] The consequences of poor adherence are poor outcomes and increased health care costs.[1]

CONCEPTS

Literacy

The simple version is that literacy has been considered the ability to read and write. As society becomes more complex, the definition has expanded. The United Nations Educational, Scientific and Cultural Organization (UNESCO) defines it as the "ability to identify, understand, interpret, create, communicate and compute, using printed and written materials associated with varying contexts."[2] For this chapter, we define *literacy* as the "ability to read, understand and interact with text information."

Health Literacy

The Patient Protection and Affordable Care Act of 2010, Title V, defines *health literacy* as the degree to which an individual has the capacity to obtain, communicate, process, and understand basic health information and services to make appropriate health decisions.[3] The WHO use a similar definition—the ability to access, comprehend, evaluate, and communicate information to promote, maintain, and improve health in a variety of settings across the life course.[1]

Physical Literacy

Physical literacy has been defined by The International Physical Literacy Association as "the motivation, confidence, physical competence, knowledge and understanding to value and take responsibility for engagement in physical activity." Whitehead[4] has written on the philosophical underpinnings of physical literacy, describing it as the extent to which an "individual moves with poise, economy and confidence in a wide variety of physically challenging situations. Furthermore, the individual is perceptive in 'reading' all aspects of the physical environment, anticipating movement needs or possibilities and responding appropriately to these, with intelligence and imagination." In her book on the topic, she provides a definition similar to that adopted by the International Physical Literacy Association, although it emphasizes the life course rather than personal responsibility: "as appropriate to each individual's endowment, physical literacy can be described as the motivation, confidence, physical competence, knowledge and understanding to maintain physical activity throughout the life course."[4]

Fidelity

Fidelity may be defined as the extent to which delivery of an intervention adheres to the treatment protocol or program model originally developed.[5] This relates to the extent to which individual therapists deliver the intervention as proposed by developers or as tested in research studies. Rehabilitation interventions are typically complex or multimodal and often have a theoretical or mechanistic foundation that is thought to provide the therapeutic benefit. These are considered the active ingredients, and testing the delivery of these can be just as important as testing the active ingredients or chemical composition in drugs.

Patient or Participant Uptake

Patient or participant uptake is defined as the extent to which the target recipient demonstrates that she or he has taken up or received the intervention that was delivered.

Decisional Balance

Decisional balance refers to when people assess the positive and negative consequences of choosing a new behavior.

(Hand Therapy) Adherence

The WHO report on adherence to long-term therapies defined *adherence* as "the extent to which a person's behavior—taking medication, following a diet, and/or executing lifestyle changes, corresponds with agreed recommendations from a health care provider."[1] Adapting definitions of adherence to therapy leads to this definition: the extent to which a person can implement and maintain behaviors (lifestyle, activity modifications, devices or orthoses) and self-administered therapeutic interventions (exercises, medications, devices, modalities) that have been recommended and agreed upon with a health care provider. This latter is in line with the WHO definition but is more relevant to hand therapy in that it emphasizes both implementation and maintenance of a behavior because hand therapy interventions must be maintained over time.

Patient Preference

Within the context of evidence-based practice, patient values and preferences have been defined as "the collection of goals, expectations, predispositions, and beliefs that individuals have for certain decisions and their potential outcomes." In the context of this chapter, *patient preference* is defined as "the individual's opinions and preferred choices about his or her health care as influenced by their goals, priorities, expectations, beliefs, history, life situation, culture, gender, and societal influences."

Shared Decision Making

Shared decision making (SDM) has been defined as "an approach where clinicians and patients share the best available evidence when faced with the task of making decisions, and where patients are supported to consider options, to achieve informed preferences."[6] The National Institute of Health and Care Excellence (NICE) defines SDM as "when health professionals and patients work together. This puts people at the center of decisions about their own treatment and care. During shared decision making, it's important that care or treatment options are fully explored, along with their risks and benefits, different choices available to the patient are discussed and a decision is reached together with a health and social care professional."[7] A more simple and direct definition is "the conversation that happens between a patient and her or his health care professional to reach a health care choice together."

Patient-Centered Care

The Institute of Medicine defines *patient-centered care* as "providing care that is respectful of, and responsive to, individual patient preferences, needs and values, and ensuring that patient values guide all clinical decisions." Stewart and associates[8] defined patient-centered care as a five-step process in which the health provider (1) explores the patient's main reason for the visit, concerns, and need for information; (2) seeks an integrated understanding of the patient as a whole person; (3) finds common ground on the problem and its management; (4) engages in health promotion; and (5) supports the continuing relationship. Although a systematic review found inconsistency in how patient-centered care has been defined, three core themes were identified: (1) patient participation and involvement, (2) the relationship between the patient and the health care professional, and (3) the context where care is delivered.[9]

Evidence-Based Practice

Evidence-based practice recognizes the integration of three pillars: clinical research, clinical expertise, and patient values and preferences. A common definition as by Sackett[9a] is "the conscientious, explicit, and judicious use of current best evidence in making decisions about the care of individual patients. The practice of evidence-based medicine means integrating individual clinical expertise with the best available external clinical evidence from systematic research. By individual clinical expertise we mean the proficiency and judgment that individual clinicians acquire through clinical experience and clinical practice." A consensus definition of the Sicily Statement[10] defined *evidence-based practice* as "decisions about health care are based on the best available, current, valid and relevant evidence. These decisions should be made by those receiving care, informed by the tacit and explicit knowledge of those providing care, within the context of available resources." The major paradigm shift that the evidence-based medicine movement instigated was a greater focus on clinical research for making clinical decisions and more rigorous evaluation of the quality of clinical research in deciding how much confidence should be placed in the conclusions. As a result, two common misconceptions are that evidence-based practice dictates decisions based on research and that without high-quality research studies to support a specific course of action, it cannot be undertaken.

THE CONTINUUM OF LITERACY TO ADHERENCE

It is apparent that the concepts so far in this chapter are integral and interdependent and that adherence is a process that moves through stages that engage these elements iteratively. This process is described conceptually in Fig. 105.1, which demonstrates the steps, modifiers, and principles involved in this continuum.

Health literacy begins before the patient interacts with the health care professional and continues beyond the shared decisions that form the individual treatment plan to the implementation and maintenance of that plan that is ultimately reflected as adherence. A patient cannot adhere to an intended intervention unless she or he understands it and has engaged in an informed decision. A patient cannot implement the plan unless it was delivered with fidelity and taken up as intended. Nor can patients adhere over time unless they have the skills to manage obstacles and adaptation of the plan.

The process starts with the patient assessment, which informs the therapist's clinical decision making about what intervention plan should be implemented. Clinicians formulate a framework and expectations for a treatment plan based on their experience, expertise in clinical assessment, and toolbox of treatment strategies. Pattern recognition, understanding the patient's circumstances, scope of practice, skills acquired during professional or postprofessional training, and knowledge of the best evidence are integrated to develop potential options that will meet the patient's needs or presenting problem. This is consistent with the principles of evidence-based practice, specialization, and patient-centered care.

The clinician's ability to communicate and the patient's health literacy are critical components of ensuring that effective interaction occurs to affect the patient's decisional balance. Patients cannot make rational choices if they do not understand the options or recommendations, including the potential benefits and drawbacks of different choices. Literature on shared decision making emphasizes how health care choices should be made conjointly, and philosophically, many clinicians agree with the principles of shared decision making. However, barriers to shared decision making for clinicians include the context, time constraints, and patient characteristics.[11] Shared decision making may be more relevant for long-term decisions, especially in chronic conditions compared with acute management in which decisions have to be made more quickly and the nature of the injury may direct the need for specific actions.[12] For example, therapists may take a more directive consent-based process when demonstrating range of motion exercises to a patient coming out of a cast and may take on a more

shared decision-making approach when developing self-management programs for a patient with hand arthritis. There are barriers to shared decision making on the patient side, which include difficulty in understanding the clinical condition, its natural history, and the consequences of different decisions. The power imbalance patients experience with clinicians is a recognized barrier.[13] For this reason, therapists have to be cautious about assuming implied consent or that decisions are "shared" during their patient interactions because a lack of engagement in therapy often occurs when the therapist and patient are not "on the same page." Although there is a substantial body of literature on shared decision making, most of the evidence supports improved satisfaction with the process of care, whereas limited evidence is available for the effect on outcomes.[14]

The process of being "on the same page" throughout the clinical interaction is part of what is called the *therapeutic alliance*.[15] Therapeutic alliance has been described as the working relationship or positive social connection between the patient and the therapist and is established through collaboration, communication, therapist empathy, and mutual respect.[16] Our scoping review of therapeutic alliance indicated that congruence, connectedness, communication, expectations, and individualized therapy were common themes across the research on therapeutic alliance.[15] Managing the professional relationship in a way that leverages these dimensions to promote therapeutic alliance is a major factor in adherence.

There is some overlap in concepts between therapeutic alliance and patient-centered care, although the former focuses on the therapeutic relationship and the latter on the clinical process. When we analyzed responses from patients with distal radius fractures using patient-centered care tools, we found that two factors emerged: clinician–patient dialogue, representing communication components of patient-centered care, and clinician–patient alliance, representing partnership components of patient-centered care.[17] The presence of these factors during early fracture management had a small but significant effect on patient outcomes 1 year after fracture.

A major benefit to the movement in patient-centered care has been recognition of the need to "tailor the treatment to the patient's lifestyle, not the other way round."[18] One of the thought leaders of patient-centered care, Moira Stewart,[19] has laid out steps for clinical

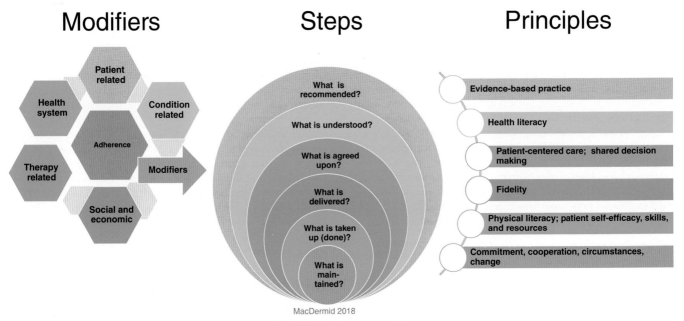

MacDermid 2018

Fig. 105.1 Adherence model.

interactions that are patient centered that have been implemented with family physicians. She suggested that patient-centered care "(a) explores the patients' main reason for the visit, concerns, and need for information; (b) seeks an integrated understanding of the patients' world—that is, their whole person, emotional needs, and life issues; (c) finds common ground on what the problem is and mutually agrees on management; (d) enhances prevention and health promotion; and (e) enhances the continuing relationship between the patient and the doctor."[19] Patient-centered care processes support a therapeutic alliance. Improvements in the therapeutic alliance between hand therapist and patient are expected to improve adherence,[15,20] as is patient-centered care. Both emphasize the importance of establishing a clear understanding of the patient's needs during the initial assessment and coming to the common understanding about the problem and how it should be managed. The inclusion of prevention and health promotion encourages hand therapists to think beyond the immediate problem, to think about the person and his or her health trajectory. Obviously, this is critical for family physicians, but it is also increasingly being recognized as a role for hand therapists. For example, it is not enough to teach people how to regain motion after a distal radius fracture. Rather, hand therapists should think about the person's overall bone health, secondary fracture prevention, and how this fracture might be a learning moment to address longer term bone health issues.[21] This indirectly may affect adherence when the patient understands the overall value of the treatment plan.

An often overlooked component of the process is ensuring that clinicians implement interventions the way they were intended. Because documentation of the detail of interventions is often limited in clinical trials, clinicians may implement interventions inappropriately while believing they are being evidence based. For example, clinicians may be aware that systematic reviews suggest that exercise is effective for lateral elbow tendinopathy. However, the dosage and type of exercise evaluated in the clinical trials demonstrating this effect must be replicated to achieve this benefit. Many systematic reviews of hand therapy management support the use of education in different clinical conditions. However, what are the core concepts that need to be delivered during education for different conditions, and what strategies are most effective in delivering this education? It can be challenging to ensure that consistent core content and optimal delivery methods are used in educational interventions because this is often poorly documented. However, these issues are central to fidelity.

Even when clinicians do an optimal job of delivering an intervention with complete fidelity and optimize their communication strategies, it is not always possible to ensure that patients fully take up the delivered intervention. Health literacy, physical abilities, physical literacy, patient self-efficacy, stress reactions, resiliency, and other patient skills and resources influence what they understand and retain from the intervention delivered. Consent is not something that occurs at a single point in time, but rather is a continuous process. Although patients may initially agree to the concept of a treatment program, as they become more aware of what it fully means in their life, they may modify their intentions. Commitment to elements of the treatment program is constantly being challenged as patients encounter competing priorities in their life. Lack of time, other responsibilities, responses to the therapy, and the recovery process all influence sustained implementation. The extent to which adherence is maintained outside of the clinic and over time relates to the initial commitment, the ongoing therapeutic alliance that develops between clinicians and their patients, circumstances that arise, and the therapeutic effects that patients attribute to their treatment program.

MODIFIERS OF ADHERENCE

The modifiers are those described by the WHO in five domains related to the: patient, health condition, health system, therapy, and socioeconomics.[1] O'Brien[22] has discussed these factors specifically in relation to hand therapy. Many of these factors are modifiable and hence can be secondary treatment targets within the treatment plan. Conversely, nonmodifiable factors may lead to adjustments in the treatment plan.

Patient-Related Factors

A wide range of patient related factors are potential modifiers of adherence. These factors include attitudes, beliefs, expectations, personal resources, problem-solving abilities, self-efficacy, physical literacy, health literacy, and others. A variety of negative factors have been identified, including forgetfulness, psychosocial stress, anxiety, low motivation, inadequate knowledge, lack of perceived need for treatment, negative beliefs around the efficacy of the treatment, nonacceptance of the disease, disbelief in the diagnosis, lack of risk perception, inability to understand instructions, low treatment expectations, hopelessness, negative cognitions, dissatisfaction with previous health care, and feelings of stigmatization.[1] A systematic review of the factors that related to adherence to lifestyle modifications in obese patients indicated that barriers to behavior change include poor motivation, social pressures, environmental factors, lack of time, health and physical limitations, negative thoughts or moods, socioeconomic constraints, gaps in knowledge or awareness, and lack of enjoyment of exercise.[20] Facilitators are often less studied, but the same review indicated that a better body mass index, early success, better baseline mood, being male, and older age were all facilitators of behavior change. A 2017 systematic review that focused on adherence to home-based therapies reported that adherence was better in patients who had greater self-efficacy, self-motivation, social support, intentions, and previous adherence to physical therapies.[23] It is noteworthy that many of these characteristics can be assessed using standardized tools, or they may be revealed during the history taking. Thus, these prognostic factors can be used to identify the risk of nonadherence during an initial assessment, allowing therapists to start an early process of inquiry and problem solving to address potential barriers to adherence. That is, assessment of adherence potential should be considered a core element of patient assessment and should help the hand therapist develop an adherence promotion plan that is reevaluated based on results of formal monitoring of adherence.

Patients' competency to do exercise, beliefs around exercise, physical capabilities, experience with exercise, and other factors discussed in the physical literacy research are also likely to influence hand therapy interventions, particularly those involving exercise. These concepts are common in health promotion literature,[4] where they are applied to the goal of keeping people active, but are equally relevant for adherence to therapeutic regimens and home programs. Hand therapists likely have experience where it is easier to obtain adherence and positive treatment benefits from home programs when managing a patient who is motivated, who clearly understands the rationale for the therapeutic exercises being demonstrated, who exercises regularly, who is confident that exercises are usually beneficial, and who quickly gains proficiency in performing exercises as instructed. Conversely, those with low self-efficacy about their ability to exercise, who lack exercise experience, or who have negative attitudes toward exercise (e.g., fear of movement) are likely to face substantial barriers in achieving the goals of a home program.

The components of physical literacy[4] include motivation and confidence, physical competence, knowledge and understanding, and engagement in physical activity. *Motivation and confidence refers* to an individual's enthusiasm for, enjoyment of, and self-assurance in adopting a physical activity (or exercise program). We know that previous exercise experience has a positive effect on adherence.[24] *Physical competence* refers to an individual's ability to develop movement skills and patterns and the capacity to experience a variety of movement intensities and durations. These are important patient capabilities that affect hand therapy because therapeutic exercises often require very specific movements (e.g., tendon-gliding exercises, recruitment of transferred muscles, or reinnervated motor units). Patients who have previously engaged in more complicated motor planning are likely to have the ability to replicate therapeutic exercises as instructed by the hand therapist. Fidelity in exercise performance facilitates therapeutic benefits and minimizes pain, both of which promote adherence. *Knowledge and understanding* relates to the ability to identify and express the essential qualities that influence movement, understand the health benefits of an active lifestyle, and appreciate appropriate safety features associated with physical activity in a variety of settings and physical environments. For example, in hand therapy home programs, patients who require balance training for secondary fracture prevention must implement the training safely at home after instruction in the clinic by the therapist. Patients whose gender or cultural behavioral expectations discourage participation in physical activity or those who choose not to engage in physical activity are less likely to effectively engage in a home program. Engagement in physical activities for life includes behavioral aspects that manifest as taking personal responsibility for exercise or activity. Those with poor physical literacy skills may present with involuntary nonadherence but may become adherent with more intensive instruction and feedback.

Although patient related factors are important, they are often overemphasized as the primary determinant of adherence without considering the other four dimensions outlined by the WHO. O'Brien[25] found that age and gender did not consistently relate to adherence to hand orthoses but noted that the research was very limited. A number of studies[26] have suggested that poor adherence is related to negative illness cognitions, beliefs that exercise will worsen their condition (fear avoidance), pain catastrophizing (magnification, helplessness, rumination), or low self-efficacy. These patients may not believe they can manage the problem, that the treatment is unlikely to be beneficial, or that their case is hopeless regardless of what they do. Unfortunately, some literature on the relationship between psychological factors and adherence or outcomes can unintentionally blame the patient for failure to recover rather than a focus on what strategies can be used to mitigate barriers to recovery.[26] Furthermore, the literature has often underemphasized that psychological features are transient pain- or stress-related behaviors that can dissipate with physical treatment.

Although the literature has focused on negative predictors, recognition and facilitation of positive predictors is equally important. High self-efficacy, problem-solving abilities, positive cognitions, positive attitudes toward exercise, and resiliency are positive traits that can facilitate adherence. Promotion of these protective factors can be enabled by therapists.

In separate papers, we discussed in detail how to apply social cognitive factors and self-efficacy theory to hand therapy using RACE[27] and the LEARN[28] approaches. In the RACE approach, the hand therapy assessment identifies psychosocial barriers such as helplessness and negative cognitions and modifies the treatment approach to include four key strategies: **r**educe the pain stimulus and achieve pain control, **a**ctivate through achievable goals and meaningful activity, **c**ognitive reshaping, and **e**mpowerment.[27] We further described how self-efficacy theory could be translated into specific treatment and adherence strategies in the LEARN paper.[28] The patient's self-efficacy expectations are derived from four principal sources of information: (1) performance accomplishments, (2) vicarious experiences, (3) verbal persuasion, and (4) physiological state. Self-efficacy can be enhanced by leveraging these resources and using related techniques such as modeling, desensitization, and self-instructed performance. The LEARN approach suggests: **l**earn exercise or activity using techniques to enhance performance accomplishment, **e**ncourage or cue using a variety of verbal persuasion techniques (e.g., expectations for improvement, attainable goals, demonstrating progress on outcome measures), **a**ddressing unpleasant symptoms (e.g., acknowledge, treat, and address coping), **r**einforcement or **r**ole models (e.g., visuals or classes in which success is modeled), and **n**egating disability (resolving barriers, using current abilities).

Therapy- and Therapist-Related Factors

Much of the focus on adherence has been on patient factors, not therapist factors. One of the key recommendations of the WHO is that health professionals should be trained in adherence.[1] Therapist factors include competence, interpersonal skills, communication skills, ability to build therapeutic alliance, knowledge, hands-on skills, biases, beliefs, and expectations. As an example of how therapist attitudes can influence the patient's behavior, a study looking at lifting performance during a physical therapy interaction found that therapists who scored high on kinesiophobia resulted in patients lifting less in both patients with and without kinesiophobic beliefs.[29] Therapists who are overly cautious may unconsciously reduce adherence or progress. Therapist skills in assessment and management of adherence are modifiable factors in improving adherence, and even a brief workshop on adherence can provide new skills.[30] Depending on the patient and problem, the therapist may need to alter their role. A caregiver role may be more needed when specific clinical skills are needed (e.g., wound care, orthotic fabrication). When minimal intervention is needed, the role may be as a consultant, providing a discrete unit of education. Where patients have signs of helplessness, the role may be as a coach who encourages and directs but avoids promoting dependency.

Characteristics of the therapy also influence adherence. Complex, demanding, uncomfortable, and time-consuming home programs are unlikely to be adhered to because of the negative immediate consequences of adherence. Conversely, positive aspects of the therapeutic interaction can enhance adherence. Patients report that when therapists notice their progress, it is an important motivator to maintaining adherence.[31] Hand therapists develop expertise in knowing how much force or repetition is indicated based on the injury tissue responses. Overly aggressive therapy that causes pain or swelling is not only ineffective but also undermines the patient's confidence in the therapist and inevitably results in poor adherence. Strategies that make home programs more enjoyable, more convenient, and more effective are likely to improve adherence. Therapists who are skilled at matching the home program to the patient's abilities, lifestyle, and expectations are likely to obtain better adherence.

Health Condition–Related Factors

Features of the health condition and associated comorbidities can also influence adherence. Some health conditions are highly variable, and adherence during acute episodes may be vastly different than during more stable periods. Patients who have severe illnesses may not focus on a more minor health problem. Certain comorbidities such as depression, dementia, drug abuse, brain injury, alcoholism, or mental health issues can directly affect adherence through the communication channels discussed earlier. Multiple studies have shown that patients with comorbidities have poorer outcomes with upper extremity surgery and therapy. Because therapists cannot modify most comorbid health conditions, they must adjust treatment plans and expectations.

Health Care System Factors

A variety of factors that determine how care is provided can have impact on adherence. Clinicians who are required to see high volumes of patients in a short period of time may not have sufficient time to fully develop a therapeutic relationship, to use best practices in patient education, to assess the potential for adherence, or to fully address adherence barriers. Lack of appropriate training of health care providers either in providing best practice or on optimizing adherence can be a barrier to achieving adherence. Health care systems, employee benefit plans, and supplemental health coverage influence what services patients receive and the perceived value of those services. Lack of access to tests, equipment, or services can create negative expectations or outcome potential. Inadequate instruction and monitoring may be a barrier to adherence. Conversely, the knowledge that therapy services are not available may encourage patients to stick to their home program because there are few therapeutic alternatives.

Social and Economic Factors

Economic factors influence the patient's competing demands and resources. Patients with limited resources may not be able to afford therapy sessions, orthotics, or assistive devices. Economic constraints are highly variable across different health care systems, countries, economies, and political contexts. These effects are compounded by the individual economic constraints of the patient. Patients may not be able to afford to take time off from work, may not have benefits, may have poor health care coverage, may have limited transportation, and experience other barriers based on their economic status. Social roles as caregivers may affect the extent to which people are able to attend or engage in therapy.

Social factors such as gender or racial biases can affect the care offered and undermine the therapeutic alliance, which negatively affects adherence. Clinicians may not even be aware that they are biased in their clinical decision making based on these factors. For example, surgeons were four times more likely to offer knee replacement to male patients compared with matched female standardized patients.[32] Similar biases have been shown with respect to pain management in which gender influences perceived need and drugs provided. Bias undermines the therapeutic alliance and its impact on adherence.

Social factors can also influence how patients perceive their hand therapists. Patients can also have gender biases. The extent to which the patient respects the clinician as an authority or expert is likely to have an impact on her or his adherence. A variety of societal attitudes about how people should behave, the meaning of illness, pain behaviors, and religious views affect adherence through multiple mechanisms.

MEASURES OF ADHERENCE

A variety of measures have been used to assess adherence. The type of measure often depends on the nature of the intervention and the context. A 2017 systematic review of a variety of measures that have been used to assess adherence to home rehabilitation found generally low-quality evidence. The review focused on different elements of adherence to home rehabilitation programs, including frequency, duration, intensity, accuracy, and general.[33] This review found the most evidence on adherence diaries, which are used both in clinical practice and research, and concluded that there was moderate validity and acceptability of using adherence diaries.

As technology solutions are increasingly used in hand therapy it is increasingly possible to embed usage measures. However, this approach, although convenient, is also subject to pitfalls because the assumption that "the more, the better" is not necessarily true.[34] The importance of assessing the intended use was emphasized in a recent review of adherence in technology interventions.[34] This reinforces the need to consider fidelity and uptake when assessing adherence. Diaries have limitations because they assess counts and are subject to reporting bias. A wide variety of adherence measures have been used in clinical trials, but many are neither feasible for clinical practice nor relevant to hand therapy. The Sport Injury Rehabilitation Adherence Scale[35] is brief and feasible but is slanted to sports rehabilitation. Based on the need for a brief hand therapy–relevant tool, the author devised an adherence tool with versions for therapist or patients ratings (Fig. 105.2). These can be used in isolation or to evaluate the concordance of clinician and therapist perceptions. It can be important to assess this discordance because previous studies have shown that patients' and therapists' perceptions differed significantly on 24 of the 33 aspects of adherence.

OPERATIONALIZING ADHERENCE IN CLINICAL PRACTICE

Understanding and leveraging the factors and processes that contribute to adherence, discussed in this chapter, is the first step in improving adherence and outcomes. Clinicians can evaluate the potential for adherence during their initial assessment and check for breakdowns during each clinical interaction. It is likely that multiple strategies will be needed to optimize adherence.[22] Social interventions might include building self-management skills and capacity building within the local community. The health care team and system should integrate adherence management in their processes of care (e.g., continuity of care, consistent messaging, eliciting patient perceptions, and considering patient priorities). Ensuring that therapy is comfortable and meaningful, informing patients of what to expect, ensuring adequate pain management, and providing exemplars of problem solving promote better adherence. As therapists evaluate patients' psychological status and comorbid health conditions, they should consider how these might affect adherence and then adapt their programs as needed. Therapists should develop skills in cognitive techniques that help patients think positively about their recovery. Cognitive reshaping strategies can promote self-efficacy and optimism, reinforce the patient's responsibility for his or her recovery, and counter negative thoughts that might be barriers to hand therapy participation. For example, the use of less threatening, medicalized, or frightening words[22] is one strategy that can be used to affect how patients interpret their clinical condition. Strategies must be broad in spectrum, have a motivational-behavioral focus, and be provided in combination to optimize the impact on adherence.[25,36]

Perhaps the single most important aspect of promoting adherence is effective communication. There is a broad body of literature on communication that can be drawn on to support adherence. A key strategy is the use of teach back. Teach back is an iterative process by which therapists can chunk information, have the patient explain what she or he has heard, and then correct any misconceptions or areas that were unclear. The importance of this simple strategy is emphasized in the Agency for Healthcare Research and Quality's 2001 report, "Making Health Care Safer," which stated, "Asking that patients recall and restate what they have been told is one of 11 top patient safety practices based on the strength of scientific evidence." Teach back is not a test of the patient but rather a test of the effectiveness of the communication and can be an effective way for therapists to learn how to be better communicators. After presenting a chunk of information therapists, explore using nonthreatening probes such as: "Tell me how you will describe

Adherence Assessment—Clinician

I think that this patient _____

	Not at all	A little	Quite a bit	Mostly	Always	Does not apply
1. Performs their exercise as instructed						
2. Has modified their activity (as instructed)						
3. Is using splints/orthotics/aids correctly						
4. Is engaged in their current therapy						
5. Will follow their home program						

Therapy Adherence Assessment—Patient

I have been able to do the following (as instructed by my therapist):

	Not at all	A little	Quite a bit	Mostly	Always	Does not apply
1. Do my exercises						
2. Change my activity						
3. Use my splints or aids						
4. Put full effort into my therapy						
5. Complete my therapy at home						

Fig. 105.2 Adherence assessment.

this to your family when you get home" or "Can you tell that back to me, so I will know if I missed anything?"

The author and her trainee (Folarin Babatunde) have developed an approach to adherence called SIMPLIFY. The elements integrate the principles and evidence in the literature into key themes (see Critical Points Box), which summarize many of the concepts discussed in this chapter. A nonexhaustive list of strategies is in the Critical Points Box. Overall, this chapter emphasizes that adherence assessment and management must be fully integrated into the therapy assessment, treatment, and evaluation plan.

REFERENCES

1. World Health Organization. *Adherence to Long-term Therapies: Evidence for Action.* 2003:211. Available from: http://www.who.int/chp/knowledge/publications/adherence_full_report.pdf.
2. Education U, Position S. *UNESCO Education Sector Position Paper: Plurality of Literacy and its Implications for Policies and Prorgrammes [Internet].* Paris; 2004. Available from http://unesdoc.unesco.org/images/0013/001362/136246e.pdf.
3. U.S. Department of Health and Human Services. *National Action Plan to Improve Health Literacy*; 2010. Washington, DC.
4. Whitehead M. The concept of physical literacy. *Phys Lit Throughout Lifecourse.* 2010:10–20.
5. Mowbray CT, Holter MC, Teague GB, Bybee D. Fidelity criteria : development , measurement , and validation. *Am J Educ.* 2003;24:315–340.
6. Elwyn G, Laitner S, Coulter A, Walker E, Watson P, Thomson R. *Implementing Shared Decision Making in the NHS. BMJ [Internet].* BMJ Publishing Group Ltd; 2010:341. Available from: http://www.bmj.com/content/341/bmj.c5146.
7. National Institute for Health and Care Excellence. *Shared Decision Making [Internet].* 2018. Available from: https://www.nice.org.uk/about/what-we-do/our-programmes/nice-guidance/nice-guidelines/shared-decision-making.
8. Stewart M, Brown J, Weston WW, McWhinney IR, McWilliam CL, Freeman TR. *Patient-centered Medicine: Transforming the Clinical Method.* 2nd ed. Radcliffe Medical Publishing; 2003.
9. Alison K, Amy M, Katherine B, Kathryn Z. What are the core elements of patient-centred care? A narrative review and synthesis of the literature from health policy, medicine and nursing. [Internet]. *J Adv Nurs.* Wiley/Blackwell (10.1111); 2012;69:4–15. Available from: https://doi.org/10.1111/j.1365-2648.2012.06064.x.
9a. Sackett DL. Evidence-based medicine. *Semin Perinatol.* 1997;21:3–5.
10. Dawes M, Summerskill W, Glasziou P, Cartabellotta A, Martin J, Hopayian K, et al. Sicily statement on evidence-based practice. *BMC Med Educ.* 2005;5:1–7.
11. Légaré F, Ratté S, Gravel K, Graham ID. Barriers and facilitators to implementing shared decision-making in clinical practice: update of a systematic review of health professionals' perceptions. *Patient Educ Couns.* 2008;73:526–535.
12. Joosten EAG, DeFuentes-Merillas L, De Weert GH, Sensky T, Van Der Staak CPF, De Jong CAJ. Systematic review of the effects of shared decision-making on patient satisfaction, treatment adherence and health status. *Psychother Psychosom.* 2008;77:219–226.
13. Joseph-Williams N, Elwyn G, Edwards A. Knowledge is not power for patients: a systematic review and thematic synthesis of patient-reported barriers and facilitators to shared decision making. *Patient Educ Couns Elsevier Ireland Ltd*; 2014;94:291–309.
14. Aubree Shay L, Lafata JE. Where is the evidence? A systematic review of shared decision making and patient outcomes. *Med Decis Mak.* 2015;35:114–131.
15. Babatunde F, MacDermid J, Macintyre N. Characteristics of therapeutic alliance in musculoskeletal physiotherapy and occupational therapy practice: a scoping review of the literature. [Internet]. *BMC Health Serv Res.* 2017;17:375. Available from: http://bmchealthservres.biomedcentral.com/articles/10.1186/s12913-017-2311-3.
16. Marilyn C. *Therapeutic Relationships.* 2006;19:33–56.
17. Constand MK, MacDermid JC, Law M, Dal Bello-Haas V. Patient-centered care and distal radius fracture outcomes: a prospective cohort study analysis. [Internet]. Elsevier Ltd *J Hand Ther.* 2014. [cited 2016 Jul 4];27:177–183; quiz 184. Available from: http://www.ncbi.nlm.nih.gov/pubmed/24874854.
18. Aronson JK. Compliance, concordance, adherence. *Br J Clin Pharmacol.* 2007;63:383–384.

19. Stewart M. Towards a global definition of patient centred care. The patient should be the judge of patient centred care. *Br Med J.* 2001;322:444–445.

20. Hall AM, Ferreira PH, Maher CG, Latimer J, Ferreira ML. The influence of the therapist-patient relationship on treatment outcome in physical rehabilitation: a systematic review. *J Am Phys Ther Assoc.* 2010;90:1099–1110.

21. Dewan N, MacDermid JC, MacIntyre NJ, Grewal R. Therapist's practice patterns for subsequent fall/osteoporotic fracture prevention for patients with a distal radius fracture. *J Hand Ther.* 2018.

22. O'Brien L. The evidence on ways to improve patient's adherence in hand therapy. *J Hand Ther Hanley Belfus.* 2012;25:247–250.

23. Essery R, Geraghty AWA, Kirby S, Yardley L. Predictors of adherence to home-based physical therapies: a systematic review. *Disabil Rehabil.* 2017:519–534.

24. Burgess E, Hassmén P, Pumpa KL. Determinants of adherence to lifestyle intervention in adults with obesity: a systematic review. *Clin Obes.* 2017;7:123–135.

25. O'Brien L. Adherence to therapeutic splint wear in adults with acute upper limb injuries: a systematic review. *Hand Ther.* 2010;15:3–12.

26. MacDermid JC, Valdes K, Szekeres M, Naughton N, Algar L. The assessment of psychological factors on upper extremity disability: a scoping review. *J Hand Ther.* 2017.

27. Mehta S, MacDermid J, Tremblay M, Mehta SMJTM. The implications of chronic pain models for rehabilitation of distal radius fracture. *Hand Ther.* 2011;16:2–11.

28. Dewan N, MacDermid JC, Packham T. Role of a self-efficacy-based model of intervention: the LEARN approach in rehabilitation of distal radius fracture. *Crit Rev Phys Rehabil Med.* 2013;25:241–259.

29. Lakke SE, Soer R, Krijnen WP, Schans CP van der, Reneman MF, Geertzen JHB. Influence of physical therapists' kinesiophobic beliefs on lifting capacity in healthy adults. *Phys Ther.* 2015;95. 1224–1223.

30. Babatunde FO, MacDermid JC, MacIntyre N. A therapist-focused knowledge translation intervention for improving patient adherence in musculoskeletal physiotherapy practice. [Internet] *Arch Physiother.* 2017;7:1. Available from: http://archivesphysiotherapy.biomedcentral.com/articles/10.1186/s40945-016-0029-x.

31. Macdermid JC, Walton DM, Miller J, ICON. What is the experience of receiving health care for neck pain? [Internet] *Open Orthop J.* 2013 [cited 2016 Jul 4];7:428–339. Available from: http://www.ncbi.nlm.nih.gov/pubmed/24155803.

32. Borkhoff CM, Hawker GA, Kreder HJ, Glazier RH, Mahomed NN, Wright JG. Patients' gender affected physicians' clinical decisions when presented with standardized patients but not for matching paper patients. *J Clin Epidemiol.* 2009;62:527–541.

33. Frost R, Levati S, McClurg D, Brady M, Williams B. What adherence measures should be used in trials of home-based rehabilitation interventions? A systematic review of the validity, reliability, and acceptability of measures. [Internet]. Elsevier Inc *Arch Phys Med Rehabil.* 2017;98:1241–1256. e45 Available from: https://doi.org/10.1016/j.apmr.2016.08.482.

34. Sieverink F, Kelders SM, Gemert-Pijnen V. Clarifying the concept of adherence to ehealth technology: systematic review on when usage becomes adherence. *J Med Internet Res.* 2017;19.

35. Kolt GS, Brewer BW, Pizzari T, Schoo AMM, Garrett N. The sport injury rehabilitation adherence scale: a reliable scale for use in clinical physiotherapy. *Physiotherapy*; 2007.

36. McLean SM, Burton M, Bradley L, Littlewood C. Interventions for enhancing adherence with physiotherapy: a systematic review. *Man Ther.* 2010:514–521.

106

Client-Centered, Bio-occupational Framework for Orthotic Intervention

Pat McKee, Annette Marie Rivard

OUTLINE

CRITICAL POINTS

- The Client-Centered, Bio-occupational Framework for Orthotic Intervention guides therapists to address the (1) biological and (2) occupational (functional) goals of the client.
- Goals are achieved by providing an optimally usable, well-engineered orthosis through a holistic, client-centered, professional practice process that considers personal attributes and unique environmental contexts.

- Usability is enhanced by optimizing comfort, appearance, and convenience and using a less-is-more approach.
- Monitoring, modifying, and evaluating outcomes are essential processes for ensuring orthotic usability while potentially providing evidence of orthotic efficacy and the continuous improvement of practice guidelines.
- The ultimate goal of orthotic intervention is to enable participation in occupations that are important and meaningful to the person.

INTRODUCTION TO THE FRAMEWORK

We contend that the application of our Client-Centered Bio-occupational Framework for Orthotic Intervention achieves optimal benefit for hand therapy clients. This framework guides the therapist to address the (1) biological and (2) occupational (functional) needs of the client by providing an optimally usable, well-engineered orthosis through a holistic, client-centered, professional practice process that considers persons' unique social and physical environmental contexts. The ultimate goal is to enable participation in activities that are important and meaningful to the person.[1,2]

Orthotic intervention, as it is commonly described in hand therapy literature (including most chapters in this book), tends to be predominated by discussions of orthoses being used, largely in the acute stages of treatment, to address biological (anatomical and physiological) disorders of the upper extremity. With the publication of the revised International Classification of Functioning, Disability and Health (ICF) published by the World Health Organization (WHO) and the move to a more social model of rehabilitation, hand therapists are increasing their focus on enabling activity and participation from a more holistic (occupational) perspective and thus supporting the importance of orthoses in nonacute stages of rehabilitation.[3,4] The ICF defines function as the outcome of a complex and dynamic interaction between the components (1) *body structures and functions* (e.g., joints, muscles, nerves, range of motion [ROM], strength), (2) *activities* (tasks or actions performed by an individual, e.g., grasping, holding), (3) *participation* (involvement in life situations, e.g., self-care, meal preparation, child care, work tasks, playing a sport), (4) *environmental factors* (physical, social, and attitudinal), and (5) *personal factors* (age, coping style, social background).[4-7]

Although the ICF is useful for guiding therapeutic approaches, it does not explicitly consider the concepts of persons' values, what is meaningful to them, and the social roles that affect their participation in occupations important to them.[8] We assert that these concepts are essential to the orthotic intervention process to ensure usability of the orthosis (which we discuss later) and optimal outcomes from the intervention.

An occupation-based approach to hand therapy considers and addresses all components of the ICF and promotes the use of occupation as a framework within which biomechanical approaches should be applied.[4] It ensures careful consideration of the person and her or his occupational roles, needs, and goals.

The Client-Centered Bio-occupational Framework for Orthotic Intervention goes beyond addressing biological needs, promoting a holistic view that considers the complete client picture. What does the individual want and need to do in the short and long terms? What orthotic interventions are required to optimally continue, or return, to play, recreation, work, school, one's household, or daily living activities?

The appropriateness of the Client-Centered Bio-occupational Framework for Orthotic Intervention is supported by the US Medicare Part B directive, which states that "OTs and PTs must include information on personal factors, the living environment, activities, and roles of patients in the formulation of the treatment plan" and that "demonstrated improvement in functional outcomes is mandated to receive reimbursement."[3] We will illustrate this framework with client stories. The word "story" or narrative rather than "case" is a deliberate attempt to acknowledge the individual with a life full of personal meaning. *Narrative-based medicine*, a coin termed by Greenhalgh[8a] in 1999, balances the science of evidence-based medicine with the art of clinical proficiency and judgment. Because hand injury cannot be separated from the personal experiences that give the problem its meaning, narratives or stories help therapists to consider how the hand condition impacts the lives of our clients. Details emerge through clients' stories that open new avenues for problem solving, leading to more effective hand therapy assessment and interventions. Individual stories are compelling and memorable and have much to teach us. Cooper[9] found that clients' adherence to hand therapy guidelines was greater when they are encouraged to tell their stories.

The Client-Centered, Bio-occupational Framework for Orthotic Intervention presented here outlines six principles that are explicitly aimed at orthotic intervention that enables current or future activity and participation while minimizing biological harm. We assert that orthotic intervention must be individualized and client-centered, with consideration of the individual's unique biological and occupational goals, personal attributes, and environmental contexts. The client stories throughout this chapter illustrate how the interaction and communication between the therapist and client influences the outcome as much as the actual orthotic device does. One intervention protocol does not fit all. The best outcomes occur when orthotic interventions are creatively designed with client input and holistic consideration of the individual's unique circumstances.

SHELLEY'S STORY

This story, beginning in 2001 and continuing until the time of this writing, is adapted from McKee and Rivard[2] (2011) and discusses a client who experienced a closed head injury causing hemiplegia. The bio-occupational orthotic intervention goals were to control wrist spasticity and enable participation in paracycling.

In 2001, Shelley, a physical therapist who ironically worked in hand therapy, was injured in a mountain biking accident at 32 years of age. Despite wearing a helmet, she sustained a severe head injury and was in a coma for 6 weeks. After several months in an acute-care hospital and then a rehabilitation facility, she was discharged home with mild cognitive impairment, spastic right-sided hemiplegia, and dysarthria. Although her cognition and speech steadily improved over the years, the spastic hemiplegia did not.

Shelley returned to cycling within 1 year of her accident, using a modified recumbent tricycle. All the power for cycling came from her unaffected lower extremity. She wore an ankle–foot orthosis made by an orthotist and had many assistive devices to enable her to live independently (Fig. 106.1A). She also used a hiking stick to help her walk.

Seven years after the injury, Shelley decided to have injections of botulinum toxin to suppress the spasticity in her right upper and lower extremities. This caused her right hand to become flaccid and unable to grip the handlebar. She expected that she would need to wait about 3 months for the effects of the botulinum toxin to wear off. However, the provision of a prefabricated Benik Grip Assist Glove[10] enabled Shelley to fasten her hand to the tricycle handlebar. She was able to apply the grip assist independently but with some difficulty and was delighted that she could immediately resume cycling. However, in warm weather, the black neoprene glove was uncomfortably warm to wear, causing her hand to sweat and subsequently slide off the handlebar, which was unsafe.

A new, custom-made grip assist was created that better suited Shelley's individual context and needs (Fig. 106.1B and C). Four new features addressed the problems of excessive warmth and hand sliding and facilitated donning: (1) $\frac{1}{16}$-in, 1.6-mm-thick neoprene (compared with Benik's $\frac{1}{4}$-in, 6.4-mm thickness); (2) beige rather than black color; (3) hook-and-loop attachment to the handlebar; and (4) easier-to-manage strapping. Shelley was able to continue her healthy, active lifestyle; fulfill her passion to cycle; and return to using a convenient and pleasurable form of transportation.

In 2008, Shelley set a goal to compete in the Paralympic cycling events in London in 2012 and acquired a custom-made three-wheeled racer to begin training. However, she found that her hyperextending right thumb interphalangeal (IP) joint was catching on the zipper of her pants or her leg when she was riding, causing pain and preventing her from exerting full effort (Fig. 106.2A). The thumb problem also made it difficult to securely grip the handlebar of her tricycle. She first tried a prefabricated Oval-8 orthosis and then a custom-made sterling silver figure-8 "ring" orthosis, individualized to reduce pressure over the dorsum of her thumb proximal phalanx (Fig. 106.2B and C). She preferred the aesthetics of the latter but made use of both.

After an adverse reaction, injections of botulinum toxin were discontinued, causing the flexor spasticity to return. Shelley's cycling coach wanted her spastic, flexed wrist (Fig. 106.3A) to be positioned in the same degree of extension as her unaffected wrist to improve upper arm comfort, body alignment, and leg thrust.

Shelley and her coach brought her racing tricycle into the hand therapy clinic to see the issue in context and to ensure that the orthosis fit both her limb and the tricycle when she was riding. Various circumferential prefabricated wrist orthoses were tried, but none could control her wrist position because of the strong flexor spasticity. The goal was met with a custom thermoplastic orthosis, molded from a rigid-when-cold $\frac{1}{8}$-in (3.2-mm) -thick thermoplastic (Fig. 106.3B and C) designed in collaboration with Shelley and her coach. The final contours were achieved while Shelley's hand was positioned on the handle grip of the tricycle. In addition, the orthosis was spot heated to contour to the shape of her muscles as they contracted while she rode her tricycle. Shelley could independently apply the orthosis, and the dorsal-based design allowed her to lever her flexed wrist into extension (Fig. 106.4 and Video 106.1). The orthosis had a long forearm trough—longer than the typical $\frac{2}{3}$ length proximal to the wrist—to ensure adequate control of the spastic wrist muscles to correct the flexed wrist posture.

For the first time since her injury, Shelley was able to use her affected arm to help steer, which meant that she did not need to rely on her left hand to both steer and brake at the same time. A concurrent benefit was improved body alignment, which eliminated pain and improved the affected lower extremity thrust. She began to ride faster, which improved her Paralympic hopes (Fig. 106.5). Shelley personalized her orthosis with Canadian flags on the straps. Listen to Shelley explain how much the wrist orthosis has favorably affected her cycling ability (Video 106.2).

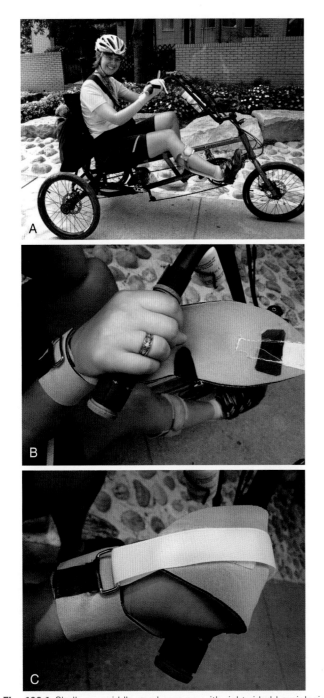

Fig. 106.1 Shelley, a middle-aged woman with right-sided hemiplegia from a traumatic head injury. **A,** Riding her recumbent tricycle while wearing the custom-made grip assist made from 1/16-in (1.6-mm) thick neoprene with hook-and-loop fasteners and an ankle–foot orthosis **B,** Dorsal view of neoprene grip assist before fastening the panel that goes over the fingers. **C,** Dorsal view of neoprene grip assist after fastening the finger panel, holding the hand onto the handlebar. (© P. McKee. All rights reserved.)

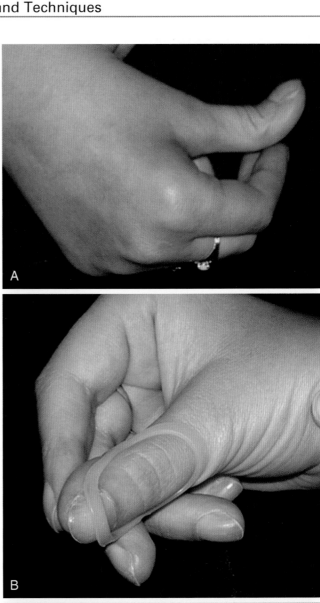

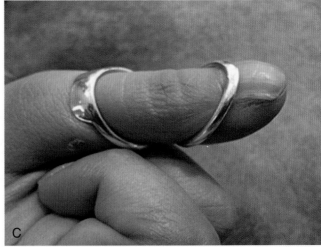

Fig. 106.2 Shelley's right thumb and orthotic intervention. **A,** Hyperextending thumb interphalangeal (IP) joint. **B,** Thumb IP hyperextension corrected with an Oval-8 orthosis from 3-Point Products, Inc. (Annapolis, MD). **C,** Thumb IP hyperextension corrected with a silver ring style orthosis. Note the expanded surface area over the proximal phalanx to reduce pressure. (© P. McKee. All rights reserved.)

In her own words: "The brace that I wear on my wrist allows me to steer with my right hand so I am a two-handed person on the trike. It's really nice because other people [who are hemiplegic] have their hand strapped up inside their cycling shirts, so then they have only one hand to use on the trike. But I have two hands on the trike and that makes me

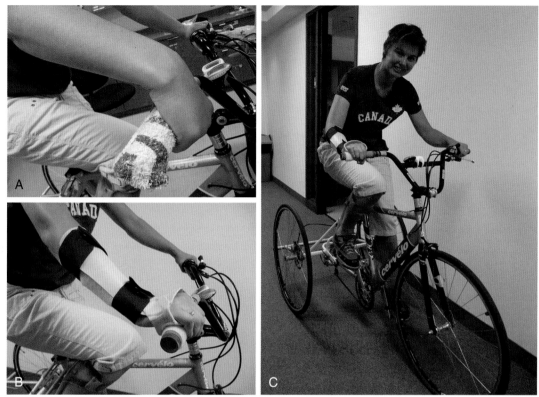

Fig. 106.3 Shelley's right wrist and orthotic intervention. **A,** Flexed wrist position caused by spasticity. **B** and **C,** Wrist position corrected with a dorsal forearm-based wrist orthosis. (© P. McKee. All rights reserved.)

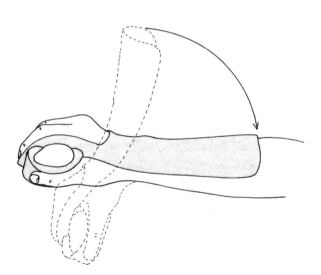

Fig. 106.4 Using a dorsal forearm–based wrist-hand orthosis to lever the wrist into extension. (From McKee P, Morgan L. *Orthotics in Rehabilitation: Splinting the Hand and Body.* Philadelphia: FA Davis; 1998:14. © Pat McKee; used with permission.)

feel safer and stabilizes me on the handles. The grace of riding is made better by the brace."

Shelley's words draw attention to the fact that the only time that she can use both upper extremities is when she is on her trike, using her wrist orthosis. After many months of use, Shelley's dorsal-based wrist orthosis began to crack from exposure to ultraviolet light and required frequent repairs. When Shelley qualified to compete in

the 2012 Paralympics in London, her hand therapist advised her to get a new, more durable, wrist orthosis (of high-temperature thermoplastic) from an orthotist, made to ensure that it would not fail in competition. When presented with this request, the orthotist announced that he could not take a cast of Shelley's arm while it was properly positioned while gripping the handlebar. He overcame the obstacle by casting Shelley's therapist-made wrist orthosis to create the required positive mold on which to form the high-temperature wrist orthosis.

Shelley triumphantly competed in the 2012 Paralympics wearing her new wrist orthosis and was the fastest woman in her class (Video 106.3). Since 2012, Shelley has gone on to compete in numerous international events, getting faster and winning medals, most notably a silver medal at the 2015 Parapan Am Games and a bronze medal at the 2016 Rio Paralympics. She usually wears her therapist-made wrist orthosis during training and her orthotist-made orthosis during competitions.

Shelley's story illustrates the application of the Client-Centered Bio-occupational Framework for Orthotic Intervention. As we discuss the principles of the framework, we will exemplify them using this story and others. Shelley's wrist orthosis addressed her biological needs (post–head injury spasticity) by controlling the post–head injury spasticity to better position her wrist, thereby addressing her occupational needs—to optimally ride her adapted tricycle to be a competitive paracyclist. To ensure optimal usability, the orthotic design needed to be easy to apply and remove. The orthosis was designed and fabricated meeting professional practice responsibilities of client education, monitoring, and modifying.

WHAT IS AN ORTHOSIS?

An orthosis (splint) is a prefabricated or custom-made device applied to biological structures to optimize *body function and structures* to

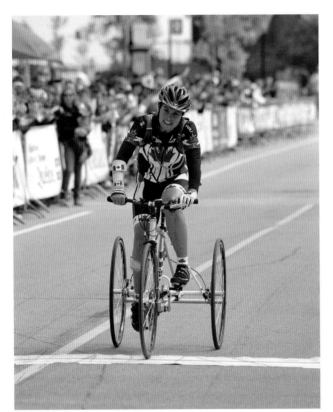

ultimately promote current or future *activities and participation* in roles important to the individual.[1] As previously discussed, "body functions and structures" and "activities and participation" are key concepts influencing health, as described in the ICF published by the WHO.[5]

An orthosis is a type of wearable health device (WHD).[11] Other such WHDs, which many readers can personally relate to, include eyeglasses and hearing aids. Users of these devices seek to have their biological needs (impaired vision or hearing) addressed in a manner that enhances participation in daily activities, with optimal usability and appearance and aesthetics. For example, some individuals select eyeglasses that are rimless and thus minimally obvious; others choose designer frames that make a noticeable statement about their style. Users of hearing aids generally choose devices that are minimally visible. If we keep these considerations in mind, we can perhaps better address the orthotic needs of our clients and enhance adherence to their orthotic regimen.[11]

Orthoses are most commonly made from low-temperature thermoplastics, as was Shelley's dorsal forearm–based wrist orthosis. However, recent years have seen an increasing use of neoprene and other soft materials to create more usable and wearable devices, again seen in Shelley's story and as discussed in Chapter 110). Custom-made orthoses include those made from sterling silver, such as Shelley's silver ring thumb orthosis, which are popular with clients who prefer the aesthetics of a device that looks like jewelry. There is also an increasing array of prefabricated orthoses available, such as Shelley's plastic Oval-8 orthosis and the Benik Grip Assist. Today, therapists and their clients have a large range of orthotic options. Also, as we read in Shelley's story, at times it might be more appropriate for an orthotist to make the orthosis.

Orthotic intervention (splinting), an integral part of hand rehabilitation for several decades, is the process of client evaluation,

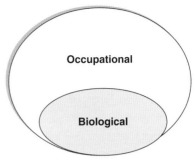

establishment of objectives, and provision of an orthosis to ultimately enhance participation in life occupations.[1]

USING A BIO-OCCUPATIONAL LENS

We use the analogy of eyeglasses to describe a bio-occupational lens, which is essential to the Bio-occupational Framework. Those who wear bifocal eyeglasses that provide both distance and close-up visual assistance should readily grasp this concept.

According to Robinson and coworkers,[12] "Hand therapy merges occupational therapy and physiotherapy approaches to treatment" and as such "should recognize the benefits of … prescriptive exercise programs and physical agents modalities … as well as occupation as a therapeutic mechanism" (p. 294). They refer to this as a duality of focus that embraces "an occupational perspective on health and incorporates interventions that are grounded in the key principles of the profession" while addressing the body structures and functions approach that hand therapy demands. Similarly, Fisher proposed that therapists consider practice along a continuum that at one extreme focuses mechanistically and at the other focuses on authentic, client-chosen occupations in a naturalistic context.[12a,13] Gillen and Gruber[13] assert that "occupation-focused thinking on the part of the practitioner remains possible, even in very medically oriented services," as in hand therapy (p. 41).

With respect to our analogous bifocal, bio-occupational lens (Fig. 106.6), the close-up "reading" part of the lens focuses on the individual's biological needs, generally described in terms of a diagnosis such as fracture, nerve injury, arthritis, spasticity, and so on. The distance part of the lens focuses on the individual's occupational needs and unique circumstances. It is a holistic view that considers the complete client picture—what this individual wants and needs to do in the short and long terms, addressing barriers to optimally continue, or return to, work, school, household, or daily living activities.

As with eyeglasses, in which the lenses are mounted in a frame, we propose that the bio-occupational lens is framed by professional practice responsibilities—one of the principles. in our framework.

PRINCIPLES OF THE FRAMEWORK

This Framework has six key principles, which will be discussed in the following order:
1. Ensure client-centeredness.
2. Identify and address biological goals and minimize biological harm.
3. Identify and address occupational goals.
4. Optimize usability.

5. Apply sound design and fabrication guidelines.
6. Meet professional practice responsibilities.

Principle 1. Ensure Client-Centeredness

Client-centeredness "embraces a philosophy of respect for, and partnership with people receiving services."[14] As illustrated in Shelley's story, client-centeredness was essential to the positive outcomes in all aspects of orthotic intervention.

When we describe our intervention as *assessing for a splint* or *splinting a patient or client*, then the provision of an orthosis becomes the focus, and the process can be very technical, without sufficient consideration of client-specific context and circumstances. Concerns for biological structures may dominate the process, and important occupational goals can be overlooked. In addition, this language suggests, a paternalistic approach in which we are doing something to the client and in which his or her knowledge and expertise may not be fully respected nor solicited.[12]

In contrast, we propose that optimal benefit from orthotic intervention is achieved through our Client-Centered Bio-occupational Framework for Orthotic Intervention that explicitly addresses both the client's biological needs and occupational goals with consideration of his or her unique circumstances. The framework involves (1) identifying and addressing the biological factors that underlie the occupational barriers to optimal participation and (2) designing orthoses using a client-centered approach, which often requires creativity. This requires holistic consideration of the client, including his or her physical, cognitive and affective attributes, occupational goals, and environmental contexts.[6,14,15] The Client-Centered Bio-occupational Framework for Orthotic Intervention ensures that the central therapeutic aim of orthotic intervention remains that of enabling current or future occupational performance, rather than simply "providing a splint."

A client-centered approach challenges us to modify our language and terminology, as discussed earlier, and advocates for the careful selection of assessment tools and outcome measures.[6] Routine use of function-based, client-centered assessments promotes optimal collaboration with the client and a focus on occupational rather than biological outcomes. Examples include the Canadian Occupational Performance Measure (COPM)[6,12,15] and the Patient-Rated Wrist and Hand Evaluation.[4] These measures have the added benefit of providing evidence of orthotic efficacy. When results are shared with clients, recovery becomes more relevant and discernible by the client.[14]

In a client-centered orthotic intervention process, both the therapist and the client make important contributions. The therapist contributes knowledge of pathology, tissue healing, biomechanical and orthotic principles, and characteristics of various materials, as well as technical fabrication skills. With encouragement from the therapist, the client contributes personal information about her or his situation and how it affects occupational performance. This process seeks to identify and address the client's unique occupational and biological concerns and develop an orthotic intervention plan in which options are offered and appropriate outcome measures are used.

Our client Peggy expressed the following sentiments, "I'm grateful to my therapist for listening to what I needed and adapting the orthosis to meet my needs. It's important to individualize the approach for each person and not to assume that everyone is the same."[16]

Consider Psychosocial Factors

Fess[17] eloquently articulates the importance of psychosocial considerations: "Injured extremities are attached to an individual being, each with his/her own set of physical and emotional parameters.

Psychological factors including, but not limited to, peer pressure, secondary gain, dysfunctional family life, pending legal action, or substance abuse may negatively influence splint compliance. Identifying and adapting to the client's emotional issues may be more challenging that dealing with the physical injury."

Wilton and Dival[18] emphasize the importance of considering factors unique to the client, including his or her attitudes, lifestyle, and living and working environment, to avoid failure of even the "the very best splint." Psychosocial factors pertaining to orthotic usability are unique to each individual and vary with different cultural groups.

Psychosocial adjustment to using an orthosis is unique to each individual and varies in different cultural groups. For example, individuals with long-term, progressive conditions may become accustomed to ongoing medical intervention and thus accept an orthosis more readily than those confronted with sudden trauma. Alternatively, individuals who require long-term intervention may develop "gadget intolerance" and resist additional devices.

The reaction of family, friends, peers, and strangers to the orthosis may also affect psychosocial adjustment to the orthosis. Sometimes clients are too self-conscious or embarrassed to wear an orthosis in the presence of others. At other times, family members or friends are uncomfortable when accompanying the person who is wearing a visible orthosis in public.

ORTHOTIC PEARL: HOW TO BE CLIENT-CENTERED

- Use a holistic approach considering the whole client picture, addressing (1) personal factors (physical attributes, age, cognition, affect, psychosocial factors, and, when appropriate, spiritual beliefs), (2) unique context (environment, culture), and (3) occupational goals.
- Recognize that the client has expert knowledge of his or her own situation and its effect on his or her occupations.
- Individualize the intervention.
- Use functional outcome measures.
- Offer options when appropriate.
- Facilitate psychosocial acceptance.

JIM'S STORY

This story, adapted from McKee and coworkers[19] (2012), discusses a client with psoriatic arthritis. The bio-occupational orthotic goals were to reduce pain, correct contractures, and restabilize joints to enhance participation in daily and work activities.

Jim was first seen at age 52 years, 18 months after the onset of psoriatic arthritis. He presented with joint malalignment and pain (5.5 of 10), which restricted participation in simple daily activities such as holding a toothbrush and turning doorknobs and taps. Ulnar subluxation (drift) of the long, ring and small finger metacarpophalangeal (MCP) joints was apparent, along with swelling of thumb carpometacarpal (CMC) and finger MCP joints. A 25-degree limitation in MCP extension, observed when Jim attempted to place his hand flat on the table, was attributed to intrinsic tightness (Fig. 106.7A). Biological goals were to support inflamed joints, relieve pain, correct contractures, and restabilize joints by promoting tissue elongation and resorption. Occupational goals were to enable participation in self-care and work activities.

He was fitted with a custom-made finger–MCP and thumb–CMC stabilizing orthosis. Individual finger supports applied a gentle radial-ward force to correct the ulnar drift (Figs. 106.7B and 106.8). The

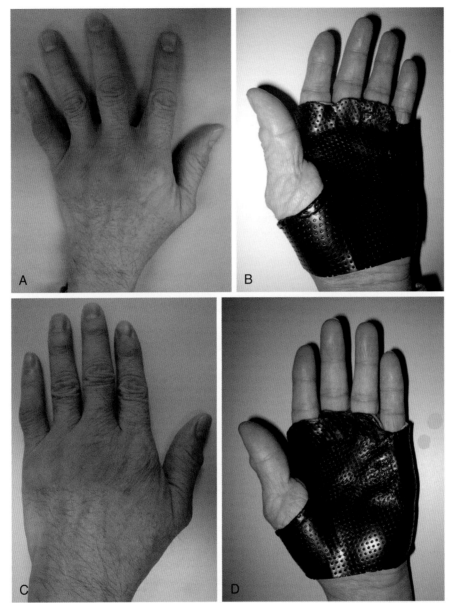

Fig. 106.7 Jim, a 52-year-old man with psoriatic arthritis. **A,** Left dominant hand at the outset of orthotic intervention showing marked ulnar drift of long, ring and small finger metacarpophalangeal (MCP) joints and mild MCP flexion contracture. **B,** Custom-made finger–MCP and thumb–carpometacarpal stabilizing serial-static orthosis molded from 1/16-in (1/6-mm) -thick thermoplastic. Individual finger supports provide a gentle radial-ward force to correct ulnar drift. **C,** After 10 days of day and night orthotic use showing decreased MCP ulnar drift and flexion contracture. **D,** Orthosis after remolding to position finger MCPs in an increased radial direction. (© P. McKee. All rights reserved.)

MCP joints were positioned in 30 degrees of flexion to provide volar support and facilitate active stretch of the lumbricals and interossei without interfering with functional hand use. He wore it day and night, removing it several times daily for intrinsic muscle stretching and ROM exercises.

At his 10-day follow up, Jim's joint pain was less, and ulnar drift severity had diminished by 10 degrees in the ring finger. The MCP flexion contracture had reduced from 25 to 0 degrees, and he was able to place his hand flat on the table (Fig. 106.7C). His serial static orthosis was remolded, repositioning the finger MCP joints in an increased radial direction (Fig. 106.7D). He continued with his original wearing regimen for 6 months and then decided to wear the orthosis at night only.

Approximately 14 months after his first orthotic fitting, Jim returned for a new custom-molded orthosis that provided increased correction of the ulnar drift. At 27 months, he was still using the hand orthosis at night. He reported decreased pain (1.5 of 10), which only occurred after stressful hand activities. At that visit, the orthosis was remolded to provide further correction of the ulnar drift. He could now do many activities that were previously very painful and difficult.

Two and a half years after his first orthotic fitting, Jim reported: "I am amazed how the orthosis has helped my hand by stopping the progression of the ulnar drift and gradually achieving correction. It seems to work like the braces that I wore to straighten my teeth when I was younger. I continue to wear the hand orthosis at night, like the

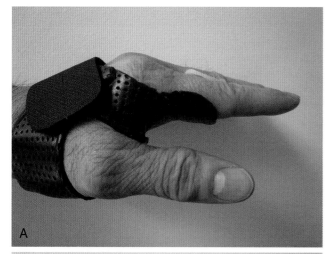

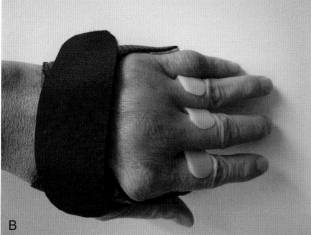

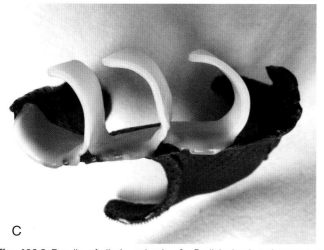

Fig. 106.8 Details of Jim's orthosis. **A,** Radial viewing demonstrating about 30 degrees of metacarpophalangeal flexion, providing volar support while facilitating active stretch of lumbricals and interossei. **B,** Dorsal view showing finger supports. **C,** Finger supports individually bonded to the base to provide corrective radial force to each finger. (© P. McKee. All rights reserved.)

orthodontic retainer I wore on my teeth at night, to hold the corrected position of the fingers."

In the 8 years since the first orthotic fitting, Jim returned periodically to the hand therapy clinic for replacement of his orthosis

after the thermoplastic cracked. At the last visit, Jim was wearing his orthosis occasionally at night. He proudly reported that since retiring, he had the time and sufficient joint stability and hand strength to undertake projects such as building a fence, shed and deck, as well as gardening and landscaping. Upon reflection, Jim stated "without the orthosis I don't know that I would be able to do the things I want to do. It gave me a second chance to participate in important, enjoyable activities that I thought would never again be possible."

The biological goals of Jim's serial static finger MCP joint stabilizing orthosis were to relieve pain, arrest progression of the ulnar drift, and if possible correct ulnar and flexion contractures and achieve joint stabilization. This was achieved by applying a low tensile force to promote elongation of contracted tissues on the ulnar side of the finger MCP joints while creating slack in the lax tissues on the radial side to promote resorption. The latter was important to restore joint stability. In addition, active intrinsic muscle stretching that was facilitated by orthotic positioning of the MCP joints reduced intrinsic muscle tightness, thus reducing the MCP joint flexion contractures. Prolonged stress on the cartilage was avoided by frequent removal of the orthosis for ROM and intrinsic muscle strengthening exercises.

The Client-Centered Bio-occupational Framework for Orthotic Intervention guided the collaborative orthotic process, ensuring that Jim's orthosis met both his biological needs (pain relief, joint stabilization, and preservation) and occupational needs (ability to continue to work and return to leisure activities).

Principle 2. Identify and Address Biological Goals and Minimize Biological Harm
Biological Goals
By using the Client-Centered Bio-occupational Framework for Orthotic Intervention, the hand therapist can influence how current and potential biological factors can affect activity and participation.

These factors relate to the ICF's body structure and function.[5] Biological goals address restoration or maintenance of optimal health, integrity, stability, mobility, and function of neuromusculoskeletal tissues (Table 106.1). In Shelley's story, biological and physical issues were numerous and included hand flaccidity, hyperextending thumb IP joint, and inability to maintain wrist extension while bike riding, which in turn caused neck and upper extremity pain. In Jim' story, the biological goals to improve joint alignment and relieve pain greatly influenced the orthotic intervention.

Acute injuries often require prompt, biologically focused intervention to restore the integrity of the injured tissues. In these time-sensitive circumstances, orthotic intervention is focused on promoting optimal conditions for healing to restore tissue integrity and function and may impose unavoidable, but temporary, occupational hindrance. For example, surgically repaired lacerated finger flexor tendons should be protected with an orthosis designed to restore intact, freely gliding tendons. Thus, for several weeks, the orthotic intervention may impose greater restriction of hand function than the actual injury does. Enabling future occupational performance is the long-term goal.

If soft tissue contracture is the biological problem requiring orthotic intervention, as in Jim's story, it is essential to identify the specific structures responsible for the limited mobility: joint capsule, ligaments, intrinsic muscles, or extrinsic muscles and tendons. After the range-limiting tissues or structures have been identified, the orthosis can then be designed to target corrective forces at the specific tissues or structures. See Chapter 109 for further discussion.

TABLE 106.1 Biological Considerations

Identify and Address Biological Goals	Minimize Biological Harm, Including:
• Promote healing (e.g., burn, skin graft, fracture, injured tendon, ligament, or nerve) • Preserve or restore optimal tissue length and joint flexibility • Compensate for weak or paralyzed muscles • Protect against (re)injury or degeneration • Relieve pain and inflammation • Stabilize joints or tendons • Prevent or correct deformity • Optimize tendon–nerve glide • Optimize lymphatic function • Apply tissue-specific corrective forces	• Pressure points causing injury to skin or compression of nerves • Burns caused by molding overheated thermoplastics to the skin • Failure to protect injured structures during the healing process • Undue stress to tendons or joints, causing inflammation because of poor design, joint positioning, or inappropriate dynamic or static progressive force • Adverse effects of immobilization, including disuse atrophy and contracture • Muscle fatigue • Skin maceration • Adverse skin reactions • Edema • Sleep disturbance

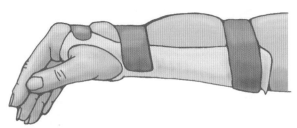

Fig. 106.9 The consequence of strap fixation when the limb has marked edema. The tissue fluid accumulates between the straps. (From McKee P, Morgan L. *Orthotics in Rehabilitation: Splinting the Hand and Body.* Philadelphia: FA Davis; 1998:14. © Pat McKee; used with permission.)

ORTHOTIC PEARL: IDENTIFY AND ADDRESS BIOLOGICAL PRIORITIES

When time-sensitive, acute biological needs are identified, restoration of biological integrity is the focus of orthotic intervention, and current occupational needs may be temporarily compromised to ultimately achieve future occupational performance.

Minimize Biological Harm

The orthotic intervention process should ultimately make some positive contribution to the individual's life. If the orthosis fails to achieve its intended outcome, at the very least, it should minimize biological harm. Avoidable harmful consequences are listed in Table 106.1.

To be specific, biological structures must not be compromised by, among other things, pressure points that result in skin breakdown, diminished circulation, or nerve compression. Vigilance is especially important if sensation is impaired because of conditions such as nerve injury, stroke, or spinal cord injury. Consider the presence of, or potential for, edema, which poses a serious threat to joint mobility and tendon excursion.

Efforts to control edema are a fundamental component of rehabilitation, especially when it involves the hand. Because edema tends to fluctuate, the orthosis should be molded when edema is greatest; an orthosis that is a little too loose (after edema subsides) is preferable to one that is too tight (if edema increases). Using a thinner thermoplastic or one that is more flexible when cool allows easy "cold adjustment" to spread apart the sides of the orthosis to accommodate increased edema or squeeze in the sides of the orthosis to accommodate decreased edema. The therapist can teach these techniques to the client or caregiver. Straps may be unsuitable when edema is severe (Fig. 106.9) and should be replaced with bandage fixation.

To minimize edema while the orthosis is worn, encourage the client to:
• Elevate the limb whenever possible.

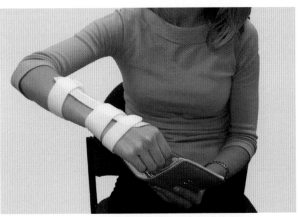

Fig. 106.10 Radial wrist–thumb orthosis prevents wrist flexion; thus, undesirable, compensatory shoulder elevation occurs when attempting to remove a card from a wallet. (© P. McKee. All rights reserved.)

• Move unrestricted joints to actively contract the muscles; this enlists the skeletal muscle pump to assist venous blood return from the limb.

When an orthosis is designed to apply tensile forces to reduce a soft tissue contracture (as in Jim's story), the magnitude of the force should be low and prolonged to stimulate growth and subsequent lengthening of the contracted tissues. If the magnitude of the corrective force is excessive, the resulting trauma will elicit pain and a counterproductive inflammatory response[19] as discussed in Chapter 109.

Although it is important to minimize the potential for secondary pathology as a result of orthotic intervention, in some circumstances, it may be necessary to accept some negative consequences to achieve the desired outcomes. For example, range-restricted orthotic positioning of the wrist and fingers after surgical repair of lacerated finger tendons usually causes some loss of ROM (see Chapters 31 and 33). This is generally viewed as an acceptable consequence, and contractures can be addressed after the tendons are fully healed.

To prevent pressure points, note the location of bony prominences over which the thermoplastic is to be formed. Before the molding process, pad the bony prominences with a thin layer of self-stick padding. After molding, either transfer the padding to the inside of the orthosis or discard it to leave a space between the bony prominence and the thermoplastic. This prevents injury and enhances comfort.

Immobilizing one joint increases stress on adjacent joints, which could become inflamed or subluxed, especially if those joints are arthritic.[20] Examples include the negative effects of wrist immobilization on hand, elbow, and shoulder function.[20] When the wrist is immobilized with an orthosis, the client must use compensatory shoulder elevation (Fig. 106.10), which can lead to proximal muscle fatigue and pain. Therapists

TABLE 106.2 Factors that Enhance Usability

Appearance	Convenience	Comfort	Less-Is-More
• Lack of construction defects (e.g., pen marks, rough edges, and surface impressions) • Lack of soiling of thermoplastic, straps, and stockinette • Appearance that is aesthetically acceptable to client, family, or caregiver • Minimal visibility (if possible)	• Acceptable wearing regimen • Durability of all materials, including straps • Easy to apply and remove • Easy to clean and resistant to soiling • Easy to adjust, if necessary • Easy to understand • No unnecessary restriction of function • When appropriate, provide stability rather than immobilization • Tolerable amount of compensatory motions	• No pressure points • Tolerable amount of compensatory motions • No discomfort from the orthosis • No new discomfort from muscle fatigue • No adverse skin reactions • Acceptable amount of perspiration and warmth • Acceptable weight of orthosis; consider age and strength of the client	Minimal: • Size, weight, and rigidity of the orthosis • Visibility of the orthosis • Amount of skin enclosed • Extent of motion restriction • Thickness (weight) of orthotic materials • Complexity of straps and adjustable components • Care requirements (e.g., easy to clean)

should inquire about concomitant pathology proximal or distal to the wrist before providing an orthosis that limits wrist joint mobility.

ORTHOTIC PEARL: IF POSSIBLE, AVOID WRIST IMMOBILIZATION

Daytime use of an orthosis that restricts wrist mobility promotes compensatory shoulder elevation that can cause harmful muscle pain and fatigue and imposes occupational hindrance. Whenever possible, avoid wrist immobilization, choosing instead a hand-based orthosis.

As eloquently stated by Brand, "by its very presence on the hand, a splint is doing harm, inhibiting free movement and use of the hand. It is justified only if the specific good that it will do compensates for the general harm and restriction."[21]

SAMUEL'S STORY

This story was contributed by Marie Eason Klatt, CHT (personal communication, September 25, 2017).[22]

Five-year-old Samuel was referred to hand therapy because he was having difficulty with daily living and play activities involving fine prehension. Bilaterally, his thumb IP joints were hypermobile, causing extreme IP hyperextension when attempting to pinch and grasp with his thumb (Fig. 106.11A). An assessment revealed that (1) Samuel seemed to have difficulty activating his flexor pollicis longus (FPL) muscles and that (2) because of hypersensitivity, he avoided contacting objects with the volar side of his distal phalanges. He had difficulty managing buttons and zippers, playing electronic games, and holding pencils and crayons. The therapist also observed knee and elbow hypermobility. It was hypothesized that hypersensitivity had developed because of the lack of regular sensory input to the pulp of the distal phalanx and that maladaptive pinch and movement patterns were interfering with the acquisition of fine prehension skills.

To encourage activation of the FPL muscles, Samuel was provided with bilateral custom-molded hand-based thumb IP-stabilizing orthoses, molded from 2.4-mm (³⁄₃₂-in) thick thermoplastic (with 1.6-mm closed-cell foam padding over the dorsum) and a padded strap (Fig. 106.11B). The orthoses prevented IP hyperextension while allowing active IP flexion. He was encouraged to use his thumbs in usual child activities. He was given a home progressive desensitization program using textiles and particles.

After 1 month of wearing the hand-based thumb IP-stabilizing orthoses and doing the desensitization program, the hypersensitivity had resolved, Samuel was able to activate the FPL muscles, and he was using the pulp of his distal phalanx with pinching. He was now independently dressing, and his printing skills had improved.

At the 8-month follow-up visit, the hand-based thumb orthoses were replaced with custom-molded figure-8 thumb IP extension-blocking orthoses to use for fine prehensile activities. The hand-based orthoses were still used during outdoor play and gym classes (Fig. 106.11C).

At 10 months, Samuel's increased hand size allowed the custom-molded figure-8 orthoses to be replaced by prefabricated thumb IP extension-blocking Oval 8 orthoses (Fig. 106.11D), which he wore for all functional activities. The hand-based thumb orthoses were discontinued.

At 14 months, orthotic intervention was discontinued because Samuel demonstrated normal movement patterns and was able to stabilize his thumb IP joints during resisted prehensile tasks (Fig. 106.11E). Pinch strengths were equal bilaterally. Although passive thumb IP joint hypermobility was still present bilaterally, it had ceased to be a functional issue.

Children are often referred to occupational therapy for difficulties with handwriting. Samuel's story illustrates how orthoses that are comfortable and acceptable and that enable activities that the child wants and needs to do enhance the acquisition of fine prehension skills, including handwriting. Samuel learned to activate his FPL tendons, and hypersensitivity subsided. This story demonstrates that early intervention for joint hypermobility in children can mitigate its impact on the development of skills and how orthotic intervention and desensitization can facilitate favorable neuroplasticity.

Principle 3. Identify and Address Occupational Goals

What Is Occupation?

Occupations are "things that people do to occupy life for intended purpose, such as paid work, unpaid work, personal care, care of others, leisure play, recreation, and subsistence."[23]

The stories of Shelley, Jim, and Samuel illustrate how therapists consciously or unconsciously apply the Client-Centered Bio-occupational Framework for Orthotic Intervention to address factors of human structure and function to ultimately help individuals to engage in meaningful and relevant occupations. Jim's orthosis enabled him to continue working and do the leisure activities that gave him personal satisfaction. Samuel's orthoses were essential to his development of hand skills and participation in play activities. Shelley's quote draws attention to the fact that the only time that she can use both upper

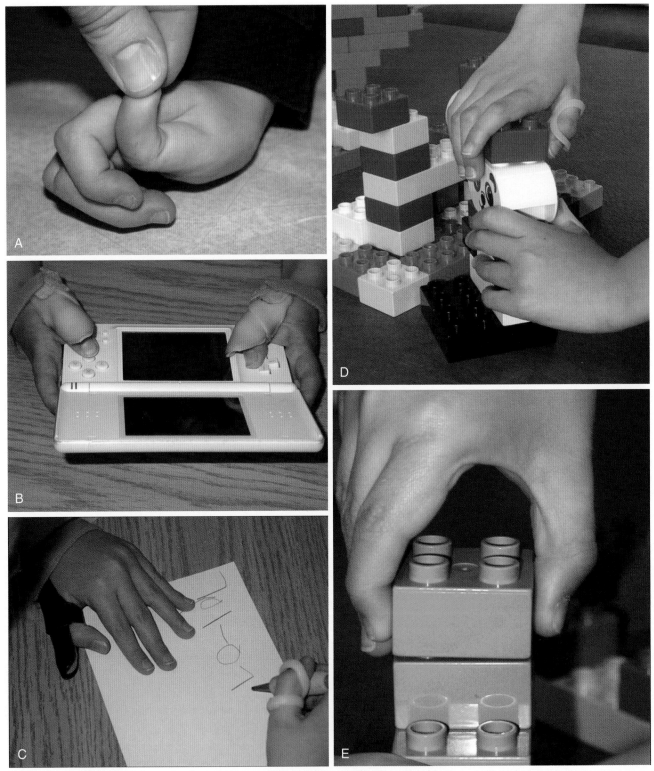

Fig. 106.11 Samuel, a 5-year-old boy with instable thumbs. **A,** Thumb interphalangeal (IP) joint hyperexten-sion instability. **B,** Bilateral hand-based thumb stabilizing orthoses. **C,** Hand-based thumb orthosis on left hand and figure-8 thermoplastic thumb IP-extension blocking orthosis; the latter was introduced at 8 months. **D,** Bilateral Oval-8 orthoses introduced at 10 months. **E,** After 14 months, stable thumbs no longer require orthotic stabilization. (© M. Eason Klatt. All rights reserved.)

extremities is when she is on her trike using her wrist orthosis. Her orthosis helped her to achieve her goal of becoming an internationally successful paracyclist.

As the stories exemplify, an important part of the orthotic interven-tion process is identifying the individual's unique occupational needs in context and then developing a plan in partnership with the client or caregiver. Orthotic intervention should enable the individual to do what he or she wants to, needs to, or is expected to do. The unique occupational demands of musicians which are addressed by creative, individualized orthotic solutions are presented in Chapter 117. To help identify goals that are important and meaningful to the client, Hannah and Cheng (see Chapter 83) recommended using evaluations such as the COPM and the Patient Specific Functional Scale.

Several publications specifically encourage an increased focus on occupation in hand therapy,[19,20,24] whereas "occupation-based orthotic intervention," a term coined by McKee and Rivard[25] in 2007 has now been adopted and emphasized by those who previously used the term "occupation-based splinting."[26]

One client expressed it well: "Orthoses can immediately give a person back much of their function. I didn't realize how much of my life I had abandoned because I wanted to avoid pain. Much of the activities were leisure-based like badminton, basketball, yoga and pilates. Having the range of activities to choose from again has been so motivating and provided more chances for successful life changes."[1]

Principle 4. Optimize Usability

Orthotic usability refers to the effectiveness, efficiency, and satisfaction with which users can participate in activities in their various environments while wearing their orthosis. As the client stories illustrate, to optimize usability, an orthosis must be comfortable, convenient, and effective and must impose minimal occupational hindrance (Table 106.2).

Clients' stories exemplify how attention to the characteristics of the individual's environment enhances usability. When Shelley was competing in hot outdoor temperatures, the low-temperature thermoplastic of her therapist-made orthosis became soft and deformed. When Samuel was playing outside, he wore his hand-based thumb orthoses rather than the digit-based ones because the latter were more likely to fall off and get lost in that context.

Usability was the driving force behind the development of Silver Ring Splints (SIRIS) by occupational therapist Cynthia Garris. When she developed rheumatoid arthritis, a personal need for hand orthoses led Cynthia to design comfortable, effective, usable, and attractive thumb and finger orthoses that look like attractive jewelry. Beginning in the mid-1980s, custom-made silver ring-style orthoses became commercially available through the Silver Ring Splint Company (Charlottesville, VA).[27] Shelley herself, and many others, benefitted from Cynthia's innovation.

McKee and Rivard[28] discussed a client named Mildred with thumb IP joint arthritis who was fitted with a protective thumb-based orthosis to enable her to carry out daily living activities without pain. During a follow-up visit, Mildred revealed that she was not using it. As her therapist explored the nonuse, she learned that Mildred was simply concerned about getting the orthosis wet or soiled. When her therapist realized that she had neglected to educate Mildred about the care of the orthosis, she provided instructions explaining how to clean it. In a subsequent follow-up contact, Mildred was found to be using the orthosis as recommended, thereby preventing joint stress during household activities.[27]

Client-centeredness is not evident when outcomes are discussed in terms of compliance.[9] *Compliance* refers to the client's (or caregiver's) adherence to the prescribed regimen. Unfortunately, to some extent, the term has become synonymous with obedience, and a client who is labeled noncompliant is often viewed as uncooperative or lacking motivation.

To enhance the likelihood of orthotic use, we propose a paradigm shift. Instead of asking: "Is the individual compliant with the orthotic regimen?" ask: "Is the orthosis usable for individual?" In asking this question, the therapist better recognizes her or his responsibility to be client-centered. With a little education, Mildred was comfortable using her orthosis. With a collaborative approach, the design of Shelley's orthoses ensured optimal usability that facilitated participation in activities that were important and meaningful to her.

Factors that might predict the usability of orthoses may be similar to those that affect use of assistive technologies. Wielandt and coworkers[29] found three strong predictors of devices being used 4 to 6 weeks after introduction. These were (1) participants' perceptions of its durability, dependability, and appearance; the awkwardness of its use; the fatigue of its use; and the extent to which it caused embarrassment and pain; (2) the presence or absence of clients' anxiety about their condition and the interventions being proposed; and (3) clients' ability to recall their training. The authors reported that usability and actual usage of assistive technologies are improved when clients' opinions are considered and client choice is encouraged.[29]

As the client stories illustrate and the literature supports, the reasons why an orthosis is not used include lack of education, degree of discomfort, inconvenience, or the occupational hindrance it imposes. When the client is a child or a dependent adult, the involvement of family members and caregivers adds another dimension to the process. The durability of the orthosis is important to ensure long-term usability. Fabrication of a durable orthosis begins with planning for materials that will last and careful construction that includes firmly attaching components, such as hook fastener and outriggers, so they do not detach.

ORTHOTIC PEARL: FACTORS THAT DETRACT FROM USABILITY

- Discomfort
- Inconvenience—excess occupational hindrance
- Difficulty with donning and doffing
- Lack of understanding of its purpose or how to use it
- Lack of client or caregiver "buy-in" to the orthotic intervention
- Negative perceptions about disability and illness
- Client or family embarrassment caused by appearance of orthosis; fear of being "identified as disabled"
- Cultural beliefs
- Lack of durability
- Unsatisfactory appearance
- Too complicated for the user

Optimize Comfort

Because discomfort adversely affects how long and how regularly a client wears an orthosis, it is vital that an orthosis should, at least, cause no pain. Pain can arise from pressure points or other undue stress applied to tissues, indicating that the orthosis is causing some degree of biological harm. Furthermore, immobilization of one or more joints interferes with the natural patterns of movement and results in compensatory motions on the part of the client that can produce muscle fatigue and joint pain, as discussed earlier (see Fig. 106.10).[20]

Optimize Convenience

Restricted mobility of pain-free joints imposes a degree of inconvenience that limits the usability of an orthosis. As the client stories demonstrate, client input is important to ensure that the orthoses suit the person's lifestyle, especially if they are required for long-term use. Samuel's story demonstrates that one orthotic design might not be suitable in all environments.

Unless removal of an orthosis is contraindicated, ensure that the client understands how to and is physically able to apply and remove the orthosis and understands when it is to be worn. For clients with poor prehension because of weak or painful hands, consider the mode of fixation. An overlap strap is easy to make by cutting a length of strap material and attaching it to hook fastener. To facilitate manipulation of overlap straps, cut a hole in the end of the loop fastener strap (Fig.

106.12). A D-ring closure makes it easier to cinch an orthosis snugly in place.

It is important to seek the most convenient option that will best enable the client to maintain as much occupational performance as possible while addressing biological goals.

To design orthoses that impose the least possible inconvenience for the client or caregiver, a clear understanding of both the client's occupational roles and the environments in which he or she functions is required. When current occupational performance is temporarily compromised to achieve long-term goals, the client or caregiver also must clearly understand the goal of orthotic intervention as well as the consequences of not wearing the orthosis.

However, even an orthosis designed to enhance current occupational needs is likely to represent varying degrees of inconvenience. As such, an orthosis is not unlike a prescribed medication in that each may have adverse as well as positive effects. The suitability and usability of an orthosis is very individual and depends on which effects are most compelling—the benefits achieved by the orthosis or the inconvenience and discomfort imposed by it. Obviously, if the client does not use the orthosis, then the identified goals will not be achieved.

Whether the goal is to enable current or future occupational needs, it is important to design an orthotic intervention that imposes the least possible occupational hindrance to the client or caregiver.

Paul Brand observed: "We may be specialists in treating a single limb with a specific instrument, but we must be guided by the whole individual—body, mind, spirit—who has to decide to what extent he or she is prepared to place the whole person at the service of one of the digits and restrict his or her whole freedom and activity to improve a single joint" (p. 1817).[21]

Optimize Appearance

Unlike other interventions in hand rehabilitation, orthotic intervention results in an individualized device that meets specific biological and occupational needs that the client wears outside the clinic. Thus, the appearance of the orthosis deserves careful attention. For example, concert pianist Catherine (described in the 2011 edition of this book) insisted that for performances, she needed a thumb CMC-stabilizing orthosis that looked professional and was aesthetically pleasing.[16] The acceptable orthosis was achieved through a client-driven, iterative process (Fig. 106.13).

The device becomes a part of the client's personal environment and, like clothing, is seen by others. Most clients prefer their orthoses to be inconspicuous and not to draw attention. Possible exceptions include young or athletic clients for whom an orthosis may symbolize something they value. Thermoplastics, neoprene, and hook-receptive fasteners are available in a wide range of colors and, in some cases, patterns.

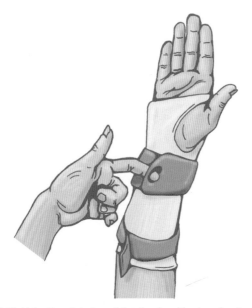

Fig. 106.12 Volar thumb-hole wrist orthosis with strapping techniques to make it easier for a client with poor prehension to grasp the strap (a long proximal strap and a hole in the wrist strap). (From McKee P, Morgan L. *Orthotics in Rehabilitation: Splinting the Hand and Body*. Philadelphia: FA Davis; 1998:14. © Pat McKee; used with permission.)

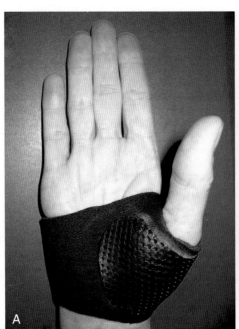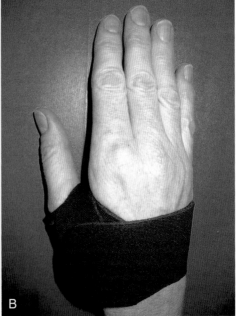

Fig. 106.13 Circumferential hand-based thumb carpometacarpal stabilizing orthosis made from black 1/16-in (1.6-mm) thick thermoplastic and bonded black 1/8-in (3.2-mm) thick neoprene. **A,** Volar view. **B,** Dorsal view. (© P. McKee. All rights reserved.)

Black thermoplastics (see Fig. 106.13) are becoming increasingly popular with youths and adults, whereas children may prefer a combination of brightly colored thermoplastics and strapping materials.

Cosmetic defects such as pen marks, rough edges, impressions of the fabricator's hands on the surface of the orthosis, and soiling greatly detract from the appearance of orthoses. Light-colored thermoplastics, particularly if they are uncoated, quickly become soiled when they are used to make functional hand orthoses. Coated and antimicrobial thermoplastics are more soil resistant and easier to clean; soiling is less apparent on dark-colored thermoplastics. Soiling of light-colored hook-and-loop fastener straps and stockinette, worn under an orthosis, is also unattractive.

An orthosis is a product of our therapeutic intervention that will be on display, representing our profession and us individually, and as such should meet exemplary standards. Efforts to optimize appearance should not be viewed as time consuming and unimportant. For Susie, "how the orthosis looked made a huge difference for me."[1] If not putting in the required time results in the client not wearing the orthosis, then the time used to fabricate it is truly wasted.

Use a Less-Is-More Approach

Less is more is a phrase originating in the 1940s and is attributed to the architect Ludwig Mies van der Rohe to describe minimalism in form and design.[29] Many of the guiding principles presented here can be favorably affected by adopting this guideline. The client stories confirm that it can serve as a sound guiding principle when designing and fabricating orthoses. We propose that orthotic design should follow a minimalist approach with regard to size, weight, and rigidity of the orthosis; visibility of the orthosis; amount of skin enclosed; number of restricted joints; thickness of the thermoplastic; complexity of straps and adjustable components; and ease of maintenance.

In Shelley's story, a simple, easy-to-apply orthosis was fabricated, ensuring that it did not exceed her cognitive capacity (see Fig. 106.3B). Over time, Samuel's orthoses became progressively smaller and therefore less visible and restrictive.

As a general rule, unless rigidity is required of the orthosis to control spasticity (as in Shelley's story), create an orthosis that is as lightweight as possible while providing adequate support. This is particularly important for children and adult clients with muscle weakness or fatigue. The weight of the orthosis is determined primarily by the thickness and degree of perforation of the thermoplastic.

Increased orthotic rigidity can be increased in two ways. Use a thicker thermoplastic, but this adds additional weight to the client's limb and additional stress to the therapist's hands to cut, mold, and cold adjust. Alternatively, the therapist can use molded contours in a thinner thermoplastic to make the orthosis more rigid.

ORTHOTIC PEARL: USE A LESS-IS-MORE APPROACH

Design, fabricate, and finish an orthosis to impose the least amount of inconvenience and visibility possible. *Less* can achieve *more* in terms of outcomes that are satisfactory to the client.

Principle 5. Apply Sound Design and Fabrication Principles

Applying sound design and fabrication guidelines during the planning and fabrication of an orthosis is essential to ensuring that orthoses are effective, usable, comfortable, and durable and do no harm. These

TABLE 106.3	Sound Design and Fabrication Guidelines
Appropriate length of lever arms
Optimal force distribution through appropriate surface area
Conformity to body contours
Optimal rigidity, controlled by contours and material characteristics
Padding of bony prominences before molding
All corners rounded, including straps and hook fastener tabs
No unnecessary restriction of uninvolved joints
Create a compact, minimally conspicuous design with all elements as close to the hand as possible

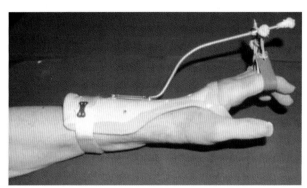

Fig. 106.14 Poor orthotic design. The proximal end of this dynamic orthosis for radial nerve injury is lifting away from the limb because the lever arm is too short and the strap is too narrow. It lacks a wrist strap; the edges are covered with moleskin, which will become smelly and shabby, and there is no extension stabilization for the metacarpophalangeal joints. Made by the first author circa 1975. (© P. McKee. All rights reserved.)

tenets, summarized in Table 106.3, are briefly discussed below and in Chapter 109.

Optimize Surface Area to Improve Distribution of Forces

If the area of force application is too small, as shown in Fig. 106.14, high localized pressure results, causing discomfort and possible skin irritation. Increasing the surface area of the orthosis improves the force distribution and increases comfort. This applies to both straps and the trough of the orthosis.

The trough of the orthosis needs to be sufficiently deep so that the limb is well seated and the orthosis fits securely. If the trough is too shallow, the limb will "overflow" the sides of the trough, and the straps will need to be applied tighter to secure the orthosis in place. As a general rule, the trough should extend slightly more than halfway up the sides of the limb. However, if the trough is too deep and the material is inflexible, the orthosis will be difficult to apply and remove. An exception to this guideline for trough depth is the circumferential orthosis, which encircles the body part.

Conformity to Contour

The thermoplastic should conform to the contours of the body, without any gapping. Material that does not contact the body serves no purpose and should be removed. Using thermoplastics that are more conforming and malleable when warm enhances conformity. Straps should also conform to the body contours to enhance comfort and increase the distribution area of the securing force. When thermoplastic is molded over bony prominences, it must conform to the contours to prevent pressure points over these sensitive areas. Alternatively, pad bony prominences before molding the orthosis. Using padded strap materials enhances

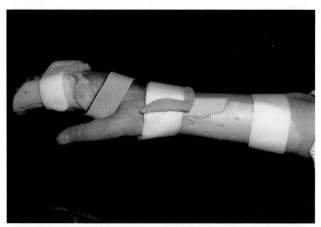

Fig. 106.15 Volar forearm–based wrist–finger orthosis illustrating strap pad on the wrist strap and neoprene hand strap. (© P. McKee. All rights reserved.)

strap conformity. This is particularly important for the straps that apply force over a bony prominence, such as the head of the ulna.

Round All Corners

All corners should be rounded to improve the aesthetics of the orthosis and to eliminate sharp square corners that could injure the skin. Hook fastener patches with rounded corners are less likely to peel off than those with square corners, thus enhancing orthotic durability.

Flare the Proximal Weight-Bearing Edge

Many functional activities are performed with the forearm pronated. As a result, it is common to bear weight on the forearm trough of an orthosis when one is seated at a table. To prevent the proximal edge from causing a pressure point, it should be very slightly flared. Avoid an excessive flare of the forearm trough because it creates a ridge that makes it more difficult to apply and remove sleeves and can irritate other parts of the body.

Lever Arm

As a general rule, to optimize the mechanical advantage of an orthosis, use the longest lever arm possible without restricting the motion of other joints. With some exceptions, forearm-based orthoses should extend approximately two thirds of the way up the forearm from the wrist (Fig. 106.15). Lengthening the forearm trough further than two thirds restricts elbow flexion, and the proximal edge will irritate soft tissues above the elbow. Conversely, a lever arm that is too short results in poor stabilization of affected joints and the tendency to apply increased force through the straps to compensate (see Fig. 106.14).

An exception is illustrated in Shelley's dorsal forearm–based wrist orthosis that exceeded the two-thirds guideline (see Fig. 106.3B). In her situation, the longer lever arm effectively controlled wrist flexor spasticity and was acceptable because she did not need to flex her elbow while riding her tricycle. Another exception is a circumferential orthosis, either prefabricated or custom made. Generally, the increased surface area allows sufficient wrist control with a shorter lever arm.

Straps

Straps are an integral component of the orthosis. Their width, location, orientation, and conformity of contour greatly contribute to the comfort and usability of the orthosis and make the difference between effective and ineffective intervention. As shown in Figure 106.15, to be optimally effective, a volar forearm–based orthosis requires a counter-force centered directly over the target joint axis (i.e., wrist). Thus, the

wrist strap applies the key force to keep the wrist positioned within the orthosis. To maximize the distribution of this force and thereby enhance comfort, use a strap that is 1.5 or 2 inches (3.8–5 cm) wide.

Durability of strap components is essential to ensuring long-term usability of the orthosis. With extended use, padded strapping materials lose their sensitivity to hook fastener; standard loop fastener is more durable. Use padded materials to make a strap pad, which is attached to a loop fastener strap (see Fig. 106.15). Of particular importance is ensuring that the hook fastener adheres well because if it peels off, the orthosis becomes immediately unusable.

Facilitating strap attachment and removal was previously discussed and illustrated in Figure 106.12.

Dynamic and Static Progressive Components

Orthoses designed to influence biological structures through the application of forces, for example, to correct contractures or assist specific movement(s), often require the attachment of additional components. Such components, including outriggers, hinges, springs, pulleys, screws, nylon line, and elastic cord, can be either prefabricated or custom made.

It is important that these be lightweight, easy to adjust (if appropriate), durable, firmly bonded, and comprehensible for the user. They must also impose the least amount of occupational hindrance. In addition, the direction of pull and magnitude of force must be carefully considered.

When possible, the outrigger should be as close to the hand as possible, unlike in Figure 106.14. This creates a more compact, less conspicuous orthosis and positively affects usability. All these characteristics enhance effectiveness and usability. Read more in Chapter 108.

Principle 6. Meet Professional Practice Responsibilities

Hand therapists, by virtue of their licensing or certification status, are accountable for the effectiveness of their interventions. As such, orthotic intervention is not method driven (i.e., defined by tasks or procedures) but rather focused on client need, based on sound theory and subject to continual evaluation of outcomes.[30]

Although it is clear that hand therapy practice contexts (e.g., institutional, private practice, insurance funded) influence orthotic intervention processes, regulated health care professionals are expected to comply with established practice standards and codes of ethics. These include adherence to the practice competencies and processes established by professional bodies and regulatory agencies. Competencies include therapists' knowledge and skills, client education, monitoring and modifying one's interventions, and evaluating outcomes, as outlined in Table 106.4 and described next. Also required is "conscientious, explicit, and judicious use of current best evidence in making decisions" (p. 272).[30]

Therapist's Knowledge and Skills

An essential trait of professional practice is specialized knowledge, both theoretical and technical.[30] Licensed professionals are responsible for ensuring that they possess the knowledge and skills required for their positions.

Therapists who provide orthotic intervention must have sound knowledge of anatomy and physiology, pathology, wound healing, biomechanics, human occupation, orthotic materials, and mechanical principles of orthotic fabrication. Also required are skills in activity analysis, client assessment and education, and fabrication techniques (see Chapter 108).Maintaining currency in this knowledge and skill set is an obligation of professional practice. Continuously assessing and developing professional skills and applying current research evidence ensures best practice.[14,31]

TABLE 106.4 Professional Practice Responsibilities			
Develop and Maintain Specialized Knowledge and Skills	Provide Comprehensive Client or Caregiver Education About:	Monitor and Modify:	Evaluate Outcomes:
• Anatomy and physiology • Pathology • Wound healing • Body biomechanics • Human occupation • Orthotic materials • Mechanical principles • Activity analysis • Assessment • Client education • Design principles and fabrication skills • Outcome measuring	• Objectives of orthotic regimen and consequences of nonuse • Correct application and removal of orthosis • Wearing schedule and circumstances when it can be removed • Care of the orthosis • Indications of poor fit (e.g., pressure points) that need prompt attention	• To verify and evaluate effectiveness at meeting occupational and biological goals • To verify and evaluate whether orthosis is being used and explore reasons for nonuse or incorrect use • To make adjustments and repairs (e.g., to relieve pressure points and ensure adequate mobility of joints that should be unrestricted) • To clarify use and care of orthosis	• To assess whether occupational and biological goals have been achieved • To gather evidence concerning efficacy of orthotic intervention • To contribute to the body of professional knowledge

Provide Comprehensive Client or Caregiver Education

The client or caregiver must clearly understand the rationale for the orthosis, when to wear it, how to put it on and make adjustments, how to care for it, and when and how to contact the therapist. The therapist must reassure the client that feedback and inquiries are welcome. Thus, it is essential to provide clear verbal education as well as written instructions. As discussed earlier, this education was initially lacking for Mildred.

Use everyday language and avoid jargon or anatomical terms. If there is a language barrier, a translator should be enlisted. Consider the client's level of education, literacy, and comprehension. Ensure that the client or caregiver knows how to, and is physically able to, apply and remove the orthosis and manage the straps or other modes of fixation. Comprehensive education enhances usability.

Pain relief provides a compelling incentive for an orthosis to be worn. However, in many circumstances, pain relief is not the primary goal of the orthosis, and occupations may be temporarily hindered to promote optimal healing. In these situations, it is especially important to clearly explain biological goals of orthotic intervention. For example, therapists understand that surgically repaired lacerated finger tendons must be protected with an orthosis that limits hand function for several weeks to prevent tendon rupture (see Chapters 31 and 33). However, the client or caregiver may not appreciate the consequence of not wearing an orthosis without an explanation using clear language aimed at the listener's comprehension level.

If adverse reaction by others is likely to occur, try to provide education about the objectives of orthotic intervention to significant individuals in the client's social environment. It is important to enlist their support to optimize usability of the orthosis.

Monitor and Modify

Monitoring and modifying are essential to the orthotic intervention process.[32] *Monitoring* involves ongoing evaluation and collaboration with the client or caregiver to determine whether the intervention process is meeting biological and occupational goals, as illustrated in the client stories. It can help identify whether the client is using the orthosis and explore reasons for nonuse. Monitoring also helps determine whether additional education or clarification is required.

Modifying the orthosis is indicated when the monitoring process identifies problems that are interfering with usability, such as discomfort from pressure points or unnecessary restriction of joint motion. Modifications are also required, as seen with Jim when the condition changes or when a child grows, as seen with Samuel. Also personal, occupational, or environmental situations change, or an orthosis may not be meeting expectations.

Unfortunately, a number of client-related or institutional factors may present barriers to monitoring and orthotic modification. For example, the client may deem it too inconvenient or costly to return to the clinic. In this case, the therapist should consider alternative strategies, such as telephone follow-up or referral to a therapist closer to the client's home. Organizational policies or funding restrictions (e.g., insurance companies), as well as human resource issues, can also restrict monitoring. Advocating to employers about the vital nature of monitoring and how it contributes to more effective interventions may be required.

ORTHOTIC PEARL: MONITOR AND MODIFY

Optimal benefits of orthotic intervention may not be realized if monitoring and modification do not occur.

Evaluate Outcomes

Explicit evaluation of outcomes identifies the extent to which biological and occupational goals have or have not been achieved. If goals have not been met, the therapist and client can collaborate to revise the intervention plan. Evaluating outcomes also fulfills the basic professional responsibility to assess the orthotic process for the purpose of continuous program improvement. This helps ensure that future clients will receive the best possible care. Finally, outcome evaluation assists with gathering evidence to demonstrate the effectiveness of our interventions and to contribute to the professional body of knowledge, which, again, benefits future clients.

SUMMARY: ACHIEVING BETTER OUTCOMES

The provision of an orthosis cannot be taken lightly. Orthoses have a great influence on activity and participation by way of both their positive and negative effect on biological structures.

Therapists are perpetually challenged to apply expert knowledge, creativity, and problem-solving skills to meet the unique requirements and preferences of each client using available resources and despite the limitations of their work environment.

Collaboration with the client throughout the assessment, intervention, monitoring, and modification processes and use of the Client-Centered Bio-occupational Framework for Orthotic Intervention, help to optimize outcomes. This approach involves identifying and addressing the biological issues that underlie occupational barriers to optimal participation and considering the complete client picture.

The principles of the Client-Centered Bio-occupational Framework for Orthotic Intervention are explicitly aimed at providing orthoses that enable current or future activity and participation while minimizing biological harm and occupational interference. Orthoses can benefit clients only if they are actually worn. Thus, orthoses should be comfortable, lightweight, aesthetically pleasing, and convenient to use. Usability is enhanced by optimizing comfort, appearance, and convenience and using a less-is-more approach. Monitoring, modifying, and evaluating outcomes are essential processes for ensuring orthotic usability while potentially providing evidence of orthotic efficacy and the continuous improvement of practice guidelines.

ORTHOTIC PEARL: EXERCISE IN EMPATHY

When students are learning orthotic skills, a useful exercise is to have them wear a hand orthosis fabricated by a fellow student for a 24-hour period. They will experience first-hand (pun intended) how having one or more joints immobilized can affect function. Also apparent are discomfort from pressure points, the attention that the orthosis attracts in public, and the heat and perspiration retained by the orthotic material. This experience reinforces the importance of:

- Optimal joint positioning
- No unnecessary restriction of joint motion or function
- Optimal appearance, comfort, and convenience
- Discreet design
- Environmental considerations when selecting materials and design
- Considering cultural and spiritual factors

Superior outcomes are achieved when the central aim of orthotic intervention is to enable current or future occupational needs rather than merely provide an orthosis. Orthoses that are thoughtfully designed with client input, carefully constructed, monitored, and modified as needed can make a difference in a person's life by relieving pain, stabilizing joints, protecting vulnerable tissues, and enabling valued occupations. This in turn promotes physical and emotional well-being.

We respectfully leave the final words to Dr. Paul Brand: "The art of the therapist is to remain poised, flexible and responsive to the input of science and technology on one hand and the human values of the patient on the other."[21]

ACKNOWLEDGMENTS

The authors wish to thank Marie Eason Klatt for providing Samuel's story and our clients who very kindly allowed us to use their stories and provided quotes.

REFERENCES

1. McKee P. Bio-occupational orthotic approach. In: Jacobs M, Austin N, eds. *Orthotic Intervention for the Hand and Upper Extremity: Splinting Principles and Process.* 2nd ed. Philadelphia: Wolters Kluwer / Lippincott Williams and Wilkins; 2013:119–121.
2. McKee PR, Rivard A. Biopsychosocial approach to orthotic intervention. *J Hand Ther.* 2011;24(2):155–163.
3. Winthrop Rose B, Kasch MC, Aaron DH, Stegink-Jansen CW. Does hand therapy literature incorporate the holistic view of health and function promoted by the world health organization? *J Hand Ther.* 2011;24(2):84–88.
4. Weinstock-Zlotnick G, Bear-Lehman J. How therapists specializing in hand therapy evaluate the ability of patients to participate in their daily lives: an exploratory study. *J Hand Ther.* 2015;28(3):261–268.
5. World Health Organization. International Classification of Functioning, Disability and Health (ICF); 2017. Available at: http://www.who.int/classifications/icf/en/. Accessed 11/27, 2017.
6. Langer D, Luria S, Maeir A, Erez A. Occupation-based assessments and treatments of trigger finger: a survey of occupational therapists from Israel and the United States. *Occup Ther Int.* 2014;21(4):143–155.
7. Hansen AØ, Cederlund R, Kristensen HK, Tromborg H. The effect of an occupation-based intervention in patients with hand-related disorders grouped using the sense of coherence scale: study protocol. *Hand Therapy.* 2016;21(3):90–99.
8. Hemmingsson H, Jonsson H. The issue is. An occupational perspective on the concept of participation in the International Classification of Functioning, Disability and Health - Some critical remarks. *Am J Occup Ther.* 2005;59(5):569–576.
8a. Greenhalgh T. Narrative based medicine in an evidence based world. *BMJ.* 1999;318:323.
9. Cooper C. Special Issue: Narratives in hand therapy. *J Hand Ther.* 2011;24(2):132–139.
10. H-200 Grip Assist Glove. Available at: https://www.benik.com/adults/wrist/h-200. Accessed Nov/22, 2017.
11. Bush P, ten Hompel S. An integrated craft and design approach for wearable orthoses. *Design for Health.* 2017;1:86–104.
12. Robinson LS, Brown T, O'Brien L. Embracing an occupational perspective: occupation-based interventions in hand therapy practice. *Aust Occup Ther J.* 2016;63(4):293–296.
12a. Fisher AG. Uniting practice and theory in an occupational framework. *American Journal of Occupational Therapy.* 1998;52(7):509–521.
13. Gillen A, Greber C. Occupation-focused practice: challenges and choices. *BR J Occup Ther.* 2014;77(1):39–41.
14. Mulligan S, White BP, Arthanat S. An examination of occupation-based, client-centered, evidence-based occupational therapy practices in New Hampshire. *OTJR Occupation, Participation and Health.* 2014;34(2):106–116.
15. Colaianni DJ, Provident I, DiBartola LM, Wheeler S. A phenomenology of occupation-based hand therapy. *Aust Occup Ther J.* 2015 06;62(3):177–186.
16. McKee P, Rivard A. Foundations of Orthotic Intervention. In: Skirven T, Osterman L, Fedorczyk J, Amadio P, eds. *Rehabilitation of the Hand and Upper Extremity.* 6th ed. Philadelphia: Elsevier; 2011:1565–1580.
17. Fess EE. Design principles. In: Fess EE, Gettle KS, Philips CA, Jansen JR, eds. *Hand and Upper Extremity Splinting: Principles and Methods.* 3rd ed. St. Louis: Elsevier Mosby; 2005:210–236.
18. Wilton JC, Dival TA. *Hand Splinting: Principles of Design and Fabrication.* London: W.B. Saunders; 1997.
19. McKee P, Hannah S, Priganc VW. Orthotic considerations for dense connective tissue and articular cartilage - the need for optimal movement and stress. *J Hand Ther.* 2012;25(2):233–243.
20. Liu C, Chiang H, Chen K. The compensatory motion of wrist immobilization on thumb and index finger performance-kinematic analysis and clinical implications. *Work.* 2015;50(4):611–619.
21. Brand PW. The forces of dynamic splinting: ten questions before applying a dynamic splint to the hand. In: Mackin EJ, Callahan AD, Osterman AL, Skirven TM, Schneider L, Hunter JM, eds. 5th ed. Philadelphia: Elsevier; 2002:1811–1817.
22. Eason Klatt M. Orthotic intervention for thumb hypermobility: a case study and new orthotic design. *J Hand Ther.* 2008;21(4):420.
23. Christiansen CH, Townsend ES. *Introduction to Occupation: the Art and Science of Living.* 2nd ed. Upper Saddle River, NJ: Pearson Education; 2010.
24. Amini D. Occupational therapy interventions for work-related injuries and conditions of the forearm, wrist, and hand: a systematic review. *Am J Occup Ther.* 2011;65(1):29–36.
25. McKee P, Rivard A. Occupation-based orthotic intervention. In: Townsend EA, Polatajko HJ, eds. *Enabling Occupation II: Advancing an Occupational Therapy Vision for Health, Well-being & Justice through Occupation.* Ottawa: Canadian Association of Occupational Therapies; 2007:172–174.

26. Amini D. Occupation-based orthotic intervention. In: Coppard B, Lohman H, eds. *Introduction to Orthotics; A Clinical Reasoning and Problem-Solving Approach*. 4th ed. Philadelphia: Elsevier; 2015:13–25.

27. About SIRIS. Available at: http://www.silverringsplint.com/about/. Accessed Nov/30, 2017.

28. McKee P, Rivard A. Orthoses as enablers of occupation: client-centred splinting for better outcomes. *Can J Occup Ther*. 2004;71(5):306–314.

29. Wielandt T, McKenna K, Tooth L, Strong J. Factors that predict the post-discharge use of recommended assistive technology (AT). *Disabil Rehabil Assist Technol*. 2006;1(1-2):29–40.

30. Craik J, Davis J, Polatajko HJ. Introducing the Canadian Practice Process Framework (CPPF): Amplifying the context. In: Townsend EA, Polatajko HJ, eds. *Enabling Occupation II: Advancing an Occupational therapy Vision for Health, Well-Being and Justice through Occupation*. Ottawa: Canadian Association of Occupational Therapists; 2007:229–246.

31. Dy LB, Yancosek KE. Introducing purposeful activity kits in a hand rehabilitation practice: Effects on clinical practice patterns and job satisfaction among occupational therapy practitioners. *Hand Therapy*. 2017;22(1):3–12.

32. Craven J. Mies van der Rohe - What is Neo-Miesian? 2017. Available at: https://www.thoughtco.com/mies-van-der-rohe-neo-miesian-177427. Accessed 11/28, 2017.

107

Relative Motion Orthoses: The Concepts and Application to Hand Therapy Management of Finger Extensor Tendon Zone III and VII Repairs, Acute and Chronic Boutonnière Deformity, and Sagittal Band Injury

Wyndell H. Merritt, Julianne Wright Howell

OUTLINE

CRITICAL POINTS

Simulated Relative Motion Extension or Relative Motion Flexion PENCIL Test

The "pencil test" is a practical way to simulate a relative motion flexion (RMF) or relative motion extension (RME) orthosis. Simply place a pencil or tongue depressor above (RMF) or below (RME) the proximal phalanx of the affected digit and opposite for the neighboring digits and observe while the digit is flexed and extended for the desired response. If the index or small are the affected digit, the pencil can be balanced by weaving it in the same way (above or below) as the affected digit using the central two digits for support. The pencil test is a quick and useful tool to simulate the relative motion positions during hand examination to decide if either position offers the desired response or as an "exercise device" to position the MCP joint in relative flexion–extension or during wide-awake local anesthesia and no tourniquet surgery to guide the choice of orthosis and postoperative instruction details.[3,17,57]

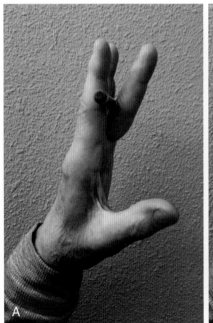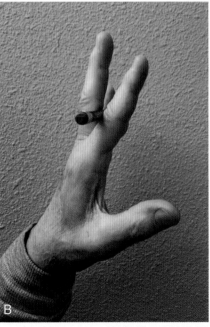

The figure shows the simulated relative motion orthosis "pencil test **(A)** RMF and RME **(B)** for the long finger.

The concept of relative motion (RM) is not new; it was proposed in the late 1970s as an idea to mobilize extensor tendon zones V and VI repairs.[1–3] The idea of active finger motion controlled by an orthosis was suggested to minimize the morbidity of tendon adhesions and joint stiffness seen after 4 to 6 weeks of immobilization. The original 1978 RM orthosis design permitted active motion of only the metacarpophalangeal (MCP) joints.[3,4] Over the past 40 years, the orthosis design, concept, and nomenclature have evolved, and use has expanded into therapy management for a variety of hand conditions.[3] RM orthoses have been known by many names, such as the Wyndell Merritt splint,[5–7] immediate controlled active motion (ICAM, an acronym chosen to emphasize that it is active motion rather than dynamically assisted passive motion),[2] yoke splint,[8,9] border digit splint,[10] sagittal band bridge splint,[11,12] and most recently in conversation, the RM orthosis. Today, the preferred terms are *relative motion extension (RME)* and *relative motion flexion (RMF)* to highlight the relative position of the affected digit's MCP joint and minimize confusion.[3,13] The RME and RMF orthoses are finger based; the RME orthosis positions the MCP joint of the affected finger(s) in 15 to 20 degrees *more extension* relative to that of the neighboring MCP joints, and the RMF orthosis positions the affected digit's MCP joint(s) in *greater flexion* relative to that of the neighboring MCP joint(s), which are in 15 to 20 degrees less flexion. RME is widely used after extensor tendon zone IV to VII repair and for surgical and nonsurgical management after sagittal band injury[1,2,11,12,14] (Fig. 107.1). RMF has been advocated to restore balance to the extensor mechanism after acute and chronic boutonnière and after extensor tendon zone III repair[15–17] (Fig. 107.2). Most recently, a scoping review of worldwide experience using the RM concept was published by Hirth and coworkers,[3] who pointed out the versatility of this concept, which can apply to three orthotic purposes: "protective, adaptive and exercise." This chapter reviews some established and some expanded uses of this concept. The RM concept is attractive because of its small size,[3] low-profile design that is simple and inexpensive to fabricate,[2,7,11,18] less morbidity because of decreased rehabilitation time,[1,2,18–20] early functional hand use,[2,21–23] earlier return to work,[1,2,18–24] improved patient compliance,[3,6] and less financial investment for care.[19]

The goal of this chapter is to establish the framework for understanding the RM concept. To do so, the authors have included relevant anatomy and biomechanics, clinical studies, illustrations, photos, and videos.

RELATIVE MOTION: THE METACARPOPHALANGEAL JOINT AND THE "QUADRIGA EFFECT"

The Relative Motion concept is simple.

WH Merritt[25]

Four types of finger orthoses are commonly described: static, dynamic, serial static, and static progressive.[26] The RM orthosis differs in that it takes advantage of the relationship between a single muscle shared by extrinsic extensor or flexor tendons to use what has been called the "quadriga effect" by positioning the affected digit's MCP joint in relative extension or flexion to its neighbors for safe early active motion and functional hand use. The RM concept provides a simple management technique that safely permits active finger motion with decreased tension of the repaired or ruptured tendon, thus reducing repair adherence, reducing unfavorable joint capsule and collateral ligament remodeling, and likely increasing the strength of the repair.

Understanding the quadriga effect and its application to RME and RMF is important in achieving effective results. Verdan[27] introduced this term for a complication that can occur after single-digit amputation, causing adjacent fingers to lose flexion. He named this the *syndrome of the quadriga*, resulting when the extensor tendon is sutured to the flexor digitorum profundus (FDP) tendon over an amputation stump. As a result, the performance of the FDP, a single muscle shared by multiple tendons, is hampered by the suture to create a relative length difference between the tendons, placing slack in the adjacent flexor profundi tendons and thus limiting active finger flexion.

Although Verdan's description was only of profundi tendons to caution surgeons not to suture the extensors to the flexors over an amputated stump, the extensor digitorum communis (EDC) tendons also arise from a single muscle and have multiple juncturae tendinae and intramuscular connections between the four digits, allowing similar quadriga features, evidenced when one attempts to extend the ring finger while in a fisted position.

Quadriga is the name the Romans gave their two-wheeled chariot with equidistant reins used by the charioteer to control the four horses during the Roman and Greek Olympic races, explaining Verdan's choice of terminology (Fig. 107.3A). In the human hand, the charioteer's body is like the FDP or EDC muscle; the reins of the four horses are compared to the flexor or extensor tendons. To control the horses, the charioteer wraps the reins around his trunk so that with a twist of his body, the harnessed horses are pulled as one.[27] Although Verdan originally described the quadriga effect as an analogy for complications, this relationship can be advantageous. RME applies the principles Verdan described in the flexor profundi to the common extensor to produce a useful extensor "quadriga effect" designed specifically to protect extensor tendon repairs and sagittal band injuries. Although the extensor indicis proprius (EIP) and extensor digitorum minimi (EDM) are not single muscles shared by multiple tendons, management with RME works conceivably because the excursions of the independent extensor tendons match the excursions of the common extensor tendons with all sharing intramuscular and juncturae tendinae connections.[28,29]

Sharma and coworkers[30] measured elongation of repaired tendons of cadavers with and without the RME orthosis, validating the protective benefit of the orthosis throughout the full range of motion (ROM) of the fingers, including making a fist. These authors' results aligned with our clinical experience to confirm that tendon repairs are protected by the relative position of the MCP joints, demonstrating the least amount of elongation was measured in the experimental MCP joint position of RME neutral, and there were also no tendon ruptures in the RME orthosis–protected digits, even with full motion, but the repairs without the orthosis did gap.[30] This protective function of the RME orthosis was easily demonstrated by our 1978 cadaver study using only a "single weak" 6-0 nylon suture for tendon repair and repeated at the 2003 meeting of the American Society of Hand Therapists (ASHT) (Video 107.1). However, it is even more convincing in the emergency department, when under local anesthesia, a "single weak" 6-0 nylon suture is placed in an extensor tendon repair and a tongue depressor is positioned beneath the proximal phalanx to simulate an RME orthosis followed by active flexion and extension of the fingers without rupture.

In the 1978 cadaver study, composite finger and wrist flexion pulled on the single 6-0 nylon suture, although it did not rupture. Therefore, our original recommendation was to immobilize the wrist and interphalangeal (IP) joints, allowing active movement of only the MCP joints within the RME orthosis. Simply stated, the RM concept is all about the relative position of the MCP joints to one another. When the affected digit's MCP joint is positioned in

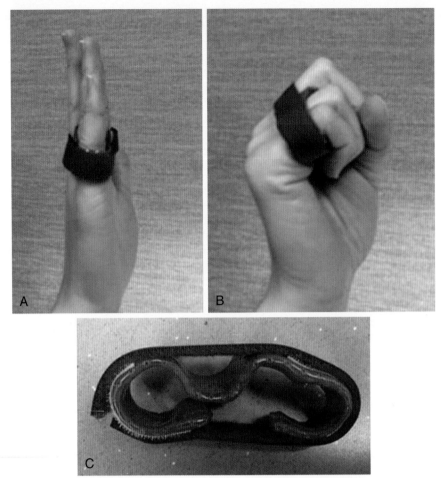

Fig. 107.1 A–C, Relative motion extension orthosis for the long finger. (© 2018 JW Howell, PT, MS, CHT.)

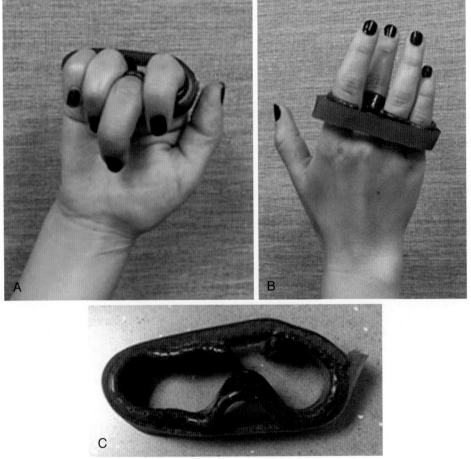

Fig. 107.2 A–C, Relative motion flexion orthosis for the long finger. (© 2018 JW Howell, PT, MS, CHT.)

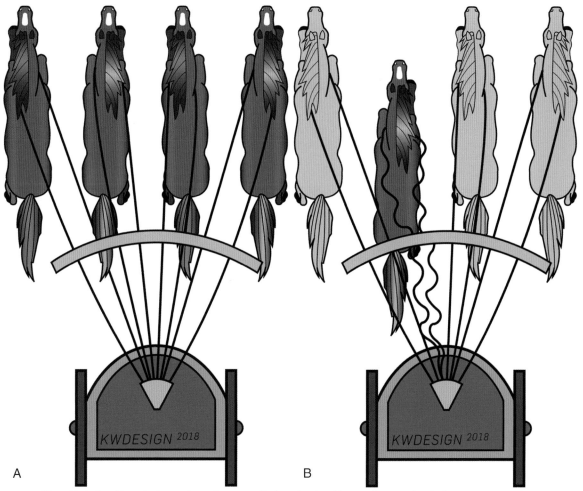

Fig. 107.3 Quadriga chariot analogy. Four equal-in-length reined horses (four tendons) share a common charioteer (muscle). All reins are of equal length, resulting in equal reining (**A**) and one rein on slack (**B**; 15–20 degrees RME position in humans). As the charioteer pulls, the relatively longer reins predominate, while the slack rein and horse remain on lax tension. (© *2018 KW Design.* Contact Katie Wright of KW Design; Wright.design.illustration@gmail.com.)

relatively more extension, a length difference is created between the repair and its neighbor tendons, resulting in less tension on the repair. As the digits *actively* flex, the equidistant neighboring tendons, united by their interconnections, pull the shared EDC muscle distally to maintain the "quadriga effect" throughout the ROM. As demonstrated by the chariot analogy, when all reins are the same, equal reining results. If one rein is put on slack (as in a 15- to 20-degrees RME position in humans) when the charioteer pulls the reins, the relatively longer reins predominate, unloading the shorter rein so that the horse on the slack rein remains on lax tension (Fig. 107.3B).

RELATIVE MOTION EXTENSION

Long Extensor Tendon Lacerations in Zones IV to VII

Before 1980, active finger motion after extensor tendon repair was a bold idea. Subsequent to cadaver observations, the RME orthosis was designed to verify that motion was safe for the repaired extensor tendons. The original edition of the RME orthosis was a finger-based orthosis that positioned the MCP joint of the affected digit in relatively more extension with the IP joints immobilized

and was secured to the wrist orthosis with a strap.[3] In the second edition of the RME orthosis, the wrist remained immobilized at 25 to 30 degrees of extension, and all digits were allowed full motion, except the MCP joint of the affected digit, which was positioned in 20 to 25 degrees relatively more extension. In 1986, the RM concept and this second edition orthosis were published in a textbook reviewing advances in tendon management, as a "new approach to splinting extensor tendon zones V-VI."[19] Robinson and coworkers[21] reported successful use of this new approach in 23 patients at the 1986 meeting of the ASHT. Concurrently, with additional experience and the successful management of many more patients, the third edition of the RME orthosis reduced the MCP joint relative position to 15 to 20 degrees.[1,2] At this same time, RME use was expanded to the management of extensor tendon zones IV and VII and sagittal band repairs.[1,2]

The absence of reported secondary surgeries to release adhesions and stiff joints is a direct result of early active motion and early tendon excursion achieved by the RME orthosis.[2,6,7,20,21,33-36] Actual measurements of the amount of tendon excursion permitted by the RME orthosis have not been formally studied. Evans and Burkhalter[35] previously measured normal extensor tendon excursion intraoperatively, concluding that 30 to 40 degrees of MCP joint flexion produced 5 mm of safe—and what they believed sufficient—extensor tendon excursion to obviate adhesions. Lalonde's[32] excellent video demonstrates a patient under wide-awake local anesthesia, no tourniquet, technique (WALANT) moving actively through full finger motion except the 15 to 20 degrees limited by the RME orthosis with total excursion measured as 8 mm, exceeding the 5 mm suggested to limit adhesions (Video 107.2). Although much has been written about the strength of various extensor tendon repair techniques and suture material, these seem far less relevant than selecting an orthosis that permits safe early active motion. This notion aligns with the authors' experiences in that some patients with infected extensor lacerations have been successfully managed with no repair whatsoever; they have been treated with only the RME orthosis.[2,25]

The largest clinical series was published in 2005 under the acronym ICAM (immediate controlled active motion) by Howell and associates,[2] who reported on 20 years of experience with the RME and wrist orthoses in 140 patients with 190 extensor tendon zone IV to VII simple ($n = 89$) and complex ($n = 51$) injuries. Since that publication, Hirth and associates'[3] scoping review recognized the growing worldwide acceptance of the RM concept, citing six therapy programs that managed a total of 226 patients with both the RME and wrist orthoses and seven programs that used the RME-only orthosis for 145 patients with zone IV to VI repairs. Because usage of the RME-only orthosis without the wrist orthosis is relatively new and various authors have changed some of the original program details, review of these studies is worthwhile[6,7,20,23,24,33-36] (Table 107.1). In one study, the author reports better ROM and fewer extensor lags in the wearers of the RME-only orthosis than those wearing both orthoses.[6] Others instruct patients not to simultaneously fist and flex their wrists to avoid passive tension on the repair.[24] Another used the RME-only orthosis when repairs were distal to the juncturae tendinum in zones IV-V, otherwise these authors used both orthoses when the repair was proximal to the junctura and/or involved the EDM in zones IV to VI.[20] Two case reports confirmed that patients with multi-tissue injuries benefitted from a single orthosis fabricated to combine both the RME and RMF positions for adjacent finger usage, safely avoiding complex trauma complications.[14,16] Since 2005, a count of the global literature for extensor tendon repairs in zones IV to VI by author JWH shows approximately 203 patients with 212 repairs reported in 207 zones have been managed by the RME-only orthosis (see Table 107.1). However, since 2005, 246 patients with 266 tendon repairs reported in 252 zones have been managed with the combined wrist and RME finger orthoses (Table 107.2). Seemingly, the RME-only orthosis is being more extensively used, so these numbers will continue to change as therapists have greater experience using the finger-based orthosis to manage extensor tendon repairs. For now, it is important to keep in mind how the evidence for management of extensor tendon repairs with the RME-only orthosis varies by zone. To date, these reports suggest that zone IV repairs are well protected by the finger orthosis only. The 137 tendon repairs reported for zone V that have been successfully managed suggest that substantial evidence is accumulating. In zone VI, although the RME-only orthosis numbers are growing, program changes made by various authors have affected interpretation, and in zone VII, there is no evidence for use of the RME-only orthosis.

The original ICAM program described for management of zone IV to VII repairs has been altered by the various authors[6,10,20,23,24,33-36] (see Tables 107.1 and 2). A current update to the RME program for management of zone IV to VII extensor tendon repairs has been compiled by the authors in Box 107.1. The one rule, however, that

has remained consistent is that at least one EDC or EIP or EDM tendon must remain intact to use the RME program. Most begin using the RME orthosis within 5 to 7 days of repair with inclusion of a wrist orthosis dependent on the zone of injury and therapist's preference. Some require another orthosis for overnight, and some add a wrist orthosis if an extensor lag is present initially.[10,24,33] In the original ICAM study, workers safely returned to work in an average of 18 days wearing both the RME finger and wrist orthoses, Hirth and colleagues'[2,24] workers returned wearing the RME orthosis only by 3.3 weeks. These early return-to-work times have not been matched, which may be a result of restrictions appended by others to the original ICAM program, such as no driving or light use only. Collocott and coworkers[23] described the dilemma between the employer and the injured worker when the worker is advised to return to work under such provisions of no driving or no more than light duty use, for which the employer has no such work available or orthosis wear is not permitted on the worksite.

Of primary importance, no tendon ruptures have been reported by use of the RME-only orthosis or the combined wrist and finger RME orthoses. There have been only a few minor complications mentioned such as suture irritation, edema, and superficial skin infections, all of which resolved.[2,3,14,20,23,24]

The number of therapy sessions has decreased from seven sessions reported in the 2005 ICAM report to four to six sessions.[2,3] Studies that have compared the RME-only orthosis with dynamic, early active motion, and immobilization programs found recovery of ROM substantially easier at 3 to 4 weeks for the RME group. However, by 3 months, all programs had comparable motion.[20,23,24] Measurement of ROM remains the most widely used method for reporting results of extensor tendon repair management. However, because there is no universal grading system or designated time to measure, comparison among studies is difficult.[3] Authors who report on grip strength make comparison with the opposite hand, which show an 85% recovery by week 8 and 100% by week 12.[3] Assessment of patient's hand function with the Sollerman Hand Function Test has been compared between RME-only orthosis users and those assigned to another early active motion program wearing a wrist–hand–finger static orthosis with the IP joints free. At 1 month after surgery, those wearing the RME-only orthosis had significantly better Sollerman Test and QuickDASH (Disability of the Arm, Shoulder and Hand) scores of function and total active motion and less loss of flexion and at 8 weeks were found more satisfied with the RME-only orthosis.[23]

Sagittal Band Injuries and Rupture: Acute and Chronic

The long extensor tendon in zones IV and V over the MCP joint level is maintained in a central position by deep and superficial fibers of the sagittal bands, which arise from the volar plate, flexor tendon sheath, proximal annular pulley, and intermetacarpal ligaments and form a retinacular tunnel that attaches to the extensor hood to stabilize the long extensor tendon during active motion. The MCP joint is extended through this sagittal band lasso noose, lifting up on the proximal phalanx. If this "ring" is broken by sagittal band disruption, the tendon may dislocate to a position between the metacarpal heads, and active extension will fail from the flexed MCP joint position.

Ryan and Murray[37] classified sagittal band injuries into three types, all of which can benefit from RME orthotic management. Type 1 is a contusion without tear or instability of the sagittal band. Type 2 involves tearing of the sagittal band tunnel, sometimes with painful snapping of the extensor tendon but without complete

TABLE 107.1   Relative Motion Extension Orthosis Only Studies Since 2005 Shown by Zone and Author Changes to the Original Immediate Controlled Active Motion Program for Extensor Zones IV to VI

Reference (Year)	Patients (n)	Zone IV	Zone V	Zone VI	Changes to Original ICAM Program, Including No Wrist Orthosis
Berry et al[6] (2008)	14	1	11	2	No further changes
Hirth et al[24] (2011)	23	—	21	2	*Added*: night WHFO *Advice*: no combined finger and wrist flexion
Burns et al[7] (2013)	2	—	2	—	*Inclusion criteria*: only simple injuries *Advice*: no heavy lifting in RME orthosis
Izadpanah et al[33] (2015)	55	20	30	5	*Inclusion criteria*: only simple injuries; zone IV proximally only and zone VI to distally only
Svens et al[20] (2015)[a]	13	1[b]	12[b]	—	*Orthotic use*: 4 wk *Added*: WHO for all EDM[b] repairs and all zone VI repairs (see Table 107.2)
Turner[34] (2015)[c]	31	4[d]	18[d]	9[d]	*Added*: WHO or WHFO when extensor lag initially present *Inclusion criteria*: zone IV proximal only and zone VI to distally only
Collocott[23] (2016)	22	—	15	7	*Added*: night WHFO *Inclusion criteria*: only simple injuries except 2 digits with multiple repairs in both zones V and VI *Advice*: no combined fist and wrist flexion, driving, and specific activities
Pilbeam (C. Pilbeam, written communication March 2018)	8	1	7	0	*Inclusion criteria*: zones IV and V only *Added*: WHO for all EDM and zone VI–VII repairs (see Table 107.2)
Pilbeam (C. Pilbeam, written communication March 2018)	35	11[e]	21[e]	7[e]	*Added*: night splint not routine; added on occasion if extensor lag developed
Approximate RME orthosis only (203 patients with 212 tendon repairs reported in 207 zones)		**38**	**137**	**32**	

[a]One participant had two injured fingers.
[b]Three small finger repairs noted in one group, so numbers are approximate.
[c]Audit of 56 patients; extensor tendon detail available on 31 patients.
[d]Wrist orthosis when extensor lag initially present, so numbers are approximate.
[e]A total of 43 tendon repairs in 35 patients and 39 zones.
EDM, Extensor digiti minimi; *ICAM*, immediate controlled active motion; *RME*, relative motion extension; *WHFO*, wrist–hand–finger orthosis; *WHO*, wrist–hand orthosis.

TABLE 107.2   Relative Motion Extension + Wrist Orthoses: Studies Since 2005 Shown by Zone and Author Changes to Original Immediate Controlled Active Motion Program for Extensor Zones IV to VI

Reference (Year)	Patients (n)	Zone IV	Zone V	Zone VI	Author Changes to Original ICAM Program
Howell et al[2] (2005)	135	4	112	9	Not applicable; original ICAM program
Berry et al[6] (2008)	7	2	3	2	*Orthotic use*: worn an average of 45 days
Blakeway[36] (2013)	1		1		No changes to original ICAM program
Altobelli et al[35] (2013)[a]	5	1	5		*Added*: night WHFO
Svens et al[20] (2015)[b]	50	2	35	12 5	*Orthotic use*: work 6 wk by 45 patients in 49 zones and in 5 zone VI repairs worn 4 wk
Pilbeam[18] (2016)[c]	25	5	18	2	*Added*: prefabricated WHO substituted for custom WHO
Pilbeam (2018)[d] (written communication, March 2018)	23	1	8	15	*Inclusion criteria*: zones VI–VII and all EDM repairs (C)
Approximate RME + wrist orthosis (246 patients with 266 tendon repairs reported in 252 zones)		**25**	**182**	**45**	

[a]Two tendon repairs in one patient.
[b]A total of 48 fingers involved in 45 patients in 49 zones.
[c]A total of 29 tendon repairs in 25 patients.
[d]A total 35 tendon repairs in 23 patients in 24 zones because 1 patient was combined zone V–VI repair.
EDM, Extensor digitorum minimi; *ICAM*, immediate controlled active motion; *RME*, relative motion extension.

BOX 107.1   Use of Relative Motion Extension With or Without the Wrist Orthosis: An Update From the Original ICAM Program for Managment of Extensor Tendon Zones IV to VII[2,a]

0–10 days postoperative: RME with or without wrist orthoses; zone VII modifications[a]

Exercise in RME orthosis: active hook fist and composite finger flexion/extension

Advice: light functional hand use (10 lb/4.5 kg)

Avoid combined fist with wrist flexion

11–14 days postoperative: RME with or without wrist orthosis

Exercises in RME orthosis: continue finger exercises; add isolated wrist motion

Advice: light to medium functional hand use (10–20 lb/4.5–9 kg)

Avoid combined fist with wrist flexion *except zone VII*

2–3 wk postoperative: RME with or without wrist orthosis

Exercise in RME orthosis: continue finger exercises, add fist with wrist flexion

Advice: light to medium functional hand use (10–20 lb/4.5–9 kg)

3–6 wk postoperative: RME orthosis only, all zones

Advice: medium to unrestricted functional hand use (20 lb/9 kg)

Consider: wrist orthosis only without RME orthosis for zone VII

4–8 wk postoperative: at clinician's discretion discontinue all orthoses and therapy

Advice: medium to unrestricted functional hand use for work or sports

Zone VII modification[a]

0–10 days: fabricate orthosis with wrist in neutral to 20 degrees flexion for maximum zone VII tendon excursion

11–14 days: if tendon tethers or lags, add wrist exercises wearing RME orthosis; flex wrist 35 degrees then gently fist; extend wrist to neutral with fingers fully extended

[a]Offered as a guideline only; does not imply mandatory protocol.
ICAM, Immediate active controlled motion; *RME,* relative motion extension.

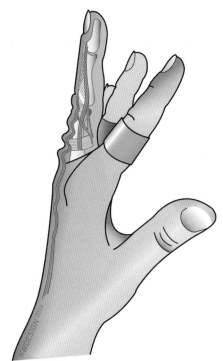

Fig. 107.4 Relative motion extension position demonstrating slack in common extensor, sagittal band, and extensor hood. (© *2018 KW Design.* Contact Katie Wright of KW Design; Wright.design.illustration@gmail.com.)

Acute Sagittal Band Injury

For a patient with a typical acute sagittal band rupture, extension is possible when the EDC tendon is out of the intermetacarpal space and only redevelops when full flexion is attempted. Evidence is variable about how late conservative management can be effective for patients with complete tendon dislocation. Peelman and associates[12] used the RME orthosis after sagittal band rupture and found better success (95%) when patients were treated within 3 weeks of injury and a significant decrease (62%) in success after 6 weeks. The authors' experience has been that if there is still inflammation present at 6 weeks, there is a better chance for success with this orthosis technique, and when wearing the orthosis, most patients soon reported pain relief. Pain is frequently relieved with use of an RME orthosis as opposed to buddy taping, which has been reported to remain painful even after 1 year of taping.[39] It should be noted that when extensor tendon subluxation is constant and occurs without pain, swelling, or other inflammatory manifestations, nonsurgical measures can be expected to fail.[1]

Nonsurgical management of sagittal band injuries with the RME orthosis is relatively new for hand therapists, so a synopsis of the following studies is worth review. Several authors have successfully used a three- or four-finger RME orthosis design to position painful digits in 25 to 35 degrees of relative extension full time for 6 to 8 weeks.[11,12] In one large study of nonrheumatoid patients with sagittal band injury, traumatic or atraumatic onset did not affect the results in the acute (<3 weeks' onset) and subacute (3–6 weeks' onset) groups if treatment started within 6 weeks of onset of symptoms. The length of orthotic management ranged from 3 to 16 weeks, with pain resolved in most, although tendon subluxation was not always corrected. There were equal numbers of patients within the traumatic and atraumatic onset groups who eventually chose to have surgery.[12] The trend has been for most reports to exclude

dislocation. Type 3 consists of tendon dislocation into the groove between the metacarpal heads, most frequently to the ulnar side. Ishizuki[38] described superficial and deep sagittal band layers, suggesting that spontaneous sagittal band rupture observed in patients with connective tissue disorders might involve only the superficial layer, whereas traumatic dislocation most likely involves both layers. A healing sagittal band is well protected by the RME orthosis only because it prevents the fully flexed MCP joint position that leads to dislocation, maintaining the injured extensor tendon sagittal band complex in a more lax tension than its neighboring digits. The orthosis protectively places the injured or repaired extensor retinacular system as well as the proximal extensor hood on slack (Fig. 107.4). When the RME orthosis is used with the affected digits in relatively more MCP extension, tension from the pull of the EDC is reduced as a result of the "quadriga effect," allowing for safe active ROM. Contouring the sides of the RME orthosis during fabrication to hug the finger keeps it protected and centralizes the tendon. Use of the RME orthosis during the healing phase allows for the early active motion necessary to limit adhesion formation and to guide remodeling.[1–3,14] rheumatoid patients from RME orthosis use after sagittal band rupture. However, our experience has been that rheumatoid patients with sagittal band injuries benefit from the RME orthosis when used as "protective" orthoses, provided the sagittal band rupture is the only problem and not accompanied by the presence of MCP joint volar subluxation and ulnar translocation of the flexor tendons. However, when RME orthoses are used as "adaptive" orthoses to improve hand function, even with these coexisting problems, patients with rheumatoid arthritis certainly do benefit.[1,3]

In the authors' experience, the RME program for nonsurgical management of acute sagittal band ruptures should be individualized to each patient, with the relative angle of extension of the affected digit MCP joint determined by observing the stability of the extensor tendon during active motion (Video 107.3). If more stability is needed, the orthosis can be modified by contouring the trough of the orthosis to hug the digit or by widening the volar aspect of the orthosis to reduce the arc of proximal interphalangeal (PIP) joint flexion or include the digit radial to the affected digit until pain and subluxation observed during movement is gone. If these adaptations do not provide the desired stability, a wrist orthosis can be tried to eliminate the destabilizing forces noted to occur during concurrent finger and wrist flexion with ulnar deviation.[39] The RME orthosis provides protective stability, so patients are encouraged to functionally use their hands, and wear should be full time for at least 6 weeks and for some as long as 3 months before surgery is considered. Although not common, some patients unknowingly remove their RME orthoses during sleep, interfering with sagittal band healing. To avoid this, fabrication of a less easily removed orthosis for nighttime wear may be required, or the RME orthosis may be taped to the hand overnight.

Chronic Sagittal Band Injury and Ruptures

Patients with chronic sagittal band ruptures and failed nonsurgical management require surgical reconstruction. The typically published conventional techniques have two common features: (1) to stabilize the ruptured side (usually ulnar) by reefing, grafting, or transferring tendon slips with the proper tension to centralize the tendon and (2) to immobilize the hand for 6 to 10 weeks followed by an intensive therapy program to recover motion. Merritt and coworkers[1] first described the use of the RME orthosis only for chronic sagittal band rupture in an older adult patient with rheumatoid arthritis, who, depending on which way her finger pointed, subluxed the tendon to either the radial or ulnar side, likely because of repeated steroid injections. This obviated the typical reconstruction techniques to stabilize the rupture side, so a juncturae tendinum graft pulley passed through the metacarpal head was used to centralize the EDC. Postoperatively, the dilemma to avoid adherence by means of early motion without rupture was solved by using the RME orthosis for 6 weeks, also permitting functional use of her hand and recovery of normal ROM without further subluxation.[1]

Subsequently, 23 patients with similar sagittal band reconstructions have been reported, with equivalent results achieved using various centralized tendon grafts, including half of the flexor carpi ulnaris; half of the EIP; the juncturae tendinum; and most frequently, the palmaris longus, passing the centralized graft through a drill-hole tunnel in the metacarpal head followed by 6 weeks of RME orthosis management.[40] It is likely any of the published techniques for correcting chronic sagittal band rupture can be successfully managed with the RME-only orthosis (Videos 107.4 and 104.5).

RELATIVE MOTION FLEXION

Relative Motion Flexion Orthosis for Boutonnière Deformity: "Winslow's Diamond"

Boutonnière deformity has remained the most difficult of extensor tendon management problems, with acute injury intervention typically requiring 2 to 4 months out of work and the chronic fixed boutonnière deformity a conundrum that often defies any acceptable correction with current surgical or nonsurgical technique. Chronic deformity occurs largely because when first seen after injury, the deformity is frequently not present, and the diagnosis is not apparent without a careful, knowledgeable physical examination. *The best treatment of boutonnière deformity is to avoid the deformity* by early diagnosis and treatment. The authors believe that emergency department and immediate care physicians, primary care providers, hand surgeons, and hand therapists all need to be knowledgeable about the clinical tests that will reveal the occult boutonnière injury (Elson's, modified Elson's, and Boyes' tests).[25] Any time the boutonnière injury diagnosis is in doubt, use of the RMF orthosis offers the ability to continue normal hand function during recovery and is a safe-protective alternative, worn full time until confirmation by clinical assessment, ultrasound, or magnetic resonance imaging (MRI).

The 18th century Danish-born French anatomist Jacob B. Winslow (1669–1760) described the *tendinous rhombus* that later became known as "Winslow's diamond,"[41] which represents the dynamic relationship between the extrinsic and intrinsic muscle contributors to the extensor mechanism. This tendinous diamond encircles the PIP joint, making it critical not only to balanced IP joint extension but also to potential use of the RMF orthosis to manage boutonnière injury (Fig. 107.5).

Biomechanical engineers have offered complex computerized mathematical studies of Winslow's diamond relationships, citing the importance of the position of the MCP and PIP joints on tendon forces in the isolated digit. There has been little or no attention given to the significance of how changing the position of the MCP joints relative to each other alters the force relationship of the extrinsic flexor and extensor muscles and as a result causes an important IP joint response because of the dynamics of Winslow's diamond.[41-45]

Boutonnière deformity provides a unique opportunity for the RMF orthosis to provide simultaneous useful "quadriga effect" from both flexor and extensor extrinsic motor systems. The first opportunity to provide the "quadriga effect" comes from the flexor side in the profundi and the lumbrical muscles arising from the radial side of the profundi tendons. Although controversial, Kaplan[46] and Brand[47] both regarded the lumbrical as the principal extensor of the IP joints. Although not as powerful as the interossei, the lumbrical has four times greater excursion required for IP joint amplitude of motion and is more volarly positioned as it passes from beneath the deep transverse metacarpal ligament, giving it a greater angle for flexion leverage. Additionally, there is suggestion that it may provide sensory–motor feedback to position the IP system.[45] Zancolli's[48] electromyographic studies confirm that the lumbrical remains active throughout digital extension, whereas the interossei is only intermittently active. He found that the powerful interossei are most active when there is need for forceful IP joint extension such as to stabilize the MCP joint in flexion against the powerful pull of the long extensors through its lateral slips and the lumbrical on the lateral bands.[47] This becomes apparent if one palpates the first dorsal interosseous muscle; then weakly extends the index finger IP joint; and then without changing the position of the MCP joint, more forcefully extends the IP joint to feel firm contractions of the

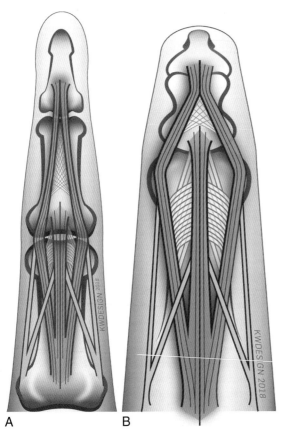

Fig. 107.5 Winslow' diamond. **A,** "Cinched diamond" with the proximal interphalangeal (PIP) joint in extension with lateral bands positioned dorsal medially. **B,** "Relaxed diamond" with the PIP joint in flexion with lateral bands positioned laterally volar. (© *2018 KW Design.* Contact Katie Wright of KW Design; Wright.design.illustration@gmail.com.)

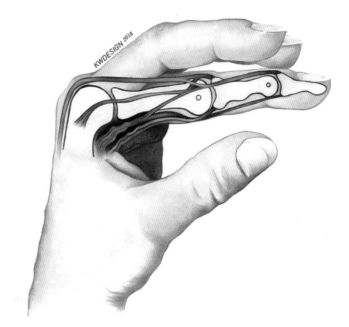

Fig. 107.6 Simultaneously beneficial "quadriga effect." Relative motion flexion position with the flexor digitorum profundus–lumbrical on slack and the extrinsic common extensor tensioned. (© *2018 KW Design.* Contact Katie Wright of KW Design; Wright.design.illustration@gmail.com.)

interosseous muscle. In the absence of interosseous function, one sees MCP joint hyperextension as in the fourth and fifth digits of an ulnar palsied hand. Because lumbricals arise from the profundi, placing an MCP joint in 15 to 20 degrees greater flexion relaxes that profundus tendon compared with its neighbors because of their common muscle, thereby also relaxing the lumbrical at its origin (Fig. 107.6). In boutonnière deformity, the lumbrical appears to be the principal deforming force to pull the lateral bands below the PIP joint axis of rotation, attenuating the residually weakened horizontal and oblique extensor hood fibers and injured triangular ligament of Winslow.

Under normal conditions, the extensor hood fibers and Winslow's triangular ligament function to restrain the lateral band–conjoined tendon complex above the axis of PIP joint rotation as the complex shifts volar and lateral during flexion of the PIP joint, as described by Winslow.[41] In boutonnière deformity, the central slip attachment is absent, and the lateral bands are abnormally positioned below the joint axis of rotation, which allows the extrinsic extensor to pull the MCP joint into hyperextension and by way of the lateral slip attachments to the now relocated lateral band–conjoined tendon complex to cause PIP joint flexion and distal interphalangeal (DIP) joint hyperextension unless the RMF orthosis is used to alter the extrinsic extension force acting on the MCP and IP joints. Because the MCP joint of the affected digit is positioned in greater flexion, a simultaneously useful "quadriga effect" is created to relax pull of the long extensor–lateral slips and profundus–lumbrical muscle pull on the lateral bands. In fact, when the

digit is placed in the RMF position, provided it is not a fixed boutonnière deformity, the lateral bands will dorsally reposition with active extension of the IP joints.

The second opportunity for the "quadriga effect" comes from the dorsal hand through the EDC tendons and their important trifurcation proximal to the PIP joint, the central slip inserting into the base of the middle phalanx and the lateral slips joining the combined interossei and lumbrical lateral bands to ultimately form the conjoined tendon that crosses the DIP joint to unite distally as the terminal tendon. Winslow[41] described the dynamics of this encircling "diamond" that normally separates and widens when the PIP joint is flexed and the EDC tendon is relaxed and then with PIP extension relocates centrally in a "cinching" fashion as the intrinsic and extrinsic tendons muscles actively contract (see Fig. 107.5). However, the lateral slips of the extrinsic long extensor tendon are quite capable of extending the IP joints alone without any intrinsic function. This is evidenced in complete ulnar nerve palsy when a dorsal blocking orthosis is used to position the palsied fourth and fifth digits in equal or greater MCP joint flexion relative to the radial digits and the lateral slips of the engaged long extensor produces IP joint extension in the affected digits. This same response can be created by the RMF orthosis when there is complete disruption of the central slip, extensor hood, and triangular ligament as long as the lateral band position remains correctable and the slack in Winslow's loop is compensated by placing the affected MCP joint(s) in 15 to 20 degrees greater flexion.

The relative position of the MCP joints creates a simultaneously beneficial quadriga effect in the muscles of the extrinsic long extensor as well as the lumbrical via its origin from the profundus (see Fig. 107.6). Importantly, these beneficial differences in forces persist throughout the full range of active motion as permitted by the RMF orthosis because of the quadriga effect. The fact that the lumbrical origins of the fourth and fifth digits are bimodal does not seem to adversely influence the successful use of the RMF orthosis for these digits. A possible reason could be the powerful counterforce dispersed from the EDC through the lateral slips into the lateral band–conjoined tendon by the RMF orthosis.

Isolated disruption of the EDC's central slip insertion into the middle phalanx alone does not cause boutonnière deformity, as evidenced by the Fowler procedure, which carefully divides this central attachment from underneath the extensor hood to rebalance the extrinsic–intrinsic relationship for chronic mallet deformity.[49] A boutonnière deformity does not result from this procedure because the surrounding extensor hood and Winslow's triangular ligament remain intact. Often after an acute boutonnière injury, the extent of extensor hood and triangular ligament of Winslow injury varies so that deformity may occur immediately or later. Provided enough of these structures remain intact to restrain the lateral bands dorsal to the PIP joint axis of rotation, the patient will be able to fully extend the PIP joint. However, if not protected after the PIP joint injury, the volar pull of the lumbrical will gradually attenuate these injured structures until the PIP joint "buttonholes" into the boutonnière deformity unless extrinsic and intrinsic muscle activity is counterbalanced by the RMF orthosis. This is why so many patients with boutonnière injury present initially with apparent normal ROM, only to progress to the deformity in subsequent weeks if undiagnosed and improperly managed.

The requirements for boutonnière deformity were defined by a recent innovative cadaver model.[50] In this model, Grau and colleagues[50] divided various combinations of Winslow's ligament, extensor hood fibers, and the central slip. After dividing the central slip, a "modest" amount (2.4 degrees) of PIP joint extension was lost. However, missing from their model was lumbrical input, known as an important contributor to full PIP joint extension after a Fowler procedure. After further division of the extensor hood and Winslow's ligament, a "marked" (29.2-degree) loss of PIP joint extension resulted; however, a boutonnière deformity was not created until all three structures were divided and the PIP joint was flexed to greater than 35 degrees.[50] It appears that if an RMF orthosis had been introduced into the study, the boutonnière deformity could have been avoided. A similar example was demonstrated at the 2003 ASHT meeting when all three structures were divided and the PIP joint flexed and extended with and without the RMF orthosis (see Video 107.1).

Acute Boutonnière Deformity

When patients present with an inability to extend the PIP joint or have painful full extension, it is important to determine whether the pain or loss of extension is attributable to disruption of the central slip, extensor hood, or Winslow's triangular ligament (boutonnière deformity); a flexion contracture preceded by a pulley or volar plate injury (pseudo boutonnière); or a skin or Dupuytren's cord contracture.

Elson's test[51] and the modified Elson's test[52] are used to examine for early central slip involvement after acute closed boutonnière injury. The Boyes test is often more useful for late deformity, although at times, it can identify boutonnière before deformity.[53] Elson's test requires full flexion of the PIP joint over a table edge and assessment of the patient's ability to extend the PIP joint and then observation for any extension force at the DIP joint. If the central slip is disrupted, PIP joint extension will be weakened, and the DIP joint may extend if the conjoined lateral bands have not slipped volarly. The modified Elson test offers visible evidence of volar displacement of the lateral bands by comparing the affected finger with the noninjured finger. This is done by placing the dorsal surface of the same digit of the opposite hand against the middle phalanx of the injured digit, keeping both PIP joints flexed to 90 degrees and requesting the patient to

extend the DIP joints. If the lateral bands have shifted volarly, there will be greater extension seen in the DIP joint of the injured digit.[52]

The Boyes test can be useful in acute injury, especially if there is some deformity. To perform this test, the PIP joint is first held in passive extension by the examiner while active and passive motion of the DIP joint is observed; second, the PIP joint is flexed, and DIP joint motion is compared. Volarly displaced lateral bands are verified if the DIP joint has less active and passive flexion when the PIP joint is extended compared with when the PIP joint is flexed.[53] In some acute patients, however, the result of the Boyes test might be negative if the lateral bands easily slide above and below the axis of rotation and full passive PIP extension is still possible.[25] However, in *chronic* boutonnière deformity, when lateral bands have become adherent, the Boyes test is usually the most useful provided the DIP joint remains supple. In the chronic stage, when the lateral bands become adherent, the DIP joint component of the test is restricted, so Elson's test may not be of value. It is important that use of these tests is done to also separate PIP joints that have lack of extension because of flexor pulley or volar plate damage or stenosing tenosynovitis (pseudoboutonnière) from those with central slip, extensor hood, and Winslow's triangular ligament involvement (boutonnière deformity). On examination, it is our experience that injuries to the volar PIP joint structures will test negative on the Elson and Boyes tests. Because of the flexor tendon restriction, only limited success will be achieved with use of the RMF orthosis because the relaxation of the flexor tendon is only temporary, with no correction of the primary problem. Unfortunately, late flexor tendon contracture or chronic extensor boutonnière deformity often has the same fixed ankylosed DIP joint that prohibits accurate clinical testing. MRI or ultrasound study can confirm whether the deformity originates from the dorsal or volar structures. In general, ultrasound seems preferable if extensor injury is likely,[54] and MRI may better determine the cause of flexor injury.

The authors find the "pencil test" is a simple way to simulate either the RMF or RME orthosis. This is done by placing a pencil, cotton-tipped applicator, or tongue depressor above (RMF) or below (RME) the proximal phalanx of the injured digit compared with the neighboring digits followed by active flexion and extension of the digit[17] (see the Critical Points box). This simulated RME–RMF pencil test is useful, for example, when examining an acutely injured PIP joint or the painful digit[55] or during intraoperative assessment using the simulated orthosis to determine how much active motion is safe.

Relative motion flexion is a fairly new orthotic management program with no established protocols. Various management techniques are used by different hand therapists and hand surgeons, although the anatomic rationale remains the same. Success requires the patient to understand the value of wearing the RMF orthosis full time after early diagnosis to avoid developing a boutonnière deformity or advancing an established deformity. If the early finger deformity is supple and easily correctable in the RMF position, the only requirement is to wear the RMF orthosis full time for 6 weeks, all the while moving the fingers through ROM and functionally using the hand. Therapy needs are minimal for a supple, orthosis-corrected deformity, needing only to be monitored to ensure compliance and recovery of motion and for orthosis adjustment.[25] Individualized therapy management is required in patients whose digits have developed DIP hyperextension or early volar PIP joint remodeling. Author WHM suggests that if the RMF orthosis is applied immediately after injury on fingers with supple PIP joints, DIP joint hyperextension will be corrected simply by wearing the RMF orthosis and using an orthosis to block

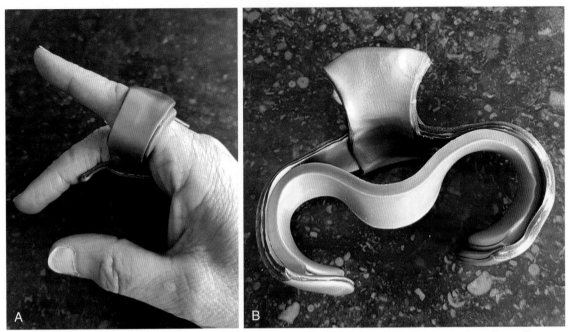

Fig. 107.7 A, Relative motion flexion (RMF) orthosis with flexion block attachment for the long finger. **B,** Flexion block attachment *(orange)* and RMF orthosis *(blue).* (Photo and orthosis design courtesy of © 2018 Gwendolyn van Strien, LPT, MSc.)

DIP joint hyperextension while allowing DIP joint flexion. In an acute boutonnière deformity, author JWH initially limits PIP joint flexion so as to not interfere with dorsal repositioning of the lateral bands. This is in contrast to author WHM, who encourages full active flexion any time full active extension has been achieved in the RMF orthosis.

Fingers in which DIP joint hyperextension is accompanied by a PIP joint extension lag (although the joint is passively supple) may require both a DIP hyperextension block and RMF orthosis until extrinsic–intrinsic balance is restored. In the course of acute boutonnière assessment, author JWH applies the RMF orthosis–simulated "pencil test" to get a sneak preview before fabricating the RMF orthosis. For example, when "pencil tested," the desired response in a supple PIP joint is that it actively extends to at least 20 degrees of neutral with minimal DIP joint hyperextension and has full passive extension. This indicates that the digit is a perfect candidate for the RMF orthosis worn full time for 6 weeks. However, if during the pencil test a similar supple digit achieves less than 20 to 30 degrees of active PIP joint extension (and there is no volar joint injury history), author JWH would add an RMF attachment to limit PIP joint flexion initially to 35 degrees, worn full time until active PIP extension improves to at least −20 degrees of neutral (Fig. 107.7). As active PIP joint extension continues to improve, the flexion block attachment can be either adjusted to allow more flexion or eliminated altogether with the RMF orthosis worn for at least another 6 weeks as determined by the therapist. It is common for some patients to not tolerate wearing the RMF orthosis at night, often removing it, so it may be necessary to use a static PIP joint extension orthosis for nighttime comfort and to better protect the finger. Patients with generalized joint hypermobility may require an additional orthosis to limit hyperextension of the DIP joint, worn together with the RMF orthosis to restore the extrinsic–intrinsic balance necessary for full PIP joint extension.

An acute open boutonnière surgical repair should be done under the Lalonde WALANT technique[32] using local anesthesia with epinephrine

because the delicate intrinsic–extrinsic balance is difficult to restore without the patient's active "awake" cooperation; this also provides the opportunity to apply the RMF position while in surgery to determine how much PIP joint flexion is safe for the repair (Video 107.6). After acute inflammation has subsided a few days after surgery, therapy to fabricate and fit the RMF orthosis, educate, and manage motion recovery with full-time orthosis wear is suggested for 6 to 8 weeks.

Chronic Boutonnière Deformity

Chronic boutonnière deformity has been an unresolved problem. In fact, any better active PIP joint extension than −20 degrees is considered an "excellent" result, and because of poor surgical results, no surgical effort is recommended if extension is no worse than −30 degrees.[56] The conundrum regarding inconsistent surgical outcomes was addressed in a recent literature review, with the authors concluding that "hand surgeons disagree not only on the best surgery, but even if surgery makes the finger better at all."[57] Historically, nonsurgical management of patients with chronic boutonnière deformity has been restricted to intermittent serial casting with prolonged immobilization producing variable results with significant morbidity and frequent recurrent deformity. There is, however, wide agreement that before any other definitive treatment is considered, all digits with fixed PIP joint flexion contractures should be serial casted to gain as much passive PIP joint extension as possible, with at least −20 degrees recommended and as much recovery of DIP flexion as possible.

Jarrell and Merritt,[58] in their series of acute and chronic boutonnière deformities, serially casted all 15 chronic cases for an average of 2.5 weeks to achieve −20 degrees or less of passive PIP joint extension. Serial casting was followed by 3 months of full-time RMF orthosis wear, and therapy management required an average of 7.5 therapy sessions. In their series, the initial passive PIP joint extension in the chronic boutonnière deformities averaged −29 degrees (ranging from zero to −55), and final measures in these patients with chronic boutonnière deformities were rated as "excellent" by Steichen and Strickland[56] standards. In this group, an unforeseen average increase in combined IP joint ROM of 35.9 degrees was realized as a result of gains in both extension and flexion. Jarrell[58] stated that the most common reason for patients to return to therapy was to replace well-worn broken orthoses, which led her to routinely provide a second replacement orthosis. Although in this series, adequate PIP joint extension was achieved with serial casting, it is conceivable that if a PIP joint remains stiff and cannot be passively corrected to at least −20 degrees of PIP joint extension, a surgical release and reconstruction under WALANT followed by postoperative use of an RMF orthosis could offer greater success.

Chronic boutonnière deformity encompasses a wide spectrum of injury and chronicity for therapists to manage. Some patients are sent to therapy to prepare for surgical correction; for others, therapy is the final attempt to maximize digit function. To individualize management, an essential piece of the puzzle includes a "functional assessment" undertaken by a hand therapist regarding the patient's functional and emotional needs. For example, if the PIP joint active extension lag can be passively improved to 30 to 35 degrees, some will be satisfied and willing to wear an RMF orthosis indefinitely as an "adaptive" orthosis, but others will be dissatisfied. Some may experience functional improvement from passive correction of the IP joint deformity contractures but find no value in wearing an RMF orthosis full time. Awareness through functional assessment of the patient's goals will improve outcome acceptance. By definition, a chronic boutonnière deformity involves soft tissue changes of variable IP joint stiffness. Recovery of the 20/20 goal: 20 degrees of active DIP joint flexion and at least −20 degrees of passive PIP joint extension before RMF orthosis use is ideal and may be achieved with serial casting. Usually therapist preference determines the approach; choices include as a serial cast for both IP joints or a PIP joint cast worn with a progressive static DIP joint flexion orthosis. Often a piece of the boutonnière posture is MCP joint hyperextension; to counteract this, an RMF orthosis can be paired with the IP joint cast or orthosis. In the most challenging chronic boutonnière cases, author JWH prefers to reach the 20/20 goal and at least 30 degrees of active PIP joint extension before active PIP joint flexion in the RMF orthosis. When these guiding parameters are achieved, the transition from PIP joint casting into RMF orthosis wear should be therapist guided to individualize the program. For successful transition, the therapist and patient will need to determine how much PIP joint flexion is safe. One criterion is to use the patient's sense of "tightness" during IP

joint flexion, usually felt over the dorsal middle phalanx at about 30 to 40 degrees flexion of each IP joint. Author JWH limits PIP joint flexion by adding an attachment to the RMF orthosis to block flexion but allow extension (see Fig. 107.7). Subsequently over the next few weeks, the flexion block is pared down, guided by the feeling of tightness and goniometric measurement. Keeping realistic therapy goals in mind is important when managing patients with chronic deformities; few will have a perfect result. More realistically, the goal may be to recover "functional PIP joint motion." Functional PIP joint motion has been observed to be −23 degrees of extension and 87 degrees of flexion,[59] which aligns with the Steichen-Strickland classification result of excellent as −20 degrees of extension and 80 degrees of flexion and good −30 degrees of extension and 70 degrees of flexion.[56] It has been the author's (JWH) experience that management of the chronic boutonnière deformity accompanied by these stiffer soft tissue changes may require 3 to 6 months of limited therapy to maximize therapy results for the purpose of monitoring motion, education, and ensuring proper orthotic fit and function. For patients who chose to manage their chronic boutonnière long term, a custom-made commercially available jewelry-type orthosis and a static PIP extension orthosis for night wear might be needed.

Repaired Central Slip Extensor Tendon Zone III

Several therapy programs have been suggested for use after extensor tendon zone III central slip repair, including short-arc active motion,[60] a dynamic-assist orthosis,[61] a combination of a static PIP joint extension and an RMF orthoses,[62] and the RMF orthosis. The value and simplicity of the RMF program is that after repair, the patient wears the orthosis full time for 4 to 6 weeks while able to functionally use the hand and simultaneously exercise the finger. The RMF orthosis protects the repaired central slip in many ways. Early postoperative therapy management requires knowing how much PIP joint flexion is safe for the repair. If at the time of WALANT surgery author WHM determines that full flexion was easily achieved in the RMF position, postoperatively, he encourages full PIP joint ROM in the RMF orthosis. When no surgeon guidelines have been provided or motion has not been observed under WALANT, author JWH is guided by the important marker of 35 degrees of PIP joint flexion coupled with the patient's feeling of "tightness." RMF orthosis fabrication can include either the PIP joint flexion block attachment (see Fig. 107.7) or a dorsal static PIP joint extension addition (Fig. 107.8).

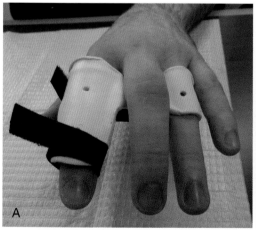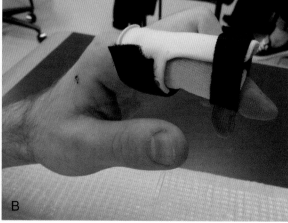

Fig. 107.8 A, Relative motion flexion (RMF) orthosis modified with dorsal static interphalangeal (IP) joint extension component and guide strap used for central slip repair. **B,** Strap-guided early active progressive IP joint flexion–extension within the three-finger design RMF orthosis. (Photo and orthosis design courtesy of © 2018 Clyde Johnson PT, CHT.)

The suggested angle for PIP joint flexion postoperative progression is at least 75 degrees at week 4 and at least 100 degrees and discontinuation of the orthosis by week 6. Pairing active DIP joint flexion–extension as the PIP joint is held extended while wearing the RMF orthosis benefits tendon excursion and repair healing (Fig. 107.9). Through experience, author JWH has observed extensor lags of 15 to 20 degrees to resolve with full-time wear of the RMF orthosis; however, greater than 20-degree lags require detective work because a central slip is not a requirement for PIP joint extension, other critical dorsal structures may have been injured, or there is lateral band adherence, indicating a need for more PIP joint flexion and DIP joint flexion–extension exercises.

SUMMARY

Our goal for this chapter was to review the rationale for the RM concept used as a "protective orthosis" in hand therapy management of extensor tendon zone III to VI repairs, sagittal band injuries, and acute and chronic boutonnière deformity. Although beyond the scope of this chapter, RM has other applications as a "protective" orthosis such as in tendon transfers after attrition ruptures in caput ulnae syndrome and Vaughn-Jackson syndrome,[25] flexor tendon[63] and digital nerve repair,[3] skin grafting,[3] intrinsic transfers,[3] intrinsic musculotendinous injury,[55] and finger joint arthroplasty.[3] As an examination tool, the simulated RMF–RME pencil test is used to evaluate undetermined finger joint pain[3] and to sneak preview the quadriga effect before orthosis fabrication.[3] When used as an "exercise" orthosis, it is most often used to improve ROM after such conditions as Dupuytren's surgery or collagenase injection,[25] a mild flexion PIP joint contracture,[3,25] extensor hood adherence with PIP joint extension lag[3,25] (Fig. 107.10), MCP joint flexion that overpowers IP joint flexion,[64] or PIP joint hyperextension by stretching tight intrinsic muscles.[3]

Finally, one of the most exciting RM orthotic applications is what Hirth and coworkers[3] described as the "adaptive" orthosis category, which has been used to manage rheumatoid arthritis finger deformities and the muscle imbalances of ulnar nerve palsy, cerebral palsy, Parkinson's disease, and after C5 to C6 discectomy.[3,64] The authors look forward to further expansion that may provide deformity prevention such as for PIP joint strains, burned digits, adolescent hypermobile fingers, and early inflammatory arthritis. Many of these conditions require orthotic design originality and development of materials that are work or sport friendly, safe to be worn with open wounds, soft for

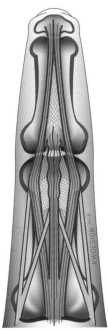

Fig. 107.9 Exercise for zone I to III proximal and distal lateral band excursion and application of controlled on/off stress to the central slip done by holding the proximal interphalangeal joint in extension as the distal interphalangeal joint is actively flexed and extended. (© *2018 KW Design*. Contact Katie Wright of KW Design; Wright.design.illustration@gmail.com.)

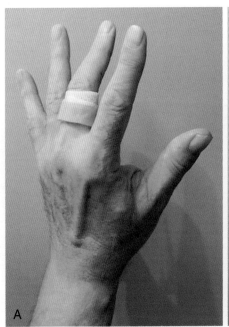
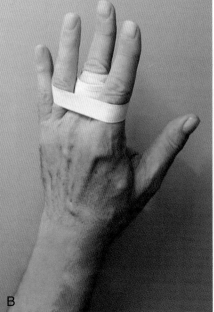

Fig. 107.10 A, Proximal phalanx (P1) long finger fracture brace with proximal interphalangeal joint extension lag. **B,** P1 fracture brace used in combination with the soft version, a three-finger design relative motion flexion orthosis used as an "exercise orthosis" for extensor lag correction. (Photo and orthosis design courtesy of © 2018 Dr. Lynne Feehan, BScPT, MSc, PhD.)

fragile skin, and aesthetically appealing for long-term wearers, all the while being compatible and focused on preserving useful hand function.[65,66] Refer to Video 107.7 for practical tips for fabrication of RM orthoses.

ACKNOWLEDGMENTS

The authors thank Sandra Robinson and Melissa Hirth for their invaluable insights in strengthening the content of this chapter and to recognize their major contributions to the concept of RM.

REFERENCES

1. Merritt WH, Howell JW, Tune R, et al. Achieving immediate active motion by using the relative motion splinting after long extensor repair and sagittal band ruptures with tendon subluxation. *Operative Tech Plast Reconstr Surg.* 2000;7:31–37.
2. Howell JW, Merritt WH, Robinson SJ. Immediate controlled active motion following zone 4-7 extensor tendon repair. *J Hand Ther.* 2005;18(2):182–190.
3. Hirth MJ, Howell JW, O'Brien L. Relative motion orthoses in the management of various hand conditions: a scoping review. *J Hand Ther.* 2016:405–432.
4. Merritt WH. Complications of hand surgery. In: Greenfield LJ, ed. *Complications in Surgery Trauma.* Philadelphia: Lippincott; 1984:852–885.
5. Saldana MJ. *Early Relative Motion Rehabilitation of Proximal Extensor Tendon Lacerations Using the "Wyndell Merritt" Splint.* Paper presented at: American Association for Hand Surgery Annual meeting 1997; Phoenix, AZ.
6. Berry N, Tonozzi J, Neumeister MW. AAHS concurrent scientific paper session B. Analysis of limited Wyndell Merritt splint for extensor tendon injuries to hand immobilization. *Hand.* 2008;3(2):170.
7. Burns MC, Derby B, Neumeister MW. Wyndell Merritt immediate controlled active motion (ICAM) protocol following extensor tendon repairs in zone IV-VII: review of the literature, orthosis design and case study-a multimedia article. *Hand.* 2013;8:17–22.
8. Robinson SJ. What is ICAM? *ASHT Times.* 2012;17:4–5.
9. Minchin K. "Soft yoke" to replace thermoplastic yoke for ICAM protocol. *AHTA Newsletter.* 2014;98:64.
10. Retallack L. *A review of the Effectiveness of the Border Digit Splints in the Treatment of Extensor Tendon Repairs Zones V & VI [Diploma]:* Diploma, Occupational Therapy. Perth; Western Australia: Curtin University of Technology; 2002.
11. Catalano LW, Gupta S, Ragland R, et al. Closed treatment of the non-rheumatoid extensor tendon dislocations at the metacarpophalangeal joint. *J Hand Surg.* 2006;31:242245.
12. Peelman J, Markiewitz A, Kiefhaber T, et al. Splintage in the treatment of sagittal band incompetence and extensor tendon subluxation. *J Hand Surg. Br.* 2015;40:287–290.
13. Merritt WH. What's in a name? "ICAM versus "relative motion" splints: What should we call these immediate active motion splints? *Hand Surg Q Fall.* 2012;8.
14. Hirth MJ, Howell JW, O'Brien L. Two case reports-use of relative motion orthoses to manage extensor tendon zones III and IV and sagittal band injuries in adjacent fingers. *J Hand Ther.* 2017;30:546–557.
15. Howell, JW Merritt WH. *Extensor Tendon Repair and Management with Immediate Controlled Active Motion.* Paper presented at: American Association for Hand Surgery Annual Meeting; Tucson, AZ: January 11-14, 2006.
16. Hirth MJ. *A Single Case Study of Relative Motion Extension Splinting & Relative Motion Flexion Splinting.* Paper presented at: American Association for Hand Surgery Annual Meeting; Kauai, HI: January 8-11, 2014.
17. Howell JW. Therapist's Corner- Relative motion flexion. In: *American Association for Hand Surgery.* Hand Association News. 2016.
18. Pilbeam C, Ellis J, Arundell M. Extensor tendon repairs zones 4 to 8: a year's prospective comparison audit of early active motion and immediate active motion regimes. Proceedings of IFSSH 2016, Buenos Aires, Argentina. *Hand.* 2016; suppl, Sept 26 101S–102S.
19. Rosenblum NI, Robinson SJ. Advances in flexor and extensor tendon management. In: Moran C, ed. *Hand Rehabilitation.* 1st ed. New York: Churchill Livingstone; 1986:17–44.
20. Svens B, Ames E, Burford K, et al. Relative active motion programs following extensor tendon repair: a pilot study using a prospective cohort and evaluating outcomes following orthotic interventions. *J Hand Ther.* 2015;1:11–19.
21. Robinson SJ, Rosenblum NI, Merritt WH. A new splint design for immediate active motion following extensor tendon repair. New Orleans: Paper presented at: American Society for Hand Therapists (ASHT) Conference 1986; February 14th-16th
22. Collocott SJF, Kelly E, Ellis RF. Optimal early active mobilization protocol after extensor tendon repairs in zones V-VI: a systematic review of the literature. *Hand Therapy.* 2017. online.
23. Collocott SJF. Can relative motion extension splinting (RMES) provide earlier return to function than a controlled active motion (CAM) protocol? *A Randomized Clinical Trial.* Unpublished thesis; Auckland University of Technology: 2016.
24. Hirth MJ, Vennett k, Mah E, et al. Early return to work and improved range of motion with immobilization splinting for zones V and VI extensor tendon repairs. *Hand Ther.* 2011;16:86–94.
25. Merritt WH. Relative motion splint: active motion after extensor tendon injury and repair. *J Hand Surg Am.* 2014;39:1187–1194.
26. Amadio PC, Shu AY, The Stiff Finger. In: Wolfe SWW, Hotchkiss RN, Pederson WC, Kozin SH (eds). Green's Operative Hand Surgery. 6th ed, Philadelphia, Pa Elsevier-Churchill-Livingstone; 2011:364.
27. Verdan C. Syndrome of quadriga. *Surg Clin North Am.* 1960;40:425–426.
28. Elliott D, McGrouther DA. The excursion of the long extensor tendons of the hand. *J Hand Surg Br.* 1986;11:77–80.
29. Leijnse JNAL, Carter S, Gupta A, et al. Anatomic basis for individuated surface EMG and homogeneous electrostimulation with neuroprostheses of extensor digitorum communis. *J Neurophysiol.* 2008;100:64–75.
30. Sharma JV, Liang NJ, Owen JR, et al. Analysis of relative motion splint in the treatment of zone VI extensor tendon injuries. *J Hand Surg Am.* 2006;31:1118–1122.
31. Evans RB, Burkhalter WE. A study of the dynamic anatomy of extensor tendons and implications for treatment. *J Hand Surg Am.* 1986;11:774–779.
32. Lalonde D. Advantages of WALANT for extensor tendon repair. In: Lalonde D, ed. *Wide Awake Hand Surgery.* 1st ed. Boca Raton, FL: CRC Press; 2016:209.
33. Izadpanah A, Abrams M, Murray K et al. *A Modified Merritt Splint in Zone IV, Zone V and Distal Zone vi Extensor Tendon Injuries: Nine Years Rehabilitation Experience in a Single Center.* Paradise Island, Bahamas: Poster presentation at: American Association for Hand Surgery Annual meeting; 2015.
34. Turner S. *An Audit of the use of the Merritt Yoke Relative Motion Splint for Extensor Tendon Repair.* Paper presentation at: British Association of Hand Therapists Annual Conference; Liverpool, England: 2015.
35. Altobelli GG, Conneely S, Haufler, et al. Outcomes of digital zone IV and V and thumb zone TII to TIV extensor tendon repairs using a running interlocking horizontal mattress technique. *J Hand Surg Am.* 2013:1079–1083.
36. Blakeway M. New directions for extensor tendon management: the immediate controlled active motion (ICAM) regime-a case report. New Delhi, India: Poster presentation at: 9th Triennial Congress of the International Federation of Societies for Hand Therapy; March 4-8, 2013.
37. Ryan GM, Murray D. Classification of treatment of closed sagittal band injuries. *J Hand Surg Am.* 1999;19:590–594.
38. Ishizuki M. Traumatic and spontaneous dislocation of extensor tendons of the long finger. *J Hand Surg (Am).* 1990;15:967–972.
39. Young CM, Ryan GM. The sagittal band: anatomic and biomechanical study. *J Hand Surg Am.* 2000;25:1107–1113.
40. Nigro L, Merritt WH. *A Novel Approach for Chronic Sagittal Band Rupture Permitting Immediate Active Motion and Hand Use During Recovery.* Williamsburg, VA: North Carolina Society for Surgery of the Hand Annual meeting 2017.
41. Winslow JB. *Exposition Anatomique de La Structure Du Corps Humain.* Paris: Guillaume Desperezet, Jean Desessarte; 1732.
42. Valero-Cuevas F. An integrative approach to biomechanical function and neuromuscular control of the finger. *Biomechanics.* 2005;38:673–684.

43. Cipra BA. Applied math enters the digital age. *SIAM News.* 2007.

44. Lee SW, Chen H, Towles JD, et al. Effect of finger posture on the tendon force distribution within the finger extensor mechanism. *J Biomech Eng.* 2008;130:1–25.

45. Wang K, McGlinn, Chung KC. A biomechanical and evolutionary perspective in the function of the lumbrical muscle. *J Hand Surg Am.* 2014;39:149–155.

46. Kaplan EB. *Functional and Surgical Anatomy of the Hand.* 2nd ed. Philadelphia: EB Kaplan, ED. JB Lippincott, Co; 1965:209.

47. Brand PW. Mechanics of individual muscles at individual joints. In: Brand PW, ed. *Clinical Mechanics of the Hand.* 1st ed. St Louis: CB Mosby Co; 1985:288–289.

48. Zancolli E. In: Zancolli, ed. *Structural and Dynamic Bases of Hand Surgery.* 2nd ed. Philadelphia: Lippincott Co; 1979:33.

49. Bowers WH, Hurst LC. Chronic mallet finger, the use of Fowler's central slip release. *J Hand Surg Am.* 1978;3:374–376.

50. Grau L, Baydoun H, Chen K, et al. Biomechanics of the acute boutonniere deformity. *J Hand Surg Am.* 2018;43:80.e1–e6.

51. Elson RA. Rupture of the central slip of the extensor hood of the finger: a test for early diagnosis. *J Bone and Joint Surg.* 1986;68B:229–231.

52. Schreuders TAR, Soeters JNM, Hovius SER, et al. A modification of Elson's test for the diagnosis of an acute extensor central slip injury. *British J of Hand Ther.* 2006;11:111112.

53. Boyes JH. Intrinsic muscles of the fingers. In: *Bunnell S revised by Boyes ed. Bunnell's Surgery of the Hand.* 4th ed. Philadelphia: JP Lippincott; 1964.

54. Soni P, Stern CA, Foreman KB, et al. Advances in extensor tendon diagnosis and therapy. *Plastic Reconstructive Surg.* 2009;123:52e–57e.

55. Lalonde DH, Flewelling LA. Solving hand/finger pain problems with the pencil test and relative motion splinting. *Plast Reconstr Surg Glob Open.* 2017;5(10):e1537.

56. Steichen JB, Strickland J, et al. Results of surgical treatment of chronic boutonniere deformity: an analysis of prognostic factors. In: Strickland J, Steichen JB, eds. *Difficult Problems in Hand Surgery.* 1st ed. St Louis: CV Mosby; 1982:62–69.

57. To P, Watson JT. Boutonniere deformity. *J Hand Surg Am.* 2011;36:139–142.

58. Jarrell K, Merritt WH. A Paradigm shift in the managing acute and chronic boutonniere deformity: the relative motion concepts that permits immediate active motion and hand use. *Submitted to J Plastic Surgery.* 2017.

59. Bain GI, Polites BG, Higgs RG, et al. The functional range of motion of the finger joints. *J Hand Surg Eur.* 2014;23:1–6.

60. Evans RB. Early active short arc motion for the repaired central slip. *J Hand Surg Am.* 1994;19:991–997.

61. Maddy LS, Meyerdierks EM. Dynamic extension-assist splinting of acute central slip lacerations. *J Hand Ther.* 1997;1997:206–212.

62. Howell JW, Peck F. Rehabilitation of flexor and extensor tendon injuries in the hand: current updates. *Injury.* 2013;44:397–402.

63. Chung B, Thanik V, Chiu D. Relative motion flexion splinting for flexor tendon repairs: proof of concept. *Annual meeting of the American Association for Hand Surgery.* Paradise Island, Bahamas; January 21-24, 2015.

64. Robinson SA, Gyovai JE, Howell JW. The versatility of the immediate controlled active motion yoke (ICAM). Abstract. *J Hand Ther.* 2004;17:78–79.

65. Feehan L. *IC18: Better Results with Extensor Injuries and Late Deformities (Boutonniere, Swan Neck, Mallet and Extensor Lag).* San Francisco: American Society for Surgery of the Hand 72nd annual meeting; 2017:7–9.

66. Ishiguro T, et al. Tension-reducing early mobilization for reconstruction of ruptured extensor digitorum communis tendons. *J Japanese Society of Hand Surgery.* 1989;3:509512.

108

Orthoses for Mobilization of Joints: Principles and Methods

Elaine Ewing Fess

CRITICAL POINTS

- There are no rote solutions for orthotic intervention to combat pathologic conditions of the hand and upper extremity. Orthoses must be created individually to meet the unique needs of each patient.
- Mobilization orthoses can be used (1) to correct contractures and increase passive motion or (2) to substitute for lost active motion, thereby enhancing functional use of the hand and extremity.
- The expanded American Society of Hand Therapists Splint/Orthosis Classification System (ESCS) allows consistent and improved communication among medical personnel and

- elevates the art of orthotic fabrication to a level that supports the advancement of knowledge and improved patient outcomes.
- The principles of mobilizing joints through orthotic intervention must be observed to ensure the efficacy of the orthosis.
- A hand or upper extremity orthosis requires ongoing reevaluation and adjustment as the target joint (or joints) improves to ensure that principles of fit are maintained.

Although significant advances have been made in materials and techniques over the decades, application of external devices to alter upper extremity deformity is not a contemporary concept. One of the earliest descriptions of an orthosis comes from ancient Egypt circa 2750 to 2625 BC, and numerous examples are found from the mid-1600s. Surprisingly, the primitive appearance of many of these 15th-century devices belies their relative sophistication of design.[1,2] Obvious predecessors to current orthoses, these inventions often provided serial adjustment in tension through mobilizing forces applied with leather strings, chained loops, or metal screws (Fig. 108.1).

Today's thermoplastic materials facilitate the construction and fitting phases of orthosis preparation, but these technologic advancements have not automatically led to better understanding of orthosis design and use. Far too often, an orthosis is exactingly reproduced from a picture without understanding of the underlying pathologic conditions of the hand or upper extremity and the realistic goals expected of the orthosis. Furthermore, without the application of the principles of mechanics, design, fit, and construction and without use of outriggers and mobilization assists that must be applied correctly, effective results cannot be achieved. Unfortunately, any "cookbook" approach to orthotic fabrication is predisposed to ending in frustration, failure, undue expense, and loss of time for the patient. Of paramount importance is the understanding that there are no rote orthotic fabrication

solutions to combating pathologic conditions of the hand and upper extremity. Orthoses must be created individually to meet the unique needs of each patient, as evidenced by designs that incorporate the variable factors of anatomy, physiology, kinesiology, pathology, rehabilitation goals, occupation, vocation, and psychological status.

OBJECTIVES OF MOBILIZATION ORTHOSES

Mobilization orthoses may be used (1) to correct existing deformity through application of gentle forces that gradually cause collagen realignment and tissue growth and the concomitant increased passive range of motion (PROM) or (2) to substitute for lost active motion, thereby enhancing functional use of the hand or upper extremity.[2]

Correction Orthoses

If full joint motion is not present, an orthosis is applied to first decrease existing deformity. Orthoses designed to improve passive joint motion are usually temporary and should be constructed of materials that are easily altered because configuration changes must be made as range of motion (ROM) improves (Fig. 108.2).

Control Orthoses

Requiring full passive joint motion, control or substitution orthoses may be fabricated of more durable, less adjustable materials because of their expected protracted time of use. It is essential to clearly understand the differences between these two basic groups of mobilization orthoses. By selecting an inappropriate design option, one may create an orthosis that is ineffective or that actually contributes to the existing

Although the terms *splint* and *orthosis* are used interchangeably throughout this chapter, *orthosis* is the preferred, more current terminology.

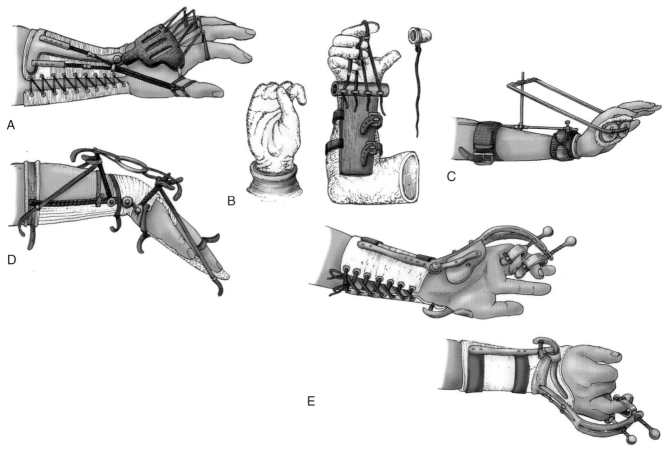

Fig. 108.1 A, Wrist extension, index–small finger metacarpophalangeal joint extension, thumb carpometacarpal joint radial abduction mobilization orthosis, type 2 (11). **B,** Index–small finger flexion mobilization orthosis, type 1 (13). **C,** Wrist extension mobilization orthosis, type 0 (1). **D,** Wrist extension mobilization orthosis, type 6 (16). **E,** Wrist extension, ring–small finger metacarpophalangeal–proximal interphalangeal joint extension mobilization orthosis, type 0 (5). (Numbers in parentheses indicate number of joints affected by the orthosis.) Orthoses for mobilization of hand–upper extremity joints is not a new concept. These orthoses were described between 1647 and 1927. (From Fess EE. A history of splinting: to understand the present, view the past. *J Hand Ther.* 2002;15:97-132.)

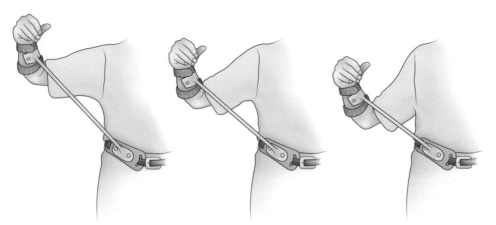

Fig. 108.2 Shoulder abduction and external rotation mobilization orthosis, type 3 (4). Shoulder abduction and external rotation may be increased through lengthening of the connector bar. (Orthosis design courtesy of McClure and Flowers. From Fess EE, Gettle KS, Philips CA, Janson JR. *Hand and Upper Extremity Splinting, Principles and Methods.* 3rd ed. St. Louis: Mosby/Elsevier; 2005.)

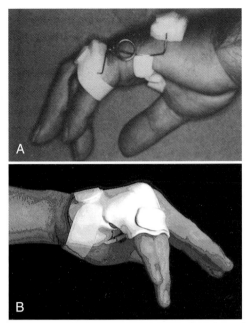

Fig. 108.3 Both A and B orthoses have identical functions. They both replace lost intrinsic muscle flexion by limiting finger MCP extension. Simultaneously, they allow extrinsic extensor muscle action to be directed to finger IP joints, thereby decreasing propensity for IP flexion contractures. Both A and B have the same ESCS name: Ring–small finger metacarpophalangeal joint extension restriction; interphalangeal joint extension torque transmission orthosis, type 0 (6). Requiring passive mobility of joints, these substitution orthoses prevent joint contractures and enhance functional use of the hand in an ulnar nerve injury. (From Fess EE, Gettle KS, Philips CA, Janson JR. *Hand and Upper Extremity Splinting, Principles and Methods*. 3rd ed. St. Louis: Mosby/Elsevier; 2005.)

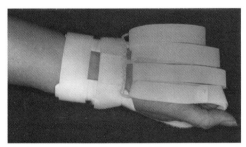

Fig. 108.4 Index–small finger flexion mobilization orthosis, type 1 (13). Designed to improve joint motion, this orthosis does not allow functional use of the hand during wearing periods. (From Fess EE, Gettle KS, Philips CA, Janson JR. *Hand and Upper Extremity Splinting, Principles and Methods*. 3rd ed. St. Louis: Mosby/Elsevier; 2005.)

pathologic condition. Control or substitution orthoses commonly do not incorporate the types of forces necessary to alter fixed deformity (Fig. 108.3); conversely, correctional orthosis designs may temporarily impede functional use of the hand or extremity (Fig. 108.4). Therefore, it is imperative that an orthosis design accurately reflects the purpose for which the orthosis is intended.

CLASSIFICATION OF MOBILIZATION ORTHOSES

A clear and accurate orthotic language is essential to practice, research, and teaching. Traditional orthotic terminology is riddled with inconsistencies, inadequacies, and nonsensical verbiage. Historically, orthoses have been classified according to a myriad of methods, including eponym (e.g., inventor or place of origin), acronym, purpose of application, configuration, power source, material, anatomic site, and colloquial jargon. One of the most commonly used classification systems has been that of grouping orthoses according to inherent structural characteristics, resulting in two major subdivisions. "Static" orthoses have no moving components and are used to provide support and immobilization, whereas "dynamic" orthoses use traction devices such as rubber bands, springs, or cords to apply corrective forces to stiffened joints. With the advancement of experience and knowledge in orthoses, the value of using "static" orthoses to improve ROM through consecutive configuration changes was recognized, and the term "static progressive" orthosis was introduced. Unfortunately, this method of grouping orthoses into three categories is primitive and antiquated. As a means of communication, it is analogous to "You Tarzan, me Jane." Its limitations are increasingly apparent as practitioners and researchers struggle to better define the devices they create.[3–5]

Development of a Taxonomy

In 1981, Fess and coworkers[6,7] devised a descriptive orthosis classification system based on three criteria: (1) orthosis forces, (2) anatomic site, and (3) kinematic intent. This system described orthoses according to the how, what, and why of design and purpose, grouping similarly functioning orthoses regardless of traction type, material, surface of application, or configuration. This was an important first step toward establishing a true classification system, but it required considerable development and refinement.

American Society of Hand Therapists Splint/Orthosis Classification System and Expanded Classification System

In 1986, the American Society of Hand Therapists (ASHT) conducted a survey of splint and orthosis nomenclature usage among its members and found that considerable differences existed even in this highly specialized group. To address this problem, a special splint and orthosis Nomenclature Task Force of nationally and internationally recognized hand and upper extremity orthotic fabrication experts was established by the ASHT Board in 1989. This task force was given the charge "to conclusively settle the problems of existing splinting nomenclature." The result of their work, the ASHT Splint/Orthosis Classification System (SCS),[8] was published in 1992. Later, in what became known as the Expanded ASHT Splint/Orthosis Classification System (ESCS), an additional purpose category (torque transmission) and two entirely new descriptor groups for prostheses and orthosis–prosthesis were identified by Fess and coworkers[2] as they applied the classification system to more than 1100 orthosis illustrations included in the third edition of their splinting and orthotic fabrication book that subsequently was published in 2005.

Both the SCS 8 and ESCS[2] categorize orthoses according to a series of six descriptive criteria: (1) articular or nonarticular, (2) anatomic focus, (3) kinematic direction, (4) primary purpose, (5) type or number of secondary joint levels, and (6) total number of joints included in the orthosis (Fig. 108.5). These six criteria combine to form a "sentence" that clearly and definitively describes an orthosis. Paralleling grammatical sentence structure, each element of the orthosis "sentence" defines a distinctly separate orthosis element.

For the first criterion, orthoses are considered to be either *articular* or *nonarticular*, depending on whether or not they affect joint motion. With the exception of a few specialized, two-point pressure, coaptation orthoses (e.g., fracture braces, pulley orthoses),[2] the majority of orthoses operate as three-point pressure systems,[2] directly influencing joint motion. Because most orthoses are articular in nature, the designation of articular is assumed for all orthoses in this category. Therefore, the

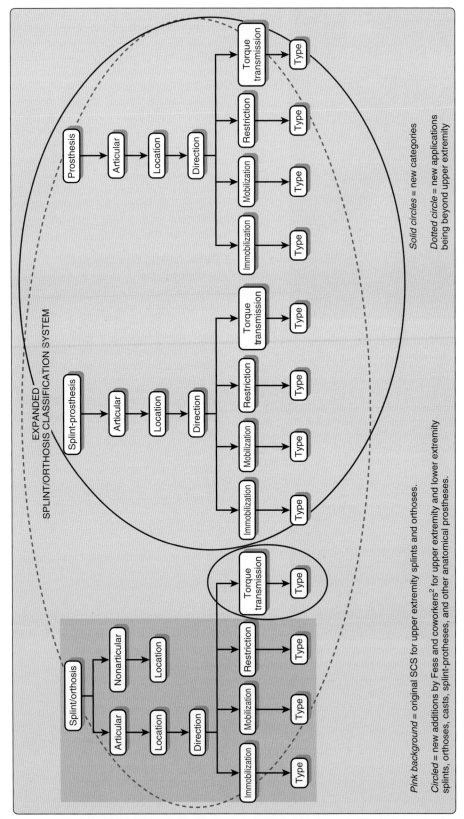

Fig. 108.5 An extension of the original American Society of Hand Therapists (ASHT) Splint/Orthosis Classification System (SCS), the Expanded ASHT Splint/Orthosis Classification System (ESCS) adds an additional purpose category (torque transmission) and allows descriptives for prostheses and splint-prostheses.

word *articular* is not included in the SCS/ESCS sentence. In contrast, nonarticular orthoses are always designated as such in an SCS/ESCS sentence (e.g., nonarticular humeral orthosis). All of the orthoses discussed in this chapter fall into the articular category. Articular is assumed rather than specified in their respective SCS/ESCS names.

The second criterion is *anatomy*. The *primary* joints affected by an orthosis are defined by the second of the six descriptors (e.g., shoulder, elbow, forearm; wrist, index, long, ring, small, thumb carpometacarpal [CMC] joint, metacarpophalangeal [MCP] joint, interphalangeal [IP] joint). If all the joints of a segment are considered primary joints, then the segment is named instead of the individual joints involved (e.g., finger, thumb). An example is that if all four proximal interphalangeal (PIP) joints are included as primary joints in an orthosis, the anatomy sentence descriptor would be *Index-small finger PIP joint*.

The third criterion, *direction*, delineates the kinematic course into which the primary joints or segments are moved or positioned (e.g., flexion, extension, radial deviation). Continuing with the example, if the desired direction is flexion, the SCS/ESCS sentence becomes *Index-small finger PIP joint flexion*.

Purpose, the fourth criterion, designates whether an orthosis is intended to immobilize, mobilize, restrict motion,[8] or transmit torque[9] to primary joints or segments.[2] If the purpose of this example orthosis is mobilization, then the sentence is expanded to become *Index-small finger PIP joint flexion mobilization orthosis*.

The fifth descriptor, *type*, identifies the number of secondary joint levels included in an orthosis. Whereas the first four criteria are intuitive, type addresses the mechanical function of an orthosis. It is less obvious but no less critical than are the first four criteria. Without type, the classification system falls apart. In defining the type, it is important to understand that secondary joints are not named per se, nor are they counted individually. Only the number of secondary-joint longitudinal levels is counted in the orthosis "sentence." This is in direct contrast to primary joints that are specifically named. Secondary joints often are included to anchor orthoses or to control or eliminate undesirable motion of joints other than the primary-focus joints or segments. Secondary joints are not the joints to which corrective forces of an orthosis are aimed. For example, in the previously used orthosis example, the wrist and MCP joints may be included to eliminate wrist tenodesis effect and to stabilize the MCP joints. This allows corrective forces to be directed to the primary PIP joints and eliminates unwanted dissipation of force at the two proximal-joint levels, the wrist level, and MCP joint level. In this example, two secondary joint levels, the wrist and MCP joint, are included; therefore, the orthosis would be considered a type 2 orthosis. The example orthosis sentence is further expanded to *Index-small finger PIP joint flexion mobilization orthosis, type 2*. If no secondary joint levels are included in an orthosis, it is classified as type 0; one secondary joint level is a type 1; three secondary joint levels are type 3; and so on.

The final descriptor, *total joint count*, is included at the end of the SCS/ESCS sentence in parentheses. This last criterion of the orthosis sentence explicitly counts the number of joints affected by the orthosis. Contrary to type, in which only the joint levels are counted, all primary and secondary joints are tallied individually in the total joint count number. In this orthosis example, there are four primary joints (the PIP joints), and there are five secondary joints (the wrist and four MCP joints), for a total count of nine joints. The number 9 is included at the end of the sentence in parentheses. The finished orthosis sentence reads *Index-small finger PIP joint flexion mobilization orthosis, type 2 (9)*.

Although many orthosis designs and configurations may fit the orthosis sentence mentioned, all function in the same manner. Note that it makes no difference in the SCS/ESCS if an orthosis is applied volarly, dorsally, or laterally or from what material it is constructed because design options such as surface of application or material do not influence the intent or function of the orthosis. If it is absolutely critical to convey design options, these specifications may be added at the end of the sentence following a colon. This example might then read *Index-small finger PIP joint flexion mobilization orthosis, type 2 (9): elastic traction*, or if surface of application is vital to communication, the sentence may be written as *Index-small finger PIP joint flexion mobilization orthosis, type 2 (9): volar application*.

If the colloquial term "wrist cock-up" is used in a referral, confusion may ensue. Is the purpose of the orthosis to immobilize, to mobilize, or to restrict wrist motion, or is it intended to transmit torque to digital joints? One can only guess. In contrast, using the SCS/ESCS, a "wrist cock-up" may be more scientifically described as:

A. Wrist extension immobilization orthosis, type 0 (1)
B. Wrist extension mobilization orthosis, type 0 (1)
C. Wrist flexion restriction orthosis, type 0 (1)
D. If its purpose is to transmit torque to the fingers as in an "exercise" orthosis, it is an Index-small finger extension and flexion torque transmission orthosis, type 1 (13).

In A through C, the wrist is the primary joint, and no secondary joint levels (type) are included in the orthosis. However, in D, the wrist is the secondary joint, and the finger joints are primary joints, although they (finger joints) are not included within the physical boundaries of the orthosis. Compare the total joint count for orthoses A through D. It immediately becomes apparent that D is a very different functioning orthosis from A through C; furthermore, A through C differ in function from each other. Note that not one design option is included in A to D, yet the essential facts about these orthoses are known. It is even possible to speculate associated diagnoses for these orthoses, an impossibility when confronted with the ubiquitous "wrist cock-up" moniker.

A final example, the extension portion of an MCP joint arthroplasty orthosis, is classified as an *Index-small MCP joint extension and radial deviation mobilization orthosis, type 1*. The wrist is included as a secondary joint, whereas the MCP joints are primary joints. Although many different orthosis designs fit into this classification, they all function in the same manner.

As noted at the beginning of this section, many earlier classification methods disintegrate and ultimately fail when required to describe current orthotic fabrication practice. With the SCS/ESCS method of grouping, orthoses are not categorized according to deficient terminology but rather according to specific intent of application. A serial cast applied to extend the ring finger PIP joint is classified as a *Ring finger PIP joint extension mobilization orthosis, type 0 (1)*. The archaic and limited descriptors "static," "dynamic," and "static-progressive" are not used in the SCS/ESCS. Furthermore, perplexing eponyms, acronyms, and colloquial jargon are eliminated, as are ineffectual configuration and material groupings.

Although the ramifications of using an accurate orthosis classification are readily apparent in these examples, the positive consequences of exactly describing orthoses are not restricted to clinical applications. In research, the SCS/ESCS allows orthoses with identical functions but different designs to be compared in clinical trials. For example, elastic and inelastic traction design options may be compared to orthoses with the same classification. Language is the key to professional evolution. The more defined splint and orthotic language is, the better the potential becomes for advancing knowledge and improving patient outcomes.[3,4]

The power of the SCS/ESCS lies in the fact that communication among medical personnel is vastly improved through definition of the important functional aspects of orthoses and through elimination of the confusion caused by colloquial or regional orthosis jargon. Design options such as type of traction (elastic, inelastic), surface of application, material, and outrigger configuration are deemphasized and left to the expert judgment and creativity of those who fabricate orthoses. Use of the SCS/ESCS is an important element to firmly elevate the art of orthotic intervention to a solid science foundation by requiring those who fabricate orthoses to fully understand the intricacies of orthosis function and by discouraging cookbook approaches. Through its inherent characteristics that require in-depth knowledge of anatomy, kinesiology, physiology, and pathology, the SCS/ESCS transitions those who use the system from a technical to a professional echelon.

ASSESSMENT

Assessment provides a foundation for orthotic intervention programs by delineating baseline factors from which orthoses can be individually created and progress can be monitored. The evaluation process involves gathering and integrating information derived from many sources. A finished orthosis should not only reflect anatomic, kinesiologic, physiologic, and pathologic requirements but should also meet the patient's psychological and socioeconomic needs. Astute observation, detailed interviews, careful inspection, and concise measurement guide upper extremity specialists in creating orthosis designs that are uniquely adapted to meet specific requirements.

Using instruments proven to be reliable and valid, measurements of extremity mass, temperature, ROM, strength, sensibility, and dexterity provide concrete numeric data about given components of hand and upper extremity function. These measurements are essential to establishing, monitoring, and evaluating[9] orthotic intervention and exercise programs. Often exhibiting rapid change, a healing hand or upper extremity must be constantly and carefully monitored so that therapists can direct appropriate and efficient adaptation of orthoses and exercises.

PHYSIOLOGIC FACTORS

Orthotic intervention is one of the most effective means of improving the passive mobility of stiffened joints (Figs. 108.6 and 108.7). When used appropriately, orthoses produce gradual rearrangement or lengthening of the pericapsular structures and an elongation of adhesions through directed gentle traction. Therefore, it is important to thoroughly understand the stages of wound healing and how they apply to specific tissues. The careful integration of these concepts into orthotic intervention and exercise programs provides the foundation on which efficacious therapeutic intervention is based. Dictated by the rate of healing and the method of repair of healing tissues after injury, orthotic programs must be designed to judiciously use and manipulate the physiologic process of collagen formation.[2,6,7]

The evidence for soft tissue remodeling may be found in research regarding cellular response to mechanical tension-stress.[1] Beginning in the late 1940s, Paul W. Brand recognized the importance of tissue remodeling, and as a researcher and educator, he continued to emphasize this concept to the hand and upper extremity rehabilitation community.[10] Although the subspecialty of plastic surgery is especially attuned to this arena because of its involvement in tissue expansion endeavors, other specialty areas are also investigating the biochemical elements of tissue growth. When tension-stress is applied to soft tissues in the form of an orthosis or tissue expander, changes occur in the collagen network alignment. Two types of tissue deformation exist. *Mechanical creep* (stretch) involves a temporary longitudinal reorganization of collagen from its relaxed random pattern to a parallel pattern in the direction of the applied tension-stress. When the fibers are parallel, no additional change in tissue length occurs without creating microscopic tissue tearing. A simple analogy is pulling fabric on its bias to its elastic limit. The fabric elongates to a certain length, and if the limit of the fabric bias is exceeded,

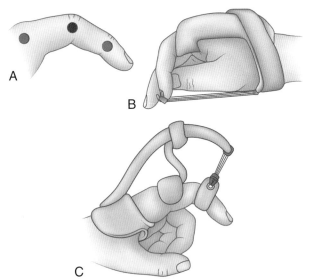

Fig. 108.6 A, Directing mobilization forces to problematic joints is technically more difficult when normal or less stiff joints are situated proximally or distally *(blue dots)* to the more stiff joint(s) *(red dot)* for which an orthosis is applied. **B,** Index finger interphalangeal joint flexion mobilization orthosis, type 1 (3). **C,** Index finger proximal interphalangeal (PIP) joint extension mobilization orthosis, type 1 (2). Although **B** and **C** have different kinematic directions, the two orthoses function mechanically in a similar manner. To prevent dissipation of the PIP joint mobilization force, both orthoses control position of the proximal, normal metacarpophalangeal (MCP) joint, preventing MCP joint flexion and MCP joint extension, respectively. (From Fess EE, Gettle KS, Philips CA, Janson JR. *Hand and Upper Extremity Splinting, Principles and Methods.* 3rd ed. St. Louis: Mosby/Elsevier; 2005.)

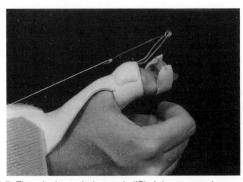

Fig. 108.7 Thumb interphalangeal (IP) joint extension mobilization orthosis, type 3 (4). This orthosis controls secondary joint level (wrist and thumb carpometacarpal and metacarpophalangeal joints) positions while providing a mobilization force to the thumb IP joint. (From Fess EE, Gettle KS, Philips CA, Janson JR. *Hand and Upper Extremity Splinting, Principles and Methods.* 3rd ed. St. Louis: Mosby/Elsevier; 2005.)

the fabric tears. In contrast, *biological creep* involves generation of new tissue through mitotic activity—that is, tissue growth.

When tension-stress is applied to living tissue over a prolonged period of time, a cascade of biochemical actions gives rise to biologic creep (tissue growth), including but not limited to generation of growth factors, cytoskeletal structures, and protein kinases. Although not fully understood, changes that occur at the cellular level involve the following events: cell attachment to the matrix decreases, membrane ruffling occurs, extracellular collagen is produced, sensitivity to insulin increases, growth factors are generated, ion channels are stimulated, and signaling molecules induce the cell nucleus to divide. Cells strive for equilibrium (Fig. 108.8),[11] and both amplitude and

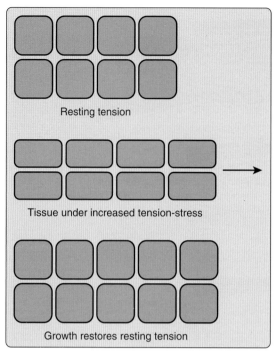

Fig. 108.8 Mechanical tension-stress stimulus initiates the tissue remodeling process. (From Fess EE, Gettle KS, Philips CA, Janson JR. *Hand and Upper Extremity Splinting, Principles and Methods.* 3rd ed. St. Louis: Mosby/Elsevier, 2005; originally from De Filippo RE, Atala A. Stretch and growth: the molecular and physiologic influences of tissue expansion. *Plast Reconstr Surg.* 2002;109:2450-2462; adapted from http://www.plasticsurgery.org.)

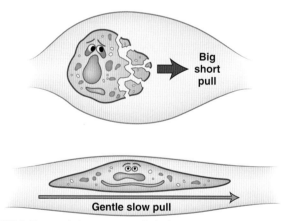

Fig. 108.9 Too much force over too little time creates tearing of soft tissues, resulting in increased inflammatory response and additional scar formation. (From Fess EE, Gettle KS, Philips CA, Janson JR. *Hand and Upper Extremity Splinting, Principles and Methods.* 3rd ed. St. Louis: Mosby/Elsevier; 2005.)

duration are critical to the outcome of application of tension-stress. Gentle tension-stress over a protracted time creates cell proliferation (Fig. 108.9). Conversely, forceful stretch over a short period of time leads to cell damage, increased inflammatory response, and increased scar formation.

PRINCIPLES OF USING MOBILIZATION ORTHOSES

Basic rules apply to all phases of orthosis preparation regardless of the purpose of application and ultimate orthotic configuration.[2,6,7] These principles define fundamental elements that contribute to the creation

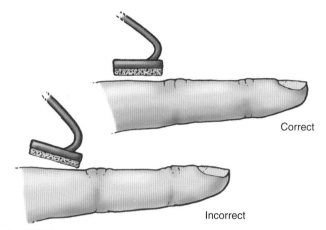

Fig. 108.10 To reduce pressure, narrow orthosis components should be fitted carefully to achieve contiguous contact between orthosis part and hand. (From Fess EE, Gettle KS, Philips CA, Janson JR. *Hand and Upper Extremity Splinting, Principles and Methods.* 3rd ed. St. Louis: Mosby/Elsevier; 2005.)

of an effectively working orthosis that is comfortable, durable, and cosmetically acceptable and that successfully meets individual patient requirements. Failure to incorporate these principles may result in orthoses that are eventually discarded because they are uncomfortable and ineffective or, worse, orthoses that, if worn, cause additional damage to the extremity through pressure sores, attenuation of ligaments, compression or distraction of joint surfaces, or inappropriate application of force direction or magnitude to healing structures. The decision to apply mobilizing forces to an injured or diseased upper extremity is a serious consideration; it should involve close communication between the physician, the therapist, and the patient. Furthermore, it is important that the goals of orthosis application be realistic and that all those involved thoroughly understand and accept the responsibilities of such an endeavor.

Mechanical Principles

Because orthotic intervention consists of external application of forces to the extremity, an understanding of basic mechanical engineering concepts is an essential prerequisite to the design, construction, and fitting of all hand and upper extremity orthoses. Pressure from an orthosis on the extremity can be controlled or diminished by widening the area of force application and by increasing the mechanical advantage of lever systems. Clinically, this means that orthoses that are longer and wider are more comfortable, and a contiguous fit of narrow components over bony prominences is of paramount importance (Fig. 108.10).

Elimination of the translational component of an applied force by maintaining a 90-degree angle of approach to the segment being mobilized (Fig. 108.11) is also of utmost importance when designing and fitting orthoses. This allows the full magnitude of the rotational force to be directed toward correcting the joint deformity and excludes force components that cause compression or distraction of the articular surfaces. In addition, understanding of torque and the integrated effects of reciprocal parallel forces allows identification and control of the magnitude of corrective and stabilizing forces as they relate to the placement of specialized orthosis parts. The relative degree of passive mobility of successive joints also plays an important role in orthosis design. If mobilizing forces are dissipated at normal or less involved joints, the potential for increasing passive motion of stiff joints within the same longitudinal segment is diminished considerably. Therefore, mobilization orthoses must be

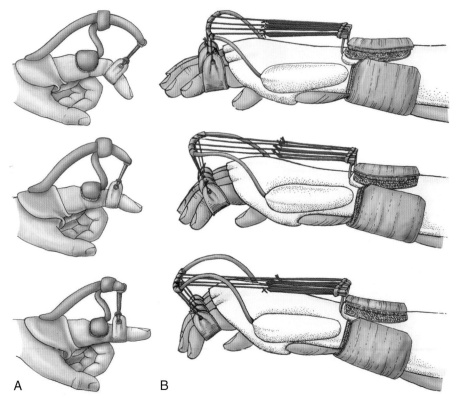

Fig. 108.11 A 90-degree angle of the dynamic assist to the mobilized segment must be maintained as passive joint motion changes. **A,** High profile. **B,** Low profile. (From Fess EE, Gettle KS, Philips CA, Janson JR. *Hand and Upper Extremity Splinting, Principles and Methods.* 3rd ed. St. Louis: Mosby/Elsevier; 2005.)

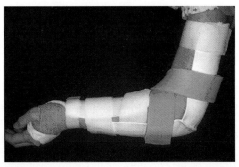

Fig. 108.12 Forearm supination or pronation mobilization orthosis, type 2 (3). Incorporation of the elbow and wrist as secondary joints focuses mobilization forces on the forearm. (Orthosis design courtesy of Paul Van Lede, OT, MS, Orfit Industries, Wijnegem, Belgium. From Fess EE, Gettle KS, Philips CA, Janson JR. *Hand and Upper Extremity Splinting, Principles and Methods.* 3rd ed. St. Louis: Mosby/Elsevier; 2005.)

designed to apply corrective forces to only joints that lack passive motion (Fig. 108.12).

Excessive shear stress leads to tissue breakdown and ulceration. Understanding the effects of shear on soft tissue is also imperative in successfully designing, constructing, and fitting orthoses. High-shear effects may be avoided by rounding orthosis edges, by keeping pressures low through contiguous fit, and by eliminating unwarranted motion and friction. Finally, for a more effective method of increasing orthosis durability than the retrospective trussing of layers of plastic, orthotic material strength may be increased by designing contour into the orthosis. Mechanical principles determine an orthosis' effectiveness, comfort, and durability ord should be carefully incorporated into the design, construction, and fitting phases of orthosis preparation.

Principles of Using Outriggers and Mobilization Assists

Regardless of their external configuration, orthoses that are designed either to improve motion of stiff joints or to substitute for loss of active motion must have a means of generating and directing forces. Depending on the purpose of orthosis application, these forces either apply prolonged gentle pull to influence collagen alignment of stiffened joints or move passively supple joints to enhance hand and upper extremity function.

The two key words associated with application of force to mobilize stiffened joints are *prolonged* and *gentle.* Orthoses designed to improve passive ROM must be worn for sufficient time to allow collagen realignment and tissue growth to occur. Wearing an orthosis for 1 or 2 hours a day is insufficient time for tissue growth to take place. For example, it would not be unusual for a patient to be instructed to wear his or her orthosis continuously except for exercise sessions when the orthosis is removed for 10 minutes of exercise, every 2 or 3 hours throughout the day. Wearing schedules must, of course, be modified to meet the specific requirements of each situation, but the concept of the application of traction over a long period of time is fundamental. The second word, *gentle,* is of equal importance. Forces that are too great create microscopic tissue tears, causing further injury, pain, increased inflammatory response, and additional scar formation. The devastating and debilitating cyclic pattern of forceful traction (through orthotic intervention or manipulation), tissue injury, pain, inflammation, and production of additional scar must be avoided at all costs.

When mobilization assists are used to apply traction to stiff joints, identification, control, and maintenance of force magnitude are critical. Generally speaking, forces between 100 and 300 g are thought to be acceptable to generate tissue remodeling of the small joints of the hand. It has been shown that experienced hand therapists adapt the amount of pull within this range to accommodate variations in diagnosis and physiologic timing.[2] Larger upper extremity joints lacking PROM, such as the wrist, elbow, and shoulder, respond more quickly to somewhat greater prolonged gentle forces.[12,13] Actual measurement of force magnitude for substitution or control orthoses is not necessary because the joints being moved are supple, and the required force is that which is sufficient to move the segments into desired postures. As myoelectric control becomes more sophisticated, robotic hand or upper extremity orthoses will add important functional capacity for patients. This emerging field provides exciting potential for patients requiring substitution orthoses.[14]

The range of forces generated by a mobilization assist depends on inherent physical properties of its base material and on the specific design of the assist. Forces created by rubber bands depend on thickness, length, and quality of rubber; springs rely on gauge, tensile strength, and diameter and length of coils. Shelf life also influences some mobilization-assist materials. The physical properties of a mobilization assist should be correlated with patient requirements and with orthosis design. For example, an assist that requires frequent adjustment would not be an appropriate choice for a patient who has difficulty returning to the clinic, and an assist that depends on considerable length to provide consistent tension would be inappropriate for a hand-based orthosis design.

Independent studies by Gyovai and Howell,[15] Boozer and coworkers,[16] and van Velze and Farmer[17] show that not only must one know the force magnitude of the mobilization assist used on an orthosis, but one also must understand that a frictional component exists between the interface material of the mobilization assist and the outrigger fulcrum in all low-profile outrigger designs. This friction component affects the force required to bring the positioned segment into position for substitution orthoses or the magnitude of corrective force applied to a stiff joint, as well as the active opposing finger forces required to overcome the pull of the mobilization assist. A simple formula may be used to define the effects of this friction. For example, if A is the force required to effect tissue growth at a stiff joint and B is the amount of friction between the outrigger and the mobilization assist interface, then $A + B = C$, in which C is the total amount of pull the mobilization assist (rubber band or spring) must generate to overcome the frictional component and apply A amount of corrective force to the joint. Because C will always be greater than A because of the added frictional component B, muscle strength to oppose the force of C must be greater than C. Clinically, this means that patients fitted with low-profile outrigger design orthoses need greater muscle strength than patients fitted with high-profile outriggers in which friction between the outrigger and the mobilization assist is nonexistent. High-profile outrigger designs have only the force of the mobilization assist A to consider. If weakness opposite to orthosis pull is an important patient factor, a high-profile outrigger design is preferable.

Mechanical and fit principles also must be applied in conjunction with principles of using mobilization assists. A mobilization assist should apply force in a direction that is 90 degrees to the segment being mobilized[18] (bone angle of rotation [BAR])[2] and perpendicular to the axis of joint rotation (JAR).[2] Pressure on attachment devices such as finger cuffs and nail hooks should be monitored carefully and maintained at minimum levels, and friction and shear must be avoided.

Design Principles

The principles of design may be divided into two basic groups: general considerations and specific considerations. General principles incorporate broad concepts that result in an orthosis that is practical for both the patient and the therapist, whereas the more specific guidelines are concerned with the unique pathologic conditions exhibited by individual patients. Factors such as age, ability to accept responsibility,

independence, and occupational and avocational demands contribute to the overall design of an orthosis, as do anticipated use time and prescribed exercise regimens.[19,20] Orthoses should allow maximum function and sensation and should be as simple in design and appearance as possible. Construction time also should be within reason. Specific principles of design individualize orthoses to the existing requirements of pathology, anatomy, physiology, and kinesiology. Clinicians must consider the following questions: Is the orthosis intended to substitute for absent active motion, or is it designed to correct existing deformity? Will elastic or inelastic forces be more effective? What orthosis components are required to control which joints, and what type of mobilizing forces will provide the greatest potential for increasing passive and concomitant active motion of stiff joints? Which mechanical principles should be used to increase effectiveness, comfort, and durability? These and many other questions must be anticipated and answered before design concepts reach the finality of pattern construction.

Component designing[2] lends an organized and rational approach to creating orthoses that meet individual patient needs. Problems are identified, and orthosis parts are mentally assembled to control or diminish the projected pathologic situation. This approach requires that the designer be fully cognizant of the uses and ramifications of each orthosis component. For example, low-profile outriggers have been shown to lose adjustment more quickly than do high-profile outriggers (Fig. 108.13). However, this is a potential problem only if one is dealing with correctional forces. If the purpose of an orthosis is to substitute for active motion, full passive joint motion is a prerequisite, and the need for sequential adjustments to accommodate motion improvements is nonexistent. Low-profile outriggers are appropriate design options for control or substitution orthoses because sequential adjustments are not needed. Conversely, high-profile outriggers provide longer increments of near 90-degree angle of pull than do the low-profile designs, indicating that for correctional orthoses, the higher design option will require fewer adjustments as improvements in motion are gained. Whether this is an important concept in the designing of a correctional orthosis entirely depends on the patient's capacity to return to the clinic for adjustments, expenses incurred for adjustments, and the time demands of the therapist's caseload.

Orthosis designing should never be approached in a rote or routine manner. Although patients may have similar diagnoses, the pathologic conditions presented are unique, as are each patient's intellectual and emotional capacities to deal with injury and dysfunction. Therapists must approach each case anew to attain maximum rehabilitation potential, using orthoses designed efficaciously, realistically, and practically for all involved.

Construction Principles

Observing proper construction principles and selecting equipment and methods appropriate to the materials used will help ensure the durability, cosmesis, comfort, and usefulness of the finished orthosis.[2] Orthosis corners should be uniformly rounded, edges smoothed, joined surfaces stabilized, rivets finished, and straps and padding secured. Mechanical principles should be analyzed and incorporated to enhance durability and comfort, and careful adherence to safety precautions when working with orthotic fabrication equipment is important. The equipment and the type and temperature of heat should be selected to meet the demands of the orthotic material used. Failure to adhere to construction guidelines may result in orthosis disuse because of patient discomfort, lack of acceptance, or orthosis breakage from mechanical failures, all of which represent loss of time and needless expense for both the patient and the members of the rehabilitation team. Therapist time to construct an orthosis is also an important consideration. Orthoses are not "edifices" to their creators. Selecting designs and materials that allow efficient and efficacious construction decreases therapist time fabricating orthoses.

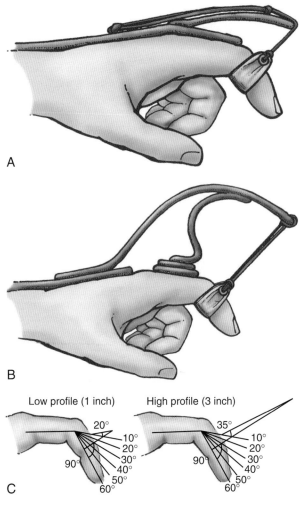

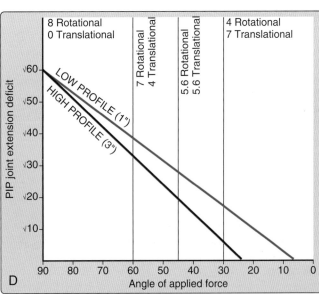

Fig. 108.13 Schematic representation of a low-profile outrigger **(A)** and a high-profile outrigger **(B)**. Comparison of low- and high-profile outriggers indicates that as passive motion improves, the high-profile design maintains a better angle of pull without adjustment than does the low-profile design **(C** and **D)**. *PIP,* Proximal interphalangeal.

Three-dimensional (3D) printing as a method of constructing orthoses and orthotic components is a relatively new concept, and a plethora of orthotic designs are available on "maker" websites. Although 3D printed orthoses may facilitate construction phases, attaining the superior fit afforded by thermoplastic orthoses that are fitted directly to extremities is seriously lacking at this time. As computer-aided design software programs become more sophisticated, this issue may be less problematic in the future.[21-23]

Principles of Fit

Fitting principles may be divided into four groups: (1) mechanical, (2) anatomic, (3) kinesiologic, and (4) technical. Mechanical factors include use of forces that are perpendicular both to the bone being mobilized (BAR)[2] and to the axis of the joint (JAR).[2] When traction is applied simultaneously to several joints within a digit, care must be taken to ensure that the pull is perpendicular to the rotational axis of each joint. In addition, pressure reduction through contiguous fit and application of lever systems in fitting orthosis components is important. Anatomic factors encompass the use of skin creases as guidelines for orthosis boundaries, identification and adaptation to bony prominences, support of longitudinal and transverse arches, understanding of ligamentous stress, and proper alignment of orthosis and anatomic joint axes. A hand or upper extremity in motion presents a multiplicity of differing external configurations and internal muscle dynamics as it moves through various planes. Kinesiologic considerations,[5] which include kinematic and kinetic principles, are very important to orthosis design and fitting phases. Orthosis parts must be fitted to allow motion, and they must be placed appropriately to control or augment motion, depending on individual requirements. Technical considerations emphasize efficiency and include developing patient rapport, developing work skills, and adapting methods to the materials used. An orthosis must be reevaluated continually to ensure a proper fit. As the hand or extremity heals and motion improves, the therapist must recognize changes that occur, incorporating appropriate adaptations into the orthosis as needed. Failure to do so will invariably render the orthosis less effective, impeding the advancement of the rehabilitation process.

CONCLUSION

Mobilization orthoses play an important role in the rehabilitation process of the diseased or injured hand or upper extremity. Providing correctional or substitutional forces, mobilization orthoses are designed and fitted according to specific requirements unique to each patient. Orthotic intervention programs also must be augmented with appropriate exercise routines and activities that encourage functional use of the extremity. Orthoses alone do not produce the active motion necessary for hand or extremity use. It is the astute combination of passive motion, provided through orthotic endeavors, and active exercise programs aligned with patient occupational and vocational needs that forms the foundation for hand and upper extremity rehabilitation techniques, allowing the patient to return to a productive life.

For additional information, readers are referred to Chapter 111 by Paul W. Brand, FRCS, in the fifth edition of *Rehabilitation of the Hand and Upper Extremity*, which is included in the online supplemental elements of this seventh edition. Using practical and easy-to-understand examples, Brand is a superb "translator" of the often difficult concepts relating to tissue remodeling and applied orthotic concepts. His chapter, "The Forces of Dynamic Splinting: Ten Questions Before Applying a Splint to a Hand,"[24] addresses the following questions:

1. How much force?
2. Through what surface?
3. For how long?

4. To what structures?
5. By what leverage?
6. Against what reaction?
7. For what purpose?
8. Measured by what scale?
9. Avoiding what harm?
10. Warned by what signs?

Brand's chapter is a classic that should be read by all those that employ orthotic intervention to improve hand and upper extremity function.

Judith Bell-Krotoski, MA, OTR, CHT, FAOTA, and Donna Breger-Stanton, MA, OTR, CHT, FAOTA, both of whom worked with Brand at the US Public Health Service National Hansen's Disease Hospital, Carville, LA, expand further on Brand's original chapter in the sixth edition of *Rehabilitation of the Hand and Upper Extremity*, Chapter 123.[25] A companion recommended work is Bell-Krotoski's Chapter 125 on tissue remodeling and contracture correction, also included in the sixth edition.[26]

REFERENCES

1. Fess EE. A history of splinting: to understand the present, view the past. *J Hand Ther.* 2002;15(2):97–132.
2. Fess EE, Gettle K, Philips C, Janson R. *Hand and Upper Extremity Splinting: Principles and Methods.* 3rd ed. St. Louis: Mosby; 2005.
3. Borkholder CD, Hill VA, Fess EE. The efficacy of splinting for lateral epicondylitis: a systematic review. *J Hand Ther.* 2004;17(2):181–199.
4. Fess EE. *Orthosis Classification According to Escopdex Taxonomy: are There Predictable Diagnosis-Specific Patterns to Orthotic Therapeutic Intervention? [Capstone]: Department of Occupational Therapy.* Post-Professional OTD Program. Indiana University; 2016.
5. Cha YJ. Changes in the pressure distribution by wrist angle and hand position in a wrist splint. *Hand Surg Rehabil.* 2018;37(1):38–42.
6. Fess EE, Gettle KH, Strickland JW. *Hand Splinting Principles and Methods.* St. Louis: Mosby; 1981.
7. Fess EE, Philips CA. *Hand Splinting Principles and Methods.* 2nd ed. St. Louis: Mosby; 1987.
8. American Society of Hand Therapists A. *Splint Classification System.* Chicago: The Society; 1992.
9. Teo SH, Ng DCL, Wong YKY. Effectiveness of proximal interphalangeal joint-blocking orthosis vs metacarpophalangeal joint-blocking orthosis in trigger digit management: a randomized clinical trial. *J Hand Ther.* 2018.
10. Brand PW, Hollister A. *Clinical Mechanics of the Hand.* 3rd ed. St. Louis: C. V. Mosby Co; 1999.
11. De Fillipo RE, Atala A. Stretch and growth: the molecular and physiologic influences of tissue expansion. *Plast Reconstr Surg.* 2002;109(7):2450–2462.
12. Saremi H, Chamani V, Vahab-Kashani R. A newly designed tennis elbow orthosis with a traditional tennis elbow strap in patients with lateral epicondylitis. *Trauma Mon.* 2016;21(3):e35993.
13. Nowotny J, El-Zayat B, Goronzy J, et al. Prospective randomized controlled trial in the treatment of lateral epicondylitis with a new dynamic wrist orthosis. *Eur J Med Res.* 2018;23(1):43.
14. Ryser F, Butzer T, Held JP, Lambercy O, Gassert R. Fully embedded myoelectric control for a wearable robotic hand orthosis. *IEEE Int Conf Rehabil Robot.* 2017;2017:615–621.
15. Gyovai J, Howell J. Validation of spring forces applied in dynamic outrigger splinting. *J Hand Ther.* 1992;5:8–15.
16. Boozer JA, Sanson MS, Soutas-Little RW, et al. Comparison of the biomedical motions and forces involved in high-profile versus low-profile dynamic splinting. *J Hand Ther.* 1994;7(3):171–182.
17. van Velze C, Farmer H. Low-profile dynamic splints: a solution to the friction problem. *J Hand Ther.* 1993;6(4):308–312.
18. Bai Z, Shu T, Hao Y, Niu W. An alternative static progressive orthosis for forearm pronation and supination. *J Hand Ther.* 2018.
19. Davison PG, Boudreau N, Burrows R, Wilson KL, Bezuhly M. Forearm-based ulnar gutter versus hand-based thermoplastic splint for pediatric metacarpal neck fractures: a blinded, randomized trial. *Plast Reconstr Surg.* 2016;137(3):908–916.
20. Saito K, Kihara H. A randomized controlled trial of the effect of 2-step orthosis treatment for a mallet finger of tendinous origin. *J Hand Ther.* 2016;29(4):433–439.
21. Baronio G, Harran S, Signoroni A. A critical analysis of a hand orthosis reverse engineering and 3D printing process. *Appl Bionics Biomech.* 2016;2016:8347478.
22. Baronio G, Volonghi P, Signoroni A. Concept and design of a 3d printed support to assist hand scanning for the realization of customized orthosis. *Appl Bionics Biomech.* 2017;2017:8171520.
23. Portnova AA, Mukherjee G, Peters KM, Yamane A, Steele KM. Design of a 3D-printed, open-source wrist-driven orthosis for individuals with spinal cord injury. *PLoS One.* 2018;13(2):e0193106.
24. Brand PW. The forces of dynamic splinting: Ten questions before applying a dynamic splint to the hand. In: Mackin EJ, Callahan AD, Skirven TM, Schneider LH, Osterman AL, eds. *Rehabilitation of the Hand and Upper Extremity.* 5th ed. Vol. 2. St. Louis: Mosby, Inc.; 2002:1811–1817.
25. Bell-Krotoski JA, Breger-Stanton D. The forces of dynamic orthotic positioning: Ten questions to ask before applying a dynamic orthosis to the hand. In: Skirven TM, Osterman AL, Fedorczyk JM, Amadio PC, eds. *Rehabilitation of the and Upper Extremity.* 6th ed. Vol. 2. Philadelphia: Elsevier Mosby; 2011:1581–1587.
26. Bell-Krotoski JA. Tissue remodeling and contracture correction using serial plaster casting and orthotic positioning. In: Skirven TM, Osterman AL, Fedorczyk JM, Amadio PC, eds. *Rehabilitation of the and Upper Extremity.* 6th ed. Vol. 2. Philadelphia: Elsevier Mosby; 2011:1599–1609.

109

Tissue Remodeling and Contracture Correction Using Serial Casting and Orthotic Intervention

Karen S. Schultz

OUTLINE

CRITICAL POINTS

- When applied as close to 24 hours a day as possible, the technique of comfortably holding tissues at the "ends of their elastic limit"—not stretching—results in soft tissue remodeling.

PATHOMECHANICS: THE INEVITABILITY OF GRADUALNESS

Used correctly, serial application of orthoses or circumferential casts increases the length of shortened tissues and the range of motion (ROM) of contracted joints in a nontraumatic way. This approach holds the shortened tissue or the contracted joint at the end of its available length or ROM for a prolonged period of time. Through serial application of a cast or orthosis, the tissue gradually elongates, resulting in correction of joint and soft tissue contractures and muscle–tendon unit tightness.[1,2]

Serial plaster orthotic positioning or casting for contracted joints or soft tissues began with Paul Brand, MD, in his use of plaster casting of clubfeet in children. He began to understand that the deep tissue scarring and later tissue contraction resulting from the high-force application involved with traditional methods of treatment failed to achieve the goal of creating supple joints with functional ROM. Brand found that frequent successive recasting resulted in correction of the deformity—and a healthy joint! The great success of this method motivated Brand to apply the technique to the interphalangeal (IP) joints of severely clawed hands.

Brand established The New Life Center, in Vellore, India[2–4] to treat patients with Hansen's disease (leprosy). These patients often presented with IP joint flexion contractures caused by the ulnar and median nerve impairment that results from Hansen's disease. The technique of serial casting met with equal success in these patients, many of whom were thought to be unable to benefit from medical intervention. The technique

has continued to demonstrate success in improving the flexibility of any small or large contracted joint or soft tissue. It effectively lengthens the skin and contracted soft tissue, *including vessels and nerves* and muscle–tendon units, for single or multiple joints. Plaster's conforming properties make it ideal for orthotic positioning because it distributes forces throughout the length of the cast, minimizing points of pressure under the cast. Although plaster conforms to extremities better than any other material now available, the circumferential application of other products has demonstrated their value as well. Materials that feature fabric impregnated with thermoplastic as well as thin thermoplastic and neoprene often provide sufficient conformity and pressure distribution.[5,6]

GROWTH, NOT STRETCH

The serial casting and positioning technique that Brand described changes tissue length via remodeling rather than progressive "stretch." Forceful stretching of soft tissue can cause tissue damage, resulting in inflammation and secondary scar formation. To accomplish remodeling, the successful method holds the contracted joint or tissue in a lengthened position for a significant period of time, often several days. The mechanical stimulus of tension stimulates the contracted tissues to gradually elongate.[7] Ideally, this tension holds tissue at the maximum possible length. In the best case scenario, the clinician removes the cast or orthosis at frequent intervals and repositions the joint or soft tissue at the newly achieved greater length (Fig. 109.1). This serial casting or

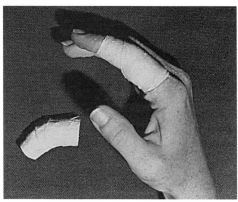

Fig. 109.1 Progressive casting of the index proximal interphalangeal joint into extension.

positioning method gradually corrects the joint, soft tissue, or muscle–tendon unit contracture over a period of days or weeks. In support of this approach, Eppenstein and associates[8] documented research demonstrating that low-load, long-duration tension optimally reduces the risk of tearing soft tissue. Importantly, it increases residual elongation and provides more permanent realignment of collagen fibers into a more parallel orientation.

Steve Kolumban,[9,10] a therapist working with Brand at the Christian Medical College and Hospital in Vellore, India, compared night orthotic positioning with "regular physiotherapy technique" in 24 outpatients with contractures of the IP joints. "Regular physiotherapy" consisted of wax baths, oil massage, and exercise (passive and active assistive). At the end of the study, the group with the orthotic positioning had significantly superior results. The percentages of degrees straightened from the total possible number were 45.7% with orthotic positioning and 0.9% without it. Of the 25 fingers in the group without orthotic positioning, *12 joints ended with a greater contracture than that with which they began.*

Later Kolumban[11] compared cylinder serial plaster casting with elastic tension orthotic positioning. The study matched fingers from both groups into pairs of six variables: age, contracture angle, joint resiliency (the continuum of soft to hard end feel), length of the finger, length of orthotic positioning, and applied straightening force. Both methods of positioning applied a straightening force of 250 g. At the end of the study, the results showed *a strong indication that the casting was superior to dynamic positioning.* Of 26 patients with 52 contracted IP joints, the percentage of degrees straightened from the total possible with serial cylinder plaster casting was 47.8% and with elastic tension orthotic positioning was 34.9%. Importantly, the involved tissues sustained no injuries (many of the patients had anesthetic hands) resulting from the plaster casting. The elastic tension orthotic positioning group experienced seven injuries.

Ugurlu and Özdogan[12] analyzed the effects of plaster serial casting in the treatment of proximal interphalangeal (PIP) joint flexion contractures in patients with rheumatoid arthritis and juvenile idiopathic arthritis. Their retrospective case-series reviewed the data from 18 patients (49 fingers) treated with serial casting over a 14-year period. They analyzed angular changes in the finger joints and compared them statistically using t-tests. The serial casting resulted in significant (26.8 degrees; $P < .001$) reduction in the PIP joint extension loss. Small but statistically significant losses in flexion were associated with these gains ($P < .001$). The magnitude of the initial extension loss was the only factor to explain the amount of motion gained ($P < .001$; $r^2 = 0.38$). They concluded that serial casting is an effective method to correct flexion contractures in PIP joints in selected patients with arthritis.

Hand surgeons in England adopted the technique and used it for joint and tendon contractures due to war injuries.[13] Brand brought the technique to the United States in the treatment of patients with Hansen's disease when he relocated to the US Public Health Service Hospital in Carville, Louisiana, in 1966. He continued to teach it in his worldwide tours and lectures. Under his direction at the New Orleans US Public Health Service Hospital for seamen in 1973, Bell-Krotoski used the serial cylinder casting technique for IP joints of the hand and developed a method to make the casts removable. In 1976, having relocated to the Hand Rehabilitation Center (now the Philadelphia Hand to Shoulder Center), Bell-Krotoski introduced the casting techniques to the center's therapists and physicians. Subsequently, these clinicians successfully applied the approach for patients with a wide variety of conditions resulting in joint contractures of the hand, including arthritis, reflex sympathetic dystrophy, postsurgical Dupuytren's contracture, congenital contractures, sequelae of ulnar nerve injury, joint dislocations, burns, skin grafts, boutonnière deformities, swan-neck deformities, and contractures after fractures and tendon repairs.

Brand and Kolumban, as well as Eppenstein and coworkers, emphasized the importance of pre- and postcasting measurements and using fixed repeatable positions for measurement. The clinician should address the position of proximal and distal joints during evaluation. For example, if the clinician records active and passive finger extension before casting with the wrist in neutral, she or he should use the same position for measurement postcasting. In assessing finger stiffness and contracture, Brand used passive controlled tension measurements with the wrist in flexion, neutral, and extension to differentiate joint contracture versus muscle–tendon unit tightness. Before using serial casting or orthotic positioning, a therapist should determine the underlying cause of the limitation, whether bone–cartilage abnormality, periarticular structure contracture, deep or superficial scar, muscle contracture, muscle–soft tissue imbalance, nerve injury, or spasticity.

INDICATIONS FOR SERIAL PLASTER CASTING OR ORTHOTIC POSITIONING

Serial casting or orthotic positioning for progressive tissue remodeling works on large joints and on muscle–tendon units. This approach has demonstrated consistent effectiveness with small joint contractures, in which other forms of positioning often fail. Most therapists know that if active exercise alone can achieve a full ROM, then the joint does not require an orthosis. A skilled therapist can use specific exercise and positioning or teach the patient to use these to maintain or restore active movement and joint balance. Patients with mild contractures often experience successful ROM correction with a simple augmentation to therapy consisting of a static night orthosis or a mobilization orthosis. But for more significant contractures, serial casting usually works better than other forms of orthotic positioning. The cast maintains tension in the tissues for 24 hours a day to effect a change in length of the tissue.[14]

Unless the joint demonstrates a bony block or lack of congruity, serial casting can successfully reestablish passive range of motion (PROM) with old, fixed deformities. Other orthotic positioning approaches will not provide good outcomes. In fact, it is indicated when the use of elastic traction fails. Circumferential orthosis management of IP joint contractures has many advantages over three-point pressure, elastic tension methods.

The nature of elastic tension orthoses can generate less effective results for improving PROM. This approach challenges clinicians to readily and precisely adjust the elastic force so that it creates a tolerable tension that places tissue at maximum length but does not stress beyond it. The elastic component that generates the amount of force needed to remodel scar tissue may continue to shorten to the point where it tractions the joint beyond its currently available end range. Although initially this amount of tension might appear desirable and the logical solution to lengthen tissue, in fact, it is not. Stressing tissue beyond maximum available length causes pain and ultimately creates microtears in tissue and increased scar formation. Edema, heat, erythema, pain, and stiffness indicate the occurrence of microtrauma from excess tension. These microtears, in turn, undergo the normal phases of wound healing—inflammation, fibroplasia, and maturation. As the scar matures, it contracts and further limits PROM. Currently, the only elastic tension exception that consistently results in good outcomes is the Punsola-Izard design of a custom neoprene tube orthosis.[6] The exact reasons for this success are unknown, but the excellent pressure distribution as well as the ideal force application may explain its efficacy.

In addition to the challenge of setting an initial force that will create the desired outcome, elastic tension orthoses require ongoing monitoring that circumferential designs do not. An elastic tension mobilization orthosis requires the therapist or patient to continually check the orthosis to ensure that it creates the desired force vector. Rubber bands and even springs attenuate, creating the need to change them. Even finger-based elastic tension orthoses have a higher profile than circumferential designs, limiting hand function during wear.

ADVANTAGES OF CASTING FOR TISSUE REMODELING

Well-applied circumferential casting never increases swelling and often decreases it because the cast provides well-distributed compression and keeps the joint still for periods of rest. In contrast, elastic tension mobilization orthoses can cause an increase in swelling when the tissue does not tolerate the force or if the finger cuff or straps do not adequately distribute pressure. Because casting does not forcefully stretch the tissue, it does not increase pain and often decreases pain. This is particularly important in patients with complex regional pain syndrome (CRPS), for whom even a slight increase in pain constitutes a step in the wrong direction. Clinicians can apply plaster directly over lacerations and ulcers. Particularly with insensitive fingers, the use of the casting technique facilitates healing without further trauma. Plaster allows the skin underneath to breathe and does not macerate the skin if applied directly. The plaster allows some air to the wound and absorbs tissue exudates. Fabric and thermoplastic casting tapes also allow air to circulate. Therapists can apply other circumferential materials over open wounds, but they should use a dressing such as sterile petrolatum gauze dressing over the wound and under the casting material.

CONTRAINDICATIONS FOR SERIAL PLASTER CASTING OR ORTHOTIC POSITIONING

As with any treatment approach, the therapist must carefully consider the nature of the problem before applying the cast or orthosis. Patients with PROM limitations owing to soft tissue abnormalities that will not respond to low-load, prolonged stress such as fibrosis and preoperative Dupuytren's contracture should not receive a cast. Joint limitation caused by heterotopic ossification, exostosis, or loose body will also not benefit from casting. The circumferential design of the cast allows mobilization of a joint that might not be a candidate for conventional splinting (e.g., in the case of some forms of joint instability and acute inflammation). However, avascular necrosis, infection, unstable fracture, marked demineralization, myositis ossificans, and stress across healing structures without adequate blood supply or adequate tensile strength remain contraindications to cast application.

SERIAL CYLINDRICAL CASTING METHOD: PLASTER OF PARIS

Tissue Preconditioning

Clinical experience supports more rapid achievement of increased ROM when the clinician preconditions the joint (lengthens periarticular structures) just before casting. One or more of the following techniques have clinically demonstrated efficacy: compression or massage for edema reduction, heat combined with stretch, joint mobilization, active and passive exercise, and therapeutic activities (Fig. 109.e1).

Materials and Preparation for Serial Casting of Proximal Interphalangeal Joint Flexion Contractures

Making a PIP joint extension cast from plaster of Paris (POP) requires the following materials:

- POP[15] cut into 2½-inch strips, folded in half (two types are available: fast setting with a 5- to 8-minute set time and extra-fast setting with a 2- to 4-min set time)
- Small clean bowl
- Warm water
- Plaster scissors
- Splint or cast trimmers
- Tissues
- Petroleum jelly
- Synthetic cast padding
- Drapes to protect work surfaces and the patient's clothes

Thermal Effect of Plaster During Setting

One needs to be aware of the thermal effect of plaster during setting. Generally, temperature peaks between 5 and 15 minutes after cast application. Heat produced is somewhat relative to the number of layers used. In a recent study by Ahmed and Carmichael,[16] the temperature produced in vivo by current casting techniques and materials was assessed. The highest temperature reached with 40°C water was 39.5°C, which was reached twice: once with Johnson & Johnson Fast Set Plaster with 5 layers of plaster and 3 layers of soft roll and once with DeBusk Classic Synthetic Casting Tape of 10 layers with 1 layer of soft roll. They concluded that under the clinically applicable conditions described in this study, using the materials tested and with a normal vascular supply, it is unlikely that temperatures high enough to cause a burn will be produced. However, they caution that good clinical judgment is advised if a patient reports a cast feels too hot.

Another study by Hutchinson and Hutchinson[17] evaluated factors that contribute to the elevated temperature beneath a cast and, more specifically, the differences of modern casting materials, including fiberglass and prefabricated splints. Outcomes revealed that material type, cast thickness, and dip water temperature played key roles regarding the temperature beneath the cast. Faster setting plasters achieved peak temperature quicker and at a higher level than slower setting plasters. Thicker fiberglass and plaster casts led to greater peak temperature levels. Increasing dip water temperature led to elevated temperatures. The thickness and type of cast padding had less of an effect for all materials. With a definition of thermal injury risk of skin injury being greater than 49°C they found that thick casts of extra-fast-setting plaster consistently approached dangerous levels (>49°C for an extended period). A cast of extra-fast-setting plaster, 20 layers thick, placed on a pillow during maturation, maintained temperatures above 50°C for more than 20 minutes. They concluded that clinicians should be cautious when applying thick casts with warm dip water. The greatest risk of thermal injury occurs when thick casts are allowed to mature while resting on a pillow.

Position and Technique for Serial Casting of Proximal Interphalangeal Joint Flexion Contractures

Before making the cast, decide on patient and finger positions.. Be sure the patient understands the materials, technique, and rationale for cast application. Prepare and position the patient as follows:

1. Remove any rings from the target finger(s).
2. Seat the patient, placing the elbow of the affected extremity on a firm but padded surface.
3. Hold the finger being casted at the distal phalanx, leaving the distal interphalangeal (DIP) joint crease free. Pull the finger into IP extension, using axial traction, while the patient pulls the hand away from the traction force by extending the wrist or bending the elbow. At the same time, stabilize the metacarpophalangeal (MCP) joint in approximately 90 degrees of flexion. The force must take the PIP joint to maximum available extension without causing pain. The use of a tissue or Coban around the distal phalanx will help provide traction to maintain firm prehension (Fig. 109.2).
4. Sustain the traction force until the cast sets. Some differing opinions (level 5 evidence) exist with regard to the amount of force a therapist should apply during casting. Bell-Krotoski[18] opines that force application could result in joint and skin irritation and potentially cause more joint stiffness; she advocates for gradually increasing tension with successive casts after the patient demonstrates tissue tolerance.

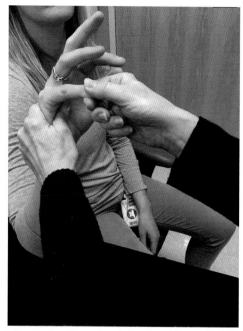

Fig. 109.2 Positioning the patient's hand and finger for PIP joint traction. (Copyright © 2019 K.S. Schultz.)

SKIN TOLERANCE

Clinical experience shows that casting will consistently create some erythema over the dorsum of the PIP joint. If the patient presents initially with erythema of the dorsal aspect of the PIP joint or if this develops over a period of time in the cast, casting may still continue. To minimize this skin response, the therapist strategically applies a small amount of padding. Bell-Krotoski[18] described a technique using "clouds"—wisps of cast padding—to protect vulnerable tissue (Figs. 109.e2 and 109.e3). To make the "cloud," pull a small fluff of cast padding from the roll. To keep the "cloud" in place during cast fabrication, apply petroleum jelly over the area where the padding will go. With the padding over the dorsum of the PIP, the normal casting procedure can begin.

Thin fluffs of cotton or cast padding placed at the distal and proximal volar edges of the cast can help patients with fragile skin tolerate a cast. Therapists may find that they can apply this volar edge padding after they finish making the cast. The therapist must be sure that the padding stays in place during cast fabrication. Bulkier approaches to padding the cast usually do not have a satisfactory result.[18]

Options For Cast Fabrication

Bell-Krotoski[18] originally described using a single strip of plaster approximately 1 inch wide. Another technique uses a double strip (a wider strip folded in half). The therapist can choose to make the cast all in one piece wrapped distally from the base to the tip of the finger or in two pieces cut from the 1-inch-wide plaster in 12- to 15-inch lengths. This chapter describes several options for cast fabrication.

Option 1

To begin the cast fabrication process, coat the finger with petroleum jelly, which protects against the drying effects of the plaster (Fig. 109. e2). Tear off a small wisp of synthetic cast padding and apply it to the dorsum of the PIP joint (see Fig. 109.e3). Dip the length of plaster into the water; then run the POP between two fingers to remove excess water (Fig. 109.e4). Allowing the plaster strip to lie on a paper towel will remove excess water, making it easier to handle and wrap while minimizing drip. Taking care to avoid the fragile skin of the finger web, place the POP strip as far proximally as possible on the proximal phalanx. Wrap all the way around the proximal phalanx twice and then begin to spiral distally, overlapping the previous layer halfway, or by about ¾ inch (Fig. 109.3). With the finger wrapped with POP, use a continuous rotary motion of the fingers to coax the material down onto the finger (Fig. 109.e5). To allow the DIP joint to move freely, end the POP approximately ³⁄₃₂ inch proximal to the DIP joint flexion crease but extend the cast fully to the DIP joint dorsally (Fig. 109.4). Some therapists prefer to use tissues to assist with the casting process in the following manner: with one hand, hold the tip of the finger with a tissue (this helps the therapist maintain prehension of the fingertip). With the other hand, use another tissue in a rotary fashion around the cast to absorb additional water from the POP. Caution: Avoid point pressure against the material at all times (Fig. 109.e6). Be sure to maintain PIP joint axial traction during the entire process until the cast sets (Fig. 109.5). Marking the final end edge of the plaster facilitates removal (Fig. 109.6).

Option 2

Bell-Krotoski[18] described the following plaster application procedure.

Start with folding the gauze plaster edge that will first be in contact with the finger about the width of the finger (Fig. 109.7). Begin wrapping from the base of the finger in an overlapping fashion (see Fig. 109.3). Then reverse, fold the gauze plaster edge the width of a finger, and start the second wrapping from the tip of the finger to just beyond the level of the PIP joint. In this way, the last bit of cast material can often be placed just under the PIP joint for a little extra support (while not making the cast too thick). If it is desirable to be able to remove the cast, the very tip of the cast can be left open.

In either method, just before the strip of plaster is applied to the hand, a slight fold on the edge of the plaster strip will make a smooth rather than a rough edge against the finger web and volar distal edge of the cast. This slight fold will help with smoothness and durability for any cast edge. End the plaster wrap just proximal to the DIP joint crease to permit later DIP joint movement.

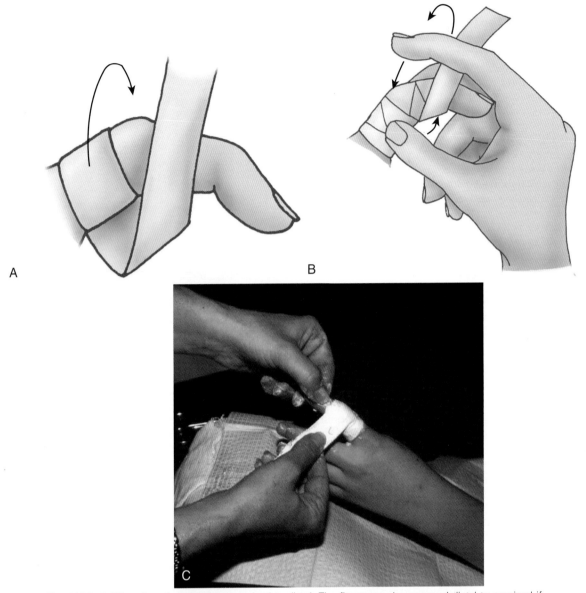

Fig. 109.3 A, Wrapping of plaster from proximal to distal. The finger may be wrapped distal to proximal if desired, but this is usually not necessary because plaster is for positioning of the joint only and wrapping should not compress tissue. **B,** Wrapping of finger while it is being supported in position. **C,** Maintain traction on finger as you wrap distally. (Part C copyright © 2019 K.S. Schultz.)

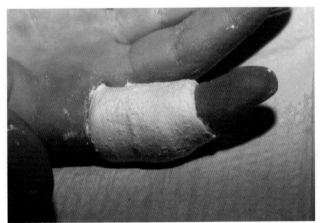

Fig. 109.4 To allow the distal interphalangeal (DIP) joint to move freely, end the Plaster of Paris approximately ³⁄₃₂ inch proximal to the DIP joint flexion crease but extend the cast fully to the DIP joint dorsally. (Copyright © 2019 K.S. Schultz.)

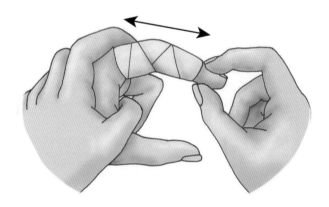

Fig. 109.5 Positioning of finger for traction. Care should be taken to avoid point pressure on the plaster. Maintain proximal interphalangeal joint axial traction during the entire process until the cast sets.

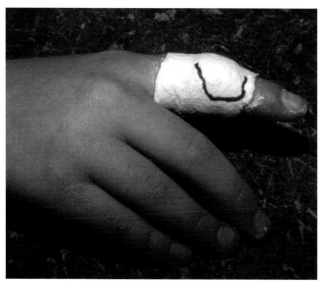

Fig. 109.6 Marking the final end edge of the plaster facilitates removal. (Copyright © 2019 K.S. Schultz.)

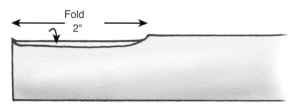

Fig. 109.7 Plaster strip 1 inch wide (cut from 2-inch-wide plaster). Start with folding the gauze plaster edge that will first be in contact with the finger about the width of the finger.

DISTAL INTERPHALANGEAL JOINT INCLUSION AND EXCLUSION

If the therapist deems that the patient should perform active DIP flexion–extension, the cast is ended just proximal to the DIP joint. Indications for DIP active range of motion (AROM) include:

- Increasing flexor digitorum profundus (FDP) excursion
- Increasing DIP flexion via exercise, especially after central slip injury
- Helping to rebalance the extensor mechanism via excursion of the extensor mechanism
- Maintaining or increasing oblique retinacular ligament (ORL) length

The cast may include the DIP joint in the case of DIP joint flexion contracture. Lengthening the cast to the tip of the finger increases the mechanical advantage for PIP joint extension. To block DIP joint hyperextension, the therapist can add a dorsal DIP joint "block" to the finger serial cast (Fig. 109.8).

Check and Revision

Assessment of the cast following its application is essential. Inspect the palmar joint crease at the MCP joint and be sure the patient can flex the MCP joint without the proximal–palmar end of the cast pressing into the joint crease. If this occurs, push or roll the damp plaster back away from the crease or use a safe scissors or tool to carve out some of the material to allow unimpeded movement. Next, check the DIP crease to be sure that the DIP joint can fully flex. Again, either push or roll the damp plaster back away from the crease or use trimmers to

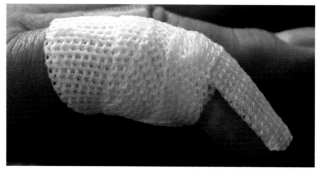

Fig. 109.8 Dorsal block included in this proximal interphalangeal joint cylinder cast to encourage distal interphalangeal joint flexion and block hyperextension. (Copyright © 2019 K.S. Schultz.)

trim the cast if needed. Finally, check the webspaces and contour or trim as needed (Fig. 109.9). Tools such as a Kirschner wire (K-wire) cutter pose a minimal risk to the patient's skin. Under optimal conditions, the cast will not need trimming. Observe the cast closely for any signs of indentation along the substance of the cast. If indentation is evident, remove the cast and start over (see Fig. 109.e6).

If the cast appears unsatisfactory after making it, the therapist can remove the plaster and begin again with fresh supplies. It may be possible to raise the end of the POP cast and unwind it (see Fig. 109.6), or the patient can soak the POP cast off in warm water. Alternately, the clinician can use a K-wire cutter to cut into the plaster either at the proximal or distal end to help remove it.

SERIAL CYLINDRICAL CASTING METHOD WITH FABRIC-BASED THERMOPLASTIC TAPES

Materials and Preparation

Making a QuickCast or OrfiCast PIP extension cast requires the following materials[19]:

- Cast tape
- Hairdryer (long-nosed, 1600-Watt dryer)
- Splint or cast trimmers
- Towel
- Petroleum jelly or hydrating cream
- Cast padding
- Tincture of benzoin (optional)

The hair dryer must deliver a powerful airflow. This type of dryer heats the tape effectively and quickly. Long-nosed dryers will not shut off when hot air funnels back into the dryer end. Short-nosed dryers shut down when hot air returns into the nose, which often occurs when heating the material. Some therapists soften the tape in hot water. Moisture on the tape decreases its ability to bond to itself and can make the cast fabrication more challenging. Caution: Use of a heat gun may result in overheating the material as well as discomfort or burns to the fabricator's fingers.

To begin the cast fabrication process, cut the amount of casting material needed for the finger length. This quantity of material depends on the length and circumference of the finger and the number of joints incorporated into the orthosis (Fig. 109.e7). These fabric-based casting tapes require two layers of material proximally and distally. The material should overlap by half as the tape spirals up the finger, creating two layers along the entire cast.

Precondition the finger as described earlier in this chapter (see Fig. 109.e1). Positioning for casting tapes is virtually the same as that for POP (see Fig. 109.2), with a few exceptions.

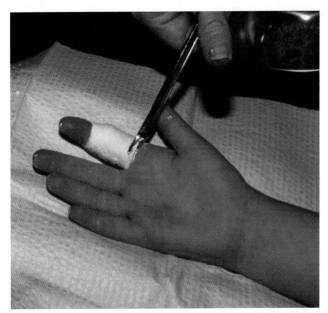

Fig. 109.9 Check webspaces and flexion creases. Trim and smooth as indicated to avoid skin irritation. (Copyright © 2019 K.S. Schultz.)

Cast Fabrication

Cut the casting tape and place it flat on a towel. Set the hairdryer to the hottest setting and highest airflow. Hold the dryer directly above the tape, almost touching it (Fig. 109.e8). The therapist can apply the cast tape as soon as it softens. QuickCast II sets up so fast that it sometimes requires two strips to cast a long or large finger. OrfiCast has a longer working time. This author (KSS) prefers to hold the OrfiCast at both ends and evenly stretch the material, causing it to become slightly narrower. After the OrfiCast encapsulates the finger, it will not shrink back down and cause overcompression.

Taking care to avoid the fragile skin of the finger web, place the tape as far proximally as possible on the proximal phalanx. Use the same application method as for the double-thickness POP cast (see Fig. 109.3). As with plaster, avoid point pressure against the QuickCast at all times (see Fig.109.e6).

Check and Revision

Smooth cast edges prevent skin irritation. Observe the cast closely for any signs of indentation along the substance of the cast. If the cast appears unsatisfactory, simply unwind the material, being careful not to stretch it widthwise. With the tape removed from the finger, simply repeat the heating process and reapply the same material. Unwinding the material becomes quite difficult after the tape fully hardens. The cast will set up quickly, in 1 minute or less.

HELPFUL TECHNIQUES FOR FINGER CASTING

Cast Removal

Both the patient and the therapist must be familiar with techniques for cast removal. The patient should leave the clinic only after indicating a clear understanding of how to and how *not* to remove the cast.

Mark the distal end of the POP or cast tape with a pen; this will help with cast removal in an emergency and help assure patients that they can unwind the cast (see Fig. 109.6). The therapist must instruct the patient not to seek cast removal with a cast saw because of the absence of padding.

In the case of a contracture of 30 degrees or less, the patient will most likely be able to pull off the cast. For patients with unstable MCP joints (e.g., with rheumatic disease), the patient will have to stabilize the proximal phalanx before pulling off the cast. If the joint is too

tender or swollen or if the contracture is more severe, then the cast removal is more involved.

The patient can immerse the casted finger in the warmest tolerable water to soften the POP and unwind the cast (Fig. 109.e9). Squeezing the cast from side to side also helps with cast removal. Soaking, unwinding, and squeezing sometimes work for casting tape as well, but with these materials, the patient must be able to tolerate very warm to hot water. The patient should soak the cast in the warmest water tolerable for 1 to 2 minutes for casting tape and 5 minutes or longer for POP. With the distal flap of the casting material raised, unwrapping the cast becomes possible. The patient may need to resoak several times before the cast becomes removable. The therapist or patient can soak the cast to soften it partially and then use a safe tool or cast scissors specifically designed for finger serial casts to cut it off.

The therapist may choose one of two approaches to cut the cast for removal. Bell[20] described cutting a window over the dorsal aspect of the cast along the proximal phalanx. With this section of the cast removed, the patient can usually slip off the cast (Fig. 109.10). Another option involves creating a univalve in the cast with a longitudinal cut along either the radial–palmar or the ulnar–palmar border (Fig. 109.11). The location for these cuts has two advantages. The palmar skin has more subcutaneous padding than the dorsal skin, and the volar approach avoids the PIP condyles. Cutting over a bony prominence usually creates discomfort for the patient.

The tape technique has three options for removal: pulling it off, softening it in very hot water, or cutting it off. After the material has set, the patient may be able to pull off the cast. If the patient has lost a great deal of edema—which frequently happens after several hours in a cast—simply pulling will remove the cast. Often, right after cast application, the tape sticks to the skin. Although this helps secure the cast, the stickiness makes removal more difficult. Running water over the cast will reduce this tackiness and release the cast.

If the patient cannot pull off the cast, immersing it in *very* hot water will often soften it enough to allow for it to be unwrapped. Not all patients will be able to tolerate the water temperature required to soften the tape. A patient with an insensate hand is not a candidate for this approach.

The third option for cast removal involves use of tools, including K-wire cutters or sharp scissors that have blunted tips. A therapist may send a patient home with a clinic-provided safe tool (K-wire cutter, suture scissors or wire snips with blunted tips). Getting a deposit from the patient for the tool helps to ensure the patient will return it. Cut along the lateral or volar surface of the finger where the skin has more subcutaneous padding. Caution: Do not use a hairdryer to reheat the cast tape while it is on the finger. The heat can cause great discomfort and may damage tissue. The most commonly used finger casting techniques lack any insulating lining to protect the patient's skin.

Securing the Cast in Place

Sometimes the patient will have trouble keeping the cast on. This occurs most frequently with fingers that are approaching full extension and with initially edematous fingers at the time of cast application that have since lost volume. This author has found three techniques helpful for maintaining cast position on the finger when the proper casting technique does not result in a secure cast:

1. **Additional material.** The therapist can cut an additional piece of material, laminate it to the proximal end of the cast, and continue wrapping through the first webspace and around the palm (Fig. 109.12).
2. **Nonadhesive wrap.** The patient can wrap the cast and adjacent skin with self-adherent nonadhesive wrap, such as Coban. As an alternative to a simple wrap around the finger, the patient can apply the wrap around the cast and then through the palm (Fig. 109.13).

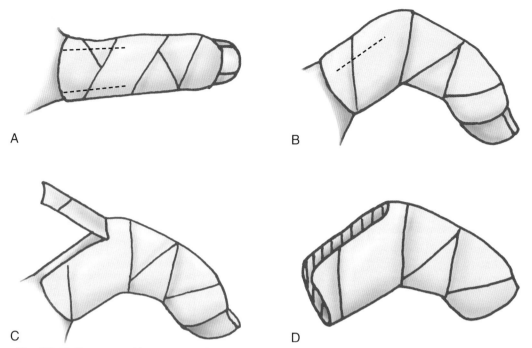

Fig. 109.10 Cast removal for a severely flexed interphalangeal joint. **A,** Dorsal view. **B,** Lateral view. **C,** Flap. **D,** Cast.

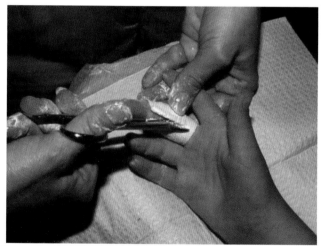

Fig. 109.11 A longitudinal cut along either the radial–palmar or the ulnar–palmar border can be made for removal of cast. (Copyright © 2019 K.S. Schultz.)

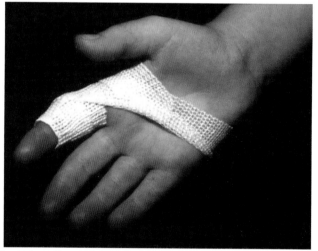

Fig. 109.12 If needed, to secure the cast in place, an additional piece of material can be laminated to the proximal end of the cast and wrapped through the first webspace and around the palm. (Copyright © 2019 K.S. Schultz.)

3. **Tincture of Benzoin.** Also known as Tough Skin, this iodine- and alcohol-based liquid product creates a tacky surface on the skin. The cast maker can dab a tiny amount on the skin before the cast is applied. Rubbing alcohol removes the tincture when desired. Before trying this, determine first that the patient does not have an allergy to iodine.

Protecting Adjacent Fingers

Sometimes the finger adjacent to the casted finger becomes irritated from rubbing against the cast. To prevent this or to relieve it when it occurs, the patient may cover the adjacent finger with Moleskin, a bandage (Band-Aid), or light Coban wrap. The patient may also cover the cast with a nonabrasive material such as finger tubular stockinette, Coban, or a finger cot. When using a finger cot, air will not circulate, so the therapist must instruct the patient in precautions for this approach.

Precautions for Finger Casting
Material Tolerance

If the patient does not tolerate the cast tape directly against the skin or if additional padding is desired, the therapist may apply one or more layers of tubular finger bandage to the finger before making the cast. In the case of wounds or the use of padding, the patient must avoid getting the finger wet. Techniques for keeping the finger dry in a cast range from putting a plastic bag around the whole hand to cutting a finger from a surgical glove and placing it over the cast (Fig. 109.e10).

Therapists' reports of POP intolerance are virtually nonexistent. In 40 years of clinical practice using POP, this author (KSS) has seen one possible case of POP sensitivity. Bell-Krotoski (personal communication, 1999) noted that she has never seen a case of POP intolerance despite many years of use. Reporting the rarity of contact sensitivity to POP, Tribuzi[21] noted a study that describes this problem.[22]

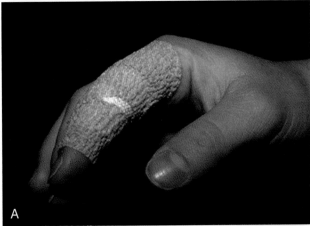

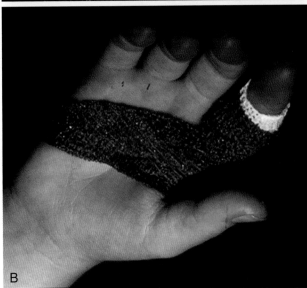

Fig. 109.13 A, To secure the cast in place, Coban can be used to wrap the cast and adjacent skin. **B,** As an alternative to a simple wrap around the finger, the patient can apply the wrap around the cast and then through the palm. (Copyright © 2019 K.S. Schultz.)

Casting Over Wounds

Each clinician must use professional judgment when the finger has open wounds. A therapist can apply POP casts directly over open wounds and over dressings. However, when using casting tape, the wound must have a dressing.[23] A thin dressing offers the advantages of better pressure distribution, less bulk for the patient to contend with, and a more secure cast. A layer or two of a petroleum gauze such as Xeroform may be all the wound needs. The person applying the cast must take care to keep the dressing in place during cast application.

Padding

The outline of the finger casting procedure above does not include the use of padding except for the "cloud" or wisp of cast padding placed at the dorsum of the PIP joint. Therapists often question the reason for minimizing cast padding. Direct pressure to skin does not create the most damaging force to the skin. Rather, shear force, when the skin moves in a lateral direction relative to an edge or normal pressure, generates the greatest skin insults. Plaster without padding will conform and adhere slightly to the skin, preventing shear force under the cast when the fingers move. If skin irritation develops in the cast, then therapist must critically review his or her own casting technique.

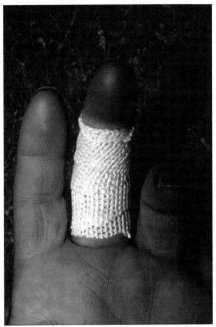

Fig. 109.14 Vascular compromise evident in color change of fingertip with this tightly applied finger cast. The cast must be removed and reapplied less tightly. (Copyright © 2019 K.S. Schultz.)

Indications for Cast Removal

The therapist must thoroughly instruct the patient in symptoms that signal an ill-fitting cast. A poorly made cast can compromise nerve, vascular structures, or skin. Vascular compromise, if not dealt with, can cause skin breakdown. Sharp cast edges—proximally or distally—can also compromise skin integrity. Point pressure directly against a digital nerve can cause a neuropraxia. The symptoms that signal vascular compromise are tingling, numbness, unusual pain, color change, unusual coolness, and persistent throbbing. Tingling, numbness, and unusual pain signal pressure on a nerve. Unusual pain and red skin just proximal or distal to the cast indicate skin compromise from sharp edges.

Sensory Compromise

Casting a patient with sensory compromise places an even greater responsibility on the therapist to make a well-fitting cast. A patient with numbness will not have the primary signal (pain) to warn of problems. However, Brand's initial casting population suffered extreme sensory compromise from Hansen's disease and did extremely well with POP casting. The pressure-distributing nature of the circumferential cast makes it appropriate for this at-risk population. Still, the therapist must strongly emphasize the potential risks to the patient and teach him or her to inspect the skin regularly to check for problems that the nervous system may miss.

Vascular Compromise

With the cast complete, the therapist must inspect the color of the fingertip. It may appear slightly darker red than the adjacent fingers or can change color so much as to appear purplish, which indicates difficulty with venous outflow (Fig. 109.14). Although very rare, the finger may also become white or dusky, indicating difficulty with arterial inflow. The patient must remain in the clinic until the color of the finger normalizes. Usually, the discoloration occurs after the initial cast fabrication, and the problem does not recur with subsequent casts. The therapist applying the cast must use her or his best judgment to determine whether the color of the finger means that the cast can stay on or that it requires removal. A sustained color change can signal unsustainable focused pressure against major arteries or veins. The patient must receive instructions regarding removal of the cast at home if symptoms persist.

Casting Regimen

The frequency of cast changes varies with the characteristics of the patient. Diagnosis, severity and duration of contracture, and wound and sensory status all help determine the number of times a week or month a therapist schedules the patient for a cast change. Often, the issues of geography, financial status, patient schedule, and motivation have more impact on the regimen than the medical factors.

Additional reasons warrant expedited cast change or recheck, especially after the first cast application:

- To check on patient tolerance
- To teach hygiene with the cast in place
- To inspect skin or wound
- To address the looseness of the cast caused by reduced edema

Some patients seem to benefit from less frequent cast changes, whereas others have the best results with more frequent cast changes. Theoretically, the more frequent cast changes captures the new end range and therefore will have better results, enhancing the mechanical signal to the tissue to remodel.[1] Brand and Bell-Krotoski advocated for keeping the cast in place 24 hours a day and changing it every other day (see Fig. 109.1).

At this time, no evidence exists to support a specific regimen. Turner and associates[24] studied the effect of serial plaster casting with clubfeet and concluded that more frequent cast changes correlated with higher level of PROM change. Flowers and LaStayo[14] found that the amount of increase in PROM of a stiff joint is proportional to the amount of time the joint is held at its end range, or total end range time. As a therapeutic model, their study used serial casting for joint positioning. Their results demonstrated that holding a PIP joint at maximum extension for 6 days versus 3 days yielded twice as much ROM gain.

Despite these findings, there are still many unanswered questions such as: At what point does remaining in a single cast—or at a given end range—result in *maximum* PROM gain? At what point does the stress in the tissue relax such that it is no longer being held at its "maximum" length? At some point, tissue remodeling occurs with an increase in length of the contracted tissue that will not progress unless the cast is changed and the joint positioned at its new, more extended end range. Even if the tissue were to increase proportionally past 6 days, as Flowers and LaStayo[14] suggest, would it not increase *even faster* if the new end range were captured before 6 days? These questions deserve future study.

The therapist determines whether to focus solely on one direction of motion—either flexion or extension—or to allow brief joint mobilization at the time of cast removal and replacement. Some literature recommends changing the cast at least twice a week and allowing AROM during the cast change treatment session to maintain full joint mobility.

Clinically, this author (KSS) has found that allowing flexion when the goal is casting to increase passive and active extension seems to lead to greater extensor lags and less PROM gain in extension than continuous focus on extension only. The patients who have demonstrated functional flexion before casting have not—in this author's experience—lost flexion after many months of extension positioning. In the vast majority of these casts, the DIP joint was left free to flex and extend. This AROM may have contributed to flexion maintenance. Yet we have only suggestive evidence that FDP excursion produced this clinical finding.

Ongoing improvement indicates continuation of the casting procedure. When measurements plateau, the therapist may consider modifying the treatment plan or discontinuing the approach. Treatment modification may consist of longer duration heat and stretch before recasting; trial with modalities reputed to soften scar tissue such as vibration, continuous ultrasound, or iontophoresis; or changing the cast at different intervals. The joint's failure to improve suggests referral to a hand surgeon.

When the joint achieves the ROM goal, the patient can wear the final cast as a removable retainer until after that period of time when joint contracture tends to recur or the clinician may choose to fabricate a thermoplastic orthosis as a final "cast," but it lacks the same high level of conformity as plaster or casting tape. The therapist works with the patient to design a weaning process. The patient *gradually* decreases time in the extension orthosis and increases time with functional hand use. The patient and therapist monitor the joint PROM and AROM—extensor lag—to determine how to progress the program. This "balancing act" between flexion and extension requires judgment, patience, and patient compliance.

An additional orthosis used to block the MCP joint in flexion has proven invaluable for helping to establish and then maintain PIP joint ROM in extension and minimize extensor lag. A therapy regimen can couple such an orthosis with the extension cast or neoprene tube. Several designs have proven effective to block the MCP joint into flexion, including the hand-based gutter, the "figure 8" (Fig. 109.15A and B), and the yoke or relative motion orthosis (see Chapter 107) (Fig. 109.15C and D). As always, the therapist and patient determine which design is most effective and allows hand use for activities of daily living (ADLs).

REMOVABLE CYLINDER CASTS

Occasions will arise when the patient must have the ability to remove the serial cylinder cast for exercise. The most obvious cases involve diagnoses that have the potential to result in tendon adhesions if the patient does not perform AROM. For example, after tendon reconstruction or when the patient can attend therapy only infrequently, the removable cast becomes essential.[18,20,25]

The therapist can make the cast removable if it is removed and replaced immediately after the material firmly sets. After the material becomes rigid, one should grasp along the length of the cast and gently loosen and remove it from the finger (Fig. 109.e11) *Cast removal at this point is essential to make it removable for exercise of the joint.* The therapist should continually check the finger and cast for points of pressure. The therapist should clean the excess plaster off the finger, optionally apply a light coat of lanolin to the finger, and replace or allow the patient to replace the cast. A coating of nail polish on top of the dry cast will add strength and prevent breakdown of the plaster as the cast is repeatedly removed and reapplied to the finger. Note that the application of nail polish may affect air circulation.

If swelling or joint contours of the IP joint prevents easy removal of the cast, the therapist can make a small cut (Fig. 109.e12) or window (see Fig. 109.10) in the dorsoradial portion of the cast at the proximal phalanx. The cut extends toward the IP joint until pulling on the cast releases it. With the cast off the finger, the therapist can trim the edges. The therapist can then replace the cast, wrapping the slit or window in the cast with tape so the finger joint does not lose position (Fig. 109.16).

PLASTER CASTING FOR DORSAL PROXIMAL INTERPHALANGEAL JOINT WOUNDS OR WEBBED FINGERS

Paul Brand, MD, developed an alternative casting method with a hand-based extension for casting a dorsal PIP joint wound or casting for improved ROM with webbed fingers. This technique provides increased cast stabilization. A wound over the dorsum of the PIP

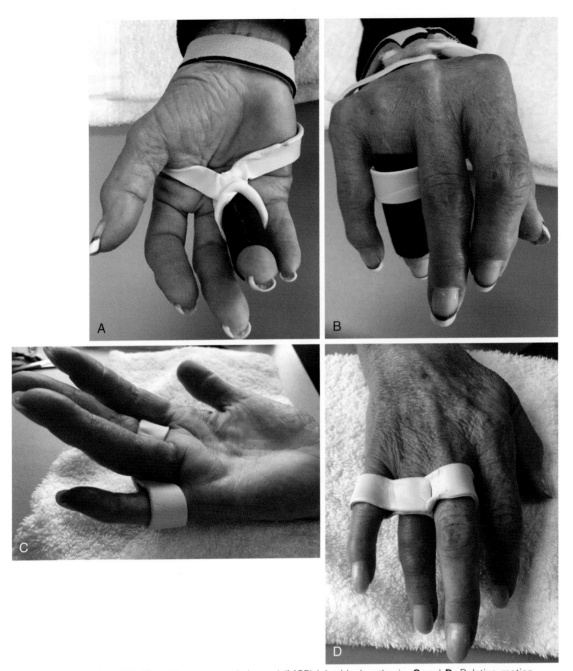

Fig. 109.15 A and **B,** Figure-8 metacarpophalangeal (MCP) joint block orthosis. **C** and **D,** Relative motion orthosis both used to block MCP joint extension and promote active proximal interphalangeal (PIP) extension (reverse blocking for PIP joint extension). The MCP joint extension block orthosis can be used to prevent or improve a PIP joint extensor lag when the extension cast or neoprene tube is being weaned. (Copyright © 2019 K.S. Schultz.)

joint necessitates the application of a dressing. Because the dressing decreases the plaster contact with the skin, the padding and plaster cast will shift and cause shear pressure with finger use. Webbed fingers decrease the length of the proximal phalanx that the cast contacts. Inadequate length of the proximal portion of the cast will allow it to rotate forward on the finger, causing additional pressure over the DIP joint. A plaster or thermoplastic volar extension including the volar MCP joint will increase support and prevent dorsal PIP joint pressure (Fig. 109.e13).

After dressing the wound lightly, a volar extension strip is added, made of six layers of plaster, casting tape, or thermoplastic, along the length of the finger, extending to the proximal palmar crease. The

plaster will stick to the finger and dressing. This adherence helps to evenly distribute pressure. External to the cast, this additional plaster or thermoplastic palmar support, will often stick to the plaster, especially if attached to the plaster while hot, and eliminate pressure in the palm. This palmar extension method of casting works particularly well for IP joint wounds, including dorsal PIP joint burns that often involve the extensor mechanism. When the therapist removes and replaces the cylinder cast, the volar slab can be left in place, limiting movement at the PIP joint.

After the plaster sets, a cylinder of plaster around the finger is made, including the slab, in the same wrapping fashion as for cylinder casting. Care should be taken to ensure that the proximal edge of the plaster

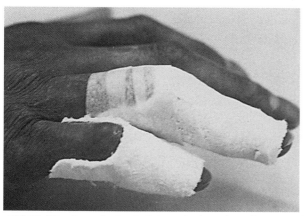

Fig. 109.16 After the patient puts the cast back on, it can be secured at the proximal phalanx with a small strip of paper tape

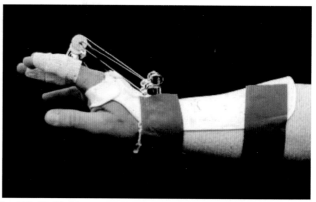

Fig. 109.17 Clinicians can coordinate plaster casting with other forms of orthotic positioning and intervention. (Copyright © 2019 K.S. Schultz.)

does not dig into the palm when the fingers flex. When the clinician identifies a pressure problem, an additional extension is made that encompasses the palm and inhibits MCP joint flexion before making the cylinder cast. Because the therapist applies the cylinder plaster cast after the slab has set, the slab can be left in place and can be cut and the cast peeled off the slab. When used for wounds such as burns, the cast seeks to maintain rather than increase ROM and to limit movement of the joint except when absolutely necessary.

CASTING FOR CORRECTION OF MORE THAN ONE JOINT IN TWO PLANES OF MOVEMENT: FLEXION AND EXTENSION

Clinicians can coordinate plaster casting with other conventional forms of orthotic positioning (Fig. 109.17). This coordinated approach facilitates treatment of fingers that require correction at more than one joint and in two planes of movement. Swan-neck deformities, boutonnière deformities (see Fig. 109.8), IP joint flexion contractures secondary to nerve injuries, and CRPS exemplify these types of finger joint problems.

The technique for casting a swan-neck deformity involves two separate staged casts. The first positions the DIP joint in maximum tolerated extension; the second cast positions the PIP joint to block PIP hyperextension into flexion (Fig. 109.e14).

In the case of a boutonnière deformity, the PIP joint is casted in maximum extension. With PIP joint extension, the lateral bands are slackened, allowing increased flexion of the DIP joint for casting during a second stage.

Brand also described the use of casting to block motion or transfer motion to other joints in the same or another plane of movement.[2,18,20] An immobilization orthosis, although deemed "static," may "dynamically" function to shift motion to joints adjacent to the casted joint during hand movement. For example, casting only the DIP joint for a stiff PIP joint allows the full power of the FDP to act on the PIP joint and enhance efforts at PIP joint flexion (Fig. 109.e15). After intrinsic tendon transfers, the patient often demonstrates undesired flexion at the IP joints with early attempts at activating the transfers. Casting and restricting IP joint motion enhance tendon transfer training and MCP joint flexion (Fig. 109.e16).

The postoperative phase of a central slip repair or a boutonnière deformity reconstruction necessitates casting of the PIP joint exclusively. The cast minimizes PIP joint flexion and so protects the repair or reconstruction. The cast leaves the DIP joint free, allowing DIP joint

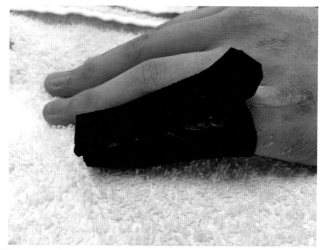

Fig. 109.18 The custom circumferential neoprene tube, designed by hand therapist Vicenç Punsola-Izard, generates the ideal elastic tension to correct the contracture. In addition, it gently compresses the finger to manage scar and edema while it also provides warmth. (Copyright © 2019 K.S. Schultz.)

flexion exercise. Active and passive DIP flexion promotes early limited gliding of the reconstructed or repaired extensor mechanism, encourages normal length of the ORL, and balances the forces acting on the PIP and DIP joints for flexion and extension.

ELASTIC TENSION DIGITAL NEOPRENE ORTHOSIS

Seeking a more effective approach to managing IP joint flexion contractures, Vicenç Punsola-Izard, PT, CHT, MsC, PhD(c), designed the custom Elastic Tension Digital Neoprene Orthosis (ETDNO)[6] (Fig. 109.18). A physiotherapist and hand therapist from Barcelona, Punsola-Izard has been developing this alternative approach to managing IP joint contractures less than 45 degrees for several years. This custom circumferential neoprene tube generates the ideal elastic tension to correct the contracture, gently compresses the finger to manage scar and edema, and provides warmth.

CIRCUMFERENTIAL THERMOPLASTIC TUBE ORTHOSIS

The tube orthosis (designed by Pattie Paynter, OTR, CHT) provides close conforming thermoplastic circumferential positioning of the PIP or DIP joint. Indications for this approach include:

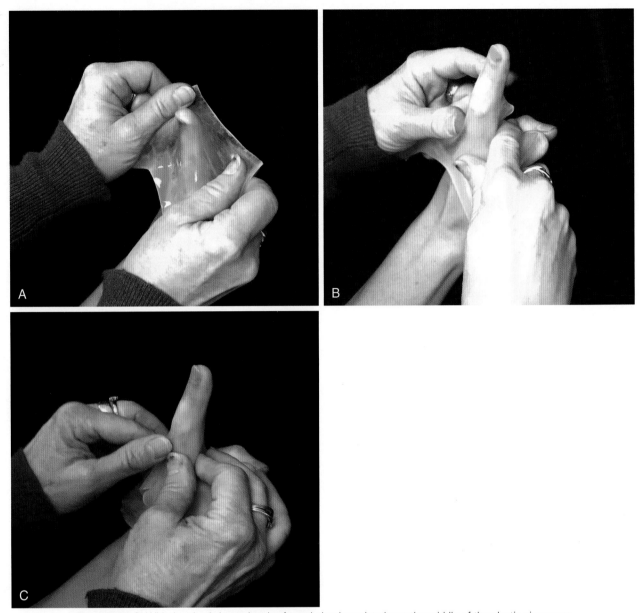

Fig. 109.19 A, With the plastic heated and softened, the therapist places the middle of the plastic piece over the tip of the finger. **B,** Then, holding the plastic piece with as much evenly distributed pressure around the proximal edges as possible, the plastic is pulled down over entire length of the finger. **C,** The clinician should take care to avoid wrinkles in the material. (Copyright © 2019 K.S. Schultz.)

- Maintenance of PIP extension after serial casting, elastic tension orthosis, or static progressive orthosis management has been discontinued
- Immobilization of the PIP joint to minimize flexor tendon glide and resolve inflammation (trigger finger management for patients who require PIP joint control to prevent triggering)
- Blocking orthosis for focus on isolated DIP or isolated PIP flexion
- Protective orthosis over cysts and nodes of the PIP or DIP joints (or both)

Paynter described fabrication with a 2- × 2-inch (5- × 5-cm) piece of ¹⁄₁₆-inch (1.6-mm) thick, smooth thermoplastic in the classic elastic family of plastics[25a] that are characterized by elasticity and stretch but with full memory of the polymers. She recommends practicing with the patient to be sure of positioning and understanding. The patient must know that the plastic will feel warm. The patient needs to stabilize the entire kinetic chain of forearm, wrist, and finger.

With the plastic heated and softened, the therapist places the middle of the plastic piece over the tip of the finger. Then, holding the plastic piece with as much evenly distributed pressure around the proximal edges as possible, the plastic is pulled down over entire length of the finger (Fig. 109.19). The clinician should to take care to avoid wrinkles in the material. The plastic contacting the finger will be ultra thin. After sliding the hardened orthosis off the finger, the excess plastic is trimmed away from the base. Usually one will want to open the tip or the pad of the finger and attend to additional trimming about flexion creases and webspaces (Fig. 109.e17). If heat is used to contour edges, caution must be observed because the ultra-thin plastic will transmit heat quickly, risking the loss of orthosis shape and contours.

If the patient cannot slide the orthosis on and off the finger because of bony contours, the therapist may want to univalve it. The patient can then secure the device with any type of tape or with a hook-and-loop tape strapping system.

The therapist and patient should establish a wear and care regimen together. To clean the inside of the orthosis, the patient should use isopropyl alcohol and a small brush or cotton applicator; exterior cleaning involves a cleaner such as Softscrub or toothpaste. The wear schedule will depend on the purpose of the orthosis.

When the orthosis' goal is to maintain PIP extension after treatment for flexion contracture, the patient will start off wearing the "retainer" for most of the day. The therapist monitors contracture recurrence and extensor lag changes as time without PIP joint extension positioning increases. If the patient loses extension quickly and the extensor lag increases with minimal time with the finger free, then the patient will need to spend more time in the retainer orthosis.

CASTING WITH SOFTCAST

Softcast (3M Scotchcast Softcast, St. Paul, MN) offers another alternative for casting. Unique in the world of casting materials, Softcast remains somewhat flexible and never sets rigidly, as do fiberglass and POP. In addition, although the material does adhere to itself, with a moderate pull, Softcast unwraps much like an Ace bandage. These characteristics offer two major advantages. First, because it never becomes rigid, clinicians can use Softcast for patients who will benefit from slightly flexible immobilization. Second, Softcast does not require a cast saw for removal, so clinicians can use it for patients who cannot tolerate a saw or who may need to remove the cast on their own.

Clinicians either apply Softcast directly to the skin or over a stockinette liner. After the package is opened, there is a relatively short working time to apply the material. Softcast immediately expires; this necessitates discarding any unused material. The rigidity of Softcast improves with the addition of layers; however, this makes the cast heavier and bulkier. Placing a plaster strut underneath the Softcast increases overall rigidity.

CASTING OF OTHER JOINTS AND MUSCLE–TENDON UNITS

Clinicians can use the technique of plaster casting described in the serial cylinder casting section for PIP joint contractures on any joint, muscle–tendon unit, or other soft tissue contractures. Muscle–tendon unit contractures usually require slab casting to incorporate the full length of the muscle–tendon unit in the cast. Casts to lengthen finger flexor muscle–tendon unit shortening involve two stages: a set volar slab (six to eight layers) followed by a circumferential cast (one to two layers). The clinician fabricates the plaster slab for the volar wrist and forearm over light padding or stockinette. To secure the volar slab, plaster is then applied circumferentially about the dorsal aspect of the forearm without padding. Just as in the serial cylinder finger casting technique, the sticking of the cast to the skin helps distribute point pressure and holds the position exactly for tissue remodeling to occur.

Serial Plaster Slabs

Serial-static plaster orthoses have many applications in the management of complex hand injuries. A patient may be referred for serial casting after tendon transfer surgery to serially adjust the positioning of the fingers and wrist when the transfers are initially too tight. Volar plaster slabs effectively reduce extrinsic flexor tendon tightness, and dorsal plaster slabs combat extrinsic extensor tendon tightness (Figs. 109.20 and 109.e18).[2,21] Clinicians use either volar or dorsal slabs for MCP and wrist joint tightness depending on the direction of tightness. For example, the application of a volar slab with the wrist positioned in maximum extension will decrease a limitation in wrist extension secondary to a volar wrist scar contracture. A dorsal slab with the MCP joints positioned in maximum flexion will improve MCP

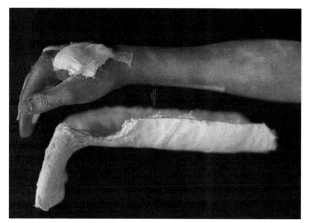

Fig. 109.20 Early postoperative cast orthosis.

joint flexion. A plaster orthosis that positions the MCP joints in extension and the PIP and DIP joints in flexion will reduce tightness of the intrinsic muscle–tendon units. Serial casting of the thumb webspace can correct contracture between the first and second metacarpals.

Extrinsic Muscle–Tendon Unit Tightness

Extrinsic muscle–tendon unit tightness occurs after many types of injuries, including extensive soft tissue injury to the hand or wrist, crush injury, tendon and nerve laceration, replantation, and fracture. It can also occur as a sequela to protective positioning. Although the therapist has several treatment options for minimizing the muscle–tendon unit shortening, the POP stretcher is one of the most effective. The advantage of plaster lies primarily in its extreme rigidity. The initial plaster costs little. However, if the patient requires many serial adjustments, the price of the material, including setup and cleanup, may equal or even exceed the cost of thermoplastic material. The serial static orthotic fabrication process involves progression of the orthosis shape to position the tissue at ever-greater lengths.

The superior drape and ability of POP to distribute pressure allow the shortened tissue to withstand higher forces (Brand, personal communication, 1988). The limitations in the amount of force that an orthosis can generate relates to skin tolerance. However, well-distributed force at the orthosis–skin interface allows the shortened target tissue to withstand higher loads.[2] Some theorize that higher loads may have the potential to increase tissue length faster. Thus, plaster provides the opportunity to increase PROM faster than materials that do not conform as well and demonstrate less efficient load distribution.

Serial Static Plaster of Paris Casting to Lengthen Shortened Muscle–Tendon Units and Scar Tissue

Materials and Preparation

The following are needed to fabricate a POP cast (stretcher):

- Approximately 6 to 10 layers of extra-fast-setting POP cut from rolls or strips—width and number of strips depends upon size of arm. (A recent study by Vieira and associates[26] found that the use of 10 layers for positioning orthoses is advisable because it was found to have better correlation between mechanical strength and weight compared with orthoses fabricated from 6 to 8 layers.)
- Stockinette
- Additional POP strips for finishing
- Warm water
- Clean bowl
- Plaster scissors
- Tissues

- Drapes to protect work surfaces and the patient's clothes
- Finger loops of vinyl with line attached or flexible surgical drain tubing (the necessity of finger loops becomes apparent when flexor tightness differs significantly among the digits)
- Cast padding (optional)
- Draped arm wedge—foam or solid (optional)
- Banding metal, thermoplastic strips, or additional POP strips for reinforcement (optional)
- Paper tape or other finishing material (optional)

Gather the required materials and equipment. Protect surfaces from plaster drippings with disposable, waterproof covers. Both the therapist and patient should protect their clothing with drapes or aprons and should remove their watches and rings.

To determine the amount of POP required for the cast, measure the greatest width of the extremity, generally the palm or proximal forearm. Be sure to include the drape of the material halfway down the forearm or palm in the measurement. To determine POP strip length, measure the length from the longest fingertip to two thirds of the way up the forearm (Fig. 109.e19). Round the corners of the plaster. Lay the plaster down on the hand to determine the location of the thenar eminence. Cut a slit in the plaster at the midway point of the thenar eminence. This area is turned back to leave the thumb free, and the overlap will reinforce this thinner part of the splint.

If using precut plaster strips and working with a large or long arm, two sets of layered plaster can be overlapped to achieve desired length and width. Another approach for incorporating the thumb involves, a 3- × 4- × 2-inch section of plaster gauze that the therapist intersperses in the layers of plaster before wetting the plaster.

Method

Tissue Preconditioning. As for finger casting, gains in PROM of the forearm occur more rapidly and change to a greater magnitude after preconditioning. Note that patients with sensory compromise may not be candidates for tissue preconditioning with heat.

Position and Technique. Be sure the patient understands the materials, technique, and rationale for cast application. Position the patient and prepare the tissue as follows:

1. Clean and dry the area of the arm to be casted.
2. Seat the patient and place the affected extremity on a firm but padded surface (a foam wedge serves well) with the forearm supinated and position the additional joints as indicated.
3. Determine extension priority: fingers versus wrist. For example, for finger flexor muscle–tendon unit tightness, you will start with the wrist in neutral (or even slight flexion) and place the MCP and IP joints in maximum available extension. When the fingers demonstrate full passive extension, begin progressing the wrist into extension while maintaining digit extension until the target joints achieve full composite extension. In contrast, the therapist may want to position the wrist into maximum extension first and then the fingers. Because clinicians can use the technique of serial plaster fabrication for any joint or soft tissue contracture, applications vary widely. For example, one can cast the MCP joints into flexion using a modified circular casting technique (Fig. 109.e20).[21]
4. To position the fingers, especially if the flexor tightness varies significantly between the digits, place vinyl finger slings or loops with line attached or place flexible surgical drain tubing over the fingertips and have the patient place the fingers under traction into maximum tolerable extension. Caution: Avoid point pressure at all times.

Applying the Plaster of Paris Cast and Stretcher. As the process begins, keep in mind that even with extra-fast-setting plaster, the therapist will have adequate time to contour the POP to the arm. The POP will set in 3 to 5 minutes. Tribuzi[21] described the application

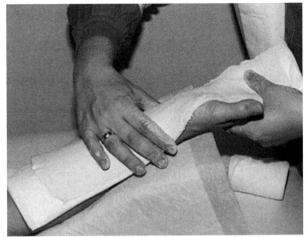

Fig. 109.21 Placing plaster directly on the arm, which has had cast padding applied.

of padding or stockinette before applying the POP. Bell-Krotoski[18] describes applying stockinette or cast padding to the arm prior to molding so it becomes incorporated into the plaster slab (Fig. 109.21). When adding padding after the slab cures, one must use great care because it adds bulk and can become a source of pressure rather than alleviating it. (Incorporation of silastic gel or elastomer padding sometimes works, but they occlude air; Fig. 109.e21.)

Using care to fully saturate all of the POP, immerse all the strips as a group into the water for 5 to 10 seconds. Remove the POP as a unit and gently squeeze along the length of the strips to remove excess water. Laying the plaster on a paper towel will also help to decrease water content. Smooth the plaster while unfolding it. Place the wet plaster on the patient's arm and over the fingers (or fingers in the slings if used). Leave the tips of the fingers visible to observe circulation. Unless the stretcher also incorporates the thumb, cut a slit in the plaster at the midway point of the thenar eminence.

Using all of the POP layers as a single unit, mold the POP to the arm, carefully contouring the forearm, palm, fingers, and spaces between the fingers. Avoid pressure application to the POP. The person positioning the fingers controls the finger and wrist joint angles, and the person forming the stretcher simply follows the shape and position of the hand and arm. Apply uniform tension and maintain the position of the wrist and fingers during molding and setting of the plaster. *If the ROM of each finger differs significantly, the plaster can be cut longitudinally between the fingers to position the fingers at different angles.*

After the POP sets up, remove it from the arm. Although the plaster feels dry on the surface, deeper layers may still be moist. At this point in the fabrication process, the slab will still have enough moldability to permit edge smoothing by hand or with plaster scissors. To increase the rigidity of the orthosis, the therapist may add reinforcement using thermoplastic or banding metal. The reinforcement bar should extend over most of the length of the stretcher. Additional strips of POP secure the reinforcements to the POP base. Trim rough edges. Overlap the plaster with the cast padding or stockinette. If one uses tape, it will need to adhere back onto itself because it does not stick to wet plaster. Thin Elastoplast (Beirsdorf-Jobst, Inc., Rutherford College, NC) can create a finished edge.

Securing the Plaster of Paris Stretcher. With the final POP stretcher revisions complete, the patient puts it on and wraps it into place with an elasticized bandage (Ace wrap). Clinicians have also described using two-sided Velcro, a bias-cut stockinette, or a roll of thin plaster to secure the plaster. The therapist must carefully instruct the patient in proper wrapping technique to avoid vascular compromise and to avoid creating "windowpane" edema. To start the wrap, the patient tucks the end of the wrap in between the index finger and POP stretcher and then starts wrapping proximally in a figure-8 or spiral fashion. The addition of D-ring hook-and-loop straps can reinforce the wrist or finger position.

If the arm underwent preconditioning before stretcher fabrication, the therapist must instruct the patient how to apply the cast when the lengthened tissue returns to its shorter length. In this situation, when first applied, the arm will not fit perfectly into the stretcher. The patient will have to readjust the wrap over time as tissue again lengthens. Some patients do not tolerate this readjustment process well, and for these patients, it may be best to avoid tissue preconditioning. Patients with sensory compromise need to fit into the stretcher when they first put it on. Without excellent skin contact, inadequate pressure distribution results and creates a risk of skin injury.

Check and Revision. Check the stretcher for sharp edges, cracks, and pressure areas. Hot water application can help with edge rounding. A pair of sharp plaster scissors will also effectively contour edges. If cracks appear in the plaster, apply warm water to the cracked area and add two or more strips of plaster. These strips do not need to be the length of the whole splint but must be long enough to adhere well and give adequate reinforcement.

Check the amount of tension the plaster stretcher exerts. Observe the color of the fingertips for adequate circulation. If positioning seems to require wrist flexion, the clinician must monitor for median nerve compromise. Prolonged wrist hyperflexion is contraindicated in almost every case.

Plaster Slab Removal. Because securing of the plaster slab usually involves wrapping or strapping it into place, removal is not an issue. The clinician can remove a circular or two-stage cast by cutting the thin layer of circular plaster or having the patient soak the casted hand in warm water to soften the cast and then unwrapping it or cutting it with scissors.

Cast and Stretcher Regimen. When a patient demonstrates the ability to lift out of the stretcher by 5 degrees at the target joint(s), the time has come for a new stretcher. This makes the decision about progressing a stretcher much easier than for a serial cast.

The therapist assesses the characteristics of each patient and then works with the patient to determine a safe and effective wearing schedule. The patient with a stretcher secured with additional plaster wrap wears it 24 hours per day. With a removable stretcher, the patient should initially wear it for a trial period of 20 to 30 minutes to determine skin tolerance. With tolerance established, the patient can gradually increase time in the orthosis. Patients often demonstrate the ability to wear the stretcher at night during sleep. This achieves 6 to 8 hours of end-range positioning and then leaves the extremity free during the day for exercise and function. With the goal to wear the stretcher during sleep, the therapist may want to decrease the amount of stretch placed on the tissue during stretcher fabrication or may want to avoid preconditioning before fabrication.

For a patient who cannot sleep while wearing a stretcher, the therapist must achieve a balance between stretcher wear, ADLs, and exercise. The more the patient wears the stretcher, the faster the patient will reach the therapeutic goals. A minimum amount of time in the stretcher (which depends on the individual patient) must occur for it to have any effect.[27] The therapist may consider combining other orthoses or POP finger casts with stretchers. Applying the finger orthoses or casts before stretcher fabrication may help achieve optimal IP joint position.

STRATEGIC CASTING OF A CHRONICALLY STIFF HAND

The management of a patient with chronic stiffness of multiple joints of the hand and upper extremity can seem overwhelming. The strategic casting of specific joints of the stiff hand and leaving other joints free for self-mobilization via AROM has proven effective when other approaches have failed.[28-30] Often the clinician notes chronic, unresponsive edema, stiff joints and dysfunctional patterns of movement (e.g., wrist flexion with finger flexion rather than wrist extension with finger flexion). Theoretically, the casting facilitates the lymphatic system, helps reeducate the patient to perform functional movement patterns, and allows the patient to focus on a few stiff joints at a time.[28-29] Although the casting of stiff joints such as the wrist and MCP joints in one position for a significant time may seem to contradict basic philosophies about how to mobilize joints, this approach has demonstrated effectiveness. Readers are referred to Chapter 28 for more information on casting motion to mobilize stiffness.

MEASUREMENT AND DOCUMENTATION OF CHANGE

Clinicians quantify improvement in soft tissue mobility and joint ROM for all joints with ROM and torque angle measurements[31] before the application of the plaster cast or orthosis. Torque-angle range of motion (TAROM) refers to controlling the amount of force when measuring passive joint ROM to maximum end range.[32] If one clinician applies a different force than another, then the amount of ROM achieved will vary. Using TAROM to perform an evaluation results in consistent outcomes. After each cast removal, the clinician records measurements before application of the next cast. In this way, the therapist documents change in ROM and evaluates treatment efficacy.[2,4,9,14]

SUMMARY

Casting is a powerful treatment technique. The circumferential approach to orthosis management has many benefits, including improved pressure distribution and minimized sheer force and migration. Even patients with cognitive and sensory impairment can benefit from casting. Plaster casting for tissue remodeling is a relatively safe, cost-efficient, and effective method of treating contracted tissues intrinsic and extrinsic to the joint, including joints with a hard end feel. Although the goal of casting often focuses on improvement in joint ROM, the benefits have wider ramifications. Not only can serial casting remodel tissue, but it can also "rebalance" the hand when it reestablishes improved tendon gliding caused by adhesion lengthening or reorients structure position relative to a joint's axis of rotation. Therapists can also combine casting with more complex mobilizing orthoses.

The family of casting products continues to increase, offering patients and clinicians more options. Familiarity with the characteristics of each product helps the therapist choose the material that best meets the patient's needs. Circumferential and noncircumferential casting techniques to serially increase PROM require skills that are unique to this modality. Continued innovation in the use of casting will benefit patients in new and effective ways.

Clinicians must pay special attention during the application of the plaster orthosis or cast to avoid pressure points while positioning the joint or joints in the desired position. Measurements of the change in the tissue length or joint ROM with each successive cast or orthosis change is essential to evaluate the efficacy of the technique and to determine continuation of treatment. Continued clinical research is needed to further define the indications, parameters, and outcomes of serial casting and thermoplastic orthotic intervention for contracture correction of joints and muscle–tendon units.

ACKNOWLEDGMENT

Judy Bell Krotoski was the primary author on this chapter for the first six editions of this text. This chapter is a posthumous collaboration between Judy's previous substantial work and this author's (KSS) desire to add to and update the existing practice.

REFERENCES

1. Brand PW, Beach RB, Thompson DE. Relative tension and potential excursion of muscles in the forearm and hand. *J Hand Surg.* 1981;6:209–219.
2. Brand PW, Hollister A. *Clinical Mechanics of the Hand.* 2nd ed. St Louis: Mosby; 1993.
3. Brand PW. The reconstruction of the hand in leprosy. *Ann R Coll Surg Engl.* 1952;11:350–361.
4. Brandsma JW, Brand PW. Quantification and analysis of joint stiffness. In: *Proceedings of the International Conference on Biomechanics and Clinical Kinesiology of Hand and Foot.* India: IIT Madras; 1986.
5. Beasley J. SoftOrthoses: indications and techniques. In: Skirven TM, Oserman AL, Fedorczyk JM, Amadio PC, eds. *Rehabilitation of the Hand.* 6th ed. Philadelphia: Mosby; 2011:1618.
6. Punsola-Izard V, Rouzaud JC, Thomas D, et al. Le collage en tension dans les orthèses dyanmiques en materiau neoprène. *Chirurgie Main.* 2001;20:231–235.
7. Williams PE, Goldspink G. J Anat. Changes in sarcomere length and physiological properties in immobilized muscle. 127(3):459–468.
8. Eppenstein P, Hill J, Philip P, et al. *Casting Protocols for the Upper and Lower Extremities.* Gaithersburg, M: Aspen; 1999.
9. Kolumban SL. *The Use of Dynamic and Static Splints in Straightening Contracted Proximal Interphalangeal Joints in Leprosy Patients: A Comparative Study.* Washington, DC: Paper read at the forty-seventh annual conference of the American Physical Therapy Association; 1960.
10. Kolumban SL. *Master's Thesis.* New York: University; 1967.
11. Kolumban SL. The role of static and dynamic splints, physiotherapy techniques and time in straightening contractures of the interphalangeal joints. *Lep in India.* 1969:323–328.
12. Ugurlu U, Özdogan H. Effects of serial casting in the treatment of flexion contractures of proximal interphalangeal joints in patients with rheumatoid arthritis and juvenile idiopathic arthritis: a retrospective study. *J Hand Ther.* 2016;29:41e50.
13. Parry W. *Rehabilitation of the Hand.* 4th ed. London: Butterworth; 1981.
14. Flowers KR, LaStayo P. Effect of total end range time on improving passive range of motion. *J Hand Ther.* 1994;7:150–157.
15. Johnson & Johnson. *Plaster of Paris Bandages, their Composition, Manufacture and Modes of Application.* New Brunswick, NJ: Johnson & Johnson; 1927.
16. Ahmed SS1, Carmichael KD. Plaster and synthetic cast temperatures in a clinical setting: an in vivo study. *Orthopedics.* 2011 Jan 1;34(2):99.
17. Hutchinson MJ, Hutchinson MR. Factors contributing to the temperature beneath plaster or fiberglass cast material. *J Orthop Surg Res.* 2008 Feb 25;3:10.
18. Bell-Krotoski JA. Plaster cylinder casting for contractures of the interphalangeal joints. In: Mackin EJ, Callahan AD, Skirven TM, et al., eds. *Rehabilitation of the Hand and Upper Extremity.* 5th ed. St. Louis: Mosby; 2002:1826–1837.
19. Schultz KS. Casting techniques. In: Jacobs ML, Austin N, eds. *The Hand Splinting Process: A Comprehensive Manual.* 2nd ed. Philadelphia: Lippincott Williams and Wilkins; 2003:245–266.
20. Bell JA. Plaster casting in the remodeling of soft tissue. In: Fess EE, Philips CA, eds. *Hand Splinting: Principles and Methods.* 2nd ed. St. Louis: Mosby; 1987.
21. Tribuzi SM. Serial plaster splinting. In: Mackin EJ, Callahan AD, Skirven TM, et al., eds. *Rehabilitation of the Hand and Upper Extremity.* 5th ed. St. Louis: Mosby; 2002:1828–1837.
22. Staniforth P. Allergy to benzalkonium chloride in plaster of Paris after sensitization to centrimede. *J Bone Joint Surg.* 1980;62B:500–501.
23. Brand PW, Yancey P. *The Gift of Pain: Why We Hurt and What We Can Do About It.* Grand Rapids: Zondervan Publishing; 1997.
24. Turner J, Quiney F, Cashman J, et al. The effectiveness of sustainable serial casting for clubfoot deformity in a low resource setting. *Malawi Med J.* 2018;30(1):37–39.
25a. Austin N. Equipment and materials. In: Jacobs MA, Austin MN (eds). *Orthotic Intervention for the Hand and Supper Extremity: Splinting Principles and Process,* 2nd ed. Hagerstown, MD: Wolters Kluwer Health; Lippincott Williams and Wilkins, 2014; p 95.
25. Bell JA. Plaster casting of contractures of the interphalangeal joints. In: Hunter JM, Schneider LH, Mackin EJ, Bell JA, eds. *Rehabilitation of the Hand.* 1978;59:644–651.
26. Vieira GC, Barbosa RI, Marcolino AM, Shimano AC, Elui VMC, Fonseca MCR. Influence of the number of layers of paris bandage plasters on the mechanical properties specimens used on orthopedic splints. *Rev Bras Fisioter São Carlos.* 2011;15(5):380–385.
27. Flowers KR, Michlovitz SL. Assessment and management of loss of motion in orthopedic dysfunction. In: *Postgraduate Advances in Physical Therapy.* Alexandria, VA: APTA; 1988.
28. Colditz J. Preliminary report on a new technique for casting motion to mobilize stiffness in the hand. *J Hand Ther.* 2000a;13:68–73.
29. Colditz J. *Presentation Outline: Therapist's Management of the Stiff Hand.* Philadelphia: Paper presented at the Surgery and Rehabilitation of the Hand Symposium; 2000b.
30. Glasgow C, Tooth LR, Fleming J. Mobilizing the stiff hand: combining theory and evidence to improve clinical outcomes. *J Hand Ther.* 2010;23(4):392.
31. Breger-Lee D, Bell-Krotoski J, Brandsma WJ. Torque range of motion in the hand clinic. *J Hand Ther.* 1990;3(1):7–13.
32. Flowers KR, Pheasant SD. The use of torque angle curves in the assessment of digital joint stiffness. *J Hand Ther.* 1988;1:69–75.

110

Soft Orthoses: Indications and Techniques

Jeanine Beasley, Dianna Lunsford

OUTLINE

CRITICAL POINTS

- Orthotic positioning of the hand is both an art and a science.
- A variety of upper extremity conditions may benefit from soft orthoses.
- Soft orthoses are preferred by many patients, which may improve wearing compliance.
- A variety of materials and fabrication techniques are used for soft orthoses.

Orthotic positioning of the hand is both an art and a science. The definition of an orthosis according to Oxford Dictionaries is "an artificial support or brace for the limbs or spine."[1] Depending on the condition, the goals, and the patient's requirements, an orthosis made of soft materials can be the treatment of choice. Soft orthoses can be flexible, semiflexible, or rigid, depending on the properties of the material and the combination of materials used. The materials used in fabrication are limited only by the therapist's imagination. Various products are available, and more are being developed (Table 110.1). Some examples include neoprene, foam, Lycra, Velcro, leather, Coban, and Moleskin. The requirements of the patient and condition must also be considered in the design of the orthosis. Many patients find soft orthoses more easily tolerated, therefore improving compliance and facilitating wear during activities of daily living (ADLs). Several studies have found that patients prefer soft orthoses to more rigid designs, improving adherence.[2–4] It is important to remember that some patients may not be able to tolerate some of the materials used in soft orthoses. Neoprene, as noted by Stern and colleagues,[5] can cause allergic contact dermatitis and malaria rubra (i.e., prickly heat) in some patients. Patients should also be screened for latex allergies even though less than 1% of the population is currently reported to have a latex allergy.[6] Many of the materials used by therapists are available in latex-free options. Patients should be instructed to discontinue orthotic use if skin irritation occurs and to contact their therapist or physician. This chapter highlights some examples of soft orthoses that have been applied to specific conditions commonly seen in the clinic. This is by no means a complete list but is meant to provide guidelines and suggestions for soft orthosis application and other creative options.

COMMON CONDITIONS FOR SOFT ORTHOSES

Carpal Tunnel Syndrome

Patients with carpal tunnel syndrome (CTS) can have higher intratunnel pressures, resulting in increased pressure on the median nerve.[7] The position of the wrist changes the configuration of the carpal tunnel, which can increase symptoms in the median nerve distribution.[8] Using a sonographic evaluation, Kuo and colleagues[9] reported that the lowest carpal tunnel pressure is with the wrist in neutral for most individuals. An orthosis can keep the wrist in a near-neutral position to decrease these symptoms.[10] Many soft commercial wrist orthoses are a combination of metal stays, fabric, and Velcro. Care must be taken in fitting these prefabricated orthoses to ensure that the wrist is placed in a near-neutral position by adjusting the metal stays. Proximal migration of the lumbricals into the carpal tunnel during digital flexion can increase pressure on the median nerve. Apfel and colleagues[11] recommend an orthosis that also limits digital flexion by 75%. A soft orthosis that includes the digits may be helpful while sleeping to decrease symptoms. The MANU is an orthosis designed to keep the lumbricals out of the carpal tunnel (Fig. 110.1). Two studies demonstrated a reduction in symptoms and improved hand function when the MANU orthosis was worn while sleeping.[12,13] Exposure of the hand to vibration has also been reported to increase carpal tunnel symptoms.[14] Antivibratory gloves (Fig. 110.2) and tool adaptations can be helpful in decreasing these symptoms.

Postoperatively, some patients have persistent pain, aching, or incision site sensitivity. This has been referred to as *pillar pain*.[15] Soft orthoses have been used to protect the tender incision site. Use of padded gloves during activities may reduce pillar pain (Fig. 110.3). Elastic sleeves such as Tubigrip to secure silicone or mineral gel sheeting can also be used while sleeping to soften incisions and scars. A release to the transverse carpal ligament results in increased width of the carpal arch, which may contribute to pillar pain.[16] Cupping the hand by decreasing or bridging the distance between the thenar and hypothenar eminences can be comforting to some patients with the application of a soft orthosis (Fig. 110.4) or by using Kinesio Tex Tape (Fig. 110.5). The taping or orthosis may provide gentle support, allowing gradual adjustment to the new position of the carpal bones.

TABLE 110.1   Product Information

Company	Website or Email Address	Product(s)
3-Point Products Inc	www.3pointproducts.com	3ppBuddy Loops, Wrist P.O.P. 3ppThumSpica Plus-hybrid orthosis
AGF Orthopaedic Devices srl	www.agfmanu.com	MANU Carpal Tunnel Orthosis
Ali Med	www.alimed.com	Dynamic Digit Extensor Tube
Benik Corporation	www.benik.com	Neoprene orthoses
Bullseye Brace	https://bullseyebrace.com	Bullseye Wrist Brace
Ergodyne	www.ergodyne.com/home.aspx	Ergodyne Proflex gloves
Kinesio Holding Corp	https://kinesiotaping.com	Kinesio Tex Tape
Medical Modifications	Karenrozelle@gmail.com	Custom neoprene elbow orthosis
North Coast Medical, Inc	www.ncmedical.com	Comfort Cool thumb CMC restriction orthosis, Count'R Force Radial Ulnar Wrist Brace, Contour Foam, neoprene, iron-on Velcro, and iron-on seam tape
Performance Health	https://www.performancehealth.com	Coban, Rolyan Hand-Based In-line Splint, neoprene proximal interphalangeal extension orthoses, Moleskin, Cica-Care, Rolyan Fabricform CarpalGard Wrist Support, Rolyan Temper Foam, R-Securable II Strapping Material
RBJ Athletic Specialties	lionpawwristsupport.com	Lion Paw Wrist Supports
Second Skin	www.secondskin.com.au	Dynamic Arm Splints: Lycra sleeves
Tiger Paws	www.tigerpawwristsupports.com	Tiger Paw Wrist Supports

CMC, Carpometacarpal.

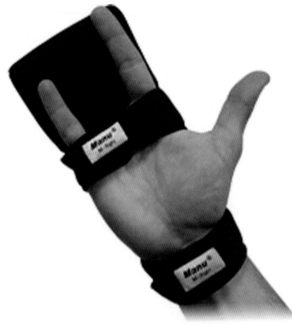

Fig. 110.1 Apfel and colleagues[11] recommend an orthosis that limits digit flexion by 75%. This can decrease pressure on the nerve by preventing the lumbricals from entering the carpal tunnel area during digit flexion.[11] A soft orthosis that includes the digits may be helpful while sleeping to decrease symptoms. The MANU is a soft orthosis designed to keep the third and fourth digits in extension to help prevent the lumbricals from entering the carpal tunnel area. Two studies demonstrated reduced symptoms and improved hand function when the orthosis is worn at night.[12,13] (Used with permission from AGF Orthopaedic Devices.)

Cubital Tunnel Syndrome

The second most common nerve entrapment in the upper extremity is ulnar neuropathy or cubital tunnel syndrome.[17] The cubital tunnel is narrowed with elbow flexion, increasing ulnar nerve symptoms in some patients. A soft orthosis that limits or prevents elbow flexion at

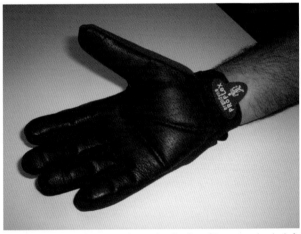

Fig. 110.2 Padded gloves such as the Proflex Glove can be helpful in decreasing vibration during activities of daily living in patients with carpal tunnel syndrome symptoms. These gloves have also been found to be helpful after carpal tunnel surgery in patients with sensitive scars or pillar pain. (Used with permission from Ergodyne.)

night while sleeping has been used to increase patient comfort and decrease symptoms (Fig. 110.6). Apfel and colleagues[18] tested several soft orthoses from commercial manufacturers as well as the use of a folded or rolled bath towel. All of the orthoses limited elbow flexion to less than 90 degrees in their cadaver model.[18] A simple soft orthosis can be made with a paper plate placed on the anterior elbow and secured with an elastic bandage (Fig. 110.7A and B) or upholstery foam secured with Tubigrip (Fig. 110.7C and D). Another more durable option is the use of a sports shin guard or kneepad placed on the anterior aspect of the elbow to limit flexion (Fig. 110.8A). During ADLs, many patients with cubital tunnel report tenderness at the ulnar groove near the medial epicondyle. They also may have a positive Tinel's sign, indicating a possible nerve compression. Pain and sensitivity can be ameliorated by wearing protective elbow pads during daily activities (Fig. 110.7D and 110.8B). Some clinicians encourage patients to wear the padding posteriorly during ADLs and anteriorly at night to restrict elbow flexion.

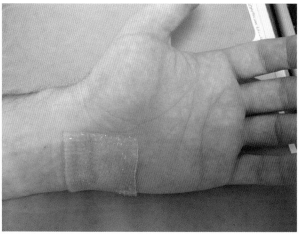

Fig. 110.3 Soft orthoses or wraps can help secure silicone pads or mineral gel sheeting when used to soften scars. Here a Cica-Care pad is applied to the scar. It gently adheres to the skin, and some patients prefer a soft overwrap or orthosis to support the area. (Used with permission from Performance Health.)

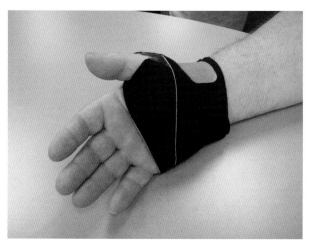

Fig. 110.4 The CarpalGard wrist support helps to gently cup the palm and may decrease pain in patients reporting pillar pain after carpal tunnel release. This position may assist in supporting the carpal bones after release of the transverse carpal ligament. (Used with permission from Performance Health.)

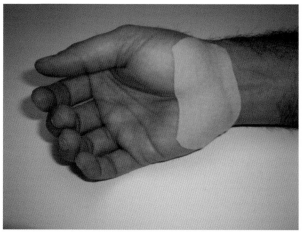

Fig. 110.5 Kinesio Tex Tape (Kinesio Holding Corp) applied to bridge the base of the thenar and hypothenar eminences can help to cup the base of the hand. This may decrease pillar pain in patients after release of the transverse carpal ligament.

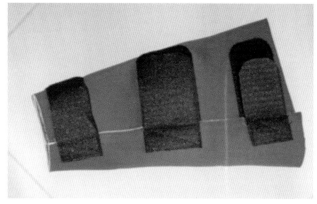

Fig. 110.6 This custom-fabricated neoprene sleeve can be worn at night to prevent elbow flexion, increasing patient comfort and compliance. (Fabricated by Medical Modifications and used with permission.)

de Quervain's Tenosynovitis

Tenosynovitis of the first dorsal compartment, also known as de Quervain's tenosynovitis, involves inflammation of the tendon and sheath of the extensor pollicis brevis and abductor pollicis longus musculotendinous units. Conservative treatment includes immobilization of the wrist and thumb.[19] A recent systematic review indicates that there is moderate evidence to support the use of immobilization along with a steroid injection.[20] Some patients may object to wearing a rigid orthosis and may prefer to attempt treatment with a soft orthosis. A reduction in stress to the inflamed tendons may be achieved with a hybrid orthosis (Fig. 110.9) that combines rigid and soft materials (3ppThumSpica Plus-hybrid orthosis from 3-Point Products, Inc). This may reduce the load of the inflamed tendons and restrict active range of motion. As symptoms improve, a custom-sewn neoprene or Lycra sleeve can provide gentle compression and light support for repetitive activities (Fig. 110.10). This may be helpful for individuals involved in repetitive activities such as musicians.

Lateral and Medial Epicondylitis

Inflammation, degeneration, or pain at the origin of the wrist extensor muscles near the lateral epicondyle has been referred to as tennis elbow or lateral epicondylitis. Golfer's elbow or medial epicondylitis refers to the same condition at the origin of the flexor–pronator muscles at the medial epicondyle. In both cases, wrist and elbow orthotic positioning has been used to rest the structures and decrease pain.[21] Some patients reject rigid orthoses in favor of smaller forearm bands or counterforce straps available from several manufacturers. Soft forearm bands have been found to decrease the force at the extensor carpi radialis brevis (ECRB) origin.[22,23] One study noted this force was reduced by approximately 13% to 15%.[24] A newer strap option was identified by one author advocating for pressure to be both horizontal as well as vertical on the ECRB origin.[25] Care must be taken to avoid a possible radial nerve compression caused by bands applied too tightly. It is important to monitor the patient's symptoms after application of a forearm band. The band should be discontinued if symptoms increase, and more rigid orthotic positioning of the wrist or elbow (or both) may be needed.

Carpometacarpal Joint Osteoarthritis

Many patients with thumb carpometacarpal (CMC) osteoarthritis (OA) demonstrate a deformity that includes metacarpal adduction with subluxation of the CMC joint, metacarpophalangeal (MCP) joint extension or hyperextension, and interphalangeal joint flexion[26] (see Chapters 85, 87, and 88). Orthotic positioning for pain reduction and joint protection in this condition include gently positioning opposite

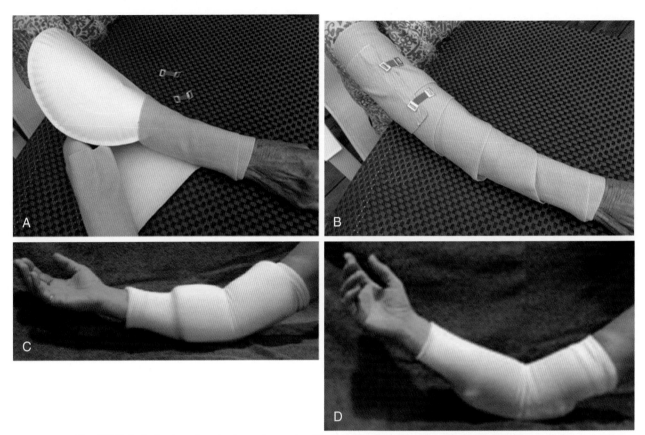

Fig. 110.7 A, A simple soft orthosis can be made with a paper plate placed on the volar elbow. **B,** It is then secured with an elastic bandage. **C,** It can also be made of upholstery foam secured with Tubigrip, **D,** The foam can be placed dorsally to protect the elbow during waking hours. (Part C and D concepts and photos courtesy of Joni Armstrong, OTR, CHT.)

that of the deformity in patients who are passively correctable.[27] This position includes MCP joint flexion, metacarpal abduction, and stabilization of the thumb metacarpal on the trapezium.[28] Some patients request a flexible option for daily activities. The Comfort Cool prefabricated orthosis (Fig. 110.11) was reported by Weiss and colleagues[29] to decrease pain and reduce first CMC joint subluxation. This soft orthosis was preferred by patients over the short opponens thermoplastic orthosis. A study by Hermann and coworkers[30] in 2014 demonstrated that a soft, prefabricated orthosis decreased pain while it was worn. One example of a hybrid neoprene–thermoplastic thumb CMC stabilizing orthosis was designed by McKee to treat this condition (Fig. 110.12). The McKee custom-made hybrid neoprene–thermoplastic thumb stabilizing orthosis (used with permission) is made of ⅛-inch (3.2-mm) thick neoprene and ¹⁄₁₆-inch (1.6-mm) -thick thermoplastic material. The neoprene is secured to the thermoplastic with seam tape. This orthosis gently abducts the metacarpal and stabilizes the CMC joint, gently positioning the thumb opposite of the deformity. The absence of pain during pinch activities while wearing the orthosis is one way to assure that the fit is correct. Radiographs can also be used to assure proper joint alignment in the orthosis.

Rheumatoid Arthritis: Metacarpophalangeal Joint Ulnar Deviation and Palmar Subluxation

Ulnar deviation and palmar subluxation of the MCP joints is the most common deformity seen in rheumatoid arthritis (RA).[31] Orthoses for the rheumatoid hand and wrist have been reported to decrease pain and improve the grip strength by placing the joints in gentle alignment.[32] Callinan and Mathiowetz[3] reported increased adherence when

a hybrid orthosis was made of soft materials with a ¹⁄₁₆-inch volar thermoplastic insert to immobilize the wrist. Soft orthoses can also be worn for daytime activities to allow manipulation of objects. Gilbert-Lenef[33] designed an orthosis (Fig. 110.13) that uses R-Securable II strapping material (Performance Health), which improves alignment and decreases the MCP joint ulnar deviation position. A prefabricated neoprene alternative is also commercially available (Fig. 110.14). Some patients with RA may have difficulty adducting their fifth digit because of disruption of the extensor mechanism and intrinsic weakness. A simple adduction strap to the fifth digit can facilitate MCP alignment during ADLs (Fig. 110.14B). It is important to remember that the digits should not be forced into alignment with these soft orthoses. Forcing digits can cause tilting of joint surfaces instead of smoothly gliding into proper position, as described by Brand.[34] Tilting of joint surfaces can cause additional damage and bring about the wearing away of joint surfaces (see Chapter 85). Another gentle intervention with this condition includes the use of simple stretch gloves that are worn while sleeping. These gloves have been found to be helpful in decreasing morning stiffness and pain.[35]

Instability of the Distal Radioulnar Joint

The distal ulna is normally prominent dorsally in pronation and less prominent in supination. Chronic instability of the distal radioulnar (DRU) joint from a variety of conditions can result in even more dorsal prominence of the distal ulna and can cause pain during forearm rotation.[36] Using an orthosis to brace the area can assist with stability and may reduce pain.[37] Orthotic positioning that provides a dorsal restraint of the distal ulna and a volar counterforce to the distal radius can conservatively

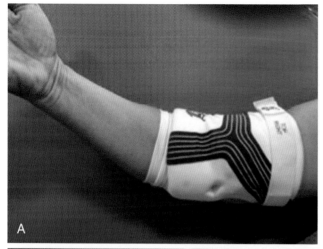

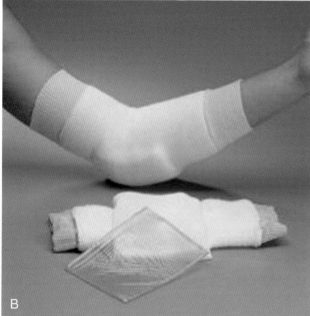

Fig. 110.8 A, Sports kneepad or shin guard can be used on the anterior elbow to limit elbow flexion. **B,** Rolyan Elbow/Heel Protector with gel pad can protect the sensitive posterior elbow in cases of cubital tunnel syndrome. At night, the gel pad can be placed volarly to restrict elbow flexion with the goal of decreasing ulnar nerve compression symptoms. (Courtesy of Performance Health; used with permission.)

manage this condition (Fig. 110.15). This method provides stability to the DRU joint while decreasing pain. The therapist can determine whether this type of orthosis will be helpful if, when examining the patient, he or she manually depresses the distal ulna and finds decreased pain during forearm rotation. Elastic materials are helpful in maintaining a more constant pressure as the patient pronates and supinates. Foam padding can be added to the inside of a prefabricated wrist orthosis or wrist wrap as a quick solution that will add gentle compression to the distal ulna and radius. Patients with long-term discomfort can experience significant pain reduction when the DRU joint is supported in this manner. Other orthoses are commercially available, including the 3-Point Pressure Wrist P.O.P. Splint, which applies compression over the distal ulna and a counterpoint of pressure under the distal radius for stability (Fig. 110.16). The orthosis is applied correctly when pain is reduced with pronation and supination of the forearm. Another option to provide gentle dorsal force over the ulna without pressure to the ulnar head is the Bullseye Brace wristband to assist with the ulnar-sided wrist pain (Fig. 110.17).

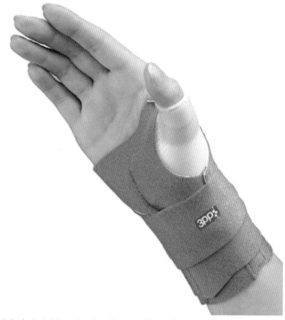

Fig. 110.9 A hybrid orthosis, the 3ppThumSpica Plus-hybrid orthosis, which combines soft and hard materials, may be beneficial in the treatment of de Quervain's tendonitis to reduce stress of inflamed tendons in the first dorsal compartment. (Used with permission from 3-Point Products.)

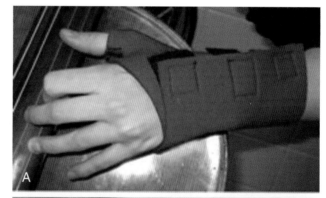

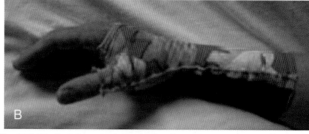

Fig. 110.10 A, A forearm-based orthosis custom sewn out of neoprene for a patient with de Quervain's tenosynovitis. This can help to prevent extremes of motion and is particularly helpful for musicians who are involved in high-repetition activities as they may need to continue to play their instrument. **B,** As symptoms improve, a custom-sewn Lycra sleeve can provide gentle compression and light support for repetitive activities. (Courtesy of Joni Armstrong, MS, OTR, CHT; used with permission.)

Indications for Buddy Tapes

Buddy tapes are another type of soft orthosis that provide support for a variety of conditions, such as collateral ligament injuries, staged tendon repairs, and proximal interphalangeal (PIP) joint deviation caused by OA. Adapting buddy tapes to provide appropriate

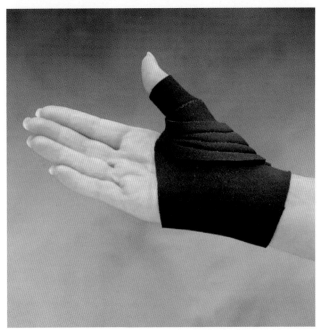

Fig. 110.11 The Comfort Cool thumb carpometacarpal (CMC) joint restriction orthosis has a strap to support and compress the CMC joint while gently positioning the metacarpal in abduction. (Courtesy of North Coast Medical, Inc; used with permission.)

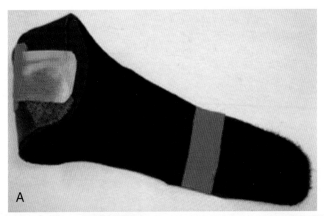

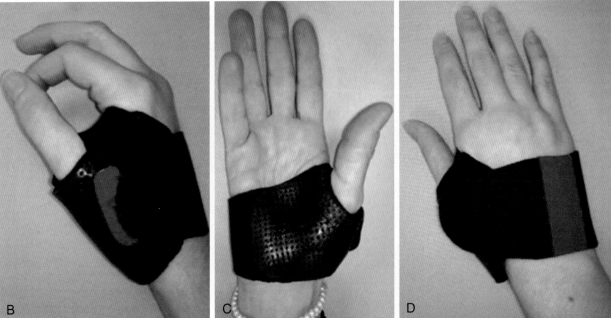

Fig. 110.12 A, The McKee custom-made hybrid neoprene-thermoplastic thumb stabilizing orthosis is made of ⅛-inch (3.2-mm) -thick neoprene and 1/16-inch (1.6-mm) -thick thermoplastic. **B,** The neoprene is secured to the thermoplastic with seam tape (indicated in *red*). **C** and **D,** This orthosis gently abducts the metacarpal and stabilizes the carpometacarpal joint, gently positioning the thumb into a position opposite that of the deformity. (Provided by and copyright of Pat McKee; used with permission.)

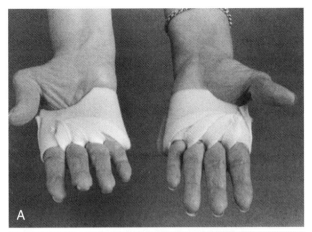

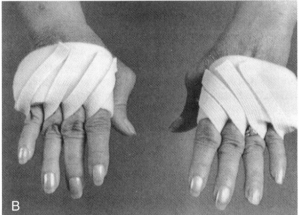

Fig. 110.13 A, Gilbert-Lenef designed a soft antiulnar-deviation orthosis fabricated of Durable II strapping material (volar view). **B,** Dorsal view. (From Gilbert-Lenef L. Soft ulnar deviation splint. *J Hand Ther* 1994;7:29-30; used with permission.)

digital alignment can be accomplished by adding felt or padding (Fig. 110.18). Buddy tapes can be made of a variety of soft materials. Care should be taken to apply buddy tapes correctly, especially with different digit lengths.

Orthotic Positioning of the Athlete's Hand

Athletes are often anxious to return to competition as soon as possible and may need to wear an orthosis during the sport. The challenge is to allow adequate time for healing before returning to the activity.[38] Some rigid orthoses may harm an opponent if they are used in practice or competition. A rigid orthosis on the athlete's hand may not be accepted by the conference referee or permitted by various leagues. During the final phases of healing injuries, soft casts or neoprene orthoses can be helpful.[39] Athletes who may benefit from a soft orthosis include gymnasts with tendon inflammation and wrist pain caused by repetitive weight bearing on an extended wrist. Some of these gymnasts use a soft orthosis called the Lion Paw (RBJ Athletic Specialties, lionpawwristsupport.com) or Tiger Paw (Tiger Paws, http://www.tigerpawwristsupports.com), which support yet limit full wrist extension (Fig. 110.19). A complete examination is needed in these cases to rule out other conditions that may need specific treatment.

Neoprene Digit Extension Orthoses

Tube-shaped digit extension neoprene orthoses are commercially available in a variety of sizes. These orthoses are designed to increase PIP joint extension by means of volar stays or seams (Fig. 110.20). These orthoses can be helpful in treating patients who need increased PIP extension but cannot tolerate pressure to the skin across the dorsal PIP joint. A soft orthosis may assist in reducing these pressures and be more comfortable than some rigid orthoses. In all cases, these orthoses should be monitored to avoid skin irritation and possible skin breakdown.

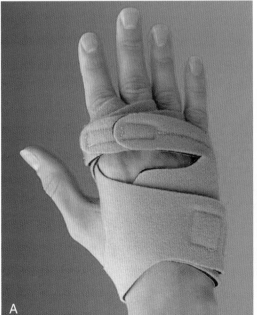

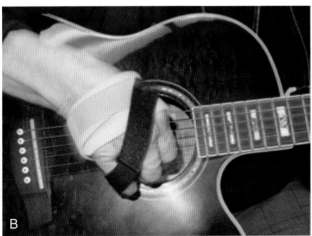

Fig. 110.14 A, Hand-based In-Line orthosis made of neoprene is a prefabricated antiulnar-deviation orthosis. **B,** Some patients with RA may have difficulty adducting their 5th digit due to disruption of the extensor mechanism and intrinsic weakness. A simple adduction strap to the 5th digit can facilitate MP alignment during ADLs. (Part A courtesy of Performance Health; used with permission. Part B photo and concept courtesy of Joni Armstrong, OTR, CHT.)

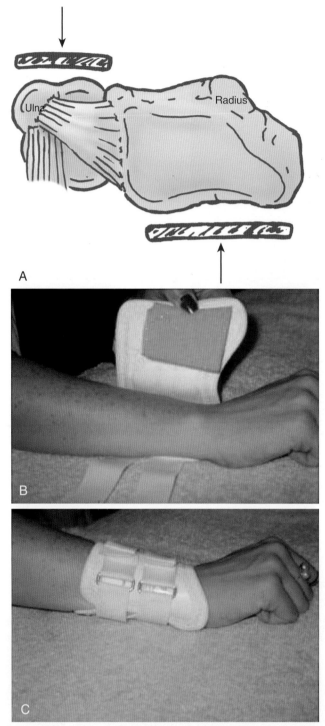

Fig. 110.15 A, Instability of the distal radioulnar joint can be supported with a soft orthosis that provides compression of the distal ulna in a volar direction and a counterforce to the distal radius in a dorsal direction. **B,** A prefabricated wrist wrap orthosis (Count'R Force; North Coast Medical) padded with Temper foam (Performance Health) at the distal ulna and volarly at the radius. **C,** This provides a gentle compressive force to stabilize the distal ulna. (Part A concept courtesy Judy Leonard, OTR, CHT. Redrawn from Melvin JL. *Rheumatic Disease: Occupational Therapy and Rehabilitation*, 2nd ed. Philadelphia: FA Davis; 1982.)

Soft Orthoses for Spasticity and Tone

Orthotic positioning of the upper extremity with spasticity and tone has unique challenges. Children with spasticity caused by cerebral palsy or other disorders can benefit from soft orthoses.[40] A soft orthosis can support the thumb and hand in a more functional position for ADLs in hopes of preventing contractures. A

study by Louwers and coworkers[41] involving children with spastic hemiplegic cerebral palsy used a soft fabric orthosis (with stays) for the wrist and thumb. The orthosis improved spontaneous use of the affected upper limb in bimanual activities with 52% of participants.[41] Spasticity and flexor tone can result in upper extremity postures that can include wrist and digit flexion, digit adduction,

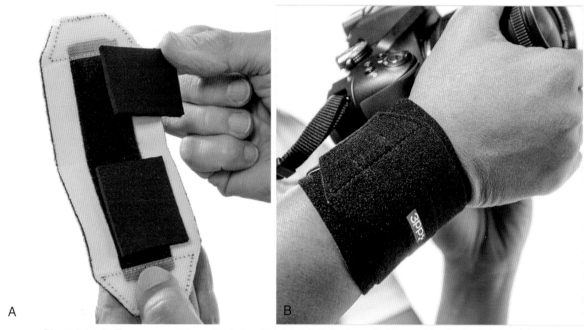

Fig. 110.16 **A,** The commercially available 3pp Wrist P.O.P. Splint is applied to provide distal radial ulnar joint stability. **B,** The orthosis applies compression over the distal ulna and a counterpoint of pressure under the distal radius increasing stability. (Used with permission of 3-Point Products.)

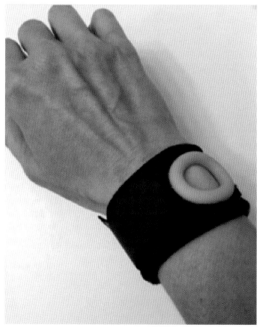

Fig. 110.17 Bullseye Brace Used to provide gentle ulnar compression without pressure on the ulnar head to decrease ulnar-sided wrist pain. (Used with permission of Bullseye Wrist Brace.)

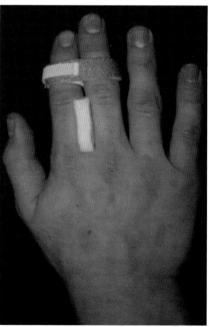

Fig. 110.18 A Foam wrap buddy loop to radially align the middle finger proximal interphalangeal joint (3-Point Products, Buddy Loops). The felt pad facilitates proper positioning.

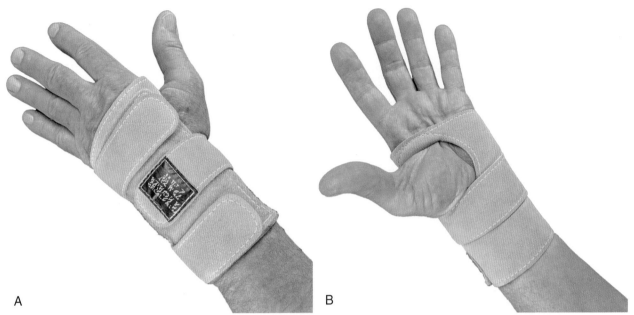

Fig. 110.19 A, Athletes who may benefit from a soft orthosis include gymnasts with tendon inflammation and wrist pain caused by repetitive weight bearing on an extended wrist. Some of these gymnasts use a soft orthosis called the Tiger Paw (Tiger Paws, http://www.tigerpawwristsupports.com). This orthosis provides support and limits full wrist extension with various foam or plastic dorsal inserts. The orthosis is customized to the individual needs of the athlete. **B,** Volar view of the Tiger Paw wrist support. (Courtesy of Tiger Paws; used with permission.)

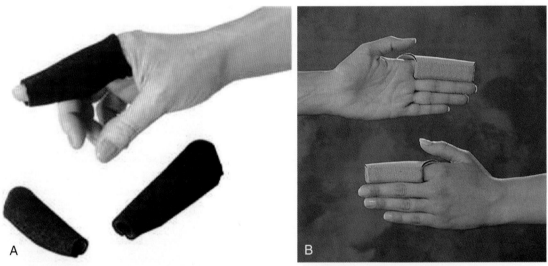

Fig. 110.20 A, A proximal interphalangeal (PIP) joint extension orthosis, the Dynamic Digit Extensor Tube with volar seam, helps extend the digit gently while minimizing dorsal PIP joint pressure. **B,** Neoprene sleeve has a volar metal stay to facilitate PIP joint extension. (Part A used with permission of Alimed. Part B used with permission of Performance Health.)

thumb adduction, and forearm pronation. Casy and Kratz[42] describe a neoprene orthosis to abduct the thumb and supinate the forearm. In cases in which just the thumb is adducted and flexed because of flexor tone, a simple neoprene thumb loop can facilitate gentle placement of the thumb in a more functional abducted position.[43] A step-by-step fabrication of a similar orthosis is included later. Several companies make prefabricated neoprene orthoses, including the Benik Corporation (https://www.benik.com), which also

has pediatric sizes. Lycra sleeves have been used in one study by Elliott and associates[44] to address upper extremity tone at the elbow as demonstrated by a pronation–flexion or supination–extension position (Fig. 110.21). The Lycra sleeve provides a low force to resist the hypertonic muscles and facilitates the agonist. The study demonstrated that wearing the Lycra arm orthosis when combined with goal directed training achieved movement goals during selected functional tasks.[44]

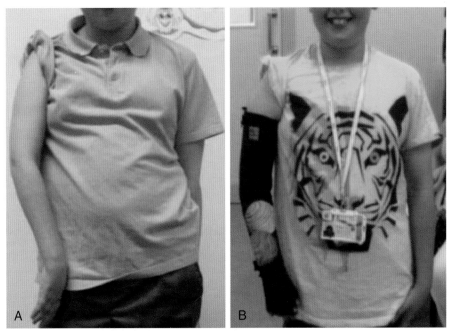

Fig. 110.21 A, Spasticity and flexor tone can result in upper extremity postures that may include wrist flexion, forearm pronation, and shoulder internal rotation. **B,** The Lycra sleeves by Second Skin provide a low force that resists the hypertonic muscle and facilitates the agonist. A study by Elliott and coworkers[42] demonstrated that wearing the Lycra arm orthosis when combined with goal-directed training achieved movement goals during selected functional tasks. (Courtesy of Second Skin; used with permission.)

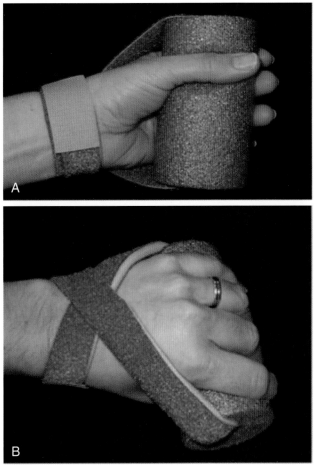

Fig. 110.22 A and **B,** A simple pool foam noodle can be adapted with an electric knife to help prevent flexion contractures of the digits with conditions such as clenched fist syndrome. (Photos and concept courtesy of Joni Armstrong, OTR, CHT.)

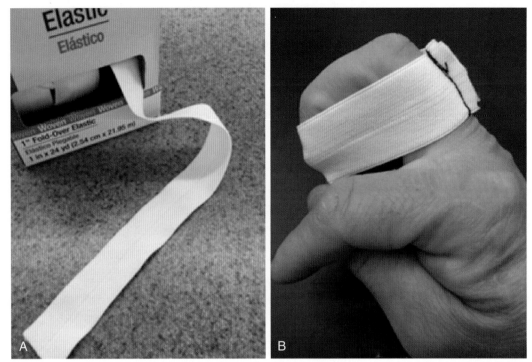

Fig. 110.23 A, Waistband elastic can be purchased by the yard. **B,** It is then sewn into an appropriately sized finger flexion band.

Soft Orthoses Fabricated Out of Nontraditional Materials

Hand therapists working in or traveling to underserved countries may find themselves, out of necessity, using nontraditional materials to fabricate orthoses. Simple designs such as the paper plate elbow extension orthosis (see earlier discussion under cubital tunnel) can be used to treat not only cubital tunnel conditions but also other conditions requiring elbow extension. A simple pool foam noodle can be adapted with an electric knife to help prevent flexion contractures of the digits with conditions such as clenched fist syndrome (Fig. 110.22). A simple elastic bandage can wrap stiff digits into a gentle fist for a few minutes several times a day to provide a low-load, prolonged stretch for passive composite digit flexion for digits 2 to 5. Additionally, waistband elastic sewn into an appropriately sized loop is an option for a single digit to assist with interphalangeal flexion (Fig. 110.23).

FABRICATION OF A THUMB NEOPRENE ABDUCTION ORTHOSIS FOR FLEXOR TONE WITHOUT SEWING

Many therapists shy away from the use of soft orthoses due to limitations in sewing skills. The following technique can be used for therapists who require an alternative approach. A neoprene soft orthosis can support the thumb with flexor tone in a more functional position for ADLs. A similar technique can also be adapted for the osteoarthritic CMC joint. Neoprene material is cut into two strips (Fig. 110.24A). One strap goes around the wrist, and one should be long enough to go through the thumb webspace to place the thumb in abduction (Fig. 110.24B and C). A Velcro hook tab is added to close the wrist strap and at the end of the thumb strap to allow initial positioning and adjustability. One end of each of the Velcro hook tabs and the base of the thumb strap are then permanently secured with iron-on seam tape (North Coast Medical, http://www.ncmedical.com) (Fig. 110.24D–F).

SUMMARY

Soft orthoses for the hand are individualized to meet the needs of the patient and consist of a wide variety of materials. Additional research is needed to determine the effectiveness of these orthoses. The advantages of lower costs, patient comfort, acceptance, and functional use of the hand during ADLs make these orthoses very desirable treatment options for many patients.

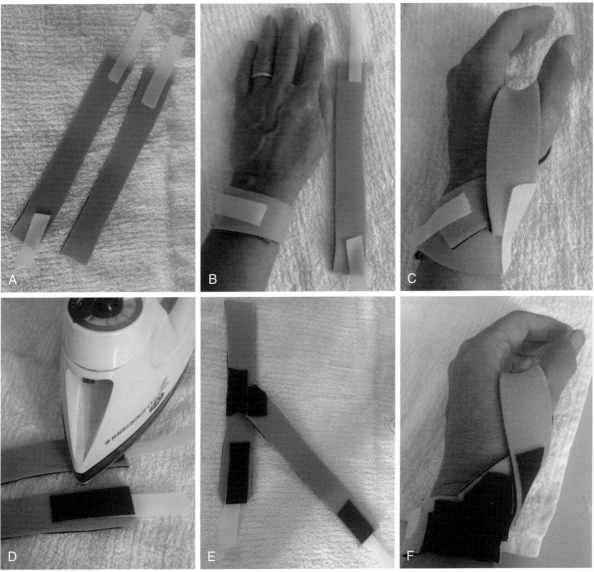

Fig. 110.24 A, The neoprene material is cut into two strips. **B** and **C,** One strap goes around the wrist, and one should be long enough to go through the thumb webspace and place the thumb in abduction. A Velcro hook tab is added to close the wrist strap and at the end of the thumb strap to allow initial positioning and adjustability. **D** and **E,** One end of each of the Velcro hook tabs and the base of the thumb strap are then permanently secured with iron-on seam tape (North Coast Medical). **F,** This thumb neoprene soft orthosis can support the thumb with flexor tone in a more functional position for activities of daily living.

REFERENCES

1. Orthotics. *Oxford Dictionaries*; 2017. [online] Available at: https://www.oxforddictionaries.com. Accessed 25 Sep 2017.
2. Weiss S, LaStayo P, Mills A, Bramlet D. Splinting the degenerative basal joint: custom-made or prefabricated neoprene? *J Hand Ther*. 2004;17(4):401–406.
3. Callinan NJ, Mathiowetz V. Soft versus hard resting hand splints in rheumatoid arthritis: pain relief, preference and compliance. *Am J Occup Ther*. 1996;50:347–353.
4. Henshaw JL, Satren JW, Wrightsman JA. The semi-flexible support: an alternative for the hand injured worker. *J Hand Ther*. 1989;2:34.
5. Stern EB, Callinan N, Hank M, et al. Neoprene splinting: dermatological issues. *Am J Occup Ther*. 1998;52:573–578.
6. Cabañes N, Igea JM, de la Hoz B. Latex allergy: position paper. *J Investig Allergol Clin Immunol*. 2012;22:313–330.
7. Gelberman RH, Hergenroeder PT, Hargens AR, et al. The carpal tunnel syndrome: a study of carpal canal pressures. *J Bone Joint Surg*. 1981;63:380–383.
8. Yoshioka S, Okuda Y, Tamai K, et al. Changes in carpal tunnel shape during wrist joint motion MRI evaluation of normal volunteers. *J Hand Surg*. 1993;18B:620–623.
9. Kuo MH, Leong CP, Cheng YF, Chang HW. Static wrist position associated with least median nerve compression: sonographic evaluation. *Am J Phys Med Rehabil*. 2001;80:256–260.
10. Weiss ND, Gordon L, Bloom T, et al. Position of the wrist associated with the lowest carpal-tunnel pressure: implications for splint design. *J Bone Joint Surg Am*. 1995;77(11):1695–1699.
11. Apfel E, Johnson M, Abrams R. Comparison of range-of-motion, restraints provided by prefabricated splints used in the treatment of carpal tunnel syndrome: a pilot study. *J Hand Ther*. 2002;15:226–233.

12. De Angelis MV, Pierfelice F, Di Giovanni P, Staniscia T, Uncini A. Efficacy of a soft hand brace and a wrist splint for carpal tunnel syndrome: a randomized controlled study. *Acta Neurol Scand.* 2009;119:68–74.

13. Manente G, Torrieri F, Di Blasio F, Staniscia T, Romano F, Uncini A. An innovative hand brace in carpal tunnel syndrome: a randomized controlled trial. *Muscle Nerve.* 2001;24:1020–1025.

14. Jetzer T, Haydon P, Reynolds DD. Effective intervention with ergonomics, antivibration gloves, and medical surveillance to minimize hand arm vibration hazards in the workplace. *J Occup Environ Med.* 2003;45(12):1312–1317.

15. Boya H, Ozcan O, Oztekin HH. Long-term complications of open carpal tunnel release. *Muscle Nerve.* 2008;38(5):1443e1446.

16. Schiller JR, Brooks JJ, Mansuripur PK, Gil JA, Akelman E. Three dimensional carpal kinematics after carpal tunnel release. *J Wrist Surg.* 2016;5(3):222–226.

17. Osei D, Groves AP, Bommarito K, Ray W. Cubital tunnel syndrome: incidence and demographics in a national administrative database. *Neurosurg.* 2017;80(3):417.

18. Apfel E, Gloria T, Sigafoos GT. Comparison of range-of-motion constraints provided by splints used in the treatment of cubital tunnel syndrome—a pilot study. *J Hand Ther.* 2006;19(4):384–392.

19. Cavaleri R, Schabrun SM, Te M, Chipchase LS. Hand therapy versus corticosteroid injections in the treatment of de Quervain's disease: a systematic review and meta-analysis. *J of Hand Ther.* 2016;29(1):3–11.

20. Huisstede BM, Gladdines S, Randsdorp MS, Koes BW. Effectiveness of conservative, surgical, and post-surgical interventions for trigger finger, Dupuytren's disease, and de Quervain's disease. A systematic review. *Arch Phys Med Rehabil.* 2017;17:31018–31023.

21. Carin D, Borkholder CD, Hill VA, Fess EE. The efficacy of splinting for lateral epicondylitis: a systematic review. *J Hand Ther.* 2004;17(2):181–199.

22. Kroslak M, Murrell GAC. Tennis elbow counterforce bracing. *Tech Should Elbow Surg.* 2007;8:75–79.

23. Walther M, Kirschner S, Koenig A, Barthel T, Gohlke F. Biomechanical evaluation of braces used for the treatment of epicondylitis. *J Shoulder Elbow Surg.* 2002;11(3):265–270.

24. Meyer NJ, Walter F, Haines B, Orton D, Daley RA. Modeled evidence of force reduction at the extensor carpi radialis brevis origin with the forearm support band. *J Hand Surg.* 2003;28A(2):279–287. 03.

25. Saremi H, Chamani V, Vahab-Kashani R. A newly designed tennis elbow orthosis with a traditional tennis elbow strap in patients with lateral epicondylitis. *Trauma Mon.* 2016;21(3):e35993.

26. Spaans AJ, van Minnen LP, Kon M, et al. Conservative treatment of thumb base osteoarthritis: a systematic review. *J Hand Surg Am.* 2015;40:16–21.

27. Bertozzi L, Valdes K, Vanti C, et al. Investigation of the effect of conservative interventions in thumb carpometacarpal osteoarthritis: systematic review and meta-analysis. *Disabil Rehabil.* 2015;37:2025–2043.

28. Aebischer B, Elsig S, Taeymans J. Effectiveness of physical and occupational therapy on pain, function and quality of life in patients with trapeziometacarpal osteoarthritis- A systematic review and meta-analysis. *Hand Ther.* 2016;21(1):5–15.

29. Weiss S, LaStayo P, Mills A, Bramlet D. Splinting the degenerative basal joint: custom-made or prefabricated neoprene? *J Hand Ther.* 2004;17(4):401–406.

30. Hermann M, Nilsen T, Eriksen CS, Barbara Slatkowsky-Christensen B, Haugen IK, Kjeken I. Effects of a soft prefabricated thumb orthosis in carpometacarpal osteoarthritis. *Scand J Occup Ther.* 2014;21(1): 31–39.

31. Combe B. Progression in early rheumatoid arthritis. *Best Pract Res Clin Rheumatol.* 2009;23(1):59–69.

32. Steultjens EEMJ, Dekker JJ, Bouter LM, Schaardenburg DD, Kuyk MAMAH, Van den Ende ECHM. Occupational therapy for rheumatoid arthritis. *Coch Database of Syst Rev.* 2004;1. https://doi.org/10.1002/14651858.CD003114.pub2.

33. Gilbert-Lenef L. Soft ulnar deviation splint. *J Hand Ther.* 1994;7:29–30.

34. Brand P. *Clinical Mechanics of the Hand.* St Louis: Mosby; 1985.

35. Ehrlich GE, DiPiero AM. Stretch gloves: nocturnal use to ameliorate morning stiffness in arthritic hands. *Arch Phys Med Rehab.* 1971;52: 479–480.

36. Zimmerman RM, Jupiter JB. Instability of the distal radioulnar joint. *J Hand Surg Eur.* 2014;39:727–738.

37. Millard GM, Budoff JE, Paravic V, Noble PC. Functional bracing for distal radioulnar joint instability. *J Hand Surg Am.* 2002;27(6):972–977.

38. Creighton DW, Shrier I, Shultz R, et al. Return-to-play in sport: a decision-based model. *Clin J Sport Med.* 2010;20:379–385.

39. Almekinders LC, Tao MA, Zarzour R. Playing hurt: hand and wrist injuries and protected return to sport. *Sports Med Arthrosc.* 2014;22(1):66–70. https://doi.org/10.1097/JSA.0000000000000010.

40. Armstrong J. Splinting the pediatric patient. In: Fess EE, Gettle KS, Philips CA, Janson JR, eds. *Hand and Upper Extremity Splinting: Principles and Methods.* 3rd ed. St. Louis: Elsevier Mosby; 2005:517–536.

41. Louwers A, Meester-Delver A, Folmer K, Nollet F, Beelen A. Immediate effect of a wrist and thumb brace on bimanual activities in children with hemiplegic cerebral palsy. *Dev Med Child Neurol.* 2011;53(4):321–326. Retrieved from http://search.proquest.com.ezproxy.gvsu.edu/docview/862237569?accountid=39473.

42. Casy C, Kratz E. Soft splinting with neoprene: the thumb abduction supinator splint. *Am J Occup Ther.* 1988;42(6):395–398.

43. Currie DM, Mendiola A. Cortical thumb orthosis for children with spastic hemiplegic cerebral palsy. *Arch Phys Med Rehab.* 1987;68(4):214–216.

44. Elliott CM, Reid SL, Alderson JA, Elliott BC. Lycra arm splints in conjunction with goal-directed training can improve movement in children with cerebral palsy. *NeuroRehab.* 2011;28(1):47–54. https://doi.org/10.3233/NRE-2011-0631.

Therapy Management of the Upper Extremity Poststroke: Understanding the Mechanisms of Motor Recovery

Rebecca L. Birkenmeier, Eliza M. Prager

OUTLINE

CRITICAL POINTS

- Numerous cognitive and physical factors contribute to motor recovery after stroke.
- Systems theory of motor control and motor learning theory are foundational concepts supporting current best practice.
- A task-oriented approach should be utilized during treatment sessions.
- High intensity practice frequency with distributed, random, variable, and whole task conditions are recommended.

- Performance feedback should be provided in a limited manner with a fading frequency.
- Evaluation should incorporate both objective, therapist administered assessments as well as self-report measures.
- Numerous intervention methods exist but therapists should select a method which follows a motor learning approach.
- Therapists are encouraged to create a client-centered, high intensity, intervention plan designed to increase the client's ability to perform daily activities.

INTRODUCTION TO STROKE AND MOTOR RECOVERY

Hand therapists traditionally treat patients with upper extremity orthopedic and peripheral nerve conditions. However, it is becoming more common for hand therapists to encounter individuals who have upper extremity impairments after stroke. Typical poststroke medical care involves acute and inpatient rehabilitation with roughly 30% of stroke survivors also receiving outpatient rehabilitation.[1] It is during the outpatient stage of care that a hand therapist may treat a patient who has experienced a stroke.

Stroke is the leading cause of long-term disability in the United States with roughly 795,000 people experiencing a stroke each year. A study by Bonita and associates[2] found that 88% of stroke survivors demonstrated hemiparesis immediately after stroke. The majority of stroke survivors experiencing hemiparesis will not recover full motor function in the limb and will continue to demonstrate impairment, activity, and participation limitations for the rest of their lives.[1,3]

Numerous longitudinal studies suggest that there is a predictable motor recovery window within the first 3-6 months poststroke.[4] Initial severity of upper extremity hemiparesis predicts future upper extremity motor impairment,[5] therefore, it is thought that during this early recovery window therapist-directed rehabilitation may have the greatest effect on function outcomes.[6]

This chapter addresses the most common deficits affecting motor function after stroke. A brief overview of the principles of neuroplasticity and the theories of motor control and motor learning are provided as a foundation for clinical decision making. Current evidence-based outpatient therapies directed at improving motor impairment are explained.

COMMON DEFICITS AFFECTING UPPER EXTREMITY MOTOR PERFORMANCE

Hemiparesis

Fifty percent of individuals who experience a stroke will have one-sided upper extremity weakness 6 months later,[5] making hemiparesis the most common movement deficit following stroke.[2,3,7] Paresis, or weakness, occurs when some motor commands are unable to successfully travel from the brain to the spinal cord via the corticospinal tracts.[7] If an individual is unable to initiate any movement at all, this is total paresis or plegia. An individual who is unable to volitionally activate motor units required for coordinated movement,[7] may demonstrate significant difficulty performing daily activities.[1,3] Poststroke hemiparesis is typically one component of upper motor neuron syndrome in which the patient experiences muscle weakness, spasticity, ataxia or decreased coordination, and apraxia or motor planning deficit.[7,8] When observing a patient with stroke, a therapist will observe that movement with the affected upper extremity is slower and less accurate than typical movement. The hemiparetic upper extremity is frequently adducted and internally rotated at the shoulder and partially flexed at the elbow. Because of the decreased movement at the shoulder and elbow, individuals will often compensate for the lack of forward reach with trunk flexion. Hand function is also frequently impaired following stroke.[9] In the recent past, it was thought that motor impairment in the upper extremity exhibited a proximal to distal gradient. The distal joints at the hand were thought to be more impaired than the proximal joints at the shoulder complex.[10] However, recent research has demonstrated that upper extremity segments demonstrate motor deficits at similar severities and that decreased hand function is a result of the limited ability of multiple upper extremity segments to coordinate movement.[10]

Spasticity

Development of spasticity after stroke is associated with severity of hemiparesis at hospital admission, left-sided hemiparesis, and a history of smoking.[3,11] Various studies report that 26% of individuals will show spasticity in the acute phase of stroke, up to 4 weeks after stroke, with 46% of stroke survivors demonstrating spasticity in the chronic phase, more than 3 months after stroke.[12,13] Although spasticity is more likely to develop later after stroke, spasticity can develop as early as 1 week poststroke.[12] Spasticity is defined as a velocity-dependent increase to stretch reflexes resulting from impaired supraspinal inhibitory signals.[8,14] It is important to note that outpatient therapists may be familiar with spinal-origin spasticity experienced by individuals with spinal cord injury or multiple sclerosis. However, cerebral-origin spasticity, experienced by individuals with stroke, differs from spinal-origin spasticity.[8] Patients exhibiting poststroke spasticity typically demonstrate the following posture in the upper extremity: shoulder adducted; forearm pronation; and elbow, wrist, and fingers in flexion.[8] Poststroke spasticity is frequently associated with upper extremity pain,[12] appears to increase in severity over time,[13] and is correlated with limitations in upper extremity function and performance.[3,8,15,16] However, not all spasticity negatively impacts the individual and requires treatment.[17] Indeed, some spasticity can replace voluntary muscle control for simple tasks such as finger flexor spasticity, which aids the individual in holding an object.[8,15]

When spasticity interferes with functional performance, a multifaceted approach including physicians, physical and occupational therapists, nurses, and caregivers is recommended.[18] Pharmacologic treatments include oral medications, an intrathecal pump, or Botox injections.[19] However, limited effectiveness of these treatments and possible side effects require thorough evaluation of the impact of spasticity on an individual's health before treatment.[20] Treatments provided or instructed by the therapist make up the majority of spasticity treatment.[20] Patient and caregiver education on the health conditions that can exacerbate spasticity symptoms, such as pressure ulcers, ingrown toenails, constipation, and urinary tract infections, are imperative to management.[15] Other treatments frequently used in the clinical setting by therapists are stretching and orthotic fabrication.[16,17] Although it is believed that stretching the spastic muscle can maintain muscle fiber length and prevent contracture, recent evidence suggests that stretching has no effect on spasticity.[21] Orthotic fabrication as a treatment modality to reduce spasticity and joint contracture is not supported in the literature as a stand-alone treatment.[3,17]

Ataxia: Decreased Coordination

Ataxia results from a stroke affecting the cerebellum or the cerebellar tracts. An individual who presents with ataxia will demonstrate limited initiation of movement, over- and undershooting of task targets, and inadequate timing of movements.[3,22] Patients with ataxia often use improper force to grasp objects because of the poor quality of movement during functional tasks. Motor learning can be impaired as well, depending on the location of the stroke in the cerebellum, such that motor gains are limited.[23] Although research on remediation of ataxia is limited, various strategies have been shown to benefit the patient. Patients should be encouraged to perform "slow and controlled" movements.[22] Decreasing the number of moving joints by stabilizing the body proximally, either by the patient or therapist, may limit ataxic interference when performing reaching tasks. A few case studies do suggest that a task-specific training (TST) approach is beneficial for improving motor impairment associated with ataxia.[24,25]

Pain

Prevalence of poststroke shoulder pain varies depending on the measurement and definition used; however, up to 84% of individuals have been found to have shoulder pain after stroke.[3] Numerous factors are thought to contribute to pain following stroke[26,28]; specific to the shoulder, these include glenohumeral subluxation[3] and spasticity.[26]

Immediately after stroke, weakness of the scapular muscles reduces the upward rotation of the scapula when in a resting position. As gravity exerts a force on the humeral head in a downward direction, the humeral head can translocate inferiorly, resulting in shoulder subluxation.[3,27] In the chronic phase of stroke, more than 3 months poststroke, capsular stiffness also contributes to shoulder pain.[3,26] It is thought that in acute stroke when subluxation contributes to shoulder pain, early attempts to reposition the humerus in the glenoid fossa using arm trays or troughs are imperative.[3,26] Passive range of motion (PROM) can help maintain the length of soft tissues making up and surrounding the joint capsule, which may reduce pain.[3,26] Evidence on taping for repositioning of the subluxed shoulder is inconclusive[3] but electrical neuromuscular stimulation is thought to increase muscle strength and reduce shoulder pain.[29–31] In patients with some motor function, weakness of scapular muscles and subluxation of the humerus prevent proper kinematics of the glenohumeral joint, leaving the glenohumeral joint vulnerable to injury and limiting functional use of the arm. Further information on the treatment of shoulder instability and stiffness can be found in Chapters 70 and 71.

Complex regional pain syndrome (CRPS) can also occur in the upper extremity after stroke.[26] See Chapters 97 and 98 for information regarding CRPS.

Impaired Sensation

Studies investigating sensory impairment following stroke indicate that roughly half of all stroke survivors have impairment in light touch and/or proprioception.[32] Interestingly, numerous studies report that stroke survivors demonstrate sensory impairment in the ipsilesional extremity as well as the contralesional extremity, though with lower prevalence.[32] Winward, Halligan, and Wade observed that in the first 6 months after stroke, proprioception was the modality with the greatest spontaneous recovery.[33] They noted that sensory recovery was variable within and among patients, indicating no pattern to somatosensory recovery as measured by the Rivermead Assessment of Somatosensory Performance.[33]

Sensory impairment is associated with reduced motor capacity, function, and quality of life after stroke.[36] Recovery of sensation is correlated with positive outcomes in arm function[36-38]; however, some evidence suggests that sensation is not an independent factor predicting upper extremity recovery, but rather individuals with more severe sensory loss also experience more severe hemiparesis.[37]

Though evidence is limited regarding the best method and dose of sensory intervention, emerging evidence indicates that for ideal motor recovery to occur, it is necessary for the patient to demonstrate intact sensorimotor connections.[39] Therefore, it is important that sensory impairment following stroke be thoroughly measured and treated.[36,39,40] Therapists must not neglect educating patients and caregivers on safety concerns associated with impaired sensation as well as cuing patients with poor attention or awareness to the sensory aspects of their tasks.[36]

Apraxia

Apraxia is common poststroke, occurring in roughly one third of survivors.[41] Apraxia results in the inability to perform purposeful, everyday movements[42] and thereby manifests as a movement deficit but cannot be explained by primary sensorimotor impairment. Rather, apraxia is a deficit in motor planning and is therefore ultimately a cognitive impairment. It occurs most frequently after left hemisphere stroke but can also occur after right hemisphere stroke.[41,42] There are many subtypes of apraxia, including ideomotor apraxia and dressing apraxia, but in general, apraxia is considered an individual's difficulty with multistep, purposeful movements that require using a tool.[43] Often, apraxia can present as what appears to the patient and therapist as an abnormal clumsiness of the hand.[43] For example, when a patient is asked to pick up a pen and sign his or her name, the patient may inappropriately grip the pen to pick it up, may struggle with how to hold the pen to write, or may hold the pen upside down and be unable to correctly reposition the pen in his or her hand. Current research suggests strategy training or gesture training to compensate for apraxia, TST, or mental practice may be the best approach to addressing apraxia in the outpatient setting.[3]

Hemispatial Neglect

Hemispatial neglect, also called unilateral body neglect, is a cognitive deficit that occurs in roughly 50% of stroke survivors.[43,44] Therapists will observe that a patient with hemispatial neglect seems to ignore one side of her or his body, typically the left side. While walking, the patient may bump into doorways or walls on the left side.[45] The patient may not use the affected arm in bimanual tasks even though he or she has the motor capacity to do so. Patients with hemispatial neglect are at risk for catching their affected arm in their wheelchair wheel or sitting such that the affected arm is in a harmful position. Treatment for hemispatial neglect can include prism adaptation, visual scanning training, virtual reality, limb activation, and mental practice.[45]

FOUNDATIONAL KNOWLEDGE OF MOTOR REHABILITATION

Recovery from stroke is thought to involve multiple mechanisms, including recovery of tissue in the peri-infarcted area, resolution of temporarily deactivated brain networks, neural plasticity, and compensatory strategies.[6]

To understand the mechanisms driving motor recovery and rehabilitation, it is important to understand the principle of neuroplasticity and the theories of motor control and motor learning.

Neuroplasticity

Neuroplasticity refers to the flexibility of the nervous system, its ability to adapt and change based on experience. Numerous animal studies have shown that the cerebral cortex is capable of reorganization as a result of sensory stimuli and learning experiences, that is, it is experience dependent.[46,47] Indeed, changes to the cortical motor map occur immediately after postinjury behavioral training.[48] After cortical injury, it has been shown that the amount of reorganization of surrounding neural tissue is proportional to the area of damage.[47] In other words, the greater the stroke damage, the greater the reorganization of surrounding tissue. Recent studies have found that behavioral training of just any kind does not promote the cortical plasticity necessary for motor learning to occur. Instead, novel tasks in which new motor challenges are overcome appears to be imperative to experience-dependent plasticity in animals and humans.[48,49] Plasticity of the human motor cortex associated with the upper extremity has been demonstrated in recent stroke studies. After receiving constraint-induced movement therapy (CIMT), participants demonstrated reorganization of injury adjacent brain areas and improved motor performance in the affected upper extremity.[50,51] Neuroplasticity is a widely accepted concept relating to acquired brain injury, such as stroke; however, plasticity-related treatment parameters such as ideal intensity of practice and time poststroke to begin treatment require further study.

Motor Control

To best treat patients with upper extremity movement disorders, the therapist must have a basic understanding of the theory behind motor control. Motor control is the "ability to regulate or direct the mechanisms essential to movement."[52] Motor control is the result of the interconnected influences of the individual, the task required, and the external environment. As such, motor control is dependent on not only the neuromuscular system but also the somatosensory and cognitive systems in the body.

Motor control theories attempt to explain the mechanisms underlying control of movement. The *reflex theory* is one of the more well-known motor control theories. It states that movement is a reflexive response to a peripheral sensory stimulus. In a sense, sensory afferents initiate movement in that they elicit a reflex, or motor response. Normal movement is considered a summation of multiple appropriate reflexes.[53] When treating a patient using the *reflex theory,* improving motor performance is dependent on using the proper sensory stimuli to evoke the desired reflex.[52,53] The *hierarchical theory* states that the central nervous system (CNS), rather than peripheral afferents, drives movement. As the name implies, the *hierarchical theory* divides motor control into levels; the highest levels are commanded by the cerebral cortex, the intermediate levels by the brainstem, and the lowest levels by the spinal cord.[53] Voluntary movement is the highest order of movement and is controlled by the cerebral cortex, whereas reflexive movements such as tonic reflexes and stretch reflexes are controlled by lower levels of the CNS.[53] Using hierarchical theory in treatment, the progress of the patient is thought to follow the hierarchy of involuntary movement to greater cortical command and voluntary movement. Therapists would need to consider methods to "block" lower order movement mechanisms, such as stretch reflexes, for cortical control of movement to appear.[53]

In contrast to the previous two theories, which propose motor control as peripherally or centrally controlled, respectively, the *systems theory* is rooted in the idea that motor control results from neither the peripheral nervous system (PNS) nor the CNS in entirety. Instead, the *systems theory* proposes that motor control is a result of the PNS and CNS exerting control at the same level. The systems theory, sometimes called the dynamic systems theory,[54] involves a complex relationship among the individual, the task, and the environment such that movement is a result of specific task goals and demands.[53] In the systems theory of motor control, feedback from the internal and external environment drives revision of the movement model, resulting in the most efficient means to accomplish a behavioral goal, the ultimate endpoint.[53] A therapist treating a patient using systems theory will need to facilitate the development of new movement models by the patient's nervous system to achieve task goals.

Two categories of treatment approaches based on motor control theory currently exist. Neurofacilitation approaches are based on the reflex and hierarchical theories of motor control, whereas the task-oriented approach is based on the systems theory of motor control. These theories provide a foundation on which a therapist can create a treatment plan and choose interventions. Traditional approaches to motor control, neurofacilitation approaches, include the Rood approach in which various sensory stimuli evoke a motor response, the Brunnstrom approach in which reflexes are inhibited and volitional movement is facilitated, proprioceptive neuromuscular facilitation (PNF) in which movement is seen as a balance between agonist and antagonist muscle groups, and the neurodevelopmental approach in which handling techniques inhibit unwanted movements.[52,54] Each of these treatment methods focuses on reducing the inappropriate movement pattern exhibited by the individual and facilitating voluntary motor control.

More recently developed is the task-oriented approach, or motor learning approach, to motor rehabilitation.[52] A task-oriented approach assumes that motor control results from the dynamic interaction of the individual, the skill, and the environment.[52-54] Important components of the task-oriented approach are attempting to perform real tasks rather than simulated tasks, using real tools and objects as part of the task, and problem solving the most effective motor movements in conditions and environments.[52,54]

Motor Learning

Whereas motor control is the study of control of movement one already has, motor learning is the study of how an individual acquires new motor skills or modifies existing motor skills.[52] Motor learning involves both explicit learning, the recalling of knowledge or facts, and implicit learning, associating a stimulus and response or procedural learning.[52] For example, a patient can verbally repeat steps of a task using explicit learning or physically practice the task such that its movements become automatic using implicit learning. Following is a brief review of motor learning theories.

In *Schmidt's schema*, Schmidt proposes a relationship between four aspects of a motor skill: initial conditions, response specifications, sensory consequences, and response outcome.[55] The relationship of these four aspects of a particular movement is strengthened as the movement is repeated, creating a "motor program." With this motor program in place, the individual can anticipate movement requirements based on the context, and variability of the task can add depth to the motor program.[52,55]

Fitts and Posner's three-stage model conceptualizes motor learning into three hierarchical stages: the cognitive stage in which movement requires a great deal of attention, is slow, inefficient, and inconsistent; the associative stage in which the best strategy for movement is repeated and the movement is refined; and the autonomous stage in which the movement becomes automatic, smooth, and efficient. The attentional demands of the motor movement are greatest during the cognitive stage and least or even absent during the autonomous stage.

Bernstein's three-stage approach also proposes the individual will move through three hierarchical learning stages from novice to advanced to expert. However, Bernstein focuses on the degrees of freedom involved in a given motor task rather than the attentional demands. He states that each joint in the body has many ways in which it can move, and typically, even more muscles that are capable of moving that joint.[53] Therefore, there are infinite ways in which a person can perform a motor movement involving multiple joints and muscles. However, the nervous system controls this problem by "freezing" the degrees of freedom. In other words, the nervous system uses certain established patterns of movement to attain a goal, thus reducing the possible moving parts in the equation. This is particularly important when learning a new motor skill. As motor performance improves, the individual or therapist can gradually "unfreeze" joints or reduce supports, allowing the individual to exert greater control over his or her own posture and movement.[52]

Gentile's two-stage model proposes that the individual first must learn the goals of a task, the relevant environmental feedback, and the best strategy to perform the task. When this is completed, the individual moves on to the second stage of learning, in which the task is either refined into a single movement pattern that is always appropriate for that task, or she or he develops a number of variable movement patterns to complete the task given variation in context.[52]

Three core principles can be drawn from the motor learning theories described. These principles guide the therapist in determining the most appropriate intensity of rehabilitation, activity characteristics, and feedback for each unique patient.

Principle 1: Practice Frequency

How much motor practice should a patient receive during a treatment session or over the course of multiple treatment sessions to maximize functional recovery?

Motor learning researchers widely accept that improvement in motor performance is dependent on the amount of practice.[56] The "power law of practice" states that there is a logarithmic relationship between the *rate* of motor improvement and the amount of potential improvement to be gained.[52] In other words, an individual will improve in skill faster when there is a lot of improvement to be made and slower when less improvement potential remains. This is in keeping with motor learning theories that propose the greatest gains in motor performance are observed in the first stage of motor learning when the learner is in the acquisition, or novice, stage.[52] Stroke studies exploring the relationship between practice frequency or intensity of practice and motor improvement, demonstrate that patients receiving high repetitions of practice show greater improvement in upper extremity motor function than control groups.[57–59] However, in a recent phase II, randomized controlled trial (RCT) frequency of practice involving 4 dose groups upper extremity did not demonstrate the dose–response effect on function witnessed in similar task-based practice studies.[60]

Principle 2: Practice Conditions

How should practice sessions be structured such that fatigue and injury do not limit recovery? Should practice be massed or distributed? Should practice be random or blocked? Should practice be constant or variable? Should practice be whole or part?

Massed practice is a treatment condition in which active time practicing a skill is longer in duration than inactive rest time between practice trials.[52] Whereas *distributed practice* is when the inactive, rest time is equal to or longer in duration than the active practice time.[52] Distributed practice has demonstrated improvements in skill acquisition in patients with stroke.[61] Additionally, distributed practice does not produce levels of fatigue that are likely to lead to injury.[52] Current thinking on this principle is that improvements seen after massed practice are temporary changes in performance, whereas with distributed practice, long-term learning actually occurs.[62] Similar to cramming for a test, massed practice may demonstrate improvement in the short term, but for retention to occur, practice must be repeated over time. Of course, there are situations in which massed practice may be useful, particularly when a patient may benefit emotionally or motivationally from even short-term success on a task.[59] When considering the complexity of the task and patient strength, endurance, attention, and cognitive limitations, massed practice may be necessary to achieve treatment session goals.[59]

Blocked practice is task practice in which the same skill is repeated for numerous trials before moving onto another task. *Random practice* involves context effects or context interference; that is, alternative skills are practiced between trials of the targeted skill such that the targeted skill cannot be, in a sense, memorized and repeated but must be problem solved anew with each trial.[52] In contrast to the repetition and memorization that occurs with blocked practice, random practice forces the individual to generate and execute a motor program with each trial which leads to greater transferability to similar tasks. However, random practice can make skill acquisition more difficult in the initial stages of motor learning. Therefore, utilizing blocked practice is appropriate when the individual is in the acquisition stage of learning, before capturing the task dynamics.[52] Therapists must consider treatment session goals, individual characteristics, and task complexity when determining whether to use blocked or random practice in a given therapy session.[52,59]

Constant practice involves trials of the same task with constant parameters for each trial. *Variable practice* involves trials of the same task in which parameters are varied with each attempt. When attempting to transfer motor learning to a new skill, individuals who participated in variable practice demonstrated better motor performance on transfer skills than those who participated in constant practice.[52,59] The degree of variability can be graded to remain client centered given the individual characteristics and the task complexity.

Finally, *part task training* is when a therapist breaks down the steps of a skill into discrete components that are practiced independently of each other. As the name implies, *whole-task training* involves attempting the entire sequence of steps in a skill with each practice attempt. Breaking down a task can make learning the components of a motor program easier, particularly if it is a complex motor program. There is also a motivational benefit to a patient when he or she is successful in therapy even if only on one component of a task.[59] When tasks are discrete, as they often are for upper extremity movement, part task practice can allow the individual to create a small, simpler motor program with success. Eventually, with practice, small motor programs can be assembled into one larger, more complex motor program. For improvement in functional skills, it is important that the whole task practiced be utilized at some point during treatment.[52,55,59]

Principle 3: Feedback

How much, when, and what kind of feedback should my patient receive?

Motor learning is enhanced by effective feedback. Feedback from within the individual, like proprioception or visual information, is called internal feedback.[56] After stroke, an individual may have impaired proprioception, impaired kinesthesia, hemispatial neglect, or cognitive deficits contributing to poor internal feedback. Information provided by a therapist or outside tool such as a scale or mirror is called *augmented* or *external feedback*. It is important to note that extrinsic feedback is not encouragement; rather, it is specifically timed information regarding the performance of a task and the outcome of a task.[52] *Knowledge of performance* feedback is provided by the therapist and relates to the quality of the movement performed (e.g., limb position or movement velocity).[52] In contrast, *knowledge of results* feedback is information regarding the success or failure of movements that contribute to the outcome of the task.[52] The best knowledge of results feedback is quantitative and provided with fading frequency.[52] In other words, more frequent feedback early in task practice and less frequent feedback later in task practice.[52] Research suggests that a delay between the task attempt and knowledge of results doesn't impact motor learning in and of itself. However, if

PRACTICE PRINCIPLES TO ENHANCE MOTOR LEARNING

Practice Frequency	High intensity therapy: the greater the task practice, the greater the motor learning
Practice Conditions Massed vs distributed Random vs blocked Constant vs variable Part vs whole	**Distributed:** task practice should be repeated with rest periods longer in duration than practice trial **Random:** perform practice trials in random sequence with other tasks **Variable:** vary the parameters (distance, direction, force) within each trial of the same task **Whole:** once patient understands dynamics of the components of the task, perform whole task practice of functional skills
Feedback	Knowledge of results feedback should be provided: In a limited manner with a fading frequency. Where possible, quantitative feedback should be provided.

other tasks or activities take place during the delay, the effectiveness of knowledge of results feedback is compromised. The initial frequency of feedback depends on the capacities of the individual, the difficulty of the task, and the environment. A more challenging or complex interaction of the individual, task, and environment might require more frequent feedback. A simple task completed in a calm and low-stress environment with a highly capable individual requires less frequent feedback. Motor learning is enhanced when the individual utilizes intrinsic feedback to problem solve new, challenging, and meaningful tasks. It is the responsibility of the therapist to provide enough knowledge of performance and knowledge of results feedback to appropriately direct the attention of the individual to components of the task, but not so much that he or she is distracted or disengaged from the task.[63,64]

EVALUATION OF THE UPPER EXTREMITY AFTER STROKE

An essential component of upper extremity evaluation is determining the individual's current level of participation in meaningful activities. A patient should have the opportunity to identify 3-5 tasks or activities that he or she has difficulty performing in the home environment. With these tasks and activities recorded in the medical record, the therapist can clearly and directly relate treatment goals to the functional challenges faced by the patient.

Best practice guidelines recommend that a comprehensive evaluation of the upper extremity is essential for the development of a client-centered treatment plan after stroke.[67] The upper extremity performance issues caused by the stroke are frequently caused by a combination of deficits. Therefore, each patient with a diagnosis of stroke who receives outpatient therapy should be evaluated for the presence and severity of numerous upper extremity deficits. A thorough outpatient poststroke upper extremity evaluation should assess paresis, spasticity, ataxia, impaired sensation, apraxia, and hemispatial neglect. See Figure 111.1 for an example of a comprehensive neuromotor evaluation. Each

Patient Name:		Date:	
Diagnosis:		Prior Level of Function:	
Social & Medical History		Prior Living Situation:	
Precautions:			

UPPER EXTREMITY STRENGTH & ROM

Note- ROM is passive unless indicated with an "A"
Use standard muscle test grades for strength
WNL= Within Normal Limits; N/T= Not Tested

Left		ROM/STRENGTH		Right	
ROM	Strength	Action		ROM	Strength
		Shoulder Flexion	180		
		Shoulder Extension	60		
		Shoulder Abduction	180		
		Shoulder External Rotation	90		
		Shoulder Internal Rotation	70		
		Elbow Flexion	150		
		Elbow Extension	0		
		Forearm Supination	80		
		Forearm Pronation	80		
		Wrist Flexion	80		
		Wrist Extension	70		
		Finger Flexion	Full		
		Finger Extension	Full		

MUSCLE TONE

❑ Normal ❑ Hypertonic ❑ Hypotonic Modified Ashworth Score: ❑ 0 ❑ 1 ❑ 1+ ❑ 2 ❑ 3 ❑ 4

UPPER EXTREMITY COORDINATION

	Left	Right	Coordination with Functional Tasks:
RAM	❑ Intact	❑ Intact	
	❑ Impaired	❑ Impaired	
FNF	❑ Intact	❑ Intact	
	❑ Impaired	❑ Impaired	

GRIP/PINCH STRENGTH

	Left	Right
Hand Dominance (Circle)		
Gross Grasp		
Tripod Pinch		
Tip to Tip Pinch		
Lateral Pinch		

VISUAL/SENSATION/PERCEPTUAL SKILLS   N= Normal   N/T= Not Tested   I= Impaired   A= Absent

	Left	Right	
Light Touch			Comments:
Sharp- Dull			Comments:
Localization of touch			Comments:
Vision/Visual Fields			Comments:
Visual Tracking			Comments:
Hearing			Comments:
R/L Discrimination			Comments:
Motor Planning			Comments:
Proprioception			Comments:
Stereognosis			Comments:
Hot/Cold			Comments:

Fig. 111.1 Two-page initial evaluation of upper extremity performance, including paresis, spasticity, ataxia, impaired sensation, apraxia, and hemispatial neglect. Other factors such as endurance and pain are also included. *ROM,* Range of motion.

ENDURANCE:	PAIN:
❑ _____ % ❑ O2 at _____ L ❑ On room air	Location:
Sitting tolerance:	❑ None ❑ Intermittent ❑ Constant
Standing tolerance:	PAIN INTENSITY: (RANK AND COMMENT AS APPROPRIATE) ╠═╪═╪═╪═╪═╪═╪═╪═╪═╪═╣ 1 2 3 4 5 6 7 8 9 10
Precautions/Contraindications:	
Equipment Recommendations:	

OUTCOME MEASUREMENT SCORES:

FUNCTIONAL PROBLEMS RELATED TO UPPER EXTREMITY MOVEMENT DEFICITS:

OTHER FACTORS INFLUENCING PERFORMANCE:

❑ Edema

❑ Subluxation

❑ Contracture

❑ Orthotic Device Required   ❑ N/A

REHAB POTENTIAL:

❑ Excellent   ❑ Good   ❑ Fair   ❑ Guarded   ❑ Poor

Comments:

Signature / Title:	Date:

Fig. 111.1, cont'd

of these impairments contributes to the motor control and performance of an individual after stroke. Function and performance-based measures should be used in addition to impairment-based measures. The results of this comprehensive upper extremity evaluation can assist the therapist in predicting a patient's anticipated improvement.[64] Properly using and interpreting assessment results can assist the therapist in developing a patient-centered treatment plan.[65,66] Additionally, these results can assist the therapist in adjusting a patient's goals such that goals are achievable but remain meaningful and relevant.[64] Because a patient's deficit severity and functional ability can change over time, it is important to recognize that evaluation after stroke is typically ongoing.[68]

Assessments Addressing Upper Extremity Motor Impairment

Therapists typically perform a series of clinical tests to determine if the client is experiencing upper extremity hemiparesis. A thorough motor impairment evaluation includes assessments of muscle strength, active range of motion (AROM), PROM, spasticity, ataxia, apraxia, and hemispatial neglect.

Assessment of Paresis. Manual muscle testing is typically used to determine the amount, location, and severity of weakness in the upper extremity.[7] Standard muscle testing is reported on a rating scale of (0–5) in which 0 indicates no movement or palpable muscle activation at a particular joint and 5 indicates normal movement.[69] After peripheral nerve injury, hand therapists frequently perform individual muscle testing. However, group muscle testing results are typically (e.g., all shoulder flexor muscles, all shoulder abduction muscles, all shoulder extensor muscles) used poststroke. A dynamometer and pinch gauge should be used to test grip and pinch strength.[68] Using a goniometer, the therapist can measure AROM and PROM deficits.

Assessment of Spasticity. Spasticity is frequently assessed using the Modified Ashworth Scale. Determining the presence of and severity of spasticity is important[8] to quantify patient outcomes. The Modified Ashworth Scale is a quick, easy-to-administer spasticity assessment appropriate for use in outpatient clinics.[70] Because cortical spasticity typically presents with flexion of the antigravity muscles, shoulder flexors and abductors, elbow flexors, and wrist flexors are typically tested. To do this, the patient is asked to lie supine while the therapist places a joint in a maximally flexed position and then quickly moves the joint to a position of maximal extension. It is intended that the PROM performed by the therapist take 1 second. If the therapist decides to test spasticity in extensor muscles, the joint is placed in a maximally extended position and then moved to a maximally flexed position. The therapist then scores the severity of the spasticity on a 0- to 4-point scale. Higher scores indicate more severe spasticity[70] (Box 111.1).

Assessment of Coordination. The ability to produce coordinated upper extremity movement is important for the accurate performance of daily activities. Patients with decreased coordination demonstrate difficulty moving a single joint in one plane. For example, when asked to flex the shoulder, a patient will also abduct the shoulder, flex the elbow and wrist, and pronate the forearm.[7] Patients with cerebellar strokes typically demonstrate ataxia, a type of decreased coordination in which they overshoot and undershoot a target.

Decreased coordination is typically assessed using a series of quick screens. Three commonly used clinical screens include finger opposition, rapid alternating movements, and the finger–nose–finger test.[7] Finger opposition is performed by instructing the patient to touch the tip of the second digit to the tip of the thumb followed by the third, fourth, and fifth digits touching the thumb. Observation of finger dexterity can determine the severity of coordination

---

BOX 111.1   Modified Ashworth Scoring[70]

0	No increase in muscle tone
1	Slight increase in muscle tone, manifested by a catch and release or by minimal resistance at the end of the ROM when the affected part(s) is moved in flexion or extension
1+	Slight increase in muscle tone, manifested by a catch followed by minimal resistance throughout the remainder (less than half) of the ROM
2	More marked increase in muscle tone through most of the ROM, but affected part(s) easily moved
3	Considerable increase in muscle tone; passive movement difficult
4	Affected part(s) rigid in flexion or extension

ROM, Range of motion.
From Bohannon RW, Smith MB. Interrater reliability of a Modified Ashworth Scale of muscle spasticity. *Phys Ther.* 1987;67(2):206-207.

---

impairment. The rapid, alternating movements screen begins with the patient seated with both elbows flexed to 90 degrees. The patient is then instructed to turn the palms up and down rapidly and simultaneously by performing pronation and supination. This test, similar to finger opposition, assesses the fractionated movement of larger more proximal joints than the fingers. Last, the finger–nose–finger test is an assessment of ataxia specifically. The patient is seated across from the therapist and asked to touch the tip of the therapist's finger, then the tip of her or his own nose, and then the therapist's finger again. This reaching and retracting movement is performed several times during which the therapist changes the location of her or his finger. For each of these screens, the therapist can compare the performance of the affected upper extremity with the unaffected upper extremity. Slow or lagging movement in the affected upper extremity indicates impaired ability to coordinate joint motion in the affected limb. Undershooting or overshooting the target indicates ataxia.

Assessments Addressing Nonmotor Factors Affecting Upper Motor Impairment

Assessment of Sensory Deficits. Sensation includes more than one modality, so it is typically assessed using more than one screening tool. The Semmes-Weinstein monofilament test is a pressure threshold test.[54] It is validated and easy to administer. (For further information regarding sensibility testing, please see Chapter 10.) Additionally, static and moving two-point discrimination tests are considered functional sensory tests. These tests classify sensation as normal, fair, poor, protective, and anesthetic.[54] Proprioception can be tested by occluding the patient's vision and, with as little tactile cues as possible, moving the patient's limb. The patient is then asked to describe the direction he or she felt the limb moving.[54] It is important to note that using the unimpaired side as a reference for testing the impaired side is not advised because of the evidence suggesting that sensory impairment after stroke is often bilateral.[32,71]

Assessment of Apraxia. Observation of functional performance is the most common way for therapists to identify apraxia. Patients with apraxia may eliminate key steps of a multistep task, complete task steps out of order, or attempt to use an inappropriate tool to complete a task.[7] If apraxia is suspected and a quantitative assessment is preferred, the 12-item Apraxia Screen of Tulia can be used.[72] The Apraxia Screen of Tulia is free to obtain and takes less than 5 minutes to administer, making it an appropriate tool for the outpatient setting. For the test, the patient is asked to perform a total of 12 gestures and receives a score of

1 (pass) or 0 (fail) according to listed parameters. A maximum score of 12 indicates no apraxia, a score of less than 9 indicates apraxia, and a score below 5 indicates severe apraxia.[72]

Assessment of Hemispatial Neglect. Hemispatial neglect is a disorder that includes visuospatial neglect and body neglect. Visuospatial neglect is typically assessed using a cancellation test such as the star cancellation. Observation of functional tasks is frequently used to determine body neglect in which a patient will not dress the left side of the body. A standardized assessment for both body neglect and visuospatial neglect is the Catherine Bergego Scale. This test is an observational performance-based evaluation of hemispatial neglect.[73] Administration takes 15 to 45 minutes depending on the severity of a patient's symptoms. Patients are scored on 10 items using a 4-point scale (0 = no neglect; 1 = mild; 2 = moderate; 3 = severe).

Assessments Addressing Upper Extremity Performance

We have reviewed several common clinical assessments designed to measure the upper extremity impairments that frequently occur after stroke. Impairment-level assessment can measure changes in deficits, but they cannot measure change in function or performance. It is critical to also use performance-based measures to capture an appropriate picture of a patient's ability to conduct daily life activities.[64]

Best practice suggests that assessment of function and performance should take place at initial evaluation and follow-up evaluations,[3,74] thereby monitoring a patient's progress over time. However, it is common for these assessments to be excluded from patient evaluation because of the additional time burden they add to the evaluation process.[64]

Assessment of function and performance can take two forms, therapist administered performance based measures or client self-report measures.[64] Performance-based measures are scored using either objective ratings by a trained therapist or time to complete the task. For a performance-based measure, a variety of upper extremity functional movements are completed during the assessment. In contrast, self-report measures rely on the patient's or caregiver's perception of his or her functional ability and performance with the impaired upper extremity.

There are a number of reliable and valid performance-based and self-report measures validated for use with the stroke population. We have chosen to include descriptions of a few of these measures used widely in clinical and research settings to assess the upper extremity. Included assessments are relatively quick to administer, require no formal training, are commercially available, and have good to excellent reliability and validity.[29,75-89]

Performance Measures

Action Research Arm Test. The Action Research Arm Test (ARAT) is a criterion-rated assessment of upper extremity activity limitations.[77,90] It includes 19 items divided into four subscales: grasp, grip, pinch, and gross movement. The items within each subtest are scored based on a 4-point ordinal scale ranging from 0 to 3 in which 0 represents no movement possible and 3 represents normal performance of the task. Item scores are summed to create subtest and total scores. A total score of 57 indicates normal movement. Reliability and validity of the ARAT have been well established. The ARAT has a low test burden and high reliability, so it is easy to use and responsive to small changes in function.[9] The ARAT can be purchased commercially or built from instructions included in research studies.[74] The ARAT is appropriate for patients with mild to severe hemiparesis.

Box and Blocks Test. The Box and Blocks Test is a reliable, valid, and quick performance assessment that measures unilateral, gross manual dexterity.[78,79,91] The patient should be seated with the assessment set

up comfortably in front of him or her on a table. Using the unaffected extremity first, the patient grasps one 1-inch block at a time from a box and transports the block over a partition, releasing it into the adjacent box. Patients are given 1 minute to transfer as many blocks as possible from one box to the other. The total number of blocks transferred is recorded as the patient's score. The test is then repeated using the affected extremity. Scores are compared to established norms. This assessment is most appropriate for individuals with some gross finger and arm movement.

Nine-Hole Peg Test. The Nine-Hole Peg Test is a quick performance assessment that measures unilateral finger dexterity.[92,93] Beginning with the unimpaired extremity, patients are timed while they place nine small pegs into a pegboard and remove them as quickly as possible. Total time, up to 120 seconds, is recorded and then compared with norms. Two consecutive trials with the unaffected extremity are completed before the affected hand is tested. The Nine-Hole Peg Test takes approximately 5 minutes to administer and is commercially available.[74] Although highly correlated to both the ARAT and Box and Blocks Tests, the Nine-Hole Peg Test is most useful for detecting small changes in finger dexterity. It is not a sufficient assessment for determining treatment planning or functional improvement in patients with more significant movement deficits.[74,79] Patients need enough finger dexterity to pinch a small peg.

Self-Report Measures

Disabilities of the Arm, Shoulder and Hand. Hand therapists are likely already familiar with the Disabilities of the Arm, Shoulder and Hand (DASH) self-report measure.[94] The DASH was developed to measure disability associated with upper extremity musculoskeletal disorders; however, when used with patients after stroke, it can be a useful measure of the change in patient perception of upper extremity function over the course of treatment.[95,96] The DASH is composed of 30 upper extremity activities typically performed on a regular basis. Items are scored from 1 (no disability) to 5 (unable to complete). A total disability score is derived by averaging the item scores and then converting this out of 5 score to an out of 100 score. This allows DASH scores to be compared with other assessments more easily. Therapists should note that 27 items on the DASH must be completed for scoring to be calculated. A higher score indicates greater perceived disability. The DASH takes 5 to 30 minutes to administer and is free to obtain from the DASH website. The QuickDASH is an 11-item self-report measure intended to provide a quicker method for assessing the properties of the full DASH. However, based on the psychometric properties of the DASH and QuickDASH, the creators recommend the full DASH be used with individual patients because the reliability is higher.

Motor Activity Log. The Motor Activity Log (MAL) is administered as a semistructured interview with the patient, caregiver, or both.[87,97] It is intended to determine how frequently and how successfully patients use their affected extremity for daily activities in the home. The MAL is available in a 28-item and a 14-item measure in which specific activity of daily living (ADL) tasks are evaluated on amount of use and quality of use using a 6-point Likert scale. Example tasks on the MAL include buttoning a shirt, brushing teeth, and using a key. Higher scores indicate better patient perceived frequency of arm use and quality of movement with the affected arm.[64]

Stroke Impact Scale. The Stroke Impact Scale (SIS), is a stroke-specific, comprehensive health measure that assesses health-related quality of life, including dimensions of emotion, communication, memory and thinking, and social role function.[88] This questionnaire is composed of 59 items broken down into eight domains: strength, hand function, mobility, ADLs, emotion, memory, communication, and social participation. The ADL and hand function subscales are the most useful for assessing upper extremity function.[64] A patient rates his or her perceived recovery in each of the domains on a 5-point scale. The total recovery item is presented in the form of a visual analog scale from 0 to 100 in which the participant is asked to rate his or her global recovery level from stroke. The SIS is administered using a semistructured interview and takes approximately 15 to 20 minutes.[88]

INTERVENTION METHODS ADDRESSING MOTOR RECOVERY AFTER STROKE

Treating poststroke hemiparesis is a complex task considering the number of deficits that can limit upper extremity recovery. Additionally, each patient presents with a unique set of impairments and degree of these impairments. Selecting the most appropriate intervention method must include consideration of the patient's current level of function as well as incorporation of the meaningful activities she or he wishes to pursue.[64,67] There is growing evidence that performing meaningful activities as part of therapy provides greater benefit for relearning skills than rote exercise or other modalities that do not encourage the patient to physically move the upper extremity.[98]

Evidence-Based Interventions

Task-Specific Training

Task-specific training is the active, repetitive practice of functional activities to regain motor function after stroke.[99,100] Also, referred to as task-oriented training and repetitive task practice, it is becoming one of the most prevalent poststroke motor interventions and can be easily paired with other upper extremity motor interventions. Earlier in this chapter, the principles of motor learning (practice frequency, practice conditions, and feedback) were presented to help guide the therapist in designing treatment tasks and activities. TST should be implemented using these motor learning principles. The extent to which TST can improve upper extremity movement is currently unknown, but nonetheless, it is reported to be the gold standard intervention choice for improving upper extremity movement resulting from hemiparesis. Several studies have found improvements in upper extremity function using TST.[63,101-103] However, two recent RCTs indicated task-specific movement training did not result in better functional outcomes than results in people who received less movement training.[60,104] This recent evidence suggests that although TST may have a positive impact as reflected on clinical measures, these improvements do not translate to increased arm use in the home setting.[105] Although strong evidence for TST is limited, the principles of TST most closely align with current practice guidelines for stroke.

Principles of Task-Specific Training. Task-specific training is intended to be an individualized approach to improving upper extremity movement following a set of principles derived from both animal models of stroke and other studies investigating movement of individuals after stroke. Lang and Birkenmeier[64] determined several principles of TST from prior literature to help guide the implementation of the intervention.

- Movement improves with repeated practice of that movement.
- Movements must be practiced numerous times to master a motor skill.
- Practicing the same task repeatedly will not be beneficial unless the task challenges current motor capabilities.

- Therapist feedback should be provided in a manner that allows the patient to problem solve the movement problem of a task and is crucial for learning to occur.
- Practicing the same task in varied settings and locations improves the patient's ability to relearn the task and generalize to other contexts.
- Practicing the task as a whole versus breaking the task into parts will help the patient learn the task better.

The 6 principles above can be broken down into 4 simple guidelines therapists can use to design a treatment task: (1) the more movement repetitions, the better; (2) the more the activity is similar to how it will be performed in real life, the better; (3) treatment activities should be difficult but not impossible to perform; and (4) therapist feedback should allow the patient to problem solve her or his performance deficits, which will lead to better relearning of the desired movement.

Matching Goals to Tasks. At the beginning of this section, an individualized, patient-centered approach to developing treatment activities was recommended. Using assessment results from the Neuromotor Evaluation (see Fig. 111.1), the therapist can pair tasks based on the patient's current abilities. During the initial evaluation, patients should be asked what goals they wish to work on, and the therapist should help guide patients to make the goals as specific as possible. For instance, it will be difficult to develop a task if the patient's stated goal is "I want my arm to move better." But therapists can probe the patient by asking, "What types of activities do you wish to do with your affected arm?" This should lead the patient to be more specific. Ultimately, the therapist should guide the patient to create a goal that is more measurable (e.g., "I want to be able to button my shirt without assistance from my spouse" vs "I want my arm to move better"). An example of how to choose a task based on assessment results is provided in Figure 111.2.

Grading Tasks. Repeatedly practicing tasks that have already been mastered takes up valuable treatment time and does not assist the patient in achieving his or her highest level of performance.[64] Likewise, practicing tasks at which he or she repeatedly fails can decrease a patient's motivation for and engagement in the therapy process. Tasks should be practiced until a plateau is reached. At this time, the task should be graded up to make the task more challenging. This process should be repeated for each of the goals the patient has identified.

Example Tasks. Table 111.1 provides an example of how to create tasks for a patient.

Constraint-Induced Movement Therapy

Constraint-induced movement therapy is a widely studied and evidence-supported treatment intervention that demonstrates favorable results compared with usual and customary care.[57,106] The CIMT protocol requires the patient to wear a constraint mitten on the unaffected hand while he or she completes daily activities with the affected hand. The original CIMT protocol has the patient perform activities for up to 6 hours per day solely using the affected upper extremity. Articles on modified CIMT have reported similar improvements for individuals who meet minimum movement criteria at the wrist and fingers.[107,108] The original CIMT protocol requires patients to have active wrist extension of at least 20 degrees and active MP and IP extension of at least 10 degrees in two digits as well as the thumb.[57] Individuals with less than the required movement may not see any benefit from participating in a CIMT protocol. Several barriers exist to implementing CIMT in standard clinical settings. First, the protocol includes 6-hour treatment sessions of intense practice. Patients participate in this intervention for 5 days a week for a total of 2 weeks.

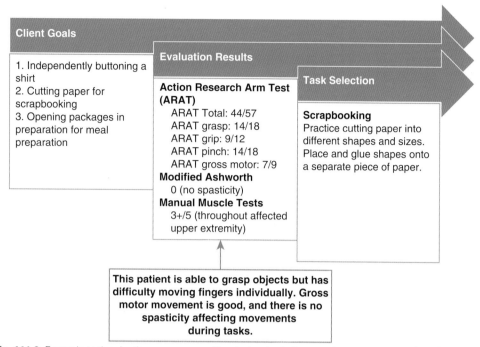

Client Goals

1. Independently buttoning a shirt
2. Cutting paper for scrapbooking
3. Opening packages in preparation for meal preparation

Evaluation Results

Action Research Arm Test (ARAT)
ARAT Total: 44/57
ARAT grasp: 14/18
ARAT grip: 9/12
ARAT pinch: 14/18
ARAT gross motor: 7/9
Modified Ashworth
0 (no spasticity)
Manual Muscle Tests
3+/5 (throughout affected upper extremity)

Task Selection

Scrapbooking
Practice cutting paper into different shapes and sizes. Place and glue shapes onto a separate piece of paper.

This patient is able to grasp objects but has difficulty moving fingers individually. Gross motor movement is good, and there is no spasticity affecting movements during tasks.

Fig. 111.2 Example task selection process used in a task-oriented approach to upper extremity rehabilitation. Choosing a motor activity appropriate for high-repetition task practice involves consideration of client goals and neuromotor evaluation results.

TABLE 111.1   Examples of Goals and Tasks Chosen to Address Them

Goal	Tasks Chosen to Address the Goal	Rationale for Chosen Task
Buttoning	Practice buttoning; practice first not wearing the shirt followed by wearing the shirt to improve fine-motor coordination.	Buttoning is important for the self-care skill of dressing. It allows individuals to be independent with a typical daily activity.
Cleaning a table	Practice cleaning a table using a washcloth.	Cleaning a table is a typical IADL task most people perform as part of their cleaning routine. Grasping a washcloth and wiping down a table works on proximal strength, grip strength, and fine-motor control.
Opening containers	Practice opening and closing containers. (Identify typical containers used in daily life.)	Opening containers is required to perform many ADLs and IADLs independently. Practice of this task allows individuals to work on improving decreased pinch and grip strength.
Playing golf	Practice putting golf ball into target hole.	Playing golf is an important leisure activity for many individuals. Putting a golf ball addresses motor impairments in grip strength, forearm strength, and proximal strength.
Typing a text message	Practice typing text messages into the patient's mobile phone.	Individuals typically use mobile phones on a daily basis. Practicing text messages addresses decreased finger control and decreased finger and hand strength.

ADL, Activity of daily living; *IADL,* instrumental activity of daily living.

During this time, a therapist works one on one with the patient as he or she performs all activities with the affected arm. Additional barriers to implementation include safety limitations because of wearing a constraint mitten, productivity standards that do not allow for the intense therapy sessions required by CIMT, and reimbursement for services.

In an effort to increase the clinical applicability of CIMT, several studies have attempted to modify the treatment to make it more feasible to perform in a clinical setting. In these studies, CIMT is performed for 30-minute sessions three times per week. The patient then wears the constraint mitten at home for an additional 5 hours. Results from these studies indicate that modified CIMT improves upper extremity hemiparesis.[107,108]

It is unclear whether CIMT is superior to other conventional upper extremity interventions of similar intensity; it may not be the constraint that promotes recovery, but rather the high levels of task practice.[109]

Strengthening and Exercise

It is common to develop an exercise program for patients to perform at home when not participating in therapy. Exercise programs focusing on strengthening the upper extremity should not be used in the absence of other functional activities. Instead, therapists should develop strengthening exercise programs as an adjunct therapy. Current evidence suggests that pairing a strengthening program with TST may be beneficial for improving movement of the upper extremity.[110,111] Hands-on interventions (stretching, PROM, and mobilization) commonly used as part of a strengthening and exercise program thought to benefit the individual with hemiparesis have limited support in the literature.[112]

Emerging Treatments
Neuromuscular Electrical Stimulation

Neuromuscular electrical stimulation (NMES) has been shown to improve movement and function of the upper extremity when used during functional tasks.[31] Though a stand alone intervention, it is most often paired with other poststroke upper extremity interventions such as task-specific training.[31] When used with poststroke patients, NMES demonstrates effectiveness in improving both spasticity and range of motion, particularly when applied to the muscles moving the wrist and digits.[113–115]

Mental Practice

Mental practice, also called motor imagery, involves imagining repeatedly moving the affected upper extremity.[116] Imagining this movement activates the same areas of the brain involved in actual movement of the limb. Mental practice can be used as a no-cost treatment that can be completed independently by the patient even when little to no volitional movement exists in the limb.[117]

Virtual Reality

As discussed in previous sections, intensive, massed practice of meaningful activities has been shown to be effective at improving arm function after stroke. Virtual reality or computer technology systems have looked to capitalize on the advantages of task-specific practice through the use of technology. Gaming systems such as the Nintendo Wii and Microsoft Kinect have allowed patients to perform multiple repetitions using real-world objects in the context of a game, thus allowing patients to perform higher intensities of desired movement. Research is limited, but preliminary studies suggest that using virtual reality to achieve high repetitions of movement of the upper extremity is a promising method for improving upper extremity function after stroke.[118]

Mirror Therapy

Mirror therapy, considered a type of mental practice, uses a mirror to convey a reflected image of the unaffected extremity to the patient's brain.[119] The mirror, placed at midline and facing the unaffected extremity, allows the patient to perform hand and arm movement with the unaffected extremity while in the reflection it appears that the affected extremity is actually moving. In addition to observing the reflection, the patient can attempt to move the affected hand and arm while observing the reflection of the unaffected side performing normal movements.[119] Mirror therapy can be useful in helping patients with minimal upper extremity movement regain enough function to participate in more intensive therapies (TST and CIMT) that have movement requirements for success. Recent research has found mirror therapy to be an effective intervention for the improvement of upper extremity function.[120] Chapter 100 provides more detail regarding mirror therapy.

SUMMARY

Regardless of the treatment intervention selected, interventions should be tailored to the individual needs of the patient.[119] The intervention should go beyond routine exercises and be directly catered to the goals the patient has identified. In most situations, it is best to simulate how the patient would typically perform the task in daily life to increase the probability that improvements in function can be generalized to the home setting.

CONCLUSION

This chapter highlights the many complexities that can occur with hemiparesis after stroke. Some have been well studied, but others still lack support. The evidence presented in this chapter highlights the current supported approaches to both evaluation and intervention following best practice guidelines identified for stroke. Therapists are encouraged to create a patient-centered, high-intensity intervention plan designed to increase the patient's ability to perform daily activities.

REFERENCES

1. Benjamin EJ, Blaha MJ, Chiuve SE, et al. Heart disease and stroke statistics—2017 update: a report from the American Heart Association. *Circulation.* 2017;135(10):e146–e603.
2. Bonita R, Solomon N, Broad JB. Prevalence of stroke and stroke-related disability. Estimates from the Auckland stroke studies. *Stroke.* 1997;28(10):1898–1902.
3. Winstein CJ, Stein J, Arena R, et al. Guidelines for adult stroke rehabilitation and recovery: a guideline for healthcare professionals from the American Heart Association/American Stroke Association. *Stroke.* 2016;47(6):e98–e169.
4. Hankey G, Spiesser J, Hakimi Z, Bego G, Carita P, Gabriel S. Rate, degree, and predictors of recovery from disability following ischemic stroke. *Neurology.* 2007;68(19):1583–1587.
5. Go AS, Mozaffarian D, Roger VL, et al. Executive summary: heart disease and stroke statistics—2014 update: a report from the American Heart Association. *Circulation.* 2014;129(3):399–410.
6. Kwakkel G, Kollen B, Lindeman E. Understanding the pattern of functional recovery after stroke: facts and theories. *Restor Neurol Neurosci.* 2004;22(3-5):281–299.
7. Sathian K, Buxbaum LJ, Cohen LG, et al. Neurological principles and rehabilitation of action disorders: common clinical deficits. *Neurorehabil Neural Repair.* 2011;25(suppl 5):21S–32S.
8. Bethoux F. Spasticity management after stroke. *Phys Med Rehabil Clin N Am.* 2015;26(4):625–639.
9. Lang CE, Beebe JA. Relating movement control at 9 upper extremity segments to loss of hand function in people with chronic hemiparesis. *Neurorehabil Neural Repair.* 2007;21(3):279–291.
10. Beebe JA, Lang CE. Absence of a proximal to distal gradient of motor deficits in the upper extremity early after stroke. *Clin Neurophysiol.* 2008;119(9):2074–2085.
11. Leathley MJ, Gregson JM, Moore AP, Smith TL, Sharma AK, Watkins CL. Predicting spasticity after stroke in those surviving to 12 months. *Clin Rehabil.* 2004;18(4):438–443.
12. Wissel J, Manack A, Brainin M. Toward an epidemiology of poststroke spasticity. *Neurology.* 2013;80(3 suppl 2):S13–19.
13. Opheim A, Danielsson A, Alt Murphy M, Persson HC, Sunnerhagen KS. Upper-limb spasticity during the first year after stroke: stroke arm longitudinal study at the University of Gothenburg. *Am J Phys Med Rehabil.* 2014;93(10):884–896.
14. Lance JW. The control of muscle tone, reflexes, and movement: Robert Wartenberg Lecture. *Neurology.* 1980;30(12):1303–1313.
15. Kheder A, Nair KP. Spasticity: pathophysiology, evaluation and management. *Pract Neurol.* 2012;12(5):289–298.
16. Francisco GE, McGuire JR. Poststroke spasticity management. *Stroke.* 2012;43(11):3132–3136.
17. Khan F, Amatya B, Bensmail D, Yelnik A. Non-pharmacological interventions for spasticity in adults: an overview of systematic reviews. *Ann Phys Rehabil Med.* 2017.
18. Yelnik AP, Simon O, Bensmail D, et al. Drug treatments for spasticity. *Ann Phys Rehabil Med.* 2009;52(10):746–756.
19. Li S. Spasticity, motor recovery, and neural plasticity after stroke. *Front Neurol.* 2017;8:120.
20. Yelnik AP, Simon O, Parratte B, Gracies JM. How to clinically assess and treat muscle overactivity in spastic paresis. *J Rehabil Med.* 2010;42(9):801–807.

21. Katalinic OM, Harvey LA, Herbert RD. Effectiveness of stretch for the treatment and prevention of contractures in people with neurological conditions: a systematic review. *Phys Ther.* 2011;91(1):11–24.

22. Bastian AJ. Mechanisms of ataxia. *Phys Ther.* 1997;77(6):672–675.

23. Hatakenaka M, Miyai I, Mihara M, Yagura H, Hattori N. Impaired motor learning by a pursuit rotor test reduces functional outcomes during rehabilitation of poststroke ataxia. *Neurorehabil Neural Repair.* 2012;26(3):293–300.

24. Richards L, Senesac C, McGuirk T, et al. Response to intensive upper extremity therapy by individuals with ataxia from stroke. *Top Stroke Rehabil.* 2008;15(3):262–271.

25. Stoykov ME, Stojakovich M, Stevens JA. Beneficial effects of postural intervention on prehensile action for an individual with ataxia resulting from brainstem stroke. *NeuroRehabilitation.* 2005;20(2):85–89.

26. Harrison RA, Field TS. Post stroke pain: identification, assessment, and therapy. *Cerebrovasc Dis.* 2015;39(3-4):190–201.

27. Gillen G. *Cerebrovascular Accident (Stroke).* 8th ed. St. Louis: Elsevier; 2018.

28. Paci M, Nannetti L, Taiti P, Baccini M, Rinaldi L. Shoulder subluxation after stroke: relationships with pain and motor recovery. *Physiother Res Int.* 2007;12(2):95–104.

29. Uswatte G, Giuliani C, Winstein C, Zeringue A, Hobbs L, Wolf SL. Validity of accelerometry for monitoring real-world arm activity in patients with subacute stroke: evidence from the extremity constraint-induced therapy evaluation trial. *Arch Phys Med Rehabil.* 2006;87(10):1340–1345.

30. Koog YH, Jin SS, Yoon K, Min BI. Interventions for hemiplegic shoulder pain: systematic review of randomised controlled trials. *Disabil Rehabil.* 2010;32(4):282–291.

31. Knutson JS, Fu MJ, Sheffler LR, Chae J. Neuromuscular electrical stimulation for motor restoration in hemiplegia. *Phys Med Rehabil Clin N Am.* 2015;26(4):729–745.

32. Carey LM, Matyas TA. Frequency of discriminative sensory loss in the hand after stroke in a rehabilitation setting. *J Rehabil Med.* 2011;43(3):257–263.

33. Winward CE, Halligan PW, Wade DT. Somatosensory recovery: a longitudinal study of the first 6 months after unilateral stroke. *Disabil Rehabil.* 2007;29(4):293–299.

34. Carey LM, Lamp G, Turville M. The state-of-the-science on somatosensory function and its impact on daily life in adults and older adults, and following stroke: a scoping review. *OTJR: Occupation, Participation and Health.* 2016;36(suppl 2):27S–41S.

35. Carey LM, Matyas TA. Training of somatosensory discrimination after stroke: facilitation of stimulus generalization. *Am J Phys Med Rehabil.* 2005;84(6):428–442.

36. Sullivan JE, Hedman LD. Sensory dysfunction following stroke: incidence, significance, examination, and intervention. *Top Stroke Rehabil.* 2008;15(3):200–217.

37. Tyson SF, Hanley M, Chillala J, Selley AB, Tallis RC. Sensory loss in hospital-admitted people with stroke: characteristics, associated factors, and relationship with function. *Neurorehabil Neural Repair.* 2008;22(2):166–172.

38. Turville M, Carey LM, Matyas TA, Blennerhassett J. Change in functional arm use is associated with somatosensory skills after sensory retraining poststroke. *Am J OccupTher.* 2017;71(3). 7103190070p7103190071–7103190070p7103190079.

39. Bolognini N, Russo C, Edwards DJ. The sensory side of post-stroke motor rehabilitation. *Restor Neurol Neurosci.* 2016;34(4):571–586.

40. Winward CE, Halligan PW, Wade DT. Current practice and clinical relevance of somatosensory assessment after stroke. *Clin Rehabil.* 1999;13(1):48–55.

41. Civelek GM, Atalay A, Turhan N. Association of ideomotor apraxia with lesion site, etiology, neglect, and functional independence in patients with first ever stroke. *Top Stroke Rehabil.* 2015;22(2):94–101.

42. Park JE. Apraxia: review and update. *J Clin Neurol.* 2017;13(4):317–324.

43. Zoltan B. *Vision, Perception, and Cognition: A Manual for the Evaluation and Treatment of the Adult with Acquired Brain Injury.* 4th ed. Thorofare, NJ: Slack, Inc.; 2007.

44. Buxbaum LJ, Ferraro MK, Veramonti T, et al. Hemispatial neglect: subtypes, neuroanatomy, and disability. *Neurology.* 2004;62(5):749–756.

45. Li K, Malhotra PA. Spatial neglect. *Pract Neurol.* 2015;15(5):333–339.

46. Nudo RJ, Milliken GW, Jenkins WM, Merzenich MM. Use-dependent alterations of movement representations in primary motor cortex of adult squirrel monkeys. *J Neurosci.* 1996;16(2):785–807.

47. Frost S, Barbay S, Friel K, Plautz E, Nudo R. Reorganization of remote cortical regions after ischemic brain injury: a potential substrate for stroke recovery. *J. Neurophysiol.* 2003;89(6):3205–3214.

48. Nudo RJ, Plautz EJ, Frost SB. Role of adaptive plasticity in recovery of function after damage to motor cortex. *Muscle & Nerve.* 2001;24(8):1000–1019.

49. Turkstra LS, Holland AL, Bays GA. The neuroscience of recovery and rehabilitation: what have we learned from animal research? *Arch Phys Med Rehabil.* 2003;84(4):604–612.

50. Liepert J, Bauder H, Miltner WH, Taub E, Weiller C. Treatment-induced cortical reorganization after stroke in humans. *Stroke.* 2000;31(6):1210–1216.

51. Wolf SL, Thompson PA, Winstein CJ, et al. The EXCITE stroke trial: comparing early and delayed constraint-induced movement therapy. *Stroke.* 2010;41(10):2309–2315.

52. Schumway-Cook A, Woollacott M, Motor Control. *Translating Research into Clinical Practice.* 5th ed. Philadelphia: Wolters Kluwer; 2017.

53. Horak FB. Assumptions underlying motor control for neurologic rehabilitation. Paper presented at: contemporary management of motor control problems: proceedings of the II STEP conference1991.

54. Pendleton HM, Schultz-Krohn W. *Pedretti's Occupational Therapy-E-Book: Practice Skills for Physical Dysfunction.* Elsevier Health Sciences; 2017.

55. Schmidt RA. A schema theory of discrete motor skill learning. *Psychological Review.* 1975;82(4):225–260.

56. Schmidt RA, Lee TD. *Motor Control and Learning: A Behavioral Emphasis.* Champaign, IL: Human Kinetics; 2005.

57. Wolf SL, Winstein CJ, Miller JP, et al. Effect of constraint-induced movement therapy on upper extremity function 3 to 9 months after stroke: the EXCITE randomized clinical trial. *JAMA.* 2006;296(17):2095–2104.

58. Harris-Love ML, Morton SM, Perez MA, Cohen LG. Mechanisms of short-term training-induced reaching improvement in severely hemiparetic stroke patients: a TMS study. *Neurorehabil Neural Repair.* 2011;25(5):398–411.

59. Muratori LM, Lamberg EM, Quinn L, Duff SV. Applying principles of motor learning and control to upper extremity rehabilitation. *J Hand Ther.* 2013;26(2):94–103.

60. Lang CE, Strube MJ, Bland MD, et al. Dose response of task-specific upper limb training in people at least 6 months poststroke: a phase II, single-blind, randomized, controlled trial. *Ann Neurol.* 2016;80(3):342–354.

61. Wu AJ, Hermann V, Ying J, Page SJ. Chronometry of mentally versus physically practiced tasks in people with stroke. *Am J Occup Ther.* 2010;64(6):929–934.

62. Krakauer JW. Motor learning: its relevance to stroke recovery and neurorehabilitation. *Curr Opin Neurol.* 2006;19(1):84–90.

63. Boyd LA, Vidoni ED, Wessel BD. Motor learning after stroke: is skill acquisition a prerequisite for contralesional neuroplastic change? *Neurosci Lett.* 2010;482(1):21–25.

64. Lang CE, Birkenmeier RL. *Upper-Extremity Task-Specific Training After Stroke or Disability: A Manual for Occupational Therapy and Physical Therapy.* Bethesda, MD: AOTA Press; 2014.

65. van Delden AL, Peper CL, Beek PJ, Kwakkel G. Match and mismatch between objective and subjective improvements in upper limb function after stroke. *Disabil Rehabil.* 2013;201335(23):1961–1967.

66. Rice DB, McIntyre A, Mirkowski M, et al. Patient-centered goal setting in a hospital-based outpatient stroke rehabilitation center. *PM&R.* 2017;9:856.

67. Wolf TJ, Nilson DM. *Occupational Therapy Practice Guidelines for Adults with Stroke.* Bethesda, MD: AOTA Press; 2015.

68. Gutman SA, Schonfeld AB. *Screening Adult Neurologic Populations: A Step-by-step Instruction Manual.* 2nd ed. Bethesda, MD: AOTA Press; 2009.

69. Kendall FP, McCreary EK, Provance PG, Rodgers MM, Romani WA. *Muscles: Testing and Function with Posture & Pain.* 5th ed. Philadelphia: Lippincott, Williams, and Wilkins; 2005.

70. Bohannon RW, Smith MB. Interrater reliability of a Modified Ashworth Scale of muscle spasticity. *Phys Ther.* 1987;67(2):206–207.

71. Carmon A. Disturbances of tactile sensitivity in patients with unilateral cerebral lesions. *Cortex.* 1971;7(1):83–97.

72. Vanbellingen T, Kersten B, Van de Winckel A, et al. A new bedside test of gestures in stroke: the apraxia screen of TULIA (AST). *J Neurol Neurosurg Psychiatry.* 2011;82(4):389–392.

73. Azouvi P, Marchal F, Samuel C, et al. Functional consequences and awareness of unilateral neglect: study of an evaluation scale. *Neuropsychological Rehabilitation.* 1996;6(2):133–150.

74. Lang CE, Bland MD, Bailey RR, Schaefer SY, Birkenmeier RL. Assessment of upper extremity impairment, function, and activity after stroke: foundations for clinical decision making. *J Hand Ther.* 2013;26(2):104–114; quiz 115.

75. Nijland R, van Wegen E, Verbunt J, van Wijk R, van Kordelaar J, Kwakkel G. A comparison of two validated tests for upper limb function after stroke: the Wolf Motor Function Test and the Action Research Arm Test. *J Rehabil Med.* 2010;42(7):694–696.

76. Van der Lee JH, De Groot V, Beckerman H, Wagenaar RC, Lankhorst GJ, Bouter LM. The intra- and interrater reliability of the action research arm test: a practical test of upper extremity function in patients with stroke. *Arch Phys Med Rehabil.* 2001;82(1):14–19.

77. Yozbatiran N, Der-Yeghiaian L, Cramer SC. A standardized approach to performing the Action Research Arm Test. *Neurorehabil Neural Repair.* 2008;22(1):78–90.

78. Chen HM, Chen CC, Hsueh IP, Huang SL, Hsieh CL. Test-retest reproducibility and smallest real difference of 5 hand function tests in patients with stroke. *Neurorehabil Neural Repair.* 2009;23(5):435–440.

79. Lin KC, Chuang LL, Wu CY, Hsieh YW, Chang WY. Responsiveness and validity of three dexterous function measures in stroke rehabilitation. *J Rehabil Res Dev.* 2010;47(6):563–571.

80. Platz T, Pinkowski C, van Wijck F, Kim IH, di Bella P, Johnson G. Reliability and validity of arm function assessment with standardized guidelines for the Fugl-Meyer Test, Action Research Arm Test and Box and Block Test: a multicentre study. *Clin Rehabil.* 2005;19(4):404–411.

81. Heller A, Wade DT, Wood VA, Sunderland A, Hewer RL, Ward E. Arm function after stroke: measurement and recovery over the first three months. *J Neurol Neurosurg Psychiatry.* 1987;50(6):714–719.

82. Sunderland A, Tinson D, Bradley L, Hewer RL. Arm function after stroke. An evaluation of grip strength as a measure of recovery and a prognostic indicator. *J Neurol Neurosurg Psychiatry.* 1989;52(11):1267–1272.

83. Parker VM, Wade DT, Langton Hewer R. Loss of arm function after stroke: measurement, frequency, and recovery. *Int Rehabil Med.* 1986;8(2):69–73.

84. Bot SD, Terwee CB, van der Windt DA, Bouter LM, Dekker J, de Vet HC. Clinimetric evaluation of shoulder disability questionnaires: a systematic review of the literature. *Ann Rheum Dis.* 2004;63(4):335–341.

85. Beaton DE, Wright JG, Katz JN, Group UEC. Development of the Quick-DASH: comparison of three item-reduction approaches. *J Bone Joint Surg Am.* 2005;87(5):1038–1046.

86. van der Lee JH, Beckerman H, Knol DL, de Vet HC, Bouter LM. Clinimetric properties of the motor activity log for the assessment of arm use in hemiparetic patients. *Stroke.* 2004;35(6):1410–1414.

87. Uswatte G, Taub E, Morris D, Vignolo M, McCulloch K. Reliability and validity of the upper-extremity Motor Activity Log-14 for measuring real-world arm use. *Stroke.* 2005;36(11):2493–2496.

88. Duncan PW, Wallace D, Lai SM, Johnson D, Embretson S, Laster LJ. The stroke impact scale version 2.0. Evaluation of reliability, validity, and sensitivity to change. *Stroke.* 1999;30(10):2131–2140.

89. Carod-Artal FJ, Ferreira Coral L, Stieven Trizotto D, Menezes Moreira C. Self- and proxy-report agreement on the stroke impact scale. *Stroke.* 2009;40(10):3308–3314.

90. Lyle RC. A performance test for assessment of upper limb function in physical rehabilitation treatment and research. *Int J Rehabil Res.* 1981;4(4):483–492.

91. Mathiowetz V, Volland G, Kashman N, Weber K. Adult norms for the Box and Block Test of manual dexterity. *Am J Occup Ther.* 1985;39(6):386–391.

92. Mathiowetz V, Weber K, Kashman N, Volland G. Adult norms for the Nine Hole Peg Test of finger dexterity. *OTJR: Occupation, Participation, and Health.* 1985;5:24–38.

93. Oxford Grice K, Vogel KA, Le V, Mitchell A, Muniz S, Vollmer MA. Adult norms for a commercially available Nine Hole Peg Test for finger dexterity. *Am J Occup Ther.* 2003;57(5):570–573.

94. Hudak PL, Amadio PC, Bombardier C. Development of an upper extremity outcome measure: the DASH (disabilities of the arm, shoulder and hand) [corrected]. The Upper Extremity Collaborative Group (UECG). *Am J Ind Med.* 1996;29(6):602–608.

95. Baker K, Barrett L, Playford ED, Aspden T, Riazi A, Hobart J. Measuring arm function early after stroke: is the DASH good enough? *J Neurol Neurosurg Psychiatry.* 2016;(6):604.

96. Davis AM, Beaton DE, Hudak P, et al. Measuring disability of the upper extremity: a rationale supporting the use of a regional outcome measure. *J Hand Ther.* 1999;12:269–274.

97. Uswatte G, Taub E, Morris D, Light K, Thompson PA. The Motor Activity Log-28: assessing daily use of the hemiparetic arm after stroke. *Neurology.* 2006;67(7):1189–1194.

98. Daly JJ, Ruff RL. Construction of efficacious gait and upper limb functional interventions based on brain plasticity evidence and model-based measures for stroke patients. *Scientific World Journal.* 2007;7:2031–2045.

99. Bayona NA, Bitensky J, Salter K, Teasell R. The role of task-specific training in rehabilitation therapies. *Top Stroke Rehabil.* 2005;12(3):58–65.

100. Hubbard IJ, Parsons MW, Neilson C, Carey LM. Task-specific training: evidence for and translation to clinical practice. *Occup Ther Int.* 2009;16(3-4):175–189.

101. Arya KN, Verma R, Garg RK, Sharma VP, Agarwal M, Aggarwal GG. Meaningful task-specific training (MTST) for stroke rehabilitation: a randomized controlled trial. *Top Stroke Rehabil.* 2012;19(3):193–211.

102. Shimodozono M, Noma T, Nomoto Y, et al. Benefits of a repetitive facilitative exercise program for the upper paretic extremity after subacute stroke: a randomized controlled trial. *Neurorehabil Neural Repair.* 2013;27(4):296–305.

103. French B, Thomas L, Leathley M, et al. Does repetitive task training improve functional activity after stroke? A Cochrane systematic review and meta-analysis. *J Rehabil Med.* 2010;42(1):9–14.

104. Winstein CJ, Wolf SL, Dromerick AW, et al. Effect of a task-oriented rehabilitation program on upper extremity recovery following motor stroke: the icare randomized clinical trial. *JAMA.* 2016;315(6):571–581.

105. Waddell KJ, Strube MJ, Bailey RR, et al. Does task-specific training improve upper limb performance in daily life poststroke? *Neurorehabil Neural Repair.* 2017;31(3):290–300.

106. Taub E, Uswatte G, Mark VW, et al. Method for enhancing real-world use of a more affected arm in chronic stroke: transfer package of constraint-induced movement therapy. *Stroke.* 2013;44(5):1383–1388.

107. Smania N, Gandolfi M, Paolucci S, et al. Reduced-intensity modified constraint-induced movement therapy versus conventional therapy for upper extremity rehabilitation after stroke: a multicenter trial. *Neurorehabil Neural Repair.* 2012;26(9):1035–1045.

108. Page SJ, Levine P, Leonard A, Szaflarski JP, Kissela BM. Modified constraint-induced therapy in chronic stroke: results of a single-blinded randomized controlled trial. *Phys Ther.* 2008;88(3):333–340.

109. Wolf SL. Revisiting constraint-induced movement therapy: are we too smitten with the mitten? Is all nonuse "learned"? and other quandaries. *Phys Ther.* 2007;87(9):1212–1223.

110. Corti M, McGuirk TE, Wu SS, Patten C. Differential effects of power training versus functional task practice on compensation and restoration of arm function after stroke. *Neurorehabil Neural Repair.* 2012;26(7):842–854.

111. Harris JE, Eng JJ. Strength training improves upper-limb function in individuals with stroke: a meta-analysis. *Stroke.* 2010;41(1):136–140.

112. Winter J, Hunter S, Sim J, Crome P. Hands-on therapy interventions for upper limb motor dysfunction following stroke. *Cochrane Database Syst Rev.* 2011;(6):CD006609.

113. Stein C, Fritsch CG, Robinson C, Sbruzzi G, Plentz RD. Effects of electrical stimulation in spastic muscles after stroke: systematic review and meta-analysis of randomized controlled trials. *Stroke.* 2015;46(8):2197–2205.

114. Pomeroy VM, King L, Pollock A, Baily-Hallam A, Langhorne P. Electro-stimulation for promoting recovery of movement or functional ability after stroke. *Cochrane Database Syst Rev.* 2006;(2):CD003241.

115. Alon G, Levitt AF, McCarthy PA. Functional electrical stimulation (FES) may modify the poor prognosis of stroke survivors with severe motor loss of the upper extremity: a preliminary study. *Am J Phys Med Rehabil.* 2008;87(8):627–636.

116. Jackson PL, Lafleur MF, Malouin F, Richards C, Doyon J. Potential role of mental practice using motor imagery in neurologic rehabilitation. *Arch Phys Med Rehabil.* 2001;82(8):1133–1141.

117. Guerra ZF, Lucchetti ALG, Lucchetti G. Motor imagery training after stroke: a systematic review and meta-analysis of randomized controlled trials. *J Neurol Phys Ther.* 2017;41(4):205–214.

118. Laver KE, Lange B, George S, Deutsch JE, Saposnik G, Crotty M. Virtual reality for stroke rehabilitation. *Cochrane Database Syst Rev.* 2017;11:CD008349.

119. Nilsen DM, Gillen G, Geller D, Hreha K, Osei E, Saleem GT. Effectiveness of interventions to improve occupational performance of people with motor impairments after stroke: an evidence-based review. *Am J Occup Ther.* 2015;69(1):6901180030p6901180031-6901180039.

120. Pérez-Cruzado D, Merchán-Baeza JA, González-Sánchez M, Cuesta-Vargas AI. Systematic review of mirror therapy compared with conventional rehabilitation in upper extremity function in stroke survivors. *Aust Occup Ther J.* 2017;64(2):91–112.

Hemiplegia: Operative Management

Michael J. Botte, Michael A. Thompson, Lorenzo L. Pacelli, M. Jake Hamer,
R. Scott Meyer

OUTLINE

CRITICAL POINTS

Recovery Periods After Neurologic Injury (Periods in Which Surgery is Avoided)
- Cerebrovascular accident (stroke): 6 months
- Incomplete spinal cord injury: 12 months
- Traumatic brain injury: 18 months

Indications for Operative Management In Hemiplegia
- The patient is beyond the period of spontaneous neurologic recovery.
- The patient is no longer improving in an aggressive hand or upper extremity therapy program.
- Problematic deformity persists (functional impairment or problems with hygiene, dressing, or positioning).

Common Deformities and Main Offending Muscles
Shoulder deformity: adduction, internal rotation, and forward flexion
    Offending muscles: pectoralis major, subscapularis, latissimus dorsi, teres major
Elbow deformity: flexion
    Offending muscles: brachioradialis, biceps brachii, brachialis

Forearm deformity: pronation
    Offending muscles: pronator teres, pronator quadratus
Wrist deformity: flexion
    Offending muscles: flexor carpi ulnaris, flexor carpi radialis, palmaris longus, digital flexors (secondary wrist flexors)
Hand deformity: digital flexion, clenched fist deformity
    Offending muscles: flexor digitorum profundus, flexor digitorum superficialis, intrinsic hand muscles
Thumb deformity: thumb-in-palm deformity
    Offending muscles: thenar muscles, adductor pollicis, first dorsal interosseous, flexor pollicis longus (FPL)

Timing After Surgery to Resume Hand or Upper Extremity Therapy
- For muscle release or recession procedures: Passive limb mobilization can be done as soon as wound healing and patient comfort permit, often within 2 weeks.
- For muscle lengthening or transfer procedures: Delay therapy for 4 to 6 weeks to allow healing of lengthened or transferred muscles; then use progressive passive and active mobilization.

Acquired hemiplegia most commonly occurs from traumatic brain injury (TBI), cerebrovascular accident (stroke), or isolated unilateral cervical spinal cord injury (SCI).[1-6] After the initial neurologic insult, there usually follows a period of neurologic recovery in which gradual and spontaneous neurologic improvement can occur.

In TBI, this recovery can last 18 to 48 months, in stroke up to 6 months, and in incomplete SCI to about 12 months (Critical Points Box). During these recovery periods, efforts are made to prevent fixed contractures through management of spasticity using a comprehensive hand and upper extremity therapy program. Useful adjuncts to the therapy program during this recovery period include intramuscular botulinum toxin injection, oral muscle relaxants, spinal Baclofen pumps, and phenol nerve blocks. Surgery to correct deformity should usually be avoided during these recovery periods because overcorrection or unnecessary surgery may result if the patient continues to improve after surgery is performed.

Despite an aggressive comprehensive hand and upper extremity therapy program, severe spasticity can still persist or lead to fixed contractures.[1-3,7-9]

INDICATIONS AND GOALS OF SURGERY

If progress is no longer continuing in an aggressive hand and upper extremity therapy program *and* the patient is beyond the period of spontaneous recovery, operative management can be considered for noxious spasticity or fixed contractures (Critical Points Box).

SHOULDER: DEFORMITY AND ASSOCIATED PROBLEMS

The most common deformity of the shoulder in hemiplegia is internal rotation, adduction, and often some forward flexion (Fig. 112.1).[2,7] The muscles contributing to this deformity usually involve the pectoralis major, subscapularis, latissimus dorsi, and teres major (Critical Points Box). The deformity leads to hygiene problems in the axilla and difficulty positioning or dressing the patient.[1,3,6,7,10-13] An algorithm for operative indications for shoulder deformity is shown in Fig. 112.1C.[2]

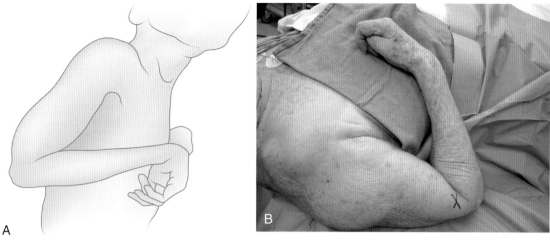

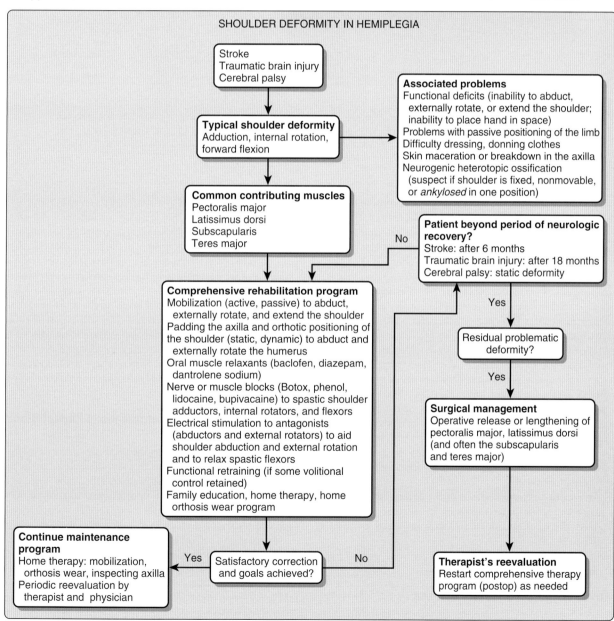

SHOULDER DEFORMITY IN HEMIPLEGIA

Stroke
Traumatic brain injury
Cerebral palsy

↓

Typical shoulder deformity
Adduction, internal rotation,
forward flexion

Associated problems
Functional deficits (inability to abduct,
  externally rotate, or extend the shoulder;
  inability to place hand in space)
Problems with passive positioning of the limb
Difficulty dressing, donning clothes
Skin maceration or breakdown in the axilla
Neurogenic heterotopic ossification
  (suspect if shoulder is fixed, nonmovable,
  or *ankylosed* in one position)

Common contributing muscles
Pectoralis major
Latissimus dorsi
Subscapularis
Teres major

No

**Patient beyond period of neurologic
recovery?**
Stroke: after 6 months
Traumatic brain injury: after 18 months
Cerebral palsy: static deformity

Yes

Comprehensive rehabilitation program
Mobilization (active, passive) to abduct,
  externally rotate, and extend the shoulder
Padding the axilla and orthotic positioning of
  the shoulder (static, dynamic) to abduct and
  externally rotate the humerus
Oral muscle relaxants (baclofen, diazepam,
  dantrolene sodium)
Nerve or muscle blocks (Botox, phenol,
  lidocaine, bupivacaine) to spastic shoulder
  adductors, internal rotators, and flexors
Electrical stimulation to antagonists
  (abductors and external rotators) to aid
  shoulder abduction and external rotation
  and to relax spastic flexors
Functional retraining (if some volitional
  control retained)
Family education, home therapy, home
  orthosis wear program

Residual problematic
deformity?

Yes

Surgical management
Operative release or lengthening of
pectoralis major, latissimus dorsi
(and often the subscapularis
and teres major)

**Continue maintenance
program**
Home therapy: mobilization,
  orthosis wear, inspecting axilla
Periodic reevaluation by
  therapist and physician

Yes   Satisfactory correction
and goals achieved?   No

Therapist's reevaluation
Restart comprehensive therapy
program (postop) as needed

Fig. 112.1 Illustration (**A**) and photograph (**B**) of upper extremity deformity of a patient with hemiplegia. Common deformities include shoulder adduction and internal rotation, elbow flexion, forearm pronation, wrist and digit flexion, and thumb-in-palm deformity. **C,** Shoulder deformity in hemiplegia: algorithm for operative indications for shoulder deformity in hemiplegia.

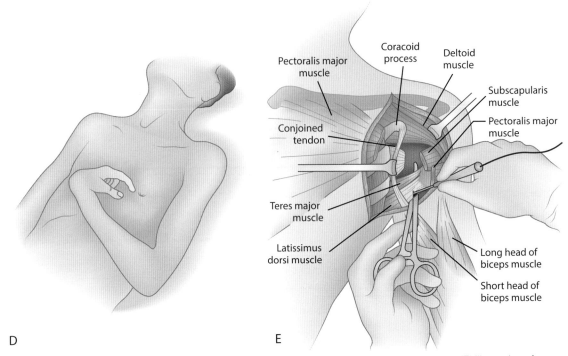

Fig. 112.1, cont'd D, Typical deformity includes shoulder adduction and internal rotation and (**E**) illustration of operative treatment for shoulder deformity releasing the pectoralis major, subscapularis, lattisimus dorsi, and teres major. (Parts A, D, and E reproduced from Keenan MAE, Kozin SH, Berlet AC. *Manual for Orthopaedic Surgery for Spasticity.* New York: Raven Press; 1993.)

In a nonfunctional limb, operative management consists of either muscle–tendon lengthening or complete release or motor neurectomy.[1,5,7] The goals of these procedures for severe deformities are to help improve hygiene and skin care, assist with dressing, and help prevent pressure sores by improving passive limb positioning.

In a limb with some retained volitional control, operative management consists of less aggressive procedures, such as selective muscle lengthening, avoiding complete release of the muscle or tendon. The goals of these procedures are to decrease the deformity and to preserve or improve function.

Additional associated problems of the shoulder include inferior subluxation from flaccid musculature (as opposed to spasticity). With lack of shoulder mobility, patients can often also develop painful adhesive capsulitis or capsular contracture.

To determine which muscles contribute to the deformity, abduct and externally rotate the arm. All but the subscapularis are clinically palpable. If the humerus resists external rotation with the arm at the side, the subscapularis is usually contributing as well.[2] Selective Botox injections to involved muscles are also helpful diagnostically in determining contributing muscles.

Surgery consists of initial release of the insertions of the pectoralis major and subscapularis muscles. If adequate correction is not obtained, the latissimus dorsi and teres major are released as well[3,10–13] (Fig. 112.1E).[2,7]

Alternatively, for mild deformities, percutaneous phenol nerve block to the pectoralis major can be useful.

Operative Technique: Shoulder Release

Place a 7-cm deltopectoral incision over the insertion of the pectoralis major muscle. Isolate the pectoralis major tendon and incise the tendon near its insertion onto the humerus (Fig. 112.1E).[2,7] Retract the anterior deltoid superiorly to expose the head of the humerus. Identify the tendon of the subscapularis as it inserts onto the humerus. Separate the tendon from the anterior joint capsule and transect the tendon near its insertion. Removal of a segmental portion of the tendon may prevent reattachment and recurrence of the deformity. Leave the shoulder capsule intact to preserve shoulder stability. If the latissimus dorsi and teres major were thought to be involved preoperatively or demonstrate myostatic contractures intraoperatively, these are also released (Fig. 112.1E).[2,7] Develop the interval lateral to the short head of the biceps and medial to the anterior deltoid. This will expose the insertion of the latissimus dorsi and teres major. Release these muscles near their insertion. At wound closure, drains are useful to prevent hematoma because of dead space created. Start an aggressive mobilization therapy program as soon as the wound healing and patient comfort permit[10–13] (Critical Points Box).

Operative Technique: Percutaneous Phenol Block to the Pectoralis Major

Percutaneous phenol block to the pectoralis major is useful for mild flexible adduction deformities that still cause difficulty in dressing or hygiene care in the axilla. The pectoralis should be noted to be palpably tight with passive abduction or external rotation of the shoulder. Although considered a temporary treatment, phenol often provides some residual long-term effect of muscle relaxation.

Position the patient in a supine position. Use a cutaneous nerve stimulator to identify the motor points of the pectoralis major muscle. Motor points represent motor branches to the muscle or areas of high concentrations of motor endplates within the muscle. Mark these points on the skin. The nerve stimulator is then attached to the hub of a hypodermic needle that has an insulated shaft but an exposed tip. An intravenous needle with its plastic catheter shield will suffice. These types of needles ensure stimulation of nerves only at the tip of the needle. A syringe containing a 5% aqueous solution of phenol is attached to the needle. The phenol solution should not undergo heat sterilization because this inactivates the phenol. Introduce the needle into the pectoralis major muscle at the motor point areas previously marked and with the electric current applied. Manipulate the needle within the muscle until a maximal contraction is elicited. Aspirate before injection to rule out vascular puncture and inject 2 mL of phenol solution. Repeat the procedure for three or four other motor points within the muscle or until adequate decrease in muscle tone is accomplished.

The percutaneous phenol block addresses only one of the four possible muscles responsible for the adduction and internal rotation deformity of the shoulder. However, it still may afford significant shoulder relaxation and allow mobilization. Repeat the block in 2 months if necessary. Although phenol blocks are often replaced by Botox intramuscular injections, they remain a valuable adjunct for refractory spasticity if Botox is not effective.

In some patients, weakness (instead of spasticity) is a predominant development in shoulder girdle muscles, involving the deltoid muscle or the rotator cuff muscles. Weakness of these muscles, which normally support and stabilize the shoulder, can result in inferior subluxation of the humerus. As the humerus "sags" inferiorly, it not only reduces function but can also apply traction on the brachial plexus. Subsequent pain or brachial plexopathy can result and cause further limb neurologic dysfunction. Mobilization and strengthening can help, but the problem can often be chronic, and spontaneous neurologic recovery does not occur. The traction effect from the weight of the arm can be reduced using a sling on the upper extremity. Alternatively, a custom orthosis can be fabricated that transfers the weight of the arm to the pelvis. The device is custom fabricated and contains a support that lies on the rim of the pelvis. The forearm is supported as it rests on the pelvis and reduces the traction on the brachial plexus. Unfortunately, there is currently no reliable operative alternative to help flaccid shoulders.

ELBOW: DEFORMITY AND ASSOCIATED PROBLEMS

Flexion is the most common deformity of the elbow, caused by spasticity of the biceps, brachialis, or brachioradialis (see Critical Points Box).[2,3,7] The major antagonist muscle is the triceps, and it cannot usually compete with the elbow flexors because of mechanical disadvantage. Associated problems of elbow flexion deformity include difficulty with active extension, poor hygiene in the antecubital fossae, risk of olecranon pressure sores or skin breakdown, and difficulty with positioning and dressing. Operative management usually consists of lengthening or release of the specific involved muscles.[1–3,6,7,14] Alternatively, motor neurectomy of the musculocutaneous nerve will address spasticity of the biceps and brachialis. Motor neurectomy of the radial nerve will address the brachioradialis. Although motor neurectomy will effectively decrease spasticity, it will not address fixed myostatic contracture. Therefore, we generally prefer operative release or lengthening of the muscles.

An algorithm for operative indications for elbow deformity is shown in Fig. 112.2A.[2]

In a nonfunctional elbow with a greater than 75 to 90 degree flexion contracture, operative release addresses the biceps, brachialis, and brachioradialis (Fig. 112.2B).[2,7] Avoid joint capsule release to preserve elbow stability. Approximately 40 degrees of correction can be expected. Further elbow extension is often limited by contracture of the joint capsule or the neurovascular structures. This residual deformity can then subsequently be further improved slowly, over time, in a postsurgery therapy program that is facilitated by the surgical elimination of the major contributing muscles (Fig. 112.2C and D).[2,7]

If there is a *functional* elbow and hand, *selective* release or lengthening is performed, addressing only the most clinically spastic or contracted of these three muscles. Muscle selection is assessed by muscle palpation, selective diagnostic intramuscular Botox injection, diagnostic lidocaine block to the musculocutaneous or radial nerves, or if available, dynamic electromyograms from a motion analysis laboratory.

Operative Technique: Elbow Flexor Muscle Release

Place a curved incision on the lateral elbow, starting at the origin of the brachioradialis, and extend the incision along the interval between the biceps and the brachioradialis. Protect the radial nerve in the interval between the brachioradialis and brachialis. Release the brachioradialis by *recession*, by releasing the muscle from its origin on the humerus (see Fig. 112.2B).[2,7] The released muscle then slides distally. Next, lengthen the biceps using a Z-lengthening in its long tendinous portion. Following the Z-incision on the biceps, access to the brachialis is provided and the muscle is lengthened with *fractional* lengthening. Fractional lengthening is accomplished by placement of multiple incisions in the tendinous portion of the muscle's long myotendinous junction (see Fig. 112.2B).[2,7] Repair the Z-lengthened biceps with 3-0 nonabsorbable suture. Placement of surgical drains minimizes hematoma when dead space is created by these procedures. Place a bulky long-arm dressing with the elbow in maximal extension without stressing the neurovascular structures. Immobilize the elbow for 4 weeks to allow healing of the lengthened muscles followed by mobilization to achieve additional correction of any residual deformity (see Critical Points Box).

In a nonfunctional elbow with less than a 75 degree contracture, a neurectomy of the motor branches can be performed.[2,3,5,6] A concomitant elbow muscle flexor release is recommended if there is a 75-degree or more deformity.[4–6] If the brachioradialis has volitional control or spasticity, this radial-innervated muscle will preserve some elbow flexion and prevent a flail or hyperextended elbow.

Operative Technique: Musculocutaneous Motor Neurectomy

Place a straight 5-cm longitudinal incision on the medial aspect of the arm, starting at the level of the pectoralis major tendon and extending distally along the interval between the biceps and the brachialis muscle. Develop the interval between these two muscles. Identify the nerve where it exits the coracobrachialis and continues between the biceps and brachialis. Confirm the identity of the musculocutaneous nerve with a nerve stimulator. Identify motor branches as the nerves enter the biceps or brachialis. Excise a 1-cm segment of motor nerve to each identifiable motor branch. Passively extend the elbow and splint in a corrected position. Mobilize the elbow as soon as wound healing and patient comfort permit.

Operative Technique: Radial Motor Neurectomy to the Brachioradialis

Place an 8-cm longitudinal incision beginning at the flexion crease of the elbow and extending proximally on a line between the biceps and brachioradialis. Develop the interval between the brachialis and brachioradialis. The lateral antebrachial cutaneous nerve is identified and protected. Identify the larger and more deeply located radial nerve. Gently dissect the laterally coursing motor branches to the brachioradialis and to the extensor carpi radialis longus and then confirm the function with a nerve stimulator. Remove a 1- to 2-cm section of the motor branches seen entering the brachioradialis.[2,3,5,6] Extend the elbow and splint in a corrected position. Initiate mobilization in 1 week or when patient comfort and wound healing permit.

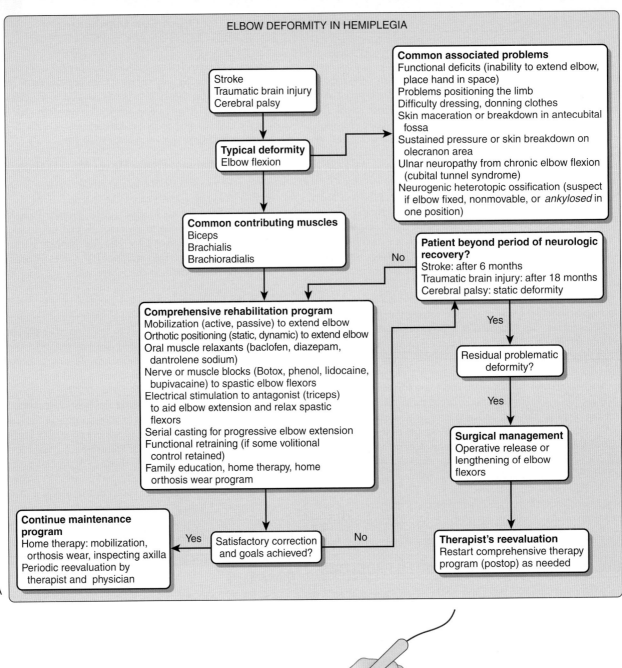

ELBOW DEFORMITY IN HEMIPLEGIA

Stroke
Traumatic brain injury
Cerebral palsy

Typical deformity
Elbow flexion

Common associated problems
Functional deficits (inability to extend elbow, place hand in space)
Problems positioning the limb
Difficulty dressing, donning clothes
Skin maceration or breakdown in antecubital fossa
Sustained pressure or skin breakdown on olecranon area
Ulnar neuropathy from chronic elbow flexion (cubital tunnel syndrome)
Neurogenic heterotopic ossification (suspect if elbow fixed, nonmovable, or *ankylosed* in one position)

Common contributing muscles
Biceps
Brachialis
Brachioradialis

No

Patient beyond period of neurologic recovery?
Stroke: after 6 months
Traumatic brain injury: after 18 months
Cerebral palsy: static deformity

Yes

Residual problematic deformity?

Yes

Comprehensive rehabilitation program
Mobilization (active, passive) to extend elbow
Orthotic positioning (static, dynamic) to extend elbow
Oral muscle relaxants (baclofen, diazepam, dantrolene sodium)
Nerve or muscle blocks (Botox, phenol, lidocaine, bupivacaine) to spastic elbow flexors
Electrical stimulation to antagonist (triceps) to aid elbow extension and relax spastic flexors
Serial casting for progressive elbow extension
Functional retraining (if some volitional control retained)
Family education, home therapy, home orthosis wear program

Surgical management
Operative release or lengthening of elbow flexors

Continue maintenance program
Home therapy: mobilization, orthosis wear, inspecting axilla
Periodic reevaluation by therapist and physician

Yes

Satisfactory correction and goals achieved?

No

Therapist's reevaluation
Restart comprehensive therapy program (postop) as needed

A

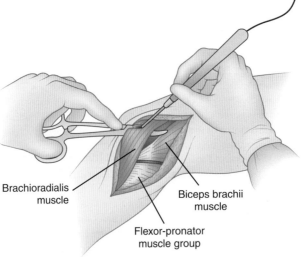

Brachioradialis muscle

Biceps brachii muscle

Flexor-pronator muscle group

B

Fig. 112.2 A, Algorithm for operative indications for elbow deformity in hemiplegia. **B,** Operative correction of the elbow flexion deformity. The brachioradialis, biceps, and brachialis are addressed. The brachioradialis does not have a long tendinous portion to lengthen by Z-lengthening and does not have substantial myotendinous junction for fractional lengthening; therefore, it is released by recession, which consists of direct release of the muscle from the humerus. The biceps, because of its long tendinous portion, is lengthened by Z-lengthening. The brachialis usually has a long myotendinous portion, which lends itself to fractional lengthening by placement of multiple incisions in the tendinous-only portion of the junction. (Part A reproduced from Keenan MAE, Kozin SH, Berlet AC. *Manual for Orthopaedic Surgery for Spasticity.* New York: Raven Press; 1993.)

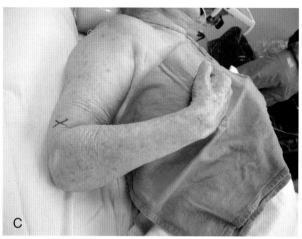 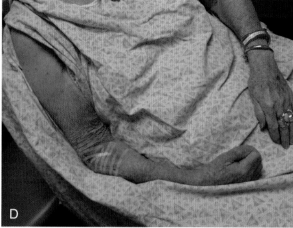

Fig. 112.2, cont'd Preoperative (**C**) and postoperative (**D**) photographs of a stroke patient with refractory elbow flexion deformity in a limb without volitional control. Despite a comprehensive rehabilitation program, flexion deformity persisted and caused problems with hygiene in the antecubital fossa and difficulty with dressing and positioning the patient. Surgery included recession of the brachioradialis, Z-lengthening of the biceps tendon, and fractional lengthening of the brachialis.

FOREARM AND WRIST: DEFORMITY AND ASSOCIATED PROBLEMS

Deformities of the forearm usually consist of forearm pronation and wrist flexion. These deformities are often accompanied by digital flexion and thumb flexion and adduction (often resulting in thumb-in-palm deformity, discussed further later). Because these deformities usually exist simultaneously, they are often treated at one operative setting (see Fig. 112.1A and B).[2,7]

Forearm pronation is caused by spasticity of the pronator teres and pronator quadratus. Flexion of the wrist is caused predominantly by the flexor carpi ulnaris (FCU) and flexor carpi radialis (FCR), with additional contributions from the digital extrinsic flexors (see Critical Points Box).

These deformities cause problems with dressing, positioning, and hygiene. A severely flexed wrist causes problems with donning a shirt or jacket. A tightly clenched fist can result in maceration of the palm or skin breakdown from the digits or fingernails pressing into the palm. Operative correction consists of multiple tendon lengthening of the extrinsic and intrinsic muscles. Additionally, corrective wrist arthrodesis can be used for severe wrist flexion associated with spasticity.[3,6,15,16]

An algorithm for operative indications for wrist and forearm deformity is shown in Fig. 112.3A.[2]

The FCU is lengthened using fractional lengthening at its broad myotendinous junction, or Z-lengthened if there is a long tendinous portion. The FCR, however, usually only has a long tendon, which lends it to lengthening by a Z-lengthening technique (Fig. 112.3B and C).[2,7]

The flexor pronator slide procedure, previously used for forearm pronation and wrist and digital flexion deformities, is an option for correction of wrist flexion, digital flexion, and forearm pronation. The procedure, however, has the disadvantage of nonselectively releasing all of the flexor muscles, including the pronator teres.[17,18] The procedure can result in overcorrection, resulting in a supinated forearm with wrist extended.

Operative Technique: Flexor Carpi Ulnaris Lengthening

Place an 8-cm longitudinal incision along the FCU tendon at the junction of the middle and distal thirds of the forearm. Protect the ulnar artery and ulnar nerve, located deep to the muscle. Expose the broad musculotendinous junction of the FCU (see Fig. 112.3B and C).[2,7] Place two to four transverse or oblique incisions through only the tendon substance proximal to the most distal insertion of the muscle fibers on the tendon. Leave the muscle fibers at this level intact. Passively extend the wrist to obtain the desired amount of lengthening. The cut portions of the tendon will gap as the muscle is lengthened, and the underlying muscle fibers preserve continuity. Immobilize the wrist for 4 weeks to allow muscle healing before mobilization.

Operative Technique: Flexor Carpi Radialis Lengthening:

Place an 8-cm incision over the distal third of the FCR muscle. Identify and protect the median nerve (with its palmar cutaneous branch) located deep and ulnar to the tendon. Protect the radial artery, located radial to the tendon. Identify the FCR and place a Z-incision in the tendon (see Fig. 112.3B and C).[2,7] Position the wrist in the desired corrected position. Repair the tendon with 3-0 nonabsorbable suture. Immobilize the wrist for 4 weeks to allow tendon healing before restarting a therapy program.

If both the FCU and the FCR are to be lengthened, place a single broad S-shaped incision over the palmar forearm to allow access to both tendons from one incision. This incision will also allow exposure of the digital flexors if needed. The palmaris longus, if present, can be completely released with removal of a section of the tendon (see Fig. 112.3B and C).[2,7]

Operative Technique: Release of the Pronator Quadratus and Pronator Teres

For pronation deformity, the pronator quadratus can be released from its attachment on the distal volar radius using the same incision as that used for wrist flexor lengthening. Retract the extrinsic flexor tendons to expose the pronator quadratus. Release the muscle sharply from the distal radius attachments. Passively supinate the forearm to achieve correction of the pronation. When released from the distal radius, the pronator quadratus will slide into a new position as the forearm is passively supinated. Release or lengthen the pronator teres from its origin on the medial epicondyle (humeral head) and the from the proximal ulna (ulnar head) if needed. Place a separate incision in the proximal volar forearm and identify the pronator teres. Identify each head of the pronator teres. Release each head to achieve correction of the deformity. Immobilize the forearm in a neutral position of rotation for 4 weeks to allow the pronator muscles to reattach in their new, lengthened position. Avoid immobilization in full supination because an overcorrected position can result.

When wrist deformity or spasticity is severe, arthrodesis can be performed in addition to wrist flexor release. Wrist arthrodesis

has the advantage of permanent correction without the future need of a supportive orthosis. Arthrodesis can also overcome severe deformities associated with severe capsular and myostatic contracture.

Operative Technique: Wrist Arthrodesis for Wrist Flexion Deformity

Initially release the FCU and FCR as described earlier through a volar incision. If flexion deformity is severe, perform a carpal tunnel release in the standard fashion. Then place a dorsal wrist incision in line with

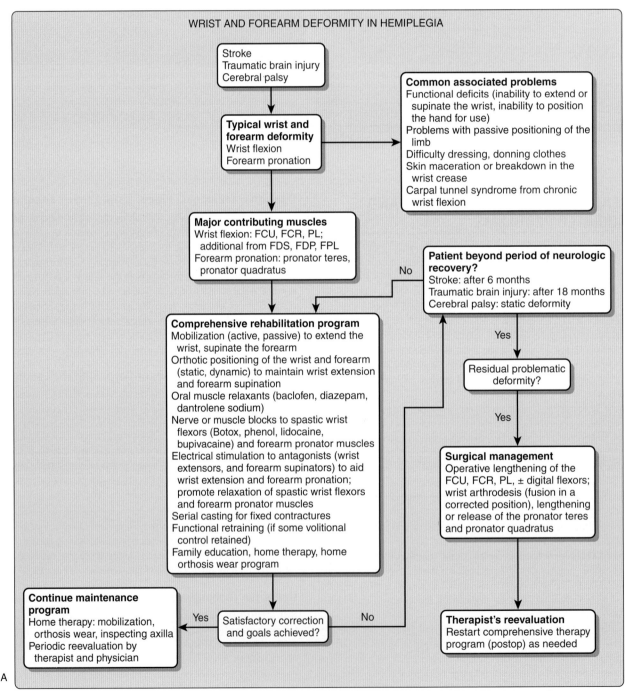

Fig. 112.3 Wrist flexion deformity in a patient with hemiplegia. **A,** Algorithm for the operative indications for wrist and forearm deformities.

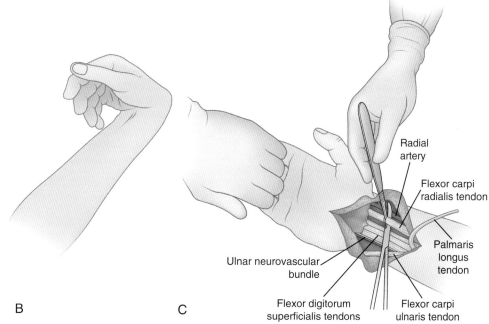

Fig. 112.3, cont'd B, Illustration of marked wrist flexion deformity. **C,** Operative lengthening of the wrist flexors, addressing the flexor carpi radialis (FCR), flexor carpi ulnaris (FCU), and palmaris longus (PL). *FDP,* Flexor digitorum profundus; *FDS,* flexor digitorum superficialis; *FPL,* flexor pollicis longus. (Reproduced from Keenan MAE, Kozin SH, Berlet AC. *Manual for Orthopaedic Surgery for Spasticity.* New York: Raven Press; 1993.)

the long finger metacarpal and Lister's tubercle. Open the extensor retinaculum between the third and fourth extensor compartments. Retract the extensor pollicis longus (EPL) radially. Elevate the second and fourth compartments off the radius subperiosteally and remove Lister's tubercle. Expose and divide the dorsal wrist capsule and ligaments in line with the third metacarpal. Then expose the dorsal aspect of the metacarpal subperiosteally. Remove the cartilage and subchondral bone of the radiolunate, radioscaphoid, lunocapitate, scaphocapitate, and capitometacarpal joints. Position the wrist in 15 degrees of extension with the shaft of the radius in line with the third metacarpal. If excessive tension is placed on the palmar tissues, perform a proximal row carpectomy. Internal fixation of the wrist is accomplished with a precontoured wrist arthrodesis fixation plate that extends from the shaft of the radius to the third metacarpal. Repair the retinaculum. Immobilize the wrist for 6 to 8 weeks or until consolidation is complete.

HAND DEFORMITIES AND ASSOCIATED PROBLEMS

The most common hand deformity is digital flexion. If severe, digital flexion deformity can result in a tight clenched fist deformity. Digital flexion results from spasticity of the flexor digitorum superficialis (FDS) and flexor digitorum profundus (FDP) and from the hand intrinsic muscles. The hand intrinsic muscles will specifically add to flexion at the metacarpophalangeal (MCP) joints. Thumb-in-palm deformity often coexists (discussed later) (see Critical Points Box).

In a clenched fist deformity, both the FDS and FDP are usually involved. Options for treatment include either fractional lengthening of each flexor tendon or individual Z-lengthening. These procedures are preferred if there is some retained volitional control. Alternatively,

if there is a severe clenched fist deformity when there is no residual volitional control, the superficialis-to-profundus transfer (STP) can be performed.[3,6,16,19,20] An algorithm for the operative indications for digital flexion deformities is shown in Fig. 112.4A.[2]

Fractional lengthening or Z-lengthening of the digital flexors is performed in moderate deformities or in limbs with some retained volitional control. The procedure is performed in the distal forearm in a similar manner to wrist flexor lengthening as described earlier[16] (Fig. 112.4B–D).[2,7]

Operative Technique: Digital Flexor Fractional Lengthening or Z-Lengthening

Place a slightly curved or longitudinal incision on the distal half of the palmar forearm. Protect the median nerve, ulnar nerve and artery, and radial artery. Expose the musculotendinous junction regions of the FDS and FDP. Fractional lengthening is performed by placing multiple incision in the tendinous portions along the musculotendinous region, proximal to the distal end of the junction, leaving muscle fibers intact to preserve continuity (see Fig. 112.4D).[2,7] The muscles are then lengthened by passively extending the digits to a desired corrected position. The incisions in the tendons will gap, but muscle fibers will remain intact and provide continuity. A 1-cm gap created by each tendon incision is usually adequate.[16] Half or full correction of digital position is usually satisfactory. Immobilize the hand for 4 weeks to allow muscle healing. Alternatively, a Z-lengthening of the individual tendons can be performed if there is a more severe deformity that may not be correctable with fractional lengthening. Place a Z-lengthening tenotomy through the tendinous portion, passively extend the digits to a desired correction, and repair the tenotomy with 3-0 nonabsorbable suture. Immobilize the digits for 4 weeks to allow tendon healing.

In a nonfunctional spastic or contracted clenched fist deformity with associated hygiene problems, the STP transfer is recommended. This transfer provides a substantial amount of extrinsic digital flexor lengthening while restricting finger hyperextension and preventing possible overcorrection. The procedure works well with a clenched fist deformity, in which adequate correction is not obtainable with either fractional or Z-lengthening.[3,19–23] The procedure does *not* improve active function but adequately addresses positioning and skin and hygiene problems.

The procedure requires adequate supination of the elbow to allow access to the palmar forearm. If severe forearm pronation exists, it is addressed before addressing digital flexion by releasing the pronator quadratus or pronator teres (discussed earlier).

Operative Technique: Superficialis-to-Profundus Transfer

Place a longitudinal, curved incision on the palmar aspect of the distal two thirds of the forearm. Identify and protect the median nerve, ulnar nerve and artery, and radial artery. Expose the FDS and FDP. Suture the tendons of the FDS together at equal length in an en masse fashion 1 to 2 cm proximal to the wrist. A straight needle can be used to pass through all tendons with the digits at equal correction; 3-0 nonabsorbable suture is used. Transect the FDS tendons distal to the level of the suture. Reflect, as one unit, the FDS. Access is now provided to the FDP. Protect the median nerve that passes between the FDS and the FDP muscle. Suture the tendons of the FDP together at equal length

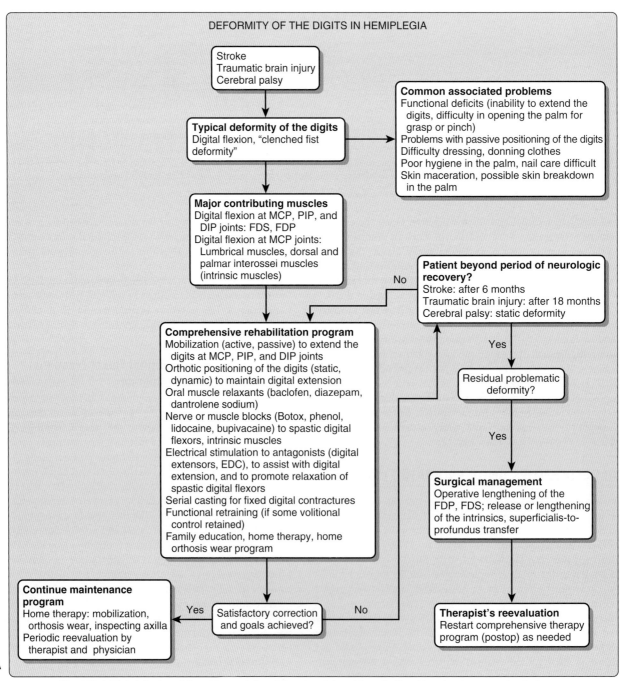

Fig. 112.4 Digital flexion deformities and thumb-in-palm deformities. **A,** Algorithm for the operative indications for digital flexion deformities.

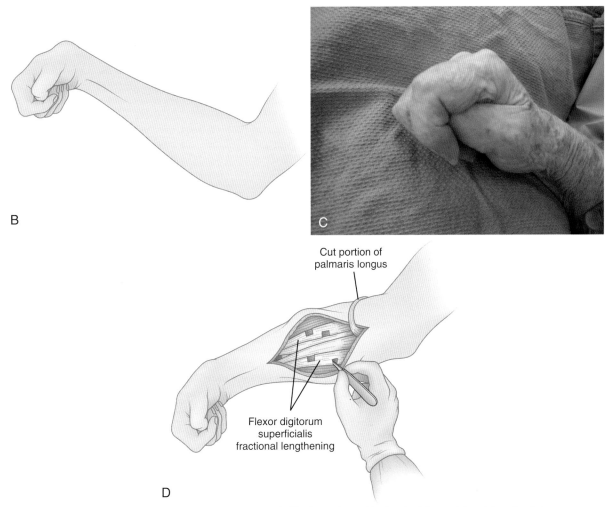

Fig. 112.4, cont'd Illustration (**B**) and photograph (**C**) of a patient with clenched fist and thumb-in-palm deformity. **D,** Illustration of operative correction of digital flexion deformities using fractional lengthening of the flexor digitorum superficialis (FDS) deformities. *DIP,* Distal interphalangeal; *EDC,* extensor digitorum communis; *FDP,* flexor digitorum profundus; *MCP,* metacarpophalangeal; *PIP,* proximal interphalangeal. (Parts B and D reproduced from Keenan MAE, Kozin SH, Berlet AC. *Manual for Orthopaedic Surgery for Spasticity.* New York: Raven Press; 1993.)

in an en masse fashion proximally in the forearm at or near the level of the musculotendinous junction; 3-0 nonabsorbable suture is used. Transect the tendons just proximal to the level of the suture. Extend the digits to the desired corrected position. Slight digital flexion should be retained to prevent possible overcorrection. Suture the proximal portion of the FDS tendons to the distal tendon portion of the FDP tendons with the digits held in the corrected position.[3,20,21] If the wrist flexors and FPL tendons are contracted, these tendons are lengthened before the STP transfer. The digits are immobilized for 4 weeks.

After release or lengthening of the FDS and FDP tendons in a clenched fist deformity, intrinsic muscle tightness or contracture may become apparent. This will be noted by residual tight or fixed flexion at the MCP joints. Evaluate for intrinsic muscle tightness by passively extending the digits at the MCP joints. Passively extending the MCP joints will place the intrinsic muscles at stretch (which normally flex the MCP joints and extend the proximal interphalangeal [IP] joints). If there is additional resistance to passive flexion of the proximal IP joints (or additional extension is noted at the proximal IP joints), there is tightness of the intrinsic muscles (Bunnell intrinsic muscle tightness test). Residual intrinsic muscle tightness that is "unmasked" at

this time can be addressed by either ulnar motor neurectomy or by intrinsic muscle lengthening or release. Ulnar motor neurectomy is useful in the nonfunctional hand, with noted intrinsic tightness and when hand hygiene is difficult. Ulnar motor neurectomy is often used in combination with extrinsic flexor lengthening or with STP transfer. Ulnar motor neurectomy will address noxious spasticity but will not completely correct an intrinsic plus deformity if there is fixed myostatic contracture of the intrinsic muscles (in which case intrinsic tendon–muscle release would be indicated, discussed later).

Operative Technique: Ulnar Motor Neurectomy

Place a 5-cm incision on the palmar ulnar surface of the hand over Guyon's canal. Identify the ulnar nerve and artery. Trace the ulnar nerve distally to the division of the motor and sensory branches. Identify the main motor branch and confirm using a nerve stimulator. Excise a segment of the nerve from the motor branch. A separate motor branch to the hypothenar muscles is often present and can be resected as well. Commence mobilization when the wound permits.[3]

For fixed myostatic intrinsic muscle contractures contributing to hygiene problems in the hand, intrinsic muscle release is warranted.

There are three separate operative procedures to consider. These are the distal intrinsic release, the proximal intrinsic release, and the interosseous muscle slide (recession) procedure.[3,6,24,25] In general, the distal intrinsic release has proven adequate and is currently our preferred method.

Operative Technique: Distal Intrinsic Muscle Release for Intrinsic Contracture

Place a 4-cm incision over the dorsum of the proximal phalanx. Dissect to the level of the extensor hood and continue dissection ulnarly and radially to expose the palmar edge of the lateral bands. Transect or resect the lateral bands, including the oblique fibers. Take care to preserve the transverse fibers of the intrinsic apparatus as well as the central and lateral slips of the extensor tendon. The digit is then passively mobilized to a corrected position. Immobilize the digits in a corrected position for 4 weeks before restarting a hand therapy program.

Operative Technique: Proximal Intrinsic Muscle Release for Intrinsic Contracture

Place a 3-cm longitudinal incision on the dorsum of the hand between the metacarpal heads and extend the incision distal to the MCP joint. Identify the tendons from the interossei and remove a 1-cm segment of tendon. The lumbrical tendons are present only on the radial side of the corresponding metacarpal and are located deep to the deep transverse metacarpal ligament. Identify the lumbrical tendons as each exits from beneath the deep transverse metacarpal ligament and remove a segment of each tendon.

The third method of intrinsic release is the intrinsic muscle slide. The procedure very effectively releases tight but functional interossei while preserving function. The procedure has been criticized as being extensive and traumatic. We have tended to avoid this procedure in favor of the distal or intrinsic release procedures described earlier.

Operative Technique: Interosseous Muscle Slide (Recession)

Place a dorsal transverse incision at the level of the midshafts of the metacarpals. Isolate and retract the digital extensors radially and ulnarly to allow visualization of the interosseous muscles. Take care to protect the branches of the superficial radial nerve and dorsal branch of the ulnar nerve. Perform a subperiosteal dissection to free the interossei from their origins on the metacarpals. Splint the digits in a corrected position. The muscles will reattach in a more distal (effectively lengthened) position. Early active mobilization is initiated when patient comfort permits.

THUMB: DEFORMITY AND ASSOCIATED PROBLEMS

Spasticity of the thumb intrinsic muscles and extrinsic flexor can lead to thumb adduction and flexion, resulting in the thumb-in-palm deformity. Several muscles can contribute to the deformity, including the thenar muscles (flexor pollicis brevis [FPB], abductor pollicis brevis [APB], opponens pollicis), the adductor pollicis, the first dorsal interosseous, and the FPL (Fig. 112.5).[2,3,7,26,27] The abductor pollicis brevis, the opponens pollicis, the superficial head of the flexor pollicis brevis, and the FPL are innervated by the median nerve. The adductor pollicis, the deep head of the flexor pollicis brevis, and the first dorsal interosseous are innervated by the ulnar nerve. In stroke and brain injury, any or all of these muscles can have varying amounts of spasticity and can subsequently result in varying degrees of the deformity

(see Critical Points Box). When the thumb is pulled into the palm, its function as an opposing force is obliterated. Hand grasp and pinch are severely impaired. Hygiene problems in the thenar crease arise. Pressure from the end of the thumb or from the nail can result in skin breakdown or a pressure ulcer in the palm. The thumb-in-palm deformity often coexists with a clenched fist deformity, thus compounding the function deficits and skin and hygiene problems.

The markedly adducted, flexed thumb is difficult to splint into a corrected position. Joint instability and hyperextension at the MCP joint may result from attempts to abduct and extend the thumb when the metacarpal is tightly adducted.

Operative management must take into consideration the specific (and often multiple) muscles contributing to the deformity. Spasticity of the thenar muscles usually results in flexion at the thumb MCP joint with a supple or extended IP joint. Spasticity of the FPL results in flexion deformity at the IP joint, with variable flexion at the MCP joint. Involvement of the adductor pollicis causes flexion at the MCP joint and adduction of the metacarpal toward the midpalm. Involvement of the first dorsal interosseous or opponens pollicis results in an adducted position of the metacarpal in the plane of the palm and tightness of the thumb webspace.

Sequential diagnostic lidocaine hydrochloride nerve blocks to the median and ulnar nerves at the wrist can assist the physical exam to differentiate contributions from the median- and ulnar-innervated intrinsic muscles. An additional lidocaine hydrochloride block to the median nerve proximal to the elbow defines involvement of the FPL. Fixed contracture (as opposed to spasticity) of the myotendinous units or joint capsule is marked by persistent deformity following nerve blocks.

An algorithm for operative indications for thumb-in-palm deformity is shown in Fig. 112.5A.[2]

Operative Technique: Thenar Origin and Adductor Pollicis Recession

Place a curved incision along the thenar crease. Extend the dissection to the base of the thenar muscles. Identify the FPB and APB at their origin from the transverse carpal ligament (Fig. 112.5B and C).[2,3,26] Elevate these muscles from their attachments on the transverse carpal ligament, taking care to protect the recurrent motor branch of the median nerve. Passively extend the proximal phalanx of the thumb, allowing the released thenar muscles to slide radially. Exposure of the opponens pollicis is then provided; release its origin in a similar fashion. Immobilize the thumb in a corrected position for 4 weeks.

If the adductor pollicis is involved, release the muscle at the time of thenar origin release. Identify the muscle in the distal aspect of the incision, deep and distal to the FPB. Release the adductor pollicis either from its origin on the third metacarpal or near its insertion (Fig. 112.5C and D).[2,3,7,26] To release the muscle from its origin, the digital neurovascular bundles and flexor tendons to the index and long fingers are identified and protected. Trace the adductor pollicis to its origin on the third metacarpal. Identify and protect the deep palmar vascular arch and the deep branch of the ulnar nerve, which pierce the adductor pollicis between the transverse and oblique heads. Release the muscle from the metacarpal. Partial release of the distal portion of the transverse carpal ligament will assist exposure of the proximal portion of the muscle.

Alternatively, the adductor pollicis can be released from its tendinous insertion (5C).[2,7] The muscle is traced radially and released. Release of the origin of the adductor pollicis has the advantage of preserving function. Release at the insertion, although technically easier, obliterates the muscle function.

Operative Technique: Release of the First Dorsal Interosseous

Place a longitudinal incision on the dorsum of the hand along the palpable ulnar margin of the thumb metacarpal. Identify and protect cutaneous branches of the superficial radial nerve. Identify the EPL tendon along the radial margin of the incision. Continue the dissection ulnar to the EPL tendon to expose the broad origin of the first dorsal interosseous from the ulnar margin of the thumb metacarpal. Release the muscle from its origin and passively abduct the thumb metacarpal into the plane of the palm to a corrected position (see Fig. 112.5D).[2,3,7,26] The insertion of the adductor pollicis can be released at this time if the incision is extended distal to the MCP joint. The tendinous insertion is visible at the ulnar margin of the base of the proximal phalanx, distal to the first dorsal interosseous muscle. Release the tendon through this tendinous portion, including release of the attachments to the ulnar sesamoid. Immobilize the thumb for 4 weeks.

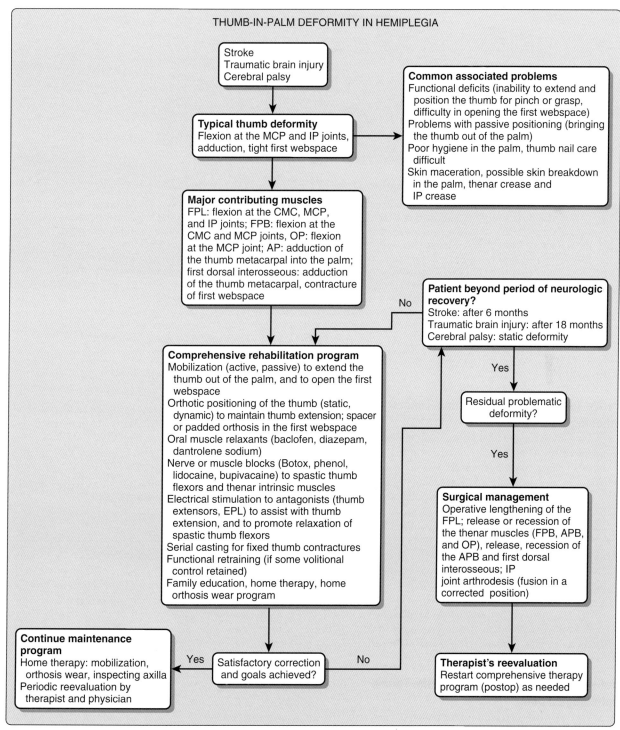

Fig. 112.5 Thumb-in-palm deformity in hemiplegia. **A,** Algorithm for operative indications for thumb-in-palm deformity.

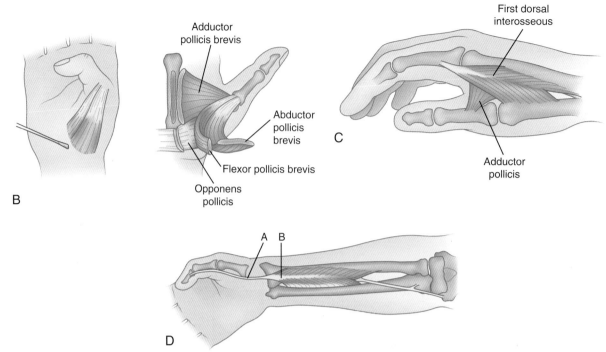

Fig. 112.5, cont'd B and **C,** Illustrations of operative release of thumb-in-palm deformity. Operative correction usually requires addressing the thenar muscles as well as the adductor pollicis and first dorsal interosseous. The thenar muscles are released from their attachments on the transverse carpal ligament. If needed, the adductor pollicis is released as well, either from its origin on the third metacarpal (**B**) or from its insertion into the proximal phalanx of the thumb (**C**). The first dorsal interosseous is released through a separate dorsal approach along the thumb metacarpal, releasing the muscle from its origin on the thumb metacarpal (**C**). **D,** If the flexor pollicis longus (FPL) contributes to the deformity, it can be either Z-lengthened in its tendinous portion *A* (if there is a relatively long tendinous portion) or by fractional lengthening in its myotendinous junction *B* (if there is a relatively long myotendinous junction). *AP,* Adductor pollicis; *APB, abductor* pollicis brevis; *CMC,* carpometacarpal; *EPL,* extensor pollicis longus; *FPB,* flexor pollicis brevis; *IP,* interphalangeal; *MCP,* metacarpophalangeal; *OP,* opponens pollicis. (B, C, and D reproduced from Botte MJ, Keenan MAE, Gellman, H et al. Surgical management of spastic thumb-in-palm deformity in adults with brain injury. *J Hand Surg.* 1989;14A:174-182.)

Operative Technique: Flexor Pollicis Longus Lengthening

Place a gently curved longitudinal incision on the distal third of the radiopalmar forearm. Identify and protect the FCR tendon, the median nerve with its palmar cutaneous branch, and the radial artery. The FPL tendon is located deep to the FCR tendon. Lengthen the tendon by either fractional lengthening in the myotendinous junction or by Z-lengthening through the tendinous portion, depending on the length of the coexisting tendon and muscle in the musculotendinous junction encountered at the time of dissection (see Fig. 112.5D).[2,7] Fractional lengthening is performed by placement of two to three incisions into the tendinous portion of the musculotendinous junction, leaving the connecting muscle fibers intact to preserve continuity of the muscle. Extend the thumb to the desired corrected position to create gaps at the incision of the tendinous portion and thereby lengthening the muscle–tendon unit. Avoid overcorrection. Residual flexion of 10 to 20 degrees at the IP joint is desirable. Immobilize the thumb in the corrected position for 3 to 4 weeks.

Operative Technique: Arthrodesis of the Thumb Interphalangeal Joint

If there is a severe, fixed contracture at the thumb IP joint, arthrodesis in a corrected position is an alternative to soft tissue release. Arthrodesis is performed in a standard fashion, placing a curved dorsal incision over the flexed IP joint. Denude the articular cartilage and subchondral bone. Position the thumb in 10 degrees of flexion and 10 degrees of pronation. Internal fixation is accomplished using smooth pins, screws, a wire loop, or small fixation plate. Immobilize the joint for 6 weeks or until fusion is evident.

If secondary webspace contracture has developed, deepen the webspace using a two- or four-quadrant Z-plasty.

SUMMARY

Despite an aggressive hand and upper extremity therapy program, refractory or fixed deformities can develop from severe, acquired spasticity. Operative management may be of benefit for these problematic deformities but is reserved for deformities that still exist after a patient is no longer spontaneously neurologically recovering from the initial neurologic insult *and* the patient has reached a plateau in an aggressive hand and upper extremity therapy program. The common deformity of shoulder adduction and internal rotation, elbow flexion, forearm pronation, wrist flexion, digital flexion with clenched fist deformity, and thumb-in-palm deformity can all usually be addressed, to some degree, with operative management. Operative management helps to correct deformity; assists with extremity hygiene, patient dressing, position, and prevention of skin maceration and pressure sores; and often improves function.

REFERENCES

1. Braun RM. Spasticity in the upper extremity. *Clin Orthop*. 1974;104:80–91.
2. Botte MJ, Kivirahk DL, Kinoshita YO, et al. Hemiplegia. In: Skirvin TM, Osterman AL, Fedorczyk JM, Amadio PC, eds. *Rehabilitation of the Hand and Upper Extremity*. 6th ed. Philadelphia: Elsevier; 2011:1659–1683.
3. Botte MJ, Keenan MAE. Brain injury and stroke. In: Gelberman RH, ed. *Operative Nerve Repair and Reconstruction*. Philadelphia: JB Lippincott; 1991:1415–1451.
4. Garland DE, Keenan MAE. Orthopedic strategies in the management of the adult head-injured patient. *J Am Physical Therapy Assoc*. 1983;63:2004–2009.
5. Keenan MAE. The orthopaedic management of spasticity. *J Head Trauma Rehab*. 1987;2:62–71.
6. Botte MJ, Keenan MAE. Reconstructive surgery of the upper extremity in the patient with head trauma. *J Head Trauma Rehabil*. 1987;2:34–45.
7. Keenan MAE, Kozin SH, Berlet AC, eds. *Manual of Orthopaedic Surgery for Spasticity*. New York: Raven Press; 1993.
8. Smyth MD, Peacock WJ. The surgical treatment of spasticity. *Muscle Nerve*. 2000;23(2):153–163.
9. Young RR. Spasticity: a review. *Neurology*. 1994;44:512–520.
10. Braun RM, West F, Mooney V, Nickel FL, et al. Surgical treatment of the painful shoulder contracture in the stroke patient. *(Am)*. 1971;53:1307–1312.
11. Braun RM, Botte MJ. Treatment of shoulder deformity in acquired spasticity. *Clin Orthop Relat Res*. 1999;368:54–65.
12. Namdari S, Baldwin K, Horneff JG, et al. Orthopedic evaluation and surgical treatment of the spastic shoulder. *Orthop Clin N Am*. 2013;44:605–614.
13. Namdari S, Alosh H, Baldwin K, et al. Outcomes of tendon fractional lengthenings to improve shoulder function in patients with spastic hemiparesis. *J Shoulder Elbow Surg*. 2012;21(5):691–698.
14. Anakwenze OA, Namadari S, Hsu Je, et al. Myotendinous lengthening of the elbow flexor muscles to improve active motion in patients with elbow spasticity following brain injury. *J Shoulder Elbow Surg*. 2013;22(3):318–322.
15. Rayan GM, Young BT. Arthrodesis of the spastic wrist. *J Hand Surg (Am)*. 1999;24:944–952.
16. Keenen MAE, Abrams RA, Garland DE, et al. Results of fractional lengthening of the finger flexors in adults with upper extremity spasticity. *J Hand Surg (Am)*. 1987;12:575–581.
17. Braun RM, Mooney V, Nickel VL. Flexor origin release for pronation-flexion deformity of the forearm and hand in the stroke patient: an evaluation of the early results in eighteen patients. *J Bone Joint Surg (Am)*. 1970;52:907–920.
18. Thevenin-Lemoine C, Denormandie P, Schnitzler A, et al. Flexor origin slide for contracture of spastic finger flexor muscles: a retrospective study. *J Bone Joint Surg (Am)*. 2013;95(5):446–453.
19. Braun RM, Vise GT, Roper B. Preliminary experience with superficialis to profundus tendon transfer in the hemiplegic upper extremity. *J Bone Joint Surg (Am)*. 1974;56:466–472.
20. Botte MB, Keenan MAE, Korchek JI, et al. Modified technique for the superficialis-to-profundus transfer in the treatment of adults with spastic clenched fist deformity. *J Hand Surg (Am)*. 1987;12:639–640.
21. Keenan MAE, Korchek JI, Botte MJ, et al. Results of transfer of the flexor digitorum superficialis tendons to the flexor digitorum profundus tendons in adults with acquired spasticity of the hand. *J Bone Joint Surg (Am)*. 1987;69:1127–1132.
22. Pomerance JF, Keenan MAE. Correction of severe spastic flexion contractures in the nonfunctional hand. *J Hand Surg (Am)*. 1996;21:828–833.
23. Heijnen CM, Franken RJP, Bevaart BJW, et al. Long-term outcome of superficialis-to-profundus tendon transfer in patients with clenched fist due to spastic hemiplegia. *Disability and Rehab*. 2008;30:675–678.
24. Harris Jr C, Riordan DC. Intrinsic contracture in the hand and its surgical treatment. *J Bone Joint Surg (Am)*. 1954;36:10–20.
25. Keenan MAE, Todderud EP, Henderson R, et al. Management of intrinsic spasticity in the hand with phenol injection or neurectomy of the motor branch of the ulnar nerve. *J Hand Surg (Am)*. 1987;12:734–739.
26. Botte MJ, Keenan MAE, Gellman H, et al. Surgical management of spastic thumb-in-palm deformity in adults with brain injury. *J Hand Surg (Am)*. 1989;14:174–182.
27. Rayan GM, Saccone PG. Treatment of spastic thumb-in-palm deformity: a modified extensor pollicis long tendon rerouting. *J Hand Surg (Am)*. 1996;21:834.

Rehabilitation of the Hand and Upper Extremity in Tetraplegia

Allan E. Peljovich, Bryce T. Gillespie, Anne M. Bryden, Kevin Malone, Harry Hoyen, Eduardo Gonzalez-Hernandez, Michael W. Keith

OUTLINE

CRITICAL POINTS

Patient Evaluation

- Repeat examinations are important to understanding an individual's particular impairments, disabilities, and abilities.
- It is important to develop a relationship with the individual patient to understand his or her particular desires and goals so as to determine what therapeutic options are reasonable and appropriate.

Principles of Nonoperative Management

- Early intervention is critical to preventing contractures.
- Treat all individuals with acute spinal cord injury as if they will improve.
- A supple hand with a good tenodesis effect is the goal of treatment.
- Maintaining shoulder and elbow mobility is critical to hand function.

INTRODUCTION

Among the most disabling aspects of traumatic tetraplegia is the loss of useful hand function. During the acute phase of a patient's injury, the focus of treatment concerns the survival of the patient. In the sub-acute phase, care is often shifted into the rehabilitation environment, where the long road to recovery, both mentally, and physically, begins. Focus here is aimed towards the long-term phase, where patient's medical and psychological systems are maintained, and he/she becomes reintegrated into society. In this final phase, patients are hopefully discharged from a full-term care facility into a more personal environment; and, just as important, into an environment that provides them with purpose and gain. During this entire process, a large and multi-disciplinary team including physicians, nurses, therapists, and social workers cares for the patient. In recent years, Model Spinal Cord centers have increasingly recognized the importance of incorporating hand and upper extremity rehabilitation into their patient care schemes. This is important considering research has documented the loss of hand function in tetraplegic patients to be among the most disabling features of their injury, and that they often regard the hope for restoration of hand function to be of paramount importance.[1-3]

As knowledge of spinal cord injury (SCI) care has improved, so too has that of hand and upper extremity restoration. We believe conceptually that to aid the patient in the long run, treatment directed to the hand and upper extremity should begin early in the acute phase of care and that this treatment extends beyond traditional concepts of exercise, splinting, and braces. In fact, true rehabilitation of a tetraplegic hand should be thought of as the judicious application of nonoperative and operative interventions tailor-made to the particular patient to maximize his or her function, bearing in mind the patient's global psychosocial and medical state.

Hand and upper extremity rehabilitation are vital in the SCI population to improving such function in people with tetraplegia. Research continues to demonstrate underuse of resources and surgical reconstruction.[4-6] A recent qualitative study identified that patients proceed stepwise through a sequence of three steps before proceeding with upper extremity reconstructive surgery. Patients must have functional dissatisfaction with their upper extremities; then become aware that reconstruction is an option; and, finally, accept to proceed with surgery. We must recognize how we can intervene during the rehabilitation process to ensure that patients are making informed decisions.[7]

This chapter examines how the pathophysiology of SCI in tetraplegia applies to hand and upper extremity function, reviews the functional deficits the patients have, and describes a comprehensive approach to rehabilitation based on the former that involves both nonoperative and operative modalities.

THE SCOPE OF THE PROBLEM

Data gathered from the National SCI Database, recently updated in 2017, indicate that the annual incidence of SCI remains approximately 54 cases per million people or about 17,5000 new cases per year, which translates to 285,000 current Americans with SCI. The incidence has increased since the last version of this chapter. Just over half of the individuals, 54.2%, are tetraplegic, and most of them have incomplete injury. The average age of a person who sustains SCI is 42 years, a trend that has increased since such statistics have been recorded. Current standard quality of care that individuals receive at the time of their injury has turned a death sentence into a long and potentially fruitful life. A person injured in their 20s who receives modern care and rehabilitation can expect to live an additional 41 years with low-level tetraplegia (C5–C8).[8] Someone in their 40s will live an additional 26 years. To this end, estimates of direct costs of SCI have been compiled, and for low-level tetraplegia, the estimated cost of the first year of injury is $779,969; each subsequent year is $114,988 and $3,499,423 in lifetime costs for a young patient. These figures do not include indirect costs of injury such as lost income, nor does it estimate the true impact of the injury on individuals' personal lives, including lower postinjury employment, reduced rates of marriage, and higher rates of divorce.[8]

Although tetraplegia is defined as the impairment from an injury to any of the cervical segments of the spine, the extent of disability is primarily determined from the specific functional level of the injury. The fifth cervical spinal cord segment is not only the most common injured level in tetraplegia, but it is also the most common level injured in all SCI (15.2%).[9] The next two most commonly injured levels are also in the cervical spine, namely the C4 and C6 segments, with both amounting to about 25% of all SCI. The remaining cervical segments comprise about 14% of all SCIs. Most individuals retain at least the ability to flex their elbows, and some can extend their wrists, but most do not retain voluntarily elbow extension, wrist flexion, or finger control. Factors that influence functional ability include whether the injury is neurologically "complete," if any cognitive impairment exists (brain injury), the age of the patient, any other upper extremity injury, the presence of uncontrolled spasticity, contractures that limit mobility, and depression.

Intuitively, the level of function and independence improves when an individual's injury is at a lower level in the cervical spine as he or she retains more function. Patients with high-level tetraplegia, with functional levels from C2 to C4, generally have no movement of the arms short of some shoulder elevation. They have some control of their neck muscles and are likely ventilatory support–dependent depending on the actual functional level of injury. Patients who retain voluntary innervation in the C5 myotome can feed themselves and perhaps even groom themselves with the aid of special adaptive equipment attached to their wrists and hands. At the C6 level, patients, with the aid of adaptive equipment, can be independent in grooming, bathing, driving, and preparing simple meals. At the C7 level, patients may be able to perform all the previous activities and be fairly efficient in daily living tasks. Importantly, if the triceps is of sufficient strength, they may be able to independently transfer themselves provided they have voluntary control of most of their shoulder musculature and, therefore can live alone with the aid of special hand and environmental adaptive equipment. With the exception of this latter patient, all patients require an able-bodied attendant nearly most of the time to help them with their daily activities. Although this is an oversimplified and generalized view of function based on level of injury, it should be readily apparent that any treatment or intervention that improves a level of function (e.g., C5 to C6) would result in a dramatic improvement in both function and independence.

TABLE 113.1 Characteristic Clinical Patterns of Motor Neuron Disease or Injury

	Upper Motor Neuron	Lower Motor Neuron
Muscles involved	Groups (myotomes) are affected	Individual muscles may be affected
Atrophy	Slight and secondary to disuse	Pronounced, ≤70%–80% of normal bulk
Muscle tone	Spasticity, hyperactive tendon reflexes, Babinski sign present	Flaccidity, hypotonia, loss of deep tendon reflexes
Fascicular twitches	Absent	May be present
EMG/NCS	Normal NCS; no denervation on EMG	Abnormal NCS; denervation present on EMG

EMG, Electromyography; *NCS*, nerve conduction study.

The extent of impairment patients experience is truly great. The spinal cord serves not only as the conduit for transmission of efferent and afferent information between the limbs and the brain but is also an important neural conduit for the bowel, bladder, respiration, temperature regulation, cardiovascular integrity, and sexual function. All of these important physiological systems are affected by the injury, and until recently, served as a common and serious cause of morbidity. The affected people are young, usually otherwise healthy, and might otherwise have expected to live long and productive lives. At the time of injury, about 57.4% are employed. The impact of injury extends well into their personal life, with sound data indicating lower rates of marriage and higher rates of divorce among patients with SCIs. The results of modern SCI care and management have dramatically improved the quantity of life, in terms of long-term survival, to a level near able-bodied individuals. Similar care has dramatically improved the quality of their lives as well, but any intervention that can improve a patient's functional ability will have a tremendous positive impact that will extend beyond activities they can perform. Patients continue to place great importance in improving hand and upper extremity function among the various components of SCI rehabilitation.[1–3] Robert Waters, a surgeon from Ranchos Los Amigos, and his colleagues[10] noted the "…the greatest potential for improvement of quality of life lies in rehabilitation and maximal restoration of upper extremity function." Clearly, attention should be directed to rehabilitating the hand and upper extremity as part of a more global approach to treating patients with tetraplegia.

PATHOPHYSIOLOGY

Traumatic SCI disrupts the neural communication that exists between the central and peripheral nervous systems at the level of the spinal cord. Traditional simplified patterns of nerve injury have been used to explain the resulting pathophysiology; SCI represents loss of upper motor–sensory neurons as opposed to peripheral nerve injuries that are lower motor–sensory neurons. Table 113.1 displays the common clinical patterns associated with these two different injury patterns. Both careful examination of a spinal cord injured patient and clinical research have documented that there is a spectrum of nerve loss associated with the injury.[11,12] It is more appropriate to think in terms of a "zone of injury" to the nervous system centered about, but not exclusively confined to, the spinal cord. This zone is three dimensional, extending in a proximal–distal plane and central–peripheral or medial-lateral-anterior-posterior plane. This is because most SCIs are caused by high-energy injury blunt trauma (motor vehicle accident, diving) in which energy is transferred to the affected bones and soft tissues in a global pattern. This is in contrast to a sharp penetrating injury (gunshot wound, laceration) in which the energy is transmitted to a more specific area of tissue. In fact, it is now believed that the extent of the neurologic damage in SCI occurs from both the initial trauma and the secondary and reactive inflammatory response.[13] Edema, venous stasis, spinal cord infarction, and the release of toxic biochemical compounds during the response to injury all combine to increase the extent of spinal injury.[13]

That the zone of injury can include both the cord and the peripheral nervous system about the neck has important implications for the individual and potential operative strategies to improve function. Above the zone of injury, the central and peripheral systems and their interconnections are intact and fully functional. Below this zone, the nerve pathophysiology resembles an upper motor neuron lesion with hyperreflexia. Within the zone of injury, however, damage can extend from the spinal cord to the level of the dorsal sensory ganglia and nerve roots. The pattern of nerve loss can be a combination of pure upper motor neuron and lower motor neuron and sensory involvement. This is the reason that two patients with two seemingly similar anatomical levels of spinal injury can have different degrees of paralysis, spasticity, and neural loss.

Coulet and colleagues[13] have elegantly demonstrated how the extent of this zone of injury can influence the presentation of a particular individual and can be located through a combination of clinical examination, spinal imaging, and electrical studies. Patients with larger zones of denervation are more prone to the development of limiting contractures and counterproductive forearm and hand posturing. In addition, if there is peripheral nerve injury within this zone, critical muscles may become permanently denervated, which has implications on the ability to perform a nerve transfer to restore function (discussed later in the chapter). On the other hand, muscles below the zone of injury, as they remain innervated, maintain a dynamic tone that helps to create an inherent balance to the forearm and hand that is functional and easier to base a reconstruction on. They theorized that by understanding a particular person's zone of injury, one might predict the person's tendency to develop, for example, a forearm supination contracture and therefore take preventive steps.[13] Although these concepts have not been universally adopted, their work is promising, clinically relevant, and could help therapists identify particular "at-risk for contracture" individuals early in the course of their injuries.

Classification systems based primarily on the functional level of injury results in too much uncertainty.[14,15] Health care providers discovered that gross motor functions conferred important prognostic information. This is because the innervation of the hand and upper extremity, from spinal roots C4 through T1, proceeds in a fairly ordered and segmental pattern from proximal to distal (Fig. 113.1), making predictions of functional loss and retention fairly reliable after the functional level of the injury is apparent. The classification system most commonly used, devised by the International Standards for Neurological Classification of Spinal Cord Injury (ISNCSCI) and known as the ASIA Impairment Scale (AIS), is based on this functional level and distinguishes the completeness of the injury and the motor and sensory integrity between the extremities.[16] In this system, the most distal myotome with manual muscle test (MMT) strength of at least 3 is the motor level; similarly, the most distal dermatome with sensation is the sensory level. Motor grade 3 was chosen because it is unambiguous, whereas motor grades 4 and 5 cannot de-differentiated when examiners of varying strength confront persons with varying strength. Despite the simplicity and general usefulness of the system, it is not precise enough from the standpoint of hand surgical rehabilitation. Patients with preserved myotomes can still vary

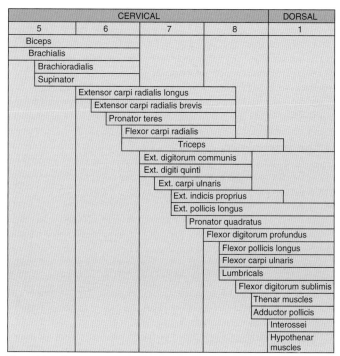

Fig. 113.1 Segmental innervation of muscles of the elbow, forearm, and hand. *Ext.,* Extensor. (From Zancolli E. Surgery for the quadriplegic hand with active, strong wrist extension preserved. A study of 97 cases. *Clin Orthop.* 1975;112:101.)

in terms of the motors with voluntary innervation. For example, a C5 patient, defined by at least grade 3 elbow flexion, may or may not have a strong, voluntary brachioradialis (BR), and a C6 patient, defined by at least grade 3 wrist extension, may or may not have a strong, voluntary extensor carpi radialis brevis (ECRB). From the standpoint of surgical restoration, these differences are very significant, which was the impetus for the International Classification for Surgery of the Hand in Tetraplegia (ICSHT) created in 1984 in Giens, France, during an international meeting of hand surgeons devoted to the care of tetraplegic patients.[14] Since that time, the classification system has undergone some modification, and its present form is shown in Table 113.2.[14] The basis for the classification is the segmental innervation of the hand, and because tendon transfers are typically considered only in muscles with at least grade 4 strength, the system supplies the physician with the potential transferable motors. This is currently the accepted classification used by most surgeons performing tetraplegic hand surgery.

PATIENT EVALUATION

Only through thorough evaluation of the patient at various points in time can one determine the appropriate goals of rehabilitation and reconstruction for that particular patient. The health care provider must develop a relationship with the patient that provides insight into the patient's own goals and desires.[7,15,17] Consideration for rehabilitation, especially surgical intervention, requires that the patient and primary caregivers understand the reconstructive options and their risks and benefits. Tendon transfer–based surgery, for example, means that the patient will be more disabled than normal for a short period after surgery while the arm is temporarily immobilized and he or she goes through a period of rehabilitation. Patients undergoing nerve-based reconstructions must understand that their recovery will take place over the course of 1 to 2 years. A patient must be motivated to improve and be cooperative throughout the postoperative phase of rehabilitation.

TABLE 113.2 Classifications

INTERNATIONAL STANDARDS FOR NEUROLOGICAL CLASSIFICATION OF SPINAL CORD INJURY (ISNCSCI): ASIA IMPAIRMENT SCALE (AIS)[16]

Spinal Cord Root Level	Functional Group at Grade 3 Strength
C5	Elbow flexors
C6	Wrist extensors
C7	Elbow extensors
C8	Finger flexors
T1	Fifth finger abduction

INTERNATIONAL CLASSIFICATION FOR SURGERY OF THE HAND IN TETRAPLEGIA (ICSHT)[18]

Group	Muscle at Grade 4 Strength
1	BR
2	ECRL
3	ECRB
4	PT
5	FCR
6	EDC and finger extensors
7	EPL and thumb extensors
8	Finger flexors
9	All except intrinsics
0	Exceptions
T+ or T-	Triceps at grade 4

"O" for ocular (no sensation) and "Cu" for cutaneous (< 10mm 2-point discrimination intact to the index finger and thumb)
BR, Brachioradialis; *ECRB*, extensor carpi radialis brevis; *ECRL*, extensor carpi radialis longus; *EDC*, extensor digitorum communis; *EPL*, extensor pollicis longus; *FCR*, flexor carpi radialis; *PT*, pronator teres; *T*, triceps. Revised in Cleveland, Ohio, at the 6th International Conference on Surgical Rehabilitation of the Upper Limb in Tetraplegia; 1998.

Similarly, the patient's general medical condition and cognition must be stable enough in order to undergo a potentially lengthy surgery and not interfere with the postoperative rehabilitation program. The success of restorations requires continual effort on the part of the patient both physically and mentally; otherwise, she or he may lose the benefits of any surgical reconstruction. Then, too, if the patient or surgeon is too overly optimistic about the results of surgery, patients will lose the motivation to continue rehabilitation and may be worse off for it. Clearly, the decision to undergo surgical restoration must not be taken likely.

Other factors must be considered as vital to the success of any restorative program.[18] Patients should be easily transferable to a wheelchair and have good trunk support and adequate seating so they can stay seated to take full advantage of any use of their upper extremities. Any restorative program should be delayed until it is apparent that no further motor recovery is predicted. This may take as long as 1 year from the time of a complete cord injury or even longer in the case of incomplete injury. In some cases in which the lesion is well defined and severe and when there is no progression, early intervention is justified. Because many of the restorative procedures involve the transfer of voluntary muscles to more effective insertions (tendon transfers), the prerequisites to successful procedures must exist, including supple joints and sufficient strength of the donor muscle. A patient who is allowed to develop joint contractures in the hands, wrists, forearms, elbows, and

shoulders will be a poor candidate for a complete restorative program that includes surgical reconstruction or even a splinting program. A muscle that is spastic and difficult to control with through therapy or medication cannot serve as a useful donor. These criteria have been established through years of experience and remain a useful tool in guiding surgeons to distinguish which patients will have a good chance of success through surgical restoration. The addition of medications, which selectively weaken spastic muscles, such as Botox, and reduce contractures, is an essential part of early management.

Physical Examination

The physical examination ultimately forms the foundation for any surgical reconstruction. The integrity and function of both the motor and sensory systems in the upper extremity must be understood. The motor system must be evaluated in its entirety, from the proximal muscles in the shoulder, to the intrinsic muscles in the hand, to determine which muscles are voluntary, spastic, or flaccid. Each muscle must be evaluated independently in order to classify the patient; and, the examiner should not discontinue the examination with what appears to be an ASIA level, all muscles should be examined because voluntary innervation may "skip" myotomes depending on whether the injury is complete or on the particular patient's neural system and zone of injury. We use the manual muscle testing (MMT) grading system that is well accepted (strength graded from 0–5). If patients do have spastic muscles, they should be assessed for the degree of spasticity and whether it is functional.[19] For example, a patient who develops spasticity of the flexor pollicis longus (FPL) muscle on voluntary wrist extension may have a strong lateral pinch that should neither be sacrificed nor necessarily augmented. At the same time, if the spasticity on the FPL is constant and severe, it cannot be used in a tendon transfer, as an electrically stimulated muscle, nor can useful lateral pinch occur without chemical or surgical release of that muscle. Uncontrolled, global spasticity is considered a contraindication to restorative surgery and fortunately is rare. The sensory examination stresses the two-point discrimination in the digits, particularly the thumb. Much has been written concerning the presence of two-point discrimination in the thumb as both a means of classifying the patient under the international system and understanding the outcomes of surgical restoration. Many authors have stressed that goals should be limited in patients who require direct visualization of grasp because they lack meaningful sensation; however, others, such as ourselves, have found that patients adapt well and prefer increased function even in the face of poor sensation.[20] The motion of the joints, both passive and active, must be ascertained. A final aspect of our motor assessment involves determining the muscles that are electrically excitable using transcutaneous electrical stimulation (TES).[12] This is because previous study has documented that up to 50% of ASIA C5 patients and 13% of C6 patients have important muscle groups that are not electrically excitable.[21]

Evaluation of the upper extremity in the patient with a new injury should begin within 48 hours of admission within the limits of precautions. The evaluation should consist of a brief social and functional history. The patient's physical appearance should be documented, identifying incisions, edema, scars, and apparent atrophy of the muscles. Examination of strength, sensation, and motion should be completed as indicated earlier. Reevaluation of the upper extremity should then take place at regular intervals, typically every 4 weeks.

Patients manifest injury very differently depending on their zone of injury. Detailed and critical examination is therefore paramount to an appropriate custom-tailored rehabilitation plan. Over time, we have come to emphasize certain aspects of the exam in formulating plans. Resting thumb and finger positions are important to note. The thumb ideally rests in a position near opposition with the fingers gently flexed, especially at the metacarpophalangeal (MCP) joint. The wrist tenodesis effect should produce a nice alignment with the thumb resting near the radial side of the index and the fingers gently flexing at the MCP and interphalangeal (IP) joints. A hand that rests with the fingers or thumb flat in the plane of the palm, including intrinsic-minus positions, is more troublesome. Thumb carpometacarpal (CMC) stability is also important to assess, especially when surgical plans are being formulated. An unstable CMC joint generally requires an arthrodesis, as does a stiff thumb flat in the plane of the hand. A stable and mobile CMC joint can be reconstructed with either an arthrodesis or an opponensplasty or adductorplasty as described by House and Shannon.[22] Some CMC joints can be left alone if the tenodesis effect of the wrist produces excellent lateral pinch alignment and the joint remains stable. Finally, it is important to pay attention to extensor lags of the proximal interphalangeal (PIP) joints. This usually indicates a stretched intrinsic tendon and central slip. If this is not corrected either by splinting or at the time of surgery, extension of the fingers may prove insufficient for grasp.

PRINCIPLES OF NONOPERATIVE MANAGEMENT

Nonoperative management of individuals begins in the early phases of recovery from SCI and continues in one form or another throughout an individual's life. Whether surgical intervention is used, nonoperative management helps to maintain hand and upper extremity function. The spectrum of this care includes physiotherapy, splinting, orthotics, and pharmacologic therapy. One of the recurring themes of this chapter is that the choice of a rehabilitation strategy must be individualized to suit the patient's general condition. In addition to variations based on the zone of injury discussed in an earlier section, each individual may present with her or his own combination of associated injuries that may include direct trauma to the hand and upper extremity. Although a nonoperative program will maintain the same principles and goals, its application will vary from individual to individual.

Forethought is critical during the early phases of injury recovery. The authors believe that a systems approach to treating the hand and upper extremity should be incorporated from the early stages of their injury. Just like programs for skin and bowel and bladder care, early attention to the hand and upper extremity is warranted. On one end of the spectrum are individuals with tetraplegia who undergo interventions designed to optimize upper extremity usage and function. On the other end of the spectrum are individuals whose potential is negated or mitigated by impairing articular contractures of the shoulder, elbow, forearm, and hand. Regardless of whether individuals in the former group undergo surgical restoration of hand function, their hand or upper extremity function will be optimized for their level of injury. Individuals in the latter group, hampered by contractures and stiffness, have a greater level of disability beyond what their level of injury would dictate. Tetraplegic individuals with a C6 level injury and an elbow flexion contracture may function at the level of a C5 patient if the contracture interferes with their ability to transfer.[23] The importance of appropriate nonoperative programs to prevent contractures and maximize function cannot be overemphasized.[24]

This means that joints should be kept supple, and multiple modalities should be incorporated, especially if stiffness is developing. These modalities include the use of more invasive measures such as intrathecal spasmolytics, injectable targeted spasmolytics (botulinum toxin), to TES, and static and dynamic splints to maintain muscle strength and supple joints. This should be prioritized regardless of whether a patient will undergo a future reconstructive procedure.

Therapeutic intervention should begin as soon as the spine has been deemed clinically and radiographically stable. With the patient's motor and sensory functioning understood, therapy can be directed to maintaining or restoring range of motion (ROM) and strength. Passive range of motion (PROM) and stretching of the muscles should be completed twice daily. The patient should assist with these exercises when volitional movement is present. Stretching should be done slowly, and joints should not be forced. Stretching the wrist and fingers in the natural tenodesis pattern should be emphasized to take advantage of the functional nature of this synergistic motion complex. The fingers and thumb should extend when the wrist is flexed and the fingers flexed and thumb opposed to the side of the index when the wrist is extended. MCP joint hyperextension should be avoided to prevent clawing and loss of the important palmar supports needed in grasp. Nighttime splints that re-create the tenodesis positions should be used. Edema in the upper extremity is one important cause of limited ROM and is minimized through daily active and PROM exercises. Retrograde massage is another useful tool, as well as proper positioning of the upper extremity in the wheelchair and in bed.

Because the strength of a muscle contraction increases as more motor units are recruited, increasing the load requirements of voluntary movements is an important component of the therapy. Weight training and endurance training, with particular emphasis on functional motions and activities, are effective in strengthening muscles. Another modality that has been shown to improve muscle strength and endurance is TES.[25] When establishing a strengthening program, it is important to begin thinking about possible surgical procedures that could be performed to increase functional independence. These muscles, if voluntary, should be incorporated into the strengthening program. Muscles that should be targeted include the posterior deltoid (PD; elbow extension transfer), the biceps (elbow extension transfer), the BR (wrist extension, thumb pinch, thumb opposition, finger extension transfers), the extensor carpi radialis longus (ECRL; finger flexion transfer), and the pronator teres (PT; thumb pinch).

ORTHOTIC POSITIONING AND ORTHOSES

Orthotic positioning is an important means of preventing deformity, enhancing function, and promoting a normal appearance of the hand. Static positioning at night and careful monitoring for tendon tightness in patterns of tenodesis can be encouraged without sacrificing supple joints. The stiff hand is almost impossible to overcome by conservative methods in a reasonable amount of time (Fig. 113.2C). These contractures must be surgically released, which can delay other procedures but realistically also limits the surgical alternatives for restoration. A supple hand without contractures is also more aesthetically pleasing and acceptable to the patient, a feature patients themselves are all too aware of (Fig. 113.2A and B).[26] We recommend that contractures be avoided and patients educated and encouraged to use functional splints during early rehabilitation.

Orthoses should be incorporated early during recovery (Table 113.3). Patients who begin to use orthoses early after their injury and realize functional gains are more likely to continue to use them. We have found certain splints to be more useful in promoting functional hand positions and diminishing the degree of contractures (see Table 113.3). Individuals with C5 and C6 motor levels have been the most challenging population to establish a successful splinting protocol. Patients with a C5 motor level (no voluntary wrist control) benefit from a dorsal wrist support with a universal cuff when performing activities of daily living (ADLs) and a splint at night for better hand position. Those with C6 motor levels (voluntary wrist extension) benefit from the use of a flexor hinge splint on the dominant hand and a short opponens splint on the opposite hand. Occasionally, patients prefer flexor hinge splints bilaterally.

Despite a carefully chosen program, however, the rate of splint use among tetraplegic patients varies from as low as 39% to as high as

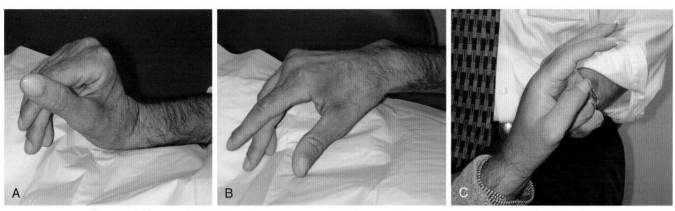

Fig. 113.2 The tenodesis pinch and grasp patterns. **A,** Voluntary wrist extension creates a natural pinch and grasp posture. **B,** Gravity-induced wrist flexion creates natural digital and thenar extension. **C,** Example of poor wrist extension tenodesis caused by contracture. Note the absence of pinch and grasp posture with voluntary wrist extension.

TABLE 113.3	Available Hand Splints Based on Level of Injury in Tetraplegia		
Level of Injury	**Splint**	**Purpose**	**Wearing Schedule**
C1–C4	Resting hand splint	Maintains the hand in a functional position; prevents deformity; maintains an aesthetically pleasing hand	When in bed, complete PROM regularly
C5	Long opponens splint	Provides a stable post against which the index finger can pinch; positions the thumb in a functional key-pinch position	As needed to increase function
	Dorsal wrist support	Protects the integrity of wrist joint; acts as a universal cuff to increase function	As needed to increase function
	Modified resting hand splint	Protects the integrity of wrist and fingers; the splint should allow wrist flexion with MCP, PIP, and DIP extension and thumb extension	When in bed
	Elbow extension splint	Prevents biceps contraction	When in bed
C6	Short opponens	Provides a stable post against which the index finger can grasp; thumb in key pinch based on the preference of the patient	As needed to increase function
	Wrist drive flexor hinge splint	Augments natural tenodesis and alignment of the fingers	As needed to increase function
	Modified resting hand splint	Protects the integrity of the wrist and fingers; the splint should allow wrist flexion with MCP, PIP, and DIP extension and thumb extension.	When in bed
	Elbow extension splint	Prevents biceps contraction	When in bed
C7	MCP block splint	Prevents hyperextension deformity of the MCP joints	As needed to increase function and decrease deformity

DIP, Distal interphalangeal; *MCP,* metacarpophalangeal; *PIP,* proximal interphalangeal; *PROM,* passive range of motion.

89%.[27] We have found that becoming brace free and more able bodied in appearance is among the major goals of patients who desire surgical reconstruction. Moberg[26] believed that as many as 60% of tetraplegic patients could benefit from traditional surgical restoration, whereas Gorman and coworkers[28] found that approximately 36% of consecutively admitted tetraplegic individuals to a rehabilitation center would qualify for traditional surgical restoration (13% met the rigid criteria for functional electrical stimulation). Careful patient evaluation addresses these issues.

PHARMACOTHERAPY AND CONTRACTURES

Muscle spasticity will be present in some patients with tetraplegia depending on their zone of injury. Some individuals will also have sustained a traumatic brain injury in addition to their SCI. Dalyan and associates[29] found that delayed admission to model SCI system, the presence of pressure ulcers, and spasticity and head injury were all associated with higher rates of joint contracture in the setting of acute SCI. The ability of a physiotherapy program alone to help manage contractures associated with spasticity is in doubt, and the ultimate consequence of spasticity is the formation of myostatic and then articular contractures, which are difficult to treat without surgical intervention.

Pharmacotherapy is often incorporated in the management of individuals who present with spasticity or contractures. Medications include spasmolytics administered orally or intrathecally (baclofen pump). Although believed to be very useful, the literature does not provide either the rationale for clear guidelines or even its efficacy.[30] The use of botulinum toxins to help with a physiotherapy program to treat spasticity before the onset of fixed contractures is also useful. These toxins cannot restore mobility to a contracted joint but can help achieve or maintain mobility when spasticity alone interferes with the effectiveness of physiotherapy.[31] As with medications, clear guidelines and applications for botulinum toxin in the setting of SCI remain unknown. In the setting of fixed myostatic or articular contractures, surgery is the only viable intervention to restore mobility.

ROLE OF ELECTRICAL STIMULATION

Transcutaneous electrical stimulation is a technique that applies electrical pulses to peripheral nerve fibers through the skin surface, causing paralyzed but innervated muscles to contract. Functional electrical stimulation (FES) involves the stimulation of the motor unit and control of useful patterns with an electrical impulse, usually applied by implanted electrodes. Although the nerves remain functional, the muscles they innervate do undergo atrophy and develop type II glycolytic metabolism. These changes can be reversed by electrical stimulation of the intact peripheral nerve branch in a conditioning and exercise program. A suprathreshold stimulus applied directly to the nerve and muscle at a frequency of 12 Hz for 8 hours a day has been effective in changing the contractile properties of muscles to a slow oxidative metabolic state, rendering them more fatigue resistant.[11] Over time, consistent exercise will yield softening of joint capsular contracture and reduction in spasticity during the stimulation. Increasing the strength of weak but innervated muscle groups, decreasing the effects of muscle atrophy, increasing muscle endurance, and increasing the ROM of tight tendons before contractures develop are among the effects of a TES program.[32,33] Several centers now incorporate TES exercise programs for lower extremities based on such research. Stimulation-induced contracture of MMT grade 2 or higher muscles can also be strengthened by electrical stimulation to functional levels of force.[21,34] Strengthening innervated but paralyzed muscles improves the efficacy of splinting programs, tendon transfers, and FES systems.[25]

We have found TES beneficial when also applied early in the rehabilitation process. We start patients with as little as 20 minutes of stimulation per day per muscle group and advance slowly to a total of 4 to 6 hours per day. Patients tolerate the program quite well and are compliant if properly motivated. Improved strength and endurance of involuntary, innervated functional muscle groups is the goal of a TES program. Muscle groups emphasized include finger flexors (median–ulnar nerve), thumb flexors–abductors (median nerve), and thumb-finger extensors (radial nerve). Based on our experience, we believe there is a valid role for its use as part of a therapy protocol that seeks to maintain motion, prevent contractures, and prevent atrophy.

PRINCIPLES OF SURGICAL RECONSTRUCTION

The ultimate goal of upper extremity rehabilitation is to provide patients with the ability to manipulate objects in space efficiently and effectively (i.e., create an "able-bodied" person's arm and hand). We must strike a balance with what is achievable, and this requires an understanding of what minimal functions will confer improvements in ability, as well as what are the reasonable goals for a particular patient. As a rule of thumb, surgical restoration improves a patient by one or two levels on the ASIA scale. Not all patients meet our strict criteria for surgical reconstruction. Dedicated and experienced multidisciplinary teams in regional referral centers are continuously working to improve on current methods and in the end restore the patients to independence, social integration, and occupation. Our current bias is that surgical restoration as outlined in this chapter should be undertaken by surgeons skilled and experienced in taking care of patients with tetraplegia and be done in concert with similarly experienced teams of physiatrists, nurses, and therapists.

Most individuals with tetraplegia are injured around the C5 and C6 levels. This means that for most, shoulder stability and mobility are voluntarily present. Elbow flexion is also present, as is forearm supination.

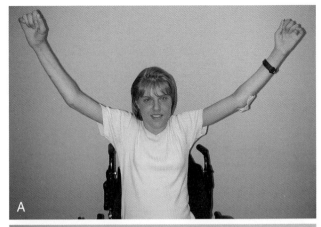
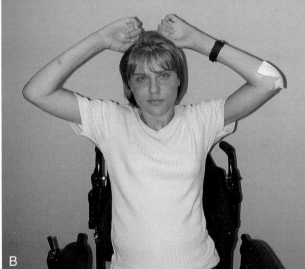

Fig. 113.3 Elbow extension restoration using the posterior deltoid to triceps tendon transfer and forearm supination contracture correction using a radial osteotomy. **A,** Antigravity elbow extension. **B,** Maintenance of elbow flexion.

Voluntary elbow extension is typically absent in these individuals. The presence of strong, voluntary wrist extension and forearm pronation depend on the actual zone of injury. Elbow extension, wrist flexion, and digital extension are not present unless the zone of injury is at or below the C7 myotome. The following discussion focuses on the average person with tetraplegia, but the same principles apply regardless of the level of injury.

The fundamental functions we seek to restore, in order of priority, include elbow extension (Figs. 113.3 and 113.4A), wrist extension, lateral pinch and release, and palmar grasp and release (Figs.113.4B and 113.5).[14,15,18] Current surgical techniques and technology do not allow us to reliably restore shoulder function yet; therefore, patients with ASIA motor levels proximal to C5 are rarely candidates for tendon transfer surgery but are still candidates for FES and some limited nerve transfers. And the former hierarchy is not absolute because some individuals may prioritize their reconstructive goals uniquely.

The combination of shoulder function and elbow extension allows patients to effectively "reach out" to manipulate objects in space in front of them and above them.[14,35] Without this ability, a patient's effective "workspace" is limited. Another way to think about this is to imagine the shoulder and elbow working in concert to transport the hand to a location in space so that it may manipulate a desired object. Better mobility, stability, and strength of the shoulder and elbow confer a large

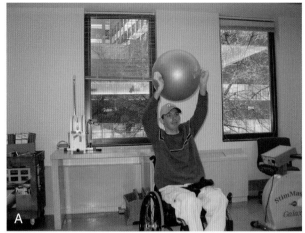

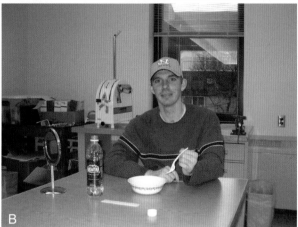

Fig. 113.4 A patient with International Classification of Tetraplegia OCu:2 who underwent bilateral elbow extension restoration using biceps to triceps transfer and lateral pinch reconstruction using brachioradialis to flexor pollicis longus transfer, carpometacarpal stabilization via arthrodesis, and thumb interphalangeal stabilization by split transfer. **A,** Demonstration of bilateral manual muscle test grade 4 elbow extension. **B,** Patient eating with fork without the need for adaptive splinting.

potential workspace for the hand. This is especially valuable in people with tetraplegia because they are fixed to a wheelchair and cannot move around their immediate space the way an able-bodied individual can. In fact, the provision of elbow extension can translate to functional abilities such as self-care, hygiene, wheelchair propulsion, and transferring; these abilities are critical to creating functional independence.[36] Wrist extension activates the natural tenodesis grasp pattern and serves as the foundation on which finger function is activated and restored (see Fig. 113.2). Surgical restoration of hand function, in fact, builds on the provision or presence of the wrist tenodesis pinch and grasp. Regarding finger function, although it would be ideal to restore all the different grasp patterns we apply subconsciously in our daily activities, lateral pinch, not opposition or tip pinch, and palmar grasp are used most commonly.[20] Because lateral pinch is used more often for ADLs, we prioritize this form of grasp over palmar grasp when both cannot be restored. Planning the reconstruction begins with a balance of the remaining voluntary, nonspastic function. And as also previously discussed, this is best suited for patients whose hands and arms are reasonably supple.

Too much can be attempted, however, and experience and research have taught us that there is occasion to "downsize" the extent of surgical restoration under certain conditions. Patients who, because of physical distance or insufficient family infrastructure, do not have easy access to their therapists and physicians will likely experience poor outcomes if the restorative regimen is complex and sophisticated. In these instances, it may better serve the patient to limit the goals of surgery to what she or he will be able to take advantage of. This is also the case for patients with brain injuries or relatively poor cognition who will rehabilitate a simpler surgical protocol with greater ease. There may be a role for nerve transfers as a preferred method of reconstruction for such people, too. At the same time, a motivated, intelligent, and well-adjusted patient will be unsatisfied with a restorative program that undercuts his or her true rehabilitative potential. We have also learned that patients will occasionally require later secondary surgery to modify "loosened" transfers, augment weak transfers, stabilize a joint that becomes functionally unstable, and so forth. Patients must also continuously use and exercise the hand and arm in maintain the muscle tone and endurance qualities necessary for successful transfers and FES systems. Finally, the surgical program should seek to accomplish as much

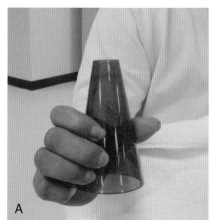

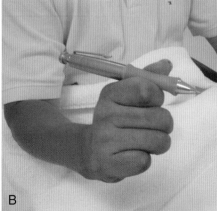

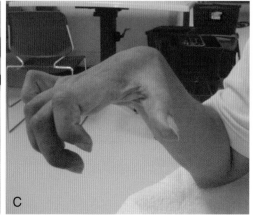

Fig. 113.5 A patient with International Classification of Tetraplegia O:Cu6 who underwent single-stage pinch and grasp restoration to augment previous nerve transfer for finger and thumb extension. **A,** Palmar grasp using the extensor carpi radialis brevis to synchronized flexor digitorum profundus used to hold a cone. **B,** Lateral pinch using the brachioradialis to flexor digitorum superficialis ring opponensplasty, pronator teres to flexor pollicis longus (FPL) pinch stabilized by FPL split transfer to hold a pen. **C,** Release phase using voluntary weak extensor digitorum communis and wrist flexion to induce tenodesis extension.

as possible as efficiently as possible. Prolonged postoperative periods of overburdening dependency will generally lead a patient and his or her family to postpone or cancel future staged procedures, which, in turn, will reduce the likelihood of success. Operative techniques and protocols should minimize immobilization and allow for early rehabilitation whenever possible. We previously discussed the hierarchical order of surgical goals, that is, elbow extension, wrist extension, key pinch, and palmar grasp. Although Table 113.4 outlines the specific procedures performed by level, there are a few generalizations that we follow in planning reconstructions. These are described next.

TREATING EACH PATIENT INDIVIDUALLY

The sequelae of the initial trauma is so varied and multifactorial that patients are truly unique in their presentations. Surgical protocols that are rigidly set to the level of injury will fail in a number of patients if these issues are not considered early in the surgical planning. In particular, spasticity and the patient's goals and desires are two specific examples of where surgical planning must be both flexible and creative. To accommodate variations in patient presentations and goals, surgeons should be aware of the various described techniques in achieving similar reconstructive goals.

Because different patterns of upper and lower motor neuron injury are clinically manifest in patients, the degree to which muscle spasticity varies considerably. Clearly, any spasticity must be controlled for a patient to be a candidate for surgery. Typically, this is achieved through therapy and pharmacy. Control at a plateau of tolerance and efficacy is the goal. The problem lies in striking a balance between the benefits and side effects of the medication. Higher levels of effective spasmolytic agents, such as diazepam, may produce muscle weakness. Side effects such as drowsiness or blunting of affect are a frequent reason patients reduce or discontinue them. Concerns about habituation or abuse have also led to fewer prescriptions. Use of implantable baclofen pumps may lead to steady-state suppression of spasticity. Since the Food and Drug Administration's (FDA's) approval of botulinum toxin in 1989, its role in the management of spastic paralysis, including tetraplegia, is increasing.

It is believed that uncontrollable spastic muscles should not be transferred and frequently need to be released to prevent severe contractures.[37] In a similar vein, the donor nerve for a nerve transfer should not come from a spastic muscle. Mildly spastic muscles, however, can be useful transfers. In addition, certain "functional" spasticity, such as contraction of the FPL with wrist extension, may be desirable and probably should not be altered.[38] Because each patient presents with unique patterns of spasticity and the ability to control it, surgical protocols must be flexible to accommodate the patient.

Surgical planning must be tailored to the patient's needs to be successful. Patients, especially those many years from their injury, develop a number of substitution maneuvers that allow them to function, sometimes with surprising independence. Some patients with level C5 (ICSHT 0–1) injuries need their biceps, in addition to their brachialis, to help propel a manual wheelchair or in weight shifts critical to preventing pressure sores. The surgeon who chooses to restore elbow extension using the biceps as a donor motor should be very cautious to ensure that no critical, patient-specific functions are lost with any of the reconstructive options.

Finally, the surgeon and patient must be cognizant of the duration of postoperative rehabilitation. During the initial period of immobilization for tendon transfers, which may last up to 3 weeks, patients become more dependent on attendant care. This places great personal stress on the patient and his or her support group, especially if the family is the primary source of help. Arrangements for care must be

secured before surgery. Newer methods to coapt tendons, as well as nerve transfers, can limit the period of immobilization to even less than 3 weeks and are appropriate to consider for the right person.[39–42]

SPECIAL CONSIDERATIONS FOR CHILDREN AND ADOLESCENTS

Children with SCIs have special needs and considerations. Their mechanism of injury varies compared with adults and includes birth trauma, infection, tumor, and child abuse. Children are also more likely to sustain traumatic SCIs without radiographic findings, a condition known as SCIWORA (SCI without radiographic abnormality). New SCI centers, especially within the Shriner's Hospitals, have developed special protocols and focus on this group of patients. The textbook by Betz and Mulcahey[43] is devoted to this patient group and is the foundation for their management. Successful rehabilitation requires extra attention to developmental status, family support, and reaction to the surgical process. Explanation and agreement is needed for the time and personal investment during periods of physical dependency, loss of mobility, and loss of personal freedom.

Children may be less tolerant of failure than adults. Children are compelled to be trusting in a complex process they may not fully understand or consent to. Their parents can be educated to understand the reconstruction and technology, but children may not fully understand the mechanisms. They are sharp critics and good observers of true progress. They are hard to satisfy. Many children expect miracles or immediate gratification and lack tolerance for months of rehabilitation. Younger children have short attention spans and need reinforcement and repetition in their training. Older children and adolescents are distracted by their social needs and conscious of cosmetic appearance, incisions, braces, and hardware. They want to be physically and visibly normal. Reconstruction that incorporates correction of paralytic posture, removes wrist braces, or improves social contact is well received.

Many children dread the return to the sick role and many have bad memories of the time they spent in the hospital at the acute injury. Overcoming their physical loss and restoring hand function must also minimize the stress of reentry to the hospital. Performing procedures in combination, as an outpatient, or in rehabilitation rather than acute care sites all contribute to better acceptance. The therapist often has the key role in preparing, guiding, and befriending the child, contributing the subjective support and continuity to recovery.

Preoperative assessment can often be accomplished in the context of play or ADLs. The functional emphasis for children will often be on accomplishments at school using pencils, artistic materials, computer access, and reading. Self-care activities are the same as for adults. Children's ingenious adaptive strategies must be understood in context of planned reconstructions because these strategies may be negatively altered.[44]

Surgical planning follows the same technical principles and priorities as with adults with notable exceptions. First, children may plateau neurologically from their complete SCIs earlier than adults. Kozin[44] suggests that earlier surgery is not only possible with children but may be very advantageous for their unique situation. Surgical challenges include the technical issues associated with smaller tendons and muscles; the presence of growth plates within the bones; and contractures and secondary bone changes associated with children, especially around the elbow, forearm, and digital MCP joints.[44] Postoperative care follows the same protocols as for adults except that longer term monitoring is required to assess the effects of growth and development, and protocols may need to be prolonged to accommodate for smaller tendons and weaker tendon transfer coaptation sites.

TABLE 113.4	Surgical Protocol by the International Classification Group
Level	**Goals of Surgery**
O/Cu:0 No muscles for transfer for the hand	**ELBOW EXTENSION** Our Approach Biceps-to-triceps transfer[73,74,76,105] Option Tendon Transfer Posterior deltoid-to-triceps transfer[106,107] Nerve Transfer Posterior deltoid nerve branch to triceps nerve branch[39,108–110] Teres minor nerve branch to triceps nerve branch[57,88,111] FES neuroprosthesis[61,62] **HAND GRASP** Options Nerve Transfer Brachialis nerve to ECRL branch[112] Brachialis nerve branch to AIN[39,57,108] FES neuroprosthesis[61,62]
O/Cu:1 BR	**ELBOW EXTENSION** As for O/Cu:0 **FOREARM PRONATION (if there is supination contracture)** Our Approach Pronation osteotomy of the radius[113] Option Biceps pronatorplasty FES to pronator quadratus **LATERAL PINCH and RELEASE** Key pinch procedure: modified because wrist extension is not present[20] Our Approach Wrist extension through transfer of the BR Natural tenodesis of fingers with wrist extension provides lateral pinch (extension and flexion augmentation if necessary) Thumb stabilization for pinch strength (CMC arthrodesis and FPL bridle transfer to IP) Option Nerve Transfer As per O/Cu:0 Consider BR nerve to AIN[114] FES neuroprosthesis
O/Cu:2 ECRL	**ELBOW EXTENSION AND FOREARM PRONATION** As previous **GRASP AND RELEASE** Standard key-pinch procedure for lateral pinch (wrist extension transfer not needed, and BR used as a donor motor)[14,18,22,47,115–117] Our Approach FPL powered by the BR Thumb stabilized by CMC arthrodesis and split FPL tenodesis Finger and thumb extension–flexion natural tenodesis augmented as necessary Option Restore key pinch and forearm pronation simultaneously[55,56] Restore palmar and lateral grasp with Zancolli two-stage reconstruction[38] Restore weak palmar grasp with ECRB to FDP via interosseous membrane[68] Intrinsic balance[51–53] Nerve Transfer Restore pinch with brachialis or BR to AIN nerve transfer Restore finger extension with supinator nerve to PIN transfer (as long as the biceps is not a donor muscle)[57,118] FES neuroprosthesis

Level	Goals of Surgery
O/Cu:3 ECRB	**ELBOW EXTENSION AND FOREARM PRONATION** As previous **GRIP, PINCH, and RELEASE** As for previous; exception is now two motors (BR and ECRL) are available for transfer Our Approach As for group 2; the thumb CMC joint can be treated by arthrodesis or dynamic opponensplasty or left alone[22] Options Alphabet procedure (single-stage pinch and grasp combined with early rehabilitation)[41,42] Consider a two-stage reconstruction to restore lateral pinch and palmar grasp (see references under O/Cu:4) Standard key pinch plus ECRL to FDP[10,22] Intrinsic balance as previous Nerve Transfer Nerve transfers for pinch and extension (see O/Cu:2) Consider ECRB nerve as a donor for pinch[119] FES Neuroprosthesis
O/Cu:4 PT	**ELBOW EXTENSION** As previous **GRIP, PINCH, and RELEASE** These patients can undergo transfers to power finger and thumb extension Our Approach Single-stage lateral pinch procedure as with O/Cu: 3 or two-stage extensor–flexor reconstruction via Zancolli (PT powers FCR) or House (PT powers FPL) methods; we prefer this method of reconstruction for groups 4-8, differences based on references[20] Options Alphabet procedure (single-stage pinch and grasp combined with early rehabilitation)[41,42] Nerve transfer approaches per O/Cu3
O/Cu:5 FCR	**ELBOW EXTENSION** As previous only if triceps power is not present because these patients may have useful voluntary elbow extension. **GRASP, PINCH, AND RELEASE** As previous; leave FCR as a powerful wrist flexor, which also augments finger extension via tenodesis effect Our Approach Some patients have a weak but present EDC; if so, can consider a single-stage pinch and grasp procedure[120] or single-stage lateral pinch procedure as earlier or two-staged pinch and grasp reconstruction as earlier Option Alphabet procedure (single-stage pinch and grasp combined with early rehabilitation)[41,42] Nerve transfer options remain the same
O/Cu:6 EDC	**GRASP, PINCH, AND RELEASE** As previous These patients may be less functional than level 5 because they may lose the finger flexion effect from wrist extension because they have voluntary finger extensors (same with group 7); this must be taken into account in planning transfers (i.e., through finger flexion and intrinsic reconstruction)[10,20] Option Single-stage grasp and pinch procedure
O/Cu:7 EPL	**GRASP, PINCH, AND RELEASE** As previous Both ulnar- and radial-sided intrinsics can be powered[20] Option Thumb adduction–opponensplasty
O/Cu:8 Finger flexors (usually stronger on ulnar side)	**GRASP, PINCH, AND RELEASE** As previous Standard opponensplasties should be performed; intrinsic reconstruction is more likely necessary because there are extrinsic flexors and extensors present to create an intrinsic minus imbalance Powered intrinsic reconstruction via ECRL or BR[38] Standard opponensplasty using EIP or EDQM[38]
O/Cu:9 Lack intrinsics	**GRASP, PINCH, AND RELEASE** As previous As with group 8, intrinsic reconstruction and opponensplasties may be required[51–53]

AIN, Anterior interosseous nerve; *BR,* brachioradialis; *CMC,* carpometacarpal; *Cu,* 10-mm static two-point discrimination of the index finger (C6 dermatome); *ECRB,* extensor carpi radialis brevis; *ECRL,* extensor carpi radialis longus; *EDC,* extensor digitorum communis; *EDQM,* extensor digiti quinti minimi; *EIP,* extensor indicis proprius; *FCR,* flexor carpi radialis; *FDP,* flexor digitorum profundus; *FES,* functional electrical stimulation; *FPL,* flexor pollicis longus; *ICSHT,* The International Classification for Surgery of the Hand in Tetraplegia; *IP,* interphalangeal; *O,* ocular feedback; *PT,* pronator teres.

Children are harder on hardware, braces, wheelchairs, and electronic components than adults. They have a sense that they will heal themselves and that someone else can repair broken things. Careful instruction is important because reconstructed limbs are not normal in their tolerance for injury, weight bearing, or use as tools.

The results of surgical reconstruction in children can be very rewarding for the automatic way they adjust to new capabilities, the generally good results they experience with surgery, and the joy to the health care team for changing their lives.

GENERAL SURGICAL TECHNIQUES

Stability, mobility, and power are all required to create movements, which in turn provide functional ability. This section focuses on the principles and concepts involved and dwells less on the actual described procedures. Table 113.4 is a list of the surgical procedures we recommend based on classification. We refer readers to the references provided to further explore the history, details, and development of these procedures and their alternatives. Case studies are provided that summarize outcomes reasonably to be expected.

Bone and Joint Procedures
Joint Releases and Mobilization

Mobility and function are mutually dependent. Whether a joint is under voluntary control or will be mobilized through surgical restoration, suppleness and ROM are critical to ability. Stiffness occasionally develops despite appropriate nonoperative care, and when contractures develop and inhibit function, the joint must be released and rebalanced.[45] Wrist flexion contractures are uncommon except in patients with spasticity of the extrinsic wrist flexors who may develop a flexion contracture. Finger and thumb contractures are usually a result of a therapeutic philosophy that creates key pinch using stiffened thumbs and fingers as a "claw." We believe that stiff fingers preclude a successful restorative program and should be avoided instead of treated.

One relatively common example of a contracture in tetraplegia is the forearm supination deformity that can develop in patients with ICSHT 0 to 2. The deformity develops from an imbalance between voluntary or spastic elbow flexors–supinators and weak elbow extenders–pronators. Poor bed positioning, neglect of the person, neglect of therapy, or a highly spastic muscle can lead to the development of a chronically supinated forearm and flexed elbow. Because most functional activities are performed with the hand and wrist pronated, this contracture is disabling. Concomitant mild to moderate elbow flexion contractures and forearm supination deformities in tetraplegia often respond to conservative measures with serial casting in extension and pronation at weekly intervals. Residual contractures must be released surgically.

Our management algorithm proceeds from conservative measures such as botulinum toxin injections, serial cast correction, and stretching for mild to moderate flexion supination contractures to a radial pronation osteotomy. If there is also an elbow flexion deformity present, we will perform anterior capsular release with associated biceps and brachialis fractional lengthening. We have found the osteotomy to be a particularly effective procedure because a functional arc of rotation is restored and maintained, the procedure is technically straightforward, and it is well suited as part of a comprehensive single-stage surgical reconstruction because no rehabilitation is required to "learn" it. The biceps pronatorplasty originally described by Zancolli[38] is an alternative procedure that both releases the deformity and rebalances the forearm by creating an active pronator.

Joint Stabilization

The individual digital rays of the hand are, in effect, a series of intercalated segments normally controlled by muscles that have multiple attachments throughout these segments to create a finely balanced and coordinated mechanism for motion. In tetraplegic patients with few voluntary motors for transfer and only a finite number that can be electrically activated with currently available implantable systems, the able-bodied finger cannot yet be re-created. Because the goals of surgery are limited to providing the fewest functions that provide the greatest abilities, joint stabilization becomes an integrated part of reconstruction. Restoring thumb flexion to create key pinch, for example, is difficult without stabilizing one or more of the three joints of the thumb ray because control of the CMC joint, in addition to the MCP and IP joints, is impossible with one or two donor motors. If the CMC joint is unstable or the MCP joint is hyperextendable, then a controlled, aligned, and strong pinch is difficult to reconstruct. Unstable CMC joints are treated with arthrodesis. Stable CMC joints can be treated by a tendon transfer or not at all.[22] A hyperextendable thumb MCP joint will need to be stabilized to create a firm pinch.[20] A common strategy that has developed is to power effective key pinch using one motor that flexes the thumb through the scaphotrapezial and MCP joint, positioned in space by stabilizing the CMC joint in opposition, and transferring the power of flexion to the thumb pulp via a stabilized IP joint. A variety of techniques are available to "hold" joints for balance and stability.

Arthrodesis. Stabilizing a joint in series through arthrodesis reduces the dissipation of torque exerted by an active motor or tendon transfer, prevents deformity from torque and subsequent joint imbalance, and aids in placing a joint or finger or thumb ray in a more functional position. In effect, arthrodeses can increase the efficiency and efficacy of voluntary, transferred, or activated motors, a beneficial situation in the tetraplegic patient. Today, through the teachings of Eric Moberg,[26] we seek to create supple hands that are more reconstructable, and importantly, more appealing to a patient reintegrating him- or herself into their community. Therefore, arthrodesis should be applied judiciously and sparingly.

Thumb CMC arthrodesis is one the most useful operations in tetraplegia hand reconstruction. By positioning the thumb in opposition, a flexion moment provided through the FPL by transfer creates a stable and effective key pinch. This procedure has been applied extensively in tetraplegic reconstruction with reliable results.[22] In select patients with low-level tetraplegia (ICSHT ≥4), House and Shannon[22] have written extensively on an alternative to CMC arthrodesis whereby an adduction–opponensplasty is constructed through two donor motors, the PT and the BR. Wrist arthrodesis is rarely ever indicated because the important tenodesis effect is lost. It is indicated to replace an external splint or if insufficient motors are available for wrist extension. Some patients select the procedure for cosmetic qualities and the strong desire to be brace free. A patient with weak ASIA C5 motor strength (ICSHT 0) who has some voluntary BR function with a MMT grade less than 4, unsuited for transfer into ECRB, may benefit from BR-to-FPL transfer, wrist fusion, and flexor digitorum profundus (FDP) and extensor pollicis longus (EPL) tenodesis. Such weaker patients are more likely to benefit from systems that stimulate the muscles externally or internally because there are too few effective donor muscles. The Freehand system was such a system, but it is no longer commercially available; fortunately, such research and investigation continue.

Split Transfers

As an alternative to arthrodesis, the split transfer (bridle transfer) technique has been described in the reconstruction of tetraplegic hands to stabilize select joints. The premise of this transfer is to balance a

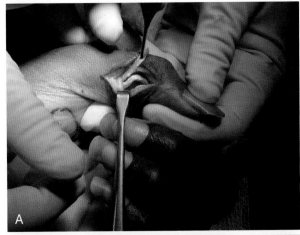

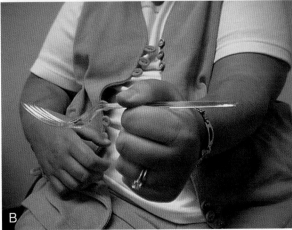

Fig. 113.6 A, Intraoperative photograph of the flexor pollicis longus (FPL) split transfer to stabilize the interphalangeal (IP) joint of the thumb. By transferring the radial half of the FPL tendon into the extensor pollicis longus, the IP joint will not hyperflex when a tendon transfer activates the FPL. **B,** Instead, the pull of the FPL will create a balanced flexion with IP joint remaining only slightly flexed such that the pulp of the thumb will rest against the side of the index finger during lateral pinch.

functionally single-axis joint with one motor, thereby converting a moment force into a balanced compressive force. Specifically, the IP joint of the thumb has traditionally been stabilized by arthrodesis or pinning when performing key-pinch procedures. This improves the efficiency and efficacy of an FPL transfer because its moment is primarily transferred to mobilizing the MCP and CMC joints (or just the MCP if the CMC is fused).[46] The irreversibility of arthrodesis and problems associated with permanent pins or screws across the joint in order to stabilize it, however, have led to the creation of a split transfer described by Mohammed and associates.[47] The radial half of the FPL at the level of the oblique pulley is transferred dorsally into the EPL proximal to the IP joint (Fig. 113.6). In the passive state, the joint remains supple. In the activated state, as through FPL activation during key pinch, the IP joint is held stable on both sides of the joint during pinch. This procedure is now our standard method of IP stabilization.

Capsulodesis

In this technique of joint stabilization, static balance is achieved by "tightening" one of the axes of any particular joint. This technique has been described in key-pinch procedures in which the volar plate of the thumb MCP is tightened if hypermobile because there is the risk for the development of volar plate laxity over time.[38] In this scenario, the

pinch force produced by the thumb becomes steadily weaker as force that should be applied through the thumb pulp is lost through a hyperextensible MCP joint. The reverse is also occasionally required, that is, a hyperflexible MCP joint may result in the thumb "missing" the index finger during pinch, and a dorsal capsulodesis may be required.[20] PIP volar capsulodesis is indicated in a hyperlax patient who develops swan-neck posturing preventing functional grip. These procedures can both be performed primarily when dysfunctional laxity is already present or secondarily if the same laxity develops from use or chronic joint imbalance from a previous reconstruction.

Dynamic Stabilization

Mobilization procedures such as tendon transfers and tenodesis provide joint stability when they serve as an antagonist to an agonist motor. For example, the BR is a more powerful donor when an extension transfer stabilizes the elbow, whether through a PD or biceps donor.[48-50] The reason is that in the absence of an elbow extension moment, the force of the BR contraction is distributed between elbow flexion and to whatever tendon it has been transferred to. In the presence of an active elbow extension moment, this same force is primarily distributed to the tendon it has been transferred to. A BR-mediated thumb adductor–opponensplasty, as described by House and Shannon,[22] also provides dynamic stabilization of the thumb CMC joint during pinch. This transfer is occasionally used in patients with midlevel tetraplegia in whom the ICSHT grade is greater than 4 and the PT is voluntary and strong enough to serve as a donor muscle for transfer. Instead of fusing the thumb CMC joint, a more dextrous thumb is created by performing an opponensplasty using the BR powered by a flexor digitorum superficialis (FDS) tendon graft. By creating the position of opposition actively, the CMC is stabilized during pinch. A tenodesis, the static equivalent of a tendon transfer, can perform a similar function. The finger extension moment provided through a tenodesis described by Zancolli or House, in which the intrinsic muscles are mimicked by a slip of the FDS tendon can similarly empower grasp strength when the finger flexors are motorized or activated.[51-53]

The basis for surgical restoration of the tetraplegic hand lies in mobilizing paralyzed joints. The next sections concerning soft tissue procedures and neuroprostheses discuss the fundamental principles.

Soft Tissue Procedures

Tenodesis. Tenodesis is a technique of creating a dynamic tethering effect of a tendon by stabilizing it proximal to the closest joint proximal to its site of insertion. As a result of this "anchoring," the tendon now "pulls" on its insertion when the joint is mobilized in an eccentric direction or motion. The result is desired active motion mediated by the tendon caused by motion of the proximal joint; in this way, voluntary wrist extension, for example, can drive thumb flexion if the FPL was tenodesed proximal to the wrist joint. The normal wrist tenodesis effect is, in fact, the foundation for motion produced by tenodesis in tetraplegia hand reconstruction. In high-level patients (ICSHT 1), no motors are available to transfer after the BR is transferred to the ECRB to create wrist extension; however, by tenodesing the FPL tendon on the distal radius in appropriate tension, wrist extension now produces a flexion moment to the thumb ray and serves as the basis for lateral pinch. Secondary procedures, such as CMC stabilization or arthrodesis, and perhaps extensor tenodesis augment the FPL tenodesis to create positioning and strength, and this is the basis for the key-pinch procedure originally described by Moberg.[26] The problem is that tenodeses tend to "stretch" over time; therefore, they are currently used in high-level tetraplegia when there is no other option and as an antagonist-balancing procedure as discussed earlier.[54]

Tendon Transfer. Tendon transfers permit relocation of available motors for loss of function. Usually a function, such as finger flexion, is distilled to the activity of one muscle, the FDP in this example. A voluntary, strong muscle and its tendon are then detached from its normal insertion and routed into the paralyzed muscle (Fig. 113.7). When the patient "learns" to isolate the contraction of the transferred muscle, the paralyzed "function" is restored. Together with tenodeses, these procedures represent the core of traditional reconstruction of the upper extremity in tetraplegia. The basic principles for transfers continue to apply:

1. Supple joints with at least a functional arc of passive motion are necessary for mobility.
2. Comparable excursion and force of contraction between the transfer with the muscle it is to replace should be present or provided.
3. Synergy, whenever possible, will facilitate reeducation. Transferring the ECRB to the FDP takes advantage of synergy. (The biceps to triceps transfer for elbow extension is a notable exception.)
4. The transfer should traverse a healthy bed of tissue to minimize scarring.
5. Stabilization of a joint, whenever a transfer spans across multiple joints increases it efficacy and efficiency, as has been clearly demonstrated with BR transfers.[48]
6. A straight line of pull from the donor motor to the recipient tendon will minimize lost strength from the transfer.
7. Side-to-side transfers allow a single motor to effect motion across several joints. The entire FDP can be activated by one donor motor.
8. The morbidity from loss of the donor motor should be none or minimal.
9. Anticipate secondary motions based on the vector of pull of the donor muscle. For example, the BR can be routed into the FPL in such a way as to create secondary pronation, if so desired.[55,56]

There is an important technical caveat with regards to setting the transfer in the appropriate degree of tension. Newer tendon coaptation techniques have been demonstrated to resist more load, and the latest protocols allow for motion within the first week of surgery.[40–42]

Nerve Transfer. A nerve transfer, analogous to a tendon transfer, involves transferring a nerve fascicle (or whole nerve) from a muscle under voluntary control into the nerve of an innervated but paralyzed muscle. In this way, the "voluntary" nerve innervates the paralyzed muscle. Prerequisites for this procedure are similar to tendon transfers, especially with regards to supple joints. And, the donor nerve and nerve fascicle must come from a healthy muscle under voluntary control that is able to be sacrificed. The recipient nerve must innervate a paralyzed muscle that has not been chronically denervated. Because many times the muscles are centrally paralyzed with SCI, many muscles below the zone of injury remain potential viable recipients. Muscles within the zone of injury, on the other hand, may have been peripherally denervated at the time of SCI, and this issue must be vetted in cases of chronic SCI because they may no longer be viable recipients.

The earliest application of this for the hand and upper extremity, other than using intercostal nerves, was using a branch of the ulnar nerve to directly innervate the nerve to the biceps for upper trunk brachial plexus injuries. This initiated investigations that continue to explore various nerve transfers applied in various settings outside of the brachial plexus, including peripheral nerve injury, peripheral nerve palsy, upper motor neuron disease, and SCI. Nerve transfer for SCI is in its nascent stage of development with regards to best applications and best indications but demonstrates promise to help augment current reconstructive strategies and for some individuals possibly represents the primary strategy.[57] Among its greatest advantages is that immobilization is not required postoperatively. Among its greatest disadvantages, especially for nerve transfers for pinch, is that it can take 1 to 2 years for patients to start to gain sufficient strength and that not all nerve transfers are successful. Tendon transfer–based reconstructions continue to form the basis of most surgeries, and the authors believe

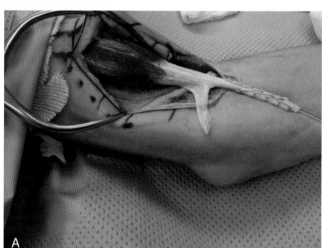
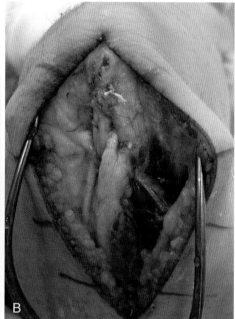

Fig. 113.7 Intraoperative photographs of the biceps-to-triceps tendon transfer. **A,** The biceps is mobilized from the surrounding skin (the hand is to the left of the photo), and fascia and muscles and then released from its insertion onto the radial tuberosity. **B,** The mobilized biceps is then routed to the posterior aspect of the elbow (the elbow is flexed, and the shoulder is toward the bottom of the photo) through the medial soft tissues, weaved through the triceps tendon, and then inserted into a drilled tunnel in the olecranon process posteriorly.

this is still the "standard" format for improving hand and arm function in tetraplegia. Nerve transfers are currently suited to augment tendon transfers (i.e., creating voluntary thumb and finger extension). Some centers exclusively rely on nerve transfers, and the rationale includes the lack of follow-up and therapeutic resources available in these centers. Continued research and technique modifications continue, and as knowledge accrues and indications become more refined, the authors believe nerve transfers will assume a greater and more reliable role for some individuals (Fig. 113.8).

Neuroprostheses. High-level SCI leaves few opportunities for reconstruction of the hand. At ASIA levels C5 and C6, the most common levels, only elbow extension and key pinch can be created using traditional reconstructive surgery and rehabilitation tools. The use of FES has expanded the options for improved function in this patient group. Neuroprostheses and their application and outcomes have been well described in the literature.[21,34,58,59] The first commercial implanted upper extremity neuroprosthesis, the Freehand System, gained FDA approval in 1997. Despite the clinically and functionally successful outcomes of the system, it is no longer commercially available. Subsequent generations of devices have been implanted with the support of grants from research agencies and foundations.

Progress continues to be made in the development of advanced neuroprosthetic systems by researchers at the Cleveland FES Center.[60] One system consists of an implantable stimulator that controls stimulation to activate 12 different muscles in the upper extremity. In addition to the traditional set of eight muscles that were controlled by the eight-channel Freehand system (typically the adductor pollicis, abductor pollicis brevis, FPL, EPL, FDP, FDS, and extensor digitorum communis and sometimes the triceps), additional options include the intrinsics, abductor pollicis longus, pronator quadratus, palmaris longus, pectoralis major, rhomboids, and extensor digiti quinti. These muscle choices are personalized to the needs and goals of the patient. In subsequent versions with 12 or more muscle stimulators, myoelectric signals, generated by the user's voluntary musculature, are used to control the functions of the neuroprosthesis. These signals are recorded via implanted electrodes and are processed within the device or transmitted out of the body via a transcutaneous link. There advantages to this new method of control compared with the previously implemented external control sources: (1) surgical implantation of the recording electrode is straightforward and results in reliable repeatable signals, (2) the recording electrode can be implanted in a wide variety of muscles facilitating the personalization of the system to the user, and (3) myoelectric control signals can be obtained from weak or partially paralyzed muscles. Therefore, myoelectric control can be used by a wide variety of patients as long as voluntary function is retained in at least one muscle or another control signal, movement, or biosignal is sensed.[60]

The current, advanced Networked Neuroprosthesis (NNP) has a greater variety of applications, the control sensors are implanted and ipsilateral to the muscles stimulated, bilateral systems are possible and have been implemented in three patients to date. A system has also been used to provide shoulder and trunk control in addition to hand control for patients with a C5 injury. The features of this advanced neuroprosthesis have even facilitated implementation in a patient who has had a stroke. In total, at the time of this publication, the advanced neuroprosthesis has been implanted in more than 13 people (19 devices).

Past indications for neuroprostheses were in candidates who are ICSHT 4; this translates to patients with ASIA motor levels C5 and C6, or lower in the spinal cord. (Criteria are discussed in the section on patient evaluation.[27]) Multiple implanted stimulators for each limb can be used to provide shoulder, arm, and hand control in patients with C4 or higher tetraplegia. We have shown that patients with ASIA level C4 or higher can benefit from FES implantation including linkage to recording devices such as Braingate, which provides brain cortical control for hand movements.[61,62]

Although not specifically been studied, we believe that patients who have ASIA C7 motor strength or greater (ICSHT ≥5 or 6) are either very functional or have very satisfactory hand performance through more traditional surgical restoration. Most of these patients have strong voluntary triceps function and may have voluntary finger and thumb

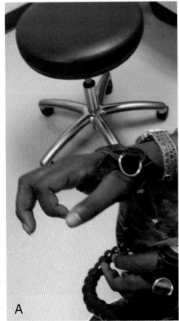
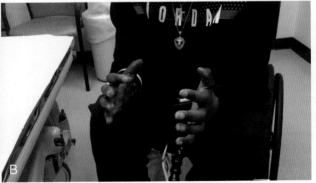

Fig. 113.8 Pinch and release in a patient with International Classification of Tetraplegia O:Cu 5 who underwent a combination of nerve transfers for finger extension and tendon transfers for pinch and grasp. **A,** Lateral pinch pattern with control of index positioning using a combination of voluntary extension of tendon transfer–mediated flexion. **B,** Active, voluntary digital extension secondary to a nerve transfer.

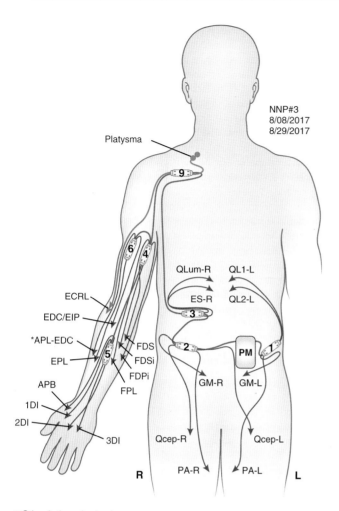

NNP#3
8/08/2017
8/29/2017

Platysma

▼ Stimulating electrodes
⬍▼ MES recording electrodes
— Network leads

Fig. 113.9 Modular networked implantable neuroprosthetic diagram for both upper and lower extremity function. *1–6,* Stimulus modules; *9,* MES module; *AbPB,* abductor pollicis brevis; *AdP,* adductor pollicis; *APL,* abductor pollicis longus; *DI,* distal interosseous; *ECRL,* extensor carpi radialis longus; *EDC,* extensor digitorum communis; *EIP,* extensor indicis; *EPL,* extensor pollicis longus; *ES,* erector spinae; *FDP,* flexor digitorum profundus; *FDS,* flexor digitorum superficialis; *FPL,* flexor pollicis longus; *GM,* gluteus maximus; *L,* left; *MES,* myoelectric signal electrode; *NNP,* networked neuroprosthesis; *PA,* posterior adductor; *PM,* power module; *Qcep,* quadriceps; *Qlum,* quadratus lumborum; *R,* right. (Redrawn from the Cleveland FES Center.)

function. It is more likely that patients in this group would benefit from simpler neuroprosthetic systems that activate fewer muscles targeted to augment voluntary procedures. Examples of this need would be to stimulate the C8 intrinsic muscles to facilitate hand opening or to stimulate C8 thumb adduction or abduction to provide additional hand grasp patterns.

Current research at the Cleveland FES Center is also addressing the need for control of other paralyzed functions through a modular NNP. This device allows expansion of neural control in a modular way for control of autonomic and lower extremity functions such as standing, assisted transfers, and walking. The enabled complexity is demonstrated in Fig. 113.9. Continued progress in miniaturization of components, coupling control signals to larger nerves, better batteries, and similar electronic progress may lead to reproduction of able-bodied function.

Important Surgical Concepts

Joint Balance. For best functional results, procedures that mobilize a joint, such as a tendon transfer, require "balance" to prevent subsequent deformity. It has been our observation, for example, that patients with ASIA motor level C6 (ICSHT 2 and 3) who have voluntary wrist extension develop a slight extension contracture over time. The extent of the contracture is limited by gravity because most functional activities are performed with the forearm pronated, and the flexion moment produced by the weight of the hand counterbalances the active wrist extensors. On the other hand, bedridden or poorly rehabilitated patients and those who are C5 or ICSHT 0 or 1 can develop severe elbow flexion–supination contractures because of the lack of an elbow extension–pronation moment to overcome a powerful or spastic biceps.[38,63] Other contractures that can develop include shoulder adduction, internal rotation contractures, and finger contractures (flexion, clawing, or extension).[64] These contractures are best prevented but can be treated by a staged surgical release. In a similar fashion, if tendon transfers or FES systems are used to power a particular joint or joints that become imbalanced as a result of surgery, contractures can also develop. Procedures that restore grasp through transfer of the ECRL or BR to the FDP without the creation of an extensor moment may result in tighter fingers.[47,65,66] The result can be the development of finger flexion contractures. This extensor can be a static force such as a tenodesis or a dynamic force such as an "antagonist" tendon transfer. Both Zancolli and House have written extensively about such principles as they apply to achieving finger function with tendon transfers.[22,38,67] An improperly balanced joint will lose function over time. The treating surgeon must bear this principle in mind to optimize results of surgery.

Which Motors (Muscles) Should Be Preserved?

Wrist Extensors (Extensor Carpi Radialis Brevis). Because wrist extension is critical to restoration, a wrist extensor is not a suitable donor motor unless there are at least two under voluntary control and of sufficient strength. This means patients must be of ICSHT 3 or greater unless one chooses to use a weak voluntary ECRB to transfer in the presence of a strong ECRL (ICSHT 2). Studies demonstrate differences between the ECRL and ECRB that are important in surgical planning. The different force vectors of the ECRL and ECRB confer different motions. The ECRL, with its insertion radial to the center of the wrist on the base of the index metacarpal, produces radial deviation along with wrist extension. The ECRB, on the other hand, with its central insertion on the base of the long finger metacarpal, produces wrist extension with minimal radial–ulnar deviation, a more balanced and desirable motion. In the absence of a full cadre of muscles to help fine tune motion, our choice of donor motor will result in either radially deviated or neutral wrist extension. As such, when transferring one of two strong and voluntary wrist extensors, the ECRL is chosen either to restore lateral pinch or palmar grasp depending on the patient's ICSHT. Similarly, when restoring wrist extension, the ECRB is the preferred recipient.[10]

We have found one situation in which transfer of the ECRB is useful. There are some patients for whom restoring palmar grasp is important, but they lack sufficient donor motors for routine protocols. In such patients undergoing surgical restoration with weak grade (MMT ≤ 3 from ≤3/5) ECRB (some ICSHT 2), transferring the ECRB to the FDP via a window in the interosseous membrane creates palmar grasp superior to a tenodesis procedure without sacrificing critical wrist extension. Haque and associates[68] reviewed our series of seven patients undergoing this transfer. The total active finger flexion averaged 122 degrees per digit, and lateral pinch and palmar grasp strength were improved. The patients did experience a variable loss of wrist extension motion, we believe, to the wrist flexion moment created by the transfer but not of wrist extension strength due loss of the weak ECRB from its transfer.

The key to performing a transfer involving the wrist extensors is determining that a patient is, in fact, ICSHT 2 versus 3. Clinical examination of the wrist extensors is not always reliable. Bean, as described by Mohammed and associates,[47] found that a groove forms in between the ECRL and ECRB in the proximal lateral forearm with the elbow in 90 degrees of flexion and resisted wrist extension when both are grade 5 of 5 strength. In addition to the usefulness of the "Bean" sign, the authors have found other reliable signs that the ECRB is 4 or greater: grade 5 wrist extension and wrist extension with minimal to no radial deviation.

Wrist Flexors (Flexor Carpi Radialis). In patients present with ICSHT of 5 or greater, the flexor carpi radialis (FCR) is of sufficient strength to be considered a potential donor motor. Zancolli and Shannon[22] and House,[38] however, advocate preservation of the FCR. They believe that the presence of an active, voluntary wrist flexor improves the finger tenodesis extension and prevents wrist extension contractures by improving wrist balance. Voluntary wrist flexion is also helpful in patients who use a manual wheelchair in weight shifts to prevent pressure sores and aids in weight transfers. Sacrificing the FCR as a donor motor incurs a high "cost," and we do not currently use the FCR as a donor motor when presented with the uncommon patient with ICSHT of 5 or greater desiring surgical restoration.

What Motors (Muscles) Are Transferable?

Deltoid. One of the original tendon transfers applied in individuals with tetraplegia involved using the posterior portion of the deltoid muscle to restore elbow extension, and the deltoid-to-triceps transfer remains a gold-standard operation (see Fig. 113.3).[26] As study demonstrates, the deltoid muscle is able to generate approximately 20% of the potential maximum isometric tension of the triceps muscle it is substituting for but has such a long excursion and an ability to maintain tension over a such large percentage of that excursion that it serves as a suitable donor.[69–71] The ability to maintain a consistent strong "pull" while the muscle fibers shorten more than makes the deltoid transfer a reliable and predictable operation. Although obtaining antigravity strength elbow extension is typical, it is more difficult to obtain strength for weight transfers, and this is borne out in clinic study. The transfer requires a bridging tendon graft to span the distance between the deltoid tendon and the triceps insertion, and this appears to predispose to stretching of the tendon transfer, which may weaken the transfer over time.[72] Extensive analysis has supported the need to maintain a strict and extended postoperative therapeutic regimen to help the transfer succeed.[72]

Biceps. Strong elbow flexion (ICSHT ≥1) in an individual translates to the presence of voluntary and strong biceps, brachialis, and BR. In 1999, the clinical efficacy of using the biceps as a donor motor to restore elbow extension in the setting of tetraplegia was published.[73] Although a nonsynergistic transfer, both studies found that patients were able to learn how to isolate the biceps contraction to activate the transfer, the postoperative regimen was simpler, and the postoperative elbow extension strength was superior to antigravity strength. Mulcahey and colleagues,[74] in a comparative study, found that the biceps transfer provided more elbow extension strength and a greater loss in elbow strength compared with a PD transfer (47% vs 32%). Peterson and colleagues[75] recently found that people undergoing elbow extension transfers had higher rates of donor muscle activation when the biceps was the donor muscle compared with the deltoid, and strength of elbow extension was significantly improved. Both procedures result in improvements in ADLs and in the achievement of self-selected goals, but the more reliable improvements have led the authors to favor using the biceps as the donor muscle for elbow extension.[76]

Because the brachialis is the primary elbow flexor, the biceps can be spared as a donor motor without sacrificing meaningful elbow flexion

strength, but it is critical to ensure that the brachialis is functional before the transfer. Individuals will lose some supination strength as well, but this may actually be desirable to prevent supination contractures and help balance a forearm that does not have a strong pronation moment (ICSHT <4). In fact, it is considered by some surgeons to be an excellent choice in the setting of a patient with a dynamic elbow flexion–forearm supination contracture because its use weakens this undesirable posturing. The biceps has gained wide acceptance for use as an elbow extension donor muscle (see Figs.113.4A and 113.7).

Brachioradialis. The BR is the most readily available and versatile muscle for reconstructive transfers in tetraplegia. Because it functions as a secondary elbow flexor and forearm pronator and because most patients have an active and strong biceps or brachialis, the BR is commonly sacrificed with minimal deficit to the patient. It is truly the workhorse muscle in tetraplegia surgery. The muscle characteristics of the BR have been studied extensively. The BR has a broad origin along the lateral epicondylar ridge, and its proximal muscle belly has significant fibrofascial tethers that limit its potential excursion. The average excursion demonstrated surgically is 41.7 mm. Typically finger and thumb extensors require 40 to 60 mm of excursion and the thumb flexor 50 to 60 mm. By releasing the proximal muscle belly from the surrounding connective tissue without detaching its origin, its excursion can be increased to 61 mm, making it a suitable donor for these latter functions.[77] The length–tension characteristics of the BR have also been investigated intraoperatively. The active force produced by the BR was found to be greater than 90% of maximal over a range of 1.5 to 2 cm centered about its resting length. Therefore, transfers of the BR should be tensioned at its resting length with the recipient "joint" mobilized in a balanced position. Intraoperative muscle stimulation is a great aid to the surgeon in making this decision. In addition, the vector of the BR transfer can create secondary motions that can be used to the benefit of an individual person. Normally a secondary forearm pronator and primary elbow flexor, the BR loses its pronation force when transferred to the FPL using the traditional approach.[55] Friden and colleagues[56] found clinically that transferring the BR dorsally though the interosseous membrane and then to the FPL improved the pronation moment without sacrificing the strength of the FPL transfer. Therefore, depending on the needs of a particular individual, especially one who tends to supinate more than desirable, altering the transfer can produce a very effective result.

Some surgeons and therapists believe that the BR is difficult to train, especially in the absence of elbow stabilization. There is certainly support for this viewpoint because previous surface electromyographic study has suggested that people have difficultly truly isolating the BR.[49] In the absence of elbow stabilization, the BR is effectively a two-joint muscle and will be a weak transfer as would be predicted under the general principles of tendon transfer surgery. Brys and Waters[48] were among the first to demonstrate how elbow stabilization by either a brace or an elbow extension transfer enhances the BR as a donor muscle. Others have demonstrated how early mobilization and task-oriented therapy dramatically improve the strength of BR-mediated transfers.[50,78,79] We currently perform an elbow extension transfer as a first-stage procedure or combined with transfers, including the BR.

Extensor Carpi Radialis Longus. The ECRL is available for transfer whenever there is a strong ECRB (ICSHT ≥3). We commonly transfer the ECRL to a synchronized FDP to restore palmar grasp. We initially create a "reverse cascade" such that all fingers flex simultaneously and equally as advocated by Hentz and Leclercq.[20] The transfer is synergistic for wrist extension and finger flexion, although the line of pull around the radial border of radius is not ideal.

Pronator Teres. We previously discussed the occurrence of supination contractures that limit the functional capacity of the patient's hand. It would seem that the presence of an active, voluntary PT would prevent these latter contractures and would be useful as an active pronator to position the hand for use. Indeed, just as for the FCR, one would tend to advocate preservation of the PT in patients with ICSHT of 4 or greater. Experience, however, has proven otherwise. Zancolli[38] favors transfer of the PT, especially to the FCR, placing emphasis on the restoration of active wrist flexion to stabilize the wrist in patients with strong wrist extension and to improve the finger tenodesis effect. In addition, we have not observed, nor have we seen reported, cases of supination contractures occurring in patients with ICSHT of 2 or greater.

Postoperative Therapy. Reconstructive surgery of the arm and hand involves a large commitment from the patient, therapist, and surgeon. Education is critical to ensure that the patient has a realistic understanding of the surgical and rehabilitation process and the time commitment involved. Better preparation before surgery will lead to better postsurgical outcomes because the patient and team will be more likely to identify potential complications such as infection, adhesions, or stretching (rupture). Additionally, thorough education will help the patient to develop realistic expectations for the surgical outcomes and allows the team to understand the patient's motivation level and goals.

GENERAL TENDON TRANSFER MANAGEMENT

After surgery, certain procedures should be used to protect the reconstructive procedures throughout the healing process. Immediately after surgery, treatment focuses on protective techniques such as casting and splinting to avoid damage to the procedures such as stretching or rupturing a tendon transfer. As time after surgery progresses, the focus shifts toward mobilization to prevent adhesions, which can limit movement. It is a complicated balance requiring consistent monitoring to prevent complications. Generally, in situations without complication, the patient can resume all normal activities, including transferring, by approximately 12 weeks after surgery.

Experience and research have illustrated the lengthy time course of recovery. Although the surgery site "heals" within a few weeks to a couple of months, it takes time for patients to both learn their new functions and incorporate their new skills into their daily lives. Patients often spend the next 3 months to 1 year learning their transfers and learning how to incorporate them into their lives. Motivation to improve is clearly the most important patient characteristic associated with a favorable result.[80] Home programs that focus on task-specific functions that activate their transfers have been beneficial.[50,81] Such programs, whether instituted as part of a postoperative program or as a "refresher" to people who had previously had surgery, have been shown to significantly increase pinch strength. The other advantage is that these programs can eliminate the need for extended supervised physiotherapy that many people would not be able to accomplish.

Immediate Postoperative Treatment

Patients undergoing tendon transfers are immobilized postoperatively to protect the tendon transfers. Early rehabilitation involves transitioning to a removable orthosis within the first week of surgery or as soon as the healing incision allows. Traditional protocols protect the transfer in a cast or nonremovable splint for up to 3 to 4 weeks before initiating motion. A joint that has been arthrodesed is protected for 6 to 8 weeks but typically in a removable splint one motion is initiated. The position of immobilization is that which prevents tension on the transferred tendons. Elbow extension transfers, for example, are immobilized in extension. Programs that emphasize early therapy tend to improve strength and outcome measures.[81,82]

In the immediate postoperative period, therapy includes educating the patient and family in precautions, proper positioning of the

extremity, edema management, and recognizing signs of infection. Instruction in ROM exercises to the noninvolved joints of the extremity is beneficial in preventing overall tightness. As soon as the transfer allows, in approximately 3 weeks traditionally and within 1 week with early protocols, protected ROM is initiated to help prevent adhesions, which would limit the transferred muscle's excursion, and to help strengthen the transfer coaptation site.

Finally, there are important logistics to consider. Power wheelchairs should be used by the patient to maintain independence of transport. Hydraulic lifts, bath accommodations, and increased attendant and family care are helpful at home or convalescent location to aid in daily living without requiring stress on the operative arm(s). Whenever possible, ADL training using the contralateral extremity (assuming unilateral reconstruction) with adaptive devices as needed maximizes the patient's independence and reduces caregiver burden. This can include simple approaches such as moving the driving controls for a power wheelchair to the opposite side to increase mobility and making changes to the patient's workspace to facilitate use of the nonoperative arm.

Mobilization Phase

The goals of therapy during the mobilization phase are to increase active movement in a controlled manner throughout the healing process while simultaneously "teaching" the patient how to activate their tendon transfers. For the first 4 to 6 weeks, precautions are instituted to (1) prevent rupture of the transferred tendon, (2) prevent elongation of the transferred muscle, and (3) protect any bony stabilization procedures. Therapy during this time focuses on (1) initiation of biofeedback techniques, (2) active contraction of the transferred tendons only, (3) supervised and gentle passive motion to maintain gliding, (4) avoidance of sudden or uncontrolled movements, (5) no pulling from a supine position to sitting using the operative arm, (6) no weight bearing on the operative arm, (7) continued orthotic positioning at night and during the day, and (8) edema control and modalities to encourage venous drainage.

On the day of cast removal, sutures are removed (nonabsorbing), and the incision sites are cleaned. The fabricated protective orthoses follow the precautions and the same principles as for immediate postoperative immobilization. The orthosis os generally set with the joints in neutral, functional positions with the coaptations in a relaxed state. For most of the extrinsic forearm donor muscles, slight wrist extension combined with digital intrinsic-plus and thumb opposition positioning generally keeps the wrist and digits in relaxed, contraction-preventing protection while keeping the transfers sites free from tension. If the BR is a donor, as is often the case, then the need to also immobilize the elbow depends on the strength of the BR transfer coaptation. In the case of elbow extension transfers, including when these are typically combined with hand grip transfers, the elbow is maintained in extension while the wrist and fingers and thumb are positioned as previously stated. Table 113.5 describes appropriate splinting positions for some of the more typical procedures.

Specifically for elbow extension transfers, patients are rehabilitated in a hinged elbow orthosis set with a flexion block during the day and a static elbow extension orthosis at night positioned at 0 to 10 degrees of elbow extension. The hinged brace allows slow progression of elbow flexion (~15 degrees per week for ≤10 days) as long as full active elbow extension is maintained. Precautions are reviewed with the patient, who is instructed in edema management and protection techniques.

In our current health care delivery system, patients are typically discharged either the same day as surgery or the day after provided they meet criteria for discharge. In one European center, they remain inpatients for just a few days when early motion protocols can be

TABLE 113.5 Various Postoperative Splints

Procedure	Daytime Immobilization	Nighttime Immobilization
Posterior deltoid to triceps	Hinged elbow brace set to desired flexion block	Static extension splint (0–10 degrees of extension)
Biceps to triceps		
BR to ECRB	Wrist cock-up splint (50 degrees of extension)	
BR to FPL	Wrist neutral position with thumb positioned lateral to index finger	
FPL tenodesis		
ECRL to FDS or FDP	Wrist neutral to 20 degrees of flexion with the fingers positioned in ~70 degrees of MCP flexion, ~70 degrees of PIP flexion, and ~ 45 degrees of DIP flexion	
PT to FDS or FDP		
EDC tenodesis	Wrist and fingers positioned in extension; thumb can be left free if no transfer	
PT to EDC		
EPL tenodesis	Thumb spica splint with wrist in ~20 degrees of extension; full MCP and IP extension	
PT to EPL		

Daytime and nighttime immobilization guidelines should follow protocols outlined in postoperative therapy section under the guidance of the surgeon. All splints initially are fabricated in a position so as not to stress the tendon transfer except for the daytime hinged elbow brace for the elbow extension transfers which are commercially available and easily adjustable. Immobilization positions may change when more than one procedure is performed.
BR, Brachioradialis; *DIP*, distal interphalangeal; *ECRB*, extensor carpi radialis brevis; *ECRL*, extensor carpi radialis longus; *EDC*, extensor digitorum communis; *EPL*, extensor pollicis longus; *FDP*, flexor digitorum profundus; *FDS*, flexor digitorum superficialis; *FPL*, flexor pollicis longus; *IP*, interphalangeal; *MCP*, metacarpophalangeal; *PIP*, proximal interphalangeal; *PT*, pronator teres.

initiated and reinforced before their discharge.[41] Ideal therapy requires at least 2 visits per week for the first several weeks from when therapy is initiated, which can then taper after about 4 to 6 weeks depending on the patients progress. Tendon transfers are generally strong enough for unrestricted activity by 2 to 3 months postoperatively, assuming an unremarkable recovery. As patients continue to incorporate their "new" arms into their daily lives, neurologic remodeling facilitates the ease of pinch, grasp, and elbow extension to where the new movements and functions become "second nature."

Weeks 1 Through 3 of Therapy Initiation (Weeks 3–6, Traditional; Weeks 1–3, Early Protocol). The priority of therapy during this time frame is muscle reeducation and active ROM. In some cases, this can mean teaching the muscle to perform a new movement without letting it default to its original movement. For example, in the case of a transfer of the BR muscle to the ECRB, the patient must initially learn to activate the BR so that it extends the wrist without flexing the elbow. After this technique is mastered, the patient is encouraged to activate the transfer at varying degrees of elbow flexion to maximize wrist extension at all elbow angles. Muscle reeducation can be improved with a variety of facilitation techniques, including biofeedback, tapping, vibration, and electrical stimulation (with surgeon approval). Active and active-assisted ROM exercises are encouraged. Light tenodesis activities are suitable for transfers to restore wrist extension or thumb pinch. PROM is gently applied to maintain joint mobility and tendon transfer coaptation site gliding. This should be discussed with the surgeon. Protective orthoses are used at all times except during exercise and bathing. In cases of retained hardware for stabilizations or fusions, fabricated rehabilitation splints that protect these joints are applied for protection while tendon transfers are mobilized. These often take the

form of hand-based thumb CMC orthoses and thumb IP splints or wraps. Soft tissue mobilization or scar management techniques can be initiated as needed as long as all incisions are well healed.

For elbow extension transfers, patients start mobilizing and learning the transfer as soon as immobilization ceases. This starts with holding the elbow in a hinged brace in extension, and 3 to 4 times a day, starting to mobilize the transfer up to about 15 degrees of flexion. Progression occurs weekly by 15 degrees until they get to 90 degrees, and then the splint is discontinued. Patients must be able to fully extend the elbow against gravity to progress, but exercising is done first with gravity eliminated. Although many patients can discontinue their splint about 4 to 5 weeks after the initiation of motion, this time could be delayed if they fail to progress. For early motion protocols, we slow the process down so that progression is limited for about 2 to 3 weeks to allow the coaptation to heal, and the brace is never discontinued before 6 weeks. During supervised sessions, the patient works with the therapist with the brace off, and the elbow in a protected position. All patients sleep in an elbow extension orthosis.

Weeks 4 Through 8 (Weeks 6–10, Traditional; Weeks 4–8, Early Protocol). Functional activities can be performed with increasing resistance. Protective positioning is only used for strenuous activities and at night. Patients begin to work on their specific preoperative goals under supervision while they continue to learn how to activate the transfers. Wound care, soft tissue mobilization, and PROM continue as needed during this time. Retained hardware in the form of pins to secure the thumb CMC arthrodesis are removed after about 8 weeks after surgery.

In the case of transfers for elbow extension, the patient may still require use of the dynamic flexion block orthosis. When the flexion progresses to 90 degrees and full elbow extension is maintained, the orthosis can be discontinued.

Three Months Postsurgery

Protective orthoses are discontinued during strenuous activities and night use. Therapy is directed to functional transfer training and push-ups for weight shifts as appropriate. Patients begin to "feel" their greater independence and learn how to apply their new functions throughout all activities in their life. Therapy focuses on continuing to work on patient-directed goals and help to strategize the "hows" of task completion with or without adaptive equipment. The process of neurological remodeling and learning continues for up to 1 year.[80]

GENERAL THERAPY GUIDELINES AFTER NERVE TRANSFERS

A specialized therapy program is imperative in patients undergoing nerve transfer surgery because the donor nerve necessarily has different motor patterns and cortical mapping in the brain than the original injured nerve it replaces. Therefore, new motor pattern cortical mapping must be established to optimize the functional outcome after surgery. The therapist must create the program based on the particular nerve transfers performed and the specific functional tasks that are part of the patient's goals. It is important to understand the time course for when reinnervation might be expected in timing the phases of therapy, especially when different nerve transfers are expected to reinnervate at different times. The posterior interosseous nerve (PIN) supinator to PIN finger–thumb extensor transfer can show signs of reinnervation within 4 to 6 months; however, a brachialis donor nerve may take 1 year or more.[39]

In general, postoperative therapy is divided into two main blocks: early-phase and late-phase rehabilitation.[83] Early-phase rehabilitation focuses on setting up the patient for optimal function until re-innervation of the target muscles can be observed. This includes maintaining ROM of the affected joints, such as the shoulder and elbow in the case of a teres minor to triceps nerve transfer. Patient education, particularly on the anatomy of the surgery, is another important factor to set realistic expectations, establish a timeline, and help with patient motivation and compliance. Patients undergoing teres minor to triceps nerve transfers can be expected to take as long as 14 to 19 months to achieve maximum recovery, although initial signs of reinnervation present much sooner. Pain and edema control are important aspects of immediate postoperative care, as are minimizing scarring in and adherence of the nerve repair through early shoulder motion. Continuous assessment for return of muscle activity, namely triceps function, sets the timeline for initiating late-phase rehabilitation.

Late-phase rehabilitation begins with evidence of target muscle (triceps) reinnervation. Successful reinnervation after nerve transfers follows a lengthy, stepwise pattern that starts with fasciculations in the recipient muscle with cocontraction of the donor muscle and ideally progresses to target muscle strength of at least MMT 3 or more. Motor reeducation is the main focus of late-phase rehabilitation, along with establishing muscle balance, by teaching the patient how to correctly recruit the newly innervated muscle, which initiates cortical remapping. Planning exercises that involve the coordinated movement of both the donor muscle and recipient muscle is a helpful strategy to help the patient learn the nerve transfer as it starts to gain strength.[84] Integrating functional, task-specific goals into this phase help build confidence and enthusiasm to continue working. The donor action is blocked after muscle strength of the recipient is sufficient (MMT 3). Strengthening and independent exercise program training typically continues for 2 years after surgery.

GENERAL NEUROPROSTHETIC IMPLANTATION THERAPY

The postoperative therapy protocols after implantation of an upper extremity neuroprosthesis are similar to those after tendon transfers. The arm is immobilized for 3 weeks after implantation, with the elbow positioned at 90 degrees of flexion and the hand in a functional position. Any voluntary tendon transfer procedures performed at the same time would change the postoperative positioning accordingly. After the cast is removed, the appropriate protective splints are applied if voluntary or FES tendon transfers were performed. If not, the participant would not need any form of immobilization. Upon cast removal, all of the electrodes are tested, and the resulting muscle responses are recorded. An exercise regimen using the neuroprosthesis is programmed for the patient. After 4 weeks of exercising with the neuroprosthesis, the patient returns and functional programming of the system begins. This may be delayed until voluntary tendon transfers are completely healed. The patient is given at least two, potentially more functional grasps to be used as a tool to complete ADLs. The most popular type of grasps programmed is lateral and palmar grasp. Additional specialty grasps are programmed based on the interests of the patient. ADLs with the neuroprosthesis follow and are guided by the interests of the patient.

OUTCOMES

A well-selected, comprehensive program of hand and upper extremity rehabilitation will have a reliably beneficial impact on patients' lives. These benefits can and have been measured in terms of improved strength of grasp and pinch; increased number of different ADLs that can be performed independently and brace free, including bowel and bladder care; and decreased need for both orthotics or braces and full-time assistant care. The impact that these improvements confer onto

the quality of life have been inferred by the high rates of satisfaction; the improved comfort level in the community; and the number of patients who develop personal interests, including vocations, education, and hobbies. The greatest benefit may be on the patients' psyche, with dramatic improvements in their self-image, confidence, and overall quality of life.[85]

Measuring the impact of a comprehensive, tailored approach to restoration of upper extremity function in the person with tetraplegia is critical for determining the benefits to patients, which ultimately affects the decision-making process for health care resource allocation. Historically, outcomes of reconstructive procedures have been measured in terms of grasp and pinch strength and ADL performance. Recent studies exploring outcomes continue to report consistent and important functional gains. Wangdell and Friden[86] looked at self-rated performance, and individuals who had undergone pinch and grasp reconstructions were now able to achieve 78% of their preoperative goals, most obtained within 6 months of tendon transfers. A couple of Scandinavian outcomes studies found improved functional ability in 73% to 81% and an overall 74% to 90% satisfaction with surgery.[87,88] Patients reported significantly higher degrees of independence with less need for attendant care and functional aids.[88] And, importantly, these benefits persist over the long term after surgery, making these reconstructions reliable over the individual's lifetime.[54]

Another group of studies explored specific gains associated with the particular components of upper extremity reconstruction. Elbow extension, for example, provided significant improvements in wheelchair maneuverability; transfers; and notably, the ability to write and reach objects.[35,89] Pinch reconstructions dramatically improved bladder care, with 75% of patients gaining the ability to self-catheterize after surgery.[90]

Results from the application of FES reveal similar successes. Among the earliest studies, patients who were ASIA C5 functioned at the level of C6 or higher without the need for adaptive tools and equipment.[91] Kilgore and associates[34] reported that the neuroprosthesis not only improved on the ability to perform functional tasks but also allowed patients to perform many activities without adaptive equipment. All five patients evaluated used the system at home, four on a regular basis. In 1999, results of subjective outcomes on 34 patients with an average 5.2 years of follow-up were reported.[27] There were high rates of general satisfaction (87%), life improvements (88%), improved ADLs (87%), increased independence (81%), and confidence (67%). Motor level correlated with success, with the best subjective outcomes noted in C5 or C5 to C6 patients. Although no longer commercially available but still studied in select academic centers, the functional benefits of an implanted neuroprosthesis are consistently demonstrated through the increased independence in ADL performance these systems confer.[92] High satisfaction with reconstructive procedures and implanted neuroprostheses has also been demonstrated by Wuolle and coworkers.[27,93]

A newer set of research studies is beginning to provide surgeons insight into the actual technical aspects of these procedures. Mulcahey and asociates[74] compared two popular procedures for restoring elbow extension and determined that the transfer of the biceps is a viable alternative to the PD to restore this function. Murray and associates[94] examined the influence of elbow angle on transfers of the BR to restore wrist extension, concluding that altering surgical tensioning can improve wrist extension when the elbow is flexed. Additional work by Lieber and coworkers[95] proposes improved surgical outcomes through the use of an intraoperative technique for measuring sarcomere length to facilitate the length setting process of the transferred muscle. Such study may soon help surgeons make intraoperative decisions regarding technical issues such as tensioning a tendon transfer to create a specific, desired effect.[96]

Despite the generally positive outcomes reported historically for reconstructive surgery in tetraplegia, these studies lack the rigor of high-quality randomized controlled trials that is urgently needed to strengthen the base of evidence of the success of these procedures. This is a phenomenon not limited to measuring outcomes after reconstructive surgery but found more globally within rehabilitation medicine. Two trends are happening concurrently in the field of outcome measurement that will improve the quality of measurement and the quality of evidence to support upper extremity reconstruction for people with tetraplegia. First, more formal attention is placed on the use of conceptual frameworks to guide the outcomes measurement process. Second, study design is more formally considered in all phases of research, from inception through publication of results. As a result, the measured effect reconstructive procedures have on all aspects of the lives of people with tetraplegia will contribute not only to the medical decision-making process in the care of this population but also to access to these treatments.

In the context of reconstructive surgery for people with tetraplegia, the International Classification of Functioning, Disability and Health (ICF) can be used to guide intervention and to structure the interpretation of outcomes measurement.[97,98] The ICF was developed by the World Health Organization in an effort to provide a standardized framework or language for discussing health and health-related states.[99] The objective of the ICF is to facilitate communication about health and health states among various health care disciplines and sciences across the world. It is a useful conceptual model that can be applied to assessment, outcome measurement, and research. The key domains of the ICF include body functions and structures, activities, and participation. Personal and environmental factors as they relate to these three domains are also considered. As such, this framework guides outcome assessment beyond just strength measurement and ADL testing and encourages the consideration of how interventions affect the patients' participation in life. Therefore, a holistic approach to measuring the outcomes after reconstructive surgery would include measures that address each domain. To date, there has not been a consensus among clinicians on which tests are preferred to measure the effects of surgery in this population. However, there are increasing efforts to achieve consensus through the collaboration of professionals in groups such as the International Group on Upper Limb Surgery for Tetraplegia and the International Campaign for Cures of Spinal Cord Injury Paralysis (ICCP).[100-102] The International Group on Upper Limb Surgery discussed measures during its 2007 meeting. Many outcome measures were debated, and agreement was reached on the use of the Canadian Occupational Performance Measure as a tool for measuring functional outcomes after upper extremity reconstruction.[103] The ICCP, although acknowledging lack of agreement among clinicians on what measures are most appropriate, recommends the Spinal Cord Independence Measure (SCIM) as a more sensitive comprehensive tool than the Functional Independence Measure.[101,104]

CONCLUSIONS

Rehabilitating a person who sustains traumatic tetraplegia from the time of injury to "reintegration into the community involves focused and dedicated care and effort on the part of a multitude of health care providers. This process seeks to both improve and maximize the quantity and quality of the individuals' life. Rehabilitation of the hand and upper extremity is an integral part of this process and should ideally begin soon after injury and at the inception of care. Using techniques from splinting, therapy, and medicine to surgery, function can be maximized and often restored or reconstructed. The impact on a patients' lives is generally beneficial and lifelong.

REFERENCES

1. Snoek GJ, MJI J, Post MW, Stiggelbout AM, Roach MJ, Zilvold G. Choice-based evaluation for the improvement of upper-extremity function compared with other impairments in tetraplegia. *Arch Phys Med Rehabil*. 2005;86:1623–1630.
2. Anderson KD. Targeting recovery: priorities of the spinal cord-injured population. *J Neurotrauma*. 2004;21:1371–1383.
3. Lo C, Tran Y, Anderson K, Craig A, Middleton J. Functional priorities in persons with spinal cord injury: using discrete choice experiments to determine preferences. *J Neurotrauma*. 2016;33:1958–1968.
4. Bryden AM, Wuolle KS, Murray PK, Peckham PH. Perceived outcomes and utilization of upper extremity surgical reconstruction in individuals with tetraplegia at model spinal cord injury systems. *Spinal Cord*. 2004;42:169–176.
5. Curtin CM, Wagner JP, Gater DR, Chung KC. Opinions on the treatment of people with tetraplegia: contrasting perceptions of physiatrists and hand surgeons. *J Spinal Cord Med*. 2007;30:256–262.
6. Curtin CM, Hayward RA, Kim HM, Gater DR, Chung KC. Physician perceptions of upper extremity reconstruction for the person with tetraplegia. *J Hand Surg [Am]*. 2005;30:87–93.
7. Dunn JA, Hay-Smith EJ, Keeling S, Sinnott KA. Decision-making about upper limb tendon transfer surgery by people with tetraplegia for more than 10 years. *Arch Phys Med Rehabil*. 2016;97:S88–S96.
8. National Spinal Cord Injury Statistical Center, Facts and Figures at a Glance. In: Birmingham: University of Alabama at Birmingham; 2017:2.
9. 2016 Annual Report - Public Version. Birmingham: University of Alabama at Birmingham; 2017.
10. Waters RL, Sie IH, Gellman H, Tognella M. Functional hand surgery following tetraplegia. *Arch Phys Med Rehabil*. 1996;77:86–94.
11. Peckham PH, Mortimer JT, Marsolais EB. Upper and lower motor neuron lesions in the upper extremity muscles of tetraplegics. *Paraplegia*. 1976;14:115–121.
12. Bryden AM, Hoyen HA, Keith MW, Mejia M, Kilgore KL, Nemunaitis GA. Upper extremity assessment in tetraplegia: the importance of differentiating between upper and lower motor neuron paralysis. *Arch Phys Med Rehabil*. 2016;97:S97–S104.
13. Coulet B, Allieu Y, Chammas M. Injured metamere and functional surgery of the tetraplegic upper limb. *Hand Clin*. 2002;18:399–412.
14. Zlotolow DA. The role of the upper extremity surgeon in the management of tetraplegia. *J Hand Surg Am*. 2011;36:929–935; quiz 35.
15. Dunn JA, Sinnott KA, Rothwell AG, Mohammed KD, Simcock JW. Tendon transfer surgery for people with tetraplegia: an overview. *Arch Phys Med Rehabil*. 2016;97:S75–S80.
16. Kirshblum SC, Burns SP, Biering-Sorensen F, et al. International standards for neurological classification of spinal cord injury (revised 2011). *J Spinal Cord Med*. 2011;34:535–546.
17. Dunn J, Hay-Smith E, Whitehead L, Keeling S. Issues influencing the decision to have upper limb surgery for people with tetraplegia. *Spinal Cord*. 2012;50:844–847.
18. Friden J, Gohritz A. Tetraplegia management update. *J Hand Surg Am*. 2015;40:2489–2500.
19. Holtz KA, Lipson R, Noonan VK, Kwon BK, Mills PB. Prevalence and effect of problematic spasticity after traumatic spinal cord injury. *Arch Phys Med Rehabil*. 2017;98:1132–1138.
20. Hentz VR, Leclercq C. *Surgical Rehabilitation of the Upper Limb in Tetraplegia*. London: W.B. Saunders; 2002.
21. Keith MW, Kilgore KL, Peckham PH, Wuolle KS, Creasey G, Lemay M. Tendon transfers and functional electrical stimulation for restoration of hand function in spinal cord injury. *J Hand Surg [Am]*. 1996;21:89–99.
22. House JH, Shannon MA. Restoration of strong grasp and lateral pinch in tetraplegia: a comparison of two methods of thumb control in each patient. *J Hand Surg [Am]*. 1985;10:22–29.
23. Grover J, Gellman H, Waters R. The effect of a flexion contracture of the elbow on the ability to transfer in patients who have quadriplegia at the sixth cervical level. *J Bone Joint Surg*. 1996;78(A):1397–1400.
24. Yarkony GM, Bass LM, Keenan 3rd V, Meyer Jr PR. Contractures complicating spinal cord injury: incidence and comparison between spinal cord centre and general hospital acute care. *Paraplegia*. 1985;23:265–271.

25. Bersch I, Friden J. Role of functional electrical stimulation in tetraplegia hand surgery. *Arch Phys Med Rehabil.* 2016;97:S154–S159.

26. Moberg E. *The Upper Limb in Tetraplegia: A New Approach to Surgical Rehabilitation.* Stuttgart: Georg Thieme Publishers; 1978.

27. Wuolle KS, Doren CLV, Bryden AM, et al. Satisfaction with and usage of a hand neuroprosthesis. *Arch Phys Med Rehabil.* 1999;80:206–213.

28. Gorman PH, Wuolle KS, Peckham PH, Heydrick D. Patient selection for an upper extremity neuroprosthesis in tetraplegic individuals. *Spinal Cord.* 1997;35:569–573.

29. Dalyan M, Sherman A, Cardenas DD. Factors associated with contractures in acute spinal cord injury. *Spinal Cord.* 1998;36:405–408.

30. Taricco M, Adone R, Pagliacci C, Telaro E. Pharmacological interventions for spasticity following spinal cord injury. *Cochrane Database Syst Rev.* 2000:CD001131.

31. Ward AB. Spasticity treatment with botulinum toxins. *J Neural Transm.* 2008;115:607–616.

32. Gerrits HL, de Haan A, Sargeant AJ, Dallmeijer A, Hopman MT. Altered contractile properties of the quadriceps muscle in people with spinal cord injury following functional electrical stimulated cycle training. *Spinal Cord.* 2000;38:214–223.

33. Sabatier M, Stoner L, Mahoney E, et al. Electrically stimulated resistance training in SCI individuals increases muscle fatigue resistance but not femoral artery size or blood flow. *Spinal Cord.* 2006;44:227–233.

34. Kilgore KL, Peckham PH, Keith MW, et al. An implanted upper-extremity neuroprosthesis. Follow-up of five patients. *J Bone Joint Surg Am.* 1997;79:533–541.

35. Wangdell J, Friden J. Activity gains after reconstructions of elbow extension in patients with tetraplegia. *J Hand Surg Am.* 2012;37:1003–1010.

36. Hoyen H, Gonzalez E, Williams P, Keith M. Management of the paralyzed elbow in tetraplegia. *Hand Clin.* 2002;18:113–133.

37. Wangdell J, Friden J. Rehabilitation after spasticity-correcting upper limb surgery in tetraplegia. *Arch Phys Med Rehabil.* 2016;97:S136–S143.

38. Zancolli E. Functional restoration of the upper limb in traumatic quadriplegia. In: *Structural and Dynamic Bases of Hand Surgery.* 2nd ed. JB Lippincott; 1979:229–262.

39. Fox IK. Nerve transfers in tetraplegia. *Hand Clin.* 2016;32:227–242.

40. Brown SH, Hentzen ER, Kwan A, Ward SR, Friden J, Lieber RL. Mechanical strength of the side-to-side versus Pulvertaft weave tendon repair. *J Hand Surg Am.* 2010;35:540–545.

41. Friden J, Reinholdt C, Turcsanyii I, Gohritz A. A single-stage operation for reconstruction of hand flexion, extension, and intrinsic function in tetraplegia: the alphabet procedure. *Tech Hand Up Extrem Surg.* 2011;15:230–235.

42. Reinholdt C, Friden J. Outcomes of single-stage grip-release reconstruction in tetraplegia. *J Hand Surg Am.* 2013;38:1137–1144.

43. Betz RR, Mulcahey MJ. *Child With a Spinal Cord Injury.* Chicago: American Academy of Orthopaedic Surgeons; 1996.

44. Kozin SH. Pediatric onset spinal cord injury: implications on management of the upper limb in tetraplegia. *Hand Clin.* 2008;24:203–213.

45. Reinholdt C, Friden J. Selective release of the digital extensor hood to reduce intrinsic tightness in tetraplegia. *J Plast Surg Hand Surg.* 2011;45:83–89.

46. Towles JD, Murray WM, Hentz VR. The effect of percutaneous pin fixation of the interphalangeal joint on the thumb-tip force produced by the flexor pollicis longus: a cadaver study. *J Hand Surg Am.* 2004;29:1056–1062.

47. Mohammed K, Rothwell A, Sinclair S, Willems S, Bean A. Upper limb surgery for tetraplegia. *J Bone Joint Surg.* 1992;74B:873–879.

48. Brys D, Waters RL. Effect of triceps function on the brachioradialis transfer in quadriplegia. *J Hand Surg [Am].* 1987;12:237–239.

49. Johanson ME, Hentz VR, Smaby N, Murray WM. Activation of brachioradialis muscles transferred to restore lateral pinch in tetraplegia. *J Hand Surg [Am].* 2006;31:747–753.

50. Johanson ME, Dairaghi CA, Hentz VR. Evaluation of a task-based intervention after tendon transfer to restore lateral pinch. *Arch Phys Med Rehabil.* 2016;97:S144–S153.

51. Arnet U, Muzykewicz DA, Friden J, Lieber RL. Intrinsic hand muscle function, part 1: creating a functional grasp. *J Hand Surg Am.* 2013;38:2093–2099.

52. Muzykewicz DA, Arnet U, Friden J, Lieber RL. The effect of intrinsic loading and reconstruction upon grip capacity and finger extension kinematics. *J Hand Surg Am.* 2015;40:96–101.e1.

53. Muzykewicz DA, Arnet U, Lieber RL, Friden J. Intrinsic hand muscle function, part 2: kinematic comparison of 2 reconstructive procedures. *J Hand Surg Am.* 2013;38:2100–2105.e1.

54. Dunn JA, Rothwell AG, Mohammed KD, Sinnott KA. The effects of aging on upper limb tendon transfers in patients with tetraplegia. *J Hand Surg Am.* 2014;39:317–323.

55. Ward SR, Peace WJ, Friden J, Lieber RL. Dorsal transfer of the brachioradialis to the flexor pollicis longus enables simultaneous powering of key pinch and forearm pronation. *J Hand Surg [Am].* 2006;31:993–997.

56. Friden J, Reinholdt C, Gohritz A, Peace WJ, Ward SR, Lieber RL. Simultaneous powering of forearm pronation and key pinch in tetraplegia using a single muscle-tendon unit. *J Hand Surg Eur.* 2012;37:323–328.

57. van Zyl N, Hahn JB, Cooper CA, Weymouth MD, Flood SJ, Galea MP. Upper limb reinnervation in C6 tetraplegia using a triple nerve transfer: case report. *J Hand Surg Am.* 2014;39:1779–1783.

58. Peckham PH, Keith MW, Kilgore KL, et al. Efficacy of an implanted neuroprosthesis for restoring hand grasp in tetraplegia: a multicenter study. *Arch Phys Med Rehabil.* 2001;82:1380–1388.

59. Keith MW, Peckham PH, Thrope GB, et al. Implantable functional neuromuscular stimulation in the tetraplegic hand. *J Hand Surg [Am].* 1989;14:524–530.

60. Kilgore KL, Hoyen HA, Bryden AM, Hart RL, Keith MW, Peckham PH. An implanted upper-extremity neuroprosthesis using myoelectric control. *J Hand Surg [Am].* 2008;33:539–550.

61. Ajiboye AB, Willett FR, Young DR, et al. Restoration of reaching and grasping movements through brain-controlled muscle stimulation in a person with tetraplegia: a proof-of-concept demonstration. *Lancet.* 2017;389:1821–1830.

62. Memberg WD, Polasek KH, Hart RL, et al. Implanted neuroprosthesis for restoring arm and hand function in people with high level tetraplegia. *Arch Phys Med Rehabil.* 2014;95:1201–1211.e1.

63. Keith M, Lacey S. Surgical rehabilitation of the tetraplegic upper extremity. *J Neuro Rehabil.* 1991;5:75–87.

64. Treanor WJ, Moberg E, Buncke HJ. The hyperflexed seemingly useless tetraplegic hand: a method of surgical amelioration. *Paraplegia.* 1992;30:457–466.

65. Colyer RA, Kappelman B. Flexor pollicis longus tenodesis in tetraplegia at the sixth cervical level. A prospective evaluation of functional gain. *J Bone Joint Surg [Am].* 1981;63:376–379.

66. Gansel J, Waters R, Gellman H. Transfer of the pronator teres tendon to the tendons of the flexor digitorum profundus in tetraplegia. *J Bone Joint Surg [Am].* 1990;72:427–432.

67. House J, McCarthy C, VanHeest A, Dahl J, Dahl A. Intrinsic balancing in reconstruction of the tetraplegic hand. In: Vastamaki M, ed. *Current Trends in Hand Surgery.* Elsevier Siene; 1995:373–378.

68. Haque M, Keith M, Bednar M, et al. Clinical Results of ECRB to FDP transfer through the interosseous membrane to restore finger flexion. In: Keith M, ed. *International Conference on Surgical Rehabilitation for Tetraplegia.* 1998. 6th ed. Cleveland, Ohio; 1998.

69. Friden J, Lieber RL. Quantitative evaluation of the posterior deltoid to triceps tendon transfer based on muscle architectural properties. *J Hand Surg [Am].* 2001;26:147–155.

70. Lacey S, Wilber R, Peckham P, Freehafer A. The posterior deltoid to triceps transfer, a clinical and biomechanical assessment. *J Hand Surg.* 1986;11:542–547.

71. Rabischong E, Benoit P, Benichou M, Allieu Y. Length-tension relationship of the posterior deltoid to triceps transfer in C6 tetraplegic patients. *Paraplegia.* 1993;31:33–39.

72. Friden J, Ejeskar A, Dahlgren A, Lieber RL. Protection of the deltoid to triceps tendon transfer repair sites. *J Hand Surg [Am].* 2000;25:144–149.

73. Kuz J, Van Heest A, House J. Biceps-to-triceps transfer in tetraplegic patients; report of the medial routing technique and follow-up of three cases. *J Hand Surg.* 1999;24:161–172.

74. Mulcahey MJ, Lutz C, Kozin SH, Betz RR. Prospective evaluation of biceps to triceps and deltoid to triceps for elbow extension in tetraplegia. *J Hand Surg [Am].* 2003;28:964–971.

75. Peterson CL, Bednar MS, Bryden AM, Keith MW, Perreault EJ, Murray WM. Voluntary activation of biceps-to-triceps and deltoid-to-triceps transfers in quadriplegia. *PLoS One*. 2017;12:e0171141.

76. Kozin SH, D'Addesi L, Chafetz RS, Ashworth S, Mulcahey MJ. Biceps-to-triceps transfer for elbow extension in persons with tetraplegia. *J Hand Surg Am*. 2010;35:968–975.

77. Kozin SH, Bednar M. In vivo determination of available brachioradialis excursion during tetraplegia reconstruction. *J Hand Surg Am*. 2001;26:510–514.

78. Friden J, Shillito MC, Chehab EF, Finneran JJ, Ward SR, Lieber RL. Mechanical feasibility of immediate mobilization of the brachioradialis muscle after tendon transfer. *J Hand Surg Am*. 2010;35:1473–1478.

79. Johanson ME, Jaramillo JP, Dairaghi CA, Murray WM, Hentz VR. Multicenter survey of the effects of rehabilitation practices on pinch force strength after tendon transfer to restore pinch in tetraplegia. *Arch Phys Med Rehabil*. 2016;97:S105–S116.

80. Wangdell J, Carlsson G, Friden J. From regained function to daily use: experiences of surgical reconstruction of grip in people with tetraplegia. *Disabil Rehabil*. 2014;36:678–684.

81. Johanson ME. Rehabilitation after surgical reconstruction to restore function to the upper limb in tetraplegia: a changing landscape. *Arch Phys Med Rehabil*. 2016;97:S71–S74.

82. Wangdell J, Bunketorp-Kall L, Koch-Borner S, Friden J. Early active rehabilitation after grip reconstructive surgery in tetraplegia. *Arch Phys Med Rehabil*. 2016;97:S117–S125.

83. Novak CB. Rehabilitation following motor nerve transfers. *Hand Clin*. 2008;24:417–423. vi.

84. Hahn J, Cooper C, Flood S, Weymouth M, van Zyl N. Rehabilitation of supinator nerve to posterior interosseous nerve transfer in individuals with tetraplegia. *Arch Phys Med Rehabil*. 2016;97:S160–S168.

85. Moberg E. Helpful upper limb surgery in tetraplegia. In: Hunter J, Schneider L, Mackin E, Bell J, eds. *Rehabilitation of the Hand*. St. Louis: The CV Mosby Co.; 1978.

86. Wangdell J, Friden J. Satisfaction and performance in patient selected goals after grip reconstruction in tetraplegia. *J Hand Surg Eur*. 2010;35:563–568.

87. Jaspers Focks-Feenstra J, Snoek G, Bongers-Janssen H, Nene A. *Long-Term Patient Satisfaction After Reconstructive Upper Extremity Surgery to Improve Arm-Hand Function in Tetraplegia*. Spinal Cord; 2011.

88. Gregersen H, Lybaek M, Lauge Johannesen I, Leicht P, Nissen UV, Biering-Sorensen F. Satisfaction with upper extremity surgery in individuals with tetraplegia. *J Spinal Cord Med*. 2015;38:161–169.

89. Lamberg AS, Friden J. Changes in skills required for using a manual wheelchair after reconstructive hand surgery in tetraplegia. *J Rehabil Med*. 2011;43:714–719.

90. Bernuz B, Guinet A, Rech C, et al. Self-catheterization acquisition after hand reanimation protocols in C5-C7 tetraplegic patients. *Spinal Cord*. 2011;49:313–317.

91. Keith MW, Peckham PH, Thrope GB, Buckett JR, Stroh KC, Menger V. Functional neuromuscular stimulation neuroprostheses for the tetraplegic hand. *Clin Orthop*. 1988;233:25–33.

92. Bryden AM, Kilgore KL, Keith MW, Peckham PH. Assessing activity of daily living performance after implantation of an upper extremity neuroprosthesis. *Top Spinal Cord Inj Rehabil*. 2008;13:37–53.

93. Wuolle KS, Bryden AM, Peckham PH, Murray PK, Keith MK. Satisfaction with upper-extremity surgery in individuals with tetraplegia. *Arch Phys Med Rehabil*. 2003;84:1145–1149.

94. Murray WM, Bryden AM, Kilgore KL, Keith MW. The influence of elbow position on the range of motion of the wrist following transfer of the brachioradialis to the extensor carpi radialis brevis tendon. *J Bone Joint Surg Am*. 2002;84A:2203–2210.

95. Lieber RL, Friden J. Implications of muscle design on surgical reconstruction of upper extremities. *Clin Orthop Relat Res*. 2004;419:267–279.

96. Lieber RL, Murray WM, Clark DL, Hentz VR, Friden J. Biomechanical properties of the brachioradialis muscle: implications for surgical tendon transfer. *J Hand Surg [Am]*. 2005;30:273–282.

97. Bryden AM, Sinnott KA, Mulcahey MJ. Innovative strategies of improving upper extremity function in tetraplegia and considerations in measuring functional outcomes. *Top Spinal Cord Inj Rehabil*. 2005;10:75–93.

98. Sinnott KA, Dunn JA, Rothwell AG. Use of the ICF conceptual framework to interpret hand function outcomes following tendon transfer surgery for tetraplegia. *Spinal Cord*. 2004;42:396–400.

99. Organization WH, ed. *International Classification of Functioning, Disability and Health (ICF)*. Geneva, Switzerland: WHO; 2002.

100. Lammertse D, Tuszynski MH, Steeves JD, et al. Guidelines for the conduct of clinical trials for spinal cord injury as developed by the ICCP panel: clinical trial design. *Spinal Cord*. 2007;45:232–242.

101. Steeves JD, Lammertse D, Curt A, et al. Guidelines for the conduct of clinical trials for spinal cord injury (SCI) as developed by the ICCP Panel: clinical trial outcome measures. *Spinal Cord*. 2007;45:206–221.

102. Tuszynski MH, Steeves JD, Fawcett JW, et al. Guidelines for the conduct of clinical trials for spinal cord injury as developed by the ICCP Panel: clinical trial inclusion/exclusion criteria and ethics. *Spinal Cord*. 2007;45:222–231.

103. Law M, Baptiste S, McColl M, Opzoomer A, Polatajko H, Pollock N. The Canadian Occupational Performance Measure: an outcome measure for occupational therapy. *Can J Occup Ther*. 1990;57:82–87.

104. Catz A, Greenberg E, Itzkovich M, Bluvshtein V, Ronen J, Gelernter I. A new instrument for outcome assessment in rehabilitation medicine: spinal cord injury ability realization measurement index. *Arch Phys Med Rehabil*. 2004;85:399–404.

105. Endress RD, Hentz VR. Biceps-to-triceps transfer technique. *J Hand Surg Am*. 2011;36:716–721.

106. Leclercq C, Hentz VR, Kozin SH, Mulcahey MJ. Reconstruction of elbow extension. *Hand Clin*. 2008;24:185–201. vi.

107. Netscher DT, Sandvall BK. Surgical technique: posterior deltoid-to-triceps transfer in tetraplegic patients. *J Hand Surg Am*. 2011;36:711–715.

108. Brown JM. Nerve transfers in tetraplegia I: background and technique. *Surg Neurol Int*. 2011;2:121.

109. Bertelli JA, Tacca CP, Winkelmann Duarte EC, Ghizoni MF, Duarte H. Transfer of axillary nerve branches to reconstruct elbow extension in tetraplegics: a laboratory investigation of surgical feasibility. *Microsurgery*. 2011;31:376–381.

110. Bertelli JA, Ghizoni MF. Nerve transfers for elbow and finger extension reconstruction in midcervical spinal cord injuries. *J Neurosurg*. 2015;122:121–127.

111. Bertelli JA, Ghizoni MF, Tacca CP. Transfer of the teres minor motor branch for triceps reinnervation in tetraplegia. *J Neurosurg*. 2011;114:1457–1460.

112. Friden J, Gohritz A. Brachialis-to-extensor carpi radialis longus selective nerve transfer to restore wrist extension in tetraplegia: case report. *J Hand Surg Am*. 2012;37:1606–1608.

113. Coulet B, Boretto J, Allieu Y, Fattal C, Laffont I, Chammas M. Pronating osteotomy of the radius for forearm supination contracture in high-level tetraplegic patients: technique and results. *J Bone Joint Surg Br*. 2010;92:828–834.

114. Bertelli JA, Ghizoni MF. Nerve transfers for restoration of finger flexion in patients with tetraplegia. *J Neurosurg Spine*. 2017;26:55–61.

115. Paul SD, Gellman H, Waters R, Willstein G, Tognella M. Single-stage reconstruction of key pinch and extension of the elbow in tetraplegic patients. *J Bone Joint Surg Am*. 1994;76:1451–1456.

116. Leclercq C. Surgical rehabilitation for the weaker patients (groups 1 and 2 of the international classification). *Hand Clin*. 2002;18:461–479.

117. Rothwell AG, Sinnott KA, Mohammed KD, Dunn JA, Sinclair SW. Upper limb surgery for tetraplegia: a 10-year re-review of hand function. *J Hand Surg [Am]*. 2003;28:489–497.

118. Bertelli JA, Tacca CP, Ghizoni MF, Kechele PR, Santos MA. Transfer of supinator motor branches to the posterior interosseous nerve to reconstruct thumb and finger extension in tetraplegia: case report. *J Hand Surg Am*. 2010;35:1647–1651.

119. Bertelli JA, Mendes Lehm VL, Tacca CP, Winkelmann Duarte EC, Ghizoni MF, Duarte H. Transfer of the distal terminal motor branch of the extensor carpi radialis brevis to the nerve of the flexor pollicis longus: an anatomic study and clinical application in a tetraplegic patient. *Neurosurgery*. 2012;70:1011–1016. discussion 16.

120. Koo B, Peljovich AE, Bohn A. Single-stage tendon transfer reconstruction for active pinch and grasp in tetraplegia. *Top in Sp Cord Inj Rehab*. 2008;13:24–36.

114

Management of the Injured Athlete

Angela Stagliano, Dana Webb

CRITICAL POINTS

- Athletes experience injuries that are unique to their individual sport. It is important to be able to recognize these common injuries at the time of initial evaluation.
- Upper extremity deep vein thromboses are common in hockey players, gymnasts, and swimmers. It is vital to differentiate their signs and symptoms from common musculoskeletal injuries.
- There are six phases of graded exercise progressions when returning to sport after a concussion. It is important to be able to

identify the stage the athlete is in to allow for safe progression to competition.
- A sports physical therapist is a key member of the multidisciplinary team, but it is important to understand the role played in the rehabilitation of the injured athlete.
- Athletes require alternative physical assessments, which should be reassessed throughout their rehabilitation process. It is important to relate these tests to their specific athletic activities.

When providing care to this specialized population, a therapist needs to have an understanding of tissue healing time frames, evidence-based postoperative protocols, body mechanics, and forces being placed on the body. Another important skill the therapist requires is creativity to "think outside the box" because specific needs vary from athlete to athlete. The therapist must have a well-rounded knowledge of sport-specific exercises, plyometrics, agility drills, multidirectional movements, and periodization. Periodization consists of planning the physical training of an athlete to peak at a particular point in time, such as the Olympic Games. When developing a plan of care, multiple additional factors must be considered, such as sport and position, outside influence that might interfere with therapy, timeline for return to practice, and timeline for return to sport. Additional challenges that the therapist may encounter include the interdisciplinary approach to treatment, psychological issues, and peer pressure.

This chapter reviews the following topics: common injuries and mechanism of injuries, injury prevention, the interdisciplinary approach to rehabilitation, various treatment strategies, return to practice, and return to sport. There is supplemental information provided on the companion website of the text that has quick links (Box e114.1) for information on concussion, bracing, and specialty equipment requirements for sports.

COMMON INJURIES IN SPORTS

Over the course of an athlete's career, one can encounter numerous types of injuries. Injuries can be as simple as a laceration, sprain, strain, or bone bruise. Some can be more complex, such as a dislocation; fracture; or tear of a ligament, tendon, or muscle. There are numerous possibilities for

the mechanism of injury, such as overuse, physiological changes in the body, or nontraumatic causes. Regardless of the mechanism of injury, rehabilitation follows the principles described throughout this text. The application of stress to the healing tissues is timed and progressed according to the phase of healing and clinical indicators observed at each phase. (Please refer to Chapter 15 for more information regarding tissue healing.) Table 114.1 lists a variety of sports with associated common injuries, potential mechanisms of injury, and risk factors.

TRENDING TOPICS

Concussion and upper extremity deep vein thrombosis (DVT) have been popular topics in sports and the news over the past few years. The heightened awareness of the long-term effects of concussions as seen in professional athletes has brought about many changes in rules and regulations, on-the-field treatments, equipment, and penalties. Additionally, upper extremity DVT is an injury that has been devastating to at least one professional hockey player each season over the past few years. This section briefly covers these two trending topics.

Concussion

A concussion is a mild traumatic brain injury (mTBI) caused by a blow to the head or body, resulting in physiological changes in function.[1] In the United States, about 1.6 to 3.8 million concussions occur every year from sports.[1,2] The common associated signs and symptoms are dizziness, sensitivity to light, double vision, blurred vision, altered visual tracking, delayed reaction time, decreased coordination, altered cognition, headaches, nausea, vomiting, and confusion.[2] The majority of

TABLE 114.1   Commonly Associated Upper Extremity Injuries or Conditions, Mechanism of Injury, and Risk Factors by Sport

Sport	Injury or Condition	Mechanism of Injuries	Risk Factors
Archery[35,36]	Shoulder impingement, overuse injuries; lacerations, punctures, contusions, abrasions, compression neuropathy of digital nerves; medial epicondylitis, median nerve compression at the wrist or elbow, de Quervain's tenosynovitis	Mishandling arrows, bowstring hitting arm	
Badmitton[37,38]	RTC tendonitis or strains, medial–lateral epicondylitis, strain or sprain of wrist or fingers	Repetitive flexion–extension of elbow, wrist, and fingers	Increased volume of participation
Baseball[39,40]	SLAP lesion, RTC tears, little leaguer's shoulder and elbow, UCL injuries, posteromedial elbow instability, ligament or muscle strains or sprains, olecranon stress fractures, wrist sprains, dislocation of phalanges, upper extremity thrombosis	Excessive amounts of pitching or catching; physical workload, playing with injuries; contact with the bat, ball, or another player	Increased repetitive trauma, poor body mechanics, increased length of training sessions, increased number of games played
Basketball[41]	Mallet finger, avulsion fractures, thumb UCL sprains, CMC sprains, TFCC sprain, distal radial–ulnar fractures; finger or thumb fractures	FOOSH, contact with the ball or another player, dunking on the rim	
Boxing[42]	Wrist, hand, or finger fractures; CMC instability	Axial load, forces placed on opponent	Increased size or strength of opponent, amateur status
Canoeing, kayaking, and rafting[43,44]	Overuse injuries of the shoulder, wrist, forearm, or hand; abrasions, contusions; dislocations	Repetitive motions while paddling with arm in overhead position, collisions with other rafters/paddles/rocks in riverbed while swimming, ejection from raft	Rapids, obstacles in water, increased current, improper equipment
Cheerleading[45,46]	Anterior GH laxity, stiffness, wrist or hand injuries	Overuse injuries, falls, or collisions	Inadequate conditioning; amateur status; inadequate supervision; level of difficulty of stunts or tumbling; landing surfaces
Crew and rowing[47]	Forearm, wrist, or hand injuries; extensor tenosynovitis; de Quervain's tenosynovitis; hand blisters; wrist sprains; rib fractures	Overuse injuries	Inadequate conditioning or stretching; muscle imbalances
Cricket[48,49]	Hook of hamate stress fracture; other wrist, hand, or finger injuries; elbow tendonitis	Gripping of bat, overuse injuries	Poor technique
CrossFit and obstacle course racing[50]	AC impingement, labral tears, RTC tears, biceps tendonitis	Improper technique, overuse injuries	Improper technique, inadequate conditioning
Cycling or mountain biking[51]	AC joint separation, GH dislocations, clavicle fracture, wrist tendinopathies, cyclist's palsy (ulnar nerve injury in Guyon's canal)	Falls, collisions with other cyclists, uneven terrain, incorrect technique	Mechanical failures, poor conditions, insufficient training
Fencing[52]	Wrist tendinopathy, lacerations, PIP joint dislocations, RTC or elbow tendinopathy, contusions, bruises	Overuse injuries	Improper technique, equipment malfunction
Field hockey[53,54]	Shoulder separations, lacerations, fractures (typically the thumb), forearm strains, finger fractures, hand or finger contusions	Collision with ball, stick, or human; overuse injuries	Increased velocity of the ball, improper physical protective equipment
Football[55]	AC joint injury, shoulder ligament sprain, subluxation, contusion, muscle or tendon strain, hand or finger fractures, labral tears, cartilage injury	Contact injuries, overuse injuries	Competition, older age
Golf[56,57]	RTC injuries, posterior shoulder instability, wrist strains, trigger finger, lateral–medial epicondylitis, hook of hamate fracture, FCU tendinopathy, de Quervain's and pisiform ligament complex syndrome	Grounding the club, overuse injuries, ejection from a golf cart	Amateur status, female gender, increased force of grip on club, improper grip material of club
Gymnastics or tumbling[58,59]	Wrist injuries, distal radius fractures, scaphoid fractures, avascular necrosis of capitate, posterior interosseous nerve compression, TFCC tears, scaphoid stress fractures, radial head fractures, RTC tendinopathy, labral tears	Falling off equipment, improper landing	Improper technique, skeletal immaturity, older age, inadequate conditioning

TABLE 114.1 **Commonly Associated Upper Extremity Injuries or Conditions, Mechanism of Injury, and Risk Factors by Sport—cont'd**

Sport	Injury or Condition	Mechanism of Injuries	Risk Factors
Handball[60,61]	Shoulder overuse injuries	Overuse injuries	Decreased total GH rotation, weakness of the external rotators and scapular dyskinesia
Ice hockey[62,63]	AC joint dislocations, GH joint dislocations, clavicle fractures, hand fractures, wrist ligament strains	Contact injuries with other players, board, or stick, falls onto the ice	Older age, improper technique
Judo[64,65]	AC joint dislocations, GH joint dislocations, ligamentous elbow injuries	Contact injuries (thrown, landed on), submission positions (arm lock), FOOSH	Improper technique, inadequate conditioning
Lacrosse[66,67]	Clavicle fractures, AC separations, SLAP tears, posterior shoulder dislocations, shoulder ligament sprains, contusions, subluxations, thumb fractures	Contact injuries with other players, stick, ball, or environment; overuse injuries	Improper technique, inadequate level of conditioning, improper equipment
Martial arts[68]	Labral tears, shoulder dislocations, AC joint separations, hand or finger fractures, wrist strains or sprains	Contact injuries with other players, falls	Improper training, older age, history of delayed healing
Ping pong[69]	Dislocations, ruptured tendons or ligaments, fractures, wrist or elbow strains	Overuse injuries, contact injuries with ball or paddle	Trying new techniques
Rafting[70,71]	Shoulder, elbow, or finger dislocations; contusions; lacerations; strains; sprains; finger fractures	Contact injuries with paddle, raft, water, or another person or object in the water	Amateur status, increased current speed
Racquet sports[37,38,72]	Scapular dyskinesia, GIRD, posterior capsule tightness, SICK scapula (shoulder dyskinesis), RTC pathology, labral tears, elbow tendinopathies, wrist tendinitis, de Quervain's tenosynovitis, ECU subluxation, ECU tendinitis	Overuse injuries, velocity of ball and swing, collisions	Inadequate conditioning, older age
Rock climbing[73]	Shoulder dislocation, finger tendon strains or tears, elbow tendonitis, shoulder muscle strains	Overuse injuries, falls	Delay in seeking medical attention, older age, climbing in indoor gym (versus outdoors)
Rollerblading[74]	Distal radius, scaphoid, and radial head injuries; concussions	Falls caused by road hazards, loss of control with the inability to stop, speed skating	Increased speed, obstacles, harder surfaces; amateur status, aggressive skating; amount of time spent skating; resistance to using personal protective equipment
Rugby[75,76]	Shoulder dislocation–subluxation, AC joint injuries, RTC injuries, concussions	Contact injuries, gym conditioning	Female gender, reduced agility, reduced speed, and tightness of the hip flexors
Sailing[44]	Overuse sprains and strains of the shoulder, head lacerations	Falls, handling lines and winches	Amateur status, increased wind speed
Skateboarding[77,78]	Forearm fractures of the radius, ulna, or both, most often the distal third of the forearm; elbow fractures	High-velocity FOOSH	Attempting increased complexity of tricks on hard surfaces
Skiing and snowboarding[79]	Clavicle and proximal humerus fractures, skier's thumb (radial stress to MCP of the thumb), anterior dislocation of the GH joint, AC joint disruption	Handle of ski pole acts as a fulcrum across the MCP, stressing the UCL; skier's step out of bindings to stop a fall (lower extremity injury risk is higher); snowboarders reach out to stop a fall (upper extremity injury risk is higher)	Catching a fall
Skimboarding[80]	Wrist fractures, elbow fractures	FOOSH when running on the beach toward the incoming waves	
Skydiving[81]	Shoulder dislocation, upper arm fracture, forearm and wrist fractures, concussion	Using a reserve parachute (bilateral arm function required), landing technique, packing and pulling a chute	Line entanglement, unlicensed, miscalculations during flight and turbulence
Soccer[82,83]	Distal radius fractures, scaphoid fractures	FOOSH, contact injuries with equipment or other players, impact of ball on hands when making a save	Goalkeeper position
Softball[84]	Shoulder strains and muscular injury, UCL injuries, facial fractures	Overuse injuries, "windmill" pitching mechanics, fielding batted balls	Pitcher position, inadequate conditioning
Strongman[85]	Shoulder strain or tear, bicep tendon injury, elbow tendon injury, cervical strain	Performing farmers walk, log press, stones, tire flip, axle work, or yoke walk	Improper technique, increased length of training sessions, lack of warm-up, preexisting conditions, load too great, poor flexibility or mobility

Continued

Sport	Injury or Condition	Mechanism of Injuries	Risk Factors
Surfing[44,86]	Head or face lacerations, cervical joint injury, cervical strain, cervical nerve injury, shoulder joint injury, shoulder muscular injury	Striking seafloor, paddling (abduction followed by adduction and internal rotation), tube riding, contact injuries with sea surface or board	Amateur status, increased hours surfed, ability to perform aerial maneuvers
Swimming and diving[87]	Shoulder entrapment or impingement, shoulder tendonitis, shoulder strain, concussion	Overuse injuries, contact injuries with surface of water	Female gender (for overuse injury), improper technique, rapid increases in frequency of training
Track and field: discus[88]	RTC tear or tendinopathy, GH dislocation, ulnar nerve traction neuritis	Overuse injuries, hyperextension with implements	Improper technique, excessive repetitions in practice, inadequate flexibility program, no coach present, inappropriate footwear, poor periodization of strength program
Track and field: hammer throw[88]	RTC tear or tendinopathy, ulnar nerve traction neuritis	Overuse injuries	Improper technique, excessive repetitions in practice, inadequate flexibility program, no coach present, inappropriate footwear, poor periodization of strength program
Track and field: javelin[88]	RTC tear or tendinopathy, UCL injury, ulnar nerve traction neuritis, pronator teres rupture	Extreme ER + abduction with cocking phase, significant valgus force through elbow in late cocking and early acceleration phase; hyperextension with implements	Improper technique, excessive repetitions in practice, inadequate flexibility program, no coach present, inappropriate footwear, poor periodization of strength program
Track and field: pole vault[89]	Elbow strain, RTC strain or tendonitis, wrist sprain, wrist tendonitis, scaphoid fracture, forearm laceration, triceps or deltoid strain, wrist contusion	Plant or takeoff phase of vaulting, overuse injuries	History of previous injury, >4 seasons of prior vaulting, advanced personal record, event timing (competition)
Track and field: shot put[88]	RTC tear or tendinopathy, pectoralis major strain, intersection syndrome, volar plate injuries	Carrying position of the wrist carries the weight in an extended position; explosive activation of pec major before release of shot put	Improper technique, excessive repetitions in practice, inadequate flexibility program, no coach present, inappropriate footwear, poor periodization of strength program
Tennis[90]	Shoulder internal impingement, SLAP tears, elbow tendinopathy, ECU tendinitis or subluxation	Overuse injuries, types of shots performed (forehand or backhand most common)	Size of the racquet, racquet material or weight, stroke biomechanics, hand grip positions
Ultimate Frisbee[91]	Separation, dislocation , or subluxation of the shoulder	Laying out (diving for the disc), contact injuries, jumping, stepping on uneven surfaces	Male gender
Volleyball[92–94]	Shoulder muscle strains; thumb, finger, or wrist ligament sprains; shoulder tendinitis; shoulder subluxation; finger fractures	Overuse injuries with swinging, spiking, blocking	
Water polo[95,96]	RTC tear or impingement, GH dislocation, AC joint separation, UCL thumb injury, de Quervain's tenosynovitis, osteochondritis dissecans of the capitellum, IP or MCP joint dislocation, cervical fracture, face laceration, ear drum perforation, facial bone fractures	Excessive ER and abduction with late-cocking phase, blocking a shot (goalie), contact with other players	Increased throwing frequency, increased shot frequency, reduced pec minor length
Water skiing and wake boarding[97]	Contusions, abrasions, lacerations, fractures, sprains, strains	Resistance to using personal protective equipment, waterway obstacles, rapid acceleration	
Weightlifting[98–100]	Osteolysis of the distal clavicle; overuse tendon injuries; anterior shoulder instability; intersection syndrome; neuropathies of the suprascapular, long thoracic, musculocutaneous, or medial pectoral nerves	Bench press produces unfavorable position for RTC	Anabolic steroid use, hypertrophy (nerve compression)
Windsurfing[101]	Fractures, lacerations, strains, sprains, abrasions, blisters, jellyfish stings	Contact injuries with equipment; jumping, uncontrolled falls	High wind speed, increased length of training sessions, boom size, boom grip size, harness use
Wrestling[102–105]	Shoulder, elbow, forearm, wrist, or hand injuries; general trauma; dislocations; subluxations; sprains; strains; fractures; neurotrauma	Contact injuries with opponent or playing surface, takedown injuries, falls, illegal maneuvers	Skeletal immaturity, amateur status

AC, Acromioclavicular; *CMC,* carpometacarpal; *ECU,* extensor carpi ulnaris; *ER,* external rotation; *FCU,* flexor carpi ulnaris; *FOOSH,* fall on outstretched hand; *GH,* glenohumeral; *GIRD,* glenohumeral internal rotation deficit; *IP,* interphalangeal; *MCP,* metacarpophalangeal; *PIP,* proximal interphalangeal; *RTC,* rotator cuff; *scapular dyskinesia/SICK scapula,* Scapular malposition, Inferior medial border prominence, coracoid pain, and dyskinesis of scapular movement; *SLAP,* superior labrum anterior and posterior; *TFCC,* triangular fibrocartilage complex; *UCL,* ulnar collateral ligament.

these symptoms resolve in 7 to 10 days. When treating an athlete who has recently sustained a concussion or has a history of multiple mTBIs, it is important to evaluate for symptoms that might influence treatment and recovery. Postconcussion syndrome (PCS) is defined as an individual presenting with cognitive deficits.[1] Cognitive deficits affect attention or memory and have at least three of the following symptoms: fatigue, sleep disturbance, headache, dizziness, irritability, affective disturbance, apathy, or personality change.[1] Persistent postconcussion symptoms pose long-term challenges and can negatively affect the athlete's quality of life because of prolonged periods of rest[3] (see https://www.ncbi.nlm.nih.gov/pmc/articles/PMC5139792/-i10 62-6050-51-9-739-b03). Current research indicates that prolonged rest may not always be the most appropriate course of treatment for patients who do not follow the normal timeline to resolve symptoms.[2] It has been found that low levels of graded exercise may benefit athletes postinjury with symptoms closely monitored.[2] Although concussed players may be asymptomatic upon return to play, the residual effects may be present when performing a skill (e.g., a baseball player lacking eye hand coordination or delayed reaction time when batting can affect his ability to make successful contact with the ball). An athlete being released to sport before the individual is completely recovered increases the chance of second-impact syndrome. Second-impact syndrome occurs when a player sustains another concussion before symptoms have resolved from the first concussion, causing rapid swelling of the brain and could be fatal.[3] It is vital that the six stages of graduated exercise are used for return to play and to prevent further injury.[4] (For additional information on the six stages of graduated exercise and return to play, please reference online supplement materials.) The most updated Zürich guidelines from 2016 Berlin International Concussion Conference are located in the online materials along with links to articles, evaluation tools, and return-to-sport protocols.

Upper Extremity Deep Vein Thrombosis

Upper extremity deep vein thrombosis (UEDVT), also known as Paget-Schroetter syndrome or effort thrombosis, is defined as a thrombosis of the deep veins of the upper extremity.[5,6] The thrombosis is caused by subclavian compression leading to a thrombus formation in the subclavian vein.[5] The common signs and symptoms of UEDVT are shoulder pain, neck pain, swelling of the arm and hand, bluish color of the extremity, pain that travels to arm or forearm, and hand weakness; occasionally, symptoms may be absent.[5,6] About 10% of all DVTs occur in the upper extremity and most of the time are asymptomatic. UEDVT usually presents in young and otherwise healthy patients, and it occurs more often in males than females. Although rare, UEDVT should be included in the differential diagnosis of overhead sports (rowers, dancers, gymnasts, swimmers, and hockey players) caused by the repetitive overhead motion, hyperabduction, hyperflexion, and extension.[6] A UEDVT can occur with postoperative surgeries (labral repairs, acromioclavicular joint reconstruction), and rapid diagnosis is essential for successful treatment. The typical treatment is anticoagulant therapy and physical therapy, which can resume 1 week after starting anticoagulant therapy, after a stable therapeutic IRN is achieved.[6,7] Therapy follows normal postoperative protocols while closely monitoring symptoms.[7] If an athlete requires prolonged use of anticoagulant therapy, return to sport can be questionable. Readers are referred to Chapter 56 for more information regarding vascular disorders.

MULTIDISCIPLINARY APPROACH

Athletes are unique individuals who each require a different type of assessment because of the nature of their training and demands of their sport. There are many unique qualities that define each athlete, including their body composition, genetics, mental well-being, and history of injuries. Because of all of these variables, a multidisciplinary approach to treatment

is vital to enhance their athletic longevity. A team approach to their recovery is vital to address each of these distinct qualities. The main goal of the health care team is to connect at-risk student athletes with providers who can help them.[8] An ideal integrative team would include a physician, physical therapist, sports psychologist, dentist, sports nutritionist, exercise physiologist, podiatrist, orthopedist, nurse, school health services, strength and conditioning specialist, and massage therapist.[9] This team is responsible for injury risk reduction, treatment of injuries, and physical examinations, also referred to as preparticipation screenings.[8]

Each member of the team is vital in recognizing the signs and symptoms of various health care concerns. For example, coaches and teammates play an important role in recognizing early signs of eating disorders because they are around the athlete most frequently. According to the National Institute of Mental Health (NIMH), early signs for eating disorders include obsessions with food, body weight, and shape.[10] Female athletes are at a higher risk for developing eating disorders; however, muscle dysmorphia is a common disorder that is more prevalent in male athletes.

Early signs for psychological conditions vary depending on the degree and severity of the disorder. Some warning signs from the NIMH include noticeable changes in mood, difficulty concentrating, engaging in high-risk activities, obsessive thinking, or a need for alcohol or drugs.[10] If these traits are noticed, the athlete should be referred to a sports psychologist to better address his or her condition. Another reason to refer an athlete to a sports psychologist is prolonged recovery after a severe injury.[11]

Athletes are always training to gain an edge on their competition. Some common ways that they are successful are through increased training hours, visualizing their performance, or film study. Some athletes turn to coaches, teammates, or performance coaches to gain an edge using supplemental nutrition.[8] Nutritionists can help athletes determine habits and eating plans to assist with their training programs. They can also help optimize performance and the athlete's health with the assistance of a professional.[11] A nutritionist can also assist with education of supplements.[11]

Strength and conditioning professionals assist with documenting and reporting athlete injuries.[12] They play a strong role in facilitating athletes to feel comfortable enough to report injuries that they may not admit to coaches or athletic trainers. They also play a key role in developing leadership traits in athletes.[13] These traits often times carry over to the field or court to allow development of a more valuable member of the team. A strength and conditioning specialist should have experience under a certified strength and conditioning specialist, as well as experience attending National Strength and Conditioning Association–endorsed clinics. They should also have a bachelor's degree in a related field, knowledge of proper weightlifting form, and spotting techniques.

When the athlete has achieved physiological healing, the medical team can declare the athlete ready to return to practice. At this time, many factors need to be considered from a psychological standpoint to make sure the athlete will be confident with her or his abilities. Research has shown a higher risk of reinjury when an athlete is not confident with his or her recovery.[13] Some other signs that an athlete is unfit for competition include fear, abnormal complaints of pain inconsistent with injury, high anxiety, moodiness, agitation, and poor judgment.[11] When these signs are displayed, the athlete should be referred to a sports psychologist to work on supportive techniques, such as imagery, positive self-talk, and mental practice to improve the ability to return to sport safely.[11]

It is also important to evaluate the self-determination of the athlete. It is essential to figure out if or why the person wants to return to sport, whether it is intrinsic motivation, for the love of the game, extrinsic motivation (e.g., fear of being replaced by another player on the team), or simply just concern for disappointing teammates.[12,13] Not every athlete wants to return to the sport after an injury; therefore, it is important to identify the athlete's goals and facilitate conversations between both coaches and parents.

FUNCTIONAL ASSESSMENTS

There are many different functional assessments a health care provider can use to perform a physical evaluation. Range of motion (ROM), strength, and posture are some of the more common assessments used by health care providers. From 2016 to 2017, there were more than 7.9 million student-athletes at the high school level, competing in various sports across the United States.[14] With this high number of competing athletes, an efficient and systematic screening tool can be helpful in identifying the at-risk population. Athletes require a more extensive evaluation, whether it is performed as a preparticipation screening or before return to practice. A battery of tests has been developed to reduce the risk of injury or to prevent reinjury by identifying at risk individuals. The Functional Movement Screen (FMS), Selective Functional Movement Assessment (SFMA), and Titleist Performance Institute (TPI) Movement Screen are a few of the more common published screening assessment tools used today.

The FMS is an assessment developed to evaluate functional mobility and functional stability. It consists of the following seven movements: overhead squat, hurdle step, in-line lunge, shoulder mobility, active straight leg raise, trunk stability push-up, and rotary stability test.[15,16] Many studies have investigated the reliability of the FMS, with fair to excellent interrater reliability.[16] Limitations in glenohumeral and scapulothoracic mobility can lead to poor performance for the overhead squat, in-line lunge, and shoulder mobility tests.[16] Limitations in trunk stability can result in poor performance during push-up and rotary stability test.[17] Each test is scored on a scale from 0 to 3, with a higher score being a complete movement without compensation or pain.[16,18] If an athlete has pain while performing any of the movements, it is recommended to perform an SFMA to identify the cause(s) of movement dysfunction. In a study of 160 National Collegiate Athletic Association (NCAA) Division 1 athletes, they found that a composite score less than 14, along with a history of previous injury, puts the athlete at a 15 times increased risk for injury compared with equal individuals.[14] The FMS has been used during the NFL and NHL combines as a part of their preassessment.[19]

The SFMA is a clinical assessment that is performed on athletes who experience pain with functional movements. It is a movement-based diagnostic evaluation that helps determine the cause of the pain through regional interdependence. This assessment includes some upper extremity tests, such as cervical ROM and combined shoulder ROM.[20] Further assessments, referred to as "breakouts," are subsequently performed based on the response to this assessment.[21] Tests are "scored" as functional and asymptomatic, functional and painful, dysfunctional and asymptomatic, or dysfunctional and painful.[21] The assessment has many layers and requires additional training to successfully perform on athletes. Compared with the FMS, this assessment is more time consuming and should be performed on an individual level.

The TPI Movement Screen is used to identify physical reasons that would impede the performance of a golfer. The movement screen includes assessments of the upper body, lower body, and trunk with special attention to ROM, balance, flexibility, and strength. There have been documented faults noted in golf swings with video analysis, which correlate with the results of the TPI Movement Screen.[22,23]

There are some other assessment tools that can be used to assess the upper extremity. One of which is the Y Balance Test–Upper Quarter (YBT-UQ). This test is performed with one hand in the middle of a "Y" while the other arm reaches in three different directions (Fig. 114.1). This test has been reported to be reliable and has demonstrated no difference from the dominant to the nondominant arm when tested.[24] The indication for this test may be in a return-to-practice environment, in which the athlete should be able to demonstrate symmetry in bilateral upper extremities.[25,26]

Another test that is similar to the YBT-UQ and the trunk stability push-up from the FMS, is called the Closed Kinetic Chain Upper Extremity Stability Test (CKCUEST).[27] This test starts in an

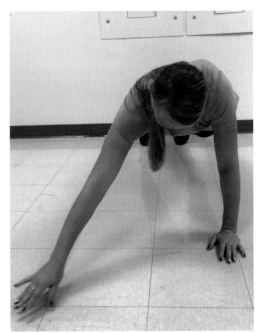

Fig. 114.1 Y Balance Test–Upper Quarter (YBT-UQ).

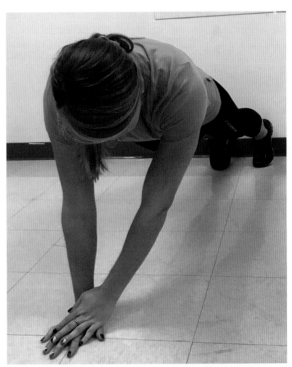

Fig. 114.2 Closed Kinetic Chain Upper Extremity Stability Test (CKCUEST).

elbow-extended plank position. The athlete would reach one hand to touch the dorsum of the other hand (Fig. 114.2). The number of times that the arms cross the body is recorded in a period of 15 seconds.[27] This test is less researched; however, a study performed on football players before the season showed that those who performed less than 21 taps were more likely to undergo a shoulder injury during the season.[27]

Traditional assessments include open kinetic chain activities, such as a 1 repetition maximal effort on the bench press.[28] The parallel-bar dip and pronated pull ups are two of the more common closed kinetic chain activities. A study performed by 15 male athletes showed that a ratio of 1.11 between dips and pull-ups exists, which may be helpful in determining readiness when returning an athlete to practice.[28]

There are some other physical performance measures that have been researched in smaller studies of athletes, measuring power and strength. Medicine balls are commonly used in training for the athletic population; an assessment by Jones and coworkers included participants tossing a 12-lb medicine ball for distance, called the seated medicine ball throw (SMBT).[24] A recent study found a strong correlation between the SMBT and isokinetic shoulder external and internal rotation and elbow strength but weak correlation with strength and YBT-UQ.[24] The other power performance measure is the seated shot put, in which the participant tosses a 4.5-kg medicine ball with two hands, or 2.72 kg for a unilateral toss.[24] The seated medicine ball toss has been used with a variety of athletic populations, including children, and was found to correlate with bench press in some female athletes.[19] Another test was the one-arm hop test, in which the participants were timed in a five-hop test onto a 10.2-cm step.[19,24] This was tested in a small sample of football players and was retested with wrestlers.[24]

REHABILITATION TECHNIQUES

A rehabilitation program requires a multifaceted approach to return the athlete to sports in an optimum time frame. This program consists of a variety of techniques that will keep the athlete engaged as well as prepare the athlete for return to sport. Each program starts with the traditional rehabilitation exercises and then progresses to more advanced exercises and finishes with sport-specific exercises. Selected strategies and techniques, including periodization, strength training, manual therapy, plyometrics, Olympic lifts, and sport-specific exercises are all discussed in this section.

Periodization

A significant challenge for therapists who work with athletes is designing an optimal training program that facilitates neural and muscular adaptation while being mindful of tissue healing constraints. By using periodization, a therapist can manipulate training variables such as intensity, duration, frequency, and skill training to meet established goals.[29] The progressive changes in the training program prevent a plateau in progress from occurring and continually challenge the athlete to achieve peak performance; helping the athlete meet her or his needs depending on offseason, preseason, midseason, or postseason. There are three cycles of periodization that occur in a program: microcycle (1 week), mesocycle (≥1 month), and macrocycle (1 year–4 years). There are four phases in which these cycles occur to create a periodization program. The phases are preparatory, transition, competition, and secondary transition. During the preparatory phase, the goal is to maximize a particular variable (i.e., strength or power), which is performed at high intensities and low to moderate volumes. At the first transition, intensity starts to decrease, and more sport-specific drills begin. Each program that is designed for an athlete must also reflect if he or she is in season or out of season. There is potential to use these various models of periodization for more "long-term" rehabilitation programs, such as labral repairs of the shoulder, rotator cuff repairs, or ulnar collateral ligament reconstructions, to see if recovery time can be improved upon or if clinical testing methods for performance can be optimized.[29] Because of a lack of communication, programming models fail to fully bridge the gap between rehabilitation and the corresponding training models of strength and conditioning that coaches use to help athletes peak for competition.[29,30] Greater knowledge of periodization models can help therapists in their evaluation, clinical reasoning skills, exercise progression, and goal setting for the sustained return of athletes to high-level competition.[30]

Traditional Therapy

Initially, the rehabilitation program is specific to the injury and surgical procedure. The application of stress to the healing tissues is timed and progressed according to the phase of healing and patient progress.

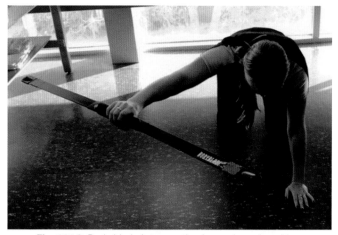
Fig. 114.3 Body blade into scaption in quadruped position.

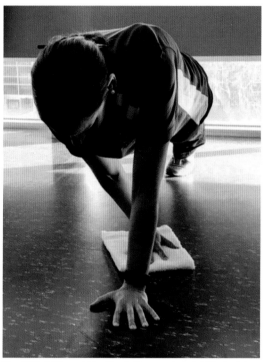
Fig. 114.4 Closed kinetic chain scapular stability training.

What is unique is that an additional phase of rehabilitation is added after healing and is directed to preparing the athlete to return to sport.

Traditional rehabilitation usually starts with the restoration of pain-free ROM across the injured joint(s) after the tissues have healed enough to tolerate this level of stress. This is usually accomplished with gentle ROM that is progressed as tolerated to include other diagnosis appropriate techniques such as joint mobilization and myofascial release of soft tissue restrictions. Additional components to focus on include postural reeducation, joint mobility, muscle and tissue mobility above and below the injury, and neuromuscular control. In the early stages of rehabilitation incorporating isometrics, stabilization and early neuromuscular control will stimulate activation and control of key muscles.[31] Neuromuscular control and stabilization can be performed in multiple-angled settings, open chain or closed chain.[31] ROM is first to be restored by body weight (thrower's 10), and then progression to elastic resistance bands (Proprioceptive Neuromuscular Facilitation [PNF] patterns), machines, free weights, and functional exercises (i.e., using the suspension trainer, body blade, sand bags, medicine balls) are used to restore the athlete's strength. Examples of these interventions

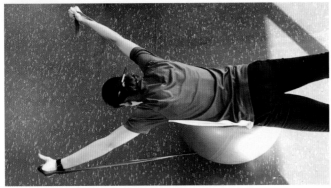

Fig. 114.5 Prone scaption on a physioball with TheraBand resistance.

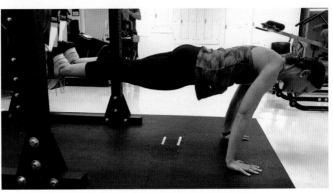

Fig. 114.8 Prone weight shifting with suspension trainer.

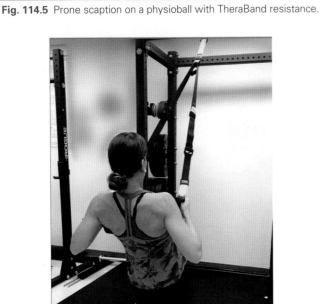

Fig. 114.6 Double arm row on suspension trainer.

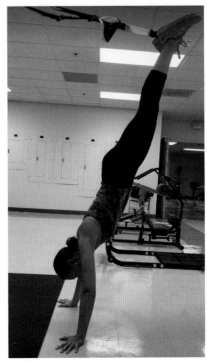

Fig. 114.9 Walk up handstand on suspension trainer.

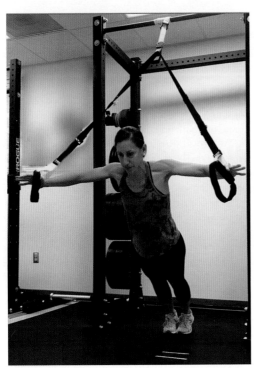

Fig. 114.7 Pectoralis flies on supsension trainer.

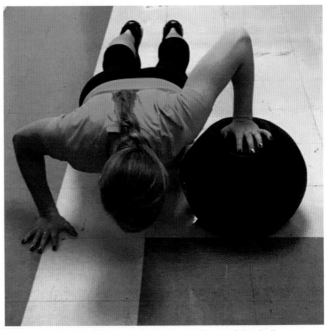

Fig. 114.10 Dynamic push-up with medicine ball.

can be seen in Figs. 114.3 to 114.11. Many different types of exercises can be performed, but the key is not to progress too quickly. For example, having an athlete perform single-arm dumbbell military press before having shoulder stability could cause further injury and develop poor form. A variety of exercise options exist, but all exercises used in the rehabilitation of an injured athlete should be taught properly with particular focus on form before advancing to the next phase of rehabilitation.

Advanced Functional Exercises

The more advanced functional and unconventional training techniques such as battle ropes, kettle bells, tires, sledgehammers, bodyweight suspension devices, and sleds have become more popular with the athletic population.[32] These different types of exercises require more in skill, technique, proper mechanics, and coordination than the conventional rehabilitation exercises. Unconventional exercises initiate the competitive drive in athletes and provide a positive mental boost.

A popular way to enhance muscle performance is through the use of plyometric training. Plyometric training is when the body goes through a quick stretching of the muscle from eccentric to concentric contraction.[32] The stretch shortening cycle requires the neuromuscular system to react quickly and efficiently after an eccentric muscle action to produce a concentric contraction for acceleration.[33,34] There are three phases to plyometrics: (1) prestretch (eccentric contraction), (2) amortization phase, and (3) shortening phase (concentric contraction).[33,34]

The prestretch phase is also known as the loading phase. During this phase, there is an increase in muscle spindle activity. There are three important factors that need to be reinforced: rate, magnitude, and duration. The transition period between the eccentric contraction and concentric contraction of the muscles is called amortization.[32,33,34] This transition period is important because a prolonged rest period can decrease the potential energy produced during the exercise. The last phase in a plyometric exercise is the shortening phase. A quick concentric contraction that allows the movement to become explosive.[32,33,34]

Plyometrics enhance excitability, sensitivity, and the reactivity of the neuromuscular system.[32,33,34] Additional benefits of using this type of exercises with athletes are increases in rate of force production, motor unit recruitment, firing frequency, and motor unit synchronization.[32,33,34] The ultimate goal is to increase the ability of the muscles to exert maximal force output in a minimal amount of time.[32,33,34] It is important to implement the appropriate types of plyometrics (upper extremity, lower extremity, core) into an athlete's rehabilitation depending on her or his sport.

Advanced Weight Training

The advanced weight training phase of rehabilitation consists of higher intensity, ballistic, and sport-specific exercise. Olympic weightlifting is a common training technique when working with elite athletes to enhance performance and facilitate or enhance the return-to-practice transition. During traditional Olympic weightlifting, there is a brief acceleration of the weight during first third of the concentric motion followed by a controlled deceleration phase.[31,34] Olympic weightlifting allows the athlete to create a strength base, from which the athlete can then progress to sport-specific activities. Ballistic training is a type of training in which an exercise is performed with acceleration (explosiveness) through the full ROM. Ballistic training requires the recruitment of the central nervous system and type II muscle fibers to produce the greatest amount of force in the shortest amount of time.[34] Using ballistic training will allow the muscles to adapt to explosive actions and reactions, as well as increase the growth and improve the recruitment of muscle fibers. Common ballistic training exercises includes bench throw, jump squat, clean, snatch, and push press. As the athlete's therapist, it is important to collaborate with the strength and conditioning coaches at this stage to work on exercise form and technique. After

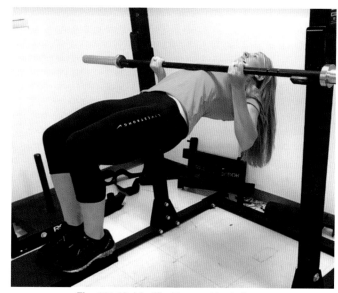

Fig. 114.11 Modified inverted barbell row.

successful completion of this phase, the athlete should have a smooth transition back to being an active member of the team.

Sports-Specific Exercises

The final phase of rehabilitation is all about sports-specific exercises and returning to practice and sport. During the final two phases, it is vital to incorporate both the athletic trainers and the strength and conditioning coaches in the rehabilitation. Incorporating athletic trainers and strength and condition coaches will help with the specific agility drills, functional assessments, sports drills, speed, and dynamic movements that are required in each sport. Another part of this phase includes different throwing protocols, hitting programs, rowing protocols, and other sport-specific requirements that an athlete will need to be able to execute with no symptoms and compensatory motions. Before the athlete can return to sport, a reassessment of initial functional tests should be performed. There are many resources that are available to keep the therapist up to date on the latest protocols and sport specific exercises in the literature. Online are quick links to in-depth manuals published by the NCAA for individual sports that contain information about protective equipment, concussion, return to play, season training, substance abuse, and much more.

ORTHOTIC INTERVENTION, TAPING, AND BRACING

During the later phases of rehabilitation after an athletic injury, attention is paid to protection of the injured joint or area of the upper extremity from repeated trauma and reinjury. Custom orthoses, prefabricated braces, and various taping techniques may be used and are designed or selected based on the specific injury, residual limitations, and vulnerable structures as well as the specific sport. Rigid or semirigid orthoses intended for use during play must comply with the rules and regulations of any applicable regulatory agencies such as the NCAA. The NCAA has posted guidelines for protective equipment for specific sports. Mandatory protective equipment is outlined as well as the rules governing special protective equipment. In general, any orthosis that might be dangerous to an opposing player is prohibited (e.g., a rigid thermoplastic orthosis or a prefabricated brace with metal stays). However, depending on the sport, hard or unyielding devices may be permitted, if covered. For example, in college football, hand and arm casts or orthoses to protect a fracture or dislocation, if covered, are permitted. The device must be covered on all exterior sides and edges with closed-cell, slow-recovery foam padding no less than ½ inch thick or a similar material of the same specifications (Fig. 114.12). In contrast, in track and field events at the college level, no taping of any part of the hand is permitted in the discus and javelin throws or for the shot put except to cover or protect an open wound. The therapist must be aware of any relevant rulings by the governing body of a sport that might affect the return-to-play phase of the rehabilitation program of the injured athlete. Collaboration with coaches and trainers is helpful and important at this stage of the process.

The specific orthosis, brace, or taping method selected may be used to provide protection against impact or to limit extremes of motion or force. For example, a dorsal wrist block orthosis (Fig. 114.13) can be used to prevent excessive wrist hyperextension in a gymnast. Taping can also be used to limit extremes of wrist flexion and extension (Fig. 114.14). To limit wrist motion in one direction, the X technique of application is used[9] (Fig. 114.15). The tape is applied in an X configuration to the volar aspect of the wrist if wrist extension is to be restricted and is applied dorsally if wrist flexion is to be restricted. Similarly, the X technique can be used to limit hyperextension of the elbow (Fig. 114.16). Taping can be used to protect an injured thumb ulnar collateral ligament (Fig. 114.17) or proximal interphalangeal joint collateral ligament (Fig. 114.18). A more specialized device is the dowel grip (Fig. 114.19) used by gymnasts to decrease the muscular contraction forces required to maintain grip.[10]

Traditional athletic taping encloses or encapsulates a joint to provide stability and restrict movement. Kinesio taping is an elastic taping method using woven cotton, highly elasticized tape that is applied to the skin with a light stretch and is significantly different from traditional taping in the method of application and functional goals. The Kinesio Taping Method focuses on applying tape over and around muscles that control specific movements and is useful for athletes returning to their sports after injuries. Chapter 103 includes a detailed review of this elastic taping method.

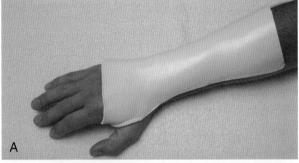

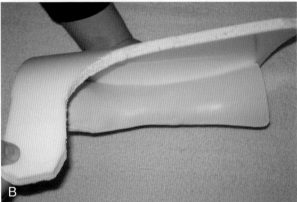

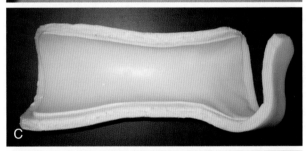

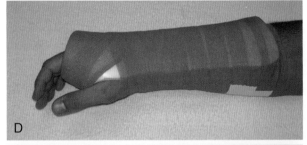

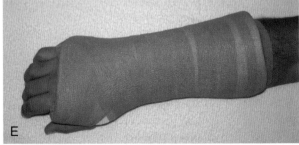

Fig. 114.12 A–E, Thermoplastic wrist orthosis covered with padding for use during play.

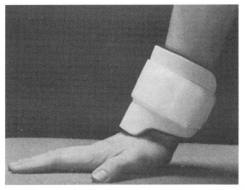

Fig. 114.13 A dorsal wrist block orthosis used to prevent excessive wrist hyperextension in the gymnast.

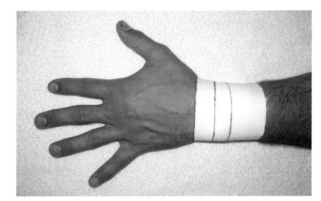

Fig. 114.14 Wrist taping to provide support and mild restriction of motion.

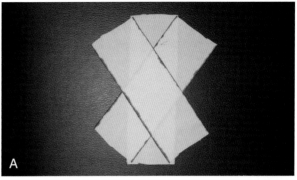

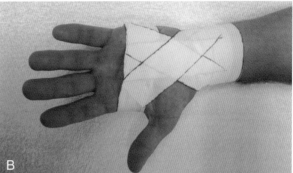

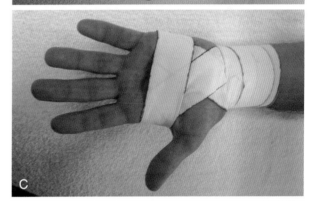

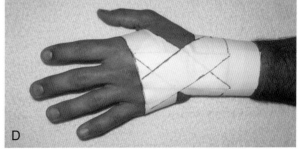

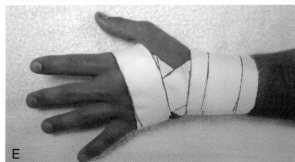

Fig. 114.15 A, X configuration of tape. **B and C,** Tape applied in an X configuration to the volar aspect of the wrist to restrict wrist extension. **D and E,** X taping is applied dorsally if wrist flexion is to be restricted.

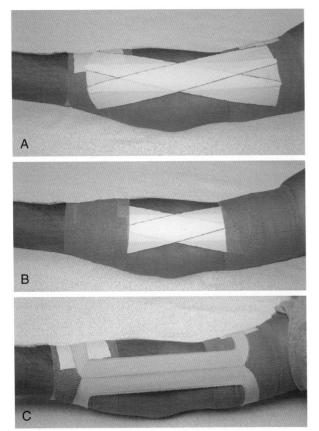

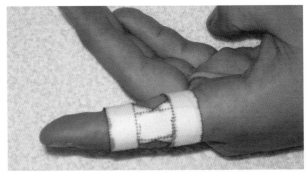

Fig. 114.18 Taping used to protect a proximal interphalangeal joint collateral ligament.

Fig. 114.16 A, The X taping technique can be used to limit hyperextension of the elbow. **B,** Distal and proximal anchors of X taping covered with 2-inch self-adherent wrap. **C,** Elastic athletic tape used as an alternative to standard white tape.

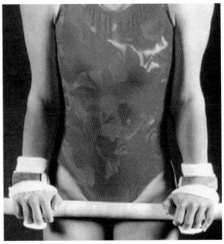

Fig. 114.19 The dowel grip used by a gymnast to decrease the muscular contraction forces required to maintain grip.

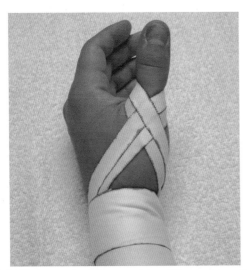

Fig. 114.17 Taping used to protect an injured thumb ulnar collateral ligament.

SUMMARY

Rehabilitation of injured athletes is challenging but rewarding. The challenge lies in designing and executing a rehabilitation program that adequately prepares the athlete for return to her or his sport and reduces the risk of reinjury. The reward lies in working with an individual who is typically motivated to return to his or her prior level of competition. Each athlete is unique, and the rehabilitation program must be tailored according to the individual' needs and requirements of the athlete. It is important for the rehabilitation professional to understand the cause of the athletic injury, as well as the demands of the specific sport to develop an appropriate and effective treatment program. Collaboration with the multidisciplinary team is helpful in achieving a positive outcome.

ACKNOWLEDGMENTS

The editors recognize the contributions of Thomas H. Bertini, Jr., DPT, ATC; Tessa J. Laidig, DPT; Nicole M. Pettit, DPT; Christina M. Read, DPT; Michael Scarneo, DPT; Michael J. Wylykanowitz, Jr., DPT; Jane Fedorczyk, PT, PhD, CHT, ATC; and Terri M. Skirven, OTR/L, CHT to this chapter in previous editions of this text.

REFERENCES

1. Leddy JJ, Sandhu H, Sodhi V, Baker JG, Willer B. Rehabilitation of concussion and post-concussion syndrome. *Sports Health*. 2012;4:147–154.
2. Sawyer Q, Vesci B, McLeod TCV. Physical activity and intermittent post-concussion symptoms after a period of symptom-limited physical and cognitive rest. *J Athl Train*. 2016;51:739–742.
3. Novak Z, Aglipay M, Barrowman N, Yeates KO, et al. Association of persistent post-concussion symptoms with pediatric quality of life. *JAMA Ped*. 2016;170:345–353.
4. Wasserman E, Abar B, Shah M, Wasserman D, Bazarian J. Concussions are associated with decreased batting performance among Major League Baseball players. *Am J Sports Med*. 2015;43:1127–1133.
5. Roche–Nagle G, Ryan R, Barry M, Brophy D. Effort thrombosis of the upper extremity in a young sportsman: Paget–Schroetter syndrome. *Br J Sports Med*. 2007;41:540–541.
6. Bushnell BD, Anz AW, Dugger K, Sakryd GA, Noonan TJ. Effort thrombosis presenting as pulmonary embolism in a professional baseball pitcher. *Sports Health*. 2009;1:493–499.
7. Durant TJS, Swanson BT, Cote MP, et al. Upper extremity deep venous venous thromboembolism following arthroscopic labral repair of the shoulder and biceps tenodesis: a case report. *Int J Sports Phys Ther*. 2014;9:377–382.
8. Starr LM. *An Interdisciplinary Sports Medicine Team Model for Sunshine State Conference Athletic Programs*. Applied Dissertation, Nova Southeastern University; 2013.
9. Prentice WE. Arnheim's principles of athletic training: a competency-based approach 2006:12. National Institute of Mental Health.
10. Manske R, Tyler T. The SPTs Sports Certified Specialist Examination Preparatory Course.
11. Talpey SW, Siesmaa EJ. Sports injury prevention: the role of the strength and conditioning coach. *Stren Cond J*. 2017;39:14–19.
12. Voight M, Hickey A, Piper M. The leadership techniques and practices of elite collegiate strength and conditioning. *Sport J*. 2017. Accessed Online at: www.thesportjournal.org in 11/2017.
13. FMS Scoring Criteria. Accessed Online at: https://www.functionalmovement.com/system/FMS.
14. 2016-17 High School Athletics Participation Survey. Available At: www.nfhs.org/participationstatistics/pdf/2016-17_participation_survey_results.pdf.
15. Cook G, Burton L, Hoogenboom BJ. Functional movement screening: the use of fundamental movements as an assessment of function-part 1. *Int J Sports Phys Ther*. 2014;9:396–409.
16. Cook G, Burton L, Hoogenboom BJ. Functional movement screening: the use of fundamental movements as an assessment of function-part 2. *Int J Sports Phys Ther*. 2014;9:549–563.
17. Garrison M, Westrick R, Johnson MR, Benenson J. Association between the functional movement screen and injury development in college athletes. *Int J Sports Phys Ther*. 2015;10:21–28.
18. Gulgin HR, Schulte BC, Crawley AA. Correlation of Titleist Performance Institute (TPI) level 1 movement screens and golf swings faults. *J Strength Cond Res*. 2014;28:534–539.
19. SFMA. Available at: www.functionalmovement.com
20. Goshtigian GR, Swanson BT. Using the selective functional movement assessment and regional interdependence theory to guide treatment of an athlete with back pain: a case report. *Int J Sports Phys Ther*. 2016;11:575–595.
21. Lorenz D, Morrison S. Current concepts in periodization of strength and conditioning for the sports physical therapist. *Int J Sports Phys Ther*. 2015;10:734–747.
22. Gorman PP, Butler RJ, Plisky PJ, Kiesel KB. Upper quarter y balance test: reliability and performance comparison between genders in active adults. *J Strength Cond Res*. 2012;26:3043–3048.
23. Westrick RB, Miller JM, Carow SD, Verber JP. Exploration of the Y-balance test for assessment of upper quarter closed kinetic chain performance. *Int J Sports Phys Ther*. 2012;7:139–147.
24. Jones M, Lorenzo D. Assessment of power, speed, and agility in athletic, preadolescent youth. *J Sports Med Phys Fitness*. 2013;53:693–700.
25. Pontillo M, Spinelli BA, Sennett BJ. Prediction of in-season shoulder injury from preseason testing in Division I collegiate football players. *Sports Health*. 2014;6:497–503.
26. Coyne JOC, Tran TT, Secomb JL, Lundgren L, Farley ORL, Newton RU, Sheppard JM. Reliability of pull up and dip maximal strength tests. *J Australian Strength and Conditioning*. 2015;23:21–27.
27. Tarara DT, Fogaca LK, Taylor JB, Hegedus EJ. Clinician-friendly physical performance tests in athletes part 3: a systematic review of measurement properties and correlations to injury for tests in the upper extremity. *Br J Sports Med*. 2016;50:545–551.
28. Borms D, Maenhout A, Cools AM. Upper quadrant field tests and isokinetic upper limb strength in overhead athletes. *J Athletic Training*. 2016;51:789–796.
29. Hoover DL, VanWye WR, Judge LW. Periodization and physical therapy: Bridging the gap between training and rehabilitation. *Phys Ther Sport*. 2016;18:1–20. https://www.ncbi.nlm.nih.gov/pubmed/26679784.
30. Kisner C, Colby LA. *Therapeutic Exercise: Foundations and Techniques*. 6th ed. Philadelphia: F.A. Davis Company; 2012:529–550, 578–585.
31. Singla D, Hussain ME, Moiz JA. Effect of upper body plyometric training on physical performance in healthy individuals: a systematic review. *Phys Ther Sport*. 2017;11:1466–1483.
32. Turgut E, Cinar-Medeni O, Colakoglu FF, Baltaci G. "Ballistic Six" upper-extremity plyometric training for the pediatric volleyball players. *J Strength Cond Res*. 2017;8:17–35.
33. Swanik KA, Thomas SJ, Struminger AH, Bliven KC, Kelly JD, Swanik CB. The effect of shoulder plyometric training on amortization time and upper-extremity kinematics. *J Sport Rehab*. 2016;25:315–323.
34. Magee DJ, Manske RC, Zachazewski, Quillen WS. *Athletic and Sports Issues in Musculoskeletal Rehabilitation*. St. Louis: Elsevier; 2011:385–400.
35. Palsbo SE. Epidemiology of recreational archery injuries: implications for archery ranges and injury prevention. *J Sports Med Phys Fitness*. 2012;52(3):293–299.
36. Rayan GM. Archery-related injuries of the hand, forearm, and elbow. *South Med J*. 1992;85(10):961–964.
37. Miyake E, Yatsunami M, Kurabayashi J, Teruya K, et al. a prospective epidemiological study of injuries in Japanese national tournament-level badminton players from junior high school to university. *Asian J Sports Med*. 2016. 1;7(1):e29637.
38. Park J, Lee Y, Kong ID. Ultrasonographic changes of upper extremity tendons in recreational badminton players: the effect of hand dominance and comparison with clinical findings. *Br J Sports Med*. 2017;51:370.
39. Saper MG, Pierpoint LA, Liu W, Comstock RD, Polousky JD, Andrews JR. Epidemiology of shoulder and elbow injuries among United States high school baseball players: school years 2005-2006 Through 2014-2015. *Am J Sports Med*. 2017 1;2:546–560.

40. Li X, Zhou H, Williams P, et al. The epidemiology of single season musculoskeletal injuries in professional baseball. *Orthop Rev.* 2013;5(1):243–247.

41. Ito E, Iwamoto J, Azuma K, Matsumoto H. Sex-specific differences in injury types among basketball players. *J Sports Med.* 2014;6:1–6.

42. Loosemore M, Lightfoot J, Palmer-Green D, Gatt I, et al. https://www.ncbi.nlm.nih.gov/pubmed/?term=Bilzon%20J%5BAuthor%5D&cauthor=true&cauthor_uid=26192194: Boxing injury epidemiology in the Great Britain team: a 5-year surveillance study of medically diagnosed injury incidence and outcome. *Br J Sports Med.* 2015;49(17):1100–1107.

43. Franklin RC, Leggat PA. The epidemiology of injury in canoeing, kayaking and rafting. *Med Sport Sci.* 2012;58:98–111.

44. Nathanson AT, Young JM, Young C. Pre-participation medical evaluation for adventure and wilderness watersports. *Clin J Sport Med.* 2015;25:425–431.

45. Jacobson NA, Morawa LG, Bir CA. Epidemiology of cheerleading injuries presenting to NEISS hospitals from 2002 to 2007. *J Trauma Acute Care Surg.* 2012;72(2):521–526.

46. Laudner KG, Metz B, Thomas DQ. Anterior glenohumeral laxity and stiffness after a shoulder-strengthening program in collegiate cheerleaders. *J Athl Train.* 2013;48(1):25–30.

47. Thornton J, Vinther A, Wilson F, Lebrun C, et al. Rowing injuries: an updated review. *Sports Med.* 2016.

48. Dhillon MS, John R, Dhillon H, Dhillon S, Prabhakar S. Hamulus stress fracture in a batsman: an unusual injury in cricket - a case report and review of literature. *J Orthop Case Rep.* 2017;7(3):25–30.

49. Ahearn N, Bhatia R, Griffin S. Hand and wrist injuries in professional county cricket. *Hand Surg.* 2015;20(1):89–92.

50. Summitt RJ, Cotton RA, Kays AC, Slaven EJ. Shoulder injuries in individuals who participate in crossfit training. *Sports Health.* 2016;8(6):541–546.

51. Aleman KB, Meyers MC. Mountain biking injuries in children and adolescents. *Sports Med.* 2010;40(1):77–90.

52. Chen TL, Wong DW, Wang Y, Ren S, Yan F, Zhang M. Biomechanics of fencing sport: a scoping review. *PLoS One.* 2017;12(2):e0171578.

53. Agel J, Harvey EJ. A 7-year review of men's and women's ice hockey injuries in the NCAA. *Can J Surg.* 2010;53(5):319–323.

54. Dick R, Hootman JM, Agel J, Vela L, Marshall SW, Messina R. Descriptive epidemiology of collegiate women's field hockey injuries: National Collegiate Athletic Association Injury Surveillance System, 1988-1989 through 2002-2003. *J Athl Train.* 2007;42(2):211–220.

55. Dick R, Ferrara MS, Agel J, et al. Descriptive epidemiology of collegiate men's football injuries: National Collegiate Athletic Association Injury Surveillance System, 1988-1989 through 2003-2004. *J Athl Train.* 2007;42(2):221–233.

56. Murray AD, Daines L, Archibald D, et al. The relationships between golf and health: a scoping review. *Br J Sports Med.* 2017;51(1):12–19.

57. Woo SH, Lee YK, Kim JM, Cheon HJ, Chung WH. Hand and wrist injuries in golfers and their treatment. *Hand Clin.* 2017;33(1):81–96.

58. Benjamin HJ, Engel SC, Chudzik D. Wrist pain in gymnasts: a review of common overuse wrist pathology in the gymnastics athlete. *Curr Sports Med Rep.* 2017;16(5):322–329.

59. Kay MC, Register-Mihalik JK, Gray AD, Djoko A, et al. The epidemiology of severe injuries sustained by National Collegiate Athletic Association Student-Athletes, 2009-2010 Through 2014-2015. *J Athl Train.* 2017;52(2):117–128.

60. Giroto N, Hespanhol junior LC, Gomes MR, Lopes AD. Incidence and risk factors of injuries in Brazilian elite handball players: a prospective cohort study. *Scand J Med Sci Sports.* 2017;27(2):195–202.

61. Andersson SH, Bahr R, Clarsen B, et al. Risk factors for overuse shoulder injuries in a mixed-sex cohort of 329 elite handball players: previous findings could not be confirmed. *Br J Sports Med Published Online First.* 2017.

62. Mosenthal W, Kim M, Holzshu R, Hanypsiak B, Athiviraham A. Common ice hockey injuries and treatment: a current concepts review. *Curr Sports Med Rep.* 2017;16(5):357–362.

63. Mölsä J, Kujala U, Myllynen P, Torstila I, Airaksinen O. Injuries to the upper extremity in ice hockey: analysis of a series of 760 injuries. *Am J Sports Med.* 2003;31(5):751–757.

64. Akoto R, Lambert C, Balke M, Bouillon B, Frosch KH, Höher J. Epidemiology of injuries in judo: a cross-sectional survey of severe injuries based on time loss and reduction in sporting level. *Br J Sports Med.* 2017;47(19):37–48.

65. Pocecco E, Ruedl G, Stankovic N, et al. Injuries in judo: a systematic literature review including suggestions for prevention. *Br J Sports Med.* 2013;47(18):1139–1143.

66. Kerr ZY, Lincoln AE, Dodge T, Yeargin SW, et al. Epidemiology of youth boys' and girls' lacrosse injuries in the 2015-2016 seasons. *Med Sci Sports Exerc.* 2017.

67. Gardner EC, Chan WW, Sutton KM, Blaine TA. Shoulder injuries in men's collegiate lacrosse, 2004-2009. *Am J Sports Med.* 2016;44(10):2675–2681.

68. Farkash U, Dreyfuss D, Funk S, Dreyfuss U. Prevalence and patterns of injury sustained during military hand-to-hand combat training (Krav-Maga). *Mil Med.* 2017;182(11).

69. Kamonseki DH, Cedin L, Habechian FAP, Piccolomo GF, Camargo PR. Glenohumeral internal rotation deficit in table tennis players. *J Sports Sci.* 2017;17:1–5.

70. Attarian A, Siderelis C. Injuries in commercial whitewater rafting on the New and Gauley rivers of West Virginia. *Wilderness Environ Med.* 2013;24(4):309–314.

71. Franklin RC, Leggat PA. The epidemiology of injury in canoeing, kayaking and rafting. *Med Sport Sci.* 2012;58:98–111.

72. Stuelcken M, Mellifont D, Gorman A, Sayers M. wrist injuries in tennis players: a narrative review. *Sports Med.* 2017;47(5):857–868.

73. McDonald JW, Henrie AM, Teramoto M, Medina E, Willick SE. Descriptive epidemiology, medical evaluation and outcomes of rock climbing injuries. *Wild Env Med.* 2017;28:185–196.

74. Mirhadi S, Ashwood N, Karagkevrekis B. Review of rollerblading. *Trauma.* 2015;17:29–32.

75. Rizi RM, Yeung SS, Stewart NJ, Yeung EW. Risk factors that predict severe injuries In University Rugby Sevens Players. *J Sci And Med In Sport.* 2017;20:648–652.

76. Booth M, Orr R. Time-loss injuries in sub-elite and emerging rugby league players. *J Sports Sci Med.* 2017;16:295–301.

77. Zalavras C, Nikolopoulou G, Essin D, et al. Pediatric fractures during skateboarding, roller skating and scooter riding. *Am J Sports Med.* 2005;33:568–573.

78. Forsman L, Eriksson A. Skateboarding injuries of today including commentary by Svanstrom L. *Brit J Sports Med.* 2001;35:325–328.

79. Laver L, Pengas IP, Mei-Dan O. Injuries in extreme sports. *J Ortho Surg Res.* 2017;12:1–8.

80. McKenna MJ, Riccio AI, Sciarretta KH. Orthopaedic injuries associated with skimboarding. *Am J Sports Med.* 2009;37:1425–1428.

81. Westman A, Bjornstig U. Injuries in Swedish skydiving. *Brit J Sports Med.* 2007;41:356–364.

82. Ostojic S. Comparing sports injuries in soccer: influence of a positional role. *Res Sports Med.* 2003;11:203–208.

83. Boyd K, Brownson P, Hunter J. Distal radial fractures in young goalkeepers: a case for an appropriately sized soccer ball. *Brit J Sports Med.* 2001;35:409–411.

84. Lear A, Patel N. Softball pitching and injury. *Cur Sports Med Reports.* 2016;15:336–341.

85. Winwood PW, Hume PA, Cronin JB, Keogh JWL. Retrospective injury epidemiology of strongman athletes. *J Strength Cond Res.* 2014;28:28–42.

86. Furness J, Hing W, Walsh J, et al. Acute injuries in recreational and competitive surfers. *Am J Sports Med.* 2015;43:1246–1254.

87. Kerr ZY, Baugh CM, Hibberd EE, et al. Epidemiology of national collegiate athletic association men's and women's swimming and diving injuries from 2009/2010 To 2013/2014. *Br J Sports Med.* 2015;49:465–471.

88. Meron A, Saint-Phard D. Track and field throwing sports: injuries and prevention. *Cur Sports Med Rep.* 2017;16:391–396.

89. Rebella G. A prospective study of injury patterns in collegiate pole vaulters. *Am J Sports Med.* 2015;43:808–815.

90. Dines JS. Tennis injuries: epidemiology, pathophysiology, and treatment. *J Am Acad Ortho Surg.* 2015;23:181–189.

91. Swedler DI, Nuwer JM, Nazarov A, et al. Incidence and descriptive epidemiology of injuries to college ultimate players. *J Athl Train.* 2015;50:419–425.

92. Agel J, Palmieri-Smith R, Dick R, Wojtys E, Marshall S. Descriptive epidemiology of collegiate women's volleyball injuries: National Collegiate Athletic Association Injury Surveillance System, 1988-1989 Through 2003-2004. *J Athl Train.* 2007;42:295–302.

93. Stickley CD, Hetzler RK, Freemyer BG, Kimura I. Isokinetic peak torque ratios and shoulder injury history in adolescent female volleyball athletes. *J Athl Train.* 2008;43:571–577.

94. Reeser J, Verhagen E, Briner W, Askeland T, Bahr R. Strategies for the prevention of volleyball related injuries including commentary By Knobloch K. *Brit J Sports Med.* 2006;40:594–600.

95. Miller AH, Evans K, Adams R, Waddington G, Witchalls J. Shoulder injury in water polo: a systematic review of incidence and intrinsic risk factors. *J Sci Med Sport.* 2017. Available At: Http://Dx.Doi.Org/10.1016/J.Jsams.2017.08.015.

96. Spittler J, Keeling J. Water polo injuries and training methods. *Cur Sports Med Rep.* 2016;15:410–416.

97. Hostetler SG, Hostetler TL, Smith GA, Xiang H. Characteristics of water skiing-related and wakeboarding-related injuries treated in emergency departments in the United States, 2001-2003. *Am J Sports Med.* 2005;33:1065–1070.

98. Raske A, Norlin R. Injury incidence and prevalence among elite weight and power lifters. *Am J Sports Med.* 2002;30:248–256.

99. Haupt H. Upper extremity injuries associated with strength training. *Clin Sports Med.* 2001;20:481–490.

100. Keogh J, Hume P, Pearson S. Retrospective injury epidemiology of one hundred one competitive Oceania power lifters: the effects of age, body mass, competitive standard, and gender. *J Strength Cond Res.* 2006;20:672–681.

101. Chalmers DJ, Morrison L. Epidemiology of non-submersion injuries in aquatic sporting and recreational activities. *Sports Med.* 2003;33:745–770.

102. Yard E, Collins CL, Dick RW, Comstock RD. An epidemiologic comparison of high school and college wrestling injuries. *Am J Sports Med.* 2008;36:57–64.

103. Powell J, Barber-Foss K. Injury patterns in selected high school sports: a review of the 1995-1997 seasons. *J Athl Train.* 1999;34:277–284.

104. Agel J, Ransone J, Randall D, et al. Descriptive epidemiology of collegiate men's wrestling injuries: National Collegiate Athletic Association Injury Surveillance System, 1988-1989 through 2003-2004. *J Athl Train.* 2007;42:303–310.

105. Jarrett G, Orwin J, Dick R. Injuries in collegiate wrestling. *Am J Sports Med.* 1998;26:674–680.

115

Clinical Conditions in Patients with Breast Cancer

Bryan Anthony Spinelli

OUTLINE

CRITICAL POINTS

- Patients diagnosed with breast cancer are at risk for experiencing upper body morbidity (pain, impaired shoulder range of motion, axillary web syndrome, adhesive capsulitis, rotator cuff disease, lymphedema) and cancer-related fatigue.
- After breast cancer treatment, patients may experience nociceptive pain from surgical incisions or muscle injury or neuropathic pain from nerves within the surgical field being injured.
- A structured exercise program is recommended for patients after breast surgery to restore shoulder function while minimizing risk for complications.
- Physical examination for breast cancer–related lymphedema includes Stemmer's sign, visual inspection, pitting examination, and examination for tissue texture changes.
- Recommended objective measures for breast cancer–related lymphedema include circumferential measurement, water displacement, and bioimpedance spectroscopy.

- Complete decongestive therapy is a conservative treatment strategy for breast cancer–related lymphedema that includes skin care, manual lymphatic drainage, compression therapy, and exercise.
- Evidence supports the use of intermittent pneumatic compression (IPC) devices for treatment of breast cancer–related lymphedema; however IPC devices are not recommended as sole treatment.
- Therapists' role in the management of cancer-related fatigue includes patient education (pattern of fatigue, self-monitoring, energy conservation, sleep hygiene) and exercise prescription.
- Exercise programs should be individualized, taking into consideration side effects of cancer and its treatment (i.e., limitations from surgery or radiation, bone metastasis, anemia, thrombocytopenia, neutropenia).

INTRODUCTION

Breast cancer accounts for approximately 15% of all new cancer cases diagnosed annually in the United States.[1] Long-term survival has improved over the past few decades because of earlier detection and improvements in medical management.[2] However, many patients experience side effects or persistent long-term effects because of the nature of the treatments for breast cancer that can negatively impact quality of life. This chapter provides an overview of breast cancer treatment and select problems experienced by patients who undergo breast cancer treatment that are amendable to rehabilitation.

BREAST CANCER TREATMENT

Treatment options for breast cancer include surgery, radiation, chemotherapy, endocrine therapy, and biologic therapy.[3] A patient diagnosed with breast cancer may receive one or a combination of these treatments, depending on a number of factors that include tumor histology, primary tumor characteristics, axillary lymph node status, tumor hormone receptor and *HER2* status, genetic testing, presence or absence of metastatic disease, comorbidities, age, menopausal status and patient preference.[3] A description of the treatment options for breast cancer is provided next.

Surgery

Surgery is the mainstay of invasive breast cancer treatment for local and regional control.[4] Two primary surgeries for local control are breast-conserving surgery and mastectomy. Breast-conserving surgery (i.e., lumpectomy, wide local excision, and partial mastectomy) involves removal of the tumor with a margin of healthy surrounding tissue. Mastectomy is a more extensive surgical procedure for patients who are not candidates for breast conserving surgery or prefer mastectomy over breast-conserving surgery.[5] Types of mastectomy include simple mastectomy, skin-sparing mastectomy, modified radical mastectomy, and radical mastectomy. A simple mastectomy refers to complete removal of the breast, overlying skin, and nipple–areolar complex.[5] For patients undergoing mastectomy with breast reconstruction, a skin-sparing mastectomy is performed.[5] This procedure involves removal of all breast tissue but preserves sufficient skin overlying the chest wall.[5] A skin-sparing mastectomy may be performed with or without preservation of the nipple. A modified radical mastectomy involves complete removal of the breast along with the overlying skin and axillary lymph node nodes, whereas a radical mastectomy includes removal of all breast tissue, pectoralis major and minor muscles, and axillary lymph nodes.

For patients who undergo mastectomy, there are a number of breast reconstruction options. Categories of breast reconstruction include autologous tissue, implant, or combined. A common autologous tissue breast reconstruction is the transverse rectus abdominis musculocutaneous (TRAM) flap. A pedicled TRAM flap involves transferring abdominal tissue to the chest wall by tunneling the tissue under the upper abdominal skin. A free TRAM flap involves removing the abdominal tissue and its blood supply, which is then connected to either the thoracodorsal or internal mammary vessels. Other procedures involving abdominal tissue include muscle-sparing TRAM flap, deep inferior epigastric perforator flap, and superficial inferior epigastric artery flap. A gluteal artery perforator flap or transverse upper gracilis flap are alternate breast reconstruction options that do not involve the abdominal tissue. Instead of using autologous tissue, breast reconstruction can be performed using different types of breast implants. The implant is usually placed underneath the pectoralis major muscle. Rather than placing the implant at the time of mastectomy, a tissue expander may be placed, which will require a second surgery at a later date. The expander is inflated to stretch the tissue to accommodate the size of the permanent breast implant by injecting saline into the expander every few weeks. Another breast reconstruction option that involves both autologous tissue and an implant is a latissimus dorsi musculocutaneous flap.

Some breast cancer surgical procedures may be performed that involve removal of axillary lymph nodes. Removal of axillary lymph nodes and determining the presence of cancer is important for determining prognosis and need for additional treatments. The axillary lymph nodes can be divided into three levels based on their location in relationship to the pectoralis minor muscle. Level I refers to lymph nodes that are lateral to the pectoralis minor. Level II lymph nodes are beneath the pectoralis minor. Level III lymph nodes are medial to the pectoralis minor. Individuals may have up to 60 axillary lymph nodes.[6]

Sentinel lymph node biopsy (SLNB) and axillary lymph node dissection (ALND) are two axillary surgeries used for the staging and treatment of breast cancer. An SLNB is performed by injecting a radiolabeled colloid and blue dye near the location of the tumor. The surgeon uses a device to identify the sentinel lymph node(s), which is the lymph node or nodes where the radiolabeled colloid and blue dye was transported. These lymph nodes are sent to pathology to determine whether the cancer has spread to the regional nodes. Depending on the extent of lymph node spread or other clinical factors, an ALND may be recommended, which typically involves the removal of all the lymph nodes in levels I and II.

Radiation Therapy

Radiation therapy uses types of energy such as photons or other particles to kill cancer cells by directly damaging DNA or indirectly through the creation of free radicals. Radiation may be delivered from outside the body (external beam) or from inside the body (brachytherapy). External-beam radiation therapy is a standard adjuvant treatment for most stages of invasive breast cancer in patients who undergo breast-conserving surgery.[3] The radiation treatment field typically includes the whole breast and may include the regional lymph node regions (infraclavicular, supraclavicular, internal mammary, axillary) depending on factors such as extent of nodal metastasis. Patients undergoing whole-breast irradiation with or without regional lymph node irradiation typically receive radiation daily for a total of 5 to 6 weeks.[3] Some patients diagnosed with early stage breast cancer may receive accelerated partial breast irradiation, which involves delivering radiation to only the region around the primary tumor. With accelerated partial breast irradiation, patients may receive radiation twice a day over 1 week.[4] For patients after mastectomy, radiation therapy may be indicated in those who present with factors suggesting intermediate to high risk of local-regional recurrence.[4]

Chemotherapy

Chemotherapy uses one or more drugs to kill cancer cells by targeting different phases of the cell cycle. Chemotherapy may be given before surgery (neoadjuvant) or after surgery (adjuvant). Chemotherapy is commonly administered intravenously through a vein or port-a-catheter that is inserted surgically underneath the skin, typically at the superior aspect of the anterior chest. Chemotherapy agents are typically prescribed in combination and are delivered in cycles every specified number of weeks. The side effects of chemotherapy agents vary based on the drug.

Endocrine Therapy

Tumors of the breast are tested for the presence of hormone receptors (estrogen and progesterone) upon diagnosis. If the tumor is considered hormone receptor positive, endocrine therapy is routinely recommended. Endocrine therapy includes classes of drugs such as selective estrogen receptor modulators (SERMs) and aromatase inhibitors (AIs). These drugs reduce disease recurrence rates and improve overall disease-free survival.[3] Side effects of both tamoxifen and AIs include hot flashes, night sweats, and vaginal dryness.[3] Patients taking tamoxifen have an increased risk of endometrial cancer and deep vein thrombosis (DVT) or pulmonary embolus, whereas patients taking AIs may experience muscle or joint pain and osteoporosis.[3]

Biologic Therapy

Biologic therapy uses the body's immune system to destroy cancer cells or specific antibodies that bind to the cancer cell to prevent tumor growth. Biologic therapy is used in patients with breast cancer whose cancer cells are *HER2* positive, which is a gene that assists in controlling how cells grow, divide, and repair. Trastuzumab is a humanized monoclonal antibody commonly used to treated *HER2*-positive breast cancer.[3] Trastuzumab is known to be cardiotoxic and cause congestive heart failure.[7] Patients receiving trastuzumab may also experience anemia, neutropenia, fatigue, nausea or vomiting, and diarrhea.[7]

UPPER BODY MORBIDITY

Patients diagnosed with breast cancer are at risk for upper body morbidity because of the nature of breast cancer and its treatments. Pain, impaired shoulder range of motion (ROM), and breast cancer–related lymphedema are common problems experienced by patients diagnosed with breast cancer that can negatively impact health-related quality of life. The following sections discuss these upper body problems likely to be seen by rehabilitation professionals.

Pain

Shoulder and arm pain has been reported to affect up to 68% of patients after breast cancer surgery.[8] Pain after breast cancer treatment may be directly-related to the cancer and its treatment or indirectly caused by treatment-related changes causing secondary health conditions or exacerbation of preexisting conditions.

The majority of patients after breast cancer surgery will experience acute postoperative pain.[9] They can also experience nociceptive or neuropathic pain. Nociceptive pain after breast surgery may occur from surgical incisions or muscle injury. For example, a window may be made in the pectoralis muscle and underlying rib to access blood vessels for anastomosis during a free flap breast reconstruction.[10] The pectoralis major may be used to create a submuscular pouch during a breast implant reconstruction procedure, which can involve separating the muscle attachments of the serratus anterior from the ribs and medially dissecting the pectoralis major toward the sternum, leaving the superior attachments intact.[11] Surgeons may retract the lateral aspect of the pectoralis major medially during ALND to expose the pectoralis minor muscle and allow dissection of any interpectoral lymph nodes.[12] The pectoralis minor muscle is retracted to expose and remove the level II and III axillary lymph nodes.[12] Thus, surgical trauma may lead to muscle spasm and hypertonicity, contributing to postoperative nociceptive pain.

Depending on the breast cancer surgery performed, a number of different nerves (i.e., intercostobrachial, long thoracic, thoracodorsal, lateral pectoral, and medial pectoral nerves) can be injured, causing neuropathic pain. The most common nerve injured during mastectomy and axillary surgery is the intercostobrachial nerve, which provides sensation to the shoulder and upper arm.[11] Neuropathic pain is often described as a burning, hot, shooting, electric shocks, pricking, numbness, tingling, and pins and needles. The prevalence of neuropathic pain in patients after breast cancer treatment has been reported to range from 14.2% to 27.2% for studies using screening questionnaires and 24.1% to 31.3% for studies using the Neuropathic Pain Special Interest Group of the International Association for the Study of Pain proposed criteria for neuropathic pain, which uses information from history and subjective complaints, clinical examination, and diagnostic testing to classify the likelihood of neuropathic pain.[13]

The following clinical guidelines have been suggested to differentiate among nociceptive, neuropathic, and central sensitization types of pain in patients after cancer treatment. First, clinicians should examine for the presence of neuropathic pain by (1) identifying if a lesion or disease of the nervous system is likely and (2) determining if pain is limited to a plausible neuroanatomical distribution and supported by both clinical examination and diagnostic tests.[15] Clinical examination of somatosensory function can include assessing touch, pain sensibility, vibration, and thermal sense.[15] Touch can be assessed using a piece of cotton wool or soft brush, whereas pain sensibility can be assessed using a wooden tooth pick.[15] Thermal sense of a 40°C warm object and 20°C cold object may be assessed, and vibration sense can be assessed using a 128-Hz tuning fork.[15] Clinicians should assess for somatosensory alterations such as allodynia (pain caused by a stimulus that does not usually provoke pain) and hyperalgesia (decreased pain threshold or increased intensity of pain sensation induced by noxious stimulation), which are findings consistent with neuropathic pain.[15]

Several tools have been used to screen patients for neuropathic pain.[15] One screening tool that has been validated in patients with breast cancer is The ID Pain, which is a patient-reported screening tool designed to differentiate between nociceptive and neuropathic pain.[16] The ID Pain consists of six items in which patients are asked if pain (1) feels like pins and needles, (2) feels hot or burning, (3) feels numb, (4) feels like electrical shocks, (5) is made worse with the touch of clothing or bed sheets, and (6) is limited to joints.[16] Items 1 through 5 are scored 1 if a patient responds "yes," and "yes" to item 6 is scored −1.[16] Patients with a history of breast cancer who score 2 or more on the ID Pain are four times more likely to have a diagnosis of neuropathic pain.[16]

If neuropathic pain is not suspected or if mixed pain is suspected, clinicians should attempt to determine nociceptive or central sensitization contribution to pain.[17] Central sensitization can be considered if (1) pain experience is disproportionate to the nature or extent of injury and (2) pain pattern is not neuroanatomically plausible.[17] If criterion 1 is met but criterion 2 is not met, it has been suggested that the presence of altered sensitivity to environmental factors (bright light, cold or heat, noise, stress, weather) and chemical stimuli (odors, pesticides, medication) would suggest central sensitization mechanism.[17] Administering the Central Sensitization Inventory (CSI) is a second proposed option for determining central sensitization mechanism in patients after cancer treatment.[17] The CSI includes a Part A and Part B. Part A of CSI consists of 25 items related to common symptoms associated with central sensitization.[18] Each item is scored using a 5-point Likert scale in which "never" is 0 points and "always" is 4 points.[18] The total score of Part A is the sum of all responses and ranges from 0 to 100.[18] Part B of the CSI, which is not scored, asks if one has been previously diagnosed with central sensitivity syndrome or related disorders.[18] A cut score of 40 out of 100 on Part A of the CSI was found to have a sensitivity of 81% to 82.8% and specificity of 54.8% to 75% for distinguishing patients with and without central sensitization pain.[19,20] Because of the relatively high number of false positives using CSI as a screening tool for central sensitization pain, combining the CSI with a comprehensive clinical examination has been suggested for identifying central sensitization pain in patients after cancer treatment.[17] Another proposed use of the CSI involves classifying patients based on the severity of central sensitization symptoms to guide clinical decision making.[21] Five proposed severity levels include subclinical (0–29), mild (30–39), moderate (40–49), severe (50–59), and extreme (60–100).[21]

Persistent pain after breast cancer treatment is relatively common. In studies investigating the prevalence of persistent pain after breast cancer surgery, the median prevalence was 37.5% (interquartile range, 30%–51%).[22] Predictors of persistent pain after breast cancer surgery include receiving radiation therapy, undergoing ALND, being of young age, having greater acute postoperative pain, and having preoperative pain.[22] Postmastectomy pain syndrome (PMPS) is a persistent pain disorder affecting patients after breast cancer surgery.[23] PMPS is typically described as pain after breast surgery that is (1) neuropathic in nature; (2) persistent for longer than 3 months; and (3) localized to the breast, chest wall, axilla, or arm of the affected side. Several psychosocial factors such as anxiety, depression, stress, sleep disturbance, and catastrophizing are believed to be associated with PMPS.[23]

Clinical measures of pain can be classified as either unidimensional or multidimensional. Unidimensional measures of pain typically assess the intensity of pain and not the descriptive quality of pain or its impact. Recommended unidimensional measures of pain for patients with a history of breast cancer include the visual analog scale (VAS) and numeric pain rating scale (NPRS).[24] For the VAS, patients place a mark along a 10-cm line with the words "no pain" at one end and "pain as bad as it can be" the other end.[24] A minimally clinically important difference of 9 to 11 mm has been established in patients with breast cancer.[24] For the NPRS, patients are asked to rate their pain from 0 to 10, in which 0 indicates "no pain" and 10 indicates "most severe pain" or "most pain imaginable."[24] A 2 point change on the NPRS has been reported to be clinically meaningful across multiple patient populations, and a rating of 5 or more at worst in patients after breast surgery has been considered clinically meaningful because of impact on health-related quality of life.[24]

Two recommended multiple dimensional pain scales are the McGill Pain Questionnaire (MPQ)–Short Form and Brief Pain Inventory–Short Form.[24] The MPQ–Short Form consists of 15 words (11 sensory and 4 affective descriptors of pain) from the original MPQ, which are rated on an intensity scale as 0 = none, 1 = mild, 2 = moderate, or 3 = severe.[24] A total score (range, 0–45) and two subscale scores (sensory [range, 0–33] and affective [range, 0–12]) can be calculated.[24] The MPQ–Short Form has been used in a number of studies for assessing pain in patients diagnosed with breast cancer.[24] The smallest detectable difference for a Norwegian version of the MPQ–Short Form in patients with musculoskeletal pain was found to be 11.9 points for the total score, 8.8 points for the sensory score, and 4.8 points for the affective score.[25] A greater than 5-point change has been reported to represent a clinically important change for the MPQ-Short Form Total Score.[25] A modified version of the MPQ-Short (SF-MPQ-2) has been developed and determined to be a valid measure of pain in young and older persons with cancer-related pain.[26] The SF-MPQ-2 includes the 15 items from the MPQ-Short Form along with 7 additional items.[27] The response format was modified from the 4-point Likert scale to an 11-point NRS (0 = none; 10 = worst possible).[27] The SF-MPQ-2 consists of four subscales: continuous descriptors (throbbing, cramping, gnawing, aching, heavy, and tender), intermittent descriptors (shooting, stabbing, sharp, splitting, electric shock, and piercing), neuropathic descriptors (hot or burning, cold or freezing, pain caused by light touch, itching, tingling or "pins and needles," and numbness), and affective descriptors (tiring or exhausting, sickening, fearful, and punishing or cruel).[27,28]

The Brief Pain Inventory (BPI)–Short Form was developed for persons diagnosed with cancer because of the amount of time needed to complete and score the original BPI.[24] The BPI-Short Form has been used in studies to assess pain in patients diagnosed with breast cancer.[24] The BFI-Short Form consists of 11 items (4 pain severity; 7 pain interference) in which a 0 to 10 numeric rating scale is used to respond to items (0 = "no pain/does not interfere" to 10 = "pain as bad as you can imagine/completely interferes").[29] Four subscale scores can be derived: pain severity (average of pain severity items), overall pain interference (average of interference items), activity-related pain interference (average of interference items related to general activity, walking and work), and mood-related pain interference (average of interference items related to relations, mood, enjoyment).[30] The minimal important difference for the BPI-Short Form has been reported to be 1.2 points for the Pain Severity Score, 1.5 points for the Overall Pain Interference Score, 1.6 points for the Activity-related Pain Interference Score, and 1.5 points for the Mood-related Pain Interference Score.[24,30]

Impaired Shoulder Range of Motion

Up to 67% of patients who underwent breast cancer surgery and radiation have been found to demonstrate impaired shoulder ROM.[8] Typically, limited shoulder ROM is found for abduction, flexion, and abduction and external rotation.[31] Limited shoulder ROM has been found to be related to ALND, greater number of lymph nodes removed, cording, seroma, mastectomy, body mass index (BMI) greater than 25, and older age.[31]

Many patients experience impaired shoulder ROM within the first month after surgery with mainly shoulder abduction, flexion, and external rotation being limited.[9] This is not surprising because, as previously mentioned, many patients after breast surgery experience pain and are at risk for muscle trauma because of the nature of the surgical procedures. Greater reductions in shoulder abduction at 1 month have been found to be associated with being nonwhite, having received neoadjuvant chemotherapy, having a mastectomy, having an ALND, and having less preoperative shoulder ROM.[32] Decreased participation in exercise preoperatively, having received neoadjuvant chemotherapy, experiencing higher breast pain, having an ALND, placement of a surgical drain, and less preoperative ROM has been found to be associated with decreased shoulder flexion at 1 month.[32]

Because of the likelihood that patients demonstrate impaired shoulder ROM after breast surgery, it is suggested that therapists use goniometry to assess passive and active shoulder ROM.[33] Therapists should assess all planes of shoulder motion, including flexion–extension, abduction–adduction, internal rotation–external rotation, and horizontal abduction/horizontal adduction.[34] To ensure consistency

of goniometric measurements, it is recommended that therapists standardize and document measurement technique and patient position.[33] If possible, preoperative assessment of shoulder ROM should be performed.[34] Preoperative assessment would allow for more accurate identification of patients who experience ROM loss after breast cancer surgery, especially patients who undergo bilateral surgical procedures.

Exercise interventions have been shown to be beneficial for addressing shoulder ROM after breast surgery.[35] Patients who perform early exercise postoperatively may demonstrate better short-term recovery of their shoulder ROM.[35] However, similar recovery has been demonstrated in patients who performed delayed exercise after completion of their exercise program.[35] Additionally, patients who perform early exercise may be at risk for seroma formation and increased wound drainage.[35] Of note, the majority of studies investigating early versus delayed exercise in patients after breast cancer surgery were conducted more than 15 years ago when patients were more likely to receive more invasive surgical procedures.[36] Therefore, there is controversy as to when to start an exercise program after breast cancer surgery.[34] The timing and type of exercises recommended for patients after breast surgery may be influenced by the type of surgical interventions performed. Different early exercise prescriptions should be considered for patients who undergo breast-conserving surgery and SLNB compared with patients who undergo mastectomy with immediate breast reconstruction and ALND. It is important for clinicians and patients to speak to the surgeons before initiating an exercise program early after surgery to avoid complications. Early complications after breast surgery include cellulitis, flap necrosis, abscess, wound dehiscence, seroma, and hematoma.[37] Exercise precautions may be necessary to reduce risk of postoperative complications, particularly for patients who undergo breast reconstruction.[37] Typically, the plastic surgeon will provide activity recommendations for the first 4 to 6 weeks for patients after breast reconstruction to reduce the risk of complications such as bleeding, loss of circulation, and tissue necrosis.[34]

Although a number of studies support the benefit of exercise after breast cancer surgery, no definitive recommendations can be made on the timing, content, and intensity of exercises.[35] A structured and progressive exercise program has been suggested for patients after breast cancer surgery to restore shoulder function while minimizing the risk of complications.[37] A reasonable approach would be to delay certain exercises during the first week after surgery or until the drains have been removed. During the first week after surgery, patients could be instructed on deep breathing; elbow, wrist, and hand active range of motion (AROM) exercises; and posture and scapular exercises.[34,35] Deep breathing can be performed sitting or lying supine. Patients can be instructed to take a deep breathe in through their nose for approximately 3 to 4 seconds, letting the chest and abdomen expand, and then slowly exhale through the mouth for approximately 4 to 6 seconds.[34] Deep breathing can assist with pain management, relaxation to reduce anxiety associated with breast cancer diagnosis and treatment, and maintenance of normal chest movement.[38,39] Elbow, wrist, and hand AROM exercises (i.e., active elbow flexion–extension, wrist circles in clockwise and counterclockwise directions, digit flexion–extension) may help promote lymph flow after surgery and reduce postoperative swelling.[39] Exercises can be performed for 10 to 25 repetitions and repeated three to five times per day.[39] Posture and scapular exercises may (1) facilitate return of motion without negatively affecting tissue healing and (2) reduce the risk of inactivity and protective posturing that may lead to adaptive tissue shortening.[34,38] Posture and scapular exercises may include chin tucks (cervical retraction), active scapular retraction, shoulder shrugs or active scapular elevation, and shoulder rolls. Each exercise may be performed 5 to 10 times and repeated two to five times per day. After 7 to 10 days or when drains have been removed,

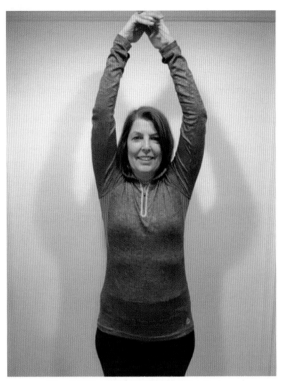

Fig. 115.1 Self-assisted shoulder flexion.

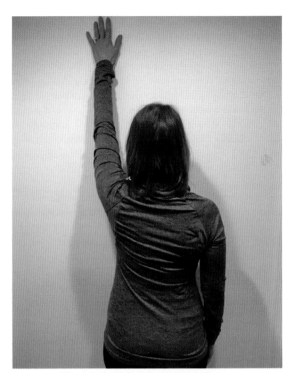

Fig. 115.3 Wall slide shoulder flexion.

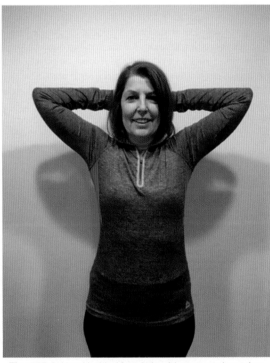

Fig. 115.2 Hand behind head shoulder external rotation.

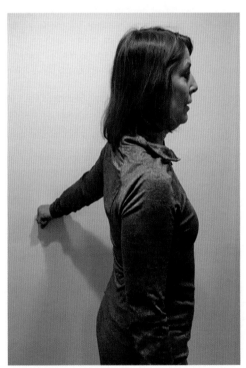

Fig. 115.4 Wall pectoralis stretch. (The modified version involves flexing the elbow and placing the forearm on a wall to reduce tension on the biceps.)

the exercise program can be progressed to include above-shoulder-level mobility exercises.[38] Types of exercise prescribed to improve shoulder mobility may include active, passive or active-assisted shoulder ROM, and stretching. Exercises designed to improved shoulder mobility after breast cancer surgery may include self-assisted shoulder flexion (Fig. 115.1), supine or standing active shoulder abduction, supine or standing hand behind head shoulder external rotation (Fig. 115.2), wall slide flexion (Fig. 115.3), self-assisted hand-up-the-back internal rotation,

lower trunk rotation with affected shoulder positioned at 90 degrees of abduction, and doorway or wall pectoralis muscle stretch (Fig. 115.4). Each exercise can be performed 5 to 10 times and repeated two to five times per day. Each exercise should be performed slowly until a gentle stretch is felt by the patient. Patients can hold each stretch for 5 to 30 seconds depending on the level of tissue irritability. Patients should be instructed to perform their exercise program until shoulder mobility has fully recovered. When they have regained their shoulder mobility and full use of their arms, patients should be instructed to continue the exercise program at least once a day. Patients after breast surgery have been found to demonstrate shoulder ROM impairments that do not become evident until 3 to 12 months after surgery.[40] Therefore, continued performance of an exercise program addressing shoulder mobility is important in patients after breast surgery, especially those who receive radiation therapy.

In a study in which approximately 70% of patients received radiation therapy, patients after breast cancer surgery demonstrated improvement in ROM over the first 4 to 6 months postsurgery followed by a period of time when a decline in ROM occurred up to 10 months, and then improvement was noted by 12 months.[32] This time frame in which a decline in ROM was found is around the time chemotherapy and radiation are typically completed (8–9 months after surgery).[40] Patients who receive radiation therapy are more likely to demonstrate impaired shoulder ROM, especially if the axilla is included within the radiation field.[31] Impaired shoulder ROM in patients who receive radiation could be due to muscle hypertonicity and fibrosis in muscles and other soft tissues exposed to radiation affecting tissue flexibility.[41] A number of shoulder muscles are located within the radiation field. The pectoralis muscles are exposed to high doses of radiation when the whole breast is irradiated, irrespective of beam arrangement.[41] Increased radiation dose to portions of the latissimus dorsi and teres major muscles occur if the radiation field encompasses the axillary and supraclavicular regions.[41] The infraspinatus, subscapularis, supraspinatus, teres minor, and trapezius muscles are exposed to 48 Gy of radiation in significantly more patients treated with directly opposed field technique compared with tangent field technique.[41]

Impaired pectoralis flexibility may be a contributing factor to impaired shoulder ROM in patients after breast cancer treatment. As previously mentioned, pectoralis muscle trauma may occur from surgery, leading to hypertonicity and spasm. Limiting arm motion secondary to pain or fear of complications and protective posturing may lead to further pectoralis tightness.[42] Additionally, radiation therapy has been shown to alter collagen synthesis,[43] and soft tissue fibrosis may develop within the radiation field, affecting the flexibility of tissues in the shoulder region.

There is no standardized clinical assessment of pectoralis major muscle flexibility. However, computer simulation modeling has shown that shoulder forward elevation places the highest level of percent strain (change in length divided by resting length with arm by side in neutral rotation) on the sternal portion (52%) and abdominal portion (55%) of the pectoralis major muscle.[10] A lower level of strain on the clavicular portion (22%) compared with sternal and abdominal portions of the pectoralis major muscle occurs during shoulder forward elevation.[10] The greatest strain on the clavicular portion of the pectoralis major was found during combined motions such as shoulder abduction to 90° followed by external rotation (33%) and shoulder extension followed by external rotation (41%).[10] The amount of pectoralis major strain across the abdominal, sternal, and clavicular portions of the pectoralis major during shoulder external rotation with the arm by the side was shown to range from 10% to 27%.[10] The lowest level of strain across all portions of the pectoralis major muscle occurred during flexion to 90 degrees (−21% to 15%).[10] Understanding these levels of strain during various arm movements is important for clinicians to know in order to assess tissue flexibility and safely prescribe an exercise program to effectively improve shoulder ROM after breast surgery.

The prevalences of pectoralis tightness have been reported to be 8.9% at 3 months, 12.3% at 6 months and 8.7% at 12 months after breast surgery.[44] In this study, pectoralis tightness was defined as a limitation of shoulder forward elevation and horizontal abduction by more than

10 degrees with no limitation in shoulder external rotation.[44] Patients who undergo mastectomy and receive radiation therapy may be more likely to demonstrate impaired pectoralis flexibility.[44] Altered pectoralis minor length may occur in patients after breast cancer surgery as well.[45] The pectoralis minor muscle originates at the third through fifth ribs and inserts at the coracoid process. Pectoralis minor length has been assessed in patients after breast cancer surgery using the following methods: (1) the distance from the table to lateral aspect of acromion while the patient is positioned supine[45] and (2) the distance from the inferior aspect of the fourth rib to the coracoid process.[46]

Studies have investigated length changes of the pectoralis minor during shoulder motions.[47,48] Muraki and coworkers[48] found that portions of the pectoralis minor lengthen approximately 40% to 50% at 150 degrees of passive shoulder flexion and scaption compared with the neutral position. Additionally, greater length changes of the pectoralis minor were shown to occur during horizontal abduction at 90 degrees of external rotation and during scapular retraction at 30 degrees of flexion compared with scapular retraction at 0 degrees of flexion.[48] Umehare and associates[49] found slightly different results in the greatest amount of pectoralis minor lengthening was found to occur during sidelying horizontal abduction at 90 degrees and 150 degrees of shoulder elevation compared to side-lying scapular retraction at 0 degrees, 30 degrees, 90 degrees, and 150 degrees of flexion. Last, Borstad and Ludewig[47] found greater length change of the pectoralis minor to occur during a unilateral self-stretch followed by a supine manual stretch compared with a sitting manual stretch. The self-stretch was performed standing with arm positioned at 90 degrees of shoulder abduction, 90 degrees of elbow flexion, and the palm and forearm flat against a surface (doorframe, wall) and having the person rotate the trunk away from the elevated arm.[47] The supine manual stretch was performed by having the examiner apply a posterior directed force at the coracoid process while the arm was positioned at 90 degrees of shoulder abduction and external rotation and 90 degrees of elbow flexion.[47] The sitting manual stretch was performed with the patient's arm by side and having the examiner apply a posterior directed force at coracoid process with one hand while stabilizing the inferior angle of scapulae with the other hand.[47]

Greater improvements in shoulder horizontal abduction ROM were found after performing a 4-week pectoralis stretching program at 90 or 135 degrees of shoulder abduction compared with pectoralis stretching performed at 45 degrees of shoulder abduction in patients diagnosed with pectoralis muscle tightness after breast surgery.[50] The stretching program involved (1) stretching the pectoralis muscles using a T-bar in a supine position and rotating the trunk and (2) a corner stretch. Each stretch was held for 15 seconds and performed 5 to 10 times, 3 times per day.[50] In individuals without history of breast cancer, active scapular retraction at 60 degrees of scapular plane elevation (held for 20 seconds and repeated 3 times with 10 seconds of rest between repetitions) has been found to increase pectoralis minor length immediately after stretching.[51]

A screening tool to identify patients with history of breast cancer who are experiencing impaired upper extremity function has been developed.[52] One of the questions of this screening tool asks patients if they are having any difficulty moving their arms or necks.[52] Patients who answered "yes" were found to demonstrate less shoulder motion when reaching overhead and behind the back compared with their unaffected side.[52] Patients who answered "yes" were shown to demonstrate worse self-report of upper extremity pain and disability as measured by the Disabilities of Arm, Shoulder and Hand (DASH) questionnaire.[52]

In summary, impaired shoulder motion is a common problem experienced by patients after breast cancer surgery because of postsurgical pain and muscle injury. Radiation therapy may contribute to impaired shoulder motion due to soft tissue fibrosis causing impaired soft tissue flexibility. Therapists should be aware of other common pathoanatomic causes of upper body pain and limited motion after breast cancer treatment, including axillary web syndrome (AWS), adhesive capsulitis, and rotator cuff disease (RCD).

Axillary Web Syndrome

AWS is a condition that may occur in patients who undergo SLNB or ALND. The frequency of AWS has been reported to range from 0.6% to 85.4% in patients after axillary surgery.[53] AWS is characterized by observable or palpable cordlike structure underneath the skin that may present in the axilla and extend down the medial aspect of arm beyond the antecubital fossa to the forearm, wrist, or base of the thumb.[53] The cordlike structure may be tender to palpate and become more prominent during shoulder abduction. AWS can present as a single cord or multiple cords. AWS can occur at the lateral chest wall, breast, and abdominal wall regions as well.[53] The cause of AWS has been reported to be lymphovenous trauma, stasis, and hypercoagulation.[53,54] Tissue sampling of the cords has revealed dilated thrombosed lymphatics, thrombosed superficial veins, or both.[54] Another theory is surgical incision through the skin and subcutaneous tissues leads to the development of scar tissue and fibrous cords.[14]

Axillary web syndrome typically occurs within the first 3 months after surgery.[53] Figueira and associates[55] found that 86.1% of patients with AWS developed cords within 30 days of surgery with the majority of patients experiencing AWS within the first week (66.1%). Lauridsen and coworkers[56] found similar results in AWS being present in 57% of patients at 1 week after surgery. AWS will resolve in the majority of patients by 3 months after surgery.[53,54] However, the resolution of AWS has been reported to range from 3 weeks to 1 year after surgery.[53] Although AWS is not common, clinicians should be aware that it can occur months after surgery and even reoccur.[53] Cases of AWS recurrence have been reported after chemotherapy and radiation.[57] Other triggering events for AWS may include trauma or an intense bout of exercise.[58]

Risk factors for AWS include being of younger age, having a lower BMI, and extent of surgery.[53] A higher incidence of AWS has been found in patients who undergo ALND compared with SLNB.[59] Patients who underwent SLNB have been found to have a 68% lower risk of developing AWS.[59]

Symptoms reported by patients with AWS include pain, pulling, and tightness.[53] These symptoms are typically better at rest with the arm by the side and worse during arm motions such as shoulder flexion or abduction. Depending on the extent of AWS, other upper extremity motions involving the elbow and wrist may exacerbate symptoms. However, the presence of pain during arm movement is not a unique feature of AWS in patients after breast surgery. Koehler and coworkers[60] found no difference in pain during arm movement in patients with and without AWS within 12 weeks of surgery, suggesting that patients experience pain after breast surgery for other reasons besides AWS. Additionally, impaired sensation is a common complaint of patients with AWS. Bergmann and associates[59] found that 81% of patients with AWS experienced numbness in the intercostal brachial nerve distribution compared with 53% without AWS. Nevola Teixeira and associates[61] found that 47% of patients with AWS demonstrated disturbed sensation in the arm or chest wall compared with 15% of patients without AWS.

Impaired shoulder ROM is another common finding associated with AWS. The typical pattern of impaired shoulder ROM is shoulder abduction and flexion being more limited than external rotation at 0 degrees of abduction and hand-behind-back internal rotation. Patients with AWS have been reported to demonstrate 111 to 139 degrees of active shoulder flexion and less than 90 to 132 degrees of active shoulder abduction.[53] On average, less shoulder ROM is found in patients with AWS (~110 degrees of shoulder abduction at 2 weeks postsurgery and 130 degrees at 4 weeks postsurgery) compared with patients without AWS (~135 degrees at 2 weeks postsurgery and 150 degrees at 4 weeks postsurgery).[60] Passive and active shoulder ROM are typically equally limited (i.e., 135 degrees of active abduction and 138 degrees of passive abduction) in patients with AWS.[60] When assessing shoulder abduction ROM, clinicians should pay close attention to compensatory strategies. Patients with AWS may flex the elbow to alleviate tension being placed on the cord during shoulder abduction. Patients with AWS have been found to demonstrate impaired elbow ROM.[53]

Interventions for AWS include therapeutic exercises, manual therapy, and thermal modalities.[53] Exercises prescribed to restore shoulder mobility in patients with AWS commonly include active-assisted and active shoulder ROM exercises.[53] Specific ROM exercises prescribed for patients with AWS may include supine forward elevation with a dowel, supine or standing active abduction, pendulums, or self-assisted exercises with a pulley.[53] Additional flexibility exercises may include stretching of the pectoralis major and minor, trapezius, subscapularis, and latissimus dorsi muscles along with lower trunk rotation with shoulder abducted to 90 degrees and shoulder flexion and abduction against-wall stretches.[53] Other types of exercise that may be beneficial for patients with AWS include nerve gliding and stretching.[62] Daily or regular performance of exercise is typically recommended; however, there is a lack of detailed description of the therapeutic exercise protocols used in studies related to AWS.[53] The exercise prescription for patients with AWS should be dependent on severity of pain. For example, patients with moderate to high levels of pain should be instructed in gentle ROM exercises with holding the end position for a shorter duration of time (1–5 seconds). When the level of pain decreases, exercises may be progressed by instructing to hold the end-range position for longer periods of time.

A number of manual therapy techniques used to treat patients with AWS have been reported in the literature (myofascial release, cord stretching, cord massage, passive skin traction, manual soft tissue techniques, cord release and traction, cord manipulation, or cord mobilization).[53] One manual technique involves clinicians pushing down on the cord with one thumb while slowly stretching the cord with the other thumb or fingers.[62] Another manual technique involves clinicians stretching or elongating the cord as if "playing a stringed instrument."[62] Clinicians may perform gentle skin stretching techniques in the region of the cord by gliding the soft tissue longitudinally in superior and inferior directions, transversely in medial and lateral directions, and rotationally in clockwise and counterclockwise directions without allowing the hand to slide over the skin.[63] All of these manual techniques may be performed at different angles of shoulder abduction to increase or decrease tension on the targeted tissue.[64] Clinicians should be aware that an audible snapping or popping sound may occur followed by an increase in amount of ROM. However, a patient may experience a crackling and burning sensation along with increased tightness and soreness within 24 to 48 hours after palpable or audible release of cords.[65] Most therapists agree that treatment should not be aggressive because of the inflammatory nature of AWS, so the goal of treatment should not be to "break up" or "pop or snap" the cords.[62] Other manual techniques used to treat AWS that do not involve cord or skin stretching include scapular mobilization and pectoralis muscle soft tissue mobilization.[62,66] Furthermore, scar massage may be performed if adequate healing has occurred and restrictions are noted. Scar massage techniques may include cross-friction scar massage as well as skin rolling and vertical lifting of scar.[53,65,67]

Manual lymphatic drainage (MLD) may be performed by clinicians to address the pain and inflammation associated with AWS. In a study that compared therapy with therapy plus MLD, no significant difference was found in visible cording among groups at 4 weeks; however, the group that received MLD demonstrated a more significant decrease in pain than the group of patients that did not receive MLD.[66] Therapy in this study consisted of stretching exercises, strengthening exercises, and 30 minutes of manual therapy (soft tissue mobilization techniques and stretching for tight cords; shoulder abduction, elbow extension, forearm supination, and wrist extension stretching; scapular mobilization; and passive ROM exercises).[66]

Topical heat has been a suggested treatment for AWS.[67] However, topical heat should be applied with caution because of the risk of burns in patients with compromised sensation and risk of lymphedema with excessive or prolonged heat exposure.[53] Suggested strategies to reduce the risk of adverse effects with heat include performing hot–cold sensation testing, frequent skin inspection, using extra padding, and prescribing shorter treatment duration times of 8 to 10 minutes.[53,67] Having patients take a warm shower rather than applying heat to the area has been suggested as an alternate strategy.[53,67] Additionally, with regard to cords that may be present within the field of radiation, applying topical heat to recently irradiated tissue has been documented as a precaution or contraindication.[68] Clinicians should weigh the risks and benefits for using any physical agent including topical heat in patients with AWS.

Patients who undergo breast cancer surgery should be educated on the signs and symptoms of AWS. Patients should be instructed to speak to their health care providers if AWS is suspected to ensure timely referral to rehabilitation services. A screening tool for AWS has been developed that has a sensitivity of 94%, a specificity of 91%, a positive prevalence value of 86%, a negative prevalence value of 96%, and an accuracy of 92% for diagnosing AWS.[61] The AWS screening tool consists of five questions related to difficulty moving the arm, visual perception of AWS, tactile perception of AWS, feeling of tension, and feeling of swelling.[61] A response of "yes" on questions about difficulty moving the arm, visual and tactile perception of swelling, and feeling of tension is scored 1 point each, and the sensation of swelling is scored 1 point for a "no" response.[61] A total score of greater than 3 is considered positive for presence of AWS.[61]

Adhesive Capsulitis

Adhesive capsulitis or frozen shoulder is a condition characterized by painful and impaired shoulder ROM.[69] Up to 10.3% of patients have been reported to develop adhesive capsulitis within 12 to 18 months after breast cancer surgery.[44,70] Risk factors for adhesive capsulitis in patients diagnosed with breast cancer include being 50 to 59 years of age, undergoing mastectomy or mastectomy with reconstruction, and having a history of thyroid surgery.[70] The difference between adhesive capsulitis and other causes of impaired shoulder ROM after breast surgery is the finding of multidirectional loss of active and passive shoulder motion, with external rotation being the most impaired, especially when the arm is adducted.[44,69] Other findings of adhesive capsulitis include limitations in shoulder external rotation and internal rotation that worsen when the arm is abducted and hypomobility of glenohumeral joint glides or accessory motions.[69]

A detailed description of the evaluation and treatment of adhesive capsulitis can be found in Chapter 70. Conservative treatment of adhesive capsulitis may include patient education, joint mobilization, exercise, and biophysical agents (i.e., ultrasound, phonophoresis, shortwave diathermy, moist hot pack, electrical stimulation, iontophoresis, laser therapy).[69,71] Therapists need be aware of the concerns for use of certain biophysical agents in patients diagnosed with breast cancer. The concerns for using some biophysical agents with patients diagnosed and treated for cancer include (1) increased tumor growth at primary site or metastatic spread of cancer, (2) increased toxic effect of adjuvant treatments such as chemotherapy and radiation, and (3) increased risk for complications or injury caused by impaired sensation.[68] The presence of cancer is considered a contraindication for biophysical agents that have the potential to alter metabolic activity or blood flow in or around the area affected by cancer.[72] However, there is controversy as to whether a history of cancer is a contraindication versus precaution for use of some biophysical agents.[72] Transcutaneous electric nerve stimulation has been used for the management of chronic pain after breast cancer treatment and bone pain associated with metastasis in patients diagnosed with breast cancer.[73] Low-level light therapy (LLLT) has been used in patients diagnosed with breast cancer to address breast cancer–related lymphedema, oral mucositis, radiodermatitis, chemotherapy-induced peripheral neuropathy, and osteonecrosis of the jaw.[74] However, more research has been suggested to investigate the long-term safety of LLLT because of concerns for its effect on increasing cancer cell proliferation.[74] The use of deep heating biophysical agents such as ultrasound and diathermy is more controversial and generally contraindicated in patients diagnosed with cancer because of concern for increased tumor growth and development of local recurrence.[68] Although the use of ultrasound and diathermy in patients with a history of breast cancer has been published in the literature, the safety with respect to risk of recurrence and metastasis was not reported.[75,76] Of note, an increased risk for local recurrence was reported in rats that received ultrasound postoperatively.[77] Therapists should consider the following factors when determining the appropriateness for using biophysical agents with patients who have a history of cancer: site and stage of cancer, time since cancer diagnosis and treatment, last cancer screening, any acute or late effects of cancer and its treatment, and comorbidities.[78]

Rotator Cuff Disease

Rotator cuff disease is believed to be a common source of shoulder pain in patients treated for breast cancer[79]; however, the incidence is not well understood. It has been theorized that breast cancer treatments and the associated impairments place patients at greater risk for RCD.[80] Patients, after breast cancer treatment, may demonstrate postural deficits because of protective guarding and pectoralis muscle tightness secondary to surgical trauma and radiation fibrosis.[80] Postural deficits are believed to contribute to the development of RCD by influencing the relationship between the humeral head and glenoid fossa during arm motions, thus leading to abnormal physical stress to tissues in the subacromial space.[80] Altered scapulothoracic motion is believed to cause mechanical impingement of the rotator cuff tendons, causing pain and pathology.[81] After breast cancer treatment, patients may demonstrate altered scapulothoracic motion caused by pain, soft tissue tightness, or impaired muscle performance.[80] Additionally, patients may develop lymphedema of the upper extremity. Increased interstitial fluid associated with lymphedema causes the weight of the arm to increase, resulting in a greater load being placed on the rotator cuff, which could contribute to tension overload within the rotator cuff tendons.[80] Therapists should perform a thorough clinical examination of the shoulder to identify relevant impairments contributing to shoulder pain in patients diagnosed with breast cancer. A detailed description of the diagnosis and treatment of RCD can be found in Chapter 71.

Breast Cancer–Related Lymphedema

Breast cancer–related lymphedema (BCRL) is an abnormal accumulation of interstitial fluid, containing proteins and cellular material, caused by an impaired lymphatic system occurring secondary to the treatment for breast cancer. Patients treated for breast cancer may experience lymphedema of the hand, arm, breast, torso, or combination of these areas. It has been estimated that one in five patients will develop upper extremity lymphedema after breast cancer treatment, although the incidence has varied considerably among studies (0%–94%) likely because of differences among treatments received, measurement methods, and length of follow-up.[82] As with upper extremity lymphedema, a wide range (0%–90.4%) exists for the incidence of breast edema.[83] Fewer studies have investigated the incidence of torso lymphedema after breast cancer treatment. One study found that 14% of patients reported swelling at the side of the chest, whereas 10% experienced swelling in the back.[84] Therapists should be aware that BCRL can occur any time after breast cancer surgery. However, the majority of patients will develop BCRL of the upper extremity within 2 to 3 years after breast cancer surgery.[82] It should be noted that edema experienced by some patients within the first year of treatment may be transient because not all patients who demonstrate upper extremity edema present with edema at long-term follow up.[85] Additionally, breast edema may increase during and after radiation therapy but return to baseline by 12 months in most patients.[86] However, BCRL may progress gradually if not treated, leading to negative health consequences or reduced quality of life.

The following sections provide an overview of the anatomy of the lymphatic system, lymphatic drainage pattern of the upper quadrant, pathophysiology of edema, differential diagnosis of edema, BCRL risk factors, stage of lymphedema, diagnosis of BCRL, and treatments strategies for BRCL.

Lymphatic System Anatomy

The lymphatic system consists of lymphatic tissues (lymph nodes, spleen, thymus, tonsils) and vessels (lymph capillaries, precollectors, collectors, trunks, ducts). The lymphatic tissues are part of the body's defense system, whereas the lymphatic vessels function to form and transport lymph to the venous system. Lymph is the fluid and substances (water, proteins, fat, cells, and particles) that enter the lymphatic vessels from the interstitial space. Lymph capillaries are the initial lymphatic vessels responsible for absorbing lymph into the lymphatic system. Lymph capillaries are located throughout the body except for the central nervous system and tissues that lack blood supply. Lymph capillaries of the superficial system originate near blood capillaries and cover the entire surface of the body. Lymph capillaries are closed tubelike structures in the interstitial space that are formed by a single layer of continuous or overlapping endothelial cells. Fibers called anchoring filaments connect the lymph capillaries to the surrounding tissues. When fluid leaves the blood capillaries, there is an increase in volume of interstitial fluid that causes tension to be placed on the anchoring filaments, which opens the junctions created by the overlapping endothelial cells. Fluid then moves into the lymphatic system because pressure is lower in the lymph capillary than in the interstitial space. The endothelial junctions close when the pressure in the lymph capillary exceeds the pressure in the interstitial space. Fluid will then move into the precollectors, which are larger lymphatic vessels that connect the lymph capillaries to the lymph collectors. Lymph collectors contain valves and the segment between a pair of valves is termed a lymphangion. The wall of a lymphangion contains smooth muscle and contracts to transport fluid from a distal to proximal lymphangion. Lymphangions contract about 10 to 12 times per minute at rest.[87] The contraction rate of a lymphangion is influenced by temperature, muscle activity, joint motion, diaphragmatic breathing, arterial pulsation, tissue hormones and external stretch on lymphangion wall.[87] Lymph collectors transport fluid to lymph nodes and lymphatic trunks. Fluid enters the lymph node via

afferent collectors and leaves via efferent collectors. Lymph nodes have a protection function (filter foreign material), immune function (store lymphocytes), and fluid equilibrium function (reabsorb water). Lymphatic trunks or ducts are the largest lymphatic vessels and have a similar structure and function as lymph collectors. Fluid is transported to the venous system via the right lymphatic duct and thoracic duct near the right and left venous angles, respectively. The right lymphatic duct receives fluid from the right head and neck region, right upper torso, and right upper extremity, whereas the thoracic duct receives fluid from the left head and neck region, left upper section of torso, left upper extremity, bilateral lower sections of the torso, and bilateral lower extremities.

Patients after breast cancer treatment are at risk for developing lymphedema of the upper extremity, breast, and torso. Understanding the lymphatic drainage pattern of the torso and upper extremity is fundamental for clinicians to recognize the regions of the body where patients are at risk for developing lymphedema and perform certain treatment techniques to reduce lymphedema.

Lymphatic watersheds separate the body into regions or territories. The sagittal watershed separates the body into two equal halves. The upper horizontal watershed separates the head and neck from the torso and arm, whereas the lower horizontal watershed separates the torso into upper and lower regions. The arm is separated from the torso by the axillary watershed.

Lymph collectors within each territory transport fluid to a specific group of lymph nodes called regional lymph nodes. Therefore, the regional lymph nodes are responsible for draining fluid from a specific adjacent region of the body. The regional lymph nodes for the upper torso and upper extremity are the axillary lymph nodes. There are lymphatic vessels that connect adjacent regions (left and right upper torso regions; ipsilateral upper and lower torso regions). These lymphatic pathways are called interterritorial anastomoses and enable fluid to be transported between adjacent regions of the body. The anterior axilloaxillary and posterior axilloaxillary anastomoses provide connections between the upper torso regions. The axilloinguinal anastomoses provide connections between ipsilateral upper and lower torso regions on both sides of the body.

Lymphatic Drainage Pathway of the Breast and Upper Extremity

Most lymph vessels of the breast transport lymph to the axillary lymph nodes; however, lymphatic drainage pathways to the parasternal lymph nodes, epigastric region, supraclavicular region, and intercostal spaces do exist.[88] The upper extremity has a superficial and deep system responsible for transporting lymph to the axillary lymph nodes. The superficial system is responsible for transporting lymph from the skin and subcutaneous region, whereas the deep system transports lymph from muscles and joints. The superficial system of the upper extremity can be divided into hand, forearm, and upper arm regions. The hand has five groups of lymphatic vessels: radial, ulnar, descending, ascending, and central.[88] The radial, ulnar, and descending vessels located at the palm travel to the dorsal hand, whereas the ascending vessels from the palm form the median forearm vessels.[88] The central vessels are deep and receive lymph from the central palm.[88] The superficial system of the forearm has three regions: median, radial, and ulnar.[88] The median vessels receive lymph from the palm and join the radial and ulnar vessels at the middle third of the forearm.[88] The radial and ulnar vessels are a continuation of the radial and ulnar vessels of the hand and join together at the elbow.[88] Ulnar vessels may connect with lymph nodes at the cubital fossa or ascend along the brachial artery.[88] The upper arm has three regions: medial, dorsolateral, and dorsomedial.[88] The medial upper arm vessels are a continuation of the forearm vessels and transport lymph to the axillary lymph nodes.[88] The dorsolateral upper arm vessels transport lymph from the dorsolateral area of the shoulder and upper arm to the level III axillary lymph nodes or supraclavicular lymph nodes.[88] Long and short variations of the dorsolateral upper arm vessels have been described, in which the long variation may receive lymph from the radial forearm vessels and the short variation may transport lymph from the dorsolateral upper arm to the median upper arm bundle.[88] The dorsomedial upper arm vessels transport lymph from the dorsomedial area of the shoulder and upper arm to the axillary lymph nodes.[88] The vessels of the deep system typically follow the arteries of the hand, forearm, and upper arm, eventually ascending along the brachial artery towards the axillary lymph nodes.[88] The deep system of the shoulder has vessels that follow the anterior and posterior circumflex, subscapular, and suprascapular arteries and transport lymph to the axillary lymph nodes, excluding the supraclavicular vessels, which transport lymph to the supraclavicular lymph nodes.[88]

Pathophysiology of Edema

The human body is mostly composed of water located within cells (intracellular) and outside of cells (extracellular). About one third of the body's water is located extracellularly with about 25% of the water being within the vascular system (intravascular space) and 75% being outside of the vascular system (interstitial space).[87,89] Fluid and other substances are constantly moving between the intravascular and interstitial spaces. The fluid located in the intravascular space is called blood or plasma, whereas fluid in the interstitial space is called interstitial fluid. Fluid exchange between the intravascular and interstitial spaces is influenced by the following physiologic forces: blood capillary pressure, colloid osmotic pressure of plasma, colloid osmotic pressure of interstitial space, interstitial fluid pressure, and permeability of the blood vessel wall.

The hydrostatic pressure of the blood (blood capillary pressure) is greater than the hydrostatic pressure of the interstitial fluid (interstitial fluid pressure) that effectively causes fluid to filter out of the vascular system (filtration). Differences in concentration of proteins between the intravascular and interstitial spaces influences fluid equilibrium because fluid travels from an area of low concentration of proteins to an area of high concentration. The concentration of proteins is greater in the vascular system, indicating that the colloid osmotic pressure of plasma exceeds the colloid osmotic pressure of the interstitial space, which would effectively lead to fluid being reabsorbed back into the vascular system. However, the amount of fluid that is filtered out of the vascular system exceeds the amount of fluid being reabsorbed, causing a net filtration.

Edema develops if the net filtration exceeds the lymphatic system's transport capacity. Net filtration will increase if blood capillary pressure increases because of expansion in plasma volume resulting from renal failure, medications, or pregnancy.[89] Additionally, increased blood capillary pressure occurs from obstruction caused by central (e.g., heart failure, cardiomyopathy) or peripheral (e.g., DVT, chronic venous insufficiency) cardiovascular diseases.[89] Net filtration will occur as well with conditions that decrease colloid osmotic pressure of the plasma (e.g., nephrotic syndrome, liver failure) or increase colloid osmotic pressure of the interstitial space (lymphatic system disorders).[89] Finally, the permeability of the blood vessel wall effects the movement of substances, including proteins, between the intravascular and interstitial spaces, thus impacting colloid osmotic pressures. Increased permeability of the blood vessel wall is a significant factor for edema caused by infections, allergic reactions, and burns.[89]

The body has passive and active mechanisms to protect against the development of edema.[88] Passive protection against edema occurs when interstitial fluid volume increases, and there is a subsequent increase in interstitial fluid pressure along with a decrease in colloid osmotic pressure, which effectively decreases filtration and increases reabsorption.[88] However, the rise of interstitial pressure is dependent on the capability of the interstitial space to become larger or stretch, meaning interstitial fluid pressure will only increase slightly when fluid volume increases if the interstitial space has a greater ability to extend.[88] Active protection against edema refers to the lymphatic system's ability to compensate for an increased net filtrate.[88] The transport capacity of the lymphatic system is about 10 times greater than the lymph flow under normal conditions.[88] Increase in interstitial fluid volume causes more lymph to be formed because of greater tension being placed on the anchoring filaments and 2) faster lymph transport because of increased contraction rate of the lymphangions.[87,88]

Breast Cancer–Related Lymphedema Risk Factors

Risk factors for BCRL can be categorized as disease related, treatment related, or personal factors. Strong risk factors for upper extremity BCRL have been reported to include having an ALND, greater number of lymph nodes removed, a mastectomy, and a higher BMI.[82] The presence of metastatic lymph nodes, receiving radiation and chemotherapy, and not participating in regular physical activity have been reported to be moderate risk factors for upper extremity BCRL.[82] Other risk factors reported in the literature include air travel, blood drawn from at risk arm, blood pressure measurements taken on at risk arm, extreme temperatures (i.e., sauna use), and infection.[90] However, there is limited high-level evidence suggesting that lifestyle factors such air travel, blood drawn from at risk arm, blood pressure measurements taken on at risk arm, and extreme temperatures are significant risk factors for developing BCRL.[90] Additionally, there is some evidence indicating that taxane-based chemotherapy is a risk factor for upper extremity BCRL, especially in those who receive docetaxel-based chemotherapy.[91] With respect to developing edema of the breast, the following risk factors have been identified: irradiated breast volume, radiation boost volume, use of photon boost, higher density of breast tissue, larger tumor, postoperative infection, and diabetes.[83] There is conflicting evidence for age, BMI, breast size, chemotherapy, and hormonal therapy being risk factors for breast edema.[83]

Differential Diagnosis of Edema

Lymphedema is a health condition characterized by edema in a specific region of the body where the lymphatic system is not functioning optimally. Edema located in the upper quadrant after breast cancer treatment is not always lymphedema. A number of health conditions can cause either generalized (entire body) or localized (specific region of body) edema. Besides BCRL, possible causes of localized edema of the upper extremity, breast or torso include DVT of the upper extremity, superior vena cava (SVC) syndrome, erysipelas or cellulitis, malignant lymphedema, and inflammatory breast cancer.

Deep vein thrombosis of the upper extremity involves the formation of fibrin clots within the subclavian, axillary, and brachial veins.[92] Pain, edema, skin discoloration, cyanosis, and dilation of superficial veins are signs and symptoms associated with DVT of the upper extremity.[93] Less common findings include weakness and paresthesia.[93] Risk factors for DVT of the upper extremity include malignancy or placement of central venous catheter, peripherally inserted central catheter, or cardiac pacemaker.[93]

The SVC returns blood from the head, arms, and torso to the heart. Obstruction of blood flow through the SVC causing facial and neck edema, upper extremity edema, cough, dilated veins, or dyspnea is referred to as SVC syndrome.[94] Patients may report that symptoms are worse lying supine compared with sitting or standing.[95] Additional signs and symptoms of SVC syndrome that may indicate a need for immediate medical attention include high-pitched breath sounds (because of concern for laryngeal edema and airway obstruction), headaches, dizziness, confusion, and decreased alertness (because of concern for cerebral edema), and syncope (because of concern for diminished cardiac reserve).[94,95]

Erysipelas and cellulitis are infections of the skin and subcutaneous tissues. Erysipelas is a superficial infection of the upper dermis and superficial lymphatics, whereas cellulitis affects deeper tissues.[96] Signs and symptoms of erysipelas and cellulitis include pain, redness, warmth, and edema.[96] Systemic signs and symptoms may include fever, chills, malaise, and palpable regional lymph nodes.[96] Erysipelas and cellulitis can lead to serious complications and can be life threatening, so immediate medical attention is required if erysipelas or cellulitis is suspected.

Tumor obstruction or spread to the regional nodes can negatively affect lymph transport, causing edema. This is referred to as malignant lymphedema, which typically differs in clinical presentation from nonmalignant BCRL. Malignant lymphedema is often characterized by a sudden onset of edema with rapid progression, greater proximal edema, skin changes, severe pain, paresthesia, and weakness.[87]

Inflammatory breast cancer is a less common type of invasive breast cancer.[97] Signs and symptoms of inflammatory breast cancer may include a rapid onset of breast erythema, edema, or warmth with or without an underlying palpable mass.[98] Patients may report breast pain, tenderness, and itchiness as well.[97]

Staging of Lymphedema

The severity of BCRL can be classified by stage based on clinical presentation. Stage 0 is considered subclinical lymphedema because edema is not visible, but lymphatic transport is impaired.[99] Patients may report symptoms consistent with BCRL in stage 0.[99] In stage I, edema is visible and subsides with elevation.[99] Pitting may be present.[99] Stage II is characterized by edema that no longer subsides with elevation; pitting is present.[99] In stage III, pitting is absent and skin changes such as thickening, deposition of fat and fibrosis, or warty overgrowth may have developed.[99]

Diagnosis of Breast Cancer–Related Lymphedema

The diagnosis of lymphedema is often based on patient-reported symptoms, physical examination, and objective measures. Symptoms of BCRL may include aching, fatigue, firmness, numbness, puffiness, soreness, stiffness, tightness, and tingling.[100] These symptoms may be early indicators of BCRL and precede visible signs of BCRL.[100] Edema is the primary sign of BCRL, which may be detected clinically by an increase in size of a body part, loss of visualization of anatomical architecture, deviation from normal anatomical contour, changes in tissue texture, and pitting.[101] Objective measures commonly used in clinical practice to assess BCRL include bioimpedance spectroscopy (BIS), water displacement, and circumferential measurement.

Bioimpedance spectroscopy has been recommended to be used to diagnose stage 0 or I lymphedema.[102] BIS can detect increased extracellular fluid up to 10 months before the onset of clinical signs or symptoms of swelling.[103] BIS uses either a single- or multifrequency device to measure fluid in a limb by determining the resistance of an electrical current passed through the body. The ImpediMed Hy-Dex DF50 (ImpediMed Ltd, Queensland, Australia) is an example of a single-frequency BIS device (50 kHz). A multifrequency BIS device approved by US Food and Drug Administration is the ImpediMed L-Dex U400 (ImpediMed Inc, Carlsbad, CA), which has a frequency range of 3 to 1000 kHz.[102] Normal BIS impedance ratios range from 0.935 to 1.139 if the at-risk side is the patient's dominant arm or 0.862 to 1.006 if the at-risk side is the nondominant arm.[102] Impedance measurements obtained from the ImpediMed L-Dex U400 are converted to a Lymphedema Index Value (L-Dex). Normal L-Dex scores range from −10 to 10 with a score of greater than 10 indicating the presence of lymphedema.[102] When preoperative scores are not available, an L-Dex score of 7.1 has been recommended to be used as a diagnostic criteria for lymphedema.[102] BIS is not approved for use in patients who are pregnant or have a pacemaker or other implanted electronic device.[104] Additionally, BIS may not capture tissue changes associated with late-stage lymphedema.[102]

Water displacement involves submerging a patient's limb in a volumeter filled with water, causing water to be displaced into an adjacent container. The amount of water in the container is measured in milliliters and represents the volume of the patient's limb. It should be noted that water displacement is contraindicated in patients with skin breakdown because of concerns for cross-contamination and infection.[103]

Patient position, measurement technique, and water temperature should be standardized when performing water displacement.[103] Patients can be standing or sitting during measurement. The entire upper extremity may not be able to be fully immersed in water because of the length of the arm and size of volumeter, so determining the upper boundaries of the immersed limb is important. Possible upper boundaries of the immersed limb include 65% of the distance from the elbow (olecranon) to the shoulder (acromion) or 15 cm below the acromion.[103] Acceptable water temperatures have been reported to range from 28°C to 30°C.[103]

The standard error of measurement for water displacement has been found to range from 27.2 to 117.0 mL.[103] The minimally detectable changes were found to be 154.3 mL and 189.5 mL for the left and right arms, respectively.[105] The at-risk side being more than 200 mL larger than the contralateral side and more than a 10% interlimb difference have been recommended as diagnostic criteria for BCRL using water displacement.[102]

Circumferential measurement using a tape measure is a clinically feasible method to assess limb size (Fig. 115.5). By determining the

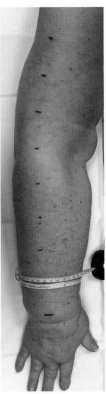

Fig. 115.5 Circumferential measurements of the upper extremity.

girth of the limb at specified increments, the volume of the limb can be calculated by using a geometric formula. Either a frustum or cylinder method can be used to calculate the volume of the limb. The frustum method assumes the limb represents a cone shape rather than a cylindrical shape, which may be a more accurate representation of the patient's limb.[102] However, both methods can overestimate the volume of the limb with the cylinder method overestimating the size of the limb by more than 5% and frustum method by at least 100 mL.[102] The cylinder method formula is

$$V = \tfrac{1}{4}\pi \sum (h)\left(C^2\right)$$

in which h is the length of each segment and C is circumference at fixed point. The formula for the frustum method is:

$$V = 1/12\pi \sum (h)\left(C^2 + Cc + c^2\right)$$

in which h is the length of each segment (i.e., 3 cm, 4 cm) and C and c are the circumferences at two adjacent points.

When performing circumferential measurement, the clinician must not only consider the geometric formula but also the starting point of measurement, the distance between fixed points along the limb, and patient position.[103] The starting point of measurement may be tip of the third digit, base of the third digit, or the ulnar styloid; thus measurement can include or exclude the fingers and hand.[103] A variety of distances along the length of arm to the axilla can be used as fixed points including every 3, 4, 5, 6, 9, 10, 15, or 20 cm.[103] Patient position can influence circumferential measurement; therefore, it should be documented and standardized to reduce measurement error. A common position for circumferential measurement of the upper extremity involves the patient being seated with arm supported on table, shoulder flexed or abducted to 90 degrees, elbow extended, and forearm pronated.

The standard error of measurement (SEM) using every 3, 6, and 9 cm as fixed points has been found to range from 120 to 130 mL for the cylinder method and 114 to 116 mL for the frustum method.[106] Using every 10 cm as fixed points, the SEMs for the frustum method were found to be 93 mL for the affected arm volume, 85 mL for the difference in arm volume (volume affected – volume unaffected), and 0.07 for interlimb ratio (volume affected/volume unaffected).[107] Circumferential measurement has been recommended for the diagnosis of stage I or greater lymphedema.[102] A limb volume ratio of 1.04 and 5% or greater volume change compared with preoperative measurements have been recommended as diagnostic criteria for BCRL.[102]

Other criteria for BCRL based on limb size reported in the literature include a greater than 2 cm difference between arms, greater than 10% volume difference between arms, greater than 10% relative volume difference, greater than 10% relative volume change, or greater than 10% weight-adjusted volume change.[108] It is possible that any one of the mentioned limb size diagnostic criteria could result in a missed diagnosis because BCRL may be present but fail to meet the defined threshold. Therefore, a thorough history and physical examination is essential for diagnosing BCRL.

Physical Examination. Physical assessment of patients with BCRL may include examination for presence of Stemmer's sign, visual inspection, pitting examination, and examination for tissue texture changes. Examination for Stemmer's sign involves the clinician assessing the ability to pinch and lift the skin of the patient. Stemmer's sign is commonly assessed at the dorsal aspect of each phalanx and dorsal aspect of hand. A positive Stemmer's sign is the inability or difficulty in lifting the skin often compared with the contralateral side. Although a positive Stemmer's sign suggests BCRL, a negative

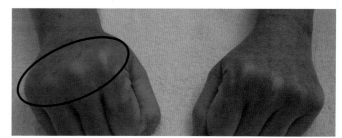

Fig. 115.6 Obscuration of anatomical architecture of the metacarpophalangeal joints.

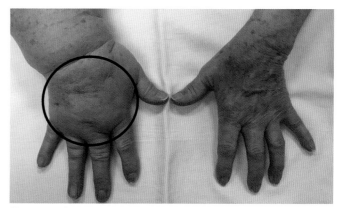

Fig. 115.7 Obscuration of anatomical architecture of the extensor tendons.

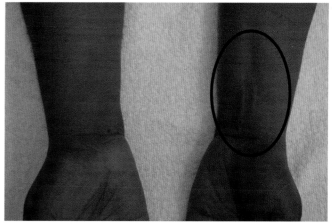

Fig. 115.8 Obscuration of anatomical architecture of the flexor tendons.

test result does not rule out lymphedema because hand swelling does not always occur in patients with BCRL. Therefore, a comprehensive assessment of the entire upper extremity, breast, and torso is required.

Clinicians may visually inspect for signs of BCRL by assessing for obscuration of anatomical architecture, deviation from normal anatomical contour, and presence of peau d'orange. Assessment for obscuration of anatomical architecture involves clinicians visually inspecting for asymmetry of anatomical structures between the at-risk and contralateral sides. Clinicians may visually inspect the metacarpophalangeal (MCP) joints (Fig. 115.6), extensor tendons at the dorsal aspect of the hand (Fig. 115.7), flexor tendons at the wrist (Fig. 115.8), ulnar styloid process, and olecranon process (Fig. 115.9). Loss of ability to visualize the anatomical structure compared to the contralateral side would be a sign of BCRL. In this author's experience, swelling may lead to an obscuration of anatomical architecture

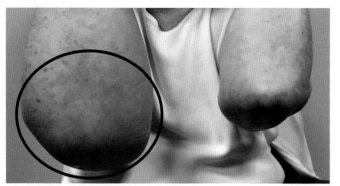

Fig. 115.9 Obscuration of anatomical architecture of the olecranon process.

Fig. 115.11 Pitting edema.

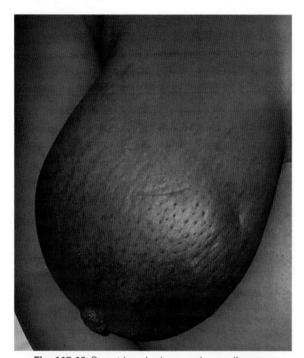

Fig. 115.10 Breast lymphedema and peau d'orange.

before significant changes in circumferential measurements, suggesting visual inspection may have value for early detection of BCRL, especially when preoperative measurements are not available. Deviation from normal anatomical contour occurs as BCRL progresses. Clinicians may assess for asymmetry in anatomical contour between the at-risk and contralateral limbs by visually inspecting the dorsal aspect of the hand, wrist–forearm region, and upper arm region. Normally, the dorsal aspect of the hand appears relatively flat; however, the dorsal aspect of the hand may appear raised with severe BCRL of the hand. With respect to the wrist and forearm, the forearm circumference is typically about twice the size of the wrist circumference. Severe BCRL of the wrist may cause the wrist and forearm to appear as a cylindrical shape, whereas a significant visual difference in the wrist and forearm ratio may occur with severe BCRL of the forearm. A visual sign of BCRL of the upper arm is an increase in the convexity of the posterior–medial aspect of the upper arm compared with the contralateral side. Peau d'orange refers to the skin resembling the skin of an orange. Peau d'orange or dimpling of the skin occurs with noticeable edema and fibrosis and is a common sign of breast edema (Fig. 115.10).

Pitting examination involves the clinician applying sustained pressure to the skin and subcutaneous tissues with his or her finger or thumb. Pitting is defined as a visible indentation in the skin that remains after the applied pressure is released (Fig. 115.11). An absence of visible indentation is considered nonpitting. Additionally, clinicians may evaluate the depth of indentation or recovery time for the skin to return to pre-pressure state to grade the severity of pitting. The traditional assessment of pitting has used a 1+ to 4+ grading system in which 1+ is slight pitting, no visible distortion, disappears rapidly; 2+ is a somewhat deeper pit, no readily detectable distortion, disappears in 10 to 15 seconds; 3+ has a noticeably deep pit, the easily identifiable depression, may last more than 1 minute, the dependent extremity looks full and swollen; and 4+ has a very deep pit, which, lasts 2 to 5 minutes, and the dependent extremity is grossly distorted.[109] Since an adaptation of this grading system was shown to have low to moderate reliability, it has been suggested to rate edema as non-pitting or pitting.[110]

Soft tissue changes may occur in patients with BCRL because of fluid stasis and resultant inflammation. Clinicians should examine for soft tissue texture changes by palpating the skin and subcutaneous tissues. Clinicians may rate tissue texture as "normal," "spongy," "firm," or "hard."[110] Palpable soft tissue texture changes may represent edema or deposition of fat and fibrosis associated with BCRL. Examination for tissue texture changes and pitting should be performed in the regions where patients are at risk for developing BCRL. These regions include the upper extremity (i.e., digits, dorsal hand, palm, wrist, forearm, elbow, and upper arm), torso (i.e., posterior torso and lateral torso), and breast (i.e., upper inner quadrant, lower inner quadrant, upper outer quadrant, lower outer quadrant) on the side treated for breast cancer.

Treatment Strategies for Breast Cancer–Related Lymphedema

Complete Decongestive Therapy. Complete decongestive therapy (CDT) is a conservative multimodal treatment for BCRL that includes skin care, MLD, compression therapy, and exercise. CDT is a two-phase intervention. The goals of phase I (intensive or reduction phase) are to reduce the amount of edema, improve skin integrity, and educate the patient on self-care strategies. The goal of phase II (maintenance phase) is for the patient with BCRL to maintain improvements achieved during phase I of treatment by performing self-care strategies.

The skin care component of CDT involves educating patients on monitoring and caring for their skin. Patients may be instructed to care for their skin by washing and applying moisturizer daily. Patients should monitor for skin breakdown. If noted, general recommendations may include keeping the area clean and dry along with applying a dressing to promote healing and reduce risk of infection. Patients should be educated on the signs of infection such as worsening of edema, redness, warmth, pain, and flulike symptoms. Patients should be instructed to seek immediate medical attention if signs or symptoms of infection are noted.

Manual lymphatic drainage is a manual techniques designed to reduce edema by increasing lymph production, increasing lymphangion contraction rate, and reversing lymph flow.[87] MLD involves hand movements performed by clinicians to stretch the skin in a specific direction. The principles of MLD include (1) use of light pressure, (2) slow movements (~1 stroke/sec), (3) repetitive movements (at least 7 strokes per area), and (4) movements performed in a proximal to distal sequence. Hand movements or strokes performed by clinicians have a "working" phase and a "relaxation" phase. The "working" phase is believed to cause tension on the anchoring filaments of the lymph capillaries and increase the amount of fluid going into the lymphatic system. Increased lymphangion contraction rate is believed to occur as well because of the smooth muscle in the wall of the lymph collectors being stimulated. The "resting" phase refers to when the hand is passively moved back to the starting position by the elasticity of the skin. Types of MLD strokes include stationary circle, pump, scoop, and rotary. Clinicians can perform additional MLD techniques to the abdominal region and to address soft tissue fibrosis. Contraindications for MLD can be classified as general or region specific. General contraindications include cardiac edema, renal failure, acute infection, DVT, bronchial asthma or bronchitis, and active malignancy (relative).[87,88] Contraindications to MLD to the neck include carotid–sinus syndrome, atherosclerosis, and hyperthyroidism.[87,88] Pregnancy, dysmenorrhea, aortic aneurysm, recent abdominal surgery, inflammatory conditions of the intestines, and diverticulosis are contraindications to abdominal MLD.[87,88] An MLD sequence for a patient with BCRL of the right extremity can be found in Fig. 115.12.

Compression therapy is a crucial component of CDT for the treatment of BCRL. Compression therapy decreases the amount of fluid filtering out of the vascular system, increases venous and lymphatic return, improves muscle pump function, increases reabsorptive surface, and softens fibrotic tissue.[87,88] Types of compression strategies used in CDT include compression bandaging (Fig. 115.13) and compression garments (Fig. 115.14). Compression bandaging involves applying multiple materials to the upper extremity to reduce BCRL by creating a compression gradient that is greater distally to facilitate movement of fluid back toward the heart. Bandaging materials may include stockinette, gauze bandages, padding material, foam, and short-stretch bandages (Fig. 115.15). Stockinette and soft padding are used to protect the skin. Gauze bandages are applied to the digits. Foam (Fig. 115.16) may be applied to the upper extremity to soften tissue fibrosis, protect bony prominences or sensitive areas, and provide more even distribution of pressure. Short-stretch bandages are preferred over long-stretch bandages because of the difference in extensibility and elasticity, which affects the amount of resting and working pressure. *Resting pressure* refers to the amount of pressure exerted by the bandage without muscle contraction or joint movement. Working pressure is the amount of pressure exerted by the bandage during muscle contraction or joint movement. A short-stretch bandage can be extended approximately 60% of the original length, whereas a long-stretch bandage can extend approximately 140% of the original length.[87] Short-stretch bandages have a lower resting pressure than long-stretch bandages but a higher working pressure. To maximize comfort and reduce the risk of tourniquet-like effect constricting veins and lymph vessels, short-stretch bandages with a lower resting pressure are desired because patients may be instructed to wear compression bandages while sleeping.[87] A higher working pressure is beneficial because an adequate counterforce or resistance during muscle contraction or joint movement can facilitate fluid transport and prevent fluid from accumulating.[87]

Compression garments are medical-grade sleeves, gloves, or gauntlets used to maintain improvements achieved during phase I of CDT. Compression garments may be prescribed, instead of compression bandaging, to address subclinical or early stage BCRL. When selecting a compression garment, clinicians must decide on the type of knit (i.e., circular or flat), size (i.e., ready-made or custom), and compression level (i.e., 20–30 mm Hg or 30–40 mm Hg). Factors clinicians should consider when selecting a compression garment for a patient with BCRL include the patient's response to compression bandaging, the shape of the limb, patient preference, physical limitations, and cost.[87] Compression garments are worn during waking hours only; they are not typically worn while sleeping because of their elasticity and high resting pressure. Patients may be instructed to self-bandage or wear bandaging alternative devices if compression is required while sleeping to control BCRL. Bandaging alternative devices are less elastic than compression garments and may be more appropriate for patients who experience significant fluctuations of their lymphedema, including patients with malignant lymphedema. Various types of bandaging alternative devices are available for patients with BCRL. Examples of bandaging alternative devices can be found in Fig. 115.17.

With respect for breast and torso lymphedema, a short-stretch bandage such as Isoband (BSN Medical, Charlotte, NC) could be circumferentially applied around the torso (Fig. 115.18). However, alternate compression strategies for the breast and torso are typically recommended, including a well-fitting bra, sports bra, compression bra, compression vest, or camisole top. Foam inserts can be fabricated as well (Fig. 115.19). Clinicians should be cautious with the use of compression therapy with patients who have hypertension, cardiac arrhythmias, renal failure, congestive heart failure, decreased or absent sensation, partial or complete paralysis, mild to moderate peripheral artery disease, and malignant lymphedema.[87] Cardiac edema, acute infection, and severe peripheral artery disease are contraindications for compression therapy.[87]

Exercise as a component of CDT is performed while wearing compression to facilitate fluid movement to the vascular system. Clinicians should design individualized exercise programs, taking into consideration any comorbidities or limitations. Exercise programs may have patients perform AROM in a proximal to distal sequence then repeat in reverse order. An example of an exercise program may include 5 to 10 repetitions of the following exercises: cervical rotation, cervical lateral flexion, shoulder rolls, shoulder shrugs, shoulder elevation, elbow flexion–extension, wrist circles in each direction, and digit flexion–extension.

Intermittent Pneumatic Compression Devices. Intermittent pneumatic compression (IPC) devices are recommended as an adjunct to CDT rather than the sole intervention for treatment of BCRL.[111] Patients may be instructed to use an IPC device for 1 hour one or two times per day. IPC devices can be classified as single-chamber, multichamber, or advanced compression system. Single-chamber IPC devices are not optimal for BCRL management because the devices do not apply a pressure gradient; the devices consist of a single cuff that applies pressure to the upper extremity.[111] Multichamber IPC devices have from 4 to 36 chambers with higher pressure in the distal chambers and lower pressure in proximal chambers; thus creating a pressure gradient.[111] Advanced compression systems may have only 1 to 2.5 chambers active at a time, which simulates the distal-to-proximal direction used during MLD.[111] Additionally, advanced compression systems may include a truncal chamber to assist with proximal lymphatic drainage.[111] Evidence supports the use of IPC pressures ranging from 30 to 60 mm Hg.[112] A sustained pressure of 60 to 70 mm Hg is suggested as the maximum pressure because of concern for lymph vessel damage if pressures are too high or sustained for too

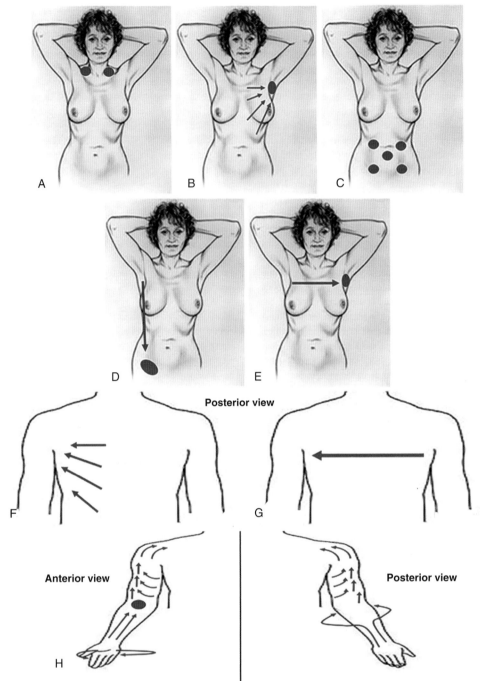

Fig. 115.12 Manual lymphatic drainage sequence for a patient with breast cancer–related lymphedema of the right upper extremity. **A,** Short neck sequence: stationary circles at supraclavicular fossa and shoulder region. **B,** Contralateral axillary lymph nodes: perform stationary circles over the contralateral axillary lymph nodes and along the normal lymphatic drainage pattern of contralateral upper torso region. **C,** Abdominal sequence: gentle circular strokes along direction of colon; diaphragmatic breathing with manual hand pressure. **D,** Ipsilateral inguinal lymph nodes: perform stationary circles over the ipsilateral inguinal lymph nodes; establish the axilloinguinal anastomosis by performing strokes along the lateral aspect of torso from the axillary lymph nodes to the inguinal lymph nodes. **E,** Anterior axilloaxillary anastomosis: establish the posterior axilloaxillary anastomosis by performing strokes over the sternum from the ipsilateral axillary lymph nodes to contralateral axillary lymph nodes. **F,** Posterior torso: perform strokes according to normal lymphatic drainage pattern of the contralateral upper torso. **G,** Posterior axilloaxillary anastomosis: establish the posterior axilloaxillary anastomosis by performing strokes over the shoulder blade region from the ipsilateral axillary lymph nodes to contralateral axillary lymph nodes. **H,** Anterior and posterior deltoid region: perform stationary circles directing fluid proximally. Lateral upper arm: perform strokes directing fluid proximally. Medial upper arm: perform strokes directing fluid toward lateral aspect of arm. Cubital fossa: perform stationary circles. Perform strokes at the elbow, forearm, and hand directing fluid according to a normal lymphatic drainage pattern as previously described. (Source for parts A, B, C, D, and E National Cancer Institute.)

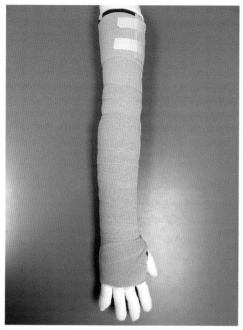

Fig. 115.13 Upper extremity compression bandage.

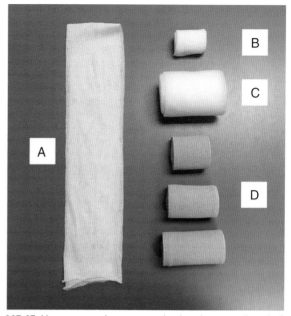

Fig. 115.15 Upper extremity compression bandage supplies. **A,** Stockinette. **B,** Gauze bandage. **C,** Soft padding. **D,** Short-stretch bandages (6, 8, and 10 cm).

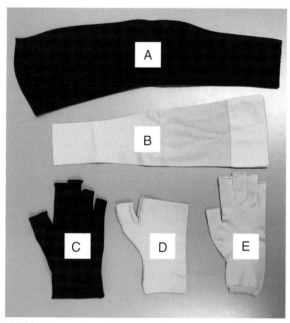

Fig. 115.14 Upper extremity compression garments. **A,** Custom compression sleeve. **B,** Ready-made compression sleeve. **C,** Custom flat knit compression sleeve. **D,** Ready-made compression gauntlet. **E,** Ready-made compression glove.

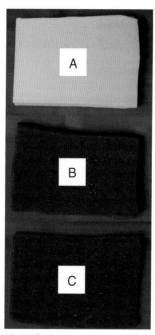

Fig. 115.16 Foam options. **A,** Komprex (Lohmann & Rauscher, Milwaukee, WI). **B,** Gray foam , ½ inch. **C,** Gray foam – ¼ inch.

long of a period of time.[111,112] Because of the concern for proximal accumulation of edema with the use of IPC devices, it has been suggested that clinicians and patients monitor for increased edema and tissue fibrosis above the location where the compression sleeve ends.[112]

CANCER-RELATED FATIGUE

Cancer-related fatigue (CRF) is defined as a "distressing, persistent, subjective sense of physical, emotional, and/or cognitive tiredness or exhaustion related to cancer or cancer treatment that is not proportional to recent activity and interferes with usual functioning."[113] CRF is one of the more common side effects experienced by patients treated for breast cancer that can negatively impact function and quality of life.[114] Up to 91% of patients treated for breast cancer have been reported to experience CRF.[114] CRF may be more likely to occur in patients who receive radiation therapy and chemotherapy.[114] CRF may continue for months and even years after treatment.[115]

CRF is often caused by more than one problem (i.e., pain, depression or anxiety, lack of sleep, poor nutrition, anemia, or other medical conditions), requiring multiple health professionals (physicians,

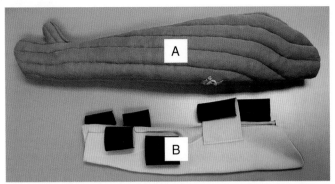

Fig. 115.17 Bandaging alternative devices. **A,** JoviPak Arm Sleeve (BSN Medical, Charlette, NC). **B,** Circaid JuxtaFit Essentials Upper Extremity (mediUSA, Whitsett, NC).

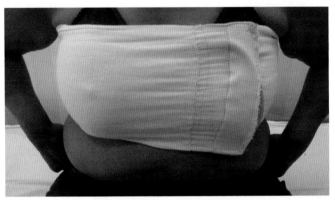

Fig. 115.18 Isoband wrap for breast and torso lymphedema.

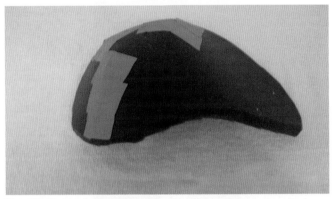

Fig. 115.19 Bowl-shaped foam insert for breast and torso lymphedema.

nurses, social workers, nutritionists) being involved to address any medical condition that may be causing or worsening fatigue.[113] The therapist's role in the management of CRF can include patient education (pattern of fatigue, self-monitoring, energy conservation, sleep hygiene) and exercise prescription.

Patient Education

Patients should be educated about fatigue and its known pattern during and after treatment. The pattern of fatigue is dependent on the type of cancer treatment the patient is receiving.[113] For patients receiving chemotherapy, fatigue has been found to peak 2 to 7 days after chemotherapy administration and then tends to decline throughout the chemotherapy cycle but does not return to pretreatment levels.[116,117] The intensity of fatigue may increase with each cycle of chemotherapy.[116,117] For patients receiving radiation, fatigue gradually increases

during treatment and then slowly decreases over the next 4 months after treatment.[118]

To minimize the effects of fatigue, patients could be educated on daily self-monitoring of fatigue levels, sleep, rest, activity, and other symptoms in a journal.[113,119] A list can then be made prioritizing usual activities to identify valued activities or activities that need to be completed.[119] Maintaining a journal helps to identify times of peak energy so activities can be planned accordingly, within a structured routine, and an energy-conservation plan can be implemented to manage valued activities and minimize the interference of fatigue.[119]

Energy conservation is defined as the deliberately planned management of one's personal energy resources to prevent their depletion.[113] Energy conservation involves balancing rest and activity during times of high fatigue to maintain the ability to perform activities and meet one's needs.[116,119] Energy-conservation strategies include taking additional rest periods along with reducing effort (sitting down to accomplish tasks or holding objects close to the body when carrying), prioritizing (eliminating or reducing tasks that may not be important or not need to be completed), delegating (allowing family members or friends who offer help to complete tasks), pacing (avoiding rushing behaviors; attending to one activity at a time), planning (thinking ahead, balancing hard activities with easier activities, scheduling activities during times of peak energy), and organizing (moving items used frequently closer).[116] For example, patients may be provided the following recommendations regarding cleaning or performing housework: only clean one room per day, use a rolling chart or apron with large pockets to carry supplies from room to room, keep extra supplies on every floor, take trash out in small bags to avoid heavy lifting, and stop working before they get too tired.

Patients should be educated on proper sleep habits.[113] They should go to bed when tired and at approximately the same time each night and should attempt to wake at the same time each morning. An environment favorable to sleep is dark, quiet, and comfortable.[113] Patients should be educated on factors that may impact sleep such as watching TV and computer or cell phone usage immediately before bed.[113] In addition, they should be educated on the possibility that ingesting caffeine, alcohol, or high-sugar foods before bed may negatively impact sleep.[113] Daytime naps may be helpful in replenishing energy but may hinder sleep at night; therefore, patients should avoid long and late afternoon naps so as to not interfere with night-time sleep quality.[113]

Physical Activity and Exercise

Physical activity and exercise have been recommended as a nonpharmacologic strategies for the management of CRF both during and after cancer treatment.[113] Although the terms *physical activity* and *exercise* are often used interchangeably, there are distinct differences. Physical activity is "any bodily movement produced by the contraction of skeletal muscle that results in a substantial increase in caloric requirements over resting energy expenditure."[120] Exercise is "a type of physical activity consisting of planned, structured, and repetitive body movements" designed to address impairments, improve function, and improve fitness and health.[120]

More physical activity has been found to be associated with less fatigue in patients diagnosed with breast cancer.[121] Patients diagnosed with breast cancer should avoid inactivity and return to normal activities as soon as possible after surgery.[122] However, certain activity restrictions may be recommended immediately after breast surgery. For example, patients with drains may be instructed to limit arm motions to below 90 degrees of shoulder elevation until drains have been removed.[38] During the first few weeks after surgery, patients may be advised to use their affected arm normally during tasks such as combing hair, getting dressed, and eating but may be instructed to avoid lifting more than 5 lb.[34,123]

Recent systematic reviews have shown that exercise reduces CRF.[124-126] Exercise has been shown to be effective in reducing CRF both during and after cancer treatment.[126] A greater effect of exercise on CRF in patients with solid tumors compared with hematologic and mixed malignancy types has been reported.[126] Exercise has been reported to significantly reduce CRF in survivors of breast cancer.[124] Both home-based and supervised exercise programs have been shown to reduce CRF.[126] The benefit of exercise has been reported to not significantly differ by type of exercise (aerobic, walking, mixed).[126] Greater reductions in CRF have been reported to occur with moderate-intensity (3–6 metabolic equivalents; 60%–80%, 1-repetition maximum) resistance exercise compared to lower intensity or aerobic exercise of any level of intensity.[124] The intensity of aerobic exercise has been found to be negatively associated with fatigue reduction, meaning moderate-intensity exercise had a greater effect on reducing fatigue than high-intensity exercise across mixed cancer types.[127] However, no significant dose–response for exercise intensity (high intensity >80% maximal heart rate) and CRF has been reported in breast cancer survivors who perform supervised exercise.[125] Greater reductions in CRF have been reported in exercise interventions performed for more than 28 weeks, nearly 3 sessions per week, and lasting 40 minutes per session in breast cancer survivors who perform supervised exercise.[125] However, duration and frequency have been reported to have no effect on magnitude of CFR reduction in studies across mixed cancer types and delivery methods.[124]

Resistance Exercise Prescription

Resistance exercise offers many health benefits for patients diagnosed with breast cancer, including (1) increased muscle strength, (2) improved body composition, (3) reduced fatigue, (4) improved emotional well-being, (5) improved physical function, and (6) improved quality of life.[128] Resistance exercise is generally considered safe both during and after breast cancer treatment; however, exercise programs may need to be adapted based on the timing and type of cancer treatments received and stage of disease.[122] The American College of Sports Medicine (ACSM) Exercise Guidelines for Cancer Survivors recognizes the need to allow adequate time to heal after surgery and state the number of weeks required as high as 8 weeks.[122] Patients receiving chemotherapy may be immune compromised or experience anemia and thrombocytopenia and may require exercise program modification.[122] Exercise programs need to be altered for patients with advanced cancer such as bone metastases to reduce risk of fracture.[122] Increased risk of fracture in patients on hormonal therapy or those diagnosed with osteoporosis should be considered as well when prescribing an exercise program.[122] Therefore, exercise prescription should be individualized, taking into consideration side effects of cancer as well as treatment, pretreatment, current fitness level, and any medical comorbidities.[122]

Historically, after breast cancer surgery and radiation therapy, patients were discouraged from participating in resistive exercise because of the concern for increasing risk of developing lymphedema; however, research supports the safe and efficacious use of resistive exercise in patients treated for breast cancer.[129] Patients who perform resistive exercise may actually have reduced risk of developing or exacerbating BCRL.[129] There is no discrete upper limit for the amount of weight or resistance that patients diagnosed with breast cancer should use. Significantly greater strength gains without risk of increased lymphedema symptoms have actually been reported to occur when patients perform moderate- to high-intensity exercise compared with no exercise.[130] However, patients with BCRL have been shown

to demonstrate a greater likelihood of experiencing a musculoskeletal injury compared with patients at risk for BCRL.[131] The ASCM's guidelines recommend that patients diagnosed with breast cancer seek care to address arm or shoulder problems before performing upper body exercise.[122]

Resistive exercise programs performed by patients after breast surgery as described in the literature have been performed two or three times per week for up to 24 months.[128,132] Intensity of upper body exercises ranged from low (0.5 lb) to high (8-repetition maximum).[132] Training volume ranged from 8 to 12 repetitions per exercise for two or three sets.[132] The timing of progressive resistive exercise may be appropriate within 4 to 6 weeks after surgery.[133] The initial use of light weights (1–2 lb) has been suggested if progressive resistive exercises are initiated soon after surgery.[133]

A reasonable approach would be to instruct patients to initiate a resistive exercise program at a low intensity (1–3 lb or smallest resistance level) and progress slowly. This may reduce the risk of injury or exacerbating lymphedema. The resistance level may be increased by the smallest increment after the patient is able to perform the exercise for consecutive sessions without a change in lymphedema symptoms.[134,135] To monitor for development or exacerbation of lymphedema, patients should be instructed to inspect for any changes in size, appearance, or texture of the arm, breast, or torso. Patients may experience lymphedema symptoms before visible edema occurring; therefore, patients should be should be educated on common symptoms associated with lymphedema. Common lymphedema symptoms include sensations of aching, firmness, numbness, puffiness, soreness, stiffness, tightness, or tingling.[100,136] If patients diagnosed with breast cancer experience changes in symptoms or swelling, a reduction or avoidance of upper body exercise should be considered until the issue has been resolved or controlled.[122]

Screening for Cancer-Related Fatigue

All patients diagnosed with breast cancer should be screened for CRF at regular intervals.[113] The National Comprehensive Cancer Network Guidelines for CRF suggests using a numeric rating scale (0–10) to screen for CRF, in which 0 indicates "no fatigue" and 10 indicates "worst fatigue imaginable."[113] If CRF is mild (rating of 1–3), patients should receive education and general management strategies for CRF.[113] If CRF is moderate (rating of 4–6) or severe (rating of 7–10), a more thorough history and examination is recommended for the assessment of treatable contributing factors.[113]

REFERENCES

1. Siegel RL, Miller KD, Jemal A. Cancer statistics, 2018. *CA Cancer J Clin.* 2018;68:7–30.
2. Miller KD, Siegel RL, Lin CC, et al. Cancer treatment and survivorship statistics, 2016. *CA Cancer J Clin.* 2016;66:271–289.
3. WJea Gradishar. *NCCN Clinical Practice Guidelines in Oncology Breast Cancer Version 4.2017. NCCN.org.* National Comprehensive Cancer Network, Inc; 2017.
4. McDonald ES, Clark AS, Tchou J, Zhang P, Freedman GM. Clinical Diagnosis and Management of Breast Cancer. *J Nucl Med.* 2016;57(suppl 1):9S–16S.
5. LaCross JS. Surgical management of breast cancer. *JAAPA.* 2015;28:47–48, 50–2, 4–5.
6. Boughey JC, Donohue JH, Jakub JW, Lohse CM, Degnim AC. Number of lymph nodes identified at axillary dissection: effect of neoadjuvant chemotherapy and other factors. *Cancer.* 2010;116:3322–3329.
7. OncoLink Rx. Trustees of the University of Pennsylvania, 2018. Accessed February 27, 2018.

8. Lee TS, Kilbreath SL, Refshauge KM, Herbert RD, Beith JM. Prognosis of the upper limb following surgery and radiation for breast cancer. *Breast Cancer Res Treat.* 2008;110:19–37.

9. Verbelen H, Gebruers N, Eeckhout FM, Verlinden K, Tjalma W. Shoulder and arm morbidity in sentinel node-negative breast cancer patients: a systematic review. *Breast Cancer Res Treat.* 2014;144:21–31.

10. Steginck-Jansen CW, Buford Jr WL, Patterson RM, Gould LJ. Computer simulation of pectoralis major muscle strain to guide exercise protocols for patients after breast cancer surgery. *J Orthop Sports Phys Ther.* 2011;41:417–426.

11. Vadivelu N, Schreck M, Lopez J, Kodumudi G, Narayan D. Pain after mastectomy and breast reconstruction. *Am Surg.* 2008;74:285–296.

12. Kuerer HM. *Kuerer's Breast Surgical Oncology.* New York: McGraw Hill Companies; 2010.

13. Ilhan E, Chee E, Hush J, Moloney N. The prevalence of neuropathic pain is high after treatment for breast cancer: a systematic review. *Pain.* 2017;158:2082–2091.

14. Piper M, Guajardo I, Denkler K, Sbitany H. Axillary web syndrome: current understanding and new directions for treatment. *Ann Plast Surg.* 2016;76(suppl 3):S227–S231.

15. Haanpaa M, Attal N, Backonja M, et al. NeuPSIG guidelines on neuropathic pain assessment. *Pain.* 2011;152:14–27.

16. Reyes-Gibby C, Morrow PK, Bennett MI, Jensen MP, Shete S. Neuropathic pain in breast cancer survivors: using the ID pain as a screening tool. *J Pain Symptom Manage.* 2010;39:882–889.

17. Nijs J, Leysen L, Adriaenssens N, et al. Pain following cancer treatment: guidelines for the clinical classification of predominant neuropathic, nociceptive and central sensitization pain. *Acta Oncol.* 2016;55:659–663.

18. Mayer TG, Neblett R, Cohen H, et al. The development and psychometric validation of the central sensitization inventory. *Pain Pract.* 2012;12:276–285.

19. Neblett R, Cohen H, Choi Y, et al. The Central Sensitization Inventory (CSI): establishing clinically significant values for identifying central sensitivity syndromes in an outpatient chronic pain sample. *J Pain.* 2013;14:438–445.

20. Neblett R, Hartzell MM, Cohen H, et al. Ability of the central sensitization inventory to identify central sensitivity syndromes in an outpatient chronic pain sample. *Clin J Pain.* 2015;31:323–332.

21. Neblett R, Hartzell MM, Mayer TG, Cohen H, Gatchel RJ. Establishing clinically relevant severity levels for the central sensitization inventory. *Pain Pract.* 2017;17:166–175.

22. Wang L, Guyatt GH, Kennedy SA, et al. Predictors of persistent pain after breast cancer surgery: a systematic review and meta-analysis of observational studies. *CMAJ.* 2016;188:E352–E361.

23. Belfer I, Schreiber KL, Shaffer JR, et al. Persistent postmastectomy pain in breast cancer survivors: analysis of clinical, demographic, and psychosocial factors. *J Pain.* 2013;14:1185–1195.

24. Harrington S, Gilchrist L, Sander A. Breast cancer edge task force outcomes: clinical measures of pain. *Rehabil Oncol.* 2014;32:13–21.

25. Strand LI, Ljunggren AE, Bogen B, Ask T, Johnsen TB. The Short-Form McGill Pain Questionnaire as an outcome measure: test-retest reliability and responsiveness to change. *Eur J Pain.* 2008;12:917–925.

26. Gauthier LR, Young A, Dworkin RH, et al. Validation of the short-form McGill Pain Questionnaire-2 in younger and older people with cancer pain. *J Pain.* 2014;15:756–770.

27. Dworkin RH, Turk DC, Revicki DA, et al. Development and initial validation of an expanded and revised version of the Short-form McGill Pain Questionnaire (SF-MPQ-2). *Pain.* 2009;144:35–42.

28. Lovejoy TI, Turk DC, Morasco BJ. Evaluation of the psychometric properties of the revised short-form McGill Pain Questionnaire. *J Pain.* 2012;13:1250–1257.

29. The Brief Pain Inventory: User Guide. 2009. Accessed February 27, 2018, at https://www.mdanderson.org/research/departments-labs-institutes/departments-divisions/symptom-research/symptom-assessment-tools/brief-pain-inventory.html.

30. Kaufman B, Wu Y, Amonkar MM, et al. Impact of lapatinib monotherapy on QOL and pain symptoms in patients with HER2+ relapsed or refractory inflammatory breast cancer. *Curr Med Res Opin.* 2010;26:1065–1073.

31. Hidding JT, Beurskens CH, van der Wees PJ, van Laarhoven HW, Nijhuis-van der Sanden MW. Treatment related impairments in arm and shoulder in patients with breast cancer: a systematic review. *PLoS One.* 2014;9:e96748.

32. Smoot B, Paul SM, Aouizerat BE, et al. Predictors of altered upper extremity function during the first year after breast cancer treatment. *Am J Phys Med Rehabil.* 2016;95:639–655.

33. Perdomo M, Sebelski CA, Davies C. Oncology section task force on breast cancer outcomes: shoulder and glenohumeral outcome measures. *Rehabilitation Oncology.* 2013;30:19–26.

34. Wilson DJ. Exercise for the patient after breast cancer surgery. *Semin Oncol Nurs.* 2017;33:98–105.

35. De Groef A, Van Kampen M, Dieltjens E, et al. Effectiveness of postoperative physical therapy for upper-limb impairments after breast cancer treatment: a systematic review. *Arch Phys Med Rehabil.* 2015;96:1140–1153.

36. McNeely ML, Campbell K, Ospina M, et al. Exercise interventions for upper-limb dysfunction due to breast cancer treatment. *Cochrane Database Syst Rev.* 2010:CD005211.

37. McNeely ML, Binkley JM, Pusic AL, Campbell KL, Gabram S, Soballe PW. A prospective model of care for breast cancer rehabilitation: postoperative and postreconstructive issues. *Cancer.* 2012;118:2226–2236.

38. Galantino ML, Stout NL. Exercise interventions for upper limb dysfunction due to breast cancer treatment. *Phys Ther.* 2013;93:1291–1297.

39. American Cancer Society. *Exercises after Breast Cancer Surgery;* 2017, at https://www.cancer.org/cancer/breast-cancer/treatment/surgery-for-breast-cancer/exercises-after-breast-cancer-surgery.html.

40. Springer BA, Levy E, McGarvey C, et al. Pre-operative assessment enables early diagnosis and recovery of shoulder function in patients with breast cancer. *Breast Cancer Res Treat.* 2010;120:135–147.

41. Lipps DB, Sachdev S, Strauss JB. Quantifying radiation dose delivered to individual shoulder muscles during breast radiotherapy. *Radiother Oncol.* 2017;122:431–436.

42. Cheville AL, Tchou J. Barriers to rehabilitation following surgery for primary breast cancer. *J Surg Oncol.* 2007;95:409–418.

43. Rodemann HP, Bamberg M. Cellular basis of radiation-induced fibrosis. *Radiother Oncol: Journal of the European Society for Therapeutic Radiology and Oncology.* 1995;35:83–90.

44. Yang EJ, Park WB, Seo KS, Kim SW, Heo CY, Lim JY. Longitudinal change of treatment-related upper limb dysfunction and its impact on late dysfunction in breast cancer survivors: a prospective cohort study. *J Surg Oncol.* 2010;101:84–91.

45. Yang EJ, Kang E, Jang JY, et al. Effect of a mixed solution of sodium hyaluronate and carboxymethyl cellulose on upper limb dysfunction after total mastectomy: a double-blind, randomized clinical trial. *Breast Cancer Res Treat.* 2012;136:187–194.

46. De Groef A, Van Kampen M, Verlvoesem N, et al. Effect of myofascial techniques for treatment of upper limb dysfunctions in breast cancer survivors: randomized controlled trial. *Support Care Cancer.* 2017;25:2119–2127.

47. Borstad JD, Ludewig PM. Comparison of three stretches for the pectoralis minor muscle. *J Shoulder Elbow Surg.* 2006;15:324–330.

48. Muraki T, Aoki M, Izumi T, Fujii M, Hidaka E, Miyamoto S. Lengthening of the pectoralis minor muscle during passive shoulder motions and stretching techniques: a cadaveric biomechanical study. *Phys Ther.* 2009;89:333–341.

49. Umehara J, Nakamura M, Fujita K, et al. Shoulder horizontal abduction stretching effectively increases shear elastic modulus of pectoralis minor muscle. *J Shoulder Elbow Surg.* 2017;26:1159–1165.

50. Lee SY, Sim MK, Do J, Jeong SY, Jeon JY. Pilot study of effective methods for measuring and stretching for pectoral muscle tightness in breast cancer patients. *J Phys Ther Sci.* 2016;28:3030–3035.

51. Viriyatharakij N, Chinkulprasert C, Rakthim N, Patumrat J, Ketruang B. Change of pectoralis minor length, and acromial distance, during scapular retraction at 60 degrees shoulder elevation. *J Bodyw Mov Ther.* 2017;21:53–57.

52. Bulley C, Coutts F, Blyth C, et al. A Morbidity Screening Tool for identifying fatigue, pain, upper limb dysfunction and lymphedema after breast cancer treatment: a validity study. *Eur J Oncol Nurs.* 2014;18:218–227.

53. Yeung WM, McPhail SM, Kuys SS. A systematic review of axillary web syndrome (AWS). *J Cancer Surviv.* 2015;9:576–598.

54. Moskovitz AH, Anderson BO, Yeung RS, Byrd DR, Lawton TJ, Moe RE. Axillary web syndrome after axillary dissection. *Am J Surg.* 2001;181:434–439.

55. Figueira PVG, Haddad CAS, de Almeida Rizzi SKL, Facina G, Nazario ACP. Diagnosis of axillary web syndrome in patients after breast cancer surgery: epidemiology, risk factors, and clinical aspects: a prospective study. *Am J Clin Oncol.* 2017.

56. Lauridsen MC, Christiansen P, Hessov I. The effect of physiotherapy on shoulder function in patients surgically treated for breast cancer: a randomized study. *Acta Oncol.* 2005;44:449–457.

57. Torres Lacomba M, Mayoral Del Moral O, Coperias Zazo JL, Yuste Sanchez MJ, Ferrandez JC, Zapico Goni A. Axillary web syndrome after axillary dissection in breast cancer: a prospective study. *Breast Cancer Res Treat.* 2009;117:625–630.

58. Welsh P, Gryfe D. Atypical presentation of axillary web syndrome (AWS) in a male squash player: a case report. *J Can Chiropr Assoc.* 2016;60:294–298.

59. Bergmann A, Mendes VV, de Almeida Dias R, do Amaral ESB, da Costa Leite Ferreira MG, Fabro EA. Incidence and risk factors for axillary web syndrome after breast cancer surgery. *Breast Cancer Res Treat.* 2012;131:987–992.

60. Koehler LA, Blaes AH, Haddad TC, Hunter DW, Hirsch AT, Ludewig PM. Movement, function, pain, and postoperative edema in axillary web syndrome. *Phys Ther.* 2015;95:1345–1353.

61. Nevola Teixeira LF, Veronesi P, Lohsiriwat V, et al. Axillary web syndrome self-assessment questionnaire: initial development and validation. *Breast.* 2014;23:836–843.

62. Black J, Green D, McKenna C, Squadrito J, Taylor S, Palombaro KM. Therapists' perspectives and interventions in the management of axillary web syndrome: an exploratory study. *Rehabil Oncol.* 2014;32:16–22.

63. Fourie WJ, Robb KA. Physiotherapy management of axillary web syndrome following breast cancer treatment: discussing the use of soft tissue techniques. *Physiotherapy.* 2009;95:314–320.

64. Lewis PA, Cunningham JE. Dynamic angular petrissage as treatment for axillary web syndrome occurring after surgery for breast cancer: a case report. *Int J Ther Massage Bodywork.* 2016;9:28–37.

65. Black Lattanzi J, Zimmerman A, Marshall LM. Case report of axillary web syndrome. *Rehabil Oncol.* 2012;30:18–21.

66. Cho Y, Do J, Jung S, Kwon O, Jeon JY. Effects of a physical therapy program combined with manual lymphatic drainage on shoulder function, quality of life, lymphedema incidence, and pain in breast cancer patients with axillary web syndrome following axillary dissection. *Support Care Cancer.* 2016;24:2047–2057.

67. Kepics JM. Physical therapy treatment of axillary web syndrome. *Rehabil Oncol.* 2004;22:21–22.

68. Pfalzer LA. Physical agents/modalities for survivors of cancer. *Rehabil Oncol.* 2001;19:12–24.

69. Kelley MJ, Shaffer MA, Kuhn JE, et al. Shoulder pain and mobility deficits: adhesive capsulitis. *J Orthop Sports Phys Ther.* 2013;43:A1–31.

70. Yang S, Park DH, Ahn SH, et al. Prevalence and risk factors of adhesive capsulitis of the shoulder after breast cancer treatment. *Support Care Cancer.* 2017;25:1317–1322.

71. Georgiannos D, Markopoulos G, Devetzi E, Bisbinas I. Adhesive capsulitis of the shoulder. Is there consensus regarding the treatment? A comprehensive review. *Open Orthop J.* 2017;11:65–76.

72. Bellow JW, Michlovitz SL, Nolan Jr TP. *Michlovitz's Modalities for Therapeutic Intervention.* 6th ed. Philadelphia: F.A. Davis Company; 2016.

73. Cheville AL, Basford JR. Role of rehabilitation medicine and physical agents in the treatment of cancer-associated pain. *J Clin Oncol.* 2014;32:1691–1702.

74. Robijns J, Censabella S, Bulens P, Maes A, Mebis J. The use of low-level light therapy in supportive care for patients with breast cancer: review of the literature. *Lasers Med Sci.* 2017;32:229–242.

75. Lindblad K, Bergkvist L, Johansson AC. Evaluation of the treatment of chronic chemotherapy-induced peripheral neuropathy using long-wave diathermy and interferential currents: a randomized controlled trial. *Support Care Cancer.* 2016;24:2523–2531.

76. Sousa MAG, Cecatto RB, Rosa CDP, Brita CMM, Battistella LR. Ultrasound therapy and transcutaneous electrical neuromuscular stimulation for management of post-mastectomy upper limb lymphedema. *Act Fisiatr.* 2014;21:189–194.

77. Ferreira da Rezende L, Silva da Costa EC, Guimaraes Moraes Schenka N, Almeida Schenka A, Uemura G. Effect of continuous and pulsed therapeutic ultrasound in the appearance of local recurrence of mammary cancer in rats. *J BUON.* 2012;17:581–584.

78. Alappattu M, Harrington S, Pfalzer LA. *Current Evidence for Use of Physical Agents in Rehabilitation Oncology: Fact vs. Fiction.* Indianapolis: Combined Sections Meeting of the American Physical Therapy Association; 2015.

79. Stubblefield MD, Keole N. Upper body pain and functional disorders in patients with breast cancer. *PMR.* 2014;6:170–183.

80. Ebaugh D, Spinelli B, Schmitz KH. Shoulder impairments and their association with symptomatic rotator cuff disease in breast cancer survivors. *Med Hypotheses.* 2011;77:481–487.

81. Lawrence RL, Braman JP, Laprade RF, Ludewig PM. Comparison of 3-dimensional shoulder complex kinematics in individuals with and without shoulder pain, part 1: sternoclavicular, acromioclavicular, and scapulothoracic joints. *J Orthop Sports Phys Ther.* 2014;44:636–645. A1–A8.

82. DiSipio T, Rye S, Newman B, Hayes S. Incidence of unilateral arm lymphoedema after breast cancer: a systematic review and meta-analysis. *Lancet Oncol.* 2013;14:500–515.

83. Verbelen H, Gebruers N, Beyers T, De Monie AC, Tjalma W. Breast edema in breast cancer patients following breast-conserving surgery and radiotherapy: a systematic review. *Breast Cancer Res Treat.* 2014;147:463–471.

84. Bosompra K, Ashikaga T, O'Brien PJ, Nelson L, Skelly J. Swelling, numbness, pain, and their relationship to arm function among breast cancer survivors: a disablement process model perspective. *Breast J.* 2002;8:338–348.

85. Kilbreath SL, Lee MJ, Refshauge KM, et al. Transient swelling versus lymphoedema in the first year following surgery for breast cancer. *Support Care Cancer.* 2013;21:2207–2215.

86. Wratten CR, O'Brien PC, Hamilton CS, Bill D, Kilmurray J, Denham JW. Breast edema in patients undergoing breast-conserving treatment for breast cancer: assessment via high frequency ultrasound. *Breast J.* 2007;13:266–273.

87. Zuther JE, Norton S. *Lymphedema Management: The Comprehensive Guide for Practitioners*; 2013.

88. Foldi M, Foldi E, Strobenreuther R, Kubik S. *Foldi's Textbook of lymphology for Physicians and Lymphedema Therapists.* Munchen, Germany: Elsevier GmbH, Urban & Fischer Verlag; 2012.

89. Cho S, Atwood JE. Peripheral edema. *Am J Med.* 2002;113:580–586.

90. Asdourian MS, Skolny MN, Brunelle C, Seward CE, Salama L, Taghian AG. Precautions for breast cancer-related lymphoedema: risk from air travel, ipsilateral arm blood pressure measurements, skin puncture, extreme temperatures, and cellulitis. *Lancet Oncol.* 2016;17:e392–405.

91. Nguyen TT, Hoskin TL, Habermann EB, Cheville AL, Boughey JC. Breast cancer-related lymphedema risk is related to multidisciplinary treatment and not surgery alone: results from a large cohort study. *Ann Surg Oncol.* 2017;24:2972–2980.

92. Czihal M, Hoffmann U. Upper extremity deep venous thrombosis. *Vasc Med.* 2011;16:191–202.

93. Heil J, Miesbach W, Vogl T, Bechstein WO, Reinisch A. Deep vein thrombosis of the upper extremity. *Dtsch Arztebl Int.* 2017;114:244–249.

94. Wan JF, Bezjak A. Superior vena cava syndrome. *Emerg Med Clin North Am.* 2009;27:243–255.

95. Rachapalli V, Boucher LM. Superior vena cava syndrome: role of the interventionalist. *Can Assoc Radiol J.* 2014;65:168–176.

96. Krasagakis K, Valachis A, Maniatakis P, Kruger-Krasagakis S, Samonis G, Tosca AD. Analysis of epidemiology, clinical features and management of erysipelas. *Int J Dermatol.* 2010;49:1012–1017.

97. Taghian A, El-Ghamry MN, Merajver S. *Inflammatory Breast Cancer: Clinical Features and Treatment.* Waltham, MA: UpToDate; 2018. Post TW.

98. Dawood S, Merajver SD, Viens P, et al. International expert panel on inflammatory breast cancer: consensus statement for standardized diagnosis and treatment. *Ann Oncol.* 2011;22:515–523.

99. International Society of Lymphology Advisory Committee. The diagnosis and treatment of peripheral lymphedema: 2013 Consensus Document of the International Society of Lymphology. *Lymphology*. 2013;46:1–11.

100. Fu MR, Axelrod D, Cleland CM, et al. Symptom report in detecting breast cancer-related lymphedema. *Breast Cancer (Dove Med Press)*. 2015;7:345–352.

101. Cheville AL, McGarvey CL, Petrek JA, Russo SA, Thiadens SR, Taylor ME. The grading of lymphedema in oncology clinical trials. *Semin Radiat Oncol*. 2003;13:214–225.

102. Levenhagen K, Davies C, Perdomo M, Ryans K, Gilchrist L. Diagnosis of upper-quadrant lymphedema secondary to cancer: clinical practice guideline from the oncology section of APTA. *Rehabil Oncol*. 2017;35: E1–E18.

103. Perdomo M, Davies C, Levenhagen K, Ryans K. Assessment measures of secondary lymphedema in breast cancer survivors. *Rehabil Oncol*. 2014;32:22–35.

104. Shah C, Vicini FA, Arthur D. Bioimpedance spectroscopy for breast cancer related lymphedema assessment: clinical practice guidelines. *Breast J*. 2016;22:645–650.

105. Taylor R, Jayasinghe UW, Koelmeyer L, Ung O, Boyages J. Reliability and validity of arm volume measurements for assessment of lymphedema. *Phys Ther*. 2006;86:205–214.

106. Sander AP, Hajer NM, Hemenway K, Miller AC. Upper-extremity volume measurements in women with lymphedema: a comparison of measurements obtained via water displacement with geometrically determined volume. *Phys Ther*. 2002;82:1201–1212.

107. Czerniec SA, Ward LC, Refshauge KM, et al. Assessment of breast cancer-related arm lymphedema—comparison of physical measurement methods and self-report. *Cancer Investigation*. 2010;28:54–62.

108. Ancukiewicz M, Miller CL, Skolny MN, et al. Comparison of relative versus absolute arm size change as criteria for quantifying breast cancer-related lymphedema: the flaws in current studies and need for universal methodology. *Breast Cancer Res Treat*. 2012;135:145–152.

109. Ball JW, Dains JE, Flynn JA, Solomon BS, Stewart RW. *Seidel's Guide to Physical Examination*. 8th ed. St. Louis: Elsevier Mosby; 2015.

110. Spinelli B, Kallan MJ, Zhang X, et al. Intra- and Interrater reliability and concurrent validity of a new tool for assessment of breast cancer-related lymphedema of the upper extremity. *Arch Phys Med Rehabil*. 2019;100:315–326.

111. Feldman JL, Stout NL, Wanchai A, Stewart BR, Cormier JN, Armer JM. Intermittent pneumatic compression therapy: a systematic review. *Lymphology*. 2012;45:13–25.

112. Chang CJ, Cormier JN. Lymphedema interventions: exercise, surgery, and compression devices. *Semin Oncol Nurs*. 2013;29:28–40.

113. Berger AMea. *NCCN Clinical Practice Guidelines in Oncology: Cancer-Related Fatigue Version 2.2018*. National Comprehensive Cancer Network, Inc.; 2018.

114. Runowicz CD, Leach CR, Henry NL, et al. American Cancer Society/ American Society of Clinical Oncology Breast Cancer Survivorship Care Guideline. *J Clin Oncol*. 2016;34:611–635.

115. Fabi A, Falcicchio C, Giannarelli D, Maggi G, Cognetti F, Pugliese P. The course of cancer related fatigue up to ten years in early breast cancer patients: What impact in clinical practice? *Breast*. 2017;34:44–52.

116. Barsevick AM, Whitmer K, Sweeney C, Nail LM. A pilot study examining energy conservation for cancer treatment-related fatigue. *Cancer Nursing*. 2002;25:333–341.

117. Schwartz AL, Nail LM, Chen S, et al. Fatigue patterns observed in patients receiving chemotherapy and radiotherapy. *Cancer Investigation*. 2000;18:11–19.

118. Hofso K, Rustoen T, Cooper BA, Bjordal K, Miaskowski C. Changes over time in occurrence, severity, and distress of common symptoms during and after radiation therapy for breast cancer. *J Pain Symptom Manage*. 2013;45:980–1006.

119. Barsevick AM, Dudley W, Beck S, Sweeney C, Whitmer K, Nail L. A randomized clinical trial of energy conservation for patients with cancer-related fatigue. *Cancer*. 2004;100:1302–1310.

120. Nobel M, ed. *ACSM's Guidelines for Exercise Testing and Prescription*. 10th ed. Philadelphia: Wolters Kluwer Health; 2018.

121. Ehlers DK, Aguinaga S, Cosman J, Severson J, Kramer AF, McAuley E. The effects of physical activity and fatigue on cognitive performance in breast cancer survivors. *Breast Cancer Res Treat*. 2017;165:699–707.

122. Schmitz KH, Courneya KS, Matthews C, et al. American College of Sports Medicine roundtable on exercise guidelines for cancer survivors. *Med Sci Sports Exerc*. 2010;42:1409–1426.

123. *Exercises After Breast Cancer Surgery*. The American Cancer Society; 2017. (Accessed February 27, 2018 at. https://www.cancer.org/cancer/ breast-cancer/treatment/surgery-for-breast-cancer/exercises-after-breast-cancer-surgery.html).

124. Brown JC, Huedo-Medina TB, Pescatello LS, Pescatello SM, Ferrer RA, Johnson BT. Efficacy of exercise interventions in modulating cancer-related fatigue among adult cancer survivors: a meta-analysis. Cancer epidemiology, biomarkers & prevention : a publication of the American Association for Cancer Research, cosponsored by the American Society of Preventive Oncology 2011;20:123–133.

125. Meneses-Echavez JF, Ramirez-Velez R, Gonzalez-Jimenez E. Effects of supervised exercise on cancer-related fatigue in breast cancer survivors: a systematic review and meta-analysis. *BMC Cancer*. 2015;15:1069.

126. Tomlinson D, Diorio C, Beyene J, Sung L. Effect of exercise on cancer-related fatigue: a meta-analysis. *Am J Phys Med Rehabil*. 2014;93:675–686.

127. Dennett AM, Peiris CL, Shields N, Prendergast LA, Taylor NF. Moderate-intensity exercise reduces fatigue and improves mobility in cancer survivors: a systematic review and meta-regression. *J Physiother*. 2016;62:68–82.

128. Dieli-Conwright CM, Orozco BZ. Exercise after breast cancer treatment: current perspectives. *Breast Cancer (Dove Med Press)*. 2015;7:353–362.

129. Keilani M, Hasenoehrl T, Neubauer M, Crevenna R. Resistance exercise and secondary lymphedema in breast cancer survivors-a systematic review. *Support Care Cancer*. 2016;24:1907–1916.

130. Nelson NL. Breast cancer-related lymphedema and resistance exercise: a systematic review. *Journal of Strength and Conditioning Research / National Strength & Conditioning Association*. 2016;30. 2656–2365.

131. Brown JC, Troxel AB, Schmitz KH. Safety of weightlifting among women with or at risk for breast cancer-related lymphedema: musculoskeletal injuries and health care use in a weightlifting rehabilitation trial. *The Oncologist*. 2012;17:1120–1128.

132. Dos Santos WDN, Gentil P, de Moraes RF, et al. Chronic effects of resistance training in breast cancer survivors. *Biomed Res Int*. 2017;2017:8367803.

133. Harris SR, Schmitz KH, Campbell KL, McNeely ML. Clinical practice guidelines for breast cancer rehabilitation: syntheses of guideline recommendations and qualitative appraisals. *Cancer*. 2012;118:2312–2324.

134. Schmitz KH, Ahmed RL, Troxel A, et al. Weight lifting in women with breast-cancer-related lymphedema. *N Engl J Med*. 2009;361:664–673.

135. Schmitz KH, Ahmed RL, Troxel AB, et al. Weight lifting for women at risk for breast cancer-related lymphedema: a randomized trial. *JAMA*. 2010;304:2699–2705.

136. Fu MR. Breast cancer-related lymphedema: symptoms, diagnosis, risk reduction, and management. *World J Clin Oncol*. 2014;5:241–247.

116

Focal Hand Dystonia

Nancy N. Byl, Jonathan Kretschmer, Alison McKenzie

OUTLINE

CRITICAL POINTS

- Although the etiology of focal hand dystonia (FHD) is still considered idiopathic, there is agreement that the phenotypic presentation has a multifactorial etiology.
- FHD includes involuntary end-range twisting and posturing of the fingers and wrist caused by co-contractions of agonists and antagonists.
- Endotypically, patients with FHD lack normal homeostatic plasticity, exhibit aberrant learning, have somatosensory challenges, and demonstrate excessive excitation with inadequate inhibition.
- Signs and symptoms of FHD are variable, and confirmation of the diagnosis may take years.
- The onset of FHD may initially manifest as an abnormality in the quality of sound produced by a musical instrument, increased errors in the performance of a specific target task, unusual fatigue, sense of weakness, or involuntary excessive movement of one or more digits.
- Although classifications for FHD remain somewhat controversial, hand dystonias are typically classified as *simple dystonia* (e.g., involving only the hand or impacting a single task), *dystonic dystonia* (e.g., abnormal hand movements disrupt multiple hand tasks), or *progressive dystonia* (e.g., dystonia involving more than one body segment such as the hand and the arm).

- Hand dystonia can also be classified by occupation (e.g., writer's cramp, musician's cramp).
- Ruling in the diagnosis is based on a comprehensive *clinical* assessment.
- There is no single, specific clinical or neuroimaging test to diagnose FHD.
- Intervention must be oriented toward management rather than cure.
- Successful management needs to be comprehensive and personalized, ranging from education, priming the nervous system to learn, to brain retraining.
- Behavioral retraining of the brain must follow evidence-based principles of neuroplasticity.
- Type one evidence supports the benefits of repeated botulinum toxin injections to weaken overexcited muscles.
- Sensorimotor rehabilitation interventions improve self- and clinician-rated subjective assessments of physical performance, but improvement in objective measurements of movement dysfunction may be lacking.
- Research evidence is weak regarding the effectiveness of different behavioral intervention strategies.
- More research is needed to understand the etiology and the most effective prevention and remediation strategies for treating patients with FHD.

INTRODUCTION

Repetitive strain injuries, or *cumulative trauma disorders*, are commonly reported in individuals who perform stressful jobs that demand accurate, repetitive fine-motor movements such as typing, playing a musical instrument, keyboarding on a computer, working in an assembly line, or writing. Some individuals manage the challenge by creating a healthy lifestyle, managing stress, taking regular time off work, integrating regular breaks at work, or modifying the ergonomics of performance. When ergonomic issues cannot be resolved, inflammation and pain can develop or, in some cases, unusual, disabling, painless involuntary movements of the hand may begin to compromise performance. These involuntary movements can be referred to as *focal hand dystonia (FHD)*. FHD is hypothesized to be caused by an accumulation of intrinsic stressors (e.g., genetics, neurophysiology, abnormal anatomic structures, behavioral characteristics) and extrinsic factors (e.g., environment, type of work, expectations, finances, stress).

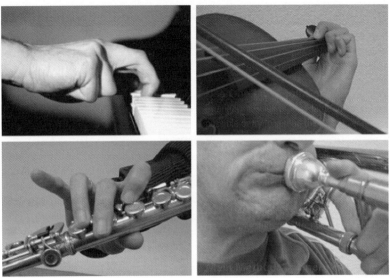

Fig. 116.1 Typical patterns of dystonic posture in a pianist (**A**), a violinist (**B**), a flutist (**C**), and a trombone player (**D**). (From Altenmuller E, Jabusch HC. Focal hand dystonia in musicians: phenomenology, etiology and psychological trigger factors. *J Hand Ther.* 2009;22:145.)

This chapter reviews the definitions, etiology, diagnosis (history, examination, ruling in the diagnosis), treatment goals, intervention strategies, effectiveness of management, future research needs, and resources associated with FHD. The aims of this chapter are to (1) increase awareness of FHD among health care professionals specializing in the hand and upper limb; (2) encourage clinicians to participate in educational programs to prevent hand dystonia and other repetitive strain injuries; (3) enable clinicians to make an early diagnosis of hand dystonia; (4) prepare multidisciplinary clinicians to provide patient education, support, and encouragement for recovery; (5) encourage physicians and therapists to help patients prime the nervous system to learn as well as develop creative, innovative, insightful, and effective learning-based retraining programs to maximize normal neural adaptation, quality of life, and independent function; and (6) challenge clinicians to participate in multidisciplinary clinical and translational research studies to better understand the etiology and improve the effectiveness of treatment for hand dystonia.

DEFINITION AND CLASSIFICATION OF FOCAL DYSTONIA

An ad hoc committee of the scientific advisory board of the Dystonia Medical Research Foundation agreed on the following definition of dystonia: *dystonia* is a syndrome including sustained and repetitive muscle contractions that cause twisting, end-range abnormal postures.[1] A dystonia that involves a particular body part (e.g., hand, neck, foot) is called a *focal limb dystonia*. When the limb dystonia occurs only during the performance of a target task, it is called *task-specific* or *action dystonia*. Albanese and colleagues[1] further define action dystonia as involuntary posturing (dystonia) superimposed on a voluntary movement. The majority of patients with task-specific *limb* dystonia have problems with the *upper* limb. However, recently, with increased emphasis on fitness and running, foot and leg dystonia (or runner's dystonia) are becoming more common.[2]

There are a variety of ways to classify focal dystonia. However, there is no universal agreement.[3] Albanese[3] classified focal dystonia into the following groups: cranial dystonia (including blepharospasm), oro-mandibular dystonia, spasmodic torticollis (cervical dystonia), truncal dystonia, writer's cramp, and other occupational or task-specific

dystonias. Fig. 116.1 provides photographs of four typical patterns of hand dystonia in musicians.

In task-specific dystonia, the tasks affected usually require (1) highly repetitive fine-motor movements; (2) extreme motor precision; (3) interplay between conscious or at least "feedback-related" modulation; or (4) a repetitively executed motor plan.[4] Although the involuntary movement dysfunction is not painful, muscle cramping can be uncomfortable. Unfortunately, task-specific FHD can bring an abrupt halt to a promising occupational, professional, or performance career.[5,6]

In 1833, Bell was the first to refer to hand dystonia as *scrivener's palsy.* In 1861, Duchenne described a similar disability in French workers. Limb dystonias may also be referred to as "action dystonias" and are often classified by occupation (e.g., musician's dystonia, golfer's "yip", writer's cramp, keyboarder's cramp, hairdresser's dystonia, table tennis dystonia).[7–9]

In addition to the classification of limb dystonias by occupation, a focal limb dystonia can be further subdivided into three additional categories: *simple cramp* (abnormal movements in relation to a single task or a single body part), *dystonic cramp* (abnormal movements in relation to more than one task), and *progressive (complex or dystonic) cramp* (abnormal movement that begins in relation to a single task or a single limb that later impacts the performance of other tasks or other body parts). A higher proportion of those who develop progressive or complex dystonia most commonly have an initial onset of dystonia of the right hand.[10] Neurologists have also noted some patients develop *mirror dystonia* on the uninvolved side. Mirror dystonia is thought to represent motor overflow to the unaffected limb when the affected limb performs the target task.[11]

It is estimated repetitive motion disorders of the upper limb may develop in up to 1% of musicians. Individuals such as writers, computer users, data entry workers, and programmers are similarly at risk.[12] Focal dystonia is more common in men.[13] Initially, writer's cramp was considered the most common type of hand dystonia. Today, it is equally common to see patients with keyboarders or musicians dystonia. Among musicians, brass players, plucking musicians (e.g., guitarists), and woodwind players have the highest relative risk for developing FHD.[14–16] More high-quality epidemiologic studies are needed to clarify the incidence and prevalence of FHD.[17]

ETIOLOGY OF FOCAL HAND DYSTONIA

Over the past 20 years, basic and clinical research studies have provided increased insight into the etiology of focal dystonia. Although the cause of FHD is still considered idiopathic, there is consensus that the problem is multifactorial.[17-20] Intrinsic factors interact with extrinsic factors to produce the clinical phenotype of FHD. For some individuals, intrinsic factors may be the strongest contributor (e.g., genetics, neurophysiologic dysfunction, anatomic restrictions, sensory deficits, aberrant homeostatic plasticity). For others, extrinsic factors such as excessive repetition, trauma, stress, poor lifestyle, certain personality characteristics (e.g., perseveration, perfectionism, phobias), and particularly poor hand biomechanics[21] may contribute to the development of the FHD phenotype.

Endophenotypic Factors

Genetics

A common intrinsic factor leading to the development of dystonia is genetics. There are known familial genes associated with primary general dystonia.[22,23] Although to date, no specific gene has been identified for focal *hand* dystonia, new genes for focal dystonia are being discovered all the time. Commonly, patients with a genetic etiology for dystonia have a receptor abnormality for dopamine binding in the putamen.[24] This can decrease the dopamine normally secreted in rewarded, repetitive, associative, and nonassociative learning behaviors. Despite a unilateral presentation of hand dystonia, abnormal neurophysiologic measures are reported bilaterally, reinforcing the possibility of a genetic risk factor.[25] Interestingly, approximately 30% of individuals with FHD have a distant relative with a movement disorder (e.g., Parkinson's disease, general dystonia, Alzheimer's disease).

In Germany, a gene has been identified in a family in whom many members develop a focal cervical dystonia. All those with cervical dystonia had the gene, but cervical dystonia did not develop in *all* family members with the gene. None of the family members reported a FHD. Another interesting gene is the *DYTI* gene detected in Ashkenazi Jewish families. Although some family members with the DYTI gene develop a generalized dystonia, others develop a focal dystonia, and others are dystonia free. Thus, the genes associated with *focal* dystonia have been classified as genes of "low penetrance."

Basal Ganglia–Thalamocortical Dysfunction

Researchers report specific dysfunction in the basal ganglia–thalamocortical motor circuit in patients with dystonia.[25] Within the basal ganglia, the striatum receives major inputs from the motor cortex. The output modems include the globus pallidus (internal segment), substantia nigra, and pars reticulata. Direct and indirect pathways connect to the input and output nuclei. Except for one excitatory projection, all pathways interconnecting the basal ganglia nuclei are inhibitory. Dystonia could result from either excessive activity in the direct striatum–globus pallidus (internal segment) pathway or from reduced activity in the indirect striatum–globus pallidus (external segment) pathway.[26] Focal dystonia is sometimes considered a prototype of a hyperkinetic disorder resulting from an imbalance of excitation and inhibition in the globus pallidus.[25] On the other hand, repetitive practice alone can also modify structure.[27,28]

Hypoactivity of inhibitory pathways could also result from reduced basal ganglia output or reduced activity in the motor thalamus. Interestingly, the putamen and the pallidum[29] show evidence of hypermetabolism in patients with general dystonia as well as some patients with hand dystonia. The involvement of the putamen may explain why a pallidotomy can reduce the severity of symptoms in patients with generalized dystonia and some with hand dystonia.

Inadequate Inhibition

Lack of inhibition at multiple levels of the nervous system seems to be a fundamental problem in the genesis of generalized and focal dystonia. The nervous system requires a balance between excitation and inhibition of neural circuits to facilitate smooth, coordinated motor control. A variety of forms of inhibition are used to control the precision and smoothness of movement, particularly in the hand, in which individual finger movements require selective and specific activation of muscles. Interestingly, repetitive finger practice can reduce surround inhibition.[30]

Reciprocal inhibition allows for the control of muscles around a single joint. Lack of reciprocal inhibition at the spinal and peripheral level leads to co-contractions of antagonistic muscles (characteristic of patients with hand dystonia).[31] In patients with FHD, moving intended fingers is associated with the firing of unnecessary adjacent fingers. Electromyographic (EMG) technology has documented muscle overactivity along with inappropriate co-contractions, prolongation of EMG bursts into muscle groups outside the intended movement, abnormal H reflexes, and abnormal long latency reflexes. These signs can also be interpreted as a reflection of a loss of *reflex* inhibition. The loss of reflex inhibition is consistent with the clinical deterioration of fine, graduated movements observed in patients with hand dystonia.

Using transcranial magnetic stimulation (TMS) as a diagnostic neurophysiological strategy, abnormal *cortical* inhibition has been demonstrated bilaterally, even in patients with unilateral FHD. Both inhibitory interneuronal activity and surround inhibition are reported as abnormal in patients with FHD. *Surround* inhibition allows selective control of individual muscles by simultaneous inhibition of surrounding muscles. The indirect pathway of the globus pallidus plays a major role in *surround inhibition*. Dysfunction of *inhibitory* interneurons that use γ-aminobutyric acid as a neurotransmitter could further mediate the abnormal *surround* inhibition at the cortical level.

Anatomic Musculoskeletal Limitations

In the population, some people have tight joints, muscles, nerves, and fascia (e.g., neural tension around the brachial plexus, restrictions in the retinaculum in the hand). These restrictions do not necessarily cause FHD, but it is common to find limitations in end-range finger spread, forearm pronation–supination, and shoulder rotation in patients with FHD. It is possible that anatomic restrictions put a patient at risk for the development of pain syndromes, weakness, or a hand dystonia, particularly under conditions of stressful, highly repetitive practice.[32]

Leijinse and Hallet[21] proposed a musculoskeletal etiologic model of FHD in which defects in the musculoskeletal system combined with environmental factors such as overuse may lead to FHD. In this model, the assumption is the acquisition of instrumental techniques requires high levels of physiologic movements under high performance demands in the face of ergonomic limitations of the instrument and individual anatomy. This model predicts the development of focal dystonia is preceded by gradual changes in playing techniques over a long period of time.

Based on this musculoskeletal hypothesis, ineffective or physiologically infeasible playing movements must be modified by voluntary (teaching) or involuntary (systemic) feedback. If the movement modifications do not converge to allow an individual to use muscle synergies that satisfy all constraints, movement modifications will continue until overcompensated muscle synergies are produced. Antagonists of the intended movements are recruited, and dystonic symptoms develop. Based on this model, musculoskeletal limitations should be addressed in the individual hand to resolve peripheral conflicts between constraints and tasks. Leijinse and Hallet[21] suggest that early remediation of the musculoskeletal limitations could prevent the dystonia, and neurologic retraining would be unnecessary.

In a posttraining anatomic study of nonhuman primates with behaviorally induced FHD, one monkey had an anatomic defect of the profundus tendon, with adhesions on the middle and distal segments of the fourth digit on the trained side and of the third digit on the untrained side. On the side trained at a highly repetitive, attended, stereotypical task, movement dysfunction developed in 5 weeks, significantly earlier than in the other monkeys. The somatosensory representation of the hand was degraded, particularly the receptive fields for D4. However, on the untrained side, there were no signs of involuntary motor control or somatosensory degradation of the third digit. If biomechanical demands on the hands are not stressful, movement dysfunction might not develop, even when anatomic restrictions are present.

Abnormal Motor Preparation

A striking characteristic of FHD is its task specificity. At onset, symptoms are manifested only when the patient performs a specific task (e.g., writing, playing an instrument, using a keyboard). This specificity may affect only certain passages, not all aspects of performance. This interesting task specificity was initially thought to be psychiatric in origin.

Some researchers report a deficiency in the preparation or organization of established motor programs in patients with FHD.[33,34] For example, using neuroimaging techniques, underactivity of motor areas has been reported during writing in patients with writer's cramp. Interestingly, Stinear and Byblow[34a] observed defective intracortical inhibition only during voluntary movements, never at rest. Other researchers report differences in set shifting in patients with FHD compared with control participants and abnormal sequential learning. Still others such as Frucht[34b] also observed that task-specific musician's dystonia seemed to begin *after* motor skills had been acquired rather than during skill acquisition. This suggests those with musicians dystonia do not have a problem of motor learning but rather a corruption of acquired, complex motor programs.

Sensory Abnormalities

Although FHD is characterized as a movement disorder, there is evidence of dysfunction in cortical sensory processing.[35] Cortical somatosensory receptive fields are abnormally enlarged and disorganized in patients with hand dystonia.[36] In patients with unilateral FHD, bilateral difficulty with discriminating sensory stimuli has been measured in both the spatial and temporal domains.[37,38]

Sensory processing may play a modulatory role in dystonia. For example, a sensory trick such as touching, holding, or taping can quiet the dystonic symptoms in an involved digit. On the other hand, tonic vibration can lead to a worsening of dystonia, whereas anesthetic blocks can relieve symptoms. In terms of intervention, sensory retraining in the form of tactile discrimination practice, including reading Braille, stereotactic matching tasks, and interpreting information drawn on the skin,[37-39] has been shown to decrease involuntary motor movements.

There is also evidence of abnormal sensorimotor integration and sensory gating in patients with FHD. For example, Cheng and coworkers[40] noted altered tactile and auditory feedback in patients with musicians dystonia. Nowak and colleagues[40a] also evaluated the impact of sensorimotor integration problems in patients with writer's cramp and musician's cramp by studying the adaptive grip forces (e.g., used when lifting a new object) or adjusting grip force when anticipating or reacting to a change in load force (e.g., when catching a weight). Interestingly, patients with FHD and normal control participants showed similar predictive grip force adjustments to expected changes in object load. On the other hand, patients with dystonia produced grip force overshoot during the initial lift and had a shorter latency of grip force

response than control participants after an unexpected load increase. The researchers proposed that patients with dystonia appear to have a greater level of preparatory motor activity or a disinhibited spinal reflex response compared with healthy control participants. They also suggested the increased grip force measured was likely attributable to a prelearned phenomenon rather than a primary disorder of sensorimotor integration.

Unfortunately, no studies have documented neurosensory processing competencies or abnormalities in patients before the onset of hand dystonia. Thus, it is unclear whether somatosensory and sensorimotor dysfunction predispose a patient to dystonia under conditions of stressful repetitive hand use or whether repetitive, nearly simultaneous overuse of the hands degrades the somatosensory hand representation and leads to involuntary dystonic movements. In basic science primate and rat studies, repetitive overuse was associated with bilateral peripheral and central inflammatory responses as well as changes in somatosensory, sensorimotor, and motor areas of the brain, even when the training involved only one side and the hand dystonia was unilateral.[40]

Side of Involvement

Retrospectively, six patients with typist's cramp and five cases of writer's cramp located in the PubMed database were evaluated. The data were compared between patients with simple dystonia (dystonia in only one specific task) and those with dystonia or progressive dystonia (dystonia in several or new tasks). The initially affected right hand ratio was significantly higher in dystonia or progressive dystonia groups than in the simple dystonia group ($P = .015$). The affected hand is usually the one associated with the amount of daily routine use, but if it is the right hand, it may also be a predictor for the progression of dystonia.[10]

Maladaptive Homeostatic Plasticity

The central nervous system (CNS) is plastic. New motor skills are acquired throughout one's lifetime. With sensory, motor, and mental learning, the plasticity of the nervous system changes circuitry to accommodate new skill development. These changes in synaptic connections and circuitry occur with maturation but can also be purposely driven by learning-based training activities in a dynamic environment. However, plasticity is not infinite. Furthermore, although plasticity is usually controlled by homeostatic mechanisms, it seems that plasticity can potentially be excessive, leading to loss of control and destabilization. In patients with focal dystonia, there is some evidence homeostatic mechanisms may be abnormal.

Quartarone and colleagues[41] hypothesized patients with dystonia had an impairment in the ability to keep cortical excitability within a normal physiologic range. Usually, anodal stimulation enhances the inhibitory effect of TMS in terms of corticospinal excitability and cathodal stimulation reverses the aftereffects of TMS, producing an increase in corticospinal excitability. In patients with writer's cramp, after preconditioning with transcranial direct current stimulation (tDCS), there were no consistent changes in corticospinal excitability after TMS stimulation. Quartarone and colleagues[41,41a] interpreted these findings to mean that the homeostatic mechanisms stabilizing excitability levels were impaired in patients with writer's cramp, reinforcing excessive corticospinal excitability.

Another interpretation of the aberrant plasticity findings is that patients with focal dystonia have an exceptionally adaptive nervous system. Neural changes may exceed the neural operating limits. This abnormally enhanced plasticity could explain the abnormal organization of the sensory, sensorimotor, and motor maps with loss of motor control of the hand in patients who develop FHD following repetitive hand use.[42-44]

It is also possible that aberrant plasticity may be generated by an environmental trigger. For example, practice and repetition usually lead to improved performance. Positive feedback and behavioral rewards increase acetylcholine, dopamine, and other modulatory neurotransmitters to generate continual positive neural adaptation. However, because of competition between neuronal pathways, neural adaptation is not infinite. When something changes in the practice cycle (e.g., modification of the equipment or technique, task complexity, time on task), there may be a marked change in behavior. Increased investment of time may lead to deterioration rather than improvement in performance. As the operative movements become faster, the temporal inputs become nearly simultaneous, losing their individual differentiation. At some point, stereotypic repetition can lead to a degradation in the response. The more the practice, the more the fatigue and the more the patient begins to sense some emergent incoordination. Finally, the fingers seem to develop a life of their own, uncontrollably curling when performing the target task.[42]

Cortical networks engage both excitatory and inhibitory neurons by strong input perturbation. Within a given cortical area, cortical pyramidal cells cannot be effectively re-excited by another perturbation for tens to hundreds of milliseconds. These integration times are dictated primarily by the time for recovery from inhibition, which dominates poststimulus excitability. The cortex continues to define its representation of the temporal aspects of behaviorally important inputs by generating more synchronous representations of sequenced input perturbations or events. These time constants both govern and limit the ability to "chunk" (i.e., to separately represent by distributed coordinated discharge) successive events within its processing channels.

Researchers such as Bara-Jimenez and colleagues[36] propose the abnormal reorganization of the cortex in patients with FHD may not be based on rigidly learned highly repetitive movements. Rather, a congenital or remote acquired abnormal cortical deficit might explain some of the abnormal reorganization. Experience-based reshaping of cortical representation can be mediated by dynamic plastic operations of the brain, with subject–environment interactions affecting the organization of the somatosensory cortex.

Exophenotypic Factors

Repetitive Use

The common association between highly skilled manual performance and the development of FHD is suggestive of an environmental contribution (e.g., repetitive use).[43] The theory is that although practice and repetition generally have a positive effect on learning, it is possible that when the repetition is excessive or even associated with some peripheral damage, it can have a negative effect on the nervous system, including involuntary movements and impaired timing.[44–46,46a]

Goal-directed, repetitive movements are known to drive measurable change in structure, neuroenzymes, myelination, and function. Selective spatial and spectral cell assemblies have sharp segregation and result in more complex, efficient behaviors. These event-by-event complex signal representations are highly plastic. Positive adaptive learning can also be measured as an increase in the size of the cortical representation; smaller receptive fields; increased efficiency, amplitude, and density of evoked responses; and distinct, orderly representations. (See Box 116.e1 for a summary of the principles of neuroplasticity.) Because fine-motor control of complex and simple finger movements requires accurate feedforward and feedback information from the primary sensory cortex and related pathways, the dystonia that can develop in individuals involved in high levels of repetitive fine-motor work could represent a type of negative integrative neural adaptation.

A primate and a rat model were created to study the effects of repetition and hand dystonia. The outcomes of these studies led to the" learning-based sensorimotor learning hypothesis." In the nonhuman primate studies by Byl and colleagues,[46b,46c] significant dedifferentiation of the sensory representation of the hand followed training with highly repetitive, stereotypical digital opening and closing movements of the hand. In these primates, the receptive fields increased in size, with the evoked neural response engaging a broadened neuronal network across adjacent digits and across dorsal and glabrous surfaces. This degradation in representation was associated with a decrease in accurate and specific motor control (Figs. 116.e1 and 116.e2). More recently, in human studies using magnetoencephalography, the same researchers not only confirmed the degradation in topography but also documented problems in timing and spatial processing in the somatosensory (S1 and S2), premotor, and motor cortices in the ipsilateral and contralateral hemispheres of the affected and unaffected digits in patients with dystonia.

Using a learning-based rat model to study peripheral inflammation associated with repetition under different force conditions, Barbe and colleagues,[46d] Elliot and colleagues,[47] and Coq[47a] and colleagues also documented a progressive model of dysfunction in motor control with excessive repetition. The dysfunction began with a cascade of peripheral inflammation of the heavily used extremity that crossed over midline to the opposite side and then centralized. As the repetitive movements continued, a noticeable, inefficient movement dysfunction in feeding was observed in the reaching hand. Clinically, the rat lost dexterity, and a scooping strategy was noted. Then aberrant cortical changes were measured (decreased differentiation of the digits) in the somatosensory, sensorimotor, and motor cortices in the rats developing the inefficient hand strategy of scooping for food. Other researchers have also reported a change in somatosensory cortical topography after repetitive motor movements. A low current stimulation of the motor cortex excessively excited the neurons and fired agonists and antagonists across the wrist and the digits.

Sanger and Merzenich[47b] translated the learning-based sensorimotor hypothesis into a computational model to explain the changes in topography and the abnormal motor output in individuals in whom FHD developed (Fig. 116.e3). This model explains several features of focal dystonia: (1) symptoms develop in otherwise healthy individuals in response to highly attended repetitive movements, (2) evolution of symptoms is variable in terms of time, (3) symptoms appear only during the performance of a target-specific task, (4) dystonic movements persist despite stopping the task, (5) symptoms can be decreased but not remediated with dopamine-depleting drugs or botulinum toxin, and (6) evidence of abnormalities in motor and sensory cortical representations of the dystonic limb.

In this model, gain can be increased by expanding or even shrinking the sensory cortical representation of a limb as a result of adaptation to repetitive use or specific increased, simultaneous firing; coupling of multiple sensory signals; and voluntary co-activation of muscles. The loop through the deep nuclei, including the cortex, basal ganglia, and thalamus, combined with the sensorimotor loop gain, contributes to instability. If only certain mechanical models of the sensorimotor loop are unstable, a focal dystonia, rather than a generalized dystonia, can develop.

Based on this computational model of FHD, treatment must decrease the imbalance in the loop gain. A permanent solution requires redifferentiation of cortical and subcortical representations to release excessive gain. Retraining may not be possible in the context of severe dystonia without temporarily breaking the cycle. Botulinum toxin injections may be one way to stop the abnormal muscle firing at the periphery. Another approach is to increase the variability of practiced movements so there are many uncorrelated movement components, each with only a few relevant sensory neurons. This is comparable with behaviors uncoupling the pathologically coupled modes.

Trauma

Focal dystonia can develop after an insult such as trauma, disease, vascular insufficiency, or anatomic restriction. For example, dystonic movements have been reported in patients after a fall on an outstretched arm, a head injury,[48] a cervical neck injury, a degenerative condition associated with radiculopathy, a neurovascular entrapment of the thoracic outlet, or an entrapment of the ulnar nerve at the elbow. In some of these unique traumatic cases, surgical intervention resolved the dystonia.

Psychological Risk Factors

For years, psychological factors were believed to be the underlying cause of focal dystonia. However, in the 1980s, Sheehy and colleagues[48a] suggested that focal dystonia was related to a neurologic pathological mechanism rather than psychological factors. Altenmuller and colleagues[5,49] including Bauer,[50] compared the personality characteristics of musicians with dystonia with musicians with chronic pain. These researchers administered a variety of personality inventories and questionnaires regarding competence and control orientation, anxiety disorders (stage fright, panic attacks, free-floating anxiety), phobias (agoraphobia, social phobia, and specific phobias such as acrophobia, claustrophobia), life satisfaction, perfectionism, and social orientation. In addition, they asked patients to self-rate their anxieties and perfectionism before and after the onset of dystonia or pain.

Anxieties were significantly more common in patients with dystonia and chronic pain than in normal healthy musician control participants. Those with dystonia admitted that the anxieties had been present before the onset of the movement dysfunction. Musicians with dystonia had more problems with social phobias than healthy musicians and those with chronic pain. In addition, even before the onset of dystonia, musicians with FHD reported significantly greater perfectionism than control participants or those with chronic pain. These findings suggest the psychological features contribute to the development of the dystonia rather than representing a psychoreactive response to the disorder.[5,49-54] On the other hand, dystonia does not develop in all patients with psychological dysfunction.[49]

CLINICAL PRESENTATION: FOCAL HAND DYSTONIA

The onset of the signs and symptoms of FHD is variable. Clinicians must be alert to the possible diagnosis of FHD when a musician, a computer programmer, a dentist or a dental hygienist, or a person working on an assembly line seeks medical care because of pain and vague motor control problems. In musicians, the problem may initially manifest as a decrease in the quality of sound produced by their musical instruments (e.g., a deterioration of vibration in a violinist), increasing errors in well-learned repertoires, unusual fatigue or sense of weakness, or involuntary or excessive movement of a single digit or multiple digits.[51-54] Initially, the symptoms are subtle and virtually indistinguishable from the normal variations seen in the execution experienced by all musicians.

The clinician should look for co-contractions of flexors and extensors when the patient performs the target task but are not present when performing other tasks. Some patients may also demonstrate a variety of subtle abnormalities. Subtle changes may be self-reported or observed, such as a reduced arm swing, loss of smooth, controlled grasping, a physiologic tremor, or hypermobility of the interphalangeal (IP) joints but decreased range of motion (ROM) in proximal joints (e.g., shoulder abduction, external rotation). One might also observe limitations in finger abduction and forearm rotation paired with neurovascular tension, compression neuropathy, or poor posture.[53-55] Most patients

with hand dystonia can describe a sensory trick to minimize the dystonia. Most do not describe problems in sensory discrimination.

The initial presentation often varies by the type of hand dystonia. For example, Frucht[54] analyzed 1000 individuals with musician's dystonia. He reported that the patients had a mean age of 35.7 years (standard deviation, 10.6) at onset with a male predominance of 80%. Although both hands were affected in 4% of the patients, the problem was primarily unilateral with the right hand affected in 64% of cases. Flexion of one or more fingers was the most common phenotype (54%). If the dystonia primarily affected one finger, the third finger was the most commonly affected followed by the index and ring fingers. In cases with multiple affected fingers, there were four frequent patterns: (1) combination 4, 5 (32%); (2) combination 3, 4 (17%); (3) combination 3, 4, 5 (17%); and (4) combination 2, 3 (10%). Isolated extension was less commonly reported (13%), and a combination of flexion and extension was seen in 17%. Side of involvement varied by type of musician. For example, although the right hand was predominantly affected in keyboard players (77%), for 78% of plucking string players (guitar, lute), 68% of bow string players, and 81% of flutists, the left hand was predominantly affected. There was no left–right hand bias in woodwind, percussion, and brass players. These findings suggest the hand performing the more complex musical tasks was the most predisposed to dystonia.

In the history of these musicians with dystonia, Frucht[54] reported that the dystonia usually began in one finger and spread to adjacent fingers, rarely skipping a finger. The ulnar side of the hand (involving the wrist and fingers 4 and 5) was disproportionately affected. The ulnar side of the hand experiences challenging ergonomics because of the design of the musical instrument as well as the technical burdens required for positioning the hand and stabilizing the wrist to activate individual finger movements. Frucht[54] also described correlations between physiologic patterns, dystonic phenotype, and the musical instrument. For example, whereas flexion of the *right* fourth and fifth fingers was common in pianists, flexion of the *left* fourth and fifth fingers was common in violinists. Flexion of the *right* third to fifth fingers was commonly reported in guitarists, whereas isolated extension of digit 3 on the right was common in woodwind players. Frucht[54] noted that after a phenotype was established in a given patient, the pattern rarely varied, even if the patient took an extended break from playing his or her instrument.

Musicians with dystonia demonstrate different patterns of sensory, motor, and musculoskeletal presentations than those with writer's cramp.[12] For example, in a study by McKenzie and colleagues,[13] there were significant differences in measures of musculoskeletal, sensory, and motor performance for patients with writer's cramp compared with patients with musician's cramp. Patients with musician's cramp had a higher level ($P < .05$) of functional independence and better ROM but more neural tension and less strength in the affected upper limb than patients with writer's cramp. Compared with participants with writer's cramp, on the affected side, participants with musician's cramp demonstrated greater ($P < .05$) accuracy on graphesthesia, kinesthesia, and localization but less accuracy and speed in stereognosis. Cimatti and coworkers[55a] reported patients with writer's cramp had a reduced response to high frequency oscillation. No between-group differences were noted in motor performance.

Rosenkranz and colleagues[55b] reported differences in pathophysiologic responses and sensorimotor reorganization in patients with musician's dystonia compared with patients with writer's cramp. Applying a vibration stimulus to measure effects on cortical excitability and short latency intracortical inhibition, these researchers reported vibration increased the amplitude of excitability and decreased the short latency intracortical inhibition in healthy nonmusicians. In patients with writer's cramp, vibration had no measurable effect on either excitability or inhibition. In patients with musician's cramp, vibration strongly reduced short latency intracortical inhibition. The lack of response to sensory vibration in patients with writer's cramp may suggest sensory processing plays less of a role in provoking pathologic, dystonic changes than in patients with musician's cramp.

RULING IN THE CLINICAL DIAGNOSIS OF FOCAL HAND DYSTONIA

Signs and symptoms of focal dystonia usually begin slowly, with the hand initially feeling thick and then uncoordinated in a few specific movements (e.g., alternating or sequential movements) while retaining the ability to do other movements.[55] Although the motor dysfunction is readily apparent to the patient, the changes are subtle and difficult for the clinician to observe or measure. Thus, it may take years to confirm a clinical diagnosis of focal dystonia. Occasionally, the signs and symptoms of hand dystonia can appear more acutely (e.g., a motor vehicle accident; a fall on an outstretched arm; or a final, competitive musical performance).

Wilson and colleagues and Wagner[55c–55f] proposed occupational hand cramps are characterized as a sustained and functionally significant loss of a previously attained manual skill, satisfying all of the following conditions:

1. The affected skill is impaired by movements in which there are errors in timing, force, or trajectory associated with stereotypical tonic postures or cramping sensations that are absent at rest.
2. Abnormal movements are initiated by the attempt to exercise a specific motor skill within a characteristic context and may fail to develop except under those conditions.
3. Skill loss at the outset cannot be explained by diminished practiced efforts.
4. Degraded movements cause the individual to function at a reduced level of skill despite any masking strategies adopted to disguise or circumvent the problem.
5. The movement abnormality persists despite resolution of any and all antecedent inflammatory, toxic, traumatic, myopathic, and neuropathic abnormalities.

History

The first step in evaluating a patient with hand dystonia is to ask for a self-reported medical history, including a thorough report on the patient's history of drugs, surgery, pain, and neuromusculoskeletal symptoms (including what makes the signs better or worse). Then it is important to inquire about a family history of dystonia or other movement disorder, a previous arm or hand injury, job requirements associated with a high level of stress and repetition, lifestyle issues, chronic pain, inflammation, or a medical problem such as a cardiovascular accident or a head injury. Psychological stress, high motivational drive, commitment to professional success, and negative expectations about recovery should also be reviewed.[49,50,56]

Neuromusculoskeletal Examination

All patients need a complete neurologic and musculoskeletal examination with all findings objectively recorded.[55] Even though hand dystonia involves the upper limb, it is a good ideal to ask the patient about any issues with mobility, balance, and falling.[56,57] Both upper limbs should be evaluated, including (1) ROM and strength, (2) neurovascular entrapment (neural tension),[48] (3) peripheral nerve signs and symptoms,[47] (4) somatosensory function,[37–39] (5) sympathetic signs,[47] (6) pain severity,[37,47] and (7) severity of dystonic signs and symptoms. As part of the examination, patients should be videotaped while performing their target task.[58] These videos can serve as a baseline to measure change over time. If available, high-speed three-dimensional video images, MIDI technology, and kinematic motion analysis can augment force, timing, and acceleration data. These tools are not usually available in the outpatient clinic.

Motor Control Examination

Hochberg and colleagues[58] recommend carefully defining the abnormal movements. For example, these clinicians suggest describing which fingers are most involved, relationship of IP finger flexion and metacarpal–phalangeal extension, degree of ulnar deviation, amount of pronation or supination of the forearm, and if there are noticeable movements of the elbow or shoulder with voluntary hand use.[59] Biofeedback may help assess whether contraction of the flexor muscles of the wrist and fingers drive the contraction of the finger and wrist extensors or vice versa.

Some patients with hand dystonia may have a specific peripheral neuropathy (e.g., compression of the nerve caused by trauma, neurovascular trauma, degenerative joints, neural degeneration of the dorsal horn, or dorsal root or autoimmune etiology). Goldman and colleagues[57] provide a thorough review of the signs and symptoms of peripheral nerve compression and FHD (Table 116.e1). A patient with a peripheral neuropathy is more likely to have painful migratory muscle cramping, fasciculations, nocturnal pain, sensory deficits in the distribution of the sensory nerve, and weakness in muscles innervated by the involved nerve. The muscles involved are often two-joint muscles, with the spasm more likely to occur when the muscles are too short or too long. Neuropathies could create some postural alterations, with movement disturbances related to weakness of the muscles. Goldman and colleagues[57] differentiated compression neuropathy mostly in terms of tetany (muscle hypercontractility), muscle spasm (cramps), fasciculations, pain, decreased sensation, decreased strength, limb posture, and movement disturbance. Compared with patients with a peripheral neuropathy, patients with FHD usually do not have radicular pain, weakness, or fasciculations. However, if the muscle co-contractions are maintained over a long period of time, vasoconstriction may occur, and muscle cramping can become painful (Table 116.e2). A patient's emotional state may make it harder to distinguish between a peripheral neuropathy and other common central movement disorders.

There are no unique fine-motor tests to use for patients with FHD. However some researchers and clinicians have used the Motor Performance Test series.[60,61] With this test, it is possible to reliably assess steadiness, line tracking, aiming, tapping, and inserting pins. It is common for patients with hand dystonia to have normal fine-motor skills except for the involuntary movements during task-specific performance.[59]

It is also important to carefully differentiate between motor signs of hand dystonia and other central movement disorders such as spasticity and rigidity (see Table 116.e2). Spasticity and rigidity can be distinguished from dystonia based on muscular resistance, speed of passive motion, presence of a fixed end-range posture, patterns of muscle activation, and reflexes. Spasticity can be characterized by a velocity-dependent resistance to passive motion, particularly in postural righting muscles. The stretch reflex is exaggerated. Slow positioning may inhibit the tone. Classically, in spasticity, quick limb movements through the ROM produce a resistive, clonic, or sudden catch (e.g., stops to the motion followed by a release after stopping) rather than smooth, easy passive motion. Commonly, the spastic muscles in the upper limb include the shoulder abductors; shoulder internal rotators; forearm pronators; and elbow, wrist, and finger flexors.

On the other hand, rigidity tends to be independent of the speed of passive movements or position. Rigidity involves a co-contraction of the

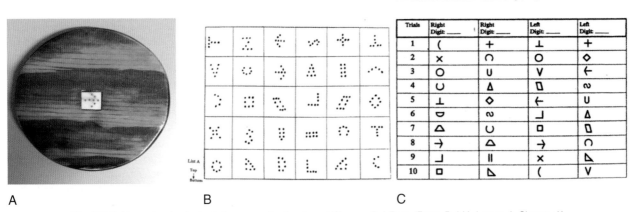

Fig. 116.2 Example of a test of stereognosis: the Boczai-Cheney-Byl Test. (From Byl N, Leano J, Cheney K. The Byl-Cheney-Boczai Sensory Discriminator: reliability, validity, and responsiveness for testing stereognosis. *J Hand Ther.* 2002;15:315–330.)

flexors and extensors that block voluntary movement (e.g., co-contractions limit wrist extension and finger spread). Usually patients have difficulty initiating movements, but when started, they can proceed, particularly if the movement is rhythmical. The co-contractions restrict not only movement range but also movement variability. There is some evidence of excessive inhibition in patients with rigidity. Positioning does not seem to help relieve the rigidity. The stretch reflex may be decreased rather than increased.

Dystonia is distinguished from spasticity and rigidity by the presence of co-contractions of the flexors and extensors, leading to end-range twisting motions. Stretch reflexes are normal. Patients with hand dystonia are more likely to demonstrate tetany with a maximum contraction, disturbances in sensorimotor integration, strength deficits in wrist flexors and extensors, and intrinsic muscles with motor control problems only at target-specific tasks. In addition, patients with dystonia have the ability to use a sensory trick to inhibit the dystonic movements.

Sensory Examination

A good sensory examination is critical for patients with FHD. For the sensory examination, sharp–dull discrimination, detection of light touch threshold as measured with the Semmes-Weinstein monofilaments, and two-point discrimination[62] should be performed even though the test results are commonly normal. More time should be spent on cortical sensory discrimination testing such as localization, graphesthesia, stereognosis, and kinesthesia as well as temporal and spatial processing. Patients with focal dystonia may demonstrate increased abnormal dystonic posturing or abnormal perception of arm movements on the involved side after tonic, maintained movements. However, patients with focal dystonia may experience a reduction in dystonic posturing and potentially improved motor accuracy and efficiency of fine motor control after a cutaneous or a proprioceptive stimulus. It is still not clear whether the motor dysfunction is primarily related to a sensory problem or directly related to errors of processing in the movement pathways (Box 116.e2).

Unfortunately, standardized cortical sensory tests are limited. Some are standardized for children, and the therapist needs to be certified to administer the test (e.g., the Sensory Integration Praxis Test).[62] Today there are some new standardized tests available to document localization, kinesthesia, graphesthesia, and stereognosis skills (Box 116.e3). Byl and associates[62a] designed a simple clinical instrument to grade stereognosis referred to as the Boczai-Cheney-Byl Test (BCB Test), which can be easily constructed for clinic use (Fig. 116.2).

Another new sensory test is the Manual Tactile Test (MTT).[63,64] The MTT requires patients to perform three tasks to sort objects by weight, coarseness, and shape. It was originally normed on patients with a peripheral neuropathy of the hand but is also applicable for other patients with other hand impairments and can be easily fabricated to use in the clinic. In addition, a new sensory, sensory motor, and perceptual motor and cognitive screening battery will be available soon online from PositScience[65] (https://www.brainhq.com/?lead_id=-google-search-text-home Brand_(US_CAN_UK_AUS_SAF_NZ)&g-clid=EAIaIQobChMIz4XP8orG1gIVzl9-Ch2tUQwhEAAYASAAE-gLfnfD_BwE). This battery measures six sensory motor processes: timing, tapping, visual discrimination (seeing and spotting), hearing, and speech discrimination. The sensory motor battery was designed to screen for early evidence of sensory, motor, and cognitive decline in older adult patients, but it has the potential to provide similar information for patients with well-established hand dystonia (Fig. 116.3).

It is important to recognize that sensory systems are interindependent. There is generalization of training across sensory systems. This may be important when planning treatment. If the somatosensory system is hypersensitive and creates dystonic movements when working with tactile stimuli, it may be necessary to begin retraining with auditory or visual stimuli.

Electromyography Testing

Dynamic EMG testing can be included as part of the diagnostic workup for hand dystonia. It is common to detect a peripheral neuropathy of the ulnar, median, or musculocutaneous nerve in a patient with hand dystonia, particularly for individuals with previous upper limb trauma or excessive forceful repetitions[47] or individuals with recurrent subclinical neck pain. EMG changes in conduction may be noted even before weakness or sensory changes are detected. The electromyogram can also document co-contractions of antagonists and agonists, muscle recruitment with excessive force, a consistent maximum contraction over time, and slow turn on/off of selective muscle firing. The inability to hold a consistent firing pattern can be used to determine whether a muscle should be injected with botulinum toxin.

Chronic Pain Assessment

Patients with chronic pain of the upper limb can have associated degradation of the sensory and motor cortices, with some developing movement challenges in the hand consistent with dystonia.[66] However, although pain is not usually the primary complaint of patients with FHD, it is still important to evaluate pain as part of the evaluation and rehabilitation program. The most common self-rated measurement instrument for rating pain severity is the visual analog scale. This scale is appropriate to use for patients with hand dystonia. This scale includes either rating pain on an ordinal scale of 0 to 10 or drawing the severity on a 10-cm line.[67]

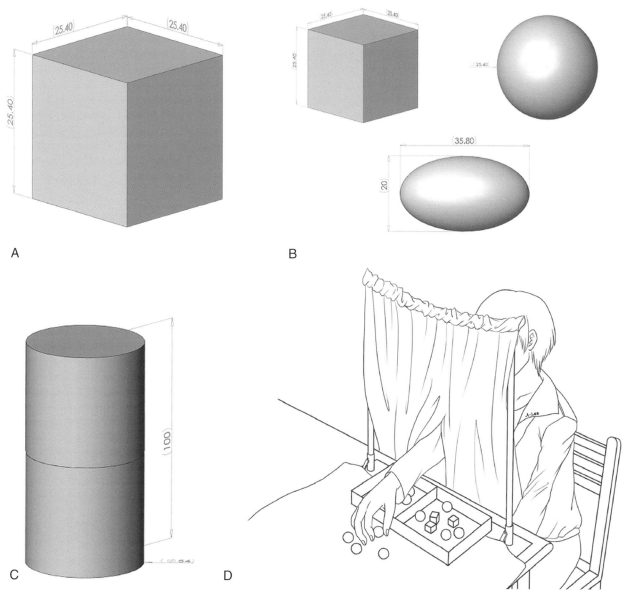

Fig. 116.3 Manual Tactile Test (MTT). **A,** Test for roughness differentiation. **B,** Test for stereognosis. **C,** Test for barognosis. **D,** Setup for the MTT. (From Hsu H-Y Kuo Y-K, Jou I-M. Diagnosis From Functional perspectives: usefulness of a manual tactile test for predicting precision pinch performance and disease severity in subjects with carpal tunnel syndrome. *Arch Phys Med Rehabil.* 2014;95:717-725 and Hsu HY, Kuo LC, Kuan TS, et al. Determining the functional sensibility of the hand in patients with peripheral nerve repair: feasibility of using a novel manual tactile test for monitoring the progression of nerve regeneration. *J Hand Ther.* 2017;30:65-73.)

Severity of Dystonia

A number of standard scales are available to quantify the severity of general and focal dystonia.[68–71] The most common dystonia scales include the Burke-Fahn-Marsden Scale (Fig. 116.e4), the Global Rating Scale (Fig. 116.e5), the Toronto Western Spasmodic Torticollis Rating Scale (Fig. 116.e6), the Unified Dystonia Rating Scale (Fig. 116.e7) with the Arm Dystonia Disability Scale (ADDS) (Fig. 116.e8),[71a,71b] the Writer's Cramp Rating Scale (WCRS) (Fig. 116.e9),[71a,71c] and a kinematic assessment tool (not scale).[71d,71e] Except for the kinematic analysis, the dystonia scales are all ordinal scales. The ADDS is the only dystonia scale that specifically targets the hand. The ordinal scale for the items on the ADDS includes 0, normal; 1, mild difficulty in playing or writing; 2, moderate difficulty in playing or writing; and 3, marked difficulty in playing or writing. It is difficult to objectively determine mild from moderate to marked difficulty (see Fig. 116.e8). The Writer's Cramp Rating Scale (see Fig. 116.e9) is appropriate for patients having difficulty writing. In a recent meta-analysis of randomized trials assessing the effectiveness of botulinum neurotoxin, the trials for arm and hand dystonia did not include a validated outcome measurement tool.[69]

There are also some unique rating scales for those with a history of overuse[70,71] and for musicians with dystonia.[72,73] Technical musical performance can be rated on an ordinal scale according to the Tubiana and Chamagne Scale.[72,73] This scale uses the following ordinal assignment: 0, unable to play; 1, plays several notes but stops because of blockage or lack of facility; 2, plays short sequences without rapidity and with unsteady fingering; 3, plays easy pieces but avoids difficult passages for fear of motor problems; 4, beginning to do some performance; and 5, returns to concert performances. It is important to note that good performance is a high score, and poor performance is a low score (just the opposite of the other scales). Patients should also be asked to self-report the severity of their dystonia as well as subjectively assess the effects of treatment based on a percentage scale by subtracting their pretreatment motor performance from the posttreatment performance or rating the success of their treatment on an ordinal or a nominal scale (e.g., excellent, very good, fairly good, poor, none). Patients should also complete an evaluation of function to reflect how much the impairment from the dystonia is interfering with their functional independence.[73a]

Despite the shortcomings of the scales, dystonia severity ratings have been correlated with other movement kinematics.[68] Mean stroke frequency is significantly reduced in musicians and writers with dystonia. General drawing movements showed a greater decrease in stroke frequency than handwriting movements. During circle drawing, mean vertical peak velocity was more variable in patients with FHD compared with control participants, but there were no significant differences in vertical pressure. This may indicate an impaired ability to maintain the reproduction of the same kinematic pattern over time. It is also possible the increase in vertical writing pressure with writing reflects a compensatory effort to stabilize the pen. Zeuner and associates[71a,73b] reported excessive pressure down and excessive grip in patients with writer's cramp but normal pressure when making circles.

Kinematic measures and individual scores on the ADDS and Toronto Western Spasmodic Torticollis Rating Scale were not correlated.[68] The lack of correlation should not be surprising given that ADDS, the Toronto torticollis scale, and kinematic analyses probe different aspects of motor impairments and different body parts. The ADDS characterizes how dystonia affects a set of fine manual tasks, whereas the torticollis scale scores the manifestation of cervical dystonia during handwriting. Therefore, the clinical scores and kinematic analysis of handwriting provide complementary insights into the motor impairments of patients with hand dystonia. Future studies need to address which combination of clinical scores and kinematic measures are needed to determine the most appropriate method to quantify and measure change in impairment in response to treatment for patients with writer's and musician's cramp.[68]

For patient with writer's cramp, a video should be made during writing. A writing test is the only way to objectively distinguish patients with writer's cramp and healthy age-matched control participants. In patients with writer's cramp, fine-motor skills and psychological–personality traits did not separate them from healthy control participants. The writing sample should include a sentence that the patient must write 10 times at the normal writing speed. Ideally, the patient should be able to compete this in 3 minutes (e.g., "Every good man should come to the aid of their country"). From the writing sample, the speed of writing should be recorded (e.g., number of times patient lifts the pen, letters per second, mean frequency of up and down strokes, mean velocity [mm/sec] and mean distance [cm] of the writing on the paper). The onset time for degraded writing should also be recorded. In addition, the difference in amplitude of the letters at the beginning and the end of the writing session should be determined. The legibility of writing can also be graded (excellent, good, fair, poor, illegible). New force sensor feedback units are being developed commercially that can be placed on a pen to allow grading of the force of the grip and the pressure down on the pen when writing.[74] A recent study reported on the use of pressure-sensitive inking pen available in Europe that can be used to write on a piece of ruled paper fixed to a digitizing tablet.[74]

Psychosocial Assessment

Some studies report psychological differences in patients with hand dystonia, and others do not.[75] For example, some researchers report patients with focal dystonia have difficulty with shifting mindsets, increased perseveration, and obsessive compulsivity that reflect complex

---

> **BOX 116.1 Clinical Diagnosis of Focal Hand Dystonia**
>
> **Key Points Regarding Diagnosis**
> - Some patients may have clear evidence of aberrant learning or excessive plasticity.
> - Some individuals may appear to develop hand dystonia after trauma.
> - Maximizing return of function requires a comprehensive team effort with the patient taking leadership; the physician providing support and medical management; and therapists creating and overseeing learning-based training, performance techniques, and sensorimotor processing.
> - It may take years to make the diagnosis.
> - Management is possible; complete recovery is less common.
> - Neuroimaging correlated with clinical research will help improve our understanding of focal hand dystonia and effective intervention strategies.

neurophysiologic dysfunction (dorsolateral, orbitofrontal, and motor frontostriatal areas). In musicians, studies confirm the presence of anxiety, perfectionism, and phobias as risk factors for the development of hand dystonia. Thus, it may be helpful to administer a personality inventory, a questionnaire on anxiety, and perhaps some standard questioning on perfectionism. This may highlight some of the personality risk factors that could contribute to the development of dystonia but may also help guide comprehensive intervention to remediate the dystonia.[44]

Categorizing personality type in patients with hand dystonia may help guide intervention strategies through counseling and stress management. There are a variety of personality inventories to help classify personality types. Many personality tests can be taken online. One online self-test identifies 16 factors common to individuals with a type A personality[76] (Box 116.1). Another psychological inventory classifies personalities in terms of tendencies for managing internal and external expectations.[77] Four tendencies have been identified: obligers, rebels, questioners, and upholders.[77] Physical and occupational therapists should not have to administer psychological tests intended to diagnose psychopathology such as the Minnesota Multiphasic Personality Inventory. If such in-depth personality testing is needed, the therapist should refer the patient to a psychologist.

Radiographs and Neuroimaging

Neither a radiograph of the hand nor a magnetic resonance image (MRI) of the hand is generally ordered by the physician to make the diagnosis of FHD unless there is a history of an injury; a structural biomechanical problem; signs and symptoms of a soft tissue lesion (e.g., ganglion, cyst, ligamentous tear, fibrosis of the retinaculum, trigger finger); or a question of a stroke, brain tumor, or structural anomaly (see Tables 116.e1 and 116.e2). Patients who need to be cleared of other neurologic pathology should be referred to a neurologist (Box 116.2).

On the other hand, advances in noninvasive imaging have expanded the opportunities to understand the neuropathophysiology of dystonia. Detailed brain anatomy and unusual deviations in volume, density, morphology, and temporal and spatial processing in cortical and subcortical structures can be examined with electroencephalography, positive emission tomography, MRI, and functional MRI (fMRI).[24,51,78-86] For example, with basic MRI and fMRI paired with TMS, several cortical abnormalities have been noted in patients with FHD: (1) a reduction in cortical blood flow and abnormal transient asymmetry in movement-related cortical potentials,[78,56-58] (2) asymmetrical muscle response to double-pulsed magnetic stimulation,[51] and (3) asymmetry in the tonic vibration reflex after intramuscular lidocaine. Diffusion tensor imaging measures water diffusion across myelinated CNS structures to reconstruct the white matter tracts, with the expansion of gray matter volume

BOX 116.2   Checklist to Clinically "Rule in" the Diagnosis of Focal Hand Dystonia

Physical or Historical Findings	Yes = 1	No = 0	Description
1. Normal neurologic examination except for involuntary movements			
2. Task specificity of abnormal movements			
3. Poor hand ergonomics (e.g., hypermobility of IP or MCP joints, difficulty stabilizing thumb, excessive ulnar wrist deviation)			
4. Type A personality characteristics			
5. Can use sensory tricks to control abnormal movements			
6. History of high stress (e.g., personal, work related)			
7. History of high levels of repetitive work			
8. Cortical sensory discrimination problems discovered in the examination			
9. Hypersensitivity or signs of central sensitization			
10. Genetic factors (e.g., family history of movement disorders, Ashkenazi Jewish family with known *DYT1* gene)			
11. Previous or recent upper limb or hand trauma			
12. History of chronic pain			
Total score (maximum 12 points)			

IP, Interphalangeal; *MCP*, metacarpophalangeal.

noted in the putamen of patients with dystonia).[24] In highly active brain regions, positron emission tomography (PET) and fMRI provide indirect measures of neural activity through the consumption of oxygen. For example, compared with control participants, patients with writer's cramp demonstrate an increase in the amplitude of the blood oxygen level–dependent signal in the fMRI in the basal ganglia.[59,79,80] Using PET, hypermetabolism has been noted in the frontal cortex and the basal ganglia in patients with dystonia.[21] Spectroscopy (a special advanced application of MRI) can identify biochemical markers such as neurotransmitters (e.g., γ-aminobutyric acid and glutamate). Although proton magnetic resonance spectroscopy provides evidence of mitochondrial dysfunction as the pathophysiology of primary dystonia, in one study of 14 patients with primary FHD, no statistically significant differences were found in any of the measured brain metabolites.

Functional imaging methods such as electroencephalography (EEG) and magnetoencephalography (MEG) can record brain activity through changes in the electrical current or changes in the magnetic fields across the scalp. MEG studies are noninvasive and can be safely used to look at cortical organization in humans.[1,60,61,79–82] MEG studies confirm sensory, sensorimotor, and motor degradation of and beyond the affected body part in patients with FHD.[12,34,35,41,83] The size of the sensory receptive fields are enlarged, the separation of the digit representations are reduced, and the digital receptive fields are altered in their sequential order.[84] Furthermore,

MEG cutaneous stimuli delivered to the digits produce somatosensory evoked fields with decreased amplitude and longer duration in the contralateral hemisphere of the affected hand for both the early (S1) and late (S2) responses.[62,81,82] However, in S2, both earlier and higher amplitude responses have been measured in the ipsilateral and contralateral hemispheres of patients with unilateral hand dystonia.[81,82] These variations in the somatosensory evoked responses can be seen in Fig. 116.e10 to 116.e13. After sensory stimuli were delivered to the digits, the somatosensory evoked potentials in patients with dystonia were disorganized, with a reduced amplitude, excessive oscillations, and early peak responses.[36,81,82] In addition, although the poststimulus somatosensory responses for digits 1 to 5 (D1–D5) were progressively ordered medial to lateral and inferior to superior, there was significant overlap across dorsal and lateral surfaces, between digits, and across segments within digits.[36,84] Sanger and colleagues[84a] also quantified the overlap in the somatosensory evoked responses after simultaneous stimulation of adjacent digits in normal participants and participants with hand dystonia. When stimulating D2 and D3, the magnitude of the response in normal participants was equivalent to a serial addition of the response of the individual digits alone, but in patients with FHD, the response of simultaneous stimulation was less than the addition of each digit stimulated individually. These findings suggest overlap and redundancy between adjacent digits, similar to the overlap recorded electrophysiologically in a behavioral monkey model, supporting the sensorimotor learning hypothesis.[35,36]

When a patient with hand dystonia performs a motor task or receives magnetic stimulation to the affected digits, M1 cortical activity in regions such as the premotor cortex (PMC) and supplementary motor area has a variable response.[42,85,86] In some cases, the M1 response is reduced.[86] In other studies, excessive plasticity in the motor cortex is noted with excitation generalizing beyond the specific task.[41] This is confusing but may suggest the possibility of an endophenotypic disorder. Unfortunately, we do not have comparative MRI data on patients before they develop a FHD.

Atypical Types of Dystonia

From the history and the examination, it is important to rule out psychogenic dystonia (also referred to as *functional dystonia*).[87] In functional dystonia, there is abnormal, unintended movement or positioning of the body caused by the nervous system not working properly. Functional dystonia can cause movement symptoms in the face, neck, shoulder, torso, or limbs. Functional dystonia is often seen in individuals with psychiatric disorders or exposure to psychological stressors. The onset of symptoms is often preceded by an injury, illness, or emotionally stressful event. Functional or psychogenic dystonia is a real and disabling condition, not deliberate.[87–89] Patients should not be viewed as crazy or hysterical. There is dysfunction of the nervous system, but it is not caused by neurologic damage or disease. Psychogenic (functional dystonia) has some distinguishing features:

- *Facial spasms:* There may be intermittent facial spasms, fixed facial movements, or one side of the mouth pulling down. These spasms may come and go, but the facial muscles function normally between episodes.
- *Blepharospasm:* Individuals with functional dystonia may have episodes of sudden blinking or sustained closure of the eyes. The blepharospasm may involve both eyes or occur with spasms on one side of the face.
- *Fixed postures:* Some patients with functional dystonia present with a fixed posture, typically in a limb, hand, or neck or shoulder. The fixed posture is not unique to functional dystonia because it can also be observed in patients with secondary dystonia caused by an injury.
- *Dysautonomia:* It is important to check for pain and dysautonomic symptoms (difference in skin temperature, skin color, sweating, or

swelling) in patients with functional dystonia. The clinician must carefully rule out complex regional pain syndrome.

- *Episodic*: Functional dystonia may occur in episodes or attacks. Although paroxysmal dyskinesis can also be episodic, the episodes of functional dystonia may last varying lengths of time (e.g., seconds to days) and can involve variable, abnormal movements in the torso or the limbs. Episodes of functional dystonia may be preceded by uncommon triggers inconsistent with organic hand dystonia.[88]

Neurologists report the importance of distinguishing focal psychogenic and organic dystonia based on PET during task performance.[89] In organic dystonia, there is an abnormal increase in blood flow in the primary motor cortex and the thalamus but decreased cerebellar activity. In psychogenic dystonia, there is an abnormal increase in blood flow in the cerebellum and basal ganglia but decreased blood flow in the motor cortex.[89] If the diagnosis is likely psychogenic dystonia, the patient should be referred to a psychiatrist, psychologist, or neurologist for management. In some cases, physical or occupational therapy, cognitive behavior therapy, or oral medications such as antidepressants can be helpful.[90]

During the history, it is also important to rule out paroxysmal exercise-induced dystonia.[91] Paroxysmal exercise-induced dystonia tends to occur intermittently. It is triggered by intense exercise and is more common in young people (2–30 years). Paroxysmal exercise-induced dystonia has a genetic component and is likely to spread beyond the hand. Sometimes the dystonia persists after the triggering activity ends and ultimately may appear without intense or prolonged repetitive exercise.

In summary, at this time, there is no one clinical test to administer to rule in or rule out the diagnosis of FHD (see Box 116.1). A considerable amount of research is still needed to correlate the diagnosis of a focal, especially a task-specific, hand dystonia with a specific gene, consistent anatomic restrictions, a generalized imbalance of neurophysiologic mechanisms, or an interaction between brain regions and endophenotypic risk factors. It is important to remember that expensive neuroimaging techniques may rule out brain pathology as the cause of the dystonic movements, but they do not necessarily rule in the diagnosis of FHD. The diagnosis of FHD is still based on a thorough clinical history and physical examination. The ultimate diagnosis of FHD will be based on an interaction of intrinsic and extrinsic factors. The clinician might assess the risk factors to more effectively "rule in" the diagnosis of FHD (see Box 116.2). When a patient demonstrates the majority of the risk factors, the sensitivity and specificity of making the diagnosis could be enhanced (Box 116.e4). Other characteristics may need to be included to confirm the diagnosis of hand dystonia, particularly in musicians (Box 116.e5). From the perspective of a physical or occupational therapist, there may be signs and symptoms that need further medical workup (Box 116.3). Continuing to clarify the pathology of FHD through MEG, fMRI, and MRI combined with diffusion tension imaging of anatomical connectivity may help individuals prevent developing the disorder as well as help clinicians recognize the diagnosis earlier and more effectively patients with treat hand dystonia.

TREATMENT FOR FOCAL HAND DYSTONIA

The treatment for FHD varies by patient characteristics, lifestyle issues, musculoskeletal findings, and personality factors as well as integration and interpretation of the different etiologies of hand dystonia. The treatment must be specific to the type of dystonic movements presented, task specificity, occupation associated with the hand dystonia (e.g., writer's cramp, musician's cramp, keyboarders dystonia, golfer's yip), side of involvement, and presence of other secondary dystonias

---

BOX 116.3 When to Refer the Patient with Hand Dystonia to a Neurologist

Rule Out Other Diagnoses	Follow up on Findings from the History of Physical Examination
• Multiple sclerosis	• Abnormal or pathologic reflexes
• Parkinson's disease	• Spasticity or increased tone
• Amyotrophic lateral sclerosis	• Resting tremor
• Posterior lateral sclerosis	• Tremor with all purposeful movements
• Stroke	• Peripheral neuropathy
• Chronic reflex pain syndrome	• Freezing of gait
• Essential tremor	• Rigidity
• Brain tumor	• Hemiparesis
• Psychogenic dystonia	• Abnormal cardiovascular signs
• Exertional dystonia	

(e.g., cervical torticollis, truncal dystonia, blepharospasm, runner's dystonia, psychogenic dystonia, paroxysmal exercise-induced dystonia).[91] Given the multifactorial origin of hand dystonia, the management must be comprehensive. The whole person and the family are affected by the problem, both physically and mentally. Unfortunately, most patients with a focal dystonia come to see health professionals after a long list of previous, usually ineffective therapies. These patients are frustrated and discouraged.

Uniquely, musicians are extraordinarily motivated to pursue and comply with treatment. Musicians are completely dependent on their hands for performance. When problems of motor incoordination initially appear, most musicians respond by practicing harder or engaging in slow, deliberate practice to consciously control individual finger and hand movements. When these techniques do not work, the musician frequently becomes depressed and discouraged. Most do not suspect a diagnosis of hand dystonia.

Goals for Management

At this time, the primary goal is to *manage rather* than *cure* FHD. The goals must be clearly stated and accepted by all team members, including the patient and the family. The management process begins by establishing an appropriate health care team who must educate the patient and family. Then it is necessary to prime the nervous system to learn and then retrain the brain (Box 116.4).

Establish a Team and Educate the Patient and Family

The biopsychosocial model of clinical management has been clearly demonstrated to be the most successful approach to the management of activity-related musculoskeletal movement disorders, including FHD. In this model, the interactions of physical impairments, personal psychological factors, and psychosocial factors are recognized and targeted for treatment in a holistic approach to care.[44] Biopsychosocial management programs require a team. At a minimum, the team must include the physician, a physical or occupational therapist, a psychologist, and an appropriate coach (e.g., ergonomist, teacher, trainer). The physician is usually the critical, coordinating team member. The physician must confirm the diagnosis and rule out other potential pathologies that could be contributing to the dystonia. As indicated earlier, this may require further diagnostic testing. Ideally, the physician should be a neurologist and a movement disorders specialist. If the patient has other health problems, it will be important for the patient to maintain a close relationship with a primary care physician.

BOX 116.4 **Goals and Objectives for Intervention for Patients with Hand Dystonia**

- Establish a team (physician, health care, work management, support staff).
- Educate the patient and the family about the etiology of focal dystonia and encourage a positive attitude regarding recovery.
- Prime the nervous system for learning.
  - Stop the abnormal movements.
  - Establish a positive lifestyle (e.g., good nutrition, perform comprehensive exercises, improve posture, do breathing for relaxation, improve balance and postural righting, get adequate sleep, stay hydrated, avoid smoking and alcohol, manage stress, reduce anxiety, improve ergonomics of hand use, engage in counseling as appropriate).
  - Quiet the hypersensitivity of the nervous system.
  - Integrate medical intervention strategies as recommended by the physician (prescription medications, rTMS, TDCS, fatigue therapy, immobilization).
- Retrain the brain: sensorimotor rehabilitation.
  - Follow the principles and guidelines of neural adaptation and neural plasticity.
  - Use mental and guided imagery to substitute for physical training.
  - Match the patient to the best sensorimotor training strategy
  - Retrain sensory discrimination.
  - Work on sensory motor activities.
  - Train to perform non–task-specific activities with and without enhancement of mirrors or biofeedback (without dystonic movements).
  - Retrain components of task specific activities (without dystonic movements).
  - Retrain at target specific tasks (simple to complex, slow to fast) without dystonic movements.

rTMS, Repetitive transcranial magnetic stimulation; *TDCS,* transcranial direct current stimulation.

BOX 116.5 **Activities to Prime the Nervous System for Retraining**

Stop the abnormal movements.
- Use sensory tricks.
- Fatigue the involved muscles.
- Try remote ischemic limb conditioning to increase oxygen delivery.
- Cool the extremity.
- Mentally rehearse performing movements normally.

Quiet the nervous system.
- Rock in a rocker; swaddle self like a baby while rocking.
- Mentally rehearse quieting the nervous system.
- Go to a quiet place to relax.
- Participate in general meditation or movement programs (e.g., yoga, Alexander work, Feldenkrais, Pilates, Nia).

Establish a positive health and wellness program.
- Integration of a strong exercise and physical activity program
- Good nutrition
- Adequate hydration
- Avoid smoking and excessive alcohol intake.
- Get adequate sleep (e.g., 7–8 hours of quality sleep).
- Integration of stress management techniques
- Learn something new each day and engage in regular cognitive brain training strategies (e.g., crossword puzzles, puzzles, Scrabble, Suduko, sensory and perceptual motor training [positscience.org; brain games]).

Correct hand ergonomics and biomechanics.
- Evaluate and minimize anatomic restrictions.
- Work on performance ergonomics with an expert tutor in a professional area.
- Use hand in functional position (e.g., wrist in neutral position, let surface open hand, keep hand in functional position preserving normal arches, move fingers from the MCP joint, use forearm and shoulder rotation to lift and place fingers).
- Use slow-twitch muscles as much as possible (e.g., intrinsic hand muscles, forearm pronators–supinators, scapular stabilizers).
- Integrate technology or use orthoses if needed to help minimize involuntary movements.
- Increase sensory awareness with voluntary movements and maximize sensory accuracy.

MCP, Metacarpophalangeal.
Data from Byl NN, McKenzie A. Treatment effectiveness of patients with a history of repetitive hand use and focal hand dystonia: a planned, prospective follow-up study. *J Hand Ther.* 2000;289–301.

The health care team must be in agreement about the goals and objectives of the patient. The team members need to educate the patient and the family about the etiology of FHD and set a positive environment for successful management. Effective *management* of the dystonia should be the focus even though some individuals with FHD claim they have achieved a cure. Education must include a discussion of the etiology of hand dystonia, a review of management strategies, the importance of compliance with a healthy lifestyle and behavioral training, and the known effectiveness of the different approaches to management.

Prime the Nervous System to Learn (Box 116.5)

The CNS in adaptable across the life span.[65,92,93] Individuals need to be receptive to the possibility of modifying the nervous system. Each individual with hand dystonia must be willing to make important lifestyle changes and commit to engaging the brain in learning activities to maximize brain health and the potential to change.

Stop the Abnormal Movement. Priming the nervous system to learn must begin with stopping the repetition of the abnormal movements. This may require using sensory tricks, taking a break from performing the target tasks, seeking help from appropriate health professionals or coaches, considering the redesign of the instrument, and using mental practice and imagery to perform the target tasks without abnormal movements.[94–96] If the abnormal movements are repeated more than the normal movements, it decreases the opportunity to restore normal topography of the brain and normal motor control.

Quiet the Nervous System. In the face of excessive excitation and reduced inhibition, it is necessary to focus on quieting the nervous system through physical, mental, and relaxing activities. In some cases, the centralized hypersensitivity is associated with chronic pain, and in other cases, it is associated with motor dysfunction such as dystonia. It may be possible to quiet the nervous system by going to a relaxing place, meditating, using stress management, wrapping tightly in a warm blanket, cooling down, or rocking in a rocker or a swing. Stopping and quietly taking some deep breaths can be effective during stressful moments. Sometimes increased awareness of the neural hypersensitivity is the beginning of learning to control it.

Create a Positive Lifestyle for Healing and Retraining. Each patient with hand dystonia must critically analyze her or his lifestyle behaviors.[42–44,47] With a healthy lifestyle, the brain is better prepared for retraining. The activities recommended for positive physical and brain health include:

- Establishing a regular aerobic, balance, posture, strengthening, and flexibility exercise program to maintain cardiopulmonary function and mobility of muscle, fascia, and neural tissue (three to five times per week for 45 minutes consistent with the Department of Health and Human Services).[90,91]
- Eating a healthy diet of fruits, vegetables, and protein and potentially eliminating glutens and lactose (Box 116.e6).[97,98]
- Maintaining adequate hydration (e.g.,8–10 glasses per day of noncaffeinated fluids to maximize oxygen delivery to the nervous system).
- Adapting strategies to manage and potentially reduce the effects of stress (e.g., diaphragmatic breathing, relaxation techniques, counseling, mindfulness courses, meditation).
- Getting adequate sleep (7–8 hours/night), preferably without medications.
- Reducing unnecessary trauma to the hands by integrating biomechanically healthy hand techniques in activities of daily living (e.g., maintaining the arches of the hand, using the intrinsic muscles, letting the surface of an object provide the sensory stimulus to open the hand, integrating forearm rotation to depress and lift the fingers, minimizing excessive use of the finger flexors and extensors).
- Initiating an ergonomic analysis of the workstation and tool design as well as analyzing the unique demands imposed by excessive repetitions or unusual mechanics imposed by different instruments used in job performance.[32,37,42,44]
- Establishing a positive attitude with expectations to improve.

Medical Management Strategies

The medical management program is part of preparing the nervous system to learn. After the diagnosis of FHD is confirmed and other diagnoses are ruled out, the physician must determine the need for medications, repetitive TMS or tDCS, fatigue therapy, or orthopedic surgery if anatomic defects are present as well as determine if deep brain stimulation (DBS) should be considered.

Medications. Anticholinergic medications may improve the foundation for retraining. Some physicians recommend cannabinoids to help facilitate relaxation and control pain.[99] Most commonly, physicians recommend botulinum toxin to weaken the dystonic muscles in patients with hand dystonia.[100]

The treatment of focal dystonia was revolutionized with the approval of botulinum toxin in the late 1980s. Botulinum toxin is most commonly used for cervical dystonia, blepharospasm, and spasmodic dysphonia. However, botulinum toxin is also used with patients with hand cramps. The toxin should be injected by experienced physicians usually performed under EMG guidance.[100] The botulinum toxin is injected into the overactive muscles to peripherally block the neurotransmitter acetylcholine at the neuromuscular junction.[53] The biological activity of the toxin usually extends to 2.5 to 4.5 cm, restricting its specificity and potentially intruding into areas that are not preferred. The effects of the injection usually last for a couple of months. Most patients require the injections to be repeated every 3 to 4 months as the effects of the toxin wear off. Usually patients experience mild weakness for a couple of weeks after the injection and then enjoy greater benefit when the weakness dissipates and the clinical benefit remains. There is some evidence that, over time, botulinum toxin exerts effects peripherally as well as centrally. The primary benefits of the injection are based on subjective or clinical ratings. Type Ia evidence supports the benefits of weakening muscles with botulinum toxin. However, although a 75% improvement with botulinum toxin injections may be beneficial for a patient with blepharospasm, cervical torticollis, or even writer's cramp, a 75% recovery is usually insufficient for a concert artist, a computer programmer, or an engineer to return to work. Thus, those with musician's dystonia rarely elect the treatment of botulinum toxin.

Transmagnetic Stimulation and Transcranial Direct Current Stimulation. These are noninvasive methods to stimulate the brain and to modulate its function.[101-116] TMS is based on the application of a magnetic field outside the scalp to induce an electric field, which can excite or inhibit neurons and create action potentials. tDCS consists of applying a weak constant electric current to modulate brain excitability without inducing the generation of action potentials. Repetitive TMS (rTMS) or tDCS can be applied over selected cortical regions to modulate specific cortical–subcortical networks. The hypothesis is dystonia results from a reduction in the inhibitory mechanisms and cortical overactivity. Thus, rTMS or tDCS (or both) could potentially increase inhibition and decrease hyper excitability.

Current neuroimaging studies of patients with writer's cramp have noted a reduction in the activation of the primary motor cortex and hyperactivity of areas of the frontal nonprimary motor areas. Intervention with TMS targets decreasing the excitation of the nonprimary motor areas (e.g., PMC and supplementary motor area) to potentially decrease dystonic symptoms. Subthreshold, low-frequency (0.2-Hz) rTMS appears to improve inhibitory actions of the cortex as well as improves motor control. Pascual-Leone and colleagues[116a-116c] also demonstrated rTMS could modulate muscle responses during acquisition of new fine-motor skills. Murase and colleagues[116d] reported stimulation of the primary motor cortex (PMC) not only significantly improved the quality and efficiency of handwriting in patients with writer's cramp but also decreased pen pressure and a prolonged silent period in patients with writer's cramp. Stimulation of other sites or using a sham coil in the patient group revealed no physiologic or clinical changes. Hyperactivity of the PMC neurons in patients with FHD may suggest secondary to decreased excitability of the motor cortex.[101] Thus, rTMS could be a supplement to other sensorimotor treatment strategies. Chen and colleagues[116e] also studied the effects of low-frequency rTMS over the lateral PMC. These researchers reported that positive rTMS induced lasting changes in regional activation and function. Repeated paired associative stimulation of the median nerve in normal participants followed by 20 to 25 msec of TMS of the hand area of the motor cortex was correlated with a prolonged increase in the size of MEPs in median nerve–innervated hand muscles. These effects of rTMS on cortical excitability appear to be dependent on the frequency and intensity of the stimulation. Low-frequency (<1 Hz) rTMS decreased cortical excitability, whereas high-frequency (>5 Hz) rTMS increased cortical excitability.

rTMS treatments have been effective with patients with musicians cramps.[106] In one case study of a violist, a symphony player with uncontrollable flexion of D3 who had tried all other intervention strategies and was still not able to play, received five consecutive sessions of TMS while seated in a comfortable chair (each session including a total of 1200 biphasic pulses in two 10-minute trains of 600 pulses separated by a short interruption of about 1 minute delivered at a rate of 1 Hz). A figure-of-8 coil (9-cm external diameter) was placed 3 cm anterior to the motor hot spot over the right hemisphere of the first dorsal interosseus of the left hand. Stimulation intensity was set to 90% of motor threshold of the relaxed first dorsal interosseus muscle, which was 64% of maximum stimulator output. After treatment, the patient reported an 80% improvement and was able to play the viola with ease with only slight troubles in the movement of his fingers. After 4 months, the patient experienced a recurrence of symptoms, and a new series of TMS was applied. This again led to significant improvement. The improvement was consistent for 6 months.[105,106] Although there has been a trend for improvement after rTMS and retraining, because of small numbers of participants and other limitations of methodology, documentation of improvement was not statistically significant.

Transcranial direct current stimulation (tDCS)[109–116] is an alternative to rTMS to modulate cortical excitability in patients with FHD. Both rTMS and tDCS have minimal risks for adverse events and are low cost. However, responses to tDCS are even more inconsistent than TMS. For example, Rosset-Llobet and coworkers[110,111] reported improvement in motor control after tDCS in patients with task-specific hand dystonia. Bradnam and coworkers[112] reported anodal transcranial direct current stimulation to the cerebellum improved handwriting and cyclic drawing kinematics. However, no improvements were measured after cathodal tDCS over the affected M1 area in patients with musician's dystonia.[113–115] However, a single session of simultaneous stimulation of pianists with cathodal tDCS to the affected MI and anodal tDCS of the unaffected M1 was associated with temporary improvement in musician's dystonia.[116]

In another study, tDCS combined with bimanual mirror retraining over 2 successive days was correlated with a reduction in the severity of dystonia.[117] The kinematic measures differentiating the groups included: mean stroke frequency during handwriting, fast cyclic drawing, and average pen pressure during light cyclic drawing. It has been suggested the therapeutic benefits may also be correlated to the severity of the dystonia. Some researchers suggest tDCS could prime the effects of rTMS, minimizing the differences between control participants and those with FHD. Anodal cerebellar tDCS reduced handwriting mean stroke frequency and average pen pressure, increased speed of writing, and reduced pen pressure during fast cyclic drawing, but kinematic measures did not change. Large randomized trials with homogeneous patients with writer's cramp are needed to verify the benefits of tDCS.

Deep Brain Stimulation. Deep brain stimulation is effective for the treatment of patients with severe generalized dystonia, but it is not used regularly for the treatment of focal dystonia.[117] A few studies report on the usefulness of stereotactic stimulation for patients with medication-refractory focal dystonia of the neck (cervical dystonia).[118] There is no literature regarding the use of pallidal surgery (ablation or DBS) for FHD. However, thalamotomies of the ventralis oralis anterior thalamus contralateral to the affected hand or thalamic DBS have been performed in Korea and Japan for patients with musician's cramp. Although the procedures were not blinded, surgeons report uniformly good results.[119,120]

In India in 2017, the international news media reported an interesting case of a guitarist with musician's cramp who successfully received brain stimulation during active musical performance in the operating room.[121] As the patient played the guitar, the neurosurgeon performed radiofrequency ablation surgery in the areas of the brain associated with the dystonia during his musical performance. After the surgery, the patient was able to play the guitar without dystonia. In this "N of 1," it is too early to know if the procedure is associated with long-term positive outcomes.

Behavioral Retraining Strategies for the Brain (Sensorimotor Retraining Strategies)

Based on the etiology of maladaptive homeostatic plasticity or aberrant plasticity of the brain as the etiology of FHD,[36,41] behavioral interventions are deemed necessary to restore normal sensory and motor function through plasticity processes (Box 116.6).[92,93] The first challenge is to match the training strategy with the patient (sensory, sensorimotor, motor, task practice, forced use, one-handed performance, biomechanical stability, imagery, taping, or a combination of strategies) (Box 116.7). The second challenge is to determine how the retraining programs should be designed to most efficiently and effectively minimize the abnormal movements and restore normal neuronal connectivity and adaptation. Third, the clinician and the patient need to determine what strategies will maximize the effectiveness of neural plasticity (Box 116.e7).

BOX 116.6 Principles of Plasticity for Retraining Brain Plasticity

- *Use it:* Stay active and keep challenging learning; failure to regularly engage specific and general brain functions in learning something new can lead to serious degradation.
- *Try to improve performance:* Engage in training behaviors that drive efficiency or new effectiveness of old and new specific brain functions.
- *Be specific in your training:* The training experience must match the desired outcomes; the new connections driven by neural plasticity are dictated by the nature of the training.
- *Repetition, repetition, repetition:* Learning requires repetition; learning must be reinforced, progressed in difficulty, and spaced over time.
- *Training must be intense:* Plasticity changes require sufficient intensity of training to ensure that new connections and pathways are durable.
- *Match training to outcomes:* To facilitate neural adaptation, the training must be salient and consistent with the outcome behavior desired.
- *Age is important:* Training-induced plasticity occurs most readily in a young brain, but neural adaptation continues across the life span after learning-based training.
- *Transfer learning:* Neural adaptation in response to one training experience can also enhance acquisition of similar behaviors and adaptation in other experiences and other parts of the body.
- *There can be interference:* Plastic changes after one training experience may interfere with the acquisition of changes in similar systems.
- *Expect improvement:* Patient expectation can facilitate the outcomes of training; patients who expect to get better can enhance their learning
- *Feedback is necessary:* Feedback and reinforcement allow modification of training behaviors, correcting errors, and improving accuracy of learning.
- *Make learning fun:* Learning activities must be interesting, motivating, and fun.
- *Add elements of surprise to practice:* When something unusual is added, it can help people remember.

Data from Kleim JA, Jones TA. Principles of experience-dependent neural plasticity: implications for rehabilitation after brain damage. *J Speech Lang Hear Res.* 2008;51:S225-S239.

BOX 116.7 Strategies for Learning-Based Behavioral Retraining for Focal Hand Dystonia

Immobilization
Fatigue therapy
Desensitization therapy
Slow Down Exercise
Balanced Hand
Constraint Use, Forced Use, Sensory Motor Retuning
Learning-based sensorimotor retraining
Braille training
Transcutaneous nerve stimulation
Intensive practice
Retraining Writing with Feedback
Imagery
Developmental strategies
Biomechanical training
Supervised musical practice
Kinesio Taping

Furthermore, the clinician must consider the constraints to implementing learning-based training.

Different rehabilitation strategies have been tried to manage hand dystonia. Even though the theoretical hypothesis may be correct, there are significant constraints to implementing learning-based training. There is the challenge of patient compliance. Then there is convincing a patient to take a break from performing the target task. Next is to challenge the patient to stop the abnormal movements. Then there is the challenge of convincing the patient to engage in specific progressive repetitive training. To complicate matters, in today's health care environment, ongoing supervised treatment sessions are difficult to have covered by health insurance. Despite these limitations, even if the dystonia cannot be cured, management strategies usually have a positive impact on quality of life.[122]

Immobilization

Inactivity-dependent neuroplasticity is one approach to remediate the effects of maladaptive plasticity in focal dystonia. Inactivity of a limb (no motor movement) can induce effects at multiple levels of the motor system. Prolonged immobilization is known to be associated with changes in skeletal muscle properties (e.g., muscle atrophy, strength reduction, ratio of type I and II muscle fibers) as well as bone demineralization. In a group of healthy control participants, Hortobagyi and colleagues[122a] reported a significant reduction of type I and II fibers with an increase in the dysregulation in myosin gene expression after immobilization. It has been suggested that prolonged reduction in muscular activity could induce a restriction of motor neuron firing (e.g., lowering firing rates and reducing afferent inputs). In addition to peripheral and spinal changes, immobilization may reduce the representation of the immobilized part on the motor cortex. After finger immobilization, Facchini and colleagues[122b] reported reduced motor evoked potentials (MEPs) as measured by TMS. Kaneko and colleagues[122c] also reported reduced MEP amplitudes during motor imagery during arm immobilization. More recently, Huber and colleagues[122d] reported only 12 hours of arm immobilization in normal participants could induce plastic changes in the sensorimotor cortex (e.g., depression of somatosensory evoked potentials and MEPs). Thus, in patients with FHD, the hypothesis is plastic cortical changes related to immobilization could lead to transient improvement in motor control by decreasing cortical motor size and cortical excitability and preparing the limb for retraining.

In the initial trials of immobilization and hand dystonia, immobilization was applied in a small patient group with *early*-onset dystonia. The affected hand was immobilized in a cast for 10 days. The immobilization was associated with a "remediation" of the hand dystonia. Badarny and associates[122e] also reported improvement in writer's cramp after hand immobilization. Priori and colleagues[122f,122g] followed their pilot study with a multisite randomized clinical trial in the United States and Europe for patients with established hand dystonia. The trial was terminated early because some patients experienced an increase in the signs and symptoms of their dystonia. Thus, immobilization therapy is no longer recommended.

Fatigue Therapy

In Italy, a group of researchers hypothesized that improvement in motor control for patients with limb dystonia might occur after creating a state of motor fatigue. In normal participants, fatigue transiently reduced and reshaped motor cortical areas, including a reduction in motor output. Thus, this technique was initiated with a small group of patients with FHD. It was hypothesized that fatigue might decrease the dystonia and prime the nervous system for relearning. The effect of fatigue was temporary.

Desensitization

As part of the discussion on etiology, there is thought to be some hypersensitization in FHD with sensorimotor injuries potentially inducing abnormal movement synergies.[123,124] It has been shown that it is possible to modulate cortical motor pathways with sensorimotor training and paired associative tactile stimulation. This has served as a foundation for a desensitization program for the treatment of FHD.

In France, Tubiana[124a] developed a four-stage treatment program specifically for musicians. This program is based on desensitization or deprogramming of the acquired "bad habits." In this program, there is an attempt to restructure the body image, selectively improve muscle differentiation and relaxation, individually retrain the muscles, and then provide technical retraining on the instrument. Usually, postural and shoulder imbalances are found along with the hand dystonia. These imbalances must also be addressed in treatment.

Slow Down Exercise

Sakai[124b,124c] reported on a systematic retraining exercise program called Slow Down Exercise. This program was designed specifically for musicians. In a small group of patients with musician's dystonia, he documented a decrease in mistakes in pianists who tried this strategy.

Negative Reinforcement

Liversedge and Sylvester[124d] developed a negative reinforcement protocol for treating typists with writer's cramp. They focused on breaking down the primary manifestations of the motor dysfunction to identify the sensorimotor aspects that needed to be treated. The patient held a metal stylus and inserted it in holes of decreasing size, traced a flat zigzag on a metal plate, or wrote with a pen that reacted to excessive pressure from the thumb. When a "mistake" was made, an electric shock was delivered to the palm. An apparatus was rigged for a typist so that a shock was received when the fingers curled into the palm. Six patients were treated, and all improved significantly, with improvement maintained for varying periods (weeks to months of follow-up).

Restoration of Physiologic Posture and a Balanced Hand

Chamagne[124e] outlined a four-part program of rehabilitation that has been successful for his own rehabilitation as well as for others with FHD. Part 1 focuses on reestablishing a balanced, stable posture with gravity. Part 2 involves the integration and function of the upper limb with a balanced posture. This part focuses on balancing the scapula and the head on the trunk as well as on breathing. Part 3 focuses on strengthening the muscles of the scapular girdle, forearm, and hand (wrist, finger extensors thumb opposition, hand intrinsic muscles). Part 4 includes retraining on the instrument to restore control of the pressure of the digits to actuate the desired sound. This may be the longest part of the rehabilitation process. This part may require dynamic and resting orthotic positioning to improve biomechanical control.

Constrained-Use Paradigms

Constrained-use paradigms have been used in stroke rehabilitation programs.[125,126] When the unaffected side is constrained, the patient is forced to use the affected side in all daily activities. For FHD, this strategy has been studied within several case studies and small pilot studies.[126] The therapy is based on the principles of neuroplasticity. It has been referred to as *sensory motor retuning*. The specific guiding principles are to (1) determine the most dystonic finger; (2) avoid constraining the most dystonic finger; (3) identify the adjacent fingers that constrain the independent use of the dystonic finger; (4) constrain the uninvolved fingers in a position that is similar to the normal resting angle used in performing the target task; (5) perform selected exercises with the dystonic finger; (6) progressively increase the speed at which the dystonic finger is required to move in concert with the other fingers and then progressively decrease the constraint of adjacent digits, expecting more exacting requirements of the dystonic finger (shaping); (7) generalize the daily practice needed to sustain patient motivation to the target task; (8) practice intensively (i.e., massed practice) but not to the point that it creates excessive fatigue or increases the dystonic movement postures; and (9) outline a home practice program.

In the Candia paradigm,[126] the movement of the affected extremity was restricted for 2 weeks; then the most affected extremity received intensive training for 6 hours per day for 10 weekdays. The treatment included identifying one finger as the main focal dystonic digit and one or two other digits as secondarily involved in performing the target-specific task. An orthosis was created to specifically free the digit exhibiting the main dystonic symptoms and control the adjacent digits, with the orthosis having the flexibility to release other digits to participate with the dystonic finger. Extensive practice was directed toward performing individual alternating and sequential movements (all possible permutations) of the focal dystonic finger in coordination with immobilizing and then freeing the movements of the other fingers. The patient performed these exercises for 10 minutes in an ascending and then descending order, with continuous repetitions. Then a 2-minute rest was instituted after the sequence of movements of two or three fingers. Five such blocks were carried out in an hour.

Performance was paced by a metronome, starting at a medium tempo (60 beats per minute), then speeded up, and gradually decreased in rate. The speed sequencing was then reinitiated with the goal of having the subject generate faster and faster and then slower and slower, alternating movements in successive sequences (shaping). This was fatiguing. After completion of the first five blocks, the orthosis was removed, and the participants were given a 10-minute rest. Then they received four more 10-minute blocks of exercises with 2 minutes of rest between blocks. Various permutations of possible finger movement were used.

After the specific motor training, participants were encouraged to play their instruments without the orthosis. They played approximately 10 bars from a self-selected musical piece (15–30 seconds). If they could not do this, they were encouraged to try again. After two successful repetitions, they were asked to play a different 10-bar segment and then asked to play portions of musical pieces for longer and longer duration until they had played for a period of 15 minutes (excluding rest intervals). The complexity and duration of the practice within the performance period without the orthosis were based on the therapist's judgment. Success encouraged more success and continued performance. After a rest of 5 minutes, if the participant was not too fatigued, the orthosis was replaced, and a second series of alternating digital maneuvers was performed for half the time taken by the first series. This regimen was continued for 8 consecutive days.

On the last treatment day, the participants were given the orthosis constructed for them and asked to practice for 1 hour daily over a period of 1 year posttherapy. The participants were also instructed to do the repertoire for 10% of the usual and customary practice time without the orthosis. This period was increased by 10% in each succeeding month if there was no deterioration in the level of motor control. Based on this strategy, guitarists were more likely to improve motor control than pianists or other artists.

Learning-Based Sensorimotor Training

With the growing evidence supporting the presence of abnormal differentiation of the hand in the somatosensory, sensorimotor, motor, and premotor cortices in patients with FHD as a consequence of lack of homeostatic plasticity or aberrant plasticity, the challenge has been to determine the best way to redifferentiate the brain and restore motor

coordination and voluntary motor control without over practicing the abnormal movements.[127] Learning-based sensorimotor training (LBST) was outlined to integrate the principles of neuroplasticity based on the behavioral strategies of goal-directed, attended, repetitive, rewarded, progressive practice (see Box 116.5).[128,129] Initially, the patient is encouraged to take a break from performing the tasks that create the dystonia and focus on reflecting back in time when the target task was performed easily with joy and confidence and no movement challenges. Simultaneously, patients are requested to replace physical practice with mental practice. In addition, in all functional activities, the patient is asked to focus on using the hand in a functional, biomechanical position while appreciating the "sensory aspects" of functional activities rather than the motor output associated with the task.

Learning-based sensorimotor training challenges patients to improve the accuracy of discriminating sensory information for all somatosensory modalities (e.g., superficial tactile (cutaneous) receptors [rapid and slowly adaptive], deep touch, muscle afferents and Golgi tendon organs, vibration reinforced with auditory discrimination training or visual discrimination training). Tactile training should be performed bilaterally with the patient's eyes closed. Stimuli must be explored actively such as locating a tactile input (e.g., localization) and searching, discriminating, and matching objects (stereognosis). Patients can carry games, coins, puzzles, shapes, and other objects in their pockets to constantly challenge sensory exploration, trying to match pairs or sort by size or shape. Patients can also practice sensorimotor behaviors by learning to read Braille. It is also important for the patient to externally receive static and dynamic stimuli to the skin in the temporal and spatial domain (e.g., graphesthesia).

The sensory tasks must be performed without increasing muscle tension. If muscle co-contractions are triggered during sensory discrimination training, the sensory tasks should shift to the unaffected side and then back to the affected limb. When the stimuli can be accurately discriminated on the affected hand within the constraints of the central hypersensitivity, then stimulation should be delivered to the affected hand with the patient in unusual positions (e.g., lying prone). The site of the stimulation should initially target the finger pads but ultimately proceed to all finger segments, starting with the less dystonic fingers and progressing to the most dystonic fingers.

Focusing on sensory-motor retraining is the next step, with the sensation and recognition of the object driving the handling of the object. Objects should be assembled that are associated with familiar tasks (pens, pencils, paint brushes, musical instruments, keyboards, screwdrivers, screws or washers, hammers, drinking glasses, shoes with laces, locks, cups, cards, chips). The surface may be altered in terms of coarseness to decrease grip force. The patient should pick up the object and put it into a functional position using the least pressure possible. When ready, the instrumental tasks should be briefly performed (e.g., writing, hammering, painting). Eventually, sensory motor training needs to be performed with the target instrument associated with the dystonia.

When sensory processing accuracy of the affected limb is improved and motor tension reduced, the patient should begin to explore the sensory interface of the *target* instrument. It is critical for the patient to be able to touch and handle the instrument without creating abnormal movements or tension. Again, it may be necessary for the patient to assume different positions when initiating the exploration of his or her instrument. For example, a guitarist may be able to hold the guitar and touch the strings without involuntary muscle contractions when he is lying on his back but not while sitting. A person may be able to use a pen and write on a pad placed on a chair while lying on her stomach but not when writing a check at the store.

Initial instrument handling might start by simply dropping the digits on a key or a string. It might include rotating the forearm back and forth (pronation and supination) to bring the fingers in contact with a

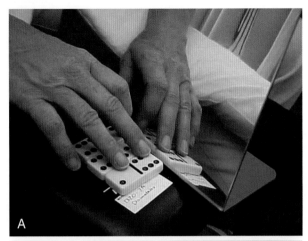

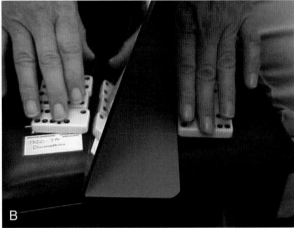

Fig. 116.4 Pictures of mirror imagery. **A,** The right, unaffected hand is placed in front of a mirror. The mirror image of the right hand looks like the left affected hand. **B,** The affected and unaffected hands perform the same task simultaneously. The patient watches the mirror images and receives positive mirror feedback that the hand is moving normally.

string or a key or lift the fingers off. The patient can progress to sequentially dropping down alternating fingers. As part of this training, the patient should also work on restoring graded movements (e.g., lightly holding the hand or digits on a moving record; lightly holding the fingers near the blades of a small portable plastic fan without stopping the movement of the blades; or moving the hand smoothly in different directions over a moving surface, e.g., the moving belt of a treadmill).

With the fingers resting on the target instrument, initial practice at the target task should begin with mental imagery of playing the instrument rather than physical performance. Normal movements can also be reinforced with visual, mirror, and motor imagery. Imagery can strengthen the pathways for normal movement and relearning of the task. For example, on a flat surface with the unaffected hand in front of the mirror and the affected hand behind the mirror, the patient can practice picking up and putting down objects and then performing some simple tasks (e.g., writing). During these activities, the patient observes the mirror image of the unaffected hand. It should look like the affected hand is working normally (Fig. 116.4). One way to check this reality is to ask the individual to make a letter that has direction (e.g., a "b"). Look on the paper on both sides of the mirror and in the mirror to check if the " b" is correct in the mirror. This requires the "b" to be backwards on the paper to actually look like a "b" in the mirror. The instrument can also be integrated into mirror therapy by placing the mirror between two computer keyboards (one completely rotated 180 degrees) or by placing a mirror directly on the piano keyboard.

When starting to perform target-specific movements, afferent muscle biofeedback can be used to increase awareness of the presence of co-contractions and the ability to move one digit at a time. For example, if the electrodes are placed on the extensors of the wrist and fingers and the patient practices moving the finger into flexion from the base joint (using the lumbricals to flex the metacarpophalangeal [MCP] joint), the objective is to keep the antagonists (finger and MCP extensors) quiet during MCP flexion The palm may need to be facing up with the dorsum of the hand resting on a surface. Or it may be necessary to create an open area for the target finger while the adjacent fingers are resting down on a surface to keep them quiet while the patient focuses on the movement of individual digits. After the patient learns to flex one MCP joint at a time without contracting the extensors, then it is time to practice turning other muscles on and off (e.g., extend the wrist or the fingers and quickly quiet and release). The biofeedback can also include a simple sensory input (e.g., using tape on the dystonic fingers, lightly pulling the hair on the dorsum of the dystonic hand, wearing gloves) or hearing a regular auditory stimulus to drive simple movements (e.g., using a metronome).

Diaphragmatic breathing paired with good posture, trunk alignment, hand posture, and biomechanics of the hand are extremely important as the precursors for the patient to begin practicing components of the target task and ultimately the complete target task. Avoiding excessive adduction of the thumb, excessive ulnar deviation of the wrist, and hyperextension of IP joints is requisite to setting the stage for safe hand use. Sometimes it is helpful to educate patients about the benefit of using slow-twitch fibers (e.g., intrinsic muscles of the hand and forearm pronators–supinators) instead of fast-twitch fibers (e.g., wrist–finger flexors and extensors).

Patients should progress to performing partial task components accurately and smoothly at different speeds before proceeding to perform the complete target task. If the patient cannot perform any components of the task without triggering the abnormal movements, the patient should try to do the task with the unaffected side or even the foot on the affected side. Well-learned, nearly automatic rhythmic tasks (e.g., walking, skipping, writing, singing, playing a musical instrument, typing) are mapped on the cortex by both function and geographic location. Thus, when retraining, it may help to drive cortical changes by activating the *functional* map by having the patient perform the task with a different extremity (e.g., write with the foot instead of the hand). Musical performance should start with practicing simple movement sequences and then new music. Well-learned repertoires should be avoided. On the computer, unfamiliar finger sequences should be practiced by resting all fingers down and using pronation and supination to lift and depress the keys.

The exact amount of training needed to restore normal topography is unknown. Based on animal research, daily training for 1 to 1.5 hours or twice daily in 30-minute sessions for 8 weeks was sufficient to degrade the topography of the digits. A similar training intensity or even more intense training may be needed to restore the differentiation of the digits. If abnormal dystonic movements continue, then retraining may take even more normal repetitions. Within these constraints, case reports and small clinical trials provide initial evidence in support of LBST as a safe, effective intervention strategy to enable patients to improve motor control and return to work.[12,39,129] Training activities for patients to follow at home are summarized in Boxes 116.e8 and 116.e9.

Braille as a Sensorimotor Retraining Strategy

In patients with writer's cramp, Zeuner and colleagues[129a,129b] studied the isolated benefits of Braille training in terms of improving writing ability. In these studies, patients were not instructed in general exercise, posture, physical strengthening, or broad-based sensory retraining. Instead, patients trained and practiced Braille reading for 8 weeks, 30 to 60 minutes daily. This was done under supervision. Patients made significant gains and continued to improve for up to 1 year if they continued to practice Braille reading as a sensory task.

In another study, Zeuner and colleagues[129c] used target-specific motor training instead of Braille reading (e.g., writing practice). Focusing on trying to decrease abnormal overflow of movement to fingers not involved in a task, a motor training program was developed for individualized finger movement. Ten patients with writer's cramp participated in the motor training program. Evaluation was based on the Fahn-Marsden dystonia scale, patient self-report of improvement, kinematic analysis of handwriting, and response to TMS and EEG. Clinical improvement of dystonia was significant (Fahn dystonia scale), and 6 patients reported an improvement in writing. The handwriting analysis showed a trend for improvement in simple exercises after training. There were no changes in cortical excitability measured by TMS or EEG. Thus, Braille training for 4 weeks led to mild subjective improvement and some objective improvements in handwriting, but it was not sufficient to reverse motor cortex abnormalities measured by TMS and EEG.

Zeuner and colleagues[129d] compared the benefits of general fine-motor retraining and those of task-specific handwriting for patients with writer's cramp. Participants were randomly assigned to two types of retraining: one group of patients trained with drawing and writing movements using a pen attached to the bottom of a finger orthosis, and the second group used therapeutic putty to train fine-motor finger sagittal and horizontal movements without doing drawing and writing movements. Training lasted for 8 weeks, 30 to 60 minutes daily. Before the retraining started, the affected hand and forearm were immobilized for 4 weeks to facilitate the responsiveness to retraining. Dystonia was assessed during handwriting using the Writer's Cramp Rating Scale. Although no clinical improvement was observed immediately after immobilization, 8 weeks of retraining was associated with a reduction in task-specific dystonia relative to baseline ($P < .005$). The more severely affected patients benefited most. There were no correlations between disease duration and the individual treatment response. Retraining also improved hand function, as indexed by the ADDS ($P < .008$). Kinematic handwriting analysis showed retraining lowered vertical force level and enhanced the fluency of handwriting. The researchers concluded retraining does not need to specifically focus on the task affected by dystonia to be clinically effective.

Zeuner and colleagues[129b] hypothesized more than 8 weeks of Braille reading would be needed to restore writing skills. Ten patients with writer's cramp who had practiced Braille reading for 8 weeks (30–60 minutes daily) were encouraged to continue Braille practice after the 8 weeks. Over time, the 10 participants significantly improved spatial acuity (grating orientation discrimination task) and reduced dystonia severity (Fahn scale). Interestingly, three patients (self-selected) continued with the Braille training for up to 1 year. These 3 subjects showed even further improvements in the grating orientation discrimination task, writing a standard paragraph, and self-rating dystonia scales. Although there was no random assignment, and the participants who decided to continue practice were completely self-selected, it is possible ongoing sensory Braille training may be a good maintenance strategy for patients with writer's cramp.

Transcutaneous Electrical Nerve Stimulation

Based on the hypothesis of sensory dysfunction in patients with FHD, transcutaneous electrical nerve stimulation (TENS) can be a part of sensory retraining. It is conceivable that TENS could remodel the balance of excitatory and inhibitory relationships in the CNS. If activation of large-diameter muscle afferents could restore the balance between agonist and antagonist muscles, then voluntary fine-motor movements at the target task could be enabled. In a randomized, placebo-controlled study including 10 patients with simple writer's cramp, Tinazzi and colleagues[129e] documented improvement of motor control in patients with hand dystonia after a 2-week period of TENS treatment. The researchers raised questions about the lasting qualities of this type of sensory retraining (e.g., may be limited to ~3 weeks).

Intensive Practice

It appears that the basic mechanisms of motor learning are intact in patients with hand dystonia given exceptional performance can be achieved with intensive practice.[130] However, dystonia may represent a corruption in learned motor programming. Thus, the resolution of the training-induced dysfunction depends on progressive retraining (practice) to correct the imbalance. This progressive retraining could include general fine-motor practice or task-specific training. In either case, the individual must begin at the level of the impairment and progress to restore function.

Different sensorimotor training strategies may fit into more than one classification of retraining. Sensory motor retuning (a variant of constraint-induced movement therapy) is one form of forced, intensive, task-specific practice. Individual fingers are trained to perform controlled movements while other fingers are positioned with an orthotic device to prevent movement.[127] Based on this paradigm, in one research paradigm, pianists experienced significant improvement in dystonic features and cortical redifferentiation. Similarly, without an orthotic device, after intensive target-specific and nonspecific target practice (30–40 min/day), Zeuner and colleagues[130a] reported a significant decrease in the severity of hand dystonia. Fatigue training is one form of priming the nervous system to learn. Pesenti and colleagues[130b] demonstrated fatigue could "temporarily" decrease dystonia and improve function, but they did not study the effectiveness of repeating the fatigue paradigm over time to permanently remediate the dystonia.

Retraining Handwriting

In 1994, Mai and Marquardt[130c] developed a handwriting retraining program. Practice of integrated handwriting motor exercises was facilitated with the use of an altered pen, a change in the grip of the pen, and the use of a writing pad. This strategy was also applied by Schenk and colleagues.[130d] This approach led to permanent improvements in the kinematic handwriting measures.

Later, Baur and colleagues[131,132] studied the direct effect of a modified pen grip (e.g., pen held between the proximal phalanges of the index and middle fingers). This modified pen grip was associated with a significant reduction in writing pressure and grip force but no change in writing performance. Although continued practice with alternative pen grips continued to reduce pressure and grip force, these methods did not document a complete reversal of the writing disorder.

Biofeedback has generically been used in rehabilitation to retrain general and neurophysiologic processing (e.g., decrease muscle spasm in areas of pain, increase muscle contractions in areas of weakness, lower blood pressure and heart rate). In focal dystonia, the goal of biofeedback is to provide information to the patient about the status of muscle contractions with the objective to enhance voluntary task performance, smooth fine-motor movements, change grip force, and decrease downward surface pressure during writing. If there are two channels, the aim is to simultaneously train a patient to turn "on" a specific set of muscles or to turn "off" a specific set of muscles. Ideally, the biofeedback system can be set to be more or less sensitive to the underlying firing of the muscles. No studies on the use of biofeedback alone for FHD could be located. Rather, biofeedback is usually adjunctive to other retraining strategies.

In terms of handwriting, most patients are unaware of the forces exerted. Neurodevelopmental sensory dysfunction might contribute to this unawareness. Thus, while writing, direct grip force feedback might be very helpful for patients with writer's cramp.[131-139] Based on the original handwriting retraining for writer's cramp by Mai and Marquardt,[139a] auditory grip force feedback was added to the retraining strategy. In one study of seven right-handed subjects with isolated writer's cramp of the right hand (54.3 ± 18.0 years of age with a mean duration of writer's cramp of 12.6 ± 16.9 years) and normal touch sensibility (two-point discrimination), Mai and Marquardt[139a] initiated handwriting retraining based on the principles of neuroplasticity. The goal was to reduce inappropriate writing strategies (decrease pressure on the pen and the writing surface as well as overflexion or overextension of the finger joints or wrist). Each individual was evaluated and matched to the appropriate motor exercise. Participants were instructed to softly bend and stretch the fingers before or interspersed with writing to improve the mobility of finger joints. Participants were specifically asked to reduce the force of the pen grip and draw lines quickly from left to right to enhance arm transport. External writing conditions were also changed as necessary to decrease the dystonia (e.g., writing on the lap instead of on the desk or writing with eyes closed). Patients started by writing letters and progressed to words and sentences. Patients participated in 7 hours of training (60 minutes per session). Five of them trained for 2 weeks, and two patients trained for 7 weeks. A conventional pen was used for 50 minutes, and a writing stylus was used the last 10 minutes. The writing stylus had sensors to measure grip force and provided auditory grip force feedback. The goal was to hear a pleasant low-frequency tone (Fig. 116.5). In addition to force measurements, the Fahn dystonia scale was administered along with a self-rated scale for subjective writing performance and pain. Average grip force during handwriting in healthy controls varies from 5 to 20 N.[133] Even in normal healthy participants, increased tone was noted with increasing grip force levels.

Training writing using biofeedback with and without botulinum toxin has been reported to be effective.[131,132-139] Within just one session, patients with writer's cramp can reduce their grip force to within normal limits. After completing the supervised training sessions, the mean writing pressure decreased in the patients, with the posttreatment values more than three times smaller than the pretreatment values. Interestingly, although participants could do the practice exercises using a normal grip force level most of the time and the grip force diminished on the pen with general writing, the change in pen gripping force in usual writing was not statistically significant. Pain decreased in six of seven participants. Patients subjectively reported improvement in writing performance, and the script generally improved in legibility and quality. However, the writing frequency and fluency and the Fahn scores did not change significantly. There was a high negative correlation between the Fahn score and pain before and after training (−0.93)

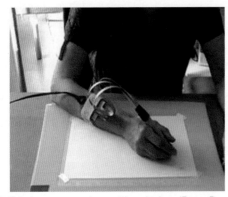

Fig. 116.5 Grip-force-measuring writing device. (From Baur B, Furholzer W, Marquardt C, Hermsdorfer J. Auditory grip force feedback in the treatment of writer's cramp. *J Hand Ther.* 2009;2:163-171.)

but a high positive correlation between subjective performance and the Fahn score.[131,132] Bleton and coworkers[139] provided feedback about posture, tension and alignment to effectively improve writing.

Mental Imagery (Graded Motor Imagery and Mirror Imagery)

There is evidence mental imagery allows an individual to recruit about 30% of the neurons normally recruited when actually performing a task. In addition, when the task cannot be performed normally, mental imagery and practice can be executed without creating the abnormal movements involved in physical practice. Furthermore, it is known that in cases of FHD resulting from overuse and after loss of a limb (e.g., the hand or the arm), the topography of the hand is disorganized. Mental imagery, mirror imagery and graded motor imagery may be strategies to help restore the sensory and motor topography.[140-143] Although imagery has been commonly used to rehabilitate patients with chronic pain, in many of the behavioral retraining strategies, imagery is also integrated as part of the paradigm.[129,144]

Biomechanical Retraining

Leijinse and coworkers[21] propose that FHD could be prevented by recognizing biomechanical limitations in the hand that may be anatomical as well as musculoskeletal. They propose that if these biomechanical restrictions are addressed early, individuals could potentially minimize the risks for dystonia by trying to correct the mechanical limitation. This could include counseling to select another career other than music.

Kinesio Taping

Kinesio taping can be used as adjunct treatment to increase proprioception for patients with FHD. This can increase sensory input, potentially improve stability, decrease pain, and potentially enhance sensory feedback to recover voluntary motor control.[97] Sensory input can increase awareness of a body part, but there is no evidence this maintained, static sensory treatment is sufficient to retrain the topographic reorganization of the brain in FHD.

Intensive Practice and Behavioral Retraining for Musicians

For musicians, supervised, intensive musical practice has been used to enable them with hand dystonia to return to musical performance.[145-152] Supervised practice is frequently combined with medications (botulinum toxin), kinematic feedback, and other behavioral training strategies, including imagery, body awareness training,[161] and forced use.[141] The practice must integrate new findings about the limitations and benefits of repetitive practice.[153-156] When biomechanical, safe, repetitive practice strategies are integrated into management and prevention programs, the prognosis for prevention as well as treatment of FHD is improved.[157]

Developmental Strategies

Some strongly suggested the benefits of neurodevelopmental training to retrain from involuntary, dystonic hand movements. These strategies range from participating in group movement therapies (e.g., Nia, yoga, Pilates, Alexander) to specific neurodevelopmental training. (e.g., Joaquin Farias[158]) or dancing.

CLINICAL EVIDENCE-BASED RESEARCH: EFFECTIVENESS OF BEHAVIORAL TRAINING

Although rehabilitation strategies based on the principles of neuroplasticity have the potential to improve outcomes in the treatment of patients with FHD, there have been no large randomized clinical trials, systematic reviews, or meta-analyses to confirm the unique benefit of any one sensorimotor retraining strategy nor the achievement of

100% recovery. The research trials generally included a small sample size, which leads to challenges of representativeness of participants as well as poor inferential statistics.[146] A brief meta-analysis of musician's dystonia by Kretschmer[145] included individual treatment protocols[40,111,127,129] and treatment combinations.[107,109,110,113,144] Six studies were level 2c or higher, and eight studies were level 4.[144] Patients and clinicians reported gains in performance post rehabilitation (effect size of 3.2 for patient perception and 2.9 for clinician perception) (Fig. 116. e14).[145] Unfortunately, objective measures of gains in voluntary, quality motor control were not documented (effect size, 0.45).

Managing practice and training for elite performance as well as restoring brain connectivity in the face of a movement disorder are based on attended, progressive practice sufficient to improve expert fine-motor skills while avoiding neuromusculoskeletal overload.[153] If a musician spends up to 10,000 lifetime hours practicing to maintain performance over an average of 16 years, would a patient with FHD have to spend an average of 625 hours a year (52 hours per month) of deliberate practice over 16 years to retrain her or his brain? Or could an individual with a movement disorder try to stop or minimize the abnormal, involuntary movements and safely engage in balanced but deliberate training over a period of 3 to 12 months (e.g., 1875–7500 hours) to restore normal motor control?

Relative to work in the occupational and sports domains, it is important to determine the length of the training sessions by considering peripheral and central issues as well as the recommended healthy work-to-rest ratio[154] and acute-to-chronic workload ratio.[155] The physical and mental requirements for the task must be modified by the intensity, duration, and type of movement activities involved.[156,157] Individual and environmental conditions must then be integrated.

To determine what is "too much" training is a complex, challenging undertaking that is seriously impacted by the strenuous nature of the task, the load and forces included in the task interact with compromised sleep, diet, and hydration; exposure to stressors; pain; expectations; experience; tradition; teacher, employer, or coach guidelines; rigid timelines; planning; and fatigue.

In a study by the Australian National Academy of Music (ANAM),[158] moderate-length practice sessions (e.g., 100 minutes) were scheduled three times a day interspersed with two short breaks (e.g., 20-30 minutes). This took place over 360 minutes per day (e.g., 6 of 8 hours). The work-to-rest ratio was approximately 3.3. Participants were asked to self-monitor fatigue and other effects of the training schedule. With this schedule, there was a dramatic drop in physical injuries and an improvement in self-reported concentration and energy.[158] Maybe this type of practice is needed to retrain the brain for patients with FHD.

Despite the limitations of available research, some individuals claim to be cured of FHD. The majority of individuals and clinicians report some improvement after treatment without necessarily demonstrating objective gains. A summary of specific effectiveness studies validating different behavioral intervention strategies can be found online for this chapter.

RECOMMENDATIONS FOR RESEARCH

A thorough review of priorities for research in limb- and task-specific dystonia was published by a leading group of researchers and clinicians experienced in movement disorders in 2017 in *Frontiers in Neurology* (Table 116.1) This summary should be reviewed by clinicians who manage patients with focal dystonia. The professionals propose that the true prevalence of focal limb dystonia is not known and is likely underestimated.

TABLE 116.1 Priorities for Research in Limb- and Task-Specific Dystonia

Key Research Areas	Clinical Features of Upper and Lower Limb Dystonia	Peripherally Induced Dystonia	Limb- and Task-Specific Dystonia Pathogenesis	Therapy in Focal Limb Dystonia
Specific priorities	• Develop clinical diagnostic criteria for upper and lower limb dystonia (consider heterogeneity) • Clarify relationships among dystonia, tremor, and dystonic tremor • Clarify relationship between dystonia and mirror dystonia • Systematically characterize clinical characteristics of patients with isolated limb dystonia who may progress to PD or other related degenerative condition • Try to characterize genetic and environmental influences on the development of musician's dystonia	• Compare clinical and neurophysiological characterizations of patients with peripherally induced dystonia with those with focal idiopathic limb dystonia and healthy control participants • Investigate patients with preexisting dystonia after peripheral injury or immobilizations to identify factors that might exacerbate underlying dystonia and peripherally induced dystonia (epidemiologic, phenomenologic, neurophysiologic, imaging)	• Distinguish cause from effect in physiology and imaging studies • Develop a diagnostic battery using neurophysiologic and imaging tests and whether one test could be sufficient for all types of dystonia • Identify therapeutic targets • Understand the variability and reproducibility of PAS and other noninvasive measurement tools in healthy participants compared with patients with dystonia • Standardize study protocols to minimize variability across studies • Determine how abnormal plasticity affects specific parietal–premotor pathways and how this may relate to spread of dystonia beyond a task or limb	• Refine role of BoNT therapy and develop new formulations with and without therapeutic modalities • In terms of rehabilitation, determine appropriate controls; understand neurophysiological rehabilitation effects; and determine the ideal frequency, duration, and longevity needed for symptom management • Determine the duration of benefits after rehabilitation

BoNT, Botulinum toxin; *PAS*, paired associative stimulation; *PD*, Parkinson's disease.
From Pirio Richardson S, Altenmüller E, Alter K, et al. Research priorities in limb and task specific dystonias. *Front Neurol.* 2017;8:1-16.

The pathophysiology of limb dystonias have commonalities with other dystonias (e.g., loss of inhibition in the CNS and loss of normal regulation of plasticity [homeostatic plasticity]). Imaging studies suggest abnormalities in anatomical networks involving the cortex, basal ganglia, and cerebellum. This review of research concluded that it will be important for future research to distinguish cause from effect in terms of neurophysiology. In addition, because of the variability in presentation, there is no specific therapy for the treatment of limb dystonia. Although botulinum toxin is most commonly recommended to help weaken overexcited muscles, rehabilitation techniques could improve outcomes. Unfortunately, small samples sizes, lack of randomization, and insufficient comparative studies minimize a clear direction for the application of rehabilitative, noninvasive, and invasive therapeutic modalities to enable quality motor learning and restoration of motor control in patients with limb dystonia. High priority must be directed to the development of diagnostic criteria for limb dystonia, more precise phenotypic characterization, and innovative clinical trial designs that consider clinical heterogeneity in individuals with limb dystonia. Although large, controlled, longitudinal, randomized clinical trials are needed to better define the parameters of intervention and to maximize neural adaptation for FHD, this type of research will be difficult because of the small numbers of individuals with FHD in any one geographical area.

Resources for Patients with Focal Hand Dystonia

A variety of resources are available to help patients who have hand dystonia. Some of these organizations have support groups that meet in person. In other cases, it is possible to establish links for online support. In addition, a variety of foundations can help patients find a physician or other team members, including a "coach"[159] or a teacher knowledgeable in treating patients with dystonia (e.g., Dystonia Medical Research Foundation). These resources are constantly changing, and it is important for clinicians to frequently go online to PubMed to check on new trials reporting on new, effective, evidence-based intervention strategies (Box 116.e10).

SUMMARY

Focal hand dystonia can be a very disabling condition. At this time, there is no consensus regarding the etiology of FHD. FHD commonly develops after an accumulation of multifactorial risks ranging from endophenotypic to exophenotypic factors. The prevalence of the problem is largely underestimated, and it may take years to diagnose. Although patients with FHD have measurable dedifferentiation of the hand representation in the somatosensory, sensorimotor, motor, and premotor cortices as well as changes in the cerebellum, putamen, and basal ganglia, each patient presents with different specific signs and symptoms.

It is important to create a team to work with the patient with hand dystonia as well as the family. It is critical for each individual to prime the nervous system for learning by stopping the abnormal movements, understanding the disorder, establishing a positive lifestyle, managing stress, and setting a positive attitude for retraining. Although medications such as botulinum toxin can help weaken the overactive muscles, the weakness may not be helpful for professional musicians. Brain retraining is essential for recovery. The goal of intervention is healthy management of the condition with the ability to return to productive work. A variety of learning-based behavioral intervention strategies have been tried with some success. Unfortunately, there have been no large randomized clinical trials to confirm the benefit of one strategy over another. Patients raise many questions about remediating their dystonia. At this time, most questions cannot be precisely answered, and a cure is rare. Continued basic science and clinical research are needed to improve the prevention, the diagnosis, and the effective management of patients with FHD.

REFERENCES

1. Albanese A, Bhatia K, Bressman SSB, et al. Phenomenology and classification of dystonia; a consensus update. *Mov Disord*. 2013;28(7):863–873.
2. Katz M, Byl NN, San Luciano M, Ostrem JL. Focal task-specific lower extremity dystonia associated with intense repetitive exercise: a case series. *Parkinsonism Relat Disord*. 2013;8. https://doi.org/S1353-8020(13)00267-8. 10.1016/j.parkreldis.2013.07.013. [Epub ahead of print].
3. Albanese A. How many dystonias? Clinical evidence. *Frontiers in Neurology*. 2017;8(18):1–11.
4. Jinnah HA. The focal dystonias: Current views and challenges for future research. *Mov Disord*. 2013;28(7):926–943.
5. Jabusch HC, Altenmuller E. Epidemiology, phenomenology and therapy of musician's cramp. In: Altenmuller E, Kesselring J, Wiesendanger M, eds. *Music, Motor Control and the Brain*. Oxford: Oxford University Press; 2006:265–282.
6. Torkamani M, Jahanshahi M. Neuropsychological and neuropsychiatric features of dystonia and the impact of medical and surgical treatment. In: Troster A, ed. *Clinical Neuropsychology and Cognitive Neurology of Parkinson's Disease and Other Movement Disorders*. New York: Oxford University Press; 2014:455–483.
7. Giorelli M, Zimatore GB. *Hairdresser's Dystonia: An Unusual Occupational Dystonia*. Tremor Other Hyperkinet Mov (N Y); 2013:3.
8. Le Floch A, Vidailhet M, Flamand-Rouviere C, et al. Table tennis dystonia. *Mov Disord*. 2010;25:394–397.
9. Dhungana S, Jankovic J. Yips and other movement disorders in golfers. *Mov Disord*. 2013;28:576–581.
10. Ham JH, Kim SJ, Song SK, et al. A prognostic factor in focal hand dystonia: typist's cramp cases and literature review. *J Neurol Sci*. 2016;371:85–87.
11. Sitburana O, Jankovic J. Focal hand dystonia, mirror dystonia and motor overflow. *J Neurol Sci*. 2008;266:31–33.
12. Altenmuller E, Baur V, Hofmann A, et al. Musician's cramp as manifestation of maladaptive brain plasticity: arguments from instrumental differences. *Ann N Y Acad Sci*. 2012;1252:259–265.
13. McKenzie AL, Goldman S, Barango C, et al. Differences in physical characteristics and response to rehabilitation for patients with hand dystonia: musician's cramp compared to writers' cramp. *J Hand Ther*. 2009;22:172–181.
14. Frucht SJ. Focal task-specific dystonia-from early descriptions to a new, modern formulation. *Tremor Other Hyperkinet Mov (N Y)*. 2014;4:230.14.
15. Groussard M, Viader F, Landeau B, et al. The effects of musical practice on structural plasticity: the dynamics of grey matter changes. *Brain Cogn*. 2014;90:174–180.
16. Steeves TD, Day L, Dykeman J, Jette N, Pringsheim T. The prevalence of primary dystonia: a systematic review and meta- analysis. *Mov Disord*. 2012;27:1789–1796.
17. Chang FCF, Frucht SJ. Motor and sensory dysfunction in musician's dystonia. *Current Neuropharmacology*. 2013;11:41–47.
18. Lin PT, Hallett M. The pathophysiology of focal hand dystonia. *J Hand Ther*. 2009;22:109–113.
19. Belvisi P, Suppa A, Marsili L, et al. Abnormal experimental and behaviorally induced LTP like plasticity in focal hand dystonia. *Exp Neurol*. 2013;240:64–74.
20. Moore AP, Gallea C, Horovitz SG, Hallett M. Individuated finger control in focal hand dystonia: an fMRI controlled study. *Neuroimage*. 2012;61(4):823–831.
21. Leijinse JN, Hallett M, Sonneveld GH. A multifactorial conceptual model of peripheral neuromusculoskeletal predisposing factors I task-specific focal hand dystonia in musicians: etiologic and therapeutic implications. *Biol Cybern*. 2015;209(1):109–123.

22. Schmidt A, Klein C. The role of genes in causing dystonia A. *Eur J Neurol.* 2010;17(suppl 1):65–70.

23. LeDoux MS, Xiao J, Rudzinska M, et al. Genotype-phenotype correlations in THAP1 dystonia: molecular foundations and description of new cases. *Parkinsonism Relat Disord.* 2012;18:414–425.

24. Hebert E, Borngräber F, Schmidt A, et al. Functional characterization of rare RAB12 variants and their role in musician's and other dystonias. *Genes.* 2017;18;8(10):E276.

25. Peterson DA, Sijnowski TJ, Poizner H. Convergent evidence for abnormal striatal synaptic plasticity in dystonia. *Neurobiol. Dis.* 2010;37:558–573.

26. Zeuner KE, Knutzen A, Granert O, et al. Increased volume and impaired function: the role of the basal ganglia in writer's cramp. *Brain and Behavior.* 2015;5(2):e00301. https://doi.org/10.1002/brb3.301 (1–14).

27. Groussard M, Viader F, Landeau B, et al. The effects of musical practice on structural plasticity: the dynamics of grey matter changes. *Brain Cogn.* 2014;90:174–180.

28. Walter U, Buttkus F, Benecke R, et al. Sonographic alteration of lenticular nucleus in focal task-specific dystonia of musicians. *Neurodegener Dis.* 2012;9:99–103.

29. Granert O, Peller M, Jabusch HC, Altenmuller E, Siebner HR. Sensorimotor skills and focal dystonia are linked to putamenal grey-matter volume in pianists. *J Neurol Neurosurg Psych.* 2011;82:1225–1231.

30. Kang SY, Hallett M, Sohn YH. Synchronized finger exercise reduces surround inhibition. *Clin Neurophysiol.* 2012;123:2227–2231.

31. Granert O, Peller M, Jabusch HC, Altenmueller E, Hartwig R, Seibner HR. Sensorimotor skills and focal dystonia are linked to putaminal grey-matter volume in pianists. *J Neurol Neurosurg Psychiatry.* 2011;82:1225e1231. https://doi.org/10.1136/jnnp.2011.245811.

32. Austin N. The wrist and hand complex. Chapter 9. In: Levangie P, Norkin C, eds. *Joint Structure and Function: A Comprehensive Analysis.* 5th ed. Philadelphia: FA Davis; 2011:305–350.

33. Sivadasan A, Sanjay M, Alexander M, Devasahayam SF, Srinivia BR. Utility of multi-channel surface electromyography in the assessment of focal hand dystonia. *Muscle Nerve.* 2013;48(3):415–420.

34. Houdayer E, Beck S, Karabanov A, et al. The differential modulation of the ventral premotor-motor interaction during movement initiation is deficient in patients with focal hand dystonia. *Eur J Neurosci.* 2012;35:478–485.

34a. Stinear CM, Byblow WD. Impaired modulation of intracortical inhibition in focal hand dystonia. *Cereb Cortex.* 2004;14:555–561.

34b. Frucht SJ. Focal task-specific dystonia in musicians. *Adv Neurol.* 2004;94:225–230.

35. Quartarone A, Rizzo V, Terranova C, et al. Sensory abnormalities in focal hand dystonia and non-invasive brain stimulation. *Front Hum Neurosci.* 2014;8:956.

36. Bara-Jimenez W, Shelton P, Hallett M. Spatial discrimination is abnormal in focal hand dystonia. *Neurology.* 2000;55:1869–1873.

37. Kimberley TJ, Borich MR, Arora S, Siebner HR. Multiple sessions of low-frequency repetitive transcranial magnetic stimulation in focal hand dystonia: clinical and physiological effects. *Restor Neurol Neurosci.* 2013;31(5):533–542.

38. Avanzino L, Tinazzi M, Ionta S, Fiorio M. Sensory-motor integration in focal dystonia. *Neuropsychologia.* 2015;79:288–300.

39. Avanzino L, Martino S, Martino J, et al. Temporal expectation in focal hand. *Brain.* 2013;136:444–454.

40. Cheng FP, Grossbach M, Altenmuller EO. Altered sensory feedbacks in pianist's dystonia: the altered auditory feedback paradigm and the glove effect. *Front Hum Neurosci.* 2013;7:868.

40a. Nowak DA, Rosenkranz K, Topka H, Rothwell J. Disturbances of grip force behavior in focal hand dystonia: evidence for a generalized impairment of sensory-motor integration? *J Neurol Neurosurg Psychiatry.* 2005;76:953–959.

41. Quartarone A, Bagnato S, Rizzo V, et al. Abnormal associative plasticity of the human motor cortex in writer's cramp. *Brain.* 2003;126:2586–2596.

41a. Quartarone A, Rizzo V, Bagnato S, et al. Homeostatic-like plasticity of the primary motor hand area is impaired in focal hand dystonia. *Brain.* 2005;128:1943–1950.

42. Altenmüller E, Baur V, Hofmann A, Lim VK, Jabusch HC. Musician's cramp as manifestation of maladaptive brain plasticity: arguments from instrumental differences. *Ann N Y Acad.* 2012;1252:259–265.

43. Rozanski VE, Rehfuess E, Botzel K, Nowak D. *A Systematic Review of Extensive Music-Practice as a Risk Factor for Musician's Dystonia; Review Protocol* 2013. www.klinikum.uni-muenchen.de/Institut-und-Poliklinik-fuer-Arbeits-SozialundUmweltmedizin/download/inhalt/publikatonslisten/Rozanski-studienprotokolleonline.pdf.

44. Altenmüller E, Jabusch HC. Focal dystonia in musicians: phenomenology, pathophysiology, triggering factors, and treatment. *Med Probl Perf Artists.* 2010;25:3–9.

45. Kadota H, Nakajima Y, Miyazaki M, et al. An fMRI study of musicians with focal dystonia during tapping tasks. *J Neurol.* 2010;257:1092–1098.

46. Schmidt A, Jabusch HC, Altenmuller E, Kasten M, Klein C. Challenges of making music: what causes musician's dystonia? *JAMA Neurol.* 2013;70:1456–1459.

46a. Groussard M, Viader F, Landeau B, et al. The effects of musical practice on structural plasticity: the dynamics of grey matter changes. *Brain Cogn.* 2014;90:174–180.

46b. Byl NN, Merzenich M, Jenkins W. A primate genesis model of focal dystonia and repetitive strain injury: I. Learning-induced de-differentiation of the representation of the hand in the primary somatosensory cortex in adult monkeys. *Ann Neurol.* 1996;47:508–520.

46c. Byl NN, Merzenich MM, Cheung S, et al. A primate model for studying focal dystonia and repetitive strain injury: effects on the primary somatosensory cortex. *Phys Ther.* 1997;77:269–284.

46d. Barbe MF, Barr AE, Gorzelang I, Arnin M, Gauglan JP, Safadi FF. Chronic repetitive reaching and grasping results in decreased motor performance and widespread tissue responses in a rat model of RSI. *J Ortho Res.* 2003;21:167–176.

47. Elliot MD, Barr AE, Clark BD, et al. High force reaching task induces widespread inflammation, increased spinal cord neurochemical and neuropathic pain. *Neuroscience.* 2009;158:922–931.

47a. Coq JO, Barr AE, Strata F, Byl N, Barbe M. Peripheral and central changes combine to induce motor behavioral deficits in a moderate repetitive task. *Exp Neurol.* 2009;220(2):234–245.

47b. Sanger TD, Merzenich MM. A computational model of the role of sensory representations in focal dystonia. *J Neurophysiol.* 2000;84:2458–2464.

48. Frei K. Posttraumatic dystonia. *J Neurol Sci.* 2017;379:183–191.

48a. Sheehy MP, Rothwell JC. Marsden CD. Writer's cramp. *Adv Neurol.* 1988;50:457–472.

49. Altenmueller E, Jabusch H-C. Focal hand dystonia in musicians: phenomenology, etiology, and psychological trigger factors. *J Hand Ther.* 2009;22:144–154.

50. Baur V, Jabusch HC, Altenmuller E. Behavioral factors influence the phenotype of musician's dystonia. *Mov Disord.* 2011;26:1780–1781.

51. Van der Stein MC, VanVugt FT, Keller PE, Altenmuller E. Basic timing abilities stay intact in patients with musicians dystonia. *Plos One.* 2014;25(9):e 9290b. https://doi.org/10.1371/journal.pone.0092906. e Collection 2014.

52. Hofman A, Grossbach M, Baur V, Hermsdoefer J, Altenmueller E. Musician's dystonia is highly task specific: no strong evidence for everyday fine motor deficits in patients. *Med Prob Perform Art.* 2015;30(2):38–46.

53. Jankowski J, Schee F, Paus S, et al. Abnormal movement preparation in task specific focal hand dystonia. *Plos One.* 2014;8(20):e78234. https://doi.org/jo.1371/journal.pne.0078234collection2013.

54. Frucht SJ. Focal task specific dystonia of the musicians' hand—a practical approach for the clinician. *J Hand Ther.* 2009;22:136–142.

55. Srivanitchapoom P, Shamim EA, Diomi P, et al. Differences in active range of motion measurements in the upper extremity of patients with writer's cramp compared with healthy controls. *J Hand Therapy.* 2016;29(4):489–495.

55a. Cimatti A, Schwartz DP, Bourdain F, et al. Time-frequency analysis reveals decreased high-frequency oscilllations in writer's cramp. *Brain.* 2007;130(Pt 1):198–205.

55b. Rosenkranz K, Williamon A, Butler K, et al. Pathophysiological differences between musician's dystonia and writer's cramp. *Brain.* 2005;128:918–931.

55c. Wilson F, Wagner C, Homberg V. Biomechanical abnormalities in musicians with occupational cramp/focal dystonia. *J Hand Ther*. 1993;6:298–307.

55d. Wilson F, Wagner C, Hömberg V, Noth J. Interaction of biomechanical and training factors in musicians with occupational cramps/focal dystonia. *Neurology*. 1991;4:291–292.

55e. Wagner C. Determination of finger flexibility. *Eur J Appl Physiol*. 1974;32:259–278.

55f. Srivanitchapoom P, Shamim EA, Diomi P, et al. Differences in active range of motion measurements in the upper extremity of patients with writer's cramp compared with healthy controls. *J Hand Ther*. 2016;29:489–495.

56. Berman BD, Hallet M, Herscovitch P, Simonyan K. Striatal dopaminergic dysfunction at rest and during task performance in writer's cramp. *Brain*. 2013;136(Pt 12):3645–3658.

57. Goldman SB, Brininger TL, Antczak A. Clinical relevance of neuromuscular findings and abnormal movement patterns: a comparison between focal hand dystonia and upper extremity entrapment neuropathies. *J Hand Ther*. 2009;22:115–123.

58. Hochberg F, Harris S, Blattert T. Occupational hand cramps: professional disorders of motor control. *Hand Clin*. 1990;6:417–428.

59. Schuhfried GmbH, Modling, Austria version 6.34.001; https://www.schuhfried.com/test/MLS

60. Hoffman A, Grossback B, Baur V, Hermsdorfer J, Altenmuller E. Musician's dystonia is highly task specific: no strong evidence for everyday fine motor deficits in patients. *Med Probl Perform Art*. 2015;30(1):138–146.

61. Furuya S, Toinaga K, Miyaszki F, Altenmuller E. Losing dexterity: patterns of impaired coordination of finger movements in musician's dystonia. *Scientific Reports*. 2015:1–14| 5:13360. https://doi.org/10.1038/srep13360.

62. Dellon A. *Somatosensory Testing and Rehabilitation*. Bethesda, MD: Dellon Institutes for Peripheral Nerve Surgery; 2016.

62a. Byl N, Leano J, Cheney K. The Byl-Cheney-Boczai Sensory Discriminator: reliability, validity, and responsiveness for testing stereognosis. *J Hand Ther*. 2002;15:315–330.

63. Hsu HY, Kuo LC, Jou IM, Chen SM, Chiu HY, Su FC. Establishment of a proper manual tactile test for hands with sensory deficits. *Arch Phys Med Rehabil*. 2013;94(3):451–458. https://doi.org/10.1016/j.apmr.2012.07.024. Epub 2012 Aug 9.

64. Hsu Kuo LC, Kuan TS, Yang HC, SU FC, Chiu HY, Shieh SJ. Determining functional sensibility of the hand in patients with peripheral nerve repair: feasibility of using a novel manual tactile test for monitoring the progression of nerve regeneration. *J Hand Therapy*. 2017;30:65–73.

65. https://www.brainhq.com/?lead_id=google-search-text-home. Brand_" title="https://www.brainhq.com/?lead_id=google-search-text-home Brand_">https://www.brainhq.com/?lead_id=google-search-text-home Brand_(US_CAN_UK_AUS_SAF_NZ)&gclid=EAIaIQobChMIz4X-P8orG1gIVzl9-Ch2tUQwhEAAYASAAEgLfnfD_BwE.

66. Albanese A, Del Sorbo F, Comella C, et al. Dystonia rating scales: critique and recommendations. *Mov Disord*. 2013;28:874–883.

67. Delrobaei M, Rahimi F, Mallory E, et al. Kinematic and kinetic assessment of upper limb movements in patients with writer's cramp. *J Neuroeng Rehabil*. 2016;13:15. https://doi.org/10.1186/s12984-016-0122-0.

68. Albaneze A. Botulinum neurotoxins for the treatment of focal dystonias: review of rating tools used in clinical trials. *Toxicon*. 2015;107:89–97.

69. Erro R, Hirschbichler SJ, Ricciardi L, et al. Mental rotation and working memory in musician's dystonia. *Brain Cogn*. 2016;69:124–129.

70. Cheng FP, Eddy ML, Ruiz MH, Grobhach M, Altenuller EO. Sensory feedback-dependent neural de-orchestration: the effect of altered sensory feedback on musician's dystonia. *Restor Neural NeuroScience*. 2015;34(2):55–65.

71. Peterson DA, Berque P, Jabusch HC, et al. Rating scales for musician's dystonia: the state of the art. *Neurology*. 2013;81:589–598.

71a. Zeuner KE, Peller M, Knutzen A, et al. How to assess motor impairment in Writer's Cramp. *Mov Dis*. 2007;22(8):1102–1109.

71b. Fahn S. Assessment of the primary dystonias. In: Munsat T, editor. *The Quantification of Neurologic Deficit*. Boston: Butterworths; l989:241–270.

71c. Wissel J, Kabus C, Wenzel R, et al. Botulinum toxin in writer's cramp: objective response evaluation in 31 patients. *J Neurol Neurosurg Psychiatry*. 1996;61:172–175.

71d. Wilson F. Digitizing digital dexterity: a novel application for MIDI recordings of keyboard performance. *Psychomusicology*. 1992;11:79–95.

71e. Delrobaei M, Rahimi F, Mallory E, et al. Kinematic and kinetic assessment of upper limb movements in patients with writer's cramp. *J Neuroeng Rehabil*. 2016;13:15.

72. Armouzandah A, Grossbach M, Hermsdorfer J, Altenuller E. Pathophysiology of writer's cramp: an exploratory study on task-specificity and non-motor symptoms using an extended fine-motor testing battery. *J of Clin Mov Dis*. 2017;4:13. https://doi.org/10.1186/s40734-017-0060-4.

73. *WACOM Intuos3 A4 Oversize with GRIP Pen*; WACOM Europe, Krefeld, Germany.

73a. Fung S, Byl N, Melnick M. Reliability and sensitivity of a new functional evaluation tool. *Eur J Rehabil*. 1996;7:154–187.

73b. Zeuner KE, Knutzen A, Pedack L, Hallett M, Deuschl G, Volkmann J. Botulinum neurotoxin treatment improves force regulation in writer's cramp. *Parkinsonism Relat Disord*. 2013;19:611–616.

74. Voon V, Butler TR, Ekanayake V, et al. Psychiatric symptoms associated with focal hand dystonia. *Mov Disord*. 2010;25(13):2249–2262.

75. http://www.statisticssolutions.com/16-personality-factors/.

76. Rubin Gretchen. *The Four Tendencies*; 2016.

77. Butcher JN. *A Beginners' Guide to the MMPI-2*. 3rd ed. 2011. USBB867-1-4388-0922-4.

78. Quartarone A, Rizzo V, Terranova C, et al. Sensory abnormalities in focal hand dystonia and non-invasive brain stimulation. *Front Hum Neurosci*. 2014;956(8):1–5. https://doi.org/10.3389/fnhum.2014.00956. eCollection 2014.

79. Jin SH, Hallett M. Abnormal reorganization of functional small world networks in focal hand dystonia. *PlosOne*. 2011;6(12). e Epub 2011.

80. Dolberg R, Hinkley LB, Homma S, Zhu Z, Byl NN, Nagajaran SS. Amplitude and timing of somatosensory cortex activity in task specific focal hand dystonia. *Clinical Neurophysiology*. 2011;122(12):2441–2451.

81. Hinkley LBN, Webster R, Byl NN, Nagarajan SS. Neuroimaging characteristics of patients with focal hand dystonia. *J Hand Ther*. 2009;22:125–134.

82. Weiss D, Gentner R, Zeller D, Nagel A, Reunsberger S, Rumpf JJ, Classen J. Focal hand dystonia: lack of evidence for abnormality of motor representation at rest. *Neurology*. 2012;78(2):122–128.

83. Dresel C, Li Y, Wilzeck V, Castrop F, Zimmer C, Haslinger G. Multiple changes of functional connectivity between sensorimotor areas in focal hand dystonia. *J Neurol Neurosurg Psychiatry*. 2014;85 911:1245–1252.

84. Houdayer E, Beck S, Karabanov A, Poston B, Hallett M. The differential modulation of the ventral pre-motor interaction during movement initiation is deficient in patients with focal hand dystonia. *Eur J Neuroscience*. 2012;35(2):478–485.

84a. Sanger TD, Tarsy D, Pascual-Leone A. Abnormalities of spatial and temporal sensory discrimination in writer's cramp. *Mov Dis*. 2001;16:94–99.

85. Newby R, Alty J, Kempster P. Functional dystonia and the borderland between neurology and psychiatry: new concepts. *Mov Disord*. 2016;31:1777–1784.

86. Ioannou CI, Furuya S, Altenmuller E. The impact of stress on motor performance in skilled musicians suffering from focal dystonia: Physiological and Psychological characteristics. *Neuropsychologica*. 2016;85:226–236.

87. Schrag AE1, Mehta AR, Bhatia KP, et al. The functional neuroimaging correlates of psychogenic versus organic dystonia. *Brain*. 2013;136(Pt 136):770–781. https://doi.org/10.1093/brain/awt008.

88. https://www.dystonia-foundation.org/what-is-dystonia/forms-of-dystonia/psychogenic-dystonia/more-on-psychogenic-dystonia. Beginning treatment and foundation of plasticity.

89. Jinnah HA, Factor SA. Diagnosis and treatment of dystonia. *Neurol Clin.* 2015;33:77–100. https://doi.org/10.1016/j.ncl.2014.09.002. http://www.neurologic.theclinics.com. note Videos of various dystonias accompany this article at http:// www.neurologic.theclinics.com/.

90. Department of Health and Human Services Healthy People 2000.

91. Fletcher GF, Balady G, Blair SN, Blumenthal J, Caspersen C, et al. Statement on exercise: benefits and recommendations for physical activity programs for all Americans. *Circulation.* 1996;94(4):857–862.

92. Merzenich M, Wired Soft. *How the New Science of Brain Plasticity Can Change your Life.* LLD, San Francisco: Parnassus Publishing; 2013.

93. Kleim JA, Jones TA. Principles of experience-dependent neural plasticity: implications for rehabilitation after brain damage. *J Speech Lang Hear Res.* 2008;51:S225–239.

94. Pelosin E, Avanzino L, Marchese R, Stramesi P, Bilanci M, Trompetto C. KinesioTaping reduces pain and modulates sensory function in patients with focal dystonia: a randomized crossover pilot study. *Neurorehabil Neural Repair.* 2013;27(8):722–731.

95. Thieme H,N, Rietz C, Dohle C, Borgetto B. The efficacy of movement representation techniques for treatment of limb pain-A systematic review and meta-analysis. *J of Pain.* 2016;17(2):167–180.

96. Castrop F, Dresel C, Hennennlotter A, Zimmer C, Haslinger B. Basal ganglia premotor dysfunction during movement imagination in writer's cramp. *Mov Disord.* 2012;27(11):1432–1439.

97. Bredeson DE. *The End of Alzheimer's Disease.* 1st ed. Penguin Random House; 2017.

98. Perlmutter D. *Grain Brain.* New York: Little, Brown and Company; 2013.

99. Koppel BS, Brust JCM, Fife T, et al. Systematic review: Efficacy and safety of medical marijuana in selected neurologic disorders report of the guideline development subcommittee of the *American Academy of Neurology.* 2014;82:1556–1563.

100. Lungu C, Karp BI, Alter K, Hallett M. Long term follow up of botulinum toxin therapy for focal hand dystonia: outcomes at 10 years or more. *Mov Disord.* 2011;26(4):750–753.

101. Vymazal J, et al. Repetitive TMS of the somatosensory cortex improves writer's cramp and enhances cortical activity. *Neuro Endocrinol Lett.* 2010;31:73–86.

102. Bharath RD, Biswal BB, Bhaskar MV, et al. Repetitive transcranial magnetic stimulation induced modulations of resting state motor connectivity in writer's cramp. *Eur J Neurol.* 2015;22(5):796–805.

103. Kimberley TJ, Borich MR, Arora S, Siebner HR. Multiple sessions of low-frequency repetitive transcranial magnetic stimulation in focal hand dystonia: clinical and physiological effects. *Restor Neurol Neurosci.* 2013;31:533–542.

104. Havrankova P, Jech R, Walker ND, Operto G, Tauchmanova J, Vymazal J, et al. Repetitive TMS of the somatosensory cortex improves writer's cramp and enhances cortical activity. *Neuroendocrinology Lett.* 2010;31(1):73–86.

105. Kimberley TJ, Borich MR, Carey JR, Gillick B. Focal hand dystonia individualized intervention with repeated application of repetitive transcranial magnetic stimulation. *Arch Phys Med Rehabil.* 2015;96(suppl 4):S122–128.

106. Kieslinger K, Yvonne Höller Y, Jürgen Bergmann J, Golaszewski S, Staffen W. Successful treatment of musician's dystonia using repetitive transcranial magnetic stimulation. *Clin Neurol Neurosurg.* 2013;115:1871–1872.

107. Kimberley TJ, Schmidt RL, Chen M, et al. Mixed effectiveness of rTMS and retraining in the treatment of focal hand dystonia. *Front Hum Neurosci.* 2015;9:385.

108. Kimberley TJ, Di Fabio RP. Visualizing the effects of rTMS in a patient sample: Small N vs. group level analysis. *PLoS ONE.* 2010;5(12):1–5. [e15155 https://doi.org/10.1371/journal.pone.0015155].

109. Furuya S, Nitsche MA, Paulus W, Altenmuller E. Surmounting retraining limits in musicians' dystonia by transcranial stimulation. *Ann Neurol.* 2014;75:700–707.

110. Rosset-Llobet J, Fabregas-Molas S, Pascual-Leone A. Transcranial direct current stimulation improves neurorehabilitation of task-specific dystonia: a pilot study. *Med Probl Perform Art.* 2014;29:16–18.

111. Rosset-Llobet J, Fabregas-Molas S, Pascual-Leone A. Effect of transcranial direct current stimulation on neurorehabilitation of task-specific dystonia: a double-blind, randomized clinical trial. *Med Probl Perform Art.* 2015;30:178–184.

112. Bradnam LV, Graetz LJ, McDonnell MN, Ridding MC. Anodal transcranial direct current stimulation to the cerebellum improves handwriting and cyclic drawing kinematics in focal hand dystonia. *Fron Hum Neurosci.* 2015;28:266. https://doi.org/10.3389frnhum 2015 00286. eCollection 2015. PID 26042019.

113. Buttkus F, Weidenmuller M, Schneider S, Jabusch HC, Nitsche MA, Paulus W, et al. Failure of cathodal direct current stimulation to improve fine motor control in musician's dystonia. *Mov Disord.* 2010;25:389–394.

114. Buttkus F, Baur V, Jabusch HD, de la Cruz Gomes-Pellin M, Paulus W, Nitsche MA, et al. Retraining and transcranial direct current stimulation in musician's dystonia-a case report. *Restor Neurol Neurosci.* 2011;29:85–90.

115. Benninger DH, Lomarev M, Lopez G, Pal N, Luckenbaugh DA, Hallet M. Transcranial direct current stimulation for the treatment of focal hand dystonia. *Mov Disord.* 2011;26:1698–1702.

116. Furuya S, Nitsche MA, Paulus W, Altenmuller E. Surmounting retraining limits in musicians' dystonia by transcranial stimulation. *Ann Neurol.* 2014;75:700–707.

116a. Pascual-Leone A, Horvath JC, Robertson EM. Enhancement of oral cognitive abilities through noninvasive brain stimulation. Cortical Connectivity: Brain Stimulation for Assessing and Modulation Cortical Connectivity and Function. 207–249. https://doi.org/10.1007/978-3-642-32767-4_11.

116b. Davila-Perez P, Pascual-Leone A, Cudeiro J. Effects of transcranial static magnetic stimulation on Motor cortex evaluated by different TMS waveforms and current directions. *Neuroscience.* 2019;413:22–30.

116c. Eldaief MC, Press DZ, Pascual-Leone A. Transcranial magnetc stimulation in neurology. A Review of established and prospective applications. *Neurol Clin Pract.* 2013;3(6):519–526.

116d. Murase N, Rothwell JC, Kaji R, et al. Subthreshold low-frequency repetitive transcranial magnetic stimulation over the premotor cortex modulates writer's cramp. *Brain.* 2005;128(1):104–115.

116e. Chen R, Classen J, Gerloff C, et al. Depression of motor cortex excitability by low-frequency transcranial magnetic stimulation. *Neurology.* 1997;48:1398–1403.

117. Quartarone A, Rizzo V, Terranova C, et al. Sensory abnormalities in focal hand dystonia and non-invasive brain stimulation. *Front Hum Neurosci.* 2014;8:956.

118. Voolkmann J, Mueller J, Deuschl G, Kuhn AA, Krauss JK, Poewe W, et al. Pallidal neurostimulation in patients with medication-refractory cervical dystonia: a randomized, sham-controlled trial. *Lancet Neurol.* 2014;9:875–884.

119. Horisawa S, Taira T, Goto S, Ochial T, Nakajima T. Long term improvement of musician's dystonia after stereotactic ventro-oral thalamotomy. *Ann Neurol.* 2013;74:648–654.

120. Asahi T, Koh M, Kashiwazaki D, Kuroda S. Stereotactic neurosurgery for writer's cramp: report of two cases with an overview of the literature. *Stereotact Funct Neurosurg.* 2014;92:405–411.

121. http://edition.cnn.com/2017/0722/health/india-guitar-brain-surgery/index.html.

122. Lee A, Eich C, Loannou CI, Altenmuller E. Life satisfaction of musicians with focal dystonia. *Occup Med (Lond).* 2015;65(5). https://doi.org/10.1093/occmed/kqv038.

122a. Hortobagyi T, Dempsey L, Fraser D, et al. Changes in muscle strength, muscle fiber size and myofibrillar gene expression after immobilization and retraining in humans. *J Physiol.* 2000;524:293–304.

122b. Facchini S, Romani M, Tinazzi M, Aglioti SM. Time-related changes of excitability of the human motor system contingent upon immobilization of the ring and little fingers. *Clin Neurophysiol.* 2002;113:367–375.

122c. Kaneko F, Murakami T, Onari K, et al. Decreased cortical excitability during motor imagery after disuse of an upper limb in humans. *Clin Neurophysiol.* 2003;114:2397–2403.

122d. Huber R, Ghilardi MF, Massimini M, et al. Arm immobilization causes cortical plastic changes and locally decreases sleep slow wave activity. *Nat Neurosci*. 2006;9:1169–1176.

122e. Badarny S, Meer J, Drori T, Zivziner S, Honigman J. Writer's cramp treated with hand immobilization. *Mov Disord*. 2002;17:1020.

122f. Priori A, Pesenti A, Cappellari A, et al. Limb immobilization for the treatment of focal occupational dystonia. *Neurology*. 2001;57:405–409.

122g. Pesenti A, Barbieri S, Priori A. Limb immobilization for occupational dystonia: a possible alternative treatment for selected patients. *Adv Neurol*. 2004;94:247–254.

123. Karabanov A, Jin SH, Joutsen A, et al. Timing-dependent modulation of the posterior parietal cortex-primary motor cortex pathway by sensorimotor training. *J Neurophysiol*. 2012;107:3190–3199.

124. Santello M, Lang CE. Are movement disorders and sensorimotor injuries pathologic synergies? When normal multi-joint movement synergies become pathologic. *Frontiers in Human Neuroscience*. 2015;8| Article 1050 | 1. https://doi.org/10.3389/fnhum.2014.01050.

124a. Tubiana R. Prolonged neuromuscular rehabilitation for musician's focal dystonia. *Med Probl Perf Artists*. 2003;18:166–169.

124b. Sakai N. Slow down exercise for the treatment of focal hand dystonia in pianists. *Med Probl Perform Art*. 2006;21:25–28.

124c. Sakai N, Liu MC, Bishop AT, An K-N. Hand span and digital motion on the keyboard: Concerns of overuse syndrome in musicians. *J of Hand Surgery*. 2006;31:830–835.

124d. Liversedge LA, Sylvester JD. Conditioning techniques in the treatment of writer's cramp. *Lancet*. 1955;4:1147–1149.

124e. Chamagne R. Functional dystonia in musicians: Rehabilitation. *Hand Clinic*. 2003;19:309–316.

125. Kwakkel G, Veerbeek JM, van Wegen EE, Wolf SL. Constraint-induced movement therapy after stroke. *Lancet Neurol*. 2015;14(2):224–234. https://doi.org/10.1016/S1474-4422(14)70160-7. Review. PMID: 25772900.

126. Flor H, Diers M. Sensorimotor training and cortical reorganization. *Neurorehabilitation*. 2009;25: 17–19.

127. Furuya S, Altenmuller F. Acquisition and reacquisition of motor coordination in musicians. *Ann NY Acad Sci*. 2015;1337:118–124.

128. Byl N, Barbe M, Byl CA. Repetitive stress pathology: soft tissue. In: Magee DJ, Zachazewski JE, Quillen WS, eds. *Pathology and Intervention in Musculoskeletal Rehabilitation*. Canada: Saunders, Elsevier; 2014.

129. Byl N, Archer E, McKenzie A. Effectiveness of a home program of fitness and learning-based sensorimotor and motor training. *J Hand Ther*. 2009;22:183–198.

129a. Zeuner KE, Moloy FM. Abnormal reorganization in focal hand dystonia; sensory and motor training programs to retrain cortical function. *NeuroRehabilitation*. 2008;23:43–53.

129b. Zeuner KE, Bara-Jimenez W, Noguchi PS, Goldstein SR, Dambrosia JM, Hallet M. Sensory training for patients with focal hand dystonia. *Ann of Neurol*. 2002;51(5):593–598.

129c. Zeuner KE, Shill HA, Sohn YH, et al. Motor training as treatment in focal hand dystonia. *Mov Disord*. 2005;20:335.

129d. Zeuner KE, Peller M, Knutzen H, et al. Motor retraining does not need to be task specific to improve writer's cramp. *Mov Disord*. 2008;23(16):2319–2327.

129e. Tinazzi M, Farina S, Bhatia K, et al. TENS for the treatment of writer's cramp dystonia: a randomized, placebo-controlled study. *Neurology*. 2005;64:1946–1948.

130. Krullaards RL, Pel JJM, Snijders CJ, Kleinrensink G-J. The potential effects of a biofeedback writing exercise on radial artery blood flow and neck mobility. *International J of Biomedical Science*. 2009;5(2):192. https://www.researchgate.net/publication/236909900. Accessed Aug 17, 2017.

130a. Zeuner KE, Baur B, Siebner H. Therapy of sensorimotor dysfunction of the hand: focal hand dystonia. In: Nowak DA, Hermsdoerfer J, eds. *Sensorimotor Control of Grasping: Physiology and Pathophysiology*. Cambridge, UK: Cambridge University Press; 2009.

130b. Pesenti A, Priori A, Scarlato G, Barbieri S. Transient improvement induced by motor fatigue in focal occupational dystonia: the handgrip test. *Mov Disord*. 2001;16:1143–1147.

130c. Mai N, Marquardt C. Treatment of writer's cramp: kinematic measures as an assessment tool for planning and evaluating training procedures. In: Faure C, Keuss P, Lorette G, Vinter A, eds. *Advances in Handwriting and Drawing: A Multidisciplinary Approach*. Paris: Europia; 1994:445–461.

130d. Schenk T, Baur B, Steidle B, Marquardt C. Does training improve writer's cramp? An evaluation of a behavioral treatment approach using kinematic analysis. *J Hand Ther*. 2004;17:349–363.

131. Baur B, Furholzer W, Jasper I, et al. Effects of modified pen grip and handwriting training on writer's cramp. *Arch Phys Med Rehabil*. 2009;90(5):867–875. 69,137,239.

132. Baur B, Furholzer W, Marguardt C, Hermsdorfer J. Auditory grip force feedback in the treatment of writer's cramp. *J Hand Ther*. 2009;22:163–171.

133. Hermsdörfer J, Marquardt C, Schneider AS, Fürholzer W, Baur B. Significance of finger forces and kinematics during handwriting in writer's cramp. *Human Movement Sci*. 2011;30(4):807–817.

134. Atashzar SF, et al. Effect of kinesthetic force feedback and visual sensory input on writer's cramp, in *Proc. Int. IEEE/EMBS Conf. Neural Eng.* 2013:883–886.

135. Atashzar SF, Shahbazi M, Ward C, et al. Haptic feedback manipulation during botulinum toxin injection therapy for focal hand dystonia patients: a possible new assistive strategy. *IEEE Transactions on Haptics*. 2016;9(4):523–535.

136. Zeuner KE, Knutzen A, Pedack L, Hallett M, Deuschl G, Volkmann J. Botulinum neurotoxin treatment improves force regulation in writer's cramp. *Parkinsonism and Related Disorders*. 2013;19:611e616.

137. Schneider A, Baur B, Fürholzer W, Jasper I, Marquardt C, Hermsdörfer J. Writing kinematics and pen forces in writer's cramp: Effects of task and clinical subtype. *Clinical Neurophysiology*. 2010;121(11):1898–1907.

138. Schneider AS, Fürholzer W, Marquardt WC, Hermsdörfer JJ. Task specific grip force control in writer's cramp. *Clinical Neurophysiology*. 2014;125:786–797.

139. Bleton JP, et al. Somatosensory cortical remodeling after rehabilitation and clinical benefit in writer's cramp. *J Neurology Neurosurgery Psychiatry*. 2010;82:574–577.

139a. Marquardt C, Mai N. A computational procedure for movement analysis in handwriting. *J Neurosci Methods*. 1994;52:39–45.

140. Bowering KJ, O'Connell NE, Tabor A, et al. The effects of graded motor imagery and its components on chronic pain: a systematic review and meta-analysis. *J Pain*. 2013;14(1). (January):3–13. Available online at www.jpain.org www.sciencedirect.com.

141. Dohle C, Pallen J, Nakaten A, Just J, Rietz C, Karbe H. Mirror therapy promotes recovery from severe hemiparesis A randomized controlled trial. *Neurorehabilitation and Neural Repair*. 2009;23(3):209–2017.

142. Thieme H, Mehrholz J, Pohl M, Behrens J, Dohle C. Mirror therapy for improving motor function after stroke. *Cochrane Database Syst Rev*. 2012;3:CD008449. https://doi.org/10.1002/14651858.CD008449.pub2. Review. Review. PMID:22419334.

143. Bowering KJ, O'Connell NE, Tabor A, Catley MJ, Moseley GL, Stanton TR. The effects of graded motor imagery and its components on chronic pain: a systematic review and meta-analysis. *J of Pain*. 2013;14(1):3–13.

144. Berque P, Gray H, Harkness C, et al. A combination of constraint-induced therapy and motor control retraining in the treatment of focal hand dystonia in musicians. *Med Probl Perform Art*. 2010;25: 149–161.

145. Kretschmer J. *Unpublished Doctoral Project-UCSF/SFSU Graduate Program in Physical Therapy*; 2016.

146. Straus SRW, Glasziou P, Haynes RB. *Evidence-Based Medicine: How to Practice and Teach EBM*. 3rd ed. Edinburgh: Churchill Livingstone; 2005.

147. Rosenkranz K, Butler K, Williamon A, et al. Regaining motor control in musician's dystonia by restoring sensorimotor organization. *J Neurosci*. 2009;29:14627–14636.

148. van Vugt FT, Boullet L, Jabusch HC, et al. Musician's dystonia in pianists: long-term evaluation of retraining and other therapies. *Parkinsonism Relat Disord*. 2014;20:8–12.

149. de Lisle R, Speedy DB, Thompson JMD, et al. Effects of pianism retraining on three pianists with focal dystonia. *Med Probl Perform Art.* 2006;21:105–111.

150. Jabusch HC, Zschucke D, Schmidt A, et al. Focal dystonia in musicians: treatment strategies and long-term outcome in 144 patients. *Mov Disord.* 2005;20:1623–1626.

151. Woldendorp KH, vanGils W. One-handed musicians–more than a gimmick. *Med Probl Perform Art.* 2012;27(4):231–237.

152. Maidhof C, Kastner T, Makkonen T. Combining EEG, MIDI, and motion capture techniques for investigating musical performance. *Behav Res Methods.* 2014;46:185–195.

153. Ackerman BJ. *How Much Training is too Much?* 2017:61–62.

154. Combes A, Dekerle J, Bougault V, Daussin FN. Effect of work: rest cycle duration on fluctuations during intermittent exercise. *J Sport Sci.* 2017;35(2):7–13.

155. Hulin BT, Gabbett TJ, Caputi P, et al. Low chronic workload and the acute:chronic workload ratio are more predictive of injury than between-match recovery time: a two-season prospective cohort study in elite rugby league players. *Br J Sports Med.* 2016;50:1008–1012.

156. Halson SL. Monitoring training load to understand fatigue in athletes. *Sports Med.* 2014;44(S2):139–147.

157. Kok LM, Huisstede BMA, Douglas TJ, Nelissen RGHH. Association of arm position and playing time with prevalence of complaints of the arms, neck, and/or shoulder (CANS) in amateur musicians: a cross-sectional pilot study among university students. *MPPA.* 2017;32(1):8–12.

158. *Australian Ballet: Injury Management and Prevention Programme.* Cot; 2007. Available at: https://s3-ap--southeast-2.amazonaws.com/tab-website-images/content-images/mMedical_Team/InjuryManagementand-PreventionProgramme.pdf. Accessed 1 Mar 2017.

159. Richardson SP, Altenmuller E, Alter K, et al. Research priorities in limb and task-specific dystonias. *Frontiers in Neurology.* 2017;8:1–16.

160. http://ndb.nal.usda.gov/.

161. Waissmann F, Orsini M, Nascimento OJM, Leite MAA, Pereira JS. Sensitive training through body awareness to improve the writing of patients with writer's cramp. *Neurology International.* 2013;5(24):84–88.

117

Assessment and Treatment Principles for the Upper Extremities of Instrumental Musicians

Katherine Butler

CRITICAL POINTS

- Performance-related issues such as excessive training, change in instrument, increased demands of repertoire, pressures in the workplace, lack of or inconsistent work, and instrument quality are discussed.
- Nonmusical activities and factors that can affect musicians such as environmental factors and anatomic variations are mentioned.
- Assessment and treatment techniques are explored, with a particular focus on tendinopathies, hypermobility, task-specific

dystonia, work-related upper limb disorders or nonspecific arm pain, nerve entrapment syndromes, and ganglions.
- Professional musicians give "tips and tricks" regarding their instrument.
- General treatment principles for musicians are explored. These include orthotic intervention, musical ergonomics, and resuming playing after an injury.
- Surgical intervention and the musician are considered.

Musicians' hands are vital to their musical performance. Musicians often have to perform to the limit of their abilities physically, emotionally and spiritually. They use rapid, complex, coordinated movements and are frequently required to play for long periods of time with poor facilities, less than ideal environments, and under pressure. They can injure themselves or acquire injuries that can lead to difficulties or an inability to play their instruments.

Musicians' medicine has become an increasingly popular specialization over the past 20 years, with at least eight textbooks relating to this topic published in English. Professional groups and organizations have been established in numerous countries to research preventive measures and evidence-based treatments for musicians. Each country has specific circumstances (e.g., health care system, financial support available, and perceived medical need) that influence the administration structure of the performing arts organizations. Encouragingly, there is growth in international cooperation, assisted by the development of international conferences,[1] which means that multicenter research projects are being undertaken.

Specialist assessment and rehabilitation techniques are required when dealing with this patient group. An understanding of the instrument and the type of music played is imperative. An area of specialization that has come to the fore in musicians' medicine is hand therapy.

The focus of performing arts medicine should be prevention. Wynn Parry[2] made a detailed analysis of 1046 musicians he assessed (Fig. 117.1) and found that 48% of this group presented with clear-cut pathologies. Of the structural disorders, four broad bands were evident: old injuries (22%),

tenosynovitis (12%), hypermobility (9%), and focal hand dystonia (5%). In the remaining 52%, few physical signs could be found, and the symptoms were vague and generalized and caused by performance-related issues such as incorrect practice or technique when playing their instrument.

PERFORMANCE-RELATED ISSUES

When a musician presents with a nontrauma related condition, careful analysis and consideration are required. Hand surgeons and therapists

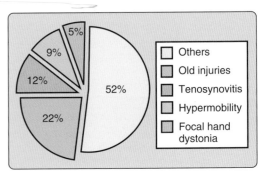

Fig. 117.1 Percentage breakdown of specific versus nonspecific diagnosis for injured musicians. (Data from Wynn Parry CB. Managing the physical demands of musical performance. In: Williamon A, ed. *Musical Excellence Strategies and Techniques to Enhance Performance.* Oxford, UK: Oxford University Press; 2004:41-60.)

may be able to assist with providing an anatomical diagnosis for a painful condition in a musician's hand or arm.[3,3a] There can be issues developing from:

- Excessive playing
- Change in instrument
- Increased demands of repertoire
- Pressures in the workplace
- Lack of or inconsistent work
- Quality of instrument

Excessive Training

An abrupt increase in practice or performance time is perhaps the most common risk factor for musicians of all levels.[4] This can occur while preparing for a recital or competition, at a summer festival, during the holiday seasons when musical performances may have an increased demand (e.g., Christmas, Easter, and over the summer for weddings), or when an amateur decides to intensify her or his study. Newmark and Lederman[5] carried out research on musicians at a conference. Only two players were professional musicians, and 73% (79 of 109) did not practice regularly, had a rapid increase in playing time, and were predisposed to overuse injuries. Of those affected by the significant increase in practice time, 61% (48 of 79) developed new playing-related complaints, and 34% (27 of 79) experienced problems even without a significant increase in playing time. The authors comment that musicians should view themselves as athletes, be more attentive to their physical limitations, condition their bodies, work at preventing overuse injuries, and implement a graded plan to increase playing time. More recently, Robitaille, Tousignant-Laflamme, and Guay reported that a sudden increase in playing time that was experienced by bowed string instrument players taking part in an intensive music camp related to an increase in playing-related musculoskeletal pain.[5a]

When managing training in elite performers, preventing musculoskeletal overload and overuse-related injuries has an important role. It is estimated that at least 10,000 hours, with an average of 16 years systematic training, is required for musicians to reach their peak performance.[5b] With this in mind, healthy practice techniques that decrease the chance of developing conditions are imperative. Musicians frequently overpractice, and although the whole of the individual's body and mind can be affected, most injuries are seen in the hands and upper limbs. While practicing for long periods of time, the instrumentalist may begin to use suboptimal body mechanics, which most frequently affect the hands and arms.[3] Training errors often include failure to take at least a 5- or 10-minute break every hour of practice. Practice of physically difficult or awkward passages should be limited to short segments of 2 to 3 minutes each within a practice session.

Musicians often think of warm-up sessions being on their instrument, with practicing scales, studies, and easy pieces, but physical warm-up and cool-down sessions before and after playing are desirable with the neck, shoulders, and arms being the areas of focus.[6,7,7a] If the musician plays an instrument that requires him or her to sustain a constrained posture, such as the violin, viola, or flute, these sessions are particularly important. Warming up is a protective strategy that musicians should use to prevent performance-related injury.[8] The upper limbs and neck should be gently moved through range, and most musicians benefit from flexing and extending their hips while maintaining a neutral spine because this encourages movement at the hips rather than at the spine while practicing and performing.[7] For wind players, thoracic rotation can help get the thoracic cage mobile before performance, which can optimize breathing capacity. Much time is spent with patients discussing "graded return to play" programs and practice techniques, which are discussed later in the chapter.

Change in Instrument, Teacher, or Musical Style

Instrument changes can alter the demands on the musicians' body. Some examples of this are:

- Increasing the size of the instrument (e.g., moving from the violin to the viola)
- Increasing the length of the finger board and finger span (e.g., moving from the electric bass to the string bass)
- Increasing the force required for sound production (e.g., moving from the synthesizer to the acoustic piano)
- Decreasing the hand span and finger spacing (e.g., moving from the flute to the piccolo)
- Increasing weight of the instrument and hand span (e.g., moving from the bassoon to the contrabassoon)
- Increasing the requirements for upper extremity reaching (e.g., moving from a standard to an "extended" drum set).

These changes may predispose the musician to injury, especially if combined with an abrupt increase in playing time. The solution is to decrease the intensity of practice when such a change is made and then to gradually build to the desired level of play. A change in teacher or style of music being played may require alterations to technique, which could require an increase in the intensity of practice.

Increased Demands of Repertoire

A change in repertoire can be problematic if the demands of the piece are more than the musician's ability or if the music must be learned in a pressured environment (e.g., getting ready for an audition or if deputizing for another musician at short notice). An increase in playing time with muscular tension and more pressure exerted through the digits can result in pain, weakness, muscle strains, and at times altered sensation.

Pressures in the Workplace

Relationships with coworkers in orchestras, quartets, bands, and jazz ensembles are not always smooth, and this can cause stress, anxiety, depression, sleep disturbances, and increased muscular tension and can result in people having to take time out of the work environment.

Some anxiety related to performance is natural and to be expected because going out on stage requires confidence. A performance may be facilitated by a certain level of anxiety but can be ruined by a debilitating level.[9,9a] A survey of more than 2000 orchestral musicians showed that 27% of musicians reported using beta-blockers at some stage, with particular prevalence among brass players.[10] Second to musculoskeletal conditions, stage fright is the most commonly reported problem, and people affected by this may need counseling and coaching to help manage the condition.[11] Performance anxiety is most likely multifactorial, and the symptoms, management techniques, and treatments are unique for each individual. A recent overview of research literature relating to performance anxiety highlighted that combining behavioral and cognitive therapies is the most promising way of reducing music performance anxiety, and, in turn, improve the quality of the music performance. The authors stated that the most popular approaches for managing physical symptoms included relaxation techniques, deep breathing exercises, yoga, meditation, Alexander technique, and a healthy lifestyle. They went onto say that the techniques most commonly reported to manage cognitive symptoms included cognitive restructuring, setting realistic goals, psychotherapy, and systematic desensitization.[11a] Some musicians find psychotherapy or relaxation techniques useful, while others rely on beta-blockers, smoking, drinking, and the use of nonprescription drugs as a "way of coping" with stress and anxiety.

Lack of or Inconsistent Work

There are often far too many musicians for the number of jobs available, and therefore many people who have dreamt of performance careers may never have these desires fulfilled. Some musicians are fortunate to find themselves in paid employment with potential benefits such as health care, pension, and holiday pay included in their salaries. Other musicians may either choose to or must work in a freelance capacity. Some people like to work this way because it provides them with a variety of work and the ability to choose when and with whom they work. However, others work in this manner because they have not managed to secure a full-time post. This can result in stressful situations of not knowing if they will get work in or too much work coming in all at once. Frequently, freelance musicians are called in at very short notice to cover someone who has taken ill, and therefore they may have the added stress of having to sight read the music and of being "judged" by the people sitting around them.

Quality of Instrument

Leaking keys or valves on a poorly maintained wind instrument can result in increased fingertip pressure required to produce a clean sound. Bridges on string instruments that are too high can increase the force needed to depress the strings. Bows for stringed instruments that need rehairing can cause the musician to press too hard to produce the required sound. A piano in poor condition may require more force to achieve the desired dynamics and subtleties in sound, color, light, and shade. Animal studies have shown that highly repetitive motor movements can contribute to degradation in an area of the brain called the somatosensory cortex.[12] However, if the speed and force of the repetitive motor task is varied and interspersed with regular other activities, the changes in the hand cortical representation and loss of motor control can be minimized.[12] Therefore, it is important to maintain instruments in top playing condition so the energy required to get the desired performance is not excessive.[13] Musicians need to intersperse practice and playing with other activities to decrease the chances of developing medical conditions.[14]

NONMUSICAL ACTIVITIES AND FACTORS

Although musicians may have excellent technique and practice habits, they can sustain trauma from nonmusical activities. These injuries need to be managed within the context of their instrument and the demands placed on their hands. Sports such as volleyball and martial arts are correlated with a particularly high incidence of hand injuries.[15,16] Other hand-intensive activities that may cause problems include knitting, needlepoint, woodworking, fly tying and fishing, skiing, rock climbing, writing, and computer use.

Environmental Factors

Cold temperatures can have several adverse effects on musicians' limbs. There is a decrease in cutaneous sensitivity that may lead to the use of excessive fingertip pressure, an increase in joint fluid viscosity, slowing of nerve conduction velocity, and diminished blood flow because of vasoconstriction. These effects may occur despite increased muscular demands. Players must guard against these effects by whatever means available, including wearing thermal underwear, layering clothes, using fingerless gloves, or placing a heater in the practice studio.

Anatomic Variations

Anatomic variations range from the obvious to the subtle. Obvious ones, such as small stature or hand size, can be a problem when playing large or awkward instruments or certain pieces of music

---

TIPS AND TRICKS FROM THE PROFESSIONALS

Classical Pianist Alisdair Hogarth, Soloist and Artistic Director of The Prince Consort

Physical approach to the piano:

- Practice in a variety of ways: loud, soft, fast, slow, in rhythms, staccato, and legato. Make difficult passages harder so the original feels easy (e.g., turn a one-octave leap into a two-octave leap just for practice).
- Warm up using a balanced program of hand exercises away from the piano (tendon gliding, therapeutic putty, and gentle lengthening exercises).
- Practice technical work every day so that all techniques are visited every couple of days. This improves stamina and reduces technical practice required when learning new pieces.
- Understand that sometimes you can't be "relaxed" when playing; it is important to know when to exert your muscles and when to relax them.
- Lots of physical technical issues can be solved through rethinking fingering and considering redistributing the notes between the hands (e.g., playing a left-hand note with the right hand).

Common pitfalls when playing the piano:

- Finger joints and knuckles collapsing
- Lack of strength and stamina in the hands, arms, and upper body
- Lack of flexibility in the wrist
- Lack of independence and coordination in the fingers (e.g., ability to press keys with certain fingers while holding others down)

Classical Guitarist Mark Ashford, Head of Guitar Royal Birmingham Conservatoire

It is important that guitarists do not fixate on what is happening in the small joints of their fingers but that they acknowledge and really focus on their posture and use of the larger muscle groups. It could be viewed that these are the "engine" that drive all the smaller cogs.

Incredibly slow practice thinking of the points below is vital to emulate this on the concert platform.

1. Breathing through the music
2. Letting go in the shoulders especially
3. Feeling that your legs and feet are completely grounded
4. Weight of the arms are in complete support of the hands and fingers
5. Fingers are then free to move as they will. A feeling of effortlessness as the right-hand fingers move through the strings and the left-hand fingers push with just the right amount of pressure on the fretboard. This will ensure a clean sound can be produced safe in the knowledge that all the previous points are well established.

Jazz Saxophonist Adam Waldmann, Kairos 4Tet Bandleader and Composer

1. Make sure there aren't any embouchure issues that can initiate tension at the beginning of the chain such as biting or too much pressure on the reed.
2. Try to play with "neutral" wrists (no or as little flexion) whenever possible. Try to eradicate any "holding" behaviors such as hunched or raised shoulders and keep your chin pointing forward rather than up or down.
3. Make your stance flexible and fluid, evenly distributing your weight rather than focusing your weight on one leg or point. Keep your knees bent, not locked.
4. Work on core strength as well as wrist, arm, and finger strength. Include stretching in your daily routine and seek assistance for any physical issues as soon as they arise.

(Continued)

Jazz Saxophonist Adam Waldmann, Kairos 4Tet Bandleader and Composer—cont'd

5. Try a neck strap that takes the weight off the neck such as a Sax Holder or Marmaduke.
6. Make it your primary objective to listen intently while giving any performance, perhaps focusing attention on a specific instrument in the band. This can help take the focus away from you, which can relieve personal tension and performance anxiety and let you play "in the moment," which often leads to a much better and more relaxed music making.

Classical Violinist Jack Liebeck, Soloist and Professor of Violin at The Royal Academy of Music, London

1. Look for the most natural approach. Hold the violin in a neutral position with the chin gently resting on the chin rest, not clamping it.
2. Play with relaxed neutral joints because this allows the muscles and tendons to move in multiple directions. Problems can occur when muscles or tendons are at their limit because this can create tension and strain, which destroys the sound. The bowing arm's elbow should not be too high, and gravity rather than muscle power should create the weight with the bow. The elbow is merely a facilitation joint that connects the hand to the body, and it should not be used to force the bow down on to the string. A relaxed and flexible neck is essential rather than clamping down on the chin rest, and the left shoulder should not grip onto the shoulder rest. Practicing while rocking the head from side to side is useful to enable this flexibility.
3. Flexibility from the fingertips to the shoulder is an important aspect of the left hand. Movements into higher left-hand positions that are robotic, taking place at only one speed, are not only unmusical but can also induce tension. Shifts on the finger board should be viewed as a gentle breath rather than a sudden gulp of air.
4. If pain is felt when playing, the situation needs to be evaluated. Is it caused by overextension, playing for too many hours, or tension?
5. Listen to your body is the number one rule.

Classical Flautist Katie Bedford, Flautist and Professor of Flute at the Royal College of Music, London

As flautists, we are at risk of various problems arising from tension of the upper back, arms, and neck caused by the arms being raised and head turned for long periods of time. It is important to achieve an ease of sound and technique while also keeping the neck and shoulders free of tension.

Practice Tips

- Try to always warm up your upper body with some gentle stretching or yoga before and after playing. I have found this incredibly important to improve awareness of posture and to avoid pain when playing for an extended period.
- When lifting the flute to play, start by holding it as you would a clarinet and ensure you do not move your head to the flute. Instead, while turning your head to the left (feel you are lifting up as you turn, like you are unscrewing a bottle top), lift your arms and bring the flute to you while maintaining enough space between your arms so as not to restrict your breathing.
- Slow practice is essential to avoid unnecessary tension, especially with technically demanding passages. It is important to maintain a good technique by the regular practice of scales and studies to avoid the need for excessive repetition of passages that put strain on the wrists, which then also leads to tension and pain elsewhere.
- Try to keep the wrists as neutral as possible without flexing the hands or fingers and maintain a slight bend in all your fingers to avoid "locking" the joints.
- It is also important to practice without the instrument because there is a lot that can be done by listening and studying the score, which again avoids unnecessary repetition and limits the time spent in the same position.

Classical Flautist Katie Bedford, Flautist and Professor of Flute at the Royal College of Music, London —cont'd

Common Pitfalls

- Shoulder and neck pain from raising the shoulders up and shortening the neck by pushing the chin forward to play
- Wrist pain arising from tightly gripping the instrument, especially when playing technically demanding passages. Try to maintain a relaxed hold and think about lifting the fingers up rather than pressing down. This is particularly important with trills and other fast passages.
- Tension in the face and jaw; forming a tight embouchure with the flute pressed hard against the lip, which then leads to a tight and restrictive sound and possibly increased tension in the upper body.
- Shallow breathing by "gasping" for the air and lifting the shoulders and chest. It is essential to regularly practice long, straight notes and simple melodies with and without vibrato to achieve a good support of the sound with the diaphragm and breathing.
- Slouching while sitting or standing to play. Angle your feet or chair when sitting or standing to the right so that you don't compromise your posture and to ensure you always feel grounded.

composed by persons with unusually large or flexible hands, such as Paganini or Rachmaninoff. An example of this can be seen in Figure 117.2.

A troublesome subtle variation is positive ulnar variance,[17] which can cause an impingement syndrome when playing instruments that require ulnar deviation—for example, certain fingers in the piano, harp, matched grip with the drums, the left hand in the trumpet, and at the end of the up-bow passage in stringed instruments. For musicians playing these instruments, accessory tendons in the first dorsal extensor compartment can predispose them to de Quervain's disease.

Tendinous interconnections between the flexor digitorum superficialis of the fourth and fifth fingers can lead to severe problems if they occur in the left hand of violinists or violists (Fig. 117.3).[18] Cervical ribs may cause problems on the left side in string bass players or musicians who are required to flex or rotate the neck while playing instruments-such as the viola, violin, or flute.

CLEAR-CUT PATHOLOGIES AFFECTING MUSICIANS

Tendinopathies

Tendinopathies are a common degenerative rather than inflammatory condition. Histopathologic surgical specimens show a lack of inflammation.[19–22] The term *tendinopathy* should be used rather than *tendinitis*, *tendinosis*, *paratendinitis*, or *tenosynovitis* because this term refers to the primary symptomatic tendon disorder and has no implication of pathology.[23] The cause of tendinopathy is unclear, but three broad ideas cover possible methods of development:

- **Mechanical:** Perhaps the tendon has been overloaded, causing damage to the extracellular matrix, which in turn has caused a failed healing response in the tenocytes.[24,25]
- **Vascular:** Tissue hypoxia may decrease the viability of tendon cells, and as the tendon reperfuses, oxygen free radicals are released, possibly leading to a pathologic tendon. Free radicals are associated with aging,[26,27] neurodegenerative diseases,[28] chondral and meniscal lesions,[29] and tendon degeneration in rats.[30] If this hypothesis is valid, then the possibility of treating tendinopathies with antioxidants is raised.

(Continued)

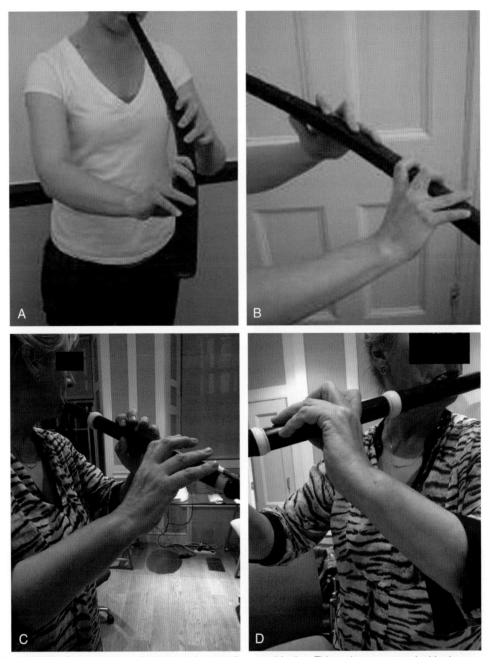

Fig. 117.2 A, Cornetto player displaying wrist and elbow positioning. This patient presented with ulnar nerve symptoms and intrinsic muscle strain in both hands, probably caused by long-term awkward positioning of both upper extremities due to constraints of the instrument. **B,** Small hand size with limited finger span, resulting in intrinsic muscle strain. **C,** A baroque flute with few keys may mean that unusual finger and wrist positions are unavoidable. The right wrist has to extend, and the ring and small fingers have to assume an intrinsic-minus position to cover the open holes and operate the key. **D** Left wrist hyperextension and radial deviation are hard to avoid while playing. (A and B, K Butler 2009; C and D, K Butler 2018.)

- **Neural:** There may be a neurogenic origin to diseased tissues because mast cell degranulation, and release of substance P have been implicated and found in degenerative tendons.

Butler and Sandford[23] outline the intrinsic and extrinsic factors that can lead to the development of tendinopathies.

Intrinsic factors include:

- **Age:** Tendinopathies mostly affect people older than 30 years of age.
- **Nutrition:** Tendinopathies predominately affect people with poorer nutrition levels.

- **Anatomic variations:** Tendinopathies affect people with extra-long tendons or individuals who have two tendons in one tendon sheath.
- **Joint laxity:** Hypermobile patients are more frequently affected.
- **Gender:** Women are more often affected than men.
- **Systemic disease:** Patients with diabetes are more commonly affected.

Extrinsic factors include:

- **Occupation:** if you work in confined spaces or perform repetitive movements

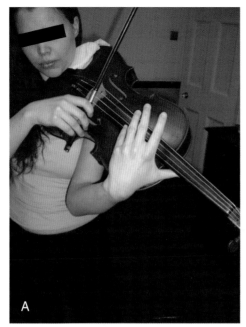
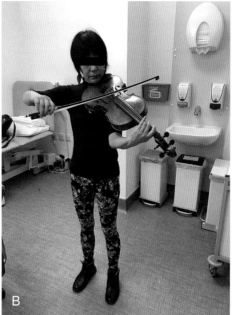
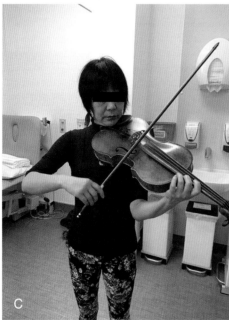

Fig. 117.3 A, The wrist flexion and forearm hypersupination required to reach the higher positions on the viola. **B** and **C,** The size of the instrument relative to the individual can influence the ease of playing and the possibility of the musician being predisposed to developing medical symptoms. (A, K Butler 2009; B and C, K Butler 2018.)

- **Sports or hobbies:** if forceful repetitive movements or sustained postures are required[31]
- **Physical load:** if heavy loads are required to be repeatedly moved
- **Equipment:** if the equipment is not well maintained, of poor quality, or inappropriate to the individual
- **Rapid increase in workload:** if the workload is intense, fast paced, and pressurized
- **Environment:** if the environment is too cold, too hot, cramped, or pressured

De Quervain's Disease

Most commonly, pianists, clarinetists, and oboists develop de Quervain's disease, which is a stenosing tenovaginitis of the abductor pollicis longus and extensor pollicis brevis.[32] These two muscles commonly share a tendon sheath, and although the tendons are entirely normal and no inflammation is present, a cross section of the fibro-osseous channel shows diminishment of the channel and fibrotic thickening of the extensor retinaculum.[20] Clinical examination shows swelling, thickening, and pain of the first dorsal compartment. There is pain on resisted thumb extension and abduction, weak pinch grip,[33] and the Finkelstein test is positive. There are no reliability studies for this test, but it is commonly used in the clinical setting.[34] Differential diagnosis for de Quervain's disease includes first carpometacarpal (CMC) joint osteoarthritis, scaphoid fracture, intersection syndrome, superficial radial nerve irritation (Wartenberg's syndrome), and central referral.[23]

Trigger Finger and Trigger Thumb

Triggering of the right thumb can occur in soprano saxophone players and upper stringed instrumentalists (violin and viola). Thickening of the flexor tendons, nodule formation, or stenosing of the flexor tendons may hinder the tendon to pass smoothly through the pulley system, resulting in a classic "trigger finger or thumb." Instrumentalists often report that they can flex their fingers into the palm but that they have trouble extending their fingers from this position. Often patients report a snapping or popping sensation as they try to overcome the resistance into extension.

A nodule may be felt on the tendon in one or more fingers and often a nonsteroidal antiinflammatory drug (NSAID), rest, wearing a night orthosis, and ultrasound therapy can reduce the tendon and synovial swelling or thickening and result in a full recovery. Sometimes steroid injections are required, and if these are successful and the patient presents with further triggering, then further injections are given, beyond the point at which one would normally resort to surgery in nonmusicians.[35] If surgery is required, then the principle concern is bow stringing of the released tendons, and the surgical approach needs to be carefully considered.

Other tendinopathies include lateral and medial elbow pain and carpal tunnel syndrome (CTS), which are discussed later in the chapter.

Treatment Principles for Tendinopathies

Patient education, ergonomic advice, activity modification, biomechanical considerations, electrotherapy, acupuncture, cooling, strengthening, muscle-lengthening exercises, myofascial release, trigger point therapy, orthotic positioning, administration of NSAIDs, local steroid injections, and surgery are all possible treatments for symptomatic patients. Activity analysis is imperative when assessing and treating musicians.

Patient Education

The patient with a tendinopathy or muscular strain who rests just enough to keep playing but manifests lingering symptoms can develop a chronic condition that flares up repeatedly until adequate rehabilitation is received. Requirements for adequate rehabilitation include full range of motion (ROM), minimum pain on palpation of the muscle bellies or tendon origins and insertions, reasonable normative maximum grip strength, good endurance rates, and high levels of coordination. The musician must be aware that the length of the healing process is in months rather than weeks and that the key to getting better and staying better is to modify the way the task is being performed because this may be predisposing to the condition.

Activity Modification and Ergonomic and Biomechanical Considerations

Some awkward postures are probably unavoidable, but some are related to poor instrumental ergonomics and technical difficulties.[36] Marked wrist deviation[37] and excessive fingertip loading can lead to increased tissue stresses[38] and elevated pressures in the carpal tunnel.[39,40] The use of excessive force, whether it be gripping drumsticks, pressing down on strings or keys, or clenching a violin between neck and shoulder, increases the risk of soft tissue injury.[41] Carrying heavier instruments can strain the hands, neck, and back. An accordion can weigh up to 16 kg and is usually carried by hand (Fig. 117.4). Using wheels or backpack-style straps on cases can effectively reduce the carrying load placed on the limbs (Fig. 117.5). Instruments such as the harp and drum kit usually require transportation in a car.

Many adaptive devices and cases have been specifically designed to decrease joint strain, distribute the load of the instrument, or protect instruments and yet be lighter and more ergonomically sound. Some examples of such supports are shown in Figure 117.6.

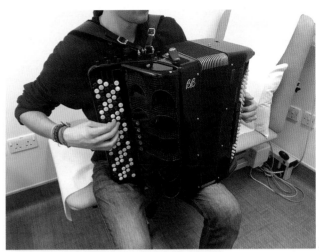

Fig. 117.4 An accordion can weigh up to 16 kg and is either carried by hand or in a wheeled case. (K Butler 2018.)

Computer Use

Computer use is ubiquitous, often ergonomically unsound, and frequently intense, especially among students. The musician must be counseled to minimize computer use, especially during periods of intensified musical activity. Optimal ergonomic positioning while at the computer should be enforced for all patients, and keyboard shortcuts should be used whenever possible to decrease the total number of keystrokes made during a session at the computer.

Here are some general concepts that are readily accepted when using a computer keyboard and mouse:

- Keep the wrists neutral.
- Don't rest the wrists while typing.
- Move the whole arm while keying.
- Avoid stretching the fingers to reach keys that are far away.
- Keep fingers curved and relax the thumb.
- Use a light touch.
- Keep fingernails short.[42]
- Avoid double clicking as much as possible when using a mouse.

Myofascial Pain and Stretching

Myofascial pain may be caused by overactivity of motor endplates in muscles, which results in distinct referral patterns of pain. For example, a tender point or trigger point in the brachioradialis can refer to the elbow, thumb, and dorsum of the hand. Treatment can include trigger pointing, soft tissue massage, muscle-lengthening exercises, cooling using a cold pack, acupuncture, home acupressure, and activity modification (e.g., how to carry items, sleeping positions that assist in decreasing symptoms). See Figure 117.7 for examples of possible forearm flexor and extensor muscle-lengthening exercises.[43,44]

These muscle-lengthening exercises can be useful for most musicians; however, it is important that the joints are not taken into an overextended or hypermobile range. While doing these exercises, the elbow must be slightly flexed, the wrist not taken beyond a 85-degree angle, and there must never be any force exerted through the fingers. The idea of "lengthening" rather than "stretching" is useful because the exercises can be used initially as a treatment for tight forearm flexor and extensor muscles, but in time, they can be used prophylactically and as a warm-up and cool-down before and after playing. It is important to discuss with the musician that overstretching can be as harmful as not stretching at all. Frequently, musicians are seen forcing their joints into extreme positions before a concert or during a rehearsal, especially if they are feeling some symptoms. Regular gentle lengthening of forearm

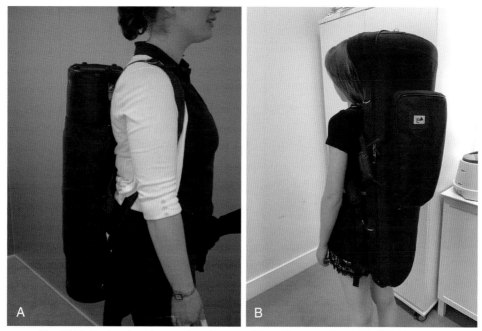

Fig. 117.5 Backpack-style case for a bassoon (**A**) and for a trombone (**B**). (K Butler 2018.)

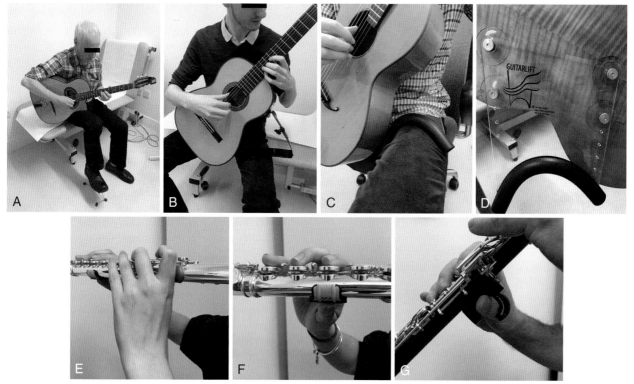

Fig. 117.6 Rather than using a footstool (**A**), an Ergoplay support (**B**) can be attached to the classical guitar, enabling both feet to be kept on the floor and the use of a more neutral pelvis, spine, and optimal arm placement. The Guitarlift (**C** and **D**) attaches securely to the instrument and can be inclined to hold the guitar slightly to the left rather than at the center of the body, which can aide in reducing back pain. Flute gels (**E**) or Bo-Pep finger supports can assist in maintaining the left index finger metacarpophalangeal joint in a more neutral position and decreasing pressure on the radial digital nerve. A Thumbport (**F**) can facilitate and enhance a balanced right hand position by providing additional support, especially if the flautist has a short or hypermobile thumb, A Ton Kooiman thumb rest (**G**) can be used for clarinet or oboe players to decrease the load placed through the right thumb. (K Butler 2018.)

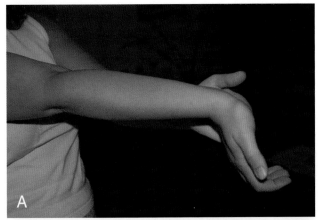

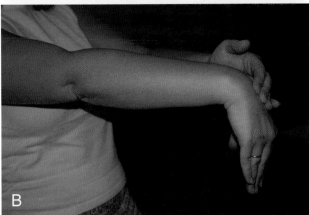

Fig. 117.7 A, Forearm flexor lengthening exercise. With the elbow slightly bent inwards to about 5 degrees and your palm facing upward, gently move your wrist backward using your own muscle strength until you feel a lengthening. Then, with the other hand, gently pull the wrist farther backward, but not more than 85 degrees, by placing light pressure in the palm. Hold this position for 30 seconds. **B,** Forearm extensor lengthening exercise. With the elbow slightly bent inward to about 5 degrees and your palm facing downward, gently bring the wrist and fingers in toward yourself using your own muscle strength until you feel a lengthening. Then with the other hand, lightly push on the back of your wrist, bringing it farther toward you. Hold this position for 30 seconds. (K Butler 2009.)

muscles can assist in preventing symptoms from occurring or decrease symptoms if they have been triggered by a particularly challenging rehearsal or performance.

HYPERMOBILITY

Musicians seem to have a higher incidence of hypermobility than the population at large.[2] Although some exhibit a "full-blown" benign hypermobility syndrome (Marfan's or Ehlers-Danlos syndrome), it is more frequent that the laxity is limited to the upper limb (shoulder, elbow, wrist, thumb, and fingers) and sometimes only one joint (e.g., the metacarpophalangeal [MCP] joint of the thumb). A higher incidence of hand and arm pain can often be associated with having significant finger joint laxity.[45] Proximal interphalangeal joints are classified as hypermobile if there is 15 degrees or more extension beyond 180 degrees.[46] Hypermobility has a strong genetic link, so it is important to ask about other family members who may be affected while taking the medical history. However, playing a musical instruments may aggravate the condition.

Increased range can be very advantageous to musicians such as string players and pianists. Indeed, some very virtuosic players such as Paganini

and Liszt were hypermobile. Larson and colleagues[47] studied 660 musicians and concluded that hypermobility in the fingers, thumb, and wrist may be an asset when playing repetitive motions on instruments such as the flute, violin, or piano. This author went on to say, however, that hypermobility may be a limitation when the joints are required to be stabilizers—for example, knee joints for timpanists who stand to play. Larson and coworkers[48] showed that musculoskeletal symptoms associated with practice and performance may be caused by the lack of hypermobility of some joints involved in intensive repetitive movement. Participants who played instruments requiring repetitive motion reported fewer symptoms in their joints if they were hypermobile.

Jull[49] states that for many musicians, hypermobility is an impediment. The weakness in muscle power and increased vulnerability of the associated joint can lead to an increased propensity for these musicians to develop injuries or chronic "overuse" syndromes and can lead to premature OA.[11] There is evidence to suggest that hypermobile joints have a decreased sensitivity to proprioception,[2,49a] so musicians may exert more force than necessary on keys or strings, thus increasing the possibility of chronic strain.

Hypermobility and the Role of Hand Therapy

Patients are routinely assessed for hypermobility in the initial examination using the nine-point Beighton score,[49a,50,50a] which involves the following features. If 4 or more points are reached, the participant is said to have generalized hypermobility[51,52]:

- Dorsal flexion of the fifth MCP joint at 90 degrees: 1 point for each hand (2 possible points)
- Ability to appose the thumb to the radial aspect of the forearm: 1 point for each thumb (2 possible points)
- Hyperextension of the elbow beyond 10 degrees: 1 point for each elbow (2 possible points)
- Hyperextension of the knee by 10 degrees: 1 point for each knee (2 possible points)
- The ability to put the hands flat on the floor with the knees extended when bending forward: 1 possible point

Assessment on the instrument is imperative because hyperlaxity may be more evident while the musician is playing (Fig. 117.8). Brandfonbrener[53] consistently found a correlation between musicians with hand and arm pain and the presence of joint laxity. Whether the hypermobility is the primary cause of symptoms, joint protection advice is always provided. Specific exercises can be helpful, and many adaptive ways of performing tasks can be incorporated into the patient's lifestyle.

Advice and adaptive task performance can prevent injuries from developing and ensure that performers are more able to have a fulfilling and less painful time, especially when playing their instruments. Patients can benefit greatly from a rehabilitation program to improve muscle power.[11,54] The stability-strengthening exercises encourage co-contraction of the muscles surrounding a joint. Isometric strengthening and proprioception exercises both on and away from the instrument can assist in achieving this goal (Fig. 117.9).

When exercising away from the instrument, initial stability exercises include isometric muscle contraction in a pain-free range while wearing a support. Later in the rehabilitation phase, exercises can be progressed to include concentric and eccentric strengthening. Isometric strengthening exercises on the instrument can be a useful tool (e.g., exercises in the neutral joint position while holding the bow, string instrument, or clarinet).[55] Proprioception exercises and retraining such as tapping exercises and weight-bearing exercises in a neutral position should be performed first with the eyes open and then with the eyes closed. After months of performing strengthening exercises, symptoms can improve, and it is common to detect an improvement in ligament

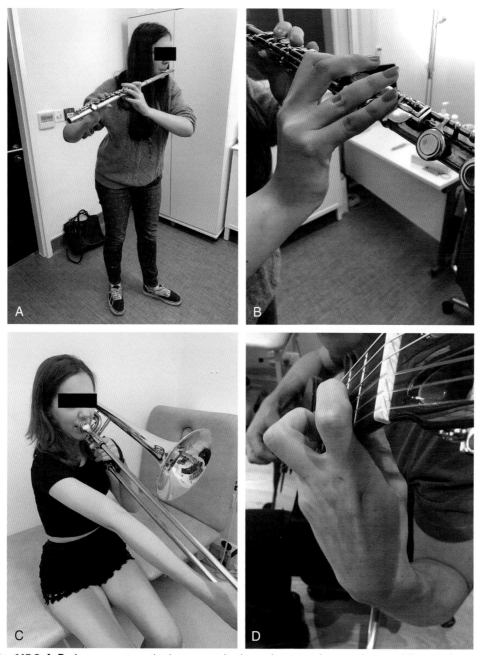

Fig. 117.8 A–D, Assessment on the instrument is always important because hypermobility may become more evident. The whole body has to be taken into consideration when assessing a hypermobile musician because the knees, spine, pelvis, and neck can all have an impact on the patient's ability to function in daily life as well as the ability to play their instrument. (K Butler 2018.)

tautness with joint translation testing. It is encouraging for the musician to be told that biomechanical dysfunction can be improved.

The intrinsic and extrinsic muscles of the hand are frequently stressed to compensate for joint instability.[53] Strengthening exercises using therapeutic putty can be useful when treating hypermobile patients. It is important that the patient is aware that it is the positioning and accuracy of movements through and against the resistance of the putty and not the "brute force" that is being exerted while doing these exercises. Many people can have flareups of their symptoms up by being overvigorous or doing these exercises incorrectly. The goals are to retrain movement patterns and strengthen the muscles that support the joints in a functional position for specific instruments; therefore, putty exercise programs can vary according to the instrument that

the individual plays. Treatment must focus on stability-strengthening exercises, temporary supports, sensorimotor retraining to improve proprioception, and patient education regarding good practice habits and healthy joint use.[55] Temporary supports to maintain the joint in a neutral position are useful for playing, and the patient should be gradually weaned as strength increases and symptoms decrease. Supports can include light thermoplastic orthoses, neoprene wraps, wrist braces, Lycra finger sleeves, or a Coban wrap. It may take many months for stability strength to improve enough for a modified playing schedule to be instigated. Temporary orthoses or wraps may need to be worn for some time. Exercises must be continued until enough muscle strength has been gained or orthotic use continued until a neutral joint position can be maintained.

Stability Exercises
for the hand and wrist

These exercises do not involve any movement but are static and resisted.
Support the length of your forearm on a table.
You should feel resistance rather than pain, and only use 10% pressure initially
and then gently increase the pressure to a maximum of 50% effort.
Hold each position for 5–10 seconds, increase as tolerated up to 30 seconds.

Forward bending

With the palm of your hand
facing down and your hand
forming a light fist, push your
forearm into the table and feel
the resistance right up into
your upper arm.

Repeat ___ times ___ per day

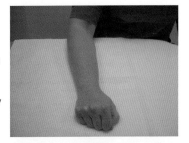

Backward bending

With your affected wrist in a
neutral plane and whilst
forming a light fist, place your
unaffected hand over the
back of the wrist and resist
the backwards movement.

Repeat ___ times ___ per day

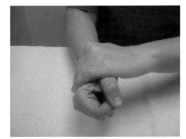

Side to side

Rest your hand and forearm
with the little finger in contact
with the table. Make a light fist
and push the side of your
forearm into the table.

Repeat ___ times ___ per day

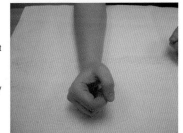

Rest your hand and forearm
with the palm facing the table
and make a light fist. Resist
movement toward the thumb
with the palm of the other
hand.

Repeat ___ times ___ per day

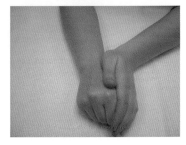

Turning

Rest your hand and forearm
with the little finger in contact
with the table, resist against
your affected side using your
other hand. Place your
unaffected hand over the base
of your wrist. Imagine you are
turning your palm down
toward the table and resist this
movement without moving the
wrist.

Repeat ___ times ___ per day

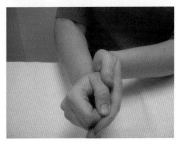

Fig. 117.9 Patient handout showing stability exercises for the wrist and forearm. (K Butler 2009.)

TASK-SPECIFIC DYSTONIA

Dystonia is a syndrome characterized by involuntary prolonged muscle contractions that can lead to sustained twisting postures.[56–58] Three criteria are used in classifying this syndrome: age of onset, cause, and distribution of symptoms.[59,60] Onset before 28 years of age is classified as early and after this age is classified as late-onset dystonia. Cause can be divided into idiopathic (no obvious effects on the brain) or symptomatic (often the basal ganglia are affected, resulting in more generalized symptoms).[61] Distribution of symptom manifestation can be:

- **General:** Symptoms manifest in all extremities, including the trunk.
- **Hemi:** Symptoms are focused on one side of the body.
- **Segmental:** A segment of the body is affected.
- **Focal:** A single body part is affected.

Any part of the body can be affected by focal dystonia, including the neck, eyelids, vocal cords, or hand.[62,63,63a]

Task-specific dystonia (TSD) is a subtype of dystonia in which an abnormal posture occurs during the performance of a specific, usually highly skilled task, such as playing a musical instrument (musician's dystonia) or writing (writer's dystonia) (Fig. 117.10). It can be very disabling, especially for professional musicians, with up to 62% of affected patients unable to continue their performance careers.[64]

The pathophysiology and etiology of TSD are not completely understood. It is thought likely to be related to sensorimotor system alterations potentially caused by interaction between the continued repetitive practice of a highly skilled movement in the face of imposed intrinsic (e.g., fatigue or injury) or extrinsic (alterations in technique or mechanical demands) changes. Correspondingly there is experimental evidence for both motor and sensory dysfunction (e.g., altered inhibition within motor cortical areas and alterations in the delineation of the sensory homunculus representing the affected part) as well as a wider cognitive context, which includes an abnormal attentional focus during performance, anxiety, and perfectionism.[65] An influence of genetic risk factors is suggested by the preponderance for males to develop task-specific dystonia (4M:1F in musicians dystonia),[65a] and a positive family history of task-specific dystonia in a proportion of cases.[65b] A multicenter genome-wide study has identified arlysulfatase G as a locus which may confer risk for teas-specific dystonia of the hand.[65c]

Existing medical treatments such as oral medications (e.g., trihexyphenidyl) and botulinum toxin injections are limited in their long-term efficacy.[66,87] There is an increasing interest in using specific rehabilitative techniques, which include sensory reeducation,[67–71] sensory motor retuning,[72–76] mirror therapy,[77] and slow down exercise treatment.[78] While controlled studies of each of these individual techniques are not available a recent study indicated that there is moderate evidence

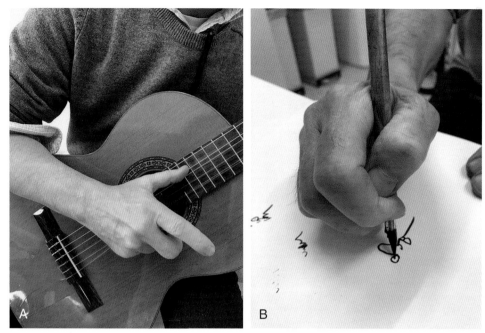

Fig. 117.10 Task-specific dystonia has two main forms: musician's dystonia (**A**) and writer's dystonia (**B**). (K Butler 2018.)

to support the effectiveness of neuromuscular re-education programs on reducing abnormal movements for the musician affected by task specific dystonia. However, further research is required to evaluate the effectiveness of such programs using reliable and valid outcome measures and study methods which provide a higher level of evidence.[78a]

Task-Specific Dystonia in Musicians

Task-specific dystonia in musicians is a painless focal isolated dystonia that tends to be task-specific and of late onset. Symptoms can include lack of coordination, cramping, and tremor[79,79a] and tend to be specific to the individual and related to the instrument played rather than hand dominance.

Patients can respond to sensory tricks and, if they do, this is usually a good indicator of how successful hand therapy will be. *Sensory tricks* can be used to "fool" the brain and give a "nonsense" feedback loop that breaks the fixed link in the sensory motor loop for a short period.[62,63a,80,81] Often the novelty is only effective for a short time until the brain recalibrates to an automatic pattern, which is the dystonic one. Coban, Blu-Tack, latex gloves, and orthoses can all be used as sensory tricks (Fig. 117.11).

The estimated prevalence of TSD among professional musicians is about 2% to 10%,[82–84] which is higher than that of writer's cramp (0.1%) in the general population.[85] TSD is overwhelmingly more common in classical rather than pop, rock, or jazz musicians. The high percentage of TSD in this population reflects the specific demands of continuous repetition made by classical music.

Treatments

At present, there is no cure for dystonia, and many of the treatments available have significant limitations. Current treatments include oral medication such as trihexyphenidyl, botulinum toxin injections, surgery, rehabilitative therapies, and supportive approaches. Butler and Rosenkranz[14,86] published two papers that clearly outline many of the treatments that have been researched and undergone clinical trials.

The rehabilitative approaches include:
- **Sensory reeducation:** focuses on sensory discrimination.
- **Sensory–motor retuning (SMR):** combines both the sensory and motor aspects of TSD.

- **Multidisciplinary approach:** includes hand therapy and combines the sensory and motor aspects of TSD.
- **Limb immobilization:** interrupts motor performance and decreases afferents from the limb.
- **Supportive approaches:** can include assistive devices, instrument modification, Alexander technique, and psychotherapy. There is a strong clinical impression within a very experienced group of treating practitioners that some personality abnormalities and a strong psychological trait is correlated with patients who develop TSD.

The mechanisms by which TSD develops in musicians need to be identified. Treatment must assist in reestablishing sensory–motor control. A comprehensive therapy program with an aggressive sensory reeducation element can improve sensory processing and motor control of the hand. SMR is of value for treating TSD in pianists and guitarists. Scientific research investigating preventive measures and appropriate treatments for TSD is essential. Collaboration and a multidisciplinary team approach to prevention, treatment, and research are imperative and will be of benefit to all.

A classical guitarist when diagnosed with TSD said:

Playing the guitar had been the most important part of my life but also my main source of income. It was my job, my career and my chosen way to communicate with others.
I felt devastated by the idea of having to consider giving it up.

A recent feasibility study by Butler and coworkers[87] assessed the utility and compliance of several subjective and objective outcome measures in patients going through a unique mixed rehabilitative approach combining several specific and general therapies. Fifteen patients were recruited (musician's dystonia = 8, writer's dystonia = 7) with complete data sets collected for twelve people. The program comprised of a maximum of six treatment sessions plus daily home exercises over a 6-month period. Baseline, 3- and 6-month medical reviews were undertaken with a number of self-report measures taken at each of these sessions. Task performance was video-recorded at baseline and 6 months and interviews exploring participant experiences of the intervention were carried out at 6 months. The sensory motor rehabilitation program that was designed and implemented

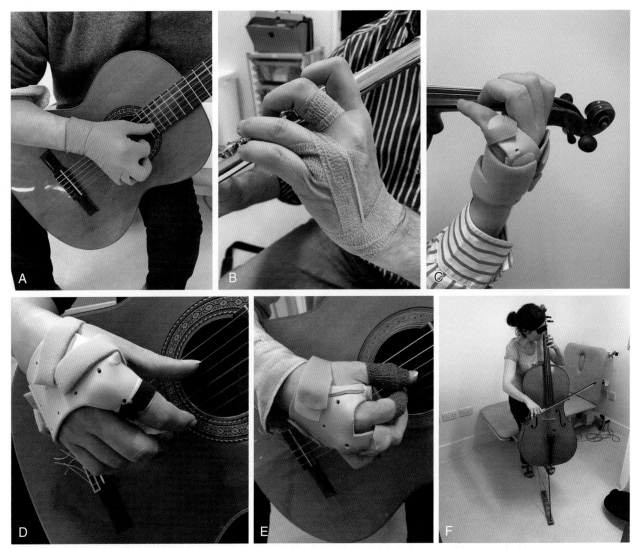

Fig. 117.11 Sensory tricks can include playing with a latex glove on (**A**), Coban tape (**B**), dorsal blocking orthoses to limit hyperextension of the compensatory finger (**C**), a combination of Coban and splint (**D** and **E**), or changing the relationship of the body to the instrument (**F**) (e.g., this cellist is standing to play, and the altered playing position means the body is being used as a sensory trick). (K Butler 2018.)

included sensory re-education, sensory motor returning, mirror therapy, slow-down exercise treatment, soft tissue massage, ultrasound therapy, forearm muscle stretches, shoulder exercises, and hand strengthening exercises (putty.) The study showed that this rehabilitation intervention is feasible to deliver and acceptable, with high retention and adherence, and supports the development of controlled trials in this area. Qualitative interviews showed three main themes: the negative impact of dystonia, individuals respond differently to treatment techniques, and persistence and time are required when undertaking rehabilitation.

Some poignant quotes from the study reflect the marked impact the condition can have on people's emotional well-being and the negative impact on their professional lives:

I feel I have a hole inside me. I am completely gutted that I can't play the piano like I used to.

My playing is getting worse and my hand movements "do not flow" and my repertoire is limited and I have "no enjoyment when playing now."

I cannot perform any more or demonstrate in lessons. Playing is hard work, it knocks me out, and I do not loosen up as the time progresses—it becomes painful.

A further study by Butler and asssociates[88] showed that people affected with musician's dystonia (MD) reported a change in technique, slow practice, and focusing on using larger movements when playing were the three most effective treatments for managing and treating their symptoms with orthoses, sensory tricks, and sensory reeducation also being noted as beneficial.

WORK-RELATED UPPER LIMB DISORDER OR NONSPECIFIC ARM PAIN

The term *overuse injury* has been defined as a condition that occurs when any biologic tissue is stressed beyond its physical or physiologic limits. The common presenting complaints are pain and stiffness but may also include swelling and diminished coordination and function. Some histologic studies have revealed pathologic but nonspecific changes.[89] There is no clear evidence that musicians suffer true overuse with tissue damage, as seen in athletes, and the experimental evidence used to argue this point in musicians is not strong.[90,90a]

The clinician needs to be careful to assess the patient thoroughly with respect to diagnosis and then to review for nonspecific arm pains. The diagnosis of *nonspecific arm pain* should not be a blanket term for patients for whom no specific diagnosis can be made.

Classification and Grading

Work-related upper limb disorders (WRULDs), overuse, or nonspecific arm pain injuries can be classified as acute or chronic. An acute injury follows a specific incident, such as overpracticing a difficult passage. The musician may experience pain or stiffness during practice or the following day. A chronic injury usually has a more insidious onset. The limb becomes progressively more painful and dysfunctional over time.

Fry[91] has developed a five-category grading system:

Grade 1: pain at one site only while playing

Grade 2: pain at multiple sites

Grade 3: pain that persists well beyond the time that the musician stops playing

Grade 4: all the above plus activities of daily living (ADLs) begin to cause pain

Grade 5: all the above plus all daily activities that engage the affected body part cause pain

Most injuries fall into categories 1 to 3.[92] The earlier the symptoms are recognized and treated, the sooner the recovery is likely to occur and the more complete it is likely to be. Unfortunately, the prevalence of injury can be quite high, especially among professional orchestra members. A survey of more than 2000 orchestra members revealed 76% of those surveyed had significant physical problems.[10] Subtle loss of motor control or technique may be one of the earliest signs of overuse.[93]

Treatments for Nonspecific Arm Pain

The cornerstone of treatment is pain avoidance, also known as relative rest.[94] Other treatment modalities will usually be inadequate unless relative rest is strictly observed. It is important to emphasize to musicians that they must *not* avoid playing altogether but equally that they must *not* play for long periods of time. The patient needs to become highly aware of pain-producing activities, whether they are musical, nonvocational, or ADL. The patient must learn to avoid, or at least modify, activities to minimize the number of daily painful "twinges."

Hand therapists can assist in giving advice about joint protection and energy conservation techniques. These principles are similar to those used for patients with osteoarthritis and rheumatoid arthritis (Box 117.1).

Principles of joint protection and energy conservation can be used to preserve the patient's joints and reduce pain levels. It is a "style of life" that after it has been learned becomes second nature. It is not designed to make life complicated but rather to encourage independence. These principles are also very important to implement if the patient is hypermobile.

All previous treatment methods mentioned in this chapter apply to musicians who experience nonspecific arm pain. The playing position, the "interface" (relationship between the instrument and the musician's body and vice versa), and general levels of fatigue all need to be assessed and relevant modifications made because they all affect symptoms and healing.

NERVE ENTRAPMENT SYNDROMES

Digital Compression Neuropathies

Digital compression neuropathies occur when the digital nerves are compressed between the hard instrument and the phalanx. Many different instrumentalists can present with these symptoms:

- Percussionists, especially players of double-mallet instruments, such as the xylophone, vibraphone, and marimbas
- The index fingers of those using traditional drumsticks
- The left index finger of flutists
- The right index finger of violin, viola, and cello players, from pronation forces against the bow stick

- The right thumb tip in cellists where it presses against the "heel" or "frog" of the bow (i.e., the end part of a stringed instruments bow that encloses the mechanism responsible for tightening and holding the bow hair ribbon)

Coban wrapped around the bow, stick, or the finger works especially well to protect the digital nerve. The use of a foam pad, Lycra, or silicon sleeve such as Silipos or an orthosis can also assist with not only decreasing the symptoms but also retraining proprioception while playing the instrument.

It may be necessary, depending on the severity of the condition, to reduce playing time. Misdiagnosis is common, and clinicians can often be misled by the presence of index finger paresthesia into considering CTS. Electrodiagnostic testing can be useful to clarify the diagnosis, especially with "double-crush" syndromes, in which the patient may have multiple sites of entrapment, such as the cervical, brachial, or carpal regions. This highlights the importance of observing the musician playing the instrument. When practical and possible, musicians are always assessed with their instrument, and frequently, treatment sessions involve the use of the instrument as a rehabilitative tool.

Carpal Tunnel Syndrome

Carpal tunnel syndrome can be classified as bona fide and non–bona fide. Winspur[95] wrote about three classification subgroups for musicians with CTS.

- Classic idiopathic CTS, or bona fide CTS caused by increased pressure within the carpal tunnel.
- Wrist flexor tenosynovitis with carpal tunnel-like symptoms. These symptoms usually emerge after intense practice or prolonged performance. The symptoms are not present when the musician has a break from playing, is on holiday, or limits playing. Examination shows boggy swelling at the wrist, and the flexor tendons are commonly swollen, nodular, and tender. Nerve conduction studies (NCSs) are normal, and Phalen's test produces discomfort but no paresthesia. Treatment for flexor tenosynovitis of the wrist is conservative, and NSAIDs with or without an injection of nonabsorbable steroid into the carpal canal can be of great value. If NCS results are abnormal, then surgery may be indicated, but it should be considered as a last resort.[95a,96]
- Acute positional CTS symptoms[97,98] can be caused by positioning the wrist in flexion while playing, and thus symptoms may only occur during the act of making music. In Figure 117.12, you can see the amount of wrist flexion used by this guitarist to gain access to the lower strings; sustaining this position can lead to CTS-like symptoms and can in turn cause trauma to the median nerve if the playing position and schedule is not modified adequately.

Diabetes, thyroid disease, peripheral neuropathy, and fluid retention associated with pregnancy can be predisposing factors. CTS symptoms may also be caused by cervical symptoms, and thus upper limb tension testing may be necessary and appropriate to differentiate the source of the compression.

Wrist orthoses can be useful for decreasing pressure on the nerve and retraining wrist positioning while playing.[98a,98b] The orthosis should hold the wrist in a neutral position of 0 to 5 degrees of extension. Most commercial orthoses hyperextend the wrist considerably more than this, thus possibly raising the pressure in the carpal tunnel. The palmar aluminum strips can easily be flattened out to achieve a neutral position. The orthoses should be worn at night for those who complain of nocturnal or early morning paresthesias. If positional paresthesias occur during the day, the orthoses may be also worn then but should be removed hourly for gentle, active ROM exercises to prevent stiffness. Depending on the severity of the symptoms, it may be necessary to use a full-length resting orthosis because wrist orthoses leave the fingers free to pinch and grip, which can lead to raised carpal tunnel pressures.

BOX 117.1 Patient Handout on Joint Protection and Energy Conservation Techniques

Main Methods of Joint Protection
1. Use joints in a good position.
2. Avoid activities that do not allow for a change in position.
3. Respect pain.
4. Avoid tight grips or gripping for long periods.
5. Avoid actions that may lead to joint deformity.
6. Use large joints when possible.

Use Joints in a Good Position
Joints work best in certain positions. When they are used in the wrong position, such as twisting, extra force is placed through the joint and the muscles are unable to work as well, eventually causing pain and deformity. Try to consciously use "soft" joints whenever possible, for example, holding the elbow about 5 degrees bent inward and resting against your body rather than locking it out into the end of range or over straightened position. Often it is a good idea to place the index finger next to the thumb so your hand is used more like a paddle with the palm lightly holding items such as a steering wheel or supermarket cart because this helps in decreasing excessive grip through the fingers and thumb.

Avoid Activities That Don't Let You Change the Position of Your Hand
When you are in a position for a long time, your muscles get stiff and can pull joints into bad positions. The muscles also get tired quickly, so the force is taken up by the joint and not the muscles, thereby leading to pain and damage.

Respect Pain
The nature of arthritis means that you may always have pain. If pain continues for hours after an activity has stopped, this means that the activity was too much and should have been changed or stopped sooner. Your therapist will talk to you about the many ways of dealing with pain, such as the use of orthoses, saving energy, learning relaxation methods, planning the day ahead, or using equipment or gadgets to help you with certain activities.

Avoid Tight Grips or Gripping for Long Periods
Gripping tightly increases your pain and may damage your joints further. It is better to avoid it if possible. If you grip something that is small or narrow, it can require greater power to hold and manipulate it. More power usually means an increase in pain and an increase of forces through the joints. Some examples of how to decrease strain on joints include:
- Using thicker or padded pens for writing
- Resting books on a table or book rest
- Using a chopping board with spikes to secure vegetables
- Using nonslip mats under bowls to hold them
- Allowing hand washing to drip dry rather than wringing it out
- Relaxing your hands regularly during activities such as knitting or writing
- Building objects up using foam tubing or special grip aids
- Increasing the grip ability on a slippery object such as a shiny pen or toothbrush by using Elastoplast or Coban tape
- Many items have been ergonomically designed and can be purchased from supermarkets and department stores.

Avoid Activities that Could Lead to Deforming Positions
Some directions of force can be more detrimental than others to the hand. Damage to your joints could lead to deformities in your hand, such as your fingers appearing to drift in the direction of your little finger (ulnar deviation) or your individual fingers bending or straightening in unusual positions (swan-neck deformity). Activities can be changed to avoid these.
- When turning taps or opening and closing jars, use the palm of your hand and use one hand to open and the other to close. Remind others not to close them too tightly.

- Use a flat hand when possible such as when dusting or wiping.
- Try to use lightweight mugs with large handles rather than small teacups so pressure is not put on just one or two fingers.

Use One Large joint or Many Joints
Stronger muscles protect large joints, so it is better to use large joints when possible or try to spread the force over many joints.
- Use the palms of your hands and not your fingers when you carry plates or dishes.
- When standing up from a chair, try to rock gently forward and use your leg muscles to stand up rather than pushing from your knuckles or wrists.
- Carry light bags from a strap on your shoulder rather than your hands.
- Use your buttocks or hips to close drawers or move light chairs.
- Use your forearms to take the weight of objects when carrying, not your hands.

Main Methods of Energy Conservation
1. Balance rest and activity.
2. Organize and arrange space.
3. Stop activities or parts of them.
4. Reduce the amount of weight you take through your joints.
5. Use equipment that saves energy.

Balance Rest and Activity
It is important to balance your rest and activity to allow your joints to rest and repair. Stop before you feel tired or are in pain and avoid activities that you can't stop when you need to.
- Try to plan ahead. Write a weekly or daily diary with activities in red and rest times in blue. Think about what you need to do and space out the harder activities over time.
- Activities such as vacuuming, ironing, and cleaning windows mean that you are doing the same movements lots of times and keeping the hand in the same position for long periods of time. Try to do them for very short periods, or when possible, get someone else to do them for you.

Organize and Arrange Space
Prepare your work areas so you have everything you need for that activity. Store items you use often in places that are easy to reach and keep things in small refillable containers rather than large, heavy jars.

Stop Activities or Parts of Them
- Use clothes that are easy to care for.
- Make the bed on one side and then the other.
- Soak dishes before washing them and let them drip dry.
- When possible, use tinned, frozen, or prepared foods.
- Hang items within easy reach.
- When possible, get someone else to help with activities.

Reduce the Amount of Weight You take Through Your Joints
- Consider using wheeled trolleys rather than carrying things.
- Slide pans when possible and use a wire basket or slotted spoon to drain vegetables.
- When you buy new equipment, make sure it is lightweight.
- Use a teapot or kettle tipper and fill the kettle using a lightweight jug.

Use Equipment that Saves Energy
Your therapist will discuss with you some of the things that are available to buy.
Automatic washing machines, frost-free freezers, and food processors are all energy-saving devices, and simple things such as sharp knives use less pressure and therefore less energy.

(Continued)

BOX 117.1 Patient Handout on Joint Protection and Energy Conservation Techniques—cont'd

Should I Exercise My Hands?

It is important to maintain the amount of movement you have in your joints so that you are able to use your hands as much as possible. You may find that without regular exercise, your hands feel weak, and activities become more difficult. Exercise can help to relieve pain, keep bones and muscles strong, and keep your joints moving. Strong muscles around your joints can help keep them in a good position, but do not overdo your exercises or use weights or resistance because this may harm your joints.

Do I Need to Wear an Orthosis?

Your therapist will talk to you about wearing an orthosis. They can be used to rest a joint and allow the muscles around it to relax. This can help reduce swelling and pain. Orthoses can also be used to prevent deformities around the joint or stop existing deformities from worsening. It is often advisable to wear one during activity to support a joint and restrict movement.

There are various types of orthoses, and your therapist may provide you with more than one.

A thermoplastic resting orthosis can be made, which because of its strength, can also be used during activity to restrict movement around the joint. Softer orthoses made from neoprene are also available that allow more movement.

Other therapy tools that people have found useful are Lycra gloves worn at night and hot or cold gel packs. Your therapist will talk about your symptoms and your daily activities.

© Butler 2018.

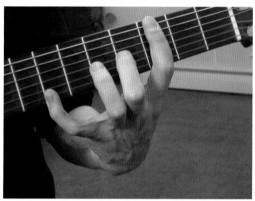

Fig. 117.12 The extreme wrist flexion and finger abduction assumed by some players to access the lower strings and play certain chords on the instrument can cause acute positional carpal tunnel syndrome. (K Butler 2009.)

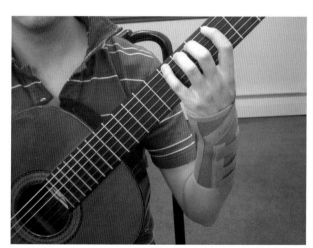

Fig. 117.13 Using a wrist orthosis to retrain wrist position and encourage larger movements of the elbow and shoulder when accessing the lower strings on a classical guitar. (K Butler 2009.)

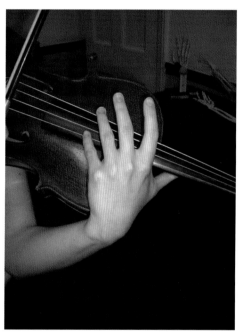

Fig. 117.14 A combination of elbow flexion and flexor carpi ulnaris contraction in the left upper limb of a viola player can lead to cubital tunnel symptoms. (K Butler 2009.)

Cubital Tunnel Syndrome

The boundaries of the cubital tunnel are the medial epicondyle anteriorly, the ulnohumeral ligament laterally, and the fibrous arcade formed by the two heads of the flexor carpi ulnaris (FCU) posteromedially. A fibrous band from the olecranon to the medial epicondyle forms the roof of the tunnel. The pertinent clinical biomechanical features are a 55% narrowing of the cubital tunnel along with a marked increased pressure during elbow flexion.[99,100] In vivo, additional pressure may be caused by FCU muscle contraction.[36] The latter is evidenced by the high incidence of cubital tunnel syndrome in the left hands of string players,[100] in whom a combination of elbow flexion and FCU contraction is found (Fig. 117.14).

Piccolo players' right and left arms and the left arms of cellists are at high risk of developing cubital tunnel syndrome because they are required to play with extreme elbow flexion for extended periods.

The most common clinical findings are a positive Tinel's sign over the cubital tunnel. With the patient's elbow fully flexed and the wrist held in a neutral position, the examiner taps over the nerve with her

Musical technique should be evaluated to minimize extremes of wrist position. Biofeedback may be used for neuromuscular reeducation to reduce grip force and fingertip loading. Orthoses can be useful for retraining wrist position. For example, guitarists can benefit from using a wrist orthosis while playing to retrain a more neutral wrist position and facilitate use of larger joints such as the elbow or shoulder (Fig. 117.13).

or his finger (not a reflex hammer). A positive elbow flexion test can produce paraesthesia in the ulnar aspect of the hand. The examiner should document in the medical notes the length of time it takes for the symptoms to appear because this is an objective marker and can assist in evaluating symptom history and treatment effectiveness.

Weakness in the abductor digiti minimi is also a common presenting feature in cubital tunnel syndrome.[101]

Although electrodiagnostic testing may be helpful in evaluating the severity of the condition, results may be negative, even in the face of florid symptoms.[102] One must always treat the patient, not the test.

The mainstay of treatment is prevention of sustained or repetitive elbow flexion and when possible to decrease or eliminate the need to go into the hypermobile range. Sometimes using a shorter bow can help string players learn a new position because it decreases their ability to go into a position that allows a hyperextended elbow. A soft elbow pad or semirigid night orthosis is usually tolerated better than rigid ones.

When returning to the instrument a gentle resumption of elbow flexion and FCU contraction must be observed (see the section Resuming Playing After an Injury) Oral medications such as NSAIDs or gabapentin may be very helpful. Injection of soluble corticosteroids can be helpful but must be done with caution to avoid intraneural injection. Sometimes these patients require a surgical release with or without transposition depending on the surgical finding and the playing position. After surgery, instrument-focused rehabilitation is imperative.

Radial Nerve Neuropathies

Although uncommon, sensory radial neuropathy should be mentioned in passing because it is often mistaken for de Quervain's disease or nonspecific arm pain. Patients with this neuropathy may display a positive Finkelstein's test result, paresthesias over the dorsum of the radial side of the hand, and have a Tinel's sign over the radial aspect of the forearm where the nerve emerges between the tendons of the extensor carpi radialis longus and brachioradialis. When the forearm is pronated, these tendons "scissor" the nerve between them.[104] As the terminal branches go to the dorsum of the thumb, ulnar deviation with thumb adduction stretches the already compromised nerve. This combination of forearm pronation, ulnar deviation, and thumb adduction occurs with upbowing as the bow hand approaches the strings. During practice, the bowstroke can be limited to minimize the offending position. Tight watchbands may contribute to the problem, and the bands should be loosened or the watch removed.

GANGLIONS

Scapholunate wrist ganglions are the most common type and do not usually require surgical treatment. However, they can be symptomatic when stretching periarticular tissues, especially with instruments that require extremes of wrist flexion or extension.[35] Surgery should be a last resort because there is a risk of leaving the patient with decreased ROM. Aspiration is commonly performed; however, there is a 50% recurrence rate after this procedure.

A more effective method is to rupture the ganglion. The clinician fills a 10-mL syringe with a mixture of half sterile water and half 2% lidocaine. The skin is anesthetized by using Fluori-methane spray. Using an 18-gauge needle, lidocaine is injected until the ganglion ruptures. This may require quite a bit of force. The thick viscous gel spreads subcutaneously over the dorsum of the hand and is reabsorbed in a few days. A compression dressing with sterile gauze and Coban should be applied and left in place for 1 or 2 days. Wrist active ROM exercises should be commenced as soon as possible after this procedure to minimize any decrease in range.

GENERAL TREATMENT PRINCIPLES FOR MUSICIANS

Standard therapeutic modalities such as cooling, compression, electrotherapy, orthotic positioning, exercise, sensory reeducation, postural reeducation, acupuncture, environmental assessment, examination of technique, holistic approach, breathing, myofascial release, and nerve glides can be useful when treating musicians; however, when possible, the instrument should be used as the therapeutic tool.

Instrument-specific rehabilitation techniques such as the use of surface electromyographic biofeedback while the patient is playing the instrument can help detect the presence of excessive muscular activity[106] in the forearm flexors, extensors, or trapezius muscles. Levy and colleagues[108] carried out electrical studies on the biceps, deltoid, trapezius, and sternomastoid muscles of violinists while they played two sections of music. As the musician's neck dimensions increased, the shoulder rest was more likely to promote diminished electrical activity from the tested muscles, and thus the investigators demonstrated that the shoulder rest had a great effect on muscles used to support the violin and that with proper rest musculoskeletal injuries might be decreased.

Video feedback may be used to increase awareness of posture and technique and is complementary to biofeedback. In video feedback, the patient faces a video monitor and plays his instrument while the therapist gives postural cues.[17] The video camera is placed at various angles, allowing the musician to see his or her posture from several perspectives. The camera can record the session for further study and review. When possible, the patient is assessed on and off the instrument because sometimes the difficulty will only become evident when the musician is in the playing position or demonstrating playing.

Orthotic Intervention

Various types of orthoses are available, and it may be appropriate for the patient to have more than one during the day depending on the activity being performed.

Functional Thumb Metacarpophalangeal Joint Extension Blocking Orthosis

Hyperextension of the first MCP joint is commonly observed in people with hypermobility and arthritis and in professionals such as musicians[2] and hand therapists.[109,111] This may be caused by decreased stability of the first CMC joint or MCP joint,[110] which subsequently leads to degenerative changes. Butler and Svens[111] present an alternative orthosis based on Van Lede's[112] anti–swan-neck orthosis for fingers, which restricts MCP joint extension of the thumb (Fig. 117.15). This orthosis can be very useful for retraining awareness of joint positioning on the instrument and while writing. It can decrease joint strain and in time assist in increasing the strength of the muscles surrounding the joint and thus aid joint stability.

Osteoarthritis and the Thumb Carpometacarpal Joint

A thermoplastic resting orthosis can restrict joint movement while functional tasks are being performed. This orthosis can also be worn while sleeping. Softer orthoses made from neoprene allow more movement and provide some warmth to the affected area. Other therapy tools that osteoarthritis patients can find useful are Lycra compression gloves worn at night and hot or cold gel packs.

Functional Orthoses

After an ulnar nerve injury, hyperextension at the MCP joints and an adducted thumb can render the hand dysfunctional. With careful

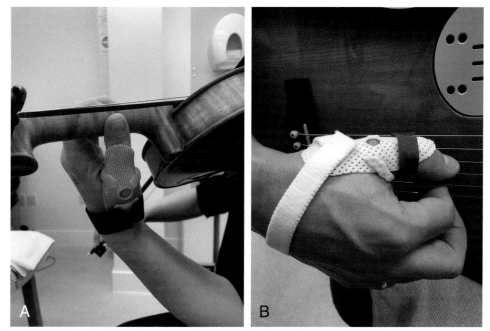

Fig. 117.15 A functional thumb metacarpal extension blocking orthosis can be used to block hyperextension of the metacarpophalangeal (MCP) joint while still allowing full flexion of the carpometacarpal, MCP, and interphalangeal joints. This orthosis can be used in many functional tasks such as playing a musical instrument, writing, or by hand therapists while working.[111] (K Butler 2018.)

orthotic positioning, ADLs and a graded return-to-play program can commence (Fig. 117.16). Prefabricated wrist orthoses can be used to retrain wrist position while playing the instrument (see Fig. 117.13). Neoprene orthoses can be worn to support a joint or area and limit some movement while increasing proprioceptive awareness and warmth. A thermoplastic reinforcement can be added to increase support or further limit movement. These orthoses can be a useful way for a musician to gradually progress from a wrist orthosis to a neoprene orthosis to no orthosis.

Dynamic Orthoses

Injury may result in a lack of full ROM. This can limit the possibility of certain positions on the instrument. After surgery, certain structures may need protection while they heal. If the therapist wants to promote gentle motion, then dynamic positioning is often the most appropriate means (Fig. 117.17). Figure 117.18 is a dynamic extension splint with a radial deviation pull to assist in retraining finger positioning while playing after a finger fracture. Figure 117.19 shows a dynamic MCP joint extension orthosis with radial pull that a pianist used during the daytime while performing functional tasks as well as in a graded return-to-play program. She was supplied with a resting orthosis with an ulnar border build-up to wear at night. This patient had a 35-year history of rheumatoid arthritis, and she was finding playing increasingly difficult. A crossed intrinsic transfer with synovectomy was performed, and she commenced light playing after 4 days of surgery, with the orthosis on. She commented: "I have been amazed with the results, as I have not been able to play like this for 20 years. I did not think this improvement was possible. My finger is articulating in a crisp way. My husband can hear the difference already as well." Getting the patient back on the instrument as soon as is reasonably possible and anatomically safe is integral to the whole healing of a musician.

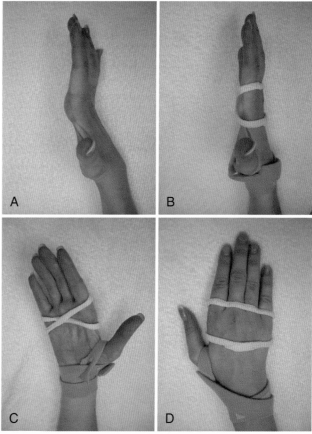

Fig. 117.16 A–D, After an ulnar nerve injury, an Orfit metacarpophalangeal joint blocking orthosis and Velfoam thumb abduction strap can assist in allowing a gentle return-to-play schedule. (K Butler 2009.)

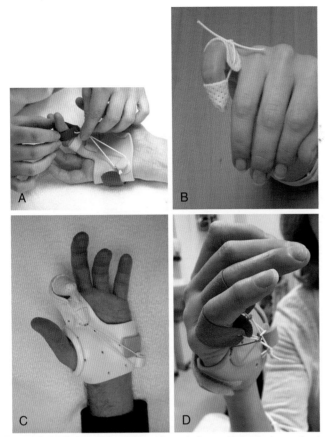

Fig. 117.17 A, Dynamic proximal interphalangeal joint flexion orthosis. **B** and **C,** Dynamic composite proximal and distal interphalangeal joint flexion orthosis. **D,** Dynamic metacarpophalangeal joint flexion orthosis. (A-C, K Butler 2009; D, K Butler 2018.)

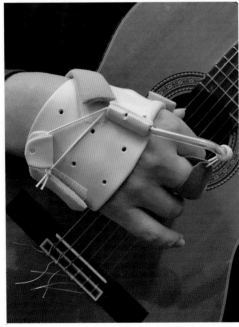

Fig. 117.18 Dynamic extension orthosis with radial pull for the middle finger of a guitarist to retrain finger positioning on the instrument. (K Butler 2018.)

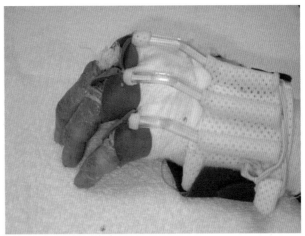

Fig. 117.19 Dynamic metacarpophalangeal joint extension orthosis with radial pull that a pianist used 4 days after cross intrinsic transfer with synovectomy. (K Butler 2009.)

MUSICAL ERGONOMICS

Musical Instrument Modifications

Guitars, violas, and violins have been designed that use lighter or less material and altered shapes with the goal of permitting the use of a more optimal ergonomic position when playing. Some electric guitars and violins finesse this problem altogether by virtually eliminating the body of the instrument.

The lower "bout" of the acoustic guitar (the part where the right forearm crosses the instrument) also can present a physical obstacle, resulting in either excessive right wrist flexion or protraction of the right shoulder for the right hand to access the strings. The larger the body size of the guitar or the smaller the player, the bigger the problem. By altering the position of the guitar, a more neutral wrist and elbow position can be gained therefore limiting extreme pressure of the right forearm onto the instrument.

For the soloist or short double bass player, the instrument should be selected with sloping shoulders if one does a lot of playing in the high positions (e.g., soloists). This minimizes impingement of the left forearm against the sharp edge of the instrument or thrusting the left shoulder forward to avoid forearm impingement when reaching down the neck.

The bassoon can be designed and made with levers and extended keys to decrease an excessive span of the fingers and thus prevent development of an intrinsic muscle strain.

Reduction of Static Loading

Static loading, which occurs when the weight of a tool is sustained and supported by the hand, has long been recognized as an etiologic factor in workers' injuries. Industry has addressed this by developing ways to suspend tools to remove the weight from the hand. This approach has also worked for musical instruments. Adding an end pin to the cello relieved the player from supporting the instrument by grasping it with the legs. End pins have also been successfully used in the bassoon, English horn, and tuba. The end pin for the last two instruments has been modified into a ball that rests on the chair between the thighs.

Several devices available on the market relieve the right thumb strain so common to oboe and clarinet players. Freeing the right hand also allows alternative fingerings that may be more efficient. Lightweight, height-adjustable posts that attach to the thumb rest and are supported on the seat between the player's legs can be very useful.

A small support can be applied to the body of the flute to take the strain off the left index finger to remind the player not to press this finger into the instrument and to the right thumb to support the instrument and decrease joint strain (see Fig. 117.6E and F).

The bassoon is best supported by using a body harness that clips onto the instrument. Seat and neck straps that are attached to the instrument are commonly used. If using a seat strap, quite a bit of weight is still required to be supported by the left hand because of the leftward inclination of the instrument, and there is torque on the left hand because it must counteract the tendency of the instrument to roll outward. Neck straps place a lot of force through the neck and can encourage a forward head position, which can affect breath control and sound production.

Key Modifications

Many instruments can be modified to make playing them more comfortable and safer.

The levers that operate the valves on the French horn can be lengthened to provide greater leverage and widened to provide increased contact area.

A hooklike device can be soldered onto the upright post of a trombone, significantly decreasing the stretch required for the left index finger to support the mouthpiece. The post itself can be wrapped with Coban to prevent digital nerve compression.

The location of the flute keys can be customized to fit the player's hand, and the cluster of keys worked by the right little finger can be angled in toward the finger, thereby reducing strain between the fourth and fifth fingers. The keys operated by the left fourth and fifth fingers can be lengthened to achieve a more neutral left wrist position. A flute with a U head can be useful for children, or covering the open holes of a flute after injury to the hand can facilitate ease of return to play, and in time the keys can be "unblocked" and open holes can be used again as the patient recovers and gains confidence. In addition to these modifications, children can benefit from disks being soldered to the keys for the right index, middle, and ring fingers to reduce the distance between keys, thus reducing hand strain (http://flutelab.com/flutelab.com/adaptive-wind-wind-instruments).

Although left-hand problems outnumber right-hand problems in flutists, quite a few players have had strain and physical tension in the base of the right thumb and the muscles pertaining to this area.[115] One could argue that this most likely represents an error of technique, with the person using an excessive amount of tension in the right hand or incorrect placement of the right thumb. However, certain intrinsic balance problems with the instrument benefit from the enhanced stability attained with the use of orthoses or "rests."

Discomfort may arise from the very small area of contact between the edge of the right thumb and the flute when the hand is held in the "natural" position, with the ulnar edge of the thumb facing the pad of the index finger. This is the position the thumb falls into when the hand is relaxed. This position concentrates the force from the flute over a small bony area of the thumb, which does not have a very high pressure tolerance. The common solution to this problem is to supinate the thumb so that the soft pad contacts the flute. Achieving and maintaining this position requires muscular force. Increased muscular tension in the thumb and hand may not only cause pain and injury but also may inhibit dexterity.

A thumb port can distribute pressure from the flute over a wider area of the thumb, thus allowing the thumb to be comfortably held in the natural position, and it encourages stability by positioning the weight of the rods to fall through the base of support, thus preventing the flute from rolling inward.

Adaptive Equipment for Musicians with Physical Disabilities

Musical instruments can be modified or adapted to increase the ease of playing them if the individual has a physical or mental disability. French horns, normally played with the left hand, have been built to accommodate left upper extremity amputees. Adaptive prosthetic terminal devices have been fabricated[116] to allow holding of the trombone, and drumsticks and metal picks have been affixed to the end of the prosthesis to allow guitar playing (Fig. 117.20).

For people with quadriplegia or severe neurologic impairments, sip and puff controls can be adapted to the computer and used in conjunction with several musical software packages to allow composition and playback.

RESUMING PLAYING AFTER TIME AWAY FROM THE INSTRUMENT

The treatment of musicians' injuries has two distinct phases. Reducing pain or symptoms is the first stage. The second consists of a structured protocol for returning to full musical activity. If the player has had to stop or significantly reduce playing during the pain reduction phase, a structured protocol for return to play is essential to decrease the chances of repeated relapses. In this protocol, the musicians perform their specific tasks but start out at a greatly reduced level of time and intensity. Injured musicians are often anxious about being away from their instrument and miss playing so much that they return to playing prematurely and suffer disastrous consequences. Fry (1986) quotes Poore (1887) on this[117]:

> The most important point in treatment is rest. The excessive use of the hand must be discontinued, and it is often necessary to insist on this rather forcibly. Piano playing, if not prohibited altogether, must only be practiced to a degree short of that which causes pain or annoyance. It is often difficult to restrain the ardor of these patients in the matter of playing. Directly they feel in a small degree better, they fly to the piano; and I have known the progress of more than one case very seriously retarded by the undoing, as it were, of the good effect of rest by an hour's injudicious and prohibited practicing.

It is critical that the treating clinical team be fully educated in both the psychological and practical aspects of guiding their patients through the difficult and often treacherous stages of resuming full musical activities to avoid the despair that can accompany setbacks, treatment failure, or career abandonment. Musicians should be reassured that they are not going to lose their technique during a few weeks' rest and that they can put their "time out" to good use by working on music theory, harmony, sight reading, solfège, mental practice, silent practice, critical listening to recordings, or learning something about the business aspects of music and career promotion.

Only in extreme cases must musicians completely refrain from playing their musical instruments. It is usually sufficient to reduce the intensity or time of playing, select a less taxing repertoire, or take more frequent breaks. It may be necessary, however, to cancel or postpone performance commitments, exams, or auditions.

If one hand is injured, the player can sometimes continue to do some playing with the unaffected side.

It is not necessary to be completely asymptomatic before beginning the return-to-play program. A person who is not yet ready or able to deal with the physical instrument can go through the motions of playing without the instrument, what Menuhin referred to as "shadow playing."[118] It is preferable that the recovering player have the endurance to

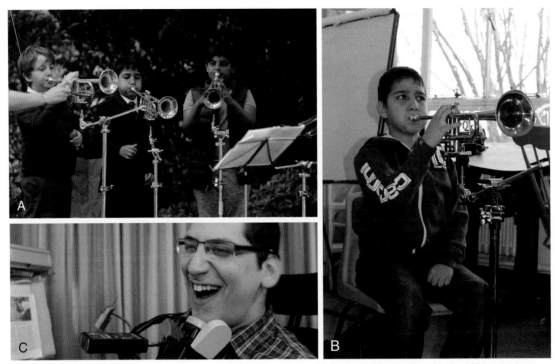

Fig. 117.20 Many adaptations can be made to instruments, which can enable people with disabilities to play and not be excluded from making music.

shadow play comfortably for 10 minutes or so before beginning to play the actual instrument.

The Return-to-Play Schedule

When the person is ready to return to the instrument, a detailed return-to-play schedule is reviewed. It is inadequate for the clinician merely to advise a player who is ready to return to playing to "go back little by little." This is too vague and open to misinterpretation. The value of a written schedule is that it minimizes the risk of overdoing things. Even if they believe that they can do more, players must be advised to strictly adhere to the schedule. The use of a clock or timer is more than helpful; it is critical because the patient often fails to recognize overexertion during the musical activity. The pain can often evolve only hours later.

Depending on the severity of the injury or the length of time taken away from the instrument, the musician may begin cautiously with a single 2- to 3-minute period, or even less, and see how he or she feels later that day and the next day. It may be necessary to grade the return to play even more and to instigate miming or performing the movements required to play the instrument without even holding the instrument. For example, a violinist may move the left arm up into the playing position three or four times an hour each hour during the waking day to rehabilitate and "remind" the body about the playing position. Shadow playing can be the next stage in a graded return-to-play program. In this, for example, the violinist moves the fingers over the strings but does not depress the strings onto the violin. In time, light pressure may be applied to the strings and then half pressure, full pressure, gentle vibrato, and in time full vibrato. Grading of positions played and strings played on stringed instruments can also be a way of increasing the difficulty and technical requirements for the playing position.

To return the musician back to her or his preinjury performance level can take a long time. The graded return-to-play program provides an outline for how to achieve this. A gentle, encouraging approach by the treating medical professional is often necessary to keep the musician in good spirits and to facilitate a gentle pace of return to play. If the musician rushes return to play, he or she can in turn cause an increase in symptoms and may require reverting to a lower level of playing.

A brief physical warm-up and cool-down should precede and follow playing, and if there is still some pain or discomfort, the sore part may be cooled with a cold pack for 10 minutes or so after the playing session. It must be emphasized that the cold pack is taken from the fridge and not the freezer so that tissues are cooled rather than frozen!

The return-to-play schedule can and should be modified to suit the individual player. In addition to the warm-up and cool-down, the musician should begin with slow, easy pieces or études. A metronome at a medium setting may be used, and gradually tempos can be increased notch by notch every few days. The musician should also gradually work down toward slower tempos because the control required to play slowly can be very demanding as well. With time, the player gradually resumes more technically difficult material. Thus, the progression is really in three dimensions: gradually increasing duration, tempo, and technical difficulty of the material.

The schedule (Table 117.1)[94] is divided into play and rest periods. Each level represents a unit of time, usually from 3 to 7 days, although this can be adjusted to meet individual needs. The musician should be comfortable at a given level before progressing to the next level. The play periods gradually increase with each level, and the rest periods gradually decrease. However, the play periods do not increase beyond about 50 minutes, and the rest periods do not fall below 5 to 10 minutes. If the injury has been severe, the musician would probably progress even more slowly.

If pain reappears after progressing to the next level, the player should drop back one or two levels until the symptoms subside. If absolutely necessary, the player may need to stop for a day or two before resuming playing. If the player encounters difficulty progressing, it may be necessary to do a mini progression, changing only one vertical column every 3 to 4 days. For example, if the musician is at level 4, rather than increasing all the play and rest periods at a single time to level 5, an alternative would be to increase only the first play period to level five, leaving the remainder of the play and rest periods at level 4. After a few more days, the second play period is increased, then the second rest period decreased, and so forth. In this fashion, the player may be able to make steady, albeit slow, progress and this in turn will hopefully assist in avoiding or decreasing levels of discouragement and depression. In the sample program, level 10 represents about 4 hours of playing time. A performer who requires more than this would simply keep adding more play and rest periods, as shown, until achieving the desired goal. Before returning to work in an orchestra or ensemble, it is usually recommended that the musician is playing for at least 3 hours of personal practice throughout a day with minimum symptoms being reported.

To assist in decreasing the disruption in the flow of practice, the musician can record the practice session and critically review what was just practiced during the break periods.

A "Healthy Practice Habits" handout (Box 117.2)[55] can be helpful when reintroducing patients to their instruments after an injury or time away for any reason. This can also be used as an educational tool to assist in preventing injuries and as a way of mapping progress. Sometimes a clock may be used so the musician can time practice sessions carefully and not overdo it by accident. After a period of not playing, musicians must return with a slow graded progression in duration, tempo, and complexity of playing, and they may require psychological support.[119,120]

Instrument-Specific Rehabilitation Protocols

To provide care on a sophisticated level, it is necessary to modify the concept of return to play to address specific injuries and instruments. Here are a few examples of the principle of instrument-specific return-to-play protocols.

Harpist

A harpist with left shoulder strain initially avoids passages with low notes. This is because the left shoulder must flex forward and protract to reach the lower bass strings, thus placing increased strain on the anterior deltoid.

TABLE 117.1 Returning to Play

Levels (3–7 Days at Each)	Play	Rest	Play	Rest	Play	Rest	Play	Rest	Play
1	5	60	5						
2	10	50	10						
3	15	40	15	60	5				
4	20	30	20	50	10				
5	30	20	25	40	15	45	5		
6	35	15	35	30	20	35	10		
7	40	10	40	20	25	25	15	50	10
8	50	10	45	15	30	15	25	40	15
9	50	10	50	10	40	10	35	30	20
10	50	10	50	10	50	10	45	20	30

Etc.

- Start with slow and easy activity or pieces. Gradually progress to faster, more difficult tasks or pieces.
- In general, perform a maximum of 50 minutes of continuous work or play with a minimum of 10 minutes of rest.
- *Warm up* before playing!
- If pain occurs at any level, drop back to level of comfort until able to progress without pain.

From Norris RN. *Musician's Survival Manual.* St. Louis: ICSOM; 1993.

BOX 117.2 Healthy Practice Habits for Musicians

Early Recognition
- Take the first sign of an injury seriously; it may not be necessary to completely stop playing.

Frequent Breaks when Practicing
- Practice only as long as you can maintain concentration; stop if feeling discomfort or fatigue.
- Take a 3-5 minute "macro-break" every 30 minutes (e.g., water, breathing or stretch break) so your muscles are more responsive.
- Take frequent "mico-breaks" for a few seconds with one hand off the instrument.

Warm Up Before Practicing
- Warm up *away from the instrument* such as adhering to a short fitness regimen before playing.
- Warm up *at the instrument* with easy music concentrating on slow perfection.
- Find easy postures and positions (e.g., use cues such as "relax the thumb" or "free up the elbow").

Cool Down After Practicing
- Cool down *away from the instrument.*
- Stretching and icing overworked areas of the body may be necessary.

Maximize Playing Time in Good Posture
- Adjust seat and music stand for optimal posture.
- Keep wrists and thumbs in their neutral position as much as possible.
- Good posture on stage communicates *command* and *presence.*

Technical Awareness
- A technical problem may have a musical solution (e.g., evaluate phrasing or fingering).
- Extreme fatigue can indicate something is wrong technically.
- Volume and resonance can be produced with muscle release and gravity without excessive tension.

Instrument Supports
- Neck straps, harnesses, floor stands, customized chin rests, individualized thumb stops or keys, instrument posts, backpack-style carrying cases, or wheels on instrument cases are available.

Mental Training
- Strive to *reduce* practice time before a performance and increase mental training.
- Score read *away* from the instrument.
- Use visualization to hear and see your performance.[120]

Fitness and Relaxation
- Choose fitness activities that you enjoy, have minimal risk of injury, and help alleviate your particular muscle imbalances (professional advice may be required).
- Allow yourself some relaxation time.

Piccolo

Piccolo players recovering from cubital tunnel syndrome should commence practicing on the flute because the elbows are more extended on this instrument.

String Players

A cellist or bassist with a left shoulder strain is recommended to commence the graded return-to-play program primarily with thumb position (down toward the bridge), in which the deltoid is more relaxed than in the first position (up by the tuning pegs), which requires shoulder abduction. Because the thumb position requires less elbow flexion, it is also advisable for a cellist recovering from cubital tunnel syndrome.

String players with de Quervain's tenovaginitis of the right wrist should avoid using the proximal third of the bow, playing at the heel, because the wrist assumes an increased flexed and ulnar-deviated position as the hand approaches the strings on the upbow.

A cellist with right rotator cuff injury should initially avoid bowing out to the tip of the bow, especially on the two treble strings,[121] to avoid abduction and internal rotation, which aggravates impingement of the cuff. A violinist or violist with the same problem, on the other hand, begins on the two treble strings because reaching for the lower strings with the bow necessitates humeral abduction, often above shoulder height, which can aggravate rotator cuff impingement.

Guitarists

Guitarists with left hand or shoulder problems could place a capo (a rubber-coated steel bar that clamps across the strings) on the third fret, thus decreasing the stress of supination with external rotation that occurs when playing on the first three frets. Because the distance between the frets decreases as one goes higher up the neck, the finger abduction required for chords or intervals is also lessened. Guitarists can change to lighter gauge strings as a way of grading their return-to-play program.

Pianists

A pianist recovering from a hand or shoulder problem might avoid using the thumb on the black keys or crossing to the opposite side of the keyboard to avoid wrist ulnar deviation and shoulder adduction. It may be easier for the pianist with painful forearm overuse to resume playing on a synthesizer or electronic keyboard because the key depression requires less force.

SURGERY

Surgery on musicians must be entered into cautiously—either all other treatment options should have been attempted first, or surgery must be the only appropriate treatment indicated. Importantly, the interface must be assessed and altered as necessary before surgery for most conditions. Surgery is often seen as the last treatment option available to a musician.

Winspur[122] reports that of the musicians presenting with recognizable orthopedic or rheumatologic conditions in the upper limb 4% to 6% are candidates for surgery. Nonsurgical treatment should always be tried first, and it should not be forgotten that in some situations, adjustment or modification of the instrument or playing technique (the interface) may solve the problem rather than surgery.

The implications of surgery are profound for musicians, whose hands are their livelihood. Thus, respect for their hand and career must be paramount. Accurate diagnosis, analysis of need and disability, and precision in planning all need to be carefully considered to ensure optimal outcome of surgery. In acute trauma, techniques that permit early return to function (e.g., rigid fixation of fractures and early rehabilitation) are often advantageous. Electrodiagnostically documented carpal or cubital tunnel syndrome and ligamentous injuries leading to instability that have not responded to activity modification or nonoperative therapy can be considered appropriate indications for surgery in the musician's hand.[123]

Winspur[35,96,122] states that four areas must be identified and specifically addressed when planning surgery on a musician's hand:

1. The incisions must avoid critical tactile areas.
2. Repair should be anatomic whenever possible.
3. Adjustment must be considered for any anticipated anatomic compromise to the musician's specific musical needs.
4. The surgery should allow for an early return to limited playing.

A large series of professional musicians operated on by a single surgeon are presented by Butler and Winspur.[124] These are the results from that study:

- A total of 127 of 130 musicians operated on returned to full-time professional work or could complete their final-year music college examinations.
- Piano players appear to take the longest to initially return to their instrument (3.3 weeks), and string players appear to take the most time to fully rehabilitate (11 weeks), that is, to return to full playing on their instrument.
- Trauma appears to be the most difficult condition from which to initially recover, with patients taking an average of 5.2 weeks to return to part-time playing.
- Full return to play took the nerve-release group an average of 17 weeks, the arthrodesis and arthroplasty groups 13 weeks, and the trauma group 12.7 weeks.
- The most common medical condition requiring surgery in the series was nerve compressions (32.3%).
- Of the musicians undergoing hand surgery, 35.4% played the piano or organ as their primary instrument.
  For three patients, the surgery was deemed unsuccessful:
- One was misdiagnosed with CTS despite abnormal NCS results. This patient had multilevel cervical disk disease and required spinal surgery. This patient could return to teaching but not performing at a professional level after spinal surgery.
- One young pianist had a hypermobile thumb and was lost to follow-up. Early surgical results appeared to be unsatisfactory after a synovectomy.
- One patient with a hypermobile distal radial ulnar joint did not return to full-time professional performance levels and now only does some teaching because of a recurrent dislocating extensor carpi ulnaris.

These important points must be considered when working with musicians who may require surgical intervention:

- All other treatment options must be attempted first.
- Surgery must only be considered when the condition interferes with playing.
- Surgery must be strongly indicated, and the pros and cons of the surgery must be discussed clearly with each patient in respect to lifestyle, level of performance, and the demands of the instrument.
- A specialized, multidisciplinary, and instrument-focused approach is necessary when rehabilitating musicians.[55]

The following conclusions can be drawn from this large series of 130 professional musicians, all of whom were operated on by a single surgeon:

- The musical instrument must be used as the rehabilitative tool for the player to gain confidence levels, ROM, desensitization, strength, and psychological support during the rehabilitation phase, and thus strong surgical techniques that can withstand early return to play must be implemented when appropriate and indicated.

- *Do not* operate on hypermobile painful joints but rather used other therapeutic devices, such as positional orthoses, to assist this patient group.
- Appropriate surgical intervention will not end a musician's career, provided it is performed properly, for the correct reasons, and with postoperative instrument-focused hand therapy available.

SUMMARY

There has been an increase in focus on health issues that relate to performing artists in recent years. There is frequently hand and arm pain in this patient group. Their playing conditions and life-styles are often not conducive to ergonomically sound approaches to performance, and general living standards can vary greatly. Rapid repeated movements are often required, and frequently, unusual postures are held for extended periods of time. Overuse while playing, practicing, and performing is common in music students and experienced performers alike. Musicians are often perfectionists who are striving for excellence in their field, and they are usually ill-prepared for the physical and emotional demands that may be placed on them in their student and professional lives. When assessing and treating this group, early assessment and accurate diagnosis are imperative. Happily, surgical intervention is not usually required, and holistic approaches to practice schedules, an ergonomic approach to playing, and relevant warm-up and cool-down exercises can assist the musician's return to playing with much less pain or discomfort. When possible, the musical instrument should be used as a rehabilitative tool. A specialized multidisciplinary approach to rehabilitation is advantageous and necessary when working with musicians. Prevention of injury is the primary aim of performing arts medicine. Scientific research and practical advice regarding minimizing the effects of performance and playing on the musician's bodies must be our focus, as well as educating the wider community about these strategies. In this way, we can all enjoy a wide variety of music and musical expression, and performers can enjoy the experience of playing their instruments and sharing music with the audience, with minimal tension and pain in their bodies.

REFERENCES

1. Winspur I, Tubiana R. The musician's hand. *Hand Clin*. 2003;19(2): 343–353.
2. Wynn Parry CB. Managing the physical demands of musical performance. In: Williamon A, ed. *Musical Excellence Strategies and Techniques to Enhance Performance*. Oxford, UK: Oxford University Press; 2004:41–60.
3. Butler K. Musicians and hand therapy. *ISM Music J*. 2005:142–146.
3a. Butler K. Helping Hands. *Classical Music Magazine*. 2018:68–69.
4. Buckley T, Manchester R. Overuse injuries in non-classical recreational instrumentalists. *Med Probl Perform Art*. 2006;21:80–87.
5. Newmark J, Lederman RJ. Practice doesn't necessarily make perfect: incidence of overuse syndromes in amateur instrumentalists. *Med Probl Perform Art*. 1987;2:142–144.
5a. Robitaille J, Tousignant-Laflamme Y, Guay M. Impact of changes in playing time on plating-related musculoskeletal pain in string music students. *Medical Problems of Performing Artists*. 2019;33(1):6–13.
5b. Ackerman BJ. How much training is too much? *Medical Problems of Performing Artists*. 2017;33(1):61–62.
6. Hoppmann, Richard A. Musculoskeletal problems of instrumental musicians. In: Sataloff RT, Brandfonbrener AG, Lederman RJ, eds. *Performing Arts Medicine*. 3rd ed. Science and Medicine; 2010:207–227.
7. Ackermann BJ. Therapeutic management of the injured musician. In: Sataloff RT, Brandfonbrener AG, Lederman RJ, eds. *Performing Arts Medicine*. 3rd ed. Science & Medicine; 2010:247–269.
7a. Watson A. Prevention. In: Winspur I, ed. *The Musician's Hand a Clinical Guide*. London: JP Medical Ltd; 2018:151–171.
8. Zara C, Farewell VT. Musicians' playing-related musculoskeletal disorders: an examination of risk factors. *Am J Ind Med*. 1997;32:292–300.
9. Powell DH. Treating individuals with debilitating performance anxiety: an introduction. *J Clin Psychol*. 2004;60(3):801.
9a. Evans A. Performance psychology. In: Winspur I, ed. *The Musician's Hand a Clinical Guide*. London: JP Medical Ltd; 2018:173–183.
10. Fishbein M, Middlestadt SE, Ottati V, et al. Medical problems among ICSOM musicians: overview of a national survey. *Med Probl Perform Art*. 1988;3:1.
11. Wynn Parry CB. Musicians' hand and arm pain. In: Winspur I, ed. *The Musician's Hand a Clinical Guide*. London: JP Medical Ltd; 2018:3–13.
11a. Zhukov K. Current approaches for management of music performance anxiety. *Medical Problems of Performing Artists*. 2019;34(1):53–60.
12. Byl NN, Merzenich MM, Cheung S, Bedenbaugh P, Nagarajan SS, Jenkins WM. A primate model for studying focal dystonia and repetitive strain injury: effects on the primary somatosensory cortex. *Phys Ther*. 1997;77(3):269–284.
13. Hoppman RA. 'Instrumental musicians' hazards. *Occup Med*. 2001;16(4):619–631.
14. Butler K, Rosenkranz K. Focal hand dystonia affecting musicians. Part 1: an overview of epidemiology, pathophysiology and medical treatments. *Br J Hand Ther*. 2006;11(3):72–78.
15. Amadio PC. Epidemiology of hand and wrist injuries in sports. *Hand Clin*. 1990;6:379–381.
16. Dawson WJ. Hand and wrist injuries. In: Grabois M, ed. *Physical Medicine and Rehabilitation*. Malden, Mass: Blackwell Science; 2000.
17. Dommerholt J, Norris RN. Physical therapy management of the instrumental musician. *Orthop Phys Ther Clin North Am*. 1997;6:185–206.
18. Norris RN. The 'lazy' finger syndrome. In: Torch D, ed. *The Musician's Survival Manual*. St Louis: ICSOM; 1993.
19. Potter HG, Hannafin JA, Morwessel RM, et al. Lateral epicondylitis: correlation of MR imaging, surgical, and histopathologic findings. *Radiology*. 1995;196(1):43–46.
20. Clarke MT, Lyall HA, Grant JW, Matthewson MH. The histopathology of dequervain's disease. *J Hand Surg [Br]*. 1998;23-B(6):732–734.
21. Read HS, Hooper G, Davie R. Histological appearances in post-partum de Quervain's disease. *J Hand Surg [Br]*. 2000;25B(1):70–72.
22. Kleinbart FA., McElroy H. Low back and lower extremity injuries in dancers. In: Sataloff RT, Brandfonbrener AG, Lederman RJ, eds. *Performing Arts Medicine*. 3rd ed. Science & Medicine; 2010:285.
23. Butler K, Sandford F. Tendinopathies of the hand and wrist. *AOCP*. 2007;1:4–24.
24. Davenport TE, Kulig K, Matharu Y, Blanco CE. The EdUReP model for nonsurgical management of tendinopathy. *Phys Ther*. 2005;85(10):1093–1103.
25. Soslowsky LJ, Thomopoulos S, Tun S, et al. Neer Award 1999. Overuse activity injures the supraspinatus tendon in an animal model: a histologic and biomechanical study. *J Shoulder Elbow Surg*. 2000;9(2):79–84.
26. Harman D. Aging: a theory based on free radical and radiation chemistry. *J Gerontol*. 1956;11(3):298–300.
27. Harman D. The aging process. *Proc Natl Acad Sci USA*. 1981;78(11):7124–7128.
28. Barnham KJ, Masters CL, Bush AI. Neurodegenerative diseases and oxidative stress. *Nat Rev Drug Discov*. 2004;3(3):205–214.
29. Haklar U, Yüksel M, Velioglu A, et al. Oxygen radicals and nitric oxide levels in chondral or meniscal lesions or both. *Clin Orthop Relat Res*. 2002;403:135–142.

30. Radák Z, Ogonovszky H, Dubecz J, et al. Super-marathon race increases serum and urinary nitrotyrosine and carbonyl levels. *Eur J Clin Invest*. 2003;33(8):726–730.

31. Szabo R. Show me the evidence. *Am Soc Surg Hand*. 2008;33A:150–156.

32. Coldham F. The use of splinting in the non-surgical treatment of de Quervain's disease: a review of the literature. *Br J Hand Ther*. 2006;11(2):16–23.

33. Fournier K, Bourbonnais D, Bravo G, et al. Reliability and validity of pinch and thumb strength measurements in de Quervain's disease. *J Hand Ther*. 2006;19(1):2–10, quiz 11.

34. Finkelstein H. Stenosing tendovaginitis at the radial styloid process. *J Bone Joint Surg*. 1930;12a:509–540.

35. Winspur I. Specific conditions. In: Winspur I, ed. *The Musician's Hand a Clinical Guide*. London: JP Medical Ltd; 2018:31–55.

36. Norris RN. Applied ergonomics: adaptive equipment and instrument modification. *Md Med J*. 1993;42:271–275.

37. Bejjani FJ, Ferrara L, Tomaino CM, et al. Comparison of three piano techniques. *Med Probl Perform Art*. 1989;4:109.

38. Hillberry BM. Dynamic effects of work on musculoskeletal loading. In: Gordon M, ed. *Repetitive Motion Disorders of the Upper Extremity*. Rosemont, Ill: American Academy of Orthopaedic Surgeons; 1995.

39. Gelberman RH, Hergenroeder PT, Hargens AR, et al. The carpal tunnel syndrome: a study of carpal tunnel pressures. *J Bone Joint Surg*. 1981;63A:380–383.

40. Rempel D. Musculoskeletal loading and carpal tunnel pressures. In: Gordon M, ed. *Repetitive Motion Disorders of the Upper Extremity*. Rosemont, Ill: American Academy of Orthopaedic Surgeons; 1995.

41. Wolf FG, Keane MS, Brandt KD, Hillberry BM. An investigation of finger joint and tendon forces in experienced pianists. *Med Probl Perform Art*. 1993;8:84.

42. Jansen CW, Patterson R, Viegas SF. Effects of fingernail length on finger and hand performance. *J Hand Ther*. 2000;13(3):211–217.

43. Simmons DG, Travell JG, Simons LS. *Myofascial Pain and Dysfunction. The Trigger Point Manual Volume 1. Upper Half of Body*. 2nd ed. Lippincott Williams & Wilkins; 1999.

44. Hardy M, Woodall W. Therapeutic effects of heat, cold, and stretch on connective tissue. *J Hand Ther*. 1998;11(2):148–156.

45. Furuya S, Nakahara H, Aoki T, Kinoshita H. Prevalence and casual factors of playing-related musculoskeletal disorders of the upper extremity and trunk amongst Japanese pianists and piano students. *Med Prob Perform Art*. 2006;21:112–118.

46. Brandfonbrener AG. Etiologies of medical problems in performing artists. In: Sataloff RT, Brandfonbrener AG, Lederman RJ, eds. *Performing Arts Medicine*. 3rd ed. Science and Medicine; 2010.

47. Larson LG, Baum J, Mudholkar GS. Hypermobility: features and differential incidence between the sexes. *Arthritis Rheum*. 1987;30:1426–1430.

48. Larson LG, Baum J, Mudholkar GS, Kollia GD. Benefits and disadvantages of joint hypermobility among musicians. *N Engl J Med*. 1993;329:1079–1082.

49. Jull JA. Examination of the articular system. In: Boyling J, Palastanga N, eds. *Grieve's Modern Manual Therapy*. 2nd ed. Edinburgh: Churchill Livingstone; 1994:511–524.

49a. Keer R, Butler K. Physiotherapy and occupational therapy in the hypermobile adult. In: Hakim A, Keer R, Grahame R, eds. *Hypermobility, Fibromyalgia and Chronic Pain*. London: Churchill Livingstone Elsevier; 2010:143–161.

50. Beighton P, Solomon L, Soskolne C. Articular mobility in an African population. *Ann Rheum Dis*. 1973;32:413–418.

50a. Butler K. Regional complications in joint hypermobility syndrome: The hand. In: Hakim A, Keer R, Grahame R, eds. *Hypermobility, Fibromyalgia and Chronic Pain*. London: Churchill Livingstone Elsevier; 2010:207–216.

51. Hakim AJ, Malfait F, De Paepe A. The heritable disorders of connective tissue: epidemiology, nosology and clinical features. In: Hakim A, Keer R, Grahame R, ed. *Hypermobility, Fibromyalgia and Chronic Pain*. London: Churchill Livingstone Elsevier; 2010:3–17.

52. Hoppmann, Richard A. Musculoskeletal problems of instrumental musicians. In: Sataloff RT, Brandfonbrener AG, Lederman RJ, eds. *Performing Arts Medicine*. 3rd ed. Science and Medicine; 2010:207–227.

53. Brandfonbrener A. The epidemiology and prevention of hand and wrist injuries in performing artists. *Hand Clin*. 1990;6(3):365–377.

54. Wynn Parry CB. Prevention of musician's hand problems. *Hand Clin*. 2003;19(2):317–324.

55. Warrington J. The hand therapist's contribution to the rehabilitation of the musician's hand. In: Winspur I, ed. *The Musician's Hand a Clinical Guide*. London: JP Medical Ltd; 2018:117–134.

56. Hofmann A, Grossbach M, Baur V, Hermsdorfer J, Altenmuller E. Musician's dystonia is highly task specific: no strong evidence for everyday fine motor deficits in patients. *Med Probl Perfom Art*. 2015:38–46.

57. Altenmuller A, Jabusch HC. Focal dystonia in musicians: phenomenology, pathophysiology, triggering factors, and treatment. *Med Probl Perfom Art*. 2010:3–9.

58. Altenmuller E, Ioannou CI, Lee A. Apollo's curse: neurological causes of motor impairments in musicians. *Prog Brain Res*. 2015;217:89–106.

59. Fahn S, Bressman SB, Marsden CD. Classification of dystonia. *Adv Neurol*. 1998;78:1–10.

60. Fahn S, Marsden CD, Calne DB. Classification and investigation of dystonia. In: Marsden CD, Fahn S, eds. *Movement Disorders 2*. London: Butterworth; 1987.

61. Fahn S. Concept and classification of dystonia. *Clin Nueropharmacol*. 1998;9(2):S37–S48.

62. Berardelli A, Rothwell JC, Hallett M, et al. The pathophysiology of primary dystonia. *Brain*. 1998;121:1195–1121.

63. Deuschl G, Hallett H. Focal dystonias: from occupational cramp to sensorimotor disease that can be treated. *Aktuel Neurol*. 1998;25:320–328.

63a. Altenmuller E, Lee A, Ioannou CI. Musician's dystonia. In: Winspur I, ed. *The Musician's Hand a Clinical Guide*. London: JP Medical Ltd; 2018:135–149.

64. Peterson DA, Berque P, Jabusch HC, et al. Rating scales for musicians' dystonia. *Neurology*. 2013;81:589–598.

65. Sadnicka A, Kassavetis P, Parees I, et al. Task-specific dystonia: pathophysiology and management. *J Neurol Neurosur Psychiatry*. 2016:1–7.

65a. Altenmüller E, Jabusch HC. Focal hand dystonia in musicians: phenomenology, etiology, and psychological trigger factors. *J Hand Ther*. 2009;22:144–154; quiz 55.

65b. Schmidt A, Jabusch HC, Altenmüller E, et al. Etiology of musician's dystonia: familial or environmental? *Neurology*. 2009;72:1248–1254.

65c. Lohmann K, Schmidt A, Schillert A, et al. Genome-wide association study in musician's dystonia: a risk variant at the arylsulfatase G locus? *Mov Disord*. 2014;29:921–927.

66. Karp BI, Cole RA, Cohen LG, et al. Long-term botulinum toxin treatment of focal hand dystonia. *Neurology*. 1994;44:70–76.

67. Byl N, Merzenich MM, Jenkins WM. A primate genesis model of focal dystonia and repetitive strain injury: I. Learning induced dedifferentiation of the representation of the hand in the primary somatosensory cortex in adult monkeys. *Neurology*. 1996;47:508–520.

68. Byl N, Wilson F, Merzenich MM, et al. Sensory dysfunction associated with repetitive strain injuries of tendonitis and focal hand dystonia: a comparative study. *J Orthop Sports Phys Ther*. 1996;23:234–244.

69. Byl NN, McKenzie A. Treatment effectiveness for patients with a history of repetitive hand use and focal hand dystonia: a planned, prospective follow-up study. *J Hand Ther*. 2000;13:289–299.

70. Byl NN, McKenzie A, Nagarajan SS. Differences in somatosensory hand organization in a healthy flutist and a flutist with focal hand dystonia: a case report. *J Hand Ther*. 2000;13:302–309.

71. Byl N, Topp KS. Focal hand dystonia. *Phys Ther Case Rep*. 1998;1:39–52.

72. Taub E, Miller NE, Novack TA, et al. Technique to improve chronic deficit after stroke. *Arch Phys Med Rehabil*. 1993;74:347–354.

73. Taub E, Uswatte G, Pidikiti R. Constraint-induced movement therapy: a new family of techniques with broad application to physical rehabilitation - a clinical review. *J Rehabil Res Dev*. 1999;36:1–21.

74. Candia V, Elbert T, Altenmüller E, et al. Constraint-induced movement therapy for focal hand dystonia in musicians. *Lancet*. 1999;353:42.

75. Candia V, Schafer T, Taub E, et al. Sensory motor retuning: a behavioural treatment for focal hand dystonia of pianists and guitarists. *Arch Phys Med Rehabil*. 2002;83:1342–1348.

76. Candia V, Wienbruch C, Elbert T, et al. Effective behavioural treatment of focal hand dystonia in musicians alters somatosensory cortical organisation. *Proceedings of the National Academy Science USA*. 2003.

77. Ramachandran VS, Hirstein W. The perception of phantom limbs. *Brain*. 1998;121:160–163.

78. Sakai N. Slow-down exercise for the treatment of focal hand dystonia in pianists. *Med Probl Perform Art*. 2006;21:25–28.

78a. Enke AM, Poskey GA. Neuromuscular re-education programs for musicians with focal hand dystonia—a systematic review. *Medical Problems of Performing Artists*. 2018;33(2):137–145.

79. Jankovic J, Shale H. Dystonia in musicians. *Semin Neurol*. 1989;9:131–135.

79a. Altenmuller E, Lee A, Ioannou C. Musician's Dystonia. In: Winspur I, ed. *The Musicians Hand a Clinical Guide*. London JP Medical Ltd; 2018:135–149.

80. Hallett M. Is dystonia a sensory disorder? *Ann Neurol*. 1995;38(2):139–140.

81. Lederman RJ. Focal dystonia in instrumentalists: clinical features. *Med Probl Perform Art*. 1991;6:132–136.

82. Jabusch HC. Epidemiology, phenomenology and therapy of musician's cramp. In: Altenmüller E, ed. *Music, Motor Control and the Brain*. Oxford: Oxford University Press; 2006.

83. Brandfonbrener AG. Musicians with focal dystonia: a report of 58 cases seen during a ten-year period at a performing arts medicine clinic. *Med Probl Perform Art*. 1995;10(4):121–127.

84a. Lim VK, Altenmüller E, Bradshaw JL. Focal dystonia: current theories. *Hum Movement Sci*. 2001;20:875–914.

84b. Poore GV. Clinical lecture on certain conditions of the hand and arm which interfere with the performances of professional acts, especially piano-playing. *Br Med J*. 1:441–444.

85. Nutt JG, Muenter MD, Melton IJ. Epidemiology of dystonia in Rochester, Minnesota. *Adv Neurol*. 1988;50:361–365.

86. Butler K, Rosenkranz K. Focal hand dystonia affecting musicians. Part 2: an overview of current rehabilitative treatment techniques. *Br J Hand Ther*. 2006;11(3):79–87.

87. Butler K, Sadnicka A, Freeman J, Anne-Marthe Meppelink et al. Sensory-Motor Rehabilitation Therapy for Task Specific Task Specific Dystonia: a Feasibility Study. *Hand Therapy*. 2018;23(2):53–63.

88. Butler K, Rosenkranz K, Freeman J. *Task Specific Dystonia – a Patients' Perspective*. In review.

89. Fry HJH. Overuse syndrome: a muscle biopsy study. *Lancet*. 1988;1:905.

90. Winspur I. Controversies surrounding "misuse", "overuse", and "repetition" in musicians. *Hand Clin*. 2003;19(2):325–329.

90a. Winspur I. The misuse syndrome. In: Winspur I, ed. *The Musician's Hand a Clinical Guide*. London: JP Medical Ltd; 2018:191–197.

91. Fry HJH. The treatment of overuse injury syndrome. *Md Med J*. 1993;42:277.

92. Fry HJH. Overuse syndrome of the upper limb in musicians. *Med J Aust*. 1986;144:182.

93. Fry HJH. Instrumental musicians showing technique impairment with painful overuse. *Md Med J*. 1992;41:899.

94. Norris RN. Overuse injuries. In: Torch D, ed. *The Musician's Survival Manual*. St Louis: ICSOM; 1993.

95. Winspur I. Nerve compression. In: Winspur I, ed. *The Musician's Hand a Clinical Guide*. London: JP Medical Ltd; 2018:71–88.

95a. Youl B. Nerve conduction testing. In: Winspur I, ed. *The Musician's Hand a Clinical Guide*. London: JP Medical Ltd; 2018:89–91.

96. Winspur I, Warrington J. The instrumentalists' arm and hand – surgery and rehabilitation. In: Sataloff RT, Brandfonbrener AG, Lederman RJ, eds. *Performing Arts Medicine*. 3rd ed. Science and Medicine; 2010:229–246.

97. Dawson WJ. Carpal tunnel syndrome in instrumentalists. *Med Probl Perf Art*. 1999;14:25.

98. Rempel D, Keir PJ, Smutz WP, Hargens A. Effect of fingertip loading on carpal tunnel pressure. *Trans Orthop Res Soc*. 1994;19:698.

98a. Butler K. Getting a grip. *International Piano Magazine*. 2019:66–67.

98b. Butler K. Preventing injuries in guitarists—part 4. *Acoustic Magazine*. 2011:76–78.

99. Apfelberg DB, Larson SJ. Dynamic anatomy of the ulnar nerve at the elbow. *Plast Reconstr Surg*. 1973;51:76.

100. Charness ME, Barbaro NM, Olney RK, Parry GJ. Occupational cubital tunnel syndrome in musicians. *Neurology*. 1987;37:115.

101. Charness ME. Unique upper extremity disorders in musicians. In: Kasdan M, ed. *Occupational Disorders of the Upper Extremity*. New York: Churchill Livingstone; 1992.

102. MacLean IC. Carpal tunnel syndrome and cubital tunnel syndrome: the electrodiagnostic viewpoint. *Med Probl Perform Art*. 1993;8:41.

103. Deleted in review.

104. Dellon AL, McKinnon SE. Radial sensory nerve entrapment in the forearm. *J Hand Surg [Am]*. 1986;11A:199.

105. Deleted in review.

106. Philipson L, Sorbye R, Larsson P, Kaladjev S. Muscular load levels in performing musicians as monitored by electromyography. *Med Probl Perform Art*. 1990;5:79.

107. Deleted in review.

108. Levy CE, Lee WA, Brandfonbrener AG. Electromyographic analysis of muscular activity in the upper extremity generated by supporting the violin with and without a shoulder rest. *Med Probl Perform Art*. 1992;7:103–109.

109. Bozentka DJ. Pathogenesis of osteoarthritis. In: Mackin EJ, Callahan AD, Skirven TM, Schneider LH, Osterman AL, eds. *Evaluation of the Hand and Upper Extremity*. 5th ed. St Louis: Mosby; 2002:1637–1645.

110. Alter S, Feldon P, Terrono AL. Pathomechanics of deformities in the arthritic hand and wrist. In: Mackin EJ, Callahan AD, Skirven TM, Schneider LH, Osterman AL, eds. *Evaluation of the Hand and Upper Extremity*. 5th ed. St Louis: Mosby; 2002:1545–1554.

111. Butler K, Svens B. A functional thumb metacarpal extension blocking splint. *J Hand Ther*. 2005;18(3):375–377.

112. Van Lede P. Minimalistic splint design: a rationale told in a personal style. *J Hand Ther*. 2002;15:192–201.

113. Deleted in review.

114. Deleted in review.

115. Norris RN. Clinical observations on the results of the 1991 National Flute Association survey. *Flutist Q*. 1996;21:77.

116. Hooper G, Pillet J. Instrument playing and severe hand deformity. In: Winspur I, ed. *The Musician's Hand: A Clinical Guide*. London: Martin Dunitz; 1998.

117. Fry HJH. Overuse syndrome in musicians 100 years ago: a historical review. *Med J Aust*. 1986;145:620.

118. Menuhin Y. *The Complete Violinist*. New York: Summit Books; 1986.

119. Tubiana R. Musicians' focal dystonia. In: Tubiana R, Amadio PC, eds. *Medical Problem of the Instrumentalist Musician*. 1st ed. London: Martin Dunitz; 2000:329–342.

120. Connolly C, Williamon A. Mental skills training. In: Williamon A, ed. *Musical Excellence Strategies and Techniques to Enhance Performance*. 1st ed. Oxford: Oxford University Press; 2004:221–245.

121. Caillet R. *Shoulder Pain*. 3rd ed. Philadelphia: FA Davis; 1990.

122. Winspur I. Surgical indications, planning and technique. In: Winspur I, ed. *The Musician's Hand a Clinical Guide*. London: JP Medical Ltd; 2018:93–103.

123. Amadio PC. The role of surgery. In: Tubiana R, Amadio PC, eds. *Medical Problems of the Instrumentalist Musician*. London: Martin Dunitz; 2000:421–431.

124. Butler K, Winspur I. Retrospective case review of time taken for 130 professional musicians to fully return to playing their instruments following hand surgery. *Hand Ther*. 2009;14:69–74.

118

Psychosocial Aspects of Arm Health

Carrie Barron, David Ring, Ana-Maria Vranceanu

OUTLINE

CRITICAL POINTS

- Symptoms and limitations arise in part due to pathophysiology and in part to mindset (thoughts and emotions) and circumstances.
- A substantial proportion of the variation in symptom intensity and magnitude of limitations is accounted for by stress (e.g., financial, job, housing, health, family), distress (e.g., symptoms of depression or anxiety), and less effective coping strategies (e.g., catastrophic thinking).
- Behavioral (e.g., avoidance), social (e.g., secondary gain), and cultural factors are also important.
- Medically unexplained symptoms (somatic symptom disorders) or abnormal weakness or movement (functional neurologic disorders) are common. One may also see self-inflicted problems (factitious disorders). These more extreme manifestations of normal human illness behavior help us understand our patients. Although it is not particularly useful to attempt to categorize patients, it is helpful to be aware that these psychosocial aspects of illness are encountered to some degree in every person.
- Treatment strategies that account for and address the psychosocial aspects of musculoskeletal illness (e.g., cognitive behavioral therapy) can help reduce symptom intensity and magnitude of limitations.
- Effective communication strategies and compassion bring out people's most effective coping strategies and enhance recovery. It is important to take care with what we say and how we say it.

INTRODUCTION

All human experiences, especially pain and injury, create thoughts and emotions. All experiences are psychological. Attention to the emotional, relational, and behavioral aspects of illness improves health.

Clinicians who attend to the emotional aspects of recovery have an advantage: the physical situation often improves when the psychosocial situation is addressed. A person's reaction to injury is as important as the injury itself to resiliency, recovery, satisfaction, and outcome. The hand specialist's insight into, and support of, the patient's subjective experience has a positive and meaningful impact on both parties.

In hand illness, the subjective does not correlate well with the objective. Psychological and sociological factors account for much of the variation in the degree of limitation and symptoms. For a clarification of terms, disease is objective pathophysiology and impairment (e.g., a stiff joint, and malaligned bone, diminished two-point discrimination).[1] Nociception is the stimulation of nerves that convey information about tissue damage to the brain. Pain is the subjective perception that results from nociception, filtered through a person's genetic makeup, physiological and psychological status, social milieu, and unique lens.

Health is determined by how a person and his or her social network perceive, respond to, and live with injury or disease.[2] The details in a patient narrative can reveal useful information about coping strategies, options for self-care, and ongoing health. The hand specialist can elicit the story with genuine interest and compassion, creating an open conversation. It is the quality of the conversation that matters, not the duration. Use a few choice words to convey technical expertise and have the patient do most of the talking.

Anticipating the psychology of illness in all forms of care decreases stigma. We should never lose site of the fact that all experiences have associated thoughts and feelings. When a patient asks, "Are you saying its all in my head?" it reflects stigma and the false mind–body dichotomy, and it often indicates that the patient has taken offense. Because hope is often pinned on an outward fix for a physical problem delivered by a powerful other, inward exploration may be grating. But disappointment and temporary despair in response to disease or injury are normal and expected.

We can all use a hand when facing a challenge. That challenge might morph into growth: an opportunity to uncover dormant strengths, new interests, and untapped talents. All clinicians can help with adaptation. Some people might fall into a deeper depression or stubbornly ineffective coping strategies that might benefit from stronger interventions and specific expertise from psychologists or social workers. There is a continuum with regard to adaptation, resiliency, and function in the face of impairment. Some people pick up and move on relatively easily, whereas others might be more caught in the conundrum of this change. Hand specialists are familiar with some of the psychosocial factors associated with arm pain. Secondary gain such as active litigation, disability claims, worker's compensation disputes, and opioid misuse disorder are familiar influences on illness. Symptoms of depression, less effective coping strategies such as catastrophic thinking, and symptoms of heightened illness concern (i.e., health anxiety or hypochondriasis) are also common and important, but hand specialists may not be as comfortable and familiar with these aspects of normal human illness behavior. It is helpful to become facile with them. Disproportionate symptoms and limitations with little or no objective impairment are often an expression of psychological angst or inner rancor.

DEPRESSION, CATASTROPHIC THINKING, AND HEALTH ANXIETY

Pain intensity and magnitude of limitations are influenced by catastrophic thinking, heightened illness concerns, and depressed feelings.[3] For instance, a person who tends to worry about minor matters may dwell on worst-case scenarios and tend to misinterpret symptoms. This "catastrophic thinking" involves a tendency to magnify, feel helpless about, and ruminate on the problem, the nociception in particular. Those with notable heightened illness concern may see a benign issue as a sign of serious pathology despite repeated assurances to the contrary. Symptoms of depression reflect a downward spiral. A person with substantial symptoms of depression may become self-critical ("It's my fault"), feel pessimistic ("Everything goes wrong"), or feel hopeless ("I will never get over this"). Pain may elicit or intensify symptoms of depression. Pain may also be the somatic manifestation of symptoms of depression.[4] Negative thinking increases symptoms and limitations.

There are questionnaires that quantify psychological phenomena. Symptoms of depression can be quantified with the Center for the Epidemiologic Study of Depression (CESD)[5] scale, the Beck Depression Inventory (BDI),[6] or the Depression Subscale of the Patient Health Questionnaire (PHQ).[7] These measures inquire about typical symptoms of depression, and they vary in terms of their emphasis on the somatic versus emotional and cognitive components of depression. Although major depression is a discrete diagnosis, these scales measure depressive traits or symptoms along their spectrum, all meriting attention.

The Pain Catastrophizing Scale (PCS)[8] is a 13-item measure of catastrophic thinking in response to nociception. It has three subscales: magnification (belief that pain will worsen), helplessness (a sense of impotence), and rumination (preoccupation with the pain). Catastrophic thinking is one of the strongest predictors of pain intensity and magnitude of limitations.

Health anxiety (hypochondriasis) can be assessed with the Health Anxiety Inventory,[9] Whitley Index,[10] and Somatic Symptoms Inventory (SSI).[11] The latter assesses the extent to which patients experience nausea, vomiting, hot or cold spells, heart pounding, heavy arms, and other bodily symptoms. The Health Anxiety Inventory and Whitley Index assess degree of worry about health and serious illness. Health anxiety seems particularly relevant in nonspecific, activity-related pains.[15]

Validated measures might facilitate the clinician's ability to address sensitive topics. Empathy and effective communication strategies gain trust and help people open up. Multidisciplinary teams including surgeon and nonsurgeon specialists, hand therapists, and social workers or behavioral medicine specialists are prepared to address all opportunities for helping people get and stay healthy.[12]

SECONDARY GAIN

Some circumstances—conscious or unconscious—make it beneficial to be ill. For instance, being ill can help with a legal dispute, lead to disability payments, or garner attention. This so-called secondary gain can increase symptoms and limitations.

Early psychodynamic theories described secondary gain as emotional conflict manifesting in psychosomatic pain. Current theories suggest that secondary gain is a learned behavior reinforced by environmental factors. For example, a doting spouse, job escape, or general sympathy can encourage the continuation of an illness state. Unconscious forces motivate the situation. It is not a deliberate manipulation of others. Deep down, attention may be so enticing that one holds on to the pain. If the safe and nurturing holding environment fills an unsatisfied need, it can be hard to relinquish, even if pain is the price.

Patients who feign sickness or exaggerate a condition to secure money or time off likely have a different character structure. Malingering is a conscious activity that can belie lack of conscience.

According to the social-learning theory model of pain, pain is paradoxically self-protective. If aid and sympathy are forthcoming, pain behavior is reinforced. The desire for nurture can lead to ongoing pain. Fordyce[13] argued that if secondary gains push pain past the normal healing period, the pain becomes persistent. Desirable consequences of pain might be sympathy, release from responsibilities, opioid prescriptions, and monetary compensation. But this can backfire. Anger and rejection ensue when family and friends get tired and frustrated. Taking on the patient's daily tasks, managing medical bureaucracy, and battles for benefits; seeing opioid misuse and dependency unfold; and dealing with side effects can deplete even the most altruistic caregiver. Genuine, skillful discussion of the consequences of secondary gain contributes to healing. It can circumvent persistent symptoms and limitations. Direct confrontation in the context of a trusting relationship can be useful for some. For others, a slower process allows a nondefensive acceptance, reckoning, and ultimate resilience.

PUZZLING OR DISPROPORTIONATE SYMPTOMS OR LIMITATIONS

Psychosocial factors are particularly important when a patient's problem is puzzling. Clinicians often see uncharacteristic, nonanatomical, or disproportionate symptoms. Inconclusive or contradictory examinations and diagnostic procedures are indicative of puzzling pain.[14,15] It is important to stay puzzled. Medically unexplained symptoms (somatic symptom disorder) and weakness or movement (functional neurologic disorder) are common. Self-inflicted problems are also seen (factitious disorder). It may not be helpful to try to categorize people, but it is helpful to recognize that these are aspects of normal human illness behavior encountered—to some extent—in each person we care for.

Immediate action with typical biomedical means can be counterproductive. Procedures and modalities may enter the mind as treatment options because they are our well-honed, reliable tools; it is what we do. We know the diagnostic criteria, and we apply them. Well versed in categories and formulas, we might not consider, "What else could this be?" Maybe whatever it is has not yet taken its place in the lexicon of knowable ailments. We can't place it.

For many people, especially eager and able problem solvers, being puzzled is uncomfortable. Wanting the person to fit a clear category with an established mode of action is natural. One may be tempted to dismiss confounding information in order to have the satisfaction of action. But the wrong action can have consequences for both the specialist and the patient. Complications, complaints, and even legal battles might follow. Taking a step back and embracing the liminal space is useful because it decreases risk and creates opportunity. If one cannot heal with steel, there are other options. Approaching illness from a biopsychosocial rather than a purely biomedical approach improves health and peace of mind. Curiosity, human connection, ease with uncertainty, conversation, and the elucidation of inner stress can help.

Puzzling hand and arm conditions reflect the interrelation between medical and psychological factors. In the next section, we discuss factitious disorders, in which medical symptoms are consciously produced, and somatization disorder, in which bodily symptoms express psychological conflict.

Factitious Disorders

Factitious disorders involve deliberately producing, feigning, or exaggerating symptoms. There is a motivation to assume the sick role for attention, not time or money.[16] Patients may go to surprising extremes. They hurt themselves to elicit symptoms or alter diagnostic tests (e.g., contaminating a urine sample) to acquire treatment or hospitalization. Factitious disorders can involve the self or another. A mother may subject a healthy child to contamination and painful treatments for attention, sympathy, and leniency—for herself. In the mind of the perpetrator, this intense emotional succor feels otherwise unobtainable.[17] Those with factitious disorders deny responsibility, which perpetuates the compulsion, even after being caught.[18] If they were able to own or experience their actions as harmful, they probably would not act. The drive for gratification can be so great that it blinds the mind and stifles conscience.

It is uncommon to meet a person with a full-blown factitious disorder, but elements of fabrication or exaggeration are common.[19] Specific named disorders in the hand realm include clenched fist disorder, factitious lymphedema, and Secrétan syndrome. But there are myriad ways to self-inflict or fabricate illness.

The factitious components are particularly challenging for hand specialists. As pragmatists, our style is to observe details, determine a diagnosis, and offer a straightforward treatment. If signs and symptoms do not make sense, whether they are consciously feigned or unconsciously driven, we are in a confounding dilemma. Stopping to consider the psyche helps. Learning what we can about the patient's inner state can lead to an answer. Our interest, curiosity, empathy, and rapport may do much to alleviate symptoms in some patients. Others with extensive needs might do well with the support of a behavioral health expert.

Clenched fist or finger syndrome is a condition in which the arm is healthy but one, a few, or all the fingers are in a flexed posture, often with the distal interphalangeal joints straight or even hyperextended. Often, the index finger and thumb are not involved, thereby allowing the patient useful hand function. Clenched fist syndrome is probably somewhere between a factitious disorder (conscious) and a functional neurologic disorder (unconscious).[20] The diagnosis can be confirmed by anesthetizing the patient and demonstrating much more limited fixed contracture. A variation on this theme is a stiff index finger that will not bend except under anesthesia.

Unexplained swelling of the hand or arm may be a result of surreptitious application of a tourniquet. Popular apparatuses include ACE bandages, sphygmomanometer cuffs, rubber bands, or pieces of string. Placing the extremity in a cast that makes it impossible to apply a tourniquet usually allows the swelling to subside. The swelling that accompanies factitious lymphedema (caused by intermittent application of a tourniquet) usually has a broken windowpane pattern of collateral lymphatic circulation distal to the site of tourniquet obstruction. Ruptured lymph channels caused by recurrent lymph stasis and direct constriction may also appear. The size and distribution of the lymphatics are normal, and there is no abnormality of the lymph nodes.[21]

Hand specialists will encounter self-inflicted wounds such as self-cutting, cigarette burns, stab wounds, subcutaneous injection of feces and substances, and even bite wounds. Clinicians must discriminate between the deliberate self-inflicted wound and the accidental one in patients with other types of mental problems such as a hand that is damaged by accidental intraarterial injection by a drug addict.

When distress is expressed by self-cutting, there may be dozens or even hundreds of lacerations or scars on the forearms and hands. The lacerations usually involve only the epidermis but occasionally are deeper. Self-cutting is common in patients with borderline personality disorder and is usually conceptualized as means of coping with intense psychological pain as well as need for attention.[16]

Secrétan syndrome (also known as peritendinous fibrosis or posttraumatic hard edema) is a condition caused by the patient repeatedly striking the dorsum of the hand with a blunt object or against a blunt object, causing diffuse swelling. The origin may be secondary gain or as a conversion reaction and is best treated with nonoperative care and psychiatric counseling.[22]

People with factitious disorder often have a history of multiple illnesses, treatments, and operations. They may go from one medical facility to the next seeking interventions. They may know more about their proposed ailment than the consulting physician. Satisfaction is derived from manipulating the clinician. If discovered, they are not daunted because the intense drive for attention causes them to continue the façade. Patients with multiple carpal tunnel operations may represent a variant of this condition.

Somatic Symptom Disorders

These disorders involve physical symptoms that appear to be a medical condition, but the symptoms are not fully explained by pathophysiology.[16] Prevalence rates are as high as 97% in some cohorts of people with persistent low back pain in an inpatient rehabilitation setting.[23]

The symptoms are not a function of an underlying medical condition, or, when a medical condition is present, symptoms are in excess of what is normally expected from the interview, examination, or laboratory findings.[16] The process of somatization is conceptualized as the focusing of attention on internal stimuli and development of sensory amplification[11] along with denial of psychological or interpersonal difficulties,[24] resulting in an increase in somatic symptoms that remain partly or completely unexplained by objective disease processes.

Illness anxiety disorder (formerly referred to as hypochondriasis) represents a preoccupation with fears of having or the idea that one has a serious disease based on a misinterpretation of bodily symptoms. This preoccupation persists despite appropriate medical evaluation and reassurance, and it causes notable distress or impairment in social or occupational function.[16] Although few patients meet the full criteria for the diagnosis of illness anxiety disorder, exaggerated concern about a medical or perceived medical condition is common. Pain is concerning, but most people are able to put their worries to rest with reassurance. Others are difficult to soothe, and they continue to believe that the clinicians "missed something." There is evidence that health anxiety is an important contributor to persistent pain.[25]

Functional Neurologic Disorders

Formerly known as conversion disorder, functional neurologic disorders are abnormalities of numbness, strength, or movement that are unexplained by pathophysiology. An example is nonepileptic seizures. These are recognized somatic expressions of psychological distress. Patients with unexplained hand weakness or posturing may have elements of functional neurologic disorder.

Applying these Concepts to Upper Limb Problems

There are several diagnoses used by hand specialists that have minimal or no objective, verifiable pathology and may represent somatic symptom disorders or functional neurologic disorders. Biopsychosocial approaches may provide the most effective treatment of these conditions.

Repetitive strain injury, writer's cramp, and focal dystonia are biomedical labels for medically unexplained, activity-related symptoms and signs. In the absence of identifiable pathophysiology, it is possible that these labels might represent social constructions (i.e., things that exist in a society because the members of that society agree to behave as if it exists). The shared phenomenon may reflect a leaning of the collective unconscious or cultural intuition, the need to contain an anxiety or uncertainty via naming, or a tendency to turn an expectable inconvenience into a catastrophe in a stressful situation.

Other upper limb pain conditions with little or no objectively verifiable pathophysiology might prove to be biomedical social constructions for what are actually somatic symptom disorders include radial tunnel and pronator syndromes; electrophysiologically normal thoracic outlet, carpal tunnel, and cubital tunnel syndromes; dynamic scapholunate instability; and occult dorsal ganglion. These conditions are similar to other nonspecific medical conditions such as the commonly comorbid fibromyalgia and chronic fatigue syndrome.

Persistent nonspecific arm pain correlates with symptoms of depression and health anxiety and is associated with less effective coping strategies such as catastrophic thinking. Although hand specialists recognize this, they may not have protocols in place for addressing these psychosocial phenomena. They may be uncomfortable with affects and emotions or even fear them. Patients can become angry at the idea of psychological causes and say, "I am in pain, and you are saying it is all in my head!" This is a tense or even wrenching moment for both parties. Hand specialists benefit from developing a way to help patients receive the idea that the mind–body connection impacts all conditions and human beings. It does not mean that one is psychologically impaired.

Considering both medical and psychological factors helps patients get and stay healthy. One can avoid unnecessary medical procedures, alleviate psychological distress, and enhance quality of life. Medical labels may serve the patient's need to have a physical rather than the psychosocial explanation of their illness.[11,26,27] Although such a label avoids dreaded stigmatization, the benefit is short lived. Administration of tests and procedures reinforce a "sick role" and do not address core issues or true etiologies. Although the process may be complex and seemingly intangible, acceptance and adaptation are possible for many people. This approach breeds personal resiliency—better mood and stronger body, even if it is a different body. Capacity, peace of mind, pride, and hope result from interventions that elicit a patient's inner healer—his or her form of personal resiliency.

Complex regional pain syndrome (CRPS) is another puzzling condition that may be best conceptualized as part somatic symptom disorder and part functional neurologic disorder.[28] Lack of understanding of basic pathophysiology, and disagreement on definition and diagnostic criteria add to the confusion.[29] The most recent definition and diagnostic criteria are vague (thereby allowing for overdiagnosis) and internally inconsistent (it is arguable that criterion 4 [not otherwise explainable] is never met).[29] Disuse, with or without injury, can create the other symptoms and signs of this disorder. And the disuse correlates with catastrophic thinking.[30,31]

It is possible that CRPS is a biomedical social construction that attempts to explain the expected physical manifestations of common psychosocial aspects of human illness behavior.[29]

THE PSYCHOLOGY OF THE CLINICIAN

The clinician's experience, habits, beliefs, attitudes, cultural norms, and social leanings influence diagnostic and treatment recommendations.[32,33] Discomfort with psychological phenomena, a hypertrophied belief in one's own knowledge and technical abilities, and even well-intentioned etiquette can interfere with effective intervention.[34] We may fear insulting the patient or being a target of her or his anger.

Although a healthy confidence accompanies expertise, overzealous self-esteem can cause one to miss important clues. One common assumption is that psychosocial issues will resolve when the physical ailment is addressed. But caution is warranted because this mindset risks missed diagnosis or undertreatment of important opportunities for improved mood or more effective coping strategies. In other words, the reverse concept—that treatment of the psychosocial aspects of illness may adequately reduce symptoms and limitations—is also true. One is also at risk of misdiagnosis of patient preferences given that the psychosocial aspects of illness can reinforce misconceptions that lead patients to choose options that are not consistent with their values.[35,36]

Health providers often use intuition, experience, and comfortable habits rather than evidence to guide practice.[37] Humans invented the scientific method to decrease errors of judgment. The belief that intense pain is strongly associated with more severe pathology is erroneous and even dangerous. It is important to catch compartment syndrome and necrotizing fasciitis, but unnecessary invasive and risky treatments may lead to iatrogenic harm and even litigation. Medical and surgical interventions can ultimately worsen illness, in part by medicalizing it (reinforcing the tendency to think passively and seek treatments from powerful others rather than adapting to changes and uncertainty by cultivating resiliency), even if they often achieve a transient placebo effect (indirect activation of innate mechanisms such as endorphins and prompting of resiliency).[38]

Specialists often have the perspective that everything is fixable, as do many patients. Although this may create optimism or cement a sense of mastery in both the patient and doctor, it can backfire. It is important to be honest about the diagnostic and therapeutic limits of modern medicine while remaining supportive and hopeful.

Another pitfall is a paternalistic decision-making process. An exploration of subjective experience allows patients to express the inner life, be heard, and feel valued, which are inherently soothing. Integration of the patient's values and preferences into the treatment approach seeds trust, compliance, respect, and satisfaction with care. Finding a way to draw upon the physician's expertise and ability to enlighten while honoring the values of the patient is an art of medicine.[39]

Although we may be proud of our knowledge, sometimes facts, logic, data, or evidence will not move patients with fixed mindsets. It is best to try to meet them where they are. This can create greater receptivity as well as rapport. Denial of modern medicine's limits; desire to please via prescriptions, surgeries, or injections; and difficulty with managing psychological factors can compromise health.

Often, it is only after several ineffective interventions and surgeries that patients are referred for psychological treatment. This can feel like failure for both parties. Gently addressing psychological phenomena from the get-go can circumvent problems. Frame it with the idea that all human experiences are psychological—we all have feelings, stressors, and a unique mind–body connection.

It is true that some personalities are more challenging than others. Some people have an inner condition wherein they do not feel satisfied or cared for no matter what they are provided. It can be a challenge to inform a person with high rancor or low satisfaction that a procedure is not suitable or ethical to offer. It would behoove specialists to develop methods of management for frustrated gratifications in the name of medical ethics.

If hand specialists look beyond mechanical causes and cures for symptoms and limitations and address psychosocial phenomena, they are more empowered. It can help to communicate clearly, empathically, genuinely, and confidently that psychosocial factors and mind–body interplay impact us all. Another useful intervention is to convey that you are standing with the patient. Communicating "we" will find the best path for "you" is powerful.

THE PSYCHOLOGY OF THE PATIENT

People are not passive responders to physical sensations. Rather, we seek to make sense of experience. We appraise our condition by matching sensations to personal cognitive schemas based on our past experience and present knowledge base.

Some people are more able than others to shift positions in the face of objective facts. Rather than cognitive fusion (thoughts are facts), there is cognitive flexibility.[40] The way we understand our condition determines whether a sensation is seen as evidence of a concerning disorder or a discomfort that can be moved to the background. Our experience of injury is always tied to our uniquely constructed reality—the story that we tell ourselves.

When information is ambiguous, people rely on attitudes and beliefs conjured by past experiences, current information, personal culture, or input from family and friends. Time spent on the personal story is well spent as sorting through subjectivities is key for pain intensity and disability.[41,42]

Pain that is interpreted as ongoing tissue damage when it is actually a condition that will improve (e.g., enthesopathy), an age-related change that is adaptable (e.g., arthritis), or even a healthy part of the healing process (e.g., a stretching exercise) leads to greater symptoms and limitations. Patients who believe that their pain will forever hinder achievement of their goals may take a fatalistic, passive approach to their health. Cognitive factors impact illness in two interrelated ways: (1) they influence mood and coping efforts, and (2) they affect physiological activity associated with pain, such as muscle tension[43] and production of endogenous chemicals.[44]

Self-efficacy, or the belief in one's ability to successfully achieve a desired outcome, is a cognitive factor strongly associated with less pain and fewer limitations. Compromised self-efficacy belies a common set of cognitive errors that affect pain intensity, affective distress, and magnitude of limitations.[45,46] A cognitive error is a negatively distorted belief about oneself or one's situation. The most common cognitive errors in patients limited by pain are catastrophic thinking (rumination, magnification and helplessness), overgeneralization (assumption that current issues will apply to future events), personalization (feeling that the event is imbued with personal meaning or responsibility), and selective abstractions (selectively attending to negative aspects of an experience).

The effectiveness of automatic coping strategies and feelings of hope and confidence vary among individuals. Studies have found that those that keep to their routine despite pain and those that find distractions and ways to put pain in the background are better able to adapt. Their active coping strategies move them forward. Passive coping strategies, such as excessive dependence on others and on external treatments and overly restricted activity, lead to even greater pain intensity and symptoms of depression.[47]

The affective component of pain includes many different emotions, but they are primarily negative in quality. Substantial symptoms of depression often accompany substantial limitations due to pain.[48] Negative thinking, low self-efficacy, and high health anxiety can result from and reinforce symptoms of depression. Posttraumatic stress disorder can develop in people with pain triggered by traumatic injuries.

Frustrations from persistence of symptoms, unknown etiology, treatment failures, worker's compensation nongratification, dwindling finances, and fractured family relations can breed anger. Anger affects pain via increased arousal mechanisms, which interferes with pain acceptance and treatment adherence.

Anxiety about harm engenders avoidance of movement, which then exacerbates pain. Uncertainty, misperception of danger, and physiological changes triggered by a fight-or-flight response are common when people experience pain. These too, are associated with more severe limitations and greater pain intensity.[49] Movers heal faster! The belief that one can continue to function despite pain protects against troubling psychological states, and it can be fostered in the clinical encounter with sensitive communication.

The patient's experience of illness and health care providers is influenced by prior experience and social and cultural transmission of beliefs across generations. Ethnic and gender differences have an impact. Positive outcomes may be more possible if the physician explores how a particular family, community, or cultural belief system is operating in a given patient. For example, children respond to care, providers, symptoms, and injury based on their parents, culture, and social environment. These influences determine whether they will be fearful, measured, hopeful, or self-efficacious in the face of symptoms.

Pain behaviors affect experience with pain, pain intensity, disability, and persistence. Behaviors that are reinforced are maintained, and those that are not reinforced are stopped.[13] Grimaces to communicate pain or holding an arm to avoid additional pain are often maintained if reinforced by a doting spouse or health care provider. Too much empathy or coddling can backfire, even if well intended. Escape from pain through the use of drugs, excess rest, avoidance of undesirable activities, or work may offer immediate gratification but undermine health in the long run.

"Movers heal faster" warrants repeating. It is a mantra that people can use to counteract the stories their minds tell that reinforces maladaptive coping strategies. Avoidance of activity can reinforce and perpetuate persistent pain. In acute pain, reducing an activity may, on occasion, accelerate the healing process. However, getting stuck in this habit can lead to anticipatory anxiety about pain and muscle tension via fight-or-flight responses, which may serve as conditioned stimuli for pain (i.e., after healing ends, pain persists). A downward spiral sets in. More and more activities are seen as aversive and are avoided, contributing to deconditioning. Persistent avoidance of activities also prevents disconfirmation of the predicted pain. The opportunity to learn that pain does not imply permanent damage, disability, or defect is repeatedly lost. Anxiety exacerbates fear, avoidance, and assumption of the worst. Some anxiety is healthy, but too little or too much can cause problems. Pain avoidance preserves the belief that activity will cause pain and further injury and prevents the corrective experience of moving, which ultimately reclassifies pain and increases function.

There are subtle yet potent factors that impact the pain experience. The Internet and media can offer erroneous information that might reinforce maladaptive beliefs about symptoms, tests, and treatments. By reinforcing the idea that maintaining youth or having no discomfort is desirable, people are drawn into purchases or procedures that can create a persistent anxious mindset or a never-ending quest for the ideal. Accepting normal age-related changes and incomplete healing processes associated with pain can lead to greater inner peace. Media can interfere with good care by encouraging patients to choose doctors who overpromise and underperform but supply immediate gratification rather than supporting a healthier process that involves delayed gratification, adaptation, and resilience.

WORKING WITH OTHER EXPERTS

Teams that include both psychosocial and biomedical expertise are useful for the most common nonspecific pain conditions such as backache and headache[50-52] and for discrete painful conditions such as arthritis.[53] In addition to surgeons, nonoperative specialists, and hand therapists, a complete hand care team would also include psychologists or social workers. For some complex conditions, it might also be helpful to have health promoters or navigators (people who help patients understand what they need to do to get well and coordinate the efforts needed). The role of each provider depends on each individual's opportunities and preferences.

Some hand and arm diseases are poorly understood and not completely treatable (e.g., arthritis, advanced peripheral neuropathies). There are also several illnesses with no measurable pathophysiology. Adapting to uncertainty, discomfort, and limitations is difficult. It is even more difficult in the face of stress, distress, and less effective coping strategies. Although this might seem like common sense, hand specialists have been slow to implement multidisciplinary treatment teams or become facile with psychological phenomena.

Science supports the critical role of psychologists—and strategies based on psychology—in the treatment of pain.[54] Governing bodies such as The Joint Commission, the Commission on the Accreditation of Rehabilitation Facilities, and several professional organizations (American Pain Society, American Academy of Neurology) suggest that the psychologist's role is underappreciated and seen as potentially offensive. The key is effective communication strategies to increase the appeal of attention to mental and emotional health.

When all aspects of the patient's story and situation are understood and addressed, people get better. They feel more resilient, able, and hopeful. High-quality care requires our patients to be proactive, savvy, inquisitive, and communicative. Even if a healing process involves pain, a sense of empowerment increases when people have agency. Part of care is to protect and encourage this agency, self-efficacy, independence, and can-do, whatever alteration has ensued, whatever the new circumstances may be. Multidisciplinary teams benefit from developing effective communication strategies and working to uncover each patient's form of personal resilience.

Research shows that the first visit to an orthopedics department is a strong predictor of the course of illness in pain patients.[55] Unnecessary tests or procedures or overinterpretation of test results is not advisable, although it can be tempting to seek objective data or to be able to name a problem or assign a cause. Incidental or age-related findings that do not correspond with the symptoms usually do not benefit from a specific diagnosis or diagnostic and therapeutic interventions. Reinforce how the patient can speed up recovery by getting back into his or her routine even if it is uncomfortable, finding ways to stay hopeful and engaging in mood-enhancing activities from conversation to listening to music to watching favorite movies.

Because of the interrelation between physical and psychosocial factors in the manifestation of disease, many patients benefit from meeting with a behavioral medicine specialist for a brief consult. This serves to elicit and reinforce effective coping skills. Misconceptions about pain and medical treatments are prevalent, and a short conversation about these issues is often enough to place the patient on a healthy path. Based on the initial evaluation, some patients may continue to meet with a behavioral medicine specialist. Others may be equipped for coping on their own. If a treatment plan and set of goals are put in place at the end of the first visit, along with a list of written recommendations, recovery can begin.

PATIENT ACTIVATION

Research suggests that patient participation in decision making results in greater patient satisfaction, improved outcomes, and acceptance and adherence to treatments.[56-58] Decision making involves at least two participants—the clinician and the patient. It also can involve family members, relatives, friends, and multiple health providers.[59] This makes for a layered process. Processing and parsing out the multiple perspectives are important. The plethora can confuse or tax the patient and treatment team. For example, a specialist's advice that remaining active in painful activities is advisable may run counter to the primary care provider's recommendation to rest. Different opinions will arise. The patient's confusion and uncertainty can be alleviated by coordination of the providers and an enlightening discussion that elucidates and prioritizes his or her own values as well as the best-known course of treatment.

All parties, from clinicians to patient to family members, participate in the process of ensuring that preferences coincide with values. Research shows that patient comfort with sharing opinions and participating in the decision-making process varies. Level of assertion depends on personality style, contextual factors, social desirability, and cohort effects.[60] The importance of developing a rapport and using communication strategies that encourage the patient to become comfortable sharing, inquiring, and opining cannot be overstated. Disclosing preferences and asking questions about culture, family, and intuition allows for informed assessment of treatment alternatives and choices. This is an emotional process and an exploration as opposed to just an information transfer. In the shared-decision model, collaboration and open exchange result in a decision based on insight, enlightenment, and personal values.

Patients may bring in information from acquaintances, media, and other health providers. The provider brings sincere interest in helping the patient and an informed idea about the best course of treatment. The patient and the health care provider both bring values and subjectivities. The physician's self-awareness of biases, strengths, flaws, and draws is useful. Such insight holds us in check or allow us to go forth in ways that best serve the patient while taking care of ourselves. By acting in accordance with what we can do best while honoring a personal code of ethics, all win.

After a processing of information and leanings, parties agree on a plan. The decision may be to engage in treatment plan pronto. It may be to suspend a decision or to agree to disagree. The patient might seek other health opinions. Agreement may not mean that both parties are sure that this is the best treatment—only that both parties endorse implementation. The health provider, for example, may believe that a patient should delay surgery until he or she is feeling less vulnerable or until time for natural healing has passed. Yet he or she may accept the patient's decision to proceed with surgery as part of a negotiation. The patient is informed that the there are risks, such as persistent symptoms, or that time might be a better healer, but the patient's preferences are honored. Unless a physician believes this, he or she cannot do the procedure in good conscience. The shared decision-making model differs from the paternalistic and informed models. In these, responsibility for the decision lays with the health provider or patient, respectively, whether or not the other accepts the decision.

EFFECTIVE COMMUNICATION STRATEGIES

Helping patients identify their preferences based on their values rather than misconceptions, adhere to best current evidence, and find work on optimal mindset appealing depend on a strong relationship with the hand specialist. The key to a trusting relationship is effective communication strategies. Health providers whose communication styles are more collaborative (less dominant) receive higher satisfaction ratings than health providers who communicate in a paternalistic or authoritative manner.[58]

Health providers should be mindful of biases, both their own and those of the patient. Patients and clinicians have theories about what is best, based perhaps on evidence or on reports from colleagues, family, friends, or the media. Both providers and patients may experience *self-serving bias*, or information that disproves one's beliefs is dismissed and information that is consistent with a belief is prioritized. For example, Sue views pain as a sign of damage. She may not be able to accept that she can experience pain with an intact elbow. She may repeatedly say or assume that her elbow hurts and she can't, won't, or shan't use it, or it will deteriorate. Her inner narrative, history, and subjectivities dictate her "truth." This narrative is so powerful that it can cause Sue to dismiss, deny, and refute expert advice and even facts. Clinging to or repeating a familiar tale can provide psychological comfort even if it interferes with good health. If the health provider is staunch in his or her own message and does not empathize with Sue or judges or even shows frustration or disdain, disharmony can unfold. Such conflict can keep Sue from becoming open to more adaptive ways to understand her situation.

Even if you are an expert, you still have to contend with resistances in the patient. These resistances are there for a reason, even though the reason may be unclear or seem unfounded. Logic and expertise may not be as effective as acknowledging a person's thoughts and emotions. Just listen to the story and nod without agreeing, disagreeing, or assessing. This makes it easier to convey what you want to convey in the end. It may seem paradoxical that honoring what seems irrational creates receptivity for a "rational" intervention. Sensitive communication involves effective use of pauses, silence, and nonverbal communication in addition to thoughtful and practiced word choice.

Words with relatively negative connotations, such as "tear," "injury," or "overuse," are more likely to adhere in a mind than words with a positive connotation.[61] When clinicians use the word "tear" to refer to the expected developments of aging, there may be inadvertent reinforcement of misconceptions and maladaptive strategies. Instead, use truthful words with a positive message. Avoiding medicalization of pain conditions that are a part of normal human development whether permanent (e.g., arthritis) or temporary (lateral epicondylitis) is useful. Clarification that many conditions are genetic and developmental and not the result of "overuse" or "injury" can relieve guilt, regret, or self-blame. "I did something wrong. I caused this. If only . . ." creates a debilitating inner dialogue.

The key elements of good communication are trust, empathy, and confidence in the health care provider.[62] Clinicians can make efforts to listen, grasp, and appreciate. Clinician allies may be more helpful than experts and technicians whose unexpected advice may sometimes feel adversarial. Skillful listening serves as treatment. Listen without interruption at the beginning, summarize the patient's statements with his or her own words, legitimize the patient's concerns by restating them, and express empathy ("This must be difficult for you" or "Wow, you certainly withstood a lot").[63] Normalize the situation ("I have seen this often. Most people in your situation react the same way, but it passes"). Instead of making assumptions about what the patient would like you to do, offer options and elicit preferences. Before addressing divergences between best evidence and patient preconceptions, heightened illness concern, misconceptions, or catastrophic thinking, make a "deposit in the patient's emotional bank account." Gain trust and confidence. Foster a reciprocal human connection before introducing information that could create contention and discomfort.

Patients like to know that their hand specialist has expertise. The clinician's confidence in his or her skills can impact the patient's confidence and trust. Share that you have treated similar patients. Give a good explanation of symptoms. Relay the shortcomings of diagnostic and treatment strategies. The clinician who instills hope creates empowerment. Instead of "I don't know what's going on" or "I have nothing to offer you," try "Let's make sure we understand your situation as best we can. I am going to ask you several questions. Even if we cannot answer all of them, we will learn a whole lot more about what we can do and which possibilities are best for you" or "We have helped many patients like you, and with our whole team involved, we feel confident that we can help you, too."

Awareness of the stigmatization of the psychological and sociological aspects of illness is useful. There are delicate ways to introduce the idea that much of the pain could be from stress: "Who wouldn't be stressed? It makes complete sense that you have pain. So many people express stress in the body. Of course, you are not mentally ill! I do not know anyone who could not use support some of the time or all of the time. We have a great person here who can help you sort out this and that if you want. Up to you. It could really help. People seem to really like spending time with him." Good communications skills require an emphasis on positive truths.

Choice of words and the way in which they are delivered influences whether people accept, adhere, and have a good treatment outcome. Patients fare better if their provider is committed, energized, respectful, and real. The ability to celebrate gains (even small ones) does much. Sit down, even if it is only for a few minutes, maintain eye contact, and convey warmth. Return calls. Compassion and professional integrity in the first visit may be the strongest therapeutic agent. But things do not always go well.

Interactions with patients who have prominent psychosocial issues can be frustrating. Sad or anxious patients are one thing, but hostile, angry, accusing, and vengeful patients are another. You may have provided what you thought was a very compassionate and professional treatment only to find out that a complaint was registered. Some people are measured, and others feel easily violated. In other words, it could be you, but hopefully, it is not you if you take a rigorous self-inventory now and again to understand your triggers. If you have to explain yourself or apologize in what feels like a senseless accusation, tension, guardedness, and even a diminished sense of calling can take hold. People with alcohol and drug concerns, patients who have had negative interactions with providers in the past, and patients with limited financial resources (particularly in high-stress situations) can be difficult. Managing the physician–patient relationship well can help. Usually listening and trying to understand the patient diminishes stress and frustration, but sometimes people are provoked by what they perceive as scripted empathy or imagined neglect. If you do not offer what they were seeking, you may be experienced as abandoning them. Lowering one's voice in response to a patient with an aggressive voice, listening attentively with no interruptions, and not becoming defensive can help. Do not get into a battle of wills. Sometimes you have to set a boundary: "With all due respect, Mrs. ———, I very much want to help you, but it appears that our conversation is not moving in a useful direction. I can refer you to this person, but other than what I offered you, which is in line with my ethics and experience, I am not sure we can do much more here."

Requesting permission to examine or warning of coming discomforts demonstrates respect: "This part of the examination can be painful, but it is very important. May I proceed?" Most often, your natural empathy will serve you well: "Can we discuss some of the things that are making you feel uneasy?" Your desire to enlighten posed as a question is also likely to enhance the encounter: "Would you like to hear some of the advantages and disadvantages associated with the test or procedure?"

Cooper and others[64,65] provide suggestions for how to navigate communication in which patients resist participation in the shared-decision model. In this situation, the health provider must refrain from acting as an expert telling the patient what to do. Communication requires a two-way conversation. A statement such as: "You should do these exercises" may lead to defensiveness in patients, whereas an open question such as: "What can you do today that, in your experience, will make it better?" may help the patient think about her or his condition in a different way. Taking responsibility for recovery engenders the self-efficacy that is so useful for mood and progress. For instance, say, "Even a few minutes of exercise will help" rather than, "It's going to be hard to make time for all these exercises." There may be less resistance to a future visit with "You may be ready to try new exercises next week" rather than "We have to add these new exercises right now, or you will deteriorate." Use statements such as, "You know your hand; show me what feels okay for you" rather than "I will teach you how to treat your hand." Such approaches reinforce the patient's resilience, independence, self-esteem, and self-mastery.

Offering options may also work well with difficult or resistant patients. For example, instead of "You have to exercise 5 repetitions 5 times a day," try "Some people prefer to do 5 reps 5 times a day; others do 3 reps 10 times a days. You can see what works best for you. Your body will tell you. Or you can see what suits on a given day." The patient benefits from taking control of the healing process, with the physician's support and encouragement. A statement such as "It can be extremely helpful to elevate your arm" is better than "I need you to elevate your arm."

Remarks that help the patient envision him- or herself in a vitalized, capacious position may increase confidence and motivation. Imagination and visualization are powerful tools. A statement such as "You still can't hold a golf club. I really don't know when you will" with a shaking head is negative, whereas "In the future, when you hold your golf club . . ." encourages, empowers, and enlivens. Build trust and confidence to instill motivation and confidence. You might say, "I'm going to have you start with this exercise and do 10 repetitions. How does that sound to you?" This conveys your confidence while respecting the patient's view and valuing her or his way of doing things. Curiosity is a form of caring. Flexibility in your approach makes room for theirs. However, denying or diminishing your knowledge base, expertise, or experience is not natural, nor does it put the patient at ease. Your delivery can convey humility, curiosity, concern, and a wish to find a way for and with the patient while preserving your identity as an expert.

ASSESSMENT AND TREATMENT

Pain can trigger "worst-case" thoughts with consequent rumination, magnification, and helplessness; health anxiety (intense worry about pain and health that is resistant to reassurance); fear avoidance (avoidance of activities that cause pain for fear of reinjury or causing more damage); and affective reactions that include frustration, irritability, anger, depression, and anxiety. If the negative thoughts persist, distress and disability, as well as physiological arousal may continue despite resolution of all or most of the nociception—a persistent pain syndrome.[66]

Cognitive behavioral therapy (CBT) is a well-researched, scientific treatment approach that specifies how thoughts (beliefs, attitudes), behaviors, feelings, and sensations are interrelated. The key element of CBT and its derivatives is identification of a patient's thoughts when they are experiencing pain—thoughts that create avoidance, emotional distress, and greater physical symptoms. Identifying a person's specific and unique negative automatic thoughts about pain and medical treatments is the crux of successful CBT. Helping patients understand mind and body interplays and overcome stigma and skepticism to see how the treatment can help them is part of the process.

Delivering CBT in an orthopedic practice allows intervention early in the experience of pain, which is known to help prevent transition to persistent pain, saves patient resources and time, facilitates communication and planning, limits long wait times or lost motivation to seek care, and may improve the outcome.

Most patients presenting to a hand specialist will correct maladaptive cognitions and resolve emotions with time and compassionate care, particularly if the specialists have incorporated psychological expertise and effective communication strategies into their care. But having formal CBT immediately available is useful for patients that need additional help.

SUMMARY

Psychosocial factors present important opportunities to improve and maintain musculoskeletal health. Hand specialists can learn effective communication strategies and take care to understand and optimize mental health. Psychologists and social workers that join the team will need to understand the medicine well enough to confidently recognize unhelpful cognitive errors. Comprehensive biopsychosocial treatment is more effective than traditional biomedical treatment and may lead to a better use of resources, decreased limitations, and increased comfort and quality of life.

REFERENCES

1. Mechanic D. Illness behavior. An overview. In: McHugh S, Valis TM, eds. *Illness Behavior: A Multidisciplinary Model.* New York: Plenum Press; 1986:101–110.
2. Turk DC, Monarch E. Biopsychosocial perspective on chronic pain. In: Gatchel DTR, ed. *Psychological Approaches to Pain Management.* New York, London: Guilford Press; 1999.
3. Pincus T, Burton K, Vogel S, Field AP. A systematic review of psychological factors as predictors of chronicity/disability in prospective cohorts of low back pain. *Spine.* 2002;27:109–120.
4. Dersch J, Mayer T, Theodore BR, et al. Do psychiatric disorders first appear preinjury or postinjury in chronic disabling occupational spinal disorders? *Spine.* 2007;32:1045–1051.
5. Radloff LS. The CES-D scale: a self-report depression scale for research in the general population. *Appl Psychol Meas.* 1977;1(3):385–401.
6. Beck AT, Mendelson M, Mock J, Erbaugh J. An inventory for measuring depression. *Gen Psychiatry.* 1961;4:561–571.
7. Spitzer RL, Kroenke K, Williams JB. Validation and utility of a self-report version of PRIME-MD: the PHQ primary care study. *JAMA.* 1999;10:1737–1744.
8. Sullivan MJL, Bishop S, Pivik J. The pain catastrophizing scale: development and validation. *Psychol Assess.* 1995;7:524–532.
9. Salkovskis RK, Warwick HMC, Clark DC. The health anxiety inventory: development and validation of scales for the measurement of health anxiety and hypochondriasis. *Psychol Med.* 1978;32:843–853.
10. Pilovsky J. Dimensions of hypochondriasis. *Br J Psychiatry.* 1967;113:89–93.

11. Barsky AJ, Klerman GL. Psychiatric comorbidity in DSM-III-R hypochondriasis. *Arch Gen Psychiatry.* 1992;49:101–118.

12. Jensen MP. Correlates of improvement in multidisciplinary treatments for chronic pain. *J Consult Clin Psychol.* 1994;62:172–179.

13. Fordyce WE. *Behavioral Methods for Chronic Pain and Illness.* St Louis: Mosby; 1967.

14. Ring D, Kadzielsky J, Malhotra L, et al. Psychological factors in idiopathic arm pain. *J Bone Joint Surg Am.* 2005;87:374–380.

15. Vranceanu AM, Safren S, Ring D. Psychiatric illness predicts disability and idiopathic arm pain. *Clin Orthop Relat Res.* 2008;466(11):2820–2826.

16. American Psychiatric Association. *Diagnostic and Statistical Manual of Mental Disorders.* 5th ed. 2013. Washington, DC.

17. Eisendrath SJ. Factitious illness: a clarification. *Psychosomatics.* 1984;25(2):110–113.

18. Johnson RK. Psychological evaluation of hand pain. In: Kasdan ML, ed. *Occupational Hand and Upper Extremity Injuries and Diseases.* 2nd ed. Philadelphia: Hanley & Belfus; 1998.

19. Guziec L, Harding M. Case of a 29-year-old nurse with factitious disorder: the utility of psychiatric intervention on a general medical floor. *Gen Hosp Psych.* 1994;16(1):47–53.

20. Zeineh W, Seidenstricker M. The clenched fist syndrome revisited. *Plast Reconstr Surg.* 2008;121(3):149e–150e.

21. Smith RJ. Factitious lymphedema of the hand. *J Bone Joint Surg Am.* 1975;57(1):89–94.

22. Moretta DN, Cooley JR. Secretan's disease: a unique case report and literature review. *Am J Orthop.* 2002;31:524–527.

23. Polatin PB, Kinney RK, Gatchel RJ, et al. Psychiatric illness and chronic low back pain. *Spine.* 1993;18:66–67.

24. Osterweis M, Kleinman N, Mechanic D. *Pain and Disability. Clinical, Behavioral, and Public Policy Perspectives.* Washington, DC: National Academy Press; 1987.

25. Hadjistavropoulos HD, Hadjistavropoulos T. The relevance of health anxiety to chronic pain: research findings and recommendations for assessment and treatment. *Curr Pain Headache Rep.* 2003;7:98–104.

26. Szabo RM, King KJ. Repetitive strain injury. Diagnosis or self-fulfilling prophecy. *J Bone Joint Surg Am.* 2000;82:1314–1322.

27. Hadler NM. Fibromyalgia and the medicalization of misery. *J Rheumatol.* 2003;30:1668–1670.

28. Nelson DV, Novy DM. Psychological characteristics of reflex sympathetic dystrophy versus myofascial pain syndromes. *Reg Anesth.* 1996;21:202–208.

29. Ring D, Barth R, Barsky A. Evidence-based medicine: disproportionate pain and disability. *J Hand Surg Am.* 2010;35(8):1345–1347. https://doi.org/10.1016/j.jhsa.2010.06.007. PubMed PMID: 20684932.

30. Teunis T, Bot AG, Thornton ER, Ring D. Catastrophic thinking is associated with finger stiffness after distal radius fracture surgery. *J Orthop Trauma.* 2015;29(10):e414–e420. https://doi.org/10.1097/BOT.0000000000000342. PubMed PMID: 25866942.

31. Roh YH, Lee BK, Noh JH, Oh JH, Gong HS, Baek GH. Effect of anxiety and catastrophic pain ideation on early recovery after surgery for distal radius fractures. *J Hand Surg Am.* 2014 November;39(11):2258–64. e2. doi:10.1016/j.jhsa.2014.08.007. Epub 2014 Oct 3. PubMed PMID: 25283489.

32. Teunis T, Janssen S, Guitton TG, Ring D, Parisien R. Do orthopaedic surgeons acknowledge uncertainty? *Clin Orthop Relat Res.* 2016 June;474(6):1360–1369. https://doi.10.1007/s11999-015-4623-0. Epub 2015 Nov 9. Erratum in: Clin Orthop Relat Res. 2016 Jun;474(6):1530-1. PubMed PMID: 26552806; PubMed Central PMCID: PMC4868176.

33. Janssen SJ, Teunis T, Guitton TG, Ring D. Science of Variation Group. Do surgeons treat their patients like they would treat themselves?. *Clin Orthop Relat Res.* 2015;473(11):3564–3572. https://doi.org/10.1007/s11999-015-4304-z. PubMed PMID: 25957212; PubMed Central PMCID: PMC4586191.

34. Vranceanu AM, Beks RB, Guitton TG, Janssen SJ, Ring D. How do orthopaedic surgeons address psychological aspects of illness? *Arch Bone Jt Surg.* 2017;5(1):2–9. PubMed PMID: 28271080; PubMed Central PMCID: PMC5339350.

35. van Hoorn BT, Wilkens SC, Ring D. Gradual onset diseases: misperception of disease onset. *J Hand Surg Am.* 2017;42(12):971–977.e1. https://doi.org/10.1016/j.jhsa.2017.07.021. Epub 2017 Sep 9. PubMed PMID: 28899587.

36. Mallette P, Zhao M, Zurakowski D, Ring D. Muscle atrophy at diagnosis of carpal and cubital tunnel syndrome. *J Hand Surg Am.* 2007;32(6):855–858. PubMed PMID: 17606066.

37. Hageman MG, Guitton TG, Ring D. Science of Variation Group. How surgeons make decisions when the evidence is inconclusive. *J Hand Surg Am.* 2013;38(6):1202–1208. https://doi.org/10.1016/j.jhsa.2013.02.032. Epub 2013 May 4. PubMed PMID: 23647639.

38. Kaptchuk TJ, Miller FG. Placebo effects in medicine. *N Engl J Med.* 2015;373(1):8–9. https://doi.org/10.1056/NEJMp1504023. PubMed PMID: 26132938.

39. Vranceanu AM, Cooper C, Ring D. Integrating patient values into evidence-based practice: effective communication for shared decision-making. *Hand Clin.* 2009;25(1):83–96, vii. https://doi.org/10.1016/j.hcl.2008.09.003. PubMed PMID: 19232919.

40. Özkan S, Zale EL, Ring D, Vranceanu AM. Associations between pain catastrophizing and cognitive fusion in relation to pain and upper extremity function among hand and upper extremity surgery patients. *Ann Behav Med.* 2017;51(4):547–554. https://doi.org/10.1007/s12160-017-9877-1. PubMed PMID: 28213633.

41. DeGood DE, Tait R. Assessment of pain beliefs and pain coping. In: Turk DC, Melzak R, eds. *Handbook of Pain Assessment.* 2nd ed. New York: Guilford Press; 2001:320–345.

42. Jensen MP, Turner J, Romano JM, Karoly P. Coping with chronic pain: a critical review of the literature. *Pain.* 1991;47:249–283.

43. Flor H, Turk DC, Birbaumer N. Assessment of stress related psychophysiological responses in chronic pain patients. *J Consult Clin Psychol.* 1985;35:354–364.

44. Bandura OL, Taylor CB, Gauthier J, Gossard D. Catecholamine secretion as a function of perceived coping self-efficacy. *J Consult Clin Psychol.* 1987;53:406–414.

45. Smith TW, Follick MJ, Ahern DK. Cognitive distortion and psychological distress in chronic low back pain. *J Consult Clin Psychol.* 1986;54:573–575.

46. Smith TW, Milano RA, Ward JR. Helplessness and depression in rheumatoid arthritis. *Health Psychol.* 1990;9:377–389.

47. Lawson K, Reesor KA, Keefe FJ, Turner JA. Dimensions of pain-related cognitive coping: cross-validation of the factor structure of the Coping Strategy Questionnaire. *Pain.* 1990;43(2):195–204.

48. Turner JA. Coping and chronic pain. In: Bond MR, Woolf CJ, eds. *Proceedings of the Sixth World Congress on Pain.* Amsterdam: Elsevier; 1985:219–227.

49. Vlaeyen JWS, Kole-Snijder A, Boeren RGB, van Eek H. Fear of movement/(re)injury in chronic low back pain and its relation to behavioral preference. *Pain.* 1995;62:363–372.

50. Bruce BK, Townsend C, Hooten WM, et al. Chronic pain rehabilitation in chronic headache disorders. *Curr Neurol Neurosci Rep.* 2008;8(2):94–99.

51. Flor H, Fydrich T, Turk DC. Efficacy of multidisciplinary pain treatment centers: a meta-analytic review. *Pain.* 1992;49:221–230.

52. Gatchel RJ, Okifuji A. Evidence-based scientific data documenting the treatment and cost-effectiveness of comprehensive pain programs for chronic non-malignant pain. *J Pain.* 2006;7:779–793.

53. Keefe FJ, Williams DA, Gil KM, et al. Pain coping skills training in the management of osteoarthritic knee pain: a comparative study. *Behav Ther.* 1990;21:49–62.

54. Simon E, Folen RA. The role of the psychologist on the multidisciplinary pain management team. *Prof Psychol Res Pr.* 2001;32(2):125–134.

55. Malmivaara A, Hakkinen U. The treatment of acute low back pain—bed rest, exercises, or ordinary activity? *N Engl J Med.* 1995;332(6):351–355.

56. Gwyn R, Elwyn G. When is a shared decision not (quite) a shared decision? Negotiating preferences in a general practice encounter. *Soc Sci Med.* 1999;49(4):437–447.

57. Elwyn G, Hood K, Robling M, et al. Achieving involvement: process outcomes from a cluster randomized trial of shared decision making skills development and use of risk communication aids in general practice. *Fam Pract.* 1991;21(4):337–346.

58. Kaplan SH, Greenfield S, Gandek B, et al. Characteristics of physicians with participatory decision-making styles. *Ann Int Med.* 1996;124(5):497–504.

59. Charles C, Gainy A, Whelan T. Decision-making in the physician-patient encounter: revisiting the shared treatment decision-making model. *Soc Sci Med*. 1999;49:651–661.

60. Strull WM, Lo B, Charles G. Do patients participate in medical decision making? *JAMA*. 1984;152:2990.

61. Lang E, Koch T, Berbaum K, et al. Can words hurt? Patient-provider interactions during invasive procedures. *Pain*. 2005;114(1,2):303–309.

62. Schofield NG, Green C, Creed F. Communication skills of health-care professionals working in oncology—can they be improved? *Eur J Oncol Nurs*. 2008;12(1):4–13.

63. Branch WT, Malik T. Using windows of opportunity in brief interviews to understand patient concerns. *JAMA*. 1993;269:1667–1668.

64. Cooper C, Graff WS, Evarts JL. Psychological techniques to promote patient participation. *Paper Presented at: American Society of Hand Therapists' Annual Meeting, 2007; Phoenix, AZ.*

65. Rosen S. *My Voice Will Go with You: The teaching Tales of Milton H. Erickson*. New York: Plenum Press; 1982.

66. Sharp TJ. Chronic pain: a reformulation of the cognitive-behavioral model. *Behav Res Ther*. 2001;39:787–800.

119

The Injured Worker: Onsite Evaluation and Services

Susan A. Emerson, Denise Finch

OUTLINE

CRITICAL POINTS

The cause of musculoskeletal disorders is most commonly thought to be multifactorial and can relate to:
- Exposure to occupational risk factors
- Exposure to nonoccupational risk factors
- Personal risk factors

Job hazard risk factors and use of risk assessment tools:
- Provide a means to identify and quantify physical risk factor exposure at work.
- Enhance knowledge regarding risk factors; this can be used to teach clients about how to reduce or avoid exposures in work and home activities.
- Can inform interventions in the clinic and modifications for return to work and reinjury prevention.

Job analysis may assist the physician and employer with accurate and comprehensive information:

- To identify and quantify essential functions, including physical job demands
- That may be helpful for structuring treatment, job modifications, and return to work

Work injury management is a:
- Coordinated effort between providers as well as the employer, workers' compensation agents, and the employee, which is critical for positive stay-at-work or return-to-work outcomes.

Ergonomics
- Ergonomic principles focus on designing work, tools, and spaces considering human capacities and limitations.
- Ergonomic concepts combined with clinical evaluation provide opportunities to maximize work capacities and minimize injury or reinjury.

INTRODUCTION

Work-related upper extremity musculoskeletal disorders (UEMSDs) may be referred to as "cumulative injuries or disorders," "overuse syndrome," "repetitive injuries," or "repetitive strain injuries."[1] Practitioners working with clients experiencing UEMSDs engage in the clinical reasoning process to evaluate the tissue pathology or disorder, select interventions and outcome measures, and identify expected outcomes for their clients. Inherent to this process is an understanding of factors that may contribute to the musculoskeletal disorder (MSD).[2] Along with a thorough clinical examination of the injured tissue and functional impairments, further inquiry may include:
- Identifying exposure to occupational and nonoccupational risk factors of force, repetition, posture, static posture, contact stress, vibration, or cold temperature

- Identifying work methods or psychosocial risk factors (job satisfaction, job stress, job control) in the workplace that may increase the risk of injury
- Identifying evidence related to type of work, industry, or non–work-related activity, and incidence of specific MSDs. For example, does the client work in an environment with higher incidences of MSDs such as heavy construction or manufacturing?[3] Or does the person engage in nonoccupational tasks such as sports or hobbies that result in exposure to physical risk factors?
- Clarifying the frequency of performance of the work or other activity, task-specific physical demands, and duration of performance
- Identifying personal risk factors related to age, obesity, arthritis, diabetes, and so on
- Understanding the physical environment to allow informed suggestions for ergonomic adjustments

MUSCULOSKELETAL DISORDERS

Musculoskeletal disorders are generally described as injuries or conditions that involve structures of the musculoskeletal system of the body such as tendons, bones, muscles, ligaments, nerves, discs, and blood vessels. Common diagnoses include muscle strains or sprains, carpal tunnel syndrome (CTS), lateral or medial epicondylitis, and rotator cuff tendinitis.[4,5] See Box 119.1 for more examples. MSDs may be classified as occupationally or nonoccupationally related based on the suspected source of injury. However, there is disagreement on the degree of importance of various risk factors as well as the potential impact and interaction of occupational and nonoccupational risk factors.[6] Furthermore, the determination of work relatedness is complicated with both medical and legal contributions. Although the etiology of MSDs is considered to be multifactorial,[6,7] determining whether it is predominately occupationally or nonoccupationally related influences which insurance system (workers' compensation vs personal health insurance) will assume responsibility for payment of necessary treatment.

The dilemma of determining the contribution of personal risk factors versus the work-related risk exposure and its impact on care and benefits after an injury is illustrated by the following scenario. A 45-year old woman who is obese and has diabetes presents at your clinic with symptoms of CTS. You are reviewing the evidence and find that in a sample of approximately 3000 workers in the United States, CTS was associated with age older than 35 years, female gender, obesity, prior upper extremity disorder, recreational hand use, and other medical conditions such as diabetes.[8] However, her work involves high hand force and long-duration exposure to the combined risk factors of force and repetition, which are known work-related risk factors for CTS.[9,10] Furthermore, although the Bureau of Labor Statistics (BLS) states that MSDs are considered work related if "an event or exposure in the work environment either caused or contributed to the resulting condition or significantly aggravated a preexisting injury or illness,"[5] each US state further defines the threshold of what constitutes a work-related injury as part of the workers' compensation legislation or rules.[11] These definitions are significant because if injury is determined to be work related, the worker may be entitled to benefits through the workers' compensation system, possibly including lifetime medical care related to the injury or compensation for functional loss. This is in contrast to primary health care insurance, which may pay for only some therapeutic interventions but not provide compensation for any long-term loss of function or capacity to work.

For therapy practitioners, the challenge of understanding the cause is often related to identifying the most effective interventions and expected outcomes. For example, if the injury is related to a physical risk factor at work, reducing exposure to that risk should improve symptoms. If the injury is suspected to be related to a movement pattern such as a bent wrist during a tennis swing that creates an eccentric contraction of wrist extensors that are now on stretch, changing the method of holding the racket may be critical to recovery and reinjury prevention.

Regardless of the cause, MSDs result in more disability and absenteeism than any other group of diseases[12] and impact productivity, and personal, social, and economic activities. A wide variety of data are available regarding MSDs and upper extremity disorders. For example, Murray and coworkers[13] reported that MSDs (exclusive of low back strain) were one of 30 diseases or illnesses that contributed to health loss in the United States. They also reported that MSDs were one of the top 10 disease or illness categories that increased more than 30% from 1990 to 2010. Of further note, musculoskeletal conditions (including fractures, strains, and sprains) affected one of every two people or 54% of the US adult population in 2012, and rotator cuff tears were found in 22% of the general population older than 65 years old.[14] More specific to work related injuries, nearly 350,000 workers in the United States in 2014 experienced upper extremity MSDs.[15] Approximately 40% of those cases were hand injuries, the highest percentage among upper extremity injuries. In fact, injuries and illnesses related to the shoulder resulted in more days out of work than any other upper extremity disorders, with a median of 26 days out of work.[15] In Washington state, workers' compensation data demonstrated that approximately 50% of MSDs were upper extremity related.[3] Of these, high rates of hand injuries were noted in management of companies or enterprises, finance and insurance, information and professional, scientific, and technical service work categories.

Additional data regarding incidence rates for work related upper extremity MSDs in the United States can be found in BLS data sources, state databases, and workers' compensation insurance claim data. Data specific to types or frequency of injury in various work environments are also available on the BLS website, as well as through database searches, systematic reviews, and epidemiologic analyses.

Work-Related Musculoskeletal Disorders

As of 2011, the BLS defined work-related musculoskeletal disorders (WRMSDs) by specific diagnoses, along with exposure-related terminology: "musculoskeletal system and connective tissue diseases and disorders, when the event or exposure leading to the injury or illness is overexertion and bodily reaction, unspecified; overexertion involving outside sources; repetitive motion involving microtasks; other and multiple exertions or bodily reactions; and rubbed, abraded, or jarred by vibration."[5] Whereas the first part of the BLS definition focuses on diagnosis-related conditions, the second portion describes events and exposures that may contribute to the cause of the disorder. The term "overexertion" implies that the actions exceed body capacities in some way. "Repetitive motion involving micro-tasks" implies joint motion or muscular use in a specific repeated task cycle. These distinctions become significant to define, identify, categorize, and consider the impact of task related physical risk factors to the specific MSD.

Common physical risk factors can be found in Box 119.2. These risk factors have been identified through a number of epidemiologic studies that have investigated the relationship of various job task requirements (e.g., repetition, force, posture) with the development of adverse medical conditions such as MSDs in work populations. The National Institute of Occupational Safety and Health (NIOSH) conducted a major review of epidemiologic evidence generated between 1970 and 1997 to analyze the associations between physical risk factors and the development of WRMSDs.[16] The results of this review are available in the publication titled, "Critical Review of Epidemiological Evidence for Work-Related Musculoskeletal Disorders of the Neck, Upper Extremity and Back." The evidence of work relatedness was classified as "strong," "evidence for," "insufficient," or "no effect." Strong evidence was defined as "a causal relationship is very likely between

---

BOX 119.2 Occupational Physical Risk Factors Related to Upper Extremity Musculoskeletal Disorders[6,16]

- Forceful exertions
- Awkward or extreme postures
- Sustained exertions or postures
- Repetitive exertions
- Contact stress
- Low temperatures
- Vibration

BOX 119.3 Upper Extremity Musculoskeletal Disorders and Risk Factors: Evidence Summary (Partial) by the National Institute of Occupational Safety and Health, 1997[16]

- Neck and shoulder: strong evidence associating posture; moderate evidence related to repetition and force.
- Shoulder: moderate evidence associating posture and repetition; insufficient evidence related to force and vibration.
- Elbow: strong evidence related to combination of repetition, force, and posture; moderate evidence related to force; insufficient evidence related to repetition and posture.
- Hand and wrist, carpal tunnel syndrome: strong evidence related to combination of risk factors; moderate evidence related to repetition, force and vibration; insufficient evidence for relationship to posture.
- Hand and wrist, tendinitis: strong evidence for combination of risk factors; moderate evidence for relationship to repetition, force, and posture.

BOX 119.4 Occupational and Nonoccupational Risk Factor Summary for Carpal Tunnel Syndrome Based on Melhorn and Coauthors,[6] Review of Literature from 1997 to 2014

Occupational risk factors for CTS:
- Very strong evidence for:
  - Forceful work
  - Combination of risk factors such as force and repetition or force and posture
  - Highly repetitive work or in combination with other factors
- Conflicting evidence for highly repetitive work alone
- Insufficient evidence
  - Keyboarding activities
  - Length of employment
- Low or some evidence
  - Job satisfaction
  - Vibration

Nonoccupational risk factors for CTS:
- Very strong evidence
  - Age: risk increases with age
  - High BMI increases risk
  - Female gender increases risk
  - Biopsychosocial factors
  - Diabetes
  - Comorbidity: history UEMSDs, inflammatory arthritis, thyroid disease, diabetes
  - Genetics
- Some evidence
  - Carpal tunnel or wrist size
- Nonoccupational activities such as gardening or knitting

BMI, Body mass index; *CTS,* carpal tunnel syndrome; *UEMSD,* upper extremity musculoskeletal disorder.

---

intense and/or long duration exposure to a specific risk factor . . . a positive relationship has been observed between exposure to the risk factor and the MSD in at least several studies in which the chance, bias, and confounding could be ruled out with reasonable confidence" (p. xii). "Evidence for" or moderate work relatedness was described as "some convincing epidemiologic evidence exists for causal relationship using the epidemiologic criteria of causality for intense and/or long duration exposure to a specific risk factor" (p. xii). Understanding that "intense and/or long duration exposure" was listed as a qualifier in most cases, some of the major findings are summarized in Box 119.3. If considering the evidence from this review to determine the association between work tasks, risks factors and MSDs, the reader must be aware of study design issues common to these types of epidemiologic studies, including inconsistent description or measurement of risk factors (e.g., repetition, force or posture), misclassification of diagnoses or inconsistent diagnostic criteria, use of reported symptoms as diagnosis, lack of control groups, lack of generalizability of data collected for a specific work population or setting, sample size, and confounding modifiers such as age or other disease such as diabetes.[16,17]

More recently, the *AMA Guides to the Evaluation of Disease and Injury Causation,* by Melhorn and coworkers[6] compiled and reviewed the literature generated from 1997 through 2014 regarding UEMSDs and their relationship to occupational and nonoccupational risk factors. This resource provides summaries of the evidence relative to specific diagnoses including ganglions, de Quervain's disease, painful elbow, CTS, and other upper extremity nerve compressions, as well as shoulder tendinopathy, impingement, and rotator cuff tears. These results, along with the 1997 NIOSH findings and more recent study findings, can be used to inform practice. For example, Box 119.4 summarizes the findings of Melhorn and colleagues[5] regarding occupational and nonoccupational risk and CTS, including a determination that there is insufficient evidence to associate keyboarding with CTS. Mediouni[18] further reported that keyboarding did not have a strong association with the development of CTS. Rempel[9] concluded that nonoccupational risk factors for CTS must also be considered in conjunction with job-related physical risk factors. When treating clients who have CTS or other UEMSDs, this information helps us to understand possible exposures, plan corrective actions, and optimize treatment outcomes.

Defining Risk Factors

Risk factors are environmental, behavioral, or biological attributes or experiences to which exposure increases the probability that disease or disorder will occur and if absent or removed decreases that probability.[6,19] Although MSDs may be associated with work and nonwork activities (sports, hobbies, home maintenance), work-related MSD injuries are typically viewed as a dynamic interaction among employee, equipment, product and components, tools, and work motions.[20] If a temporal relationship exists between the onset of symptoms and exposure to occupational risk factors, it is possible but not certain that the exposure could contribute to the development of the WRMSD.[21] Exposure can also "bring out" symptoms of a condition but not be fully responsible for the development of a condition.[6] For example, if an employee reaches overhead to activate a switch and feels a pop in his shoulder and a rotator cuff tear is diagnosed, the process of reaching did not cause degeneration of the tissue, but it may be considered a terminal event. With many MSDs, it would be unusual that exposure to a single risk factor over time would be sufficient cause of the development of most MSDs unless the exposure is extreme.[21,22] Much of the research in WRMSD development has identified that exposure to multiple risk factors results in a higher probability for the development of injury[9,23] or disease, and in most cases, the exposure must be more than random or occasional,[1,19,24] or it would be considered traumatic, not cumulative.

Although there is agreement that understanding the job and quantity of exposure to associated risk is important in determining the contribution of work-related exposure to the development of MSDs, there is no standard method to achieve this assessment.[25,26] Furthermore, caution is advised when considering injury risk based on a descriptive job title or even a single task. A thorough and objective work task evaluation or risk assessment that provides qualification of posture, force and frequency, and duration of exposure relative to the most current evidence can prove most useful. The detailed information that is used to examine the potential for occupational risk contribution assists in directing the patient and employer in how to reduce risk factors to prevent or to help optimize recovery if injury has occurred.

Personal Risk Factors

Common personal risk factors or issues that affect individual susceptibility include age, body mass, sex, genetics, metabolic disorders such as rheumatoid arthritis, diabetes, thyroid disease, smoking, body mass index, conditioning, psychosocial issues, and general health condition.[27-29] Personal risk factors may affect the individual's ability to tolerate and recover from exposure to nonoccupational and occupational risk factors. Several studies have demonstrated a high association between the incidence of various MSDs and personal risk factors,[9,30,31] leading to the conclusion that personal risk must be considered and addressed relative to the development of MSDs.

Nonoccupational Risk Factors

Exposure to physical risk factors can occur through a variety of nonoccupational activities such as participation in sports activities[19,23,32]; performance of home tasks and hobbies such as cleaning or gardening[33]; and use of handheld devices such as tablets, laptops, and cell phones.[34] In addition, studies have shown a prevalence of upper limb and neck pain and disorders in the general population, as high as 50%, without a known or identified cause.[35] Discussing nonoccupational and personal risk factors with the patient is helpful to ensure that treatment concepts address these risk exposures along with work-related exposures to optimize recovery.

Occupational Risk Factors

Occupational risk factors most commonly associated with work-related UEMSDs are listed in Box 119.4. With exposure to occupational and nonoccupational risk factors, soft tissue may be stressed and experience fatigue failure[26] and if unable to adequately recover from that stress, injury to the tissue may occur.[19] Researchers have suggested that muscle fatigue increases the possibility of inflammation, microtrauma, and compensatory motion patterns or postures that may contribute to an imbalance of the body's ability to accommodate to the stress or trauma and repair the tissue.[22,36] Rodgers'[22] work provides an understanding of the interactions among effort intensity, continuous effort time and frequency of effort,[12] and potential contribution to muscle fatigue. Tissue fatigue and MSD risk was also addressed by Gallagher and associates,[26] who completed a literature review on the interaction of force and repetition and concluded that the rate of tendon damage was directly related to the level of loading. Although low force loading may be tolerated over thousands of cycles, when high force was applied to a tendon,

damage to tissue was quite quick and predictably inevitable. Force levels less than 30% of maximum strength, even applied with high rates of repetition, were not expected to result in anything more than minor damage to tissue. The authors also pointed out that awkward or extreme postures may result in increased exertion and thus a decrease in the tolerance for repetitive performance of the motion. Although the specific amount of time needed for recovery is not well identified, it is clear that exposure to tasks that combine high repetition with high force requires increased rest time between exertions over the course of a shift to allow tissue recovery and prevent injury.

Additional considerations relative to exposure include total duration of task performance, frequency of exposure, exposure to environmental heat and cold, specific work methods, and temporal relationship to the time of symptom onset. Psychosocial job components are also important to consider and might include work organization, job pace, job control, and job satisfaction. For example, Thiese and associates[37] found strong associations between job related physical risk factors such as repetition and force and multiple psychosocial factors.

Understanding the definitions of the various types of risk factors and their potential contribution to UEMSDs improves the therapist's capacity to help the patient and other stakeholders consider opportunities to reduce or prevent risk exposure. The next section provides additional details regarding physical risk factors.

Awkward Postures

The range of motion (ROM) available at the joints of the upper extremity provides adaptability to allow limb positioning for function. Without full ROM, the ability to position the arm and hand and manipulate objects is altered or limited. However, if any joint in the upper quarter is used at an extreme or non-neutral position too frequently, with high force, or for too long a period of time, tensile or compressive forces may be exerted on soft tissues surrounding the joint, and injury may occur.[26] Gallagher and associates[26] also note that frictional stress from tendons sliding against adjacent structures can stimulate an inflammatory process and that some awkward postures may decrease blood flow, increase pressure around the tissue, or result in increased force requirement for the task performed. Although risk may be associated with positions at the extreme range available to a given joint, awkward or end-range postures are not always high risk. For example, movement out of the position of concern may provide adequate tissue recovery time to prevent a deleterious effect. In addition, the end range for the distal interphalangeal joint is full extension but is considered a "safe" position for that joint, as is work with the shoulder in 0 to 20 degrees of flexion.[37] Examples of tasks involving awkward postures are shown in Figure 119.1.

Postures that result in stress to soft tissue passing over a joint or stressful muscular contractions can also contribute to risk. Muscle fatigue occurs when gravity impacts joint position and muscle contraction is needed to maintain that position. For example, reaching forward to 90 degrees of shoulder flexion without arm support requires 10% of shoulder muscle strength.[1] Using forceful hand grip to hold a tool with the wrist in flexion and typing with the wrist in extension are examples of positions that decrease muscle efficiency and may lead to potential injury if the function occurs with sufficient frequency or for prolonged duration.

To capture postural and movement components, work can be systematically observed, photographed, and videotaped[8] to document the awkward position, movement patterns, and speed of motion when employees perform a work task. Goniometers are used to measure the exact joint position and the frequency of the motion can be determined by counting the number of repetitions at the joint of concern within each work cycle performed per unit time. Specific definitions of threshold postures by joint have been defined and are outlined on Table 119.1 (see risk factors and definitions row).

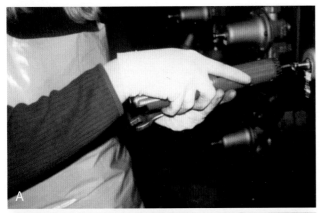

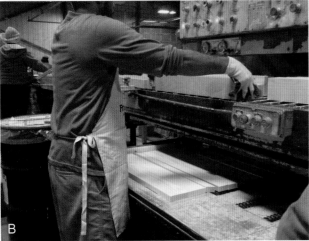

Fig. 119.1 Awkward postures. **A,** Horizontal use of an inline tool. **B,** Awkward reach for parts.

Static or Sustained Postures

When a body part maintains the same posture through the work cycle for prolonged periods of time without movement, the posture may be considered static or sustained. Terms such as *static effort, static posture, isometric contraction,* and *static exertion* may be used to describe this risk.[1] Static postures are of particular concern if the employee is not able to change the posture during work performance. Examples include sustained grip to hold a tool or part for machine operation or sustained shoulder flexion needed to reach a keyboard that is too far away from the torso as shown in Figure 119.2. Static postures can result in a buildup of lactic acid and decreased oxygen to the muscle. If the posture occurs frequently and without periods of time when the muscle relaxes to no activity or zero effort for 1 to 10 minutes,[1,22] tissue recovery from the stress of sustaining the posture may not occur. If there is force associated with the posture such as holding the weight of an object that is not supported[24] or holding the shoulder in more than 20 degrees of abduction or flexion without support, the tolerance for the position may be decreased.[37,38] The higher the required force to maintain the posture, the lower the time the posture will be tolerated. The variability of these issues may directly affect the concern and risk for injury.[1]

Evaluation of static postures using photographs helps to document the position of the employee while performing the task. Actual measurement of the joint position on the worker or from photographs can provide more specific information. Determination of the time spent in the sustained posture with use of a stopwatch during live or videotaped work performance identifies the duration of exposure to the posture. The number of times the joint moves into the static position per work cycle can be determined to quantify actual exposure and recovery time. For example, if a machine operator produces 100 parts per shift, must reach with 45 degrees of shoulder flexion into the machine to remove a part, and must reach again to place the next part into the machine, 45 degrees of shoulder flexion occurs 200 times per shift, or 26.6 times per hour in a 7.5-hour working shift. If the time spent in the machine to place or remove the part is 1 second, the employee spends 3.3 minutes per shift in 45 degrees of shoulder flexion. This quantification helps to accurately describe the exposure to the position of concern rather than relying on the perceived duration and frequency per the employee, supervisor, or employer. Alternately, an employee at a computer workstation where the keyboard is high and too far away may spend most of the 7.5-hour shift in 45 degrees of static shoulder flexion with the arm weight supported on the table, requiring constant activation of the upper trapezius muscles and parascapular muscle stretch. The latter position can be described as sustained shoulder flexion of 45 degrees for more than 6 hours per shift or 80% of the shift. By contrast, the machine operator spends less than 1% of the shift reaching into a machine.

Force

The exertion required to move or handle an object can be called "force." Force may occur as an external action or motion as when moving an object (Fig. 119.3A) or an internal action as when a force is applied to tissue (Fig. 119.3B), also described as contact stress.[1] In either case, if the force exceeds the ability of the involved tissue to accommodate, an injury may occur. Hagberg and associates[1] suggest that chronic tendon compromise may be related to permanent deformation of the structure, fraying from mechanical overuse, synovial shearing, or nutritional compromise. The critical dose exposure or exact tolerance to these loads is not known, although laboratory studies have demonstrated that biological changes in animal models occur with force application over time.[39,40] However, a definitive translation of laboratory data to industrial exposure has not been made.

When evaluating external force in job analysis, it is important to distinguish between the weight of an object and the force to move it. Often and ideally, an employer provides systems and equipment to assist the worker so that the full weight of an object is not directly handled or managed by the employee. For example, moving a client weighing 250 lb in a wheelchair may require 8 to 10 lb of force on a linoleum floor because of the wheels used on the mechanical device or the wheelchair. In the same environment, if the nursing home or rehabilitation facility has a "zero lift" policy, it is probable that the best work practice mandates use of a sit-to-stand lift or Hoyer lift to move patients. With these devices, a Licensed Nursing Assistant (LNA) can move a fully dependent resident with 10 to 12 lb of push–pull force instead of applying force equal to the patient's weight.

If an object is handled or held by the upper limbs and hands without the assistance of a tool or device to absorb some of the load, the weight of the object should be determined and documented, as well as the distance the object or tool is held from the body, the distance of vertical or lateral movement, or the distance the object is carried[41] to determine the safety of the lift. Most employers have scales available for shipping or weighing parts that can be used to determine object weights, or weights of many tools can be found on applicable websites. If the employee moves an object with push or pull, a force gauge can be employed. Force required can be measured on all surfaces on which the item may be moved as force requirements differ from carpet to linoleum or up ramps versus flat surfaces.

Sometimes the force may vary, or it is not possible to obtain a measurement of the force required. In these situations, the worker can be asked to pinch or grip a hydraulic gauge using the effort he or she feels

TABLE 119.1 Selected Evaluation Tools for Upper Extremity Risk Evaluation

Tool / INFO	OSHA Basic Screening and Ergonomic Assessment Checklist[49,59]	Washington State Checklists[24]	Rapid Upper Limb Assessment (RULA)[38]	Rapid Office Strain Assessment (ROSA)[61]	Moore Garg (Job Strain Index)[57]	ACGIH HAL-TLV[44]
Purpose	Simple qualitative screening tool to identify areas of MSD risk or concern. Additional assessment suggested if risk identified	Qualitative screening tool using a performance approach to work evaluation. Caution and hazard zone checklists	Semiquantitative posture-driven screening tool survey to identify risk factors and prioritize jobs with risk exposure. Additional assessment suggested if risk identified	Posture-driven quantitative risk assessment of computer workstations. Relates affected body parts to equipment	Quantitative job analysis method with industrial focus. Emphasis is on intensive repetitive jobs	Basic general assessment for monotasks done for 4 hr
Body part or application	Whole body in sections: • Hand, wrist, and arm • Back, trunk, and hip • Leg, knee, and ankle	Whole body: • Neck • Shoulder and arm • Hand and wrist • Back and legs	Whole body: • Trunk • Proximal arm • Distal arm • Wrist	Whole body: (may be useful to separate right and left)	Distal upper extremity: • Elbow • Forearm • Wrist • Hand	Distal upper extremity: • Hand • Wrist • Forearm
Environment or task application	General industry and office setting	General industry and office	General industry	Specific to office environments and workstation components	General industry: hand-intensive repetitive jobs. No specific office component	General industry and office. Used for monotask performed at least 4 hr
Risk factors and definitions used in study	**Repetition:** same motions every few seconds or same cycle with affected body part >2 times/min, 2 consecutive hr/day. **Force:** grip: >10 lb/hand >2 hr/day; pinch: 2 lb/hand >2 hr/day. **Contact stress:** using hand as hammer >10 times/hour >2 hr/day. **Lifting:**>75 lb once, >55 lb >10 times/day, >25 lb specific heights >25 times/day. **Push/pull:**>20-lb force >2 hr/day	**Repetition:** same motion little/no variation every few seconds >6 hr; >2 hr with high force/awkward posture. **Force:** grip: >10 lb or hold 10-lb object; pinch: 4 lb or hold 2-lb object; posture and repetition affect threshold. **Posture:** wrist: >30 degrees flexion, >45 degrees extension, ulnar deviation: >30 degrees. **Lifting:** separate calculator	**Repetition:** 4 times/min. **Static:** >1 min. **Posture:** trunk: 0–60 degrees; Neck: 20–60 degrees, >60 degrees; Proximal arm: shoulder flexion 20–45 degrees, 45–90 degrees, and >90 degrees, extension >20 degrees; Distal arm: elbow flexion >100 degrees; Wrist: flexion-extension >15 degrees. **Force:** load: 4.4 lb; 4.4–22 lb; >22 lb	**Posture:** pictorial reach, neck flexion, lower extremity position, wrist >15 degrees of extension. **Contact stress:** not specifically defined. **Duration:** <30 min, up to >4 hr per day	**Repetition:** "efforts/minute" 5-point scale from <4 to ≥20. **Posture:** 5-point scale: "perfectly normal to near extreme". **Force:** Borg 5-point scale: "light to near maximal". **Duration:** 5-point scale: <1 hr to ≥8 hr. **Speed:** 5-point scale: very slow to very fast	**Repetition:** VAS defined scale from 0–10. **Force:** VAS and Moore-Garg scales. **Duration:** monotask at least 4 hr per shift

	Col 1	Col 2	Col 3	Col 4	Col 5	Col 6
Outcome measure or scoring	• Threshold: "yes" or "no" for each body part	• Threshold: yes/no: "caution" or "hazard exists" • Can identify for body part specific	• Thresholds identified and defined • Whole-body numeric score calculated • Cannot calculate for separate body part	• Threshold identified • Workstation score calculated and compared with threshold	• Threshold identified • Numeric score calculated and compared with threshold • Right and left separate	• Threshold identified • Numeric score calculated and compared with threshold • Right and left separate • Short application time (<5 min) • No instrumentation needed
Strengths	• Preliminary • Quick assessment • Minimal training required; ergonomics experience	• Preliminary • Quick	• Preliminary • Quick • Examines posture and muscular effort • Minimal training required, 1 hr suggested	• Quick evaluation • Addresses interface with chair, keyboard, mouse, monitor, phone • Minimal training; ergonomics experience	• Scored • Allows comparisons between jobs • Score combines risk issues	
Limitations	• No quantitative number on level of hazard for comparison • Does not quantify recovery time	• No quantitative number on level of hazard for comparison • Does not quantify recovery time • Minimum 4-hr training recommended; ergonomics training	• Primarily postural • No specific office component • Looks at single posture or average posture • Duration of exposure not considered • No hand or finger postures considered • Does not quantify recovery time	• Office environment only • Posture focus • Does not quantify recovery time	• Hand, wrist, elbow only • No contact stress, vibration • Does not quantify recovery time • Minimum 4-hr training recommended; ergonomics training	• Monotask at least 4 hr • Limited to hand and wrist • Does not consider posture or contact stress • Minimum 2-hr training recommended; ergonomics training

ACGIH, American College of Government Industrial Hygienists; *HAL*, hand activity level; *MSD*, musculoskeletal disorder; *OSHA*, Occupational Safety and Health Administration; *TLV*, threshold limit value; *VAS*, visual analog scale.

is exerted in the task to mimic force used. Winnemuller and coworkers[42] used this method to assess the required force for pinch and grip tasks. Each worker in the study performed three grip trials, with the worker performing the task between each trial, and the results were averaged. Another method to assist with force determination is with the use of psychometric scales such as the Borg Exertion scale[43] or the Hand Force Scale[44] (Fig. 119.4). These scales require employee estimates of the force exertion to perform a specific task. Multiple employees should be interviewed and observed and the minimum, maximum, and average force defined. If hand grip or pinch is involved, employee grip and pinch strength can also be measured and compared with VAS results to determine an estimate of the percent of muscle force used. If one employee estimates a higher force application, the work method should be observed or other contributing factors assessed to determine methods to decrease the percent of force being used. Documenting the method of data collection is helpful to discern between objectively and subjective or psychometric data.

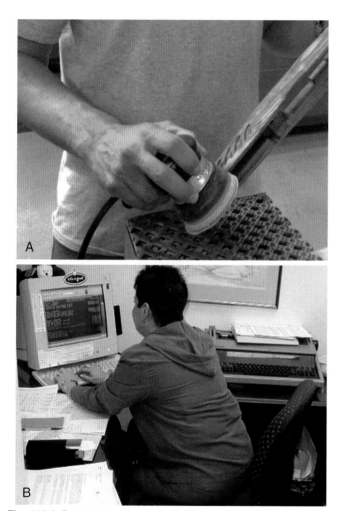

Fig. 119.2 Sustained postures. **A,** Holding sander. **B,** Reaching for a keyboard.

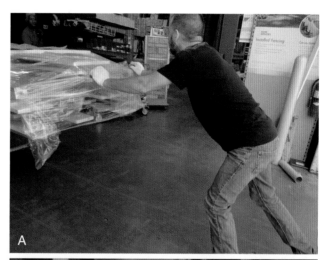

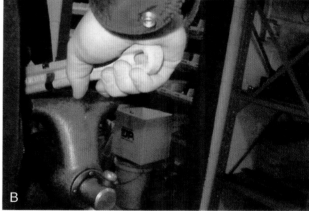

Fig. 119.3 Force to move a large object (**A**) and contact stress using a tool with force (**B**).

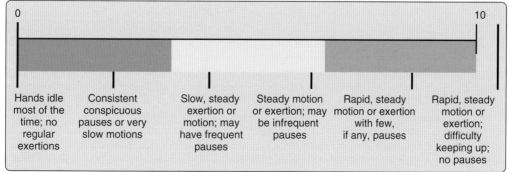

Fig. 119.4 Ten-point visual analog scale used to assess repetition. (From ACGIH. 2006 Threshold Limit Values for Chemical Substances and Physical Agents and Biological Exposure Limits. Cincinnati, OH: American Conference of Governmental Industrial Hygienists; 2006; Latko WA, Armstrong TJ, Foulke JA, et al. Development and evaluation of an observational method for assessing repetition in hand tasks. *Am Ind Hyg Assoc J.* 1997;58:278-285.)

Force requirements may increase with use of gloves.[45,46] Poorly fitting gloves or gloves that are stiff or thick increase the finger flexion force needed to flex the material and manipulate an object. If the glove material is slippery, the worker must use more force to maintain contact with the surface being handled. Alternately, properly sized gloves, gloves with tactile surfaces, and gloves that have joint sections may enhance contact, prevent slippage, and not add to required force.

The position of a joint in relation to force application should be considered. For example, wrist postures of 20 to 35 degrees of wrist extension or 7 degrees of ulnar deviation increases strength requirements for hand grip.[1] Grip type, grip span, and work behaviors can also have an impact on hand force application. It should be noted that force application occurs regularly in daily life, sports, and activities of daily living. The frequency, duration, and available recovery time in the work setting will assist in determining the significance of forceful use and application in the work environment relative to normal daily use and injury causation.

Contact Stress

Contact stress can be considered a specific type of force application. It is defined as forceful external contact between a location of the body with an external object.[1] The most vulnerable areas include the lateral sides of fingers, the palm of the hand over the medial and ulnar nerve, and the volar elbow along the superficial course of the ulnar nerve. Observation of the tools and employee's hands or areas suspected of being affected by contact stress may reveal finger blanching or tissue demarcation after time spent in a work process or holding a work tool. Finger wraps, personally padded tools, pillows or padding added to support devices or chairs, and observation of work method may reveal the source of contact stress and suggest corrective actions that should be considered. If padding or an orthosis is added as a therapeutic intervention, it must be carefully reviewed to assure that additional risk is not introduced. For example, the use of elevated mouse pads may result in force application to the distal forearm or proximal palm if the employee "anchors" on the rest when moving the mouse.[47] Contact stress includes low force such as resting the forearm on a chair armrest or high force if using the palm of the hand as a hammer to seat a tire hubcap or push on a tool such as a pill crusher in a nursing home. Care should be taken to note the exact location of the stress relative to tissues of concern. For example, an employee may describe "resting on his elbow" at the workstation as a cause of cubital tunnel, but observation reveals that he actually rests on the olecranon but holds the elbow in maximum flexion. The duration of sustained elbow flexion, an extreme posture, and resulting traction on the ulnar nerve in the cubital tunnel may hold more significance than the elbow resting on the work surface.

Repetition

Repetition is part of nearly every risk assessment, and in the authors' experience, it is frequently cited as the primary work hazard or risk factor by medical providers, patients, and the common press. However, high repetition alone does not always result in significant tissue damage.[26] Walkers, runners, and musicians regularly perform highly repetitive exertions for extended periods of time, and although injury may occur, it cannot be assumed that it will inevitably occur, particularly if optimal tools and proper technique are used. The relationship between repetitive motion and WRMSDs is equivocal at best,[8,9,23,25] and careful scrutiny should be applied to understand the degree of repetition that may occur, the amount of recovery time, the presence of force, and the influence of posture. For example, Garg and Kapellusch[25] found an association between exposure to a combination of high force or awkward posture with high repetition and development of MSDs, but no significant association was found with tasks that require high repetition or non-neutral posture alone. Similarly, Harris-Adamson and

coworkers[23] reported no significant increase in CTS rate when considering hand repetition rate independent of force, but activity that was both forceful and repetitive was associated with increased risk. Because of the wide variety of motions, forces, and postures assumed in work performance, defining "repetition" relative to injury is challenging, and no single metric for defining or assessment of repetition has been identified.[25]

Repetition has been identified as a contributor to upper limb pain and injury for centuries. As early as the 15th century, monks transcribing and handwriting Bibles described writer's cramp from holding writing instruments all day.[48] In the late 20th century, studies used various descriptors in an effort to evaluate and substantiate the contribution of repetitive motion to MSDs. Repeated hand cycles, amount of hand activity, production standards, velocity of motion, number and duration of micropauses, and hand activity rating scales are some descriptors. Based on these studies and their outcomes and in an effort to be able to compare jobs, more specific definitions have become the foundation of risk assessments and can be found in Table 119.1. Most definitions reflect the number of exertions over time or the number of times the hand holds, manipulates, or assembles parts or handles tools. Hagberg and colleagues[1] defined repetition as the same work element, action, or activity repeated many times and work that has an element of monotony or invariability reflecting the cyclical use of the same tissue. It is important to note the difference between a *repetitive task* and *repetitive tissue use*, the latter of which leads to patterns of use that may result in muscle fatigue or tendon strain because of a lack of recovery. Repetitive use of the same tissue does not apply to all tasks, particularly if a task is complex or has a long cycle with numerous smaller work elements. Some work tasks can be described in fundamental cycles or a work cycle with a definitive start and end that is repeated. If a fundamental cycle occurs repeatedly and frequently for periods of at least 2 hours without interruption, the task may be defined as repetitive.[49] But many jobs have no clear fundamental cycle and may involve too many varied work elements or too much variation in how the tasks are performed or how the task is performed from hour to hour or day to day to be defined as repetitive relative to tissue stress. The Hand Activity Level[44] provides a means to describe hand repetitions (see Fig. 119.4). An example of a task with varied hand use is an LNA in a nursing home who works with residents throughout the day to assist with personal care, providing nourishment (meals and snacks), cleaning and setting up rooms, moving them to and from activities, and transferring them to and from bed and chairs. While busy during the entire shift and doing the same tasks for five to eight residents, there is no one fundamental cycle that occurs repeatedly using the same tissue with minimal or limited recovery time (Fig. 119.5A–C). By contrast, an employee sanding parts may handle 50 to 60 parts per hour in exactly the same manner, one part after another (see Fig. 119.5D). The fundamental cycle for the sander includes the subelements of pick up part, hold to wheel, visually inspect part, hold to wheel, hand file a bur, and inspect and package the part done over and over. Periodically, the employee may have to document the process, get new parts, and remove packaged parts, but the same fundamental cycle is repeated 50 to 60 times per hour for the whole shift with very little variation or opportunity for the hands to pause or change motions. This task would expose many upper quarter tissues to repetitive motions or stress.

Because the sander has what could be considered repetitive tissue use exposure, the need for recovery time could increase if extremes of posture or force are also involved in the sanding process. The higher the stress on the tissue, the fewer cycles needed to result in tissue failure.[26] Understanding the interaction of frequency and force allows the therapist to question the patient about exposure and help identify methods to reduce risk. If an employee is able to rotate to a task that involves more inspection or a subassembly function with light finger

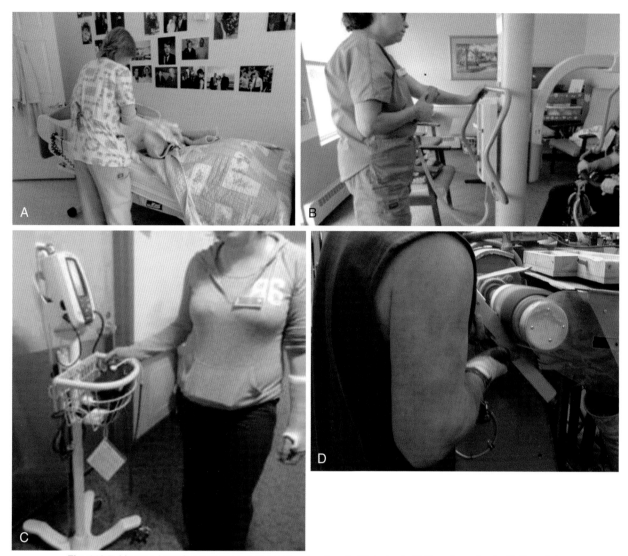

Fig. 119.5 Licensed nursing assistant varied task examples. **A,** Make beds. **B,** Transfer patients. **C,** Complete vital signs. **D,** Sander with the same task for the entire shift.

use and no extreme posture, recovery time for tissue used may occur. Optimal rotation frequency should be determined based on the ratio of load to no load.[1] Rodgers[36] stated that dynamic recovery could occur if a very light task followed 10 minutes of very heavy hand use. Other methods that may assist with reducing repetition include job enlargement and rotation, work organization, reduction in extra motions or motion economy, and use of mechanical aids.

Rather than relying on the patient's perception of repetition or injury risk to gather the more in-depth information about job requirements, the therapist can question the patient with open-ended questions that do not assume risk.[50] If the patient describes a typical work shift with one task that is done repeatedly all day, the number of parts completed or work cycles performed can begin to identify repetition rate for the work task. Within the work task, the number of work elements can be defined. The patient can then simulate the motions that occur to perform the work elements of concern. The number of tissue exertions and amount of time spent in the exertion or position can be calculated to determine the duration of exposure and recovery time that occurs through the cycle. Alternately, if it is difficult to identify one work cycle that occurs throughout the shift, it may be that the job has tasks that are repeated but do not have a high repetitive rate of tissue stress. Therefore, other contributors to injury should be suspected and

sought. Questions that can be asked to assist with these decisions are found in Table 119.2.

Vibration

Evidence of the causative effect of exposure to vibration and the development of UEMSDs is equivocal.[25,28] The discussion about this risk factor as a contributor to a specific injury requires examination of the literature and a clear understanding of the work-specific exposure to ensure proper determination. Hand-arm vibration syndrome related to segmental vibration exposure, as compared with whole-body exposure, is the diagnostic term often used in texts and studies[1,51,52] and may include symptoms involving the vascular, neurologic, and musculoskeletal systems.[53] It is thought that the hand acts as a dampener, absorbing the vibration and affecting the blood supply to the digits.[52] Vibration from a handheld tool may also change function of the mechanoreceptors and lead to more forceful gripping to handle and control the tool.[1]

With regard to MSDs, Harris-Adamson and colleagues[23] did not find an association with CTS incidence and vibration exposure in their cohort of 2474 workers. They attributed this to possible misclassification because of imprecise measures of vibration and lack of information about the type of handheld tool used by study subjects. Alternately, Fan

TABLE 119.2 Job-Related Questions for Patients to Improve Understanding of Tasks	
Generic Questions	
What is the purpose of your job?	
What are the separate tasks performed each day (list tasks by time through the shift to identify steps or all things normally done)?	
What percentage of the shift do you spend on each task?	
How many . . . ?	
How much (e.g., weight, force)?	
What tools do you use?	
What tasks do you do only occasionally, not every day?	
Job-Specific Questions Examples	
Grinder	LNA
How many parts do you make a shift?	How many patients do you care for a shift?
How much time do you spend on each part?	How much time do you spend on each task with one patient normally?
What is your main posture when grinding (demonstrate)?	What might be different sometimes? How often is it different?
Demonstrate the motion used to grind most of the time, some of the time, rarely?	Do you have lift assist devices (list them)?
What is the heaviest thing you handle (actual weight if possible), and how often do you handle it?	What is the heaviest thing you push or pull?
What do you handle most often, and how much does that weigh?	Do you push wheelchairs on linoleum, on carpet, or up and down ramps?
Do you push or pull anything?	
How much force do you use to . . (use Borg scale or comparison to ADL task)?	

ADL, Activity of daily living; *LNA,* licensed nursing assistant.

and coworkers[8] found an association between CTS and hand vibration work done by quarry or rock drillers, stonemasons, and forestry workers. Bovenzi and coworkers[53] also found an association with peripheral neurosensory disorders in their study participants who used bush and chain saws, stone workers grinders and polishers, and inline hammers. These researchers also identified that use of a vibratory handheld tool is commonly associated with exposure to other risk factors such as forceful gripping, contact stress, long duration of holding, and possibly low temperature. Understanding the specific work and types of tools as well as the duration and frequency of exposure can assist with evaluating the contribution of vibration to injury. To mitigate symptoms, efforts should be made to reduce exposures and institute engineering controls, but the actual measurement of the level of vibration exposure is complicated and may require advanced skills and sophisticated tools.

Temperature

Work in a cold environment can impact hand function by its effect on soft tissues of the upper extremity, and because use of gloves to keep the hands warm, may interfere with tactile sensation and increase the required grip force.[1] Cold exposure can occur because of work in a cold environment, exposure to exhaust from handheld tools, holding cold products, and immersion in cold fluids or refrigeration containers. In a study of work in refrigerated cold rooms at 40°F, Ceballos and coworkers[54] reported that workers were uncomfortable and required personal protective equipment. Muller and coworkers[55] noted that a decrease in fine dexterity performance on the Purdue Pegboard test in a cold environment compared with testing in a room temperature environment did not predict function in a cold environment. Dexterity and force are affected by use of gloves, particularly if bulky or mitten-style gloves are required. NIOSH[56] suggests the use of specific types of gloves to protect the hands that still allow fine motor performance, as well as rotation out of cold environments every 2 hours.

RISK AND JOB HAZARD ASSESSMENT TOOLS

Work risk or job hazard assessment tools have been developed over many years in an effort to provide quantitative or qualitative work

evaluation with goals of identifying jobs associated or not associated with the development of MSDs,[57] screening jobs to determine need for more in-depth evaluation and urgency for intervention,[38] allowing comparison between jobs to assist with prioritizing abatement and modification,[20] and predicting and evaluating efficacy in risk exposure reduction after abatement. With their understanding of anatomy, physiology, kinesiology, and activity analysis, occupational and physical therapists with expertise in hand therapy and additional training in ergonomics have a unique combination of skills to provide credible and comprehensive job hazard analysis that may assist physicians when making decisions about causation in developing interventions plans.

Many hazard assessments result in scores that reflect if a job is "safe" or "hazardous,"[24,56] "low" or "high" risk,[44] or needing "additional evaluation."[38] Hazardous jobs are considered ones in which workers are at increased risk for WRMSD because of sufficient exposure to risk factors, whereas safe jobs are ones in which the exposure is acceptable or safe for at least 75% of the working population.[25] A safe job does not mean that there is no exposure, but there is a lack of specific data on acceptable levels for safe exposure or a quantifiable relationship between exposure to risk factors and development of disease.[25] Physicians may be asked to determine causation of MSDs, and patients often ask therapists questions about the cause of MSDs. To address these questions, a comprehensive job description and risk assessment is considered superior to use of the worker's job title or self-report of exposure.[10]

Work or risk assessment tools document job tasks and related risk factors. They may include documentation of the job purpose, task sequence, component tasks or job elements, subtasks or motions, and possibly micromotions[45] (see http://www.denix.osd.mil/ergoworkinggroup/assessmenttools). This information allows the examiner to determine work cycles and specific task steps and objectively measure exposures when possible. After the job is well understood, the appropriate MSD injury risk assessment tool can be chosen and used to analyze the job tasks.

Most risk assessment tools can be categorized as qualitative, semiquantitative, or quantitative.[58] A list of frequently taught and cited tools can be found in Table 119.1. Qualitative assessment tools generally review each work element to determine the degree to which the employee may be exposed to a work hazard. A number of qualitative assessment tools have been proposed, and each generally has a specific focus or method for use.[24,49,59] Qualitative tools often have a yes/no threshold indicating whether risk exposure exists as part of the job performance. The assessment may indicate which work element contains what hazard with the objective of assisting the employer and worker with quick identification of possible hazards to assist with developing methods to decrease exposure.

Quantitative tools are based on biomechanical models and an assumption that there is a relationship between a risk factor associated with work performance and the development of a WRMSD.[25] Quantitative tools result in a score that generally can be compared with a threshold or limit value that would indicate if exposure occurs and at what level. If the assessment results in a score or comparison to thresholds that reflect a concern, further evaluation may be suggested or ergonomic abatement can be considered to decrease exposure and reduce the risk score.

To select the proper tool, it is important to understand the goal of the specific assessment tool and its intended application, as well as how the tool relates to a specific diagnosis, body part, or type of task. Because occupational and physical therapists have grounded understanding of anatomy, movement, and injury and activity analysis, they are uniquely qualified to understand assessment tools with minimal training. Qualitative tools require little training or expertise, but a thorough review of the documented purpose of the evaluation and any specific issues related to use should be attained. In contrast, most quantitative tools are intended for professional use and require some training.[58] Although none of these tools requires formal certification for use, a solid understanding of the purpose of and how to apply a specific assessment tool can be gained in various ergonomics courses, review of associated literature, and application in an appropriate setting and with professional supervision. The "Strengths" and "Limitations" rows of Table 119.1 provide information on training suggestions, and the American Industrial Hygienists Association[58] Ergonomic Assessment Toolkit provides further information on training, as well as additional tools that could be used. No one tool applies to all jobs, and appropriate use of the tools is important, particularly if decisions on employment and abatement investment are to be based on the outcome of the evaluation.

Occupational Safety and Health Administration Basic Screening Tool and Ergonomic Assessment Checklist

The Occupational Safety and Health Administration (OSHA) was a driving force encouraging hazard assessment and use of screening and job hazard risk surveys in the late 1990s when developing a proposed ergonomic standard for prevention of WRMSDs. Although the standard was never implemented, the science behind it became the foundation for the development of many risk assessment tools. The original screening tool is still available[49] and has also been modified to an Ergonomic Assessment Checklist[59] intended to assist employers with initial screening of job tasks and identification of potential hazard exposure. Both tools address the whole body and incorporate common risk factors. They are easy and quick to administer and require only a basic understanding of MSD hazards to determine if risk is thought to be present. Both checklists are scored yes/no with a "yes" indicating that further evaluation should be pursued to better understand the possible exposure.

Washington State Caution and Hazard Zone Checklists

The Washington State Department of Labor and Industries developed two checklists to screen jobs relative to hazard exposure in general industry and the office. The Caution Zone and Hazard Zone checklists are qualitative, easy to administer, performance-based initial screening tools.[60] They rely on observation of "movements and postures that are a regular and foreseeable part of the job, occurring more than one day per week, and more frequently than one week per year," thus eliminating "outlier" activities as causal factors for MSD injury. The checklists are designed to evaluate the whole job, but if there are multiple significant components to a job, each component task could be examined separately. There is a lifting calculator and hand–arm vibration calculator available as well. The Caution Zone Checklist should be completed initially, and if any activity is identified as at risk, the more detailed Hazard Zone Checklist should be completed. With easy-to-view diagrams for each category, minimal training and expertise is required to use these assessment tools, and these assessments also serve as a good base from which to determine if additional more in-depth evaluation is needed.

Rapid Upper Limb Assessment

The Rapid Upper Limb Assessment (RULA) is a semiquantitative screening, posture-based survey that scores postures of the neck, trunk, upper arms, lower arms, wrists, and legs and is applicable for general industries.[38] In addition to posture, force and duration of exposure are also considered to determine risk exposure. The tool should be used to examine single identified postures associated with specific work tasks. The specific posture, whether extreme or average, and whether the right or left extremity should be identified as evaluated to avoid confusion about the outcome. The final score is summated and compared with four categories of action levels that could indicate the need for additional evaluation. There is no specific component for the office, but specific postures at the office could be evaluated to determine need for correction. The evaluation form has drawings of the positions being considered, and although relatively easy to administer, some training is required. It is quite general with regard to the hand, so additional evaluation may be needed for wrist and hand concerns. The original study was validated for both general industry and office, but no subsequent studies have examined the reliability and validity of this assessment tool.

Rapid Office Strain Assessment

The ROSA is a posture-based semiquantitative assessment designed to provide data about risk exposure that addresses the interaction of the employee with the office equipment, including the chair, desk height, keyboard, mouse, and phone.[61] This tool also considers the duration of the employee's exposure to less than optimal positioning related to equipment use. The tool is quick to complete and uses pictures and scoring boxes to quantify observations. The evaluator observes the employee at the computer workstation; conducts a brief interview; and subsequently scores each work, equipment, and posture component. Section scores are then combined for a single score that can be compared with a threshold risk level. The developers found moderate correlations between ROSA scores and employee discomfort scores,[61] providing a quantifiable threshold from which to identify areas of greatest risk and determine the urgency for intervention. The scores can be used to compare pre- and postabatement scores to ensure that corrections effect a reduction in risk exposure. Intertester and intraobserver reliability were also found to be good for most components and similar to studies of other posture-based tools.[62]

Strain Index

The Strain Index is an involved quantitative assessment tool that examines the relationship between exertional demands of a job (physical stress), including intensity of the work, duration of work performance (percentage of job cycle), frequency of hand exertions per minute, posture, speed of work, and duration of task per day.[57] Each of these variables is scored and a multiplier applied to result in a score that relates to identified hazard levels. It is intended for use with the distal upper extremity, wrist, and hands and applies to highly repetitive jobs in a variety of industrial settings. Biomechanical, physiological, and epidemiologic principles were considered in the development of the tool, and it has been well studied relative to intertester reliability and predictive validity. Originally developed and evaluated in a pork processing plant, it has also been applied more broadly in other manufacturing settings.[63] The tool relies on observation by trained raters who understand the principles of the categories evaluated and the scoring method.

American College of Government Industrial Hygienists Threshold Limit Values for Hand Activity Level

The American College of Government Industrial Hygienists (ACGIH) is a professional organization of industrial hygienists and safety and health professionals that developed threshold limit values (TLVs) for chemical substances and physical agent exposure, including hand activity levels (HALs). The intention of the TLVs for HALs is to identify unacceptable levels of employee exposure to hand activity and force associated with monotask performance.[44] Monotask is defined as a job that requires performing the same set of motions or exertions repeatedly for 4 or more hours per day. The assessment also considers risk issues of frequency, force, and speed of movement. Using VASs with descriptors for hand activity rate and force, the evaluator observes and rates hand use and motion and considers recovery time. The activity level scale ranges from 0, "hands idle most of the time; no regular exertions" to 10, "rapid steady motions/difficulty keeping up or continuous exertion" (see Fig. 119.4). The force scale descriptors range from 0, "no force at all (0%MVC)" to 10, "greatest imaginable force (100% MVC)." A combined calculated score results in a level of exposure of (1) unacceptable: above the TLV: "workplace changes should be investigated to reduce exposure"; (2) borderline: between the TLV and action limit: "workplace changes should be considered where feasible to reduce exposure/medical surveillance of workers should be used"; or (3) below the action limit: "acceptable exposure, monotask is probably safe." A graphic of the scores relative to the TLV and action limit can be used and is helpful to visualize the outcome of the evaluation relative to threshold definitions. The HAL for TLV has been widely used, validated,[44,64] and administered along with or compared with results from other risk assessments.[33,65]

JOB ANALYSIS AND JOB DESCRIPTIONS: THE CHALLENGE OF GATHERING JOB INFORMATION

Understanding work demands is an important process when considering factors that may contribute to the development of WRMSDs.[2] In the clinical reasoning process, particularly as it relates to treatment of work-related injuries, incorporating information regarding what work activities are performed, how they are performed, and for how long provides potentially useful information to understand the mechanism of injury and develop the most effective treatment program. Although therapists may approach issues of daily function and sports with sound clinical reasoning, the issues of work are often poorly addressed and inadequately understood,[2] and there is no single method of evaluation that is recommended or applicable to all work tasks.[66] Because how and from whom work data is gathered may influence the evaluation, clinical reasoning process, and subsequent treatment, therapists should

consider the source and objectivity of data provided. For example, in the clinic, therapists are often reliant on patient descriptions of work tasks, but self-report may not be a reliable method of obtaining work task information, particularly as it relates to critical work elements, associated injury risk, and the degree of exposure.[6,19,42] Spielholz and coworkers[67] noted that employee self-report of exposure to physical risk factors was unreliable and imprecise. They used an intermethod comparison among self-report questionnaires, observational video analysis, and direct measurement to evaluate posture, repetition, force, and movement velocity and suggested that scientific measurement of exposure was more precise than self-report. The authors found that the mental workload required between jobs, experience expectations of conditions, and motivational factors could affect employee estimates of duration of exposure to risk. In another study about risk exposure, Winnemuller and coworkers[42] compared risk assessments of four job types performed by an ergonomist, supervisors, and employees. Risks were specifically defined, pictorial diagrams were provided, and a questionnaire used to assist with the evaluations. The study found that supervisors identified the presence of risk 81% of the time compared with the ergonomist's assessment, and employees identified risk 77% of the time. Both supervisors and employees overestimated the amount of keying performed, with the employees overestimating keying by almost 50%.

As an alternate to employee descriptions, the employer may provide a written job description typically used for hiring and periodic performance review, but these job descriptions generally describe employment qualifications, general task information, and performance standards. This information may provide discussion points with the patient regarding job demands, but it often lacks specifics about physical demands or risk exposures necessary to identify issues of causality, possible job modifications, and issues that may inform treatment planning. A hierarchy of exposure data outlined by Hegman and coworkers[10] suggests that the best way to obtain optimal data about a job and how it affects an individual is to have a professional who is skilled in job assessment review the job, observe the patient doing the job tasks, and take necessary measurements related to the patient and job tasks.

As a result of variations in work environments and demands, limitations associated with subjective reports of job demands, and difficulties with job descriptions, visiting the worksite can be of value. Working with the employee and employer, the therapist can develop a more detailed job description, such as an employee-specific task-based job description or a functional job description (FJD). Employee-specific, task-based job descriptions can be of value to define work tasks that the employee normally performs, identify alternate duties that may be offered, determine ways to meet physician-described restrictions, and assist with modifying and grading work tasks to accommodate work capacities and facilitate recovery. This type of evaluation focuses on issues related to the injured body part(s), modified work, and the return to work process for the patient. In contrast, a very detailed job description that is not specific to one employee or patient and contains whole-body data and other physical, cognitive, and behavioral data may be called an FJD.[36,66,68]

Employee-Specific Task-Based Job Description

A well-informed therapist with an understanding of job task analysis and risk related to WRMSDs may be able to go to the worksite to develop an employee-specific job description before an employee returns to work. This assists the physician with an understanding of the tasks an employee will perform and allows for accommodation before the employee starts the alternate duty position.

The employee-specific task-based job description may begin with a purpose statement that describes the objective of the job task and leads to a mental image of the intent and probable methods of performing the expected outcome of the position.[68] Descriptions of work hours, the work environment, and personal protective equipment should be included. If there is one primary task that is performed, the specific steps taken to perform that task would be outlined. If there are numerous tasks, they can be listed and steps for each task outlined, particularly if the affected body part is involved in task performance. For example, an office worker with wrist tendinitis may copy and sort paperwork, fold paperwork and stuff envelopes, and then spend the remainder of the shift doing a wide variety of tasks on the computer. The posture of the wrist in each task and frequency of motion to extremes or positions of concern would be the focus of the analysis and discussion. Photographs of the worker and affected body postures are helpful documentation of observed issues and can provide justification for suggested changes to tools or work method.[2] Tasks that are done rarely or not as a regular part of the expected job functions can be listed as additional tasks, with the frequency or duration of completion defined and any issues related to the involved body part identified. For alternate work, the varied tasks off the computer could be spread out through the day or additional noncomputer tasks added to allow varied hand use and to enlarge the job.

Job demands in an industrial environment where a large number of different parts can be produced by one machine operator are quite different from the demands of the office. In nonoffice, industrial settings, if all the parts involve the same steps or motions, the steps to perform the task can be listed once and the variations identified. Particular points to be considered and documented could include the length of the production cycle; the number of motions performed by the affected body part; any pause or recovery time that occurs in the work cycle; forces needed to handle, move, or hold parts or tools; and the types, size, and weight of the tools used.

When employees are asked to work on different machines or at differing operations, comparison of the physical demands between the processes or machines can be helpful. A chart listing the physical demands side by side can assist the employer, physician, and patient in understanding if the demands are essentially the same or if there are substantive differences that may affect the employee's ability to safely return to a specific job or perform the tasks required. Specific definitions of terms used should be provided to ensure that all parties understand the implications of the terms. Common definitions of these terms can be found in Table 119.3.

If unable to visit the worksite, the therapist may want to question the patient using clinical reasoning to obtain objective, helpful job-related data. Questions could involve the job purpose, the number of tasks performed each day, the time spent on each task, the production expectation, the time per part completed or work cycle, and the size and weights of items handled. A complete list of suggested questions is found in Table 119.2. The exact line of questioning will vary with the type of job, and leading questions that suggest risk should be avoided. Instead, questions should be open ended to ascertain what the employee's perspectives are regarding problem areas or job tasks that are going well. An employee who sands parts and who produces 200 parts per shift might be questioned about posture, position of machinery, and hand motions associated with the task. Conversely, an LNA is expected to provide a variety of services to eight patients assigned to her care each shift. The line of questioning to understand job tasks and potential exposure to risk factors is quite different. For the LNA, the discussion may include questions about job sequences, time in each task for each resident, lift assist devices available, and variations in work method with each resident. A call to the employer can then verify the tasks and data provided and identify areas of discrepancy or concern.

TABLE 119.3 Handling Definitions

Handling Method	Definition
Lift[24,49,59]	Using hands and arms, completely supporting weight, raise and lower item; weight >2 kg (4.4 lb)
Carry[24,49,59]	Transporting object in hands, arms, shoulders; weight >2 kg (4.4 lb); usually bilateral unless unable to use two hands or designed for one hand
Push and pull[24,49,59]	Exerting force on an object with hands or other body part; weight >2 kg (4.4 lb), so that object is held in position or moves forward against force
Gripping[24,49,59]	Closing fingers and thumb around object; includes power grip, hook grip, squeezing firmly
Finger dexterity[24,49,59]	Manipulating or fingering small objects; not computer data entry
Reaching forward[24,49,59]	Extending the arm away from the body to the front, side, or back with >15 degrees of shoulder motion from neutral
	Forward flexion or abduction of the hand(s) and arm(s) within 0–90 degrees of ROM from the shoulder or extension within 0–50 degrees ROM from the shoulder
Reaching overhead[24,49,59]	Extending the hands above the head or elbows above the shoulder
	Forward flexion or abduction of the hand(s) and arm(s) >90 degrees from the shoulder
FREQUENCY[111]	
Not present	0 hr/8-hr day
Occasional: maximum hours per 8-hr day	Activity or condition exists up to one third of the time, or 2 hr, 40 min per 8-hr day
Frequent: maximum hours per 8-hr day	Activity or condition exists from one third to two thirds of the time, or 5 hr, 20 min per 8-hr day
Constant: maximum hours per 8-hr day	Activity or condition exists two thirds or more of the time per 8-hr day

ROM, Range of motion.

Functional Job Descriptions

With the advent of the Americans with Disabilities Act (ADA), the need for comprehensive FJDs has been identified.[36] Not only must the FJD separate essential from marginal functions and physical demands, but it may also include evaluation and documentation of the sensory, behavioral, and cognitive demands of a job.[69] FJDs can be used to assist with hiring, determine readiness for return to work after personal or work-related injuries or disabilities, define alternate or light duty and reasonable accommodations, provide post offer preplacement screens, and address other issues related to hiring and employee placement.[69,70] Because the FJD is developed to describe tasks not specific to one employee, this evaluation is typically completed with observation of and discussion with several employees to ensure understanding of variations in methods of performance.[36] Duston and coworkers[70] encourage development of comprehensive job descriptions, stating that "an outdated or incomplete job description may be worse than none at all."

BOX 119.5   Questions to Determine Essential versus Marginal Functions

Essential
- Does the position exist to perform this function?
- How many employees are available to perform the task?
- Is the task highly specialized?
- How much time is spent performing the task?
- What is the consequence of not performing the function?
- How does collective bargaining affect the function?
- Are current or prior employees required to do the function?
- What is the employer's judgment about the function?

Marginal Duty Considerations
- Always list some
- Tasks always done by all or most employees
- Not performing does not create hardship or safety issue for other employees
- Not doing task does not change basic nature of the job
- Can include "other duties as assigned"

BOX 119.6   Example Items to be Measured for Job Descriptions

- Heights of work surfaces, shelves, controls, and displays
- Reach distances and angles
- Carry distances
- Lifting heights
- Shape and size of objects handled
- Weights of items handled and tools used
- Handle diameters
- Force to move items
- Force applied to tools
- Temperatures

As with the employee-specific task-based evaluation, the FJD can begin with a purpose statement that allows the reader to have a clear understanding of why the job is done and what some of the physical demands might be. Typical or essential job tasks should be identified and separated from marginal functions, which may also be referred to as nonessential functions or exceptional tasks. Job tasks are considered essential if an employee must be able to perform the task with or without reasonable accommodation, but the final decision about essential versus marginal job tasks is that of the employer. The Equal Employment Opportunity Commission (EEOC) defined specific task related issues that employers should consider when determining if a task is essential or marginal (Box 119.5).[68–70] An estimate of the amount of time spent on each task and if it is done every day or less frequently than daily may be defined. Information about training requirements, if other employees do or do not perform the task, and issues of collective bargaining all contribute to the determination of essential versus marginal work element decisions.

Balogh and coworkers[71] suggested that "direct technical measurement" should be used to objectively confirm subjective descriptions of the work environment and physical demands for FJDs. Items that might be measured for any type of job description are listed in Box 119.6. If workers handle items of many sizes, the smallest, largest, and most common will assist with defining the work demand. The specific tools used and items handled should be listed. If information about the tool (e.g., weight, vibration output, intended use) is not readily available at the worksite, the information can be obtained from manufacturers. The frequency of tool use helps to define duration and potential exposure to awkward or extreme posture, force, and vibration. Forces needed to move items should be measured with force gauges and documented. For example, the force to push a wheelchair with a 250-lb patient on linoleum can be measured with a push/pull gauge and compared with the force needed on carpet or up a ramp. Documentation of the availability of assistive devices such as suction lifts and powered forklifts in manufacturing, or sit-to-stand or Hoyer devices in nursing environments is particularly important, as are the type of keyboard and position of and type of mouse devices in office settings. Photographs of tools and workstations are helpful for readers to better understand and envision the work environment and tools and consequently the postures used to accomplish the task.

As the data are gathered, a clear understanding of physical demands and frequency of performance begins to evolve. Comments can accompany any part of the report to enhance the understanding of how the job is performed and what physical demands are expected. For example, if a shipping employee is required to pack and move 20 boxes per hour weighing up to 50 lb, we imagine this to be a physically demanding job. However, if there is a suction lift to assist with lifting boxes, the employee may only very light lift boxes once or twice an hour. Without this clarification, it appears that the employee handles heavier boxes more often than may in reality occur because the lift is available. In contrast, a piece of equipment may be present but not consistently usable because it is not made for the application or is in disrepair. Because FJD reports can be lengthy, summary lists of the normal physical demands may be provided to physicians, or shorter forms may be used for specific applications.

SYSTEMS, PERSONNEL, AND THE INJURED WORKER: COORDINATING EFFORTS TO INFLUENCE SUCCESS AT WORK OR RETURN TO WORK

An employee with a work injury or suspected work injury may encounter and interact with a number of systems, including the employer, medical care, and insurance. Each system has its own processes, personnel, and desired outcomes relative to work injuries. As the primary communicator, the injured worker, who is out of work or experiencing significant work capacity limitations, may manage communications with five or more people. The multiple systems and personnel, including therapy practitioners, are all potential stakeholders in the management and successful outcome of treatment of the WRMSD (Table 119.4), and all have various roles, possibly not understood by the worker. The course of recovery may be inhibited or supported as the multiple systems, and personnel within these systems interact with each other and the client.

Consider this scenario:
- A worker reports elbow pain to his supervisor. The supervisor instructs him to fill out an incident report.
- Human resources or a safety or occupational health nurse speaks to the worker to gather more data about the symptoms and the work tasks.
- The employee sees a medical provider associated with the employer or workers' compensation carrier.
- The employee describes the symptoms and the type of work he completes.

- A physician or health care provider determines that the elbow pain is likely work related based on the worker's description of the job tasks performed.
- The employee returns to work with information about work-relatedness and restrictions.
- The employee returns to his work tasks. The supervisor and coworkers may expect him to continue with normal work. The employee has to explain why he can't do certain things but may not have the language to do so. The employee may not have the power to change his work tasks to accommodate the restrictions.
- The supervisor may not understand how to accommodate restrictions and tells the employee to do the best he can.
- The worker's symptoms do not improve, and he returns to the physician and reports he is no better and that the work cannot be modified.
- The physician perceives the employer to be uncooperative, may take the worker out of work, and the employee becomes discouraged or feels the employer is not doing everything they can to help him.

Although this may not represent every upper extremity work injury scenario, it may be familiar to therapists who treat patients with work-related injuries. With the employee as the manager of communications and perhaps negotiating between four or more stakeholders, there is tremendous potential for miscommunication and misperception, potentially resulting in higher costs and poorer work outcomes.

The cost burden for treatment and lost wages of MSDs is significant with an $874 billion (5.7% of the US gross domestic product) price tag in 2012.[72] Efforts to coordinate care, improve communication among stakeholders, and address the psychosocial needs of employees with injuries offer potential solutions to facilitate return to work can help to reduce the economic impact and improve the quality of life of people experiencing MSDs.[73,74] Of particular concern are workers who are not working because of their work-related injuries. A plan to address work participation and rehabilitation can be instrumental in providing an understandable, clear path for all stakeholders. Durand and associates[75] proposed a six-step process to address return to work and work absence management with identified roles of stakeholders. These steps include (1) time off and recovery period, (2) initial contact with the worker, (3) evaluation of the worker and her job tasks, (4) development of a return-to-work plan with accommodations, (5) work resumption, and (6) follow-up of the return-to-work process. Potential barriers to return to work such as difficulty with communication, negative attitudes (employer or employee), and poor coping skills[7] should be identified. Furthermore, functional adaptations to address these issues should be included in the treatment plan. With a rehabilitation path, roles, and goals identified, the stakeholders listed in Table 119.4 may be more likely to understand how their expertise can facilitate tissue healing, continued work participation, or resumption of work participation for the person experiencing a work injury.

The importance of addressing communication and coordination efforts was investigated by Dowd and colleagues[74] in a study of nearly 1900 employees with work-related injuries. They developed a program that included employer–physician communication and coordination of employer–physician efforts to retain or resume work participation. The program resulted in a savings of $490 per employee, mostly in medical costs, per year. In a systematic review of early return-to-work interventions, a positive association was found between interventions initiated within the first 6 weeks of the return-to-work process and reduced time out of work.[76] Hardison and Roll[77] examined the results of early interventions for workers out of work in a general occupational rehabilitation program. They found that the number of visits and the use of work simulation was significantly (<0.001) associated with improved return-to-work outcomes. Relative to workplace interventions, Cancelliere

and colleagues[73] and Hoefsmit and colleagues[76] identified a number of features that were associated with positive return-to-work results, including multidisciplinary teams, specific return-to-work plans, reduction in exposure to potentially aggravating risk factors, use of graded activities related to work tasks, work modifications, early return to work, and treatment during work hours. Last, Anderson and associates[78] studied the value of providing information and education to workers with chronic low back and upper body pain. They concluded that providing workers with information about their health condition, methods to self-manage their condition while at work and at home, and tailored physical activity were all important to workers' ability to actively participate in the process of recovery and successfully return to work routines.

ERGONOMICS

Ergonomics is commonly described as "fitting the work to the worker." For therapy practitioners working with injured patients, using ergonomics to suggest changes to the height of a keyboard tray or the type of mouse or to modify a tool or work routine to reduce exposure to a risk factor could be considered as a part of the intervention strategy. However, these changes are only a small part of ergonomics. Ergonomics is an expansive discipline that addresses design and intervention and encompasses a wide variety of topics related to human capacity and interface with environments, including physical, cognitive, and organizational ergonomics.[79] For example, areas of interest and study include anthropometrics, vision, health care, agricultural ergonomics, ergonomics for children, and educational environments as well as musculoskeletal ergonomics. The International Ergonomics Association (IEA) defines ergonomics as

> Ergonomics (or human factors) is the scientific discipline concerned with the understanding of interactions among humans and other elements of a system, and the profession that applies theory, principles, data and methods to design in order to optimize human well-being and overall system performance. Practitioners of ergonomics and ergonomists contribute to the design and evaluation of tasks, jobs, products, environments and systems in order to make them compatible with the needs, abilities and limitations of people.[79]

The expected impact of ergonomics for those with and without injuries is that improved matching of capacity and demands will result in successful human function, fewer injuries, and more consistent output.

US Government Departments and Resources

In the United States, two governmental agencies provide structure and resources for ergonomics and workplace safety: (1) OSHA and (2) NIOSH. In 1970, US legislation efforts created OSHA.[80] This department operates through the US Department of Labor and is responsible for promoting and ensuring safe workplaces and work practices. OSHA creates safety-related standards and regulations with the expectation that employers will provide a safe workplace. Employer responsibilities include following standards, keeping accurate records of work injuries, informing employees of potential hazards, and not retaliating against employees for exercising their rights under OSH Act of 1970. Currently, OSHA does not have a national ergonomic standard regulating employer management of ergonomic risks. However, employers have a duty to provide a safe workplace and to consider ergonomic hazards and abatements as part of their duties to meet OSHA regulations. For example, the OSHA General Duty Clause[81] states,

TABLE 119.4	**Interactive Systems within Workers' Compensation Model**	
System	**Personnel Examples**	**Roles or Function Examples**
Employee	• Construction vs office worker • Manager vs production line worker	• Parent • Breadwinner • Worker
Employer	• Company owner(s), chief operating officer, chief financial officer • Human resources manager • Occupational health nurse • Occupational health physician, provider • Ergonomics consultant or person • Safety personnel • Department managers • Supervisors • Coworkers • Labor union representatives	• Maintain records of work attendance, pay wages, purchase workers' compensation insurance, provide and manage health care insurance options (if offered) as per local and federal labor laws • Maintain work environments and equipment, follow local and federal safety and health guidelines applicable to the industry • Employer-based occupational health providers may provide initial evaluation and care of injuries and/or coordinate workplace efforts to reduce time out of work and promote recovery • Employer provides work within restrictions or may interfere with ability of employee to return to work
Workers' compensation insurance	• Insurance adjuster who estimates the potential cost of the case • Case manager interfaces with various therapy, medical providers, employer, and client to facilitate efficient and cost-effective delivery of care	• Coverage purchased by employer to pay for lost wages and medical care for injured workers • Employers may be "self-insured," which means they pay the claims, usually through a third-party workers' compensation insurer • For federal employees, the DFEC handles workers' compensation • Depending on the injury and the state or federal guidelines, employees may be entitled to compensation for permanent injuries or impairments • Coverage may be restricted to a certain number of visits or certain service providers • Local laws regarding workers' compensation vary from state to state
Private health insurance	• Does not typically assign a case manager	• Paid for by employer and employee • May not cover all costs, resulting in increased employee stress and possible failure to report difficulty with work performance
Medical providers or therapy providers	• Primary care provider • Specialty provider (hand surgeon, physiatrist, orthopedist) • Independent medical examiner • Occupational therapist or physical therapist	• Provide evaluation and treatment services • May provide services independently or as part of a referral network such as a hospital system or managed care network • May or may not understand workplace requirements and issues
Managed care providers	• Case managers	• Independent local providers or national groups providing local services • Responsible for interfacing with various therapy, medical providers, employer, and client to facilitate delivery of care to resolve injury in an efficient and cost-effective manner

DFEC, Division of Federal Employees' Compensation.

(a) Each employer --

(1) shall furnish to each of his employees employment and a place of employment which are free from recognized hazards that are causing or are likely to cause death or serious physical harm to his employees;

(2) Shall comply with occupational safety and health standards promulgated under this Act.

(b) Each employee shall comply with occupational safety and health standards and all rules, regulations, and orders issued pursuant to this Act which are applicable to his own actions and conduct.

OSHA provides free consultation services to assist employers in efforts to comply with standards that are in place. OSHA has also published a number of industry-specific guidelines to prevent or reduce work injuries. These guidelines provide programming suggestions to maximize the impact of injury prevention and ergonomic modification efforts, including identifying management support, involving workers, and identifying hazards. Table 119.5 provides a list of resources and websites including these guidelines.

NIOSH was also created as a result of the OSH Act of 1970.[80] It is an arm of the Centers for Disease Control and Prevention. NIOSH supports the creation and translation of research related to occupational safety and health practices to create a safer, healthier work environment. Examples of resources available from NIOSH can be found in Table 119.5.

In addition to these resources, NIOSH launched the Total Worker Health (TWH) program in 2011 to focus on changes at the population level to integrate workplace interventions related to safety and health, employment, and the work environment to enhance the health and well-being of workers.[82] While treating work injuries, the primary focus of intervention for the individual worker is typically on the physical work-related hazards such as force or repetition and the immediate effect on the injured tissue. However, for that individual and for the work population, other workplace factors such as wages, stress at work, workload, and access to paid leave may influence worker's health, recovery, and return to work as well as work performance and community participation. TWH recognizes work as a social determinant of health and

TABLE 119.5	**Ergonomic Resources and Sites**
Resource:	**Available at:**
OSHA Basic Screening tool	https://www.osha.gov/FedReg_osha_pdf/FED20001114.pdf page 589-590
OSHA Ergonomic Assessment Checklist	https://www.osha.gov/dte/grant_materials/fy14/sh-26336-sh4/Ergonomic-Assessment-Checklist.pdf
Washington State caution and hazard zone screening tools	http://www.lni.wa.gov/SAFETY/SPRAINSSTRAINS/TOOLS/DEFAULT.ASP
Rapid Upper Limb Assessment	http://ergo.human.cornell.edu/ahrula.html
Rapid Office Strain Assessment	http://ergo.human.cornell.edu/ahROSA.html
Moore Garg Strain Index	http://health.usf.edu/publichealth/eoh/tbernard/ergotools
ACGIH TLV for Hand Activity Level	http://personal.health.usf.edu/tbernard/HollowHills/HALTLVM15.pdf
ACGIH Ergonomic Toolkit: lists common assessment tools with information about application and validation	https://www.aiha.org/get-involved/VolunteerGroups/Documents/ER-GOVG-Toolkit_rev2011.pdf
OSHA guideline: "Prevention of Musculoskeletal Injuries in Poultry Processing"	https://www.osha.gov/Publications/OSHA3213.pdf
OSHA guideline: "Guidelines for Retail Grocery Stores"	https://www.osha.gov/ergonomics/guidelines/retailgrocery/retailgrocery.html
OSHA: "Computer workstation e-tool": evaluation checklist and information about work postures, workstation setup, equipment, and organization of work	https://www.osha.gov/SLTC/etools/computerworkstations
Upper limb musculoskeletal Disorders Consortium resources: list of articles related to upper extremity injuries, risk factors, and injury prevention conducted by NIOSH researchers	https://www.cdc.gov/niosh/topics/ergonomics/upperlimb.html
Poultry industry workers information: hazard evaluation, outcomes, and resources for poultry processing work	https://www.cdc.gov/niosh/topics/poultry/default.html
Data regarding incidence and risks related to CTS in poultry processing plants	
Guide To Selecting Non-Powered Hand Tools: Provides resource for avoiding musculoskeletal injuries and information about hand tool selection, including recommended tool circumferences, weights, and uses	https://www.cdc.gov/niosh/updates/upd-11-3-04.html
A strategy for industrial power hand tool ergonomic research: design, selection, installation, and use in automotive manufacturing	https://www.cdc.gov/niosh/pdfs/95-114.pdf
Preventing musculoskeletal disorders in sonography	https://www.cdc.gov/niosh/docs/wp-solutions/2006-148/pdfs/2006-148.pdf
Ergonomic checkpoints: practical and easy-to-implement solutions for improving safety, health, and working conditions	http://www.ilo.org/global/publications/ilo-bookstore/order-online/books/WCMS_120133/lang--en/index.htm
Practical ergonomic information and solutions, including images and programming suggestions; ergonomic quality in design guidelines: focuses on the process of product development to meet the needs of the user	http://www.iea.cc/project/EQUID.pdf
Abstracts and articles published in *Applied Ergonomics*	https://www.journals.elsevier.com/applied-ergonomics/recent-articles
Total Worker Health (TWH)	https://www.cdc.gov/niosh/docs/2012-146/pdfs/2012-146.pdf
Human Factors and Ergonomics Society	https://www.hfes.org
International Ergonomics Association	http://www.iea.cc
Board of Certification in Professional Ergonomics	http://www.bcpe.org
OSHA Computer workstation e-tool	https://www.osha.gov/SLTC/etools/computerworkstations/index.html

ACGIH, American College of Government Industrial Hygienists; *CTS,* carpal tunnel syndrome; *NIOSH,* National Institute of Occupational Safety and Health; *OSHA,* Occupational Safety and Health Administration; *TLV,* threshold limit value.

attempts to address these issues from an organizational standpoint by integrating environmental health and safety, health promotion, disease and injury management, disability management, employee assistance, and group health insurance services. It is the intent that this coordinated approach will address both employee health and well-being, as well as work-related issues in the work environment, rather than provide services or interventions through separate or isolated programs. In terms of ergonomics, TWH programming integrates ergonomic efforts into a broader health promotion policy or approach. A research compendium describing the relevant issues and research supporting TWH is available at https://www.cdc.gov/niosh/docs/2012-146/pdfs/2012-146.pdf. The rationale for combining occupational health and safety and health promotion and the value and economics of TWH are discussed providing an excellent foundation for understanding how the health of the US workforce can be addressed in a more holistic way.

Ergonomics and Human Factors

For those interested in pursuing education in ergonomics or human factors, degree programs are available through a number of universities in the United States and abroad. For therapy practitioners interested in advancing their knowledge, the Human Factors and Ergonomics Society (HFES) (https://www.hfes.org) and the IEA (http://www.iea.cc) provide resources and membership opportunities. The HFES produces several publications related to ergonomics and conducts annual conferences that focus on disseminating evidence-based and innovative ergonomic content. The IEA also conducts conferences, has 23 technical committees that focus on specific areas of ergonomics, and has several publications of interest. The Board of Certification in Professional Ergonomics (BCPE) (http://www.bcpe.org) also provides an internationally recognized certification in ergonomics and outlines knowledge domains and certification types and requirements. Web addresses for these and other ergonomics resources can be found in Table 119.5.

Ergonomics and Computer Workstations

Computers are ubiquitous in home and work environments.[83] Despite controversies and inconsistencies regarding the relationship between computer keyboard or mouse use and WRMSDs such as CTS or tension neck syndrome,[84–86] computer work may present a number of potential symptom aggravators related to office equipment design, workstation setup, postures and movements used, types of tasks and duration of movement or sustained awkward posture, lack of movement, or specific task performance methods. Devices to consider include desktop-style computer workstations with full-sized keyboards, mouse, and screen(s); laptops with or without a separate mouse input device; tablets; and smartphones. Users may complete computer tasks, including data entry, email, writing code, drawing, gaming, image manipulation or editing, analyzing data, or surfing the Internet. Each task may require different types of input devices, frequency or intensity of use, or workspaces and therefore may require specific attention if symptoms present and have a suspected association with the device-related activity. For example, in a study comparing keystrokes, mouse clicks, mouse movement, and average typing rates, Wu and coworkers[87] reported significant differences in the type and duration of computer tasks between university administrators and computer-aided design draftsmen. The authors concluded that estimates of computer use time do not adequately describe tasks, particularly when assessing computer use–related risk factors and MSDs. Considering these findings, careful examination of the work tasks completed, along with workstation components, resulting postures, and actual work methods associated with work at the station must be included when evaluating office tasks. This information combined with ergonomic guidelines and current evidence related to office equipment, postures, and injury can help guide clinical decisions and interventions to prevent injury, address risk factors, and decrease symptom aggravators related to MSDs.

Computer workstation ergonomics guidelines such as the American National Standards Institute (ANSI)/HFES 100-2007 Human Factors Engineering of Computer Workstations[88] provide information to plan and design workspaces and equipment and to guide equipment choice and implementation. The standard can be applied for moderate to intensive computer users in typical office spaces. It provides information related to workstation heights, arrangement, equipment features, and suggested work postures and is intended to address the anthropometric needs of 90% of the North American population.[88] Individual work techniques, specific MSDs, and the full range of work requirements are not addressed by the standards. Therefore, person-specific equipment, posture, and work task adjustments may be needed for those with needs caused by injury, disability, or disease.

In general, the recommended upper extremity posture at a computer includes relaxed shoulders, elbows near the body, and forearms about parallel to the floor with the wrists straight.[89] Frequent movement and positional changes are suggested rather than trying to create a fixed, "perfect" posture. Whether the person is sitting upright, partially reclined, or standing, the workstation should provide opportunities to easily reposition and move the body with optimal joint position to access the keyboard as shown and described[8,88,92] in Box 119.7. Careful

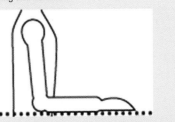

BOX 119.7   Optimal Upper Quarter Posture for Computer Workstation

- Elbow flexed 70 to 135 degrees
- Elbows flexed between 90 and 120 degrees
- Shoulder abduction at ≤20 degrees
- Shoulder flexion at ≤25 degrees
- Wrist flexion and extension angles at <30 degrees
- Head forward facing and not tilted

examination of the interplay among all the workstation components is needed to ensure that proper position of one part or one change does not adversely affect the entire system.

When a therapist is asked to assist with home or workplace computer workstation abatements, a sequential list of questions to ask and information about optimal computer workstation setup is of assistance. The OSHA e-tool[89] and the ROSA[34] evaluation are useful to obtain pertinent information and educate the patient. When an onsite evaluation is not possible, it may be helpful to obtain video or photos of the work equipment setup and postures. Studies related to remote office ergonomic evaluation are sparse. In a recent study of 23 computer workstation assessments, Liebregts and colleagues[62] evaluated the use of the ROSA to identify MSD risk at computer workstations from photographed information and compared the scores with the in-person results. Although interrater reliability was fairly good to excellent, there were sources of error related to estimates of hand–wrist joint angles from the photographs. They concluded that more study of this method was needed but that it held promise. It is the experience of the authors that if a clinician cannot visit the worksite, photographs, possibly video, and use of an assessment survey or tool will provide better data than a verbal description from the patient alone.

OFFICE ERGONOMIC DATA FOR WORKSTATION SETUP

The ANSI/HFES 100-2007[88] and OSHA e-tool[89] identify four reference postures for computer users: standing, upright sitting, declined sitting, and reclined sitting (Fig. 119.6). The positions represent work posture options for computer users to accommodate individual user styles and comfort. To access these varied postures, the interaction between the user and the individual work components can be evaluated, including the adjustability of the chair, desk, keyboard, and monitor. Changes in one component of the workstation can affect the other components and the ability to vary work position. The therapist and the user should understand this relationship and consider when and how to change components to better address comfort, work posture, and work performance.

The chair is the base of support for the body interfacing with computer workstation components, and because most employees sit at least some of the time, proper sitting posture should be carefully examined. The OSHA Computer Workstation e-tool guides the evaluator through a chair evaluation to determine if it is adjustable for height, back height and angle, seat pan depth, arm rest position, and stability.[27,89] Each of these features may influence sitting posture, back and leg support, and access to the work surface.

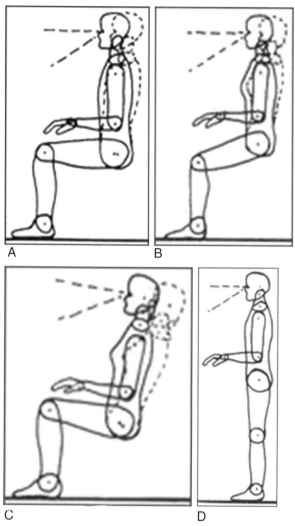

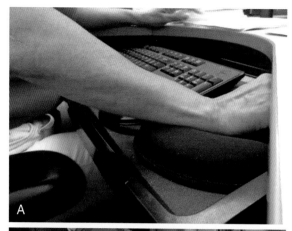

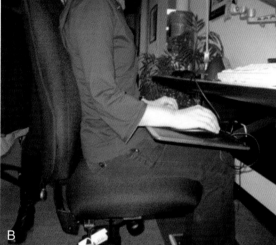

Fig. 119.7 A, Non-neutral wrist posture with a low keyboard at a positive tilt. **B,** Neutral wrist posture with an optimal keyboard height and negative tilt.

Fig. 119.6 A–D, Stand and sit postures suggested by the Occupational Safety and Health Administration.[89]

The location of the keyboard and resulting body postures is significant. Baker and Moehling[90] found that keyboard height discrepancies were significantly associated with musculoskeletal discomfort. To accommodate body dimensions for 5th percentile women to 95th percentile men, the following keyboard support height ranges are suggested (measure from floor to top of support surface)[88]:

- For seated work, adjustments from 22 to 28.3 inches
- For standing work, adjustability from 37.4 to 46.5 inches
- For adjustable sitting to standing height, adjustability from 22 and 46.5 inches

With the rising interest in standing computer workstations, it is critical to provide adequate adjustability when seated or standing to ensure that the keyboard is at about elbow height. Adjustable keyboard trays or adjustable height tables that include adjustments from about 22 to 28 inches for seated work and up to 46.5 inches for standing height provide greater opportunity for adjusting keyboard position to fit the user as compared with a fixed surface such as a standard desk, which is typically 28.5 to 30 inches high.

Although users may work on flat surfaces, use of a negative or backward tilt keyboard tray position has yielded some benefits in terms of more neutral wrist postures, carpal tunnel pressure, and comfort.[91,92] Figure 119.7A illustrates undesirable wrist postures when the keyboard tray is too low and at a positive tilt, whereas Figure 119.7B depicts placement of the keyboard in a negative incline and with the wrists neutral. In a small laboratory-based study, Woods and Babski-Reeves[93] found that placing the keyboard at about elbow height improved wrist postures and muscle activity. Rempel and coworkers[91] suggested avoiding wrist extension greater than 30 degrees and ulnar deviation greater than 15 degrees when typing for long hours to positively influence pressure in the carpal tunnel. They identified that the keyboard slope, use of split keyboards, and having the keyboard at a proper height all resulted in more neutral wrist postures. In addition, Gelberman and coworkers[94] performed a cadaver study that reported reduced pressure of the ulnar nerve at the cubital tunnel with the elbow in 90 degrees or more of extension. The negative tilt keyboard tray and posture option may be helpful to consider when treating persons experiencing wrist or cubital tunnel symptoms.

Keyboard and mouse design parameters such as key size, height, and force to depress keys or mouse buttons are important considerations in the design of input devices and are beyond the scope of this chapter but are specifically described by ANSI/HFES 100-2007 standards.[89] Traditional, straight-front keyboards, and flat mice remain readily available in the workplace and for retail purchase. Adjustable, curved, or split keyboards are easily accessed for purchase on the Internet and may be advertised as "ergonomic" but should be carefully examined in light of employee stature, job functions, and specific needs.[27] Most of these keyboard styles are designed to alter wrist deviation or reduce the degree of forearm pronation to improve comfort or reduce risk of injury,[91] but not all are appropriate for every user. In a small study, Baker and Cidboy[95] reported that three different curved keyboards influence wrist and forearm postures differently. Ripat and colleagues[96] reported that for workers experiencing symptoms and provided with an ergonomic keyboard, improved symptoms and function were sustained at the 30+ month mark. Although these results are interesting, there is little evidence to suggest that one particular style of keyboard will prevent MSDs in the majority of settings and with most types of computer work. If computer work is primarily based on mouse input, changing the keyboard would not be a priority. For the hand therapy practitioner, if changing the degree of wrist deviation or forearm pronation is needed to reduce suspected symptom aggravators, it may be helpful to try different keyboard styles with the client to find the best person-specific solution. As noted previously, the height of the keyboard or mouse relative to elbow height may represent a more significant influence on overall posture and comfort and should be considered along with keyboard selection.

Mouse input devices include traditional mouse devices, touch pads, trackballs, and other manually controlled devices for cursor management. Mouse input devices require significantly different motions and postures compared with keyboard use. Furthermore, average mouse use is estimated to be nearly three times higher than keyboard use.[97] Additionally, in a large study of nearly 2000 office workers, self-reported mouse use more than 4 hours a day was associated with increased discomfort and MSDs.[98] The frequency and duration of mouse use are of concern because increased mouse use has been associated with greater risk of MSDs than computer keyboard use.[98,99] The location of the mouse should be beside the keyboard at the same height to ensure that motions and postures recommended by ANSI/HFES 100-2007 standards[88] are achieved. Elevated wrist pads were not found to provide benefit in reducing pressure in the carpal tunnel[47] and may lead to increased pressure if the employee rests the wrist on the rest while typing, potentially creating contact stress on the volar palm and distal volar wrist.

Alternative mouse input devices and their location on the keyboard support surface are potential sources of abatement for high-risk postures, but evidence to support one type of alternate device is limited. In one study, no change in carpal tunnel pressure was noted with use of a vertical mouse,[47] and in another study,[100] the use of an alternative mouse did not produce a significant reduction in incidences of MSDs in a group of engineers. However, Conlon and coworkers[100] did conclude that use of a forearm support board may be helpful in reducing upper extremity symptoms for those using the mouse more than 20 hours per week. Options such as positioning the mouse closer to the keyboard, using a keyboard without a number pad, or even placing the mouse to the left of the keyboard can reduce the degree of wrist deviation and shoulder flexion and abduction to better meet postural recommendations. Careful assessment of the frequency and duration of mouse use and the location of the device, as well as postures and movements used to operate the device provides necessary data to inform potential computer workstation modifications for users experiencing symptoms.

Computer monitor position is an important consideration for neutral cervical spine position when at the computer workstation and is of particular concern with the use of dual monitors and laptops. It is recommended that monitors be at least 20 inches away from the user and be in line with the user's head, neck, and torso to keep the neck close to or in neutral when viewing the screen.[89,101] The height of the monitor should be such that the employee does not look up at the monitor (Fig. 119.8) but looks straight ahead at the monitor. This can require a lower height for an employee viewing the screen with multifocal lenses, and if the station is used by multiple employees,

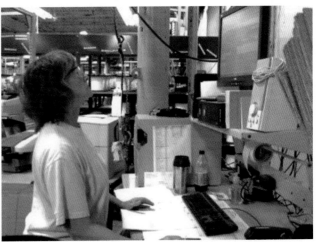

Fig. 119.8 Non-neutral cervical posture because of bifocal use with monitor that is too high.

height-adjustable monitor arms may be needed to accommodate all employees. OSHA[89] warns that a monitor that is too high can result in poor neck, shoulder, and back positioning, causing fatigue to muscles stabilizing the head. Font size can cause employees to lean forward and move into cervical extension to read some documents. With an aging population, neck position is important, and adjustability is needed. With the advent of the use of dual monitors, repeated cervical rotation to look back and forth, or static cervical rotation can occur when working from one monitor not aligned with the keyboard and chair. Employees should be encouraged to set the monitor used most often in line with the keyboard and sitting posture and adjust the chair and keyboard location if use of the second screen increases. If both monitors are used equally, they may be best centered with the keyboard and the user's body. If an employee works from a laptop for most of the shift at the office, the monitor may be too low or the keyboard too high. Optimally, the employee would dock the laptop and have a separate monitor and keyboard to achieve the ideal interface posture.

Sit–stand computer workstations have generated significant discussion because of data indicating that increased sedentary activity increases overall mortality risk along with general interest in improving overall health.[102–105] However, the Saidj and associates[105] study of Danish men found that sitting for leisure activity had a greater negative effect on cardiovascular risk factors than sitting at work; combined sitting at work and for leisure produced greater effects than either category alone.

Although standing is seen as a solution to reduce the duration of seated work, standing can be more tiring, increase stress to the circulatory system, and contribute to back pain, lower extremity edema, and cramping.[106–108] However, alternating between sitting and standing may help to improve comfort and reduce cardiovascular risk.[102] Based on the mixed and evolving body of evidence, efforts to vary work postures and increase movement during the work day can be a goal for clients. Movement out of sitting can be in the form of some periods of standing, stretching, or walking to meetings. Instituting work routine changes such as replacing seated meetings with standing or walking meetings or phone calls can also promote movement. Even with movement, improved overall health habits and sit–stand postures that meet ergonomic guidelines for work at the computer remain as important factors to address.

The ANSI/HFES 100-2007 standards[88] and the OSHA e-tool[89] provide guidance suggesting that optimal upper quarter posture for standing should mimic that suggested for sitting. The keyboard should be

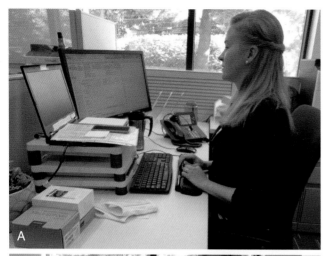

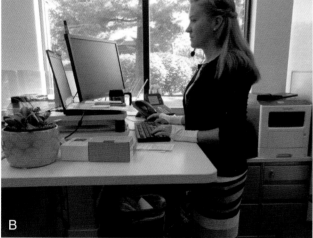

Fig. 119.9 A and B, Sit–stand station providing optimal postures for both work positions.

located at about elbow height to encourage neutral wrist positioning, shoulders relaxed, and neck in neutral. To achieve this, both the sitting and standing desk height must be slightly less than or at floor-to-elbow height (Fig. 119.9). Training users to use the equipment and in selecting postures cam be helpful improving comfort, changing positions more frequently, and attaining postures within recommended guidelines.[109,110]

There is a plethora of available equipment for the office for work conducted in seated or standing positions. Specific brands and styles may be less of a concern than whether the chosen product addresses the issue of concern, improves overall function and interface, and does not result in consequent aberrant postures or functions. As noted earlier in this section, sitting and standing options should accommodate the keyboard and screen heights for people from the 5th to 95th percentiles. For example, an electric height-adjustable table that moves from about 23 to 48 inches may provide many options to fit a wide array of users. In contrast, some tabletop add on equipment to create standing work positions may place the keyboard and monitor too high for seated computer work and should be evaluated for user fit and function before installation. If the employee must write on documents as a regular part of the work tasks, an adequate surface on which to write at the proper height for standing must be present. It is important that the employee be able to move from sit to stand with minimal effort and without requiring awkward or forceful postures to move the station from one height to another. For users experiencing upper extremity disorders, squeezing levers, applying upward or downward force, or reaching forward while lifting and pulling or pushing may be more problematic than using electric height-adjustable tables. When equipment is chosen to meet individual needs, sound clinical practice applies and should include justification for the equipment relative to patient need, reevaluation of the equipment and its interface with the employee, work methods, posture, and discussion about any other abatements that should be considered. This will help to ensure that unanticipated postures or issues have not resulted and that any consequent issues are addressed to prevent discomfort and ensure optimal positioning. Proper footwear and floor mats may also be needed to prevent fatigue and back pain when standing.[110]

SUMMARY

The intent of this chapter is to provide hand therapists with additional tools and knowledge to meet the needs of their clients experiencing WRMSDs. Understanding the language, definition, and evidence related to injury risk factors is emphasized to create a more precise discussion of the mechanism of injury as well as selection of intervention methods or solutions to reduce exposures. Hazard assessment tools and job analysis considerations provide additional detail to consider when determining work modification or abatements. Finally, it is important to consider both occupational and nonoccupational risk factors to create a more holistic view of the client's injury mechanism, inform intervention planning, and manage the recovery process.

REFERENCES

1. Hagberg M, Silverstein B, Wells R, et al. *Work Related Musculoskeletal Disorders (WMSDs): A Reference Book for Prevention*. London: Taylor & Francis; 1995.
2. Hutting N, Oswald W, Staal J, et al. Physical therapists and importance of work participation in patients with musculoskeletal disorders: a focus group study. *BMC Musculoskelet Disord*. 2017;18:196–213.
3. Marcum J, Adams D. Work-related musculoskeletal disorder surveillance using the Washington State workers' compensation system: recent declines and patterns by industry, 1999-2013. *Am J Ind Med*. 2017;60:457–471. https://doi.org/10.1002/ajim.22708.
4. OSHA. Ergonomics Overview. Available at: https://www.osha.gov/SLTC/ergonomics/. Accessed February 14, 2018.
5. Bureau of Labor Statistics[BLS]. *Injuries, Illnesses, Fatalities: Occupational Safety and Health Definitions*; 2016. Available at: https://www.bls.gov/iif/oshdef.htm. Accessed December 27, 2017.
6. Melhorn JM, Talmage JB, Ackerman III WE, Hyman MH. Introduction. In: Melhorn JM, Talmage JB, Ackerman III WE, Hyman MH, eds. *AMA Guides to Evaluation of Disease and Injury Causation*. 2nd ed. Chicago: American Medical Association; 2014:1–13.
7. Horsley R. Factors that affect the occurrence and chronicity of occupation-related musculoskeletal disorders. *Best Pract Res Clin Rheumatol*. 2011;25:103–115.
8. Fan JZ, Harris-Adamson C, Gerr F, et al. Associations between workplace factors and carpal tunnel syndrome: a multi-site cross sectional study. *Am J Ind Med*. 2015;58:509–518. https://doi.org/10.1002.ajim.22443\.
9. Rempel D, Gerr F, Harris-Adamson C, et al. Personal and workplace factors and median nerve function in a pooled study of 2396 US workers. *JOEM*. 2015;57:98–104.
10. Hegmann KT, Thiese MS, Oostema SJ. Causal associations and determination of work-relatedness. In: Melhorn JM, Talmage JB, Ackerman III WE, Hyman MH, eds. *AMA Guides to Evaluation of Disease and Injury Causation*. 2nd ed. Chicago: America Medical Association; 2014:105–114.
11. Melhorn JM, Akerman WE, Glass LS, Deitz DC. Understanding Work-relatedness. In: Melhorn JM, Talmage JB, Ackerman WE, Hyman MH, eds. *AMA Guides to the Evaluation of Disease and Injury Causation*. 2nd ed. Chicago: American Medical Association; 2014:15–104.

12. Cote J, Nygomo S, Stock S, et al. Quebec research on work related musculoskeletal disorders: deeper understanding for better prevention. *Ind Relat*. 2013;68(4):643–660.

13. Murray CJ, Atkinson C, Bhalla K, et al. U.S. Burden of Disease Collaborators. The state of US health, 1990–2010: Burden of diseases, injuries, and risk factors. *JAMA*. 2013;310:591–608. https://doi.org/10.1001/jama.2013.13805.

14. Fehringer E, Gunfeng S, Vanoeveren L, et al. Full thickness rotator cuff prevalence and correlation with function and comorbidities in patients 65 years and older. *J Shoulder Elbow Surg*. 2008;17:881–885.

15. Bureau of Labor Statistics, U.S. Department of Labor. *The Economics Daily, Type of Injury or Illness and Body Parts Affected by Nonfatal Injuries and Illnesses in 2014*; (Dec. 2, 2015). Available at: https://www.bls.gov/opub/ted/2015/type-of-injury-or-illness-and-body-parts-affected-by-nonfatal-injuries-and-illnesses-in-2014.htm.

16. National Institute for Occupational Safety and Health [NIOSH]. Musculoskeletal Disorders and Workplace Factors: A Critical Review of Epidemiological Evidence for Work-Related Musculoskeletal Disorders of the Neck, Upper Extremity and Back. DHHS(NIOSH) Publication No. 97-141. Cincinnati, OH: NIOSH.

17. daCosta JT, Baptista JS, Vaz M. Incidence and prevalence of upper-limb work related musculoskeletal disorders: a systematic review. *Work*. 2015;51:635–643. https://doi.org/10.3233AVOR-152032.

18. Mediouni Z, Bodin J, Dale AM. Carpal tunnel syndrome and computer exposure at work in two large complementary cohorts. *BMJ Open*. 2015;5:e008156.

19. Putz-Anderson V. *Cumulative Trauma Disorders: A Manual for Musculoskeletal Diseases of the Upper Limbs*. Bristol: Taylor & Francis; 1990.

20. Canadian Centre for Occupational Health and Safety. Risk Assessment. Available at: https://www.ccohs.ca/oshanswers/hsprograms/risk_assessment.html. Accessed December 29, 2017.

21. Centers for Disease Control and Prevention. *Introduction to Epidemiology CDC: Lesson 1-Section 8*; 2012. Retrieved from https://www.cdc.gov/ophss/csels/dsepd/ss1978/lesson1/section8.html. Accessed December 28, 2017.

22. Rodgers SH. Job evaluation in worker fitness determination. *Occup Med: State Art Rev*. 1988;3(2):219–238.

23. Harris-Adamson C, Eisen E, Kapellusch J, et al. Biomechanical risk factors for carpal tunnel syndrome: a pooled study of 2474 workers. *Occup Environ Med*. 2015;72:33–41.

24. Washington State Caution/Hazard Zone Checklists. Available at: http://www.lni.wa.gov/safety/SprainsStrains/evaltools/HazardZoneChecklist.PDF. Accessed February 24, 2018.

25. Garg A, Kapellusch J. Job analysis techniques for distal upper extremity disorders. *Rev Hum Fact Ergon*. 2011;7:149–196.

26. Gallagher S, Heberger J. Examining the interaction of force and repetition on musculoskeletal disorder risk: a systematic literature review. *J Hum Fact Ergon Soc*. 2013;55:108–124.

27. Dimberg L, Laestadius J, Ros S, et al. The changing face of office ergonomics. *Ergon Open J*. 2015;8:38–56.

28. Melhorn JM, Talmage JB, Ackerman WE, Hyman MH, eds. *AMA Guides to the Evaluation of Disease and Injury Causation*. 2nd ed. Chicago: American Medical Association; 2014.

29. Nathan PA, Istvan JA, Meadows KD. A longitudinal study of predictors of research-defined carpal tunnel syndrome in industrial workers: findings at 17 years. *J Hand Surg (Br)*. 2005;30:593–598.

30. Lozano-Calderon S, Anthony S, Ring D. The quality and strength of evidence for etiology: example of carpal tunnel syndrome. *JHS*. 2008;33a:525–538.

31. Tashjian RZ. Epidemiology, natural history and indications for treatment of rotator cuff tears. *Clin Sports Med*. 2012;31:589–604.

32. Wilk KE, Macrina LC, Cain EL, et al. Rehabilitation of the overhead athletes elbow. *Sports Phys Ther*. 2012;4:404–414.

33. Garg A, Kapellusch J, Hegmann K, et al. The strain index (SI) and threshold limit value (TLV) for hand activity level (HAL): risk of carpal tunnel syndrome (CTS) in a prospective cohort. *Ergonomics*. 2012;55:396–414.

34. Sharan D, Mohandoss M, Rameshkumar R, Jose J. Musculoskeletal disorders of the upper extremities due to extensive usage of hand held devices. *Ann Occup Med*. 2014;26:22.

35. Eltayeb S, Stall JB, Kennes J, et al. Prevalence of complaints of arm, neck and shoulder among computer office workers and psychometric evaluation of a risk factor questionnaire. *BMC Musculoskeletal Disord*. 2007. Available at: https://bmcmusculoskeletdisord.biomedcentral.com/articles/10.1186/1471-2474-8-68.

36. Rodgers SH. A functional Job evaluation technique, in Ergonomics. edited by J.S. Moore and A. Garg, Occupational Medicine: State of the Art Reviews. 199;7(4):679–711.

37. Thiese SM, Hegmann KT, Kapellusch J, et al. Associations between distal upper extremity job physical factors and psychosocial measures in a pooled study. *BioMed Res Int*. 2015. Available at: https://doi.org/10.1155/2015/643192.

38. McAtamney L, Weisse NE. RULA: a survey method for the investigation of work-related upper limb disorders. *Appl Ergon*. 1993;24(2):91–99.

39. Nevaiser A, Andarawis-Puri N, Flatow E. Basic mechanisms of tendon fatigue damage. *J Shoulder Elbow Surg*. 2012;21:158–163.

40. Andarawis-Puri N, Flatow E. Tendon fatigue in response to mechanical loading. *J Musculoskelet Neuronal Interact*. 2011;11(2):106–114.

41. Waters T, Putz-Anderson V, Garg A. *Applications Manual for the Revised NIOSH Lifting Equation*. US Department of Health and Human Services; 1994. Available at: https://www.cdc.gov/niosh/docs/94-110/pdfs/94-110.pdf.

42. Winnemuller LL, Spielholz PO, Daniell WE, Kaufman JD. Comparison of ergonomist, supervisor, and worker assessments of work-related musculoskeletal risk factors. *J Occup Environ Hyg*. 2004;1:414–422.

43. Borg G. Perceived exertion as an indicator of somatic stress. *Scand J Rehab Med*. 1970;2:92–98.

44. Drinkaus P, Sesek R, Bloswick D. Job level risk assessment using task level ACGIH hand activity level TLV scores: a pilot study. *J Occup Safety Ergo (JOSE)*. 2005;11:263–281.

45. Ergonomics Working Group. 2nd Chapter: Work Site Analysis. Available at: http://www.denix.osd.mil/ergoworkinggroup/assessmenttools/.

46. Willms K, Wells R, Carnahan H. Glove attributes and their contribution to force decrement and increased effort in power grip. *Hum Fact*. 2009;51:797–812.

47. Schmid AB, Kubler PA, Johnston V, Coppieters M. A vertical mouse and ergonomic mouse pads alter wrist position but do not reduce carpal tunnel pressure in patients with carpal tunnel. *Appl Ergon*. 2015;47:151–156.

48. Personal communication. *Guttenburg Museum, Mainz Germany*. 2017.

49. OSHA Basic Screening tool: https://www.osha.gov/FedReg_osha_pdf/FED20001114.pdf page 589-590. Accessed February 7, 2018.

50. Horsley R. Factors that affect the occurrence and chronicity of occupation-related musculoskeletal disorders. *Best Pract Res Clin Rheumatol*. 2011;25:103–115.

51. Helander M. *A Guide to the Ergonomics of Manufacturing*. London: Taylor & Francis; 1995:77–78.

52. Grandjean E. *Fitting the Task to the Man: A Textbook of Occupational Ergonomics*. 4th ed. London: Taylor & Francis; 1991.

53. Bovenzi M, Prodi A, Mauro M. Relationships of neurosensory disorders and reduced work ability to alternative frequency weightings of hand-transmitted vibration. *Scand J Work Environ Health*. 2015;41:247–258.

54. CeballosD, Mead K, Ramsey J. Recommendations to improve employee thermal comfort when working on 40°F refrigerated cold rooms. *J Occup Environ Hyg*. 2015;12:D216–D221.

55. Muller MD, Ryan EJ, Kim CH, et al. Test-retest reliability of Purdue Pegboard performance in thermoneutral and cold ambient conditions. *Ergonomics*. 2011;54(11):1081–1087.

56. Ramsey J, Musolin K, Ceballos D, et al. Evaluation of Ergonomic Risk Factors, Thermal Exposures and Job Stress at an Airline Catering Facility NIOSH Health Hazard Report HETA 2011-0131-3221. 2014; Report No. 2001-0131-3221. Available at: https://www.cdc.gov/niosh/hhe/reports/pdfs/2011-0131-3221.pdf. Accessed December 29, 2017.

57. Moore JS, Garg A. The strain index: a proposed method to analyze jobs for risk of distal upper extremity disorders. *Am Ind Hygiene Assn J*. 1995;56:443–458.

58. AIHA Ergonomic Committee. Ergonomic Assessment Toolkit. Retrieved December 9, 2017. Available at: https://www.aiha.org/get-involved/VolunteerGroups/Documents/ERGOVG-Toolkit_rev2011.pdf.

59. OSHA. Ergonomic Assessment Checklist. Available at https://www.os-ha.gov/dte/grant_materials/fy14/sh-26336-sh4/Ergonomic-Assess-ment-Checklist.pdf. Accessed February 8, 2018.

60. Washington State Department of Labor and Industries. Evaluation Tools. Available at: http://www.lni.wa.gov/SAFETY/SPRAINSSTRAINS/TOOLS/DEFAULT.ASP. Accessed December 9, 2017.

61. Sonne M, Villalta D, Andrews D. Development and evaluation of an office ergonomic risk checklist: ROSA – Rapid office strain assessment. *Appl Ergon.* 2012;43:98–108.

62. Liebregts J, Sonne M, Potvin JR. Photographic-based ergonomic evaluations using the Rapid Office Strain Assessment (ROSA). *Appl Ergon.* 2016;52:317–324.

63. Stevens E, Gordon AV, Stephens JP, Moore JS. Inter-rater reliability of the strain index. *J Occup Environ Hyg.* 2004;1:745–751.

64. Bonfiglioli R, Mattioli S, Armstrong T, et al. Validation of the ACGIH TLV for hand activity level in the OCTOPUS cohort: a two-year longi-tudinal study of carpal tunnel syndrome. *Scan J Work Environ Health.* 2013;39(2):155–163.

65. Kapellusch JM, Silverstein BA, Bao S, et al. Risk assessments using the strain index and the TLV for HAL, part II: multi-task jobs and preva-lence of CTS. *J Occup Environ Hyg.* 2017;14(12):1011–1019. https://doi.org/10.1080/15459624.2017 .1366037.

66. Lysaght R. Job analysis in occupational therapy: stepping into the com-plex world of business and industry. *AJOT.* 1997;51(7):569–575.

67. Spielholz P, Silverstein B, Morgan M, et al. Comparison of self-report, video observation and direct measurement methods for upper extremity musculoskeletal disorder physical risk factors. *Ergonomics.* 2001;66:588–613.

68. Job Accommodation Network. Job Descriptions in Accommodation and Compliance Series. Available at: https://askjan.org/media/downloads/JobDescriptionsA&C.pdf. Accessed March 3, 2018.

69. The U.S. Equal Employment Opportunity Commission. The ADA: Your responsibilities as an employer. Available at: https://www.eeoc.gov-/facts/ada17.html. Accessed August 28, 2017.

70. Duston RL, Russel KS, Kerr LE. *A Guide to Writing Job Descriptions Un-der the Americans with Disabilities Act.* College and University Personnel Association; 1992.

71. Balogh I, Orbsrk P, et al. Self-assessed and directly measured occupation-al physical activities – influence of musculoskeletal complaints, age and gender. *Appl Ergon.* 2004;35:49–56.

72. United States Bone and Joint Initiative. *The Burden of Musculoskel-etal Diseases in the United States (BMUS).* 3rd ed. Rosemont, IL: 2014. Available at http://www.boneandjointburden.org. Accessed on March1, 2018.

73. Cancelliere C, Donovan J, Stochkendahl MJ, et al. Factors affecting return to work after injury or illness: best evidence synthesis of sys-tematic reviews. *Chiropr Man Therap.* 2016;24:32. Available at: http://doi.org/10.1186/s12998-016-0113-z.

74. Dowd B, McGrail M, Lohman WH, et al. The economic impact of a disability prevention program. *JOEM.* 2010;52:15–21.

75. Durand MJ, Corbiere M, Coutu MF, et al. A review of the best work-absence management and return-to-work practices for workers with musculoskeletal or common mental disorders. *Work.* 2014;48:579–589.

76. Hoefsmit N, Houkes I, Nijhuis F. Intervention characteristics that facili-tate return to work after sickness absence: a systematic literature review. *J Occup Rehabil.* 2012;22:462–477.

77. Hardison ME, Roll SC. Factors association with success in an occupa-tional rehabilitation program for work related musculoskeletal disorders. *AJOT.* 2017;71. 7101180010p1-7101180010p12.

78. Andersen LN, Juul-Kristensen B, Sørensen TL, et al. Efficacy of tailored physical activity or chronic pain self-management programme on return to work for sick-listed citizens: a 3-month randomised controlled trial. *Scand J Public Health.* 2015;43:694–703.

79. IEA. Definition and domains of ergonomics. Available at: http://www.iea.cc/.

80. OSHA. OSHA at a Glance. Available at: https://www.osha.gov/Publica-tions/3439at-a-glance.pdf.

81. Occupational Health and Safety Administration[OSHA]. Standards and Enforcement. Available at: https://www.osha.gov/pls/oshaweb/owadisp.show_document?p_id=3359&p_table=OSHACT.

82. National Institute for Occupational Safety and Health [NIOSH]. National occupational research agenda. Proposed national Total Worker Health agenda for public comment (draft). Available at: http://www.cdc.gov/niosh/docket/review/docket275/pdfs/NationalTWHAgendaFinalDraft9_5_14.pdf.

83. Tornquist E, Hagberg M, Hagman M, et al. The influence of working con-ditions and individual factors on the incidence of neck and upper limb symptoms among professional computer users. *Int Arch Occup Environ Health.* 2009;82:689–702.

84. Shiri R, Falah-Hassani K. Computer use and carpal tunnel syndrome: a meta-analysis. *J Neurol Sci.* 2015;349:15–19.

85. Melhorn JM, Martin d, Brooks CN, Seaman S. Upper Limb. In: Melhorn JM, Talmage JB, Ackerman WE, Hyman MH, eds. *AMA Guides to the Evaluation of Disease and Injury Causation.* 2nd ed. Chicago: American Medical Association; 2014:243–356.

86. Waersted M, Hanvold TN, Veiersted KB. Computer work and musculo-skeletal disorders of the neck and upper extremity: a systematic review. *BMC Musculoskeletal Disord.* 2010;11. Available at: https://bmcmusculo-skeletdisord.biomedcentral.com/articles/10.1186/1471-2474-11-79.

87. Wu H, Liu Y, Chen H. Differences in computer exposure between univer-sity administrators and CAD draftsman. *Appl Ergon.* 2010;41:849–856.

88. Human Factors and Ergonomic Society. *Human Factors Engineering of Computer Workstations.* Santa Monica, CA: Human Factors and Ergo-nomics Society; 2007.

89. OSHA. Computer workstation E-tool. Available at: https://www.osha.gov/SLTC/etools/computerworkstations/index.html.

90. Baker N, Moehling K. The relationship between musculoskeletal symp-toms, postures and the fit between workers' anthropometrics and their computer workstation configuration. *Work.* 2013;46:3–10.

91. Rempel D, Keir P, Bach J. Effect of wrist posture on carpal tunnel pres-sure while typing. *J Orthopaedic Res.* 2008:1269–1273.

92. Hedge A, Morimoto S, Mccrobie D. Effects of keyboard tray geometry on upper body posture and comfort. *Ergonomics.* 1999;42:1333–1349. https://doi.org/10.1080/001401399184983.

93. Woods M, Babski-Reeves K. Effects of negatively sloped keyboard wedges on risk factors for upper extremity work-related musculoskeletal disor-ders and user performance. *Ergonomics.* 2005;48(15):1793–1808.

94. Gelberman RH, Yamaguchi K, Hollstien SB, et al. Changes in interstitial pressure and cross-sectional area of the cubital tunnel and of the ulnar nerve with flexion of the elbow: an experimental study in human cadav-ers. *J Bone Joint Surg Am.* 1998;80:492–501.

95. Baker N, Cidboy E. The effect of three alternative keyboard designs on forearm pronation, wrist extension, and ulnar deviation: a meta-analysis. *AJOT.* 2006;60(1):40–49.

96. Ripat J, Giesbrecht E, Quanbury A, Kelso S. Effectiveness of an ergonom-ic keyboard for typists with work related upper extremity disorders: a follow-up study. *Work.* 2010;37(3):275–283.

97. Richter JM, Slijper HP, Over EAB, et al. Computer work duration and its dependence on the used pause definition. *Appl Ergon.* 2008;39:772–778.

98. Ijmker MA, Huysmans BM, Blatter AJ, et al. Should office workers spend fewer hours at their computer? A systematic review of the liter-ature. *Occup Environ Med.* 2007;64:211–222. https://doi.org/10.1136/oem.2006.026468.

99. Huysmans MA, IJmker S, Blatter BM, et al. The relative contribution of work exposure, leisure time exposures and individual characteristics in the onset of arm-wrist-hand and neck-shoulder symptoms among office workers. *Int Arch Occup Environ Health.* 2012;85:651–666.

100. Conlon CF, Krause N, Rempel DM. A randomized controlled trail evaluating an alternative mouse and forearm support on upper body dis-comfort and musculoskeletal disorders among engineers. *Occup Environ Med.* 2008;65:311–318.

101. Canadian Centre for Occupational Health and Safety. Positioning the monitor 2018. Available at: http://www.ccohs.ca/oshanswers/ergonom-ics/office/monitor_positioning.html.

102. Graves L, Murphy R, Sheperd S, et al. Evaluation of sit-stand workstations in an office setting: a randomized controlled trial. *BMC Public Health.* 2015;15:1145. https://doi.org/10.1186/s12889-015-2469-8.

103. Chau JY, Grunseit AC, Chey T, et al. Daily sitting time and all-cause mortality: a meta-analysis. *PLOS ONE.* 2013;8(11):e8000. https://doi.org/10.1371/journal.pone.0080000.

104. Chricton GE, Alkerwi A. Association of sedentary behavior time with ideal cardiovascular health: the ORISCAV-LUX study. *PLOS ONE.* 2013;9(6):e99829. https://doi.org/10.371/journal.pone.0099829.

105. Saidj M, Jorgensen T, Jacobsen RK, et al. Separate and joint association of occupational and leisure-time sitting with cardio-metabolic risk factors in working adults: a cross-sectional study. *PLoS ONE.* 2013;8:e70213. https://doi.org/10.1371/journal.pone.0070213.

106. Smith P, Ma H, Glazier RH, et al. The relationship between occupational standing and sitting and incident hear disease over a 12-year period in Ontario, Canada. *Br J Sports Med.* 2016;0:1–9.

107. Coenen P, Willenberg L, Shi JW, et al. Associations of occupational standing with musculoskeletal symptoms: a systematic review with meta-analysis. *BJSM.* 2016;52(3):176–183.

108. Bahk JW, Kim H, Jung-Choi K, et al. Relationship between prolonged standing and symptoms of varicose veins and nocturnal leg cramps among women and men. *Ergonomics.* 2012;55(2):133–139.

109. Lin MY, Catalano P, Dennerlein JT. A psychophysical protocol to develop ergonomic recommendations for sitting and standing workstations. *Hum Fact.* 2016;58(4):574–585.

110. Robertson MM, Ciriello VM, Garabet AM. Office ergonomics training and a sit-stand workstation: effects on musculoskeletal and visual symptoms and performance of office workers. *Appl Ergon.* 2013;44:73–85.

111. US Department of Labor, Office of Workers Compensation. *Work Capacity Evaluation Musculoskeletal Conditions*; 2014. Available at: https://www.osha.gov/FedReg_osha_pdf/FED20001114.pdf.

120

Work Performance: Clinic-Based Assessment and Intervention

Michael J. Gerg, Vicki Kaskutas

OUTLINE

CRITICAL POINTS

- Clinicians should have an understanding of work as an occupation and realize that work is one of the most important daily activities that an adult will want to return to after an upper quarter injury.
- Early identification of the patient's work tasks is necessary to plan interventions that will facilitate successful return to work or determine inability to return to the preinjury job.
- Work-oriented activities and interventions facilitate the reinstatement of the injured person's identity as a worker.
- The ideal work-oriented rehabilitation setting promotes health and well-being while accomplishing the program goals for each participant.

It is hard to quantify how much we use our hands in life—our hands help us perform required daily activities, express our feelings, be creative, enjoy life, and interact with the world. Much of this book is dedicated to rehabilitation of a multitude of conditions that affect the hand and upper extremity. This chapter addresses rehabilitation's role in addressing work across the wide spectrum of hand and upper extremity conditions. The Occupational Therapy Practice Framework (OTPF) defines work as "Labor or exertion; to make, construct, manufacture, form, fashion, or shape objects; to organize, plan, or evaluate services or processes of living or governing; committed occupations that are performed with or without financial reward."[1] In addition to job performance, the OTPF describes employment interests and pursuits, employment seeking and acquisition, retirement preparation and adjustment, and volunteer exploration and participation as areas of work that occupational therapists should address.[1]

Work is an essential role for most Americans. The benefits of work extend far beyond the financial rewards; we learn skills, gain competence, develop self-efficacy, cultivate relationships, and often earn essential benefits, such as health care insurance. Work imposes structure and routine; it provides many people with meaning. Of course, work can have some detrimental effects such as fatigue and interruptions in sleep, interference with family and leisure roles, development of chronic conditions due to repetitive motions, stress, environmental exposures, and the possibility of injury and even death.

Employers rely on their employees to work their scheduled shift, competently perform work activities, maintain an expected level of quality, and work as safely as possible. Employers must follow federal and state laws regarding discrimination of protected groups (race, religion, sex, age, disability, pregnancy, veteran), workers' compensation, workplace safety and health, family and medical leave, and vocational rehabilitation.[2] In addition, most employers have policies and procedures in place to address workers' attendance and tardiness, inability to meet quality or productivity requirements, safety infringements, and modified duties for temporary illness or injury.

When a worker becomes a patient because of an injury or illness that affects the hand or upper extremity, functional impairments, pain, or inability to maintain work roles at the levels expected by the employer can result. These effects of the hand or upper extremity condition are similar whether work was the causative factor or not; temporary or permanent work disability can result. There is good evidence to support that the longer the period of time that an injured worker is off from work and away from the worker role because of an inability to perform the preinjury job, the less likely he or she will ever return to work[3] regardless of if the injury was work related or not.[4] The loss of the ability to work can have long-lasting devastating effects on the patient and his or her family, friends, and significant others. This chapter will help hand rehabilitation professionals address patients' struggles regarding work, whether it is a temporary interruption because of an inability to use the injured extremity, a recurring problem caused by fluctuating symptoms or abilities, or a permanent condition that will impose long-term work disability.

According to the Hand Therapy Certification Commission[5] (https://www.htcc.org/consumer-information/the-cht-credential/who-is-a-cht), 86% of certified hand therapists (CHTs) are occupational therapists. The OTPF is the official document defining the profession's perspective and guiding practice in conjunction with evidence within an identified area of practice.[1] "The overarching statement describing occupational therapy's domain of practice is achieving health, well-being, and participation in life through engagement in occupations."[1] Work is one of the eight occupations that occupational therapists "have an established body of knowledge and expertise."[1] In addition to job performance, the occupation of work includes employment interests and pursuits, job seeking and acquisition, retirement preparation and adjustment, and volunteer exploration and participation. The other 14% of CHTs are physical therapists and are guided by the 2013 Vision Statement for the Physical Therapy Profession (http://www.apta.org/Vision), which states that physical therapists evaluate and address individuals' movement system to "diagnose impairments, activity limitations, and participation restrictions; and provide interventions targeted at preventing or ameliorating activity limitations and participation restrictions."[6] Whether a therapist delivering treatment to patients with hand or upper extremity conditions is a CHT, occupational therapist, physical therapist, or licensed therapy assistant these statements support the concept that intervention should expand beyond our patients' diagnosis, structural impairments, or functional limitations to address our patients' ability to engage in meaningful activities and occupations to participate fully in life. Because work is integral to most adults' lives, it is essential for hand therapists to address work with their patients early and throughout the treatment continuum.

UNDERSTANDING THE REFERRAL QUESTION

Hand therapists typically address work performance when a patient on their caseload has an interruption in their ability to work; the patient is unable to work, working a restricted work schedule or performing partial work duties, or experiencing an increase in symptoms when working. Common questions the therapist should consider when addressing work with an existing patient include what portions of the job can the patient do and not do at this time, how much and which functions can be restored through therapy, what types of compensations can the patient use to improve work task tolerance, what methods and habits interfere or support work performance, and what workplace modifications (work tasks, environmental changes, altered schedule) would improve work performance. This chapter and Chapter 119 help prepare hand therapy practitioners to address these areas of practice.

Hand therapists may also be referred a patient with a work-related hand or upper extremity condition to address a deficit in work performance exclusively. For example, the therapist may be asked to perform a functional capacity evaluation (FCE) to quantify the patient's abilities to perform his or her job, to identify factors in the workplace that may be causing a patient's symptoms or condition, or to perform a preplacement postoffer screening before employment. This chapter and Chapter 119 address these areas to some degree; however, additional training is suggested for hand therapists who do not have experience in these areas because many policy and legal implications may need to be considered.

UNDERSTANDING THE PATIENT'S CURRENT AND PAST MEDICAL HISTORY

As with all patients seen by occupational or physical therapists, a thorough understanding of the patient's current and past medical history is essential before evaluation and intervention. Traditionally, a hand therapist has intricate knowledge of a patient's diagnosis and surgical procedures resulting in the referral to therapy plus an awareness of other health conditions and past medical history. Because many jobs require total-body effort, the therapist must also have a thorough understanding of concomitant and past health conditions, previous and current treatment for these conditions (including medications), and long-standing resultant impairments or restrictions that could impact the patient's ability to work. When the therapist can access the medical record, this information is readily available; however, this is often not the case in a hand therapy clinic. The therapist can request the patient's medical record, but it may not be accessible before seeing the patient. It is prudent to discuss concomitant and past health conditions with the patient and to gain an understanding of the patient's perceptions of the effects of these conditions on current function and ability to work.

In addition to asking patients to recall their medical conditions, it is recommended that a health history checklist that covers the body systems be administered. Most clinics have a patient reported health history form that is commonly used. The Patient Health Questionnaire is a commonly used survey of symptoms (http://www.phqscreeners.com), but it does not provide a health history. The Work Ability Index, a validated self-report instrument presented later in this chapter, includes a checklist of current health conditions that can be used to gather a health history. Patients report accidents, conditions of the musculoskeletal, cardiovascular, respiratory, neurologic, sensory, genitourinary, digestive, endocrine, and metabolic systems, mental health, accidents, tumors, blood diseases, and birth defects. The patient marks whether the condition has been diagnosed by a physician or if it is the patient's opinion. The full instrument is available at http://www.ageingatwork.eu/resources/health-work-in-an-ageing-europe-enwhp-3.pdf.

When making return-to-work recommendations, the therapist must consider the effects of these other health conditions as well as the hand or upper extremity condition for which the referral was made.

The therapist must remain mindful of the referring physician's orders and any restrictions or protocols that are in place. Hand therapists traditionally maintain close contact with the referring physician, which is especially important when addressing work as the physician may not be aware of the physically demanding tasks the therapist may need to perform to simulate the job demands. It is best to ask referring physicians for limits in the physical stresses applied to recovering structures, especially when surgery has been performed. The therapist can provide the referring physician with the job requirements to facilitate development of more accurate and specific restrictions for therapy.

UNDERSTANDING THE PATIENT'S JOB

To address work with a patient with a hand or upper extremity condition, the therapist must understand the patient's work activities, work environment, and work methods. Being aware of the demands of the job is important during evaluation, treatment planning and delivery, and discharge. The Occupational Information Network (O*NET) (https://www.onetonline.org) is a great place to begin learning about a patient's job. O*NET provides access for nearly 1000 occupations in the US economy (US Department of Labor, https://www.onetcenter.org/overview.html). Simply type in the patient's job title in the occupation quick search region of the website; it is best to do this with the patient at your side so he can help you choose his occupation and identify which of the identified tasks he routinely performs. A quick search for the job title "construction

TABLE 120.1	US Department of Labor Physical Demand Strength Rating of Work			
	Occasional (0%–33%)	Frequently (33%–66%)	Constantly (<66%)	Energy Requirements (MET)
Sedentary	10 lb	Negligible	Negligible	1.5–2.1
Light	20 lb	10 lb	Negligible	2.2–3.5
Medium	20–50 lb	10–25 lb	10 lb	3.6–6.3
Heavy	50–100 lb	25–50 lb	10–20 lb	6.4–7.5
Very heavy	>100 lb	>50 lb	>20 lb	>7.5

MET, Metabolic equivalent of tasks.

laborer" identified 26 tasks (ranging from controlling traffic to operating a jackhammer), 129 tools or technologies used (e.g., ladders and saws), 23 abilities (including manual dexterity and static strength), 17 work activities, and 37 detailed work activities. O*NET allows tasks to be displayed by level of importance, relevance, or frequency; abilities and activities can be displaced by importance or level. The US Department of Labor has historically classified the physical demand strength rating into five categories based on the level and frequency of forces exerted[7] (Table 120.1). Although this is a very general and old classification system, it is still used in work rehabilitation.

After the therapist has an understanding of the patient's job title from the generic perspective provided by O*NET, information about the specific tasks, activities, tools, technologies, and environments at the patient's workplace can be explored. A quick internet search can help the therapist envision the patient's job. For example, to learn about concrete finishing, the therapist can watch a video showing workers raking and floating a concrete driveway, view images of different concrete finishing machines and look up the weight, dimension, and vibratory forces generated by a concrete finishing machine similar to what the patient uses at work. The patient should be asked to provide details about his or her job tasks, equipment, environment, and work schedule. It is best to get input from the patient's employer also. The therapist can contact the employer to request a written job description, discuss return-to-work options, and arrange a work visit if needed. Some employers have functional job descriptions with specific measurements of the physical demands of the job, such as "lift an 80-lb sandbag from floor to 4-feet up to 50 times per day." Because many employers or job settings do not have adequate functional job descriptions, generic job descriptions such as those on O*NET and input from the patient and supervisor (if possible) are used. In addition, the clinician uses her or his best judgment.

Before any discussion with an employer representative, it is best to get the patient's written approval. It is suggested that the therapist include the patient in employer conversations that may necessitate disclosure of health-related information to prevent the therapist from having to disclose health-related information governed by Health Insurance Portability and Accountability Act of 1996 (HIPAA). This includes the patient's past, present, or future physical or mental health or condition, and details regarding provision of health care to the patient (US Department of Health and Human Services, http://www.hhs.gov/ocr/privacy/hipaa/understanding/summary/privacysummary.pdf). In addition to needing to understand the job, the hand therapist may want to be aware of the risk for musculoskeletal disorders (MSDs) associated with specific job duties. There are many job-related assessments to quantify these ergonomic risks for MSDs. Readers are referred to Chapter 119 of this book and Thomas Bernard's website (http://health.usf.edu/publichealth/eoh/tbernard/ergotools) for more information.

EMPLOYMENT POLICIES TO CONSIDER WHEN ADDRESSING WORK

There are many federal, state, and other applicable policies that hand therapists must understand when addressing work with their patients. Hand therapists are well aware that they must comply with HIPAA (https://www.hhs.gov/hipaa/for-professionals/index-.html), the Centers for Medicare and Medicaid Services (https://www.cms.gov/Medicare/Billing/TherapyServices/index.html), their professions' code of ethics, and their employer's and facility's policies. Most hand therapists are also aware of workers' compensation laws, which mandate that when an employee sustains injury, illness, or death in the course of employment, the employer must pay for medical costs, lost wages, and in most states, permanent partial disabilities incurred.[7a] Workers' compensation laws vary from state to state (https://www.expertlaw.com/library/comp_by_state/index.html). Vocational rehabilitation is a federally mandated act that provides individuals with disabilities vocational guidance, training, occupational adjustment, and placement services linked to a vocational objective goal. Vocational rehabilitation is provided at the state level, so policies vary by state (https://www.csavr.org/state-vr-directors). The Social Security Administration administers the Supplemental Security Income (SSI) and Social Security Disability Insurance (SSDI) programs for adults with disabilities who are unable to engage in any substantial gainful activity (work performed for pay) because of a medically diagnosed physical or mental impairment that lasts for at least 1 year (https://www.ssa.gov/planners/disability). The Ticket to Work Program is a federally mandated program that assists SSI and SSDI beneficiaries to obtain employment (https://www.ssa.gov/work/). The Occupational Safety and Health Act oversees workplace safety.

All employers must comply with the Occupational Safety and Health Administration's (OSHA's) general industry standards, plus there are specific construction, maritime, and agricultural standards (https://www.osha.gov/law-regs.html) and industry-specific resources (https://www.osha.gov/dcsp/compliance_assistance/industry.html). Currently, 24 states have state-mandated safety and health plans (https://www.osha.gov/dcsp/osp/statestandards.html) that must be at least as stringent as the federal OSHA requirements. It is important for clinics addressing work to ensure that equipment used in job simulations comply with OSHA standards. For example, their ladder weight limits and climbing standards must be followed, and personal protective equipment must be available.

Because work evaluation can be considered an employment test, therapists performing evaluations that are being used to make return-to-work decisions must comply with employment discrimination laws enforced by the Equal Employment Opportunities Commission (https://www.eeoc.gov/laws/index.cfm). We will review several of these discrimination laws in this chapter.

Title VII of the Civil Rights Act of 1964 prohibits employment discrimination based on race, color, religion, sex, or national origin (US Equal Employment Opportunity Commission, https://www.eeoc.gov/laws/statutes/titlevii.cfm). It is important that work evaluations treat men and women equally. Strength and lift capacity assessments often demonstrate a gender bias. For example, there is a standardized lifting evaluation that continues to be reported in peer-reviewed manuscripts,[8] which uses a lighter starting load and progresses the load by 50% less for women in comparison with men.[9] This means that a woman performs twice as many lifts to reach the load required for a specific job in comparison with a man; this practice is discriminatory.

The Age Discrimination in Employment Act (ADEA) of 1967 protects individuals who are 40 years of age or older from employment discrimination (https://www.eeoc.gov/laws/types/age.cfm). The labor force participation rate of people ages 65 to 74 years increased from 17.5% in 1996 to 28.6% in 2016, and it is projected to increase to 30.2% by 2026 (Bureau of Labor Statistics, https://www.bls.gov/emp/ep_table_303.htm). As a result, work will be a primary goal for aging patients with hand or upper extremity conditions. As the body ages, physiological changes can affect strength, agility, sensory, and cardiopulmonary functions. The work evaluation protocol must have safety measures in place to monitor physiological functions, but the testing procedures must not be discriminatory toward patients older than 40 years of age.

Title I of the Americans with Disabilities Act (ADA) of 1990 and the ADA Amendments of 2008 prohibit discrimination against qualified individuals with disabilities in the private employers with 15 or more employees and state and local governments. With unemployment nearly twice as high among individuals with disabilities (US Department of Justice, https://www.ada.gov/ada_title_I.htm), it is critically important for qualified individuals to be provided with the accommodations that might be necessary to help them perform the essential functions of the job. Testing protocols, equipment, environments, and facilities used in the rehabilitation setting should not discriminate against individuals with disabilities.[2] If a patient with a hand or upper extremity condition has a qualified disability, defined as a physical or mental impairment that substantially limits one or more major life activities, the therapist must provide reasonable accommodations when performing work evaluations and interventions. Therapists can also help patients determine the types of accommodations that they may need to be successful at the workplace, as well as advocate for patients in return-to-work negotiations.

The Family Medical Leave Act (FMLA) provides private sector employers with 50 or more employees and local, state, and federal employers to provide employees with up to 12 weeks of annual unpaid job-protected leave for a serious health condition (US Department of Labor, https://www.dol.gov/whd/fmla/index.htm). FMLA also requires that group health benefits are maintained during the leave and employees are entitled to return to their same or an equivalent job at the end of their FMLA leave. Most employers' work absence policies allow for termination of an employee that has not reported for work for a specified period of time; therefore, it is critical for therapists to advise patients to apply for FMLA if they are unable to work. FMLA allows an employee to take intermittent leave or work a reduced schedule when leave is needed for medical treatment or when leave is needed to care for a spouse, child, or parent with a serious health condition (US Department of Labor, https://www.dol.gov/whd/fmla/fmla-faqs.htm).

ISSUES SPECIFIC TO THE WORKERS' COMPENSATION POPULATION

When a patient's care is covered by workers' compensation, there is a host of issues that the hand therapy professional must consider, especially when addressing work performance. Patients who are unable to work, continue to receive a portion of their wages, usually two thirds of their customary pay, plus employers must pay other workers to perform the patients' job duties during their recovery from the work injury or illness. As a result, the workers' compensation carrier or employer may apply pressure to return patients to the workplace. For example, therapy professionals may be told they can only address the affected

body part in work interventions, should watch a videotape of a patient doing a home activity or hobby similar to work, or closely attend to any inconsistencies demonstrated by the patient. Therapy professionals must never compromise their professional ethics, remembering their commitment to the patient, understanding that the functions of the entire body are often important for work, and remaining vigilant to ensure that the patient completely understands exactly the therapists' instructions and is given every opportunity to provide maximal, consistent effort. When a condition is work related, the workers' compensation representative may push the therapist to only address the injured body part, but decisions regarding a patients' ability to return to work must consider the whole patient, including all body parts and systems. The therapy professional never sacrifices a patient's safety to obtain consistent (reliable) or valid evaluation results, which is discussed in the choice of assessments section later in this chapter. It is important for documentation to be specific in workers' compensation cases because this prevents the insurance carrier from "reading between the lines" or "jumping to conclusions." For example, if there is high variability between three grip strength trials administered early in the evaluation, but as the evaluation progressed, results became more consistent, the therapist may conclude that early inconsistencies were caused by the patient's being accustomed to avoiding forceful activities during recovery and that as the evaluation progressed, the patient gained confidence with the change from the patient role to the worker role. The therapist would want to include this observation in the documentation to prevent misinterpretation of the initial inconsistency as ingenuine effort. There are benefits to working with patients on workers' compensation. It is often easier to obtain functional job descriptions, borrow tools and equipment for job simulations, get extensions for additional therapy, and engage in conversations regarding modifications needed to facilitate return to work.

CHOOSING CONSTRUCTS TO EVALUATE

Depending on the phase of rehabilitation, the hand therapist has likely performed assessments to measure pain, capillary refill, edema, skin and wound status, range of motion (ROM), tendon gliding, grip and pinch strength, isometric muscle strength, sensation, and provocative testing. Determining the constructs (areas) that need to be evaluated to address work performance builds on the results of these assessments, current and past medical conditions and ongoing interventions, and the job requirements and workplace environment. The International Classification of Functioning, Disability, and Health (ICF) has core sets that can be useful when choosing areas and assessment to administer. For example, there are ICF category core sets for acquiring, keeping, and terminating a job; remunerative employment; and work and employment (http://www.icf-core-sets.org/en/page1.php) and the ICF Core Set for vocational rehabilitation (https://www.icf-research-branch.org/download/download/11-diversesituations/109-briefi cfcoresetforvocationalrehabilitation).

Table 120.2 lists constructs that can guide the therapist in selecting areas that need to be assessed to address work performance. This list has been created with input from the OTPF,[1] the ICF (http://www.who.int/classifications/icf/en/), and the Person-Environment-Occupational Performance model.[9a] We suggest that the hand therapist develop a list of priority assessment constructs using Table 120.2 or other resources that provide an organizational taxonomy.

It is obvious that work is an occupation that must be addressed, but it is important to assess a patient's other occupations if the patient is going to be competitively employed. For a patient with an upper quarter condition to maintain competitive employment, he or she must comply with continuing education requirements, present in a clean and

TABLE 120.2   Constructs to Consider When Addressing Work

Activities and Occupations	Intrinsic or Person Factors and Body Functions	Performance Patterns	Extrinsic or Environmental Factors
Work	Psychological: emotional control, beliefs, locus of control, mood, stress	Habits	Physical
Rest and sleep		Routines	Natural
Education	Cognitive: executive function, awareness, memory, organization, metacognition, learning	Rituals	Social
Social participation		Roles	Policy
ADLs: bath or shower, toileting and toilet hygiene, dressing, feeding, functional mobility, personal care devices, personal grooming and hygiene	Physiological: skin and wound, energy, circulation		Technology
	Sensory: pain, touch, other senses		Culture
	Motor: motion, posture, manipulate, grip, pinch, reach, coordinate, lift, carry, push, pull		Virtual
IADLs: care of others, children, and pets; communication; driving and community mobility; home management; health management and maintenance	Coordinate: manipulate, fine-motor dexterity, in-hand coordination		

ADL, Activity of daily living; *IADL*, instrumental activity of daily living.

well-groomed manner, get to work on a dependable basis, toilet and eat independently, and manage his or her health needs at the workplace. For example, inadequate sleep can lead to fatigue, attention deficits, and mood interruptions. In turn, these issues can result in decreased productivity, errors, safety breaches, damage to equipment or supplies, and potential injury to self or coworker(s).

Most hand therapy practitioners have worked with patients whose psychological status interferes with recovery, whether it is an apathetic outlook, an inability to manage stress, or an external locus of control that prevents the patient from assuming responsibility for her or his recovery. Most also have treated a patient who cannot seem to learn their home program or remember exactly how they are supposed to apply their splint, or a patient who is out of breath walking from the car or has problems healing due to smoking. Most hand therapy practitioners have training and/or experience addressing psychological, behavioral, and cognitive issues with their patients, but occupational therapists may have additional background in these areas. Hand therapists will likely only perform screening assessments of these intrinsic, person, and body functions, which is consistent with physical therapy's scope of practice. The Rehab Measures website has links to standardized assessments for many of the occupation and intrinsic, person, and body functions listed in Table 120.2. Depending on the level of involvement, successful return to work can be difficult when patients experience psychological or behavioral issues. According to a recent systematic review exploring psychological problems after hand trauma, posttraumatic stress, anxiety, depression, and chronic pain can be detected 3 months postinjury.[10] Depression has been found to be present in many individuals with peripheral nerve injuries,[11] including catastrophizing in patients with hand fractures,[12] as well as symptom magnification.[13] Catastrophizing is a common irrational thought that something is far worse than it actually is (https://psychcentral.com/lib/what-is-catastrophizing/). It is essential for hand therapists to remember that these are natural phenomenon that commonly occur and that the patient is not volitionally controlling these thoughts, feelings, or states of being.

CHOOSING ASSESSMENTS TO EVALUATE TARGETED CONSTRUCTS

After the therapist has compiled the list of constructs that need to be evaluated, the assessment instrument that will be used to measure these constructs is identified. Often an assessment addresses several constructs—for example, the Disability of the Arm Shoulder Hand

(DASH) questionnaire assesses disability and provides valuable information regarding activities of daily living (ADLs), instrumental activities of daily living (IADLs), work, leisure, and pain. It is important to understand the hierarchical criteria for work assessments that have been established by the National Institute of Occupational Safety & Health (NIOSH). Because the assessments are used to make work decisions, they must possess the following characteristics in this hierarchical order: the test must be *safe* to administer, it must give *reliable* values that are quantifiable, and it must be *valid* and able predict risk of future injury or illness.

Safety

Safety is the most critical criteria that must be maintained throughout evaluation and intervention at all costs. The therapist must do everything possible to ensure that the patient's safety is maintained at all time. This presents a challenge when there is strong evidence that a task, technique, or posture presents excessive risk of injury or illness. The therapist must define safety criteria that can *never* be overlooked by staying abreast of peer-reviewed literature with the highest level of evidence. Concerning lifting, there is a wide range of issues to consider, but focus must be placed on those that have found to be predictive of injury. In this chapter, we focus on the following safety criteria: poor coupling between the hand and the load, keeping the load close to the body, twisting motions, jerking or throwing motions where the load is quickly accelerated, using the thigh to nudge the load or back hyperextension to elevate the load to heights needed, and holding the breath. Many of these criteria are included in National Institute of Occupational Safety and Health's lifting equation (https://www.cdc.gov/niosh/docs/94-110/default.html).

Coupling, defined as the hand's interface with the object being manipulated, must be considered with all patients, especially those with hand or forearm conditions. The best position for grasping objects (from a strength–length ratio to prevent active insufficiency of the extrinsic finger flexors) is with the fingers flexed to midposition, wrist extended, forearm in neutral, and a comfortable coupling between the hand and the object being lifted (Figs. 120.1 and 120.2). The research performed on manual materials handling (MMH) has been focused on the spine and back pain; very little research has been done to study the effects of lifting on the upper limb.[14] The patient's ability to keep the load close to the body throughout the entire lift should be a priority when addressing work. The amount of torque generated by a load is equivalent to the weight of the load multiplied by the perpendicular

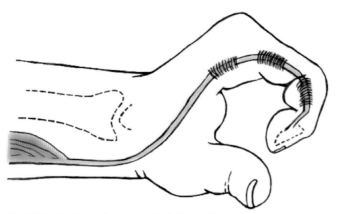

Fig. 120.1 Ideal position for extrinsic finger flexor muscles to generate force. (From http://img.medscape.com/pi/emed/ckb/orthopedic_surgery/1230552-1237885-1245758-1245824.jpg.)

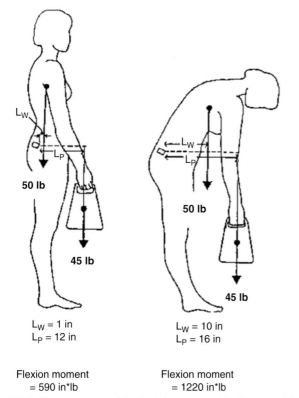

$L_W = 1$ in
$L_P = 12$ in

$L_W = 10$ in
$L_P = 16$ in

Flexion moment = 590 in*lb

Flexion moment = 1220 in*lb

Fig. 120.2 Torque generated by load increases with distance of load from the center of gravity. L_P, distance to center of gravity of body part lifted; L_W, distance to center of gravity of external load lifted.

distance between the center of gravity of the load and joint. For example, a 50-lb load generates 500 inch-lb of torque when it is held 10 inches from the glenohumeral joint, but when at held 30 inches, this same load generates 1,500 inch-lb of torque. In turn, the shoulder flexor muscles generate three times greater force to hold the load. These increased torques and forces can damage the muscles, tendons, ligaments, and cartilaginous structures in the joint.

These biomechanical factors, along with the patient's condition and medical status, are essential to consider when asking a patient to lift. For example, a person with scaphoid dysfunction may demonstrate the ability to lift loads of 50 lb or more with the wrist in neutral; however, this person will lose the ability to sustain the lift with wrist deviation. Also, a patient with lateral epicondylitis may be able to lift 25 lb in his

affected extremity when the forearm is supinated and the load is held close yet is unable to lift the load when the forearm is pronated and the load is held far from the body.

The therapist must use a wide range of methods to ensure that the patient's safety is never compromised, including continuous heart rate monitoring; patient-reported ratings of perceived exertion,[15] pain, and fatigue; observation of biomechanical factors; and other observable signs of distress, maximum tolerance, or frustration.

Reliability

Reliability is the degree to which an assessment tool produces stable and consistent results and depends on the assessment instrument that is being used, the accuracy and precision of the evaluation procedures, the therapist's ability to consistently follow the administration protocol, and the consistency of the patient's effort throughout the evaluation. Use of standardized assessment measures that demonstrate good reliability is recommended, as well as developing and following standardized administration procedures. To ensure that the patient provides consistent effort, the therapist explains the directions fully and validates that the patient fully understands the importance of providing consistent effort. The therapist closely monitors and records the patient's response to each subtest and the reason for stopping (including behaviors, statements, vital signs, grimaces, rubbing, pain ratings, and perceived exertion ratings). If the hand or upper extremity condition is work related, the worker's compensation carrier often scrutinizes the report to identify inconsistencies in the patient's effort, often termed *sincerity of effort* or *validity indicators* (which is a reliability indicator and not a validity indicator, but this term is commonly used). There are many reasons that a patient recuperating from an injury, illness, surgery, or extended time away from work may provide inconsistent effort, such as pain, fear, fatigue, medications, weight gain, muscle loss, cardiopulmonary deconditioning, decreased agility, and lack of understanding of the testing goal or procedure. When inconsistencies in patient's effort are noted, it is best to address them in the moment, repeating the instructions and repeating testing if it is safe to do so.

Validity

Validity is defined as the extent to which an assessment measures what it claims to measure; to have predictive validity, there should be content, construct, and other forms of criterion validity. The fact that most people perform their work for an entire work shift, whether it is 6, 8, or 12 hours in length, plus they must go to the workplace several days in a row, normally 5 days per week, complicates the task of performing a work evaluation. If a patient can perform simulated work for 1 hour during the three times per week therapy session, does that mean that he can work five 8-hour shifts as is required of the job? For the work assessment to be valid, it must predict actual work performance, which is very difficult to achieve. Establishing the validity of work assessments is more challenging than assessments of body functions or ADLs because the job demands vary greatly among the nearly 1000 job titles in the US economy. Because safety is more important than validity, manual material handling testing is first evaluated with objects and methods that allow for ideal coupling between the hand and patient; then objects with coupling similar to work are tested. Often the results will be very different. For example, a cement mason's status after resection of a neuroma in the digit may lift 100 lb in a crate with ideal coupling during the standardized lifting assessment but not be able to lift an 80-lb bag of cement or a 71-lb 12-inch concrete solid top block. The hand therapy practitioner must be especially vigilant when performing nonstandardized assessments because procedures and precautions are not defined as they are in standardized assessment.

SCREENING AND ASSESSMENTS REGARDING WORK

Ability to perform activities and occupations are best assessed with evaluations at the activity or occupation level. For example, patients often are able to perform their jobs at a competitive level despite structural loss (e.g., an amputation), severe ROM limitation, significant vision loss, high level of anxiety, or maladaptive habits. It is important to remember that compensatory strategies, automated methods, environmental modifications, or temporary modification of job duties can compensate for lost body structures or functions, limited performance skills, or environmental barriers. As a result, the hand therapist should *always* perform evaluations at the activity and occupation level and should base the decision regarding a patient's ability to work *more* on evaluation results of ability to perform activities and occupations than measures of body function, performance skills, or performance patterns. This is not to say that the therapist should *avoid* performing evaluations of motion, strength, or pain; in fact, the therapist *should* perform screens of the underlying body functions before asking a patient to perform a work activity or occupation. For example, screening sensory functions (vision, hearing, touch localization in upper and lower extremities) is recommended with all patients from a safety perspective, as are screens of cognition, depression, and balance. This recommendation is based on numerous expert witness cases by this chapter's authors in personal injury cases brought against therapists performing initial work evaluations or functional capacity evaluations. For example, before asking a patient to climb a ladder, the therapist should understand the patient's abilities to hear without visual cues, kinesthetically know where the extremities and trunk are in space, follow directions, flex the hip and knee to at least 90 degrees against gravity, perform eccentric contractions with one extremity against body weight, and balance while standing on one foot. Other recommendations based on this work are to strictly follow all standardized assessment procedures and your site's evaluation protocol. For example, if heart rate is to be monitored and the assessment discontinued at a certain level, it is essential to abide. If your site says that a vision screen is performed before job-simulated testing, this must be performed. This recommendation is also based on prior expert witness work.

Often the hand therapist addressing work will have already administered evaluations of the body structures (skin integrity, circulation, tendon glide), body functions (ROM, pain, sensation), and performance skills (grip strength, reaching, manipulation). These evaluations will not need to be repeated; however, other body functions and performance skills will likely need to be evaluated or at least screened. For example, an individual who is a bicycle delivery person or a construction laborer will need to have an evaluation of cardiopulmonary endurance, and a factory worker who unloads boxes from an assembly line to a pallet on a constant basis will need an evaluation of muscular endurance. If the clinician has access to an employer's functional job description or the therapist has observed the job being performed, then basic functional requirements can be determined to guide return-to-work recommendations and drive treatment goals.

It is important to note that results from patient-reported outcome measures that are routinely administered to track treatment outcomes in patients with hand and upper extremity conditions can provide information that is useful when evaluating ability to work. These include measures of upper extremity disability, such as the DASH questionnaire, the Patient Rated Wrist Hand Evaluation (PRWHE), the Patient Reported Outcomes Measurement Information System (PROMIS), and a multitude of other popular measures.[16–18] For example, the DASH score and the individual items give the hand therapist a good idea of the patient's ability to perform daily tasks and the pain levels.

Activity and Occupation Level Assessments to Evaluate Work

Given that evaluations at the activity and occupation level should be a primary focus of the hand therapist's work evaluation, we will review them first and then present evaluations of performance skills, environments, and body functions.

Disabilities of the Arm Shoulder and Hand

The DASH is a 30-item questionnaire that measures upper extremity disability.[19] The DASH questionnaire is commonly used by physicians and hand therapists; in fact, 47% of Midwestern U.S. therapists surveyed used the DASH questionnaire.[20] Items on the DASH address symptoms and ability to perform self-care, household tasks, work, sports, and hobbies. It uses a 5- to 6-point Likert scale. The DASH correlates well with other measures of disability, function, and pain (>-0.75) and demonstrates test–retest reliability that exceeds 0.95. The DASH includes optional modules for work and sports and musical instruments. Administration of the Work DASH module is strongly recommended when addressing work with a patient with a hand or upper extremity condition.

The QuickDASH is a shorter survey that consists of only 11 items and a four-question work module. The DASH and QuickDASH and administration manuals are available for download from http://dash.iwh.on.ca. Online versions are also available for purchase.

Upper Extremity Functional Index

The Upper Extremity Functional Index (UEFI) measures the impact of the patient's upper extremity function on a variety of daily activities, including work, and is easily administered in 5 minutes.[21] The UEFI uses a 5-point Likert scale and asks respondents to rate their ability to perform a variety of tasks and rate it from "Extreme difficulty or unable to perform" (0 points) to "No difficulty" (4 points). It is available in a 20-item and 15-item survey. The UEFI has demonstrated excellent test–retest reliability at 0.95 and internal consistency at 0.94. The tool has been determined to have good discriminant cross-sectional validity. An online version is available at https://www.thecalculator.co/health/Upper-Extremity-Functional-Index-(UEFI)-Calculator-955.html.

The Patient Reported Outcomes Measurement Information System (PROMIS) is a suite of person-centered measures of physical, mental, and social health in adults and children (http://www.healthmeasures.net/explore-measurement-systems/promis/intro-to-promis). Physical health measures include pain intensity, pain interference, physical function, fatigue, and interference with sleep. The PROMIS physical function, pain interference, and depression questionnaires correlate moderately with the QuickDASH questionnaire.[22] The Upper Extremity (UE) Physical Health scale measures self-reported ability to perform activities requiring use of the upper extremity including shoulder, arm, and hand activities, such as writing, using buttons, or opening containers. The full PROMIS UE includes 46 items (http://www.healthmeasures.net/index.php?option=com_instruments&view=measure&id=788&Itemid=992), and the short form includes 7 items (http://www.healthmeasures.net/index.php?option=com_instruments&view=measure&id=797&Itemid=992).

Functional Abilities Confidence Scale

The Functional Abilities Confidence Scale (FACS) is a 15-item standardized questionnaire that measures the degree of self-efficacy or confidence that a patient exhibits toward the performance of various activities or postures.[23] It asks the patient to rate the percentage of confidence that they have to perform a given activity with 0% being "not confident at all" and 100% being "completely confident." It demonstrates good test–retest reliability, internal consistency, responsiveness to change, and convergent validity.[24] This tool can be administered in

5 to 10 minutes and can facilitate patient-centered collaboration in identifying areas to focus treatment. It also can identify if there are non–upper extremity–related issues that the patient perceives that she may have (e.g., if there is an issue with the lower extremities or spine). The FACS is a free tool that can be downloaded from http://www.camb-sphn.nhs.uk/Libraries/Pain_Management_-_Scrng_Qstnrs/Functional_abilities_confidence_scale.sflb.ashx.

Work Ability Index

The Work Ability Index (WAI), an evaluation originally developed in Finland, measures an individual's capacity to work while taking into account the physical and mental demands of the job. It has been widely used throughout the European Union, has established norms, and is easy to administer. It is a self-report survey that includes 10 questions on the following 6 different dimensions:

- Current ability to work compared with the patient's lifetime best
- Work ability in relation to the job demands
- Number of diagnosed illnesses or conditions the patient currently has
- Estimated levels of impairment from illnesses and conditions
- Amount of sick time or leave the patient has taken in the past year
- Self-reported prognosis of the patient's ability to work in 2 years' time

The WAI has demonstrated validity and reliability in correlation analyses.[25] It is limited in that it does not inform the administrator with regard to the actual job demands of the patient. It is available in many different languages. Administration of the WAI can be repeated periodically during and after treatment and has been found to provide information on how the work ability of those surveyed has developed and whether action taken to promote health has had a positive impact on the patient. The WAI has been used extensively with older workers and has been found to be predictive of work disability, retirement, and mortality.[25] It can be found on page 34 of the following document: http://www.ageingatwork.eu/resources/health-work-in-an-ageing-europe-enwhp-3.pdf. There is also an online free short version available at http://www.arbeits-faehigkeit.uni-wuppertal.de/index.php?wai-online-en.

Work Productivity and Impairment Questionnaire

The Work Productivity and Impairment Questionnaire (WPAI) is a six-question survey that is completed by the patient. It was designed to assess the amounts of both absenteeism and presenteeism demonstrated by the patient because of health issues (http://www.reillyassociates.net/WPAI_General.html). The WPAI has been validated across multiple disease populations but none that are upper extremity specific. There have been validity studies done for osteoarthritis[26] and rheumatoid arthritis[27] that do substantiate the validity and reliability of this tool, but it does vary from condition to condition. The authors of the tool have made this tool available free for download on their website at http://www.reillyassociates.net/WPAI_General.html. They give permission for the tool to be adapted to fit specific diseases or health problems but not modification of the tool. This means that although the wording of the survey cannot be changed, the name of the specific condition being measured (e.g., carpal tunnel syndrome) can be used in place of the word "problem" in the survey. The authors urge anyone using this tool in outcomes research to include the study of validity in the research so that they may share it with other users of the WPAI.

Job Performance Measure

The Job Performance Measure (JPM) measures a patient's perceptions of his or her ability to perform the tasks required of his or her job.[28] The JPM is modeled after the Canadian Occupational Performance Measure (COPM) and developed by an author of this chapter and colleagues at Washington University School of Medicine in St. Louis. To identify the specific requirements of the patient's job, occupations that best represent the patient's job are searched at the O*NET website (https://www.onet-center.org/overview.html). Tasks for the target occupation are reviewed with the patient, and tasks that the patient reports routinely performing at work are recorded on the JPM. The patient's perception of his or her current ability to perform each job task is rated on the 10-point scale COPM scale, with 1 being not able to do it and 10 being able to do it extremely well. Although the JPM has not undergone rigorous psychometric testing, it has been used clinically with thousands of work rehabilitation patients. In two research studies with individuals with mild stroke, the JPM was the best predictor of return-to-work success. The JPM is included is in Appendix A and is also published elsewhere.[28]

Other Work Performance Measures

Other measures at the activity, occupation, or disability level that be useful when evaluating work in patients with hand or upper extremity conditions; however, they either require a fee to use or are specific to only one part of the upper extremity. Examples include the Shoulder Pain and Disability Index (SPADI), Shoulder Rating Questionnaire, Michigan Hand Outcomes Questionnaire (MHQ), Upper Extremity Functional Scale, Nordic Musculoskeletal Questionnaires (NMQ), and Upper Extremity Questionnaire.

JOB-SIMULATED TESTING OF WORK ACTIVITIES AND OCCUPATIONS

After performing standardized measures of the work activities and occupations, body functions, and performance skills, job simulated testing can be performed. Job simulated testing is often the most telling means of assessing where a patient's limitations will be with performing her or his work. Job-simulated tests are designed by the therapist to mimic the job demands as closely as possible. Before performing a job simulation, it is prudent to ask the patient to rate her or his perceived current ability to perform the activity and to identify barriers to performance. A simple rating scale, such as that used in the JPM, rates a patient's perception of his or her current ability to perform an activity on a scale from 0 to 10, with 0 being completely unable to perform the task to 10 being able to perform the task with no difficulty. Job descriptions, discussions with the patient and employer, worksite visits, and videotapes from the worksite and even generic videos of people using job-specific tools or equipment and performing work tasks should be used to develop the job simulations. Tools, equipment, and supplies needed for job simulations can be borrowed from the employer, purchased at the Goodwill or the Salvation Army, or brought in from the therapist's or patient's home. The therapist must ensure that equipment is safe and complies with applicable federal and state standards previously discussed. For example, an airline baggage handler who lifts in the cargo hold of a plane lifts various size and weight suitcases and arranges them similar to what is required at work while in a kneeling position. A creative clinician can develop work simulations for a variety of jobs. The work simulation establishes a baseline and can be a launching point to determine if interventions are needed.

The following practices are suggested by Innes and Straker[29,30] to increase the reproducibility and objectivity of job-simulated testing: logging a trail of processes used to reach conclusions and how conclusions were reached, detailed or thick descriptions of the findings, checking of interpretations with the patient and employer, active searching for and accounting for plausible explanation for inconsistencies, constantly refining hypotheses, negotiating recommendations with patient and employer, debriefing with peers, persistent observation, saturation of data, and triangulation of data from different sources and methods.

Job-simulated tests are non-standardized evaluations; however, a standardized evaluation can be tiered over the job simulated test. The Assessment of Work Performance (AWP) is a standardized assessment rating scale that is completed by the therapist while the patient does a performance-based job-simulated activity that the therapist has designed.[31] The AWP uses a 4-point ordinal performance scale to rate 14 skills based on performance (competent, limited, unsure, or incompetent). The 14 skills rated during the job simulation include posture, mobility, coordination, strength, physical energy, mental energy, knowledge, temporal organization, organization of space and objects, adaptation, physicality during interactions, language, relationships during interactions, and information exchange.

WORK EVALUATION AND JOB SIMULATION CASE EXAMPLE

In a case in which a phlebotomist sustained a cerebrovascular accident, her employer was not willing to allow her to return to work because she did not have any sensation in her dominant, affected hand distal to the wrist. The patient-employee insisted that she would be able to perform her job duties without the presence of sensation because she always has her eyes on the hand during the process of drawing blood (i.e., inserting the needle into the vein) and that she needed the sensation in her nondominant hand to palpate the vessels. With the patient's permission, the employer was contacted and agreed to allow the phlebotomist's job to be assessed to see if this was possible. During the job task assessment, two phlebotomists and a supervisor were interviewed and observed performing their work tasks. There was consensus that a phlebotomist does not use the sensation in the dominant hand and always visualizes the blood-drawing equipment during blood collection. The employer agreed that if the patient-employee could successfully demonstrate this during job simulation and then in live practice trials, she could return to her job. The phlebotomy department provided the therapist with needed tools (i.e., vacutainer and vials), and part of the patient's outpatient therapy regimen included working with these tools in a job simulation using fruit and then a Simulaid (a mannequin arm specially made for this purpose) and then in actual trials of drawing blood from her therapists. The patient-employee was able to safely demonstrate competence in her work tasks at all levels and was allowed to return to her work.

PERFORMANCE SKILL AND BODY FUNCTION LEVEL ASSESSMENTS TO EVALUATE WORK

Range of Motion

It is important to measure a patient's ROM during work evaluation. Because work involves the entire body, a gross active motion screen of the patient's ability to reach overhead and to the side, bend forward and backward, and squat to reach low levels is needed. More specific upper extremity measurements can be measured using goniometry. Hand therapy professionals should follow procedures documented elsewhere in this book.

Positional Tolerances

All work requires the worker to assume various static and dynamic postures within the overall context in which the work is to be performed. A job task analysis or functional job description may reveal some of these requirements (e.g., overhead reaching); however, it must be considered that an individual's body shape and size will have an influence on these postural requirements. For example, an individual with broad shoulders who performs typing at a computer keyboard

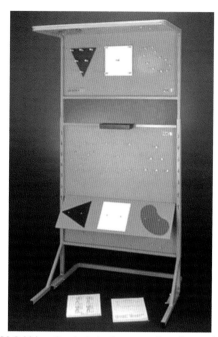

Fig. 120.3 Valpar 9: whole-body range of motion evaluation.

may have to internally rotate and abduct her shoulders and ulnarly deviate her wrists more than a smaller individual. By having a firm understanding of the postural requirements of the job and how they will be influenced by the individual's personal factors, a hand therapy practitioner can evaluate through the use of a standardized measure (if one exists), nonstandardized measure, or through work simulation. The typical postures that a hand therapy practitioner may need to evaluate are head and neck postures (i.e., head rotation, neck flexion–extension), overhead reaching, and forward reaching. Individual and composite positioning of the joints may also need to be evaluated, particularly with the distal joints because the position of the proximal joints will further dictate where the hand will need to be positioned to interface with whatever objects that it needs to access and manipulate. Having an understanding of how long the upper limb needs to be in the required position is essential to be able to assess whether or not the patient requires intervention to increase postural tolerance. Few standardized tests exist to assess upper limb positional tolerance. The Valpar 9 Work Sample–Test of Whole Body ROM (Fig. 120.3) is one that is useful because one of its four tests incorporates overhead reaching while using fine-motor control to transfer three forms that are attached to a panel with bolted nuts. Other standardized tests, such as the Purdue Pegboard test, can be used to assess for positional tolerance by setting them up in a fashion that will elicit the desired posture. However, the clinician may not score the test and refer to any normative data if there has been deviation from the test standardization. Doing so would be reporting an inaccurate result of such a test. Other activities or work simulations can be used to assess positional tolerance over a period of time. Work simulation would be the most valid means of testing positional tolerances because it is the closest that one can get to performing the actual job.

Strength Measurement

Most work activities require dynamic and static strength; therefore, it is important to include isotonic strength testing as well as isometric methods that are common in rehabilitation. Isotonic testing requires the patient to move the joint through the available ROM while wearing or holding a load. The load is increased until the maximal one

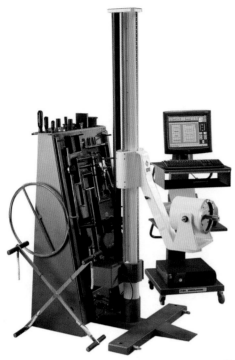

Fig. 120.4 Baltimore Therapeutic Equipment (BTE) Work Simulator II.

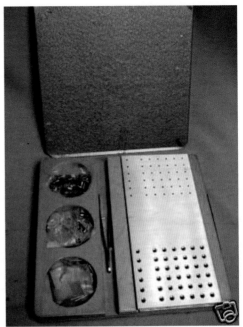

Fig. 120.5 Crawford Small Parts Dexterity Test. (From https://www.worthpoint.com/worthopedia/crawford-small-parts-dexterity-test-77752552.)

repetition maximum is achieved. Traditional manual muscle testing and grip and pinch testing are common methods to measure isometric strength of a muscle or group of muscles. Traditionally, three trials of gross grasp and lateral, palmar (three-point), and tip pinch are measured in each hand. Depending on the need, gross grasp testing can be tested on all five grip spans or just the second or third handle position (to measure the grip at the highest level of biomechanical efficiency of the hand). Results can be compared with normative data if the second handle position is used (http://www.fcesoftware.com/images/5_Grip_and_Pinch_Norms.pdf). There are several high-tech devices that can generate sophisticated isometric, isotonic, and isokinetic strength measurements. The Baltimore Therapeutic Equipment Work Simulator II (Fig. 120.4) or Primus or similar devices are available in some hand therapy settings. These devices can also be used to determine the endurance of a muscle or group of muscles acting on a joint or body part.[32]

Coordination and Dexterity

There are many standardized tests of coordination to determine if the patient has adequate dexterity to perform job tasks. When used in conjunction with work simulations, the results of these tests can be used to measure a baseline and then progress throughout the course of treatment. Depending on the type of dexterity that is needed for work, the therapist can use the Purdue Pegboard, Minnesota Rate of Manipulation, Crawford Small Parts Dexterity Test (Fig. 120.5), Bennett Hand Tool Dexterity Test (Fig. 120.6), and the Jebsen Hand Function Test (Fig. 120.7). Some manufacturers have developed standardized testing systems such as the Valpar Component Work Samples manufactured by BASES of Virginia, LLC, to measure dexterity.

The Purdue Pegboard tests the ability to pick up, manipulate, and then place small pegs in consecutive holes rapidly and accurately. Minnesota Manual Dexterity Test evaluates ability to repetitively reach, pick up, manipulate, and place medium-sized (double checker) objects with speed and accuracy. It has been found to have good validity and reliability, with even greater reliability with the three-trial administration.[33]

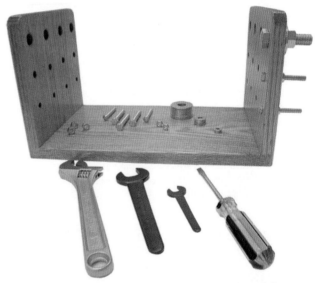

Fig. 120.6 Bennett Hand Tool Dexterity Test. (From http://lafayetteevaluation.com/products/hand-tool-dexterity.)

The Crawford Small Parts Dexterity Test (see Fig. 120.5) has two components; however, the literature is void of studies establishing solid validity and reliability for this test.[33] One study questioned the ability to use the original norm-reference values because the testing materials have changed, but normative values remain the same. The pins and collars component examines the ability to use a small hand tool (tweezers) to pick up and place small objects. The screws portion examines the ability to use a small hand tool (a screwdriver) to set small screws into prethreaded holes. The patient also must pick up, manipulate, and place a small screw.

The Bennett Hand-Tool Dexterity Test (see Fig. 120.6) provides the opportunity to observe the patient using standard hand tools (a screwdriver, a large and a small box end wrench, and an adjustable

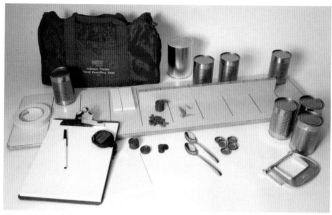

Fig. 120.7 Jebsen Hand Function Test. (From https://www.mobilitysmart.cc/media/catalog/product/cache/1/image/9df78eab33525d08d-6e5fb8d27136e95/j/e/jebsen_taylor_hand_function_test.jpg.)

wrench) to assemble and disassemble nut and bolt assemblies. The Rosenbusch Test of Finger Dexterity is the only standardized test that focuses on the ability to simultaneously hold, manipulate, and place small objects. It includes motion-time standards (MTSs) to score the patient's performance.

The Jebsen Test of Hand Function Test (see Fig. 120.7) addresses hand function related to daily living tasks. The therapist reports the normative data from the Jebsen as a mean with standard deviations. The therapist designates, via standard deviation, how far above or below the mean the worker performed. Reliability, validity, and reference values based on age have been established[33] as has criterion validity with traumatic spinal cord–injured patients. The Valpar Component Work System offers multiple workstations that evaluate a wide range of physical and cognitive work abilities and behaviors. Popular among therapists, each workstation has high face validity in that it looks like "real work" and has norms associated with it. It should be noted that the Valpar International Corporation does not sell its work samples anymore, but they are now being produced by BASES of Virginia, LLC, and can be found at http://www.basesofva.com.

Cardiopulmonary Endurance Testing

When a patient has been away from the workplace for some time, it is not unusual for his or her cardiopulmonary endurance to decline from the previous or required level to perform his job. Even though hand therapy practitioners are accustomed to working with the upper quarter, cardiopulmonary endurance is often a requirement for successful return to work. It is not unusual to consider that some form of aerobic exercise become part of a patient's work-conditioning or work-hardening program. There are a number of ways to assess aerobic capacity that range from relatively easy to complex. The YMCA Bench Step Test and Rockport Walking Test are two options for clinical use. To perform the YMCA Bench Step Test, a patient must have the motion, strength, and balance to step up and down from a 12-inch step. For the Rockport Walking Test, the patient must be able to walk for 1-mile over even terrain.

The YMCA Step Test requires the following supplies: a 12-inch high step, a metronome (a free online version is available at http://www.metronomeonline.com), and a stopwatch. The patient steps up onto the step with one foot and then the other and then down with one foot and the other, to the beat of a metronome set at 96 beats per minute. After 3 minutes, the patient's pulse is taken for 1 minute. Directions and norms are available at http://pennshape.upenn.edu/files/pennshape/YMCA-Bench-Step-Test-for-Cardiovascular-Fitness.pdf. The Rockport

Walking Test involves walking at a brisk pace over a flat, 1-mile route and record pulse and time to complete. The patient's age, sex, weight, pulse, and time are inserted into the following formula or a website (https://www.drgily.com/rockport-walk-test.php):

$$\text{Estimated VO}_{2max}\,(mL/kg/min) = 132.853 - (0.0769 \times \text{Body} \times \text{weight in [pounds]}) - (0.3877 \times \text{age [years]})$$
$$+ (6.3150 \times \text{gender [female} = 0; \text{male} = 1])$$
$$- (3.2649 \times \text{1-mail walk time [in minutes and hundredths]}) - (0.1565 \times \text{1-minute heart rate at end of mile [beats/min]}).$$

Pain Measurement

Pain is an important factor to consider when making return-to-work decisions. It is important for the hand therapist to consider many factors regarding pain during the evaluation and interventions addressing work. These include (1) the intensity, location, and quality of the pain at rest; (2) the intensity, location, and quality of the pain and what specific position or activity was the pain associated with; and (3) if the symptoms occur in a different body part or area, the intensity, location, and quality of these symptoms and what specific position or activity was the pain associated with. As with all pain reported by patients with hand or upper extremity conditions, the therapist considers potential reasons for the pain and options to allow for continuation of the activity. Developing appropriate patient education and interventions for pain modulation and management to facilitate successful return to daily activities, including work, begins with a thorough understanding of the patient's pain.

Pain is a very subjective experience that includes physical, affective, and cognitive components. Subjective rating scales such as a verbal rating of pain on a scale of 0 to 10 or the visual analog scale (VAS)[34] obtain information regarding pain intensity. It has been determined that Likert pain rating scales, such as the PROMIS Physical Function Measure (PROMIS PF), correlate well with patient outcomes.[35] The McGill Pain Questionnaire (MPQ) provides clinicians with a means to measure pain intensity on a more multidimensional level. A benefit to a multidimensional scale compared with a basic approach such as the VAS is that it provides the therapist with richer information regarding how the patient reports the experience of pain, since the context in which the pain is experienced can be defined by any number of affective, behavioral, or cognitive factors.[36] Use of a pain diagram allows the clinician to ascertain the location of the pain or discomfort (Fig. 120.8). Using symbols on the pain map can even be used to delineate the type or quality of pain experienced as in the Ransford Pain Drawing.[37] Further information regarding quality of pain can be gathered during the interview and evaluation. A discussion of work activities that either cause pain or that the patient can predict would cause pain can facilitate further investigation during work simulation activities or other assessments. Other data, such as changes in pain level (over the course of the treatment session, the course of a day, and over the course of several months), factors that increase or decrease pain, the effect pain has on sleep, and the intensity of pain, form the critical components of a pain assessment.

Many signs of pain are observable, including behavioral (e.g., rubbing or holding the affected body part, slowing of pace, facial grimacing, holding breath, groaning or crying) and physiological responses (e.g., increased heart or respiration rate, redness or flushing, clammy skin). It is important for the therapist to watch for these physical signs and to prevent patients from doing unsafe maneuvers such as the Valsalva maneuver. It is important to explore each patient's beliefs about

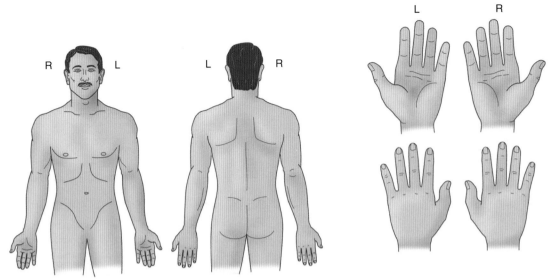

Fig. 120.8 Body diagram specifically for upper quarter pain from the Schultz upper extremity pain assessment form. *L,* Left; *R,* right. (Copyright 1993, Karen Schultz-Johnson.)

pain because her belief may not be appropriate for her condition. For example, patients with a "no pain, no gain" belief or those who have done extensive training for sports may push themselves excessively, increasing risk of injury or exacerbation of symptoms. On the other hand, patients who believe that pain is always a sign of physical damage or extreme fear of injury may not allow themselves to progress to their maximal tolerance.

Management of pain during the work evaluation is important. According to Cheung and colleagues,[38] pain is normal for up to 3 days after increased activity, symptoms increase for 24 hours after the evaluation and peak at 24 to 72 hours after evaluation, and symptoms subside or disappear 5 to 7 days after evaluation. This is common in individuals without injury or illness. Soer and colleagues[39] found that in a sample of normal, healthy volunteers administered a work evaluation, 51% experienced postevaluation pain in the thigh, 38% in the low back, 37% in the shoulders, and 36% in the upper arms. The following is recommended:

- Measure pain at baseline and after each activity.
- Observe for painful behaviors (e.g., grimace, posture, change in movement pattern, pace, stretch, rub).
- Compare symptoms and observations with baseline, self-reports, and the diagnosis to decide if they suggest advancement of the condition or are expected.
  Regarding performance limiting symptoms:
- Baseline symptoms should be understood in the context of the diagnosis and physical examination.
- Symptoms that are nonpathological responses to the task should not be criteria to stop the test.
- If new symptoms that indicate pathological response occur, stop the test and observe progression or regression of the symptoms.
- Patients are most likely not be able to work competitively with persistent symptoms.

For a full discussion of pain assessment and interventions for pain modulation, please refer to Chapter 94.

Manual Materials Handling

If a patient's job requires lifting, carrying, pushing, and pulling, the initial evaluation should assess the patient's ability to perform MMH activities up to the levels needed on the job. The evaluation should correspond to the type of MMH performed on the job per Title I of the Americans with Disabilities Act. Because most lifting, pushing, and pulling activities require dynamic movement of the object through space and there is a high risk of injury with isometric lift testing, isotonic (dynamic) evaluation of lifting is the method of choices. This is not to say that isometric force application is not important or required at work. When an object is pushed or pulled, the static coefficient of friction between the object and the surface it is being moved on must be overcome (https://www.engineersedge.com/coeffients_of_friction.htm). In addition to the coefficient of friction, computation of the amount of force needed to push or pull an object varies depending on the height of the object; the height of the person performing the push or pull; and if wheels are involved, the size, type, and service history of the wheels. As a result, clinic-based assessment of pushing and pulling rarely simulates the exact conditions at the workplace. Therapists often assess maximal isometric push and pull forces using a dynamometer designed for this purpose; however, safety measures should be in place to prevent injury. There are several approaches to testing of material handling abilities: psychophysical, isoinertial, or kinesiophysical.[40] All three approaches require the patient to lift progressively heavier loads over a specified vertical ROM, and all tests use feedback based on a predetermined scale to decide when to stop the test. The authors suggest use of a combination of these approaches when measuring MMH. In the psychophysical approach, the patient assigns a rating based on a validated rating scale similar to Borg's Rating of Perceived Exertion. When used to test lifting, the patient is asked to rate how hard it was to complete the lift or the level of effort required to complete the lift. The psychophysical approach does not mean that the patient is asked to decide when he believes he has reached the maximum, but it does mean that the patient's perceptions of difficulty or effort are taken into consideration during testing. It is irresponsible *not* to ask a patient to provide feedback after performing a strenuous task he is not accustomed to performing; in fact, asking the patient's perceptions of difficulty or effort may be better than asking about pain. It is important for the therapist to ensure that the patient understands the purpose, directions, and procedures for the lift test and the importance of providing accurate ratings.

The kinesiophysical approach involves the observation of physical efforts from low to high levels of demand to determine maximum

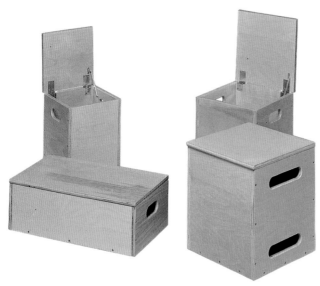

Fig. 120.9 Lift box samples.

function.[40] Because patient performance reaches a maximum gradually, the therapist can observe early signs of fatigue, incoordination, and change in body mechanics. The therapist classifies the physical changes into categories such as light, moderate, and heavy activity or slow, moderate, and rapid activity. These take into consideration physical changes that are observable as the level of work increases. *Maximum function* is defined as the greatest safe ability of a patient, either in repetitions or weight capacities. The patient may refuse to perform any further lift testing, but it is the therapist who decides the level of lifting ability based on safety as the most important criterion. To use the kinesiophysical approach, the therapist should have a significant level of training and must hone his ability to observe both gross and more subtle lifting behaviors and be able to document them.

Several such evaluations exist. The maximum isoinertial strength tests, the Progressive Isoinertial Lifting Evaluation (PILE), and the EPIC Lift Capacity Test are just a few. This type of evaluation takes the subject through a hierarchy of weights, repetitions, prehension patterns, and arcs of lift. The evaluation seeks to establish a quantification of the patient's lifting capacity, usually for comparison with future performance or with general job requirements.[41] Over the years, equipment for evaluation of lifting capacity has diversified and multiplied. Each equipment manufacturer has a recommended protocol for the evaluation of lifting capacity. Therapists also have derived their own evaluation techniques (Fig. 120.9).

Selecting Lifting Evaluation
Maximum Isoinertial Lifting Evaluations

The maximum isoinertial lifting test seeks to establish the maximum weight the patient can be able to lift from floor to waist, knee to waist, waist to shoulder, and shoulder to overhead. However, it is recommended that only the lift levels that are pertinent to the patient's job be lifted unless the test is to be performed to determine a disability rating. This test is best used for individuals who lift on an occasional (up to 33% of the workday) basis. A variety of formats can be used to perform this as described in the literature.[42] The most practical method for doing this in a clinical setting is to begin with a container for the weight that will be lifted. The object lifted should be similar in size, shape, and material quality as what will be lifted at the patient's job whenever possible because of the issues mentioned previously with prehension and coupling. The weight lifted is gradually increased in

increments of 5 to 10 lb. The therapist tests lifting at the levels that are necessary for the job. The patient lifts and lowers the load one time per increment of weight. The therapist observes the posture of the patient to assess safety and ability of the lift, monitors pain levels, and asks the patient to report on his ability if he could lift more weight. Typically, the patient is not informed of the amount of weight he is lifting so as to not negatively influence the psychophysical components of the evaluation. Throughout the evaluation, the clinician must monitor the patient's performance for safety and body mechanics. Testing can be stopped by either the therapist or patient, and the last level of safe lift would be considered the patient's functional maximum.

Progressive Isoinertial Lifting Evaluation

The Progressive Isoinertial Lifting Evaluation (PILE)[9] is a norm-referenced evaluation that measures ability to lift on a *frequent* (from 34% to 66% of the workday) basis. In the PILE, the patient lifts a box 12 times per minute from standard heights of floor to 30 inches from the floor (lumbar lift) and 30 to 54 inches from the floor (cervical lift). The initial starting weight and the incremental increases in weight are different by gender, yet the height of the surfaces is the same. For women, the initial weight lifted is 8 lb, with 5 lb added every 20 seconds. For men, the initial weight lifted is 13 lb, and 10 lb is added every 20 seconds. The patient is allowed 20 seconds to perform four lifting movements (box lift, box lower, box lift, and box lower). The endpoint for testing can be based on (1) the level of voluntary termination because of fatigue, excessive discomfort, or inability to complete the specified lifting task; (2) achievement of a target heart rate (usually 85% of age-predicted maximal heart rate); or (3) when the patient lifts a "safe limit" of his or her body weight (55%–60%).[42] In the majority of patients, the test is terminated because of the perception of fatigue, discomfort, or overexertion.[9] In older and overweight individuals, the heart rate endpoint is typically reached. Only very thin or small individuals typically reach the "safe limit" endpoint.

Limitations of the PILE relate to the fact that women are treated differently than men. For example, a woman must perform 10 lifting repetitions to get to 50 lb, whereas a man performs only 5 repetitions to get to 50 lb. Fatigue can become an issue with women because of the test design. In addition, the lifting heights are set at 30 and 54 inches, which means that shorter individuals have to lift to higher levels in comparison with their body height. As a result, the PILE may violate employment laws regarding discrimination on the basis of sex[43] and possibly racial descent. The heights for lifting are predetermined at 30 inches and 54 inches; therefore, the PILE may be more difficult for shorter people to complete, which is common among women and individuals of Asian descent. Also, the lack of a testing manual can have an effect on interrater reliability. The therapist who chooses to use this evaluation is advised that it may be contestable in a court of law because of gender bias.

EPIC Lift Capacity Evaluation

The EPIC Lift Capacity Evaluation (ELC) assessment is a proprietary, isoinertial lifting evaluation that uses psychophysical and kinesiophysical ratings. It assesses *occasional* and *frequent* lifting capacity as described by the US Department of Labor and correlates well to the revised National Institute for Occupational Safety and Health (NIOSH) Lifting Equation.[43] The ELC measures lifting capacity over three lifting heights that are linked to the patient's height: knuckle to shoulder, floor to knuckle, and floor to shoulder. Heart rate, body posture, body mechanics, and psychophysical response are evaluated to determine the recommended maximal load that can be lifted. The ELC is a proprietary system that is purchased from either http://www.mathesondevelopment.com or http://www.btetech.com. At the time of this writing, the system costs US\$4365. Matheson and colleagues[44] have demonstrated validity and

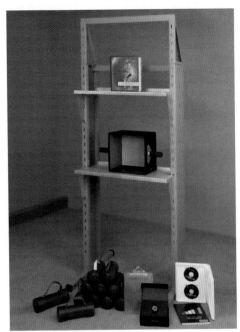

Fig. 120.10 EPIC Lift Station. (From https://www.mathesondevelopment.com/collections/fce-equipment/products/matheson-integrated-lift-evaluation-system-epic.)

reliability of the ELC and have normative data based on age and gender. Responsiveness in participants before and after conditioning treatment has been established, as well as resistance to reactivity and ability to detect sincerity of effort.[43]

Pushing, Pulling, and Carrying Evaluation

Push and pull work tasks involve a significant degree of static activity in the trunk and upper extremities. It has been estimated that nearly 50% of all MMH involves pushing, pulling, and carrying tasks.[45] As a result, an assessment of push–pull and carrying capacities should be performed if the patient performs either or both at her job. However, there is no peer reviewed, standardized assessment of these tasks available to the clinician. To date, the most comprehensive collection of psychophysical data regarding push–pull and carrying activities was provided by Stover and associates.[46] The tables provided in their work describe initial and sustained force values for pushing, pulling, and carrying tasks. Normative values of the population (10th–90th percentile) are provided by gender at various handle heights, time intervals, and distances. The therapist needs to be aware that the forces required to initiate the push or pull of an object are generally found to be approximately 15% more than the force sustaining the object in motion when it is moving. For this reason, just simply having the patient push or pull on a force gauge that is attached to the wall (i.e., an isometric test) is not as telling as actually having the patient move an object. The typical method of testing this in the clinic is to have the patient move a friction sled with weights in it. After the upper limit of the testing has been determined, the clinician can use an engineering force gauge or a dynamometer to determine the amount of force it takes to both initiate and sustain the push and pull. The "Snook Tables" can be used as a guide by the therapist to determine what the upper limit of testing should be. These tables can be found at http://www.ergonomiesite.be/documenten/trekkenduwen/Snook-tabellen.pdf. It should be noted that more recent studies have suggested that the values provided by Stover and associates[46] may be too high when considering what today's industrial worker may perceive acceptable during psychophysical

testing.[47] Pushing and pulling forces demonstrated a decrease averaging 82% and 94%, respectively, for initial and sustained forces. For this reason, directly comparing the normative data presented by Stover and associates[46] is not advised. Indirectly, however, by calculating the force required to initiate and sustain the push or pull with the friction sled, the clinician may correlate observed ability to normative data and arrive at a percentile rank for the patient. The static nature of pushing and pulling, with regard to the trunk and upper extremities, means that the aerobic capacity of the patient may also be quickly reached. It would be advisable to monitor heart rate during a repetitive push–pull evaluation to ensure that the patient's 85% of maximal, age-predicted heart rate is not exceeded. If it is, then testing should also be stopped at this point.

Similar to pushing and pulling evaluation, there exists no standardized test of carrying capacity in the peer reviewed literature. Michael Gerg suggests that the clinician have the patient simulate the type of object and distance the object is carried while in the clinic. To determine an upper limit for the carry or apply normative data for comparison, the "Snook tables" offer normative data for carrying tasks over three distances at four heights, and at seven frequencies.[46] Again, heart rate should be monitored to ensure that the patient's aerobic capacity is not exceeded.

Documenting Patient Lifting Performance

Central to the ability to document the patient's performance is the ability to biomechanically analyze the lifting task. Chaffin and Andersson[48] group the factors that define the MMH task or system as follows:
- Worker characteristics
- Material or container characteristics
- Task characteristics
- Work practices

These categories assist the therapist in structuring a report of the many complex and interrelated aspects of the patient's lifting performance. A form helps organize the necessary data from a jobsite lifting analysis.

The interaction between the following factors determines the body's response to the work demand placed on it[49]:
- Muscle contraction
- Tendon excursion
- Joint flexibility
- Joint stability
- Skin tolerance to pressure, texture, temperature, or shear
- Physiologic status to support effort (e.g., circulatory or respiratory sufficiency)
- Biomechanical status to support effort (e.g., acceleration, jerking the load, hyperextending the spine, nudging the load with the thigh)
- Sensation
- Proprioception
- Joint or soft tissue status outside of the upper extremity
- Pain experience

The therapist systematically documents this response.

These factors have been used successfully during functional capacity evaluations (FCEs) to document the important components of and observation during a lifting task. In addition to the amount of weight lifted, the therapist should note the quality of the task performance. The speed, control, and smoothness of the lift can reveal a great deal about the patient. With this information, the therapist determines several other crucial task characteristics. What muscle groups engage the load? What is the duration of the lift? What percentage of maximum voluntary contraction of a given muscle group does the lifter use during the lift? Which joints require flexibility? Which require stability? How do these designations change as the lift progresses and the load moves from one height to another?

When a worker has difficulty performing a lifting task, the therapist must identify the reason. Often this consists of recognizing the weak link in the system, which could be any one or a combination of the factors listed previously. A patient's ability or inability to problem solve and spontaneously adapt significantly affects the accomplishment of physically challenging tasks.

FUNCTIONAL CAPACITY EVALUATIONS

There are times when a hand therapist will receive a referral to perform an FCE. An FCE is defined as an evaluation of capacity for activities that is used to make recommendations for participation in work while considering the person's body functions and structures, environmental factors, personal factors, and health status.[39] As an evaluative tool, the FCE was developed in the demand for quantitative measures of individual functional capacity from the insurers, legal professionals, and regulatory agencies such as the Social Security Administration and workers' compensation boards. As an objective measurement tool, it assists in determining safe, tolerable functional levels and predicts an individual's readiness to assume or to return to specific work functions. Some people see the FCE as only evaluating mobility, strength (static and dynamic), material handling (lifting, carrying, pushing, and pulling), tolerance of positions and movements, and cardiovascular fitness[50]; however as noted in the definition, the FCE should measure the broad range of body functions and structures, environmental factors, personal factors, and health status. Statistics indicate that there is a significant financial impact of work-related injuries on society and support the need for a system of evaluation and treatment to minimize the impact of these injuries. At the time of this writing, Liberty Mutual Insurance Company[51] estimated that the total cost of workplace injuries was $59.9 billion based on data from the US Bureau of Labor Statistics (BLS) in 2015.[52] The BLS reported 2.9 million nonfatal occupational injuries and illnesses, with 1.3 million of these culminating in lost workdays, job transfers, or restrictions being placed on the worker (i.e., light duty).[53] Disability related to musculoskeletal disorders (MSDs) is one of the leading causes of limitation in the ability to perform work and accounted for more than 31% of the occupational illnesses requiring days away from work in 2015. The median days away from work for an MSD was 12 days to recuperate compared with 8 median days lost work time for all other work-related injuries.[52] An MSD is defined by the BLS as "cases where the nature of the injury or illness is pinched nerve; herniated disc; meniscus tear; sprains, strains, tears; hernia (traumatic and non-traumatic); pain, swelling, and numbness; carpal or tarsal tunnel syndrome; Raynaud's syndrome or phenomenon; musculoskeletal system and connective tissue diseases and disorders, when the event or exposure leading to the injury or illness is over-exertion and bodily reaction, unspecified; overexertion involving outside sources; repetitive motion involving microtasks; other and multiple exertions or bodily reactions; and rubbed, abraded, or jarred by vibration."[54] Most FCE referrals to hand therapists are because of an MSD.

Indications for Functional Capacity Evaluations

Typically, an FCE will be ordered for worker's compensation cases or in an accident or injury case in which there is a lawsuit or insurance settlement being sought. The FCE can and often does involve all of the assessments mentioned previously in this chapter; however, they do typically report on other areas such as consistency of effort, maximal voluntary effort (MVE), and presence of symptom magnification. It is

---

BOX 120.1 Common Indications for Functional Capacity Evaluation Referral

- Determine whether the patient can perform the physical demands of his or her previous job.
- Determine the patient's maximal level of functional capacity.
- Determine functional capacity to identify more objective job restrictions/limitations.
- Refute or rebut the results of an IME.
- Determine a patient's proclivity to perform consistently and with MVE.
- Evaluate to confirm, rule out, or discover the diagnosis.
- Determine necessary job modifications to facilitate return to work.
- Determine whether the patient would be a candidate for a work-hardening or work-conditioning program.
- Assist in determining the level of disability or loss.
- Determine functional capacity after injury from an automobile accident.

IME, Independent medical evaluation; *MVE*, maximal voluntary effort.

---

important for the therapist performing an FCE to recognize her role in coaching the patient to ensure that the patient is given ample opportunity to provide maximal, consistent effort during the FCE because inconsistencies will be interpreted by the worker's compensation insurance company as an effort to prolong benefits. The therapist must not make assumptions about functions not measured that could impact safety at the workplace, such as the ability to maintain vigilance while experiencing pain or taking a wide range of medications. Referrals for an FCE can come from a variety of stakeholders and depend the local market. Physicians, case managers, attorneys, employers, and insurance companies are typical sources of referral. At times, the referral is made at the recommendation of the treating therapist. One should be aware of state regulations as to whether a physician's prescription is required for the referral and whether precertification is required to approve the referral. The therapist needs to know the reason for the FCE; common reasons are listed in Box 120.1. When performing the FCE, the clinician will need to address the referral source's question to reach satisfactory closure of the case. The referral source questions are used to guide how the evaluation is carried out. For example, if the referral source asks what the patient's maximal level of capacity is, then the therapist must perform the evaluation to the patient's functional maximums. In contrast, if the referral source asks if a patient can return to his previous job, the therapist will only need to test the patient to just at or above the job demands of the essential duties of the job in question. It is best to ask referring physicians for limits in the physical stresses applied to recovering structures, especially when surgery has been performed.

Comparing Impairment and Disability

On occasion, the clinician performs an FCE to assist a physician in generating an impairment or disability rating. Gathering relevant information on ROM, strength, and sensation may help generate an impairment rating. The impairment rating appears as a percentage of whole-body function and often translates into a final monetary settlement for the injured patient. The impairment rating is highly structured and focuses solely on permanent, quantifiable physical loss related to the injury, disorder, or disease when the patient is considered to have reached maximal medical improvement (MMI). Impairment ratings do not take into account unique factors relating to worker vocation or overall function.

On the other hand, the determination of disability involves participation restrictions and combines the worker's impairment and the impact of the impairment on the ability to perform the preinjury

---

BOX 120.2 **Commercially Available Functional Capacity Evaluation Systems**

- BTE Hanoun (Eval-Tech, Simulator II): http://www.btetech.com/product/evaltech/
- MediGraph FCE: http://www.medigraphsoftware.com
- Arcon, FCE Software System: http://www.fcesoftware.com/home.html
- Matheson System: http://roymatheson.com
- OCCUPRO: https://www.occupro.net/
- Blankenship System: https://www.blankenshipfcesystems.com/
- Isernhagen/WorkWell System: http://www.workwell.com/functional-capacity-evaluation/
- ErgoScience Physical Work Performance Evaluation: https://www.ergoscience.com/clinics-functional-capacity-evaluation
- JobFit System based on the WorkHab FCE: http://www.workhab.com

---

job or any job. Disability considers the unique characteristics of the worker in conjunction with his or her profession to define the worker's percentage of disability and subsequent disability rating as governed by the American Medical Association's Disability Guidelines.[55] For example, consider the impact of a deficit in wrist flexion with an office worker who types at a computer keyboard most of the day and an automobile mechanic. Extreme wrist flexion is not an essential job task for most people who work at a computer workstation the majority of the day. An automobile mechanic, on the other hand, may have a much greater need for wrist flexion to access hard-to-reach areas of the vehicle during repairs. The level of disability will be higher for the mechanic than the office worker despite the same level of impairment.

Hand therapy practitioners performing an FCE that will lead to the determination of either of these ratings will need to keep the distinction between these two terms clear. The words *impairment* and *disability* appear frequently in literature and reports. However, because they have special meanings and legal implications, the clinician must use them with care and specificity.

Functional Capacity Evaluation Approaches

A clinician can choose to design or develop her own FCE format; however, the validity and reliability of such a format may be easily challenged in a court of law. It may be prudent for a clinician looking to perform FCEs to investigate FCE products that have already been developed. A multitude are available on the market, and many of them have established reliability and validity. Some of the FCE formats suggest having everyone go through the same evaluation format regardless of which body part is injured, whereas others allow the clinician to customize the evaluation to only use assessments that are pertinent to the job or the patient in question and are guided by the clinician's clinical reasoning to perform. Box 120.2 lists some available FCE products. Hand therapy practitioners are encouraged to review these various platforms and choose one that closely aligns with their treatment philosophies. Above all, clinicians should receive adequate training in whichever platform is chosen.

Functional capacity evaluations are generally performed over 1 or 2 days with an average total time of 5 to 6 hours. Follow-up contact with the patient 1 day or more after the evaluation is crucial because problems may not appear until several hours after the evaluation. The questions should address how the patient felt within the following 24-hour period. Questions should address discomfort, sleep schedule, or any other changes in activity. The patient may answer the questions by phone or may fill out a questionnaire and return it by mail, fax, or email.

Who is Qualified to Perform Functional Capacity Evaluations?

An FCE is one of the most demanding evaluations that a hand therapy practitioner could be asked to perform. The clinician providing this service must have several years of experience in the field and an in-depth background in upper extremity rehabilitation, including the following:
- Knowledge of the pathologic conditions affecting the upper extremity
- Appreciation of the range of recovery consistent with various pathologic conditions
- Comprehensive upper extremity evaluation skills, including ROM, strength, sensation, pain, coordination, dexterity, provocative testing, and soft tissue evaluation
- Ability to screen the broad range of cognitive, emotional, and sensory system functions needed for work
- Ability to establish differential diagnoses and to use physician- and therapist-provided evaluation results to rule out pathologic conditions and to determine the most likely pathology
- Knowledge of the physician- and therapist-offered interventions to be able to determine whether patient-worker has received appropriate treatment
- Knowledge of the impact that pain and medication can have on higher level cognitive functions
- Understanding of the many reasons that a person with a prolonged recovery may not provide maximal, consistent effort
- Familiarity with resources in the area to be able to refer the worker to appropriate further intervention
- Interview skills
- Ability to work with a team
- Ability to establish rapport with people
- Excellent observation skills
- Excellent documentation skills. The documentation must provide the needed information and communicate it clearly. In some cases, the documentation must hold up in court under the scrutiny of attorneys, a judge, and a jury.
- Solid background in ergonomics

Administration of an FCE is not for the novice therapist or the therapist new to upper extremity rehabilitation. The therapist performing the FCE needs to have the experience and judgment appropriate to the weight and significance that the FCE carries, which often affects a patient's financial compensation.

The Additional Areas That an Functional Capacity Evaluation Can Measure

As mentioned previously, the purpose of the FCE is to measure an individual's maximal functional performance or ability to perform the job in questions. One may ask, then, why not just perform a battery of tests in the clinic and provide the results of said tests? Because the FCE is usually a tool that is used in workers' compensation and accident tort cases and to establish disability ratings, the therapist also must be able to assess whether there was good sincerity and consistency of effort and that the test results are reflective of the patient's true functional maximums. As a result, the FCE needs to document that full effort was given and, if not, what impediments there were to giving full effort. The following describes some of the terminology that is typically used to validate an FCE's findings.

Sincerity of Effort or Maximal Voluntary Effort

Many proprietary FCE products report the patient's sincerity of effort during testing as the "reliability" or "validity" measures of the patient's ability to demonstrate that he gave full effort during testing.

It should be noted that these terms are used interchangeably and do not reflect the classic definitions of either term.[56] Lechner and colleagues[57] defined *sincerity of effort* as "a patient's conscious motivation to perform optimally during an evaluation." Sincerity of effort is often measured using heart rate monitoring and measuring coefficients of variance (CV) testing. The theory with the measurement of heart rate is that if more effort is being exerted, the patient's heart rate will increase from baseline. However, heart rate has been found to be influenced by other factors such as test anxiety, medications, and other physical conditions. As a result, the use of maximum heart rate as a measure of sincerity of effort alone is questionable.[58,59] CV testing is the statistical expression of the variation of testing trials demonstrated by the patient. It is measured by dividing the standard deviation of the trials (i.e., static grip strength testing) with the mean and is expressed as a percentage[60] with 15% being the generally accepted level of variation in testing trials. If the CV exceeds 15%, the test can be interpreted as being "invalid" and not reflective of the patient's true functional maximum. However, it has been noted that the 15% cutoff has never been validated in a controlled study.[61] To accept the CV as a valid indicator of consistency of effort, one must accept the premise that the results of repeated test trials within a brief span of time will be stable. Although this seems a reasonable assumption, many factors besides sincerity of effort could interfere with the test results. These include, but are not limited to:

- Misunderstanding instructions
- Anxiety with test taking
- Lack of familiarity with testing equipment
- Very low endurance
- Fear of reinjury
- Fear of symptoms or exacerbation of pain
- Unidentified impairment
- Learned illness behavior
- Fear of symptom exacerbation or injury
- Need to gain recognition of symptoms
- Depressive disorders
- Fatigue
- Medication and psychoactive substance effects
- Malingering syndrome
- Factitious disorder
- Conversion disorder or other somatoform disorders

It should also be noted that if the patient has a hand condition or something that would grossly affect her ability to grip with full strength that it will affect the coefficient of variance and therefore should not be used as a measure to determine MVE.

The Functional Capacity Evaluation and Documentation

The final FCE report is generally a lengthy document. If done correctly, it will be between 20 and 40 pages in length. Recipients of the document (i.e., physicians, workers' compensation claims adjusters, lawyers) are generally most interested in reading a summary of the entire evaluation. As a result, placing the summary and conclusions at the beginning of the report is generally accepted as best practice and will satisfy the needs of the referral source. In instances when a determination of fitness for duty to return to the preinjury job is sought, it is good practice to provide a job match table (Table 120.3) to demonstrate which job task components are met and which are not. If further treatment is warranted and recommended, the job match table is a valuable guide on where intervention can be focused. Additional information that will need to be provided in the summary will include:

- Patient name
- Diagnosis
- Job at the time of injury
- The reason for the referral

- Sincerity of effort findings and reliability of test results
- A summary of the evaluation results

After the summary and conclusions, the evaluation needs to include a detailed report of all of the tests or assessments that were performed. Included in this should be the results, normative data (if applicable), consistency of effort findings (if applicable), and any subjective reports from the patient if they influenced the result of the test item (e.g., reports of increased pain). The clinician needs to be aware that in the documentation of the FCE, anything in the report may be used as evidence in a legal case in support of either the plaintiff or the defense. The clinician is cautioned to be very careful in the choice of how and what to report. The clinician may have a perfectly good reason to perform an evaluation, but certain data may not be useful and may, in fact, be counterproductive to what the clinician is attempting to document for the referral source. For example, if a standardized assessment, such as the Purdue Pegboard Test, is performed to test a patient's fine-motor coordination in standing because the worker would perform his job in standing, the therapist cannot use the normative data for the Purdue Pegboard Test. By doing the test in standing, the therapist deviated from the standardization of this test, which has been normed on individuals in sitting. Doing so would call the validity of the FCE into question and could invalidate the entire evaluation when presented in a court of law. The best option in this situation is to report the test result without the normative data if the clinician is just attempting to demonstrate that the patient can perform fine-motor activities in standing. Furthermore, the clinician needs to have a proper working knowledge of acceptable terminology by medicolegal standards. For example, the terms *aggravation* and *exacerbation* are often used interchangeably by clinicians. In a court of law, however, these two terms have two vastly different meanings. In the eyes of the law, *aggravation* means "the permanent worsening of a pre-existing condition," whereas *exacerbation* means "a temporary worsening that will resolve."[62]

Initially, the writing of the FCE report takes considerable time. With practice, speed increases. The timely production of reports is crucial to the reputation of the facility and to prompt reimbursement. The following suggestions offer ideas for expediting report writing.

Many of the proprietary FCE formats have software programs that assist in the report writing process. This can be a timesaver and allow for expediting getting the report to the referral source in a timely fashion. It has been Michael Gerg's experience that use of such a software program allows for completion of the report on the same day that it is performed. For clinics where the purchase of such a proprietary system is not financially feasible, the development of a word-processed form that uses a predetermined format and common language will reduce report generation time. The organization of documentation on worksheets rather than on plain sheets of paper also saves time. When each activity and standardized test have an associated worksheet with the items of observation already noted, the therapist can easily glean information about patient performance for incorporation into the report. Rapid completion of the report after the FCE makes report writing easier than waiting several weeks because the information about the evaluation remains fresh in one's mind. Following these suggestions will help minimize the time to create the report while maintaining high quality.

INTERVENTIONS TO ADDRESS WORK

The hand therapist closely reviews the results of the initial evaluation to identify the main factors limiting the patient's ability to return to work. This includes the patient's current body functions and work abilities; the job requirements; the work environment; and applicable federal state, employer, and union policies. A multifaceted intervention

TABLE 120.3   Sample Job Match Table for a Functional Capacity Evaluation of a Patient with a Left Shoulder Labral Tear

	Essential Job Demand	Evaluation Result	Job Match
Mobility			
Sitting	Frequent (1/3 to 2/3 day)	Within functional limits; no deficits	Yes
Static standing	Occasional (<1/3 day)	Within functional limits; no deficits	Yes
Walking	Occasional (<1/3 day)	Within functional limits; no deficits	Yes
Agility			
Bending or stooping	Occasional (<1/3 day)	Within functional limits; no deficits	Yes
Above-shoulder work	Never	Restricted from performing per physician order and is limited by LUE shoulder AROM	N/A
Strength			
Lifting	10 lb (medium): frequent (1/3 to 2/3 day); lifting production materials	Able to lift ≤20 lb from the floor to and from the waist Able to lift ≤25 lb 12 inches from the floor to and from the waist Able to lift ≤15 lb from the waist to and from the shoulder Unable to lift overhead per physician order All lifting done bimanually (with both arms simultaneously) Lifting tested for occasional lifting	Yes
Dexterity			
Fine finger	Frequent (1/3 to 2/3 day)	Performs without significant increase in left shoulder pain; normative scores vary by task but are well within range for the uninjured population	Yes
Grasping: light	Constant (>2/3 day)	Within functional limits; no deficits	Yes
Grasping: firm	Occasional (≤1/3 day); ≤50 lbs bimanually	Scores are slightly less than age and sex norms (left, 43 lb; right, 52 lb)	No
Pinching	Occasional (≤1/3 day); light pinch required to manipulate parts	Three-point pinch for left hand is below average for age and sex but is functionally appropriate; all other scores are in the average range	Yes
Reaching forward	Frequent (1/3 to 2/3 day); reaching to side to access small parts	No deficit if left shoulder flexion is <90 degrees; job only requires 60 degrees of shoulder abduction	Yes
Writing	Never	Within functional limits; no deficits	N/A

AROM, Active range of motion; *LUE,* left upper extremity; *NA,* not applicable.

approach is usually necessary to achieve a favorable outcome. The reimbursement source will often guide the type of interventions that will be allowable. The hand therapist chooses interventions that are supported by evidence when such evidence is available. The American Occupational Therapy Association's (AOTA's) Practice Guidelines for Individuals with Work-Related Injuries and Illnesses[63] provide an extensive evidence-based review of intervention strategies. This document also describes in detail how to approach both evaluation and intervention with the injured worker through use of the OTPF. Note that a new edition is currently being developed.

According to the OTPF,[1] occupational therapy interventions are classified into five categories: restore/remediate, modify/adapt, maintain, prevent, and create/promote. Restorative interventions are bottom-up approaches that focus on facilitating the return of lost function, such as performing Theraputty exercises to improve grip strength, tendon gliding to facilitate ROM, repetitive weight lifting to increase lifting tolerance, or practice manipulating objects to improve coordination. Interventions to modify, adapt, or compensate are a more top-down approach that shifts the focus to modifying the activity or the process of completing the activity to the current or expected abilities of the patient. An example of this is to modify a tool handle by building it up for someone with a loss of finger flexion or decreased ability

to grip narrow items. This approach can also include modifying the work demands. For example, a patient who cannot work an entire work shift may be able to return for half days, a patient may be allowed to return to light or modified duties if available, or a temporary accommodation can be provided that modifies the work environment. Maintenance interventions are designed to preserve the current capabilities of the patient. For example, a home exercise program can be provided to maintain the current level of fitness of the injured body part or the entire patient or continuing a preinjury bicycling program to maintain cardiorespiratory status. Preventive interventions seek to decrease the likelihood of an injury occurring or reoccurring. For example, a patient with lateral epicondylitis is shown proper workplace ergonomic techniques to minimize stress on the common extensor tendon or to avoid gripping excessively hard to prevent reinjury. Interventions to create/promote assume that a disability exists and the goal is to design tools or promote practices that provide the opportunity for all involved in the same work activities to have an experience that enhances performance and decreases the risk of injury or reinjury. An example of this is to advise an employer to use a more ergonomically sound tool for all workers rather than just the injured worker. This intervention may occur more in settings where the clinician is working onsite for an employer or doing ergonomic consulting.

TABLE 120.4 Intervention Approaches and Examples of Occupation-Based Goals for Patients With Work-Related Injuries

Approach	Focus of Intervention	Examples of Occupation-Based Goals
Restore/remediate: designed to change patient variables to establish a skill or ability that has been impaired[65]	Body structure Body function Performance skills Occupation	Perform tendon-gliding exercises to allow finger to tightly grasp gun trigger. Perform finger tapping quickly and accurately to prepare to type. Lift 50-lb box from floor to waist. Accurately type monthly report.
Modify, compensate, adapt: designed to find ways to revise the task, method, or environment to support performance[65]	Body functions Performance skills Occupation Context Activity demands	Use a jar opener to compensate for grip loss on the job. Use a cart to move a load rather than carrying it. Use voice activation software for word processing. Use a tilted table top to decrease the amount of reach across a table during an assembly work task. Reduce the weight of the load lifted overhead.
Maintain: designed to provide the supports that will preserve the performance capabilities patients have regained so they can continue to meet their occupational needs	Body functions Performance skills Context Performance patterns	Perform a home or work exercise program to maintain fitness level for work. Use proper body mechanics while working at a computer workstation. Maintain clear walkways in work area to avoid falls while carrying. Develop habit of using joint protection techniques during handling tasks.
Prevent: designed to prevent performance problems by supporting body structures and functions, performance skills, environment, and habits and routines[65]	Performance patterns Context Body functions Activity demands	Perform hand and wrist stretch before work shift and hourly throughout work day. Use keyboard tray for typing tasks. Use an overhead lift device to perform all lifting tasks. Decrease the number of repetitions required on assembly line.
Create/promote: does not assume a disability is present or any factors interfere with performance designed to provide enriched contextual and activity experiences that enhance performance for all persons in the natural contexts of life[65]	Context Body functions Activity demands	Design a barrier-free workplace. Establish onsite wellness programs to promote fitness. Use assistive technology to eliminate manual material handling on the job.

Modified from Kaskutas V, Snodgrass J. *Occupational Therapy Practice Guidelines for Individuals with Work-Related Injuries and Illnesses.* Bethesda, MD: AOTA Press; 2009:28.

When designing interventions to help a patient to resume work roles, the therapist considers the degree of mismatch between the patient's current abilities to work and the abilities needed for their job. If this difference is not extreme, insurance coverage is adequate, and the patient can comply with an exercise or activity program, a restorative approach may be best. These restorative services are usually covered when billed as "therapeutic interventions." If a patient's employer has a policy limiting the length of time an employee can miss work before employment termination, there may not be adequate time to restore functions. In this case, the therapist works quickly with the patient and employer to identify compensations that allow the patient to return to work as soon as possible. This may also be the preferred intervention approach if the patient is in a financial crisis, insurance benefits are dwindling or unavailable, or the patient is experiencing negative effects from not being in the worker role. The therapist must work to ensure that the compensatory approach does not put him or his coworkers at risk of future injury or illness. Usually a combination of all approaches outlined in the OTPF is best.

The OTPF also stresses that often interventions need to be directed at the context, defined as "a variety of interrelated conditions that are within and surrounding the client; including cultural, personal, temporal, and virtual (p. S28),[1] and the environment, defined as "the external physical and social conditions that surround the client and in which the client's daily life occupations occur." The last area to mention is that the OTPF notes that interventions may need to address the patients' performance patterns, defined as "the habits, routines, roles, and rituals used in the process of engaging in occupations or activities; these patterns can support or hinder occupational performance" (p. S27).[1]

It should be noted to those that are unfamiliar with occupational therapy nomenclature that the term occupation refers to any meaningful activity that the patient engages in. The eight occupations identified in the OTPF are work, ADLs, IADLs, education, rest and sleep, play, leisure, and social participation. In the case of addressing work tasks with a patient, you are addressing one of their daily occupations. It should be noted, that the interventions that a clinician may perform could address other occupations than work but, ultimately, will support the patient in resuming her performance in the occupation of work. For example, working with a patient on tying shoes or a necktie are appropriate activities to address if wearing work boots or a tie to work are required for that person's job. Providing a spinner knob and training to facilitate the resumption of driving activities, which fall under the occupation of IADLs (community mobility), would facilitate driving to and from one's job. An extremely important IADL that must be addressed when helping a client return to work is health maintenance and management, defined as "developing, managing, and maintaining routines for health and wellness promotion, such as physical fitness, nutrition, decreased health risk behaviors, and medication routines" (p. S19).[1] A patient with impingement syndrome who maintains strength in the lower trapezius or a patient with cubital tunnel syndrome who uses a speakerphone instead of holding the phone to her ear are examples of health management roles important for patients' return-to-work plan. Teaching a patient better sleep ergonomics to minimize nerve impingement in the neck or upper extremity addresses the occupation of sleep and rest but would allow the patient to get sufficient sleep to be able to be well rested for work.

Intervention approaches and examples of occupation-based goals for patients with work-related injuries modified from the AOTA Practice Guidelines for Individuals with Work-Related Injuries and Illnesses[63] are listed on Table 120.4.

The OTPF (2014) categorizes interventions as preparatory methods and tasks, occupations and activities, education and training, advocacy, and group interventions. Preparatory methods and tasks consist of interventions that "prepare the patient for occupational performance, used as part of a treatment session in preparation for or concurrently with occupations and activities."[1] This intervention type is one that most hand therapy practitioners excel at and are comfortable with because they involve activities that include the use of physical agent modalities (preparatory methods) and exercise (preparatory task) to biomechanically improve loss of function. The activities are often rote and serve no functional purpose but improve the function of the upper extremity. However, they do not generally address specific activity. The theory behind this intervention approach is that improved biomechanical function will generalize over to the occupation(s) in which these biomechanical functions are needed. For example, working with a patient on fine-motor coordination using a pegboard activity would improve his ability to move his fingers to the keys of a computer or manipulate small screws that he has to pick up as part of his production job.

Occupations and activities interventions are described as specific interventions that are designed to meet the patient's specific therapeutic goals and address the "underlying needs of the mind, body, and spirit of the patient."[1] When a clinician decides to use these types of interventions, he is choosing to perform therapeutic activities that have some inherent meaning and purpose to the patient and address the patient's shortcomings in being able to perform specific occupations. To choose appropriate interventions from this category, the clinician needs to have an awareness of the demands of the specific activities in question. These interventions can include only parts of the work activity or a similar functional task that has the same activity demands (activity intervention) as the occupation that is being addressed. For example, a patient with lateral epicondylitis who works as a housekeeper at a hospital facility and has difficulty emptying trash cans may be asked to empty water from one bucket to another for a certain number of repetitions after being taught better body mechanics for overturning an object such as a trash can. The bucket filled with water, although not actually a trash can, can simulate the same motions as emptying the trashcan. Occupation-based activities consist of actually performing the occupation in which the patient is experiencing dysfunction. From the aforementioned example of the hospital housekeeper with lateral epicondylitis, the clinician may design and implement an intervention in which the patient actually goes around the hand clinic and empties the trashcans into a cart while practicing the proper body mechanics she was instructed on. Occupations and activities interventions require more creativity and supervision than the more rote preparatory tasks. There is no better way to assess a patient's ability to meet the demands of the job than performing tasks that simulate the work activities in question or address the same activity demands as the job in question. Observing the patient's ability to perform in these interventions acts as a means to assess progress and act as a guide in the selection of future interventions. For those familiar with the earlier editions of the OTPF, activity interventions had been called *purposeful interventions*. Another important factor that needs to be taken into be taken into consideration during occupation and activity, work-related interventions is the concept of activity gradation. Each activity or occupation intervention should be made available to the worker on a progressively more demanding basis. When designing work tasks, the therapist must maintain control over the demands of each activity. Gradation allows the worker to enhance ability within each physical demand and aptitude. Although increasing repetition and duration are valid grading approaches, simply adding to the time a worker engages in these interventions will not necessarily achieve the return-to-work goal. The therapist grades as many factors as possible, including resistance, ROM, rate, accuracy, coordination, stimuli imparted, and complexity.

Education and training interventions are used in treatment with the majority hand therapy recipients. The OTPF describes education as the imparting of knowledge to the patient, whereas training is the teaching of a concrete skill to the patient. Education and training can be differentiated from one another. The goal of education is that the patient's knowledge will be enhanced, and the goal of a training intervention is that the patient's performance will be enhanced. For example, teaching a patient who has a job in data entry about office workstation ergonomics would be an education intervention, whereas teaching the patient how to adjust a computer workstation to fit them from an ergonomic standpoint would be considered a training intervention. Advocacy is an intervention that is described as "efforts directed toward promoting occupational justice and empowering patients to seek and obtain resources to fully participate in daily life occupations."[1] Advocacy can take place in two ways. The hand therapy practitioner could advocate on behalf of the patient to the employer or referring physician or impart the information needed to the patient and work with the patient on being able to self-advocate. The choice of which of these interventions is chosen will often be determined by the referral or payment source. For example, if a patient is on workers' compensation, then the clinician would have greater access to the employer and would be able to directly interact with either the claims adjuster or the employer. On the other hand, if a patient is not covered by workers' compensation insurance, then HIPAA regulations will prohibit that interaction without the patient's consent and could possibly not be welcomed by the employer. In this case, providing the patient with the knowledge and materials that he needs will allow him to self-advocate.

Group interventions involve the clinician leading and working to promote improved function in a group setting. In a hand clinic, this approach may allow a hand therapist to group multiple patients into a treatment session of an extended duration, similar to work hardening, which is discussed in the next section. Often group interventions are delivered at the place of employment (see Chapter 119).

There are other work-specific intervention models that may be employed for the Workers' Compensation patient that may not be billable to a patient's health insurance. These interventions include work hardening and work conditioning, which are discussed next.

WORK HARDENING AND WORK CONDITIONING

The terms *work hardening* and *work conditioning* are often used interchangeably by those who provide hand therapy services, however, they are quite different. The AOTA has developed definitions that describe each.[64] *Work conditioning* is defined as "a systematic approach to restore the performance skills of workers recovering from long-term injury or illness. There is a focus on restoring the musculoskeletal and cardiovascular systems, as well as safely performing work tasks. This is typically achieved through work simulation and individualized interventions to improve physical capacity that occur 3 to 5 days per week for 2 to 4 hours per session." *Work hardening* is defined as being "similar to work conditioning; however, it is multidisciplinary and can involve psycho-medical counseling, ergonomic evaluation, job coaching and/or transitional work services. Treatment is typically provided 5 days per week for 2 to 4-plus hours per day. Patients in work-hardening programs may progress to transitional work programming by actually performing job duties at their place of employment. If necessary, final adaptations and/or reasonable accommodations can be determined during this period of transition."[64]

The objective of the work-conditioning program is to restore physical capacity and function to enable the patient to return to work. Given this definition, the pre- and postprogram examinations include history, systems review, and selected tests and measures required to identify individual work-related, systemic, neuromusculoskeletal restoration needs. It uses physical conditioning interventions and functional activities related to the work activities being performed by the patient. Often it takes place in a typical outpatient clinical setting and can be the regular length of the treatment session. The referral for work conditioning can be because of a recommendation from a FCE or is recommended by the clinician when the patient is medically stable and approaching a point in her progress that warrants that the focus of therapy shift to addressing return to work.

In contrast, the content of a work-hardening program sets it apart from other rehabilitation regimens. The content of the treatment sessions is to use work-oriented tasks to enhance performance. Work hardening involves the patient in activities that simulate the resistance, repetition, duration, and biomechanics of the occupation that the patient hopes to assume or resume. Structured and graded tasks progressively increase stamina (energy at top speed), endurance (necessary for prolonged activity), physical tolerance, productivity, and confidence in the injured worker. Relying heavily on actual task replication, work-hardening programs use the concept of specificity. It is this specificity that places stress on the injured worker in a manner that challenges the neuromuscular, respiratory, cardiovascular, and psychosocial systems that is similar to the workplace. As with work conditioning, the referral for work hardening may be prompted by the results of an FCE. The primary differences between work hardening and work conditioning is that (1) not only does the work-hardening program seek to physically prepare the worker to return to work, but it also seeks to mentally prepare them for return to work, and (2) the work-hardening program includes the involvement of multiple disciplines. Work hardening is a more holistic approach and provides the patient with access to an interdisciplinary team with the skills needed to address the medical, psychological, behavioral, physical, functional, and vocational components of employability and return to work. No guideline requires that every patient who enters the facility will receive treatment from all the core disciplines or stipulates the length of time that each of the disciplines treats the worker. Each organization individually decides how it will run its program and how much treatment a particular discipline will perform. As mentioned previously, work-hardening interventions may involve groups. The purpose of this is generally to address issues such a pain modulation or addressing the psychosocial components of return to work. Because of its inherently more holistic approach, work hardening requires a significant amount of space and staffing and is more expensive than work conditioning. As a result, they are not as prevalent as work-conditioning programs.

RETURN-TO-WORK SCHEDULES

If work is addressed in treatment from the time of initial evaluation and throughout the treatment intervention process, then the treating hand therapy practitioner will be able to provide the referring physician with input that can facilitate guiding the selection of more accurate restrictions and a viable schedule for return to work. Input may be needed from the employer on the availability of modified work and what an acceptable return-to-work schedule would consist of. It can be challenging to accurately determine if the patient will be able to perform his job duties through an entire work shift if he is only being seen for 1 hour in the clinic a few times a week. The hand therapy practitioner will need to provide input to the referral source on what is being observed in treatment. Unless the patient is being seen for work hardening, it will be impossible to predict successful return to work with accuracy. Some options can be to incorporate work simulation into the patient's home exercise program and have the patient report to the therapist what the results of these efforts are. Another option is to have the patient gradually resume work on a full-time basis. With permission from the employer, the patient may be able to begin working 25%

to 50% of his work shift for a few days to a week to gauge his response to work. If there are no issues, then increasing the time and intensity worked would be warranted.

As already mentioned, work modification may also be a possibility. For example, in a case of worker who performed housekeeping duties for a hotel chain, it was determined that the worker could perform all of her full duty tasks with the exception of cleaning the bottom of the room bathtubs because she continued to have difficulty with weight bearing on her injured upper extremity when she would bend over the tub. However, she was able to demonstrate that she could satisfactorily clean the bottom of the tub surface with a long-handled cleaning brush in the outpatient clinics tub without pain. This suggested work modification was presented to the employer, which then approved her being able to return to full-duty employment. Without the input of the hand therapy practitioner, she may not have been able to return to her job until her ability to weight bear on the involved extremity resolved.

If the patient is to continue in therapy after return to work, the therapist can monitor the patient's response to working and continue to have input regarding the work schedule and the need for work modification.

SUMMARY

The occupation of work is important to most working age adults. It is where they derive meaning for their lives as well as a source of income, and it provides security and a means to finance the pursuit of other life activities. Hand therapy practitioners need to be prepared to understand the unique facets of how they can and should address work and return to work for patients with upper quarter injuries. A variety of tools, both general and work specific, can be use by therapists to aid in facilitating the determination of return to work, work modification, or the exploration of new employment options or types that the permanently injured worker can pursue. The hand therapy practitioner has more contact with their patients than the other professionals involved in their cases (e.g., physician, workers' compensation case managers) and can drive successful outcomes with the injured worker. The intent of this chapter is to increase the awareness of these tools and concepts and provide a basic understanding of how to evaluate and implement interventions that will aid in the return to some form of employment after an upper quarter injury. Although some of the assessments and intervention types can be easily implemented from the information obtained in this chapter, other assessments (e.g., FCE) and intervention types (e.g., work hardening) may require additional training to adequately provide these services. The body of evidence for some of these assessments and concepts is outdated or lacking. When this is the case, the hand therapy practitioner must use her own clinical judgment to make informed decisions on the proper course of action when treating the injured worker in the clinic.

CASE STUDY

John is a 56-year-old union construction worker with medial epicondylitis in his dominant right upper extremity. He developed acute pain after working 12-hour shifts, 6 days per week pouring concrete. The workers' compensation physician performed a cortisone injection, made a hand therapy referral, and ordered one-handed light duty work. During the intake therapy interview 3 days later, John states that he underwent right carpal tunnel release 10 years ago and right knee arthroscopic surgery 5 years ago and takes antihypertensive medication. John has a muscular build and is about 40 lb overweight; he smokes one pack of cigarettes a day. John is married and has several grandchildren in the area. He enjoys motorcycle riding, hunting, and fishing. Upon examination, John's medial elbow is slightly inflamed, and the medial epicondyle and common flexor tendon are very tender to palpation; however, he does not exhibit tenderness proximal to the elbow. John denies numbness and tingling throughout his digits, and light touch is intact. Pain is rated as 7 with activity (lifting, pulling, wrist flexion, and so on) and decreases to 0 with rest. Active range of motion (AROM) is normal throughout the right upper limb, and strength is normal in the shoulder; however, strength testing of the wrist, elbow, and grip and pinch strength are deferred because acuity of his injury. John's DASH score is 65, with inability to perform resistive leisure activities, lifting, and opening a jar. He reports that he can perform his ADLs and drive without significant pain or difficulty.

John has participated in three therapy visits for modalities, AROM, and gentle stretching of the wrist flexors. Tenderness, pain, and edema are decreased. Eccentric strengthening to the wrist flexors and postural strengthening activities are performed. While performing modalities, the therapist asks John about his regular job duties. While he is performing some resistive activities, the therapist pulls up his job on O*NET, and together they identify his major work duties. These are written on the JPM, and his mean perceived performance rating for the seven activities listed is 4.1. Grip and pinch strength are tested to John's tolerance: grip in standardized position, 99lb left and 53lb right (42lb with the elbow extended); lateral pinch, 27lb left and 18lb right; and tip to tip pinch, 17lb left and 13lb right. Wrist extension strength is normal, but resisted wrist flexion provokes pain. Pain is rated as 5 during strength testing but remains 0 at rest. John's workers' compensation case manager is contacted to get a job description and approval to speak with John's employer. The job description is fairly close to John's. While eating lunch, the therapist watches some videos of people pouring concrete to familiarize herself with the tools, positions, and forces involved.

During the next session, the therapist has John perform some pushing and pulling activities on the Baltimore Therapeutic Equipment (BTE) work simulator against low to moderate resistance. The therapist has John push and pull on a large push broom used by the crew that cleans the clinic to simulate spreading the concrete. This is performed for 5 minutes over a tile floor, with pain rated as a 4 over the medial elbow when pulling the broom inward, whereas pushing the broom outward pain is only a 1 or 2. John mentions he has a large broom at home that he uses in the garage, so he is instructed to use the broom with pushing strokes to sweep a portion of his garage. He is anxious to wipe down his motorcycle, so the therapist has John use a hand towel to wipe down the BTE work simulator. He has a tendency to reach far from his body and wipe toward his body with his wrist in flexion, which the therapist instructs him to avoid because of the stress placed on the common flexor tendon by the wrist flexors. John seems to understand and modifies his technique accordingly. Ice is applied to the medial elbow for 10 minutes. The therapist asks John to think about other activities they could simulate in therapy.

John brings in an 8-foot 2 × 4 to his next therapy session to simulate striking off concrete. He demonstrates how he performs this task, with a pain rating of 4 experienced when using wrist flexion to perform the end of the simulated concrete finishing stroke. The therapist works with John to identify a technique that involves less wrist flexion, which brings his pain rating to a 1. The therapist puts two 3-lb cuff weights on the floor and has John pull these around in actions similar to striking off concrete. He tolerates this well. John has also brought in a hand trowel from home; surprisingly, he tolerates using the trowel in his right hand better than weight bearing through the right hand when troweling with the left hand. This cues the therapist to the need for some closed-chain activities. John reports that he is able to sweep his entire garage and wipe down his motorcycle without problems. He is frustrated doing busy work in the construction trailer at work, and his work tolerances have increased, so the therapist talks to the employer

to find out what other tasks John could do within his current abilities. The employer sends the therapist a few pictures of the tools and positions used for these activities, which appear to be within John's abilities. The therapist discusses John's progress and ability to tolerate job simulations with minimal pain with the physician, who subsequently increases the light-duty work restrictions to allow for gentle use of the right hand for 15 minutes per hour.

John returns to these more resistive work tasks and has learned enough to be able to problem solve the ways that he can work without increasing his symptoms. His grip strength has increased to 74lb and lateral pinch 18lb, wrist flexor strength is 4 of 5, wrist extension is 5 of 5, and elbow is 5 of 5. John is allowed time at work to apply ice if becomes painful midshift. He attends therapy once per week to monitor his progress and symptoms. John's JPM scores have increased to a mean rating of 7.4 and his DASH score to 20%. The therapist discusses the need for long-term self-management of his condition. She does some education regarding MSDs and techniques to decrease exposures, such as proper tool usage and neutral posture. She also includes the fact that smoking decreases the healing ability of the tissues and that a heavier extremity means that his muscles will have to work harder (gently broaching the idea of weight management). John says that he will consider her suggestions. Therapy is discontinued, and John is told to check in if his symptoms increase. He does on one occasion, and the therapist discusses strategies to help remediate his symptoms, which he later finds to be helpful. He returns to full-duty work.

REFERENCES

1. American Occupational Therapy Association. Occupational therapy practice framework: domain & process, 3rd ed. *Am J Occup Ther.* 2014:S1–S48.
2. Kaskutas V. Work incentives and policies in the United States and around the world. In: Braveman B, Page J, eds. *Work: Promoting Participation & Productivity through Occupational Therapy.* Philadelphia: FA Davis; 2012:347–364.
3. Krause N, Dasinger LK, et al. Modified work and return to work: a review of the literature. *J of Occup Rehabil.* 1998;8(2):113–139.
4. Alavi H, Oxley J. *Return to work and occupational illness and injury rehabilitation*[research report] ; 2014. Available at: http://www.iscrr.com.au/__data/assets/pdf_file/0009/297756/RTW-and-Occupational-Illness-and-Injury-Rehabilitation-A-Snapshot-Review_May-2013_Final.pdf.
5. Hand Therapy Certification Commission. Who is a certified hand therapist (CHT)? Available at: https://www.htcc.org/consumer-information/the-cht-credential/who-is-a-cht.
6. American Physical Therapy Association. Vision statement for the physical therapy profession and guiding principles to achieve the vision. Available at: http://www.apta.org/Vision/.
7. United States Department of Labor. *Dictionary of Occupational Titles.* ICPSR; 1991.
7a. Guyton G. A brief history of Workers' Compensation. *Iowa Orthop J.* 1999;19:106–110.
8. Fore L, Perez Y, Neblett R, et al. Improved functional capacity evaluation performance predicts successful return to work one year after completing a functional restoration program. *PM&R.* 2015;7(4):365–375.
9. Mayer TG, Barnes ND, Kishino G, et al. Progressive isoinertial lifting evaluation – I. A standardized protocol and normative database. *Spine.* 1998;13:993–997.
9a. Person-environment-occupation-performance (PEOP): an occupation-based framework for practice. In: Kramer P, Hinojosa J, Royeen C, eds. *Perspectives on Human Occupation: Theories Underlying Practice.* 2nd ed. Philadelphia: F.A. Davis Company; 2017.
10. Ladds E, Redgrave N, Hotton M, et al. Systematic review: predicting adverse psychological outcomes after hand trauma. *J Hand Ther.* 2017;30:407–419.

11. Novak CB, Anastakis DJ, Beaton DE, et al. Biomedical and psychosocial factors associated with disability after peripheral nerve injury. *JBJS*. 2011;93:929–936.

12. Keogh E, Book K, Thomas J, et al. Predicting pain and disability in patients with hand fractures: comparing pain anxiety, anxiety sensitivity and pain catastrophizing. *Eur J Pain*. 2010;8:113–139.

13. Moorehead JF, Cooper C. Patients with functional somatic syndromes or challenging behavior. In: Cooper C, ed. *Fundamentals of Hand Therapy: Clinical Reasoning and Treatment Guidelines for Common Diagnoses of the Upper Extremity*. 2nd ed. St. Louis: Elsevier; 2013:170–176.

14. Soares MM, Jacobs K, Silva LC, et al. Are cut out handles used when available in real occupational settings? Description of grips and upper extremity movements during industrial box handling. *Work*. 2012;41:4808–4812.

15. Borg G. *Borg's Perceived Exertion and Pain Scales*. Champagne, IL: Human Kinetics; 1998.

16. Alreni ASE, Harrop D, Lowe A, et al. Measures of upper limb function for people with neck pain. A systematic review of measurement and practical properties. *Musculoskelet Sci Pract*. 2017;29:155–163.

17. Geoghegan L, Llloyd-Hughes H, Shiatis A, et al. A systematic review of patient reported outcomes (PROM) use in studies of elective hand conditions. *Brit J Surg*. 2017;104:40.

18. Jayakumar, 2017

19. Solway S, Beaton DE, McConnell S, Bombardier C. *The DASH Outcome Measure User's Manual*. Toronto, Ontario: Institute for Work & Health; 2002:54.

20. Bohnen CL. Outcome measure use in occupational therapy for upper extremity rehabilitation: results of a survey of therapist clinical practices. *Master of Arts in Occupational Therapy Theses*. St. Catherine's University; 2011; not published.

21. Stratford PW, Binkley JM, Stratford DM. Development of and initial validation of the upper extremity functional index. *Physioth Can*. 2001;53:259–267.

22. Overbeek CL, Nota SPFT, Jayakumar P, el al. The PROMIS physical function correlates with the QuickDASH in patients with upper extremity illness. *Clin Orthop Relat Res*. 2015;473:311.

23. Williams RM, Meyers A. Functional abilities confidence scale: a clinical measure for injured worker with acute low back pain. *Phys Ther*. 1998;78:624–634.

24. Williams RM, Schmuck G, Allwood S, et al. Psychometric evaluation of health-related work outcome measures for musculoskeletal disorders: a systematic review. *J Occup Reh*. 2007;17:504–521.

25. Ilmarinen J. The work ability index (WAI). *Occupational Medicine*. 2007;57:160.

26. Bushmakin AG, Cappelleri JC, Taylor-Stokes G, et al. Relationship between patient-reported disease severity and other clinical outcomes in osteoarthritis: a European perspective. *J Med Econ*. 2011;201114(4):381–389.

27. Bansback N, Zhang W, Walsh D, et al. Factors associated with absenteeism, presenteeism, and activity impairment in patient in the first years of RA. *Rheumatology*. 2012;51(2):375–384.

28. Kaskutas V. Measuring work performance. In: Law M, Baum C, Dunn W, eds. *Measuring Occupational Performance: Supporting Best Practice in Occupational Therapy*. 3rd ed. Thorofare, NJ: Slack; 2017:201–238.

29. Innes E, Straker L. Reliability of work-related assessments, Part A. *Work*. 1999;13(2):107–124.

30. Innes E, Straker L. Reliability of work-related assessments, Part B. *Work*. 1999;13(2):125–152.

31. Sandqvist J, Törnquist K, Henriksson C. Assessment of Work Performance (AWP) – Development of an instrument. *Work*. 2006;26:379–387.

32. Myers E, Triscari R. Comparison of thee strength endurance parameters for the Baltimore Therapeutic Equipment (BTE) simulator II and the Jamar handgrip dynamometer. *Work*. 2017;51:95–103.

33. Yancosek K, Howell D. A narrative review of dexterity assessments. *J Hand Ther*. 22:258–270.

34. Huskisson EC. Measurement of pain. *Lancet*. 1974;2:1127–1131.

35. St John MJ, Mitten D, Hammert WC. Efficacy of PROMIS pain interference and Likert pain scores to assess physical function. *J Hand Surg-Am*. 2017;42:705–710.

36. Badalamente M, Coffelt L, Elfar J, et al. Measurement scales in clinical research of the upper extremity, part 1: general principles, measures of general health, pain, and patient satisfaction. *J Hand Surg*. 2013;38:401–406.

37. Ransford A, Cairns D, Mooney V. The pain drawing as an aid to the psychological evaluation of patients with low back pain. *Spine*. 1976;1:1–127.

38. Cheung K, Hume P, Maxwell L. Delayed onset muscle soreness: Treatment strategies and performance factors. *Sports Med*. 2003;33:145–164.

39. Soer R, Van der Schans CP, Groothoff JW, et al. Towards consensus in operational definitions in functional capacity evaluation: a Delphi survey. *J Occup Rehabil*. 2008;18:389–400.

40. Isernhagen S, Hart D, Matheson L. Reliability of independent observers judgements of level of lift effort in a kinesiophysical functional capacity evaluation. *Work*. 1999;12:145–150.

41. JTech Medical Industries. How to Use Tracker FCE Software to Conduct Functional Capacity Evaluations. Heber City, Utah: JTech.

42. Centers for Disease Control. *Maximal Isoinertial Strength Testing – Definition of Isoinertial Strength*. physical strength assessment in ergonomics; 1998. Available at: https://stacks.cdc.gov/view/cdc/9183.

43. Matheson LN, Mooney V, Grant JE, et al. A test to measure lift capacity of physically impaired adults, part 1: reliability testing. *Spine*. 1995;20:2119–2129.

44. Matheson LN, Verna J, Dreisingera T, et al. Age and gender normative data for lift capacity. *Work*. 2014;49:257–269.

45. Kumar W, Gerrits EHJ, Bacchus C. Symmetric and asymmetric two-handed pull and push strength of young adults. *Hum Factors*. 1995;37:854–865.

46. Stover H, Snook SH, Ciriello VM. The design of manual handling tasks: revised tables of maximum acceptable weights and forces. *Ergonomics*. 1991;34:1197–1213.

47. Ciriello V, Dempsey P, Maikala R, et al. Secular changes in psychophysically determined maximum acceptable weights and forces over 20 years for male industrial workers. *Ergonomics*. 2008;51:593–601.

48. Chaffin DB, Andersson GBJ, Martin BJ. *Occupational Biomechanics*. New York: John Wiley & Sons; 1999.

49. Schultz-Johnson KS. Upper extremity factors in the evaluation of lifting. *J Hand Ther*. 1990;3:72–85.

50. Legge J, Burgess-Limerick R. Reliability of the JobFit system pre-employment functional assessment tool. *Work*. 2007;28(4):299–312.

51. Liberty Mutual Insurance. The most serious workplace injuries cost U.S. companies $59.9 billion per year, according to 2017 Liberty Mutual workplace safety index. 2017. Available at: https://www.libertymutual-group.com/about-lm/news/news-release-archive/articles/2017-lm-wsi. Accessed: November 3, 2017.

52. Bureau of Labor Statistics. Non-fatal occupational injuries and illnesses requiring days away from work. 2015. 2016. Available at: https://www.bls.gov/news.release/osh.nr0.htm. Accessed: October 20, 2017.

53. Bureau of Labor Statistics. Employer-reported workplace injuries and illnesses, 2016. 2017. Available at: https://www.bls.gov/news.release/osh.nr0.htm. Accessed: October 21, 2017.

54. Bureau of Labor Statistics. Occupational safety and health definitions. Available at: https://www.bls.gov/iif/oshdef.htm; 2016.

55. Rodinelli RD. *American Medical Association: Guides to Evaluation of Permanent Impairment*. 6th ed. Chicago: AMA Press; 2007.

56. Owen TR, Wilkins MJ. Sincerity of effort differences in functional capacity evaluations. *J Rehabil*. 2014;80(3):53–61.

57. Lechner DE, Bradbury SF, Bradley LA. Detecting sincerity of effort: a summary of methods and approaches. *Phys Ther*. 1998;73(8):867–888.

58. Morgan M, Allison S, Duhon D. Heart rate changes in functional capacity evaluations in a workers' compensation population. *Work*. 2012;42:253–257.

59. Schapmire DW, St James JD, Townsend R, et al. Accuracy of visual estimation of effort during a lifting task. *Work*. 2011;40:445–457.

60. Townsend R, Schapmire DW, St James J, et al. Isometric strength assessment, part II: Static testing does not accurately classify validity of effort. *Work*. 2010;37:387–394.

61. Schapmire DW, St James JD. Letter to the editor. *Work*. 2011;38:197–199.

62. Field D. *The Expert Expert*. Bloomington, IN: iUniverse; 2013.

63. Kaskutas V, Snodgrass J. *Occupational Therapy Practice Guidelines for Individuals with Work-Related Injuries and Illnesses.* Bethesda, MD: AOTA Press; 2009:28.

64. American Occupational Therapy Association. Work rehabilitation. Available at: https://www.aota.org/About-Occupational-Therapy/Professionals/WI/WorkRehab.aspx; 2017.

65. Dunn W, McClain L, Brown C, Youngstrom M. The ecology of human performance. In: Neistadt ME, Crepeau EB, eds. *Willard and Spackman's Occupational Therapy*. 9th ed. Philadelphia: Lippincott Williams & Wilkins; 1998:525–535.

121

Rehabilitation Considerations for the Pediatric Client

Sarah Ashworth, Cheryl Lutz, Justine LaPierre

CRITICAL POINTS

- Child and adolescent clients differ from adults in their healing potential, safety awareness, and ability to follow instructions.
- Younger children with upper extremity differences develop compensatory strategies as they mature. These may be difficult to retrain after surgical reconstruction.
- Partnering effectively with the family unit is essential for carryover of skills and recommendations for pediatric clients. Caregivers are often relied on for accurate information about activity participation, functional impairments, and symptoms in daily life.

- A patient, playful approach to common assessment components, interventions, and orthosis management is often necessary to facilitate improvement in pediatric upper extremity conditions.
- Young clients may require support across childhood and adolescence with more complex activity demands. This may include adaptive techniques and equipment modifications to support participation in age appropriate activities of daily living and recreational activities.

THE PEDIATRIC CLIENT

Recognizing childhood as a distinct period of a person's life, with rigorous developmental demands, has been the position of Western culture since the mid-19th century.[1] In the United States today, childhood is considered the first 18 years of life. Modern developmental psychology provides qualifiable stages of psychosocial development to further define that time span.[2] Common understanding of these stages of development gives us the colloquial terminology: infant, toddler, school age, preadolescent, and adolescent. Clinicians face unique circumstances when evaluating and treating pediatric clients at any stage. Pediatric clients vary from their adult counterparts in nearly all areas given consideration. Which considerations are relevant for care in the hand clinic? Experiential knowledge largely informs the practice of the pediatric clinician when other evidence is scarce and is offered here for reference by hand therapists.

When grappling with the pertinent differences, a clinician can focus her or his lens by applying an appropriate framework to analyze the pediatric client and disability. The Occupational Therapy Practice Framework (OTPF) is one relevant option, familiar to occupational therapists in the field, intended to increase occupational engagement and thereby health status.[3] The International Classification of Function (ICF) developed by the World Health Organization in 1980 considers similar factors and their implications on one's overall state of disability and health.[4] The ICF offers a common language for the multidisciplinary team to consider disability and health outcomes. The model focuses on the relationship between body structures and body functions, health conditions, activity, participation, personal factors, and environmental factors operating within larger contextual factors.[4] Examining the whole of these elements will support hand therapists to effectively identify the specific needs of pediatric clients from evaluation through treatment planning, intervention, and discharge. Relevant considerations for pediatric practice in the hand clinic are outlined in this chapter using the ICF lens as an organizational tool.

Body Structure and Body Functions

Perhaps the most overt truth to the difference between children and adults relates to their growth. Children, by definition, have immature body structures and are physically growing. The physes of bones are open until adolescence to allow for bony growth. The ongoing maturation of the skeletal system introduces both additional risks and benefits during childhood. Greenstick fractures are a unique risk in growing bones, as are fractures to the growth plate, which risk growth arrest and limb deformity or length discrepancy, if unnoticed and untreated. External fixation may be used in pediatric clients not just for maintaining stability of a healing bone but also for lengthening procedures. A bone with a significant discrepancy can be lengthened using the advantage of the client's already growing bones and the stress of a fixator on an osteotomy site.[5]

Children have more cartilaginous tissue and more porous bones and may escape traumatic bony injury from a mechanism that would typically result in a fracture in an adult. When they do occur, traumatic injuries to bone heal more quickly in children. Stages of bony healing in a young child including the formation of callus, bridging, and clinical union can take half the time compared with in an adult.[6] Reduced healing time also leads to reduced immobilization time. This, in conjunction with more flexible connective tissues, results in less joint stiffness following immobilization in pediatric clients. Children also have a greater potential to remodel bony injuries and have increased tolerance to angulation deformity.[7] The net result, when contrasted with adults, is that fewer instances of fracture reduction, shorter immobilization time, and a decreased need for formal therapeutic intervention to combat joint stiffness are required. However, the orthopedic team may also face situations when they contemplate the advantages of a "stiff and stable" joint over unsafe instability. The most common example is reconstruction of the elbow, a hinge joint that presents significant functional limitations when unstable.[8,9] This point is further exaggerated in young children who continue to use the upper extremities frequently for weight bearing during mobility. Despite the disinclination for stiffness in children, the clinician can play a vital role in increasing the available range of motion (ROM) when a joint has undergone a significant repair or has been hampered by increased immobilization times for healing. This is particularly true for the maturing skeletal systems of adolescents.

Children may be better protected with cast immobilization compared with a removable orthosis while healing because they may be more behaviorally impulsive. It is important to carefully weigh the pediatric client and family's potential to successfully adhere to precautions and immobilization instructions to determine when and if a removable orthosis is appropriate. The child's behavior and ability to follow directions during a clinical examination with the orthopedist or hand therapist is a valuable indicator of the child's ability to comply with safety instructions. However, the clinic is only a glimpse into one context of the child's behavioral repertoire. It is also important to use clinical knowledge of developmentally appropriate behavioral expectations as well as interview with the caregiver regarding day-to-day activities, routines, and "direction following."

The nervous system of the child is another wonder of development. It has been well documented that the central nervous systems of children are extremely plastic.[10,11] This is the basis for many pursuits of clinicians working with pediatric patients. In the hand clinic, one may see the negative effects of congenital impairment or even short immobilization of a child's limb, seemingly causing a decreased cortical representation of the limb. The resultant activity patterns present with an inattention to the limb and decreased rates of incorporation of the limb into functional tasks. Intervention to promote cortical remapping is an important component of optimizing function.[12,13] The sensorimotor and somatosensory cortices are inextricably linked.[14,15] Various creative strategies can be used to bring awareness to the involved limb and begin to increase the representation on the sensory or motor homunculus.[16–18] Examples for children may be as simple as a brightly colored or noisy bracelet on the affected upper extremity, stickers placed along the limb, and sing-song play such as "Where is Thumbkin?"

The peripheral nervous system has also demonstrated remarkable adaptability in children.[11,19] For example, children who experienced median and ulnar nerve injury and subsequent repair have significantly better outcomes in long-term nerve function compared even with those who had similar injuries as adolescents.[20] Although healing and adaptation potentials are high, there are limitations to the body's ability to repair itself, even with the maximized healing potential of youth. Surgeries for peripheral nervous system repair are options up

until the point of motor endplate death. Nerve regeneration is able to take place at a rate of 1 mm a day in adults and potentially more quickly in children.[21] The possibility of surgical intervention can literally be a race against time, influenced by the physical distance between the intact peripheral nervous system and the muscle that it is meant to innervate.[22,23] Pediatric repair offers two potential advantages, one being the physical size of the client's limb and therefore the distance from sound nerve to motor endplate.[24] The second advantage is the minimization of "lost" time since the injury date. For a child who was subject to a birth injury, assuming the child presents to the microsurgeon in the first couple of weeks or months after birth, the clock has only recently begun ticking. This second advantage is not a given. The severity of a child's injury may be overlooked or his or her ability to spontaneously recover overstated. Just like their adult counterparts, timely recognition of peripheral nerve damage and referral to the qualified microsurgical professional are key to maximizing the pediatric client's potential for an optimal functional outcome.[25]

Health Conditions

The variety of health conditions encountered by the clinician in pediatric populations can generally be divided between those that are congenital and those that are acquired. Although there is also a category of injuries acquired during or soon after birth, from a practical standpoint, children experience these health conditions in a similar way to congenital conditions. From the child's earliest point of consciousness, the injury or condition was present. Thus, they have developed physically and emotionally the entirety of their lives with the health condition as an aspect of their identity.

Children with congenital conditions and their families may be well versed in the arenas of medical and therapeutic care. These children are likely receiving early intervention services, school therapy, or developmentally focused pediatric outpatient therapy services on an ongoing basis. A referral to the hand therapist will often have specific goals delineated, such as orthosis fabrication, a course of serial casting, or the initiation of postoperative rehabilitation. Another opportunity for an encounter in a hand clinic could present as more complicated tasks become developmentally appropriate and a child is suddenly having difficulty meeting these demands. Examples of such tasks may be tying shoes or playing a musical instrument.

The clinician may find that the child has independently developed compensatory strategies to complete some tasks. Children can be very creative in their problem solving. However, the additional eye of a skilled clinician can assist in identifying when strategies are adaptive or maladaptive to the client and family's goals. For example, consider a child with arthrogryposis multiplex congenita (AMC) who presents with trademark atrophied bilateral shoulder girdles and no associated active ROM available. The child may present to the clinic using momentum from the trunk to create a pendulum action at the shoulders. This is an adaptive strategy that allows the child to independently position the hands onto a tabletop for participation in activities of daily living (ADLs), instrumental activities of daily living (IADLs), or school tasks (Fig. 121.1). In contrast, there is the example of a child with AMC who has no appreciable biceps, brachialis, or brachioradialis but has been able to use a Steindler effect of the flexor pronator mass to generate limited against gravity elbow flexion. For the most functional result after flexorplasty surgical intervention, the child will need specific positioning and cueing from the clinician to complete the necessary neuromuscular reeducation of the donor muscle and diminish the use of their previous compensatory strategy. At this point in time, the previous strategy would be maladaptive even though it was likely a helpful habit for that child in the past.

Although patient and caregiver education are always an important part of skilled, therapeutic intervention, emphasis may be necessary when encountering children with acquired conditions. The "newness"

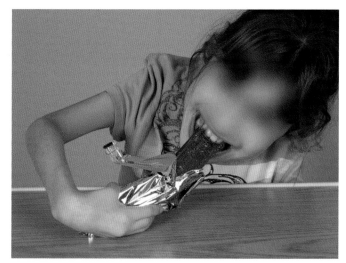

Fig. 121.1 A 10-year old girl with arthrogryposis multiplex congenita using compensatory passive elbow flexion on table top for a self-feeding activity. (Courtesy of Shriners Hospital for Children, Philadelphia.)

TABLE 121.1	**General Guide of Activities of Daily Living Skill Development**
Age	**Developing Skills**
6–12 mo	• 6–8 mo: Starts to hold bottle • 6–9 mo: Starts to pick up and self-feed finger foods; may attempt to grasp spoon • 9–13 mo: Self-feeds finger foods for significant part of meal
1–2 yr	• Pushes arms and legs into clothing • Pull off shoes and socks • Improving precision with spoon grasp, scooping, and bringing sticky foods to mouth
2–3 yr	• Doff and don open-front jacket • Unbutton large buttons • Able to use spoon with less spills; beginning fork use • Begins to participate in self-bathing
3–4 yr	• Zip and unzip connected zippers • May don pull on clothing with supervision for orientation • May be able to fasten three or four buttons
4–5 yr	• Connect open-ended zipper • Doff pull over shirt • Bathe and dry self with supervision for thoroughness
5–6+ yr	• Dress unsupervised • Beginning to tie shoes • Fasten posterior buttons and snaps • Brush teeth with supervision for thoroughness • 8+ independently prepare and complete bathing

Adapted from Shepherd J. Activities of daily living and adaptations for independent living. In Case-Smith, ed. *Occupational Therapy for Children*. 5th edition. Philadelphia: Elsevier; 2005:521-570 and Case-Smith J, Humphry R. Feeding intervention. In Case-Smith J, ed. *Occupational Therapy for Children*. 5th edition. Philadelphia: Elsevier; 2005:481-520.

of the condition implies a baseline need for education on the condition itself, treatment options, and its rehabilitation potential.[26] There may also be more acute coping concerns identifiable by the therapist and affecting participation and carryover of therapeutic interventions.[27] These are relevant considerations for both the client and the caregiver. For children with any difference, congenital or acquired, the psychosocial impact cannot be overlooked both for the child's overall health as well as for the effectiveness of therapeutic interventions. This concept is further explored in the section considering personal factors.

Activity

The seven areas of occupation are consistent throughout the lifespan. That being said, the balance among the areas, as well as the level of proficiency exhibited, varies greatly from childhood to adulthood. Pediatric clients live a rich life of stimulation to support their development. It is widely accepted that developmental milestones occur within a temporal range. Progression along a continuum rather than an overly specific timeline is most valuable.[28] However, the omnipresent use of the phrases "developmentally appropriate participation" and "developmentally appropriate level of independence" applied to task-specific goals is intended to illuminate the pediatric client's current functional deficit. Ultimately, the standard of "developmentally appropriate" implies comparison with a child's peers. Thus, a base knowledge of the norms of development can serve as a foundation for the clinician while recognizing that progression along the developmental continuum is the most relevant pursuit. Relevant skills appear in Table 121.1.

It is appropriate and necessary for children to engage in a range of activities that are not always deemed important in adulthood. Typical childhood experiences may include playing on a township tee-ball team, taking guitar lessons, and participating in a tumbling class. Many adults will remember similar activities from their own youth, whether or not they were involved in a formal organization. Yet the reflecting adults have likely not gone on to be professional baseball players, rock stars, or elite gymnasts. The physical activities themselves, cognitive demands, social interactions, and emotional regulation components are all valuable for developing bodies and minds. Participation should not be discouraged in childhood because of an impairment and, in fact, should be strongly advocated in the face of resistance.

Play is the defining occupation of childhood and children should participate in a wide variety of play activities.[29] Children require gross motor play, fine-motor play, pretend and social play, and sensory play (and various combinations thereof) to feed their development. Messy play tasks should not be overlooked as important sensory experiences for the upper extremities. Seeking toys in a bin of rice, painting with finger paints, and squeezing squirt toys in a basin of water are all valuable play experiences that are manageable in a clinic environment. Planning ahead to allow families to bring a spare set of clothes can be beneficial as well as setup considerations, including towels laid onto the floor for quicker clean-up (Table 121.2).

Participation

The clinician can play an important role in problem-solving strategies to support participation, including adaptive equipment (custom or otherwise) or adapted strategies. As the child ages and activities require increased proficiency, often the client can become his or her own subject matter expert. Preadolescents and adolescents can provide vital information related to specific challenges and illuminate their needs for adaptation. Adapted leagues and groups exist in various geographic areas. Cues from the client should serve as the guiding force for the appropriate level and venue for participation in desired activities.

Choosing activities and encouraging participation of a child in a clinic environment can present unique challenges for hand therapists. The ability to build rapport with any patient is key for a successful therapeutic relationship.[30] Setting a child at ease by engaging with her playfully is vital. Skillfully using a nuanced therapeutic use of self, such as silliness as distraction or firmness to redirect to task, is invaluable to encourage specific behavioral responses from the child. Play tasks themselves will instantly increase the child's intrinsic motivation to participate in therapeutic activities compared with rote exercise.[29] Games or competitions can be devised using creativity and supplies easily identifiable around the clinic.

TABLE 121.2   Game Time: Tips and Tools for Developmentally Appropriate Play

Infants (~birth–12 mo)	• Select items or toys that generate noise or lights to capture the attention of the youngest clients. Shiny plastic bead and rattles are popular choices. • Parents may also have a few of the child's favorite familiar toys on hand. • Be careful to introduce items that are safe to be mouthed and can be easily cleaned!
Toddlers (~1–3 yr)	• Collect items in a bucket, practicing "in" and "out" with item acquisition, grasp, and release skills. • Stack items and knock them down. • Introduce basic imaginary play concepts such as feeding a baby doll.
Preschoolers and school age (~3–11 yr)	• Imaginative play can include more complex schemas and roles for the child and clinician to play. • Introduce formal or informal games that have basic rules and structures such as turn taking. The most elementary board games are recommended for 3 years and older. • Use a preferred game or toy as the reward at the end of a treatment session.
Preadolescents and adolescents (~11–18 yr)	• Capitalize on the client's personal interests and occupations when designing therapeutic tasks to maximize compliance and efforts. • Allow the client to engage in the goal setting process for the current activity, as well as short- and long-term therapeutic goals. • Competition can serve as a positive motivating force for therapeutic activities in the clinic, against another individual, the clock, or a high score. Keeping track of personal records over the long term allows the client to objectively measure his or her progress and remain motivated.

The child's ability to differentiate between pain and discomfort and his reaction to both can affect his participation in therapeutic activity and exercise. Children have difficulty articulating their physical state of being because of developing both expressive language skills and understanding of their bodies and sensations. A child experiencing pain in a limb may not be able to specify the location or quality of the sensation. Similarly, children may use nonverbal communication skills to express both pain and discomfort. Although it is widely known that the five Ps (pain, pallor, paresthesia, paralysis, and pulselessness) indicate compartment syndrome in an adult, a child with increasing tissue pressures often does not present with a second P symptom in addition to pain.[31,32] The clinician should instead look for three As to indicate pediatric compartment syndrome: increasing anxiety, increasing agitation, and increasing analgesic requirement.[33]

The opposing consideration for hand therapists is that children may also indicate signs of distress such as fussing, crying, or even screaming when experiencing discomfort. These signs are a biologically adaptive strategy for infant survival; however, when indicating discomfort as opposed to pain, they can cause a misinterpretation and overreaction of adult concern. Common examples are a child's reaction to a passive range of motion (PROM) program or to the doffing of a cast or orthosis from a stiff joint. Client and caregiver education are most important, as is reinforcement of productive language. Considerations are expanded in the Range of Motion: Intervention section.

Carrying over behavioral techniques from the child's home environment can be an effective strategy to promote the participation of the pediatric client. This information can be ascertained during caregiver interview. Alternatively, novel strategies can be used successfully in the clinic and then may be recommended for carryover at home. Examples may include presenting limited choices or providing rewards for positive behavior (Box 121.1). Rewards can serve a dual purpose, also supporting carryover of acquired skills.[34] In any strategy used, consistency of implementation and expectations is key. Food is not recommended as a reward unless it is a natural consequence of successes in a self-feeding task. Prizes can create unrealistic and unsustainable expectations from the child and are likewise not recommended for regular rewards.

Fostering self-efficacy and intrinsic motivation via successful training is often the most valuable behavioral strategy for the promotion of participation.[35,36] When tasks are introduced, consider allowing the child to trial the task with an unaffected upper extremity or initially decrease the task demands. The concept of scaffolding, based on Lev Vygotsky's educational framework, can provide the clinician considerations for increasing demands in a realistic, stepwise fashion.[37] The teacher, or in this case clinician, must offer just the right amount of support to allow the child to achieve success and therefore increased competence[38] (Fig. 121.2). The child does not need to succeed on every attempt of the task but must experience success and solidify the skill before increasing demands. Experiencing this success before reaching the child's frustration threshold is key to ensure the child remains motivated to continue participating. The clinician must pay careful attention to the child's tolerance of frustration and ability to persevere through adversity to modulate the task appropriately. Offer children specific praise, describing the behavior they executed well.[39] Use age-appropriate language, possibly giving body parts or movements shorthand names, to build a child's awareness of the task demands being introduced and reinforced. An example when working with a child who has right hemiparesis with right upper extremity inattention may be, "I really like the way 'righty' is holding your paper while you are coloring!"

The skilled clinician's base knowledge of motor learning theories is particularly relevant when considering activities for skill acquisition in pediatric clients.[40] Bearing in mind a child's attention span and the structure of the session can guide the choice between task versus whole and massed versus distributed practice. Similarly, methods of guidance versus discovery must be carefully balanced to encourage success while allowing for the valuable experience of problem-solving natural consequences. Often a combination of principles is applied.[41] Backward chaining can be an effective strategy in pediatric intervention because it allows the child to repeatedly experience success and see the final result of the new skill.[42] This can instill natural feelings of pride and motivation to continue training for skill acquisition.

Personal Factors

The child's personal experience of her difference can have a profound impact on the impairments observed and reported to the clinician. There is a wide range in severity of health conditions, both congenital and acquired, that can affect children. However, severity is not the only predictor of perceived disability state.[43,44] The ability of the child and the caregivers to cope with the condition are relevant factors.[45] It has been described in the literature that caregivers of children diagnosed with differences experience grief for an ambiguous loss.[46,47] Formal intervention via counseling or support groups may be beneficial.[45]

BOX 121.1   Lessons from the Kid's Table

General Tips When Assessing Pediatric Clients
- Explain the assessment in age-appropriate language.
- Children with an acute injury, painful condition, or postsurgery may be particularly guarded and anxious to have affected extremity examined. Take time to build rapport.

Young Children
- Have a plan before you begin. Try to observe as much as possible during play.
- Incorporate parents' participation. They may hold an infant in supine or sidelying instead of lying on a mat for different gravity challenges. Shy children may be more willing to reach for objects from their parents presented in different planes.
- Be playful! Use small toys, stickers, or bubbles and get on their level to build trust, especially if they are painful or are anxious with strangers or medical staff. In hand clinic, often the best examinations start when we sit on the floor with a bucket of toys.
- When safe, let children touch and hold assessment tools (i.e., goniometer, measuring tape) before using the tools on them. Show them what you are going to do on parents first or let them "measure" you.
- If an infant does get upset, you may see more active movement in an affected arm. Observe but allow rest and cuddle breaks as needed.
- Small objects present a choking risk. Exercise caution and consider using age-appropriate, parent-approved edible items when suitable.

Older Kids and Teens
- Kids may try to "get it right," especially if they have been through treatment or serial examination. Ask family what is typical or provide an activity to observe so they are not focused on performing but on the task.
- Talk directly to children, not just about them with the parents. Show them their input is valued and important to the process.

Home Programs
The home program is a critical part of any therapy program. It reinforces foundational skills or techniques addressed in formal sessions to support the continuation of progress and generalization to real life. However, even the best-designed home program will fail without compliance. With pediatric clients, additional factors such as family dynamics and schedule, school and extracurricular activities, and need for supervision with program must be considered. Clearly educating the client and their caregivers on the importance and goal of the home program and making an effort to accommodate their unique situation can improve compliance.

Young Children
- Some infants' parents may believe they need the specific toys used in therapy to be effective. Educate them on the reasoning behind the activity, discuss beneficial types of toys, and show them how to use a wide variety of objects to facilitate desired interaction.
- Incorporate home program into a natural schedule (e.g., diaper changes, meals, after school or bedtime).
- Use a calendar or sticker chart to reward participation.

Older Kids and Teens
- Discuss family schedule. Work together with pediatric client and family to determine realistic ways to incorporate the program into daily life.
- Consider the importance of peer relationships. When possible, avoid additional "differences" in peer situations. This may include low-profile orthoses at school or emphasizing incorporation of the affected limb at home, with more lenience for compensation when with friends.

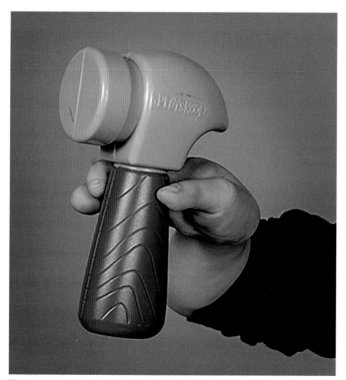

Fig. 121.2 A child with a congenital hand difference grasps a toy that was selected by the clinician to be an appropriate width and weight for success in play. The proceeding task chosen by the clinician to further challenge the child's grasping skills represent the process of "scaffolding" the skill acquisition process. (Courtesy of Shriners Hospital for Children, Philadelphia.)

As mentioned previously, a child may have a condition that predated his ability to discriminate differences between himself and his peers. Eventually, the child and his peers will recognize and have questions about the differences. It is important to remember and to remind caregivers that peer's questions are typically innocently posed in pursuit of knowledge to better understand the world around them. When a question is posited by the pediatric client or by peers, it is best to give a brief, honest answer. Leave the conversation open to further questions and dialogue. This will help shape the pediatric client's understanding of his difference and will also model how he can respond to curious peers. "That's just the way you were born" quickly turns into "That's just the way I was born." It is, however, developmentally appropriate for children to make up sensational stories about their differences. It is not important to correct the child but rather to continue to find instances to offer accurate information about his difference in a developmentally appropriate way.

It can also be difficult to address the frustration that a caregiver or child experiences when certain tasks are difficult to complete or not performed in the same manner as peers. It is important to validate the feelings of frustration and to reassure that it is "OK" to experience challenges and go through hard times. Similarly, mantras such as "practice makes progress," instead of the alternative, which references perfection, put the focus on effort and ability rather than arbitrary standards.

The reactions of peers to differences will never be completely within the control of the child or even any involved adults. In reality, children with disabilities are two to four times more likely to be bullied compared with their able-bodied peers.[48] However, children with differences can be both supported to foster resilience and provided the tools to respond to adversity.[49,50] In particular, having a "best friend" is a significant factor associated with resiliency through adversity.[51] Early social interactions should be supported to build relationships as well as the understanding and empathy of peers.[52] Most important, the child's difference should never be treated as something that needs to be disguised. Although all children strive to "fit in" with their peers, it is valuable to focus on the fact that everyone has differences rather than a façade that everyone is the same.[49,53]

Of vital importance is the consistent offering of a listening ear, acceptance, and compassion.[49,54] References in popular culture can also assist the understanding of the child and her peers; a certain cartoon fish's lucky fin is a common example from which an analogy can be drawn. "He might have a lucky fin, but he can do everything the other fish can do." There are also children's books, including *Different is Awesome*[55] and *Emmy's Amazing Hand*,[56] that can provide a developmentally appropriate storyline structure for discussing differences and abilities with children.

Environmental Factors

Working effectively with a pediatric client and family requires consideration of the environment. For the most productive session with a pediatric client in the hand clinic, the clinician must plan ahead for a developmentally appropriate setup. If there is floor space that is clean and can be cleared of furniture, it may be ideal for the clinician, child, and caregiver to work. Specialty pediatric-sized chairs offer a tailor-made option; however, environments can be improvised for smaller bodies with adjustable height benches serving as seats and tabletops. A Hi-Lo style mat is another option for tabletop surface, and the mere act of adjusting its height via the controller can serve as a motivating fine-motor activity in its own right. Choosing an area that can be secured via a door, physical positioning of the clinician and caregiver, or lap belt may be advantageous. It is helpful to have lots of activity options for participation nearby because the attention span devoted by the child on each activity may be unpredictable. Transitions between tasks can be challenging. Keeping options within arm's length of the clinician is recommended to reduce the time required to select the next activity. However, keeping additional games and activities out of the child's sight, potentially under the table or behind the clinician, can reduce distractions and maximize the time devoted to each therapeutic activity.

Safety considerations are a necessary component to planning for pediatric clients. Small toys or orthosis components (e.g., a short thumb strap) may pose a risk for a child placing them in his mouth and therefore present a choking hazard. Nontoxic supplies are always preferred. Any porous or fabric tools or toys that cannot be sanitized should be considered single use. For this reason, stuffed animals make better rewards than therapy tools. More a component of clothing safety, washable markers and paints are recommended compared with permanent alternatives when working with pediatric clients.

Ultimately, the most important environments for the carryover of skills and therapeutic successes are those outside the clinic walls. The child's home environment is arguably the most influential on the child. Consider the roles the child plays and the roles of the other family members. What is expected of the child in her day-to-day life and therefore what priorities does the family have for therapeutic goals? Families have varying values and beliefs on the important aspects of childhood and development. Cultural background may be a relevant factor in shaping these.[57–59] The caregiver's unique perspective is therefore invaluable in shaping an effective treatment plan.

A child's reliance on the family unit for care influences not only goal setting but also health.[44,60] Pediatric clients have less autonomy than adults and are often dependent, in every sense of the word, on their caregivers. This includes dependence on caregivers for the carryover of

any and all therapeutic recommendations. Consider the family's level of education on the condition and prognosis for improvements. Does their perception match that of the clinician? What is their perceived level of agency to enact positive change or to prevent further challenges? The "buy-in" of the family on intervention in the hand clinic is vital to the cause.[61,62]

Many factors can be examined by the clinician for making effective recommendations to a family. Consider other demands on the family's time and attention. A holistic approach will help set realistic expectations of participation in home exercise programs, orthotic schedules, and other recommendations to be carried over in the home. Explore what types of education and resources may be helpful. These should be multimodal and can vary widely, from support groups to peer-reviewed literature to handouts of written or pictures of instructions.[63] Use the strengths and routines of the family to develop a plan with the highest likelihood of carryover. For example, a lotion routine after bath time may be the perfect opportunity for scar massage. The inherent, multiple-times-daily interruption of a diaper change can be a good cue to complete a set of PROM stretches. Some families demonstrate a strong value of explicit therapeutic exercises in a formal exercise program, with specifics delineated on paper or even video.[64] Others respond more positively to general participation recommendations, such as implementing a half-hour-long craft activity daily. The clinician will need to discern a way to partner effectively with a child's caregiver as team members in the delivery of services to the pediatric client.[65]

Pediatric clients present to hand clinics with a variety of unique circumstances. The hand therapist, armed with information pertaining to developmental considerations, can rely on their existing skillsets to effectively evaluate, develop a plan of care, and implement interventions for each pediatric client. The following sections expand on evaluation and intervention methods for pediatric clients.

RANGE OF MOTION

Assessment

Range of motion is a basic component of any upper extremity assessment. Limitations are commonly present in both congenital and acquired upper extremity conditions. Accurate assessment is important to identify impairments and to measure progress after interventions. Goniometry with children can be challenging because of short attention spans and ability to follow directions, fearfulness, pain, and small joints sizes.

For infants and toddlers, accurate active range of motion (AROM) measurements can be difficult because of limited ability to participate, especially for the distal joints. For children who have pain or minimal tolerance for handling by the therapist, beginning with active measurements can help build rapport and allow them to understand the testing process.[66] Using age-appropriate language and demonstrating the movement can help clarify verbal instructions. Children participate more if testing is playful, such as a game of Simon Says or reaching for toys or snacks for desired motions. Shoulder and elbow motions can be measured with the parent holding a desired object to facilitate the movement. Children may be fearful of an unfamiliar tool; by allowing them to hold and examine the goniometer, they can realize it is safe.

For the smallest hands, digital PROM measurements may not be possible because of the very small size of the joints. Measuring fingertip to distal palmar crease during composite digit flexion may be a more successful and reliable option. Observation of grasping specific objects can be objectively assessed, such as a pencil or half-inch-diameter peg, can be reliably repeated to track composite digit flexion progress over time.[67] When alternative assessments are incorporated, it is imperative to include an objective component for tracking progress over time.

Measurements of PROM can also be difficult for clients who have pain, traumatic injuries, or a prolonged course of stretching with negative association. Distraction with videos, music, or sitting on a parent's lap can help relax the child, and patience may be necessary to slowly stretch to end range for accurate measurements. When a child is having a difficult time with passive assessment, prioritize the necessary movements and limit the examination; additional measurements can be obtained in a subsequent visit.[22]

Children and adolescents with ROM limitations over time often develop compensatory movement patterns to accomplish functional tasks. In children with brachial plexus birth palsy limiting overhead motion, increased trunk extension and lateral flexion is often noted with attempts to reach. In the presence of an elbow contracture, increased shoulder flexion and wrist flexion is used for hand-to-face tasks. When assessing ROM, it is also important to observe how the child has adapted to the limitation. The more ingrained this movement pattern is, the more difficult it may be to eliminate it even as improvements are made in the affected joint(s).

Intervention

When working to improve ROM deficits, a collaborative effort between the clinician, child, and family is necessary. Carryover at home is vital with any intervention to improve ROM. Caregivers need to be hands on with home exercises programs for younger children. School-aged children and adolescents often need verbal cues to complete their home programs and to monitor technique. Education in the clinic should include both the client and caregivers and be reviewed frequently.

Stretching and orthoses are often important components of the treatment plan. For children with congenital conditions who present with limited ROM (e.g., radial longitudinal deficiency or AMC), the greatest impact can be made in the first 2 years of life with a diligent stretching program. Early family education on appropriate positioning and stretching techniques to be completed multiple times throughout the day can maximize early PROM gains.[68,69] Distraction strategies can improve tolerance of stretching exercises.

Infants and younger children, during PROM exercise, often react negatively to the feeling of a muscle being put under physical tension. After determining that the reaction is due to stretching, the therapist educates the caregivers and assures them that the prescribed exercises are not causing injury to the child. The sensation can be likened to stretches completed by the parent, and the associated "pulling sensation" is related to stretching a stiff muscle after a workout. Likewise, it is important to use appropriate language in conversation with the child as well. Avoid reinforcing terms, including "pain" and "hurt," for therapeutic activities and exercises, which should not be causing these negative consequences. Rather, redirect the child to terms such as "stiff," "uncomfortable," and "stretch" when necessary.

Targeting active motion of specific joints is important to integrate gains in passive motion and eliminate compensatory patterns. With some creativity in setting up or positioning the client, many favorite games and toys can be used to facilitate repetitious ROM exercise. For children with limited shoulder flexion, painting on an easel while sitting on a low bench or simply reaching for game pieces with the trunk stabilized to reduce compensation can facilitate the desired motion. Turning a rain stick, searching for stickers placed on palmar and dorsal hand, and turning cards encourages forearm rotation (Fig. 121.3). Some children do not tolerate handling by the therapist or parent to manually stabilize adjacent joints; use of wraps, orthoses, and supportive seating can provide the same effect during an activity in a more tolerable way. A simple strip of loop strapping can be made into a belt to attach game pieces with adhesive hook to encourage repetitive internal rotation to the belly to retrieve pieces. Incorporating a rewards system

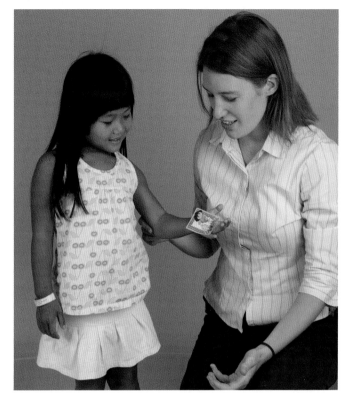

Fig. 121.3 Incorporation of sticker play to facilitate supination in a 5-year old girl with brachial plexus palsy. (Courtesy of Shriners Hospital for Children, Philadelphia.)

or counting repetitions can help the child feel more in control of the process and improve participation. Older children and teens benefit from watching their movements in a mirror to understand their compensatory movements and use the visual feedback to correct their position during exercises and activities. When maladaptive protective co-contraction is limiting motion, surface electromyographic biofeedback is a valuable tool to help normalize muscle recruitment patterns in a pain-free range.

STRENGTH

Assessment

Strength assessment is an important component of upper extremity evaluation but can be challenging with pediatric clients. Older children can participate in manual muscle testing. Begin with larger joints, basic movements, or the unaffected arm, as available, to assess the child's ability to follow the directions and exert maximum effort. Prioritize which muscles most need to be tested for children with limited attention spans for assessment. Additional testing can be completed over time.[22] A playful attitude, making testing like arm wrestling, and allowing the child to win at the end can keep him engaged. Dynamometry grip and pinch strength norms have been established as young as 6 years old.[70] Demonstrating the use of and allowing the child to see the dynamometer and pinch meter before testing can clarify verbal instructions.

For infants through preschoolers, strength is best assessed through upper extremity function.[66] Observe the weight of objects the child can grasp and how long she can maintain grasp. As she moves through appropriate developmental transitions, is she able to weight bear evenly on both arms? On the affected arm? Hang from a bar? Monitor for compensatory patterns that indicate weakness, such as the trumpeter sign in brachial plexus palsy with the arm abducted for hand-to-mouth tasks. This demonstrates weakness with external rotation, elbow flexion, or supination with hand-to-mouth tasks. Extensor digitorum communis can provide wrist extension; the long finger flexors can flex the wrist (Fig. 121.4). Some of these substitutions can be easy to miss in infants and require close and repeated examination. For children with systemic conditions, one must consider trunk control and its impact on distal function. Testing in supine or with supports for sitting can accommodate for trunk impairments and provide a better assessment of strength in the upper extremity by providing stability. This decreases the demands on the upper extremities to support upright positioning.

Intervention

Strengthening in the youngest clients should incorporate developmental transitions and weight bearing with decreasing levels of support as able. Simply reaching for toys with gravity minimized is the starting point for very weak muscles. Educating the caregivers on positioning to target muscles and movements is important for carryover at home. Weighted wrist bands as light as 0.25 lb can be placed on the child

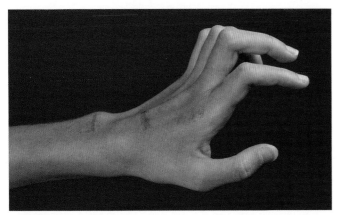

Fig. 121.4 A 12-year old child using the extensor digitorum communis to aid weak wrist extensors. (Courtesy of Shriners Hospital for Children, Philadelphia.)

during preferred play task set up to elicit desired motion. As children become more mobile and are not weight bearing with crawling, platform swings, physio balls, tunnels, and playground equipment can be used to promote strengthening. Putty or playdough (as a nontoxic option) can be incorporated for finger strengthening. Pull-apart toys, interlocking blocks, or adding hook and loop tape to favorite toys are great ways to target hand strengthening.

Older children and teens can participate in specific progressive resistive exercises with resistance bands and weights; however, these can become tedious.[71] Incorporating playful or fun activities will keep the client engaged and promote compliance with the home program. Yoga poses, virtual reality or gross movement–based video games, or sport-specific activities can be fun and promote strengthening.

DEXTERITY

Assessment

Dexterity describes using the hands to manipulate objects. This skillset is composed of a variety of grasp and release movement patterns and in-hand manipulation. These complex skills develop and are refined through childhood typically after an ulnar-to-radial and palmar-to-fingertip sequence. Assessing dexterity in a pediatric client requires consideration of the developmental level as well as all of the basic hand function components that contribute to coordinated integration of these skills, such as strength, ROM, sensation, and tone[66,67] (Table 121.3).

In the first 2 years of life, rapid changes in hand skills occur from reflexive fisting and reaching to more refined prehensile grasp patterns. More complex in-hand manipulation skills begin to emerge in the second year of life and continue refining in skill, consistency, and speed through the preteen years.[72] Observation of reflexive movements, reaching skills, grasp patterns to manipulate a variety of sized and shaped objects, and voluntary release to desired targets are valuable elements of the evaluation. Note deviations from typical patterns, such as bypassing a stiff digit, shaking or flexing the wrist to release objects, or excessive transfer of objects between hands for repositioning. Repeated assessment with the same or similarly sized

TABLE 121.3　Hand Skill Development: The First Year

0 mo	1 mo	2 mo	3 mo	4 mo	5 mo	6 mo	7 mo	8 mo	9 mo	10 mo	11 mo	12 mo
					Developmental scissors grasp • Small object pinch between adducted thumb and lateral, flexed index finger					Three-jaw chuck • Thumb and radial two digits pad to pad pinch		
				Palmar grasp • First with digits against palm • Evolves to include adducted thumb							Superior pincer • Thumb and index tip to tip pinch	
						Raking • Extends fingers, pulls object to palm	Voluntary release emerging		Inferior pincer • Small object pinch between thumb and lateral tip of extended index			
Reflexive squeeze			Ulnar palmar grasp • Grasp object placed on ulnar hand • No thumb involvement			Radial palmar grasp • Emerging thumb opposition			Radial digital grasp • Object held away from palm • First web space open	Pincer grasp • Thumb and index pad to pad pinch		

Adapted from Exner CE. Development of hand skills. In Case-Smith J, ed. *Occupational Therapy for Children.* 5th edition. Philadelphia: Elsevier; 2005:304-355 and Ho ES. Measuring hand function in the young child. *J Hand Ther.* 2010;23:323-328.

and shaped toys will improve consistency of testing.[67] Developmental motor assessments, such as the Peabody Developmental Motor Scales (PDMS-2), include fine-motor subscales that can be useful in assessing for fine-motor skill delays.[72] Ho[67] describes an approach using the developmental framework to assess hand function in children birth through 3 years. Her method includes observing grasp patterns and differences in the affected hand by using the unaffected hand as the baseline for comparison. She advocates developing a consistent set of toys to elicit each of the grasp types for more objective and reliable assessment over time.

Several standardized assessments have been tested for utility with the pediatric population for children aged 3 years and older. The Functional Dexterity Test (FDT) norms have been established for 3 to 17 years in addition to adult norms. The test consists of a peg board with 16 pegs and scores the speed in which the client can pick up (three-jaw chuck), turn each peg (in-hand rotation), and return to board (in-hand shift and release).[73] Performance is timed, and penalties are assessed for dropped pieces. The box and block test scores the number of 1-inch blocks a person can pick up, individually lift from box, and over a divider, and drop into the box on the contralateral side in 1 minute after a 15-second trial. Norms have been established for 3 years of age through adulthood.[70,74] This test relies on adequate proximal control to lift the blocks over the divider but can be useful for clients with more impaired hand function who cannot complete other available dexterity measures. The nine-hole peg test also has norms from 3 years of age through adulthood.[75] During these evaluations or through observation of manipulation during other tasks, compensatory patterns are noted. Children often want to "get it right" and after a few repeated examinations know what is being assessed. For example, clients who undergo index pollicization are trained to incorporate the new thumb in pinch–grasp patterns, and many continue to incorporate interdigital scissor pinch for certain tasks. On examination, they focus on using the thumb as trained. To get a true sense of how they are using the hand, caregiver interview or observation outside of testing tasks can be valuable.

Intervention

Games, arts and crafts, and identified ADL tasks can all be easily used to target dexterity deficits. Games can consist of making a race out of everyday items.[29] Orthoses, kinesiology taping, or buddy strapping can be helpful when trying to target a specific grasp pattern.

FUNCTIONAL ASSESSMENT

Impairments in the upper extremity impact function in self-care, school and work, and social participation. Many of the adult-based patient rated scales can be used with older adolescent clients but lack psychometric testing and applicability to younger children. Pediatric patient-reported outcome measures of global health and function that have items or subtests that assess upper extremity function include the Pediatric Outcomes Data Collection Instrument (PODCI) for ages 2 to 18 years with parent report for the younger group and parent and self-report in the older group of ages 11 to 18 years, the Pediatric Evaluation of Disability Inventory (PEDI) for ages 6 months to 7.5 years old, and the Activity Scale for Kids (ASK) for ages 5 to 15 years. The Canadian Occupational Performance Measure (COPM) can be used with children ages 6 years old and older with self or parent report. The individualized nature of the COPM makes it a valuable tool when other assessments have limited sensitivity to overall functional changes because of proficiency or adaptations with the unaffected limb in identifying meaningful deficit areas.[76]

Many children develop their own adaptations throughout childhood. This is especially true for children with congenital conditions

or who were very young when acquiring a condition. The extent of impairment needs to be considered in setting appropriate functional expectations, but motivated children often exceed these expectations. Limited participation may be caused by social considerations because it may be easier and timelier for the caregiver to provide assistance or caused by caregiver expectations that the activity is "too hard" for the child. In our practice, we often meet children who reportedly cannot don a shirt or fasten a button. When asked to try the activity, some are successful on the first attempt. Direct observation with reported deficits provides the ability to focus on the challenging components of the task.

SENSIBILITY

Assessment

Sensibility assessment in children differs widely from that with an adult population. A thorough review of adult sensibility assessment may be found in Chapter 10 on sensibility testing. What follows are pearls that may guide the clinician in successful and succinct evaluation of the child. Pediatric sensibility assessment can be quite challenging, requiring the clinician to pay careful attention to a variety of factors.[22] First, the child must be able to cooperate for the examination and have the cognitive ability to participate to achieve accurate results. Second, the examiner must be innovative, able to frame the various assessments under the guise of age-appropriate play. This minimizes fear and anxiety and promotes achievement of the evaluation goals. The examination should begin with a thorough history and then may include threshold, functional, objective and provocative tests. Finally, and most important, the clinician must use clinical observation of the appearance of the hand, incorporation of the affected limb into daily routine and play activities, preferred prehensile patterns, and the child's response to touch. When evaluating a child, always consider how questions are phrased. Avoid yes-or-no questions when possible because children often respond "yes" despite what they may feel. Instead, ask questions that facilitate a descriptive response such as, "What does it feel like?" Older children may also guess at an answer in an effort to score well on an examination. It is important to vary the test stimulus location as is appropriate for the specific test or "fake" an applied stimulus and then observe if a response is given.[77] Finally, consider the child's attention span and potential for mental fatigue. Carry out a succinct and focused examination and, when necessary, complete a portion of your assessment in a second session to assess reliability of findings.

Threshold tests assess the minimum perceivable stimulus and may include pain, temperature, touch-pressure, and vibration. With regard to children, there are several aspects that, when considered, will maximize the sensory evaluation results. First, superficial pain assessment of sharp–dull must be introduced in a positive and nonthreatening manner. It is important to avoid excessive repetitions over hypersensitive regions and save these areas for the end of the assessment to foster cooperation. Use of a "child-friendly" tool when able may ease the fear of the test and promote participation (Fig. 121.5). Similar to recommendations when measuring ROM, allowing the child to first safely explore the tool and even "test" the clinician or a stuffed animal may decrease fear and anxiety surrounding the examination. For light touch, the Semmes-Weinstein Monofilament test may be applied in older children. However, a more succinct exam such as the Weinstein Enhanced Sensory Test (WEST) is recommended for children as young as 6 years because it includes only five monofilaments, which may be rotated on one handle, each one representing a level of perceived light touch. The WEST has shown moderate to excellent test–retest reliability in normal pediatric participants[78,79] and was shown to be the most responsive sensory assessment used in a study of adults and children

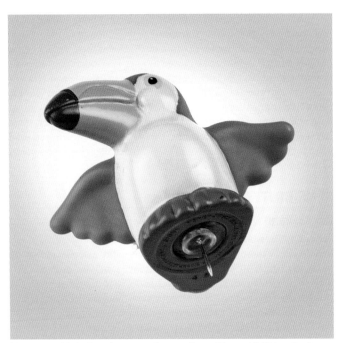

Fig. 121.5 Little People toucan figure adapted for a child-friendly sharp–dull threshold evaluation. (Courtesy of Shriners Hospital for Children, Philadelphia.)

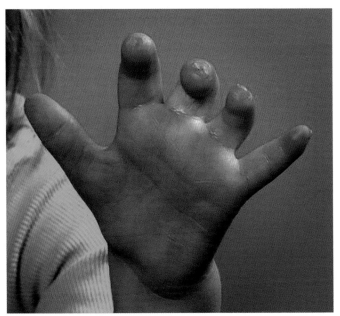

Fig. 121.6 Nail bed and digit injury secondary to self-mutilating behaviors in a 4-year-old girl with amniotic band disruption sequence. (Courtesy of Shriners Hospital for Children, Philadelphia.)

with peripheral nerve injury.[80] In a study exploring reliability of the International Standards for Neurological Classification of Spinal Cord Injury, Mulcahey and associates[81] found sensory examination (light touch and pin prick) reliable for children with spinal cord injury ages 5 years and older. Several studies have found good reliability with assessment of light touch in normal pediatric participants as young as 5 to 6 years old.[79,82,83] Select cases of 3- to 4-year-old children produced reliable results,[83] indicating that it is vital for the clinician to have a good understanding of her client's abilities and tolerance for such testing. It is important to remember that children with new injuries may have additional factors (i.e., fear, anxiety regarding injury) that may limit participation.

Functional tests evaluate the incorporation of sensibility into purposeful activity and address the impact of altered sensibility on disability. Static and moving two-point discrimination and the Moberg Pick up Test[84] are measures commonly applied with the pediatric population. Static two-point discrimination may be completed reliably in children as young as 6 to 7 years old.[82,83] The Moberg Pickup Test[84] can be used as a game wherein the child is asked to take a set of objects and place them from a table into a box. This test is repeated four times, once with each hand, without and with vision occluded. Valuable information may be gleaned from clinical observation of which fingers the child uses to acquire the objects as well as time to complete the task. The Dellon modification of the Moberg Pickup Test, which assesses stereognosis, involves asking the child to identify the objects with vision occluded.[85] For younger children, a picture of the objects may be used because object names may be difficult for the child to identify. One study of 25 children and adolescents with hemiplegic cerebral palsy found two-point discrimination, stereognosis of familiar objects, and functional assessment using the Pickup test were the most useful measures in children with cerebral palsy, with monofilament assessment and stereognosis of forms not as useful.[86]

An objective test that may be applied in children is the Wrinkle Test, developed by O'Riain.[87] In the clinic setting, the clinician may ask the caregiver if the child's hand wrinkles when in the tub or request

that they observe this at bath time. Alternatively, a brief "playtime" in a whirlpool or basin of water with age-appropriate water toys to complete the assessment will provide valuable information regarding presence and extent of wrinkling in hand. Tinel's sign is a provocative test that may also be applied to children, preferably at the end of the session because it may invoke feelings of discomfort.[88] The clinician should carefully monitor the child's nonverbal cues and, when needed, offer descriptive terminology to assist the child in describing the tingling sensation.[22]

Even in the presence of quantitative measures, clinical observations are truly the hallmark of pediatric sensory evaluation. Appearance of the hand, including sympathetic changes, caregiver report, observation of daily routine and play activities, and the child's response to touch, often tell more than any attempted formal assessment. The clinician can draw a vast amount of information regarding a nerve injury from sympathetic changes to the tissues because cutaneous sympathetic fibers travel a similar path as cutaneous sensory fibers.[89] A full description of sympathetic changes after peripheral nerve injury may be found in Chapter 10 on sensibility testing. Pay careful attention to sudomotor, vasomotor, pilomotor, and trophic changes in the affected upper extremity and document accordingly. Parents often come to the hand clinic expressing concern regarding vasomotor changes, stating, "My child's affected hand is always so cold and looks blue." It is our role as the clinician to educate families that this is common after nerve injury and is typically not cause for concern. Because lack of nerve supply impacts nutrition to all the tissues, the clinician may observe a smooth and shiny surface of the skin, finger pulp atrophy, tapered thickened nails, hair loss or finer hair, and on occasion increased hair growth. Self-mutilating behaviors such as excessive nail biting and at times inhibited nail growth may be seen in infants and very young children (Fig. 121.6). This may be caused by discomfort from nerve regeneration in cases such as obstetric brachial plexus palsy or as a result of lack of sensation. Comparison of the affected and unaffected extremity, when able, provides a clearer picture of sympathetic changes caused by an underlying nerve injury.

With regard to observation of play, children with impaired sensation may limit incorporation of the affected extremity into play activities, at times appearing to almost neglect the arm. Presentation of bimanual activities, such as hook and loop–backed play food, interlocking building toys, and craft activities such as playdough or tearing tissue paper, may facilitate the incorporation of bilateral hands for evaluation. The clinician can also attempt to elicit a response by tactile stimulation of the arm (i.e., behind the child's back or under a table). Throughout all clinical observations, be cognizant of the child's nonverbal cues. Often, the child will not verbalize discomfort or negative response to stimuli; however, the child's body language (i.e., fidgeting in chair, foot twitching, facial expressions) shows he is clearly uncomfortable (Video 121.1).

Intervention

Interventions to address sensory deficits in the pediatric population are best received when presented under the auspices of play.[66] A desensitization program may involve use of a child's favorite soft stuffed animal followed by an inside out-sock puppet, with progression over time to more noxious stimuli. Immersion interventions may include finding toy objects in colorful rice or pasta buckets and then use of the immersion materials to make a craft activity. Careful monitoring of body language during treatment interventions will guide the clinician in progression of the program. Incorporation of the child's preferences will offer the child a sense of control and promote participation. Protection of the limb is also of extreme importance in the case of nerve injury and resulting sensory impairment. This may involve orthosis fabrication to maintain proper positioning or to provide protection from self-mutilating behaviors.

ORTHOSIS CONSIDERATIONS

Orthosis fabrication with the pediatric client involves creativity and involvement of the child in the process whenever possible. Choice of orthosis and strap color may motivate the child toward increased wearing compliance. Application of decorations such as stickers, designs, jewels, or a drawing may also facilitate wear. When fabricating an orthosis, start by providing the child a piece of warm thermoplastic material to play with; this decreases the fear of the material and frames it in the light of a craft activity. Thermoplastic scraps can be reheated and offered to the patient throughout the fabrication process to provide distraction and maintain participation. When appropriate, allow the child to fabricate an orthosis for a doll or stuffed animal. This allows the child a sense of control and responsibility in the process.

Infants and young children may benefit from use of thinner or perforated materials. A variety of padding options are also available to line orthoses for infants or children with sensitive skin. Neoprene is another option, whether it is a custom neoprene thumb support or forearm rotation strap or a commercially available custom or prefabricated neoprene orthosis. Thicker, more rigid materials are recommended for protective orthoses fabricated after injury or surgery. These orthoses must be sturdy enough to endure a busy child's activity level; incorporation of a clamshell design provides additional protection. Caregivers must be educated to assure rivets and screws remain tight with a Statue of Liberty or Gunslinger orthosis. Even bulky orthoses such as these do not inhibit the typical child's active nature.

Often, children are adept at removing orthoses and various adaptations are required to facilitate increased compliance. A range of strapping alternatives may be used to increase the difficulty of independent removal. Bra hooks sewn on straps, D-ring straps applied with closure out of the child's reach, or use of a shoe string tied through holes punched in the orthosis are all viable options. The clinician may also apply adherent wrap over the orthosis, fabricate a clamshell, rivet one end of the strap to the orthosis, or recommend donning the orthosis underneath long-sleeved shirts or pajamas. For infants and toddlers, a single long "Y" strap may be used to prevent the infant from accidentally swallowing a shorter strap (Fig. 121.7).

There are many types of orthoses used in the pediatric population. Custom fabrication is often required because of the unique size and shape of each child's hand, particularly in the case of congenital differences. For an individual with a monodactylous hand, an orthosis may be fabricated to provide a post for the child to facilitate object acquisition. After a pollicization, a long opponens orthosis will provide protection during gross motor play. Children with weak finger and wrist extension may benefit from a custom pediatric dynamic finger extension orthosis that uses neoprene finger sleeves secured on a static wrist support (Benik Corporation, Silverdale, WA). This orthosis allows the child to grasp objects using active finger flexion yet promotes an open hand for the resting position, thereby facilitating acquisition of larger items. For infants or toddlers with weak wrist extensors caused by peripheral nerve injury or spasticity, a dorsal wrist orthosis allows sensory input to the palm while placing the wrist and hand in an ideal position for weight bearing or crawling activities. For older children, a wrist cockup orthosis may simulate a neutral or extended wrist position. If the child is able to carry out daily functional activities with increased ease or independence, a tendon transfer for wrist extension or a wrist fusion may be considered. After external fixator application or pin fixation for a finger fracture, a protective cover may be fabricated using thermoplastic material or neoprene to protect the child from bumping into other objects or individuals, as well as to aid in cosmesis (Fig. 121.8). For children with elbow flexion contractures, static elbow extension orthoses may be custom made using thermoplastic material or are commercially available in a neoprene version with a thermoplastic insert (Benik Corporation). For a more intense elbow extension stretch, a custom belly gutter orthosis (Fig. 121.9) may be fabricated, but it is typically recommended initially for short periods of time during the day followed by use of a static extension orthosis for night wear. Older adolescents may be fitted for a commercially available static progressive orthosis to be used in coordination with a static night orthosis to best serve the client's needs. In our practice, dynamic elbow orthoses are generally avoided for posttraumatic stiff elbows because they often encourage co-contraction of opposing muscles, ultimately limiting the client's progress. A clear wearing schedule is essential and must consider the child's daily school and sports activities as well as the caregiver's work schedule and availability to oversee the wearing regimen. A wearing schedule chart (if necessary with a rewards system included) to be displayed in a central location at home may facilitate compliance and serve as a motivator for the child. Elbow extension orthoses may also be used to facilitate increased overhead reach in children with elbow extension weakness. Application of the orthosis before targeted overhead reach activities such as easel activities, window or mirror painting, or magnetic games on the refrigerator will encourage use of the affected arm in a greater range than is feasible with the elbow free. For children who lack active and passive elbow flexion (e.g., caused by trauma or the diagnosis of AMC), a static progressive elbow flexion orthosis may be recommended. The hourglass orthosis is an excellent option for this population and may be fabricated out of 1/16-inch thermoplastic material for a smaller upper extremity (Fig. 121.10). Straps may be riveted to the orthosis to aid the caregiver in application and ensure a proper line of pull to maximize end-range passive elbow flexion. Use of a commercially available guitar tuner may also be incorporated into the design of a static progressive elbow flexion orthosis, as well as an anterior/posterior approach.[90]

ADAPTATIONS

There are also a variety of adaptations that may be fabricated to maximize a child's independence and participation in the roles of childhood. The options are limited only by the clinician's imagination and the needs of the child, but a few suggestions follow.

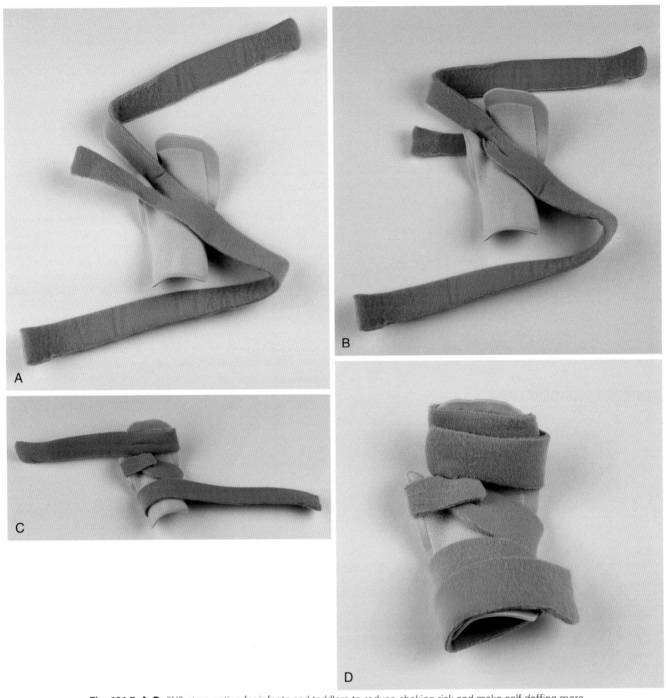

Fig. 121.7 A–D, "Y" strap option for infants and toddlers to reduce choking risk and make self-doffing more difficult. (Courtesy of Shriners Hospital for Children, Philadelphia.)

For ADLs, an array of assistive devices are commercially available. Unfortunately, many of these devices do not meet the unique needs of the pediatric population directly off the shelf. Children may be missing digits such as in radial or ulnar deficiency or have limited finger flexion ROM or strength (i.e., with AMC) for grasping the tool. Many also have shoulder or elbow contractures that limit the ability to position the tool properly for success. Simple assistive device modifications (i.e., fabrication of a universal cuff on a dressing stick, long-handled sponge, or long-handled brush) using thermoplastic or other materials may allow the child success in dressing, bathing, or grooming activities. Wall-mounted hooks, auto pump soap and shampoo dispensers, or use of wall-mounted bike rack hooks to hold a shirt for donning are all examples of using over-the-counter items to help a child in gaining independence in essential daily routine activities. Universal suction mounts are also extremely helpful in holding a variety of feeding and grooming equipment to facilitate independence (Fig. 121.11).

Sports modifications are often requested by families as children are exploring participation in team sports such as baseball or hockey as well as skills such as riding a bike. A bike handlebar modification is often

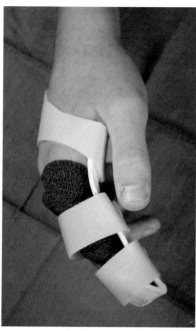

Fig. 121.8 Protective orthosis for a 15-year-old competitive swimmer, incorporating adhesive bandage and thermoplastic orthosis to protect proximal interphalangeal and distal interphalangeal Kirschner wires. (Courtesy of Shriners Hospital for Children, Philadelphia.)

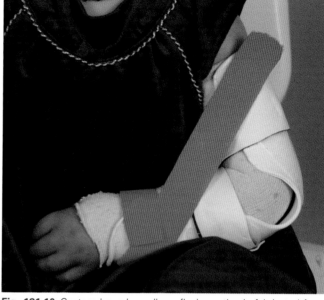

Fig. 121.10 Custom hourglass elbow flexion orthosis fabricated for a 22-month-old girl with arthrogryposis multiplex congenita after posterior elbow release and triceps lengthening. (Courtesy of Shriners Hospital for Children, Philadelphia.)

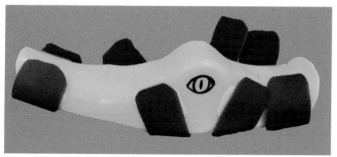

Fig. 121.9 Custom belly gutter orthosis decorated as an alligator to optimize wearing compliance. (Courtesy of Shriners Hospital for Children, Philadelphia.)

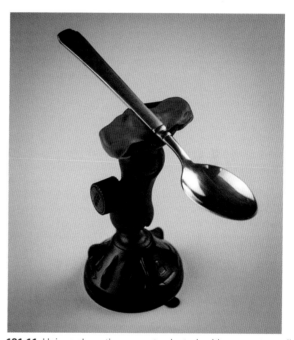

Fig. 121.11 Universal suction mount adapted with magnet to allow 7-year-old boy with arthrogryposis multiplex congenita and limited upper extremity function to self-feed. First, food is acquired by placing handle of spoon in mouth and scooping food. Spoon is then placed on magnetic portion of mount. Next, the child maneuvers the spoon with his chin or mouth as needed to place food into his mouth. (Courtesy of Shriners Hospital for Children, Philadelphia.)

requested for children with limb differences. A thermoplastic mold is fabricated in the shape of the distal residual limb and then mounted to the handlebar. The modification allows the child the ability to assist in steering with the affected limb while allowing a quick removal when required (Fig. 121.12). Custom baseball or hockey gloves may be recommended for children with symbrachydactyly. The therapist may fabricate a thermoplastic mold of the hand. The mold will then have metal or thermoplastic stays attached to it and be inserted into the glove for increased rigidity and stability.

Instrument modifications allow children with upper extremity involvement the opportunity to join their peers in exploring a variety of musical instruments in the elementary and middle school years. A custom strap or thermoplastic mold mounted on a violin bow can allow proper grip. A custom glove is another option to assist in grasping a string bow (Video 121.2). Modifications to a trombone handle may allow a child with ulnar deficiency to grasp the slide using the elbow joint in the absence of fingers. These are just a few of the endless possibilities for adaptation of musical instruments. Careful consideration of the child's upper extremity ROM, strength, movement patterns, and

interests will guide the clinician in the creation of appropriate adaptations to meet each child's unique needs. In summary, childhood is a time of exploration, and it is the role and responsibility as well as the distinct honor of the pediatric therapist to be a part of fostering the child's success.

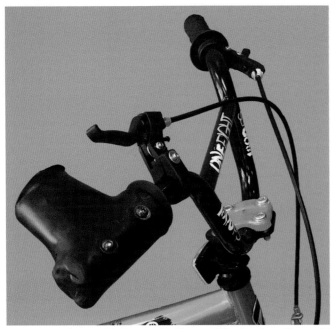

Fig. 121.12 Custom thermoplastic bike modification for a 7-year-old boy with a congenital below-elbow transverse deficiency. (Courtesy of Shriners Hospital for Children, Philadelphia.)

REFERENCES

1. Cunningham H. Chapter 3 The development of a middle-class ideology of childhood, 1500-1900. In: *Children and Childhood in Western Society Since 1500 [e-book]*. 2nd edition. Hoboken: Routledge; 2014:41. Available from: eBook Collection (EBSCOhost), Ipswich, MA.
2. Erikson E, Erikson J. *The Lifecycle Completed: Extended Version*. New York: W W Norton & Company; 1997:1–132.
3. American Occupational Therapy Association. Occupational therapy practice framework: Domain & process. 3rd edition. *Am J Occup Ther*. 2014;68:S1–S48.
4. World Health Organization. *International Classification of Functioning, Disability, and Health*. Geneva: ICF; 2001.
5. Prince D, Herzenberg E, Standard J, Paley S. Lengthening with external fixation is effective in congenital femoral deficiency. *Clin Orthop and Relat Res*. 2015;473:3261–3271.
6. Malone CA, Sauer NJ, Fenton TW, et al. A radiographic assessment of pediatric fracture healing and time since injury. *J Forensic Sci*. 2011;56:1123–1130.
7. Roth KC, Denk K, Colaris JW, et al. Think twice before re-manipulating distal metaphyseal forearm fractures in children. *Arch Orth Trauma Surg*. 2014;134:1699–1707.
8. Kozin S, Abzug J, Safier S, et al. Complications of pediatric elbow dislocations and Monteggia fracture-dislocations. *Instr Course Lect*. 2015;64:493.
9. Ladenhauf HN, Schaffert M, Bauer J. The displaced supracondylar humerus fracture: Indications for surgery and surgical options: A 2014 update. *Curr Opin Pediatr*. 2014;26:64–69.
10. Anand P, Birch R. Restoration of sensory function and lack of longterm chronic pain syndromes after brachial plexus injury in human neonates. *Brain*. 2002;125:113–122.
11. Krisa L, Murray M. The implications of injury in the developing nervous system on upper extremity function. *J Hand Ther*. 2015;28:101–105.
12. Fornander L, Nyman T, Hansson T, et al. Age- and time-dependent effects on functional outcome and cortical activation pattern in patients with median nerve injury: A functional magnetic resonance imaging study. *J Neurosurg*. 2010;113:122–128.
13. Yao J, Chen A, Kuiken T, et al. Sensory cortical re-mapping following upper-limb amputation and subsequent targeted reinnervation: A case report. *Neuroimage Clin*. 2015;8:329–336.
14. Nasir S, Darainy M, Ostry D. Sensorimotor adaptation changes the neural coding of somatosensory stimuli. *J Neurophysiol*. 2013;109:2077–2085.
15. Vahdat S, Darainy M, Milner T, et al. Functionally specific changes in resting-state sensorimotor networks after motor learning. *J Neurosci*. 2011;31:16907–16915.
16. Ostry D, Darainy M, Mattar A, et al. Somatosensory plasticity and motor learning. *J Neurosci*. 2010;30:5384–5393.
17. Izawa J, Shadmehr R, Körding K. Learning from sensory and reward prediction errors during motor adaptation (Learning from sensory and reward prediction errors). *PLoS Computational Biology [serial online]*. 2011;7:E1002012. Available at: http://journals.plos.org.
18. Mcgregor H, Cashaback J, Gribble P. Functional plasticity in somatosensory cortex supports motor learning by observing. *Curr Biol*. 2016;26:921–927.
19. Carsi M, Belen C, Anna M, et al. Transient neonatal radial nerve palsy. A case series and review of the literature. *J Hand Ther*. 2015;28:212–216.
20. Chemnitz A, Björkman A, Dahlin LB, et al. Functional outcome thirty years after median and ulnar nerve repair in childhood and adolescence. *J Bone Joint Surg Am*. 2013;95:329–337.
21. Birch R. *Peripheral Nerve Injuries a Clinical Guide*. London: Springer; 2013.
22. Ho ES. Evaluation of pediatric upper extremity peripheral nerve injuries. *J Hand Ther*. 2015;28:135–143.
23. Zhao L, Lv G, Jiang S, et al. Morphological differences in skeletal muscle atrophy of rats with motor nerve and/or sensory nerve injury. *Neural Reg Res*. 2012;7:2507–2515.
24. Gilbert A, Pivato G, Kheiralla T. Long-term results of primary repair of brachial plexus lesions in children. *Microsurg*. 2006;26:334–342.
25. Ruijs A, Jaquet J, Kalmijn S, et al. Median and ulnar nerve injuries: A meta-analysis of predictors of motor and sensory recovery after modern microsurgical nerve repair. *Plast Reconstr Surg*. 2005;116:484–494.
26. Abery BH. Family adjustment and adaptation with children with Down syndrome. *Focus Except Child*. 2006;38:2–20.
27. Bingham A, Correa V, Huber J. Mothers' voices: Coping with their children's initial disability diagnosis. *Infant Ment Health J*. 2012;33:372–385.
28. Jenni O, Chaouch A, Caflisch J, et al. Infant motor milestones: Poor predictive value for outcome of healthy children. *Acta Paediatr*. 2013;102:E181–E184.
29. Peck-Murray JA. Utilizing everyday items in play to facilitate hand therapy for pediatric patients. *J Hand Ther*. 2015;28:228–232.
30. Trombly Latham C. Conceptual foundations for practice. In: Radomski MV, Trombly Latham C, eds. *Occupational Therapy for Physical Dysfunction*. 6th Edition. Philadelphia: Wolters Kluwer Health, Lippincott Williams & Wilkins; 2008:1–20.
31. Bae D, Kadiyala R, Waters P. Acute compartment syndrome in children: Contemporary diagnosis, treatment, and outcome. *J Pediatr Orthop*. 2001;21:680–688.
32. Kanj WW, Gunderson MA, Carrigan RB, et al. Acute compartment syndrome of the upper extremity in children: Diagnosis, management, and outcomes. *J Child Orthop*. 2013;7:225–233.
33. Noonan KJ, McCarthy J. Compartment syndromes in the pediatric patient. *J Pediatr Orthop*. 2010;30:S96–S101.
34. Abe M, Schambra H, Wassermann E, et al. Reward improves long-term retention of a motor memory through induction of offline memory gains. *Curr Biol*. 2011;21:557–562.
35. Sinnott K, Biddle S. Changes in attributions, perceptions of success and intrinsic motivation after attribution retraining in children's sport. *Int J of Adolesc Youth*. 1998;7(2):137–144.
36. Chase MA. Children's self-efficacy, motivational intentions, and attributions in physical education and sport. *Res Q Exerc Sport*. 2001;72:47–54.
37. Wood D, Bruner J, Ross G. The role of tutoring in problem solving. *J Child Psychol Psychiatry*. 1976;17:89–100.
38. Maybin J, Mercer N, Stierer B. "Scaffolding" learning in the classroom. In: Norman K, ed. *Thinking Voices: the Work of the National Oracy Project*. London: Hodder and Stoughton; 1992:186–195.
39. Sutherland K, Wehby J, Copeland S. Effect of varying rates of behavior-specific praise on the on-task behavior of students with EBD. *J Emot Behav Disord*. 2000;8:2–8.

40. Burtner P, Leinwand R, Sullivan K, et al. Motor learning in children with hemiplegic cerebral palsy: Feedback effects on skill acquisition. *Dev Med Child Neurol.* 2014;56:259–266.

41. Levac D, Wishart L, Missiuna C, et al. The application of motor learning strategies within functionally based interventions for children with neuromotor conditions. *Pediatr Phys Ther.* 2009;21:345–355.

42. Apriyadi A, Efendi M, Sulthoni. The Effectiveness of backward chaining methods to improve skills in children with intellectual disability. *Jurnal Penelitian Dan Pengembangan Pendidikan Luar Biasa.* 2017;4:37–44.

43. Savage A, McConnell D, Emerson E, et al. Disability-based inequity in youth subjective well-being: Current findings and future directions. *Disabil Soci.* 2014;29:877–892.

44. Schetter D, Kazak C, Anne E, et al. Moving research on health and close relationships forward—A challenge and an obligation: Introduction to the special issue. *Am Psychol.* 2017;72:511–516.

45. Garth B, Aroni R. 'I Value What You have to Say'. Seeking the perspective of children with a disability, not just their parents. *Disabil Soci.* 2003;18:561–576.

46. Ellis J. Grieving for the loss of the perfect child: Parents of children with handicaps. *Child Adolesc Social Work.* 1989;6:259–270.

47. Willgens A, Hummel K. Uncovering a curricular model of self-care in pediatric physical therapist education. *J Phys Ther Edu.* 2016;30:55–70.

48. Houchins DE, Oakes WP, Johnson ZG. Bullying and students with disabilities: A systematic literature review of intervention studies. *Remedial Spec Educ.* 2016;37:259–273.

49. Asbjørnslett M, Helseth S, Engelsrud G. 'Being an ordinary kid' – demands of everyday life when labelled with disability. *Scand J Dis Res.* 2014;16:364–376.

50. Bjorbækmo W, Schrøder B, Engelsrud GE. My own way of moving" - movement improvisation in children's rehabilitation. *Phenomenol Pract.* 2011;5:27–47.

51. Graber R, Turner R, Madill A. Best friends and better coping: Facilitating psychological resilience through boys' and girls' closest friendships. *Br J Psychol.* 2016;107:338–358.

52. Martins I. This is my best friend Anna: Asking peers of children with cerebral palsy. *Dev Med Child Neurol.* 2015;57:18.

53. Shildrick M. *Dangerous Discourses of Disability, Subjectivity and Sexuality.* New York: Palgrave Macmillan; 2009.

54. Mortier K, Desimpel L, De Schauwer E, et al. 'I want support, not comments': Children's perspectives on supports in their lives. *Disabil Soci.* 2011;26:207–221.

55. Haack R. *Different is Awesome.* Washington DC: Mascot Books; 2015.

56. Hoffman J. *Emmy's Hand.* Morgantown: Masthof Press; 2016.

57. Mejía-Arauz R, Correa-Chávez M, Keyser Ohrt U, et al. Collaborative work or individual chores: The role of family social organization in children's learning to collaborate and develop initiative. *Adv Child Dev Behav.* 2015;49:25–51.

58. Nelson F, Masulani-Mwale C, Richards E, et al. The meaning of participation for children in Malawi: Insights from children and caregivers. *Child Care Health Dev.* 2017;43:133–143.

59. Trigwell J, Murphy RC, Cable NT, et al. Parental views of children's physical activity: A qualitative study with parents from multi-ethnic backgrounds living in England. *BMC Public Health [serial online].* 2015;15:1–11. Available at: http://eprints.leedsbeckett.ac.uk.

60. Chen E, Brody G, Miller G, et al. Childhood close family relationships and health. *Am Psychol.* 2017;72:555–566.

61. Lee P, Zehgeer A, Ginsburg G, et al. Child and adolescent adherence with cognitive behavioral therapy for anxiety: predictors and associations with outcomes. *J Clin Child Adolesc Psychol.* 2017;53:1–12.

62. Hieneman M. Positive behavior support for individuals with behavior challenges. *Behav Anal Pract.* 2015;8:101–108.

63. Kennedy D, Wainwright A, Pereira L, et al. A qualitative study of patient education needs for hip and knee replacement. *BMC Musculoskeletal Disorders [serial online].* 2017;18:1–7. Available at: https://bmcmusculoskeletdisord.biomedcentr.

64. Murphy KM, Rasmussen L, Hervey-Jumper SL, et al. An assessment of the compliance and utility of a home exercise DVD for caregivers of children and adolescents with brachial plexus palsy: A pilot study. *PM&R.* 2012;4:190–197.

65. Riley B, Lane S. Feasibility of engaging caregivers during pediatric occupational therapy services: A mixed-methods study. *Am J of Occup Ther.* 2016;70:S1.

66. Aaron DH. Pediatric hand therapy. In: Henderson A, Pehoski C, eds. *Hand Function in the Child: Foundations for Remediation.* 2nd edition. St Louis: Mosby Elsevier; 2006:367–400.

67. Ho ES. Measuring hand function in the young child. *J Hand Ther.* 2010;23:323–328.

68. Zlotolow DA, Kozin SH. Posterior elbow release and humeral osteotomy for patients with arthrogryposis. *J Hand Surg AM.* 2012;37:1078–1082.

69. Mennen U, van Heest A, Ezaki MB, et al. Arthrogryposis multiplex congenital. *J Hand Surg Br.* 2005;30:468–474.

70. Mathiowetz V, Federman S, Wiemer D. Box and blocks test of manual dexterity: norms for 6-19 year olds. *Can J Occup Ther.* 1985;52:241–245.

71. Ashworth S, Estilow T, Humpl D. Occupational therapy evaluation and treatment. In: Abzug JM, Kozin SH, Zlotolow DA, eds. *The Pediatric Upper Extremity.* New York: Springer; 2015:171–195.

72. Exner CE. Development of hand skills. In: Case-Smith J, ed. *Occupational Therapy for Children.* 5th edition. Philadelphia: Elsevier; 2005:304–355.

73. Gorgola GR, Velleman PF, Shuai X, Morse AM, et al. Hand dexterity in children: administration and normative values of the Functional Dexterity Test. *J Hand Ther.* 2013;38:2426–2431.

74. Jongbloed-Pereboom M, Nijhuis-van der Sanden MWG, Steenbergen B. Norm scores of the box and block test for children ages 3-10 years. *Am J Occup Ther.* 2013;67:312–318.

75. Wang Y, Bohannon RW, Kapellusch J, et al. Dexterity as measured with the 9-hole peg test (9-HPT) across the age span. *J Hand Ther.* 2015;28:53–60.

76. Mulcahey MJ, Kozin SH. Outcome measures. In: Abzug JM, Kozin SH, Zlotolow DA, eds. *The Pediatric Upper Extremity.* New York: Springer; 2015:57–68.

77. Greenspan JD, La Motte RH. Cutaneous mechanoreceptors of the hand: experimental studies and their implications for clinical testing of tactile sensation. *J Hand Ther.* 1993;6:75.

78. Weinstein S. Fifty years of somatosensory research: From the Semmes-Weinstein monofilaments to the Weinstein enhanced sensory test. *J Hand Ther.* 1993;6(1):11–22.

79. Thibault A, Forget R, Lambert J. Evaluation of cutaneous and proprioceptive sensation in children: a reliability study. *Dev Med Child Neurol.* 1994;36(9):796–812.

80. Rosen B, Dahlin LB, Lundborg G. Assessment of functional outcome after nerve repair in a longitudinal cohort. *Scand J Plast Reconstr Surg Hand Surg.* 2000;34(1):71–78.

81. Mulcahey MJ, Gaughan J, Betz RR, et al. The International Standards for Neurological Classification of Spinal Cord Injury: reliability of data when applied to children and youths. *Spinal Cord.* 2006;45:452–459.

82. Cope EB, Antony JH. Normal values for the two-point discrimination test. *Pediatr Neurol.* 1992;8:4.

83. Dua K, Lancaster TP, Abzug JM. Age-dependent reliability of Semmes-Weinstein and 2-point discrimination tests in children. *J Ped Ortho.* 2016;21. https://doi.org/10.1097/BPO.0000000000000892.

84. Moberg E. Objective methods for determining the functional value of sensibility in the hand. *J Bone Joint Surg Br.* 1958;40-B:454–476.

85. Dellon AL. *Evaluation of Sensibility and Reeducation of Sensation in the Hand.* Baltimore: Williams & Wilkins; 1981.

86. Krumlinde-Sundholm L, Eliasson AC. Comparing tests of tactile sensibility: aspects relevant to testing children with spastic hemiplegia. *Dev Med Child Neurol.* 2002;44(9):604–612.

87. O'Riain S. New and simple test of nerve function in hand. *Br Med J.* 1973;3:615–616.

88. Davis EN, Chung KC. The Tinel sign: A historical perspective. *Plast Reconstr Surg.* 2002;114(2):494–499.

89. Sunderland S. *Nerves and Nerve Injuries.* 2nd edition. New York: Churchill Livingstone; 1978.

90. Shultz-Johnson K. Static progressive splinting. *J Hand Ther.* 2002;15:163–178.

122

Management of Congenital Hand Anomalies

Kathleen Kollitz Jegapragasan, Wendy Tomhave, Steven L. Moran

OUTLINE

CRITICAL POINTS

The Congenital Hand Anomaly Team
- A pediatrician team leader
- Specialists on normal and abnormal child development
- Geneticists
- Social worker and social services personnel
- Occupational and physical therapists
- An orthotics and prosthetics group
- A congenital hand surgeon

Radial Club Hand
- At least 40% of children with radial club hand have some associated medical problem.
- Early stretching and orthotic intervention can aid in decreasing the severity of contracture and ease future surgical procedures.

- A radial gutter orthosis is recommended for daytime use.
- Centralization can be performed at 6 to 12 months.
- Thumb procedures are often performed at 2 to 5 years.
- Distraction of the forearm can be considered for some cases at 8 to 12 years.

Hypoplastic Thumb
- Thumb hypoplasia is often associated with radial hypoplasia.
- Stability of the thumb carpometacarpal (CMC) joint helps determine whether the thumb is salvageable.
- Pollicization is recommended for most thumbs with an unstable CMC joint

INTRODUCTION

The surgical treatment and rehabilitation of children with congenital hand deformities has substantially changed over the past 40 years. Advancements in free tissue transfer, bony reconstruction, and rehabilitation have allowed for the restoration of prehensile grasp and improved cosmesis in many children, but many defects still pose significant challenges for hand surgeons and therapists. Fortunately, children have a tremendous ability to adapt and many will thrive despite significant physical impediments. Occupational therapy, in many cases, is all that is required for affected children to perform the activities of daily living (ADLs), which will, in turn, provide them with independence in their daily activities. This chapter provides general guidelines to help with the surgeons' and therapists' interactions with patients and families. The chapter also provides an overview of the most common congenital abnormalities surgeons and therapists encounter.

INCIDENCE AND INITIAL INTERACTION WITH THE PATIENT

Assembling a Team

Congenital upper extremity anomalies occur in 0.2% of live births, but only 10% of diagnosed congenital hand anomalies are serious enough to warrant surgical intervention.[1] Children with congenital hand differences may have associated anomalies that often take precedence over the treatment of upper limb problems. The management of the hand must often be coordinated among the evaluations of many other specialists. It is often most convenient for patients and their families if the pediatric specialists are grouped close together within a specialized clinic or within the same medical facility. For this reason, the treatment of most congenital hand anomalies should be performed by hand surgeons and therapists at pediatric surgical centers.. The health care team involved with the care of the child should include:

1. A pediatrician team leader
2. Normal and abnormal child development specialist
3. Geneticists
4. Social worker and social services
5. Occupational and physical therapists
6. An orthotics and prosthetics group
7. A congenital hand surgeon

Therapy and care of these children is a team effort because no one health care provider can hope to grasp the full spectrum of the patient's problem within a single office visit. Occupational therapists, often through repeated therapy sessions, gain the best assessment of the child's ongoing hand function, needs for improved hand function, and means of adaptation. This information is often best brought to the surgeon's attention through team meetings or patient care conferences before the initiation of any surgical intervention. The goal for children with congenital hand and upper limb anomalies is to optimize the ability of the child to orient the hand in space, to provide sensate skin coverage to working digits, and to provide grasping power and precision pinch.[2]

Initial Physical Examination

Evaluation of an infant or child with a congenital anomaly can be difficult because compliance with the physical examination is often limited. We have found it much easier to provide the child with age-appropriate toys that allow the physician to examine the child's functional capabilities. Careful examination also allows the care provider to observe for compensatory patterns of activity with the affected and unaffected extremity. Laying hands on the child is necessary to evaluate joint laxity or stiffness, joint contractures, and skin deficiencies, which will determine the surgical intervention and orthotic regimen; however, this is often best reserved until late in the interview process when the child has gained some familiarity with the physician. Complete musculoskeletal examination should attempt to evaluate the entire affected and normal limb from thorax to fingers. The physician and therapist should focus on the following[3]:

1. Active range of motion (AROM)
2. Passive range of motion (PROM)
3. Manual muscle testing of the upper extremity
4. Observation of prehensile patterns
5. Sensory testing
   a. Stereognosis
   b. Two-point discrimination in older children
   c. Consideration of wrinkle test or ninhydrin test for younger children in whom a peripheral nerve injury is suspected

Often in cases of musculoskeletal impairment (hemiplegia, arthrogryposis, and cerebral palsy, which are discussed in detail elsewhere) a functional, or dynamic electromyography may be considered to better assess muscle groups and the child's volitional control of these muscle groups. Bilateral radiographs are obtained for almost all children to assess the affected and normal side and to evaluate the severity of disease and to rule out any anomalies in the "normal" side. Magnetic resonance imaging (MRI) is usually reserved for soft tissue mass, ligamentous injuries, or examination of the presence or absence of muscles and soft tissue structures. Its use is very limited because of the necessity of sedating the child for these procedures.

The overall assessment should also include an evaluation of other common musculoskeletal abnormalities, such as hip dysplasia and scoliosis. Abnormalities in facial development, lower limb development, hair growth, tooth development, and skin pigmentation should all be noted because these may be signs of a genetic syndrome or other generalized skeletal dysplasia. Evaluation of developmental progress should also be noted to assure the surgeon and therapist that the child is keeping pace with general developmental milestones.

For straightforward problems, an initial consultation may be all that is necessary before establishing a treatment plan; more commonly, however, additional visits will be required for the surgeon and therapist to fully evaluate the patient's limitations and need for any surgical intervention. Parents will also benefit from hearing the surgical and therapy plan several times in order for them to absorb the information and construct their own questions. Each visit should include an explanation of the defect, its expected effect on development, plans for intervention, timing, and alternatives to treatment. Finally parents will wish to know if this defect can be passed to other children. Often these questions should be referred to a pediatric geneticist for a full genetic analysis.[4,5]

Social Acceptance

A child with a developmental anomaly can create considerable stress for the parents and caregivers. Parents can often feel guilty and confused with regards to the exact cause of their child's deformity; they may often fear that a parental misdeed during pregnancy has caused their child's condition.[6] In addition, significant anxiety exists regarding future peer pressure and bullying that the child might experience upon entering elementary school.[7] Often, the most important thing that parents can be told is that the child's anomaly is not their fault. Helping parents work through their guilt allows them to begin to accept their child's difference and to develop an optimistic outlook regarding the child's future.

From our experience, some of the best means of helping parents and children cope with these complex issues is through the use of support groups and peer groups established independently or through specific institutions. Information about many of these groups can be obtained through the internet. Excellent resources for parents and physicians include:

- American Society for Surgery of the Hand (http://www.assh.org) under the title of "Congenital Hand Differences."
- Helping Hands Foundation (http://www.helpinghandsgroup.org): This is a nonprofit support group made up of parents who have children with upper limb differences and who are concerned with the challenges facing the child and the entire family.
- Association of Children's Prosthetic Orthotic Clinics (http://www.acpoc.org): This is an association of professionals who are involved in clinics that provide prosthetics and orthotic care for children with limb loss or orthopedic disabilities.
- Superhands (http://www.superhands.us): Superhands is a forum for anyone to learn about children who have hand or upper limb differences.

Finally, the physician should be careful with the terminology used in describing the child's congenital hand difference. It is best to use terms such as "congenital hand difference" rather than offensive terminology such as "lobster claw hand" or "club hand." Children with congenital hand anomalies may have an obvious and visible difference in arm and hand appearance. Children who are most socially adjusted are those who can explain why their hands are the way they are; the surgeon and therapist can help children formulate their responses.

UPPER LIMB CONGENITAL ANOMALIES

Development

Four weeks after fertilization, the upper limb bud develops on the lateral wall of the developing embryo. The limb develops from the migration of ectodermal and mesodermal tissue. The migration of these tissues is orchestrated through a specialized component of the ectoderm called the *apical ectodermal ridge* (AER). The AER is found in the leading edge of the limb bud and coordinates the differentiation of the underlying mesoderm (Fig. 122.1).[8–10] The limb develops in a proximal to distal direction. Injury or removal of the AER will result in a truncated limb.[11,12]

The anterior posterior axis (radioulnar relationship) of the hand is regulated by proteins that are produced in the posterior portion of the limb bud. The specialized tissue that produces these proteins has been named the *zone of polarizing activity*.[13] The specific protein signals produced in this portion of the limb bud are controlled by groups of genes, which are referred to as the *sonic hedgehog genes*. Ventral and dorsal differentiation is thought to be under the influence of bone morphogenic proteins as well as the Wnt (wingless type) signaling pathway. Wnt protein expression has been identified in the dorsal ectoderm. Expression of the Wnt protein results in a transformation in the mesoderm, causing it to form dorsal bony structures.[13–15]

Gross development is completed by the eighth gestational week, with all limb structures being present. Thus, it is during the brief time span of the fourth to eighth week of development that the majority of congenital defects are initiated. Injuries to the AER during this period will have permanent effects on all development distal to the zone if injury. Historically, congenital deformities were thought to result solely from external teratogens such as irradiation; certain infections; excessive hormone ingestion; and medications such as thalidomide, phenytoin, and warfarin; however, recent research has shown that many genetic defects are inherited or develop thorough genetic mutations or growth factor receptor abnormalities.[7,9,16] Developmental deformities that are initiated after the eighth week of development are usually the result of external trauma to the limb bud from amniotic bands, uterine wall pressure, or vascular insults.

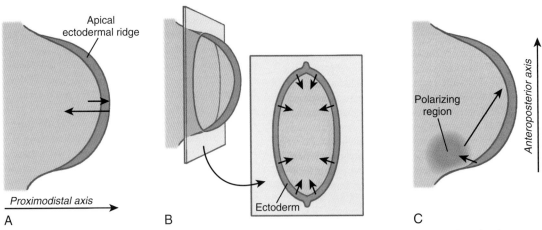

Fig. 122.1 The three interactive patterning mechanisms involved in upper limb developmental embryology. *Arrows* indicate signaling between the various tissues. **A,** Proximodistal development is determined by interactions between the apical ectodermal ridge and the underlying mesenchymal tissue. **B,** Dorsoventral patterning is determined by the surrounding ectoderm and the mesenchymal tissue of the bud. The limb has been cut along the *dotted line* as indicated, and the interactions are shown in cross-section. **C,** Anteroposterior development is mediated by interactions between the zone of polarizing activity and the mesenchymal tissue of the bud. (Redrawn From Tickle C. Experimental embryology as applied to the upper limb. *J Hand Surg* 1987;12B[3]:294-300.)

BOX 122.1 Embryologic Classification of Congenital Anomalies

1. Failure of formation of parts
   a. Transverse
   b. Longitudinal
2. Failure of differentiation of parts
   a. Soft tissue
   b. Skeletal
   c. Tumorous conditions
3. Duplication
   a. Whole limb
   b. Humeral
   c. Radial
   d. Ulnar
   e. Digit
4. Overgrowth
5. Undergrowth
6. Congenital constriction band syndrome
7. Generalized skeletal abnormalities

Classification

Attempts to uniformly classify all congenital upper limb anomalies have been ongoing since the 1800s. There are three major classification schemes used for developmental abnormalities; these are the *embryologic, teratologic,* and *anatomical* classification schemes.[17] Previously, the embryologic scheme was the most widely accepted classification scheme.[17] Within this schema, each limb deformity is classified according to its most predominant morphologic anomaly (Box 122.1). Many have argued that this classification system does not allow for categorization of all defects.[18–21] It has also been difficult to update the classification system as our understanding of congenital hand anomalies grows.[22] For example, ongoing genetic analysis has shown that many defects, although appearing clinically unique, originate from common abnormalities in limb development; an example of this can be seen in cases of central polydactyly, syndactyly, and central hand deficiency, which in animal models have been shown to develop from a common insult.[23–26]

In an effort to create a more flexible classification system in which new developments in the field of congenital hand surgery could be incorporated, Drs. Manske, Tonkin, and Oberg developed a new classification system, which was adopted in 2014 by the International Federation of Societies for Surgery of the Hand (IFSSH); this classification scheme is referred to as the Oberg-Manske-Tonkin (OMT) classification (Box 122.2).[22,27–29] This system divides anomalies into malformations, deformations, and dysplasias and cross-references any applicable syndrome. Malformations include anomalies resulting from an insult during development and are subdivided by whether they affect the entire upper limb or the hand plate only and which axis is predominantly affected. Deformations include alterations to tissues that have already been formed, such as constriction band syndrome, whereas dysplasias include abnormal organization of cells into tissues. This classification has been found to have excellent inter- and intraobserver reliability.[30]

A brief note should be made about the teratologic classification scheme. The teratologic scheme classifies anomalies on the severity of their phenotypic expression. This classification scheme, although not practical for classifying all congenital anomalies, is very helpful in classifying specific defects according to severity—for example, grade I (mild) to grade V (severe)—and is used frequently within the upper extremity. The teratologic classification scheme is used to describe radial aplasia and thumb hypoplasia described in the following sections.[31–33]

SPECIFIC CONGENITAL UPPER LIMB ANOMALIES (USING THE OBERG-MANSKE-TONKIN CLASSIFICATION)

Malformations
Transverse Deficiencies

Transverse deficiencies describe congenital amputations at various levels of the upper limb. They are classified according to the last remaining bony segment (Fig. 122.2). The OMT classification divides these into whole limb (group IA1iii) and hand plate only (group 1Biii). Transverse deficiencies occur at an incidence of one in every 30,000 births.[5] The most common transverse deficiency is through the proximal third of the forearm. Transverse deficiencies are most commonly unilateral and are sporadic in nature. The differential diagnosis for transverse

BOX 122.2 The Oberg, Manske, Tonkin (OMT) Classification of Congenital and Upper Limb Anomalies

I. Malformations
  A. Failure of axis formation or differentiation: entire upper limb
    1. Proximal–distal outgrowth
      Brachymelia with brachydactyly
      Symbrachydactyly
      Transverse deficiency
      Intersegmental deficiency
    2. Radial–ulnar (anteroposterior) axis
      Radial longitudinal deficiency
      Ulnar dimelia
      Ulnar longitudinal deficiency
      Radioulnar synostosis
      Humeroradial synostosis
    3. Dorsal–ventral axis
      Nail-patella syndrome
  B. Failure of axis formation or differentiation—hand plate
    1. Radial–ulnar (anteroposterior) axis
      Radial polydactyly
      Triphalangeal thumb
      Ulnar polydactyly
    2. Dorsal–ventral axis
      Dorsal dimelia (palmar nail)
      Hypoplastic or aplastic nail
  C. Failure of axis formation or differentiation—unspecified axis
    1. Soft tissue
      Syndactyly
      Camptodactyly
    2. Skeletal deficiency
      Brachydactyly
      Clinodactyly
      Kirner deformity
      Metacarpal and carpal synostoses
    3. Complex
      Cleft hand
      Synpolydactyly
      Apert hand
II. Deformations
  A. Constriction ring sequence
  B. Arthrogryposis
  C. Trigger digits
  D. Not otherwise specified
III. Dysplasias
  A. Hypertrophy
    1. Macrodactyly
    2. Upper limb
    3. Upper limb and macrodactyly
  B. Tumorous conditions

Reproduced with permission under STM Signatory Guidelines from Tonkin MA et al. Classification of congenital anomalies of the hand and upper limb: development and assessment of a new system. *J Hand Surg.* 2013;38A:1845-1853.

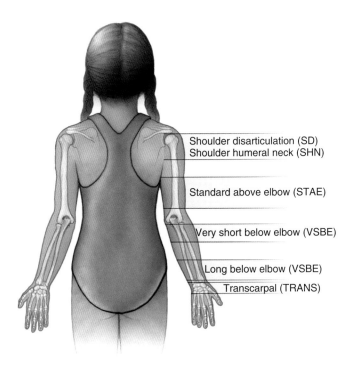

Fig. 122.2 Transverse deficiencies are classified according to the most distal remaining bone segment.

Shoulder disarticulation (SD)
Shoulder humeral neck (SHN)
Standard above elbow (STAE)
Very short below elbow (VSBE)
Long below elbow (VSBE)
Transcarpal (TRANS)

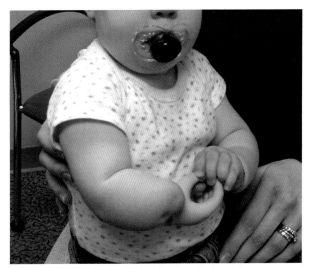

Fig. 122.3 An 8-month-old child with a long below-elbow amputation. She is holding her cosmetic prosthesis in her left hand. The child was tolerant of prosthetic wear but preferred to be without the prosthesis for all bimanual activities.

deficiency can include amnionic band syndrome (OMT classification IIA). Amnionic band syndrome may be differentiated from transverse deficiency by the presence of banding in other extremities or fingers and is not commonly a unilateral finding.[34,35] Patients with true transverse deficiencies present with well-padded amputation stumps.

Surgical intervention for unilateral cases is seldom required, and most children are fitted for a prosthesis. There is substantial controversy surrounding the optimal age for the initial fitting of a prosthesis. It has been our practice to fit children as early as 6 months of age with a passive prosthesis (Fig. 122.3). This helps with balance during the child's transition from sitting to walking as well as prosthetic acceptance. Active body-powered prostheses, including voluntary opening and closing prostheses, may be introduced at 15 months to 2 years of age.[3] Myoelectric prostheses may be considered at 3 to 5 years of age and may be preferred for school use because they are visually more

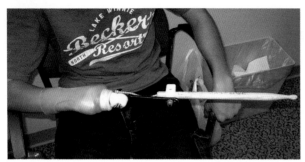

Fig. 122.4 This terminal device is designed to allow this child with a transcarpal amputation play the drums.

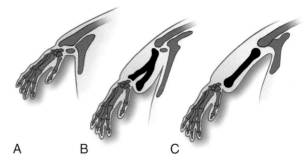

Fig. 122.5 Phocomelia classification. Type A is the most severe form of phocomelia and is used to classify children when a rudimentary hand is found attached to the clavicle or scapula. Type B presents as an absent humerus but synostotic radius and ulna attached to a rudimentary hand. Type C represents the final type where the humerus articulates with an underdeveloped hand, which has one to three digits.

acceptable; however, voluntary opening devices remain the most common form of prosthesis.

Acceptance of the prosthesis is variable, with rejection rates ranging from 10% to 32%.[36–38] Studies from the Netherlands have found that children tend to reject the prosthesis either within 3.5 years of prosthesis initiation or after 13.5 years of prosthetic use.[36] This later time period tends to correspond with puberty. Studies from Davids and colleagues have shown that initial prosthetic fitting before the age of 3 years in conjunction with occupational therapy may help in promoting long-term use of prosthetic devices.[39] Functional grading and quality of life questionnaires, when assessed in these children, are found to be near normal regardless of whether they wear a prosthesis or not.[40]

The therapist's major role in children with transverse deficiency begins at the age of 3 or 4 years; at this age, children often need help in learning to use their prosthesis with tasks such as dressing, tying shoelaces, and using buttons and zippers. Children with more proximal amputations (above the elbow) have an increased reliance on their prostheses and are more likely to become consistent users, whereas children with distal amputations are more likely to have prosthetic devices that are custom molded to aid in specific activities such as sports or for playing musical instruments[41] (Fig. 122.4). Most children should be seen every 6 months to evaluate how the prosthesis is fitting and for resizing. As the child grows, annual evaluation is still needed for prosthetic maintenance.

Intersegmental Deficiency

Intersegmental deficiencies involve portions of the longitudinal axis and include rhizomelic (humeral), mesomelic (forearm), and phocomelic deficiencies.

Phocomelia

Phocomelia is the absence of a portion of the extremity with continued distal rudimentary development of the hand. Phocomelia most commonly occurs bilaterally and was associated with perinatal ingestion of thalidomide in Europe during the 1960s, when this medication was given to pregnant women as a sedative during their first trimester.[42,43] There are three major types that are classified according to their intermediate segment. In type I, the most severe, the arm is attached directly to the shoulder. In type II, the forearm and hand attach directly to the shoulder. In type III, the forearm is absent, and the hand attaches to the humerus (Fig. 122.5).[44,45]

The hand is usually underdeveloped and often lacks the development of a thumb. Strength in the hand is decreased, but some degree of prehension is still possible.[46] Surgical intervention is rarely indicated. Patients are managed with prostheses and often adapt to performing many functions with their feet. Shoes that can be easily removed should be encouraged in these children because prehensile function with their feet is often superior to that obtained with their hands. Prosthetics are reserved for children with some hand function and who are capable of activating terminal devices. Such prosthetics are difficult to suspend from the patient's

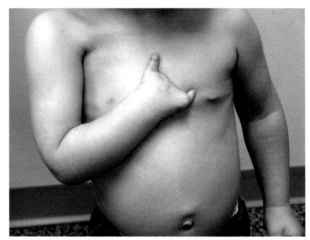

Fig. 122.6 A 4-year-old boy with Poland's syndrome as evidenced by complete absence of the pectoralis on the right, associated pectus excavatum, and symbrachydactyly.

hypoplastic shoulders but are often valuable for school activities, including writing at a desk, using scissors, and holding open books.

Surgery is usually reserved for the separation of syndactylized digits. Functional shortness of the limb is the primary problem. The hand may be incapable of reaching the face for eating or may not be long enough for self-dressing and toileting. Therapists may recommend extended tools to help a child perform self-care tasks more easily. Distraction-lengthening using external distracters may aid in increasing the length of the humerus, which may aid in the fitting of some prosthetics.[47]

Brachydactyly

Brachydactyly refers to a hand with short or hypoplastic fingers. The OMT classification places brachydactyly in group IB1, abnormal axis formation/differentiation of the hand plate in the longitudinal axis. Patients most commonly present with hypoplasia of the index through ring fingers. This deformity occurs sporadically and can often be associated with Poland's syndrome.[48] Poland's syndrome can include a variety of phenotypic presentations but should always include the absence of the sternal head of the pectoralis major muscle and a hypoplastic hand with some webbing between the fingers[49–52] (Fig. 122.6). Classification of symbrachydactyly was originally described by Pol, who divided patients into those who had evidence of Poland's syndrome and those who did not; this classification scheme has been furthered modified to describe the progression of central deficiency throughout the hand.[53,54] In most patients, the index, long, and ring fingers are

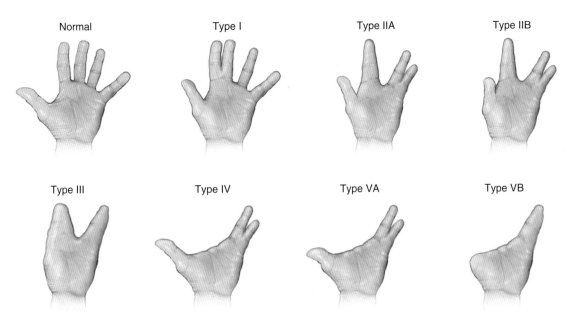

Fig. 122.7 Classification scheme for brachydactyly.

hypoplastic but present. In more severely affected individuals, there is increasing hypoplasia of the central digits with eventual absence of the index thru ring finger, including portions of the metacarpals. The thumb may be hypoplastic, unstable, and in some cases absent (Fig. 122.7). The most severely affected patients can present with complete transverse absence of the hand at the metacarpal row with only small soft tissue nubbins present with nail remnants.

Surgical management depends on the number of functioning digits. Patients with shortened fingers alone (types 1, 2 and 3; see Fig. 122.7) usually have good function, and surgery is seldom required. For patients with more severe involvement, surgical priority is always given to reconstruction of any compromise of the first webspace. Syndactylized digits should be released. As the child matures, a part-time orthosis may be used to aid with specific activities.

In hands with a deficient thumb, free vascularized toe transfer may be considered. Toe transfer can also be considered for monodactylous hands.[46,55] For fingers devoid of bony support, consideration can be given to nonvascularized toe transfer if the child is younger than 1 year of age. This technique is particularly useful for the thumb because it allows for an increase in functional length without the added complexities of a microsurgical procedure.[56–59] Nonvascularized transfers performed after the age of 1 year have little chance for ongoing physeal growth and may resorb over time.[59]

Radial Deficiency

Radial deficiency can present as a spectrum of deformity ranging from minimal wrist impairment to wrist, thumb, and elbow impairment. The incidence of radial deficiency has been estimated to be 1 in 30,000 to 1 in 100,000 births. Unilateral and bilateral cases are believed to occur at a similar frequency; however, bilateral cases occur more frequently in males at a ratio of 3 to 2.[46,60–64] Most cases of radial deficiency are associated with hypoplasia or aplasia of the thumb as well, further complicating hand function.

Associated anomalies and skeletal syndromes are extremely common with radial hypoplasia (Box 122.3) and must be excluded before any type of surgical intervention.[65] Most important is to identify any associated hematological or cardiac abnormality because these may often be life threatening. Commonly associated syndromes include the thrombocytopenia absent radius syndrome (TAR syndrome), Holt-Oram syndrome, and Fanconi's anemia.[66,67] There is also an association with

---

BOX 122.3 Syndromes Associated with Radial Hypoplasia

VACTERL (**v**ertebral anomalies, **a**nal atresia, **c**ardiac anomalies, **t**racheo-**e**sophageal fistula, **r**enal anomalies, and **l**imb abnormalities) association

Thrombocytopenia–absent radius (TAR) syndrome

Fanconi's anemia

Holt-Oram syndrome (hand and heart syndrome)

Acrofacial dysostosis (Nager syndrome)

Mandibular dysostosis (Treacher Collins syndrome)

Cornelia de Lange syndrome

Ventriculoradial dysplasia

Klippel-Feil syndrome

VACTERL syndrome (an acronym for **v**ertebral anomalies, **a**nal atresia, **c**ardiac anomalies, **t**racheoesophageal fistula, **r**enal anomalies, and **l**imb abnormalities), including the finding of radial deficiency.[68] The cardiac defects most frequently encountered in these children are atrial septal defects and ventriculoseptal defects. Associated medical problems have been noted in 40% of children with unilateral involvement and 77% of children with bilateral involvement.[65,67] Fanconi's anemia is not manifest at birth but may be identified in infancy with genetic screening, which will allow for close hematologic monitoring during the child's development.[69,70] This condition is often fatal if not treated with a bone marrow transplant. Because of the high number of associated defects, many children with radial hypoplasia require specialized cardiac monitoring while undergoing general anesthesia and thus may require all surgical procedures be conducted in a specialized pediatric center capable of monitoring these children during the peri- and postoperative periods.[68]

Radial aplasia is classified into four types based on severity (Fig. 122.8).

Type I deficiency typically presents with a minimally shortened radius compared with the ulna. Elbow function is normal. Thumb hypoplasia may or may not be present. Surgical management of the wrist in these cases is rare, and surgery, if necessary, is usually directed toward improving any abnormalities in thumb function.[71]

In type II, the radius is short and the ulna is often bowed toward the radius. The hand and wrist deviate toward the deficient radius. Radial hypoplasia usually extends into the wrist and thumb ray, evident by an absent scaphoid and underdeveloped thumb. Use of an orthosis and

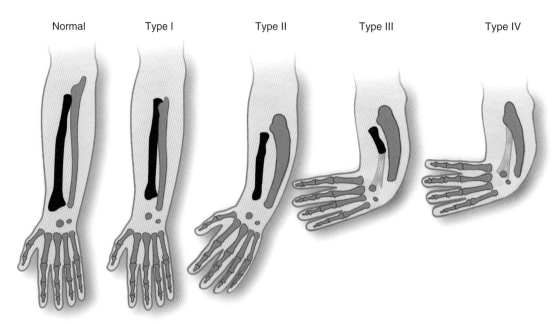

Fig. 122.8 Classification scheme for radial hypoplasia. Type I, minimally shortened radius compared with the ulna. Elbow function is normal. Type II, the radius is short, and the ulna is often bowed toward the radius. Type III, the radius is hypoplastic with absence of the distal and middle thirds. A fibrous anlage often extends from the distal radial remnant to the wrist. Type IV represents a complete absence of the radius.

stretching are often recommended in these children at an early age to attempt to limit the amount of radial deviation of the wrist. Surgery in these cases consists of procedures to correct radial bowing of the ulna and to stabilize the wrist on the ulna.

In type III, the radius is hypoplastic with absence of the distal and middle thirds. Often it is difficult to identify type III deformities when the child is very young because the proximal radial remnant may not have fully ossified. The wrist progressively moves into a pronated, flexed, and radially deviated posture. Thumb ray and radial carpal hypoplasia are often present. Children with this grade deformity often have a fibrous anlage that extends from the distal radial remnant to the carpus. This anlage must be released to allow for correction of the carpal misalignment. Children with this deformity usually undergo a centralization or radialization procedure to stabilize the wrist on the ulna bone. If the third metacarpal is centered over the distal ulna, the procedure is called *centralization*; if the index metacarpal is centered over the distal ulna, it is called *radialization.*[32]

Type IV deformities represent complete absence of the radius. Traditionally, this is believed to be the most common presentation of radial deficiency; however, Upton[46] has recently stated that the type III deformity is the most common. With type IV deformity, ulnar bowing is present, and overall ulnar growth is usually limited to no more than 60% of the contralateral side. Elbow motion is often restricted. In these children, the thumb is often absent, and the index and long fingers often lack full range of motion (ROM) and may also be hypoplastic. The one exception to this phenomenon occurs in the TAR syndrome, in which the thumb is always present but has variable function.[72] Most children with type IV hypoplasia undergo a wrist centralization procedure. In many cases, wrist centralization is preempted by soft tissue distraction for a period of 4 to 6 weeks, which substantially facilitates the centralization procedure[73,74] (see Fig. 122.9).

In adults with radial longitudinal deficiency, functional outcome has been shown to be more related to grip strength, pinch strength, and elbow and wrist ROM rather than angulation of the wrist.[75] Similarly, in children, wrist angulation was independent of performance on dexterity assessments or patient-reported outcomes scores.[76] A recent comparison of nonoperative management of modified Bayne type 3

or 4 radial longitudinal deficiency with surgical treatment offers some evidence for improved outcomes in several measures with radialization or centralization procedures.[77] The authors found surgically treated wrists demonstrated significantly better wrist alignment (hand–forearm angle of 12 degrees vs 85 degrees), long finger ROM (157 degrees vs 86 degrees), grip strength (37% of normative values vs 11.5%), and patient-rated cosmesis at a mean of 10.5 years of follow-up.

Therapy and Surgical Options for Type 2-3-4 Radial Deficiency

Stretching and use of orthoses for radial deficiencies can start at birth. The goal is to reduce the hand or carpus onto the distal ulna and prevent contracture of the wrist in radial deviation. The stretching protocol consists of progressive longitudinal distraction, ulnar deviation, and extension with stabilization of the ulnocarpal joint. The wrist is stretched as close to neutral as possible using gentle but firm passive stretching. Directing the parents to perform the stretches with each diaper change provides an easy algorithm to follow, with a forearm-based wrist and hand orthosis maintained at all other times.[71] Any improvement in ROM achieved through exercises can make future surgical correction less complex.

In addition to stretching, a radial gutter orthosis, which leaves the thumb and fingers free, is recommended during the day to maintain the correction obtained from passive manipulation. Patients with a shortened forearm and those with elbow extension limitations may require an orthosis that extends above the elbow. After passive motion is achieved, use of a day orthosis is discontinued and worn only during the night and for periods of rapid growth.

As infants, these children may have decreased weight bearing through the involved upper extremity and therefore limited crawling abilities. Children with severe deformities often have hypoplastic or stiff index fingers as well. The majority of prehension activities are accomplished through the use of the small finger. These children may need adaptive techniques or devices to maximize function and success in developmental activities such as a universal cuff to hold toys. Therapeutic activities are encouraged to improve AROM of the extremity through reaching, weight bearing, and play activities. Therapists should also monitor and engage the child in fine-motor activities as they develop.

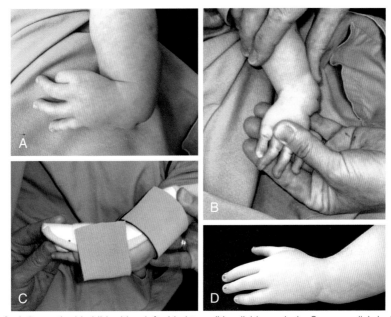

Fig. 122.9 A, A 9-month-old child with a left-sided type IV radial hypoplasia. Severe radial deviation of the wrist is present. **B,** Initial treatment begins with daily stretching and orthotic positioning. **C,** Positioning is utilized at night and during nap time. **D,** At 2 years of age, this child underwent soft tissue distraction for 6 weeks followed by wrist centralization. Soft tissue distraction allows for easier centralization of the wrist. **D,** Appearance of the limb 3 years after centralization surgery. Index finger pollicization was performed 1 year after a centralization procedure.

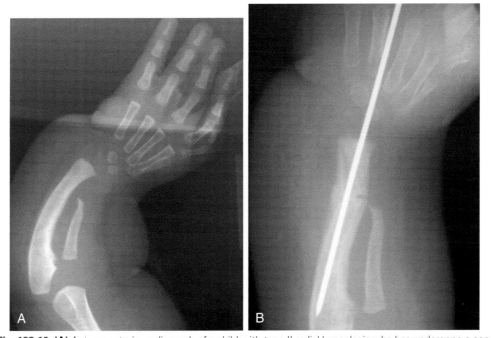

Fig. 122.10 (A) Anteroposterior radiograph of a child with type II radial hypoplasia who has undergone a centralization procedure with corrective osteotomy of the ulna and resection of the fibrous anlage. **(B)** A surgical pin is used to stabilize the wrist to the ulna. The pin in this child remained in place for 12 weeks.

Centralization and radialization have become accepted treatment options for children with type II to IV deformities. The goals of these procedures are to provide wrist stability while increasing the functional length of the forearm by placing the wrist on the distal end of the ulna. These procedures also help to improve the alignment of the flexor tendons. A temporary pin is placed across the ulnocarpal joint to stabilize the hand and wrist on the ulna (Fig. 122.10). The pin remains for a variable period of time depending on surgeon preference. During these procedures, the remaining radial tendons are often transferred to the ulnar aspect of the carpus in an attempt to rebalance the wrist and prevent recurrent contractures[78] Restoring muscle imbalance is very important for prevention of recurrence of angular deformity.[79] Recurrence of radial deviation of the wrist as the child grows has been associated with the amount of correction obtained at the initial surgery and the age at the time of initial surgery.[80,81]

Postsurgical therapy for children undergoing radialization and centralization procedures includes full-time protective orthosis use for 4 weeks after cast removal. The orthosis may be removed for hygiene and three to five times a day for ROM exercises. To help maintain the correction and minimize further ulnar bowing, a rigid night orthosis may be indicated until skeletal maturity.

The timing for surgical intervention in children with radial deficiency is a matter of some debate, but in general, wrist centralization is often performed between 6 to 12 months of age so the child will have a stable wrist for bimanual activities as well as for aiding in early ambulation. Additional procedures for thumb deficiency are usually performed before the child enters preschool at 2 to 5 years of age. Finally, distraction-lengthening of the shortened forearm may be elected at 8 to 12 years of age (Fig. 122.9).[82]

Thumb Deficiency

Thumb deficiency is often seen as a terminal extension of radial deficiency, although the OMT classification separates thumb hypoplasia limited to the hand from thumb hypoplasia associated with more proximal deficiency. Thumb hypoplasia is a condition that encompasses a varied spectrum of clinical presentation, ranging from mild hypoplasia of the thumb to complete absence or aplasia of the thumb. The sex distribution for thumb hypoplasia appears to be equal.[83] Bilateral involvement tends to predominate in better than 60% of patients followed by the right thumb involvement (21%–27%) and then left thumb involvement (12%–15%).[83,84]

Hypoplasia of the thumb has been classified by Blauth into five grades.[32] Grade I is a normal-appearing thumb; however, it is smaller in proportion to the contralateral thumb. In Grade II, there is metacarpophalangeal (MCP) joint insufficiency with joint laxity. The first metacarpal is adducted, and the MCP joint is radially deviated because of ulnar collateral ligament laxity. There is often a tight first webspace. In grade III deficiency, there is hypoplasia of the proximal portion of the first metacarpal, the degree of which can vary.[85] Grade IV represents total aplasia of the metacarpal with underdevelopment of the thumb phalanges; this is also referred to as a *floating thumb* or *pouce flottant*. Grade V presents as total absence of the thumb (Fig. 122.11).

Manske modified the Blauth classification to describe thumbs with hypoplastic metacarpals but stabile carpometacarpal (CMC) joints as type IIIA thumbs, whereas those with unstable CMC joints are classified as type IIIB (Table 122.1). This classification scheme is very practical for surgeons because type IIIB thumbs are usually not amenable to surgical correction. These children are best treated with removal of the IIIB thumb and pollicization of the index finger, whereas type IIIA thumbs can be improved after attempts at stabilization of the CMC and MCP joints.[86] The most common type of thumb hypoplasia (based on Manske's classification) is type V, representing more than 33% of cases; this is followed by Manske type IV (15%–19%), type III (16%–20%), type II (13%), and finally type I (2%–4%).[83,84] The reported incidence of type I and perhaps type II may be an underestimation because many of these children may not seek surgical treatment.[86]

Treatment options range from observation to pollicization of the index finger and typically are determined by the severity of the thumb hypoplasia. Type I thumbs require no treatment. For children with type II and IIIa hypoplasia, video-taped play sessions allow the surgeon and therapist to evaluate thumb function and the incorporation of the thumb into ADLs. Spontaneous use of the hand in a semistructured play session may uncover areas of weakness and compensation, such as difficulties with large grasp when picking up a can. Areas of concern are identified and the therapist can provide the surgeon with treatment suggestions to maximize functional use. Type II thumbs

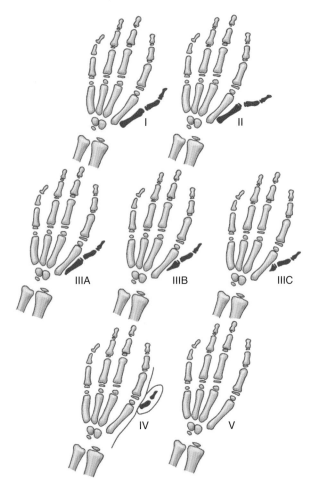

Fig. 122.11 Blauth classification of thumb hypoplasia. Thumb hypoplasia is divided into five main grades according to Blauth. Grade III is subdivided into IIIA, IIIB, and IIIC depending on the extent of aplasia of the proximal thumb metacarpal. (Modified and redrawn from Blauth W. Der hypoplastische Daumen. *Arch Orthop Unfall Chir.* 1967;62:225-246.)

TABLE 122.1 Manske's Classification of Thumb Hypoplasia

Type	Description
Type I	Minimal shortening and narrowing
Type II	Thumb–index webspace narrowing
	Hypoplasia intrinsic thenar muscles
	MCP joint instability
Type III	Type II features plus:
	IIIA: extrinsic tendon abnormalities, hypoplastic metacarpal, stable CMC joint
	IIIB: extrinsic tendon abnormalities, partial metacarpal aplasia, unstable CMC joint
Type IV	Floating thumb or *pouce flottant*
Type V	Absent thumb

CMC, Carpometacarpal; *MCP,* metacarpophalangeal.

usually benefit from stabilization of the MCP joint and centralization of the flexor and extensor mechanism. Hypoplasia of the thenar muscles may limit thumb opposition. Preoperative hand therapy in these children should include strengthening available muscles for grasp, release, and pinch. A hypoplastic thumb may be thinner and shorter than the contralateral side; in such cases, a custom thumb abduction orthosis can provide improved function and stability. A rigid thumb abduction orthosis may be indicated if the CMC joint is unstable as well. If pinch and grasp function is still limited after therapy, tendon transfers (opponensplasty) may be performed to improve oppositional strength.

Type IIIa thumbs benefit from MCP stabilization, tendon centralization, first webspace deepening, and opponensplasty (see Table 122.1). Opponensplasty in these children usually involves the transfer of the ring finger flexor digitorum superficialis (FDS) or the transfer of the abductor digiti minimi (Huber transfer). The transferred tendons are attached to the MCP joint to provide additional pinch and grip strength.[87,88] The superficialis transfer has been found to be more powerful than the abductor digit minimi transfer. In addition, the tendon end of the superficialis, when passed over or through the MCP joint, can serve to reconstruct the deficient MCP ulnar collateral ligaments[89] (Fig. 122.12). If the abductor digiti minimi muscle transfer is chosen for oppositional transfer, a tendon graft (palmaris longus) can be used to reconstruct the ulnar collateral ligament.[90–92] When multiaxial instability of the thumb MCP joint is present, joint fusion or chondrodesis can be used for joint stabilization.[86,93]

Surgical treatment for grades IIIb, IV, and V thumb hypoplasia is predominantly pollicization. Pollicization is a complex procedure involving the transfer of a finger, usually the index, to the thumb position (Fig. 122.13).[94–96] Manual dexterity of the new thumb can average up to 70% of normal controls.[95] More than 50% of patients with a pollicized index finger may continue to use a "side-to-side pinch" between the small and ring finger in stressful situations or when hand tasks are limited because of time constraints.[97] In Ogino and Ishii's[98] report, average motion of the pollicized digit was 45 degrees, and pinch strength was 55% of the intact contralateral hand. In Manske's long-term retrospective study, with an average follow-up period of 8 years, total active motion of the pollicized digit averaged 98 degrees or approximately 50% that of a normal thumb. Average grip strength was 21% of normal, and average pinch strength was as follows: opposition, 26%; apposition (i.e., lateral pinch), 22%; and tripod, 23% of the normal hand. The pollicized digit was used in the manner of a normal thumb or in modified fashion 84% of the time, with increased usage seen when handling large objects (92%) and versus small objects (77%). The time required to perform activities averaged 22% longer than the standard for a normal hand. Their results were not influenced by the age of the patient at the time of operation.[99]

Better function should be expected in children with a mobile index finger before transfer. Poorer results have been associated with grade V hypoplasia and concomitant radial deficiency. In these cases, the transferred index finger is often stiff or hypoplastic before transfer.[93,99,100]

After opponensplasty and pollicization, children are casted for 4 to 6 weeks. After cast removal, most children then go into a hand-based thumb opponens orthosis. The thumb should be positioned in maximum palmar abduction for pollicization and slight adduction after opponensplasty. Orthosis wear schedule is full time for 4 to 6 weeks, removing it three to five times daily for AROM exercises, thumb to finger opposition, and scar massage. Buddy taping the fingers can enhance functional use and discourage scissors pinch. PROM, particularly thumb extension, should be avoided to protect the new tendon transfer in cases of opponensplasty. Progressive strengthening exercises for thumb opposition and functional pinch and grasp begin at 12 weeks after surgery. At this time, rehabilitation includes stretching to maximize the thumb webspace and strengthening available muscles for grasp, release, and pinch (see Figs. 122.13 and 122.14). Soft

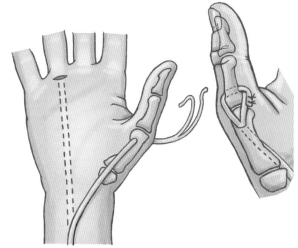

Fig. 122.12 The flexor digitorum superficialis tendon can be transferred to the thumb to aid in opposition. In addition, the tendon can also be used to stabilize the metacarpophalangeal joint, which is often unstable in cases of thumb hypoplasia. (Copyright Mayo Foundation.)

thumb opposition orthoses may be considered to improve webspace positioning, support, and function. A rigid thumb abduction orthosis may be indicated if the CMC joint is unstable to improve alignment and stability.

Although there is no universally accepted outcomes assessment to evaluate thumb function after index pollicization, there have been recent advances in this area. Timed assessments of whole-hand dexterity such as the Box and Blocks Test, the Nine Hole Peg Test, and the Functional Dexterity Test have been used in the literature as a proxy for thumb function. Although these tests are an excellent measure of activity limitation, they may not reflect the degree to which the thumb is actually incorporated into ADLs. The Thumb Grasp and Pinch assessment (T-GAP) is a newer evaluation tool designed specifically to evaluate grasp and pinch patterns and thumb use in children after index pollicization.[101] The test is performed by an occupational therapist, who video tapes the child performing nine age-appropriate tasks (Table 122.3) using whatever grasp or pinch pattern is preferred by the child. The therapist then reviews the video and classifies the predominant grasp pattern (Table 122.4). Hand skills in normally developing children begin more proximal and progress to more distal grasps, and the scoring system is designed to reflect this pattern with more mature patterns receiving higher points. Abnormal grasp patterns that exclude the thumb are also described and assigned points. Scores for each task are then summed to produce a final T-GAP score. A video of a T-GAP assessment can be viewed in the online supplementary materials (Video 122.1). The T-GAP has the advantage of allowing the child to use any grasp or pinch pattern to complete a task, including patterns that exclude use of the thumb. The assessment also defines abnormal grasp patterns such as radial scissor pinch and ulnar scissor pinch often used by children with thumb hypoplasia but rarely seen in other populations (Fig. 122.15). The assessment has shown early promise in studies of construct validity, concurrent validity, and inter- and intrarater reliability.[102]

Ulnar Deficiencies

Ulnar deficiency occurs at an incidence of 1 in 100,000 live births.[103–106] These children typically present with ulnar deviation at the wrist and subluxation and dislocation of the radial head and are lacking ulnar digits. Ulnar deficiency can be seen in families with a variable penetrance.[107] It may also be associated with other malformation syndromes,

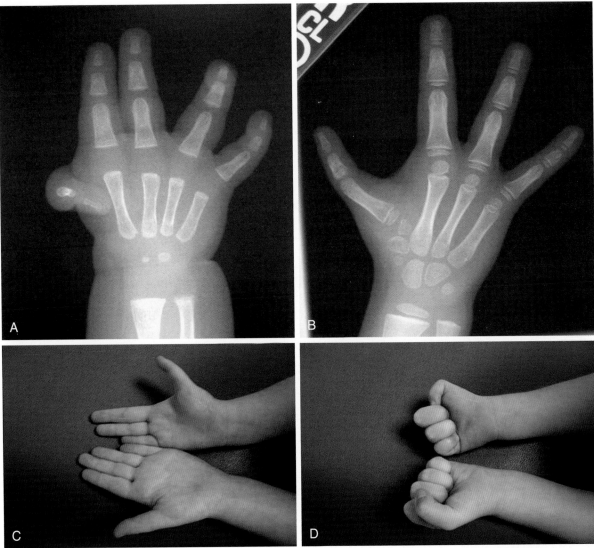

Fig. 122.13 Results of pollicization. **A,** In type IV thumb hypoplasia of the right hand in this 6-month-old girl. **B,** In this child, the index finger was pollicized to create a new thumb. Anteroposterior radiograph of the hand 3 years after surgery shows excellent position of the thumb. **C** and **D,** With acceptable range of motion at the new metacarpophalangeal and carpometacarpal joints.

including orofacial malformations, ulnar mammary syndrome, Cornelia de Lange syndrome, and femur fibula ulna syndrome.[108,109]

Ulnar deficiency is generally classified according to Bayne's classification system, which divides deformities into four grades of severity (Fig. 122.16). Type I deformity present with minimal shortening of the ulna. Wrist, elbow, and shoulder function are usually normal. These patients rarely need treatment. Patients with type II deformities, which is the most common form of ulnar hypoplasia, present with an absence of the distal or middle third of the ulna. A fibrous anlage is often present in place of the hypoplastic ulna, which can pull or tether the radius during growth, resulting in progressive radial head dislocation or radial bowing. These children will also often have deficiencies or absence of the ulnar digits (Fig. 122.17). Children with type III deformities have a complete absence of the ulna. The fibrous anlage is often absent so there is minimal deviation of the radius. The elbow is often unstable, and the radial head is dislocated. Children may also have pterygium, referring to a web contracture at the elbow. Here, as in type II deformities, ulnar deficiencies are present within the hand. Children with type IV deformities also present with complete absence of the ulna, but in addition to an absent ulna, there is a synostosis between the radius and the humerus. The hand in these children is often supinated away

from the body and positioned posterior. There is often a fibrous anlage, which results in significant radial bowing and ulnar hand deficiencies are present.[107,110–112]

Therapy for patients with mild ulnar deficiencies should begin at 6 weeks of age and includes stretching and use of a wrist and hand orthosis to promote maximum radial deviation and wrist extension. The orthosis should be worn during nap time and at night. Orthotic fabrication for all infants requires frequent follow-up visits for adjustments to maximize wrist and hand alignment. When passive correction is achieved, a night orthosis is recommended to prevent recurrence. The exercise program should include active assisted ROM and gentle PROM for the wrist and hand three to five times daily. For severe cases and those with bilateral involvement, therapists should complete a detailed evaluation to assess limitations at the elbow, forearm, wrist, and hand. Active reach should be assessed because the limb is often short and stiff at the elbow, which may affect grooming, dressing, or hygiene. Therapists may provide equipment or adaptive training to improve independence with everyday living skills.

The need for surgery in these children is usually dictated by the amount of hand deformity.[107,113,114] Children with an intact thumb and first webspace are able to perform prehensile function;

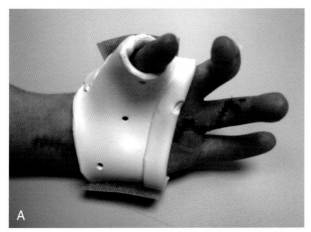

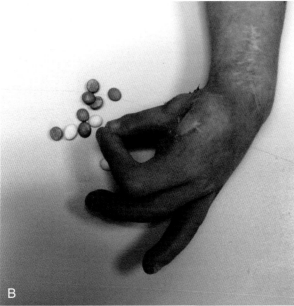

Fig. 122.14 A, After oppositional transfer—in this case, a flexor digitorum superficialis transfer—children are placed into protective thumb orthoses for 4 to 8 weeks. The orthosis here maintains some palmar abduction while maintaining a good first webspace. **B,** The orthosis is removed for gentle range of motion and strengthening exercises three to four times a day. Formal therapy sessions work on promoting fine-motor function.

TABLE 122.2 T-GAP Scoring Hierarchy	
Grasp or Pinch Type	**Point Value**
No Use of Thumb	
No grasp or pinch; passive stabilization with hand	0
Palmar grasp; fingers to palm	1
Ulnar scissor grasp; between small or ring fingers	2
Radial scissor grasp; between index or long fingers or long or ring fingers	3
Use of Thumb	
Cylindrical grasp; opposed thumb to all fingers	4
Lateral key pinch; thumb to index	5
Tip pinch; thumb to index fingertip	6
Tripod pinch; thumb to distal index or long finger	7

however, 90% of children with ulnar deficiency will not have a full complement of digits.[107,112] Syndactyly is present in more than one third of patients, and more than 50% of patients can have radial hand deficiencies, including thumb hypoplasia.[112,115] Surgery is recommended for release of the first webspace, division of syndactyly, and rotational osteotomies of the thumb to improve oppositional pinch.[106,110–116]

Polydactyly

Polydactyly is the most common congenital hand anomaly.[117] Polydactyly involving the thumb is referred to as *radial polydactyly*, and duplication that involves the little finger is referred to as *ulnar polydactyly*. Ulnar polydactyly is more commonly seen in Africans, whereas radial duplication is more common in the whites and Asians. Central polydactyly is associated with syndactyly and cleft hand, and its treatment therefore is more complex and involves treating the polydactyly, the syndactyly, the central cleft, and any accompanying thumb web tightness.

Radial Polydactyly

Radial polydactyly has an incidence of 1 in every 3000 births. Variable degrees of duplication exist and range from widening of the thumb tip to complete duplication. Classification of thumb duplication has been described by Wassel[118] with type IV representing the most common pattern (Fig. 122.18). Treatment of radial polydactyly is typically surgical and can be initiated at 6 to 9 months of age. Use of a preoperative orthosis has been found to be valuable for improving angular and rotatory deformities before surgical correction.[119] Surgery most commonly includes removal of the radial duplicate, centralization of the flexor and extensor mechanism, and correctional osteotomies for angular deviation.[120,121] The most common complications after surgery are instability at either the interphalangeal (IP) or MCP joint, growth plate injury, and surgical scarring.[122–125] Therapy after surgery usually includes scar management and night time orthosis wear for a period of 3 to 6 months. In cases in which significant reconstruction of the radial collateral ligament is required, a full-time thumb spica orthosis may be worn for 2 to 3 months for additional stability.

Triphalangeal thumb, Wassel class VII, describes a thumb that contains an extra, or third, phalanx. Radial polydactyly with triphalangism is associated with an autosomal dominant inheritance pattern and genetic mutations within the hedgehog pathway.[126–128] Surgical treatment involves correction of length, angular deformity, and web contractures. Therapy considerations for these patients depend on the extent of surgical correction required and the baseline functional status.

Central Polydactyly

Central polydactyly (duplication of the index, middle, or ring fingers) is often seen in combination with other anomalies, most commonly syndactyly. This is believed to be a heritable condition, and treatment is operative. Operative intervention is undertaken at an early age, and rehabilitation considerations in these patients depend on the extent of surgical reconstruction (Fig. 122.19).

Ulnar Polydactyly

Ulnar polydactyly is classified into types A and B. Type A represents a well-formed extra digit that articulates with the small finger metacarpal or a duplicate small finger metacarpal. Type B ulnar polydactyly describes a poorly formed digit without bony attachments to the small finger. Type B ulnar polydactyly can be inherited as an autosomal dominant trait and can be seen in the black population with an incidence

TABLE 122.3 Thumb Grasp and Pinch Assessment: 9 Goal-Specific Activities for Three Separate Age Groups

	Ages 18 Months–4 Years	Ages 5–7 Years	Ages 8–18 Years
Tip pinch	Pick up three Cheerios one at a time and release into a film container. *Score how the Cheerio is held.*	Pick up three pennies one at a time and release into a piggy bank. *Score how the penny is held.*	Thread five plastic beads onto a zip tie. *Score how the bead is held.*
Lateral key pinch	Open a zippered pencil case and remove two markers. *Score how the zipper tab is held.*	Turn a key to open a 1⅜-inch Master Padlock. *Score how the key is held.*	Turn a key to open a 1⅜-inch Master Padlock. *Score how the key is held.*
Small grasp	Pull cap off a large diameter Crayola marker. *Score how the marker is held.*	Pull cap off a small diameter Crayola marker. *Score how the marker is held.*	Remove the cap from a ballpoint pen. *Score how the pen is held.*
Medium grasp	Separate five Duplos that are stacked together. *Score how the Duplos are held.*	Turn the end of a kaleidoscope three times. *Score how the kaleidoscope is held.*	Make a telescope with a 5 × 7-inch sheet of paper and place a rubber band over it. *Score how the paper tube is held.*
Large grasp	Open a 4-oz jar of bubbles. *Score how the bottle is held.*	Twist cap from a 3-inch-diameter peanut butter jar. *Score how the container is held.*	Twist cap off from a 3-inch-diameter peanut butter jar. *Score how the container is held.*
Manipulation	Form Play-Doh into a bowl. *Score how the Play-Doh is held.*	Form Play-Doh into a bowl. *Score how the Play-Doh is held.*	Rotate a pencil three times in a handheld pencil sharpener. *Score how the pencil is held.*
Resistance	Open a drawstring bag. *Score how the bag is held when opened.*	Pull back the foam pull on a slingshot. *Score how the foam pull is held.*	Pull back the foam pull on a slingshot. *Score how the foam pull is held.*
School	Open a box of eight crayons and remove one. *Score how the crayon is held.*	Color inside a circle with a crayon. *Score how the crayon is held.*	Write name with a no. 2 pencil. *Score how pencil is held.*
Activities of daily living	Put a sock on over the toes. *Score how the sock is opened.*	Tie shoelaces into a knot. *Score how the laces are held.*	Tie shoelaces into a bow. *Score how the laces are held.*

TABLE 122.4 Manske's Classification of Cleft Hand

Type	Description	Characteristics
1	Normal first web	Normal first webspace
2a	Mild narrowing	Mild narrowing of the first web
2b	Severely narrowed	First webspace severely narrowed
3	Syndactylized	No web; thumb–index finger syndactyly
4	Merged webspace	Index finger absent, with first webspace merged with cleft
5	Absent	Thumb and radial components suppressed; ulnar ray remains

as high as 1 in 150 births.[129,130] Treatment for both types is operative and ranges from soft tissue excision to amputation of the duplicated finger with or without augmentation of the retained digit. Functional outcome is good, and rehabilitation considerations in these patients are likely to be minimal (Fig. 122.20).

Madelung's Deformity[15,18,29,67]

This deformity was previously grouped by the Swanson classification into the "other" category, whereas the OMT classification places Madelung's deformity into class IA2, indicating a malformation of the limb in the radial–ulnar axis. Madelung's deformity is an abnormality that may be isolated to the wrists, with overall decreased growth of the distal radius and with increased slope or tilt of the distal radius, because of asymmetry of the diminished growth, which is usually more significant ulnarly and volarly. This also results in an ulna that is longer than the radius, resulting in subluxation (usually dorsal, infrequently volar), ulnocarpal impaction, or both. Some cases of this deformity are random; many are associated with a generalized skeletal syndrome known as *dyschondrosteosis*. Function and appearance are seldom severe problems until adolescence, when pain, particularly with repetitive or high-intensity function, is noted. Therefore, surgical treatment traditionally has been applied late, if at all. Increasing evidence suggests early release of the more involved areas (e.g., a bony bar or an abnormal structure, such as radiolunate ligament, pronator quadratus with carpal insertions)[14] of the distal radius physis may permit growth correction. Otherwise, the surgical correction involves various types of osteotomy of the radius with bone graft interposition, often associated with shortening or removal of the distal ulna. The usual assessment and rehabilitation training are useful adjuncts to these treatments.

Central Deficiencies (Typical and Atypical Cleft Hand)

Central deficiency is used to describe a variety of deformities in which there is a deficiency within the central portion of the hand. These deformities have been referred to as "lobster" claw deformities, the split hand complex, ectrodactyly, or typical and atypical cleft hand.[131–133] Many of these children may also show evidence of central syndactyly and central polysyndactyly.[134,135]

Typical or classic cleft hand deformity can be unilateral or bilateral, and many cases express an autosomal dominant inheritance pattern. The hand cleft tends to be deep and V-shaped and may have varying degrees of syndactyly (Fig. 122.21). *Atypical cleft hand* usually presents with a phenotypic symbrachydactyly. These clefts tend to be U shaped and are unilateral and sporadic in nature. Deficiencies may include skin within the first webspace, and in severe cases, children may present with an absent thumb in addition to central elements (Fig. 122.22).[136] Multiple classification schemes have been designed to encompass all types of central deficiencies, but the authors believe the one designed by Manske can aid in the surgical decision-making process (see Table 122.4).

Indications for surgical treatment in these children is dependent on thumb function, adequacy of the first webspace, and the number of functional remaining fingers. Often typical cleft hands require no treatment. Dr. Adrian Flatt[114] has described the centrally deficient hands as functional triumphs but cosmetic disasters. In these children, the preservation of the thumb and a large webspace allows for prehension and grasp. Often cosmetic closure of the cleft can be performed in these children with little consequence to hand function.[137] Reasons to pursue surgery in these children include:

1. Flexion contractures
2. Malpositioning of the index finger ray or bridging bones at the base of the webspace
3. Deficient first webspace
4. Absent thumb

In general, most patients with central deficiency do well functionally and do not require surgery. Surgery motivated by aesthetic reasons alone may do the child a disservice by improving appearance but diminishing prehensile function. For patients considering surgery, therapists should complete a functional assessment to assess grasp and pinch function and their impact on everyday activities. These results may aid the surgeon and family with decision making when weighing the benefits of cosmetic gains versus possible loss of function.

Syndactyly

Syndactyly, or webbing between adjacent digits, is one of the most common congenital hand anomalies, occurring in one in every 2000 to 2500 births.[138] *Complete syndactyly* refers to fusion extending to the distal extent of the fingers, and *incomplete syndactyly* refers to fusion

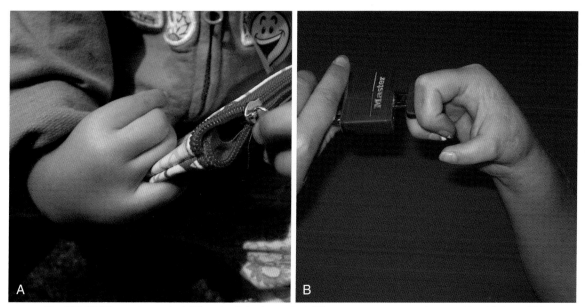

Fig. 122.15 Ulnar scissor pinch (**A**) and radial scissor pinch (**B**), two grasp patterns often used by children with thumb hypoplasia but rarely seen in other populations. (Reproduced with permission under STM Signatory guidelines from Kollitz KM, Tomhave WA, Van Heest AE, Moran SL. A new, direct measure of thumb use in children after index pollicization for congenital thumb hypoplasia. *J Hand Surg Am.* 2018;43[11]:978-986.e1.)

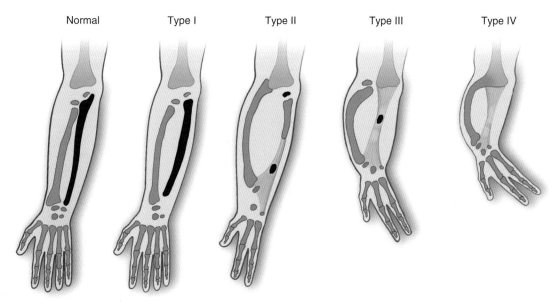

Fig. 122.16 Classification scheme for ulnar hypoplasia.

that fails to reach the distal extent of the finger. *Complex syndactyly* refers to a concomitant bony fusion between the two joined digits, whereas *simple syndactyly* refers to the absence of a bony connection. Syndactyly may occur in isolation (*pure syndactyly*) or in conjunction

with other congenital anomalies, in which it is referred to as *complicated syndactyly*. It is often seen in conjunction with brachydactyly, in which it is referred to as *brachysyndactyly*, and in central polydactyly, in which it is referred to as *central polysyndactyly*.[139] The cause of syndactyly is thought to be a failure of preprogrammed cell death, or apoptosis, during the developmental period.

Isolated incomplete pure syndactyly is most commonly encountered between the long and ring fingers.[1,140] In many cases, this may produce little functional deficit to the patient; however, when the syndactyly extends to the distal third of the proximal phalanx, it will inhibit finger abduction and potentially result in finger rotation. Greater deformity will occur if the syndactyly includes either of the border digits. Here the shorter digit will often tether the growth of the adjacent finger, resulting in bowing, loss of motion, and potential joint deformity.

The reconstructive technique can vary depending on the severity of the syndactyly, but most surgical procedures use a dorsal skin flap to reconstruct the webspace and advancement flaps from the palmar and dorsal aspect of the fingers to reconstruct some of the commissure finger skin.[141,142] Almost all children will require some skin grafting for complete coverage of the soft tissue defect. Full-thickness grafts are preferred and can be taken from the groin, antecubital fossa, medial aspect of the upper arm, or medial or lateral aspect of the malleolus. Most surgical procedures are performed between 6 months and 2 years of age.[141,143-145] Complications from surgery include scarring; "web creep," which refers to distal advancement of the finger commissure over time; finger stiffness; and skin graft loss.[146]

Long-term follow-up studies of syndactyly release show good results. Lumenta and associates[147] reported on 19 patients with 26 affected webspaces at an average of 11.5 years of follow up. Using a triangular dorsal and palmar skin flap design with full-thickness skin grafting as needed for tension-free closure, they reported webspace creep in only two webspaces. ROM, finger abduction power, and two-point discrimination were not different between affected and unaffected sides. Commissure hair growth at the onset of puberty was reported in 17 of 24 cases in which the groin was the source of full-thickness skin grafting, leading the authors to recommend a more lateral donor site at the inguinal crease. Niranjan and coworkers[148] reported web creep in 4 of 25 webspaces at

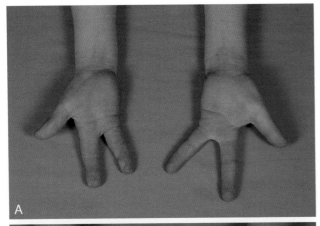
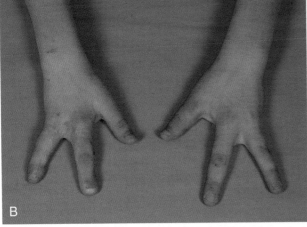

Fig. 122.17 **A** and **B,** Hand presentation in cases of ulnar hypoplasia.

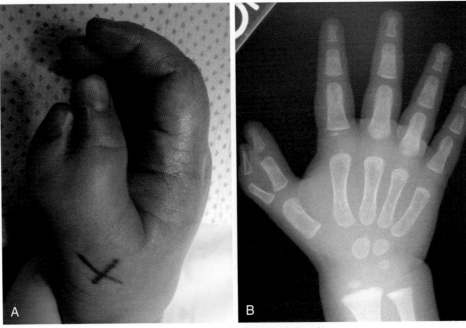

Fig. 122.18 **A** and **B,** Radial polydactyly.

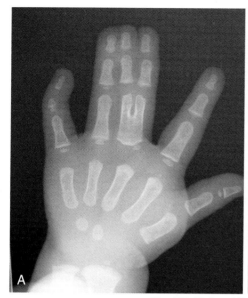
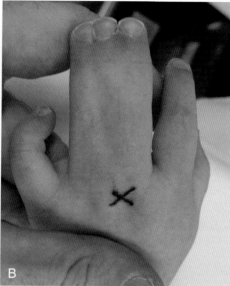

Fig. 122.19 A and **B,** Central polydactyly.

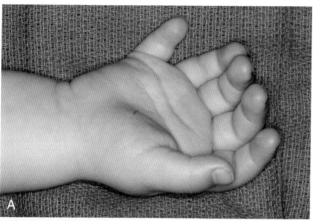
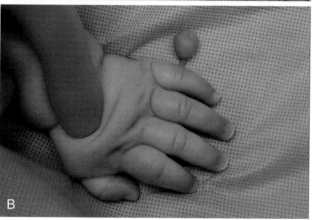

Fig. 122.20 Ulnar polydactyly type I (**A**) and type II (**B**).

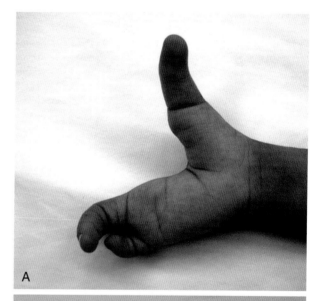
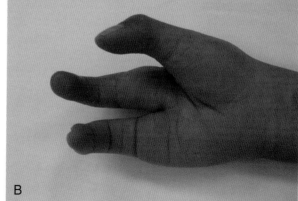

Fig. 122.21 A and **B,** Typical cleft hand deformity.

an average of 6.6 years of follow-up using a trilobed flap technique for reconstruction of the commissure. No skin grafting was required for this technique. In a 16-year follow-up study of syndactyly release of 29 webspaces with the trilobed flap technique, only two operations for webspace creep were required.[149] Twenty-two of 29 webspaces had skin thickening, and 7 reported creep up to one third of the distance from the MCP joint to the proximal interphalangeal (PIP) joint; however, no intervention was required. Overall, patients reported excellent function with a

median QuickDASH (Disability of the Arm, Shoulder and Hand) score of 2.3 points and normal sensation and dexterity.

Postsurgical therapy includes 2 to 4 weeks of casting followed by warm water soaks for gentle cleansing of the incision scar areas.

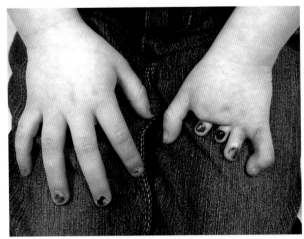

Fig. 122.22 Symbrachydactyly.

Therapy in these cases is designed to minimize scarring and prevent potential web creep. A hand-based orthosis is recommended for digits, which should have separate finger straps to control lateral deviation. For less involved digits and for young children who have difficulties with formal orthosis wear, elastomer spacers held in place with tape work well to minimize web creep and keep the digits partially abducted. Scar management is essential after initial cast removal. Special attention should be paid to ensure good wound healing in any areas of graft slough or partial graft loss, particularly in the webspace. Night orthosis wear is discontinued at 12 weeks after surgery. Additional therapy may be indicated later for bony deformities or scar problems.

Camptodactyly

Camptodactyly describes a painless flexion contracture at the PIP joint.[150] The classic presentation involves the little finger PIP joints in isolation, but additional fingers may be involved, particularly when camptodactyly is encountered as part of a syndrome.[151] The contracture usually progresses during childhood. Most deformities are thought to result from an anomalous lumbrical insertion or from an abnormal FDS tendon; however, all structures surrounding the PIP joint have been implicated in the etiology of this deformity.[152–157]

Nonsurgical treatment is recommended before any surgical intervention. Stretching, use of a removable orthosis, and serial casting can be used to improve the flexion contracture. Younger children usually require forearm-based orthoses. The duration of orthosis wear is debatable, but most regimens require at least 10 to 12 hours of wear per day until the deformity is corrected. A nighttime maintenance orthosis should continue until the time of skeletal maturity.[158–160]

Surgical release is recommended only in those cases refractory to orthosis use and with deformities greater than 40 degrees of flexion. Successful surgery requires release of all contracted structures, including anomalous lumbrical muscles and FDS tendons.[153,155] Tendon transfer is recommended for those patients who are preoperatively unable to extend the PIP joint when the MCP joint is positioned in flexion. The FDS tendon or extensor indices proprius may be used to improve active extension.[161]

Clinodactyly

Clinodactyly refers to fingers that are angled in the radial–ulnar plane. This anomaly is most common in the little finger, in which angulation is seen occurring distal to the MCP joint and directed toward the ring finger. Deviation beyond 10 degrees is considered significant. Many cases are familial; multiple digits may be involved, and there may be associated syndromes.[162,163] The anomaly develops because of abnormal longitudinal growth of the underlying phalanx. Many cases are caused by the presence of a *delta phalanx*, which describes a shortened, trapezoidal-shaped bone with a bracketed physis.[164] More recently, these abnormal physes have been described as longitudinal epiphyseal brackets to more accurately describe the shortened physis, which consists of a longitudinal composite of the proximal and distal epiphyseal ossification centers within the middle phalanx.[20]

Isolated clinodactyly of the small finger rarely warrants treatment. Use of an orthosis provides no benefit because the defect is caused by a bony problem. Surgery is indicated for severe deformities which produce shortening or angulation. Surgery involves some form of corrective osteotomy. Other alternatives include attempts at release of the tethered physis; this treatment is appropriate in patients with open physes of the longitudinally bracketed diaphysis or delta bone type.[165] Extensor tendon adhesions or contracture of the dorsal capsule of the distal interphalangeal (DIP) joint can occur postoperatively and may be benefited by rehabilitation measures, particularly stretching or static and dynamic orthosis use.

Deformations
Congenital Constriction Band Syndrome

Congenital constriction band syndrome, also known as amnionic band syndrome, congenital band syndrome, constriction band syndrome, and Streeter's disease, is characterized by partial or complete circumferential constriction around the digits or extremities[34,35] (Fig. 122.23). This congenital anomaly is present 1 in 1200 to 1 in 15,000 live births.[34] This anomaly is represented equally in males and females and is thought to be caused by adhesions developing between the amnion and developing fetus secondary to disruption of the amnionic membranes. Most deformities are seen in the extremities, but craniofacial defects and body wall defects can occur.[166,167]

The anomalies observed are diverse and can affect any limb, producing single or multiple deformities. Hand deformities can include simple rings without distal compromise, rings with distal lymphedema, rings accompanied by distal finger fusion (also known as *acrosyndactyly*) and finally congenital amputation.[2,168] Occasionally, proximal banding can produce nerve compression, vascular compromise, and muscular hypoplasia to the distal extremity. Anatomic structures proximal to the banding are normal.

Indications for operative intervention include both functional and cosmetic considerations, including distal lymphedema, nerve or vascular compromise, progressive constriction with functional impairment, and correction of syndactyly. The degree of involvement may necessitate early surgery (occasionally within the first few days of birth) if banding produces distal limb ischemia, gangrene, or lymphedematous areas become infected. The surgical possibilities for reconstruction include web release and construction; digit lengthening or augmentation; constriction band release (some of which have been found to contain amnion); debridement of fibrotic thickening; and replacement of nonfunctioning nerves, vessels, or musculotendinous units. Surgical correction includes isolated band excision with Z-plasty closure (for constriction band with distal lymphedema) to more involved reconstructions for syndactyly, nerve involvement, and short digits.[169] Cases of intrauterine endoscopic band release for impending amputation have also been reported, although this approach carries inherent risk and has not been widely adopted to date.[170–172] Rehabilitative considerations for these patients include lymphedema control, retraining, ROM, and scar management. For significant limb involvement, this may also include prosthesis fitting and training.

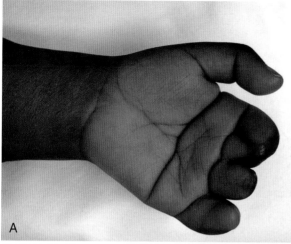

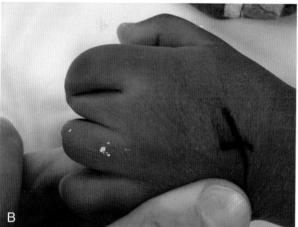

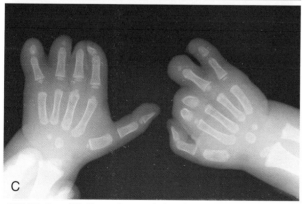

Fig. 122.23 **A** and **B,** Case of constriction ring syndrome in a 16-month-old girl. The constriction bands have resulted in distal amputations of the index through small finger and additional acrosyndactyly of the index and long finger. **C,** Additional distal amputations are seen on the radiographs of the affected and contralateral hand.

Dysplasias

Macrodactyly

Overgrowth is defined as pathologic enlargement of soft tissue parts with associated enlargement of the skeleton. When this process occurs within the hand, it is referred to as *macrodactyly* or *digital gigantism.* This anomaly is rare in the upper extremity with a reported incidence of fewer than 1% of all patients with congenital hand anomalies.[173] Phalanges, tendons, nerves, vessels, subcutaneous fat, fingernails, and skin can all be enlarged, but the metacarpals are often spared. Because of the diversity in clinical presentation, several classification systems have

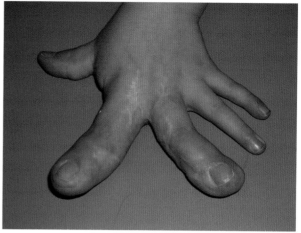

Fig. 122.24 Macrodactyly.

been proposed. Flatt has described four major types of overgrowth, with group I representing patients with lipofibromatosis, group II representing patients with macrodactyly caused by neurofibromatosis, group III representing patients with hyperostosis, and group IV representing patients with hemihypertrophy.[114,144] Although the etiology of overgrowth remains unclear, abnormal blood supply, nerve supply, and growth factors have all been implicated.

Many cases of overgrowth tend to occur within the distribution of the median or ulnar nerves[174] (Fig. 122.24). This form of macrodactyly has no known familial inheritance pattern and is usually not associated with other conditions.[173,175,176] It is unilateral in 90% of cases, males outnumber females by a 3:2 ratio, and multiple digits are affected three times as often as single digits.[176] Digits affected by macrodactyly tend to outgrow normal digits, become progressively stiff and angulated, and can interfere with overall hand function. In many cases, two-point discrimination is diminished and further limits the use of the digit.[177,178]

Surgical management depends on the patient's age and function present within the digit. Children presenting early have the best chance for improvement. In these cases, early debulking procedures, elective growth plate closure (epiphysiodesis), and closing-wedge osteotomies can be used to slow growth and correct angular deformities.[179,180] Older patients presenting with fully developed macrodactyly can be offered the surgical option of partial or total finger amputation, joint fusion, or debulking procedures as options to improve hand function.

Multiple Exostoses[73]

Multiple exostoses is considered a skeletal dysplasia in the OMT classification (group IIIB3). It is usually familial and autosomal dominant, with common involvement of multiple areas of the hands and forearms. The ulna often becomes shorter than the radius, although both bones are short compared with normal. Bowing of the radius, subluxation of the carpus, and subluxation or dislocation of the radial head are common forearm and wrist deformities and may be treated surgically. The surgical methods in use include excision, corrective osteotomy, partial physis closure, and bone lengthening. Exostoses in the hands, which are deforming, function limiting, or often traumatized, also are surgically treated by excision. Routine axial imaging of the head and spine at least once during childhood is recommended in this patient population because more than 20% of children with this syndrome may have compressive spinal or intracranial exostoses.[181] Unless symptoms warrant it, screening with MRI of the head and spine after the child has reached an age when general anesthesia is not needed has been recommended.[181] This screening strategy avoids the radiation associated with computed tomography in a population of growing children who have exostosis with the potential for malignant transformation in adulthood.

REFERENCES

1. Flatt AE. *The Care of Congenital Hand Anomalies. Ulnar Deficiencies.* St Louis: Quality Medical Publishers; 1994:411–424.
2. Moran SL, Berger RA. Biomechanics and hand trauma: what you need. *Hand Clin.* 2003;19:17–31.
3. Lutz CS, Kozin SH. Congenital differences in the hand and upper extremity. In: Burke, Higgins JP, eds. *Hand and Upper Extremity Rehabilitation. A Practical Guide.* 2006:659–688.
4. Dobyns JH. Helping parents decide what is best for their child. *Hand Clin.* 1990;6:551.
5. Dobyns JH, Wood VE, Bayne LG. *Congenital Hand Deformities.* New York: Churchill Livingstone; 1993.
6. Bradbury E. Psychological issues for children and their parents. In: Buck-Gramcko D, ed. *Congenital Malformations of the Hand and Forearm.* London: Churchill Livingstone; 1998:48–56.
7. Kozin SH. Congenital disorders: classification and diagnosis. In: Berger RA, Weiss APC, eds. *Hand Surgery.* Philadelphia: Lippincott Williams and Wilkins; 2004:1405–1423.
8. Riddle RD, Tabin CJ. How limbs develop. *Sci Am.* 1999;280:74–79.
9. Bamshad M, Watkins WS, Dixon ME, et al. Reconstructing the history of human limb development: lessons from birth defects. *Pediatr Res.* 1999;45(3):291–299.
10. Martin GR. The roles of FGF's in early development of vertebrate limbs. *Genes Dev.* 1998;12:1571–1586.
11. Summerbell D, Lewis JH, Wolpert L. Positional information in chick-limb morphogenesis. *Nature.* 1973;244:492.
12. Al-Qattan MM, Yang Y, Kozin SH. Embryology of the upper limb. *J Hand Surg Am.* 2009;34(7):1340–1350.
13. Borud LJ, Upton J. Embryology of the upper limb. In: Mathes SJ, Hentz VR, eds. *Plastic Surgery.* Philadelphia: Saunders; 2006:3–23.
14. Riddle RD, Ensini M, Nelson C, et al. Induction of the LIM homeobox gene Lmx 1 by WNT7a establishes dorsoventral pattern in the vertebrate limb. *Cell.* 1995;83:631–640.
15. Parr BA, MvMahon AP. Dorsalizing signal Wnt-7a required for normal polarity of D-V and A-P axes of the mouse limb. *Nature.* 1995;374:350–353.
16. Buck-Gramcko D. Teratologic sequence. In: Livingstone C, ed. *Congenital Malformations of the Hand and Forearm.* London: Churchill Livingstone; 1998:17–20.
17. Swanson AB. A classification for congenital limb malformations. *J Hand Surg.* 1976;1:8–22.
18. DeSmet L, Matton G, Monstrey S, et al. Application of the IFSSH (3) classification for congenital anomalies of the hand: results and problems. *Acta Orthop Belg.* 1997;63:182–188.
19. Cheng JCY, Chow SK, Leung PC. Classification of 578 cases of congenital upper limb anomalies with the IFSSH system—a 10 years' experience. *J Hand Surg.* 1987;12A:1055–1060.
20. Light TR, Ogden JA. The longitudinal epiphyseal bracket: implications for surgical correction. *J Pediatr Orthop.* 1981;1:299–305.
21. Buckwalter JA, Flatt AE, Shurr DG, Dryer RF, Blair WF. The absent fifth metacarpal. *J Hand Surg.* 1981;6:354–367.
22. Oberg KC, Feenstra JM, Manske PR, Tonkin MA. Developmental biology and classification of congenital anomalies of the hand and upper extremity. *J Hand Surg Am.* 2010;35(12):2066–2076.
23. Miura T. Syndactyly and split hand. *Hand.* 1976;8:125–130.
24. Miura T. Syndactyly and split hand. *Hand.* 1978;10(suppl):99–103.
25. Tada K, Kurisaki E, Yonenobu K, Tsuyuguchi Y, Kawai H. Central polydactyly—a review of 12 cases and their surgical treatment. *J Hand Surg.* 1982;7:460–465.
26. Ogino T, Minami A, Kato H. Clinical features and roentgenograms of symbrachydactyly. *J Hand Surg.* 1989;14B:303–306.
27. Tonkin MA, Oberg KC. The OMT classification of congenital anomalies of the hand and upper limb. *Hand Surg.* 2015;20(3):336–342.
28. Ezaki M. *IFSSH Committee on Congenital Conditions.* 2014.
29. IFSSH. *OMT Classification of Congenital Hand and Upper Extremity Anomalies.* 2015.
30. Bae DS, Canizares MF, Miller PE, et al. Intraobserver and interobserver reliability of the Oberg-Manske-Tonkin (OMT) classification: establishing a registry on congenital upper limb differences. *J Pediatr Orthop.* 2016.
31. Manske PR, McCarroll HR. Reconstruction of the congenitally deficient thumb. *Hand Clin.* 1992;8:177–196.
32. Blauth W. Der hypoplastische daumen. *Arch Orthop Unfallchir.* 1967;62:225.
33. Ogden JA, Watson HK, Bohne W. Ulnar dysmelia. *J Bone Joint Surg.* 1976;58A:467–475.
34. Moran SL, Jenson M, Bravo C. Amniotic band syndrome of the upper extremity: diagnosis and management. *J Am Acad Orthop Surg.* 2007;15:397–407.
35. Weidrich TA. Congenital constriction band syndrome. *Hand Clin.* 1998;14:29–38.
36. Postema K, van der Donk V, van Limbeek J, Rijken RAJ, Poelma MJ. Prosthesis rejection in children with a unilateral congenital arm defect. *Clin Rehabil.* 1999;13:243–249.
37. Scotland TR, Galway HR. A long term review of children with congenital and acquired limb deficiency. *J Bone Joint Surg (Br).* 1983;65B:346–349.
38. Datta D, Kingston J, Ronald J. Myoelectric prostheses for below elbow amputees: the Trent experience. *Int Disabil Stud.* 1989;11:167–170.
39. Davids JR, Wagner LV, Meyer LC, et al. Prosthetic management of children with unilateral congenital below-elbow deficiency. *J Bone Joint Surg (Am).* 2006;88:1294–1300.
40. James MA, Bagley AM, Brasington K, Lutz C, McConnell S, Molitor F. Impact of prostheses on function and quality of life for children with unilateral congenital below-the-elbow deficiency. *J Bone Joint Surg (Am).* 2006;88:2356–2365.
41. Buffart LM, Roebroeck ME, van Heijningen VG, Pesch-Batenburg JM, Stam HJ. Evaluation of arm and prosthetic functioning in children with a congenital transverse reduction deficiency of the upper limb. *J Rehabil Med.* 2007;39:379–386.
42. Taussig H. A study of the German outbreak of phocomelia: a thalidomide syndrome. *JAMA.* 1962;180:1106–1114.
43. Sulamaa A. Early treatment of congenital bone defects of the extremities: aftermath of thalidomide disaster. *Lancet.* 1964;18:130–132.
44. Swanson A. Phocomelia and congenital limb malformation: reconstruction and prosthetic replacement. *Am J Surg.* 1965;109:294–299.
45. Kay HW, Day HJ, Henkel HL, et al. The proposed international terminology of the classification of congenital limb deficiencies. *Dev Med Child Neuro Suppl.* 1975;34:1–12.
46. Upton J. Management of transverse and longitudinal deficiencies (Failure of Formation). In: Mathes SJ, ed. *Plastic Surgery.* Philadelphia: Saunders Elsevier; 2006:51–131.
47. Seitz WH, Froimson AI. Callotasis lengthening in the upper extremity: indications, techniques, and pitfalls. *J Hand Surg.* 1991;16A:932–939.
48. Miura T, Nakamura R, Horii E. The position of symbrachydactyly in the classification of congenital hand anomalies. *J Hand Surg [Br].* 1994;19:350–354.
49. Ravitch M. Poland's syndrome -a study of an eponym. *Plast Reconstr Surg.* 1977;59:508–512.
50. Mace J, Kaplan JM, Schanberger JE, Gotlin RW. Poland's syndrome. Report of seven cases and review of the literature. *Clin Pediatr.* 1972;98:98–102.
51. Al-Quattan M. Classification of hand anomalies in Poland's syndrome. *Br J Plast Surg.* 2001;54:132–136.
52. Baas M, Burger EB, Sneiders D, Galjaard RH, Hovius SER, van Nieuwenhoven CA. Controversies in Poland syndrome: alternative diagnoses in patients with congenital pectoral muscle deficiency. *J Hand Surg Am.* 2018;43(2):186. e1– e16.
53. Yamauchi Y, ed. *Symbrachydactyly.* London: Churchill-Livingstone; 1998.
54. DeSmet L, Fabray G. Characteristics of patients with symbrachydactyly. *J Pediatr Orthop.* 1998;2:158–161.
55. Vilkki SK. Advances in microsurgical reconstruction of the congenitally adactylous hand. *Clin Orthop.* 1995;314:45–58.
56. Radocha RF, Netscher D, Kleinert HE. Toe phalangeal grafts in congenital hand anomalies. *J Hand Surg.* 1993;18A:833–841.

57. Buck-Gramcko D. The role of non-vascularized toe phalanx transplantation. *Hand Clin.* 1990;6:643.

58. Carroll RE, Green DP. Reconstruction of the hypoplastic digits using toe phalanges. *J Bone Joint Surg.* 1975;57:727 (abstr).

59. Kleinert H, Brotherston M, Mesa-Betancourt F. Free toe phalangeal transfers in congenital hand anomalies. In: Gupta A, Kay SPJ, Scheker LR, eds. *The Growing Hand.* London: Churchill Livingston; 2000:1045–1048.

60. Evans JA, Vitez M, Czeizel A. Congenital abnormalities associated with limb deficiency defects: a population study based on cases from the Hungarian Congenital Malformation Registry (1975-1984). *Am J Med Genetics.* 1994;49:52–66.

61. Bod M, Czeizel A, Lenz W. Incidence at birth of different types of limb reduction abnormalities in Hungary 1975-1977. *Hum Genet.* 1983;65: 27–33.

62. Kallen B, Rahmani TM, Winberg J. Infants with congenital limb reduction registered in the Swedish Register of Congenital Malformations. *Teratology.* 1984;29:73–85.

63. Lamb DW. Radial club hand: a continuing study of sixty-eight patients with one hundred and seventeen club hands. *J Bone Joint Surg.* 1977;59A:1–13.

64. Urban MA, Osterman AL. Management of radial dysplasia. *Hand Clin.* 1990;6:589.

65. Lin A, Perloff J. Upper limb malformations associated with congenital heart disease. *Am J Cardiol.* 1985;55:1576–1583.

66. Fanconi G. Familial constitutional panmyelocytopathy. Fanconi's anemia I. Clinical aspects. *Semin Hematol.* 1967;4:233–240.

67. Wynne-Davies R, Lamb DW. Congenital upper limb anomalies: an etiologic grouping of clinical, genetic, and epidemiological data from 387 patients with "absence" defects, constriction bands polydactylies and syndactylies. *J Hand Surg.* 1985;10:958–964.

68. Quan L, Smith D. The VATER association: vertebral defects, anal atresia, T-E fistula with esophageal atresia , radial and renal dysplasia: a spectrum of associated defects. *J Pediatr.* 1973;82:104–107.

69. Goldfarb CA, Wall L, Manske PR. Radial longitudinal deficiency: the incidence of associated medical and musculoskeletal conditions. *J Hand Surg [Am].* 2006;31:1176–1182.

70. Auerbach A, Sagi M, Adler B. Fanconi's anemia: prenatal diagnosis in 30 fetuses at risk. *Pediatrics.* 1985;76:794–800.

71. Maschke SD, Seitz W, Lawton J. Radial longitudinal deficiency. *J Am Acad Orthop Surg.* 2007;15:41–52.

72. Hedberg V, Lipton JM. Thrombocytopenia with absent radii. *Am J Pediatr.* 1988;10:51–64.

73. Smith AA, Greene TL. Preliminary soft tissue distraction in congenital forearm deficiency. *J Hand Surg.* 1995;20A:420–424.

74. Nanchahal J, Tonkin MA. Pre-operative distraction lengthening for radial longitudinal deficiency. *J Hand Surg.* 1996;21B:103–107.

75. Ekblom AG, Dahlin LB, Rosberg HE, Wiig M, Werner M, Arner M. Hand function in adults with radial longitudinal deficiency. *J Bone Joint Surg Am.* 2014;96(14):1178–1184.

76. Ekblom AG, Dahlin LB, Rosberg HE, Wiig M, Werner M, Arner M. Hand function in children with radial longitudinal deficiency. *BBMC Musculoskelet Disord.* 2013;14:116.

77. Kotwal PP, Varshney MK, Soral A. Comparison of surgical treatment and nonoperative management for radial longitudinal deficiency. *J Hand Surg Eur.* 2012;37(2):161–169.

78. Manske PR, McCarroll HR JR, Swanson K. Centralization of the radial club hand: an ulnar surgical approach. *J Hand Surg Am.* 1981;6(5):423–433.

79. Kawabata H, Yasui N, Ariga K, Shirata T. Bone lengthening with the ilizarov apparatus for congenital club hands. *Tech Hand Up Extrem Surg.* 1998;2(1):72–77.

80. Geck MJ, Dorey F, Lawrence JF, Johnson MK. Congenital radius deficiency: Radiographic outcome and survivorship analysis. *J Hand Surg.* 1999;24:1132–1144.

81. Damore E, Kozin SH, Thoder JJ, Porter S. The recurrence of deformity after surgical centralization for radial clubhand. *J Hand Surg.* 2000;25:745–751.

82. Peterson BM, McCarroll HR, James MA. Distraction lengthening of the ulna in children with radial longitudinal deficiency. *J Hand Surg.* 2007;32:1402–1407.

83. Abdel-Ghani H, Amro S. Characteristics of patients with hypoplastic thumb: a prospective study of 51 patients with the results of surgical treatment. *J Pediatr Orthop.* 2004;13:127–138.

84. James MA, McCarroll HR, Manske PR. Characteristics of patients with hypoplastic thumbs. *J Hand Surg.* 1996;21A:104–113.

85. Smith P. Congenital. In: Smith P, ed. *Lister's The Hand, Diagnosis and Indications.* London: Churchill Livingstone; 2002:505.

86. Tay SC, Moran SL, Shin AY, Cooney WP. The hypoplastic thumb. *J Am Acad Orthop Surg.* 2006;14:354–366.

87. Lee DH, Oakes JE, Ferlic RJ. Tendon transfers for thumb opposition: a biomechanical study of pulley location and two insertion sites. *J Hand Surg.* 2003;28A:1002–1008.

88. Ishida O, Ikuta Y, Sunagawa T, Ochi M. Abductor digiti minimi musculocutaneous island flap as an opposition transfer: a case report. *J Hand Surg.* 2003;28A:130–132.

89. Strauch B, Spinner M. Congenital anomaly of the thumb: absent intrinsics and flexor pollicis longus. *J Bone Joint Surg.* 1976;58A:115–118.

90. Graham TJ, Louis DS. A comprehensive approach to surgical management of the type IIIA hypoplastic thumb. *J Hand Surg.* 1998;23A:3–13.

91. Glickel SZ, Malerich M, Pearce SM, Littler JW. Ligament replacement for chronic instability of the ulnar collateral ligament of the metacarpophalangeal joint of the thumb. *J Hand Surg.* 1993;18A:930–941.

92. Vasenius J, Nieminen O, Lohman M. Late reconstruction of the ulnar collateral ligament of the thumb MP joint with free tendon graft - a new technique. *J Hand Surg.* 2003;28A 1:44.

93. Lister G. Reconstruction of the hypoplastic thumb. *Clin Orthop.* 1985;195:52–65.

94. Littler JW. On making a thumb: one hundred years of surgical effort. *J Hand Surg.* 1976;1:35–51.

95. Gosset J. La pollicization de l'index (Technique chirurgicale). *J Chir.* 1949;65:403–411.

96. Buck-Gramcko D. Pollicization of the index finger; method and results in aplasia and hypoplasia of the thumb. *J Bone Joint Surg.* 1971;53A:1605–1617.

97. Kozin SH, Weiss AA, Webber JB, Betz RR, Clancy M, Steel HH. Index finger pollicization for congenital aplasia or hypoplasia of the thumb. *J Hand Surg.* 1992;17A:880–884.

98. Ogino T, Ishii S. Long-term results after pollicization for congenital hand deformities. *Hand Surg.* 1997;2:79–85.

99. Manske PR, McCarroll HR. Reconstruction of the congenitally deficient thumb. *Hand Clin.* 1992;8:177.

100. Sykes PJ, Chandraprakasam T, Percival NJ. Pollicisation of the index finger in congenital anomalies, a retrospective analysis. *J Hand Surg.* 1991;16B:144–147.

101. Kollitz KM, Tomhave W, Van Heest AE, Moran SL. A direct measure of thumb use in children after index pollicization for radial longitudinal deficiency. *J Hand Surg.* 41(9):S33.

102. Tomhave W, Kollitz KM, Moran SL. Inter- and Intra-Rater Reliability of the Thumb Grasp and Pinch Assessment (T-GAP) for children following index pollicization for congenital thumb hypoplasia. *J Hand Surg.* 2018. status: submitted.

103. Birch-Jensen A. *Congenital Deformities of the Upper Extremity.* Copenhagen: Munksgaard; 1949.

104. Swanson AB, Tada K, Yonenobu K. Ulnar ray deficiency: its various manifestations. 1984;9A:658–664.

105. Carroll RE, Bowers WH. Congenital deficiency of the ulna. *J Hand Surg.* 1977;2:169–174.

106. Broudy AS, Smith RJ. Deformities of the hand and wrist with ulnar deficiency. *J Hand Surg.* 1979;4:304–315.

107. Johnson J, Omer GE. Congenital ulnar deficiency: natural history and therapeutic implications. *Hand Clin.* 1985;3:499–510.

108. Schwabe G, Mundlos S. Genetics of congenital hand anomalies. *Handchir Mikrochir Plast Chir.* 2004;36:85–97.

109. Bambshad M, Lin RC, Wastkins WC, et al. Mutations in human TBX3 alter limb apocrine and genital development in ulnar mammary syndrome. *Nat Genet.* 1997;16:311–315.

110. Elhassan BT, Biafora S, Light T. Clinical manifestations of type IV ulna longitudinal dysplasia. *J Hand Surg.* 2007;32:1024–1030.

111. Bayne L. Ulnar club hand (ulnar deficiencies). In: Green DP, ed. *Operative Hand Surgery*. New York: Churchill Livingstone; 1982:245–256.

112. Carroll R. Congenital absence of the ulna. In: Buck-Gramcko D, ed. *Congenital Malformations of the Hand and Forearm*. London: Churchill Livingstone; 1998:449–461.

113. Blair WF, Shurr DG, Buckwalter JA. Functional status in ulnar deficiency. *J Pediatr Orthop*. 1983;3:37–40.

114. Flatt AE. *The Care of Congenital Hand Anomalies*. St Louis: Mosby; 1977.

115. Cole RJ, Manske PR. Classification of ulnar deficiency according to the thumb and first web. *J Hand Surg*. 1997;22A:479–488.

116. Marcus NA, Omer GE. Carpal deviation in congenital ulnar deficiency. *J Bone Joint Surg*. 1984;66A:1003–1007.

117. Flatt AE. *The Role of Reconstructive Surgery. The Care of Congenital Hand Anomalies*. St Louis: CV Mosby; 1977:3–7.

118. Wassel HD. The results of surgery for polydactyly of the thumb. *Clin Orthop*. 1969;64:175–193.

119. Iwasawa M, Matsuo K, Hirose T, Sakaguchi Y. Improvement in the surgical results of treatment of duplicated thumb by preoperative splinting. *J Hand Surg*. 1989;14:941.

120. Townsend DJ, Lipp EB, Chun K, Reinker K, Tuch BA. Thumb duplication, 66 years' experience—a review of surgical complications. *J Hand Surg*. 1994;19A:973–976.

121. Cheng JCY, Chan KM, Ma GFY, Leung PC. Polydactyly of the thumb: a surgical plan based on ninety-five cases. *J Hand Surg*. 1984;9A:155–164.

122. Manske PR. Treatment of duplicated thumb using a ligamentous/periosteal flap. *J Hand Surg*. 1989;14A:728–733.

123. Naasan A, Page RE. Duplication of the thumb. *J Hand Surg*. 1994;19B:355–360.

124. Horii E, Nakamura R, Sakuma M, Miura T. Duplicated thumb bifurcation at the metacarpophalangeal joint level: factors affecting surgical outcome. *J Hand Surg*. 1997;22A:671–679.

125. Kawabata H, Masatomi T, Shimada K, Kawai H, Tada K. Treatment of residual instability and extensor lag in polydactyly of the thumb. *J Hand Surg*. 1993;18B:5–8.

126. Lettice LA, Hill RE. Preaxial polydactyly: a model for defective long-range regulation in congenital abnormalities. *Cur Opin Genet Devel*. 2005;15:294–300.

127. Lettice LA, Hill AE, Devenney PS, Hill RE. Point mutations in a distant sonic hedgehog cis-regulator generate a variable regulatory output responsible for preaxial polydactyly. *Hum Mol Genet*. 2008;17:978–985.

128. Gurnett CA, Bowcock AM, Dietz FR, Morcuende JA, Murray JC, Dobbs MB. Two novel point mutations in the long-range SHH enhancer in three families with triphalangeal thumb and preaxial polydactyly. *Am J Med Genet*. 2007;143:27–32.

129. Woolf CM, Myrianthopoulos NC. Polydactyly in America negroes and whites. *Am J Hum Genet*. 1973;25:397–404.

130. Watson BT, Hennrikus WL. Postaxial type-B polydactyly. Prevalence and treatment. *J Bone Joint Surg (Am)*. 1997;79:65–68.

131. Buck-Gramcko D. Cleft hands: classification and treatment. *Hand Clin*. 1985;13:467–473.

132. Warkany J. Syndromes. *Am J Dis Child*. 1971;121:365.

133. Barsky A. Cleft hand: classification, incidence and treatment. Review of the literature and report of nineteen cases. *J Bone Joint Surg (Am)*. 1964;46:1707–1720.

134. Ogino T. Cleft hand. *Hand Clin*. 1990;6:661–671.

135. Ogino T, Minami A, Fukuda K, Kato H. Congenital anomalies of the upper limb among the Japanese in Sapporo. *J Hand Surg*. 1986;11B:364.

136. Manske PR, Halikis MN. Surgical classification of central deficiency according to the thumb web. *J Hand Surg*. 1995;20A:687–697.

137. Flatt AE. *The Care of Congenital Hand Anomalies*. 2nd ed. St Louis: Quality Medical Publishers; 1994.

138. Maccollum DW. Webbed fingers. *Surg Gynecol Obstet*. 1940;71:782–789.

139. Ogino T. Current classification of congenital hand deformities based on experimental research. In: Saffar PAP, Foucher G, eds. *Current Practice in Hand Surgery*. London: Martin Dunitz Ltd; 1997.

140. Oka I, Watanabe H, Nagumo M, et al. Incidence of congenital anomalies in the hand. *J Jpn Soc Surg Hand*. 1988;5:771–774.

141. Davis JS, German WJ. Syndactylism (coherence of the fingers and toes). *Arch Surg*. 1930;21:32–75.

142. Kojima T, HIrase Y, eds. *Congenital Disorders: Syndactyly*. Philadelphia: Lippincott Williams and Wilkins; 2004.

143. Brown PM. Syndactyly—a review and long term results. *Hand*. 1977;9:16–27.

144. Upton J. Congenital anomalies of the hand and forearm. In: McCarthy JG, ed. *Plastic Surgery, the Hand*. Philadelphia: WB Saunders; 1990.

145. Eaton CJ, Lister GD. Syndactyly. *Hand Clin*. 1990;6:555–575.

146. Percival NJ, Sykes PJ. Syndactyly: a review of the factors which influence surgical treatment. *J Hand Surg*. 1989;14B:196–200.

147. Lumenta DB, Kitzinger HB, Beck H, Frey M. Long-term outcomes of web creep, scar quality, and function after simple syndactyly surgical treatment. *J Hand Surg Am*. 2010;35(8):1323–1329.

148. Niranjan NS, Azad SM, Fleming AN, Liew SH. Long-term results of primary syndactyly correction by the trilobed flap technique. *Br J Plast Surg*. 2005;58(1):14–21.

149. Widerberg A, Sommerstein K, Dahlin LB, Rosberg HE. Long-term results of syndactyly correction by the trilobed flap technique focusing on hand function and quality of life. *J Hand Surg Eur*. 2016;41(3):315–321.

150. Smith RJ, Kaplan EB. Camptodactyly and similar atraumatic flexion deformities of the proximal interphalangeal joints of the fingers. *J Bone Joint Surg*. 1968;50A:1187–1203.

151. Krakowiak PA, Bohnsack JF, Carey JC, Bamshad M. Clinical analysis of a variant of Freeman-Sheldon syndrome (DA2B). *Am J Med Genetics*. 1998;76:93–98.

152. Ogino T, Kato H. Operative findings in camptodactyly of the little finger. *J Hand Surg*. 1992;17B:661–664.

153. Minami A, Sakai T. Camptodactyly caused by abnormal insertion and origin of lumbrical muscle. *J Hand Surg*. 1993;18B:310–311.

154. McFarlane RM, Curry GI, Evans HB. Anomalies of the intrinsic muscles in camptodactyly. *J Hand Surg*. 1983;8:531–544.

155. McFarlane RM, Classen DA, Porte AM, Botz JS. The anatomy and treatment of camptodactyly of the small finger. *J Hand Surg*. 1992;17A:35–44.

156. Engber WD, Flatt AE. Camptodactyly: an analysis of sixty-six patients and twenty-four operations. *J Hand Surg*. 1977;2:216–224.

157. Smith PJ, Grobbelaar AO. Camptodactyly: a unifying theory and approach to surgical treatment. *J Hand Surg*. 1998;23A:14–19.

158. Siegert JJ, Cooney WP, Dobyns JH. Management of simple camptodactyly. *J Hand Surg*. 1990;15B:181–189.

159. Miura T, Nakamura R, Tamura Y. Long-standing extended dynamic splintage and release of an abnormal restraining structure in camptodactyly. *J Hand Surg*. 1992;17B:665–672.

160. Hori M, Nakura R, Inoue G, et al. Nonoperative treatment of camptodactyly. *J Hand Surg [Am]*. 1987:1061–1065.

161. Kay SPJ, ed. *Camptodactyly*. Philadelphia: Churchill Livingstone; 1999.

162. Hersh AH, DeMarinis F, Stecher RM. On the inheritance and development of clinodactyly. *Am J Hum Genet*. 1953;5:257–268.

163. Wood VE, Flatt AE. Congenital triangular bones in the hand. *J Hand Surg [Am]*. 1977;2:179–193.

164. Jones J. Delta phalanx. *J Bone Joint Surg Br*. 1964;46:226–228.

165. Vickers DW. Clinodactyly of the little finger: a simple operative technique for reversal of the growth abnormality. *J Hand Surg*. 1987;12B:335.

166. Moerman P, Fryns JP, Vandenberghe K, Lauweryns JM. Constrictive amniotic bands, amniotic adhesions, and limb-body wall complex: discrete disruption sequences with pathogenetic overlap. *Am J Med Gene*. 1992;42:470–479.

167. Bamforth JS. Amniotic band sequence: Streeter's hypothesis reexamined. *Am J Med Genetics*. 1992;44:280–287.

168. Patterson T. Congenital ring-constriction. *Br J Plast Surg*. 1961;14:1–31.

169. Deleted in review.

170. Keswani SG, Johnson MP, Adzick NS, et al. In utero limb salvage: fetoscopic release of amniotic bands for threatened limb amputation. *J Pediatr Surg*. 2003;38(6):848–851.

171. Quintero RA, Morales WJ, Phillips J, Kalter CS, Angel JL. In utero lysis of amniotic bands. *Ultrasound Obstet Gynecol: The Official Journal of the International Society of Ultrasound in Obstetrics and Gynecology*. 1997;10(5):316–320.

172. Ronderos-Dumit D, Briceno F, Navarro H, Sanchez N. Endoscopic release of limb constriction rings in utero. *Fetal Diagn Ther.* 2006;21(3):255–258.
173. Wood VE. Macrodactyly. *J Iowa Med Soc.* 1969;59:922–928.
174. Kelikian H. *Congenital Deformities of the Hand and Forearm.* Philadelphia: WB Saunders; 1974.
175. Dell PC. Macrodactyly. *Hand Clin.* 1985;1:511.
176. Upton J. Failure of differentiation and overgrowth. In: Mathes SJ, ed. *Plastic Surgery*. Philadelphia: Saunders Elsevier; 2006:299–317.
177. Barsky AJ. Macrodactyly. *J Bone Joint Surg Am.* 1967;49(7):1255–1266.
178. Mirza MA, King ET, Reinhart MK. Carpal tunnel syndrome associated with macrodactyly. *J Hand Surg Eur.* 1998;23(5):609–610.
179. Tsuge K. Treatment of macrodactyly. *J Hand Surg Am.* 1985;10(6 Pt 2):968–969.
180. Akinci M, Ay S, Ercetin O. Surgical treatment of macrodactyly in older children and adults. *J Hand Surg Am.* 2004;29(6):1010–1019.
181. Ashraf A, Larson AN, Ferski G, Mielke CH, Wetjen NM, Guidera KJ. Spinal stenosis frequent in children with multiple hereditary exostoses. *J Child Orthop'* 2013;7(3):183–194.

123

Upper Extremity Musculoskeletal Surgery in the Child with Cerebral Palsy: Surgical Options and Rehabilitation

L. Andrew Koman, Zhongyu Li, Beth Paterson Smith

OUTLINE

CRITICAL POINTS

- Functional impairment affects 80% of involved hands in patients with cerebral palsy; historically, fewer than 20% are optimal surgical candidates.
- The prevention of fixed deformity in younger children with intensive therapy and neuromuscular blocking agents has increased the percentage of patients eligible for upper extremity surgery.
- Multidisciplinary evaluations provide input to improve appropriate delineation of realistic and appropriate surgical goals.
- Patients with voluntary grasp and release, good sensibility, and cognitive capability are candidates for muscle–tendon transfers to balance muscle force across selected joints.
- Patients with dystonia, rigidity, poor sensibility, fixed contractures, and cognitive impairments experience unpredictable results

after muscle–tendon transfers. However, they may benefit from arthrodeses and tendon lengthening or tenotomy.
- When used in conjunction with extensor tendon rerouting and plication, fusion of the thumb metacarpal phalangeal joint eliminates one motion segment, improves stability, enhances function, and improves appearance in a reliable manner.
- Multiple procedures involving the hand, wrist, and forearm often are required.
- Postoperative therapy is crucial. It should be instituted even while the patient is in a cast. Static and occasionally dynamic outriggers are valuable adjuncts to casting. In addition to retraining muscles after transfers, strengthening is a crucial component of postoperative care in the child or adult with cerebral palsy.

With an incidence of 2.6 per 1000 live births, cerebral palsy is the most common cause of disability in childhood. Significant functional impairment exists in 80% of the upper limbs of children and adults with upper limb involvement (hemiparesis or quadriparesis). In addition to spasticity, patients may present with pain, muscle weakness, poor sensibility, and movement disorders. Consequently, patients often demonstrate poor self-esteem, difficulty with functional activities, and deformities that impair caregiving. About 10% to 20% of affected limbs in pediatric patients with cerebral palsy may benefit from surgical intervention.[1-5] This chapter provides an overview of (1) operative options available to improve or to maintain upper extremity range of motion (ROM), prevent osseous deformity, and delay or decrease joint contracture and (2) postoperative rehabilitation strategies.

EVALUATION

History and Physical Examination

A team approach with input from the patient, caregiver(s), therapists, teachers, social workers, and other health care providers provides the optimal history. However, for many encounters, all caregivers and

health care providers are not available, and the patient may be unable to convey historical information effectively. Therefore, several visits may be required to understand functional and other needs. The use of standardized questionnaires, functional classification scales (e.g., House Scale[6]), and standardized testing regimens (e.g., Melbourne Assessment of Unilateral Limb Function[7,8]) facilitates decision making.

A complete upper extremity examination includes an assessment of active range of motion (AROM) and passive range of motion (PROM), functional capability, muscle tone, sensibility, and the effect of volitional activity on the extremity. An assessment of the impact of deformities, (i.e., thumb-in-palm, swan-neck, boutonnière, and pronation) on ROM and function is important. Voluntary control of all motor groups is assessed to distinguish dynamic from static deformities. Movement disorders are noted and recorded. If present, the magnitude of involuntary movement is noted, and the effectiveness of upper limb motor control is assessed, quantified, and recorded. Functional grasp and release is determined with the wrist in flexion and extension. If possible, the patient is observed during ambulation, standing, sitting, and recumbency, and the effect of position on posturing and motion patterns is defined. Serial evaluations are helpful to fully assess patients because factors such as the time of day, degree of anxiety, and level of fatigue can influence clinical findings.

Functional motor testing (e.g., the Jebsen's Hand Function Test) may augment the evaluation of patients with mild to moderate upper extremity involvement; however, motor testing is not practical for evaluating patients with severe involvement. Muscles being considered for transfer are assessed to determine phasic and nonphasic control. If there is a clinical concern, electromyographic evaluation is requested. Sensibility testing should include an evaluation of proprioception, stereognosis, and two-point discrimination. These tests are helpful in identifying patients who are suitable candidates for complex reconstruction procedures. Individuals with limited sensory capability are not good candidates for sophisticated surgical techniques.[9]

Diagnostic Evaluation

Radiologic studies, electromyographic data, motion analysis, and diagnostic muscle blocks may provide additional diagnostic information. Plain radiographs, computed tomography, and magnetic resonance imaging may be used to evaluate joint and osseous deformities. Surface and needle electromyography help to provide qualitative and quantitative assessments of voluntary motor recruitment and the appropriateness of motor activations.[10–12] A quantitative measure of a patient's motor performance and functional capacity can be determined from three-dimensional upper extremity motion analysis. Motor blockade produced by injection of bupivacaine or botulinum A toxin into the muscles that have been identified for surgery may serve as a diagnostic tool to predict postoperative outcomes or as an adjunct to surgical treatment.[5,13]

Selection of Surgical Candidates and Indications for Surgery

The patient, caregiver, therapist, and surgeon should formulate specific goals that they expect after upper extremity surgery. Often, involved parties cannot agree on which goals take priority. Such discrepancies must be reconciled before surgical intervention. Some of the most common goals include decreased pain, specific functional improvement, enhanced self-esteem, and facilitation of caregiver activities. To attain these goals, surgical interventions must be performed on several different joints (Table 123.1). The presence of movement disorders (e.g., athetosis, chorea, choreoathetosis, and dystonia) is a relative contraindication for tendon transfer surgery. However, these patients may benefit from arthrodesis. Furthermore, sophisticated tendon transfers should be undertaken with caution in patients who demonstrate poor or limited sensibility. The selection of an appropriate procedure(s) required to achieve both specific and global outcomes must be individualized for each patient. After a child is identified as a candidate for surgical intervention, an appropriate surgical plan, including a postoperative regimen and rehabilitation program, is formulated.

OPERATIVE PROCEDURES

Shoulder

Adduction and internal rotation shoulder deformities are common in children with cerebral palsy because of a dynamic imbalance of the internal rotators or fixed contractures of the pectoralis major, subscapularis, or joint capsule. Depending on the etiology, these deformities may be classified as dynamic, static, or combined dynamic-static. Surgery on the shoulder joint may be necessary because of dislocation, subluxation, or contractures. Deformities may occur in more than one plane. Moreover, joint incongruity with deformity of the humeral head, dysplasia of the glenoid, and arthritis of the glenohumeral articulation should be addressed. In dynamic deformities, the glenohumeral articulation is typically congruous and stable with satisfactory articular surfaces. Muscle lengthening and

TABLE 123.1 Specific Interventions (Common Choices)

Joint Area	Need	Options
Shoulder	Joint stabilization	Fusion, capsular reconstructions
	Increase external rotation	Lengthen PM or subscapularis; transfer LD and teres major
	Increase internal rotation	Lengthen or release infraspinatus or teres minor
Elbow	Stabilization	Fusion
	Increase extension	Lengthen or release biceps brachii, brachialis brachioradialis release (slide), flexor–pronator mass release, joint capsule release, humeral osteotomy, excise radial head
Forearm	Improve supination	Reroute, lengthen, or release PT; osteotomy radius ± ulna; release flexor–pronator muscle; excise radial head
Wrist	Stabilization	Fusion, tendon transfer, release, proximal row carpectomy
	Increase ROM	
	Extension	Transfers of FCU, ECU, FCR, BR, FDS, FDP
Thumb	Stabilization	Volar plate arthroplasty; fusion MCP joint
	Increase extension	Plication or transfer, EPL, APB, EPB; release or lengthen FPL
	Improve power	Reinforce EPL, reinforce FPL
	Improve abduction	Release adductor, abduction transfer, osteotomy metacarpal
Fingers	Flexion	FDS-to-FDP transfer; flexor–pronator release (slide), lengthen FDS, lengthen FDP
	Swan neck	EDC FDS tenotomy; PIP joint fusion; FDS tenodesis

APB, Abductor pollicis brevis; *BR*, brachioradialis; *ECU*, extensor carpi ulnaris; *EDC*, extensor digitorum communis; *EPB*, extensor pollicis brevis; *EPL*, extensor pollicis longus; *FCR*, flexor carpi radialis; *FCU*, flexor carpal ulnari; *FDP*, flexor digitorum profundus; *FDS*, flexor digitorum superficialis; *FPL*, flexor pollicis longus; *LD*, latissimus dorsi; *MCP*, metacarpophalangeal; *PIP*, proximal interphalangeal; *PM*, pectoralis major; *PT*, pronator teres; *ROM*, range of motion.

muscle–tendon transfer are treatment options for these patients with shoulder deformities. To manage shoulder internal rotation deformity, the pectoralis major and subscapularis may be released or lengthened by Z-plasty. In severe contractures, capsular release may also be required. Transfer of the latissimus dorsi and teres major muscles may augment external rotation power (Fig. 123.1). Patients with significant adduction and internal rotation shoulder contractures may be aided by latissimus dorsi and teres major releases in conjunction with the procedures described previously. Alternatively, a proximal or distal rotational osteotomy of the humerus may be used to improve either external rotation or internal rotation. In most cases, osteotomy is reserved for patients with arthritic or dysplastic or subluxed joints and for patients who have undergone unsuccessful tendon transfers. In patients without arthritis or significant humeral head or glenoid deformity, subluxation and dislocation may require open reduction, capsular release and/or capsulodesis, and/or humeral or glenoid osteotomy. Shoulder fusion is an option to treat patients with refractory

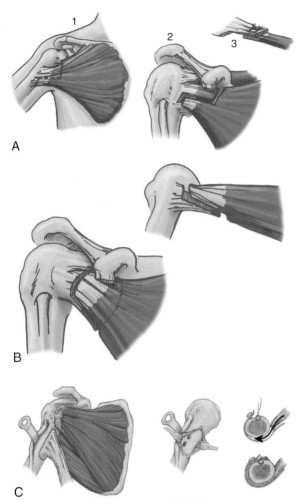

Fig. 123.1 A, In a modified L'Episcopo-Sever procedure, a Z-lengthening of the pectoralis major is performed (*1*, *2*, and *3*). Creating the Z with the distal end inferior lengthens the tendon more than the converse (*2*). The repair may be completed using grasping or mattress suture (*3*). The subscapularis is beneath the pectoralis major and is frequently contracted. **B,** By taking advantage of the orientation of the musculotendinous portion of the muscle tendon unit, an oblique cut in the transverse plane ("on the flat") allows lengthening and repair using a simple mattress suture. **C,** The latissimus dorsi and teres major may be transferred to the posterior lateral humerus using either one or two incisions. Our preference is to use the single incision in which the tendon of the latissimus and teres major are released subperiosteally as a single insertion. A subperiosteal transcircumferential plane is then created; sutures fixed to the tendon are passed and connected to two or three anchors or a bone tunnel to provide an external rotation moment. (Reproduced with permission from Koman LA, ed. *Wake Forest University School of Medicine Orthopaedic Manual.* Winston-Salem, NC: Orthopaedic Press; 2001.)

arthritic shoulder pain but must be undertaken with caution because of the attendant difficulties created in caregiving and in activities of daily living (ADLs).[14]

Postoperative Care

Casting, shoulder orthoses, and therapy are usually required after shoulder procedures. For internal rotation contracture releases and transfers, either an orthosis or a modified shoulder spica cast is applied in the operating room. The orthosis or cast is worn full time for 3 to 4 weeks. Patients may then transition to an orthosis worn only at night

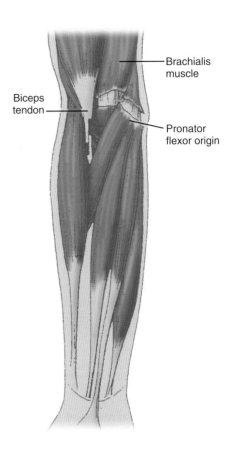

Fig. 123.2 Elbow flexion contractures between 30 and 60 degrees may be addressed surgically. The biceps tendon is Z-lengthened, and the brachialis is recessed by making cuts in the musculotendinous portion. In severe cases, the flexor pronator origin also may be released. Release of the capsule is occasionally needed (not shown). It is important to prevent elbow instability; therefore, the collateral ligaments should not be released. (Reproduced with permission from Koman LA, ed. *Wake Forest University School of Medicine Orthopaedic Manual.* Winston-Salem, NC: Orthopaedic Press; 2001.)

for an additional 3 months. At 4 weeks, AROM and PROM activities are initiated followed by strengthening activities at 6 weeks.

Elbow

Correction of an elbow flexion deformity is not required to improve functional ADLs unless the flexion deformity exceeds 30 degrees.[15,16] Deformities are typically dynamic and static, with fixed contractures of the capsule as well as the biceps, brachialis, and brachioradialis muscles. Release of the anterior elbow structures, including the lacertus fibrosis, brachialis fascia versus lacertus fibrosis, and brachialis fascia and Z-lengthening of the biceps were comparable in elbow extension, but the former lost active elbow flexion.[17] The flexor–pronator mass may also have a fixed component. Additionally, dynamic motor imbalance of the muscles about the elbow exacerbates contractures by shortening musculotendinous units. Furthermore, dysplasia and subluxation of the radial head may occur with longstanding hyperpronation deformities. In cases with milder deformities, soft tissue procedures, including lengthening of the elbow flexors, are often successful in correcting the contractures. Flexion contractures between 30 and 60 degrees may be treated in this manner (Fig. 123.2). Contractures greater than 60 degrees may require the additional release of the flexor–pronator origin or the elbow capsule. Patients with subluxation of the radial head often present with pain in addition to poor elbow ROM. These patients may benefit from resection of the radial head, which decreases pain and slightly improves forearm supination–pronation. However, patients should understand that this procedure rarely improves elbow flexion–extension capabilities. Elbow fusion is reserved for patients who experience intractable pain. Of note, elbow fusion has never been used in our patient population.

Postoperative Care

After anterior elbow release, neuromuscular blocking agents (botulinum toxin A) are injected intraoperatively for postoperative pain control and to facilitate rehabilitation. The elbow is positioned with a cast or thermoplastic orthosis in a position of comfort at 50% of the passive excursion obtained under anesthesia. Orthoses or casts are repositioned at 1- to 2-week intervals for 6 weeks to improve extension. Severe elbow deformities may require the use of additional casting or distraction using an external fixator. AROM and PROM therapy is initiated 4 weeks after surgery, and night orthoses are worn for 3 months.

Forearm

Forearm pronation deformity is usually caused by hypertonic pronator teres (PT) and pronator quadratus muscles. This deformity inhibits the handling of large objects and prevents individuals from holding objects with two hands. Dislocation of the radial head may occur as a consequence of both hyperpronation and ligamentous laxity.

Several procedures have been described to manage forearm pronation deformities, including (1) release of the flexor–pronator origin; (2) release, lengthening, or rerouting of the PT; (3) osteotomy of the radius, ulna, or both; (4) rerouting the wrist or finger flexor tendons to provide a supination moment (e.g., flexor carpi ulnaris [FCU] to extensor carpi radialis brevis [ECRB]); and (5) resection of a subluxed or dislocated radial head. Transfer of the pronator to a wrist extensor may improve wrist extension and supination.[18] In properly selected patients, transposition of the PT to the ECRB and rerouting of the PT with or without pronator quadratus myotomy is effective in the management of pronation deformity of the forearm.[19] Our experience suggests (1) an expected result is active pronation to neutral, (2) patients with a continuously active PT who have a passively correctible deformity are treated with a PT release (tenotomy), (3) Z-lengthening or fractional lengthening may be substituted for tenotomy with comparable result, and (4) patients who have noncontinuously firing or intermittent PT muscle activity undergo a rerouting procedure as the preferred surgical option at our institution (see Fig. 123.3). Ozkan and colleagues[20] describe rerouting of the brachioradialis as a successful technique to improve supination. Patients with fixed, severe deformities require radial or ulnar osteotomy procedures (or both). Radial head resection is indicated when subluxation prevents supination or causes pain. Forearm fusion (creation of a one-bone forearm) is generally not indicated in patients with cerebral palsy.

Postoperative Care

After surgery to improve supination, the patient's forearm is positioned in a thermoplastic orthosis or is casted in a neutral position or with the forearm in supination. The choice of position is determined by the observed intraoperative ROM and preoperative tone. The initial immobilization period of 3 to 4 weeks is followed by use of an orthosis at night and therapy. Therapy may include AROM and PROM, strengthening exercises, orthoses serially adjusted to improve supination, and possible neuromuscular stimulation.

Wrist

Palmar flexion of the wrist is common among patients with cerebral palsy. This deformity hinders function, produces pain, decreases sensibility (if extreme), interferes with optimal caregiver activities, or

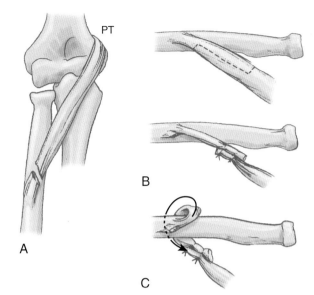

Fig. 123.3 Excessive pronation caused by hypertonicity of the pronator teres *(PT)* may be addressed by one of three surgical procedures. **A,** The tendon portion may be tenotomized. **B,** The tendon may be Z-lengthened and then sutured together to increase its resting length and decrease its force. **C,** The tendon may be Z-lengthened and rerouted by passing it around the radius to provide supination. Not shown is alternative to take the tendon off with an osteoperiosteal extension and routed around the radius and sutured to bone or itself to provide a supination moment. (Reproduced with permission from Koman LA, ed. *Wake Forest University School of Medicine Orthopaedic Manual.* Winston-Salem, NC: Orthopaedic Press; 2001.)

elicits emotional distress. Common etiologies include weak extensors, hypertonic wrist flexors, and joint contractures. Wrist joint deformities may either be fixed or dynamic, with or without osseous and cartilage deformities. Abnormal wrist postures frequently are interrelated with elbow and hand–finger deformities. Management options for wrist palmar flexion include both soft tissue and osseous procedures, depending on the severity of the deformity. Passively correctible deformities may benefit from tendon lengthening, releases, or transfers. Fixed flexion contractures with greater than 60 degrees of deformity may require a combination of tendon transfers, bony procedures, or gradual correction modalities. Gradual correction may be achieved by serial casting or by using a multiplanar, geared external fixator (i.e., Ilizarov or spatial frame).

A number of osseous procedures may be used to correct significant wrist palmar flexion, including proximal row carpectomy, radial shortening (with or without angular correction), and wrist fusion (with or without carpal resection). Patients considered for a wrist fusion should demonstrate good to excellent thumb–finger control with the wrist immobilized close to neutral. Fusion also may be considered for pain relief. Before considering a wrist fusion procedure, a careful functional evaluation of the extremity should be performed to prevent loss of the tenodesis effect on finger flexion and grasp and release.[4,21–24]

Dynamic wrist flexion deformities may be managed with tendon transfers. Assessment of tendon function to determine the appropriate tendon transfers includes both clinical and electromyographic muscle testing of the wrist during motion.[4,10,11] Muscles are noted as having phasic, nonphasic, or continuous activity. Described transfers include the transfer of the FCU to the extensor carpi radialis longus (ECRL), to the ECRB, or to the extensor digitorum communis (EDC)[10,11,25,26] (Fig. 123.4). In patients with continuous FCU activation throughout the flexion–extension arc, a transfer of the FCU to the EDC is preferable to transfer of the FCU to the ECRB–ECRL because the latter may

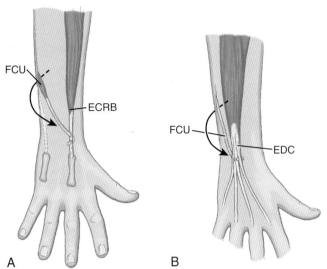

Fig. 123.4 Transfer of the flexor carpi ulnaris *(FCU)* to the extensor carpi radialis brevis *(ECRB)* (**A**) or transfer of the flexor carpi ulnaris to the extensor digitorum communis *(EDC)* (**B**) improves wrist extension. The tendon may be transferred subcutaneously to provide a supination moment or through the interosseous membrane to provide more dorsiflexion without supination. (Reproduced with permission from Koman LA, ed. *Wake Forest University School of Medicine Orthopaedic Manual.* Winston-Salem, NC: Orthopaedic Press; 2001.)

produce a wrist extension deformity.[15] The former procedure improves wrist and finger extension, permits finger flexion, and prevents wrist extension deformity by avoiding FCU overpull.[4,10] If the FCU is found to contract phasically, it may be successfully transferred to the ECRB to improve voluntary wrist extension without creating an extension deformity. In wrists that exhibit significant ulnar deviation, transfer of the FCU to the ECRL will decrease the extent of the deformity. This transfer may be enhanced by transferring the extensor carpi ulnaris (ECU) radially to the fourth metacarpal (Fig. 123.5). Concomitant contractures of the flexor carpi radialis also require Z-lengthening or fractional lengthening.[11,15]

Postoperative Care

Casting or orthotic positioning is required after wrist procedures. The wrist is positioned to protect tendon transfers or plications as well as to maintain joint position after carpectomy or arthrodesis. Therapy is initiated to prevent finger stiffness and to maintain function. After 4 weeks of full-time immobilization, AROM, PROM, and strengthening exercises are initiated. The wrist is placed in an orthosis in the optimally corrected position for a minimum of 8 hours per day. Some patients may benefit from electrical stimulation.

Thumb and Finger Deformities

Finger Flexion Deformity

Dynamic finger flexion deformity secondary to spasticity of the flexor digitorum superficialis (FDS) or flexor digitorum profundus (FDP) can be managed by augmenting power to the finger extensors or weakening the FDS. Excessive weakening of the FDS in patients who demonstrate purposeful grasp and release is not recommended.[15] A commonly used procedure is to transfer the FCU or one or more FDS tendons to the EDC. In general, either the long or ring or both flexor digitorum superficialis tendons are transferred. Similarly, power to the extensor pollicis longus (EPL) may be augmented by transfer of an FDS (usually the ring or long finger) or the brachioradialis. If an FDS tendon is transferred, it is important to maintain proximal interphalangeal (PIP)

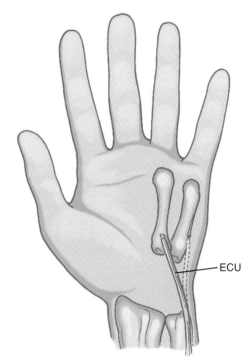

Fig. 123.5 Transfer of the extensor carpi ulnaris *(ECU)* from its insertion on the fifth metacarpal to the fourth metacarpal will decrease ulnar deviation. The extensor retinaculum should be released to allow dorsal translation of the ECU tendon. (Reproduced with permission from Koman LA, ed. *Wake Forest University School of Medicine Orthopaedic Manual.* Winston-Salem, NC: Orthopaedic Press; 2001.)

motion (especially extension) to avoid scarring of the FDS tendon and resultant flexion contractures of the PIP joint.

Fixed finger contractures result from a combination of weak finger extensors and shortened flexors. Depending on the severity of the deformity, a number of interventions may be used to lengthen the flexors. A nonoperative option involves serial muscle stretching and serial orthotic positioning after intramuscular neuromuscular blockade with botulinum A or B toxin injection(s). In mild to moderate cases treated at our institution, fractional lengthening of the individual FDS muscles is followed by injection of botulinum toxin into both the lengthened FDS and the unaffected FDP. More complex deformities may require fractional or Z-lengthening of the FDP and fractional lengthening of the FDS, in combination with intramuscular botulinum toxin A injections. In patients with severe deformities and functional or potentially functional finger flexors, a flexor–pronator slide procedure is recommended.[2,4,26,27] In patients without the potential for functional recovery, superficialis to profundus transfers decrease pain or facilitate hygiene.[23,26]

Thumb Flexion Deformity

Dynamic thumb flexion deformities can be managed by augmenting thumb extensor power. Increased extensor power is affected by using a combination of procedures, including EPL tendon plication or rerouting or reinforcement using a brachioradialis or FDS tendon. Thumb deformities typically occur concomitantly with other deformities. In addition to improving extensor power, fixed contractures of the flexor pollicis longus (FPL) muscle–tendon unit are addressed by fractional or Z-lengthening procedures. Interestingly, the contracted and spastic FPL is often weak and may need to be reinforced with either the brachioradialis or another tendon[4] (Fig. 123.6).

Thumb-in-Palm Deformity

Thumb-in-palm deformities may be caused by multiple factors, all of which must be addressed to ensure a successful outcome. Static causes of thumb-in-palm deformities include soft tissue contractures, joint instability, and contractures of the FPL or adductor pollicis. Dynamic causes include weakness of the metacarpophalangeal (MCP) joint, which may be unstable in flexion, extension, or globally.

Isolated hyperextension instability of the MCP joint may be improved by volar plate capsulodesis.[28] Combined hyperflexion and

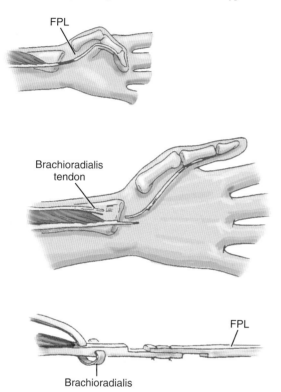

Fig. 123.6 A fixed contracture of the flexor pollicis longus *(FPL)* may be managed by Z-lengthening, as demonstrated, or more proximally by fractional lengthening (not demonstrated). Reinforcement of a weakened FPL may be achieved as demonstrated by transfer of the brachioradialis proximal to the Z-lengthening. (Reproduced with permission from Koman LA, ed. *Wake Forest University School of Medicine Orthopaedic Manual.* Winston-Salem, NC: Orthopaedic Press; 2001.)

hyperextension deformity or global instability is corrected using MCP joint fusion.[29] Additionally, MCP joint fusion enhances thumb flexor and extensor power by eliminating one motion segment and may be used in conjunction with thumb tendon transfers.[3,4,15]

Thumb adduction deformities are managed by releasing the adductor pollicis or first dorsal interosseous or by Z-plasty of these muscles (Fig. 123.7). Skin contractures can be alleviated with a four-flap Z-plasty (Fig. 123.8). Motor power to the thumb abductor may be enhanced by a number of techniques, including transfer of the brachioradialis to the abductor pollicis longus or rerouting of the EPL to the radial side of Lister's tubercle (Fig. 123.9) with or without reinforcement using an FDS tendon. As described earlier, fusion of the MCP joint improves flexor–extensor power.[15,29,30]

Deficient extensor tone with tendon attenuation may be augmented by plication of the EPL, abductor pollicis longus, or extensor pollicis brevis. Tone is increased by tendon transfers using the brachioradialis or the FDS of the ring finger. Management of FPL contractures is discussed under thumb flexion deformity (see Figs. 123.6 and 123.9).

Digital Deformities

Swan-neck deformities of the digit are caused by spasticity of either the intrinsic mechanism or the extrinsic tendons pulling against a flexed wrist. These deformities are managed by extensor tendon tenotomy, volar plate capsulodesis, FDS tenodesis, or PIP fusion.[30] Hand grip and coordination may be significantly affected by contractures of the intrinsic muscle. Although patients may benefit from intrinsic releases, improvement in function is often modest at best.[31-33]

Postoperative care. Full-time orthosis wear is implemented after surgical treatment of digital deformities. Initially, the patient is placed in an orthosis or cast designed to maintain the surgically corrected posture of the thumb and fingers and to protect tendon transfers for 3 to 4 weeks after the procedure. Subsequently, a rehabilitation program that emphasizes ROM and strengthening exercises is initiated and continued for 8 to 12 weeks. After full-time immobilization is discontinued, a nighttime orthosis that maintains the digits in the optimal position is continued for 3 months.

GENERAL POSTOPERATIVE CARE

Postoperative care is a crucial aspect that maximizes operative outcomes. A comprehensive postoperative plan should include input from

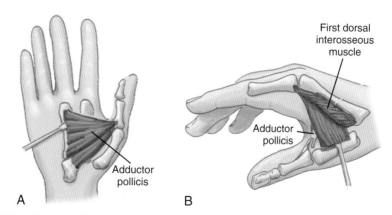

Fig. 123.7 The adductor pollicis may be released from its origin on the third metacarpal through a volar incision (**A**). Alternatively, the adductor tendon may be Z-lengthened or transferred proximally to the first metacarpal to increase the first webspace. The first dorsal interosseous may be released from the first metacarpal (**B**). (Reproduced with permission from Koman LA, ed. *Wake Forest University School of Medicine Orthopaedic Manual.* Winston-Salem, NC: Orthopaedic Press; 2001.)

therapists regarding appropriate therapy modalities and orthosis wear that will maximize surgical outcomes. The initial goal of postoperative care is to protect tendon transfers and to maintain or improve ROM.

Botulinum Toxins

Botulinum toxins are among the most potent biological agents known and have widespread utility in the management of spasticity associated

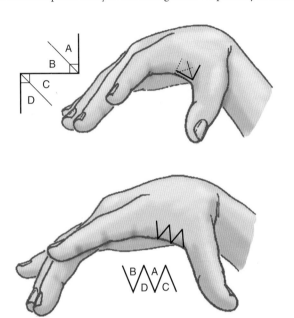

Fig. 123.8 Schematic representation of a four-flap Z-plasty. (Reproduced with permission from Koman LA, ed. *Wake Forest University School of Medicine Orthopaedic Manual.* Winston-Salem, NC: Orthopaedic Press; 2001.)

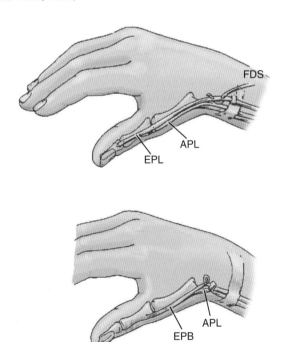

Fig. 123.9 The extensor pollicis longus *(EPL)* may be rerouted radial to Lister's tubercle, plicated, and reinforced, if necessary, with the flexor digitorum superficialis *(FDS)*. *APL,* Abductor pollicis longus; *EPB,* extensor pollicis brevis. (Reproduced with permission from Koman LA, ed. *Wake Forest University School of Medicine Orthopaedic Manual.* Winston-Salem, NC: Orthopaedic Press; 2001.)

with cerebral palsy. Both A and B toxins are approved by the US Food and Drug Administration but are *not* labeled for use in children or for the management of upper extremity spasticity in cerebral palsy. However, botulinum toxin A is labeled in Australia and New Zealand for use in the upper extremity in patients with cerebral palsy. Postoperative and intraoperative uses of toxin injections are supported by a lower extremity randomized trial, basic science data, and extensive anecdotal experience.[34]

Botulinum toxin injected directly into the target muscle produces selective partial and reversible paralysis that balances forces across joints and decreases deforming forces at repair and transfer sites and pin and plate fixation sites. Injections also help to reduce pain. Intramuscular injections are administered based upon muscle size and target receptors. Following these guidelines, botulinum toxin injections are safe and effective in appropriately selected patients. They may be used to decrease postoperative pain, protect tendon repairs, permit earlier return to active motion, and prevent overlengthening of tendons treated with fractional procedures.[35]

If botulinum toxin is used, the practitioner must recognize his or her obligation to appropriate patient follow-up and to disclosure of the advantages and disadvantages of intramuscular toxin injections. A full discussion of the use of botulinum toxin is beyond the scope of this chapter; however, after appropriate growth and, in selected patients, tendon transfer is more effective than toxin.[36]

Hand Therapy

Hand therapy by licensed occupational or physical therapists is necessary to ensure optimal postsurgical outcomes and to facilitate the rehabilitation process. During the first 3 to 4 weeks after surgery, the operative site is protected using a rigid orthosis, pins, or casts to facilitate the healing process. In addition, frequent therapist evaluations ensure maintenance of proper joint position and continued ROM exercises of the proximal and distal joints. After the initial healing phase, AROM and PROM protocols are begun, incorporating static and dynamic orthotic positioning as necessary. Strengthening becomes a crucial part of the rehabilitation process 6 to 10 weeks after surgery. Therapy sessions and a home therapy regimen are key components of this phase of the rehabilitation process.

Rehabilitation outcomes may be influenced by a number of factors, including the therapy method and regimen. Some investigators have focused on the various methods of therapy delivery. Trahan and Maloui[37] demonstrated improvement in motor function among children with cerebral palsy who underwent short, intense therapy sessions followed by longer periods of rest. They found that after short, intense therapy sessions children performed better than those who followed a traditional regimen.[37] Other studies have focused on the therapy setting and activities practiced. Therapy sessions involving performance of specific ADLs have resulted in improved outcomes as does practicing in an environment that emulates the patient's home.[38,39] In a randomized, controlled trial comparing occupational therapy with botulinum A toxin with occupational therapy alone, occupational therapy with toxin was superior.[40]

More recently, interest in constraint-induced movement therapy has increased. The practice involves forced use of the involved extremity by temporarily restraining the noninvolved extremity. The practice has been used to treat adult stroke patients. Recently, this modality has been adopted in children with cerebral palsy.[41]

Currently, it is unclear which rehabilitation method is the most effective. Investigators have evaluated various modalities and have come to divergent conclusions. Small sample size, difficulty standardizing patients, and poor study designs are some of the obstacles that are cited to explain the variation in reported findings.[37] Future multicenter trials using functional classification systems to evaluate patients both before and after surgery would help to establish evidence-based practice guidelines. For these reasons, this chapter has included only general rehabilitation guidelines after each of the various surgical sections.

SUMMARY

Although only a small percentage of children and adults with cerebral palsy are candidates for upper extremity surgery, judicious use of the surgical procedures discussed in this chapter can result in positive outcomes and improve health-related quality of life. However, proper patient selection is crucial to ensure reasonable postoperative results. Postoperative care must be coordinated with appropriately trained hand therapists for optimal results.

REFERENCES

1. Carroll RE, Craig FS. The surgical treatment of cerebral palsy. *Surg Clin North Am.* 1951;30:385–396.
2. Goldner JL. Upper extremity tendon transfers in cerebral palsy. *Orthop Clin North Am.* 1974;5(2):389–414.
3. Leafblad ND, Van Heest AE. Management of the spastic wrist and hand in cerebral palsy. *J Hand Surg Am.* 2015;40(5):1035–1040.
4. Koman LA, Gelberman RH, Toby EB, Poehling GG. Cerebral palsy. Management of the upper extremity. *Clin Orthop.* 1990;253:62–74.
5. Koman LA, Smith BP, Goodman A. *Botulinum Toxin Type A in the Management of Cerebral Palsy.* Winston-Salem, NC: Wake Forest University Press; 2002.
6. House JH, Gwathmey FW, Fidler MO. A dynamic approach to the thumb-in-palm deformity in cerebral palsy. *J Bone Joint Surg.* 1981;63A(2):216–225.
7. Johnson LM, Randall MJ, Reddihough DS, et al. Development of a clinical assessment of quality of movement for unilateral upper-limb function. *Dev Med Child Neurol.* 1994;36(11):965–973.
8. Randall M, Carlin JB, Chondros P, Reddihough D. Reliability of the Melbourne assessment of unilateral upper limb function. *Dev Med Child Neurol.* 2001;43(11):761–767.
9. Van Heest AE, House JH, Cariello C. Upper extremity surgical treatment of cerebral palsy. *J Hand Surg.* 1999;24A(2):323–330.
10. Hoffer MM, Perry J, Melkonian GF. Dynamic electromyography and decision-making for surgery in the upper extremity of patients with cerebral palsy. *J Hand Surg.* 1979;4A(5):424–431.
11. Hoffer MM, Lehman M, Mitani M. Long-term follow-up on tendon transfers to the extensors of the wrist and fingers in patients with cerebral palsy. *J Hand Surg.* 1986;1A(6):836–840.
12. Mowery CA, Gelberman RH, Rhoades CE. Upper extremity tendon transfers in cerebral palsy: electromyographic and functional analysis. *J Pediatr Orthop.* 1985;5:69–72.
13. Autti-Ramo I, Larsen A, Peltonen J, et al. Botulinum toxin injection as an adjunct when planning hand surgery in children with spastic hemiplegia. *Neuropediatrics.* 2000;31(1):4–8.
14. Landi A, Cavazza S, Caserta G, Leti Acciaro A, et al. The upper limb in cerebral palsy: surgical management of shoulder and elbow deformities. *Hand Clin.* 2004;20(3):345–347.
15. Koman LA, Smith BP, Shilt JS. Cerebral palsy. *Lancet.* 2004;15(9421):1619–1631.
16. Manske PR, Langewisch KR, Strecker WB, Albrecht MM. Anterior elbow release of spastic elbow flexion deformity in children with cerebral palsy. *J Pediatr Orthop.* 2001;21(6):772–777.
17. Gong HS, Cho HE, Chung CY, Park MS, et al. Early results of anterior elbow release with and without biceps lengthening in patients with cerebral palsy. *J Hand Surg Am.* 2014;39(5):902–909.
18. Ho JJ, Wang TM, Shieh JY, Wu KW, et al. Pronator teres transfer for forearm and wrist deformity in cerebral palsy children. *J Pediatr Orthop.* 2015;35(4):412–418.
19. Cobeljic G, Rajkovic S, Bajin Z, Lesic A, et al. The results of surgical treatment for pronation deformities of the forearm in cerebral palsy after a mean follow-up of 17.5 years. *J Orthop Surg Res.* 2015;10:106.
20. Ozkan T, Tuncer S, Aydin A, et al. Brachioradialis re-routing for the restoration of active supination and correction of forearm pronation deformity in cerebral palsy. *J Hand Surg.* 2004;29B(3):265–270.
21. Omer GE, Capen DA. Proximal row carpectomy with muscle transfers for spastic paralysis. *J Hand Surg.* 1976;1A(3):197–204.
22. Szabo RM, Gelberman RH. Operative treatment of cerebral palsy. *Hand Clin.* 1985;1(3):525–543.
23. Wei DH, Feldon P. Total wrist arthrodesis: Indications and clinical outcomes. *J Am Acad Orthop Surg.* 2017;25(1):3–11.
24. Seruya M, Dickey RM, Fakhro A. Surgical treatment of pediatric upper limb spasticity: the wrist and hand. *Semin Plast Surg.* 2016;30(1):29–38.
25. Green WT. Tendon transplantation of the flexor carpi ulnaris for pronation–flexor deformity of the wrist. *Surg Gynecol Obstet.* 1942;75:337–342.
26. Green WT, Banks HH. Flexor carpi ulnaris transplant and its use in cerebral palsy. *J Bone Joint Surg.* 1962;44A:1343–1352.
27. Golder JL. Reconstructive surgery of the hand in cerebral palsy and spastic paralysis resulting from injury to the spinal cord. *J Bone Joint Surg.* 1955;37A(6):1141–1153.
28. Filler BC, Stark HH, Boyes JH. Capsulodesis of the metacarpophalangeal joint of the thumb in children with cerebral palsy. *J Bone Joint Surg Am.* 1976;58(5):667–670.
29. Goldner JL, Koman LA, Gelberman R, Levin S, et al. Arthrodesis of the metacarpophalangeal joint of the thumb in children and adults. Adjunctive treatment of thumb-in-palm deformity in cerebral palsy. *Clin Orthop Relat Res.* 1990;253:75–89.
30. Alewijnse JV, Smeulders MJ, Kreulen M. Short-term and long term clinical results of the surgical correction of thumb-in-palm deformity in patients with cerebral palsy. *J Pediatr Orthop.* 2015;35(8):825–830.
31. Swanson AB. Treatment of the swan-neck deformity in the cerebral palsied hand. *Clin Orthop Relat Res.* 1966;48:167–171.
32. Zancolli EA, Zancolli Jr ER. Surgical management of the hemiplegic spastic hand in cerebral palsy. *Surg Clin North Am.* 1981;61(2):395–406.
33. Carlson EJ, Carlson MG. Treatment of swan neck deformity in cerebral palsy. *J Hand Surg Am.* 2014;39(4):768–772.
34. Koman LA, Mooney 3rd JF, Smith BP, et al. Management of spasticity in cerebral palsy with botulinum-A toxin: report of a preliminary, randomized, double-blind trial. *J Pediatr Orthop.* 1994;14(3):299–303.
35. Ma J, Shen J, Smith BP, et al. Bioprotection of tendon repair: adjunctive use of botulinum toxin A in Achilles tendon repair in the rat. *J Bone Joint Surg Am.* 2007;89(10):2241–2249.
36. Van Heest AE, Bagley A, Molitor F, James MA. Tendon transfer surgery in upper extremity cerebral palsy is more effective than botulinum toxin injections or regular, ongoing therapy. *J Bone Joint Surg Am.* 2015;97(7):529–536.
37. Trahan J, Malouin F. Intermittent intensive physiotherapy in children with cerebral palsy: a pilot study. *Dev Med Child Neurol.* 2002;44(4):233–239.
38. Dean C, Shepherd RB. Task-related training improves performance of seated reaching tasks after stroke. A randomized controlled trial. *Stroke.* 1997;28:722–728.
39. Duff SV, Gordon AM. Learning of grasp control in children with hemiplegic cerebral palsy. *Dev Med Child Neurol.* 2003;45(11):746–757.
40. Lidman G, Nachemson A, Peny-Dahlstrand M, Himmelmann K. Botulinum toxin A injections and occupational therapy in children with unilateral spastic cerebral palsy: a randomized controlled trial. *Dev Med Child Neurol.* 2015;57(8):754–761.
41. Gordon AM, Charles J, Wolf SL. Methods of constraint-induced movement therapy for children with hemiplegic cerebral palsy: development of a child-friendly intervention for improving upper-extremity function. *Arch Phys Med Rehabil.* 2005;86:837–844.

124

Pediatric Upper Extremity Trauma

Joshua M. Abzug, Heather Weesner, Alexandria L. Case

CRITICAL POINTS

- *Indications:* Finger fractures with malrotation, substantial deviations; substantially displaced fractures of the wrist, forearm, elbow and shoulder; all tendon and nerve lacerations
- *Priorities for surgery and therapy:* Align fractures anatomically. During tendon and nerve repair, immobilize sufficiently to prevent re-rupture.
- *Pearls:* Use observation and tenodesis during physical examination to obtain necessary information; ensure radiographs are truly orthogonal when assessing displacement.
- *Healing timelines and progression of therapy:* Most pediatric fractures and tendon and nerve injuries are completely healed within 4 to 6 weeks. Therapy is reserved for tendon and nerve injuries, as well as fractures that are not progressing as expected.
- *Pitfalls:* Failure to recognize tendon and nerve injuries in pediatric patients; failure to obtain true anteroposterior and lateral radiographs
- *Precautions:* When in doubt, children are optimally treated with prolonged immobilization.
- *Timelines for return to sports participation:* Typically, 6 to 8 weeks for fractures, with return to contact sports at roughly 3 months. Patients with tendon and nerve injuries can generally return at 3 months.

INTRODUCTION

Hand and upper extremity trauma in pediatric patients is increasing in incidence because of the increasing competitive nature of sports participation as well as the more frequent participation in high-energy recreational activities. In addition, the usual activities of children, which include frequent falls, make injuries to the upper extremity very common.

The biomechanical and physiologic properties of the growing child's bone also factor in to children frequently sustaining fractures. Longitudinal bone growth originates about the physes, or growth plates, which is biomechanically the weakest location in a child's skeleton. Injuries about the physis typically result in a fracture that involves the physis and surrounding bone. The chemical makeup of young bone also varies from that of an adult, with pediatric bone being largely composed of collagen, which diminishes the tensile strength of the bone.[1]

SALTER-HARRIS CLASSIFICATION

Salter and Harris proposed the Salter-Harris classification of pediatric fractures in 1963, and it continues to be the most widely used system for classifying physeal fractures to date.[2] There are five types within the Salter-Harris classification system. A type I fracture is a transverse fracture through the physis that does not involve ossified bone. Type II fractures pass through the physis and into the metaphysis and are the most common, with the greatest incidence of all Salter-Harris fractures. Type III fractures propagate through the physis and epiphysis. These fractures typically occur in older children and adolescents and have reported relatively low incidence rates. Type IV fractures traverse the metaphysis, the physis, and the epiphysis. These fractures have poor prognoses with regard to long-term damage to the physis. Type V fractures are very uncommon and are typically crush injuries with resultant high rates of physeal arrest.[2]

COMMON PEDIATRIC FRACTURES

Half of female children and two-thirds of male children are diagnosed with a fracture before the ages of 15 to 17 years.[3,4] The fracture incidence rates peak during adolescence with the peak incidence in the male population being slightly later in adolescence than in the female population, (14 vs 11 years, respectively).[4]

Common mechanisms of injury that result in pediatric upper extremity fractures include falling onto a shoulder or outstretched hand, contact with a ball, and direct trauma.[1] Additional factors that contribute to an increased risk of fracture include genetics, low birth weight, inadequate nutrition, and lower socioeconomic statuses.[3] The increasing involvement of children in sporting activities has been associated with an increased incidence of fractures, with unorganized sporting events being the primary cause of pediatric fractures.[3] Fortunately, many pediatric fractures typically heal quickly and produce excellent outcomes; however, this is not always the case. It is important to recognize that the ability and rates of bone healing and remodeling observed in pediatric patients have an inverse correlation with patient age.[3]

During the assessment of the pediatric upper extremity, a systemic approach to the physical examination is necessary. Consideration regarding the developmental age of the child, including their ability to follow commands, and her or his comprehension of sensation abnormalities should be factored into the assessment. For the vast majority of pediatric upper extremity injuries, plain radiographs are sufficient.[1] In the case of suspected stress fractures or concomitant soft tissue injuries, magnetic resonance imaging (MRI) may be useful.

Clavicle Fractures

Background

Clavicle fractures account for 8% to 11% of all fractures in children.[5,6] Midshaft clavicle fractures make up roughly 90% of all pediatric and adolescent clavicle fractures.[7] and are typically seen in younger children with a mean age of incidence in non-neonatal patients of 8 years.[8] The classic mechanism of injury is a fall directly onto the shoulder with the arm adducted to the side; other possible mechanisms of injury include direct trauma to the region or a fall on an outstretched hand.[8] Clavicle fractures also commonly occur during sports-related activities in older adolescents.[8]

Clinical and Radiographic Examination

Edema, ecchymosis, crepitus, and focal tenderness upon clavicular palpation are often present because of the traumatic mechanism of injury.[8,9] Patients often present with the injured arm cradled close to the body and supported by the opposite arm for stabilization.[8] Sharp fracture fragments or a severe deformity in displaced fractures may tent the skin and increase the risk of skin puncture.[9] A thorough neurovascular examination should always be performed given the close proximity of the clavicle to the subclavian vessels, apices of the lungs, and the brachial plexus.[8] A standard anteroposterior (AP) radiograph and a 45-degree cephalic tilt view are recommended to assess the fracture pattern, fracture angulation, and amount of displacement.[9]

Treatment and Therapy Considerations

Most clavicle fractures are managed nonoperatively with a sling or figure-of-8 brace for 2 to 4 weeks, whereas operatively managed fractures are immobilized for roughly 3 weeks before active range of motion (AROM) exercises are initiated.[10] Physicians often prescribe slings for immobilization because figure-of-8 braces may cause impairment of activities of daily living (ADLs), limit range of motion (ROM), and cause sleep disturbances.[10] Return to sport can typically occur 6 to 8 weeks after the injury, although return to certain collision sports may be delayed up to 4 months at the physician's discretion. Before returning to sports, an athlete should have full ROM without pain, normal strength, clinical and radiographic evidence of bony healing, and no tenderness to palpation about the fracture site. Although clavicle fractures managed nonoperatively typically heal with some degree of deformity (a bump), acceptable functional results are usually achieved.

Indications for surgical management include displaced fractures with compromised skin integrity, open fractures, and a concomitant neurovascular injury requiring a repair. Recent studies in the adult population have demonstrated that displaced midshaft clavicle fractures may be treated operatively to decrease the rate of nonunion and improve patient outcomes,[11] although a study of pediatric patients by Hagstrom and coworkers[7] found no significant difference in outcomes between patients treated operatively and nonoperatively.

The majority of patients who sustain a clavicular fracture do not require formal therapy because stiffness and pain do not usually persist much beyond the immobilization phase. If therapy is prescribed, the primary focus is to regain a pain-free arc of motion. This is done by strengthening the rotator cuff and periscapular musculature and improving the patient's posture. For patients undergoing operative management, it is recommended to initiate a scar management and desensitization program and to normalize ROM and strength of the affected extremity.

Complications

Complications resulting from surgical management of clavicle fractures are rare. However, the possible complications can be severe, including neurovascular injury and cosmetic defects.[8,10]

Proximal Humerus Fractures

Background

Proximal humerus fractures make up less than 5% of fractures in the pediatric population, with a peak incidence in adolescents around 12 years of age.[5,12] These fractures occur more often in boys than in girls.[13] Common mechanisms of injury include abuse, blunt force trauma, a fall on the affected shoulder, and traumatic births.[13,14] Salter-Harris II fractures are the most common fracture type observed in pediatric and adolescent patients.[13]

Clinical and Radiographic Examination

Children with proximal humerus fractures typically present with acute pain, notable deformity about the proximal shoulder, and the inability to move the extremity against gravity without pain. A detailed neurovascular examination is warranted because both vascular and neurologic injuries can occur.

Anteroposterior, lateral, scapula Y, and axillary views of the shoulder should be obtained. It is important for the physician to document reduction of the glenohumeral joint because fracture dislocations can occur.[15] MRI and computed tomography (CT) are not typically necessary to diagnose these injuries.

Treatment and Therapeutic Considerations

Proximal humerus fractures have abundant remodeling potential given the proximity to the proximal humeral physis, which contributes 80% of the longitudinal growth of the humerus.[16] Therefore, nonoperative management is typically accepted regardless of the amount of displacement, angulation, rotation, and translation in younger children and produces excellent outcomes.[17] The treatment options for conservative management include a sling and swathe, a shoulder immobilizer, or a coaptation orthosis for 3 to 4 weeks.

Indications for operative intervention include open fractures, fractures with associated vascular injuries, and severe angulation or displacement. Burgos-Flores and coworkers[18] reported surgical intervention occurring in proximal humeral epiphysis fractures with greater than 50% displacement of bone diameter and in those with greater than 30% in a single plane, although they comment that these thresholds should be adjusted depending on patient age to optimize functional outcomes; patients younger than 13 years of age can have greater displacement or angulation, whereas those older than 13 years of age should be treated more aggressively. A systematic review and meta-analysis by Hohloch and associates[19] found that, across the literature, proximal humerus fractures treated nonoperatively in children older than 11 years of age are at increased risk of lasting deformity, whereas those older than 13 years of age often have functional repercussions without operative management. Operative intervention involves achieving and maintaining a reduction followed by stabilization and fixation with Kirschner wires (K-wires), intramedullary (IM) nailing, or a plate and screw construct. After surgical correction, patients are placed in a sling and swathe or a shoulder immobilizer for 3 to 4 weeks, after which gentle ROM may be initiated.

The goals during formal therapy after a proximal humerus fracture are to restore proper scapulohumeral rhythm, decrease compensatory techniques with overhead movements, and regain adequate deltoid and rotator cuff strength for the patient to return to school and sports-related activities. It is important for the therapist to assess scapulohumeral rhythm and initiate scapular and joint mobilizations during treatment if warranted. Patients may also require use of visual cues in front of a mirror to decrease the use of compensatory techniques during antigravity ROM exercises. With a thorough home program and compliance in formal therapy, most children return to their normal activities after 4 to 6 weeks of formal therapy.

A systematic review of the literature by Pahlavan and colleagues[17] regarding overall outcomes for pediatric proximal humerus fractures reported that outcomes are generally excellent for both operative and nonoperative management, and the majority of patients return to unimpeded function without major restrictions or complications. This review also commented that patients treated nonoperatively have been observed to have better ROM and functional outcomes than those treated operatively, particularly in the younger pediatric population.[17]

Complications

Complications after these fractures are rare, with most patients returning to full, normal function. However, complications such as loss of reduction, malunion with varus malalignment, limb-length inequality, vascular insufficiency, fracture shortening, growth arrest, pin tract infections, hypertrophic scarring, functional ROM deficits, and axillary nerve palsies can occur.[14,17,20]

Humeral Shaft Fractures
Background

Humeral shaft fractures account for fewer than 10% of pediatric fractures of the humerus and make up roughly 2% of all traumatic fractures in children.[5,21] The highest rates of humeral shaft fractures are observed in patients younger than 3 years of age and in those older than 12 years of age.[22] In neonates, birth trauma resulting from a breech delivery or complicated birth may cause a humeral shaft fracture.[14] Humeral shaft fractures are typically caused by motor vehicle collisions, falls from ground level, or direct trauma to the affected extremity in older children.[14,15]

Clinical and Radiographic Examination

Patients typically present with the upper extremity adducted and held in a protective position secondary to pain. The majority of these fractures are accompanied by edema, ecchymosis, and tenderness about the fracture.[14,15] A thorough neurovascular examination should also be conducted because these injuries may be associated with radial nerve injuries.[15] AP and lateral radiographs of the humerus should be obtained to assess the fracture angulation and displacement.

Treatment and Therapeutic Considerations

The vast majority of pediatric humeral shaft fractures are treated with conservative management.[15,23] Mild amounts of angulation, rotation, and shortening are acceptable. Patients are immobilized for 6 to 8 weeks in a sling and swathe, a shoulder immobilizer, or a coaptation orthosis.[14,23] Weekly radiographs are obtained to monitor progress and ensure there is no substantial worsening alignment. After the fracture shows sufficient healing and callus formation, the patient may be allowed to remove the immobilization device to perform protected AROM exercises under the supervision of a therapist.[15] Patients are advised to stay out of sports for up to 3 months, depending on their age, severity of injury, and rate of healing.

Indications for operative management include open fractures, significantly displaced or irreducible fractures, concomitant vascular

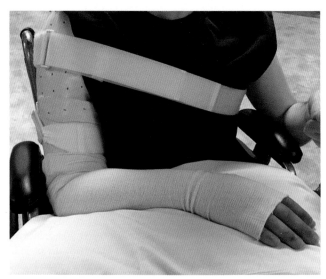

Fig. 124.1 Clinical photograph of an orthosis used to immobilize a humeral shaft fracture in a 16-year-old male patient. (Courtesy of Joshua M. Abzug.)

injuries, ipsilateral forearm or clavicle fractures, and failed nonoperative measures.[14,15,23] The most common operative interventions for humeral shaft fractures are open reduction and internal fixation (ORIF) with plate fixation, external fixation, and flexible IM nailing.[15,23] Postoperatively, patients are often placed in a Sarmiento brace, a coaptation orthosis, or a sling and swathe for 6 to 8 weeks (Fig. 124.1). Formal therapy and ROM exercises may be initiated after 4 to 6 weeks.

Therapy is recommended for patients with concomitant radial nerve palsy, those who report stiffness in the shoulder or elbow, and athletes who anticipate a rapid return to sport. For patients with a delayed return of radial nerve function, the therapeutic focus should be on the fabrication of a radial nerve palsy orthosis. For baseball players working on returning to sport, a protective orthosis that continues to protect the fracture site when batting should be fabricated in combination with specific sport-related exercises to regain the patient's ROM, strength, shoulder kinematics, and endurance (i.e., thrower's 10 program, return to pitching throwing programs). See Chapter 114 for therapy management of the injured athlete. Periscapular, rotator cuff, and deltoid strengthening therapeutic exercises should also begin at this time.

Complications

Radial nerve palsies occur in a small amount of pediatric humeral shaft fractures and can either occur at the time of injury or during attempts at manipulation maneuvers.[14] Notably, most associated nerve palsies are observed to resolve over time without requiring surgical intervention. Exploration with repair, reconstruction, or neurolysis is indicated if no recovery has occurred after 3 to 6 months.[15]

Vascular injuries are rare in association with pediatric humeral shaft fractures but require immediate evaluation and treatment, if present. Nonunion is uncommon in the pediatric population, and because of the remodeling potential and substantial amount of ROM that occurs in various planes of the shoulder, a functionally limiting malunion is also a rare finding in the pediatric population.[14]

Lateral Condyle Fractures
Background

Lateral condyle fractures represent fewer than 4% of elbow fractures in the pediatric population.[21,24,25] These fractures are commonly caused by falls onto an outstretched arm.[3,26,27]

Clinical and Radiographic Examination

Edema, lateral elbow pain, and crepitus along the fracture site are often present with lateral condyle fractures. Radiographs are essential for the diagnosis, including AP, lateral, and internal oblique views, which demonstrate the maximum amount of displacement present.[28] Some physicians will perform an arthrogram to assess the articular cartilage integrity when the epiphyseal ossification is not complete. Generally, MRI or CT scans are not necessary because they are expensive and, in the case of MRI, may require sedation.[26]

Treatment and Therapeutic Considerations

The classic nonoperative approach for fractures with less than 2 mm of displacement consists of long arm casting with the elbow at 90 degrees for 4 to 6 weeks. Weekly radiographs should be obtained for the first 2 to 3 weeks to ensure that the fracture maintains proper alignment. A recent study by Bakarman and colleagues[29] has challenged the use of this 2-mm threshold, describing improved outcomes for operative interventions even in the case of minimal displacement.

Options for operative management of lateral condyle fractures include closed reduction and percutaneous pinning (CRPP) for fractures with less than 4 mm of displacement and an intact articular cartilage hinge. After the procedure, patients are placed in a long arm cast for 4 to 6 weeks, and the pins are pulled when healing is adequate. ORIF is used for fractures with more than 4 mm of displacement, joint incongruity, or malrotation.[30] Postoperatively, patients are placed in a long arm cast for 6 weeks.

Complications

Several complications are associated with lateral condyle fractures, including malunion, physeal arrest, infection, fishtail deformity, and lateral spurring.[26] This fracture type also has a higher rate of nonunion, particularly for conservatively managed patients, because of the constant pull of the extensors on the injured region and poor distal metaphyseal circulation during casting.[31]

Bernthal and coworkers[32] performed a prospective study of 141 patients with lateral humeral condyle fractures. At the time of cast removal, patients had 44% of their ROM compared with the contralateral side; at 12 weeks, they had 84%; and at 48 weeks, they had 97%. Pediatric patients with these fractures may be referred to therapy after cast immobilization when there is substantial elbow stiffness that is not improving.

Medial Epicondyle Fractures
Background

In the pediatric population, medial epicondyle fractures account for 1% of all pediatric fractures and are predominately seen in boys.[5,33,34] The peak age of medial epicondyle fracture incidence is observed at 11 to 12 years of age.[33,34] Common mechanisms of injury include falls onto an outstretched hand with the elbow in full extension, posterior elbow dislocations, blunt trauma, and traumatic avulsions of the medial epicondyle that occur in overhead throwing athletes.[34,35]

Clinical and Radiographic Examination

Performing a thorough history regarding the mechanism of injury will be beneficial in determining the diagnosis. Observation for edema and ecchymosis along the medial aspect of the elbow should be included in the examination because this can help differentiate a medial epicondyle fracture from other differential diagnoses.[36] If a bone fragment is incarcerated in the joint, patients will often express guarding upon presentation and display substantially limited passive range of motion (PROM).

A neurovascular examination should be conducted with focus on the ulnar nerve given the proximity to the medial epicondyle. If the patient is cognizant, sensory testing should be completed. Ulnar nerve function should be documented upon initial evaluation whenever possible so it can be assessed for changes throughout the course of treatment.[36]

Standardized AP and lateral radiographs should be obtained. Most surgeons will also obtain an oblique view, which can aid in determining the amount of anterior displacement present.[37] The severity of displacement is a large contributor in the management decision, although the amount of displacement deemed "acceptable" and the recommended method in which to measure this displacement vary greatly throughout literature. A CT scan may be necessary to evaluate the displacement because fractures can appear to be nondisplaced or minimally displaced on radiographs but can have substantial anterior displacement demonstrated on CT.[37]

Treatment and Therapeutic Considerations

Conservative management consists of placing the child in a long arm cast with the elbow at 90 degrees of flexion for 3 to 4 weeks. This approach is effective for nondisplaced fractures and fractures with displacement proximal to the joint line.[36]

Open fractures and fractures with incarcerated fragments unable to be addressed via closed manipulation are the only absolute indications for surgery. Relative indications for operative management include fractures with concomitant elbow dislocations, fractures with displacement distal to the joint line, fractures with associated nerve involvement, and fractures in athletes who place high demands on the limb.[36] Substantial controversy exists within the literature regarding the amount of acceptable displacement. Many authors suggest that fractures with 2 to 3 mm or more of displacement should be surgically fixed, yet some tolerate up to 10 mm of displacement.[33,38]

Patients are placed in a long arm cast for 3 to 4 weeks with radiographs that are obtained at 1 week to ensure the maintenance of alignment. After the cast is removed, patients are instructed to begin AROM and come back for ROM checks. If the patient still has substantial deficits at the ROM check, formal occupational therapy is prescribed.[36]

Nonsurgical management of medial epicondylar fractures typically yields positive outcomes.[38] Functional results similar to those seen with operative management are achieved; nonoperative patients experience lower complication rates.[35]

Complications

Extension loss occurs more commonly in operative versus nonoperative patients, with the highest rates of decreased motion occurring in patients who required an arthrotomy to remove entrapped fragments.[33] In a study of longitudinal impacts of conservative treatment of medial epicondylar fractures, pseudoarthritis was reported in 55% of patients.[38] Ulnar nerve dysfunction has also been observed after operative treatment, particularly in patients with initial incarceration of the fragment within the joint space.[33,35,38]

Supracondylar Humerus Fractures
Background

Supracondylar fractures are the most common fractures of the elbow in the pediatric population and make up 3.3% of all pediatric fractures.[5,24] These injuries typically occur in children between the ages of 5 and 7 years, with nearly equal incidence between girls and boys.[24,39,40] Supracondylar humerus fractures are most commonly caused by falls onto an outstretched hand, with 99% of the injuries resulting in an extension-type injury and 1% in flexion-type injuries.[39]

Clinical and Radiographic Examination

The clinical examination should assess for edema, lacerations, ecchymosis, and open injuries. If substantial swelling is present, it is important to have a heightened awareness for compartment syndrome. Although it can be difficult, assessment of nerve integrity during a clinical examination is imperative because nerve injuries occur in roughly 11% of pediatric supracondylar fractures.[41] In patients with extension-type fractures, the anterior interosseous nerve (AIN) is the most commonly injured nerve, whereas the ulnar nerve is the most commonly injured in flexion-type fractures.[41,42] Notably, most associated nerve damage is transient and will resolve within a few months of initial injury.

Suspected supracondylar fractures are diagnosed with AP and lateral radiographs of the elbow. These should be assessed for fracture displacement and angulation, as well as comminution and intraarticular extension. If the determination between a fracture line and a physeal line is unclear, comparison radiographs of the contralateral elbow can be helpful. To rule out any concomitant injuries, orthogonal views of the entire upper extremity may be obtained.

Treatment and Therapeutic Considerations

Type I (nondisplaced) fractures can be treated nonoperatively in a long arm cast or an orthosis for 3 to 4 weeks, with the elbow at 90 degrees of flexion. If there is substantial edema, the cast should be initially positioned in less than 90 degrees of flexion, and the patient should be casted again after the edema subsides to achieve the full 90 degrees of flexion.

The treatment of type II (intact posterior cortical hinge) fractures is more controversial; some authors recommend CRPP of all type II fractures, others recommend CRPP of malrotated type II fractures only, and still others recommend closed reduction and casting of all type II fractures.[40,43] If a child is treated nonoperatively for a type II fracture, repeat radiographs are performed within 5 to 7 days to evaluate for worsening displacement. If an orthosis was initially placed and the alignment is maintained at the first follow-up visit, conversion to a long arm cast can be performed to permit better control of the fracture fragments without increasing the risk of compartment syndrome. Operative fixation is advised if the alignment is not maintained.

Type III (completely displaced) fractures have a high risk of concomitant neurologic and vascular injuries and are often associated with substantial edema. These are typically treated with CRPP. A reduction is considered adequate if there is neither varus nor valgus malalignment, the anterior humeral line is intact, and minimal rotation is present. Pain medications are limited to avoid sedating the child or masking signs and symptoms of an impending compartment syndrome. A non-narcotic medication, such as acetaminophen, typically provides sufficient analgesia.

Factors that determine emergent management of a supracondylar fracture include open fractures, dysvascular limbs, floating elbows, nerve lacerations, and suspicion of a compartment syndrome.

Complications

The most common complications after supracondylar fractures include transient stiffness, nerve injury, and cubitus varus.[44] Nerve injuries after supracondylar fractures often spontaneously recover within 2 months of the initial injury. If after 4 months, there are no signs of recovery, electrodiagnostic studies should be obtained to assess the injury. A study by Bashyal and associates[44] found a 4.2% complication rate for supracondylar fractures and described other possible complications, including unanticipated return to the operating room for pin removal or repeat reduction and pinning, infection, compartment syndrome, and malunion.

Compartment syndrome is another debilitating and devastating potential complication of a supracondylar fracture that must be diagnosed and addressed early for optimal outcomes to occur and avoid permanent functional impairment. Children who sustain a concomitant injury to the wrist or forearm in addition to a supracondylar fracture are at an increased risk of developing a compartment syndrome.

Return of ROM can be prolonged after a supracondylar humerus fracture. Patients undergoing formal therapy have been found to have decreased time to the return of full ROM.[45]

Elbow Dislocations
Background
Pediatric elbow dislocations make up only about 3% of pediatric elbow injuries.[46] They are seen most often in children ages 6 to 15 years old and are more common in boys.[47,48] The most common mechanism of injury is a fall onto an outstretched arm.[47,49] Posterior dislocations are observed most often, whereas anterior dislocations are considered rare in the pediatric population.[50]

Clinical and Radiographic Examination
Patients with elbow dislocations often present with a painful and swollen elbow, making it difficult to perform a through clinical examination. If a dislocation or a fracture is suspected, a physician should obtain AP and lateral radiographs. Some physicians may obtain radiographs of the contralateral elbow as a comparison. Isolated dislocations are uncommon, and therefore the radiographs must be evaluated carefully because 64% of the cases include associated fractures, which may be missed during the initial evaluation.[48] Avulsion fractures of the medial epicondyle are the most common associated injury, although injuries to the coronoid, radial head, olecranon, and lateral epicondyle may also occur.[48,50]

Treatment and Therapy Considerations
Nonoperative treatment is the most common treatment method and is appropriate for stable dislocations. Closed reductions should be followed by roughly 3 weeks of immobilization in a posterior orthosis or long arm cast.[49] Enacting a protocol for the early initiation of therapy, specifically focusing on ROM exercises, provides the best chance at decreasing elbow stiffness.

Indications for operative management include open dislocations, joint instability, incarcerated medial epicondyle or coronoid process fragments, and failure to obtain or maintain a sufficient closed reduction.[33,49,50]

Patients with an elbow dislocation are often prescribed formal therapy if they sustained a concomitant neurologic injury or if elbow or forearm stiffness is present. The goal of therapy is to restore ROM throughout the elbow, forearm, and wrist. Younger patients do not typically tolerate aggressive elbow ROM exercise because of the co-contracture of antagonistic musculature during stretching. Therefore, dynamic elbow orthoses should be avoided. Instead, the therapist must provide patients with client-centered activities to incorporate full elbow ROM activities (e.g., throwing bean bags, shooting a basketball) and forearm and wrist ROM activities (playing a card game, typing on a computer, or painting on an elevated easel). After the patient is cleared to bear weight on the joint, activities such as crab walking and playing twister may also assist a patient in regaining terminal elbow extension. Depending on the severity of the dislocation, patients may experience an elbow extension lag, although this does not generally inhibit their ability to perform any of the activities that they were engaged in preinjury.

Complications
The most common complications observed with pediatric elbow dislocations are stiffness, recurrent dislocations, arthritis, radioulnar synostosis, cubitus valgus, heterotrophic ossification, neurologic injuries, and chronic elbow instability.[49,50]

Monteggia Fractures and Dislocation
Background

A Monteggia fracture–dislocation is a radial head dislocation accompanied by a proximal ulna fracture or plastic deformation of the ulna. These are rare injuries, making up fewer than 1% of pediatric fractures, and often occur because of a fall onto an outstretched hand with simultaneous hyperpronation or hyperextension.[5,51]

Clinical and Radiographic Examination

Most children with Monteggia fracture–dislocations present with pain, edema, and deformity of the forearm and elbow. During the physical examination, palpation over the radial head is important because it may spontaneously reduce the radial head dislocation. Standard radiographs of the elbow and forearm should be obtained. The radiocapitellar line should be assessed on the lateral radiograph of the elbow; a straight line from the radial shaft through the center of the capitellum should be observed in properly aligned elbows.[51]

Treatment and Therapy Considerations

Nonoperative treatment can be effective provided that the radial head is stable after the reduction and the length of the ulna is sufficient. The most commonly used technique is a closed reduction of the ulna and radial head followed by a long arm cast. The long arm cast is typically molded in 110 to 120 degrees of flexion and full supination, keeping the limb immobilized for 4 to 6 weeks.[51,52]

Operative management is indicated for acute Bado type IV injuries (radius and ulna fractures with a radial head dislocation), open fractures, unstable reductions, and longitudinally unstable ulna fractures. A patient with a delayed diagnosis likely requires prompt surgical management because closed reductions are frequently unsuccessful.

Therapy is guided by the stability of the proximal radioulnar joint and the distal radioulnar (DRU) joint. Therapists provide education and equipment for edema control and ROM and strengthening exercises and educate patients on activities at home that can increase elbow, wrist, and forearm ROM such as ball toss, functional reaching tasks with toys, and use of gaming systems.

Complications

A delayed or missed diagnosis is the most common complication in these injuries, particularly in cases in which an orthopedic surgeon is not performing the assessment, the ulna is plastically deformed, or full-length forearm films are missing.[53] Associated deficits that commonly accompany pediatric Monteggia fracture–dislocations include posttraumatic edema, joint stiffness, hypertrophic scarring, and impaired ADL and leisure tasks. A posterior interosseous nerve (PIN) palsy is the most common nerve injury in Monteggia fracture–dislocations, although most PIN palsies are neuropraxic by nature and generally recover slowly after the radial head is reduced.[51,54] Additional complications that can occur include compartment syndrome of the forearm, chronic elbow pain and stiffness, and valgus instability.

Radial Neck Fractures
Background

Radial neck fractures account for 1% of all pediatric fractures and 5% to 10% of all pediatric elbow fractures.[5,24,55] Most occur in children between the ages of 3 and 15 years and may be associated with other injuries such as olecranon fractures, medial epicondyle fractures, and ulna shaft fractures.[36,56] The most common mechanisms of injury include a fall onto an outstretched hand while running or a fall from the monkey bars.

Clinical and Radiographic Examination

Examination will demonstrate that passive elbow flexion and extension is not as painful as forearm rotation. It is imperative to palpate the radial head and neck region of the patient because it provides contributory evidence for the physician to make the correct diagnosis.

Imaging of a suspected radial neck fracture should begin with AP and lateral views of the elbow. Superimposition of the fracture line over the ulna on radiographs may cause discrepancies during the diagnosis of minimally displaced fractures.[36] Additionally, if ossification of the epiphysis has not yet occurred, it may be difficult to discern the amount of displacement of the radial head upon inspection of the radiograph. In these instances, identification of a posterior fat pad sign on the lateral radiograph will indicate that a fracture is likely present.

Treatment and Therapy Considerations

The treatment of radial neck fractures in children varies depending on the fracture's displacement, angulation, and skeletal maturity.[56,57] The management approach algorithm should begin with closed reduction, continuing to percutaneous assisted reduction, and finally to open treatment if previous methods were unsuccessful. Most radial neck fractures are nondisplaced or minimally displaced and can be treated with closed reduction and casting with a good outcome.[36] These fractures are often immobilized in a long arm cast with the elbow at 90 degrees for 3 weeks followed by early AROM exercises to decrease the stiffness caused by immobilization.[36]

Younger children can often safely tolerate radial neck fractures with angulation of up to 30 degrees with simple immobilization, given their substantial remodeling potential. Older children and patients with fractures that have greater than 30 degrees of angulation should undergo an attempt to improve alignment.[57,58] If attempts at closed manipulation fail, then surgical management will need to be performed.[36,56]

Open reductions are reserved for cases involving comminuted fractures, fractures with a completely displaced radial head, and those in which closed reduction has failed.[55,57]

Because young children do not typically tolerate therapy that uses aggressive stretching, the therapist may be required to be creative with treatment interventions to help restore ROM. Examples of interventions include playing catch, dribbling a basketball, throwing a soccer ball, finger painting on an elevated surface, playing games (e.g., Twister, card games), and engaging in competitions using a Wii console.

Complications

The most frequent complications that arise after a pediatric radial neck fracture are restricted forearm rotation and radial head overgrowth.[58] Other complications that can occur, although rare, include injury to the PIN, heterotopic ossification, physeal arrest, radioulnar synostosis, compartment syndrome, and malunion.[55,58]

Both-Bone Forearm Fractures
Background

Diaphyseal forearm fractures are some of the most common fractures in the pediatric population and represent roughly 40% of all pediatric fractures.[24] Notably, the frequency of these injuries has increased threefold between 1997 and 2009.[59] The peak incidence occurs between 8 and 14 years of age.[59,60] The most common mechanism causing these injuries are ground-level falls, direct trauma, falls at the playground, and sporting-related activities.[59]

Clinical and Radiographic Examination

During the initial examination, it is important to inspect the skin for lacerations, edema, open injuries, ecchymosis, and tenderness to palpation throughout the elbow, wrist, and forearm region.

Deformity may or may not be noted during the physical examination, depending on the severity of the injury. A patient's AROM of the elbow, forearm, wrist, and hand should be assessed, although these may be limited secondary to pain. A thorough neurologic examination should be performed to assess the motor and sensory functions of the radial, median, and ulnar nerves.

Radiographic imaging should include true orthogonal views of the wrist, elbow, and forearm; comparison radiographs may be helpful, particularly if plastic deformation is suspected.

Treatment and Therapy Considerations

The management of these fractures depends on the patient age, type of fracture, and fracture displacement. The closer the fracture is to the distal physis, the greater the potential for remodeling, although the exact remodeling potential of these fractures remains controversial throughout the literature. Some studies have shown that children younger than 8 to 10 years of age have the ability to remodel 0 to 20 degrees of angulation without malrotation, whereas children 8 to 10 years or older tolerate less amounts of angulation.[60,61]

It is believed that 90% of pediatric both-bone forearm fractures can be successfully managed nonoperatively with closed reduction and casting.[60,62,63] Proper molding of the cast is essential to successful management. General principles of successful casting include three-point molding, adequate padding, and ample layering of casting material to maintain the molding. Patients are typically casted for 4 to 12 weeks, beginning in a long arm cast that is converted to a short arm cast or orthosis after 3 to 4 weeks[60] (Fig. 124.2). Weekly radiographs should be obtained for the first 3 weeks to ensure that the reduction is being maintained while callus formation begins.

Approximately 10% of both-bone forearm fractures are unstable and necessitate further management.[60] The most common operative interventions are closed reductions or mini open reductions, with IM nailing, and ORIF using plate and screw fixation, with each technique having both advantages and disadvantages. ORIF is indicated for comminuted fractures or fractures with late loss of reduction after closed management. Flexible IM nailing has gained popularity within the past decade because it requires shorter surgical times and has similar potential blood loss and union rates than ORIF.[62,64]

Both-bone forearm fractures can result in decreased forearm rotation and wrist ROM, which can be extremely disabling for a patient,

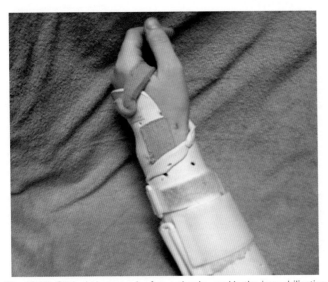

Fig. 124.2 Clinical photograph of an orthosis used in the immobilization of pediatric distal both-bone fractures. (Courtesy of Joshua M. Abzug.)

creating difficulty with self-feeding, grooming, cell phone use, and leisure activities. Therapists can incorporate play and functional activities for the pediatric population to regain their wrist–forearm ROM, strength, and endurance. Activities such as finger painting on an easel, playing basketball, playing a memory card game and flipping over cards with the injured extremity, or a beanbag toss are recommended.

Complications

Loss of reduction is the most common concern after a pediatric forearm fracture. In rare circumstances, conservative management results in malreduction that can affect a patient's ADLs. Other less common complications associated with cast immobilization include growth arrest, compartment syndrome, elbow stiffness, disuse osteopenia, muscle atrophy, and skin breakdown.[1,59] Refractures, although not often seen, can occur up to 6 months after the initial injury.[1]

Distal Radius Fractures
Background

Distal radius fractures are the most common orthopedic injury in the pediatric population.[5,21,24] The increase in incidence of these injuries in the past 40 years is hypothesized to be attributable to earlier participation in sporting events, increased body mass index (BMI), and decreased bone mineral density.[65,66] The primary mechanisms causing these injuries are falls on an outstretched limb and direct trauma to the extremity. The incidence of distal radius fractures peaks in girls 8 to 11 years of age and in boys 11 to 14 years of age.[66]

Clinical and Radiographic Examination

The clinical presentation is predicated by the severity of the initial injury. The skin should be examined carefully for open wounds, lacerations, and edema. Pain may be localized to the wrist without obvious edema or deformity. A systematic review of the bilateral elbows, hands, and shoulders should be performed to rule out any associated injuries.[67] The most common concomitant injuries include Monteggia fracture–dislocations, supracondylar fractures, and fractures of the radial neck.[68]

Posteroanterior (PA) and lateral radiographic views of the wrist are generally sufficient to make the diagnosis. Ultrasound, CT scans, and MRI can also be used for diagnostic purposes but not as frequently given that they may require sedation and exposure to larger amounts of radiation, can be time consuming, and require specialized training.[68]

Treatment and Therapy Considerations

Fractures that are nondisplaced or minimally displaced are treated effectively with a nonoperative protocol, which includes the use of orthoses or casting for 3 to 4 weeks.[67] Patients and their family members often prefer orthoses over casting because orthoses can be removed for bathing.

Substantial displacement or any rotational deformity necessitate that a closed reduction should be performed. After a closed reduction, the patient is immobilized for 3 to 4 weeks, and weekly radiographs are obtained during the first 3 weeks to ensure that proper alignment of the fracture is maintained.

Irreducible fractures, intraarticular fractures, open fractures, and floating elbows are all indications for operative management.[67] CRPP is often a successful management strategy. ORIF is reserved for open fractures, displaced intraarticular fractures, fractures with impending malunion unable to be reduced by osteoclasis, and displaced metadiaphyseal fractures that were not able to be stabilized with percutaneous pinning. Further indications for surgery include cases in which median neuropathy is present that does not improve after fracture reduction.[68]

Therapists often make patients circumferential wrist orthoses after cast removal. In most cases, formal therapy is not required unless further complications arise. Patients requiring formal therapy include those who have been immobilized for extended periods of time because of poor follow-up and those with concomitant injuries such as supracondylar humerus fractures or Monteggia fracture–dislocations. For those enrolled in formal therapy, the duration of therapy is often brief. Focus during therapy is on ROM exercises to allow a quickened return to preinjury baseline function.

Complications

Physeal arrest occurs in fewer than 7% of patients with a distal radius physeal fracture.[69] Multiple attempts at reduction increase the risk of physeal arrest. Surgical interventions should be considered in patients with a physeal arrest to decrease the likelihood of future increases of wrist pain and ulnar impaction. Radioulnar synostosis is a rare complication that often occurs in high-energy trauma.[70]

Triangular Fibrocartilage Complex Injuries
Background

The triangular fibrocartilaginous complex (TFCC) is composed of the dorsal and volar radioulnar ligaments, the ulnomeniscal homologue, the ulnolunate and ulnotriquetral ligaments, and the sheath of the extensor carpi ulnaris tendon.[67,71] The main functions of the TFCC are to stabilize the DRU joint, support ulnocarpal articulation, provide a smooth articular surface for the radius and ulna, and transmit and absorb the axial load through the ulnocarpal articulation.[67] The most common mechanisms of injury are repetitive ulnar loading, repetitive weight bearing, and falls onto an extended and pronated wrist.[71–73]

Clinical and Radiographic Examination

Children with TFCC tears typically present with ulnar-sided wrist pain that increases with forceful grip and twisting movements. For some patients, pain may only be noted with sports activities, and they may be otherwise pain free in their other daily activities.[67] Popping, clicking, and catching may also be noted with wrist and forearm rotation.[72] Most often, however, children only complain of mild amounts of pain and may not be able to localize the exact place of the pain.

Provocative tests can aid the clinician in making the diagnosis. The most common provocative tests are the TFCC compression test, the supination lift-off test, the press test, and the ulnar fovea sign test.[67,72,74] The TFCC compression test involves the physician placing an axial load while rotating the wrist in ulnar deviation; a positive test result reproduces pain or clicking along the ulnar aspect of the wrist. A supination lift test is done by instructing the patient to place his or her arms on the underside of a table and then to attempt to lift upward against the table (Fig. 124.3); a positive supination lift-off test result reproduces ulnar-sided wrist pain. The press test is done by asking patients to lift themselves out of a chair while weight bearing on the extended wrist. This test is 100% sensitive for the diagnosis of TFCC tears but is often not used during a clinical examination secondary to pain.[74] The ulnar fovea sign test is done by the examiner pressing her or his thumb into the interval between the ulnar styloid and flexor carpi ulnaris tendon.[75] A positive fovea sign is exquisite tenderness in the area. A study by Tay and associates[75] found this test to be 95.2% sensitive and 86.5% specific for TFFC tears.

Physicians may obtain bilateral plain radiographs, MRI, or MRI arthrograms to diagnose a TFCC tear, although the gold standard for diagnosis is a wrist arthroscopy.[67,76]

Treatment and Therapy Considerations

Conservative management for TFCC tears consists of activity modification, nonsteroidal antiinflammatory drugs, cryotherapy,

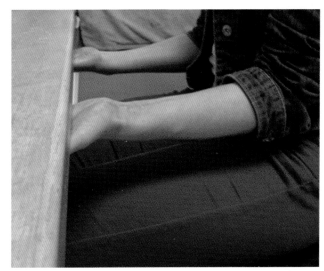

Fig. 124.3 Clinical photograph of the lift-off test for diagnosis of triangular fibrocartilaginous complex injuries. (Courtesy of Joshua M. Abzug.)

immobilization, and cessation of provocative activities. During this timeframe, the patient may be placed in a long arm cast for 3 to 4 weeks with the elbow flexed to 90 degrees and with the forearm supinated, after which they can transition to a Muenster orthosis to prevent forearm rotation for 2 more weeks.[72,77]

After the Muenster orthosis is discharged, the patient can begin formal therapy. At this time, gentle active and active-assisted ROM for the forearm and wrist, along with edema management techniques are added to the patient's treatment plan. At 12 weeks after injury, gentle strengthening exercises can be initiated.[77] A therapist should initiate isometric wrist–forearm strengthening and progress to resistance with Thera-Band and free weights to exercise the forearm and wrist. Patients should only be allowed to return to competitive sports when they are pain free during practice and have regained the appropriate ROM and strength that the particular sport or activity demands.

Operative management of a TFCC injury includes a debridement or arthroscopic repair (or both).[67] A debridement is typically used for central tears because they can be avascular in nature. Surgical repairs are performed on lesions about the peripheral TFCC, which is well vascularized. After repair, the patient is placed into a long arm cast with the elbow at 90 degrees of flexion or a sugartong orthosis.[77]

After a debridement, the focus of the first week of therapy is to control edema and regain AROM of the forearm, wrist, and hand. The therapist may fabricate a wrist orthosis; issue a Tubigrip sleeve; and initiate gentle AROM of the forearm, wrist, and hand. Leading into the second week after debridement, therapy goals include continuing with gentle ROM and scar management. Specific therapeutic interventions include scar massage; issuing an elastomer mold if the scar is hypertrophic; and continuing with AROM of the wrist, forearm, and hand. During weeks three and four post-operatively, PROM to the wrist and forearm should be initiated. A dynamic wrist and forearm orthosis, if applicable, should be fabricated to allow for terminal end ROM. At 6 weeks postoperatively, the patient may be allowed to remove the orthosis and initiate progressive strengthening of the hand, wrist, and forearm. It is important to start with the forearm supinated, working into neutral, and then progressing to forearm pronation because pronation puts the greatest stress on the TFCC.

After a TFCC repair, during the first 2 weeks after surgery, therapists may begin the initiation of retrograde massage and compressive wrapping depending on the patient and immobilization type. After about 4 to 6 weeks, a long arm orthosis in the same position as the cast should be fabricated, and gentle AROM exercises for the elbow, wrist, and forearm can begin. Therapists can initiate scar massage and issue an elastomer mold at this time if the incision scar is painful or problematic. At 8 weeks after surgery, the long arm orthosis is removed, a wrist orthosis may be fabricated, and PROM exercises for the wrist and forearm are initiated. Progressive strengthening of the wrist, hand, and forearm can begin after the patient is otherwise asymptomatic.

Complications

The most common complications for the nonsurgical management of pediatric TFCC injuries are persistent pain, joint laxity, and instability that can lead to degeneration of the articular cartilage and the need for surgical management.[67] In cases managed surgically, the most common complications are loss of fixation and recurrent DRU joint instability.[73]

Galeazzi Fractures

Background

A Galeazzi fracture is a fracture of the radial diaphysis with a disruption of the DRU joint.[78] These injuries are rare in children, observed clinically in fewer than 6% of all pediatric forearm fractures.[5,79] Because DRU joint injuries are frequently overlooked during the initial diagnosis, they are often underdiagnosed. The peak incidence occurs between the ages of 9 and 12 years of age.[79] The most common mechanism of injury for Galeazzi fractures is a fall onto an outstretched hand with simultaneous forearm rotation.[80] Other mechanisms of injury are motor vehicle accidents and electric shock.[81]

Clinical and Radiographic Examination

The clinical examination demonstrates edema and tenderness to palpation of the distal forearm. In some cases, a visible deformity along the distal forearm is observed. A patient's forearm and wrist ROM is often limited and very painful, and the patient remains guarded during the physical examination.[78]

Anteroposterior and lateral films of the forearm, wrist, and elbow are recommended for full visualization and identification of the injury, which is characterized by an angulated, shortened, and displaced fracture of the radial shaft with either joint dislocation or incongruity.[78,82] Contralateral radiographs are often helpful in the diagnosis to serve as a basis for comparison. A CT or MRI scan can be ordered to assess the disruption of the DRU joint if this is difficult to assess on plain radiographs, although these are not routinely necessary.

Treatment and Therapy Considerations

The management of Galeazzi fractures differs between adults and children. The majority of pediatric Galeazzi fractures are managed nonsurgically with a closed reduction performed under general anesthesia with guided fluoroscopy followed by immobilization of the forearm in a long arm cast for 4 to 6 weeks.[82] During casting, the forearm is held in neutral supination–pronation to allow the TFCC to heal and to maintain a good reduction of the DRU joint.[78] Children who are treated nonsurgically have excellent outcomes with very few complications, typically attaining ROM equal to the contralateral side.[82,83]

Surgical treatment in children is rarely indicated; however, possible indications for operative intervention include instances in which the initial closed reduction of the radius and DRU joint are not possible or when the alignment achieved by closed reduction is lost.[78,82] Galeazzi fractures can be managed operatively in several manners such as closed reduction with K-wire fixation, dorsal plate fixation, IM nailing, and open reduction with radioulnar transfixation. Notably, the rarity of these injuries has impacted the ability to compare the outcomes of these surgical procedures. Those patients requiring operative management are immobilized in a long arm cast in supination for 4 to 6 weeks.[82]

The surgeon may prescribe an elbow and wrist immobilization orthosis or a Muenster orthosis, both with the forearm in supination, for additional immobilization after cast removal.[84] While working through ROM exercises, it is important to educate the patient on the importance of initiating activities with the forearm in full supination, gradually working into neutral positions, and then progressing to forearm pronation given that pronation puts the most stress on the TFCC area.

Pediatric patients typically regain the full ROM in their elbows quickly after the long arm cast is removed but may struggle with regaining forearm pronation because their forearms were positioned in supination for 4 to 8 weeks. The lack of forearm pronation can cause patients difficulty with typing, texting, writing, performing schoolwork, and using utensils for self-feeding. Some patients may require static progressive or dynamic orthoses to regain full forearm ROM. Most, however, improve independently with a comprehensive home therapy program and compliance with attendance in formal hand therapy and regain their full ROM and strength within 4 to 8 weeks of cast removal.

Complications

Galeazzi fractures treated with surgery can result in complications that include persistent DRU joint instability, nerve interposition or entrapment, malunion, nonunion, infection, decreased forearm ROM, and chronic wrist pain.[80,82] The most debilitating complication of these injuries is malunion of the radius with DRU joint instability. These patients can have chronic pain, loss of grip strength, and limited forearm rotation.[78]

Scaphoid Fractures

Background

Scaphoid fractures are relatively uncommon in children, representing fewer than 0.5% of all pediatric fractures and fewer than 8% of pediatric hand–wrist fractures.[85] However, the scaphoid is the most commonly fractured pediatric carpal bone and comprises 88% of pediatric carpal fractures.[85] The scaphoid fracture incidence peaks between 12 and 16 years of age and is most commonly caused by a fall onto an outstretched wrist while participating in a sporting event.[85,86]

Recent studies have commented on a change in injury patterns presenting in pediatric and adolescent scaphoid fractures.[87,88] Increases in BMI and the popularization of extreme sports have been described as major contributing factors.[66,89] Whereas scaphoid fractures in the past were predominately of a distal pole pattern, recent studies have found that scaphoid waist fractures are now the most common location in children.[86,88] In roughly 15% of scaphoid fractures, associated injuries are reported and may include distal radius fractures, ulnar styloid fractures, capitate fractures, and bilateral scaphoid fractures.[86]

Clinical and Radiographic Examination

Patients with a suspected scaphoid fracture commonly present with tenderness about the snuffbox or over the distal pole of the scaphoid. These patients often complain of pain with active wrist motion, particularly with radial deviation.

When a scaphoid fracture is suspected, standard PA and lateral views of the wrist should be obtained, along with a PA view of the wrist in ulnar deviation. It is important to be aware that many pediatric scaphoid fractures may not be evident on radiographs up to 10 days after the injury. Common practice is to immobilize the patient with a suspected scaphoid fracture and schedule a follow-up appointment 2 weeks after the injury. MRIs and CT scans are also helpful tools to aid in the diagnosis of scaphoid fractures. MRIs are used more frequently because they are more sensitive when diagnosing acute scaphoid fractures, whereas CT scans can assist with quantifying displacement.

Treatment and Therapeutic Considerations

Cast immobilization is the standard treatment of pediatric scaphoid fractures. More than 90% of nondisplaced fractures treated with casting alone will achieve successful union and excellent patient satisfaction.[86] Conversely, only 23% of patients with chronic fractures (presenting more than 6 weeks postinjury) that are treated with closed management achieve a successful union.[86]

Three factors that will prolong cast immobilization are fracture displacement, a scaphoid proximal pole fracture, and delay in initial treatment. Patients with distal pole fractures tend to heal faster than those with scaphoid waist fracture patterns, typically demonstrating union in 6 weeks. Proximal pole fractures of the scaphoid have the longest average times to union of any scaphoid fracture pattern, requiring immobilization of up to 15 weeks.[86] Operative management is indicated for acute displaced fractures, fractures that have had unsuccessful closed management, and chronically displaced fractures. The most common operative interventions are CRPP procedures for nondisplaced fractures and K-wires or compression screws for fractures with more significant displacement or malrotation. Vascularized bone grafting, although still a treatment option, is used less frequently in the pediatric population than with the adult population.[90]

After surgery, patients should be immobilized in a short arm thumb spica cast until union is achieved and kept out of sports for 3 to 6 months. Older patients, who can typically be trusted more reliably, may be able to be transitioned to a circumferential thumb spica orthosis 4 to 6 weeks into the immobilization phase.

The majority of pediatric patients with scaphoid fractures do not require formal therapy. However, patients who have been immobilized for more than 12 weeks may be referred for therapy. These patients often have varying degrees of decreased wrist, forearm, and thumb carpometacarpal (CMC) and metacarpophalangeal (MCP) ROM, depending on the duration of immobilization. Modalities such as fluidotherapy and moist heat packs can facilitate exercises to increase ROM and decrease pain in the affected extremity. Hand therapists can also include contract–relax exercises as well as isometric wrist and forearm exercises to help regain the patient's strength, ROM, and endurance. Most patients with scaphoid fractures remain in formal therapy for 4 to 6 weeks after immobilization, regaining full ROM compared with the contralateral side and return to sports and related activities at levels similar to preinjury baselines.

Complications

Pediatric scaphoid fractures generally yield good functional outcomes. Nonunion is a chief concern, primarily in chronic fractures. Other complications, although relatively uncommon, include refracture, malunion, avascular necrosis, and persistent pain.

Hand Fractures and Dislocations

Background

Hand fractures are some of the most frequently observed injuries in the pediatric and adolescent populations, accounting for roughly 15% to 20% of all pediatric fractures.[5,91] The peak incidence is seen in children ages 9 to 14 years old, with the higher incidence observed in boys.

Clinical and Radiographic Examination

A detailed assessment of the hand should include an evaluation of the nail bed, fingers, and hand for open wounds or lacerations, edema, and ecchymosis. Observing the digital cascade of the hand also can further assess the degree of rotational deformities present. It is important to compare the contralateral hand because some children may normally experience scissoring, overlapping, or underlapping bilaterally. Isolating the flexor and extensor tendons of the affected digit is also an important evaluation tool because it may provide information about concomitant tendon injuries.

A thorough neurovascular examination should be performed to rule out any nerve damage. Monofilament and two-point discrimination testing may be difficult for children younger than 6 years of age, but for these children, the wrinkle test can be used to assess nerve function.[92] In this test, the patient submerges the involved finger in water for 5 to 10 minutes; wrinkling is absent on the volar aspect in a denervated digit.[93]

If the patient is thought to have a hand fracture, PA, oblique, and lateral radiographs of the hand should be obtained. When a phalangeal fracture is suspected, isolated finger radiographs should be taken.[94]

Treatment and Therapeutic Considerations

Metacarpal fractures often occur during physical altercations and are more common in older adolescents.[94,95] Metacarpal neck and shaft fractures are the most common in children and are treated with closed reduction and orthoses or casting in an intrinsic-plus position for 3 to 4 weeks.[94] The amount of allowable angulation depends on the digit involved and the location of the injury.[94,96] However, any rotational deformity associated with metacarpal fractures is not well tolerated and should be treated with closed reduction with or without percutaneous pinning. ORIF is recommended for intraarticular metacarpal fractures.

Proximal phalanx fractures are the most common phalangeal fracture in children and are divided into base, shaft, neck, and condylar fractures.[91,94] In the pediatric population, finger fractures occur most commonly at the base of the proximal phalanx because the physis is in this area.[95,97] The majority of proximal phalanx fractures are stable and can be treated with 3 to 4 weeks of immobilization in a gutter cast or orthosis in the intrinsic-plus position with good outcomes. However, displaced fractures can lead to a deformity in the digit and are often treated with surgical management to avoid long-term deformity. Typically, CRPP is sufficient.

Middle phalanx fractures occur less frequently and are treated in the same manner as proximal phalanx fractures. These fractures are often stable and can be treated in a cast or an orthosis if the child is believed to be able to maintain compliance.

Distal phalanx fractures are also common in the pediatric population, often affecting younger children.[94] These injuries typically occur when a child's finger gets shut in a car or house door. The majority of these injuries do not require surgical intervention and can be treated with a protective distal interphalangeal (DIP) joint orthosis or an AlumaFoam orthosis for 3 to 4 weeks. If a concomitant nail bed injury occurs, surgical management should be performed, including an irrigation and debridement and repair of the nail bed.[96] In addition, children should be placed on antibiotics because these are technically open wounds.

Hand therapists play a key role in managing pediatric hand fractures. Their knowledge in differential tissue assessment, intrinsic, extrinsic, and oblique retinaculum tightness is crucial during the treatment phase. Some of the factors influencing the initiation of therapy are the bone injured, the location of the fracture, the quantity and pattern of the fracture(s), the type of reduction and fixation, associated soft tissue injuries, and the time since the initial injury or surgical correction.

A hand therapist can fabricate the appropriate orthosis to be worn after cast immobilization. Therapists should then initiate AROM, PROM, and tendon-gliding exercises for tissue mobilization. If stiffness occurs, a differential tissue assessment is performed to determine the cause of the stiffness (intrinsic, extrinsic, oblique retinaculum tightness, or joint contracture), and the appropriate orthosis is fabricated based on the findings. For metacarpal fractures, a gutter orthosis is fabricated by the hand therapist with the MCP joints in 70 degrees of flexion and the IP joints in extension. The therapist should initiate tendon-gliding and intrinsic exercises while blocking along the affected metacarpal to decrease adherence and optimize the patient's total AROM. The orthosis most common in proximal phalanx fracture treatment is a circumferential finger orthosis with the MCP joint in 70 degrees of flexion and the interphalangeal (IP) joints in extension (Fig. 124.4). Extensor tendon gliding and differential flexor digitorum superficialis (FDS) and flexor digitorum profundus (FDP) tendon gliding are appropriate exercises to initiate within an exercise orthosis to increase total AROM in the affected digit. For middle phalanx fractures, a finger orthosis that holds the IP joints in full extension is fabricated, and the patient is instructed in FDS tendon gliding and isolated DIP flexion

exercises within the orthosis (Fig. 124.5). For distal phalanx fractures, hand therapists can fabricate a DIP extension orthosis (Fig. 124.6) or a cap orthosis over the wound dressings. DIP joint motion should then be initiated, progressing to a full arc of motion after the patient is cleared to do so by the physician.

Complications

Soft tissue complications can occur with pediatric hand fractures, including extensor tendon adherence, intrinsic muscle contracture, and dorsal incision contracture seen with metacarpal fractures. With proximal phalanx fractures, potential complications include extensor mechanism adherence and FDS adherence. Soft tissue complications to consider with middle phalanx fractures are DIP flexion contractures and FDP adherence. Distal phalanx fractures are associated with complications such as open wounds and nail bed injuries. Other complications to consider with pediatric hand fractures are infection, malunion, pin migration, and finger stiffness.

Fractures and Dislocations of the Thumb
Background

The most common mechanisms of injuries causing metacarpal fractures of the thumb are sports-related trauma and axial loading to the thumb.[93] Fractures of the metacarpal base are the most common pediatric thumb injuries.[95] MCP joint thumb dislocations occur secondary to a hyperextension injury and often times during a sports-related activity.[93]

Clinical and Radiographic Examination

Fractures of the thumb are classified in a manner consistent with that of a fracture in the metacarpal or phalanx of any other digit. MCP joint dislocations can be divided into subgroups, including incomplete dislocation, simple complete dislocation, and complex complete dislocation. Incomplete thumb MCP joint dislocations are defined as ruptures of the volar plate with partial tears of collateral ligaments. Simple, complete thumb MCP joint dislocations are defined as ruptures of the volar plate with complete disruption of the collateral ligaments. Complex complete thumb MCP joint dislocations are defined as complete ruptures of the volar plate and the collateral ligaments with joint interposition.

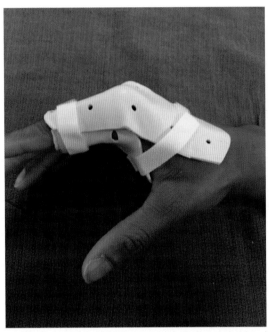

Fig. 124.4 Clinical photograph of a proximal phalanx orthosis with free flexion of the distal interphalangeal joint. (Courtesy of Joshua M. Abzug.)

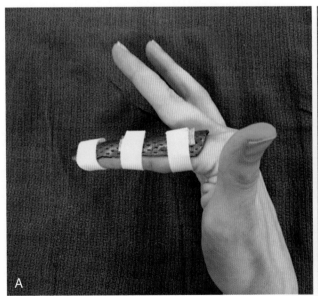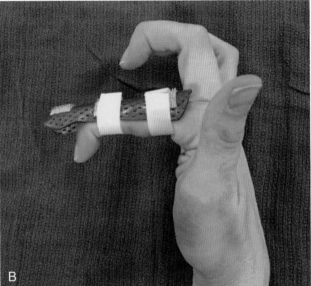

Fig. 124.5 Clinical photograph of a middle phalanx fracture orthosis. **A,** By using the most distal strap, the distal interphalangeal joint can be held in extension. **B,** By removing the most distal strap, the distal interphalangeal joint can be permitted to perform active flexion. (Courtesy of Joshua M. Abzug.)

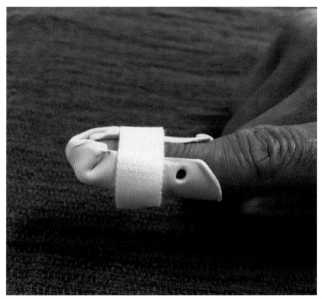

Fig. 124.6 Clinical photograph of an orthosis to immobilize fractures of the distal phalanx. (Courtesy of Joshua M. Abzug.)

Clinical and Radiographic Examination

The evaluation of a child's thumb often proves to be difficult because young children can be scared and often struggle to follow instructions. A fracture is suspected if edema, ecchymosis, deformity, or limited motion is present upon clinical examination. Detailed sensory assessment should be performed to identify possible concomitant injuries. If a fracture is suspected, then radiographs should be obtained, including AP, lateral, and oblique views.

Treatment and Therapeutic Considerations

Children have excellent remodeling potential for extraarticular fractures and therefore are often able to be treated conservatively for 3 to 4 weeks in a short arm thumb spica cast or 4-6 weeks in an orthosis with the IP joint immobilized.[93,99] After immobilization, patients should be educated on a home therapy program for wrist, hand, and thumb ROM. Formal hand therapy is not generally needed unless significant concomitant injuries were sustained. Patients are also instructed to use gaming systems and cell phones to regain thumb ROM at home.[93]

Early ROM after fixation of pediatric metacarpal fractures is controversial. Adolescents must be mature and reliable enough to be trusted with compliance for a removable orthosis to be prescribed. If the care team elects to pursue this option, early ROM can be initiated with the assistance and supervision of a hand therapist beginning 5 to 7 days after surgery, at which time a removable thumb spica orthosis can be fabricated.[93]

Thumb dislocations require immobilization in a thumb spica cast after their reduction for 3 weeks with return to sports 6 weeks from the initial injury. Open reduction may be required for complex complete joint dislocations and can be followed by an immobilization protocol similar to that of a complete thumb MCP joint dislocation.

Thumb metacarpal fractures generally heal with excellent outcomes, and patients return to normal function quickly as there is increased ROM of the CMC joint in pediatric patients that is more tolerant of malunion than in adults. Formal hand therapy is not often needed after the immobilization period because patients are able to regain thumb ROM after they resume daily activities.

Complications

Complications after thumb fractures and dislocations are rare in the pediatric population but require early management to prevent long-term sequelae. As with other injuries to the digits, infection, pin migration, and thumb stiffness are potential complications. Delay in diagnosis and treatment of thumb dislocations may result in long-term joint instability and functional ROM impairment.[99]

Nerve Palsies Related to Upper Extremity Fractures
Background

Nerve injuries are associated with 2.4% of fractures in children and are more likely to be found in upper extremity than in lower extremity fractures.[100] These injuries can be the result of the initial trauma or fracture or can occur during reduction attempts or surgical management of the fracture. Common mechanisms of initial nerve injuries include falls, high-velocity athletic injuries, and motor vehicle accidents.[101]

Certain fractures have a higher incidence of concomitant nerve injuries. For example, humerus fractures have been associated with up to a 12% incidence of nerve palsies in the pediatric population.[100] Supracondylar humerus fractures with concomitant nerve injuries have been observed in roughly 15% of such cases, with the AIN being the most commonly injured nerve.[42] Monteggia fracture–dislocations are also associated with various nerve palsies, the most common of which is a PIN palsy. PIN injuries occur most often when the radial head has anterolateral displacement, although high resolution rates are observed after the radius is reduced.[51,102]

Forearm fractures are another common pediatric injury associated with nerve palsies. Diaphyseal fractures have been noted to occur in combination with injury to the median nerve, ulnar nerve, and PINs.[101] Median neuropathy can also occur with distal radius fractures. Injuries to the ulnar nerve and AIN have been observed in conjunction with Galeazzi fractures as well.[80,101]

Clinical Examination

Diagnosis of nerve palsies can be difficult in the pediatric population, particularly when there is very little motor disturbance or sensory nerve involvement given the difficulty of assessing nerve function in young children. Young children often have difficulty verbalizing if they are experiencing numbness and struggle to comprehend most standardized sensory testing. An attempt at a sensory examination is imperative, however, for diagnosis, and both moving and static two-point discrimination testing should be attempted in patients who are cooperative.[92,101] Electrodiagnostic tests can also help establish the severity of injury, particularly if the other diagnostic studies are inconclusive or were not able to be performed.[101] This is also a difficult assessment depending on the age and development of the patient because electromyography can be a very anxiety-provoking test and is often not able to be completed without anesthesia.

Treatment and Therapeutic Considerations

Most of these injuries are neuropraxic in nature and will resolve over time without requiring surgical intervention. In cases in which the nerve function does not return within 4 months of injury, as assessed by either physical examination or electrodiagnostic testing, it is advised that surgical exploration be performed to better assess the potential for healing.[101]

Hand therapists can play an active role in pediatric patients with nerve injuries. Therapy priorities include mobility of the soft tissue and prevention of joint contractures. If muscular imbalances are observed with resultant postural deformities, orthoses can be created to help the patient compensate. These will limit excessive stretching of denervated muscles, prevent the development of substitution patterns, and maximize the patient's functional abilities for ADLs.[104] It is important during this time to provide thorough education in the necessary care of the injury to both the patient and his or her family because, given the sensory deficits, added precautions will be required in all daily activities.

An injury to the ulnar nerve at the wrist results in denervation of the intrinsic muscles of the hand, resulting in an imbalance of the extrinsic muscles overpowering the intrinsic musculature and resulting in clawing of the ring and small finger.[104] An anticlaw orthosis can be made for the ring and small fingers to block the MCP joints in slight flexion and allow the extrinsic extensor muscle to act through the dorsal hood to extend the IP joints of the fingers.

With injury to the median nerve at the level of the wrist, sensation to the volar aspect of the thumb, index, long, and radial half of the ring finger is compromised, along with motor control of the abductor pollicis brevis (APB), opponens pollicis (OP), superficial head of the flexor pollicis brevis, and first and second lumbricals. With loss of the APB and the OP and the unopposed action of the adductor pollicis a thumb webspace contracture may develop, and an orthosis can be made to maintain the webspace and prevent webspace contractures for overnight use. A daytime orthosis can also be fabricated that places the thumb in abduction for increased functional use.[104] Proximal lesions to the radial nerve result in deficits in supination and wrist and finger extension, although patients still have intact sensation over the volar aspect of the palm. Orthoses for radial nerve injuries hold the wrist and the MCP joints of all five digits in extension to allow for functional grasp and release.

Education of the patient and their support network is an important component of the rehabilitation program with particular focus on precautions that need to be observed related to the loss of sensation. For example, burns, pressure, and friction injuries that damage the skin can occur as a result of decreased or total lack of sensation.

Compartment Syndrome
Background

Compartment syndrome is caused by elevated tissue pressure in a specific osseofascial compartment, which compromises the circulation to the muscles and nerves within the compartment and can cause permanent damage to the extremity. As internal pressures rise within the affected osseofascial compartment, sensory changes occur followed by muscle weakness. Permanent and irreversible damage can occur as early as 6 to 8 hours after critical pressures are reached.

Common causes of pediatric compartment syndrome include trauma, such as fractures or crush injuries, burns, restrictive dressings or casts, vascular injuries, and bleeding disorders. The most common site in the upper extremity for compartment syndrome to occur is the forearm, which is typically associated with displaced both-bone fractures in the forearm and supracondylar fractures. Prolonged manipulation in the operating room during IM nailing poses an increased risk for developing the condition.[105] Compartment syndrome after a supracondylar fracture is very rare, often caused by casting at flexion angles greater than 90 degrees or concomitant vascular injuries.

Clinical Examination

Identification of an evolving compartment syndrome in a child is difficult given the limited ability of children to communicate in addition to potential anxiety about the evaluation. A physician may need to be creative to assess the motor and sensory neurologic function of a young patient. The physician can ask the patient to hold a crayon, reach for an object while the vision is occluded, or involve the patient's guardian(s) in the assessment to decrease the patient's stress level.

Classically, physicians are trained to look for the five Ps (pain, paresthesia, paralysis, pallor, and pulselessness) that are commonly associated with adult compartment syndrome. However, documenting the degree of pain is not always practical with children who may not be able or willing to communicate effectively. Therefore, in pediatric patients with concern for compartment syndrome, physicians should look for the three As of pediatric compartment syndrome: anxiety, agitation, and analgesia.[106,107] Particularly in young patients who have difficulty expressing themselves, those with increasing analgesic needs are thought to be at increased risk of compartment syndrome.

The diagnosis of compartment syndrome is especially difficult to make if a nerve injury occurred simultaneously with a fracture. In these cases, the sensory and motor changes that are early indications of an evolving compartment syndrome of the forearm cannot be detected if nerve function is already diminished or absent.[108,109]

Treatment and Therapeutic Considerations

The treatment of compartment syndrome is an emergent fasciotomy to relieve the internal pressures and provide the best chance for tissue and neurologic salvage. The surgeon must ensure that the individual muscles of both the superficial and deep compartments are released.[108]

After the fasciotomy, any fractures should be reduced and stabilized. When feasible, a delayed primary closure is recommended at 36 to 48 hours.[109] Throughout recovery, the patient should be placed in an orthosis to prevent contractures. After the surgical wounds are healed, hand therapy should be initiated to decrease pain, prevent soft tissue contractures, and increase muscle strength and endurance.[108] Associated fractures will also factor into the determination of the rehabilitation protocol. The recovery time for pediatric compartment syndrome can be up to 1 year.

Complications

Common associated complications after compartment syndrome and subsequent fasciotomies include stiffness and contracture of the soft tissues, although these may be combatted with early active therapy protocols.[109] Children with compartment syndrome typically experience excellent outcomes when a diagnosis is made in a timely fashion and appropriate surgical intervention is performed. However, late diagnoses can increase the risk for severe complications such as neurologic injury, infection, soft tissue necrosis, and permanent functional deficits.[108,110] Late diagnoses can also decrease the quality of the outcomes and increase the likelihood of further surgeries such as tendon lengthening, tendon transfers, and contracture releases.[106,108,110]

Flexor Tendon Injuries
Background

The incidence of flexor tendon injuries in children is roughly 3.6 per 100,000 per year.[111] These injuries are more commonly seen in boys than girls and are most often caused by falling on sharp objects such as broken glass.[111,112] The classification for flexor tendon injuries in children is the same used with the adult population. Zones II and V are the two most common injury zones in the pediatric population.[113] The age of the child plays a larger role in management than the zone of injury does. Patients with flexor tendon injuries are placed into three groups based on age: preschoolers (younger than 5 years old), children (5–10 years of age), and teenagers (11–15 years of age).[114]

Clinical and Radiographic Examination

The diagnosis of flexor tendon injuries in children is more difficult than in adults. Late presentation of these injuries and missed diagnoses of concomitant digital nerve involvement are common in children because they are often not as cooperative as adults during assessment and are not always cognizant of their fingers not working properly.[112]

A thorough history, including when the injury happened and the mechanism of injury, can give a physician important clues in making the proper diagnosis. Assessing the skin for lacerations, ecchymosis, and edema may also give information as to potential sites of tendon injury.

It is also important to assess the resting posture of the hand, the digital cascade using the tenodesis effect, and AROM of the affected digit. A flexor tendon injury is suspected if the affected digit remains in extension with simultaneous wrist extension or if a patient cannot actively isolate the tendon in question when asked to flex and extend the affected finger. A neurovascular examination should be performed, given the close proximity of the flexor tendons to the digital nerves. In cases of suspected bony involvement, radiographs should be taken.

Treatment and Therapy Considerations

For children younger than 2 years old, it is recommended that a six-strand technique be used because of the small flexor profundus.[112] Interestingly, although an increased number of strands has been correlated with improved biomechanical performance and lower rupture rates in early active protocols, Al-Qattan and associates[112] found that in children older than 5 years of age, four-strand repairs are optimal because rupture rates are lower in four-strand repairs than six-strand repairs.[115] This may be partly caused by the bulkiness associated with repairs over four strands.[115]

There is some controversy with regard to postoperative immobilization after pediatric flexor tendon repairs. Some practitioners support full immobilization for 3 to 4 weeks, whereas others advocate the implementation of early active mobilization. Factors to take into consideration when making this decision include the developmental maturity of the patient, reliability of the child, support network surrounding the child, and patient's ability to be compliant with attendance in formal hand therapy.[116] It is beneficial to have a hand therapist available at the preoperative appointment to assess the maturity level and activity level of the patient and to plan and discuss possible postsurgical rehabilitation options with the patient and his or her guardian(s). The therapist can then coordinate with the surgeon to assist in making the decision regarding postoperative management.

Patients in the preschool age group are immobilized in a long arm mitten cast with the wrist in 20 to 25 degrees of flexion, the MCP in 50 to 60 degrees of flexion, and the IP in 10 degrees of flexion for 3 to 4 weeks after a flexor tendon repair.[114,116] Because children this age often have difficulty following directions and they may unintentionally grasp within the cast, which leads to high rupture rates in this population, some surgeons prefer to place preschoolers in a long arm cast at 120 degrees of flexion with the forearm supinated, the wrist and fingers in flexion, and the palm filled with soft Webril.[114] Other surgeons apply a pulp-to-palm suture before cast application.

For children ages 5 to 10 years, current research recommends an early mobilization program under the direct supervision of a hand therapist, with immobilization in between therapy sessions. However, some surgeons may choose to immobilize for 2 to 3 weeks before initiating formal hand therapy based on the patient's risk-taking behavior and other personality traits.[114]

Teenagers can usually initiate early active mobilization provided that they are mature, have good social support, and have the ability to attend formal hand therapy.[114] The classic protocol for these patients includes application of a dorsal blocking orthosis with the wrist in neutral, MCP joints flexed to 60 degrees, and IP joints extended.[114,116] The orthosis may be removed for exercises four times a day, including synergistic exercises, passive wrist flexion with active digit extension,

and wrist extension with active digit flexion. Passive composite digit flexion should also be included in the patient's home exercise program. Despite previous research suggesting no difference in rehabilitative outcomes, a study by Nietosvaara and associates[111] on the recovery of pediatric flexor tendon injuries found that early active protocols are consistently effective in returning patients to near-normal AROM.

During the first week after immobilization, the patient and guardian(s) are instructed in passive protected extension within the orthosis and wrist active motion with relaxed digits while the orthosis is temporarily removed. During weeks 2 to 5 after immobilization, active flexion is progressed using a percentage approach; 25% of full effort is engaged during week 2, 50% during week 3, 75% during week 4, and 100% effort is engaged the week 5. The orthosis is usually weaned during the third week after the cast has been removed.[116]

Complications

The most common complications for children after flexor tendon repairs are infection, rupture, growth arrest of the distal phalanx, complex regional pain syndrome, and atrophy of the injured finger.[112,114,116] The use of two-strand repairs has been observed to have a higher rate of rupture than four-strand repairs.[112]

Extensor Tendon Injuries
Background

Within the pediatric population, extensor tendons are injured more often than flexor tendons. Common mechanisms of injury include laceration injuries by glass or knives, physical altercations, sporting accidents, and crush injuries.[113,117] Injuries at or distal to the DIP joint are most common in the pediatric population.[113]

Clinical and Radiographic Examination

Because the clinical examination of young patients is often difficult, it is important to get a thorough history from the guardian with as many details about the incident as possible, specifically, when and how the injury occurred and how it has been treated thus far. Inspection of the affected limb for gross deformity, ecchymosis, and lacerations may provide important information to aid in the diagnosis of an extensor tendon injury.[117] It is essential to attempt to assess the active ROM of the tendons in the hand. The physician should observe the patient performing activities such as playing with a toy, eating a snack, or reaching for an object. This allows the provider to gather additional information about tendon integrity in the event that the patient is uncooperative during the physical examination. Radiographs are also an integral piece of the assessment if concomitant bony injury is suspected.

Treatment and Therapeutic Considerations

For partial tendon injuries, patients can be treated with wound closure and placed in an orthosis.[117] Primary repairs are recommended for complete tendon injuries. Patients who present to clinic with old injuries can be considered for a two-stage procedure such as a tendon transfer or tendon grafting. However, these procedures often leave patients with less than optimal functional outcomes, which must be factored into the decision to operate or not to operate.[118]

Rehabilitation after extensor tendon injuries is a topic of debate among surgeons. Early AROM is generally encouraged after an extensor tendon repair, yet the literature comparing the outcomes between early active protocols and complete immobilization is sparse. The minimal amount of literature specific to the pediatric population has presented discrepancies with the adult-focused literature.[113,118] The common belief is that early active protocols limit adhesions and contractures from forming.[117] It is notable, however, that Fitoussi and coworkers[118] reported that most complications observed in their cohort of pediatric extensor tendon ruptures were associated with motion at the repair site, including complications such as ruptures of the repair or callus lengthening.

Pediatric patients are often placed in a long arm cast to ensure that the digit is securely immobilized.[117] Because recovery is much quicker in children than recovery in adults, the risk of stiffness after static immobilization is less. Static immobilization is advantageous in that the surgeon does not have to rely on the patient to be compliant with restrictions as he or she would have to be if the orthosis were removable. Children who undergo extensor tendon repairs typically describe "good" or "excellent" results on a 5-point Likert scale.[118]

Complications

Potential complications include reruction, infection, adhesion formation, joint contractures, and tendon bowstringing. (Patients with incomplete injuries or isolated injuries observe better functional outcomes than those with complete tendon ruptures or concomitant injuries.[118]) Fitoussi and coworkers[118] reported that zone I to III injuries, as well as injuries in patients younger than 5 years of age were associated with higher percentages of extension lag and "poor" or "fair" results on the Likert 5-point scale, a finding that the research team hypothesized was attributable to the difficulty of keeping patients properly immobilized.

REFERENCES

1. Carson S. Pediatric upper extremity injuries. *Pediatr Clin North Am.* 2006;53(1):41–67.
2. Salter RB, Harris WR. Injuries involving the epiphyseal plate. *J Bone Joint Surg Am.* 1963;45:587–622.
3. Arora R, Fichadia U, Hartwig E, Kannikeswaran N. Pediatric upper-extremity fractures. *Pediatr Ann.* 2014;43(5):196–204.
4. Cooper C, Dennison EM, Leufkens HG, Bishop N, van Staa TP. Epidemiology of childhood fractures in Britain: a study using the general practice research database. *J Bone Miner Res.* 2004;19(12):1976–1981.
5. Landin LA. Epidemiology of children's fractures. *J Pediatr Orthop.* 1997;6(2):79–83.
6. Hedström EM, Svensson O, Bergström U, Michno P. Epidemiology of fractures in children and adolescents. *Acta Orthop.* 2010;81(1):148–153.
7. Hagstrom LS, Ferrick M, Galpin R. *Orthopedics.* 2015;38(2):e135–e138.
8. Pecci M, Kreher JB. Clavicle fractures. *Am Fam Physician.* 2008;77(1):65–70.
9. Banerjee R, Waterman B, Padalecki J, Robertson W. Management of distal clavicle fractures. *J Am Acad Orthop Surg.* 2011;19:392–401.
10. Pandya NK, Behrends D, Hosalkar HS. Open reduction of proximal humerus fractures in the adolescent population. *J Child Orthop.* 2012;6:11–118.
11. Robinson CM, Goudie EB, Murray IR, et al. Open reduction and plate fixation versus nonoperative treatment for displaced midshaft clavicular fractures: a multicenter, randomized, controlled trial. *J Bone Joint Surg Am.* 2013;95(17):1576–1584.
12. Fernandez FF, Eberhardt O, Langedörf M, Wirth T. Treatment of severely displaced proximal humeral fractures in children with retrograde elastic stable intramedullary nailing. *Injury.* 2008;39(12):1453–1459.
13. Lefèver Y, Journeau P, Angelliaume A, Bouty A, Dobremez E. *Orthop Traumatol Surg Res.* 2014;100(suppl 1):S149–S156.
14. Bae DS. Humeral shaft and proximal humerus, shoulder dislocation. In: Flynn JM, Skaggs DL, Waters PM, eds. *Fractures in Children.* 8th ed. Philadelphia: Wolters Kluwer; 2015:784–799.
15. Shrader MW. Proximal humerus and humeral shaft fractures in children. *Hand Clin.* 2007;23:431–435.
16. Neer CS, Horwitz BS. Fractures of the proximal humeral epiphyseal plate. *Orthopedics.* 1965;41:24–31.
17. Pahlavan S, Baldwin KD, Pandya NK, Namdari S, Hosalkar H. Proximal humerus fractures in the pediatric population: a systematic review. *J Child Orthop.* 2011;5:187–194.
18. Burgos-Flores J, Gonzalez-Herranz P, Lopez-Mondejar JA, Ocete-Guzman JG, Amay-Alarcón S. Fractures of the proximal humeral epiphysis. *Int Orthop.* 1993;17(1):16–19.
19. Hohloch L, Eberbach H, Wagner FC, et al. Age- and severity-adjusted treatment of proximal humerus fractures in children and adolescents-A systematical review and meta-analysis. *PLoS One.* 2017;12(8):e0183157.
20. Dameron TB, Reibel DB. Fractures involving the proximal humeral epiphyseal plate. *J Bone Joint Surg Am.* 1969;51A:289–297.
21. Cheng JC, Shen WY. Limb fracture pattern in different pediatric age groups: a study of 3,350 children. *J Orthop Trauma.* 1993;7:15–22.
22. Curtis RJ, Dameron TB, Rockwood CA. Fractures and dislocations of the shoulder in children. In: Rockwood CA, Wilkins KE, King RE, eds. *Rockwood and Wilkins' Fractures in Children.* 3rd ed. Philadelphia: Lippincott Williams & Wilkin; 1991:829.
23. Garg S, Dobbs MB, Schoenecker PL, Luhmann SJ, Gordon JE. Surgical treatment of traumatic pediatric humeral diaphyseal fractures with titanium elastic nails. *J Child Orthop.* 2009;3(2):121–127.
24. Landin LA. Fracture patterns in children: analysis of 8,682 fractures with special reference to incidence, etiology and secular changes in a Swedish urban population, 1950–1979. *Acta Orthop Scand Suppl.* 1983;202:1–109.
25. Wilkins KE. Fractures and dislocations of the elbow region. In: Rockwood Jr CA, Wilkins KE, King RE, eds. *Fractures in Children.* Philadelphia: JB Lippincott; 1984:363–575.
26. Abzug JM, Kozin SH. Fractures Of The Pediatric Elbow I: supracondylar humerus, lateral condyle, transphyseal distal humerus and capitellum fractures. In: Herman MJ, Horn BD, eds. *Contemporary Surgical Management of Fractures & Complications. Volume 3 Pediatrics.* Delhi: Jaypee; 2014:35–69, Ch. 3.
27. Milch H. Fractures and fracture dislocations of the humeral condyles. *J Trauma.* 1964;4:592–607.
28. Song KS, Kang CH, Min BW, Bae KC, Cho CH, Lee JH. Closed reduction and internal fixation of displaced unstable lateral condylar fractures of the humerus in children. *J Bone Joint Surg Am.* 2008;90(12):2673–2681.
29. Bakarman KA, Alsiddiky AM, Alzain KO, et al. Humeral lateral condyle fractures in children: redefining the criteria for displacement. *J Pediatr Orthop B.* 2016;25(5):429–433.
30. Weiss JM, Graves S, Yang S, Mendelsohn E, Kay RM, Skaggs DL. A new classification system predictive of complications in surgically treated pediatric humeral lateral condyle fractures. *J Pediatr Orthop.* 2009;29(6):602–605.
31. Bloom T, Chen LY, Sabharwal S. Biomechanical analysis of lateral humeral condyle fracture pinning. *J Pediatr Orthop.* 2011;31:130–137.
32. Bernthal NM, Hoshino CM, Dichter D, Wong M, Silva M. Recovery of elbow motion following pediatric lateral condylar fractures of the humerus. *J Bone Joint Surg Am.* 2011;93(9):871–877.
33. Fowles JV, Slimane N, Kassab MT. Elbow dislocation with avulsion of the medial humeral epicondyle. *J Bone Joint Surg Br.* 1990;72:102–104.
34. Smith FM. Medial epicondyle injuries. *J Am Med Assoc.* 1950;142(6):396–402.
35. Farsetti P, Potenza V, Caterini R, Ippolito E. Long-term results of treatment of fractures of the medial humeral epicondyle in children. *J Bone Joint Surg Am.* 2001;83-A:1299–1305.
36. Gandhi SD, Abzug JM, Herman MJ. Fractures of the pediatric elbow II: fractures of the medial epicondyle, radial neck and olecranon. In: Herman MJ, Horn BD, eds. *Contemporary Surgical Management of Fractures & Complications. Volume 3 Pediatrics.* Delhi: Jaypee; 2014, Ch. 4.
37. Edmonds EW. How displaced are "nondisplaced" fractures of the medial humeral epicondyle in children? Results of a three-dimensional computed tomography analysis. *J Bone Joint Surg Am.* 2010;92:2785–2791.
38. Josefsson PO, Danielsson LG. Epicondylar elbow fracture in children: 35-year follow up of 56 unreduced cases. *Acta Orthop Scand.* 1986;57:313–315.
39. Cheng JC, Lam TP, Maffuli N. Epidemiological features of supracondylar fractures of the humerus in Chinese children. *J Pediatr Orthop B.* 2001;10(1):63–67.
40. Omid R, Choi PD, Skaggs DL. Current concepts review: supracondylar humeral fracture in children. *J Bone Joint Surg Am.* 2008;90:1121–1132.

41. Babal JC, Mehlman CT, Klein G. Nerve injuries associated with pediatric supracondylar humeral fractures: a meta-analysis. *J Pediatr Orthop*. 2010;30:253–263.

42. Cramer KE, Green NE, Devito DP. Incidence of anterior interosseous nerve palsy in supracondylar humerus fractures in children. *J Pediatr Orthop*. 1993;13(4):502–505.

43. Parikh SN, Wall EJ, Foad S, Wiersema B, Nolte B. Displaced type II extension supracondylar humerus fractures - do they all need pinning? *J Pediatr Orthop*. 2004;24:380–384.

44. Bashyal RK, Chu JY, Scoenecker PL, Dobbs MB, Luhmann SJ, Gordon JE. Complication after pinning of supracondylar distal humerus fractures. *J Pediatr Orthop*. 2009;29(7):704–708.

45. Costa M, Pires Mafalda, Neves C, et al. Supracondylar fracture in children. Rehabilitation in occupational therapy, Yes or No? *AIP Conference Proceedings*. 2013;1558(1).

46. Henrikson B. Supracondylar fracture of the humerus in children. A late review of end-results with special reference to the cause of deformity, disability and complications. *Acta Chir Scand Suppl*. 1966;369:1–72.

47. Lieber J, Zundel SM, Luithle T, Fuchs J, Kirschner HJ. Acute traumatic posterior elbow dislocation in children. *J Pediatr Orthop B*. 2012;21(5):474–481.

48. Carlioz H, Abols Y. Posterior dislocation of the elbow in children. *J Pediatr Orthop*. 1984;4(1):8–12.

49. Kaziz H, Naouar N, Osman W, Ayeche M. Outcomes of paediatric elbow dislocations. *Malays Orthop J*. 2016;10(1):44–49.

50. Rasool M. Dislocations of the elbow in children. *J Bone Joint Surg Br*. 2004;86:1050–1058.

51. Chin K, Kozin SH, Herman MJ, et al. Pediatric Monteggia fracture-dislocations: avoiding problems and managing complications. *Inst Course Lect*. 2016;65:399–407.

52. Wilkins KE. Changes in the management of Monteggia fractures. *J Pediatr Orthop*. 2002;22:548–554.

53. Dormans JP, Rang M. The problem of Monteggia fracture-dislocations in children. *Orthop Clin North Am*. 1990;21(2):251–256.

54. Samardzíc M, Grujicíc D, Milinkovíc ZB. Radial nerve lesions associated with fractures of the humeral shaft. *Injury*. 1990;21(4):220–222.

55. Falciglia F, Giordano M, Aulisa AG, Di Lazzaro A, Guzzanti V. Radial neck fractures in children: results when open reduction is indicated. *J Pediatr Orthop*. 2014;34(8):756–762.

56. Basmajjian HG, Choi PD, Huh K, Sankar WN, Wells L, Arkader A. Radial neck fractures in children: experience from two level-1 trauma centers. *J Pediatr Orthop B*. 2014;23(4):369–374.

57. Zimmerman RM, Kalish LA, Hresko MT, Waters PM, Bae DS. Surgical management of pediatric radial neck fractures. *J Bone Joint Surg Am*. 2013;95(20):1825–1832.

58. Chambers HG. Fractures of the proximal radius and ulna. In: Beaty JH, Kasser JR, eds. *Rockwood and Wilkins' Fractures in Children*. Philadelphia: Lippincott Williams & Wilkins; 2001:483–528.

59. Sinikumpu JJ, Pokka T, Serlo W. The changing pattern of pediatric both-bone forearm shaft fractures among 86,000 children from 1997 to 2009. *Eur J Pediatr Surg*. 2013;23:289–296.

60. Smith VA, Goodman HJ, Strongwater A, Smith B. Treatment of pediatric both-bone forearm fractures: a comparison of operative techniques. *J Pediatr Orthop*. 2005;25(3):309–313.

61. Chia B, Kozin SH, Herman MJ, Safier S, Abzug JM. Complications of pediatric distal radius and forearm fractures. *Instr Course Lect*. 2015;64:499–507.

62. Reinhardt KR, Feldman DS, Green DW, Sala DA, Widmann RF, Scher DM. Comparison of intramedullary nailing to plating for both-bone forearm fractures in older children. *J Pediatr Orthop*. 2008;28(4):403–409.

63. Zionts LE, Zalavras CG, Gerhardt MB. Closed treatment of displaced diaphyseal both-bone forearm fractures in older children and adolescents. *J Pediatr Orthop*. 2005;25:507–512.

64. Martus JE, Preston RK, Schoenecker JG, Lovejoy SA, Green NE, Mencio GA. Complications and outcomes of diaphyseal forearm fracture intramedullary nailing: a comparison of pediatric and adolescent age groups. *J Pediatr Orthop*. 2013;33(6):598–607.

65. Khosla S, Melton LJ, Dekutoski MB, Achenbach SJ, Oberg Al, Riggs BL. Incidence of childhood distal forearm fractures over 30 years: a population-based study. *JAMA*. 2003;290:1479–1485.

66. Skaggs DL, Loro ML, Pitukcheewanont P, Tolo V, Gilsanz V. Increased body weight and decreased radial cross-sectional dimensions in girls with forearm fractures. *J Bone Miner Res*. 2001;16:1337–1342.

67. Bae DS, Waters PM. Pediatric distal radius fractures and triangular fibrocartilage complex injuries. *Hand Clinics*. 2006;22:43–53.

68. Dua K, Abzug JM, Sesko Bauer A, Cornwall R, Wyrick TO. Pediatric distal radius fractures. *Instr Course Lect*. 2017;66:447–460.

69. Lee BS, Esterhai Jr JL, Das M. Fracture of the distal radial epiphysis. characteristics and surgical treatment of premature, post-traumatic epiphyseal closure. *Clin Orthop Relat Res*. 1984;185:90–96.

70. Noonan KJ, Price CT. Forearm and distal radius fractures in children. *J Am Acad Orthop Surg*. 1998;6:146–156.

71. Palmer AK, Werner FW. The triangular fibrocartilage complex of the wrist: anatomy and function. *J Hand Surg Am*. 1981;6:153–162.

72. Cornwall R. The painful wrist in the pediatric athlete. *J Pediatr Orthop*. 2010;30:S13–S16.

73. Terry L, Cooper MD, Waters M, Peter MD. Triangular fibrocartilage injuries in pediatric and adolescent patients. *J Hand Surg Am*. 1998;23A(4):626–634.

74. Lester B, Halbrecht J, Levy M, Gaudinez R. "Press Test" for office diagnosis of triangular fibrocartilage complex tears of the wrist. *Ann Plast Surg*. 1995;35:41–45.

75. Tay SC, Tomita K, Berger RA. The "ulnar fovea sign" for defining ulnar wrist pain: an analysis of sensitivity and specificity. *J Hand Surg Am*. 2007b;32:438–444.

76. LaStayo P, Howell J. Clinical provocative tests used in evaluating wrist pain: a descriptive study. *J Hand Ther*. 1995;8(10):10–17.

77. Duncan SF, Flowers CW. *Therapy of the Hand and Upper Extremity Rehabilitation Protocols*. Cham: Springer International Publishing; 2015.

78. Atesok KI, Jupiter JB, Weiss AP. Galeazzi fracture. *J Am Acad Orthop Surg*. 2011;19:623–633.

79. Walsh HPJ, McLaren CAN, Owen R. Galeazzi fractures in children. *J Bone Joint Surg*. 1987;69(5):730–733.

80. Magill P, Harrington P. Complex volar dislocation of the distal radioulnar joint in a Galeazi variant associated with interposition of the ulnar neurovascular bundle. *Eur J Orthop Surg Traumatol*. 2009;19:265–267.

81. Hostetler MA, Davis CO. Galeazzi fracture resulting from electrical shock. *Pediatr Emerg Care*. 2000;16(4):258–259.

82. Giannoulis FS, Soteranos DG. Galeazzi fractures and dislocations. *Hand Clin*. 2007;23(2):153–163.

83. Mikic ZD. Galeazzi fracture-dislocations. *J Bone Joint Surg Am*. 1975;57(8):1071–1080.

84. Jacobs MA, Austin NM. *Orthotic Intervention for the Hand and Upper Extremity: Splinting Principles and Process*. Philadelphia: Wolters Kluwer; 2014.

85. Brudvik C, Hove LM. Childhood fractures in Bergen, Norway: identifying high-risk groups and activities. *J Pediatr Orthop*. 2003;23(5):629–634.

86. Gholson JJ, Bae DS, Zurakowski D, Waters PM. Scaphoid fractures in children and adolescents: contemporary injury patterns and factors influencing time to union. *J Bone Joint Surg Am*. 2011;93(13):1210–1219.

87. Stanciu C, Dumont A. Changing patterns of scaphoid fractures in adolescents. *Can J Surg*. 1994;37(3):214–216.

88. Bae DS, Gholson JJ, Zurakowski D, Water PM. Outcomes after treatment of scaphoid fractures in children and adolescents. *J Pediatr Orthop*. 2016;36(1):13–18.

89. Larson AN, Stans AA, Shaughnessy WJ, Dekutoski MB, Quinn MJ, McIntosh AL. Motocross morbidity: economic cost and injury distribution in children. *J Pediatr Orthop*. 2009;29:847–850.

90. Waters PM, Stewart SL. Surgical treatment of nonunion and avascular necrosis of the proximal part of the scaphoid in adolescents. *J Bone Joint Surg Am*. 2002;84:915–920.

91. Young K, Greenwood A, MacQuillan A, Lee S, Wilson S. Paediatric hand fractures. *J Hand Surg Eur*. 2013;38E(8):898–902.

92. Dua K, Lancaster TP, Abzug JM. Age-dependent reliability of Semmes-Weinstein and 2-point discrimination tests in children. *J Pediatr Orthop*. 2016; Epub ahead of print.

93. Kozin SH. Fractures and dislocations along the pediatric thumb ray. *Hand Clin.* 2006;22:19–29.
94. Chew EM, Chong AK. Hand fractures in children: epidemiology and misdiagnosis in a tertiary referral hospital. *J Hand Surg Am.* 2012;37:1684–1688.
95. Hastings 2nd H, Simmons BP. Hand fractures in children. A statistical analysis. *Clin Orthop Relat Res.* 1984:120–130.
96. Cornwall R. Finger metacarpal fractures and dislocations in children. *Hand Clin.* 2006;22(1):1–10.
97. Al-Qattan MM. Juxta-epiphyseal fractures of the base of the proximal phalanx of the fingers in children and adolescents. *J Hand Surg Br.* 2002;27B(1):24–30.
98. Deleted in review.
99. Yaeger SK, Bhende MS. Pediatric hand injuries. *Clin Pediatr Emerg Med.* 2016;17(1):29–37.
100. Hanlon CR, Estes WL. Fractures in childhood, a statistical analysis. *Am J Surg.* 1954;87(3):312–323.
101. Hosalkar H, Matzon J. Nerve palsies related to pediatric upper extremity fractures. *Hand Clinic.* 2006;22:87–98.
102. Samardzic M, Grujicić D, Milinković. Radial nerve lesions associated with fractures of the humeral shaft. *Injury.* 1990;21(4):220–222.
103. Deleted in review.
104. Colditz J. Splinting the hand with a peripheral nerve injury. In: Skirven TM, Osterman AL, Fedorczyk J, Amadio PC, Schneider LH, eds. *Hunter, Mackin & Callahan's Rehabilitation of the Hand and Upper Extremity.* 5th ed. Mosby, Inc.; 2002:622–634.
105. Yuan PS, Pring ME, Gaynor TP, Mubarak SJ, Newton PO. Compartment syndrome following intramedullary fixation of pediatric forearm fractures. *J Pediatr Orthop.* 2004;24:370–375.
106. Bae DS, Kadiyala RK, Waters PM. Acute compartment syndrome in children: contemporary diagnosis, treatment and outcome. *J Pediatr Orthop.* 2001;21(5):680–688.
107. Noonan KJ, Price CT. Forearm and distal radius fractures in children. *J Am Acad Orthop Surg.* 1998;6(3):146–156.
108. Willis AA, Lochner HV. Pediatric hand and wrist injuries. *Curr Rev Musculo Skelet Med.* 2013;6:18–25.
109. Herman MJ, McCarthy J, Willis RB, Pizzutillo PD. Top 10 pediatric orthopaedic surgical emergencies: a case-based approach for the surgeon on call. *Instr Course Lect.* 2011;60:373–395.
110. Mubarak SJ, Carroll NC. Volkmann's contracture in children: aetiology and prevention. *J Bone Joint Surg Br.* 1979;61:285–293.
111. Nietosvaara Y, Lindfors N, Palmu S, Rautakorpi S, Ristaniemi N. Flexor tendon injuries in pediatric patients. *J Hand Surg.* 2006;32A(10):1549–1557.
112. Al-Qattan M. A six-strand technique for zone II flexor-tendon repair in children younger than 2 years of age. *Injury.* 2011;42(11):1262–1365.
113. Kim JS, Sung SJ, Kim YJ, Choi YW. Analysis of pediatric tendon injuries in the hand in comparison with adults. *Arch Plast Surg.* 2017;44(2):144–149.
114. Cooper L, Khor W, Burr N, Sivakumar B. Flexor tendon repairs in children: outcomes from a specialist tertiary centre. *J Plast Reconstr Aesthet Surg.* 2015;68(5):717–723.
115. Goggins T, Syme D, Murali SR. Acute flexor tendon injury and rehabilitation of hand injuries. *J Orthop Trauma.* 2014;28(4):219–224.
116. Von der Heyde R. Flexor tendon injuries in children: rehabilitative options and confounding factors. *J Hand Ther.* 2015;28(2):195–200.
117. Dwyer CL, Ramirez RN, Lubahn JD. A brief review of extensor tendon injuries specific to the pediatric patient. *Hand (NY).* 2015;10(1):23–27.
118. Fitoussi F, Badina A, Ilhareborde B, Morel E, Ear R, Pennecot GF. Extensor tendon injuries in children. *J Pediatr Orthop.* 2007;27(8):863–866.

125

Brachial Plexus Birth Palsy: Secondary Procedures to Enhance Function

Sarah Ashworth, Scott H. Kozin

OUTLINE

CRITICAL POINTS

- The mainstay for secondary brachial plexus reconstruction consists of tendon transfers about the shoulder, elbow, wrist, and hand.
- Botulinum toxin injections and joint releases can be performed for contractures about the shoulder and elbow.
- Corrective osteotomy to reposition the limb and arthrodesis to stabilize flail joints are additional techniques used in brachial plexus reconstruction.

- The physical examination should include the entire extremity, from the shoulder girdle to the hand, and must assess the muscle strength, sensory status, and joint motion.
- The range of active motion, muscle strength, and any limitations in passive motion are critical elements during formulation of a treatment strategy.
- The formulation of a list of what's in, what's out, what's available, and what's needed is the basis for the decision-making process.

Secondary reconstructive procedures for brachial plexus injuries conform to similar treatment principles regardless of the age of the patient and etiology of the brachial plexus injury. This chapter focuses on brachial plexus birth injuries that have residual deficits and are no longer candidates for nerve reconstruction.

The mainstays of treatment are tendon transfers about the shoulder, elbow, wrist, and hand. Joint releases can be performed for contractures about the shoulder and elbow. Corrective osteotomy to reposition the limb and arthrodesis to stabilize flail joints are additional techniques used in brachial plexus reconstruction. Botulinum toxin has a role in preventing or delaying shoulder joint releases in young patients and augmenting conservative management of elbow flexion contractures.

CLASSIFICATION

Brachial plexus injuries can be classified according to the level of involvement (Table 125.1). Upper plexus lesions are most common and involve the fifth and sixth cervical roots or upper trunk. These injuries are referred to as either an Erb-Duchenne or Erb's palsy.[1,2] An extended Erb's palsy also involves the seventh cervical root or middle trunk and is fairly common. Isolated lower plexus lesions are rare and referred to as a Klumpke's palsy.[3] The most severe injury is a disruption of the entire plexus—known as a global, total, or pan plexus injury.

PATIENT EVALUATION

The initial evaluation includes the history, physical examination, and imaging studies. The history should include the details of the birth, inquiry as to the presence of shoulder dystocia, and questions about associated injuries (i.e., fractures [clavicle or humerus] and Horner's syndrome). In addition, the mother should be counseled about the increased risk of repeat plexus injury in future births. The extent of the initial injury should be gleaned from the parents. Simple questions regarding movement about the shoulder, elbow, wrist, and hand will provide valuable information. The treatment rendered subsequent to the birth and any recovery of function are important facts.

The physical examination should include the entire extremity, from the shoulder girdle to the hand. The neck should also be assessed for torticollis, which can occur with a brachial plexus birth injury. The examination must assess the muscle strength, sensory status, and joint motion. The range of active motion, muscle strength, and any limitations in passive motion are critical elements during formulation of a treatment strategy. A uniform grading system for muscle strength and documentation is mandatory when evaluating a patient for surgical reconstruction. Using a brachial plexus tabulation sheet is an efficient way to record manual muscle strength and prevent inadvertent omission of important data. Muscle strength is graded from 0 to 5, enhanced by the use of a minus modifier to denote incomplete range. The sensibility of the extremity is assessed by standard measures including light touch and two-point discrimination.

TABLE 125.1   Patterns of Brachial Plexus Injuries

Pattern	Roots Involve	Primary Deficiency
Upper brachial plexus (Erb-Duchenne)	C5 and C6	Shoulder abduction and external rotation
Extended upper brachial plexus	C5, C6, and C7	Above plus elbow flexion and elbow and digital extension
Lower brachial plexus (Dejerine-Klumpke)	C8 and T1	Hand intrinsic muscles Finger flexors
Total brachial plexus lesion	C5, C6, C7, C8, and T1	Entire plexus
Peripheral brachial plexus lesion	—	Variable

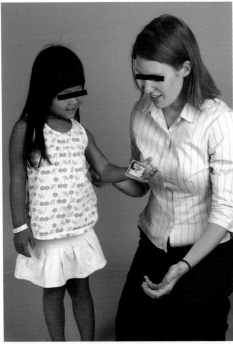

Fig. 125.1 A variety of toys, props, and games are used to examine children. (Courtesy of Shriners Hospital for Children, Philadelphia.)

Children are more difficult to examine than adults because of their limited attention span, poor ability to follow commands, and lack of cooperation. Extreme patience and repeated examinations are often required to obtain an adequate evaluation. (Fig. 125.1). Brachial plexus palsy–specific standardized assessments, including the active movement scale, Toronto scale, and modified Mallet classification (Figs. 125.2 and 125.3), can be quickly learned and administered for reliable assessment of younger children.[4] Inclusion of hand-to-belly measurement allows for greater sensitivity to changes of internal rotation of the shoulder.[5] Additional evaluation components of strength, sensibility, dexterity, and functional assessments are covered in greater detail in Chapter 121.

A baseline outcome measurement is also part of the initial patient workup and preoperative evaluation. Currently, the exact outcome tool that is appropriate for brachial plexus injuries remains unclear, and outcome measurements in children are notoriously difficult. Nonetheless, a critical evaluation of the results after brachial plexus injury or

surgery is necessary to improve future care of these patients. This task requires faithful documentation of the preoperative state and postoperative change from both subjective and objective standpoints.[6,7] The Modified Mallet classification has been shown to be a reliable instrument for assessing shoulder function in children with brachial plexus birth palsies.[8-10] The Canadian Occupational Performance Measure (COPM) is an applicable patient-reported outcome tool for children. Caregivers can report for younger children as appropriate.[11] This outcome tool also encourages discussion of realistic expectations of intervention to prevent disappointment and ensure that both the patient and the caregivers are fully educated about the potential outcome of any treatment.

ANCILLARY STUDIES

Ancillary studies can be helpful to assist in the formulation of a treatment plan. Radiographs of the injured extremity are used to assess for bony and joint alignment abnormalities in children. Limitation of passive motion should not always be assumed to be secondary to soft tissue contracture, and radiographs are required to assess joint alignment. For the shoulder, anteroposterior and axillary views are adequate in adolescent and adult patients. However, children who are skeletally immature may require advanced imaging modalities (e.g., ultrasound or magnetic resonance imaging [MRI]) to truly depict the contour of the glenohumeral joint.[12-15] Ultrasound is a valuable screening tool to assess posterior humeral head subluxation. The examination is performed in the office with the child sitting on the caregiver's lap. No sedation is required, and the shoulder can be rotated to assess the amount of subluxation in internal rotation and if the humeral head is reducible in external rotation. There have been proposed ultrasound measures to determine glenoid version; however, MRI is the most accurate imaging study of the pediatric glenohumeral joint with precise depiction of the articular cartilage and glenoid configuration.[16,17]

Electrodiagnostic tests can provide some useful information about nerve and muscle recovery when the physician is contemplating early nerve repair or reconstruction.[18,19] However, electromyography is not quantitative with respect to muscle strength and does not substitute for an astute physical examination coupled with manual muscle testing. Reinnervated muscle will demonstrate an abnormal electromyographic signal, such as increased amplitude and polyphasic waveforms. These findings indicate inherent weakness and altered contractile properties, which often preclude use of that muscle as a suitable donor for tendon transfer. Hence, electrodiagnostic tests have limited value in the decision-making process for secondary reconstructive procedures.

In recent years, motion capture analysis improvements have provided valuable information with objective measures of global shoulder motion, separating glenohumeral joint from scapulothoracic joint movements. This modality is an emerging area of data collection allowing greater insight into the kinematics of the glenohumeral joint and scapulothoracic joint concerning their relationship in overall upper extremity movements (Fig. 125.4) As this technology advances, the understanding of the shoulder joint will allow brachial plexus centers to elucidate the exact effects of interventions, such as therapy, tendon transfers, and osteotomies.[20-22]

SHOULDER

The shoulder is frequently impaired after a brachial plexus injury because most of the muscles about the shoulder are innervated by the upper plexus (C5 and C6 nerve roots). The rotator cuff and deltoid muscle are innervated by C5 and C6 and act to move the glenohumeral joint and depress humeral head motion during shoulder movement.

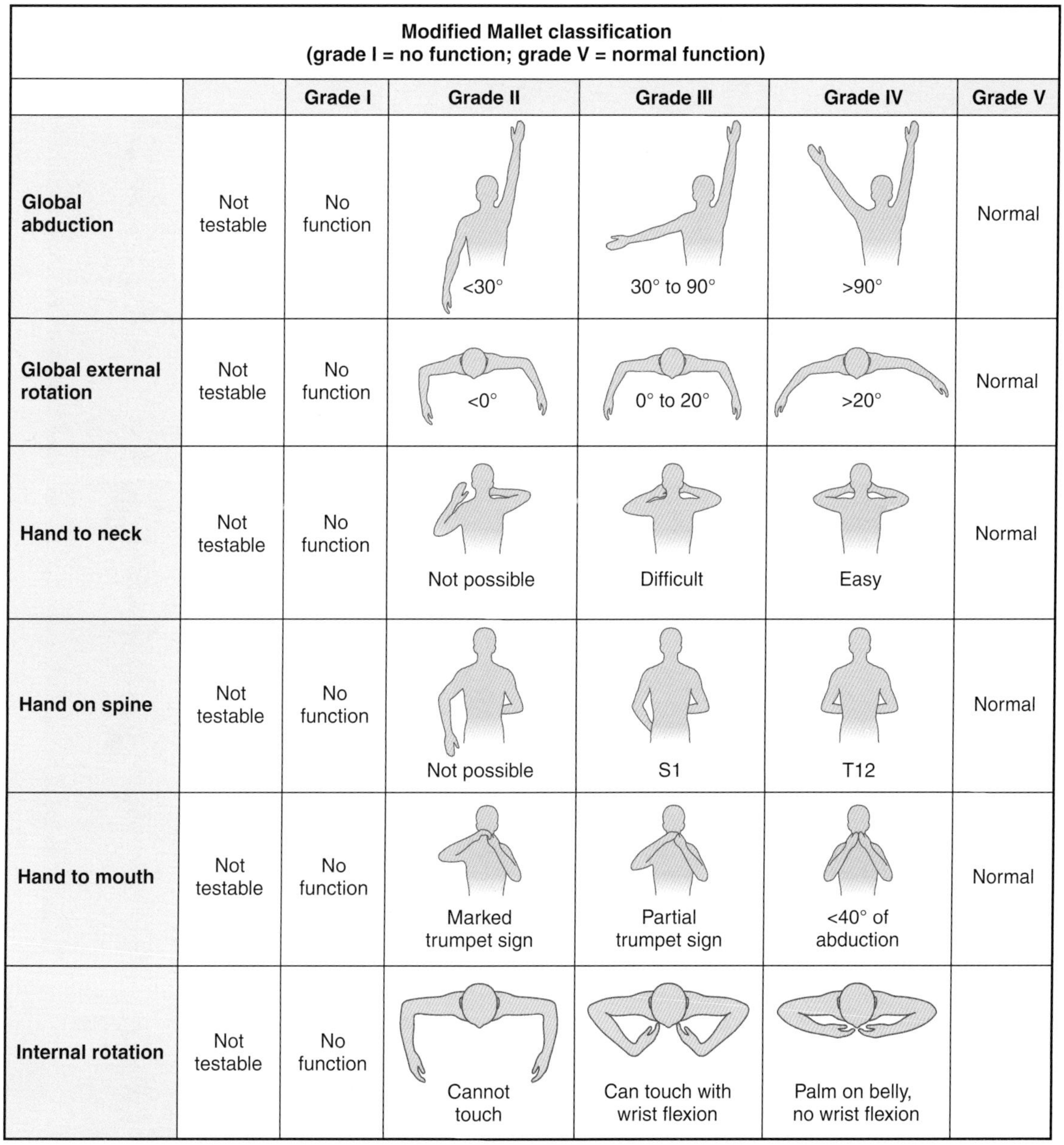

Modified Mallet classification (grade I = no function; grade V = normal function)						
		Grade I	Grade II	Grade III	Grade IV	Grade V
Global abduction	Not testable	No function	<30°	30° to 90°	>90°	Normal
Global external rotation	Not testable	No function	<0°	0° to 20°	>20°	Normal
Hand to neck	Not testable	No function	Not possible	Difficult	Easy	Normal
Hand on spine	Not testable	No function	Not possible	S1	T12	Normal
Hand to mouth	Not testable	No function	Marked trumpet sign	Partial trumpet sign	<40° of abduction	Normal
Internal rotation	Not testable	No function	Cannot touch	Can touch with wrist flexion	Palm on belly, no wrist flexion	

Fig. 125.2 Modified Mallet classification with additional internal rotation score. Grade I, no function; grade V, normal function. (Courtesy of Shriners Hospital for Children, Philadelphia.)

These muscles also maintain the concentric relationship between the humeral head and glenoid. This function and synchrony between the rotator cuff and deltoid muscles are disrupted after brachial plexus injury and impaired by incomplete nerve regeneration. Loss of abduction (deltoid and supraspinatus muscles) and a deficit in external rotation (infraspinatus muscle) are the most common problems, especially in residual brachial plexus birth palsy (Fig. 125.5). Internal rotation is usually less affected because multiple muscles (pectoralis major, latissimus dorsi, and subscapularis) are not entirely innervated by the upper plexus and maintain their ability to provide internal rotation. This resultant imbalance causes an internal rotation contracture and glenohumeral joint dysplasia (posterior humeral head dysplasia and glenoid retroversion). Therefore, an infant after brachial plexus birth palsy requires passive external rotation exercises by the parents or other caregivers to promote normal glenohumeral joint development. The scapula must be stabilized to isolate glenohumeral joint rotation (Fig. 125.6). These passive maneuvers are performed at each diaper change, and the status of the glenohumeral joint is carefully monitored. Early detection of a diminished passive external rotation with manual scapular stabilization requires a referral for formal therapy aimed at glenohumeral external rotation. An established internal rotation contracture (i.e., no external rotation) that does not respond to therapy requires urgent evaluation.[12,23] Failure to maintain external rotation will cause development of glenohumeral joint dysplasia with an irregularly shaped humeral head and corresponding deficient glenoid version (Fig. 125.7). Surgery is recommended when there is posterior humeral head subluxation that is irreducible.[9,14] The clinical test is passive external rotation with the scapula stabilized and the shoulder adducted. Negative range of motion (ROM) implies subluxation and warrants ultrasound or MRI. Release of the anterior joint capsule with or without tendon transfer can restore active external rotation and promote glenohumeral joint remodeling.[24–27] In young children (younger than 3 years of age), isolated release is often preferred followed by careful monitoring for recovery of active external rotation.

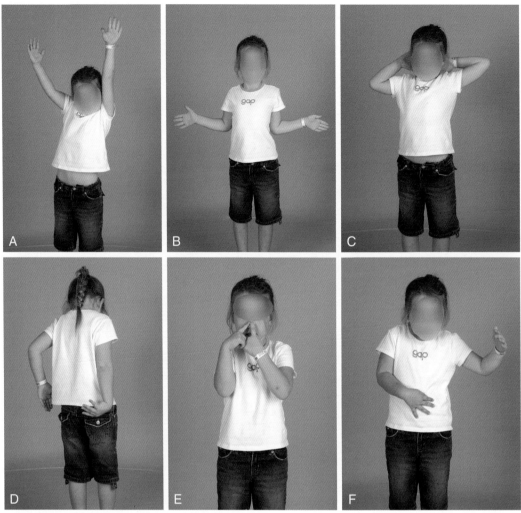

Fig. 125.3 A 3-year-old child assessed using Mallet measures after arthroscopic capsular release. **A,** Global abduction (grade IV). **B,** Global external rotation (grade IV). **C,** Hand to neck (grade IV). **D,** Hand to spine (grade II). **E,** Hand to mouth (grade IV). **F,** Internal rotation (grade III). (Courtesy of Shriners Hospital for Children, Philadelphia.)

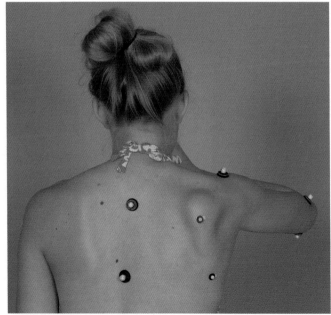

Fig. 125.4 Retroreflective marker placement to measure scapulothoracic, glenohumeral, and humerothoracic movement during modified Mallet positions with motion capture analysis. (Courtesy of Shriners Hospital for Children, Philadelphia.)

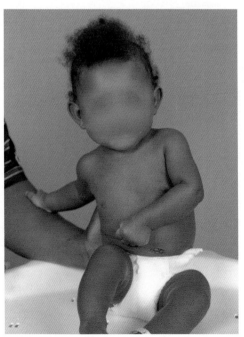

Fig. 125.5 A 6-month-old child with left brachial plexus birth palsy and deficient shoulder abduction and external rotation. (Courtesy of Shriners Hospital for Children, Philadelphia.)

With respect to internal rotation, it is important to understand the pivotal role the subscapularis muscle plays in end-range internal rotation. Weakness from the brachial plexus injury or after surgical release or lengthening to improve external rotation can result in limited ability to bring the hand to the trunk or waist (Fig. 125.8).[12,23] Baseline assessment of internal rotation motion and end-range strength is important to predict and minimize postoperative midline function limitations. When internal rotation weakness is observed, evaluation of wrist flexion strength is necessary. Surgical interventions to reduce the glenohumeral joint dysplasia or augment external rotation may jeopardize active internal rotation ROM. Wrist flexion can be used to compensate for midline activities. Weak internal rotation requires early incorporation of active midline motion and activities after surgery.

SCAPULAR WINGING

The phenomenon of scapular winging and contracture is often disconcerting to children and their families. The scapular winging is frequently attributed to nerve injury; however, the long thoracic (serratus anterior), dorsal scapular (rhomboids), and spinal accessory (trapezius) are uncommonly injured in upper and extended upper level injuries. Hence, the observed "winging" is not caused by parascapular muscle weakness. The winging is secondary to compensatory scapular movement related to glenohumeral joint contracture formation and deficient glenohumeral joint motion. Recent studies focusing on scapular contracture and position indicate that multidirectional glenohumeral joint limitations are present because of multiple factors, including motor imbalance, muscle reinnervation with decreased excursion, and muscle atrophy.[20–22,28,29] Some of these changes actually augment overall arm movement, such as the glenohumeral abduction contracture that allows greater overall arm abduction. Further research is needed to better understand the intricate factors that cause alterations in scapular movement to determine surgical and nonsurgical interventions that can prevent or improve this complex situation.

ELBOW

The elbow is frequently impaired after brachial plexus injuries, especially elbow flexion secondary to loss of the biceps and brachialis muscles (C5 and C6 nerve roots). An inability to flex the elbow is a considerable impairment because hand-to-mouth function is impossible. In patients with global injuries and minimal hand function, the affected arm uses elbow function as a support to carry objects along the forearm. The inability to flex the elbow further impairs the function of the limb. For these reasons, restoration of the functional arc of elbow motion (30–130 degrees) carries a high priority during brachial plexus reconstruction.[25] Recovery of elbow flexion secondary to nerve regeneration (natural history or surgical reconstruction) introduces a different problem. Reinnervated muscles do not grow at the same rate as intact muscle during periods of rapid skeletal growth.[29] Sheffler and colleagues[30] found 48% of their patients with brachial plexus injuries developed elbow flexion contractures of 10 degrees or greater. This contracture is exacerbated in the presence of weak triceps, but is common even when full triceps strength is present.

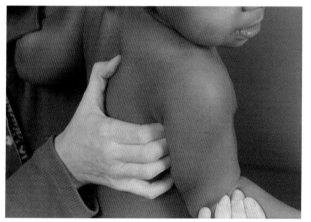

Fig. 125.6 Stabilization of the scapulothoracic joint is necessary to isolate the glenohumeral joint during external rotation exercises. (Courtesy of Shriners Hospital for Children, Philadelphia.)

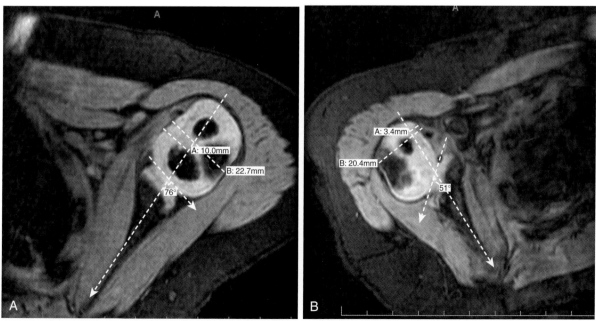

Fig. 125.7 A 4-year-old girl with right brachial plexus palsy. **A,** Normal left shoulder (percent of humeral head anterior, or PHHA, 44%; version, –14 degrees). **B,** Abnormal right shoulder with pseudoglenoid (PHHA, 16.7%; version, –39 degrees). (Courtesy of Shriners Hospital for Children, Philadelphia.)

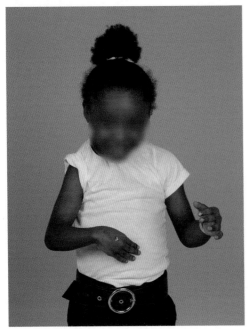

Fig. 125.8 A female patient with right brachial plexus palsy. Limited internal rotation necessitates wrist flexion for midline activities. (Courtesy of Shriners Hospital for Children, Philadelphia.)

FOREARM

Forearm rotation is often limited after brachial plexus palsies. The forearm joint is motored between muscles that provide supination and pronation. Supination is primarily an upper trunk (C5 and C6) function via the biceps and supinator muscles. In contrast, pronation is a middle and lower trunk function via the pronator teres (C7) and pronator quadratus (C8 and T1). An individual may lack supination, pronation, or both depending on the extent of injury. Although supination is important for specific tasks such as accepting change, eating, and personal hygiene, these activities are unilateral and can be completed effectively with the unaffected arm. Pronation deficiency leads to difficulty with many more bimanual tasks such as keyboarding, writing, and tabletop activities. The decision to restore forearm movement requires careful considerations of the functional limitations and potential for gains and losses.[31,32] Contraindications for improving pronation include weak or absent wrist extension, an insensate hand, and minimal finger movement. Without adequate wrist extension and finger strength, a pronated forearm limits the function of the hand as a stable carrying surface. The pronated hand becomes less functional compared with the supinated position. An insensate hand uses vision as the afferent signal, and rotation of an insensate hand into pronation increases the risk for injury owing to the inability to visualize the palmar surface of the hand.

WRIST AND HAND

Wrist and hand impairment varies with the damage to the middle and lower plexus. Upper brachial plexus lesions have a minimal effect on hand use, whereas global plexus injuries can severely hamper hand function. A definitive treatment algorithm for the wrist and hand is more difficult to formulate because of the variable clinical presentation. A detailed functional examination and manual muscle testing are the foundation for the development of a treatment paradigm. The formulation of a list of what's in, what's out, what's available, and what's needed is the basis for the decision-making process. Individualized treatment is required, and many of the principles of radial, median, and ulnar

nerve transfers are applied. The principles and techniques of these tendon transfers are covered in Chapters 43 and 44. Our preferred wrist extension transfer is discussed later in the chapter.

CONSERVATIVE VERSUS SURGICAL INTERVENTION

Conservative management is beneficial for preventing muscle tightness and subsequent joint contracture when further neurologic recovery is anticipated. Therapy interventions are also helpful to minimize joint contracture and strengthen muscles. Interventions may include active range of motion (AROM) and passive range of motion (PROM), strengthening, orthoses, kinesiology taping, electrical stimulation, muscle or sensory reeducation, and adaptive functional training. Surgical intervention is indicated when joint instability or deformity is present or when no further neurologic recovery is expected and functional deficits remain problematic for the patient.

CONTRACTURE DEVELOPMENT

The shoulder is prone to develop an internal rotation contracture, especially after brachial plexus birth palsy. Incomplete recovery after brachial plexus birth palsy often results in decreased movement and muscle imbalance about the shoulder because rotator cuff and deltoid innervation is incomplete. The internal rotators overpower the external rotators, which results in an internal rotation contracture. This constant position of internal rotation leads to early glenohumeral joint deformity as early as 3 months of age and advanced deformity by 2 years, which is characterized by increasing glenoid retroversion and posterior humeral head subluxation (glenohumeral joint dysplasia).[12,16] Children with an established internal rotation contracture and glenohumeral joint deformity are unlikely to regain optimum shoulder function without intervention.[12,23]

In patients with recovery of biceps and brachialis function, the elbow is prone to develop an elbow flexion contracture.[33] The contracture is more severe in children without triceps function. Therapy is often beneficial, especially if implemented early in the process. Nighttime orthosis use decreases the rate of progression in mild contractures and may be necessary until the child reaches skeletal maturity. Serial casting is useful in reducing more severe flexion contractures (Fig. 125.9). Botulinum toxin can be added in recalcitrant cases.[30] Established contractures are difficult to treat, and capsular release has mediocre results, with the inherent risk of losing essential elbow flexion. Therefore, an elbow release is rarely performed in patients with brachial plexus palsies.

RECONSTRUCTION OPTIONS

Shoulder

Botulinum Toxin Injection with Closed Reduction

The injection is performed under general anesthesia. With the patient in lateral decubitus position, a two-person approach is used. The examiner stabilizes the scapula while controlling the ultrasound transducer on the posterior shoulder to assess humeral head appearance and subluxation. The assistant then moves the arm into external rotation with the shoulder adducted. With a reducible shoulder, botulinum toxin injection is completed. Electrical stimulation is used before injection to verify accurate muscle placement for the pectoralis major, subscapularis, teres major, and latissimus dorsi. Immediately after closed reduction and injection, the child is immobilized with shoulder adducted and externally rotated for 3 weeks. Therapy resumes after immobilization with a focus on passive external rotation with the scapula stabilized performed multiple times per day[16,34] (Fig. 125.10).

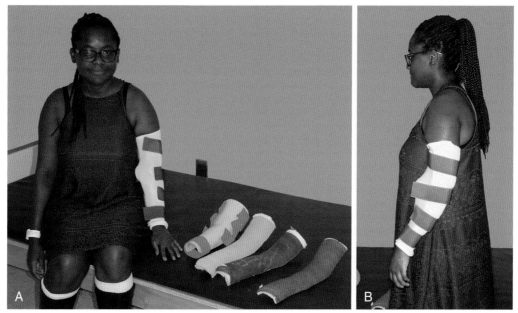

Fig. 125.9 A and **B,** A 17-year-old patient with elbow flexion contracture, treated with botulinum toxin injection to elbow flexors with a course of serial casting and static progressive and static orthoses. (Courtesy of Shriners Hospital for Children, Philadelphia.)

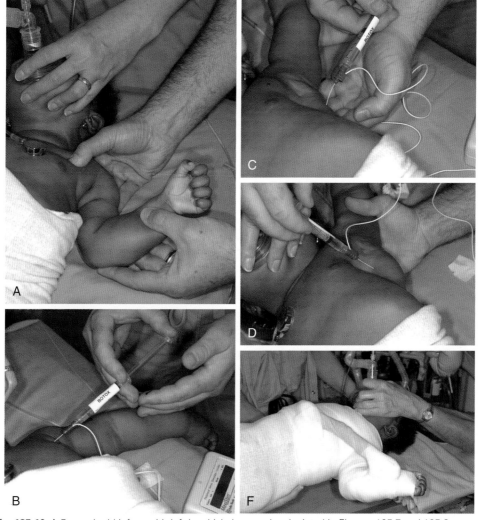

Fig. 125.10 A 5-month-old infant with left brachial plexus palsy depicted in Figures 125.7 and 125.8 treated with closed reduction and Botox injections. **A,** Successful closed reduction. **B,** Botox injection into the pectoralis major. **C,** Botox injection into the latissimus–teres major complex. **D,** Botox injection into the subscapularis muscle. **E,** Shoulder spica casting. (Courtesy of Shriners Hospital for Children, Philadelphia.)

Open Release of Internal Rotation Contracture

An anterior or axillary approach can be used. The anterior incision is performed between the deltoid and pectoralis major muscles. If the pectoralis major muscle is tight, a musculocutaneous lengthening can be performed. The subscapularis muscle is isolated and released from the underlying anterior capsule. If the contracture is resolved, then joint arthrotomy is unnecessary. Persistent contracture is usually associated with underlying joint deformity and may require anterior capsular release. The arm is positioned in 45 degrees of abduction and 40 to 50 degrees of external rotation, which is maintained by a shoulder spica cast.

The axillary approach identifies the latissimus dorsi, teres major, long head of the triceps, and posterior deltoid. The axillary nerve must be identified and protected. The long head of the triceps is traced to its origin from the infraglenoid tubercle. The subscapularis is reflected from the anterior capsule. The joint is entered and the anterior capsule released. This arthrotomy usually results in joint reduction and external rotation. Persistent tightness can be released by elevation of the subscapularis muscle from the anterior scapula and sliding the muscle, which allows additional external rotation. The surgeon, however, must avoid excessive release that will lead to impaired internal rotation and midline activities. A similar immobilization and postoperative management is used. Release of the internal rotation contracture can be combined with tendon transfer to restore external rotation at the same time or as a staged procedure after supple passive motion has been restored.

Arthroscopic Release of Internal Rotation Contracture

Arthroscopy is performed via an anterior and posterior portal.[1,12] An electrocautery is introduced through the anterior portal. The thickened superior glenohumeral ligament, the middle glenohumeral ligament, and the upper half to two thirds of the subscapularis are released (usually the upper rolled border or tendinous portion). As the release continues inferiorly, the tendinous portion of the subscapularis transitions into a more muscular portion. At this point, the release becomes isolated to the capsule, with preservation of the inferior and lateral muscular portions of the subscapularis. The electrocautery is removed and exchanged for an arthroscopic punch. The inferior glenohumeral ligament is then released to a point slightly posterior to the midportion of the axillary pouch. The axillary nerve is protected. The arthroscopic equipment is removed from the joint. The glenohumeral joint is manipulated into external rotation, both with the arm at the side and with the arm at 90 degrees of elevation. Marked improvement in external rotation is noted, often with a palpable clunk associated with glenohumeral joint reduction. Failure to achieve joint reduction or passive external rotation of less than 45 degrees with the arm in adduction requires additional arthroscopic release of the axillary pouch and the tight subscapularis.

Tendon Transfer

The latissimus dorsi or teres major tendons (or both tendons) can be transferred to the superior–posterior rotator cuff and humerus after capsular release or as a separate procedure. In children with midline weakness, the teres major is transferred, leaving the latissimus for midline function. The surgery involves releasing the tendon(s) with a periosteal sleeve. The tendon(s) are passed superficial to the long head of the triceps and secured directly to the bone using transosseous suture (Video 125.1). The tendon(s) is inserted into the bone just above the infraspinatus insertion.

When considering tendon transfers to augment shoulder external rotation and abduction, internal rotation and wrist flexion strength must also be assessed. Weakness in internal rotation may be present,

which can lead to impairment of hand-to-belly strength. Deficient midline hampers fastening pants and other vital activities for activities of daily living (ADLs) function. Wrist flexion can accommodate for mild loss of internal rotation function but must be present to accommodate for such loss. Children with middle and lower trunk involvement may have limited wrist flexion strength. For these patients, potential loss of midline must be strongly considered before shoulder surgery to enhance external rotation. Implementation of a focused exercise program to strengthen midline internal rotation and wrist flexion can be used to minimize loss and improve candidacy for reconstruction.

Other shoulder tendon transfers. Other donor tendon transfers about the shoulder are available for residual brachial plexus palsy to enhance glenohumeral abduction, external rotation, or both. Donor muscles used include the trapezius, levator scapulae, and bipolar latissimus dorsi. The upper trapezius can be transferred with a portion of the acromion to the decorticated posterolateral humerus to improve shoulder abduction. The lower trapezius can also be transferred to the infraspinatus to increase external rotation. The levator scapulae can be elongated with a fascial graft to reach the tendon of the supraspinatus and augment abduction. The latissimus can be transferred on a pedicle similar to the bipolar technique for elbow flexorplasty (see later discussion).[35] The origin is attached to the acromion and the insertion attached to the deltoid insertion on the humerus. Experience with these transfers is not extensive, and expected improvement in abduction and external rotation has been limited.[1] These tendon transfers have become far secondary options compared with the latissimus dorsi or teres major donors. In persistent cases of shoulder instability or subluxation, chondrodesis (arthrodesis with preservation of the growth plate) is preferred. A prerequisite is adequate scapulothoracic motion to allow some "shoulder" motion.

Postoperative management. Following glenohumeral joint release with or without tendon transfer, the child is placed in a shoulder spica cast with the glenohumeral joint positioned in 45 to 60 degrees of external rotation. The amount of abduction varies according to whether or not tendon transfers were performed. The arm is positioned in 30 to 40 degrees of abduction after isolated release and 100 to 120 degrees of abduction after release combined with tendon transfer (Fig. 126.11). The child continues to wear a cast for 3 weeks after isolated release and 4 to 5 weeks after tendon transfer.

After immobilization, an orthosis is fabricated to replicate the cast, with the arm abducted and externally rotated (Fig. 125.12). The orthosis is worn for sleep and weaned during the day for therapy,

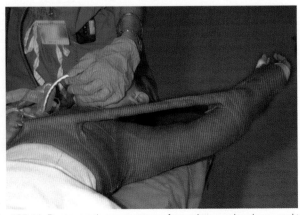

Fig. 125.11 Postoperative cast status after arthroscopic release and tendon transfers. An orthosis is fabricated that replicates the position when in the cast. (Courtesy of Shriners Hospital for Children, Philadelphia.)

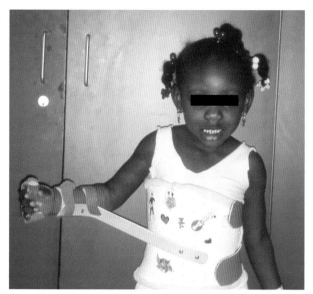

Fig. 125.12 After 4 weeks of immobilization, an orthosis is fabricated to replicate the cast with the arm externally rotated after arthroscopic release. (Courtesy of Shriners Hospital for Children, Philadelphia.)

bathing, and supervised play. For patients who quickly demonstrate fatigue with the transfer and have difficulty maintaining their active range, the orthosis may be worn more often during the day to allow for rest between exercises. On the other hand, patients who appear stiff or hesitant to move their arm out of abduction and external rotation may need more time out of the orthosis to allow for relaxation to avoid the development of contractures. The orthosis is used at night until 12 weeks after surgery. Restrictions during the mobilization and light-strengthening phases include avoiding passive internal rotation and shoulder adduction. Resistive and weight-bearing activities are also avoided.

Therapeutic intervention focuses on recruitment of the tendon transfer and active and passive shoulder abduction and external rotation. When working with children, the therapist must be creative in choosing and instituting activities to engage the patient into the desired movements (Fig. 125.13). For example, a painting activity set up on a vertical surface can be used to facilitate both external rotation and shoulder elevation. Consider changing the position of the patient for those with difficulty obtaining full abduction against gravity. Working in the supine position allows for successful active movement in a gravity-eliminated plane. Early active internal rotation and adduction are initiated to limit difficulty with midline tasks and lessen the incidence of scapulohumeral abduction contractures.

Latissimus dorsi and teres major tendon transfers can substantially improve shoulder function in patients with brachial plexus palsy. In patients with unbalanced forces around the shoulder, early tendon transfers can stop the progression of glenohumeral joint deformity. On MRI examination, isolated tendon transfers have not been shown to be effective in correcting existing glenohumeral joint deformity.[4] Combining arthroscopic glenohumeral release with tendon transfers has been successful in correcting the alignment of the glenohumeral joint and augmenting active shoulder movement when further nerve recovery is not expected (Fig. 125.14).[12]

Results. In children with glenoid dysplasia, open or arthroscopic reduction has been shown to improve joint configuration with reduction of the humeral head and improved glenoid version (i.e., the angle the glenoid makes with the plane of the scapula).[23,32] Positive changes are observed both on MRI and with clinical measurements.

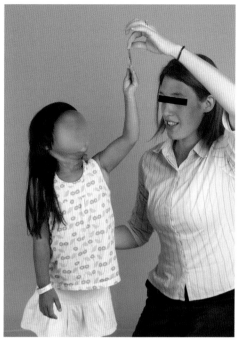

Fig. 125.13 When working with children, the therapist must be creative in choosing and setting up activities to engage the patient into the desired movements. (Courtesy of Shriners Hospital for Children, Philadelphia.)

Improvements in active shoulder ROM primarily occur with abduction and external rotation (Fig. 125.15). Limitations with internal rotation have been noted after subscapularis lengthening, which can be reduced by minimizing the amount of subscapularis release completed at the time of surgery. Importantly, superior outcomes are associated with better preoperative clinical and MRI status. This finding indicates that early recognition of glenohumeral dysplasia and timely intervention will result in better shoulder motion and improved joint alignment.[36,37]

Humeral Osteotomies

A humeral osteotomy can considerably improve an individual's function. For patients with an internal rotation contracture and advanced glenohumeral joint deformity, changing the resting position of the arm can improve activities requiring external rotation. Likewise, patients who have external rotation without internal rotation for midline tasks, such as fastening buttons or zippers on pants, would benefit from humeral osteotomy. The preoperative examination must include a careful measurement of the patient's active arc of motion and the functional goals and must consider the amount of movement that must be preserved to maintain current functional status. Simulation of both internal and external rotation activities, such as hair washing and fastening pants with passive assistance, allows the therapist to measure how much motion is required for the individual to complete each task (Fig. 125.16). The assessment must compare active arc of motion and consider the available compensatory movements, such as wrist flexion to achieve hand-to-belly movement, before giving a final recommendation regarding amount of correction.[5]

We prefer a medial arm incision along the medial intermuscular septum to hide the scar. The interval between the anterior and posterior arm musculature is developed, and the medial intermuscular septum is identified. The ulnar nerve lies just posterior to the septum, and the median nerve and brachial artery are anterior. The periosteum is incised, and reverse retractors are carefully placed anterior and posterior to the humerus.

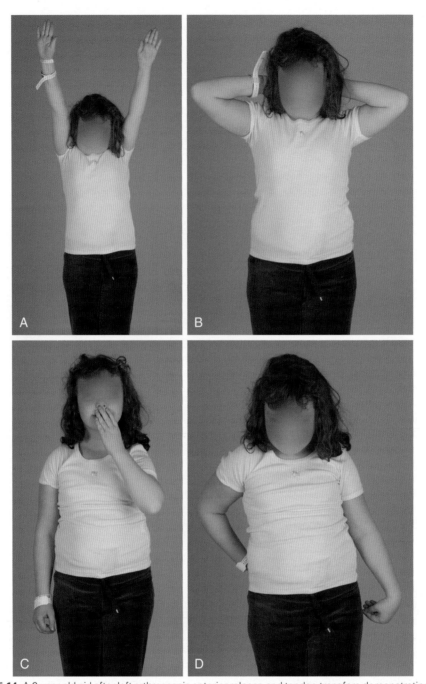

Fig. 125.14 A 6-year-old girl after left arthroscopic anterior release and tendon transfers demonstrating Mallet parameters for shoulder function. **A,** Abduction (grade IV to 170 degrees). **B,** Hand to neck (grade IV from grade II preoperative). **C,** Hand to mouth (grade IV from grade III preoperative). **D,** Hand to spine (grade II with no change from preoperative). (Courtesy of Shriners Hospital for Children, Philadelphia.)

The length of the humeral shaft necessary for osteotomy and plate fixation is exposed. The size of the plate depends on the size of the humerus. Usually, a 2.7- or 3.5-mm plate is selected with six or seven holes. The desired amount of external rotation is determined before surgery. A fine-bladed saw is selected and a transverse osteotomy performed perpendicular to the bone (Fig. 125.17). The humerus is externally rotated, and the osteotomy is reduced. The plate and screws are applied in standard fashion (Fig. 125.18). Wound closure is straightforward using absorbable sutures. The limb is wrapped in a bulky dressing from the hand to the axilla. No orthosis is used, although ample wrap is applied to "immobilize" the limb. The elbow is positioned in 90 degrees

of flexion.[38] The fingers are left free for early motion. The arm is placed into a sling when the child is walking. The dressings are removed 2 weeks after surgery and radiographs taken to ensure bony alignment.

Based on healing and patient activity level, immobilization lasts for 3 to 6 weeks. After dressing removal, a humeral fracture brace is fabricated to protect the healing bone (Fig. 125.19). The brace is worn at all times except during bathing until adequate healing is noted. Resistive activities and PROM are avoided until the bone healing is complete. Minimal therapy is required. The patient is educated on a home program of AROM and scar management. Exercises to promote new movements such as hand to ear or neck (external rotation osteotomy)

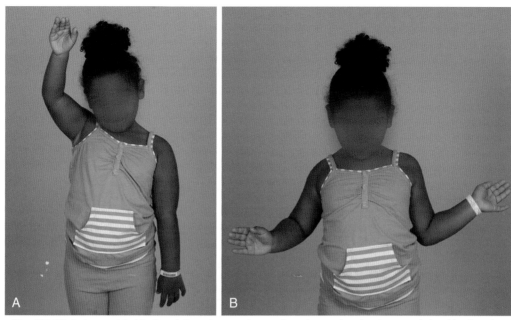

Fig. 125.15 A 4-year-old girl after right arthroscopic anterior release showing improved shoulder function. **A,** Abduction (Mallet grade IV). **B,** External rotation (Mallet grade IV). (Courtesy of Shriners Hospital for Children, Philadelphia.)

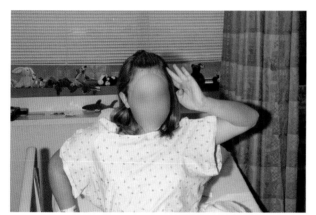

Fig. 125.16 A 14-year-old patient with internal rotation contracture and inability to touch her ear or back of her neck. (Courtesy of Shriners Hospital for Children, Philadelphia.)

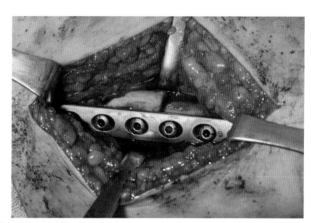

Fig. 125.18 The humerus is externally rotated, the osteotomy is reduced, and the plate and screws are applied. (Courtesy of Shriners Hospital for Children, Philadelphia.)

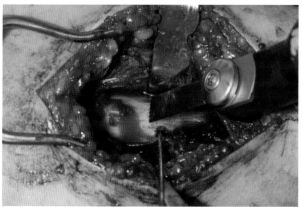

Fig. 125.17 A Kirschner wire is drilled in an oblique angle to simulate the amount of correction, and a fine-bladed saw is used for osteotomy. (Courtesy of Shriners Hospital for Children, Philadelphia.)

or hand to trunk (internal rotation osteotomy) are included. A few sessions may be necessary for the patient to adapt to the arm in the new position and maximize the functional potential.

Humeral osteotomy does not improve overall glenohumeral motion but does enhance upper extremity function by allowing the arc of shoulder rotation to be in a more functional range.[26,39] This allows the hand to be placed in a better position to accomplish certain ADLs that require external rotation, such as washing hair, placing the hand on the neck, eating, and throwing a ball (Fig. 125.20). Mallet parameters improve for the desired goals, although some reciprocal loss of motion is expected.

Elbow

Tendon Transfers for Elbow Flexion

The assessment of potential muscles for transfer is performed via inventory of available donors. There are multiple donor muscles described for elbow flexorplasty, including the latissimus dorsi, pectoralis major, triceps, and flexor–pronator muscles.[39–45] A bipolar transfer of the latissimus dorsi is the preferred donor as long as the muscle is available for transfer. The bipolar method provides a better "line of pull" and superior restoration of muscle fiber length.

The latissimus dorsi muscle is expendable, possesses adequate strength, and provides sufficient excursion for elbow flexion.[45] The other options have considerable disadvantages. The pectoralis major muscle harvest causes substantial scarring, and cosmetic concerns

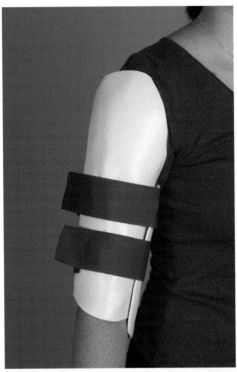

Fig. 125.19 Humeral fracture brace to protect the osteotomy and to allow elbow motion. (Courtesy of Shriners Hospital for Children, Philadelphia.)

limit its use.[42] The triceps muscle results in loss of active elbow extension, decreased workable reach space, and a substantial elbow flexion contracture.[46] The transfer or proximal advancement of the flexor–pronator muscle group, known as the Steindler procedure, provides active elbow flexion only to 90 to 100 degrees with limited strength and unwanted pronation during attempted elbow flexion.

A free muscle transfer (e.g., gracilis muscle) can be used in dire straits when there is no other donor is available, although there must be an available motor nerve to reinnervate the transferred muscle.

Latissimus dorsi transfer (bipolar technique). The patient is placed in a lateral position for harvest of the latissimus dorsi muscle and rotated into the supine position during transfer of the muscle into the anterior arm maintaining the sterile field. A longitudinal incision is made from the posterior axillary fold to the inferior aspect of the latissimus dorsi muscle. The entire muscle is mobilized, including a strip of thoracodorsal fascia and the tendinous insertion into the humerus (Fig. 125.21). The thoracodorsal nerve and vascular pedicle are isolated and protected. An anterior deltopectoral approach is performed to create a passageway for the bipolar transfer. The latissimus dorsi muscle is passed from posterior to anterior with the tendinous insertion proximal and the fascial origin distal.[1]

The latissimus dorsi muscle is passed into the arm through a subcutaneous tunnel (Fig. 125.22). The tendon of origin is secured to the coracoid via transosseous sutures and the thoracodorsal fascia woven into the biceps tendon, which can be reinforced by allograft. The transfer is placed in enough tension to create a 30-degree tenodesis effect (i.e., tension in the transfer prevents the last 30 degrees of elbow extension). The wounds are closed with drains placed in the posterior wound. A long arm splint that maintains 100 to 110 degrees of flexion and a Velpeau dressing is applied holding the arm against the side.

Postoperative management. Regardless of the muscle transfer for elbow flexion, the initial postoperative regimen is similar. The arm is placed in either an orthosis or a cast in flexion for 4 to 6 weeks' time depending on the status and effectiveness of the proximal and distal transfer sites.[47] At the time of cast removal, a posterior long

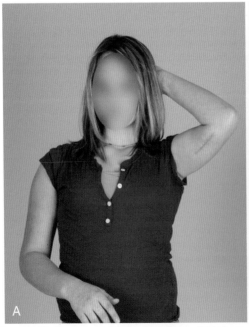 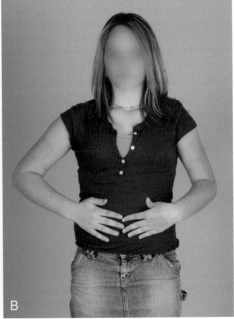

Fig. 125.20 The 6-year-old shown in Figure 125.14 after external rotation osteotomy at age 14. **A,** Improved hand to ear and neck. **B,** Mild loss on internal rotation with wrist flexion required to place the hand on the navel. (Courtesy of Shriners Hospital for Children, Philadelphia.)

arm orthosis is fabricated with the elbow flexed at approximately 110 degrees. The orthosis is primarily worn at night. The patient is also fitted with an adjustable elbow hinge brace that allows for locking flexion and extension ROM. Initially, the extension hinge is locked to 110 degrees, allowing further flexion and blocking extension beyond this point. During the early part of the mobilization phase, treatment focuses on muscle reeducation and scar management.

Muscle reeducation begins with active contraction and isolation of the transfer. To initiate recruitment, the therapist cues the patient to perform the transferred muscles' previous action. Close supervision and careful positioning of the arm in a gravity-eliminated plane are necessary to prevent elbow extension. Biofeedback allows for visual and auditory feedback when activation has occurred to further teach the patient how to isolate activation.

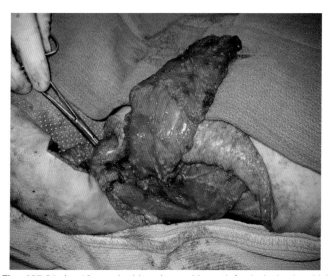

Fig. 125.21 An 18-month-old patient with an infraclavicular brachial plexus injury, absent elbow flexion, and insufficient soft tissue along the anterior arm. Latissimus dorsi muscle harvested on the thoracodorsal neurovascular pedicle before transfer beneath the pectoralis major muscle. (Courtesy of Shriners Hospital for Children, Philadelphia.)

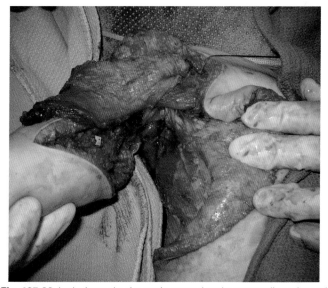

Fig. 125.22 Latissimus dorsi muscle passed under pectoralis major and into arm for restoration of elbow flexion. (Courtesy of Shriners Hospital for Children, Philadelphia.)

When activation is consistent, functional tabletop activities should be included in the program to reestablish desired movement patterns. When the patient can consistently recruit the tendon transfer, the ROM can be progressed 15 degrees each week. After achieving a 30-degree arc of motion (90–120 degrees), light resistive activities are initiated. This consists of against-gravity AROM, hand-to-mouth activities, and more challenging tabletop activities. At approximately 10 weeks with sufficient tendon excursion, patients may begin formal strengthening. Passive elbow extension is not allowed for 3 months. Tendon transfers may actually function better in patients who lack full extension. The slight elbow flexion contracture eases the initiation of active elbow flexion. The goal for end-range extension is typically 20 to 30 degrees.[48] The daytime orthosis is discontinued after the patient achieves active elbow flexion against gravity from 90 degrees to end range. Night wear of the orthosis continues until 12 weeks after surgery.

The results following elbow flexorplasties are positive with 3 of 5 to 5 of 5 muscle strength and enough active flexion for ADLs.[47,48] Patients report functional gains in unilateral and bimanual activities. Mild elbow flexion contractures are common after these procedures. In general, bipolar flexorplasties provide greater ROM than do unipolar transfers (Fig. 125.23).

Tendon Transfer for Elbow Extension

A lack of elbow extension can result from brachial plexus injury that involves the middle portion of the plexus because the triceps receives the majority of it innervation from C7. Surgical reconstruction is less commonly performed because elbow flexion is a greater priority and elbow extension can be accomplished by gravity.[49] In certain cases, elbow flexion is adequate, and the lack of elbow extension is disabling. Deficient elbow extension will decrease the patient's available workspace, especially during reaching activities that limit the ability to perform overhead tasks.

Evaluation for elbow extension transfer requires an inventory of the available muscles. Donor options include the bipolar latissimus dorsi muscle, the posterior deltoid, or the biceps-to-triceps transfer (the last two transfers are commonly used in tetraplegia). Active brachialis and supinator muscles are prerequisites to biceps transfer to maintain elbow flexion and forearm supination. The evaluation of their integrity requires a careful physical examination of elbow flexion and forearm supination strength.[50] The brachialis and supinator muscles can be palpated independent of the biceps muscle. Effortless forearm supination without resistance induces supinator function that can be palpated along the proximal radius. Similarly, powerless elbow flexion incites palpable brachialis contraction along the anterior humerus. Equivocal cases require additional evaluation to ensure adequate supinator and brachialis muscle activity.[51] We prefer injection of the biceps muscle with a local anesthetic to induce temporary paralysis and allow independent assessment of brachialis and supinator function. A free muscle transfer (e.g., gracilis muscle) can be used in dire straits when there is no other donor available, although there must be an available motor nerve to reinnervate the transferred muscle.

Tendon transfers for elbow extension are less reliable compared with tendon transfers for elbow flexion. Our results have been disappointing, and we recommend these transfers only when elbow extension is a necessity. Although the biceps to triceps transfer is effective in tetraplegia, the transfer is less predictable in brachial plexus injuries. We believe the reinnervation process after injury from the C5 and C6 nerve roots to the biceps and brachialis after brachial plexus injury negatively affects the patient's ability to fire these muscles independently. Subsequent, co-contraction negatively impacts the results after biceps to triceps transfer.

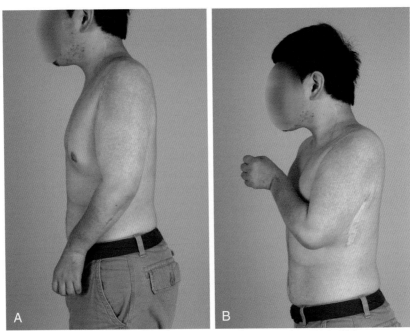

Fig. 125.23 A 12-year-old boy after bipolar latissimus dorsi flexorplasty. **A,** Elbow extension with slight contracture. **B,** Active elbow flexion. (Courtesy of Shriners Hospital for Children, Philadelphia.)

Latissimus dorsi transfer (bipolar technique). The patient is placed in a lateral position for harvest of the latissimus dorsi muscle. A longitudinal incision is made from the posterior axillary fold to the inferior aspect of the latissimus dorsi muscle. The entire muscle is mobilized, including a strip of thoracodorsal fascia and the tendinous insertion into the humerus. The thoracodorsal nerve and vascular pedicle are isolated and protected.

The latissimus dorsi muscle tendon of origin is secured to the clavicle or acromion via drill holes. The remaining muscle is passed through a subcutaneous tunnel and the thoracodorsal fascia woven into the triceps tendon, which can be reinforced by allograft. The transfer is sutured in place with the arm positioned in full extension. The wounds are closed and the arm placed in a long arm orthosis in complete extension.

Biceps transfer. The biceps tendon is routed around the medial side of the humerus and under the ulnar nerve. The musculocutaneous nerve is identified just lateral to the biceps tendon and is protected throughout the procedure. The lacertus fibrosis is incised, and the biceps tendon is traced into the forearm toward its insertion into the radial tuberosity. The biceps tendon is released and transferred around the medial aspect of the arm (Fig. 125.24).

A third 7-cm posterior incision is made over the distal third of the triceps and curved around the olecranon. The triceps is sharply split over the tip of the olecranon, and the biceps tendon is passed obliquely through the medial portion of the triceps tendon and attached to the olecranon via an osseous tunnel (Fig. 125.25). The limb is maintained in full extension, and the subcutaneous tissue and skin closed with nonabsorbable sutures. The tourniquet is deflated, and dressings and a well-padded long arm cast are applied in the operating room.[50]

Postoperative management. Regardless of the muscle transfer for elbow extension, the initial postoperative regimen is similar. The arm is placed in an orthosis or cast for 3 to 6 weeks' time depending on the status and effectiveness of the proximal and distal transfer sites. For biceps transfer, shoulder elevation above 90 degrees and extension

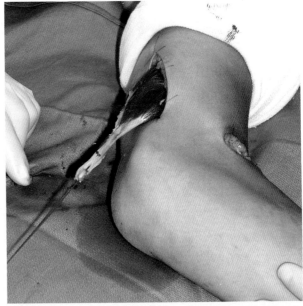

Fig. 125.24 Biceps tendon transfer for elbow extension. The biceps tendon is released from the radial tuberosity and transferred around the medial aspect of the arm. (Courtesy of Shriners Hospital for Children, Philadelphia.)

past neutral are not allowed until 6 weeks after surgery. During the immobilization phase, the patient and caregivers are educated on edema management techniques.[50]

An elbow extension orthosis in full extension is then fabricated for nighttime use. A dial-hinge brace (e.g., Breg Inc, Carlsbad, CA) is fitted for daytime use and acts as a flexion block at 15 degrees (Fig. 125.26). The brace is adjusted each week to allow an additional 15 degrees of flexion. The brace is not advanced if an extension lag develops. Tendon transfer firing is started in an antigravity plane. The medially routed

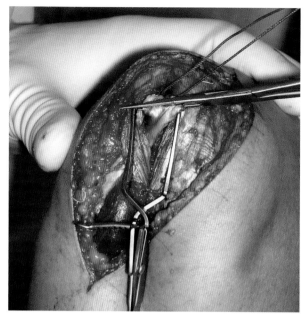

Fig. 125.25 Biceps tendon transfer for elbow extension. The biceps tendon is passed obliquely through a split in the triceps tendon and attached to the olecranon. (Courtesy of Shriners Hospital for Children, Philadelphia.)

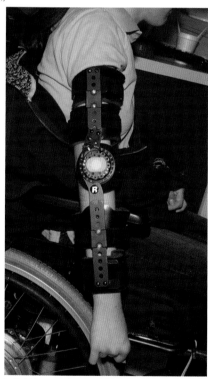

Fig. 125.26 A dial-hinge brace (e.g., Breg Inc., Carlsbad, CA) is used to monitor amount of allowable flexion. (Courtesy of Shriners Hospital for Children, Philadelphia.)

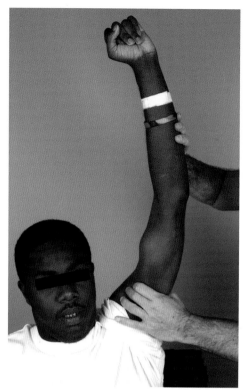

Fig. 125.27 A 16-year-old boy after biceps-to-triceps tendon transfer with strong antigravity elbow extension. (Courtesy of Shriners Hospital for Children, Philadelphia.)

degrees of elbow flexion is achieved without an extension lag. A night-time extension orthosis is maintained until 12 weeks. Strengthening is started 3 months after surgery.

Results. Biceps-to-triceps tendon transfer has been shown to effectively produce antigravity elbow extension in persons with tetraplegia (Fig. 125.27). In our series of nine patients, eight achieved 3 of 5 or greater elbow extension after tendon transfer. All patients experienced greater reachable workspace and were satisfied with their results.[50] There are no reported results in patients with brachial plexus birth injury.

Forearm
Biceps Rerouting
Biceps rerouting [46] is our preferred technique for restoration of pronation in supple supination deformities of the forearm. A Z-incision is designed with a horizontal limb across the antecubital fossa (Fig. 125.28). The biceps tendon is traced to its insertion into the radial tuberosity, and a Z-plasty of the biceps tendon is performed along its entire length to ensure sufficient tendon length for passage around the radius (Fig. 125.29). The distal Z-plasty is left attached to the insertion site, and the proximal Z-plasty is left attached to the biceps muscle belly.

The distal attachment is carefully rerouted around the radius through the interosseous space to create a pronation force (Fig. 125.30). The elbow is placed in 90 degrees of flexion and the forearm in pronation. The rerouted distal tendon is repaired back to the proximal tendon that is still attached to the biceps muscle (Fig. 125.31). A long arm cast is applied with the elbow in 90 degrees of flexion and the forearm in pronation for 5 weeks.

After 5 weeks of immobilization, the cast is removed, and rehabilitation is started. A long arm orthosis is fabricated with the elbow in a resting position with the forearm pronated and the wrist in neutral or slightly extended position (Fig. 125.32). An alternative to this is a long forearm-based

biceps can be palpated along the medial humerus during active elbow extension. Verbal prompting of active elbow flexion and forearm supination facilitates motor learning. Biofeedback may be used in patients who have difficulty with initiating the transfer or if co-contraction of antagonist muscles is occurring.

Functional ADLs are incorporated into the therapy as elbow flexion increases each week. The dial-hinge brace is continued until 90

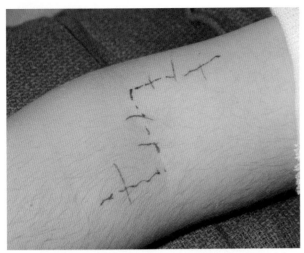

Fig. 125.28 Biceps tendon rerouting for forearm deformity. A Z-incision is designed with a horizontal limb across the antecubital fossa. (Courtesy of Shriners Hospital for Children, Philadelphia.)

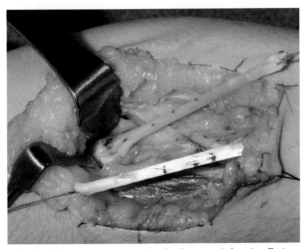

Fig. 125.29 Biceps tendon rerouting for forearm deformity. Z-plasty of the biceps tendon along its entire length to ensure sufficient tendon length for passage around the radius. (Courtesy of Shriners Hospital for Children, Philadelphia.)

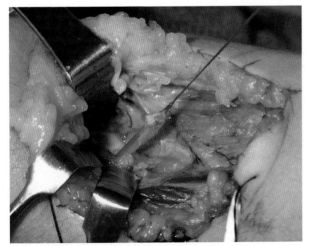

Fig. 125.30 The distal biceps tendon is rerouted around the radius through the interosseous space to create a pronation force. (Courtesy of Shriners Hospital for Children, Philadelphia.)

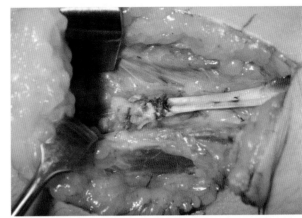

Fig. 125.31 The rerouted distal tendon is repaired back to the proximal tendon that is still attached to the biceps muscle. (Courtesy of Shriners Hospital for Children, Philadelphia.)

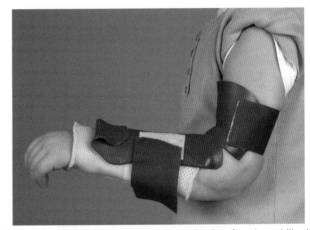

Fig. 125.32 Two-piece supracondylar orthosis after immobilization phase after biceps rerouting. (Courtesy of Shriners Hospital for Children, Philadelphia.)

orthosis that prevents supination but allows elbow motion. The orthosis is removed for bathing and the home program during the first week. The orthosis is weaned to night use only 8 weeks after surgery and discontinued at 12 weeks. During the mobilization phase, passive elbow extension and supination are avoided. Light strengthening activities for elbow flexion and pronation can be introduced 8 weeks postoperatively.[31,32]

Frequently, minimal therapy is needed after surgery. During early mobilization, the focus is on AROM, including gentle elbow extension and supination. The forearm will naturally pronate with elbow flexion. Scar management is initiated as soon as the incisional scars are closed. Self-care and other light functional activities that promote pronation, such as keyboarding, should be introduced. These are all completed as part of the home program.

The improved pronated position of the forearm enhances the patient's use of the hand for many ADLs (Fig. 125.33). A loss of supination ROM is expected and should be discussed before surgery.[32] The unaffected arm can usually compensate for hardships caused by the loss of supination.

Osteotomy of the Radius and Ulna or One-Bone Forearm

Mild rigid supination deformities can be treated with osteotomy of the radius or ulna.[32] However, severe supination deformities require osteotomy of both bones to maximize correction (Fig. 125.34). We have transitioned from combined osteotomies to the creation of a one-bone forearm as the preferred procedure for severe fixed supination deformities. The

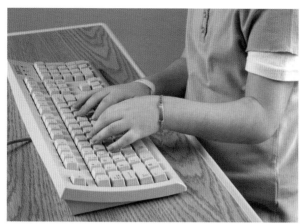

Fig. 125.33 Improved pronated position of the left forearm facilitates keyboard usage. (Courtesy of Shriners Hospital for Children, Philadelphia.)

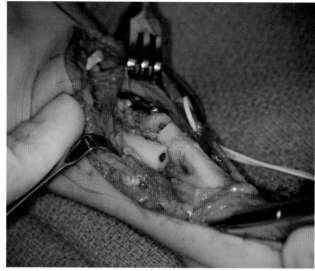

Fig. 125.35 The radius is cut distal to the ulna and manually mobilized toward the proximal ulna. (Courtesy of Shriners Hospital for Children, Philadelphia.)

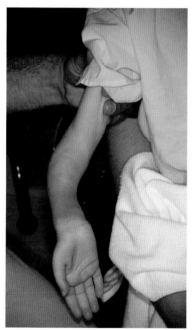

Fig. 125.34 An 8-year-old boy with residual right global brachial plexus birth palsy and fixed forearm supination deformity (Courtesy of Shriners Hospital for Children, Philadelphia.)

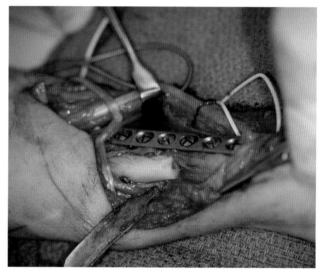

Fig. 125.36 The forearm is rotated into the desired position and the ulna secured to the distal radius using dynamic compression. (Courtesy of Shriners Hospital for Children, Philadelphia.)

paradigm shift has been due to the recurrence over time after combined osteotomies caused by persistent muscle imbalance and the ability to correct substantial deformities using the one-bone technique described below.

One-bone forearm. A curvilinear incision is made along the distal radius and proximal ulna. The volar forearm fascia is incised along the length of the skin incision. The radius is exposed via a trans–flexor carpi radialis incision. The ulna is isolated deep to the flexor carpi ulnaris and ulnar neurovascular bundle. In patients with substantial denervation, the forearm muscles have mainly been replaced by fat with only a few strands of viable muscle present.

The osteotomies are planned with the radius osteotomy 1 to 2 cm distal to the ulnar osteotomy. Proximal to the proposed ulnar osteotomy site, an appropriately sized dynamic compression plate is secured with three or four bicortical screws. The interosseous membrane is incised to allow the radius to be positioned on top of the proximal ulna. The plate is then removed, and the ulnar and radial osteotomies are performed with a fine-bladed sagittal saw. The distal ulna can be excised or simply mobilized out of harm's way.

The radius is manually mobilized toward the proximal ulna (Fig. 125.35). The plate is reapplied to the ulna. After the bones are coapted, the radius is rotated into the desired position. The reduction is held with a bone reduction clamp and the position carefully assessed. When the position is deemed acceptable, the plate is secured to the distal radius using bicortical screw fixation (Fig. 125.36). The remaining proximal radius segment is used as onlay graft across the osteotomy site. The radius is decorticated and affixed to the construct using an intraosseous suture or compression screw The subcutaneous tissue and skin are closed and a long arm splint applied. The splint is changed to a long arm cast 2 weeks after surgery. The long arm cast is worn for an additional 4 weeks. Radiographs are taken at a 2-week follow-up to ensure alignment and repeated at 6 weeks to ensure healing of the osteotomy site. A protective orthosis is then fabricated for another 6 weeks. Digital ROM exercises are started immediately after surgery. Elbow motion is begun at 6 weeks after removal of the long arm cast. The amount of correction achieved is often remarkable (Fig. 125.37).[52]

Wrist and Hand

The selection of available and appropriate donors for tendon transfer is crucial in children with residual brachial plexus palsy. As stated previously, reinnervated muscles are avoided if possible. Equally as important, every attempt is made to select a synchronous muscle because postoperative compliance in therapy is limited by age and cognition. Therefore, finger flexors for wrist extension is preferred as well as a wrist extensor for finger flexion. The main donors are the flexor digitorum superficialis (FDS) and extensor carpi radialis longus (ECRL),

respectively. When these tendons are unavailable, a search for alternative donors is needed based on the established principles of availability, expendability, synchrony, and excursion.

Flexor Digitorum Superficialis Tendon Transfer (Wrist Extension)

In the presence of adequate flexor digitorum profundus (FDP) and FDS strength in the long and ring digits, FDS transfer around the long finger metacarpal is our preferred wrist transfer. This transfer is synergistic and preserves available wrist flexion strength.

A transverse incision is made at the base of the long or ring fingers (or both). The FDS tendons are isolated from the FDP tendons. An oblique incision is then made over the distal third of the forearm, and the long and ring finger FDS tendons are isolated. The tendons are then cut distal to the suture at the base of the fingers and the tendons are passed through the carpal tunnel to the forearm incision (Fig. 125.38). The rout of passage depends on the patient. The tendons can be passed around the radial side of the forearm to enhance pronation, around the ulnar side to improve supination, or through the interosseous membrane to address only wrist extension. Passing the tendons around the long finger metacarpal is preferred (Fig. 125.39). One tendon is passed in a radial to ulnar direction and the other in an opposite direction. The wrist is placed in the desired amount of wrist extension based on the preoperative examination of digital opening and closing to set the tension of the transfer. The cast is removed 3 weeks after surgery, and a short arm orthosis is fabricated. Tendon transfer training is initiated, although the synergism of the transfer negates the necessity of substantial relearning. The orthosis daytime use is discontinued 8 weeks after surgery, often continuing night wear for an additional 4 weeks.[52]

Extensor Carpi Radialis Tendon Transfer (Finger Flexion)

The patient is placed supine on the operating room table. A longitudinal radial incision is made from the styloid to the proximal third of the forearm. Distal to the first compartment, the ECRL, and extensor carpi radialis brevis (ECRB) tendons are identified. In the proximal part of

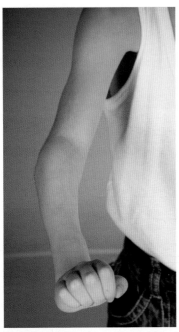

Fig. 125.37 Final position of right forearm after osteotomy site. (Courtesy of Shriners Hospital for Children, Philadelphia.)

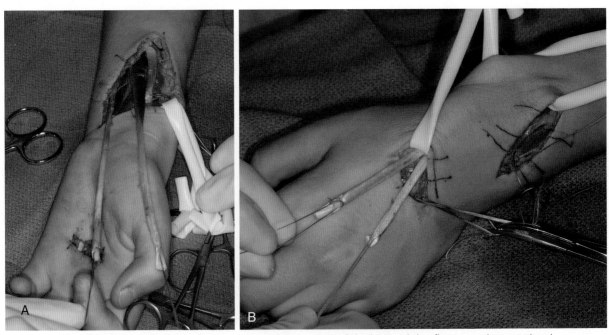

Fig. 125.38 A and B, Flexor digitorum superficialis tendons of the long and ring fingers are harvested and passed to the dorsum of the hand to prepare for transfer. (Courtesy of Shriners Hospital for Children, Philadelphia.)

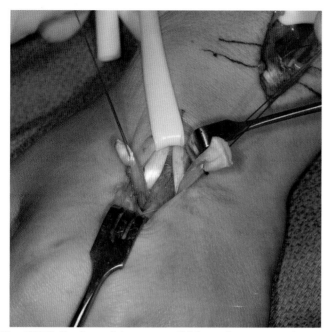

Fig. 125.39 The flexor digitorum superficialis tendons are routed around the long finger metacarpal, our preferred transfer for optimal wrist extension. (Courtesy of Shriners Hospital for Children, Philadelphia.)

the incisions, the ECRL and ECRB tendons are also isolated. The ECRL tendon is then cut as distal as possible and is passed under the first dorsal compartment.

The FDP tendons are isolated and sutured together (en masse) to set the desired finger cascade during grasp. The ECRL tendon is passed deep to the radial artery and woven through the FDP tendons. Tension is adjusted until there is finger flexion during wrist extension and tenodesis opening during wrist flexion. A short or long arm cast is applied depending on the age of the patient and the strength of the repair. The wrist is positioned in slight extension and the elbow flexed to 90 degrees with the fingers slightly flexed. This finger position is maintained with a small roll of Webril cotton cast padding. Early mobilization can be started on postoperative day 1 as long as the tendons are of adequate caliber and the transfer site is firmly repaired. The Webril is removed, and the patient is instructed to bend his or her fingers. The response is often overwhelming because finger flexion is readily initiated secondary to the synergistic actions of wrist extension and finger flexion.[52]

The cast is removed 3 weeks after surgery and a short arm orthosis is fabricated. Tendon transfer training is continued, although the synergism of the transfer negates the need for extensive relearning. The orthosis day use is discontinued eight weeks from surgery, night wear often continues for four additional weeks.[52]

Postoperative Management

After tendon transfer surgery, there are four main phases: immobilization, mobilization, light strengthening–functional training, and strengthening. Intervention during the immobilization phase focuses on edema control, pain management, and ROM of uninvolved joints. This phase typically lasts 3 to 4 weeks depending on the type of tendon transfer, the quality of the tendons, and the strength of the suture. Larger tendons can be mobilized earlier; smaller tendons require longer immobilization.

The mobilization phase begins when the cast is removed and lasts until 6 to 8 weeks after surgery. Therapy is initiated with the fabrication of a protective orthosis that maintains a tension-free position of

the tendon transfer. Resistive activities and active and passive movements that apply tension to the transfer are avoided. Treatment begins with muscle reeducation of the tendon transfer. Cues to attempt the previous action of the transferred muscle in a protected position are useful for muscle reeducation.[50] When consistent recruitment has been achieved with AROM, functional activities should be incorporated into treatment. Incorporating play activities for children or identified functional activities can make sessions more meaningful to the patient. Scar management, including massage and possible use of silicone gel sheets, should be initiated as soon as the incisions are healed.[53]

The therapist should continually examine the patient for possible complications. In addition to complications that may occur with any tendon transfer such as scarring, attenuation, or rupture, there are a few key areas to monitor after the discussed procedures. With the FDS as the donor, there is a risk of developing hyperextension at the PIP joints of the long or ring finger (or both). If present, PIP extension blocking orthoses are indicated for the donor digits. After restoration of grasp in patients with limited digital extension, there is a risk of flexor tightness developing. Many patients can maintain passive extension through wrist flexion, stretching, and activity. The development of long flexor tightness requires a night orthosis.

SUMMARY

Secondary brachial plexus palsy reconstruction requires careful evaluation of the child's upper extremity. Early intervention is warranted for joint contracture and deformity. Intervention may be additional therapy or early surgery depending on the clinical scenario. Therapy plays an integral role throughout the growth of the limb and maturation of the child. Established impairment may benefit from secondary procedures, such as tendon transfer or osteotomy, as long as the benefits outweigh the risks. The decision-making process requires thoughtful input from the surgeon and the therapist to ensure the best outcome for the patient. Communication among the patient, family, surgeon, and therapist is mandatory to develop a plan that optimizes the patient's opportunity to improve with regards to ADLs, school, work, and avocational activities.

REFERENCES

1. Kozin SH. Injuries of the brachial plexus. In: Iannotti JP, Williams GR, eds. *Disorders of the Shoulder: Diagnosis and Management.* 3rd ed. Philadelphia: Lippincott Williams & White; 2014:607–660.
2. Duchenne GB. Studies on pseudohypertrophic muscular paralysis or myosclerotic paralysis. *Arch Neurol.* 1968;19:629.
3. Klumpke A. Klumpke's paralysis:1885 [classical article]. *Clin Orthop Relat Res.* 1999;368:3.
4. Waters PM, Bae DS. Effect of tendon transfers and extra-articular soft-tissue balancing on glenohumeral development in brachial plexus birth palsy. *J Bone Joint Surg.* 2005;87A:320.
5. Abzug JM, Chafetz RS, Gaughan JP, et al. Shoulder function after medial approach and derotational humeral osteotomy in patients with brachial plexus birth palsy. *J Pediatr Orthop.* 2010;30:469–474.
6. Amadio PC. Outcomes assessment in hand surgery: what's new? *Clin Plast Surg.* 1997;24:191.
7. Hudak PL, Amadio PC, Bombardier C. Development of an upper extremity outcome measure: the DASH (disabilities of the arm, shoulder and hand) [corrected]. The upper extremity collaborative group. *Am J Ind Med.* 1996;29:602.
8. Bae DS, Waters PM, Zurakowski D. Reliability of three classification systems measuring active motion in brachial plexus birth palsy. *J Bone Joint Surg.* 2003;85-A:1733.

9. Waters PM. Comparison of the natural history, the outcome of micro-surgical repair, and the outcome of operative reconstruction in brachial plexus birth palsy. *J Bone Joint Surg.* 1999;81A:649.

10. Waters PM, Peljovich AE. Shoulder reconstruction in patients with chronic brachial plexus birth palsy: a case control study. *Clin Orthop Relat Res.* 1999;364:144.

11. McColl MA, Law M, Baptiste S, et al. Targeted applications of the Canadian Occupational Performance Measure. *Can J Occup Ther.* 2005;72(5):298–300.

12. Kozin SH, Chafetz RS, Shaffer A, et al. Arthroscopic treatment of posterior glenohumeral joint subluxation secondary to brachial plexus. *J Bone Joint Surg.* 2010;30(2):154–160.

13. Kozin SH, Chafetz RS, Barus D, Filipone L. Magnetic resonance imaging and clinical findings before and after tendon transfers about the shoulder in children with residual brachial plexus birth palsy. *J Shoulder Elbow Surg.* 2006;15:554.

14. Pagnotta A, Haerle M, Gilbert A. Long-term results on abduction and external rotation of the shoulder after latissimus dorsi transfer for sequelae of obstetric palsy. *Clin Orthop Relat Res.* 2004;426:199.

15. Waters PM, Smith GR, Jaramillo D. Glenohumeral deformity secondary to brachial plexus birth palsy: a case control study. *J Bone Joint Surg.* 1998;80A:668.

16. Kozin SH, Zlotolow DA. Advanced imaging and arthroscopic management of shoulder contracture after birth palsy. *Hand Clin.* 2012;28:541–550.

17. Donohue KW, Little KJ, Gaughan JP, et al. Comparison of ultrasound and MRI for the diagnosis of glenohumeral dysplasia in brachial plexus birth palsy. *J Bone Joint Surg Am.* 2017;99:123–132.

18. Campion D. Electrodiagnostic testing in hand surgery. *J Hand Surg.* 1996;21A:947.

19. Deletis V, Morota N, Abbott IR. Electrodiagnosis in the management of brachial plexus surgery. *Hand Clin.* 1995;11:555.

20. Russo SA, Loeffler BJ, Zlotolow DA, et al. Limited glenohumeral cross-body adduction in children with brachial plexus birth palsy: a contributor to scapular winging. *J Pediatr Orthop.* 2015;35:240–245.

21. Russo SA, Kozin SH, Zlotolow DA, et al. Scapulothoracic and glenohumeral contributions to motion in children with brachial plexus birth palsy. *J Shoulder Elbow Surg.* 2014;23:327–338.

22. Russo SA, Rodriguez LM, Kozin SH, et al. Therapeutic taping for scapular stabilization in children with brachial plexus birth palsy. *Am J Occup Ther.* 2016;70: 7005220030p1-7005220030p11.

23. Pedowitz DI, Gibson B, Williams GR, Kozin SH. Arthroscopic treatment of posterior glenohumeral joint subluxation resulting from brachial plexus birth palsy. *J Shoulder Elbow Surg.* 2007;16:6–13.

24. Hoffer MM. Closed reduction and tendon transfer for treatment of dislocation of the glenohumeral joint secondary to brachial plexus birth palsy. *J Bone Joint Surg.* 1998;80A:998.

25. Hoffer MM, Wickenden R, Roper B. Brachial plexus birth palsies: results of tendon transfer to the rotator cuff. *J Bone Joint Surg.* 1978;60A:691.

26. Phipps GJ, Hoffer MM. Latissimus dorsi and teres major transfer to rotator cuff for Erb's palsy. *J Shoulder Elbow Surg.* 1995;4:124.

27. Price AE, Grossman JA. A management approach for secondary shoulder and forearm deformities following obstetrical brachial plexus injury. *Hand Clin.* 1995;11:607.

28. Eismann EA, Little KJ, Laor T, et al. Glenohumeral abduction contracture in children with unresolved neonatal brachial plexus palsy. *J Bone Joint Surg Am.* 2015;97:112–118.

29. Nikolaou S, Peterson E, Kim A, et al. Impaired growth of denervated muscle contributes to contracture formation following neonatal brachial plexus injury. *J Bone Joint Surg Am.* 2011;93:461–470.

30. Sheffler LC, Lattanza L, Hagar Y, et al. The prevalence, rate of progression, and treatment of elbow flexion contracture in children with brachial plexus birth palsy. *J Bone Joint Surg Am.* 2012;94:403–409.

31. D'Emilio S. Preoperative and postoperative therapeutic management of the supination deformity in the pediatric brachial plexus patient. *Tech Hand Up Extrem Surg.* 2006;10:96.

32. Kozin SH. Treatment of the supination deformity in the pediatric brachial plexus patient. *Tech Hand Up Extrem Surg.* 2006;10:87–95.

33. Ho ES, Roy T, Stephens D, Clarke HM. Serial casting and splinting of elbow contractures in children with obstetric brachial plexuspalsy. *J Hand Surg.* 2010;35(7):84–91.

34. Arad E, Stephens D, Curtis CG, et al. Botulinum toxin for the treatment of motor imbalance in obstetrical brachial plexus palsy. *Plast Reconstr Surg.* 2013;131:1307–1315.

35. Itoh Y, Sasaki T, Uchinishi K, et al. Transfer of latissimus dorsi to replace a paralysed anterior deltoid. *J Bone Joint Surg Br.* 1987;69:647–651.

36. Iorio ML, Menashe SJ, Iyer RS, et al. Glenohumeral dysplasia following neonatal brachial plexus palsy: presentation of predictive features during infancy. *J Hand Surg Am.* 2015;40:2345–2351.

37. Waters PM, Bae DS. The early effects of tendon transfers and open capsulorrhaphy on glenohumeral deformity in brachial plexus birth palsy. Surgical technique. *J Bone Joint Surg Am.* 2009;91:213–222.

38. Lancaster G, Kozin SH, Porter S. The medial surgical approach to the humerus. *Techniques Hand Up Extrem Surg.* 2000;4:201–206.

39. Beaton ED, Dumont A, Mackay MB, Richards RR. Steindler and pectoralis major flexorplasty: a comparative analysis. *J Hand Surg.* 1995;20A:747–756.

40. Brooks DM, Seddon HJ. Pectoral transplantation for paralysis of the flexors of the elbow. *J Bone Joint Surg.* 1959;41B:36.

41. Carroll RE, Hill NA. Triceps transfer to restore elbow flexion: a study of fifteen patients with paralytic lesions and arthrogryposis. *J Bone Joint Surg.* 1970;52A:239.

42. Carroll RE, Kleinman WB. Pectoralis major transplantation to restore elbow flexion to the paralytic limb. *J Hand Surg.* 1979;4A:501.

43. Marshall RW, Williams DH, Birch R, Bonney G. Operations to restore elbow flexion after brachial plexus injuries. *J Bone Joint Surg.* 1988;70B:577–582.

44. Stern PJ, Caudle RJ. Tendon transfers for elbow flexion. *Hand Clin.* 1988;4:297.

45. Zancolli E, Mitre H. Latissimus dorsi transfer to restore elbow flexion: an appraisal of eight cases. *J Bone Joint Surg.* 1973;55A:265.

46. Hershman EB. Brachial plexus injuries. *Clin Sports Med.* 1990;9:311.

47. Rühmann O, Schmolke S, Gossé F, Wirth CJ. Transposition of local muscles to restore elbow flexion in brachial plexus palsy. *Int J Care Injured.* 2002;33:597–609.

48. Al-Qattan MM. Elbow flexion reconstruction by Steindler flexorplasty in obstetric brachial plexus palsy. *J Hand Surg.* 2005;30B:424.

49. Jones BN, Manske PR, Schoenecker PL, Dailey L. Latissimus dorsi transfer to restore elbow extension in obstetrical palsy. *J Pediatr Orthop.* 1985;5:287–289.

50. Kozin SH, Barus D. The evaluation and treatment of the elbow secondary to central nervous system dysfunction. *J Hand Surg.* 2006;19(2):192–205.

51. Kuz J, Van Heest AE, House JH. Biceps-to-triceps transfer in tetraplegic patients: report of the medial routing technique and follow-up of three cases. *J Hand Surg.* 1999;24A:161.

52. Kozin SH, et al. Pediatric upper extremity secondary to procedures about the elbow, forearm, wrist and hand. In: Abzug JM, Kozin SH, Zlotolow DA, eds. *The Pediatric Upper Extremity.* New York: Springer; 2015:653–682.

53. Widgerow AD, Chait LA, Stals R, Stals PJ. New innovations in scar management. *Aesthetic Plast Surg.* 2000;24:227–234.

Note: Page numbers followed by "f" indicate figures; "t" indicate tables; and "b" indicate boxes.

Interosseous muscle
   examination of, 54, 54f
   tightness, in stiff hand, 378–379
Interosseous muscle slide (recession), for hand
   deformities, 1578
Interosseous tendon(s), tendinopathy of, 513
Interphalangeal joint
   arthrodesis of, for thumb deformity, 1580
   deformity of, boutonnière, deformity caused
     by, 1206
   distal. *See* Distal interphalangeal (DIP) joint
   extension orthosis, 1173, 1173f
   proximal. *See* Proximal interphalangeal (PIP)
     joint
Interposition arthroplasty, for elbow arthritis,
   1293–1294
   rehabilitation after, 1293
   results of, 1294
Interposition vein graft(s), in replantation
   surgery, 1045, 1045f
Interscapulothoracic amputation, 1098. *See also*
   Amputation
Intersection syndrome, 67, 67f, 152, 511, 511f
Intersegmental deficiency, 1772
Interstitial fluid, 798–799
Intra-arterial injection, 787, 787f
Intraarticular fracture(s), of hand, 310–321. *See*
   also Hand fracture(s)
   at carpometacarpal joint, 318
     of thumb, 319–320, 320f
   complications of, 342
   at distal interphalangeal joint, 315–316
   early motion in, 323
     key evaluation measures for, 324
     precaution for, 323–324
     treatment techniques, 334–335, 341f
   evaluation of, 310, 324–325
   at metacarpophalangeal joint, 316–318
   at proximal interphalangeal joint, 310–315,
     311f
   rehabilitation goals for, 324–325, 325b
   therapy management of, 322–344
     differential tissue evaluation in, 324
     kinematic chain and substitute motion in,
       324, 339f
     late referral in, 342–343
     referral information in, 324
   at thumb interphalangeal joint, 315–316
   at thumb metacarpophalangeal joint, 318–319
   treatment of, 325–342
     controlled motion, 325
     dosing interventions in, 335–339
     functional activity and strengthening in, 342
     immobilization in, 327–331
     orthoses in, 325–334, 333f–340f
     orthotic modification, 325
     protected motion, 325
     time frames, 325
     universal, 325, 326t–332t
Intracarpal tunnel pressure, 721
Intraclass correlation coefficient (ICC), 173
Intramedullary fixation, of fractures, 281–282
Intraosseous ganglion, 253–254
Intraosseous wire fixation, in replantation
   surgery, 1043, 1043f
Intravenous drug abuse, abscess due to, 217–218,
   219f
Intrinsic growth capacity, activation of, in nerve
   regeneration, 573, 574f
Intrinsic hand muscle strength, in lateral
   epicondylitis, 523
Intrinsic muscle(s)
   of hand, 7–9, 8f
     examination of, 53–55, 53f–56f
     imbalance of, in synovitis of the MCP joint,
       1202

Intrinsic tendon(s)
   stiffness, surgical management of, 354
   tightness of, in swan-neck deformity, 456
Intrinsic tightness test, 55, 56f
Iontophoresis, 1427–1428, 1428f
   for lateral epicondylitis, 525
   for stenosing tendovaginitis, 501
Irreducible fractures, 1804
Irritability, classification of, 88, 88t
Ischemia
   following arterial cannulation, 786, 787f
   prolonged, as contraindication to
     replantation, 1042
Ischemic injury, of nerve, 572
Island skin flaps, for fingertip injuries, 1073
Isolated flexor digitorum profundus injuries,
   reconstructive procedures for, 485–486,
   486t, 487f
Isolated passive flexion, of proximal
   interphalangeal joint, 363
Isolation test
   serratus anterior, 98, 98f
   supraspinatus, in shoulder examination,
     107–109, 109f
Isometric contraction, 1708

J

Jeanne's sign, 53, 54f
Jebsen Hand Function Test, 1739, 1739f
Jebsen Taylor Hand Function Test (JHFT), 137,
   586
Jerk test, in shoulder examination, 104, 104f
Job analysis, 1716–1718
Job descriptions, 1716–1718
Job information, challenge of gathering,
   1716–1718
Job Performance Measure (JPM), 1736,
   1736.e1
Job simulation, work evaluation, case example
   of, 1737
Jobe's test, for rotator cuff disease, 543, 543f
Job-simulated testing, of work activities and
   occupations, 1736–1737
Joint(s)
   effects of position of, on extraneural pressure,
     681–682
   evidence for realignment of, 1454
   fusion of. *See* Arthrodesis
   of hand, 3–6
   innervation of, in hand, 1396–1397
     basal thumb, 1396–1397
     finger, 1396
     wrist, 1396
   positioning of, in prothesis control, 1108
   replacement of. *See* Arthroplasty
   scanning of, in upper quarter screening, 120,
     122f
   in tetraplegic surgery
     release and mobilization of, 1593
     stabilization of, 1593
Joint balance, in tetraplegic surgery, 1597
Joint capsule, 992–993
   of elbow, 33
   excision of. *See* Capsulectomy(ies)
   glenohumeral, pathology of, 978. *See also*
     Adhesive capsulitis
   of metacarpophalangeal joint, 4–5
     dorsal, 347
   of proximal interphalangeal joint, 5–6
Joint collapse, 486
Joint contact area and pressure, in wrist kinetics,
   27
Joint contractures. *See also* Contracture(s)
   fracture-induced, 283
Joint forces, in wrist kinetics, 27, 27f

Joint mobilization
   for adhesive capsulitis, 981–982
   distal radial fracture and, 842
   orthosis for, 384, 385f, 1511–1521, 1512f
     American Society of Hand Therapists
       Splint/Orthosis Classification System,
       1513–1516, 1514f
     assessment of, 1516
     classification of, 1513–1516
     control, 1511–1513, 1513f
     correction, 1511, 1512f
     objectives of, 1511–1513
     physiologic factors in, 1516–1517, 1516f–1517f
     principles of, 1517–1520
       construction, 1519–1520
       design, 1519, 1520f
       fitting, 1520
       mechanical, 1517–1518, 1517f–1518f
       using outriggers and assists, 1518–1519
   in pain management, 1360
Joint position sense, 1399, 1400f–1401f, 1401–1402
   definition of, 1399
   in distal radial fracture, 836
Joint protection and energy conservation
   techniques, patient handout on, 1682b–1683b
Joint range of motion, in complex regional pain
   syndrome, 1380
Joint stability, arthritis and, 1212–1213
Joint stabilizers
   dynamic, 40–41
   static, 39–40
Joint stiffness, 373. *See also* Elbow stiffness
   as complication of replantation, 1054
   evaluation of
     adherence, 378–379, 379f
     casting motion to mobilize stiffness, 376,
       376t, 376b
     joint tightness in, 378
     muscle-tendon unit tightness, 378
     skin and scar tightness, 379
   factors contributing to, 376–377
   fibroplasia stage in, 376–377
   inflammatory stage in, 376
   maturation stage in, 377
   orthotic mobilization for, 384
   prevention of, 373–376, 374t–375t
   problems of, 381
   traditional principles on, 381–383
   wound healing and, 377
Joint tightness, in stiff hand, 378
JPM. *See* Job Performance Measure
Judo, injuries associated with, 1606t–1608t
Juncturae tendinum, of extensor tendons, 445,
   445f–446f

K

Kanavel signs, in flexor sheath infections, 217,
   217f
Kapandji Index, 1270, 1270t
Kaposi's sarcoma, 262
Kase, Kenzo, 1451
Kayaking, injuries associated with, 1606t–1608t
Keloid scars, management of, 1061
Keratoacanthoma, 260, 261f
Ketamine, for complex regional pain syndrome,
   1374
Kienböck's disease, 154, 155f
Kim test, in shoulder examination, 104–105
Kinematics
   of fracture-dislocations, 887
   of wrist, 25–26
     individual carpal bone motion in, 25
     overview of, 25
     palmar flexion/dorsiflexion in, 25–26
     radioulnar deviation in, 26, 26f

Lubrication, in tendon healing, 395f, 396, 397f
  effect of, 396
Lubricin, in tendon healing, 396, 397f
Lunate
  anatomy of, 20, 20f–21f
  avascular necrosis of. *See* Kienböck's disease
  fractures of, 883
Lund Browder method, 199
Lunotriquetral ballottement test, 70
Lunotriquetral dissociation, 895–897
  diagnosis of, 896, 896f
  treatment of, 896–897, 897f
Lunotriquetral instability, 1405–1406, 1406f
  provocative tests for, 179t–180t
Lunotriquetral ligament, 152
Lupus, tenosynovitis associated with, 513
Lymph node(s), axillary, dissection of, hand
  surgery after, 794
Lymphangioma, 257
Lymphangiosarcoma, 262
Lymphangitis, 215
Lymphatic system
  anatomy of, 781, 1628
  of hand, 211
  research evidence for, 1454
  theoretical benefits of elastic tape for,
    1454–1459
Lymphatic therapies, for edema, 804–809
Lymphedema. *See also* Edema
  breast cancer-related, 1627–1635
    diagnosis of, 1630–1632, 1630f
    differential diagnosis of, 1629–1630
    physical examination of, 1631–1632,
      1631f–1632f
    risk factors of, 1629
    treatment strategies for, 1632–1635
  factitious, psychological factors in, 1696
  staging of, 1630

M

Maceration, of wound, 1076
Macrodactyly, 1785, 1785f
Macrophages, 187
  in nerve responses to injury, 572–573
Madelung's deformity, 1780
Magnetic resonance angiography (MRA)
  of thoracic outlet syndrome, 698–699, 699f
  of vascular disease, 783
Magnetic resonance imaging (MRI)
  of adhesive capsulitis, 980
  of Bankart lesion, 994
  of brachial plexus injury, 636
  of distal biceps tendon rupture, 951, 951f
  of fractures, 277, 277f
  functional, of focal hand dystonia, 1650–1651
  of hand, 1650
  of rotator cuff disease, 544, 544f
  of triceps tendon rupture, 958, 959f
  of upper extremity, 143–144, 144b
Magnetoencephalography (MEG), of focal hand
  dystonia, 1645
Maladaptive homeostatic plasticity, in focal hand
  dystonia, 1644–1645
Malignant fibrous histiocytoma, 262
Malignant melanoma, 261
Malignant peripheral nerve sheath tumors, 262
Mallet classification, modified, of brachial plexus
  injuries, 1816, 1817f–1818f
Mallet finger, 316, 452–456
  chronic, 455
    from blunt trauma, 454f
    with swan-neck deformity, 456
  clinical management of, 466
  development of, 453, 454f
  orthosis for, 316, 316f, 455f, 1174

Mallet finger *(Continued)*
  treatment of, 453–456
    for closed injury, 453–456, 455f
    for open injury, 456
Malunion
  as complication of replantation, 1054
  of fractures, 282–283, 283f
  phalangeal, 293
Management strategies, for common limb
  complications, 1110, 1110t
Manipulation, under anesthesia, for adhesive
  capsulitis, 982–983
"Mannerfelt lesion", 1197
Mannerfelt's syndrome, 1233
Manske's classification, of cleft hand, 1780t
Manual edema mobilization (MEM), 804
Manual lymphatic drainage, 1627, 1633, 1634f
  for edema, 804
Manual materials handling, 1740–1741, 1741f
Manual muscle test (MMT), 585, 1584
Manual muscular strength, 635–636
Manual resistance, 996, 996f
Manual Tactile Test (MTT), 1649f
Manual therapy
  for clinical groups, 1466–1468
    momentary pain group, 1467–1468, 1467f
    pain and stiffness group, 1467
    pain group, 1466, 1466f
    stiffness group, 1466–1467, 1467f
  efficacy of, 1462–1464
  general considerations for, 1464, 1465f
  grades of movement in, 1464–1465, 1465b
  mechanisms of, 1461–1462, 1462f
  mobilization with movement in, 1468
  randomized controlled trials of, 1463
  systematic reviews of, 1462–1464
  technique of
    available options in, 1465–1466,
      1465f–1466f
    selection of, 1464–1468
  for upper extremity musculoskeletal
    disorders, 1461–1469
Marjolin ulcer, 220, 221f
Martial arts, injuries associated with,
  1606t–1608t
Massage
  for edema, in stiff hand, 383
  friction, evaluation of, 113–114
  ice, wheal formation after, 1418–1419, 1419f
  in pain management, 1360
  retrograde, for complex hand injuries, 1063
  tendon, for stenosing tendovaginitis, 501
Massed practice, 1556–1557
Mastectomy
  radical, hand surgery after, 794
  surgery after, 1620
Matrix, definition of, 184
Matrix metalloproteinases (MMPs), 191, 197
Maturation phase, in wound healing, 198, 198f
Maximal medical improvement (MMI), 1743
Maximal voluntary effort (MVE), of functional
  capacity evaluation, 1744–1745
Maximum function, definition of, 1740–1741
Maximum isoinertial lifting evaluations, 1741
Mayfield's four stages, of progressive perilunate
  instability, 883, 884f
Mayo classification, of TFCC tears, 866, 866b
McGill Pain Questionnaire, 1344, 1344.e1f, 1381
Meal preparation, advanced prosthetic training
  for, 1108t
Measurement of Area and Volume Instrument
  System (MAVIS) III, 204
Mechanical compression, edema control with,
  after complex hand injuries, 1063
Mechanical creep, in mobilization orthosis, 1516
Mechanical debridement. *See* Debridement

Mechanical deep somatic hyperalgesia, 1434t
Mechanical dynamic allodynia, 1434t
Mechanical principles, in mobilization orthosis,
  1517–1518, 1517f–1518f
Mechanical punctate, pinprick hyperalgesia,
  1434t
Mechanical sensitivity, of peripheral nervous
  system, 1437
Mechanical static hyperalgesia, 1434t
Mechanical stimulation, positive biomechanical
  effects of, 465
Mechanoreceptors, 1394–1396, 1395f, 1396t
  free nerve endings, 1395
  Golgi-like endings, 1395
  Pacini corpuscles, 1395
  Ruffini endings, 1394–1395
  unclassifiable corpuscles, 1395–1396, 1396t
Mechanotransduction, 192
Medial antebrachial cutaneous nerve, anatomy
  of, 36
Medial collateral ligament (MCL) injury,
  provocative tests for, 179t–180t
Medial elbow pain, conservative management of,
  972–974, 972t–973t
Medial epicondyle, anatomy of, 518–519
Medial epicondylectomy, for cubital tunnel
  syndrome, 748
Medial epicondylitis
  forearm and elbow taping for, 1459
  imaging of, 149, 150f
  soft orthosis for, 1541
Medial femoral condyle flap, 1135–1136
Median nerve, 720–721
  anatomy of, 14–15, 612, 612f, 755–756
  compression of. *See also* Pronator syndrome
    in proximal forearm, 755. *See also* Pronator
      syndrome
  examination of, 55, 55f
  excursion of, 1436
  injury to, 583–584, 583f
    anatomy of, 612, 612f
    at elbow level, 583–584
    at forearm level, 583–584
    functional implications of, 584
    orthotic positioning in, 589–590, 590f
    physical examination of, 613, 613f–614f
    potential substitution patterns for, 586t
    tendon transfers for, 612–616, 612f,
      627–628
      common tendons transferred in, 628, 628t
      for high median nerve palsy, 616, 616f
      for low median nerve palsy, 613–614,
        615f
      surgical technique of, 614–616, 615f
    outcomes of, 628
    treatment of, 628, 629f
    at wrist level, 583
Median nerve palsy, tendon transfers for, with
  ulnar nerve palsy, 619
Medical-grade honey, for wound healing, 200
Medicine, narrative-based, 1479
Meissner corpuscle, response of, to denervation,
  573
Mental imagery rehearsal, 1411–1412, 1412f
Mental practice, for upper extremity poststroke,
  1564
Merkel disks, response of, to denervation, 573
Metacarpal(s)
  amputation of. *See* Amputation
  anatomy of, 1, 2f
  base of, 1–2
  fractures of, 299f, 302, 458
    early mobilization considerations in, 302,
      302f
      clinical example of, 302b, 303f
    soft tissue complications in, 302

Muscle imbalance, in rotator cuff disease, 542
Muscle inhibition
    elastic tape tension and direction for, 1453–1454
    evidence for, 1453, 1453f
    theoretical benefits of elastic taping for, 1452–1453, 1453f
Muscle length, restoration of, for nerve compression syndrome, 762
    cubital tunnel syndrome, 765
    pronator syndrome, 774
    radial tunnel syndrome, 769
    Wartenberg's syndrome, 771
Muscle performance, in scapular dyskinesis, 1017
Muscle spasticity. See also Spasticity
    in tetraplegia, 1587
Muscle strength, physical agents for, 1429, 1430.e1f
Muscle transfer, for long thoracic nerve injury, 667
Muscle weakness, in carpal tunnel syndrome, 735, 735f
Muscle-tendon units
    plaster casting of, 1535–1537, 1535f
    tightness of, in stiff hand, 378
Musculocutaneous motor neurectomy, for elbow deformity, 1571
Musculocutaneous nerve
    injury to, 672–673
    transfer of, for brachial plexus injury, 651–652, 652f
Musculoskeletal surgery, in cerebral palsy patient, 1790–1797
Musculoskeletal system
    anatomic limitations of, in focal hand dystonia, 1643–1644
    disorders of, 1705b
        awkward postures of, 1707, 1708f
        contact stress, 1712
        force, 1708–1712, 1711f
        manual therapy for, 1461–1469. See also Manual therapy
        nonoccupational risk factors of, 1707
        occupational risk factors of, 1707–1714
        personal risk factors of, 1707
        repetition, 1712–1713, 1713f, 1714t
        risk factors of, 1706–1707
        static or sustained postures, 1708
        temperature, 1714
        vibration, 1713–1714
        work-related musculoskeletal disorders, 1705–1706, 1706b
    injuries to, in complex hand trauma, 1030–1035, 1031f–1032f
Musculotendinous juncture, in tendon reconstruction, 487
Musical instrument(s)
    ergonomic modifications to, 1686
    quality of, 1670
Musicians, 1668–1693
    anatomic variations among, 1670–1671, 1672f
    carpal tunnel syndrome in, 1681–1683, 1683f
    change in instrument, 1669–1670
    cubital tunnel syndrome in, 1683–1684, 1683f
    de Quervain's disease in, 1673
    digital compression neuropathies in, 1681
    environmental factors affecting, 1670
    ergonomics for, 1686–1687
        adaptive equipment in, 1687, 1688f
        instrument modifications, 1686
        key modifications in, 1687
        reduction of static loading in, 1686–1687
    excessive training, 1669
    focal hand dystonia in, treatment of, 1679–1680

Musicians (Continued)
    ganglions in, 1684
    healthy practice habits for, 1689b
    hypermobility in, 1676–1677
        hand therapy for, 1676–1677, 1677f–1678f
        incidence of, 1676
    increased demands of repertoire, 1669
    injuries to
        resumption of practice after, 1687–1690
            instrument-specific rehabilitation protocols in, 1689–1690
            return-to-play schedule for, 1688–1689, 1689t, 1689b
            specific vs. nonspecific diagnosis of, 1668f
    lack of/inconsistent work, 1670
    myofascial pain and stretching affecting, 1674–1676, 1676f
    nerve entrapment syndromes in, 1681–1684
    nonmusical activities and factors affecting, 1670–1671, 1670b–1671b, 1673f
    nonspecific arm pain in, treatment of, 1681, 1682b–1683b
    overuse injuries in, 1680–1681
    pathologies affecting, 1671–1676
    performance-related issues for, 1668–1670
    physically disabled, adaptive equipment in, 1687, 1688f
    practice tips, 1671
    pressures in workplace, 1669
    radial nerve neuropathies in, 1684
    tendinopathies in, 1671–1674
        treatment of, 1674, 1674f–1675f
    treatment of
        general principles in, 1684–1685
        orthotic intervention in, 1684–1685
        surgical, 1690–1691
    work-related upper extremity disorders in, 1680–1681
        classification and grading of, 1681
Musician's cramp, 1644
MVE. See Maximal voluntary effort
Mycobacterial infections, 218, 219f–220f
Mycobacterium avium infection, 218, 219f
Mycobacterium intracellulare infection, 218, 219f
Mycobacterium marinum infection, 218, 219f
Mycobacterium tuberculosis infection, 218, 219f
Myelin, 569–570
Myelin-associated glycoprotein (MAG)
    in chronic nerve compression injury, 575
    in nerve regeneration, 573
Myelography, CT, of brachial plexus injury, 636
Myoelectric prosthesis, operation of
    preparation in, 1107, 1107t
    recommended muscle sites in, 1107t
Myoelectric prosthetics, in upper extremity amputation, 1083–1085, 1084f
    advanced pattern recognition algorithms in, 1085
    advantage of, 1084–1085, 1084f
Myofascial mobility, for nerve compression syndrome, 762
    cubital tunnel syndrome, 765
    pronator syndrome, 774
    radial tunnel syndrome, 769
    Wartenberg's syndrome, 771
Myofascial pain, in musicians, 1674–1676, 1676f
Myotome scan, in upper quarter screening, 120, 122f

N

Narrative-based medicine, 1479
Neck pain, 685
    neuroanatomical basis of, 1326–1328
Needle fasciotomy
    for Dupuytren's disease, 230
        intervention after, 242–243

Neer's impingement sign, in shoulder examination, 107, 107f
Negative reinforcement protocol, for focal hand dystonia, 1656
Negative-pressure wound therapy (NPWT), 202–203, 1127
Neoprene orthosis, 1539
    digit extension, 1545, 1548f
    thumb abduction, fabricated without sewing skills, 1550
Nerve(s)
    elastic limit of. See Strain
    of elbow, 34–36, 35f–36f
    fascicular patterns of, 569, 570f
    of hand, 14–16, 15f–16f, 15t
        examination of, 57–58, 58f
        injuries of, 1034
    healing of, after complex hand injuries, 1059
    lacerations of. See Nerve injury(ies)
    myelinated and unmyelinated, 569, 570f
    responses to injury, 572–573
    type of, sensory relearning and, 598–599
    vasculature of, 570–571
Nerve compression, 572, 677–684
    acute, 680
    axoplasmic transport, 679
    chronic, 575, 680–681, 681f
    double-crush phenomenon, 681
    evaluation of, 682
    histopathology of, 681
    joint position and hand loading, effects of, 681–682
    neurophysiology of, 679
    pathophysiology of, 680–681
    peripheral nervous system
        anatomy of, 677–679, 678f
        blood supply of, 679, 679f
        microanatomy of, 677–678, 678f–679f
        topography of, 678–679
    in scleroderma, 1305
    subacute, 680
    vibration in
        clinical responses to, 682
        exposure to, 682
Nerve compression syndrome(s). See also Carpal tunnel syndrome
    conservative management of
        activity modification in, 762–763, 763f
        basic principles of, 761–763
        muscle length and myofascial mobility in, 762
        neural mobilization in, 762
        orthoses and protection in, 762
    history of, 760–761, 761f
    neural mobilization for, 1441
    postoperative management of
        activity modification in, 763
        basic principles of, 763
        neural mobilization in, 763
        protected range of motion in, 763
        scar management in, 763, 763f
        sensory desensitization in, 763
    repetitive stress injuries in, 760
Nerve conduction velocity (NCV)
    in shoulder nerve injuries, 663
    in thoracic outlet syndrome, 699
Nerve entrapment syndromes
    diagnostic imaging of, 155
    in musicians, 1681–1684
Nerve fibers
    classification systems of, 1396t
    microanatomy of, 677–678, 678f
Nerve gliding exercise, for carpal tunnel syndrome, 721–722, 739
Nerve graft reconstruction, 575–576
Nerve grafting, 576, 577f

Wound contraction, 188–191, 191f
Wound healing
  after complex hand injuries, 1058
  goals of, 199–200
  phases of, 197–198
    hemostasis, 197, 197f
    inflammation, 197, 198f
    maturation and remodeling, 198, 198f
    proliferation, 198, 198f
  physical agents for, 1429–1430
  product selection for, 199–200
  stages of, stiffness in, 376–377
Wound management, 196–209
  debridement in, types of, 200–201
  edema and, 203
  in fingertip injuries, 1076, 1076f–1078f
  preferred strategy in, 214, 214t
WPAI. See Work Productivity and Impairment
    Questionnaire
Wrestling, injuries associated with, 1606t–1608t
Wright's hyperabduction test
  for brachial plexus neuropathies, 710, 710f
  for thoracic outlet syndrome, 696, 697f
Wrist, 1396
  amputation at. See also Amputation
    replantation surgery for, 1048
  anatomy of, 19–28
    bony, 19–21, 19f–21f
    joint, 21–22
    ligamentous, 22–24, 22f–23f
    tendinous, 24
    vascular, 24–25, 24f
  clinical examination of, 62–67, 65.e1t
    central dorsal zone in, 68–69, 68f–69f
    diagnostic injection in, 64–65
    history of injury or onset in, 62–63
    objective assessment in, 63–64, 64f
    radial dorsal zone in, 65–68, 66f–67f
    radial volar zone in, 72, 72.e1f, 72f–73f
    ulnar dorsal zone in, 69–72, 69f–71f,
      71f–72f
    ulnar volar zone in, 72–73, 73.e1f
    visual inspection in, 63, 63f, 63t, 63.e1f
  compression neuropathies of
    surgical management of, 720–731
    therapists' management of, 732–744
      radial, 741
      ulnar, 740–741
  disarticulation of, prosthesis for, 1097
  distal radial fracture and, 841, 841f–842f
    rotation, 841
  electric terminal device control of, 1097
  extensor tendons of, 444–445, 444f
    injury to, 444–445
    preservation of, in tetraplegic surgery,
      1597–1598
    radial, tendinopathy of, 512
  flexor, preservation of, in tetraplegic surgery,
    1598

Wrist (Continued)
  fractures of, 1406
  impairment of, after brachial plexus injuries,
    1820
  innervation of, 25
  kinematics of, 25–26, 1405
  kinetics of, 26–27
  median nerve injury at, 583
  postburn, positioning of, 1169
  radial nerve injury at, 582–583
  rheumatoid arthritis of
    classification systems for, 1201, 1201t
    end-stage deformity in, 1200
    pathomechanics of, 1197–1201
    radiographic changes in, 1200–1201
  "squeaker's", 511
  tendon pathology of, 152, 152f
  ulnar
    pain and impairment, 863–875. See also
      Triangular fibrocartilage complex
    interosseous membrane in, 867
    management of, 867–873
      algorithmic approach to, 867–873,
        868f, 869b
      articular disk tear in, 871–873, 872f,
        872b
      degenerative changes in, 870, 870b
      fractures in, 868–870, 869f–870f, 869b
      instability in, 870–871, 871f, 871b
      physical examination in, 867
      postoperative considerations in, 873
      principles in, 873–874, 874f
      tendinitis in, 871
      tenets of evaluation in, 867
      ulnar nerve compression in, 873
    midcarpal instability in, 866–867
    pisotriquetral joint in, 867
    TFCC affiliates in, 866
    TFCC articular tears in, 865, 865f
    TFCC extensor carpi ulnaris tendon
      sheath in, 866
    TFCC radioulnar ligament tears in, 866
    ulnocarpal abutment in, 865–866
  ulnar nerve injury at, 584
Wrist arthritis, 1233–1235
  diagnostic imaging of, 157–158, 157f
Wrist arthrodesis
  in tetraplegia, 1593
  total, 902–903, 902f–903f
    postoperative management of, 902–903
    preoperative management of, 902
  for wrist flexion deformity, 1575
Wrist arthroplasty
  postoperative management of, 1235–1236
    0 to 4 weeks, 1235–1236
    4 to 8 weeks, 1236
    8 to 10 weeks, 1236
  total, 903
Wrist arthrosis, in scleroderma, 1305, 1306f

Wrist block anesthesia, in fracture repair, 287
Wrist deformity, in hemiplegia, management of,
    1572–1575, 1574f–1575f
  mobilization in, 1573
"Wrist drop", 581–582, 582f
Wrist extension
  assessment of, 48, 50f
  myotome scan of, 122f
Wrist flexion
  assessment of, 48, 50f
  deformity of
    in cerebral palsy, musculoskeletal surgery
      for, 1793–1794, 1794f
    in hemiplegia, 1572
  myotome scan of, 122f
Wrist reconstruction, salvage procedure(s) for,
    901–910
  distal ulna, 904–905, 904f
  midcarpal arthrodesis, 905–909
  physical examination, 901–902
  radiocarpal arthrodesis, 905
  radiographic evaluation, 902
  total wrist arthrodesis, 902–903, 902f–903f
Wrist reflexes, 1398
Wrist sensorimotor control impairment, after
    DRFs, 1398
Wrist sprain, diagnosis of, 62
Wrist tenodesis, pattern, 379–380
Writer's cramp, 1642. See also Repetitive strain
    injury

X

Xenograft, 201
  postoperative principles for, 201–202

Y

Yard work, advanced prosthetic training for,
    1108t
Y Balance Test-Upper Quarter (YBT-UQ), 1610f
Y-condylar fractures, 277, 278f
YMCA Bench Step Test, 1739

Z

Zigzag deformity, of thumb, 1258, 1265f
Zigzag (Brunner type) incision, in surgical
    treatment of Dupuytren's disease, 234,
    234f
Z-incision, for biceps rerouting, 1829, 1830f
Z-lengthening
  for hand deformities, 1575–1576
  of tendon, 485
Zone of injury, in intraarticular hand fracture,
    322
Zone of polarizing activity (ZPA), in limb
    development, 1769
Z-plasty, for biceps rerouting, 1829, 1830f